Infectious Diseases in Immunocompromised Hosts

COVER: Adenoviruses cause various human diseases. X-ray crystallography has been used to obtain a high resolution structure of the major coat protein, hexon, and electron microscopy and image reconstruction to obtain a picture of the whole virus at lower resolution. **UPPER** The characteristic icosahedral shape of adenovirus (1; blue) is given by its 240 tooth-like hexon molecules and a penton at each of the 12 vertices. Fibers, which bind to receptors on cells to initiate infections, project from the pentons. **LOWER LEFT** The vertex region (2) shows the central penton and fiber (red) surrounded by five peripentonal hexons (white), and a further ring of ten hexons (blue). The peripentonal hexons blend from the solid molecular surface derived from electron microscopy to the stick-like internal amino acid chains revealed by X-ray crystallography. Small "cementing" molecules (purple) stabilize the virus. **LOWER RIGHT** The ~10,000 non-hydrogen atoms forming each of the three polypeptide chains in hexon (3) are shown in space-filling representation to reveal the intimate contacts between the subunits.

References

1. Stewart, P. L., Burnett, R. M., Cyrklaff, M., and Fuller, S. D., Image reconstruction reveals the complex molecular organization of adenovirus, *Cell*, 67, 145–154, 1991.
2. Stewart, P. L., Fuller, S. D., and Burnett, R. M., Difference imaging of adenovirus: bridging the resolution gap between X-ray crystallography and electron microscopy, *EMBO J.*, 12, 2589-2599, 1993.
3. Athappilly, F. K., Murali, R., Rux, J. J., Cai, Z., and Burnett, R. M., The refined crystal structure of hexon, the major coat protein of adenovirus type 2, at 2.9 = C5 resolution, *J. Mol. Biol.*, 242, 430-455, 1994.

Courtesy of Drs. John J. Rux and Roger M. Burnett, The Wistar Institute, Philadelphia. With permission by Cell Press, Cambridge, MA and Oxford University Press, London, U.K.

Acquiring Editor:	Harvey Kane
Project Editor:	Carol Whitehead
Marketing Manager:	Becky McEldowney
Cover design:	Dawn Boyd
Manufacturing:	Carol Royal

Library of Congress Cataloging-in-Publication Data

Georgiev, Vassil St.
    Infectious diseases in immunocompromised hosts / Vassil St. Georgiev.
        p.   cm. -- (CRC series on pharmacology and toxicology)
    Includes bibliographical references and index.
    ISBN 0-8493-8553-9 (alk. paper)
      1. Anti-infective agents.   2. Communicable diseases--Chemotherapy.
  3. Immunological deficiency syndromes--Complications--Chemotherapy.
I. Title. II. Series: Pharmacology & toxicology (Boca Raton, Fla.)
    [DNLM: 1. Communicable Diseases--drug therapy. 2. Communicable
Diseases--diagnosis. 3. Immunocompromised Host. WC 100 G352i 1997]
RM267.G46   1997
616.9--dc21

DNLM/DLC
for Library of Congress   97-28644
                                                 CIP

Infectious Diseases in Immunocompromised Hosts

Vassil St. Georgiev, Ph.D.

National Institute of Allergy and Infectious Diseases
National Institutes of Health
Bethesda, Maryland

CRC Press

Boca Raton   Boston   London   New York   Washington, D.C.

Pharmacology and Toxicology: Basic and Clinical Aspects

Mannfred A. Hollinger, Series Editor
University of California, Davis

Forthcoming Titles

CRC Handbook of Alcohol Addiction: Clinical and Theoretical Approaches,
    Gerald Zernig
Handbook of Immunotoxicological Methods, Leonard Ritter
Handbook of Mammalian Models in Biomedical Research, David B. Jack
Handbook of Theoretical Models in Biomedical Research, David B. Jack
Lead and Public Health Integrated Risk Assessment, Paul Mushak
CNS Injuries: Cellular Responses and Pharmacological Strategies, Martin Berry and
    Ann Logan
Lead and Public Health: Integrated Risk Assessment, Paul Mushak
Molecular Bases of Anesthesia, Eric Moody and Phil Skolnick
Receptor Characterization and Regulation, Devendra K. Agrawal

Published Titles

*Infectious Diseases in Immunocompromised Hosts,*1998, Vassil St. Georgiev
Pharmacology of Antimuscarinic Agents, 1998, Laszlo Gyermek
Handbook of Plant and Fungal Toxicants, 1997, Felix D'Mello
Basis of Toxicity Testing, Second Edition, 1997, Donald J. Ecobichon
Anabolic Treatments for Osteoporosis, 1997, James F. Whitfield and Paul Morley
Antibody Therapeutics, 1997, William J. Harris and John R. Adair
Muscarinic Receptor Subtypes in Smooth Muscle, 1997, Richard M. Eglen
Antisense Oligodeonucleotides as Novel Pharmacological
    Therapeutic Agents, 1997, Benjamin Weiss
Airway Wall Remodelling in Asthma, 1996, A.G. Stewart
Drug Delivery Systems, 1996, Vasant V. Ranade and Mannfred A. Hollinger
Brain Mechanisms and Psychotropic Drugs, 1996, Andrius Baskys and
    Gary Remington
Receptor Dynamics in Neural Development, 1996, Christopher A. Shaw
Ryanodine Receptors, 1996, Vincenzo Sorrentino
Therapeutic Modulation of Cytokines, 1996, M.W. Bodmer and Brian Henderson
Pharmacology in Exercise and Sport, 1996, Satu M. Somani
Placental Pharmacology, 1996, B. V. Rama Sastry
Pharmacological Effects of Ethanol on the Nervous System, 1996,
    Richard A. Deitrich
Immunopharmaceuticals, 1996, Edward S. Kimball
Chemoattractant Ligands and Their Receptors, 1996, Richard Horuk
Pharmacological Regulation of Gene Expression in the CNS, 1996,
    Kalpana Merchant
Experimental Models of Mucosal Inflammation, 1995, Timothy S. Gaginella
Handbook of Methods in Gastrointestinal Pharmacology, 1995, Timothy S. Gaginella
Handbook of Targeted Delivery of Imaging Agents, 1995, Vladimir P. Torchilin
Handbook of Pharmacokinetic Pharmacodynamic Correlations, 1995, Hartmut Derendorf
    and Guenther Hochhaus
Human Growth Hormone Pharmacology: Basic and Clinical Aspects, 1995,
    Kathleen T. Shiverick and Arlan Rosenbloom
Placental Toxicology, 1995, B. V. Rama Sastry
Stealth Liposomes, 1995, Danilo Lasic and Frank Martin
TAXOL®: Science and Applications, 1995, Matthew Suffness

Pharmacology and Toxicology: Basic and Clinical Aspects

Published Titles (*Continued*)

Endothelin Receptors: From the Gene to the Human, 1995, Robert R. Ruffolo, Jr.
*Alternative Methodologies for the Safety Evaluation of Chemicals
   in the Cosmetic Industry*, 1995, Nicola Loprieno
*Phospholipase A$_2$ in Clinical Inflammation: Molecular Approaches
   to Pathophysiology*, 1995, Keith B. Glaser and Peter Vadas
Serotonin and Gastrointestinal Function, 1995, Timothy S. Gaginella and
   James J. Galligan
Chemical and Structural Approaches to Rational Drug Design, 1994,
   David B. Weiner and William V. Williams
Biological Approaches to Rational Drug Design, 1994, David B. Weiner and
   William V. Williams
Direct and Allosteric Control of Glutamate Receptors, 1994, M. Palfreyman,
   I. Reynolds, and P. Skolnick
Genomic and Non-Genomic Effects of Aldosterone, 1994, Martin Wehling
Peroxisome Proliferators: Unique Inducers of Drug-Metabolizing Enzymes, 1994,
   David E. Moody
*Angiotensin II Receptors, Volume I: Molecular Biology, Biochemistry,
   Pharmacology, and Clinical Perspectives,* 1994, Robert R. Ruffolo, Jr.
Angiotensin II Receptors, Volume II: Medicinal Chemistry, 1994,
   Robert R. Ruffolo, Jr.
Beneficial and Toxic Effects of Aspirin, 1993, Susan E. Feinman
Preclinical and Clinical Modulation of Anticancer Drugs, 1993, Kenneth D. Tew,
   Peter Houghton, and Janet Houghton
In Vitro *Methods of Toxicology*, 1992, Ronald R. Watson
Basis of Toxicity Testing, 1992, Donald J. Ecobichon
Human Drug Metabolism from Molecular Biology to Man, 1992, Elizabeth Jeffreys
Platelet Activating Factor Receptor: Signal Mechanisms and Molecular Biology,
   1992, Shivendra D. Shukla
Biopharmaceutics of Ocular Drug Delivery, 1992, Peter Edman
Pharmacology of the Skin, 1991, Hasan Mukhtar
Inflammatory Cells and Mediators in Bronchial Asthma, 1990,
   Devendra K. Agrawal and Robert G. Townley

Preface

There has long been the need for a comprehensive text on drug development and treatment of infectious diseases in immunocompromised hosts. In spite of a wealth of isolated data, no single text exists in which all the essential information about the various infectious disease areas has been presented. Although we make no claim to completeness, it is hoped that this volume will fulfill that need. To achieve this goal we have endeavored to integrate both results from large-scale clinical trials and reports of single cases as well as small numbers of patients, clearly mindful that such an approach has its limitations.

The book is organized into four major parts covering bacterial, viral, parasitic, and fungal diseases affecting the immunocompromised population. Each part comprises individual infections caused not only by well known etiologic agents, but also by new and emerging species often taxonomically closely related to a major disease-producing microorganism and until recently not considered to be human pathogens (*Candida* spp. and nontuberculous mycobacteria being good examples of these). For the sake of uniformity, within each part the species have been arranged according to their taxonomic characteristics.

As the title of the book suggests, the array of diseases it includes has been broadened to encompass not only opportunistic infections exclusively associated with immunocompromised patients, but also infections commonly benign and self-resolving while affecting immunocompetent hosts but becoming fulminant or disseminated, and very often life-threatening, in immunosuppressed individuals.

As with most complex systems, the various components of the immune system function according to strict regulatory mechanisms. The immune system's response to an antigenic challenge is diverse and results in a chain of events that lead to the production of either specifically activated effector cells or humoral products, or both. The phase of the immune response associated with tissue reactions is known as cellular (cell-mediated) response; the phase involving the production of antibodies is generally referred to as humoral response. Knowledge of the intricate relations and multiple levels of interactions between various components of the immune systems is of foremost importance in our understanding of how the immune system provides protection against foreign intruders and various pathologic conditions.

In contrast to normal hosts where many infectious diseases are usually self-limited, in immunocompromised patients such infections have the potential of becoming serious illnesses characterized by high morbidity and mortality rates. There are also the opportunistic infections which occur almost exclusively in immunocompromised hosts. Usually widely distributed in the environment, the opportunistic pathogens rarely cause serious illness in normal hosts.

In this context, it is important to note that prompt and correct diagnosis of a disseminated infection may become crucial as a result of overt differences in the susceptibility to anti-infectious drugs of sometimes closely related opportunistic pathogens. While both *Pseudallescheria boydii* and *Scedosporium prolificans* have been recognized as causes of opportunistic hyalohyphomycoses in immunocompromised patients, diagnosis of disseminated disease due to *S. prolificans* has been difficult to attain since its spectrum and symptoms strongly resemble those of pseudallescheriasis and pulmonary aspergillosis. However, early positive identification of *S. prolificans* may prove to be very essential because of its extreme drug tolerance and the related poor prognosis of disseminated disease caused by this fungal pathogen.

Even though the frequency of developing infectious disease in immunocompromised patients may not be much greater than in immunocompetent hosts, the primary infection in immunocompromised hosts may develop quickly into fulminant or disseminated disease as seen in patients where severe T helper cell defects are chronic and persistently progressive. Furthermore, patients who had developed a self-limited infection when their immune system was still normal, may often experience recrudescence and dissemination after they become immunocompromised.

The information contained in this volume includes, in addition to well-planned large-scale clinical trials, reports of individual cases or treatment of small numbers of patients. When comparing large-scale clinical trials with therapies of individual cases, unquestionably a multicenter clinical therapy involving large patient cohorts is by far the better venue to evaluate therapeutic efficacy of a drug, since not only a large-scale clinical trial would provide the necessary information and clinical experience, but it will also give perspective and directions much needed for future research. On the other hand, clinical data involving limited numbers of patients or individual cases, when well documented, may become useful in evaluating the therapeutic efficacy of a drug that otherwise may go unnoticed by those involved in drug research and development or in clinical practice. However, even with its benefits, such information, because of its limited scope, should be viewed with caution when evaluating the therapeutic efficacy and/or adverse toxicity of a therapeutic modality — inevitably in such cases, individual authors will differ from one another in any way and will include their specific (sometimes divergent or controversial) interpretations. It should also be noted that in some cases of rare or emerging infections just the small number of patients and/or their distant geographic distribution would preclude any large-scale clinical trials, thereby leaving reports on treatment of individual cases as the only data available. In addition, there are also those unique cases of immunocompromised patients where an underlying condition may profoundly influence and/or even predicate the treatment of infection.

We trust that in its entirety the information contained in this volume represents a balanced and accurate account of the current status, and will serve as a useful resource for both established investigators and new researchers in the field of drug development and treatment, and will be able especially to help those clinicians who do not have easy access to medical libraries and journals. We also hope that this book will facilitate further understanding of those areas of drug development and treatment that are still not well understood. Our aim is to encourage both scientists and clinicians to explore new avenues in their search for novel, safer, and more effective therapeutic modalities against infectious diseases in immunocompromised patients.

In 1998, the *50th Anniversary* of the founding of the *National Institute of Allergy and Infectious Diseases (NIAID)* is being celebrated. During these fifty years of public service, NIAID has always been at the forefront of, and played a major role in the continuing efforts to overcome the significant socioeconomic and health burden on society caused by infectious diseases and lately by AIDS. It is our hope that the information presented in this volume will serve as a fitting tribute to the vital role and resolute commitment of this Institute in support of basic science and clinical research toward the curing of infectious diseases, as well as in the dissemination of knowledge to both health care professionals and the general public.

Vassil St. Georgiev
Bethesda, Maryland

Contents

Section I Viral Infections

Section II   Bacterial Infections

Section III   Parasitic Infections

Chapter 21   Introduction

Chapter 22   Eucoccidiida

Section IV   Fungal Infections

Chapter 28   Introduction

Chapter 29   Fungal Cell Envelope and Mode of Action of Antimycotic Agents

Chapter 36   Other Yeast-Like Fungi

Chapter 37   Fungi of the Order Moniliales

Dedicated

———————

to
Andrew David Welty

Section I

Viral Infections

Recent epidemiologic studies have shown that viral infections account for the great majority of acute infections in humans, exacting heavy toll in morbidity and greatly contributing to mortality and permanent disability, especially in infants and children, as well as in the elderly and immuno-compromised persons.

As microorganisms, the viruses represent small, obligate intracellular agents which cannot multiply outside a host cell and are capable of infecting all forms of life, including humans.

The assembled and fully infectious viral particle, known as virion, comprises only one type of nucleic acid (RNA or DNA), which in the simplest of forms is protected by a protein coat (capsid). In the more complex viruses, the genomic RNA or DNA with associated basic proteins is packaged inside the capsid. The viral capsid, together with the nucleic acid or a nucleoprotein, is called the nucleocapsid.

In the enveloped viruses, the viral capsid is surrounded by an envelope which usually contains a lipid bilayer component derived from modified host cell membrane proteins and a projecting outer layer of glycosylated proteins.

The RNA or DNA genomes contain all of the necessary genetic information to be delivered into the host cell and program the synthetic machinery of the host cell for viral replication. The protective viral coating has two major missions: to prevent viral destruction by extracellular insults, such as from nucleases, and second, to permit viral attachment to the membrane of the host cell, the negative charge of which would repel a naked nucleic acid. Once inside the host cell, the virus will start its replication by using the host cell machinery and completely depending on it for energy and synthetic requirements.

In general, viruses are difficult targets for chemotherapy because not only do they replicate inside the host cells but there is also a great similarity between host-directed and virus-directed processes, which makes it difficult for antiviral agents to differentiate. Nevertheless, it has become increasingly possible to find in the viral replication cycle distinctly specific steps that may be used as targets for highly selective chemotherapeutic agents.

1 Herpesviridae

The herpesviruses, members of the family Herpesviridae, are highly ubiquitous in nature. So far, there have been almost 100 herpesviruses isolated from mammals that are at least partially characterized, and of these 7 have been found in humans: herpes simplex virus 1 (HSV-1), herpes simplex virus 2 (HSV-2), human cytomegalovirus (HCMV), varicella-zoster virus (VZV), the Epstein-Barr virus (EBV), and human herpesvirus-6 (HHV-6) and human herpesvirus-7 (HHV-7).

The virion of a typical member of the Herpesviridae family has several characteristic features, including a core containing a linear, double-stranded DNA; an icosadeltahedral capsid (approximately 100 to 110 nm in diameter); an amorphous, occasionally asymmetric material surrounding the capsid, called the tegument; and an envelope containing viral glycoprotein spikes on its surface.

The herpesviruses have been further classified into subfamilies and genera aimed to reflect evolutionary relatedness and to help in predicting the properties and facilitate the identification of a new isolate.

The subfamily Alphaherpesvirinae consists of the genera *Simplexvirus* (HSV-1, HSV-2, circopithecine herpesvirus 1, bovine mamillitis virus) and *Varicellovirus* (VZV, pseudorabies virus, and the equine herpesvirus 1). These viruses have a variable host range, relatively short replication cycle, rapid culture growth, and the ability to destruct infected cells efficiently and to establish latent infections primarily (but not exclusively) in sensory ganglia.

The subfamily Betaherpesvirinae comprises viral species with restricted (but not nonexclusive) host range, and which have typically long reproductive cycles. The infection develops slowly in cultures, and infected cells often become enlarged (cytomegalia). These viruses may exist in a latent form in secretory glands, lymphoreticular cells, kidneys, and other tissues. Two genera, *Cytomegalovirus* (HCMV) and *Muromegalovirus* (murine cytomegalovirus), comprise the Betaherpesvirinae subfamily.

A third subfamily, Gammaherpesvirinae, comprises viruses that are specific for T or B lymphocytes, where the infection has been frequently either at a prelytic or lytic stage, but without the production of infectious progeny. Latent virus has often been demonstrated in lymphoid tissue. Two genera, *Lymphocryptovirus* (e.g., Epstein-Barr virus) and *Rhadinovirus* (herpesvirus ateles and herpesvirus saimiri), belong to this subfamily.

1.1 CYTOMEGALOVIRUS

1.1.1 INTRODUCTION

Cytomegaloviruses are ubiquitous pathogens that commonly infect animals and humans.[1-3] Their classification is based on the biological properties of host specificity, length of replication cycle, and the cytopathic effects.[4] The genera *Cytomegalovirus* (human cytomegalovirus, HCMV) together with the genera *Muromegalovirus* (murine cytomegalovirus) belong to the subfamily Betaherpesvirinae of the family Herpesviridae. A nonexclusive characteristic of the subfamily Betaherpesvirinae is a restricted host range. Their reproductive cycle is prolonged, with the infection progressing slowly in culture.[4]

Also known as betaherpesviruses, the human cytomegaloviruses are highly species-specific both for replication and pathogenesis. While some host cells are more susceptible to infection, others do not succumb to the virus but may play an important role in harboring the pathogen. The latter may persist for longer periods of time, after which it may establish latency.

The cytomegaloviruses are enveloped herpesviruses formed by an incosahedral capsid. The majority of them have large linear double-strand DNA genomes equivalent to approximately 240 kilobase pairs (or 150 million daltons).[5-11] The human cytomegalovirus (human herpesvirus V) possesses an isomerizing genome, whereas all studied animal CMVs have nonisomerizing genomes.[3] Because of its size and sequence complexity, the HCMV genome has been classified in the E group of the herpesviridae genomes (complexity of structure increasing from A to E).[4] The HCMV genome is further divided into long (L) and short (S) components, which are capable of isomerization. Since the L and S components of HCMV can invert during replication, the resulting virions may contain any one of the four isomers of the viral genome.[8]

The HCMV DNA polymerase, a 140-kDa polypeptide enzyme involved in viral DNA synthesis, is physiologically different from cellular polymerases.[12,13] Similarly to other herpesviruses,[14] the HCMV polymerase has associated with it a 3'-specific exonuclease activity that favors single-strand DNA as a substrate.[13,14] Because of its difference from cellular polymerases, inhibition of HCMV polymerase activity is a mode of action of antiviral drugs.

Probably the thousands of genetically different strains of HCMV currently in existence circulate in the general population throughout the world.[15] Humans are believed to be the only reservoir for HCMV. Cytomegalovirus infection is acquired throughout life, with over 50% of the adult population being infected by 50 years of age. While neonatal HCMV infections can be severe, in healthy populations the disease is usually asymptomatic. Transmission is carried out by direct or indirect person-to-person contact.[2,16] Among the various sources of infection, oropharyngeal secretions, cervical and vaginal excretions, spermatic fluids, urine, feces, breast milk, tears, and blood are predominant.[17-19] Oral and respiratory spread appear to be the primary routes of transmission during childhood and possibly adulthood. Multiple or large quantities of blood transfusion also convey a greater risk of both primary and recurrent HCMV infections.[2]

Infection with HCMV may be acquired throughout the year and does not appear to be seasonal or dependent on climate.[20]

HCMV infection in immunocompetent hosts[21,22] usually is benign and asymptomatic, although occasionally it may be associated with a heterophile-negative mononucleosis syndrome. In both cases there may be shedding of virus in urine and oral secretions for several months to several years after the primary infection.[23]

After primary infection, HCMV remains latent in the cells. However, similarly to other herpesviruses, HCMV can reactivate in immunosuppressed hosts. The primary HCMV infection is frequently followed by persistent and/or recurrent infections. While most often recurrent infections result from latent viral reactivation, reinfection may also occur, possibly because of the antigenic diversity of the cytomegaloviruses.[2,24]

Infected cells very often become enlarged (cytomegalia) with intranuclear inclusions similar to those produced by herpes simplex and varicella zoster virus. These cellular changes led to the term "cytomegalic inclusion disease" (CID), an early designation of the infection.[25,26] CID, which clinically is characterized as a combination of hepatosplenomegaly, jaundice, thrombocytopenia, purpura, or microcephaly,[27] is found in approximately 7% of cases of HCMV intrauterine infection. The prognosis of children with CID is poor, with high fatality rate during infancy.[28]

In severe disseminated disease, evidence of HCMV presence can be seen in virtually all organs,[2,29-32] but ductal epithelial cells are the major site of involvement. In infants and young children, salivary glands are most frequently affected.[30,32] Viruria resulting from renal infection is consistently observed in all age groups. The lungs are another organ affected by HCMV, especially in immunosuppressed older patients and bone marrow transplant recipients. Other organs, although less frequently involved in HCMV infection, include the adrenals, ovaries, bones, pancreas, and the skin.[2,29]

It is noteworthy that the term "recurrent infection" is generally used to refer to intermittent excretion of virus from single or multiple sites over a prolonged period of time, and should be differentiated from "chronic" or "prolonged excretion" of virus which characterizes certain forms of HCMV infection.[2]

In older but normal patients, the virologic and immunologic characteristics of primary HCMV infection have been best defined as a mononucleosis syndrome. IgG antibodies against HCMV-specified cellular proteins appear 2 to 3 weeks after the onset of symptoms, reach their peak within 1 to 2 months, and then persist for years.[33,34]

1.1.2 CLINICAL MANIFESTATIONS OF HCMV DISEASE

The most common clinical manifestations of CMV infection in immunocompromised hosts include chorioretinitis, gastrointestinal disorders (esophagitis, colitis, cholangitis), central nervous system (CNS) infection, pneumonitis, and adrenal gland disease.

1.1.2.1 Chorioretinitis

HCMV infection in healthy individuals is rarely manifested by ocular involvement,[35-40] and only with a handful of cases describing retinitis.[37,38] However, chorioretinitis is the most common clinical visceral presentation of HCMV infection in AIDS patients, affecting as many as 60% to 80% of the HIV-infected population.[41-45] In addition, patients with lymphoma, leukemia, and other malignancies, and organ transplant recipients receiving immunosuppressive chemotherapy are also at high risk of acquiring retinal and choroidal HCMV infections.[35,46-48]

Symptoms of HCMV retinitis include visual defects or decreased visual acuity characterized by white-colored lesions with perivascular exudates and hemorrhages.[49] HCMV retinitis may result in either serous or the more common rhegmatogenous (13.5% to 29%)[50-53] retinal detachments[54] and necrosis.[55] HCMV-induced optic neuritis has been described in lymphoma and AIDS patients.[42,51,56-58] Concomitant ocular manifestations associated with HCMV retinitis include iridocyclitis, punctate keratitis, anterior chamber cell and flare, and uveitis.[48,50,59-63] Faber et al.[64] reported the presence of retinal calcifications (focal yellow-white, plaque-like lesions and small refractile lesions) in HCMV retinitis in patients with AIDS. A persistent white border opacification on the edge of healed HCMV retinitis can often be observed in patients with AIDS undergoing systemic antiviral therapy.[65] If it is not recognized as a stable configuration, patients may undergo unnecessary reinductions with potentially toxic doses of antiviral medications.

1.1.2.2 Gastrointestinal Disease

After retinitis, HCMV-associated gastrointestinal disorders (esophagitis, gastritis/duodenitis, colitis, and cholangitis) represent the second most common site of HCMV involvement in AIDS patients (10% to 15%).[66-69] Also, patients with inflammatory bowel disease have an increased risk for developing HCMV infections of the gastrointestinal (GI) tract.[70] Other patients at risk are those with malignancies, solid organ and bone marrow transplant recipients, and patients on immunosuppressive therapy.[71]

Ulceration of the GI tract is the most common primary lesion induced by HCMV.[72] HCMV infection of columnar epithelial cells, endothelial cells, myocytes, and fibroblasts causes tissue destruction and ulceration.[73] The presence of infected endothelial cells in the small vessel walls suggests that, at least in some cases, HCMV vasculitis may be responsible for the development of necrotic ulceration.[74]

Colitis is the most common HCMV-induced GI disorder, occurring in 5% to 10% of AIDS patients. It is characterized by diarrhea, abdominal pain, weight loss, and fever.[75-77] A computerized tomography (CT) scan of the abdomen shows a thick colonic wall, producing a target spin.[78] Colitis has also been one of the sequelae of HCMV infection in transplant patients, where it can be associated with severe consequences, making its early recognition and treatment important.[79] It should be noticed that colitis may be frequently associated (up to 50% of all cases) with other pathogens, such as *Entamoeba histolytica, Campylobacter jejuni, Giardia, Cryptosporidium,* or *Mycobacterium avium intracellulare.*

Esophagitis is another manifestation of HCMV infection of the GI tract.[80] In a prospective study of 154 AIDS patients, 2.6% presented with HCMV esophagitis.[81] Esophageal symptoms were present in nearly all patients with odynophagia, and in 30% to 50% of cases of dysphagia.[82] Endoscopic findings revealed the presence of generally extensive ulceration, more often solitary than multiple, located in the middle third or distal esophagus.[81,82]

Various abnormalities of the biliary tract (e.g., cholangitis) have also been reported in association with HCMV in AIDS patients.[83] While the liver enzymes were normal or slightly higher, there were markedly elevated levels of serum-alkaline phosphatases in the majority of cases.[72]

In a prospective study, Murray et al.[84] have examined the incidence of CMV in gastroduodenal ulcerations in immunocompetent patients.

1.1.2.3   Central Nervous System HCMV Infection

The involvement of HCMV with the CNS of AIDS patients is frequent. Thus, in a consecutive study of 174 brain autopsies of AIDS patients, Mathiesen et al.[85] found 148 to be abnormal, with HCMV being the third cause of encephalitis (14.3%). The clinical diagnosis of HCMV-associated CNS disorders may be difficult because of the presence of HIV encephalopathy.[72] One diagnostic tool to distinguish HCMV encephalitis is by brain biopsy demonstrating periventricular necrosis with intranuclear or intracytoplasmic inclusions.[86]

HCMV polyradiculomyelopathy, an uncommon but distinctive clinical syndrome in HIV-infected patients,[87-101] is characterized by ascending motor weakness, areflexia, loss of sphincter control, parasthesias, and varying sensory impairments which develop subacutely in association with a polymorphonuclear pleocytosis, increased protein, and hypoglycorrhachia in the cerebrospinal fluid.[88,89,96,102] The syndrome rapidly progresses to flaccid paralysis.[97] Examination of the cerebrospinal fluid (CSF) typically reveals neutrophilic leukocytosis and an elevated concentration of protein.[87,88,93,96,103]

1.1.2.4   Pneumonitis

Compared to other immunocompromised individuals, pneumonitis is much less common in AIDS patients,[72] as well as in autologous bone marrow transplant recipients (average 0.8%).[104] Similarly to gastrointestinal infections, HCMV appears to be frequently associated with other pathogens, especially *Pneumocystis carinii.*[105] HCMV-induced pneumonitis is manifested as interstitial pneumonia with progressive dyspnea, nonproductive cough, and the presence of diffuse bilateral interstitial infiltrates.[106]

1.1.2.5   Adrenal Gland HCMV Infection

Autopsy results have indicated that infection of the adrenal gland associated with necrosis has been the most common site of HCMV infiltration.[107] Adrenal insufficiency accompanied with fatigue, hypotension, and hyponatremia are indicative of hormonal abnormalities associated with HCMV involvement.[72,108]

1.1.3   IMMUNOLOGIC RESPONSE TO HCMV DISEASE

HCMV is atypical of many viruses in that the presence of its antibodies, even neutralizing antibodies, does not imply immunity to either reactivated latent infection or reinfection. In addition,

HCMV possesses the ability to establish latency in one or more types of peripheral leukocytes, resulting in infected blood becoming a vector for transmission of the virus.

With solid organ transplant recipients there is dissociation of humoral and cell-mediated responses to HCMV infection. Thus, after initiation of immunosuppression and transplantation, the HCMV-specific cellular responses typically disappear, whereas the overall humoral response stays intact.[109] The observed loss of cellular responses correlates well with the appearance of HCMV infection.[109] Studying renal transplant recipients, Lopez et al.[110] have noticed an increase of humoral responses to HCMV infection that can compensate for depressed cell-mediated immunity.

In order to study the importance of the immune status of the donor in the development of immunity after allogeneic bone marrow transplantation, Boland et al.[111] monitored 23 HCMV antibody-positive bone marrow transplant recipients for humoral and cellular immunity to HCMV, of whom 12 had a HCMV antibody-positive and 11 a HCMV antibody-negative marrow donor. Lymphocyte proliferation to HCMV recovered significantly earlier after the transplantation in recipients of marrow from a HCMV-positive donor (10.4 weeks after surgery) compared with the recipients of marrow from HCMV-negative donors (16.7 weeks after transplantation; $p < .05$). Furthermore, while IgM responses after active infection were seen in both groups, initial IgG rises without IgM were seen only in recipients of marrow from HCMV-positive donors ($p < .05$). Lymphocyte proliferative or humoral immune responses to HCMV were not detected in any of the control group of patients consisting of HCMV-negative recipients. The results of Boland et al. provided strong evidence that T cell memory to HCMV is transferred with donor marrow from HCMV-positive donors, leading in most patients to direct IgG anti-HCMV responses and to rapid recovery of cellular immunity to HCMV.

Two distinct types of tumor necrosis factor (TNF) receptors (TNF-R) have been identified (TNF-R55 and TNF-R75). Both TNF-Rs also exist in soluble forms (TNF-sR), resulting from the release of the extracellular domains (TNF-sR55 and TNF-sR75). TNF-sR may play an important role *in vivo* as they can bind to TNF-α and prevent ligand binding to the cellular TNF-R, thus acting as naturally occurring inhibitors of TNF-α.[112] Humbert et al.[112] assayed sera from lung allograft recipients with HCMV pneumonitis for the presence of TNF-sR55 and TNF-sR75. The concentrations were compared with those from either control lung recipients displaying neither rejection nor infection, or lung recipients with allograft rejection. Both TNF-sR55 and TNF-sR75 serum concentrations were significantly higher during HCMV pneumonitis (mean values of 13.7 and 11.7 ng/ml, respectively) than during allograft rejection (3.7 and 2.6 ng/ml, respectively; $p < .001$). The TNF-sR55 and TNF-sR75 serum concentrations were also higher than in control subjects (3.6 and 1.9 ng/ml, respectively; $p < .001$). The serum TNF-α concentration was low in case of rejection or in control subjects (< 20 pg/ml). Conversely, increased levels of TNF-α were detected in the serum of 50% of patients with HCMV pneumonitis. Ganciclovir treatment of HCMV pneumonitis led to a dramatic decrease of TNF-α, TNF-sR55, and TNF-sR75 serum levels.[112]

Fietze et al.[113] also studied the role of TNF in HCMV infection in transplant recipients. Using a set of monoclonal anti-HCMV antibodies, these investigators found HCMV antigen expression in peripheral blood mononuclear cells (PBMNC), particularly in monocytes. The detection of HCMV-IE antigens and HCMV-IE DNA in PBMNC indicated that positive host cells may represent truly infected cells. Furthermore, the observed relationship between increased cytokine plasma levels (particularly following treatment by pan-T cell antibodies) and the appearance of HCMV antigens in PBMNC suggested that cytokines may play an important role in the reversal of HCMV latency. Fietze et al.[113] corroborated the latter finding by demonstrating that TNF-α was able to stimulate the activity of HCMV-IE enhancer/promoter region in the human monocytic cell line, HL-60. However, a number of cytokines (interleukin (IL)-1, IL-2, IL-3, IL-4, IL-6, IL-8, and IL-10, transforming growth factor (TGF)-β, interferon (IFN)-γ, and the granulocyte-macrophage colony-stimulating factor) did not show any enhancing effect on the HCMV promoter activity. Thus, TNF-α seems to play an important role in regulating the balance between latency and reactivation of

HCMV infection.[113] Inhibition of TNF-α release or action may represent an alternative strategy for preventing HCMV-associated morbidity in allograft patients.

To further assess the role of TNF-α on mortality in HCMV disease, Anderson et al.[114] conducted experiments in murine HCMV-infected mice. Treatment of 3-week-old Swiss Webster mice with TNF-α to infection with murine HCMV had no demonstrable effect on mortality. TNF-α treatment after infection, as expected, resulted in increased mortality; the increased mortality occurred when nonlethal doses of TNF-α were used and required virus replication. However, if mice were treated prior to HCMV infection with a combination of murine IFN-γ and murine TNF-α, the dose of IFN-γ required to achieve significant reduction in mortality was reduced by a factor >10.

Even though both the humoral and cell-mediated immunity are important in deterring infections, it appeared that in the case of HCMV, cellular responses were more important than the humoral defenses.[115] Thus, *in vitro* data by Howard and Balfour[116] demonstrated that immune lymphocytes, but not antibodies, were able to prevent the spread of herpes virus in a fibroblast monolayer culture. In further experiments,[116] mice infected with either wild-type or live attenuated murine HCMV developed both humoral and cellular immunity. However, when the mice received antilymphocyte globulin (ALG) and prednisolone during infection, the humoral immunity developed normally, whereas cellular immunity did not. Similar aberrations occurred if the mice were immunosuppressed at the time of maximum immune response to HCMV infection.[116] Translating these results to a human setting, Howard and Balfour[116] hypothesized that immunosuppressed renal transplant recipients would react in a similar fashion. This supposition was supported by several cases of transplant recipients who were able to mount responses prior to transplantation, but not after immunosuppression.[116]

Experimental evidence by van den Berg et al.[117] has shown that in renal transplant recipients, recovery from HCMV disease coincided with expansion of the CD8bright and CD56+ subset lymphocytes and with increased expression of the activation marker HLA-DR. Furthermore, primary infection was associated with activation of both subsets, whereas during secondary infection, mainly CD8bright cells responded. Progressive HCMV disease (requiring antiviral treatment) and relapse occurred in association with low numbers of activated CD8bright and CD56+ cells. Therefore, monitoring of lymphocyte activation may provide clinically useful information during the course of HCMV infections.[117]

In a further clarification of the role of cellular immunity in HCMV disease, cytotoxicity assays carried out by Starr et al.[118] using HCMV-infected fibroblast suspensions have revealed that in renal transplant recipients, natural killer (NK) cells play an important part in the response of HCMV-infected targets. There was a significant decrease in the activity of NK cells in immunosuppressed patients that returned to normal only during the late post-transplantation period. It was postulated that the observed decrease in NK cell activity was the result of immunosuppressive therapy (azathioprine, corticosteroids) as was the case in normal volunteers. In symptomatic patients, high levels of NK cell activity appeared in a temporal relationship to the reduction in doses of immunosuppressive drugs. In asymptomatic patients, however, the NK cell activity remained low, indicating the existence of other cellular or humoral factors capable of limiting the HCMV infection.[118] Charak et al.[119] have found that, both *in vitro* and *in vivo*, IL-2 promoted the generation and proliferation of NK cells in peripheral blood and bone marrow. When used in a syngeneic bone marrow transplantation setting and followed by IL-2 therapy, murine bone marrow NK cells activated with IL-2 *in vitro* (ABM) demonstrated potent graft-versus-leukemia (GVL) and anti-HCMV activities.[119] ABM cells retained their ability to reconstitute the hematopoietic system both in normal and leukemic mice. Furthermore, ABM cells can purge leukemia without loss of progenitor cell activity *in vitro*. The observed purging ability of ABM cells can be increased by IL-1, IFN-γ, and TNF-α.[119]

In addition to NK cells, the activity of two other cell subpopulations, human lymphocyte antigen (HLA)-restricted cytotoxic T cells and antibody-dependent killer cells, showed good correlation with the outcome of HCMV infection.

It has been accepted that the activity of the cytotoxic T cells is defined by the presence of appropriate surface antigens on the target cells.[120] In addition, their cytotoxic activity is further defined by the presence of HLA-A and HLA-B locus antigens on the target cell. Thus, the activity of cytotoxic T cells is conditional on the presence of both viral antigens and surface HLA antigens.

The antibody-dependent killer cells detect viral antigens on the target cells with surface Fc receptors that bind specific IgG immunoglobulins; cells in this subpopulation include both macrophages and NK cells.[120] Reviewing the effects of these cell types on the outcome of HCMV disease, Quinnan and Rook[120] found that most post-transplantation HCMV infections did occur between weeks 4 and 12 after the surgery. During that time, there was significantly more killing of matched target cells than of mismatched cells. The response was short-lived and took place during the acute stage of the infection, coinciding with the onset of viremia-associated symptoms.[120] Furthermore, Quinnan et al.[121] have observed that in the absence of a robust cytotoxic lymphocytic response, the outcome of HCMV infection in nearly all bone marrow transplant recipients was fatal; no other factor correlated as well with this outcome of HCMV infection. This finding has been corroborated by Rook et al.,[122] who reported the significance of intact responses among HCMV-specific cytotoxic lymphocytes in renal transplant recipients. In particular, cytotoxic lymphocytes detected *in vitro* at the time of HCMV infection correlated significantly with an uneventful recovery. Furthermore, Rook et al.[122] addressed two other issues, namely, (1) that HCMV infection in immunocompromised patients was frequently complicated by HCMV-associated allograft dysfunction; it is possible, therefore, that an intact HCMV-specific immune response by the organ recipient may not injure the graft and protect the kidney from HCMV infection-related damage, and (2) that immunosuppressive drugs, such as high-dose corticosteroids, can hamper HCMV-specific cytotoxicity in nonresponsive patients, making it prudent to lower the dosage to levels permitting the patient to mount a HCMV-specific response by the cytotoxic lymphocyte.[122]

The antibody-mediated responses, although thought to be significantly less involved in HCMV disease,[109,110,116,123] have been reported to still play a role. Thus, several studies have concluded that anti-HCMV IgG and IgM isotypes in transplant recipients mounted a response to HCMV infections.[124-127] O'Neill et al.[124] examined the role of anti-HCMV IgG and IgM responses to early and late HCMV antigens in renal transplant recipients with primary or recurrent HCMV infections. Anti-HCMV IgM antibody to late antigens was detected in all patients with primary HCMV infection compared to 50% of patients with reactivated HCMV infection. The results were reversed, however, for anti-HCMV IgG response to HCMV early antigens: 100% of patients with recurrent HCMV infection developed the antibody, compared to only 40% of those with primary infection. Anti-HCMV IgM antibody to early antigens was not detected in either group of patients. The presence of anti-CMV IgM to late antigens reflected an active HCMV infection, whereas its absence did not rule out the possibility of reactivated HCMV infection.[124] The reported findings were consistent with those of other studies. In further refinement of their studies, O'Neill et al.[125] measured the levels of low- and high-molecular-weight anti-HCMV IgM fractions among renal transplant recipients with either primary or reactivated HCMV infection. High-molecular-weight IgM was detected in all patients, whereas low-molecular-weight IgM was found in only 58% of patients with primary infection, and in 12.5% of patients with reactivated HCMV infection. In contrast, anti-HCMV IgM was present only in the low-molecular-weight fraction of patients with heart disease.[126] While the importance of these finding is still unclear, it may be that IgM fractions vary predictably during certain disease states.[125]

Rodriguez and Adler[127] have described differences in the response of IgG subclasses 1 through 4 to HCMV infection in HCMV-seropositive recipients of HCMV-seronegative blood transfusions. Prior to transfusion, all patients had a similar anti-HCMV IgG 1, IgG 3, and IgG 4 distribution. None of the patients studied had detectable anti-HCMV antibodies of the IgG 2 subclass. After transfusion, the patients experienced increases in one or more of the IgG 1, IgG 3, and IgG 4 subclasses. Based on these results, it has been suggested that assays for IgG subclasses may be a more sensitive indicator of HCMV infection than assays measuring total IgG.[127]

1.1.4   HCMV Infection in Immunocompromised Hosts

HCMV has long been considered to be an immunosuppressive agent capable of inhibiting the host immune response and contributing to the persistence of infection.[128] In a symptomatic primary HCMV infection, the cell-mediated immunity is depressed with T cell abnormalities most readily defined.[41] Consequently, the likelihood of cytomegalovirus infections is markedly increased in the immunocompromised host.[66,129-134] By some accounts,[129] between 46% and 80% of the immuno-compromised population may be infected. In renal allograft recipients,[135-143] the primary infections vary from 22% to 100% (average 53%) and recurrent infections from 46% to 100% (average 85%). Similar rates of infections have been seen among cardiac and bone marrow transplant recipients.[2,144-147] HCMV is the most commonly isolated opportunistic pathogen associated with hepatitis following orthotopic liver transplantation.[148-154]

To test the previously observed association between decreasing lymphocyte titers and HCMV-related death in bone marrow transplant recipients, Fries et al.[155] conducted a retrospective study of 332 HCMV-infected recipients. The data obtained suggested that, indeed, in some patients a drop in the lymphocyte counts was a consequence of HCMV infection associated with fatal HCMV disease. Whether this phenomenon can be attributed to direct infection of lymphocytes, a defective immune response, or some other mechanism remains to be determined.

Zomas et al.[156] reported unusually severe cytomegaloviremia in three patients with chronic lymphocytic leukemia (CLL) who had undergone allogeneic bone marrow transplantation from matched sibling donors. Although the number of patients was small, the severity of HCMV infection should place CLL patients undergoing allogeneic bone marrow transplantation at higher risk than patients allografted for other diseases.

While HCMV infection is frequently observed in allograft recipients, not all infected individuals will develop disease. In solid organ transplant recipients, HCMV infection develops largely when a seropositive organ containing the virus is transplanted into a recipient.[148,149] If the recipient has a preexisting immunity against HCMV, this can partially ameliorate the disease.[28,139] However, in bone marrow allograft recipients, HCMV infection usually ensues from reactivation of latent infection in the recipient.[157]

The fact that after renal transplantation most patients had become productively infected implied frequent reactivation of latent HCMV.[129,158] Reactivation occurs despite the serologic status of donors.

Due to the high rate of seropositivity (90% to 100%) among AIDS patients, HCMV was originally thought by some to be the etiologic agent of AIDS.[130,131] Approximately 40% of patients with AIDS present with HCMV visceral involvement at the advanced stage of the disease.[72,159] The most common localizations are retinitis and gastrointestinal infection, and to a lesser extent CNS disorders. When compared to HCMV infection in non-HIV immunosuppressed patients, retinitis in HIV-positive individuals is much more prevalent than pneumonitis. To this end, despite the presence of HCMV in the lungs, Millar et al.[160] found no evidence of HCMV-induced pneumonitis in AIDS patients, presumably due to the inability of the lungs to mount the T cell response necessary for immunopathology; results from mouse and human studies have lent credence to the hypothesis that the pathogenesis of HCMV pneumonitis is immunopathologically mediated.[161]

Because in AIDS patients the coexistence of multiple pathogens is frequent, the diagnosis of HCMV infection may be complicated.

The profound and progressive immune suppression caused by the human immunodeficiency virus creates optimal conditions for reactivation of a latent intracellular HCMV infection which becomes chronic with high frequency of relapses due to the progression of HIV infection over time. Also, since multiple strains of HCMV have been identified in populations at risk,[24] reinfection remains a distinct possibility.

By all accounts, HCMV has become a major opportunistic infection in AIDS patients, with autopsy studies indicating that as many as 90% of patients had active disseminated infection.[72,162]

CD4+ lymphocyte counts of less than 100×10^6/l present the highest risk for developing HCMV infection;[163] the corresponding value for CD8+ lymphocytes was less than 0.500×10^9/l.[164]

HIV and HCMV share common characteristics and clinical features. They are both lymphotropic viruses, leading to latent infection in cells, sexually and blood transmitted, and both being immunosuppressive. There is also strong evidence of transactivation between the two viruses.[165] Thus, Ghazal et al.[166] have demonstrated that interaction can occur at the single cell level by transactivation of the HIV genome by HCMV immediate-early proteins. In additon, HCMV may also augment the tropic range of HIV by expressing its Fc receptor on cells and thus allowing opsonized HIV to enter a new group of tissues, or by forming pseudotypes between the two viruses.[167] Corroborating these findings is the observation that in HIV-positive hemophilia patients[168] the risk of developing AIDS is three times higher in those with positive HCMV antibodies than in HCMV-negative patients (relative risk 3.2; $p = .02$).[169] Furthermore, the risk was independent of age, and was accompanied by the increased presence of p24 antigen, suggesting that HCMV was acting by facilitating HIV proliferation.

1.1.5 STUDIES ON THERAPEUTICS

1.1.5.1 Ganciclovir

Ganciclovir (DHPG, cytovene) is an acyclic analog of 2′-deoxyguanosine that needs to be phosphorylated in order to inhibit the viral synthesis. Its mechanism of action involves suppression of viral DNA synthesis by competitive inhibition of viral DNA polymerases and direct incorporation into viral DNA, resulting in termination of DNA elongation.

Most antiviral nucleosides (e.g., acyclovir, ganciclovir, zidovudine) depend on cellular or virus-induced thymidine kinase for the initial phosphorylation to monophosphate. Further phosphorylation to the 5′-triphosphate form will allow them to interact with the viral polymerases, and in the majority of cases to get incorporated into the viral DNA, causing the irreversible termination of DNA elongation. The viral DNA polymerase becomes inactivated during the process; for example, acyclovir and ganciclovir in their 5′-triphosphate forms will compete with deoxyguanosine triphosphate (dGTP) for incorporation into DNA. Nucleosides having this mode of action are known as suicide inhibitors; that is, once the nucleoside triphosphate-viral enzyme complex is formed, the process is irreversible and dGTP can no longer compete, leading to inactivation of the viral enzyme. Further defining the process, Reardon and Spector[170] have shown that an additional nucleotide, deoxycytidine (dCTP) is required for acyclovir triphosphate to form a dead-end complex with the viral enzyme. Selectivity is the major advantage of suicide inhibitors, since inactivation does not occur with cellular DNA polymerase α.[171]

Studies on the susceptibility of HCMV to ganciclovir have shown inhibitory concentrations (ED_{50}) ranging between 0.54 and 5.9 μM.[172] Peak plasma concentrations of 18.61 to 23.29 μM (4.75 to 6.50 μg/ml) were reached after intravenous infusion of 2.5 mg/kg of ganciclovir every 8 to 12 h, which is well above the ED_{50} values for most HCMV strains.[173] The ganciclovir levels in the CSF have been estimated to be 24% to 67% of those in plasma.[173]

The pharmacokinetics of ganciclovir in cases of severe renal dysfunction were investigated in anuric heart transplant recipients undergoing continuous venovenous hemodialysis (CVVHD).[174] Ganciclovir was administered at a dose of 5.0 mg/kg every 48 h for at least 9 d. The pharmacokinetic parameters, which were determined by high performance liquid chromatography (HPLC) of samples collected from arterial and venous blood lines and ultrafiltrate, as well as the steady-state clearance of ultrafiltration and sieving coefficient, have shown that CVVHD was highly effective in removing ganciclovir from plasma. Furthermore, CVVHD appeared to be more effective than intermittent hemodyalisis.[174] Ashton et al.[175] studied the intravitreal pharmacokinetics of ganciclovir in both rabbits and humans.

Ganciclovir, as well as acyclovir, appeared to cross the placenta at least at therapeutic levels by a simple diffusion, and this transfer was not affected by the nucleoside transport inhibitor dinitrobenzylthiosinine.[176]

The combined effect of ganciclovir and hyperimmune serum (HIS) was studied in two different rat models.[177] In immunosuppressed Brown Norway rats with a lethal generalized rat cytomegalovirus (RCMV), treatment with ganciclovir and HIS effectively reduced both mortality rate and virus titers in the liver and lungs but not in spleen. In the second model, interstitial pneumonia was established in RCMV-infected immunosuppressed Brown Norway rats after allogeneic bone marrow transplantation. Ganciclovir reduced the virus titers in the lungs but had no effect on the interstitial pneumonia. In contrast, HIS markedly decreased both the virus titers and histologic changes in the lungs. A moderate synergistic effect for the ganciclovir-HIS combination was also observed.[177]

The anti-HCMV efficacy of ganciclovir in combination with other antimicrobial agents (amphotericin B, ketoconazole, dapsone, and trimethoprim-sulfamethoxazole) have been evaluated both *in vitro* and *in vivo*.[178] When differences in three-dimensional plots for antiviral activity and cytotoxicity of ganciclovir alone and in combination were compared, the anti-HCMV activity of ganciclovir ($IC_{50} = 8.0 \mu M$; 5.0 to 9.0 μM range) was not affected by concentrations of up to 10 μM amphotericin B, 1000 μM ketoconazole, 100 μM dapsone, or 320 μM trimethoprim-sulfamethoxazole; higher concentrations were tested because of cytotoxicity. In Swiss Webster mice, the anti-CMV efficacy of ganciclovir against murine CMV was also unaffected when administered in combination with any of the four antimicrobial agents. Thus, ganciclovir alone had an ED_{50} of 7.0 mg/kg (2.0 to 12 mg/kg range), which was unaffected by daily doses of 1.0 mg/kg intravenous amphotericin B, 60 mg/kg of intraperitoneal ketoconazole, 32 mg/kg of oral dapsone, or 80/400 mg/kg of oral trimethoprim-sulfamethoxazole. The reported data indicated that ganciclovir can be administered in combination with these other antimicrobial drugs for treatment of various opportunistic infections in AIDS patients without compromising its anti-CMV efficacy.[178]

The (S)-enantiomer (SR 3772), (R)-enantiomer (SR 3773), and the (S,R)-enantiomeric mixture (SR 37745A) of ganciclovir phosphonate were evaluated for their antiviral activities against murine (MCMV)[179] and human[180] CMV. In severe combined immunodeficiency (SCID) mice infected with MCMV, SR 3773 and SR 3745A were superior to ganciclovir in extending the mean time to death, whereas SR 3772 and SR 3722 (acyclovir phosphonate) were less potent than ganciclovir. While the results of the study suggested that SR 3773 may be useful in the treatment of human CMV, its renal toxicity may be a serious drawback.[179] SR 3727A was also inhibitory to strain AD169 of human CMV — its ED_{50} value ranged from 6.0 to 17 μM for three laboratory strains of human CMV, whereas the 50% cytotoxic concentrations were over 4200 μM as determined by viable cell assay. The ED_{50} concentrations of SR 3727A against ganciclovir-sensitive clinical isolates were in the 8.0 to 47 μM range; the corresponding values against two ganciclovir-resistant strains of human CMV were 84 and 320 μM.[180]

1.1.5.1.1   Toxicity of ganciclovir

The major toxic side effect of ganciclovir is its hematoxicity, including neutropenia (40% of the cases), thrombocytopenia, or anemia (20%).[181] In order to reduce the neutropenia, Hardy et al.[182,183] have recommended the use of recombinant human granulocyte-macrophage colony-stimulating factor or human granulocyte colony-stimulating factor. Although oral ganciclovir was tolerated at doses of up to 6.0 g daily, at that dose the rate of neutropenia was higher.[184]

Another drawback of ganciclovir has been the bone marrow suppression it induced when given concomitantly with zidovudine.[185] Other side effects included confusion, fever, gastrointestinal disorders (nausea), abnormal liver function, anemia, and cutaneous rash.[50,72,186-189]

Scholz et al.[190] provided evidence for an immunosuppressive activity of ganciclovir.

Drugs that inhibit renal tubular secretion or absorption, such as probenicid, may reduce the renal clearance of ganciclovir and exacerbate its toxicity. Similarly, bone marrow suppressing agents (pentamidine isethionate, trimethoprim-sulfonamide, and amphotericin B) may inhibit bone marrow activity and spermatogenesis and further contribute to ganciclovir toxicity.

Generalized seizures have been reported in patients receiving concomitantly ganciclovir and imipenem-cilastin sodium.[35] Seizures associated with ganciclovir therapy alone were reported in a patient with AIDS and disseminated CMV disease; despite the administration of phenytoin, the seizure-like activity subsided only after discontinuing ganciclovir.[191]

1.1.5.2 Foscarnet

Foscarnet (PFA, foscavir, trisodium phosphonoformate) is a pyrophosphate analog active against a wide variety of human herpesviruses, including ganciclovir-resistant HCMV strains, by inhibiting viral DNA polymerases.[192,193] In addition, foscarnet has been shown to inhibit HIV reverse transcriptase.[194]

Contrary to ganciclovir and other nucleosides, foscarnet and other pyrophosphate analogs (phosphonoacetate; PAA) did not require prior phosphorylation in order to inhibit the viral DNA polymerase. These compounds inhibit pyrophosphorolysis competitively with pyrophosphate, but were noncompetitive with dNTPs and uncompetitive with DNA.[193]

After a single 90 mg/kg dose of foscarnet in patients with AIDS, its levels in plasma ranged from 297 to 1775 μg/ml (990 to 5920 μmol/l), with a mean value of 766 μg/ml.[195] The corresponding levels in CSF were 57 to 225 μg/ml (190 to 750 μmol/l), with a mean value of 131 μg/ml; the penetration coefficient was 0.05 to 0.72. At steady state, the mean foscarnet levels in plasma were 464 μg/ml (1553 μmol/l), whereas the mean levels in CSF were 308 μg/ml (1023 μmol/ml); the penetration coefficient was 0.66. Although the penetration coefficients were highly variable after a single administration and at steady state, the concentrations of foscarnet in the CSF were sufficient for complete inhibition of HCMV replication *in vitro*.[195] The plasma concentrations of foscarnet after twice-daily infusions of 90 mg/kg for 2 weeks showed no significant difference between day 1, day 7, and day 14; mean peak and trough concentrations on day 14 were 605 and 52 μM, respectively.[196] In all patients, the peak levels of the drug were well above those necessary to inhibit CMV. The property of foscarnet to penetrate well the blood-brain barrier would strongly bolster its use in the treatment of HCMV encephalitis.

One unique property of foscarnet has been its ability to inhibit both HIV and HCMV.[197-199] *In vitro*, the combination of foscarnet and zidovudine (AZT) produced a moderate synergistic inhibitory effect against HIV-1 at concentrations easily achieved in humans. By using partially purified HIV reverse transcriptase and human CMV DNA polymerase, Eriksson and Schinazi[198] have demonstrated significant additive interactions of various combinations of AZT-5′-triphosphate and foscarnet. The synergistic interactions in infected cells and the additive effects seen at the reverse transcriptase level have indicated that mechanisms other than the reverse transcriptase may play a role in the inhibition of HIV replication by these two compounds.[197] These *in vitro* findings suggested that concomitant administration of foscarnet to AIDS patients receiving zidovudine may be appropriate not only to treat CMV disease but also to control the HIV infection itself.

Gumbel et al.[200] conducted an *in vitro* study to establish whether liposome encapsulation of foscarnet would provide anti-HCMV efficacy comparable to that of the conventional formulation. Foscarnet was incorporated into large unilamellar vesicles of homogeneous size at a concentration of 10 mg/ml. The activity was tested against two laboratory strains (AD169 and Towne) in a plaque-reduction assay using monolayers of human foreskin fibroblasts. The IC_{50} values for encapsulated and nonencapsulated formulations in the AD169 strain were 106 and 113 μmol/l, respectively. For the Towne strain the corresponding values were 112 and 109 μmol/l, respectively. Treatment with concentrations of up to 400 μmol/l showed that foscarnet is released efficiently from the liposomes and was not toxic at the concentrations used.[200]

Utilizing a rabbit model, Sarraf et al.[201] investigated the applicability of trans-scleral iontophoresis as a technique for delivery of foscarnet to the vitreous. Using a probe tip surface area of

0.19 mm^2, a current of 1 mA, and a duration of 10 min, trans-scleral iontophoresis of 0.5 ml of a 24-mg/ml foscarnet solution was administered to normal rabbits. The vitreous aspiration was performed at 12 intervals (15 and 30 min and 1, 2, 4, 8, 16, 24, 32, 40, 48, and 60 h) after iontophoresis; the samples were analyzed by HPLC to determine the vitreous pharmacokinetics of foscarnet. A peak concentration of 200 μM was attained 4 h after iontophoresis and was well below concentrations known to cause retinal toxicity. Therapeutic concentrations of foscarnet were maintained 60 h after the iontophoresis, with no toxic effects to the anterior chamber structures; the elimination half-life was approximately 24 h. Trans-scleral iontophoresis may provide a useful and safe alternative for local treatment of HCMV retinopathy.

1.1.5.2.1 Toxicity of foscarnet

The most important side effect of foscarnet is its nephrotoxicity. It may affect as many as 50% to 60% of patients receiving continuous intravenous (IV) administration.[202] Intermittent administration[203] and concomitant saline isotonic hydration have decreased foscarnet nephrotoxicity to 15% of cases.[204,205] Electrolyte disorders induced by foscarnet have also been frequently observed. Thus, foscarnet-associated hypocalcemia is thought to be responsible for parasthesia, seizure, and nausea. It is caused by the rapid decrease of ionized calcium because of its chelation by foscarnet.[194] Hypophosphatemia and hypomagnesemia, which usually remain asymptomatic, have also been associated with foscarnet.[202,206] To this end, concomitant administration of foscarnet with antianxiety medications that may mask the symptoms of electrolyte disorders should be undertaken with caution and carefuly monitored.

Genital ulcers, due to high foscarnet concentrations in the urine, have also been reported.[207,208] Uvula and esophageal ulcerations caused by foscarnet have been discussed by Saint-Marc et al.[209]

Fan-Harvard et al.[210] have reported a possible adverse interaction between foscarnet and ciprofloxacin in patients with AIDS, HCMV retinitis, and *Mycobacterium avium* complex (MAC) infection. The incidence of seizures with foscarnet infusion has been high (13% to 15%), and is facilitated by predisposing factors, such as renal impairment, electrolyte and metabolic abnormalities, and underlying neurologic disorders. The concurrent administration of ciprofloxacin, a known epileptogenic agent, and foscarnet may predispose patients to the development of seizures and should be applied with caution.

1.1.5.3 Acyclic Nucleoside Phosphonates

HPMPC [(S)-1-(3-hydroxy-2-(phosphonylmethoxy)propyl)cytosine], an acyclic nucleoside phosphonate analog, was identified as one of the most potent and selective inhibitors of human and murine CMV.[211-216] HPMPC, which was tested in a new assay based on the enhanced esterase activity in cytomegalovirus-infected cells, specifically inhibited the viral DNA synthesis, with a very long-lasting effect. When compared to ganciclovir in a model of murine CMV (MCMV), HPMPC was far superior in preventing MCMV-induced mortality. When administered in intraperitoneally infected SCID mice as a single weekly dose of 2.0, 10, 20, or 50 mg/kg, HPMPC increased the survival period by 22, 49, 77, and 156 days, respectively. By comparison, ganciclovir at daily doses of 10, 20, or 50 mg/kg given for 5 consecutive days every week, did not delay death by more than 13, 17, and 21 days, respectively.[212]

HPMPC has also been evaluated (at 20 mg/kg as a single dose) in a murine model against rat CMV (RCMV)-induced interstitial pneumonitis secondary to allogeneic bone marrow transplantation, and its activity compared with that of ganciclovir (20 mg/kg, b.i.d. for 5 d).[213,214] HPMPC was the superior of the two drugs, leading to a complete reduction of virus titers in all organs below the detection level ($p < .01$). There was also a reduction of alveolar septal width from 6.2 μm (untreated animals) to 4.67 and 3.32 μm for HPMPC and ganciclovir, respectively.[213]

PMEDAP [9-(2-phosphonylmethoxyethyl)-2,6-diaminopurine] was also found to be highly potent in reducing the mortality rate from MCMV in both immunocompetent and immunodeficient (SCID) mice.[211]

1.1.5.4 Creatine Kinase/Creatine Phosphate Inhibitors

The creatine kinase/creatine phosphate (CK/CrP) enzyme system plays an important role in the "phosphocreatine circuit" of the cellular energy homeostasis.[217] Certain tissues of fluctuating high energy demand (e.g., brain, heart, skeletal muscle), which contain high concentrations of creatine phosphate (5 to 30 mM range),[218] utilize the natural phosphagen creatine phosphate (CrP) as a source for rapid and efficient regeneration of ATP. During this process, creatine kinase (CK) reversibly catalyzes the transfer of a high-energy phosphate bond from CrP to ADP to generate ATP. Another key function of the CK/CrP system is to produce the appropriate local ATP/ADP ratios at subcellular sites where CK is functionally coupled to ATP-consuming enzymes or processes.[217] In addition, regulation of the cellular ADP level, which affects important metabolic functions (e.g., control of mitochondrial respiration, prevention of inactivation of cellular ATPases, and prevention of the net loss of cellular adenine nucleotide pools),[219,220] may also be important for efficient viral replication.[221]

In some viral infections, human DNA viruses would normally encounter noncycling, terminally differentiated epithelial cells. In order to maximize the number of cells available for replication of viral DNA and the time spent in DNA replication, it has been hypothesized that some viruses are able to alter cell cycle controls and expression of specific proteins.[222] Thus, human CMV and adenovirus have been shown to transcriptionally activate cellular genes, and to induce the brain form of creatine kinase (CKB).[223-225] Co-transfection experiments have also demonstrated that the human CMV IE2 and adenovirus E1A gene products transactivated the CKB gene by as much as 11-fold.[224,225]

Overexpression of the brain isoenzyme of creatine kinase has been associated with several cellular proliferative processes, including response to steroid hormones (estrogen, testosterone) and signal transducers, such as phospholipase C and protein kinase C.[226-230] Overexpression of CKB has also been found in tumor growth (small cell lung carcinoma, breast and prostate cancer).[231-236]

Lillie et al.[237] and Miller et al.[238] have shown that cyclocreatine (1-carboxymethyl-2-iminoimidazolidine; CCr),[239] a cyclic analog of creatine, was able to selectively inhibit tumor growth *in vitro* and *in vivo*. The results of their studies have indicated that the CK/CrP enzyme system may well serve as a potential target for chemotherapy.

As shown in *in vitro* and *in vivo* experiments, cyclocreatine is easily phosphorylated by CK to produce cyclocreatine phosphate (CCr-P),[240,241] creating a new synthetic phosphagen pool that can partially replace CrP, the natural phosphagen,[241] but with kinetic and thermodynamic properties of CCr-P distinctly different from those of CrP.[240] For example, the phosphorus-nitrogen bond of CCr-P was more stable than that of CrP despite the structural similarity between them.[242-244] Using the V_{max}/K_m ratio as a measure of substrate quality, CCr-P is turned over 160-fold less efficiently than CrP.[240] Hence, the rate of ATP generation through the CK system was significantly reduced when CCr-P was used as the substrate.

Lillie et al.[221] evaluated *in vitro* the effect of cyclocreatine against human CMV as well as a number of other RNA and herpes viruses, providing the first example of a new class of antiviral compounds targeting the CK/CrP enzyme system. The efficacy of cyclocreatine was also evaluated *in vivo* in mouse models of HSV-2-induced vaginitis and encephalitis. In MRC-5 (normal human lung) cells, the viruses most sensitive to CCr included human CMV, varicella zoster virus, and simian CMV with ED_{50} values of 2.3, 4.0, and 5.9 mM, respectively. Against HCMV, in a single-cycle virus yield experiment in MRC-5 cells, the ED_{50} value for CCr was 4.0 mM, which was consistent with the value obtained by plaque reduction (2.3 mM). In Hs68 (human foreskin fibroblasts) cells, the ED_{50} value of CCr against human CVM was 4.6 mM. When tested against ganciclovir-resistant HCMV virus strains isolated from AIDS patients, cyclocreatine was also found active with ED_{50} values in the range of 8.5 to 10.3 mM. Overall, the *in vitro* results suggested cyclocreatine to be a selective antiviral agent with little cellular activity. Its activity appeared to be limited to herpes viruses, and particularly potent against HCMV and varicella zoster virus.[221]

1.1.5.5   DNA Topoisomerase Type II Inhibitors

DNA topoisomerases represent a class of enzymes that control and modify the topological states of DNA.[245] These enzymes are known for their ability to catalyze different types of interconversions (catenation and decatenation, and knotting and unknotting) between DNA topological isomers (topoisomers) by either: (1) temporarily breaking a DNA strand and passing another strand through the transient break (type I topoisomerases), or (2) transiently breaking a pair of complementary strands and passing another double-stranded segment (type II topoisomerases).[245] DNA topoisomerases have been found to affect many and vital biological functions, such as the replication of DNA, including DNA replication in simian virus 40 (SV40),[246] herpesvirus type I, and yeast fungi.[246-255] While both topoisomerase I and II may serve as the swivel to alleviate torsional strain produced by the movement of replication forks, the type II topoisomerase is required for the separation of newly replicated chromosomes as well as for decatenation of intertwined daughter DNA strands.[256]

Two classes of topoisomerase II inhibitors, intercalative (e.g., *m*-AMSA) and nonintercalative (e.g., VP-16, VM-26) were shown to prevent replication of human CMV DNA in tissue culture.[257] *m*-AMSA [4'-(9'-acridinylamino)methanesulfone-*m*-anisidide), a DNA-intercalative acridine derivative, induced reversible double- and single-stranded DNA breaks, the ends of which were covalently bound to topoisomerase II.[258-261] Compounds VP-16 and VM-26, two antineoplastic agents, although also specific inhibitors of topoisomerase II, did not have DNA-intercalative properties.[250,262] Benson and Huang[257] demonstrated that both *m*-AMSA and VM-26 inhibited HCMV DNA synthesis in infected confluent human embryonic lung cells. The observed anti-HCMV effect was not attributable to cytotoxic effects. Furthermore, the inhibitory activity of *m*-AMSA on the HCMV replication appeared to be distinctly irreversible. Since *o*-AMSA, a DNA-intercalative isomer of *m*-AMSA, did not inhibit topoisomerase II, the *m*-AMSA effects were not due to intercalation.[257] In addition to *m*-AMSA and VM-26 (teniposide), VP-16 (etoposide) was also shown to inhibit irreversibly HCMV replication at a drug concentration of 2.5 µg/ml, which is markedly below toxic levels to stationary phase cells.[263]

There has been a strong correlation between the magnitude of topoisomerase II activity and the effects of topoisomerase II inhibitors.[264-267] In order to more fully explain the observed anti-HCMV effect of topoisomerase II inhibitors, Benson and Huang[256] have postulated that the topoisomerase II levels in HCMV-infected cells must increase in response to infection. Indeed, they have demonstrated that not only HCMV could enhance the expression of cellular topoisomerase II, but also to require this enzyme activity for its own genomic replication. Thus, quantitation of human topoisomerase II RNA and protein levels at various times after the infection revealed that HCMV was able to induce increased intracellular levels of both topoisomerase II RNA and protein. Such accumulation began at the early stages of the infection, continued through late infection, and was not reduced by inhibition of viral DNA synthesis.[256]

1.1.6   EVOLUTION OF THERAPIES AND TREATMENT OF HCMV INFECTIONS

1.1.6.1   Management of HCMV Disease in AIDS Patients

HCMV infection is common in both homosexual and heterosexual HIV-infected patients, especially in AIDS patients with low CD4+ cell counts.[268] In an attempt to suppress HCMV viruria,

Drew et al.[269] randomly assigned symptomatic HIV-positive patients to receive zidovudine (600 mg daily) and oral acyclovir (4.8 g daily) vs. zidovudine (600 mg daily) plus placebo. The results of the study have shown that even at high daily doses (4.8 g), acyclovir failed to suppress HCMV viruria of symptomatic HIV-infected patients taking concurrent zidovudine. Acyclovir did not appear to induce ganciclovir-resistant HCMV since the ID_{50} values of isolates from the two treatment groups did not differ.[269]

HCMV retinitis in AIDS patients is often a difficult and frustrating disease to treat.[35,48,107,270-274] Therapy of HCMV retinitis should be commenced immediately to prevent rapid progression of lesions.[35,72,275-277] If left untreated, HCMV infection causes irreversible retinal necrosis ultimately resulting in loss of vision.

In patients with AIDS, central visual loss due to HCMV retinitis may present in two forms: direct macular tissue destruction, and secondary involvement as part of rhegmatogenous retinal detachment.[54] Findings by Gangan et al.[44] suggested that with appropriate treatment, the macular exudation is a reversible cause of visual impairment in patients with HCMV retinitis.

Ganciclovir[278-282] and foscarnet[283-287] are currently the drugs of choice to treat HCMV retinitis.[288-293] Their efficacy is similar, resulting in 90% to 95% response rate among patients treated for a first episode of HCMV retinitis during induction therapy (Table 1.1).[35,72] Previously, a number of therapeutic approaches have been tried, including treatments with vidarabine (adenosine arabinoside, Ara-A),[294-298] acyclovir,[43,294,295,299-301] interferon-α,[296,302,303] broad-spectrum antibiotics and antifungal agents,[35] corticosteroids,[295,304] and transfer factor.[305] All of them proved unsuccessful. Argon laser photocoagulation to the advancing edge of retinitis also resulted in failure.[306]

TABLE 1.1
Treatment of HCMV Retinitis

Drug	Regimen
Ganciclovir	5.0 mg/kg, b.i.d., for 2–3 weeks[a]
Foscarnet	60 mg/kg, t.i.d. for 2 weeks,[b] or 90–100 mg/kg, b.i.d. for 2 weeks[b]

[a] The drug is applied in 30-min IV infusions; maintenance therapy consists of once daily dose of 5.0 mg/kg.

[b] Foscarnet is applied in 90-min IV infusions with 500–1000 ml isotonic saline; maintenance therapy consists of once daily applications of 90–200 mg/kg of the drug in 90-min infusions.[449]

A number of clinical studies have documented the efficacy of ganciclovir in the treatment of HCMV retinitis.[186-188,270,278,291,307-314] In spite of that, however, retinitis recurred in nearly all cases after cessation of therapy to indicate a virustatic activity for ganciclovir.[270,300,309,311-313,315] Ganciclovir is usually administered intravenously in a 1-h period infusion with 5.0 mg/kg daily during induction therapy (Table 1.1).[35,72] Because of its renal excretion, the dosage of ganciclovir should be adjusted to compensate for renal insufficiency. The mean intravitreal concentration of ganciclovir after intravenous administration to AIDS patients with retinal detachments was 0.93 µg/ml (3.6 µM). This value, which was significantly lower than the concentration of ganciclovir required to achieve 50% of viral plaque formation for many human CMV strains, suggested that the intravenous administration of ganciclovir results in near-steady-state subtherapeutic intravitreal concentrations for many HCMV isolates.[316] This may explain the difficulty of long-term complete suppression of HCMV retinitis.

In a number of clinical trials of AIDS patients with HCMV infection, therapy with intravenous foscarnet resulted in clinical improvement in most cases and total regression in a few.[35,317-321] In immunosuppressed HIV-negative patients, such as bone marrow and renal transplant recipients, foscarnet also showed anti-HCMV efficacy.[322] The recommended induction dose of intravenous foscarnet is 60 mg/kg every 8 h (or 90 to 100 mg/kg b.i.d.) for 2 weeks, followed by a maintenance therapy of one daily dose of 90 mg/kg (Table 1.1).[35,72,323] As with ganciclovir, foscarnet is virustatic; therefore, reactivation is expected to occur once therapy is discontinued.

Patients with AIDS who had developed clinically resistant HCMV retinitis may show progression of retinitis despite extended intravenous induction single-drug therapy or alternating therapy with induction doses of ganciclovir or foscarnet. In several clinical experiments,[324-326] such patients were treated with a combination of ganciclovir and foscarnet. The recommended dosing regimen for induction combination therapy was ganciclovir (5.0 mg/kg every 12 h) and foscarnet (60 mg/kg, t.i.d.). Maintenance combination therapy was ganciclovir (5.0 mg/kg every 12 to 24 h) and foscarnet (90 to 120 mg/kg once daily). All patients exhibited a favorable response to the combination therapy, with complete healing of retinitis in 12 of 14 eyes and partial healing of retinitis with decreased border activity and a cessation of border advancement in 2 of 14 eyes. The combined drug regimen was generally well tolerated, with no significant toxic effects to require cessation of therapy.[324]

Local administration of ganciclovir can be carried out through intravitreal injection.[327-329] It is noteworthy to mention that the pars plana route for intraocular injection, which has often been used to administer anti-HCMV drugs, may result in complications such as the formation of intravitreous degranulation tissue and retinal detachment.[330]

Martin et al.[331] conducted a randomized, controlled clinical trial to assess the safety and efficacy of a 1.0 μg/h ganciclovir intraocular sustained-release implant for the treatment of previously untreated peripheral HCMV retinitis in AIDS patients. The ganciclovir implants were found to be effective. However, patients with unilateral HCMV retinitis treated with the implant were likely to develop HCMV retinitis in the fellow eye, as well as in some patients a visceral HCMV disease. Using an experimental intravitreal sustained-release device, Anand et al.[332] observed that once the device was empty of ganciclovir, reactivation of retinitis occurred in 33% of patients with subsequent stabilization of the retinitis.[333,334]

Young et al.[335] have assessed the efficacy of intravitreal administration of high-dose ganciclovir as either supplement or alternative to intravenous therapy in the treatment of HCMV retinitis in AIDS patients by measuring the visual outcome, relapse, and the complications resulting from these two treatment protocols. The results of the study showed that relapse and loss of vision occurred frequently in patients treated with intravenous ganciclovir alone or in combination with intermittent intravitreal therapy. However, patients managed with maintenance high-dose intravitreal ganciclovir alone or in combination with intravenous treatment did not relapse or lose vision, suggesting that high-dose ganciclovir given intravitreally effectively suppressed HCMV retinitis and preserved vision without adverse systemic effects.

Several surgically implantable devices for sustained intravitreal release of ganciclovir over extended periods of time have been developed.[336,337]

Akula et al.[338] applied intravitreal injection using liposome-encapsulated ganciclovir. The treatment reduced the number of intravitreal injections. While the eye did not show retinal hemorrhages or detachment, the vision declined initially but stabilized later. Weekly examination revealed neither progression of HCMV infection nor new lesions. Although retinal toxicity from intravitreal ganciclovir has been observed in animal experiments, toxicity in humans has not been reported. Diaz-Llopis et al.[339] observed complete remission of HCMV retinitis following the once-weekly intravitreal administration of liposome-entrapped ganciclovir (5.0 mg of the drug in 2 mg of lecithin).

The efficacy and tolerance of conventional (1200 μg)[340] or high-dose (2400 μg)[341] intravitreal foscarnet was studied in AIDS patients with HCMV retinitis. When a dose of 2400 μg of foscarnet was injected directly into the vitreous of two different patients, the corresponding vitreous levels were 896 μmol/l and 74.9 μmol/l at 2¾ h and 4½ h after the injection. The two patients were followed for a mean period of 16 weeks (range 8 to 28 weeks) and received a total of 304 injections. No case failed to respond or show progress.[341] Saran and Maguire[342] described a case of inadvertent intravitreous injection of a high-dose ganciclovir (40 mg/0.1 ml). Despite immediate intervention with vitreous surgery, permanent retinal damage and visual loss developed, possibly because of the high alkaline nature of the preparation, from osmotic damage, or from a direct effect of the concentrated ganciclovir.

Concurrent therapy of ganciclovir and zidovudine has been shown to significantly enhance the risk of granulocytopenia, and in most cases should be avoided.[185,343,344] Results from several *in vitro* studies have also demonstrated the presence of synergistic toxicity between ganciclovir and zidovudine.[345-347] The data by Freitas et al.,[348] which suggested that zidovudine potentiated the antiviral activity of ganciclovir against a clinical isolate of human CMV and interacted in an additive manner with a laboratory strain, have been questioned by Prichard and Shipman.[349]

However, a treatment protocol developed by Causey[350] did allow for the co-administration of zidovudine and ganciclovir under certain controlled conditions. Thus, zidovudine may be given concomitantly with ganciclovir if the absolute granulocyte counts are over 750 cells/μl. When the absolute granulocyte counts are initially below 750 cells/μl or fall below 750 cells/μl, zidovudine should be discontinued while ganciclovir is administered. Causey's protocol was designed to minimize potential toxicity by avoiding concurrent dosing with zidovudine and ganciclovir when hematologic cytotoxicity becomes evident.[350] In patients who were unable to tolerate both drugs, dideoxyinosine (ddI, didanosine) should be used in place of zidovudine;[351] alternatively, foscarnet may be used in place of ganciclovir. Carter and Shuster[352] reported that combined treatment with oral acyclovir and zidovudine cleared all clinical evidence of active HCMV retinitis.

The tolerance of neutropenia caused by ganciclovir has been increased by adjunctive therapy with granulocyte-macrophage colony-stimulating factor (GM-CSF).[353] Hardy et al.[183] have evaluated in AIDS patients the efficacy and safety of a combination of ganciclovir and GM-CSF. In phase A of the trial, patients were randomized to receive ganciclovir, 5.0 mg/kg every 12 h for 2 weeks followed by 5.0 mg/kg daily, with (n = 24) or without (n = 29) GM-CSF (1 to 8 μg/kg daily, subcutaneously) to maintain the absolute neutrophil counts between 2500 and 5000 cells/μl. In phase B, after 16 weeks, zidovudine was added to the regimen of 16 patients receiving ganciclovir plus GM-CSF and 20 patients on ganciclovir alone. At this stage, GM-CSF was added to the treatment protocol of any patient receiving ganciclovir plus zidovudine who became neutropenic. In phase A, patients in the ganciclovir plus GM-CSF group had significantly higher neutrophil counts than patients receiving ganciclovir alone (p = .0001). Overall, only 12.5% of patients treated with GM-CSF developed neutropenia compared with 45% of patients not receiving GM-CSF as part of their treatment protocol. In addition, there was a trend, although not statistically significant, for patients in the GM-CSF group to experience delayed progression of their retinitis.[183]

Several studies[293,354] have been conducted to evaluate the response to foscarnet salvage therapy in patients with HCMV retinitis who were hematologically intolerant of or resistant to ganciclovir. Thus, in a phase II dose-ranging trial,[354] these patients received an induction therapy with foscarnet at 60 mg/kg, t.i.d. for 2 weeks, followed by chronic maintenance therapy at daily doses of 60, 90, or 120 mg/kg. The salvage foscarnet therapy resulted in a longer time to retinitis progression than reported previously in historic controls who terminated ganciclovir therapy. In patients who experienced clinical resistance to ganciclovir, the foscarnet therapy appeared to control the retinitis. No significant differences in either efficacy or toxicity were observed between the different maintenance dose regimens of foscarnet.[354] Pearson et al.[355] have used intravitreal administration of foscarnet to treat HCMV retinitis in an AIDS patient.

In several rare occasions, regression of HCMV retinitis has been described following therapy with intravenous zidovudine alone (200 mg every for 4 h) for as long as active disease was present.[356-358] The mechanism of anti-CMV action of zidovudine has not been defined. The beneficial anti-HCMV effects of zidovudine, which is known for its specific anti-HIV activity, may arise from enhancement of cell-mediated immunity resulting in suppression of HCMV replication and infectivity, the inhibition of HIV replication, thereby reducing HIV-related enhancement of HCMV expression, and third, by direct suppression of HIV.[35] In another prospective, controlled study, the incidence of HCMV retinitis in AIDS patients (CD4+ cell counts under 500 cells/μl) did not decrease following combination therapy with zidovudine (500 mg/kg) and zalcitabine (dideoxycytidine, ddC) (0.02 mg/kg) as compared with therapy of zidovudine alone (500 mg/kg). However, the rates of occurrence of typical microvascular retinopathy were significantly lower in patients receiving combination therapy (26% and 56%, respectively).[359]

Spaide et al.[360] have reported the presence of frosted branch angiitis associated with HCMV retinitis. Intravenous anti-HCMV therapy, while resolving the vascular sheathing within 2 weeks, did not cure retinitis.

To provide prompt visual rehabilitation and to reduce the need for repeated operations, Regillo et al.[361] used vitrectomy with silicone oil tamponade to repair HCMV retinitis-related retinal detachment.

In AIDS patients, the therapy of HCMV pneumonitis has been less effective (50% to 60% clinical response) than that of retinitis.[72] In part, the lower response rate may be the result of a delayed diagnosis when pneumonitis is already severe.

Two AIDS patients, clinically suspected to have HCMV-associated pancreatitis, were successfully treated, one with ganciclovir (10 mg/kg daily) and the other with foscarnet (200 mg/kg daily, followed by a maintenance therapy with foscarnet at 100 mg/kg daily). No pancreatitis relapse was observed.[362]

Studies by Berman and Kim[363] suggested that while ganciclovir therapy may clinically stabilize HCMV retinitis in patients with AIDS, it did not appear to prevent the development, or be effective in the treatment, of HCMV encephalitis. However, early diagnosis of HCMV encephalitis and therapeutic regimen consisting of ganciclovir, anti-HCMV immunoglobulins, and intrathecal IFN-β led to complete recovery after 2 months.[364]

The ability to easily penetrate the blood-brain barrier and sustain virustatic concentrations in the CSF may offer foscarnet as a useful alternative to ganciclovir in the treatment of HCMV encephalitis.[195,365]

While ganciclovir has been used to treat HCMV-associated polyradiculopathy with some success,[88,91,93-96,366] in several case reports of AIDS patients already receiving antiviral therapy for HCMV retinitis, HCMV polyradiculopathy had developed because of ganciclovir-resistant strains.[97-100] In one such case, the patient developed HCMV polyradiculopathy while receiving intravenous ganciclovir at 5.0 to 7.5 mg/kg, 5 times weekly, as maintenance therapy for HCMV retinitis.[367] In a similar situation, because of worsening in the neurological status, ganciclovir 5.0 mg/kg b.i.d., IV had to be withdrawn and substituted with foscarnet (60 mg/kg, t.i.d., IV).[97] Decker et al.[368] and Karmochkine et al.[369] employed concurrent use of ganciclovir and foscarnet to treat polyradiculopathy due to cytomegalovirus in patients with AIDS.

In a retrospective study, Roullet et al.[370] analyzed 15 consecutive cases of severe HCMV multifocal neuropathy (initial numbness and painful paresthesias, followed by moderate to severe sensorimotor asymmetric neuropathy) in AIDS patients in the advanced stages of the disease (mean CD4+ counts of 18 cells/mm^3). Fourteen patients showed a marked improvement 1 to 4 weeks after starting ganciclovir or foscarnet therapy. During follow-up maintenance therapy (13 patients), the neuropathy relapsed in 3 patients.

Price et al.[371] described a case of clinically symptomatic change in the neurological status (ventriculitis and meningoencephalitis) of an AIDS patient as a result of HCMV disease. While ganciclovir therapy resulted in radiological improvement of the ventriculitis and negative HCMV cultures, there was little clinical neurological improvement noticed.

HCMV esophagitis is an important complication in AIDS patients. Wilcox et al.[372] have reported a prospective evaluation of the clinical response to ganciclovir therapy, relapse rate, and the long-term (45-month) outcome. The induction therapy consisted of daily IV ganciclovir at 10 mg/kg for approximately 2 weeks; foscarnet (60 mg/kg, t.i.d.) was given to nonresponders to ganciclovir. The complete and partial response rates were 49% and 29%, respectively, yielding a 77% overall response rate. Thirty-nine percent of all complete responders relapsed if not given maintenance therapy; in all cases relapse was manifested by recurrent odynophagia. No patient died as a direct result of HCMV esophagitis, suggesting a favorable response to induction therapy with ganciclovir. However, the long-term survival was poor, reflecting the severe immunodeficiency of the patients.

Foscarnet was also found effective in treating HCMV-related gastrointestinal disease in HIV-infected patients. Prior to 1988, it was administered as a continuous infusion of 200 mg/kg. Later, this regimen was replaced with an intermittent infusion of 60 mg/kg t.i.d. or 90 mg/kg b.i.d., with saline hyperhydration accompanying each infusion; the treatment lasted for 2 to 3 weeks.[373]

Dieterich et al.[374] have evaluated foscarnet treatment of HCMV gastrointestinal infections (esophagitis, colitis) in AIDS patients who have failed ganciclovir induction therapy (5.0 mg/kg, b.i.d. for 14 d).[375] Foscarnet at 60 mg/kg, t.i.d., was administered intravenously for 2 weeks, followed by maintenance therapy at 90 or 120 mg/kg every day with 1.0 l normal saline daily. Sixty-seven percent of patients who were evaluated before and 2 to 3 weeks after foscarnet, showed histologic improvement, whereas 74% improved clinically after a median duration of 7.5 d. Reversible nephrotoxicity occurred in 12% of patients.

Surgical treatment (resection of inflamed bowel) combined with postoperative anti-HCMV therapy led to excellent palliation and relatively favorable survival rate among AIDS patients with HCMV enterocolitis.[376] Baker et al.[70] have reported a case of CMV colitis associated with combination 5-fluorouracil-interferon-γ therapy. The patient, who developed HCMV colon inclusions, was treated successfully with ganciclovir (5.0 mg/kg) every 12 h for 2 weeks; the diarrhea resolved after approximately 8 d of therapy.

A case of adrenal insufficiency caused by HCMV infection in an AIDS patient was manifested with severe hyponatremia and hormonal abnormalities (Addison's disease). Although the administration of hydrocortisone and ganciclovir led to improvement in the patient's general clinical condition and return to normal of biochemical test results, the adrenal dysfunction was irreversible.[108]

Oral lesions associated with HCMV infections have been very rare.[377] One such case of acute periodontal HCMV disease in an HIV-infected patient has been reported by Dodd et al.[378] Initially, the clinical manifestations of the HCMV infection were indistinguishable from HIV-associated periodontal disease.

1.1.6.2 Management of HCMV Disease in Solid Organ and Bone Marrow Transplant Recipients

Acyclovir, which has displayed poor *in vitro* efficacy against HCMV, was found beneficial against HCMV infections[379] in renal,[135,136] liver,[149,380] and bone marrow[381,382] transplant recipients when given at high doses either parenterally or orally. Thus, Balfour et al.[135] have conducted a randomized, placebo-controlled trial using a high-dose acyclovir regimen to prevent HCMV disease in recipients of renal allografts. The results of the study showed that high oral doses of the drug when given during the first 3 months after the transplantation reduced both HCMV infection and disease without affecting the survival rate of either graft or patients. The greatest prophylactic benefit was observed among seronegative patients who had received a kidney from a seropositive donor.[135]

Using a similar protocol, Legendre et al.[136] carried out a case-controlled study in which 42 cadaveric kidney transplant recipients were treated prophylactically with high-dose oral acyclovir for 3 months and compared to historical controls matched for donor/recipient HCMV serological status, age, sex, and immunosuppressive therapy. Before the transplantation, the study group of patients received intravenous acyclovir (500 mg/m² over 1 h), followed by oral administration (basal dose, 800 mg, 4 times daily) from day 2 post-transplantation. In addition, all patients received 14-d induction immunosuppressive therapy. Study results have shown significantly less HCMV infection in HCMV-seropositive patients (regardless of donor HCMV serological status) in the study group compared to historical controls ($p = .005$). In contrast, there was no difference between the study group and controls in HCMV-seronegative recipients who received from a seropositive donor. With regard to HCMV disease, there was markedly less HCMV disease in HCMV-seropositive patients (regardless of the donor HCMV serological status) in the study group compared to historical controls ($p = .01$). To the contrary, there was no difference in HCMV-seronegative recipients who received an organ from a HCMV-seropositive donor between the study group and treated patients. Overall, the 3-month course of high-dose oral acyclovir reduced both HCMV infection and disease in HCMV-seropositive recipients whatever the HCMV serological status of the donor; such an effect was not observed in HCMV-seronegative renal transplant recipients receiving a HCMV-positive kidney.[136] A serious side effect of acyclovir is the neurologic symptoms (mental status disorder, involuntary movements) that resemble extension of viral infection into the CNS; renal dysfunction usually preceded neurotoxicity.[383]

Paya et al.[149] have analyzed the incidence and clinical characteristics of HCMV infection in liver transplant recipients and conducted a randomized trial to evaluate the efficacy of acyclovir and ganciclovir in the prophylaxis of HCMV infection following orthotopic liver transplantation. Symptomatic HCMV-induced hepatitis, which developed in 25% of patients, was also a major cause of death (21% of all deaths). As prophylaxis therapy, patients received either combination of ganciclovir and acyclovir (group A), or acyclovir alone (group B). Group A patients had a decreased incidence of HCMV infection mainly due to decrease in asymptomatic infection. The incidence of symptomatic infection was similar in both groups as well as when compared to control liver transplant recipients. Overall, the use of acyclovir alone did not appear to have a significant impact in reducing the incidence and severity of HCMV infection.[149]

In another study, Martin et al.[384] conducted a prospective randomized trial comparing sequential ganciclovir-high dose acyclovir to high-dose acyclovir for prevention of HCMV disease in adult liver transplant recipients. The patients were randomized to receive either high-dose oral acyclovir (800 mg four times a day) alone for 3 months after transplantation (group A), or intravenous ganciclovir (5.0 mg/kg b.i.d.) for 2 weeks followed by high-dose oral acyclovir to complete a 3-month regimen (group B). Sixty-one percent of the patients from group A developed HCMV infection as compared to only 24% from group B. Of those randomized, HCMV disease was observed in 28% of group A, but only in 9% of group B. The median time to onset for both HCMV infection and HCMV disease were longer for the ganciclovir-acyclovir group (group B) compared to the acyclovir group (group A) (78 vs. 45 d, and 78 vs. 40 d, respectively). With regard to primary HCMV infection, there was no difference in the rates between the two groups, but tissue invasive disease and recurrent HCMV disease were less frequent in the ganciclovir-acyclovir group. The overall results of this trial strongly indicated that for prevention of HCMV infection and HCMV disease after liver transplantation, a 2-week course of ganciclovir immediately after transplantation followed by high-dose oral acyclovir for 10 weeks was superior to a 12-week course of high-dose oral acyclovir alone.

Based on their results from a randomized trial with liver transplant recipients, Singh et al.[385] concluded that high-dose oral acyclovir (800 mg four times a day) is ineffective prophylaxis against HCMV disease. Instead, a preemptive, short-course therapy of intravenous ganciclovir (5.0 mg/kg, b.i.d.) for 7 d in patients with HCMV shedding was well tolerated and provided effective prophylaxis aginst subsequent HCMV disease while minimizing toxicity and cost of treatment.

Dunn et al.[386] have conducted a prospective randomized trial to appraise the efficacy of acyclovir vs. ganciclovir plus human immune globulin prophylaxis of HCMV infection after solid organ transplantation. Patients were stratified according to allograft type, age, and presence or absence of diabetes mellitus, and were then randomized to receive either long-duration acyclovir prophylaxis (800 mg orally or 400 mg four times a day, IV, for 12 weeks after transplantation or 6 weeks after any antirejection therapy), or short-duration ganciclovir (5.0 mg/kg b.i.d., IV, for 7 d after transplant or after any antirejection therapy) plus human immune globulin (100 mg, IV administration) on days 1, 4, and 7 after transplant or after any antirejection therapy. No differences in patient or allograft survival were observed between the two treatment protocols. Overall, acyclovir prophylaxis appeared to be more effective in reducing the incidence of post-transplant HCMV disease, although this effect was somewhat diminished in high-risk patients. Long-term therapy seemed to better prevent HCMV transmission or reactivation.[386]

Results from several studies suggested that combination treatment of ganciclovir and immune globulin[387] can increase the number of survivors among bone marrow transplant recipients.[388-390] In a randomized controlled trial, Snydman et al.[141] showed that passive immunization with HCMV immune globulin (HCMV-IG) reduced the incidence of HCMV-associated disease by 65% in sero-negative recipients of kidney from seropositive donors. The recommended protocol, which was chosen as a result of a pilot study,[391] consisted of randomly assigned patients receiving, IV, 150 mg/kg HCMV-IG within 72 h of transplantation, then 100 mg/kg at weeks 2 and 4 after transplantation, followed by 50 mg/kg at weeks 6, 8, 12, and 16 after transplantation. The HCMV-IG was administered initially at a rate of 15 mg/kg per hour; if there were no untoward side effects, the rate was increased to a maximum of 60 mg/kg per hour.[141] Overall, the prophylaxis with HCMV-IG was most beneficial to renal transplant recipients at high risk of HCMV-associated disease[392] and was well tolerated by patients in both this and another study involving bone marrow transplant recipients.[393]

According to studies by Przepiorka et al.,[394] ganciclovir given three times weekly was not adequate to prevent HCMV reactivation after T cell-depleted marrow transplantation to patients who were either HCMV-seropositive or had seropositive donors. Ganciclovir was administered IV at 2.5 mg/kg, t.i.d. on days −8 to −2, and at 5.0 or 6.0 mg/kg (IV, three times weekly) prophylactically from engraftment to day 100. In addition, all patients received IV immunoglobulin (500 mg/kg once weekly) and HCMV-negative or filtered blood products. G-CSF or GM-CSF was given to patients with neutropenia (neutrophil counts < 0.5 to $1.5 \times 10^9/l$). At day 120, the rates of HCMV infection and CMV disease were 58% and 36%. In another study, Engelhard et al.[395] used ganciclovir in 13 patients who underwent allogeneic T lymphocyte-depleted bone marrow transplantation, and subsequently developed severe HCMV disease without pneumonia. Ganciclovir was administered for 2 weeks, without the addition of intravenous immunoglobulins. Following therapy, the clinical manifestations subsided in most of the patients, while leukopenia, thrombocytopenia, and liver dysfunction resolved in about half of the patients. The suggested treatment was recommended especially in cases of severe HCMV disease without lung involvement and no concomitant severe graft-versus-host disease (GVHD).[395] Slavin et al.[396] have found that HCMV often persisted in the lung of bone marrow transplant patients with HCMV pneumonia despite ganciclovir treatment; ganciclovir resistance did not explain the persistence of HCMV in the lungs.

Results by Enright et al.[397] have shown that HCMV pneumonia complicating bone marrow transplantation occurred more often in allogeneic than autologous recipients. Allogeneic recipients who were at higher risk included HCMV-seropositive patients, those at an older age, those conditioned with total-body irradiation, who received antithymocyte globulin or T cell-depleted marrow, or who had HCMV viruria. The prognosis was poor for patients who were ventilator-dependent at initiation of therapy (median survival, 17 d). In contrast, patients who were ventilator-independent at initiation of therapy with ganciclovir and immunoglobulin had a median survival of over 274 d. Those patients on ganciclovir alone or acyclovir with immunoglobulin in a ventilator-independent setting had lower response (median survivals of 80 and 10 d, respectively). While less common, HCMV pneumonia in autologous patients was more severe and a prominent cause of death following bone marrow transplantation.[397]

Locatelli et al.[398] have studied HCMV infections in pediatric patients given allogeneic bone marrow transplantions, and the role of early ganciclovir treatment for HCMV pp65-antigenemia[399] for disease outcome. The development of acute GVHD, corticosteroid therapy, and the serologic status of both recipient and donor were the most important predictors of HCMV infection. All patients with pp65-positive cells were treated with ganciclovir at a dose of 5.0 mg/kg b.i.d. for 2 weeks. In patients without acute GVHD no maintenance therapy was initiated; in children with active acute GVHD, an additional therapy of ganciclovir (5.0 mg/kg daily for 2 weeks) was instituted. Overall, early short-term treatment with ganciclovir produced a complete clearing of viremia and antigenemia. Likewise, HCMV disease had completely resolved and no patient died from HCMV-related interstitial pneumonia.

The prophylactic (10 mg/kg daily during the 3rd and 4th week after surgery) vs. therapeutic (10 mg/kg daily only after clinical HCMV disease was diagnosed) use of ganciclovir after liver transplantation in adult patients was evaluated by Cohen et al.[400] in a prospective, controlled trial of 33 patients. While prophylactic ganciclovir was associated with a lower incidence of serologically diagnosed secondary infection, the development of IgM anti-HCMV antibody, and the absence of leukopenia, the frequency of clinical infections was similar in the two groups.[400]

Reinke et al.[401] examined the relationship between late-acute renal allograft rejection and asymptomatic HCMV infection. Those patients who did not respond to antirejection therapy showed an expansion of memory-type $CD8^+$ peripheral blood T cells that expressed IFN-γ and an association with clinically asymptomatic HCMV infection.[402] Therapy with ganciclovir resulted in stable and improved graft function in 17 of 21 treated patients with HCMV-associated late-acute renal rejection.[401] In a multiple regression analysis, HLA-DR7 was found to be a significant predictor of HCMV infection ($p < .005$) among renal transplant recipients; thus, HLA-DR7-positive recipients were more susceptible to CMV infection, which was also associated with administration of triple immunosuppressive therapy (cyclosporine A, prednisolone, and azathioprine).[403]

Based on clinical evidence collected from 419 cadaveric renal transplantations, ganciclovir appeared to be safe and effective in the treatment of tissue-invasive HCMV infection in such patients.[404] Ganciclovir was used effectively to treat severe HCMV disease after renal transplantation even during the rejection period.[405]

Another aspect to consider in controlling HCMV infection in solid organ transplant recipients is the nature of induction and post-transplantation immunosuppressive therapies. Lesions of HCMV-associated retinitis in immunosuppressed organ transplant recipients will often regress after tapering the immunosuppressive therapy.[48,60,298] The latter usually consists of combinations of low-dose steroids (prednisolone, 0.25 mg/kg daily), azathioprine (2.0 mg/kg daily), and cyclosporine A (dosage adjusted to reach a trough level of 100 to 200 mg/ml), and polyclonal or monoclonal (OKT3 or anti-CD7) antibodies.[406-409] As shown by Hibberd et al.,[407] therapy with the monoclonal OKT3 antibody increased the risk of HCMV disease about fivefold in HCMV-seropositive transplant recipients but did not influence the incidence of HCMV disease in HCMV-seronegative recipients. In addition, in HCMV-positive patients, OKT3 was the most important predictor of HCMV disease by multivariate analysis.[136]

1.1.6.3 Management of Neonatal HCMV Hepatitis

Human CMV has been known as one of the etiologic agents of neonatal and infantile hepatitis, although its pathogenic role has not been well defined. Numazaki and Chiba[410] have studied the natural courses of HCMV-associated liver dysfunction and assessed the efficacy of orally given glycyrrhizin to patients who had histories of prolonged liver dysfunction and poor body weight gain. Liver dysfunction clearly improved after glycyrrhizin therapy, suggesting it as an appropriate treatment for this condition.

1.1.6.4 Maintenance Therapy of HCMV Disease

Lifelong maintenance therapy with ganciclovir[188,309,311] or foscarnet[321,411-415] can slow the progression of retinitis and minimize vision loss. As an alternative to IV infusion, a capsule form of ganciclovir for oral administration has been studied.[416] The absolute bioavailability of oral ganciclovir given at a dosage of 1000 mg t.i.d. with food averaged 9%.[417] Daily doses of 3000 mg or more yielded average serum ganciclovir concentrations exceeding 0.5 µg/ml,[184] a concentration sufficient to inhibit most clinical isolates of HCMV.[418]

In an open-label, randomized trial of AIDS patients, Drew et al.[416] compared as a maintenance therapy for HCMV retinitis oral (3.0 g daily) with IV (5.0 mg/kg daily) ganciclovir. The results showed a mean time to the progression of retinitis of 62 and 57 d for IV and oral ganciclovir, respectively. Overall, oral ganciclovir was a safe and effective alternative to IV ganciclovir as maintenance therapy for CMV retinitis, and provided greater ease of administration and convenience to take. A European/Australian group has also conducted a comparative study of efficacy and safety of oral vs. IV ganciclovir for maintenance therapy against HCMV retinitis in AIDS patients.[419] The patients either received 500 mg of oral ganciclovir 6 times daily or 5.0 mg/kg of IV ganciclovir once daily infused over 1 h. The 20-week, randomized, multicenter, open-label trial also found oral ganciclovir to be an effective and safe alternative to IV administration and recommended its use as maintenance therapy for HCMV retinitis in AIDS patients.

Mastroianni et al.[420] have described two AIDS patients who developed HCMV encephalitis while receiving ganciclovir maintenance therapy for HCMV retinitis. No improvement in the neurological and virological status of the patients was observed during a further induction course of ganciclovir. The results of this study may cast doubt about the efficacy of the currently recommended ganciclovir protocols for prevention and treatment of HCMV encephalitis in AIDS patients.

AIDS patients with newly diagnosed HCMV retinitis who had just completed a 14-d course of ganciclovir induction therapy were randomly assigned to an alternating or concurrent combination regimen of chronic ganciclovir-foscarnet therapy. Each regimen used lower weekly cumulative doses of each drug than standard monotherapy maintenance treatment regimens.[421] Dose-limiting toxicity due to foscarnet has been observed in only 7% of evaluable patients, and no patients experienced dose-limiting nephrotoxicity. Although absolute neutrophil counts of less than 500 cells/µl occurred in 38% of patients, all who received adjunctive G-CSF had the neutropenia prevented. The overall results suggested that combination therapy was better than monotherapy.

In an open-labeled pilot study, Peters et al.[422] assessed the safety of alternating ganciclovir (5.0 mg/kg every other day) and foscarnet (120 mg/kg every other day) maintenance therapy for 5 to 51 weeks (median, 18.5 weeks) against HCMV infections in AIDS patients. According to this study, the alternating administration of ganciclovir and foscarnet was safe and can be used for induction and maintenance therapy.

1.1.6.5 Ganciclovir vs. Foscarnet in the Treatment of HCMV Infection

Ganciclovir and foscarnet appeared to be of similar effectiveness in halting the viral proliferation when administered as induction therapy, and preventing the progress of HCMV disease when given as maintenance therapy.[423,424] The side effects include bone marrow toxicity for ganciclovir, and renal toxicity, hypocalcemia, genital ulcers, and nausea and vomiting for foscarnet. The induction therapy usually lasts for 2 to 3 weeks, followed by lifelong maintenance treatment to prevent progression of infection, which in the case of retinitis occurs in 90% of patients within 6 weeks.[72,425]

When ganciclovir therapy is applied, in addition to monitoring serum creatinine levels and adjusting the dosage accordingly in cases of renal impairment, the neutrophil and platelet counts should also be observed every 1 to 2 d during twice-daily ganciclovir dosing, and at least once weekly thereafter, as granulocytopenia and thrombocytopenia are the most common adverse side effects of the drug.[35] Ganciclovir therapy should be withheld if the absolute neutrophil counts fall below 500 cells/mm^3. To this end, Roberts et al.[426] have addressed the issue of ganciclovir associated neutropenia during treatment of bone marrow transplant recipients, and whether the reluctance to use ganciclovir is justified. There is evidence that HCMV infection may directly or indirectly cause bone marrow suppression. In this setting, the potential benefit of ganciclovir therapy may outweigh the risk. Thus, in a retrospective review of 11 consecutive patients receiving ganciclovir for HCMV infection post-transplantation, in 10 of 13 cases the absolute neutrophil count was higher at the completion of the ganciclovir therapy than at the start of treatment, including 5 cases where the absolute neutrophil count was < 500 cells/mm^3 at the time ganciclovir was started. In only one of 13 cases was ganciclovir discontinued due to neutropenia.[426]

In the context of poor outpatient compliance, Mole et al.[427] have addressed the issue of stability of a 5-d supply of reconstituted ganciclovir used by patients undergoing lifelong parenteral maintenance therapy. Extended stability was achieved when ganciclovir was diluted with normal saline or 5% dextrose in water to final drug concentrations of 5.0 or 10 mg/ml — it remained stable for 28 d when stored both at 4°C and –22°C in polyvinyl chloride bags and at 4°C in ADFuse syringes.[427]

Compared to IV administration, local intravitreal injection of ganciclovir[307,428-430] has several advantages, namely, eliminating the need for hospitalization and catheter-associated septic risks of IV infusion, preventing the myelosuppressive effect of systemic ganciclovir, and enabling the patient to remain on concomitant zidovudine therapy.[35] The major drawback of intravitreal ganciclovir is the loss of activity against disseminated HCMV infection, and the need to repeat the injection on a regular basis (e.g., twice weekly) because of the short half-life of the drug. The primary indications for intravitreal ganciclovir therapy include the presence of severe granulocytopenia precluding the systemic use of the drug, and vision-threatening lesions of the macula and/or optic nerve, which may develop before the systemic therapy begins to take effect (often as long as 1 week after institution of systemic treatment).[35] Sanborn et al.[431] have reported the use of a surgically implanted (through the pars plana) intravitreal device that slowly releases ganciclovir. The device has a relatively short lifespan of 4 to 5 months, after which it needs to be replaced.

Like ganciclovir, the usual route of administration of foscarnet is through IV infusion. The total daily regimens of 200 mg/kg can be given by two to three infusions during 90 min of induction therapy. Data by Katlama et al.[207] have demonstrated that twice-daily administration of foscarnet at 100 mg/kg over 90 min appeared to be as effective and as well tolerated as 60 mg/kg given three times daily. As with ganciclovir, the foscarnet dosage should be adjusted for renal insufficiency, and concomitant administration of other nephrotoxic drugs (IV pentamidine, aminoglycosides, amphotericin B) should be avoided.[72]

Contrary to ganciclovir, foscarnet did not show bone marrow suppression activity.[317,321,322,432] The absence of such toxicity is of major importance in the therapeutic management of HCMV infection in AIDS patients, allowing all concomitant potentially hematotoxic drugs (co-trimoxazole, sulfonamides, pyrimethamine, and antineoplastic agents) to be used as needed in anti-AIDS therapy. Among the adverse side effects of foscarnet, elevated serum creatinine levels and development of acute renal failure,[433] infusion-site thrombophlebitis, decrease in hemoglobin, and decrease or increase in serum calcium should be closely monitored.[35]

In several studies of AIDS patients, the efficacies of ganciclovir and foscarnet were compared for induction therapy and maintenance treatment of HCMV retinitis.[434,435] While both drugs were equipotent in suppressing retinitis and preserving vision,[436] patients receiving foscarnet had a significantly longer survival rate (12 vs. 8 months). The reason(s) behind the observed reduced mortality following foscarnet therapy have not been clearly defined. However, in patients with decreased renal function (creatinine clearance of < 1.2 ml/min/kg), ganciclovir appeared to be more efficacious.[434] In an extension of the aforementioned studies, the morbidity and toxic side effects associated with ganciclovir or foscarnet IV therapy were evaluated in a multicenter, randomized trial of AIDS patients with previously untreated HCMV retinitis.[437] The following observations were made: (1) neutropenia was more common in patients receiving ganciclovir than foscarnet (34% and 14%, respectively; $p = .001$); (2) patients assigned to foscarnet reported more infusion-related symptoms (58% and 24%, respectively; $p < .001$), and in male patients, more genitourinary symptoms (36% and 16%, respectively; $p > .001$); (3) compared to the ganciclovir group, patients on foscarnet also experienced a trend toward more nephrotoxic effects (13% and 6%, respectively; $p = .082$) and electrolyte abnormalities; and (4) the incidence of seizures was similar in both groups (12% and 9% for foscarnet and ganciclovir, respectively; $p = .511$). Furthermore, mainly because of toxicity, patients assigned to foscarnet were more likely to be switched to the alternative treatment (foscarnet to ganciclovir, 46%; ganciclovir to foscarnet, 11%; $p < .001$). In 88% of the cases where a switch to alternative treatment took place, the toxic reaction resolved after the switch. In addition, the toxic reaction rarely had long-term sequelae, and based on previously reported survival benefits seen in patients treated with foscarnet, the results of the study support the use of foscarnet for initial therapy of HCMV retinitis.[437]

Bacigalupo et al.[438] have evaluated the early treatment of HCMV disease in allogeneic bone marrow transplant recipients with foscarnet (180 mg/kg daily) or ganciclovir (10 mg/kg daily). Both agents were effective in clearing HCMV antigenemia. Renal toxicity was seen in the foscarnet group, whereas myelotoxicity was the major side effect in the ganciclovir-receiving group.

An open prospective trial of combined ganciclovir and foscarnet therapy for 3 weeks was initiated in HIV-positive patients (median CD4+ cell count of 10 cells/μl) with severe HCMV gastrointestinal disease (colitis, esophagitis) and HCMV retinitis; the overall efficacy was comparable to monotherapy.[439] Weinberg et al.[440] have found that combined daily IV therapy with ganciclovir and foscarnet appeared to prolong the interval to progression and to preserve the vision in patients with recurrent HCMV retinitis. Butler et al.[441] also achieved a sustained clinical response with the combination of ganciclovir and foscarnet in an HIV-infected child suffering from aggressive CMV retinitis that progressed despite treatment with either agent alone.

1.1.6.6 Ganciclovir- and Foscarnet-Resistant HCMV Strains

With the widespread use of ganciclovir and foscarnet, HCMV-resistant strains have emerged against ganciclovir,[97-99,172,192,442-444] foscarnet,[445] and both ganciclovir and foscarnet.[446] Resistance to ganciclovir has been defined as a median effective dose (ED_{50}) of >6.0 μM.[192] Wolf et al.[447] have established that mutations in the human CMV UL97 gene conferred clinical resistance to ganciclovir. They can be detected directly in the plasma of AIDS patients with progressive HCMV disease despite ganciclovir treatment. Thus, a single nucleotide change within a conserved region of UL97 (amino acid substitution in residue 595: from leucine to serine in four, and from leucine to phenylalanine in one resistant isolate) was found in five resistant strains. A sixth resistant isolate demonstrated a single nucleotide change, leading to a threonine to isoleucine substitution in residue 659.

The evolution of resistance to ganciclovir may be explained by several mechanisms.[97] In one such hypothesis, it is postulated that AIDS patients may be coinfected with multiple strains of HCMV[24,248] that may have varying degrees of susceptibility to ganciclovir. It is also possible that long-term ganciclovir therapy was selective for a resistant strain that grew preferentially in the CNS because of its ability to maintain high CSF concentrations.

1.1.7 REFERENCES

1. Weller, T. H., The cytomegaloviruses: ubiquitous agents with protean clinical manifestations, *N. Engl. J. Med.*, 285, 203, 1971.
2. Alford, C. A. and Britt, W. J., Cytomegalovirus, in *Fields Virology*, 2nd ed., Fields, B. N., Knipe, D. M., Chanock, R. M., Hirsch, M. S., Melnick, J. L., Monath, T. P., and Roizman, B., Eds., Raven Press, New York, 1990, 1981.
3. Stinski, M. F., Cytomegalovirus and its replication, in *Fields Virology*, 2nd ed., Fields, B. N., Knipe, D. M., Chanock, R. M., Hirsch, M. S., Melnick, J. L., Monath, T. P., and Roizman, B., Eds., Raven Press, New York, 1990, 1059.

4. Roizman, B., Herpesviridae: a brief introduction, in *Fields Virology*, 2nd ed., Fields, B. N., Knipe, D. M., Chanock, R. M., Hirsch, M. S., Melnick, J. L., Monath, T. P., and Roizman, B., Eds., Raven Press, New York, 1990, 1787.

5. Geelen, J. L. M. C., Walig, C., Wertheim, P., and van der Noordaa, J., Human cytomegalovirus DNA. I. Molecular weight and infectivity, *J. Virol.*, 26, 813, 1978.

6. Geelen, J. L. M. C. and Weststrate, M. W., Organization of the human cytomegalovirus genome, in *Herpesvirus DNA*, Becker, Y., Ed., Martinus Nijhoff Medical Publishers, The Hague, 1982.

7. DeMarchi, J. M., Blankship, M. L., Brown, G. D., and Kaplan, A. S., Size and complexity of human cytomegalovirus DNA, *Virology*, 89, 643, 1978.

8. Kilpatrick, B. A. and Huang, E.-S., Human cytomegalovirus genome: partial denaturation map and organization of genome sequences, *J. Virol.*, 24, 261, 1977.

9. Lakeman, A. D. and Osborn, J. E., Size of infectious DNA from human and murine cytomegalovirus, *J. Virol.*, 30, 414, 1979.

10. Somagyi, T., Colimon, R., and Michelson, S., An illustrated guide to the structure of the human cytomegalovirus genome and a review of transcription data, *Prog. Med. Virol.*, 33, 99, 1986.

11. Stinski, M. F., Mocarski, E. S., and Thomsen, D. R., DNA of human cytomegalovirus: size heterogeneity and defectiveness resulting from serial undiluted passage, *J. Virol.*, 31, 231, 1979.

12. Huang, E.-S., Human cytomegalovirus. III. Virus-induced DNA polymerase, *J. Virol.*, 16, 298, 1975.

13. Nishiyama, Y., Maeno, K., and Yoshida, S., Characterization of human cytomegalovirus-induced DNA polymerase and the associated 3'-to-5' exonuclease, *Virology*, 124, 221, 1983.

14. Knopf, K.-W., Properties of the herpes simplex virus DNA polymerase and characterization of its associated exonuclease activity, *Eur. J. Biochem.*, 98, 231, 1979.

15. Alford, C. A., Stagno, S., Pass, R. F., and Huang, E.-S., Epidemiology of cytomegalovirus, *The Human Herpesviruses: an Interdisciplinary Perspective*, Nahmias, A., Dowdle, W., and Schinazi, R., Eds., Elsevier, New York, 1981, 159.

16. Lang, D. J., The epidemiology of cytomegalovirus infections: interpretations of recent observations, in *Infections of the Fetus and the Newborn Infant*, Vol. 3, Krugman, S. and Gershon, A. A., Eds., Alan R. Liss, New York, 1975, 35.

17. Lang, D. J. and Krammer, J. F., Cytomegalovirus in the semen: observations in selected populations, *J. Infect. Dis.*, 132, 472, 1975.

18. Reynolds, D. W., Stagno, S., Hosty, T. S., Tiller, M., and Alford, C. A. Jr., Maternal cytomegalovirus excretion and perinatal infection, *N. Engl. J. Med.*, 289, 1, 1981.

19. Stagno, S., Reynolds, D. W., Pass, R. F., and Alford, C. A., Breast milk and the risk of cytomegalovirus infection, *N. Engl. J. Med.*, 302, 1073, 1980.

20. Gold, E. and Nankervis, G. A., Cytomegalovirus, in *Viral Infections of Humans: Epidemiology and Control*, 2nd ed., Evans, A. S., Ed., Plenum Press, New York, 1982, 167.

21. Manian, F. A. and Smith, T., Ganciclovir for the treatment of cytomegalovirus pneumonia in an immunocompetent host, *Clin. Infect. Dis.*, 17, 137, 1993.

22. Blair, S. D., Forbes, A., and Parkins, R. A., CMV colitis in an immunocompetent adult, *J. R. Soc. Med.*, 85, 238, 1992.

23. Drew, W. L., Diagnosis of cytomegalovirus infection, *Rev. Infect. Dis.*, 10(Suppl. 3), 468, 1988.

24. Drew, W. L., Sweet, E. S., Miner, R. C., and Mocarski, E. S., Multiple infections by cytomegalovirus in patients with acquired immunodeficiency syndrome: documentation by Southern blot hybridization, *J. Infect. Dis.*, 150, 952, 1984.

25. Hanshaw, J. B., Cytomegalovirus, in *Virology Monographs*, Gard, S., Hallauer, C., and Meyer, K. F., Eds., Springer-Verlag, New York, 1968, 2.

26. Jesionek, A. and Kiolemenoglou, B., Uber einen befund von protozoenartigen gebilden in den organen eines heriditarluetischen fotus, *Munch. Med. Wochenschr.*, 51, 1905, 1904.

27. Stagno, S., Cytomegalovirus, in *Infectious Diseases of the Fetus and Newborn Infant*, Remington, K. S. and Klein, J. O., Eds., W. B. Saunders, Philadelphia, 1990, 2411.

28. Griffiths, P. D., Current management of cytomegalovirus disease, *J. Med. Virol. Suppl.*, 1, 106, 1993.

29. Ho, M., Pathology of cytomegalovirus infection, in *Cytomegalovirus, Biology and Infection: Current Topics in Infectious Disease*, Greenough, W. B. III and Merigan, T. C., Eds., Plenum Press, New York, 1982, 119.

30. Becroft, D. M. O., Prenatal cytomegalovirus infection: epidemiology, pathology and pathogenesis, in *Perspectives in Pediatric Pathology*, Rosengerg, H. S. and Bernstein, J., Eds., Mason Press, New York, 1981, 203.

31. Weiss, D. J., Greenfield, J. W., Jr., O'Rourke, K. S., and McCune, W. J., Systemic cytomegalovirus infection mimicking an exacerbation of Wegener's granulomatosis, *J. Rheumatol.*, 20, 155, 1993.

32. Stagno, S., Pass, R. F., Dworsky, M. E., and Alford, C. A., Congenital and perinatal cytomegalovirus infections, *Semin. Perinatol.*, 7, 31, 1983.

33. Landini, M.-P. and Michelson, S., Human cytomegalovirus proteins, in *Progress in Medical Virology*, Melnick, J. L., Ed., S. Karger, Basel, 1988, 152.

34. Hayes, K., Alford, C. A., and Britt, W. J., Antibody response to virus-encoded proteins after cytomegalovirus mononucleosis, *J. Infect. Dis.*, 156, 615, 1987.

35. Yoser, S. L., Forster, D. J., and Rao, N. A., Systemic viral infections and their retinal and choroidal manifestations, *Surv. Ophthalmol.*, 37, 313, 1993.

36. Carlström, G., Aldén, J., Belfrage, S., Hedenström, G., Holmberg, L., Nordbring, F., and Sterner, G., Acquired cytomegalovirus infection, *Br. Med. J.*, 2, 521, 1968.

37. Chawla, H. B., Ford, M. J., Munro, J. F., Scorgie, R. E., and Watson, A. R., Ocular involvement in cytomegalovirus infection in a previously healthy adult, *Br. Med. J.*, 2, 281, 1976.

38. England, A. C. III, Miller, S. A., and Maki, D. G., Ocular findings of acute cytomegalovirus infection in an immunologically competent adult, *N. Engl. J. Med.*, 307, 94, 1982.

39. Garau, J., Kabins, S., DeNosaquo, S., Lee, G., and Keller, R., Spontaneous cytomegalovirus mononucleosis with conjunctivitis, *Arch. Intern. Med.*, 137, 1631, 1977.

40. Sterner, G., Agell, B. O., Wahren, B., and Epsmark, A., Acquired cytomegalovirus infection in older children and adults: a clinical study of hospitalized patients, *Scand. J. Infect. Dis.*, 2, 95, 1970.

41. Rinaldo, C. R., Jr., Black, P. H., and Hirsch, M. S., Virus-leukocyte interactions in cytomegalovirus mononucleosis, *J. Infect. Dis.*, 136, 667, 1977.

42. Friedman, A. H., The retinal lesions of the acquired immune deficiency syndrome, *Trans. Am. Ophthalmol. Soc.*, 82, 447, 1984.

43. Holland, G. N., Pepose, J. S., Pettit, T. H., Gottlieb, M. S., Yee, R. D., and Foos, R. Y., Acquired immune deficiency syndrome: ocular manifestations, *Ophthalmology*, 90, 859, 1983.

44. Gangan, P. A., Besen, G., Munguia, D., and Freeman, W. R., Macular serous exudation in patients with acquired immunodeficiency syndrome and cytomegalovirus retinitis, *Am. J. Ophthalmol.*, 118, 212, 1994.

45. Heinemann, M. H., Characteristics of cytomegalovirus retinitis in patients with acquired immunodeficiency syndrome, *Am. J. Med.*, 92(Suppl. 2A), 12S, 1992.

46. Henderly, D. E., Freeman, W. R., Smith, R. E., Causey, D., and Rao, N. A., Cytomegalovirus retinitis as the initial manifestation of the acquired immune deficiency syndrome, *Am. J. Ophthalmol.*, 103(3 part 1), 316, 1987.

47. Moeller, M. B., Gutman, R. A., and Hamilton, J. D., Acquired cytomegalovirus retinitis: four new cases and a review of the literature with implication for management, *Am. J. Nephrol.*, 2, 251, 1982.

48. Murray, H. W., Knox, D. L., Green, W. R., and Susel, R. M., Cytomegalovirus retinitis in adults: a manifestation of disseminated viral infection, *Am. J. Med.*, 63, 574, 1977.

49. Teich, S. A. and Orellana, J., Retinal lesions in cytomegalovirus infection, *Ann. Intern. Med.*, 104, 132, 1986.

50. Freeman, W. R., Henderly, D. E., Wan, W. L., Causey, D., Trousdale, M., Green, R. L., and Rao, N. A., Prevalence, pathophysiology, and treatment of rhegmatogenous retinal detachment in treated cytomegalovirus retinitis, *Am. J. Ophthalmol.*, 103, 627, 1987.

51. Grossniklaus, H. E., Frank, K. E., and Tomsak, R. L., Cytomegalovirus retinitis and optic neuritis in acquired immune deficiency syndrome: report of a case, *Ophthalmology*, 94, 1601, 1987.

52. Teich, S. A., Orellana, J., and Friedman, A. H., Prevalence, pathophysiology, and treatment of rhegmatogenous retinal detachment in treated cytomegalovirus retinitis, *Am. J. Ophthalmol.*, 104, 312, 1987.

53. Freeman, W. R., Friedberg, D. N., Berry, C., Quiceno, J. I., Behette, M., Fullerton, S. C., and Munguia, D., Risk factors for development of rhegmatogenous retinal detachment in patients with cytomegalovirus retinitis, *Am. J. Ophthalmol.*, 116, 713, 1993.

54. Geier, S. A., Klauss, V., Bogner, J. R., Schmidt-Kittler, H., Sadri, I., and Goebel, F. D., Retinal detachment in patients with acquired immunodeficiency syndrome, *Ger. J. Ophthalmol.*, 3, 9, 1994.

55. Smit, W. M., Wagemans, M. A., Jansen, C. L., Horn, G. J. V. D., and Surachno, J. S., Acute retinal necrosis in a renal transplant recipient — an unusual manifestation of cytomegalovirus infection, *Transplantation*, 55, 219, 1993.

56. Battle, J. F., Smith, J. L., Donovan, P., Post, M. J. D., and Penneys, N., Systemic and ocular manifestations of the acquired immune deficiency syndrome (AIDS), in *Neuro-Ophthalmology Now!*, Smith, J. L., Ed., Field, Rich and Assoc., New York, 1986, 380.

57. Marmor, M. F., Egbert, P. R., Egbert, B. M., and Marmor, J. B., Optic nerve head involvement with cytomegalovirus in an adult with lymphoma, *Arch. Ophthalmol.*, 96, 1252, 1978.

58. Harkins, T. and Maino, J. H., Cytomegalovirus retinitis complicated by optic neuropathy, *J. Am. Optom. Assoc.*, 63, 21, 1992.

59. Aaberg, T. M., Cesarz, T. J., and Rytel, M. W., Correlation of virology and clinical course of cytomegalovirus retinitis, *Am. J. Ophthalmol.*, 74, 407, 1972.

60. Egbert, P. R., Pollard, R. B., Gallagher, J. G., and Merigan, T. C., Cytomegalovirus retinitis in immunosuppressed hosts. II. Ocular manifestations, *Ann. Intern. Med.*, 93, 664, 1980.

61. Hart, W. M., Jr., Reed, C. A., Freedman, H. L., and Burde, R. M., Cytomegalovirus in juvenile iridocyclitis, *Am. J. Ophthalmol.*, 86, 329, 1978.

62. Hittner, H. M., Desmond, M. M., and Montgomery, J. R., Optic nerve manifestations of human congenital cytomegalovirus infection, *Am. J. Ophthalmol.*, 81, 661, 1976.

63. Scott, W. J., Giangiacomo, J., and Hodges, K. E., Accelerated cytomegalovirus retinitis secondary to immunosuppressive therapy, *Arch. Ophthalmol.*, 104, 1117, 1986.

64. Faber, D. W., Crapotta, J. A., Wiley, C. A., and Freeman, W. R., Retinal calcifications in cytomegalovirus retinitis, *Retina*, 13, 46, 1993.

65. Keefe, K. S., Freeman, W. R., Peterson, T. J., Wiley, C. A., Crapotta, J., Quiceno, J. I., and Listhaus, A. D., Atypical healing of cytomegalovirus retinitis: significance of persistent border opacification, *Ophthalmology*, 99, 1377, 1992.

66. Jacobson, M. A. and Mills, J., Serious cytomegalovirus disease in acquired immune deficiency syndrome (AIDS): clinical findings, diagnosis and treatment, *Ann. Intern. Med.*, 108, 585, 1988.

67. René, E., Marchie, C., Regnier, B., Saimot, A. G., Vildé, J. L., Perrone, C., Michon, C., Wolf, M., Chevalier, Th., Vallot, Th., Brun-Vezinet, F., Pangon, B., Delouol, A. M., Camus, F., Roze, C., Pignon, J. P., Mignon, M., and Bonfils, S., Intestinal infections in patients with acquired immunodeficiency syndrome: a prospective study in 132 patients, *Digest. Dis. Sci.*, 34, 773, 1989.

68. van der Ende, M. E., van Buuren, A. C., Kroes, A. C., and ten Kate, F. J., Failure of antiviral therapy in AIDS-associated cytomegalovirus cholangitis, *Infection*, 20, 371, 1992.

69. Wilcox, C. M. and Schwartz, D. A., Symptomatic CMV duodenitis: an important clinical problem in AIDS, *J. Clin. Gastroenterol.*, 14, 293, 1992.

70. Baker, J. L., Gosland, M. P., Herrington, J. D., and Record, K. E., Cytomegalovirus colitis after 5-fluorouracil and interferon-alpha therapy, *Pharmacotherapy*, 14, 246, 1994.

71. Buckner, F. S. and Pomeroy, C., Cytomegalovirus disease of the gastrointestinal tract in patients without AIDS, *Clin. Infect. Dis.*, 17, 644, 1993.

72. Katlama, C., Cytomegalovirus infection in acquired immune-deficiency syndrome, *J. Med. Virol. Suppl.*, 1, 128, 1993.

73. Goodgame, R. W., Gastrointestinal cytomegalovirus disease, *Ann. Intern. Dis.*, 119, 924, 1993.

74. Tatum, E. T., Sun, P. C., and Cohn, D. L., Cytomegalovirus vasculitis and colon perforation in a patient with acquired immunodeficiency syndrome, *Pathology*, 21, 235, 1989.

75. René, E., Marche, C., Chevalier, T., Rouzioux, C., Regnier, B., Saimot, A. G., Negesse, Y., Matheron, S., Leport, C., Wolff, B., Moriniere, B., Katlama, C., Godeberge, B., Vittecoq, B., Bricaire, F., Brun-Vezinet, F., Pangon, B., Deluol, A. M., Coulaud, J. P., Modai, J., Frottier, J., Vildé, J. C., Vachon, F., Mignon, M., and Bonfils, S., Cytomegalovirus colitis in patients with acquired immunodeficiency syndrome, *Digest. Dis. Sci.*, 33, 741, 1988.

76. Gill, H. H., Shah, S., and Desai, H. G., Cytomegalovirus colitis in a patient with Castleman's disease, *J. Assoc. Physicians India*, 42, 923, 1994.

77. de Rodriguez, C. V., Fuhrer, J., and Lake-Bakaar, G., Cytomegalovirus colitis in patients with acquired immunodeficiency syndrome, *J. R. Soc. Med.*, 87, 203, 1994.

78. Colebunders, R., Desmidt, P., Fleerackers, Y., Wijnants, H., Arts, M., Corthouts, B., and Van den Ende, J., Cytomegalovirus colitis in a patient with AIDS: CT findings, *J. Belg. Radiol.*, 77, 284, 1994.

79. Etheridge, S. P., Bolman, R. M. III, and Braunlin, E. A., Cytomegalovirus colitis in a pediatric heart transplant patient, *Clin. Transplant.*, 8, 409, 1994.

80. Wilcox, C. M. and Karowe, M. W., Esophageal infections: etiology, diagnosis, and management, *Gastroenterologist*, 2, 188, 1994.

81. Connolly, G. M., Hawkins, D., Harcourt-Webster, J. N., Parsons, P. A., Husain, O., and Gazzard, B. G., Oesophageal symptoms: their cause, treatment, and prognosis in patients with the acquired immunodeficiency syndrome, *Gut*, 30, 1033, 1980.

82. Wilcox, C. M., Diehl, D. L., Cello, J. P., Margaretten, W., and Jacobson, M. A., Cytomegalovirus oesophagitis in patients with AIDS: a clinical, endoscopic, and pathologic correlation, *Ann. Intern. Med.*, 113, 589, 1990.

83. Cello, J. P., Acquired immunodeficiency syndrome cholangiopathy: spectrum of disease, *Am. J. Med.*, 86, 539, 1989.

84. Murray, R. N., Parker, A., Kadakia, S. C., Ayala, E., and Martinez, E. M., Cytomegalovirus in upper gastrointestinal ulcers, *J. Clin. Gastroenterol.*, 19, 198, 1994.

85. Mathiesen, L., Marche, C., Labrousse, F. et al., Etude neuropathologique de l'encephale de 174 patients du Sida dans un hopital parisien, de 1982 a 1988, *Ann. Intern. Med.*, 143, 43, 1992.

86. Morgello, S., Cho, E. S., Nelsen, S., Devinsky, O., and Petito, C. K., Cytomegalovirus encephalitis in patients with acquired immunodeficiency syndrome: an autopsy study of 30 cases and a review of literature, *Hum. Pathol.*, 18, 289, 1987.

87. Behar, R., Wiley, C., and McCutchan, J. A., Cytomegalovirus polyradiculoneuropathy in acquired immune deficiency syndrome, *Neurology*, 37, 557, 1987.

88. de Gans, J., Portegies, P., Tiessens, G., Troost, D., Danner, S. A., and Lange, J. M. A., Therapy for cytomegalovirus polyradiculomyelitis in patients with AIDS: treatment with ganciclovir, *AIDS*, 4, 421, 1990.

89. Eidelberg, D., Sotrel, A., Vogel, H., Walker, P., Kleefield, J., and Crumpacker, C. S. III, Progressive polyradiculopathy in acquired immune deficiency syndrome, *Neurology*, 36, 912, 1986.

90. Mahieux, F., Gray, F., Fenelon, G., Gherardi, R., Adams, D., Guillard, A., and Poirier, J., Acute myeloradiculitis due to cytomegalovirus as the initial manifestation of AIDS, *J. Neurol. Neurosurg. Psychiatry*, 52, 270, 1989.

91. Marmaduke, D. P., Brandt, J. T., and Theil, K. S., Rapid diagnosis of cytomegalovirus in the cerebrospinal fluid of a patient with AIDS- associated polyradiculopathy, *Arch. Pathol. Lab. Med.*, 115, 1154, 1991.

92. Moskowitz, L. B., Gregorios, J. B., Hensley, G. T., and Berger, J. R., Cytomegalovirus: induced demyelination associated with acquired immune deficiency syndrome, *Arch. Pathol. Lab. Med.*, 108, 873, 1984.

93. Talpos, D., Tien, R. D., and Hesselink, J. R., Magnetic resonance imaging of AIDS-related polyradiculopathy, *Neurology*, 41, 1995, 1991.

94. Fuller, G. N., Gill, S. K., Guiloff, R. J., Kapoor, R., Lucas, S. B., Sinclair, E., Scaravilli, F., and Miller, R. F., Ganciclovir for lumbosacral polyradiculopathy in AIDS, *Lancet*, 335, 48, 1990.

95. Graveleau, P., Perol, R., and Chapman, A., Regression of cauda equina syndrome in AIDS patient being treated with ganciclovir, *Lancet*, 2, 511, 1989.

96. Miller, R. G., Storey, J. R., and Greco, C. M., Ganciclovir in the treatment of progressive AIDS-related polyradiculopathy, *Neurology*, 40, 569, 1990.

97. Tokumoto, J. N. and Hollander, H., Cytomegalovirus polyradiculopathy caused by a ganciclovir-resistant strain, *Clin. Infect. Dis.*, 17, 854, 1993.

98. Ebright, J. R. and Crane, L. R., Ganciclovir-resistant cytomegalovirus, *AIDS*, 5, 604, 1991.

99. Crane, L. R. and Ebright, J. R., Cytomegalovirus polyradiculopathy caused by a ganciclovir-resistant strain, *Clin. Infect. Dis.*, 19, 365, 1994.

100. Cohen, B. A., McArthur, J. C., Grohman, S., Patterson, B., and Glass, J. D., Neurologic prognosis of cytomegalovirus polyradiculomyelopathy in AIDS, *Neurology*, 43, 493, 1993.

101. Domingo, P., Puig, M., Iranzo, A., Lopez-Contreras, J., and Ris, J., Polyradiculopathy due to cytomegalovirus infection: report of a case in which an AIDS patient responded to foscarnet, *Clin. Infect. Dis.*, 18, 1019, 1994.

102. Cohen, B. A., McArthur, J. C., Grohman, S., Patterson, B., and Glass, J. D., Neurologic prognosis of cytomegalovirus polyradiculomyelopathy in AIDS, *Neurology*, 43 (3 Part 1), 493, 1993.

103. de Gans, J., Tiessens, G., Portegies, P., Tutuarima, J. A., and Troost, D., Predominance of polymorpho-nuclear leukocytes in cerebrospinal fluid of AIDS patients with cytomegalovirus polyradiculomyelitis, *J. Acquir. Immune Defic. Syndr.*, 3, 1155, 1990.

104. Ljungman, P., Biron, P., Bosi, A., Cahn, J. Y., Goldstone, A. H., Gorin, A. H., Link, H., Messina, C., Michallet, M., Richard, C., and Verdonck, L. for the Infectious Disease Working Party of the European Group for Bone Marrow Transplantation, Cytomegalovirus interstitial pneumonia in autologous bone marrow transplant recipients, *Bone Marrow Transplant.*, 13, 209, 1994.

105. Bower, M., Barton, S. E., Nelson, M. R., Bobby, J., Smith, D., Youle, M., and Gazzard, B. G., The significance of the detection of cytomegalovirus in the bronchoalveolar lavage fluid in AIDS patients with pneumonia, *AIDS*, 4, 317, 1990.

106. Aglas, F., Rainer, F., Herman, J., Gretler, J., Hüttl, E., Domej, W., and Krejs, G. J., Interstitial pneumonia due to cytomegalovirus following low-dose methotrexate treatment for rheumatoid arthritis, *Arthritis Rheum.*, 38, 291, 1995.

107. Reichert, C. M., O'Leary, T. J., Levens, D. L., Simrell, C. R., and Macher, A. M., Autopsy pathology in the acquired immune deficiency syndrome, *Am. J. Pathol.*, 112, 357, 1983.

108. Fujii, K., Morimoto, I., Wake, A., Okada, Y., Inokuchi, N., Ishida, O., Nakano, Y., Oda, S., and Eto, S., Adrenal insufficiency in patient with acquired immunodefciency syndrome, *Endocr. J.*, 41, 13, 1994.

109. Linnemann, C. C., Jr., Kauffman, C. A., First, M. R., Schiff, G. M., and Phair, J. F., Cellular immune response to cytomegalovirus infection after renal transplantation, *Infect. Immun.*, 22, 176, 1978.

110. Lopez, C., Simmons, R. L., Park, B. H., Najarian, J. S., and Good, R. A., Cell-mediated and humoral immune responses of renal transplant recipients with cytomegalovirus infections, *Clin. Exp. Immunol.*, 16, 565, 1974.

111. Boland, G. J., Vlieger, A. M., Ververs, C., and De Gast, G. C., Evidence for transfer of cellular and humoral immunity to cytomegalovirus from donor to recipient in allogeneic bone marrow transplantation, *Clin. Exp. Immunol.*, 88, 506, 1992.

112. Humbert, M., Roux-Lombard, P., Cerrina, J., Magnan, A., Simonneau, G., Dartevelle, P., Galanaud, P., Dayer, J. M., and Emilie, D., Soluble TNF receptors (TNF-sR55 and TNF-sR75) in lung allograft recipients displaying cytomegalovirus pneumonitis, *Am. J. Respir. Crit. Care Med.*, 149, 1681, 1994.

113. Fietze, E., Prösch, S., Reinke, P., Stein, J., Döcke, W.-D., Staffa, G., Löning, S., Devaux, S., Emmrich, F., von Baehr, R., Krüger, D. H., and Volk, H.-D., Cytomegalovirus infection in transplant recipients: the role of tumor necrosis factor, *Transplantation*, 58, 675, 1994.

114. Anderson, K. P., Lie, Y. S., Low, M. A., and Fennie, E. H., Effects of tumor necrosis factor-alpha treatment on mortality in murine cytomegalovirus-infected mice, *Antiviral Res.*, 21, 343, 1993.

115. van den Berg, A. P., van Son, W. J., Tegzess, A. M., and Hauw The, T., Cellular immune activation reflects antiviral immunity and is a favorable prognostic marker in patients with cytomegalovirus infection, *Transplant. Proc.*, 25 (1 part 2), 1419, 1993.

116. Howard, R. J. and Balfour, H. H., Jr., Cell-mediated immunity to cytomegalovirus in mice and in renal transplant recipients, *Transplant. Proc.*, 11, 75, 1979.

117. van den Berg, A. P., van Son, W. J., Janssen, R. A., Brons, N. H., Heyn, A. A., Scholten-Sampson, A., Postma, S., van der Giessen, M., Tegzess, A. M., de Leij, L. H., and Hauw The, T., Recovery from cytomegalovirus infection is associated with activation of peripheral blood lymphocytes, *J. Infect. Dis.*, 166, 1228, 1992.

118. Starr, S. E., Smiley, L., Wlodaver, C., Friedman, H. M., Plotkin, S. A., and Barker, C., Natural killing of cytomegalovirus-infected targets in renal transplant recipients, *Transplantation*, 37, 161, 1984.

119. Charak, B. S., Choudhary, G. D., Tefft, M., and Mazumder, A., Interleukin-2 in bone marrow transplantation: preclinical studies, *Bone Marrow Transplant.*, 10, 103, 1992.

120. Quinnan, G. V., Jr. and Rook, A. H., The importance of cytotoxic cellular immunity in the protection from cytomegalovirus infection, *Birth Defects*, 20, 245, 1984.

121. Quinnan, G. V., Jr., Kirmani, N., Rook, A. H., Manischewitz, J. F., Jackson, L., Moreschi, G., Santos, G. W., Saral, R., and Burns, W. H., Cytotoxic T cells in cytomegalovirus infection: HLA-restricted T-lymphocyte and non-T-lymphocyte cytotoxic responses correlate with recovery from cytomegalovirus infection in bone-marrow-transplant recipients, *N. Engl. J. Med.*, 307, 7, 1982.

122. Rook, A. H., Smith, W. J., Burdick, J. F., Manischewitz, J. F., Frederick, W., Siegel, J. P., Williams, G. M., and Quinnan, G. V., Jr., Virus-specific cytotoxic lymphocyte responses are predictive of the outcome of cytomegalovirus infection of renal transplant recipients, *Transplant. Proc.*, 16, 1466, 1984.

123. Rytel, M. W. and Balay, J., Cytomegalovirus infection and immunity in renal allograft recipients: assessment of the competence of humoral immunity, *Infect. Immun.*, 13, 1633, 1976.

124. O'Neill, H. J., Shirodaria, P. V., Connolly, J. H., Simpson, D. I. H., and McGeown, M. G., Cytomegalovirus-specific antibody responses in renal transplant patients with primary and recurrent CMV infections, *J. Med. Virol.*, 24, 461, 1988.

125. O'Neill, H. J., Shirodaria, P. V., and Simpson, D. M., Low and high molecular weight cytomegalovirus-specific immunoglobulin M antibody in renal transplant patients with cytomegalovirus infections, *J. Med. Virol.*, 24, 445, 1988.

126. Iberer, F., Halwachs-Baumann, G., Rödl, S., Pleisnitzer, A., Wasler, A., Auer, T., Petutschnigg, B., Müller, H., Tscheliessnigg, K., and Wilders- Truschnig, M., Monitoring of cytomegalovirus disease after heart transplantation: persistence of anti-cytomegalovirus IgM antibodies, *J. Heart Lung Transplant.*, 13, 405, 1994.

127. Rodriguez, G. E. and Adler, S. P., Immunoglobulin G subclass responses to cytomegalovirus in seropositive patients after transfusion, *Transfusion*, 30, 528, 1990.

128. Griffiths, P. D. and Grundy, J. E., Molecular biology and immunology of cytomegalovirus, *Biochem. J.*, 241, 313, 1987.

129. Ho, M., Cytomegalovirus infections in immunosuppressed patients, in *Cytomegalovirus, Biology and Infection: Current Topics in Infectious Disease*, Greenough, W. B. III and Merigan, T. C., Eds., Plenum Press, New York, 1982, 171.

130. Drew, W. L., Conant, M. A., Miner, R. C., Huang, R. C., Ziegler, J. L., Groundwater, J. R., Gullett, J. H., Volberding, P., Abrams, D. I., and Mintz, L., Cytomegalovirus and Kaposi's sarcoma in young homosexual men, *Lancet*, 2, 125, 1982.

131. Drew, W. L. and Mintz, L., Cytomegalovirus infection in healthy and immune-deficient homosexual men, in *The Acquired Immune Deficiency Syndrome and Infections of Homosexual Men*, Ma, P. and Armstrong, D., Eds., Yorke Medical Books, New York, 1984, 117.

132. Drew, W. L., Mintz, L., Miner, R. C., Sands, M., and Ketterer, B., Prevalence of cytomegalovirus infection in homosexual men, *J. Infect. Dis.*, 143, 188, 1981.

133. Stratta, R. J., Clinical patterns and treatment of cytomegalovirus infection after solid-organ transplantation, *Transplant. Res.*, 25 (5 Suppl. 4), 15, 1993.

134. Pollard, R. B., Cytomegalovirus infections in renal, heart, heart-lung and liver transplantations, *Pediatr. Infect. Dis. J.*, 7, 97, 1988.

135. Balfour, H. H., Chace, B. A., Stapleton, J. T., Simmons, R. L., and Fryd, D. S., A randomized placebo-controlled trial of oral acyclovir for the prevention of cytomegalovirus disease in recipients of renal allograft, *N. Engl. J. Med.*, 320, 1381, 1989.

136. Legendre, C., Ducloux, D., Ferroni, A., Chkoff, N., Geffrier, C., Rouzioux, C., and Kreis, H., Acyclovir in preventing cytomegalovirus infection in kidney transplant recipients: a case-controlled study, *J. Med. Virol. Suppl.*, 1, 118, 1993.

137. Rubin, R. H., Tolkoff-Rubin, N. E., Oliver, D., Rota, T. R., Hamilton, J., Betts, R. F., Pass, R. F., Hillis, W., Szmussess, W., Farrell, M. L., and Hirsch, M. S., Multicenter seroepidemiologic study of the impact of cytomegalovirus infection on renal transplantation, *Transplantation*, 40, 243, 1985.

138. Peterson, P. K., Balfour, H. H., Marker, S. C., Fryd, D. S., Howard, R. J., and Simmons, R. L., Cytomegalovirus disease in renal allograft recipients: a prospective study of the clinical features, risk factors and impact on renal transplantation, *Medicine (Baltimore)*, 59, 283, 1980.

139. Rocha, E., Campos, H. H., Rouzioux, C., Le Bihan, C., Landais, P., Legendre, C., and Kreis, H., Cytomegalovirus infections after kidney transplantation: identical risk whether donor or recipient is the virus carrier, *Transplant. Proc.*, 23, 2638, 1991.

140. Rubin, R. H., Cosimi, A. B., Tolkoff-Rubin, N. E., Russell, P. S., and Hirsch, M. S., Infectious disease syndromes attributable to cytomegalovurus and their significance among renal transplant recipients, *Transplantation*, 24, 458, 1977.

141. Snydman, D. R., Wemer, B. G., Heinze-Lacey, B., Berardi, V. P., Tilney, N. L., Kirkman, R. L., Milford, E. L., Che, S. L., Bush, H. L., Levey, A. S., Strom, T. B., Carpenter, C. B., Levey, R. H., Harmon, W. E., Zimmerman, C. E., Shapiro, M. E., Steinman, T., Logerflo, F., Idelson, B., Schroter, G. P. J., Levin, M. J., McIver, J., Leszczynski, J., and Grady, G. F., Use of cytomegalovirus immune globulin to prevent cytomegalovirus disease in renal-transplant recipients, *N. Engl. J. Med.*, 317, 1049, 1987.

142. Burd, R. S., Gillingham, K. J., Farber, M. S., Statz, C. L., Kramer, M. S., Najarian, J. S., and Dunn, D. L., Diagnosis and treatment of cytomegalovirus disease in pediatric renal transplant recipients, *J. Pediatr. Surg.*, 29, 1049, 1994.

143. Saatci, U., Ozen, S., Ceyhan, M., and Secmeer, G., Cytomegalovirus disease in a renal transplant recipient manifesting with pericarditis, *Int. Urol. Nephrol.*, 25, 617, 1993.

144. Devine, S. M. and Wingard, J. R., Viral infections in severely immunocompromised cancer patients, *Support Care Cancer*, 2, 355, 1994.

145. Goodrich, J. M., Boeckh, M., and Bowden, R., Strategies for the prevention of cytomegalovirus disease after marrow transplantation, *Clin. Infect. Dis.*, 19, 287, 1994.

146. Kirklin, J. K., Naftel, D. C., Levine, T. B., Bourge, R. C., Pelletier, G. B., O'Donnell, J., Miller, L. W., and Pritzker, M. R., Cytomegalovirus after heart transplantation. Risk factors for infection and death: a multiinstitutional study. The Cardiac Transplant Research Database Group, *J. Heart Lung Transplant.*, 13, 394, 1994.

147. Arabia, F. A., Rosado, L. J., Huston, C. L., Sethi, G. K., and Copeland, J. G. III, Incidence and recurrence of gastrointestinal cytomegalovirus infection in heart transplantation, *Ann. Thorac. Surg.*, 55, 8, 1993.

148. Singh, N., Dummer, J. S., Kusne, S., Breinig, M. K., Armstrong, J. A., Makowka, L., Starzl, T. E., and Ho, M., Infections with cytomegalovirus and other herpes viruses in 121 liver transplant recipients: transmission by donated organ and the effect of OKT3 antibodies, *J. Infect. Dis.*, 158, 124, 1988.

149. Paya, C. V., Marin, E., Keating, M., Dickson, R., Porayko, M., and Wiesner, R., Solid organ transplantation: result and implications of acyclovir use in liver transplants, *J. Med. Virol. Suppl.*, 1, 123, 1993.

150. Paya, C. V., Hermans, P. E., Wiesner, R. H., Ludwig, J., Smith, T. F., Rakela, J., and Krom, R. A. F., Cytomegalovirus hepatitis in liver transplantation: prospective analysis of 93 consecutive orthotopic liver transplantations, *J. Infect. Dis.*, 160, 752, 1989.

151. Paya, C. V., Hermans, P. E., Washington, J. A., Smith, T. F., Anhalt, J. P., Wiesner, R. H., and Krom, R. A. F., Incidence, distribution, and outcome of episodes of infection in 100 orthotopic liver transplantations, *Mayo Clinic Proc.*, 64, 555, 1989.

152. Kusne, S., Dummer, J. S., Singh, N., Iwatsuki, S., Makowka, L., Esquivel, C., Tzakis, A. G., Starzl, T. E., and Ho, M., Infections after liver transplantation: an analysis of 101 consecutive cases, *Medicine (Baltimore)*, 67, 132, 1988.

153. Sano, K., Tanaka, K., Uemoto, S., Fujita, S., Tokunaga, Y., Inomata, Y., Ozawa, K., and Minamishima, Y., Cytomegalovirus infection in living related liver transplantation: rapid diagnosis by human monoclonal antibody staining of blood leukocytes, *Transplant. Sci.*, 4, 105, 1994.

154. Wiens, M., Schmidt, C. A., Lohmann, R., Oettle, H., Blumhardt, G., and Neuhaus, P., Cytomegalovirus disease after liver transplantation: diagnostics and therapy, *Transplant. Res.*, 25, 2673, 1993.

155. Fries, B. C., Khaira, D., Pepe, M. S., and Torok-Storb, B., Declining lymphocyte counts following cytomegalovirus (CMV) infection are associated with fatal CMV disease in bone marrow transplant patients, *Exp. Hematol.*, 21, 1387, 1993.

156. Zomas, A., Mehta, J., Powles, R., Treleaven, J., Iveson, T., Singhal, S., Jameson, B., Paul, B., Brincat, S., and Catovsky, D., Unusual infections following allogeneic bone marrow transplantation for chronic lymphocytic leukemia, *Bone Marrow Transplant.*, 14, 799, 1994.

157. Winston, D. J., Huang, E.-S., Miller, M. J., Lin, C. H., Ho, W. G., Gale, R. P., and Champlin, R. E., Molecular epidemiology of cytomegalovirus infection associated with bone marrow transplantation, *Ann. Intern. Med.*, 102, 16, 1985.

158. Betts, R. F., The relationship of epidemiology and treatment factors to infection and allograft survival in renal transplantation, in *CMV: Pathogenesis and Prevention of Human Infection*, Plotkin, S. A., Michelson, S., Pagano, J. S., and Rapp, F., Eds., Alan R. Riss, New York, 1984, 87.

159. Salmon, D., Lacassin, F., Harzic, M., Leport, C., Perronne, C., Bricaire, F., Brun-Vezinet, F., and Vildé, J.-L., Predictive value of cytomegalovirus viremia for the occurrence of CMV organ involvement in AIDS, *J. Med. Virol.*, 32, 160, 1990.

160. Millar, A. B., Patou, G., Miller, R. F., Grundy, J. E., Katz, D. R., Weller, I. V., and Semple, S. J., Cytomegalovirus in the lungs of patients with AIDS: respiratory pathogen or passenger? *Am. Rev. Respir. Dis.*, 141, 1474, 1990.

161. Grundy, J. E., Shanley, J. D., and Griffiths, P. D., Is cytomegalovirus interstitial pneumonitis in transplant recipients an immunopathological condition? *Lancet*, 2, 996, 1987.

162. Gallant, J. E., Moore, R. D., Richman, D. D., Keruly, J., and Chaisson, R. E., Incidence and natural history of cytomegalovirus disease in patients with advanced human immunodeficiency virus disease treated with zidovudine: the Zidovudine Epidemiology Group, *J. Infect. Dis.*, 166, 1223, 1992.

163. Galant, J. E., Moore, R. D., Richman, D. D., Keruly, J., Chaisson, R. E., and the Zidovudine Epidemiology Study Group, Incidence and natural history of cytomegalovirus disease in patients with advanced human immunodeficiency virus disease treated with zidovudine, *J. Infect. Dis.*, 166, 1223, 1992.

164. Fiala, M., Kermani, V., and Gornbein, J., Role of CD8+ in late opportunistic infections of patients with AIDS, *Res. Immunol.*, 143, 903, 1992.

165. Webster, A., CMV and HIV interactions, in *Progress in Cytomegalovirus Research*, Elsevier, New York, 1991, 313.

166. Ghazal, P., Young, J., Giulietti, E., Demattei, C., Garcia, J., Gaynor, R., Stenberg, R. M., and Nelson, J. A., A discrete cis element in the human immunodeficiency virus long terminal repeat mediates synergistic trans activation by cytomegalovirus immediate-early proteins, *J. Virol.*, 65, 6735, 1991.

167. McKeating, J. A., Griffiths, P. D., and Weiss, R. A., HIV susceptibility conferred to human fibroblasts by cytomegalovirus-induced Fc receptor, *Nature*, 343, 659, 1990.

168. Tegtmeier, G. E., Post-transfusion cytomegalovirus infections, *Arch. Pathol. Lab. Med.*, 113, 236, 1989.

169. Webster, A., Lee, C. A., Cook, D. G., Grundy, J. E., Emery, V. C., Kernoff, P. B., and Griffiths, P. D., Cytomegalovirus infection and progression towards AIDS in hemophiliacs with human immunodeficiency virus infection, *Lancet*, 2, 63, 1989.

170. Reardon, J. E. and Spector, T., Herpes simplex virus type 1 DNA polymerase: mechanism of inhibition by acyclovir triphosphate, *J. Biol. Chem.*, 264, 7405, 1989.

171. Furman, P. A., St. Clair, P. H., and Spector, T., Acyclovir triphosphate is a suicide inactivator of herpes simplex virus DNA polymerase, *J. Biol. Chem.*, 259, 9575, 1984.

172. Erice, A., Chou, S., Biron, K. K., Stanat, S. C., Balfour, H. H. J., and Jordan, M. C., Progressive disease due to ganciclovir-resistant cytomegalovirus in immunocompromised patients, *N. Engl. J. Med.*, 320, 289, 1989.

173. Fletcher, C., Sawchuk, R., Chinnock, B., de Miranda, P., and Balfour, H. H., Jr., Human pharmacokinetics of the antiviral drug DHPG, *Clin. Pharmacol. Ther.*, 40, 281, 1986.

174. Boulieu, R., Bastien, O., and Bleyzac, N., Pharmacokinetics of ganciclovir in heart transplant patients undergoing continuous venovenous hemodialysis, *Ther. Drug Monit.*, 15, 105, 1993.

175. Ashton, P., Brown, J. D., Pearson, P. A., Blandford, D. L., Smith, T. J., Anand, R., Nightingale, S. D., and Sanborn, G. E., Intravitreal ganciclovir pharmacokinetics in rabbits and man, *J. Ocul. Pharmacol.*, 8, 343, 1992.

176. Gilstrap, L. C., Bawdon, R. E., Roberts, S. W., and Sobhi, S., The transfer of the nucleoside analog ganciclovir across the perfused human placenta, *Am. J. Obstet. Gynecol.*, 170, 967, 1994.

177. Stals, F. S., Wagenaar, S. S., and Bruggeman, C. A., Generalized cytomegalovirus (CMV) infection and CMV-induced pneumonitis in the rat: combined effect of 9-(1,3-dihydroxy-2-propoxymethyl)guanine and specific antibody treatment, *Antiviral Res.*, 25, 147, 1994.

178. Freitas, V. R., Fraser-Smith, E. B., and Matthews, T. R., Efficacy of ganciclovir in combination with other antimicrobial agents against cytomegalovirus in vitro and in vivo, *Antiviral Res.*, 20, 1, 1993.

179. Smee, D. F., Sugiyama, S. T., and Reist, E. J., Nucleotide analogs related to acyclovir and ganciclovir are effective against murine cytomegalovirus infections in BALB/c and severe combined immunodeficient mice, *Antimicrob. Agents Chemother.*, 38, 2165, 1994.

180. Barnard, D. L., Huffman, J. H., Sidwell, R. W., and Reist, E. J., Selective inhibition of cytomegalovirus by 9-(3'-ethylphosphono-1'-hydroxymethyl-1'-propyloxymethyl)guanine, *Antiviral Res.*, 22, 77, 1993.

181. Laskin, O. L., Cederberg, D. M., Mills, J., Eron, L. J., Mildvan, D., and Spector, S. A., Ganciclovir for the treatment and suppression of serious infections caused by cytomegalovirus, *Am. J. Med.*, 83, 201, 1987.

182. Hardy, D. W., Combined ganciclovir and recombinant human granulocyte-macrophage colony-stimulating factor in the treatment of cytomegalovirus retinitis in AIDS patients, *J. Acquir. Immune Defic. Syndr.*, 4(Suppl. 1), S22, 1991.

183. Hardy, D., Spector, S., Polsky, B., Crumpacker, C., van der Horst, C., Holland, G., Freeman, W., Heinemann, M. H., Sharuk, G., Klystra, J. et al., Combination of ganciclovir and granulocyte-macrophage colony- stimulating factor in the treatment of cytomegalovirus retinitis in AIDS patients, *Eur. J. Clin. Microbiol. Infect. Dis.*, 13(Suppl. 2), S34, 1994.

184. Spector, S. A., Busch, D. F., Follansbee, S., Squires, K., Lalezari, J. P., Jacobson, M. A., Connor, J. D., Jung, D., Shadman, A., Mastre, B., Buhles, W., Drew, W. L., and the AIDS Clinical Trial Group, and the Cytomegalovirus Cooperative Study Group, Pharmacokinetic, safety and antiviral profiles of oral ganciclovir in persons infected with human immunodeficiency virus: a phase I/II study, *J. Infect. Dis.*, 171, 1431, 1995.

185. Hochster, H., Dieterich, D., Bozzette, S., Reichman, R. C., Conner, J. D., Liebes, L., Sonke, R. L., Spector, S. A., Valentine, F., Pettinelli, C., and Richman, D. D., Toxicity of combined ganciclovir and zidovudine for cytomegalovirus disease associated with AIDS, *Ann. Intern. Med.*, 113, 111, 1990.

186. Collaborative DHPG Treatment Study Group. Treatment of serious cytomegalovirus infections with 9-(1,3-dihydroxy-2-propoxymethyl) guanine in patients with AIDS and other immunodeficiencies, *N. Engl. J. Med.*, 314, 801, 1986.

187. Hooymans, J. M. M., Sprenger, H. G., and Weits, J., Treatment of cytomegalovirus retinitis with DHPG in a patient with AIDS, *Doc. Ophthalmol.*, 67, 5, 1987.

188. Orellana, J., Teich, S. A., Friedman, A. H., Lerebours, F., Winterkorn, J., and Mildvan, D., Combined short- and long-term therapy for the treatment of cytomegalovirus retinitis using ganciclovir (BW B759U), *Ophthalmology*, 94, 831, 1987.

189. Figge, H. L., Bailie, G. R., Briceland, L. L., and Kowalsky, S. F., Possible ganciclovir-induced hepatotoxicity in patients with AIDS, *Clin. Pharm.*, 11, 432, 1992.

190. Scholz, D., Arndt, R., and Meyer, T., Evidence for an immunosuppressive activity of ganciclovir, *Transplant. Proc.*, 26, 3253, 1994.

191. Barton, T. L., Roush, M. K., and Dever, L. L., Seizures associated with ganciclovir therapy, *Pharmacotherapy*, 12, 413, 1992.

192. Drew, W. L., Miner, R. C., Busch, D. F., Follansbee, S. E., Gullett, J., Mehalko, S. G., Gordon, S. M., Owen, W. F., Jr., Matthews, T. R., Buhles, W. C., and DeArmond, B., Prevalence of resistance in patients receiving ganciclovir for serious cytomegalovirus infection, *J. Infect. Dis.*, 163, 716, 1991.

193. Öberg, B., Antiviral effects of phosphonoformate (PFA, foscarnet sodium), *Pharmacol. Ther.*, 19, 387, 1983.

194. Sandström, E. G., Kaplan, J. C., Byington, R. E., and Hirsch, M. S., Inhibition of human T cell lymphtropic virus type III by phosphonoformate, *Lancet*, 1, 1480, 1985.

195. Hengge, U. R., Brockmeyer, N. H., Malessa, R., Ravens, U., and Goos, M., Foscarnet penetrates the blood-brain barrier: rationale for therapy of cytomegalovirus encephalitis, *Antimicrob. Agents Chemother.*, 37, 1010, 1993.

196. Taburet, A. M., Katlama, C., Blanshard, C., Zorza, G., Gazzard, D., Dohin, E., Gazzard, B. G., Frostegard, C., and Singlas, E., Pharmacokinetics of foscarnet after twice-daily administration for treatment of cytomegalovirus disease in AIDS patients, *Antimicrob. Agents Chemother.*, 36, 1821, 1992.

197. Schinazi, R. F., Combined chemotherapeutic modalities for viral infections: rationale and clinical potential, in *Synergism and Antagonism in Chemotherapy*, Chou, T.-C. and Rideout, D. C., Eds., Academic Press, San Diego, 1991, 109.

198. Eriksson, B. F. H. and Schinazi, R. F., Combinations of 3'-azido-3'- deoxythimidine (zidovudine) and phosphonoformate (foscarnet) against human immunodeficiency virus type 1 and cytomegalovirus *in vitro*, *Antimicrob. Agents Chemother.*, 33, 663, 1989.

199. Reddy, M. M., Grieco, M. H., McKinley, G. F., Causey, D. M., van der Horst, C. M., Parenti, D. M., Hooton, T. M., Davis, R. B., and Jacobson, M. A., Effect of foscarnet therapy on human immunodeficiency virus p24 antigen levels in AIDS patients with cytomegalovirus retinitis, *J. Infect. Dis.*, 166, 607, 1992.

200. Gumbel, H. O., Rückert, D. G., Cinatl, J., Rabenau, H., Doerr, H. W., and Ohrloff, C., In vitro anti-human cytomegalovirus activity of liposome-encapsulated foscarnet, *Ger. J. Ophthalmol.*, 3, 5, 1994.

201. Sarraf, D., Equi, R. A., Holland, G. N., Yoshizumi, M. O., and Lee, D. A., Transscleral iontophoresis of foscarnet, *Am. J. Ophthalmol.*, 115, 748, 1993.

202. Chrisp, P. and Crissold, S. P., Foscarnet: a review of its antiviral activity, pharmacokinetic properties and therapeutic use in immunocompromised retinitis patients with cytomegalovirus retinitis, *Drugs*, 41, 104, 1991.

203. Aweeka, F., Gambertoglio, J., Mills, J., and Jacobson, M. A., Pharmacokinetics of intermittently administered intravenous foscarnet in the treatment of acquired immunodeficiency syndrome patients with serious cytomegalovirus retinitis, *Antimicrob. Agents Chemother.*, 33, 742, 1989.

204. Deray, G., Katlama, C., and Dohin, E., Prevention of foscarnet nephrotoxicity, *Ann. Intern. Med.*, 113, 332, 1990.

205. Deray, G., Martinez, F., Katlama, C., Levaltier, B., Beaufils, H., Danis, M., Rozenheim, M., Baumelou, A., Dohin, E., Gentilini, M., and Jacobs, C., Foscarnet nephrotoxicity: mechanism, incidence and prevention, *Am. J. Nephrol.*, 9, 316, 1989.

206. Geahart, M. O. and Sorg, T. B., Foscarnet-induced severe hypomagnesemia and other electrolyte disorders, *Clin. Pharmacother.*, 27, 285, 1993.

207. Katlama, C., Dohin, E., Caumes, E., Cochereau-Massin, I., Brancon, C., Robinet, M., Rogeaux, O., Dahan, R., and Gentilini, M., Foscarnet induction therapy for cytomegalovirus retinitis in AIDS: comparison of twice-daily and three times daily regimens, *J. Acquir. Immune Defic. Syndr.*, 5(Suppl. 1), S18, 1992.

208. Evans, L. M. and Grossman, M. E., Foscarnet-induced penile ulcer, *J. Am. Acad. Dermatol.*, 27, 124, 1992.

209. Saint-Marc, T., Fournier, F., Touraine, J. L., and Marneff, E., Uvula and oesophageal ulcerations with foscarnet, *Lancet*, 340, 970, 1992.

210. Fan-Harvard, P., Sanchorawala, V., Oh, J., Moser, E. M., and Smith, S. P., Concurrent use of foscarnet and ciprofloxacin may increase the propensity of seizures, *Ann. Pharmacother.*, 28, 869, 1994.

211. Neyts, J. and De Clercq, E., New inhibitors of cytomegalovirus replication: in vitro evaluation, mechanism of action, and in vivo activity, *Verh. K. Acad. Geneeskd. Belg.*, 56, 561, 1994.

212. Neyts, J., Sobis, H., Snoeck, R., Vandeputte, M., and De Clercq, E., Efficacy of (S)-1-(3-hydroxy-2-phosphonylmethoxypropyl)cytosine and 9-(1,3-dihydroxy-2-propoxymethyl)guanine in the treatment of intracerebral murine cytomegalovirus infections in immunocompetent and immunodeficient mice, *Eur. J. Clin. Microbiol. Infect. Dis.*, 12, 269, 1993.

213. Stals, F. S., Zeytinoglu, A., Havenith, M., De Clercq, E., and Bruggeman, C. A., Rat cytomegalovirus-induced pneumonitis after allogeneic bone marrow transplantation: effective treatment with (S)-1-(3-hydroxy-2-phosphonylmethoxypropyl)cytosine, *Antimicrob. Agents Chemother.*, 37, 218, 1993.

214. Stals, F. S., Zeytinoglu, A., Havennith, M., De Clercq, E., and Bruggeman, C. A., Comparative effect of (S)-1-(3-hydroxy-2-phosphonylmethoxypropyl)cytosine and 9-(1,3-dihydroxy-2-propoxymethyl)guanine treatment on cytomegalovirus-induced interstitial pneumonitis in allogeneic bone marrow transplant recipient rats, *Transplant. Proc.*, 25(1 Part 2), 1248, 1993.

215. Smee, D. F., Morris, J. L., Leonhardt, J. A., Mead, J. R., Holy, A., and Sidwell, R. W., Treatment of murine cytomegalovirus infections in severe combined immunodeficient mice with ganciclovir, (S)-1-[3-hydroxy-2-(phosphonylmethoxy)propyl]cytosine, interferon, and bropirimine, *Antimicrob. Agents Chemother.*, 36, 1837, 1992.

216. Neyts, J., Balzarini, J., Naesens, L., and De Clercq, E., Efficacy of (S)-1-(3-hydroxy-2-phosphonyl-methoxypropyl)cytosine and 9-(1,3-dihydroxy-2-propoxymethyl)guanine for the treatment of murine cytomegalovirus infection in severe combined immunodeficiency mice, *J. Med. Virol.*, 37, 67, 1992.

217. Wallimann, T., Wyss, M., Brdiczka, D., Nicolay, K., and Eppenberger, H. M., Intracellular compartmentalization, structure and function of creatine kinase isoenzymes in tissues with high and fluctuating energy demands: the "phosphocreatine circuit" for cellular energy homeostasis, *Biochem. J.*, 281, 21, 1992.

218. Walker, J. B., Creatine: biosynthesis, regulation and function, *Adv. Enzymol. Relat. Areas Mol. Biol.*, 50, 177, 1979.

219. Iyengar, M. R., Creatine kinase as an intracellular regulator, *J. Muscle Res. Cell. Motil.*, 5, 527, 1984.

220. Iyengar, M. R., Fluellen, C. E., and Iyengar, C. W. L., Creatine kinase from the bovine myometrium: purification and characterization, *J. Cell. Motil.*, 3, 231, 1982.

221. Lillie, J. W., Smee, D. F., Huffman, J. H., Hansen, L. J., Sidwell, R. W., and Kaddurah-Daouk, R., Cyclocreatine (1-carboxymethyl-2-iminoimidazolidine) inhibits the replication of human herpes viruses, *Antiviral Res.*, 23, 203, 1994.

222. Braithwaite, A. W., Cheetham, B. F., Li, P., Parish, C. R., Waldron-Stevens, L. K., and Bellett, A. J. D., Adenovirus-induced alterations of the cell growth cycle: a requirement for expression of E1A but not E1B, *J. Virol.*, 45, 192, 1983.

223. Colberg-Poley, A. M. and Santomenna, L. D., Selective induction of chromosomal gene expression by human cytomegalovirus, *Virology*, 166, 217, 1988.

224. Kaddurah-Daouk, R., Lillie, J. W., Daouk, G. H., Green, M. R., Kingston, R., and Schimmel, P., Induction of a cellular enzyme for energy metabolism by transforming domains of adenovirus E1a, *Mol. Cell. Biol.*, 10, 1476, 1990.

225. Colberg-Poley, A. M., Santomenna, L. D., Harlow, P. P., Benfield, P. A., and Tenney, D. J., Human cytomegalovirus US3 and UL36-38 immediate early proteins regulate expression, *J. Virol.*, 66, 95, 1992.

226. Chida, K., Kasahara, K., Tsuneaga, M., Kohno, Y., Yamada, S., Ohmi, S., and Kuroki, T., Purification and identification of creatine phosphokinase B as a substrate of protein kinase C in mouse skin in vivo, *Biochem. Biophys. Res. Commun.*, 173, 351, 1990.

227. Chida, K., Tsuneaga, M., Kasahara, K., Kohno, Y., and Kuroki, T., Regulation of creatine phosphokinase B activity by protein kinase C, *Biochem. Biophys. Res. Commun.*, 173, 346, 1990.

228. Reiss, N. A. and Kaye, A. M., Identification of the major component of estrogen-induced protein of rat uterus as the BB isozyme of creatine kinase, *J. Biol. Chem.*, 256, 23, 1981.

229. Somjen, D., Weisman, Y., Harell, A., Berger, E., and Kaye, A. M., Direct and sex-specific stimulation by sex steroids of creatine kinase activity and DNA synthesis in rat bone, *Proc. Natl. Acad. Sci. U.S.A.*, 86, 3361, 1989.

230. Somjen, D., Zor, U., Kaye, A. M., Harell, A., and Binderman, I., Parathyroid hormone induction of creatine kinase activity and DNA synthesis is mimicked by phospholipase C, diacylglycerol and phorbol ester, *Biochim. Biophys. Acta*, 931, 215, 1987.

231. Carney, D. N., Zweig, M. H., Ihde, D. C., Cohen, M. H., Makuch, R. W., and Gazdar, A. F., Elevated serum creatine kinase BB levels in patients with small cell lung cancer, *Cancer Res.*, 44, 5399, 1984.

232. Feld, R. D. and Witte, D. L., Presence of creatine kinase BB isoenzyme in some patients with prostate carcinoma, *Clin. Chem.*, 23, 1930, 1977.

233. Gazdar, A. F., Zweig, M. H., Carney, D. N., Van Steirteghen, A. C., Baylin, S. B., and Minna, J. D., Levels of creatine kinase and its BB isoenzyme in lung cancer specimens and cultures, *Cancer Res.*, 41, 2773, 1981.

234. Homberger, H. A., Miller, S. A., and Jacob, G. L., Radioimmunoassay of creatine kinase B-isoenzymes in serum of patients with azotemia, obstructive uropathy, or carcinoma of the prostate or bladder, *Clin. Chem.*, 26, 1821, 1980.

235. Ishiguro, Y., Kato, K., Akatsuka, H., and Ito, T., The diagnostic and prognostic value of pretreatment serum creatine kinase BB levels in patients with neuroblastoma, *Cancer*, 65, 2014, 1990.

236. Thompson, R. J., Rubery, E. D., and Jones, H. M., Radioimmunoassay of serum creatine kinase-BB as a tumour marker in breast cancer, *Lancet*, 2, 673, 1980.

237. Lillie, J. W., O'Keefe, M., Valinski, H., Hamlin, H. A., Jr., Varban, M. L., and Kaddurah-Daouk, R., Cyclocreatine (1-carboxymethyl-2- iminoimidazolidine) inhibits growth of a broad spectrum of cancer cells derived from solid tumors, *Cancer Res.*, 53, 1, 1993.

238. Miller, E. E., Evans, A. E., and Cohn, M., Inhibition of rate of tumor growth by creatine and cyclocreatine, *Proc. Natl. Acad. Sci. U.S.A.*, 90, 3304, 1993.

239. Rowley, G. L., Greenleaf, A. L., and Kenyon, G. L., On the specificity of creatine kinase: new glycocyamines and glycocyamine analogs related to creatine, *J. Am. Chem. Soc.*, 93, 5542, 1971.

240. Annesley, T. M. and Walker, J. B., Cyclocreatine phosphate as a substitute for creatine phosphate in vertebrate tissues: energetic considerations, *Biochem. Biophys. Res. Commun.*, 74, 185, 1977.

241. Griffiths, G. R. and Walker, J. B., Accumulation of analog of phosphocreatine in muscle of chicks fed 1-carboxymethyl-2-iminoimidazolidine (cyclocreatine), *J. Biol. Chem.*, 251, 2049, 1976.

242. Herriott, J. R. and Love, W. E., The crystal structure of the disodium salt of *N*-phosphorylcreatine hydrate, *Acta Crystalogr.*, B24, 1014, 1968.

243. Mendel, H. and Hodgkin, D. C., The crystal structure of creatine monohydrate, *Acta Crystalogr.*, 7, 443, 1954.

244. Phillips, G. N., Thomas, J. W., Jr., Annesley, T. M., and Quiocho, F. A., Stereospecificity of creatine kinase: crystal structure of 1-carboxymethyl-2-imino-3-phosphonoimidazolidine, *J. Am. Chem. Soc.*, 101, 7120, 1979.

245. Wang, J. C., DNA topoisomerases, *Annu. Rev. Biochem.*, 54, 665, 1985.

246. Yang, L., Wold, M. S., Li, J. J., Kelly, T. J., and Liu, L. F., Roles of simian DNA topoisomerases in simian virus 40 replication in vitro, *Proc. Natl. Acad. Sci. U.S.A.*, 84, 950, 1987.

247. DiNardo, S. K., Voelkel, K., and Sternglanz, R., DNA topoisomerase II is required for segregation of daughter molecules at the termination of DNA replication, *Proc. Natl. Acad. Sci. U.S.A.*, 81, 2616, 1984.

248. Holm, C., Goto, T., Wang, J. C., and Botstein, D., DNA topoisomerase II is required at the time of mitosis in yeast, *Cell*, 41, 553, 1985.

249. Uemura, T. and Yanagida, M., Isolation of type I and II DNA topoisomerase mutants from fission yeast: single and double mutants show different phenotypes in cell growth and chromatin organization, *EMBO J.*, 3, 1737, 1984.

250. Richter, A., Strausfeld, U., and Knippers, R., Effects of VM 26 (teniposide), a specific inhibitor of type II DNA topoisomerase, on SV40 DNA replication in vivo, *Nucleic Acids Res.*, 8, 3455, 1987.

251. Edenberg, H. J., Novobiocin inhibition of simian virus 40 DNA replication, *Nature*, 286, 1059, 1980.

252. Snapka, R. M., Topoisomerase inhibitors can selectively interfere with different stages of simian virus 40 DNA replication, *Mol. Cell. Biol.*, 6, 4221, 1986.

253. Snapka, R., Powelson, M., and Styrayer, J., Swiveling and decatenation of replicating simian virus 40 genomes in vivo, *Mol. Cell. Biol.*, 8, 515, 1988.

254. Spivac, J. G., O'Boyle, D. R., and Fraser, N. W., Novobiocin and coumermycin inhibit viral replication and the reactivation of herpes simplex virus type I from the trigeminal ganglia of latently infected mice, *J. Virol.*, 61, 3288, 1987.

255. Holm, C., Stearns, T., and Botstein, D., DNA topoisomerase II must act at mitosis to prevent nondisjunction and chromosome breakage, *Mol. Cell. Biol.*, 9, 159, 1989.

256. Benson, J. D. and Huang, E.-S., Human cytomegalovirus induces expression of cellular topoisomerase II, *J. Virol.*, 64, 9, 1990.

257. Benson, J. D. and Huang, E.-S., Two specific topoisomerase II inhibitors prevent replication of human cytomegalovirus DNA: an implied role in replication of the viral genome, *J. Virol.*, 62, 4797, 1988.

258. Cain, B. F. and Atwell, G. J., The experimental antitumor properties of three congeners of the acridylmethanesulphonanisidide (AMSA) series, *Eur. J. Cancer*, 10, 539, 1974.

259. Nelson, E. M., Tewey, K. M., and Liu, L. F., Mechanism of antitumor drug action: poisoning of mammalian topoisomerase II on DNA by 4'-(9'- acridinylamino)methanesulfon-*m*-anisidide, *Proc. Natl. Acad. Sci. U.S.A.*, 81, 1361, 1984.

260. Tewey, K. M., Chen, G. L., Nelson, E. M., and Liu, L. F., Intercalative antitumor drugs interfere with the breakage-reunion reaction of mammalian topoisomerase II, *J. Biol. Chem.*, 259, 9182, 1983.

261. Zwelling, L. A., Michaels, S., Erickson, L. C., and Kohn, K. W., Protein-associated deoxyribonucleic acid strand breaks in L 1210 cells treated with the deoxyribonucleic acid intercalating agents AMSA and adriamycin, *Biochemistry*, 20, 6553, 1981.

262. Chen, G. L., Yang, L., Rowe, T. C., Halligan, B. D., Tewey, K. M., and Liu, L. F., Nonintercalative antitumor drugs interfere with the breakage-reunion of mammalian DNA topoisomerase II, *J. Biol. Chem.*, 259, 13560, 1984.

263. Huang, E.-S., Benson, J. D., Huong, S. M., Wilson, B., and van der Horst, C., Irreversible inhibition of human cytomegalovirus replication by topoisomerase II inhibitor, etoposide: a new strategy for the treatment of human cytomegalovirus infection, *Antiviral Res.*, 17, 17, 1992.

264. Deaven, L. L., Oka, M. S., and Troy, R. A., Cell cycle specific chromosome damage following treatment of cultured Chinese hamster cells with m-AMSA, *J. Natl. Cancer Inst.*, 60, 1155, 1978.

265. Deffie, A. M., Batra, J. K., and Goldenberg, G. J., Direct correlation between DNA topoisomerase II activity and cytotoxicity in adriamycin-sensitive and -resistant P388 leukemia cell lines, *Cancer Res.*, 49, 58, 1989.

266. Liu, L. F., DNA topoisomerase poisons as antitumor drugs, *Annu. Rev. Biochem.*, 58, 351, 1989.

267. Potmesil, M., Hsiang, Y.-H., Liu, L. F., Wu, H.-Y., Traganos, F., Bank, B., and Silber, R., DNA topoisomerase II as a potential factor in drug resistance of human malignancies, *Natl. Cancer Inst. Monogr.*, 4, 105, 1989.

268. Jacobson, M. A., Current management of cytomegalovirus disease in patients with AIDS, *Acquir. Immune Defic. Syndr. Human Retrovir.*, 10, 917, 1994.

269. Drew, W. L., Anderson, R., Lang, W., Miner, R. C., Davis, G., and Lalezari, J., Failure of high-dose oral acyclovir to suppress CMV viruria or induce ganciclovir-resistant CMV in HIV antibody positive patients, *J. Acquir. Immune Defic. Syndr. Human Retrovir.*, 8, 289, 1995.

270. Henderly, D. E., Freeman, W. R., Causey, D. M., and Rao, N. A., Cytomegalovirus retinitis and response to therapy with ganciclovir, *Ophthalmology*, 94, 425, 1987.

271. Merigan, T. C., Cytomegalovirus infection and treatment with ganciclovir: introduction and summary, *Rev. Infect. Dis.*, 10(Suppl. 3), 457, 1988.

272. Palestine, A. G., Rodrigues, M. M., Macher, A. M., Chan, C.-C., Lane, H. C., Fauci, A. S., Masur, H., Longo, D., Reichert, C. M., Steis, R., Rook, A. H., and Nussenblatt, R. B., Ophthalmic involvement in acquired immunodeficiency syndrome, *Ophthalmology*, 91, 1092, 1984.

273. Pepose, J. S., Holland, G. N., Nestor, M. S., Cochran, A. J., and Foos, R. Y., Acquired immune deficiency syndrome: pathogenic mechanism of ocular disease, *Ophthalmology*, 92, 472, 1985.

274. Roarty, J. D., Fisher, E. J., and Nussbaum, J. J., Long-term visual morbidity of cytomegalovirus retinitis in patients with acquired immune deficiency syndrome, *Ophthalmology*, 100, 1685, 1993.

275. Das, B. N., Weinberg, D. V., and Jampol, L. M., Cytomegalovirus retinitis, *Br. J. Hosp. Med.*, 52, 163, 1994.

276. Dhillon, B., Maclean, H., Eddyshaw, D., Cheong, I., Flegg, P., and Brettle, R., Cytomegalovirus retinitis and AIDS in Edinburgh, UK, *Int. J. STD AIDS*, 4, 339, 1993.

277. Maclean, H. and Dhillon, B., Cytomegalovirus retinitis: diagnosis and treatment, *Int. J. STD AIDS*, 4, 322, 1993.

278. Markham, A. and Faulds, D., Ganciclovir: an update of its therapeutic use in cytomegalovirus infection, *Drugs*, 48, 455, 1994.

279. Stevens, C. and Roberts, W. B., Jr., Ganciclovir: treatment of cytomegalovirus in immunocompromised individuals, *ANNA J.*, 21, 204, 1994.

280. Bachman, D. M., Treatment of CMV retinitis, *N. Engl. J. Med.*, 326, 1702, 1992.

281. Deray, G., Katlama, C., and Jacobs, C., Treatment of CMV retinitis, *N. Engl. J. Med.*, 326, 1702, 1992.

282. Skolnik, P. R., Treatment of CMV retinitis, *N. Engl. J. Med.*, 326, 1701, 1992.

283. Wagstaff, A. J. and Bryson, H. M., Foscarnet: a reappraisal of its antiviral activity, pharmacokinetic properties and therapeutic use in immunocompromised patients with viral infections, *Drugs*, 48, 199, 1994.

284. Greening, J. G., Intravenous foscarnet administration for treatment of cytomegalovirus retinitis, *J. Intraven. Nurs.*, 17, 74, 1994.

285. Wagstaff, A. J., Faulds, D., and Goa, K. L., Aciclovir: a reappraisal of its antiviral activity, pharmacokinetic properties and therapeutic efficacy, *Drugs*, 47, 153, 1994.

286. Polis, M. A., de Smet, M. D., Baird, B. F., Mellow, S., Falloon, J., Davey, R. T., Jr., Kovacs, J. A., Palestine, A. G., Nussenblatt, R. B., Masur, H., and Lane, H. C., Increased survival of a cohort of patients with acquired immunodeficiency syndrome and cytomegalovirus retinitis who received sodium phosphonoformate (foscarnet), *Am. J. Med.*, 94, 175, 1993.

287. Smith, D. G., Jr. and Handy, C. M., A protocol for foscarnet administration, *J. Intraven. Nurs.*, 15, 274, 1992.

288. Moyle, G. and Gazzard, B. G., Foscarnet or ganciclovir for treatment of AIDS and CMV retinitis, *Am. J. Med.*, 98, 319, 1995.

289. Colucciello, M., Phosphonoformate for CMV retinitis in AIDS, *Am. J. Med.*, 98, 317, 1995.

290. Balfour, H. H., Jr., Cytomegalovirus retinitis in persons with AIDS: selecting therapy for a sight-threatening disease, *Postgrad. Med. J.*, 97, 109, 1995.

291. Spector, S. A., Weingeist, T., Pollard, R. B., Dieterich, D. T., Samo, T., Benson, C. A., Busch, D. F., Freeman, W. R., Montague, P., Kaplan, H. J., Kellerman, L., Crager, M., De Armond, B., Buhles, W., Feinberg, J., AIDS Clinical Trial Group, and Cytomegalovirus Cooperative Study Group, A randomized, controlled study of intravenous ganciclovir therapy for cytomegalovirus peripheral retinitis in patients with AIDS, *J. Infect. Dis.*, 168, 557, 1993.

292. AIDS Clinical Trials Group (ACTG). Studies of ocular complications of AIDS foscarnet-ganciclovir cytomegalovirus retinitis trial. I. Rationale, design, and methods, *Control. Clin. Trials*, 13, 22, 1992.

293. Geier, S. A., Klauss, V., Matuschke, A., Kronawitter, U., and Goebel, F. D., 2.5 years survival with sequential ganciclovir/foscarnet treatment in a patient with acquired immune deficiency syndrome and cytomegalovirus retinitis, *Ger. J. Ophthalmol.*, 1, 110, 1992.

294. Bachman, D. M., Rodrigues, M. M., Chu, F. C., Straus, S. E., Cogan, D. G., and Macher, A. M., Culture-proven cytomegalovirus retinitis in a homosexual man with the acquired immunodeficiency syndrome, *Ophthalmology*, 89, 797, 1982.

295. Friedman, A. H., Orellana, J., Freeman, W. R., Luntz, M. H., Starr, M. B., Tapper, M. L., Spiglane, I., Rotterdam, H., Mesa Tejada, R., Branhut, S., Mildvan, D., and Mathur, U., Cytomegalovirus retinitis: a manifestation of the acquired immune deficiency syndrome (AIDS), *Br. J. Ophthalmol.*, 67, 372, 1983.

296. Gal, A., Pollack, A., and Oliver, M., Ocular findings in the acquired immunodeficiency syndrome, *Br. J. Ophthalmol.*, 68, 238, 1984.

297. Newman, N. M., Mandel, M. R., Gullet, J., and Fujikawa, L., Clinical and histologic findings in opportunistic ocular infections: part of a new syndrome of acquired immunodeficiency, *Arch. Ophthalmol.*, 101, 396, 1983.

298. Pollard, R. B., Egbert, P. R., Gallagher, J. G., and Merigan, T. C., Cytomegalovirus retinitis in immunocompromised hosts. I. Natural history and effects of treatment with adenine arabinoside, *Ann. Intern. Med.*, 93, 655, 1980.

299. Balfour, H. H., Jr., Bean, B., Mitchell, C. D., Sachs, G. W., Boen, J. R., and Edelman, C. K., Acyclovir in immunocompromised patients with cytomegalovirus disease: a controlled trial at one institution, *Am. J. Med.*, 73(Suppl. 1A), 241, 1982.

300. Neuwirth, J., Gutman, I., Hofeldt, A. J., Behrens, M., Marquardt, M. D., Abramovsky-Kaplan, I., Kelsey, P., and Odel, J., Cytomegalovirus retinitis in a young homosexual male with acquired immunodeficiency, *Ophthalmology*, 89, 805, 1982.

301. Schulman, J. A., Peyman, G. A., Fiscella, R. G., Pulido, J., and Sugar, J., Parenterally administered acyclovir for viral retinitis associated with AIDS, *Arch. Ophthalmol.*, 102, 1750, 1984.

302. Chou, S., Dylewski, J. S., Gaynon, M. W., Egbert, P. R., and Merigan, T. C., Alpha-interferon administration in cytomegalovirus retinitis, *Antimicrob. Agents Chemother.*, 25, 25, 1984.

303. Schuman, J. S. and Friedman, A. H., Retinal manifestations of the acquired immune deficiency syndrome (AIDS): cytomegalovirus, *Candida albicans*, cryptococcus, toxoplasmosis and *Pneumocystis carinii*, *Trans. Ophthalmol. Soc.*, 103, 177, 1983.

304. Karpe, G. and Wising, P., Retinal changes with acute reduction of vision as initial symptoms of infectious mononucleosis, *Acta Ophthalmol.*, 26, 19, 1948.

305. Rytel, M. W., Aaberg, T. M., Dee, T. H., and Heim, L. H., Therapy of cytomegalovirus retinitis with transfer factor, *Cell. Immunol.*, 19, 8, 1975.

306. Stevens, G., Jr., Palestine, A. G., Rodrigues, M. M., Macher, A. M., and Nussenblatt, R. B., Failure of argon laser to halt cytomegalovirus retinitis, *Retina*, 6, 119, 1986.

307. Cantrill, H. L., Henry, K., Melroe, N. H., Knobloch, W. H., Ramsey, R. C., and Balfour, H. H., Jr., Treatment of cytomegalovirus retinitis with intravitreal ganciclovir: long-term results, *Ophthalmology*, 96, 367, 1989.

308. Felsenstein, D., d'Amico, D. J., Hirsch, M. S., Neumeyer, D. A., Cederberg, D. M., de Miranda, P., and Schooley, R. T., Treatment of cytomegalovirus retinitis with 9-[2-hydroxy-1-(hydroxymethyl)ethoxymethyl] guanine, *Ann. Intern. Med.*, 103, 377, 1983.

309. Holland, G. N., Sidikaro, Y., Kreiger, A. E., Hardy, D., Sakamoto, M. J., Frenkel, L. M., Winston, D. J., Gottlieb, M. S., Bryson, Y. J., Champlin, R. E., Ho, W. G., Winters, R. E., Wolfe, P. R., and Cherry, J. D., Treatment of cytomegalovirus retinopathy with ganciclovir, *Ophthalmology*, 94, 815, 1987.

310. Jabs, D. A., Enger, C., and Bartlett, J. G., Cytomegalovirus retinitis and acquired immunodeficiency syndrome, *Arch. Ophthalmol.*, 107, 75, 1989.

311. Jabs, D. A., Newman, C., de Bustros, S., and Polk, B. F., Treatment of cytomegalovirus retinitis with ganciclovir, *Ophthalmology*, 94, 824, 1987.

312. Palestine, A. G., Stevens, G., Jr., Lane, H. C., Masur, H., Fujikawa, L. S., Nussenblatt, R. B., Rook, A. H., Manischewitz, J., Baird, B., Megill, M., Quinnan, G., Gelmann, E., and Fauci, A. S., Treatment of cytomegalovirus retinitis with dihydroxy propoxymethyl guanine, *Am. J. Ophthalmol.*, 101, 95, 1986.

313. Rosecan, L. R., Stahl-Bayliss, C. M., Kalman, C. M., and Laskin, O. L., Antiviral therapy for cytomegalovirus retinitis in AIDS with dihydroxy propoxymethyl guanine, *Am. J. Ophthalmol.*, 101, 405, 1986.

314. Holland, G. N. and Shuler, J. D., Progression rates of cytomegalovirus retinopathy in ganciclovir-treated and untreated patients, *Arch. Ophthalmol.*, 110, 1435, 1992.

315. Mar, E. C., Cheng, Y. C., and Huang, E.-S., Effect of 9-(1,3-dihydroxy- 2-propoxymethyl) guanine on human cytomegalovirus replication in vitro, *Antimicrob. Agents Chemother.*, 24, 518, 1983.

316. Kuppermann, B. D., Quiceno, J. I., Flores-Aguilar, M., Connor, J. D., Capparelli, E. V., Sherwood, C. H., and Freeman, W. R., Intravitreal ganciclovir concentration after intravenous administration in AIDS patients with cytomegalovirus retinitis: application for therapy, *J. Infect. Dis.*, 168, 1506, 1993.

317. Jacobson, M. A., O'Donnell, J. J., and Mills, J., Tolerance and efficacy of intermittent, intravenous (IV) foscarnet (PFA) therapy for cytomegalovirus (CMV) retinitis in AIDS patients, *4th Int. Conf. AIDS*, Stockholm (Abstr.), Bio-Data Publishers, Washington, D.C., 1988, 422.

318. Leinikki, P., Grantström, M. L., Santavuori, P., and Pettay, O., Epidemiology of cytomegalovirus infections during pregnancy and infancy: a prospective study, *Scand. J. Infect. Dis.*, 10, 165, 1978.

319. Mintz, L., Miner, R. C., and Yeager, A. S., Anticomplement immunofluorescence test that uses isolated fibroblast nuclei for detection of antibodies to human cytomegalovirus, *J. Clin. Microbiol.*, 12, 562, 1980.

320. Singer, D. R. J., Fallon, T. J., Schulenburg, W. E., Williams, G., and Cohen, J., Foscarnet for cytomegalovirus retinitis, *Ann. Intern. Med.*, 103, 962, 1985.

321. Walmsley, S. L., Chew, E., Read, S. E., Vellend, H., Salit, I., Rachlis, A., and Fanning, M. M., Treatment of cytomegalovirus retinitis with trisodium phosphonoformate (foscarnet), *J. Infect. Dis.*, 157, 569, 1988.

322. Klintmalm, G., Lönnqvist, B., Öberg, B., Gahrton, G., Lernestedt, J.-O., Lundgren, G., Ringdén, O., Robert, K.-H., Wahren, B., and Groth, C.-G., Intravenous foscarnet for the treatment of severe cytomegalovirus infection in allograft recipients, *Scand. J. Infect. Dis.*, 17, 157, 1985.

323. Katlama, C., Dohin, E., Caumes, E., Cochereau-Massin, I., Brancon, C., Robinet, M., Rogeaux, O., Dahan, R., and Gentilini, M., Foscarnet induction therapy for cytomegalovirus retinitis in AIDS: comparison of twice-daily and three-times-daily regimens, *J. Acquir. Immune Defic. Syndr.*, 5(Suppl. 1), S18, 1992.

324. Kupperman, B. D., Flores-Aguilar, M., Quiceno, J. I., Rickman, L. S., and Freeman, W. R., Combination ganciclovir and foscarnet in the treatment of clinically resistant cytomegalovirus retinitis in patients with acquired immunodeficiency syndrome, *Arch. Ophthalmol.*, 111, 1359, 1993.

325. Flores-Aguilar, M., Kuppermann, B. D., Quiceno, J. I., Dankner, W. M., Wolf, D. G., Caparelli, E. V., Connor, J. D., Sherwood, C. H., Fullerton, S., Gambertoglio, J. G., Spector, S. A., and Freeman, W. R., Pathophysiology and treatment of clinically resistant cytomegalovirus retinitis, *Ophthalmology*, 100, 1022, 1993.

326. Dieterich, D. T., Poles, M. A., Lew, E. A., Mendez, P. E., Murphy, R., Addessi, A., Holbrook, J. T., Naughton, K., and Friedberg, D. N., Concurrent use of ganciclovir and foscarnet to treat cytomegalovirus infection in AIDS patients, *J. Infect. Dis.*, 167, 1184, 1993.

327. Anand, R., Font, R. L., Fish, R. H., and Nightingale, S. D., Pathology of cytomegalovirus retinitis treated with sustained release intravitreal ganciclovir, *Ophthalmology*, 100, 1032, 1993.

328. Baudouin, C. and Gastaud, P., A modified procedure for intravitreal injections of ganciclovir in the treatment of cytomegalovirus retinitis, *Ophthalmology*, 99, 1183, 1992.

329. Melchior, W. R., Bindlish, V., and Rybak, M. J., Intravitreal ganciclovir for cytomegalovirus retinitis in AIDS patients, *Ann. Pharmacother.*, 26, 36, 1992.

330. Kreiger, A. E., Foos, R. Y., and Yoshizumi, M. O., Intravitreous granulation tissue and retinal detachment following pars plana injection for cytomegalovirus retinopathy, *Graefes Arch. Clin. Exp. Ophthalmol.*, 230, 197, 1992.

331. Martin, D. F., Parks, D. J., Mellow, S. D., Ferris, F. L., Walton, R. C., Remaley, N. A., Chew, E. Y., Ashton, P., Davis, M. D., and Nussenblatt, R. B., Treatment of cytomegalovirus retinitis with an intraocular sustained-release ganciclovir implant: a randomized controlled clinical trial, *Arch. Ophthalmol.*, 112, 1531, 1994.

332. Anand, R., Nightingale, S. D., Fish, R. H., Smith, T. J., and Ashton, P., Control of cytomegalovirus retinitis using sustained release of intraocular ganciclovir, *Arch. Ophthalmol.*, 111, 223, 1993.

333. Geier, S. A., Sadri, I., Bogner, J. R., and Goebel, F. D., Ganciclovir intraocular device and patient survival, *Arch. Ophthalmol.*, 112, 20, 1994.

334. Spaide, R. F., Ganciclovir intraocular device and patient survival, *Arch. Ophthalmol.*, 112, 19, 1994.

335. Young, S. H., Morlet, N., Heery, S., Hollows, F. C., and Coroneo, M. T., High dose intravitreal ganciclovir in the treatment of cytomegalovirus retinitis, *Med. J. Aust.*, 157, 370, 1992.

336. Smith, T. J., Pearson, P. A., Blandford, D. L., Brown, J. D., Goins, K. A., Hollins, J. L., Schmeisser, E. T., Glavinos, P., Baldwin, L. B., and Ashton, P., Intravitreal sustained-release ganciclovir, *Arch. Ophthalmol.*, 110, 255, 1992.

337. Sanborn, G. E., Anand, R., Torti, R. E., Nightingale, S. D., Cal, S. X., Yates, B., Ashton, P., and Smith, T., Sustained-release ganciclovir therapy for treatment of cytomegalovirus retinitis: use of an intravitreal device, *Arch. Ophthalmol.*, 110, 188, 1992.

338. Akula, S. K., Ma, P. E., Peyman, G. A., Rahimy, M. H., Hyslop, N. E., Jr., Janney, A., and Ashton, P., Treatment of cytomcgalovirus retinitis with intravitreal injection of liposome encapsulated ganciclovir in a patient with AIDS, *Br. J. Ophthalmol.*, 78, 677, 1994.

339. Diaz-Llopis, M., Martos, M. J., Espana, E., Cervera, M., Vila, A. O., Navea, A., Molina, F. J., and Romero, F. J., Liposomally-entrapped ganciclovir for the treatment of cytomegalovirus retinitis in AIDS patients: experimental toxicity and pharmacokinetics, *Doc. Ophthalmol.*, 82, 297, 1992.

340. Diaz-Llopis, M., Chipont, E., Sanchez, S., Espana, E., Navea, A., and Menezom J. L., Intravitreal foscarnet for cytomegalovirus retinitis in a patient with acquired immunodeficiency syndrome, *Am. J. Ophthalmol.*, 114, 742, 1992.

341. Diaz-Llopis, M., Espana, E., Munoz, G., Navea, A., Chipont, E., Cano, J., Meneza, J. L., and Romero, F. J., High dose intravitreal foscarnet in the treatment of cytomegalovirus retinitis in AIDS, *Br. J. Ophthalmol.*, 78, 120, 1994.

342. Saran, B. R. and Maguire, A. M., Retinal toxicity of high dose intravitreal ganciclovir, *Retina*, 14, 248, 1994.

343. Jacobson, M. A., de Miranda, P., Gordon, S. M., Blum, M. R., Volberding, P., and Mills, J., Prolonged pancytopenia due to combined ganciclovir and zidovudine therapy, *J. Infect. Dis.*, 158, 489, 1988.

344. Millar, A. B., Miller, R. F., Patou, G., Mindel, A., Marsh, R., and Semple, S. J. G., Treatment of cytomegalovirus retinitis with zidovudine and ganciclovir in patients with AIDS: outcome and toxicity, *Genitourin. Med.*, 66, 156, 1990.

345. Prichard, M. N., Prichard, L. E., Baguley, W. A., Nassiri, M. R., and Shipman, C., Jr., Three-dimensional analysis of the synergistic cytotoxicity between ganciclovir and zidovudine, *Antimicrob. Agents Chemother.*, 35, 1060, 1991.

346. Tian, P. Y., Croutch, J. Y., and Hsiung, G. D., Combined antiviral effect and cytotoxicity of ganciclovir and azidothymidine against cytomegalovirus infection\ in cultured cells, *Antiviral Res.*, suppl. 1 (April, 1991), 115, Abstr. No.134.

347. Medina, D. J., Hsiung, G. D., and Mellors, J. W., Ganciclovir the anti-human immunodeficiency virus type 1 activity of zidovudine and didanosine in vitro, *Antimicrob. Agents Chemother.*, 36, 1127, 1992.

348. Freitas, V. R., Fraser-Smith, E. B., Chiu, S., Michelson, S., and Schatzman, R. C., Efficacy of ganciclovir in combination with zidovudine against cytomegalovirus in vitro and in vivo, *Antiviral Res.*, 21, 301, 1993.

349. Prichard, M. N. and Shipman, C., Jr., Efficacy of ganciclovir in combination with zidovudine against cytomegalovirus in vitro and in vivo, *Antiviral Res.*, 24, 357, 1994.

350. Causey, D., Concomitant ganciclovir and zidovudine treatment for cytomegalovirus retinitis in patients with HIV infection: an approach to treatment, *J. Acquir. Immune Defic. Syndr.*, 4, 516, 1991.

351. Jacobson, M. A., Owen, W., Campbell, J., Brosgart, C., and Abrams, D. I., Tolerability of combined ganciclovir and didanosine for the treatment of cytomegalovirus disease associated with AIDS, *Clin. Infect. Dis.*, 16(Suppl. 1), S69, 1993.

352. Carter, J. E. and Shuster, A. R., Zidovudine and cytomegalovirus retinitis, *Ann. Ophthalmol.*, 24, 186, 1992.

353. Patel, H. D., Anderson, J. R., Duncombe, A. S., Carrington, D., and Murday, A., Granulocyte colony-stimulating factor: a new application for cytomegalovirus-induced neutropenia in cardiac allograft recipients, *Transplantation*, 58, 863, 1994.

354. Jacobson, M. A., Wulfsohn, M., Feingerg, J. E., Davis, R., Davis, R., Power, M., Owens, S., Causey, D., Heath-Chiozzi, M. E., Murphy, R. L., Cheung, T. W., Dieterich, D. T., Spector, S. A., McKinley, G. F., Parenti, D. M., Crumpacker, C., and the AIDS Clinical Trial Group of NIAID, Phase II dose-ranging trial of foscarnet salvage therapy for cytomegalovirus retinitis in AIDS patients intolerant of or resistant to ganciclovir (ACTG protocol 093). AIDS Clinical Trials Group of the National Institute of Allergy and Infectious Diseases, *AIDS*, 8, 451, 1994.

355. Pearson, P. A., Jaffe, G. J., and Ashton, P., Intravitreal foscarnet for cytomegalovirus retinitis in a patient with acquired immunodeficiency syndrome, *Am. J. Ophthalmol.*, 115, 686, 1993.

356. D'Amico, D. J., Skolnik, P. R., Kosloff, B. R., Pinkston, P., Hirsch, M. S., and Schooley, R. T., Resolution of cytomegalovirus retinitis with zidovudine therapy, *Arch. Ophthalmol.*, 106, 1168, 1988.

357. Fay, M. T., Freeman, W. R., Wiley, C. A., Hardy, D., and Bozzette, S., Atypical retinitis in patients with the acquired immunodeficiency syndrome, *Am. J. Ophthalmol.*, 105, 483, 1988.

358. Guyer, D. R., Jabs, D. A., Brant, A. M., Beschorner, W. E., and Green, R., Regression of cytomegalovirus retinitis with zidovudine: a clinico-pathologic correlation, *Arch. Ophthalmol.*, 107, 868, 1989.

359. Kaulen, P., Pham, D. T., Baranowski, E., and Wollensak, J., Cytomegalovirus retinitis under combination therapy with zidovudine and dideoxycytidine in advanced immunodeficiency virus infection, *Ger. J. Ophthalmol.*, 2, 412, 1993.

360. Spaide, R. F., Vitale, A. T., Toth, I. R., and Oliver, J. M., Frosted branch angiitis associated with cytomegalovirus retinitis, *Am. J. Ophthalmol.*, 113, 522, 1992.

361. Regillo, C. D., Vander, J. F., Duker, J. S., Fischer, D. H., Belmont, J. B., and Kleiner, R., Repair of retinitis-related retinal detachments with silicon oil in patients with acquired immunodeficiency syndrome, *Am. J. Ophthalmol.*, 113, 21, 1992.

362. Colebunders, R., Van den Abbeele, K., Fleerackers, Y., Bols, K., Lachenal, M., and Van Damme, L., Two AIDS patients with life-threatening pancreatitis successfully treated, one with ganciclovir the other with foscarnet, *Acta Clin. Belg.*, 49, 229, 1994.

363. Berman, S. M. and Kim, R. C., The development of cytomegalovirus encephalitis in AIDS patients receiving ganciclovir, *Am. J. Med.*, 96, 415, 1994.

364. Bamborschke, S., Wullen, T., Huber, M., Neveling, M., Baldamus, C. A., Korn, K., and Jahn, G., Early diagnosis and successful treatment of acute cytomegalovirus encephalitis in a renal transplant recipient, *J. Neurol.*, 239, 205, 1992.

365. Peters, M., Timm, U., Schurmann, D., Pohle, H. D., and Ruf, B., Combined and alternating ganciclovir and foscarnet in acute and maintenance therapy of human immunodeficiency virus-related cytomegalovirus encephalitis refractory to ganciclovir alone: a case report and review of the literature, *Clin. Invest.*, 70, 456, 1992.

366. Kim, Y. S. and Hollander, H., Polyradiculopathy due to cytomegalovirus: report of two cases in which improvement occurred after prolonged therapy and review of the literature, *Clin. Infect. Dis.*, 17, 32, 1993.

367. Jacobson, M. A., Mills, J., Rush, J., O'Donnell, J. J., Miller, R. G., Greco, C., and Gonzales, M. F., Failure of antiviral therapy for acquired immunodeficiency syndrome-related cytomegalovirus myelitis, *Arch. Neurol.*, 45, 1090, 1988.

368. Decker, C. F., Tarver, J. H. III, Murray, D. F., and Martin, G. J., Prolonged concurrent use of ganciclovir and foscarnet in the treatment of polyradiculopathy due to cytomegalovirus in a patient with AIDS, *Clin. Infect. Dis.*, 19, 548, 1994.

369. Karmochkine, M., Molina, J. M., Scieux, C., Welker, Y., Morinet, F., Decazes, J. M., Lagrange, P., Schnell, L., and Modai, J., Combined therapy with ganciclovir and foscarnet for cytomegalovirus polyradiculomyelitis in patients with AIDS, *Am. J. Med.*, 97, 196, 1994.

370. Roullet, E., Assuerus, V., Gozlan, J., Ropert, A., Said, G., Baudrimont, M., El Amrani, M., Jacomet, C., Duvivier, C., Gonzales-Canali, G., Kirstetter, M., Meyohas, M.-C., Picard, O., and Rozenbaum, W., Cytomegalovirus multifocal neuropathy in AIDS: analysis of 15 consecutive cases, *Neurology*, 44, 2174, 1994.

371. Price, T. A., Digioia, R. A., and Simon, G. L., Ganciclovir treatment of cytomegalovirus ventriculitis in a patient infected with human immunodeficiency virus, *Clin. Infect. Dis.*, 15, 606, 1992.

372. Wilcox, C. M., Straub, R. F., and Schwartz, D. A., Cytomegalovirus esophagitis in AIDS: a prospective evaluation of clinical response to ganciclovir therapy, relapse rate, and long-term outcome, *Am. J. Med.*, 98, 169, 1995.

373. Blanshard, C., Treatment of HIV-related cytomegalovirus disease of the gastrointestinal tract with foscarnet, *J. Acquir. Immune Defic. Syndr.*, 5(Suppl. 1), S25, 1992.

374. Dieterich, D. T., Poles, M. A., Dicker, M., Tepper, R., and Lew, E., Foscarnet treatment of cytomegalovirus gastrointestinal infections in acquired immunodeficiency syndrome patients who have failed ganciclovir induction, *Am. J. Gastroenterol.*, 88, 542, 1993.

375. Dieterich, D. T., Kotler, D. P., Busch, D. F., Crumpacker, C., Du Mond, C., Dearmand, B., and Buhles, W., Ganciclovir treatment of cytomegalovirus colitis in AIDS: a randomized, double-blind, placebo-controlled multicenter study, *J. Infect. Dis.*, 167, 278, 1993.

376. Soderlund, C., Bratt, G. A., Engström, L., Grützmeier, S., Nilsson, R., Sjunnesson, M., and Sandström, E., Surgical treatment of cytomegalovirus enterocolitis in severe human immunodeficiency virus infection: report of eight cases, *Dis. Colon Rectum*, 37, 63, 1994.

377. Heinic, G. S., Northfelt, D. W., Greenspan, J. S., MacPhail, L. A., and Greenspan, D., Concurrent oral cytomegalovirus and herpes simplex virus infection in association with HIV infection: a case report, *Oral Surg. Oral Med. Oral Pathol.*, 75, 488, 1993.

378. Dodd, C. L., Winkler, J. R., Heinic, G. S., Daniels, T. E., Yee, K., and Greenspan, D., Cytomegalovirus infection presenting as acute periodontal infection in a patient infected with the human immunodeficiency virus, *J. Clin. Periodontol.*, 20, 282, 1993.

379. O'Brien, J. J. and Campoli-Richards, D. M., Acyclovir: an update review of its antiviral activity, pharmacokinetics properties and therapeutic efficacy, *Drugs*, 37, 233, 1989.

380. Mollison, L. C., Richards, M. J., Johnson, P. D., Hayes, K., Munckhof, W. J., Jones, R. M., Dabkowski, P. D., and Angus, P. W., High-dose oral acyclovir reduces the incidence of cytomegalovirus infection in liver transplant recipients, *J. Infect. Dis.*, 168, 721, 1993.

381. Meyers, J. D., Reed, E. C., and Shepp, D. H., Acyclovir for prevention of cytomegalovirus infection and disease after allogeneic marrow transplantation, *N. Engl. J. Med.*, 318, 70, 1988.

382. Ljungman, P., De Bock, R., Cordonnier, C., Einsele, H., Engelhard, D., Grundy, J., Locasciulli, A., Reusser, P., and Ribaud, P., Practices for cytomegalovirus diagnosis, prophylaxis and treatment in allogeneic bone marrow transplant recipients: a report from the Working Party for Infectious Diseases of the EBMT, *Bone Marrow Transplant.*, 12, 399, 1993.

383. Adair, J. C., Gold, M., and Bond, R. E., Acyclovir neurotoxicity: clinical experience and review of the literature, *South. Med. J.*, 87, 1227, 1994.

384. Martin, M., Manez, R., Linden, P., Estores, D., Torre-Cisneros, J., Kusne, S., Ondick, L., Ptachcinski, R., Irish, W., Kisor, D., Felser, I., Rinaldo, C., Stieber, A., Fung, J., Ho, M., Simmons, R., and Starzl, T., A prospective randomized trial comparing sequential ganciclovir-high dose acyclovir to high dose acyclovir for prevention of cytomegalovirus disease in adult liver transplantation, *Transplantation*, 58, 779, 1994.

385. Singh, N., Yu, V. L., Mieles, L., Wagener, M. M., Miner, R. C., and Gaywski, T., High-dose acyclovir compared with short-course preemptive ganciclovir therapy to prevent cytomegalovirus disease in liver transplant recipients: a randomized trial, *Ann. Intern. Med.*, 120, 375, 1994.

386. Dunn, D. L., Gillingham, K. J., Kramer, M. A., Schmidt, W. J., Erice, A., Balfour, H. H., Jr., Gores, P. F., Gruessner, R. W., Matas, A. J., Payne, W. D., Sutherland, D. E. R., and Najarian, J. S., A prospective randomized study of acyclovir versus ganciclovir plus human immune globulin prophylaxis of cytomegalovirus infection after solid organ transplantation, *Transplantation*, 57, 876, 1994.

387. ASHP therapeutic guidelines for intravenous immune globulin. ASHP Commission on Therapeutics, *Clin. Pharm.*, 11, 117, 1992.

388. Reed, E. C., Bowden, R. A., Dandliker, P. S., Lilleby, K. E., and Meyer, J. D., Treatment of cytomegalovirus pneumonia with ganciclovir and intravenous cytomegalovirus immunoglobulin in patients with bone marrow transplants, *Ann. Intern. Med.*, 109, 783, 1988.

389. Emanuel, D., Cunningham, I., Jules-Elysee, K., Brochstein, J. A., Kernan, N. A., Laver, J., Stover, D., White, D. A., Fels, A., Polsky, B., Castro- Malaspina, H., Peppard, J. R., Bartus, P., Hammerling, U., and O'Reilly, R. J., Cytomegalovirus pneumonia after bone marrow transplantation successfully treated with the combination of ganciclovir and high dose intravenous immune globulin, *Ann. Intern. Med.*, 109, 777, 1988.

390. Dentamaro, T., Volpi, A., Cudillo, L., Masi, M., Tribalto, M., Sordillo, P., Salanitro, A., and Papa, G., Effective pre-emptive therapy with ganciclovir and specific immunoglobulins for CMV infection in a bone marrow transplanted patient, *Haematologica*, 77, 284, 1992.

391. Snydman, D. R., McIver, J., Leszczynski, J., Cho, S. I., Werner, B. G., Berardi, V. P., LoGerfo, F., Heinze-Lacey, B., and Grady, G. F., A pilot trial of a novel cytomegalovirus immune globulin in renal transplant recipients, *Transplantation*, 38, 553, 1984.

392. Tsevat, J., Snydman, D. R., Pauker, S. G., Durand-Zaleski, I., Werner, B. G., and Levey, A. S., Which renal transplant patients should receive cytomegalovirus immune globulin? *Transplantation*, 52, 259, 1991.

393. Bowden, R. A., Sayers, M., Flornoy, N., Newton, B., Banaji, M., Thomas, E. D., and Meyers, J. D., Cytomegalovirus immune globulin and seronegative blood products to prevent primary cytomegalovirus infection after marrow transplantation, *N. Engl. J. Med.*, 314, 1006, 1986.

394. Przepiorka, D., Ippoliti, C., Panina, A., Goodrich, J., Goodrich, J., Giralt, S., van Besien, K., Mehra, R., Deisseroth, A. B., Anderson, B., Luna, M., Tarrand, J. J., and Champlin, R. E., Ganciclovir three times per week is not adequate to prevent cytomegalovirus reactivation after T cell-depleted marrow transplantation, *Bone Marrow Transplant.*, 13, 461, 1994.

395. Engelhard, D., Naparstek, E., Or, R., Nagler, A., Shahar, M. B., Haradan, I., Baciu, H., Raveh, D., and Slavin, S., Ganciclovir for the treatment of disseminated CMV disease without pneumonia in allogeneic T-lymphocyte depleted bone marrow transplantation, *Leuk. Lymphoma*, 10, 143, 1993.

396. Slavin, M. A., Bindra, R. R., Gleaves, C. A., Pettinger, M. B., and Bowden, R. A., Ganciclovir sensitivity of cytomegalovirus pneumonia in marrow transplant recipients, *Antimicrob. Agents Chemother.*, 37, 1360, 1993.

397. Enright, H., Haake, R., Weisdorf, D., Ramsay, N., McGlave, P., Kersey, J., Thomas, W., McKenzie, D., and Miller, W., Cytomegalovirus pneumonia after bone marrow transplantation, *Transplantation*, 55, 1339, 1993.

398. Locatelli, F., Percivalle, E., Comoli, P., Maccario, R., Zecca, M., Giorgiani, G., De Stefano, P., and Gerna, G., Human cytomegalovirus (HCMV) infection in paediatric patients given allogeneic bone marrow transplantation: role of early antiviral treatment for HCMV antigenaemia on patients' outcome, *Br. J. Haematol.*, 88, 64, 1994.

399. Bacigalupo, A., Tedone, E., Sanna, M. A., Moro, F., Van Lint, M. T., Grazi, G., Balestreri, M., Frassoni, F., Occhini, D., Gualandi, F., Lamparelli, T., Tong, J., Figari, O., Piaggio, G., and Marmont, A. M., CMV infections following allogeneic BMT: risk factors, early treatment and correlation with transplant related mortality, *Haematologica*, 77, 507, 1992.

400. Cohen, A. T., O'Grady, J. G., Sutherland, S., Sallie, R., Tan, K. C., and Williams, R., Controlled trial of prophylactic versus therapeutic use of ganciclovir after liver transplantation in adults, *J. Med. Virol.*, 40, 5, 1993.

401. Reinke, P., Fietze, E., Ode-Hakim, S., Prösch, S., Lippert, J., Ewert, R., and Volk, H. D., Late-acute renal allograft rejection and symptomless cytomegalovirus infection, *Lancet*, 344, 1737, 1994.

402. Laine, L. and Bonacini, M., Esophageal disease in human immunodeficiency virus infection, *Arch. Intern. Med.*, 154, 1577, 1994.

403. Kraat, Y. J., Christiaans, M. H., Nieman, F. H., van den Berg-Loonen, P. M., van Hooff, J. P., and Bruggeman, C. A., Risk factors for cytomegalovirus infection and disease in renal transplant recipients: HLA-DR7 and triple therapy, *Transplant. Int.*, 7, 362, 1994.

404. Jordan, M. L., Hrebinco, R. L., Jr., Dummer, J. S., Hickey, D. P., Shapiro, R., Vivas, C. A., Simmons, R. L., Starzl, T. E., and Hakala, T. R., Therapeutic use of ganciclovir for invasive cytomegalovirus infection in cadaveric renal allograft recipients, *J. Urol.*, 148, 1388, 1992.

405. de Koning, J., van Dorp, W. T., van Es, L. A., van t' Wout, J. W., and van der Woude, F. J., Ganciclovir effectively treats cytomegalovirus disease after solid-organ transplantation, even during rejection treatment, *Nephrol. Dial. Transplant.*, 7, 350, 1992.

406. Debure, A., Chkoff, N., Chatenoud, L., Lacombe, M., Campos, H., Noel, L. H., Goldstein, G., Bach, J. F., and Kreis, H., One-month prophylactic use of OKT3 in cadaver kidney transplant recipients, *Transplantation*, 45, 546, 1988.

407. Hibberd, P. L., Tolkoff-Rubin, N. E., Cosimi, A. B., Schooley, T. R., Isaacson, D., Doran, M., Delvecchio, A., Delmonico, F. L., Auchincloss, H., and Rubin, R. H., Symptomatic cytomegalovirus disease in cytomegalovirus antibody seropositive renal transplant recipients treated with OKT3, *Transplantation*, 53, 68, 1992.

408. Shennib, H., Massard, G., Reynaud, M., and Noirclerc, M., Efficacy of OKT3 therapy for acute rejection in isolated lung transplantation, *J. Heart Lung Transplant.*, 13, 514, 1994.

409. Morgan, J. D., Horsburgh, T., Simpson, A., Donnelly, P. K., Veitch, P. S., and Bell, P. R., Cytomegalovirus infection during OKT3 treatment for renal allograft rejection, *Transplant. Proc.*, 24, 2634, 1992.

410. Numazaki, K. and Chiba, S., Natural course and trial of treatment for infantile liver dysfunction associated with cytomegalovirus infections, *In Vivo*, 7, 477, 1993.

411. Jacobson, M. A., O'Donnell, J. J., Brodie, H. R., Wofsy, C., and Mills, J., Randomized prospective trial of ganciclovir maintenance therapy for cytomegalovirus retinitis, *J. Med. Virol.*, 25, 339, 1988.

412. Jacobson, M. A., Causey, D., Polsky, B., Hardy, D., Chown, M., Davis, R., O'Donnell, J. J., Kuppermann, B. D., Heinemann, M.-H., Holland, G. N., Mills, J., and Feinberg, J. E., A dose-response study of daily maintenance intravenous foscarnet therapy for cytomegalovirus retinitis in AIDS, *J. Infect. Dis.*, 168, 444, 1993.

413. Jacobson, M. A., O'Donnell, J. J., and Mills, J., Foscarnet treatment of cytomegalovirus retinitis in patients with acquired immunodeficiency syndrome, *Antimicrob. Agents Chemother.*, 33, 736, 1989.

414. Le Hoang, P., Girard, B., Robinet, M., Marcel, P., Zazoun, L., Matheron, S., Rozenbaum, W., Katlama, C., Morer, I., Lernestedt, J. O., Saraux, H., Pouliquen, Y., Gentilini, M., and Rousselie, F., Foscarnet in the treatment of cytomegalovirus retinitis in acquired immune deficiency syndrome, *Ophthalmology*, 96, 865, 1989.

415. Jacobson, M. A., Maintenance therapy for cytomegalovirus retinitis in patients with acquired immunodeficiency syndrome: foscarnet, *Am. J. Med.*, 92(Suppl. 2A), 26S, 1992.

416. Drew, W. L., Ives, D., Lalezari, J. P., Crumpacker, C., Follansbee, S. E., Spector, S. A., Benson, C. A., Friedberg, D. N., Hubbard, L., Stempien, M. J., Shadman, A., and Buhles, W., Oral ganciclovir as maintenance treatment for cytomegalovirus retinitis in patients with AIDS. Syntex Cooperative Oral Ganciclovir Study Group, *N. Engl. J. Med.*, 223, 615, 1995.

417. Anderson, R. D., Griffy, K. G., Jung, D., Dorr, A., Hulse, J. D., and Smith, R. B., Ganciclovir absolute bioavailability and steady-state pharmacokinetics after oral administration of two 3000-mg/d dosing regimens in human immunodeficiency virus- and cytomegalovirus-seropositive patients, *Clin. Ther.*, 17, 425, 1995.

418. Plotkin, S. A., Drew, W. L., Felsenstein, D., and Hirsch, M. S., Sensitivity of clinical isolates of human cytomegalovirus to 9-(1,3- dihydroxy-2-propoxymethyl)guanine, *J. Infect. Dis.*, 152, 833, 1985.

419. The Oral Ganciclovir European and Australian Cooperative Study Group. Intravenous versus oral ganciclovir: European/Australian cooperative study of efficacy and safety in the prevention of cytomegalovirus retinitis recurrence in patients with AIDS, *AIDS*, 9, 471, 1995.

420. Mastroianni, C. M., Ciardi, M., Folgori, F., Sebastiani, G., Vullo, V., Delia, S., and Sorice, F., Cytomegalovirus encephalitis in two patients with AIDS receiving ganciclovir for cytomegalovirus retinitis, *J. Infect.*, 29, 331, 1994.

421. Jacobson, M. A., Kramer, F., Bassiakos, Y., Hooton, T., Polsky, B., Geheb, H., O'Donnell, J. J., Walker, J. D., Korvick, J. A., and van der Horst, C., Randomized phase I trial of two different combination foscarnet and ganciclovir chronic maintenance therapy regimens for AIDS patients with cytomegalovirus retinitis: AIDS Clinical Trials Group Protocol 151, *J.Infect. Dis.*, 170, 189, 1994.

422. Peters, M., Schürmann, D., Bergmann, F., Grunewald, T., Timm, H., Pohle, H. D., and Ruf, B., Safety of alternating ganciclovir and foscarnet maintenance therapy in human immunodeficiency virus (HIV)-related cytomegalovirus infections: an open-labeled pilot study, *Scand. J. Infect. Dis.*, 26, 49, 1994.

423. Balfour, H. H., Jr., Drew, W. L., Hardy, W. D., Heinemann, M. H., and Polsky, B., Therapeutic algorithm for treatment of cytomegalovirus retinitis in persons with AIDS: a roundtable summary, *J. Acquir. Immune Defic. Syndr.*, 5(Suppl. 1), S37, 1992.

424. Polis, M. A., Foscarnet and ganciclovir in the treatment of cytomegalovirus retinitis, *J. Acquir. Immune Defic. Syndr.*, 5(Suppl. 1), S3, 1992.

425. Palestine, A. G., Polis, M. A., De Smet, M., Baird, B. F., Falloon, J., Kovacs, J. A., Davey, R. T., Zurlo, J. J., Zunich, K. M., Davis, M., Hubbard, L., Brothers, R., Ferris, F. L., Chew, E., Davis, J. L., Rubin, B. I., Mellow, S. D., Metcalf, J. A., Manuschewitz, J., Minor, J. R., Nussenblatt, R. B., Masur, H., and Lane, H. C., A randomized controlled trial of foscarnet in treatment of cytomegalovirus retinitis in patients with AIDS, *Ann. Intern. Med.*, 115, 665, 1991.

426. Roberts, W. D., Weinberg, K. I., Kohn, D. B., Sender, L., Parkman, R., and Lenarsky, C., Granulocyte recovery in pediatric marrow transplant recipients treated with ganciclovir for cytomegalovirus infection, *Am. J. Pediatr. Hematol. Oncol.*, 15, 320, 1993.

427. Mole, L., Oliva, C., and O'Hanley, P., Extended stability of ganciclovir for outpatient parenteral therapy for cytomegalovirus retinitis, *J. Acquir. Immune Defic. Syndr.*, 5, 354, 1992.

428. Cochereau-Massin, I., Le Hoang, P., Lautier-Frau, M., Zazoun, L., Marcel, P., Robinet, M., Besingue, A., and Rousselie, F., Efficacy and tolerance of intravitreal ganciclovir in cytomegalovirus retinitis in acquired immune deficiency syndrome, *Ophthalmology*, 98, 1348, 1991.

429. Heineman, M. H., Long-term intravitreal ganciclovir therapy for cytomegalovirus retinopathy, *Arch. Ophthalmol.*, 107, 1767, 1989.

430. Henry, R., Cantrill, H., Fletcher, C., Chinnock, B. J., and Balfour, H. H., Jr., Use of intravitreal ganciclovir (dihydroxy propoxymethyl guanine) for cytomegalovirus retinitis in a patient with AIDS, *Am. J. Ophthalmol.*, 103, 17, 1987.

431. Sanborn, G. E., Anand, R., Torti, R. E., Nightingale, S. D., Cal, S. X., Yates, B., Ashton, P., and Smith, T., Sustained-release ganciclovir therapy for treatment of cytomegalovirus retinitis: use of an intravitreal device, *Arch. Ophthalmol.*, 110, 188, 1991.

432. Rindgén, O., Lönnqvist, B., Paulin, T., Ahlmén, J., Klintmalm, G., Wahren, B., and Lernestedt, J.-O., Pharmacokinetics, safety and preliminary clinical experiences using foscarnet in the treatment of cytomegalovirus infections in bone marrow and renal transplant recipients, *J. Antimicrob. Chemother.*, 17, 373, 1986.

433. Cacoub, P., Deray, G., Baumelou, A., Le Hoang, P., Rozenbaum, W., Gentilini, M., Soubrie, C., Rousselie, F., and Jacobs, C., Acute renal failure induced by foscarnet: a case, *Clin. Nephrol.*, 29, 315, 1988.

434. Studies of Ocular Complications of AIDS Research Group, in collaboration with the AIDS Clinical Trial Group. Mortality in patients with the acquired immunodeficiency syndrome treated with either foscarnet or ganciclovir for cytomegalovirus retinitis, *N. Engl. J. Med.*, 326, 213, 1992.

435. Moyle, G., Harman, C., Mitchell, S., Mathalone, B., and Gazzard, B. G., Foscarnet and ganciclovir in the treatment of CMV retinitis in AIDS patients: a randomized comparison, *J. Infect.*, 25, 21, 1992.

436. Studies of Ocular Complications of AIDS Research Group, in collaboration with the AIDS Clinical Trials Group. Foscarnet-ganciclovir retinitis trial. IV. Visual outcomes, *Ophthalmology*, 101, 1250, 1994.

437. Studies of Ocular Complications of AIDS Research Group, in collaboration with the AIDS Clinical Trials group. Morbidity and toxic effects associated with ganciclovir or foscarnet therapy in a randomized cytomegalovirus retinitis trial, *Arch. Intern. Med.*, 155, 65, 1995.

438. Bacigalupo, A., van Lint, M. T., Tedone, E., Moro, F., Sanna, M. A., Longren, M., Trespi, G., Frassoni, F., Occhini, D., Gualandi, F., Lamparelli, T., and Marmont, A. M., Early treatment of CMV infections in allogeneic bone marrow transplant recipients with foscarnet or ganciclovir, *Bone Marrow Transplant.*, 13, 753, 1994.

439. Salzberger, B., Stoehr, A., Heise, W., Fätkenheuer, G., Schwenk, A., Franzen, C., Cornely, O., and Schrappe, M., Foscarnet and ganciclovir combination therapy for CMV disease in HIV-infected patients, *Infection*, 22, 197, 1994.

440. Weinberg, D. V., Murphy, R., and Naughton, K., Combined daily therapy with intravenous ganciclovir and foscarnet for patients with recurrent cytomegalovirus retinitis, *Am. J. Ophthalmol.*, 117, 776, 1994.

441. Butler, K. M., De Smet, M. D., Husson, R. N., Mueller, B., Manjunath, K., Montrella, K., Lovato, G., Jarosinski, P., Nussenblatt, R. B., and Pizzo, P. A., Treatment of aggressive cytomegalovirus retinitis with ganciclovir in combination with foscarnet in a child infected with human immunodeficiency virus, *J. Pediatr.*, 120, 483, 1992.

442. Jacobson, M. A., Drew, W. L., Feinberg, J., O'Donnell, J. J., Whitmore, P. V., Miner, R. D., and Parenti, D., Foscarnet therapy for ganciclovir- resistant cytomegalovirus retinitis in patients with AIDS, *J. Infect. Dis.*, 163, 1348, 1991.

443. Razis, E., Cook, P., Mittelman, A., and Ahmed, T., Treatment of ganciclovir resistant cytomegalovirus with foscarnet: a report of two cases occurring after bone marrow transplantation, *Leuk. Lymphoma*, 12, 477, 1994.

444. Gerna, G., Baldanti, F., Zavattoni, M., Sarasini, A., Percivalle, E., and Revello, M. G., Monitoring of ganciclovir sensitivity of multiple human cytomegalovirus strains coinfecting blood of an AIDS patient by an immediate-early antigen plaque assay, *Antiviral Res.*, 19, 333, 1992.

445. Leport, C., Puget, S., Pepin, J. M., Levy, S., Perronne, C., Brun-Vezinet, F., and Vildé, J.-L., Cytomegalovirus resistant to foscarnet: clinicovirulogic correlation in a patient with human immunodeficiency virus, *J. Infect. Dis.*, 168, 1329, 1993.

446. Knox, K. K., Drobyski, W. R., and Carrigan, D. R., Cytomegalovirus isolate resistant to ganciclovir and foscarnet from a marrow transplant recipient, *Lancet*, 337, 1291, 1991.

447. Wolf, D. G., Smith, I. L., Lee, D. J., Freeman, W. R., Flores-Aguilar, M., and Spector, S. A., Mutations in human cytomegalovirus UL97 gene confer clinical resistance to ganciclovir and can be detected directly in patient plasma, *J. Clin. Invest.*, 95, 257, 1995.

448. Spector, S. A., Hirata, K. K., and Neuman, T. R., Identification of multiple cytomegalovirus strains in homosexual men with acquired immunodeficiency syndrome, *J. Infect. Dis.*, 150, 953, 1984.

449. Jacobson, M. A., Maintenance therapy for cytomegalovirus retinitis in patients with acquired immunodeficiency syndrome: foscarnet, *Am. J. Med.*, 92(Suppl. 2A), 26S, 1992.

1.2 VARICELLA-ZOSTER VIRUS (HERPES ZOSTER) INFECTIONS

1.2.1 INTRODUCTION

Varicella-zoster virus is one of six herpesviruses isolated from humans. The core of a typical herpesvirus contains a linear, double-stranded DNA, whereas the viral capsid is icosadeltahedral and contains 162 capsomeres with a hole running down the long axis.[1]

The varicella-zoster virus (VZV) is associated with two distinct clinical syndromes: varicella (chickenpox) and herpes zoster (shingles). While varicella is a ubiquitous and highly contagious primary infection affecting the general population (especially in childhood), herpes zoster is a less common endemic clinical condition that usually occurs in older and/or immunocompromised individuals. In the U.S., over 90% of adults have serologic evidence of previous infection by VZV and almost all carry VZV in a latent state.[2,3] During some period of life up to 20% of individuals may experience reactivation of varicella occurring as zoster.[4]

AIDS patients with CD4+ counts of 500 cells/mm^2 or less, or organ transplant recipients (especially bone marrow allograft recipients) are at significant risk of VZV infections. Furthermore, patients who have received prior repeated acyclovir treatment have the highest risk of harboring acyclovir-resistant strains.[5,6]

Herpes zoster is usually manifested with a painful vesicular eruption customarily limited to a single dermatome, although cases of generalized eruptions have also been observed. It does not associate to exogenous exposure but appears to be secondary to reactivation of VZV that remained latent after an earlier attack of varicella.[7] During varicella infection, a lifelong infection of the sensory nerve ganglion is established.[4,8-10] However unlikely though, exogenous reinfection in a partially immune host can occur.[11-15] In general, the pathogenesis and mechanism of reactivation of herpes zoster are not well understood. Predisposing factors associated with the appearance of herpes zoster are generally linked to compromised immune defenses[16] and include Hodgkin's disease and other lymphomas, immunosuppressive therapy, trauma to the spinal cord and adjacent structures, and heavy-metal poisoning.[16-19] In some instances, the host immune response is still viable enough to halt cutaneous lesions, but not the necrosis and inflammatory response in the ganglion. Such cases, known as zoster sine herpete, are characterized with radicular pain without associated skin lesions.[18,20,21]

The histopathology of herpes zoster skin lesions is identical to that of varicella, including those of disseminated disease.[22] In addition, herpes zoster is accompanied by acute inflammation of the corresponding sensory nerve and ganglion. The disease tends to be more severe in patients with malignancies, those with immune deficiencies, or those receiving immunosuppressive therapy. Cutaneous dissemination, which occurs in up to 50% of immunocompromised patients, usually does not affect the morbidity and mortality in this population. However, patients with visceral disease (particularly pneumonitis) have increased mortality rate.[7]

The most common complication of herpes zoster is the postherpetic neuralgia which occurs in nearly 50% of patients 60 years and older; it has been rarely observed in patients under 40 years. Other complications, especially in immunocompromised hosts, include chronic zoster,[23] and persistent CNS infection.[24,25] Dolin et al.[26] have found linkage between increased severity of herpes zoster and compromised status of the cell-mediated response. The presence of VZV-induced lymphocyte blastogenesis and interferon production correlated well with the ability to contain VZV reactivation.

Varicella infections are common in immunosuppressed patients, with 50% of patients developing infection after bone marrow transplantation,[27] over 20% following cardiac transplantation,[28] and up to 25% of patients receiving chemotherapy for Hodgkin's disease.[29] In fact, patients with Hodgkin's disease have been reported to have an increased risk for disseminated herpes zoster virus infection.[30-32] Chemotherapeutic regimens consisting of chlorambucil, vinblastin, procarbazine, and prednisone have been associated with increased incidence of herpes zoster infections in patients treated for Hodgkin's disease[33] — procarbazine has been suspected to be the cause behind it.[34] On several occasions in cancer patients, disseminated herpes zoster infections have been diagnosed concomitant with bacterial and/or fungal infections.[35] Varicella infections have also been reported in AIDS-related syndromes,[36] especially in Africa,[37] but it appears to be less common in patients with established AIDS in spite of their severely immunocompromised state.[38]

1.2.2 STUDIES ON THERAPEUTICS

1.2.2.1 Acyclovir

Acyclovir, a cyclic analog of 2-deoxyguanosine, was introduced into clinical practice as an antiviral drug in 1977.[39] It has a highly selective mode of action against both varicella-zoster virus and herpes simplex,[40-43] resulting in the inhibition of herpesvirus replication at concentrations 300- to 3000-fold lower than those needed to inhibit mammalian cell functions.[44] In order to exert its biologic activity, acyclovir (a nucleoside that has no antiviral properties itself) must be phosphorylated to its monophosphate form by virus-encoded thymidine kinase, an event that does not occur in an uninfected cell.[45] Subsequent di- and triphosphorylations are catalyzed by cellular enzymes resulting in the formation of acyclovir triphosphate. The latter, which is the clinically active form of the drug, is an inhibitor by competing with deoxyguanosine triphosphate as a substrate for viral DNA polymerase.[46] It is incorporated into the growing DNA chain, but because it lacks a hydroxyl group in the 3′ position further DNA elongation is halted. The viral DNA polymerase is tightly associated with the terminated DNA chain and is rendered functionally inactivated.[47] In addition, the viral polymerase has greater affinity for acyclovir triphosphate than does cellular DNA polymerase, making the antiviral activity of acyclovir selective.[48]

Acyclovir has an apparent volume of distribution of 62.5 l,[49] with less than 20% plasma protein binding.[39] The major route of elimination is through the kidney, with a total body clearance of 185 ml/min,[49] indicating that active tubular secretion is expanding the glomerular filtration [50]

Since peak serum levels of the drug after oral administration are only 1 to 2 μM and concentrations of 4 to 8 μM are often necessary to inhibit clinical isolates of VZV, oral administration of acyclovir is not advocated in immunosuppressed patients. In such cases, intravenous acyclovir is preferable to prevent the risks of progression and dissemination; the recommended intravenous dose regimens consist of 500 mg/m^2 (or 10 mg/kg) given every 8 h for 7 to 8 d (or until crusting). Because higher oral doses (800 mg) achieve greater serum levels (6 to 8 μM), they are recommended in immunocompetent patients.[51]

Heidl et al.[52] conducted a controlled clinical trial to compare the efficacy of acyclovir and vidarabine against varicella zoster in 30 immunocompromised children with malignancies. The study showed that while both drugs were effective, acyclovir was the more effective of the two in promoting cutaneous healing. Other studies[53-55] have also confirmed the superior efficacy of acyclovir over vidarabine in controlling VZV infections in immunocompromised patients.

A note of caution should be applied when acyclovir is administered orally or even intravenously at lower dosages, since acyclovir-resistant mutant strains of VZV can be readily selected in the presence of the drug.[56]

1.2.2.1.1   Acyclovir-induced neurotoxicity

In general, acyclovir is well tolerated in a wide variety of disease states, population types, and age groups.[40] However, there have been several reports of acyclovir-associated neurotoxicity[57] (confusion, hallucinations, seizures, and coma) in bone marrow transplant recipients[58] and patients with chronic renal failure.[59] In the latter case, however, when the dosage regimens of acyclovir had been reduced according to the degree of renal failure, the neurotoxicity was reversed.[60-62]

Acute neurotoxicity in patients receiving intravenous acyclovir, although infrequent, has been well documented,[57] especially in patients with renal failure.[59] Acute nephrotoxicity has also been observed in patients given oral acyclovir therapy.[63,64] Davenport and Mackenzie[50] and Beales et al.[65] have treated oral acyclovir-induced neurotoxicity in patients with herpes zoster and end-stage renal failure (undergoing continuous ambulatory peritoneal dialysis) with hemodialysis, which by removing the drug[66] effectively reduced the plasma concentrations of acyclovir. It would also seem advisable to recommend dose modification in those patients with end-stage renal failure, by either reducing the dose, increasing the dose intervals, or both.[65] A modified acyclovir regimen for intravenous route of administration has also been described.[67]

However, based on their clinical experience with patients undergoing dialysis, MacDiarmaid-Gordon et al.[68] reported that acyclovir-induced neurotoxicity can occur in spite of dose reduction and within the time-course of a standard course of treatment.

Since there is a wide overlap of serum concentrations in patients with and without neurologic side effects, the relation between CNS effects and acyclovir serum concentrations remains unclear.[57,61,69-73] Symptoms of neurotoxicity usually appear 24 to 72 h after acyclovir peak concentrations. Therefore, single drug level measurements may be of little diagnostic value.[73]

1.2.2.2   Desciclovir

Desciclovir is the 6-deoxy analog of acyclovir. It is considered to be a prodrug of the latter showing better oral bioavailability. Desciclovir was evaluated in a noncomparative open study of 20 patients with uncomplicated herpes zoster and in 10 patients with hematological malignancies.[74,75] Desciclovir displayed activity (even at doses of 125 mg, t.i.d.) similar to that of acyclovir. However, its absorption was subject to considerable interindividual variations.[75] In animal models, desciclovir showed higher chronic toxicity than acyclovir.[76]

1.2.2.3   Valaciclovir

Valaciclovir (BW256U87) is the L-valyl ester of acyclovir.[74-76] Its discovery was spurred by the need to develop prodrugs of acyclovir with improved oral bioavailability followed by rapid conversion to active acyclovir.[77,78] Compared to all of the acyclovir esters prepared, valaciclovir produced the best estimated acyclovir bioavailability of 63%,[79] thus reducing the need for multiple administration of acyclovir.[80,81] Phase I clinical trials have shown that valaciclovir hydrochloride was well absorbed and rapidly and completely metabolized to acyclovir.[82] Single doses ranging from 100 mg to 1.0 g resulted in dose-proportional increases in peak plasma concentration (C_{max}) levels of 0.8 to 5.6 µg/ml.[82,83] The 1.0-g dose produced an acyclovir peak plasma concentration of 5.0 to 6.0 µg/ml, and half-life of 2.8 h.[84] Side effects included nausea, vomiting, abdominal pain, and diarrhea; some patients have also developed neutropenia.[85]

In a preliminary study, Smiley[86] compared valaciclovir with placebo in 400 patients with herpes zoster and showed that valaciclovir was clinically effective and well tolerated. Furthermore, valaciclovir (1.0 g, t.i.d.) and acyclovir (800 mg, 5 times daily) when given orally were approximately equivalent in their ability to reduce the duration of virus shedding and to accelerate cutaneous healing.[78]

Results from a multicenter, double-blind, randomized study involving more than 1100 adult patients have confirmed that compared to acyclovir, valaciclovir reduced duration of herpetic pain by 1 to 2 weeks.[87]

1.2.2.4   Penciclovir

Penciclovir was derived from ganciclovir by replacing the ether oxygen in the acyclic side chain by a methylene group.[88] An acyclic guanine derivative, penciclovir is structurally similar to acyclovir and has a comparable spectrum of activity and mode of action. There are, however, some qualitative differences in the mechanisms of action of penciclovir and acyclovir in terms of rates of phosphorylation, stability and concentration of the triphosphate derivatives, and affinity for viral DNA polymerase.[78] Thus, penciclovir triphosphate has a high intracellular concentration and extended intracellular half-life ($T_{1/2}$), although the impact of these phenomena on its clinical efficacy are yet to be demonstrated.[89] Biochemical studies on the mode of action have revealed that penciclovir was preferentially phosphorylated in herpesvirus-infected cells to a larger degree than acyclovir.[90] Under conditions designed to represent physiological concentrations of nucleoside triphosphates found within virus-infected cells, penciclovir triphosphate (a non-obligate chain terminator) was more effective than acyclovir triphosphate (a non-obligate chain terminator) in inhibiting viral (HSV-2) DNA polymerase-mediated DNA chain elongation.[89-91]

The minimal phosphorylation of penciclovir in uninfected cells coupled with the low activity of penciclovir triphosphate against cellular DNA polymerases accounted for its low toxicity in cell cultures.[92]

Penciclovir is effective against both herpes simplex virus and VZV, but has no appreciable activity against human cytomegalovirus in spite of its structural similarity to ganciclovir.[93] *In vitro*, the activity of penciclovir against VZV is similar to that of acyclovir, with a mean EC_{50} value in MRC-5 cells of 3 to 4 µg/ml.[94] Penciclovir is not metabolized and is excreted unchanged in urine with an elimination $T_{1/2}$ of about 2 h after IV administration.[78]

The poor absorbtion of penciclovir by the gastrointestinal tract following oral administration has been circumvented by conversion into an orally bioavailable prodrug, famciclovir.[95]

1.2.2.5   Famciclovir

An approach similar to valaciclovir has been taken in the development of famciclovir (famvir), the diacetyl ester of 6-deoxypenciclovir and a prodrug of penciclovir.[78] Famciclovir is absorbed in the upper intestine and rapidly metabolized in the intestinal wall and liver to penciclovir by deacetylation and oxidation;[94] the bioavailability of penciclovir is about 77%.[96] Similarly to valaciclovir, famciclovir also reduced the duration of postherpetic neuralgia.[97] The primary elimination pathway appeared to be renal excretion of unchanged penciclovir.

In a multicenter, double-blind controlled trial, 1-week treatment with oral famciclovir (either 500 mg or 750 mg, t.i.d.) was compared to placebo.[98,99] The time to full crusting of zoster lesions was 5 d with the drug and 7 d with placebo. Furthermore, the duration of postherpetic neuralgia was 61 d in patients receiving 750 mg of famciclovir, 63 d in those taking 500 mg, and 119 d in the placebo-receiving group. In another controlled trial, oral famciclovir (administered at doses of either 250, 500, or 750 mg, t.i.d.) was compared to acyclovir (800 mg, 5 times daily) in 545 patients with herpes zoster; the time of crusting, loss of acute pain, and duration of postherpetic neuralgia were similar in all groups. While there were no significant differences among the three famciclovir dosing regimens, the primary advantage of famciclovir over acyclovir appeared to be its more convenient dosing schedule.[98,100]

The recommended dosage of famciclovir for treatment of acute herpes zoster is 500 mg, 3 times daily (every 8 h) for 1 week. Famciclovir therapy should be initiated within 72 h after the onset of rash.[98]

Side effects with famciclovir (given at doses ranging from 125 mg to 2.25 g) during clinical trials occurred no more frequently than with the placebo and included headache (9.3% of treated patients), nausea (4.5%), diarrhea (2.4%), and to a lesser extent fatigue, dizziness, abdominal pain, and dyspepsia. When studied for toxicity on testicular functions in male patients with recurrent genital herpes, famciclovir has shown no adverse side effects.[98,101] The safety of famciclovir therapy during pregnancy or breast feeding has not yet been established.[98]

Aside from fewer doses of medication per day than acyclovir, there appears to be little clinical advantage of famciclovir over acyclovir.

1.2.2.6 Sorivudine (BV-araU, SQ 32756, YN-72, Brovavir)

Sorivudine, a novel antiviral bromovinyl-substituted pyrimidine arabinosyluracil nucleoside, has been found to have significant activity *in vitro* against VZV. It was about 3000 times more active than acyclovir in the plaque reduction assay.[102] Against clinical isolates of VZV, the activity of sorivudine (EC_{50} = 0.0001 µg/ml) was at least 1000-fold better than that of acyclovir.[102] In VZV-infected cells, the drug is sequentially mono- and diphosphorylated by viral thymidine and thymidylate kinases.[103] The diphosphate form, in turn, is further phosphorylated by cellular kinases into the triphosphate. The BV-araU-triphosphate exerts its antiviral activity by inhibiting viral DNA polymerase. Contrary to acyclovir, the mode of action of sorivudine does not seem to involve its incorporation into the viral DNA and termination of chain elongation.[78]

Sherman et al.[104] studied the pharmacokinetics of sorivudine. The drug is well absorbed. Its bioavailability following oral administration was 50% to 70%, and serum and AUC levels were dose-dependent. While peak serum concentrations (1.0 to 2.0 µg/ml) were achieved with a 40-mg dose of sorivudine, the trough levels at 24 h (0.05 µg/ml or higher) were still over 10-fold higher than the EC_{50} for VZV. The elimination half-life ($T_{1/2}$) was 5 to 6 h, and the drug was excreted in the urine.

Initial clinical trials conducted in Japan have suggested clinical benefits in patients with herpes zoster at daily doses of 30 to 300 mg.[105] Thus, in a double-blind clinical study,[106] oral sorivudine (50 mg, t.i.d. for 7 d) significantly accelerated the reduction and resolution of pain, the disappearance of erythema and vesicles, and the formation of crusts in patients with herpes zoster. An open trial conducted in 55 immunocompromised patients with hematological malignancies demonstrated that at daily doses of 150 mg given over 1 week, oral sorivudine was effective in 56% of the patients as compared to only 15% of patients receiving a 1-week course at daily doses of 30 mg of the drug.[107] In other clinical trials (Europe and North America), the efficacy of sorivudine (40 mg once daily) is being compared with that of acyclovir (800 mg, 5 times daily) for the treatment of immunocompromised patients with herpes zoster, including those with HIV infection.[78]

While sorivudine has been well tolerated with few reports of short-term toxicity, there has been a potentially serious drug interaction involving its metabolite bromovinyl uracil (BVU). The latter is an inhibitor of dihydropyrimidine dehydrogenase, an enzyme required to metabolize 5-fluorouracil. Deaths have been reported to occur as a result of severe bone marrow suppression in patients receiving concurrent medication of sorivudine and 5-fluorouracil.[78] Sorivudine has been withdrawn from clinical trials in Japan following deaths after concurrent therapy with 5-fluorouracil.

1.2.2.7   Fiacitabine

Fiacitabine is a pyrimidine nucleoside analog reported to elicit potent anti-VZV activity both *in vitro* and *in vivo*.[108] When tested in a randomized, double-blind study of 34 immunocompromised patients with VZV infections, fiacitabine (200 mg/m² b.i.d. for 5 d) was superior to vidarabine (400 mg/m² daily for 5 d); adverse effects, although rare, included nausea and transient increase in aspartate aminotransferase levels.[109]

1.2.2.8   Compound BW 882C87

Compound BW 882C87 is another uracil derivative with potent and selective inhibitory activity against varizella-zoster virus.[110] Similarly to sorivudine, BW 882C87 was both mono- and diphosphorylated by VZV-encoded kinases, followed by triphosphorylation by cellular kinases. Its mode of action involves inhibition of viral DNA polymerase.[111] BW 882C87 inhibited purified, cloned VZV DNA polymerase with an IC_{50} value of 0.045 μM.

The pharmacokinetics of BW 882C87 have been studied in both healthy young[112] and elderly[113] volunteers, as well as in patients with herpes zoster.[114] Following the oral administration of a 100-mg dose, the peak plasma concentrations (C_{max}) of 1.6 to 2.1 µg/ml were reached in about 4 h,[115] and the plasma elimination half-life was approximately 12 to 15 h.[116] In healthy young persons, the C_{max} values were 5.5 and 8.9 μM following the administration of 100 and 200 mg doses, respectively.[112] After twice-daily dosing with 50, 100, and 200 mg of BW 882C87, the respective C_{max} values were 7.7, 12.6, and 24.8 μM; the corresponding half-life values were 15.1, 17.7, and 20.0 h.[114]

As compared to other 5-substituted 2'-deoxyuridine analogs, compound BW 882C87 showed lack of cellular toxicity, with IC_{50} values against various VZV strains ranging from 0.6 μM to 1.9 μM; by comparison, the corresponding values of acyclovir were 6.2 to 14 μM.[76,110] In infected MRC-5 cells, the IC_{50} of BW 882C87 ranged from 0.6 to 3.8 μM depending on the VZV strain, thus making it three to seven times more effective than acyclovir.[114] The drug was more than 80% protein-bound in human plasma.

In clinical trials with patients with VZV infection, BW 882C87 is being tested at doses of 100 to 200 mg given once or twice daily.[78]

1.2.2.9   Brivudine (BVDU)

Brivudine (BVDU) is an orally active anti-herpesvirus 2'-deoxyuridine derivative.[117-119] Similarly to other nucleoside analogs from this class of antiviral agents, the 5'-triphosphate form of BVDU interacted with the viral DNA polymerase as either inhibitor, which shut off the DNA synthesis, or a substrate which was incorporated into the DNA.[120-124]

Shigeta et al.[119] have compared the inhibitory efficacy of brivudine with a number of antiherpes compounds against five laboratory and five clinical strains of VZV in human embryoblast cultures. The IC_{50} values of BVDU ranged between 0.0002 and 0.006 µg/ml (average 0.0024 µg/ml); the corresponding average IC_{50} values of two other very active compounds, *E*-5-(2-iodovinyl)-2'-deoxyuridine (IVDU) and 1-β-D-arabinofuranosyl-(*E*)-5-(2-bromovinyl)uracil (BV-araU) were 0.0015 and 0.0013 µg/ml, respectively.

It is interesting to note that BVDU as well as other 5-(2-halovinyl) substituted uracils (IVDU and BV-araU) while active against herpesvirus type 1, did not exert activity against herpesvirus type 2. This lack of activity was likely the result of the inability of HSV-2 kinases to effectively phosphorylate these compounds.[125,126] The selective anti-VZV activity of BVDU, IVDU, BV-araU, as well as other structurally similar pyrimidine nucleoside derivatives (e.g., BVDC, BV-addU) seemed to depend on their specific phosphorylation by the virus-induced deoxythymidine (dThd) kinase. This would have explained why these compounds were virtually inactive against dThd-deficient strains of VZV.[119]

Drug serum levels of approximately 1.0 µg/ml have been measured in patients after oral administration of 7.5 mg/kg of brivudine, which is nearly 400-fold higher than the IC_{50} needed to inhibit the VZV replication in cell cultures.[127] Baba et al.[128] have developed a simple and sensitive bioassay to measure human serum and urine concentrations of BVDU based on the inhibitory effect of the drug on the VZV focus formation *in vitro*. Thus, following a single oral dose of 250 mg BVDU, serum concentrations of 1.2 to 2.2 µg/ml were attained 1 h later; at 5 and 7 h, the serum concentrations were below 0.2 µg/ml. The urinary levels of BVDU were on average 10 to 20 times higher than the serum concentrations.[128]

As with sorivudine, BVDU is rapidly degraded by pyrimidine nucleoside phosphorylases, such as deoxythymidine phosphorylase[129] to its free base (*E*)-5-(2-bromovinyl)uracil (BVU). The latter itself has no antiviral activity, but can inhibit the dihydropyrimidine dehydrogenase and thereby interfere with the metabolism of 5-fluorouracil, leading to severe bone marrow suppression. Again, caution should be applied when concomitant BVDU and 5-fluorouracil medication is administered. Brivudine itself did not affect bone marrow progenitor cell proliferation or human lymphocyte functions up to a concentration of 40 to 200 µg/ml,[130,131] which is 100-fold higher than the serum concentration reached by the drug in the serum. The clearance of BVDU from plasma is by rapid degradation to BVU and/or elimination as such by the kidney.

In a preliminary uncontrolled clinical trial, Tricot et al.[132] treated 11 severely immunosuppressed patients with hematological malignancies and disseminated or localized VZV infections with brivudine at daily oral doses of 7.5 mg/kg (divided over 4 doses a day) for 5 d. At this dosage, brivudine readily achieved plasma levels of 1.0 µg/ml, which is well above its MIC value (0.01 µg/ml) for either VZV or HSV-1. The outcome in all 11 cases was complete recovery.

Heidl et al.[133] evaluated the efficacy of brivudine vs. acyclovir in a prospective randomized study of 43 immunocompromised children with VZV infections. Acyclovir (1.5 g/m² daily, IV) was given to 22 patients, whereas 21 children received oral brivudine at daily doses of 15 mg/kg. The eruption of lesions stopped in all children within 1 to 5 d, and complete remission was achieved within 5 to 6 d after initiation of therapy. Overall, there was no difference in the efficacy of acyclovir and brivudine. Previously, Benoit et al.[134] treated 21 children with malignanices and VZV infections for 5 d with oral brivudine at the same daily regimen of 15 mg/kg; the results were similar: the existing lesions subsided promptly and the occurrence of new lesions was suppressed within 1 to 5 d after brivudine treatment was started.

When given orally to 20 adult cancer patients with severe disseminated or localized herpes zoster at daily doses of 7.5 mg/kg for 5 d, brivudine caused rapid cessation of the acute infection in all but one patient; the progression of disease was arrested in the majority of patients within 1 d of starting treatment.[135] Wutzler et al.,[136] who also used brivudine in the therapy of cancer patients with VZV infections, reported that 13 of 20 patients responded by prompt cessation of new vesicle formation, accompanied by rapid resolution of fever, crusting, and complete epithelization of cutaneous lesions. However, when treatment is started later than 48 h after the onset of initial rash, dissemination of epithelial lesions could not be prevented.[136]

The existence of a BVDU-resistant mutant has been described, although it was not selected in the presence of BVDU.[119]

Overall, when compared with acyclovir and vidarabine, brivudine may prove to be a more attractive candidate for treatment of systemic VZV infections because of its intrinsically much more potent anti-VZV activity, and oral administration; both acyclovir and vidarabine must be given intravenously in order to achieve sufficiently high blood levels.

1.2.2.10 Idoxuridine

Topical idoxuridine formulated in dimethyl sulfoxide (DMSO) was one of the first antiherpes agents used against herpes zoster. However, data from several studies proved somewhat contradictory and inconclusive.[137-141]

Idoxuridine has been associated with significant toxicity when used systemically. Because of study design deficiencies, interpretation of results has been difficult. Thus, Juel-Jensen et al.[139] suggested that 5% idoxuridine solution was generally ineffective, whereas a 40% solution applied constantly to the entire area of the affected dermatome (by soaking a piece of lint cut to shape) was significantly beneficial in alleviating acute pain and preventing the development of postherpetic neuralgia. In a subsequent study, however, Dawber[137] reported that intermittent therapy with 5% or 25% idoxuridine solution in DMSO was equally effective. More recently, Wildenhoff et al.[140] suggested that a 40% solution of idoxuridine (but not ointment) applied to lint was effective in rash healing. In a follow-up study,[138] however, the same authors concluded that 40% DMSO solution of idoxuridine had no effect overall on postherpetic neuralgia. Surprisingly, there were differences in the response to treatment among patients with trigeminal and thoracic zosters; idoxuridine shortened the duration of pain but not the sensitivity changes in the skin in the former but not the latter group.[138] The impracticality of using topical idoxuridine solution in DMSO (covering the affected dermatoma with a soaked lint for 5 d) far outweighs its benefits for treating trigeminal zoster.

Aliaga et al.[142] compared the efficacy of topical treatment with idoxuridine (40% solution in DMSO) for 4 d vs. oral acyclovir (15 mg/kg daily) given for 7 d in 171 patients with uncomplicated herpes zoster. Local idoxuridine provided better resolution of herpes zoster than acyclovir in time-to-drying of vesicles, prevention of formation of new vesicles, improvement of pruritus and hyperesthesia. There was no difference in the development of postherpetic neuralgia between the two groups.

Allergic contact dermatitis is the most serious adverse effect from idoxuridine.[143] Overall, the use of idoxuridine may be limited only to the topical treatment of uncomplicated herpes zoster in immunocompetent patients.

1.2.2.11 Vidarabine (Adenine Arabinoside)

Intravenous vidarabine at daily doses of 10 mg/kg for 5 d proved to be effective against herpes zoster in immunocompromised patients when administered within 6 d after eruption.[144] In a randomized, double-blind, placebo-controlled trial involving immunosuppressed patients, Whitley et al.[145] used a 5-d course of IV vidarabine to treat herpes zoster. There was a rapid resolution of acute pain. Four months after the initiation of treatment, the duration (but not the incidence) of postherpetic neuralgia was also reduced. However, the toxicity of vidarabine may prevent its more extensive use in herpes zoster.

In several studies involving immunocompromised adults and children with herpes zoster, the efficacies of IV vidarabine have been compared with IV acyclovir.[53,146-149] In three of these studies, acyclovir showed markedly fewer side effects and superior activity than vidarabine when evaluated in terms of period of time during which cultures were positive, developments of new lesions, and the interval until the first decrease in pain and pustule formation.[53,147] However, in a double-blind trial in 73 immunocompromised patients there has been no significant difference between acyclovir (30 mg/kg daily for 7 d) and vidarabine (10 mg/kg daily for 7 d).[146]

A combination therapy of acyclovir (15 mg/kg daily) and vidarabine (10 mg/kg daily) has been used successfully in the treatment of disseminated VZV infections in severely immunocompromised patients[150] and patients with hematologic malignancies.[151]

Among the adverse clinical effects of vidarabine, nausea, vomiting, cutaneous rash, diarrhea,[144] and bone marrow suppression have been predominant. Neurotoxic effects, such as tremors and evolution to coma, were observed in patients without renal or hepatic dysfunction.[152] In addition, Semel and McNerney[153] have described three patients exhibiting inappropriate antidiuretic hormone secretion after receiving vidarabine.

Based on clinical results, vidarabine should be considered in combination therapy with acyclovir, or when acyclovir resistance has developed during cutaneous or visceral dissemination of herpes zoster in severely immunocompromised patients[154] (see also studies with acyclovir).

1.2.2.12   Cytarabine (Cytosine Arabinoside)

Because of its toxicity, intravenous cytarabine is used rarely and only in immunocompetent patients with herpes zoster. In controlled studies conducted in immunocompromised patients, the drug was shown to be harmful.[155] Even when administered subcutaneously, cytarabine was found ineffective in the therapy of localized zoster in immunocompetent hosts leading to prolongation of rash and new symptoms.

1.2.2.13   Adenosine Monophosphate

Sklar et al.[156] desribed the use of intramuscular adenosine monophosphate (AMP) (100 mg, 3 times weekly for up to 4 weeks) in the treatment of 32 patients with herpes zoster. The results showed faster healing, decreased desquamation time, and reduced pain as compared with controls. After 4 weeks, 88% of patients remained pain-free compared with 43% in the placebo group, and no toxicity was noticed in the AMP-receiving group. However, the reported findings should be viewed with caution since serious AMP-associated toxicity is known.[157] In fact, AMP is metabolized to adenosine, which is toxic for both prokaryotic and eukaryotic cells. In addition, adenosine inhibits the maturation and proliferation of T lymphocytes, as well as monocyte transformation into macrophages.[154]

1.2.2.14   Foscarnet

Foscarnet (phosphonoacetic acid) is an inhibitor of viral DNA polymerase and acts as a chain elongation terminator. Like vidarabine, it is not dependent on phosphorylation by viral thymidine kinase (TK) to become active.[154] Foscarnet can easily penetrate the cerebrospinal fluid.[158] It attaches to the pyrophosphate binding sites of the viral DNA and RNA polymerases causing reversible inhibition of enzyme activity.[5]

Prolonged treatment with oral acyclovir in immunosuppressed patients (those with AIDS) may be responsible for acyclovir resistance due to the emergence of TK-deficient VZV strains.[6] Foscarnet has been recommended as an alternative therapy against acyclovir-resistant VZV infections.[5,159,160]

1.2.2.15   Interferon-α (IFN-α)

The use of intramuscular IFN-α has been reported in the treatment of herpes zoster in immunocompromised patients. In one such study,[161] human leukocyte IFN-α reduced both acute pain and the incidence and duration of postherpetic neuralgia. In a multicenter study of immunocompromised cancer patients, recombinant IFN-α (36 to 68 × 10^6 U daily for 5 d) was given via intramuscular injections; dissemination occurred in 17% of treated patients vs. 58% in the placebo group.[162]

Results from a trial in immunocompetent patients with herpes zoster were inconclusive and did not provide enough confidence because of design deficiencies.[163]

In a randomized trial of 127 adult patients with herpes zoster, subcutaneous recombinant human IFN-α (10 × 10^6 U daily for 5 d) was compared with systemic acyclovir (5.0 mg/kg, t.i.d. for 5 d). Both drugs proved to be effective, although side effects were more frequent with IFN-α; postherpetic neuralgia was not prevented in either group.[164]

1.2.2.16   Thymopentin

For more than a decade, thymic hormones, such as thymopoietin, have been known for their ability to shorten the course of viral infection and accelerate the restoration of T cell responses.[165,166] Thymopoietin is a small peptide comprised of 49 amino acids.[167] Its biological activity is retained in a 5-amino acid sequence (Arg-Lys-Asp-Val-Tyr) corresponding to amino acids 32–36 of the parent molecule. This pentapeptide has been synthesized and designated as thymopentin.[168] In spite of its brief half-life (30 s),[169] thymopentin is capabable of initiating long-lasting changes[170] in lymphocyte functions, especially the T cells. Cumulative clinical experience has suggested that thymopentin may be of particular value in the therapy of some recurrent viral infections, such as herpes simplex, herpes zoster, and human papillomavirus. Since herpes zoster can be especially severe in patients with secondary immunodeficiencies and immunosuppression, the immuno-stimulatory effects of thymopentin in controlling such infections may prove to be useful.

The mechanism of action of thymopentin in viral infections is mainly the consequence of its stimulatory effect on T lymphocytes. Several events will take place during that process, namely, the stimulated T helper cells will activate the B cells, which then will secrete antibodies against the virus and infected cells. In addition, interleukin-2 released from stimulated T cells will activate cytotoxic T cells and natural killer cells, which in turn will attack infected cells. Finally, IFN-γ-stimulated T cells have the ability to protect noninfected cells against the virus, and further activate B cells and tissue macrophages. The latter then again stimulate T helper cells through the release of interleukin-1.[171]

In several studies, herpes zoster seemed to be responsive to treatment with thymopentin. Because the bioavailability of thymopentin is low after subcutaneous injections,[169] this particular route of administration would preferentially stimulate T cell helper mechanisms in immuno-compromised hosts.[171]

Sapuppo et al.[172] have conducted a placebo-controlled, double-blind trial in 40 elderly patients with herpes zoster of different localization. Half of the patients were randomized to receive thymopentin subcutaneously at 50 mg three times weekly for 6 weeks; the remaining 20 patients were given placebo. Local use of gentamicin cream was allowed. All recorded clinical parameters (erythema, vesicles, pain, pruritus, duration of symptoms) showed statistically significant improve-ment in the thymopentin group over the placebo-receiving patients.

In another trial,[173] thymopentin was compared to acyclovir in patients who were recruited within 72 h of developing typical cutaneous lesions. Twenty-five patients received IV acyclovir (10 mg/kg, t.i.d.) for 5 to 7 d, and 27 were treated subcutaneously with thymopentin (50 mg, three times weekly) for 30 d. Both drugs appeared effective in promoting recovery of lesions and in alleviating pain, provided the therapy was initiated within 48 h of development of visible eruptions. In a further open study,[174] all 40 patients received acyclovir (5.0 mg/kg, t.i.d., IV) for 7 to 10 days. Twenty of them were randomly assigned to additional thymopentin therapy (50 mg, subcutaneously, three times weekly) for 6 weeks. The baseline cutaneous Merieux test and CD4/CD8-cell ratio remained normal in both groups and did not change significantly during therapy, neither was a difference in the therapeutic outcome observed among the groups.

Lomuto et al.[175] treated 53 patients with herpes zoster with thymopentin (50 mg, subcutaneously, three times weekly) for 6 weeks; for 25 patients this was the sole therapy, whereas 14 patients additionally received analgesics and 14 others received conventional therapy "A" (consisting of oral tetracyclines and antihistamines, in addition to intramuscularly given vitamin B complex, and animal polypeptides). Ninety patients receiving only therapy "A" served as controls. The mean scabbing time in the thymopentin group was 5.4 d as compared to 11.5 d in the controls, and pain alleviation was 70% in the former group vs. 20% in the controls. The outcome of treatment appeared to be independent of adding concomitant therapy to the background thymopentin regimen. There was no correlation observed between T cell subsets and the clinical response.[175] In another study[176] of 15 patients with severe herpes zoster only 2 had slight abnormal T cell subpopulations at baseline; these 2 patients with 5 others received thymopentin (50 mg, subcutaneously, three times weekly) for 4 weeks, along with conventional therapy consisting of acyclovir, vitamin B complex, levodopa, and carbamazepine. The remaining 8 patients received conventional therapy only. Even though the T cell composition normalized in the two patients with abnormal baseline values, the clinical outcomes in both groups were similar.

Based on observations in the abovementioned studies, there apppeared to be no consistent correlation between results from *in vitro* lymphocyte testing and clinical response to thymopentin.[171] Nevertheless, such consistency had been observed in individual patients with primary immuno-deficiencies where thymopentin did produce favorable clinical response.[177] The absence of definitive and predictive correlation between *in vitro* activity and clinical efficacy would determine as feasible for thymopentin treatment those patients with frequently recurring herpes zoster who do not — or insufficiently — respond to conventional therapies.[171]

1.2.2.17 Immunomodulating Drugs

Several immunomodulating drugs (inosiplex, neuramide, and cimetidine) have been evaluated for efficacy against herpes zoster.[154]

Bunta and Peris[178] have used inosiplex (isoprinosine) in the treatment of herpes zoster. The potential efficacy of the drug is apparently associated with its immunopotentiating activity on the cellular immune responses (increasing the T-lymphocyte levels, especially those of T helper cells), and the activity of natural killer cells.[179,180] In a placebo-controlled study, Payne et al.[181] did not find any significant efficacy of inosine pranobex in the treatment of herpes zoster in 38 elderly patients.

A combination therapy of methisoprinol and griseofulvin (125 mg, four times daily) was found beneficial in the rapid healing of herpes zoster; methisoprinol given alone was less potent.[182]

The efficacy against herpes zoster of neuramide given intramuscularly twice daily was compared to that of rifampicin (twice daily intramuscular injections of 250 mg, and twice daily topical application of 1% solution).[183] Both therapies controlled the symptoms of disease, although rifampicin was more effective in alleviating pain than neuramide. The rationale for using rifampicin was not clear and the study was not blinded.

Cimetidine is a H_2-receptor blocking agent with immunostimulating properties. Mavlight and Talpaz[184] reported that oral cimetidine (300 mg, five times daily for 1 week) rapidly resolved pain and reduced pruritus in four immunosuppressed cancer patients. Similarly, in a randomized, placebo-controlled trial, Miller et al.[185] found cimetidine effective in shortening the median time in pain decrease and healing. A dose regimen of 800 mg, b.i.d. for 5 d, has been recommended.[186]

1.2.3 EVOLUTION OF THERAPIES AND TREATMENT OF VARICELLA-ZOSTER INFECTIONS

Acyclovir has been the standard therapy for VZV infections for more than a decade. However, it has a relatively short half-life and poor bioavailability, necessitating the administration of high doses five times daily in order to maintain adequate plasma concentrations above the IC_{50} for VZV. Nevertheless, its systemic administration has been effective in reducing the severity of acute attack of herpes zoster.[80,187] In immunocompromised hosts, infections due to acyclovir-resistant VZV strains have attained some urgency, creating the need for alternative antiviral therapies.[188,189]

Intravenous acyclovir therapy in immunocompetent patients with herpes zoster, while acceler-ating the rate of cutaneous healing and reducing the severity of acute neuritis[190,191] has no effect on postherpetic neuralgia.[192-194] Orally administered acyclovir also reduces the severity of acute neuritis and accelerates the rate of cutaneous healing[80,81,187] (Table 1.2).

TABLE 1.2
Antiviral Therapy for Varicella-Zoster Infections

VZV Infection	Drug/Route of Administration	Dose	Duration
Immunocompromised patients	Acyclovir/IV	30 mg/kg daily, divided every 8 h (1500 mg/m^2 daily divided every 8 h for children < 12 years old)	5–7 d
	Vidarabine/IV	10 mg/kg daily, infused over 12 h	5–7 d
	Foscarnet/IV	40 mg/kg daily, divided every 8 h	5–7 d
Immunocompetent patients	Acyclovir/orally	20 mg/kg per dose, four times daily for children; 800 mg per dose, four times daily for adolescents; 800 mg per dose, five times daily for adults	5 d

In immunocompromised patients, intravenous therapy with acyclovir markedly reduced the frequency of cutaneous dissemination and visceral complications.[53,195] The treatment is intravenous at doses of 10 mg/kg every 8 h for 7 to 10 d.[41]

A pregnant HIV-positive patient with herpes zoster was treated successfully with intravenous acyclovir (800 mg every 8 h) for 10 d; at 1-year follow-up examination neither the mother nor the infant revealed any complications from the treatment.[196]

Studies by Sempere et al.[197] have shown that long-term acyclovir prophylaxis delayed but did not prevent VZV infections after autologous blood stem cell transplantation in patients with acute leukemia.

Since the absorption from the gastrointesinal tract is only 15% to 25% of the ingested dose, higher doses have been suggested for oral therapy.[198] In immunocompetent patients oral administration of acyclovir should be initiated within 48 h of the onset of rash and consist of 800 mg, five times daily for 7 d.[41] There is, however, a strong possibility that in elderly patients the pharmacokinetics of acyclovir are altered. For elderly patients with apparently normal renal function, oral acyclovir regimens of 800 mg five times daily for 7 d, would likely produce elevated trough concentrations of the drug; however, such high concentrations are not associated with significant side effects.[199] A reduction of dosage or an extended dosage interval should, however, be considered for those patients with known serious renal deficiencies, or patients receiving concomitant diuretic therapy.[199] Vidarabine may be considered as alternative therapy.[53,145,146]

In two studies, vidarabine was shown to accelerate the cutaneous healing in immunosuppressed patients, including cessation of new vesicle formation, time to total pustulation, and scabbing.[200-202] One of the most significant advantages of vidarabine therapy of herpes zoster in immunocompromised hosts is the reduced frequency of visceral complications (from 19% to 5%).[201] Beneficial results can be achieved with a 1-week course at daily doses of 10 mg/kg given intravenously at concentrations of 0.5 mg/ml over 12 h.[203] One disadvantage of vidarabine therapy is the necessity of hospitalization and intravenous administration for prolonged periods of time (12 h) because of poor solubility.

Whitley et al.[146] have compared the therapeutic activity of acyclovir (30 mg/kg daily at 8-h intervals) and vidarabine (continuous 12-h infusion at 10 mg/kg daily) in a double-blind controlled trial of 73 immunocompromised patients with disseminated herpes zoster. Both regimens were administered for 7 d. Although the acyclovir recipients were discharged more promptly than the vidarabine-receiving patients, the results of the trial indicated that the disseminated herpes zoster was amenable to therapy with either acyclovir or vidarabine.[146]

In retrospect, the currently available clinical data have established that both acyclovir and vidarabine favorably alter the clinical course of herpes zoster in immunocompromised patients.

However, the fact that it is perhaps less toxic and easier to administer has made intravenous acyclovir the drug of choice for treatment of herpes zoster in immunocompromised patients.[188]

In a double-blind, controlled, randomized trial of patients with acute herpes zoster, Wood et al.[190] compared the efficacy of 21-d vs. 7-d therapy with acyclovir, as well as the addition of prednisolone. Both the prolonged 21-d treatment and the addition of prednisolone confered only slight benefits over the standard 7-d therapy with acyclovir.

Foscarnet has been recommended for treatment of VZV infections in severely immuno-compromised patients (such as those with AIDS or bone marrow transplant recipients) when acyclovir-resistant VZV strains are present.[5,159,160] The low incidence of myelosuppression associated with foscarnet allows for the drug to be used in combination with bone marrow-toxic antiretroviral therapies, such as zidovudine. To minimize adverse effects, patients should receive adequate hydration prior to and during foscarnet therapy.[204] Nevertheless, patients should be monitored frequently for renal toxicity, electrolyte abnormalities, and alterations in the calcium/phosphorus metabolism during therapy. Chronic maintenance therapy has not been recommended in this situation.[5]

Bendel et al.[205] have reported failure of foscarnet to control disseminated visceral and cutaneous herpes zoster in an allogeneic bone marrow transplant recipient who was unable to tolerate acyclovir concurrent with steroid therapy for GVH disease.

Mallett and Staughton[206] have investigated the efficacy of flamazine (silver sulfadiazine), an anti-infective pyrimidine benzenesulfonamide derivative, against acute herpes zoster. In a double-blind, placebo-controlled trial, the drug was applied as a cream to immunocompetent patients. There was no statistical difference between the flamazine- and placebo-treated groups with regard to duration of eruption or development of postherpetic neuralgia (defined as pain lasting for more than 30 d after the onset of symptoms). However, during the first 2 weeks, fewer patients from the flamazine group required additional analgesia than the placebo-treated patients (22% vs. 65%). Previous studies have suggested that flamazine cream may be active *in vivo* against both herpes simplex and VZV, and may be useful as topical treatment of acute herpes zoster.[207,208]

In two trials with griseofulvin, the results were contradictory. While Gwiezdzinski and Protas-Drozo[209] found daily dose regimens of 500 mg for 10 d effective in 46 patients with herpes zoster, in another study,[182] doses of 125 mg (four times daily) griseofulvin were ineffective.

1.2.3.1 Herpes Zoster in Organ Transplant Recipients

Varicella-zoster infections in immunocompromised patients, such as bone marrow transplant (BMT) recipients, can be severe and frequently associated with widespread dissemination reaching mortality rates as high as 50%.[53,210,211]

Reactivation of VZV infections, which has been documented after allogeneic BMT in 30% to 40% of patients,[212] most commonly presents as zoster. Therefore, the prophylactic use of acyclovir in this population has been recommended.[213,214] Horowitz and Hankins[215] have reported the use of intravenous acyclovir (5.0 mg/kg every 8 h, for 10 d) for the treatment of disseminated herpes zoster in an allogeneic BMT recipient early in the second trimester of pregnancy (13 to 14 weeks). The patient responded with complete resolution of all herpetic lesions and no adverse effect on the infant. The successful outcome of the pregnancy appears to corroborate other observations that acyclovir use during the mid and third trimesters is safe and without undue risk to the fetus.[215]

Although fatal disseminated VZV infection after high-dose chemotherapy and autologous BMT is uncommon, Stemmer et al.[216] have described such a case in a patient who had undergone BMT for intermediate-grade non-Hodgkin's lymphoma and had received conditioning therapy consisting of cyclophosphamide (1875 mg/[m^2 · d] for 3 d), cisplatin (55 mg/[m^2 · d] as a continuous infusion for 3 d), and carmustine (600 mg/m^2 as a 2-h infusion), followed after the transplantation with 100 mg daily of prednisone (subsequently tapered to 20 mg daily).

When compared to vidarabine, acyclovir proved superior in the treatment of BMT recipients.[51,53,217]

It has been postulated that when used in organ transplant recipients receiving immuno-suppressive cyclosporin A therapy, acyclovir may adversely interact with cyclosporin A by increasing its nephrotoxicity.[53,218-221] However, based on several cases of renal transplant recipients with herpes zoster, Hayes et al.[222] found that acyclovir therapy did not interfere with the concomitant cyclosporin A medication. These results seem to contradict two earlier reports, one by Johnson et al.,[223] who suggested a slight improvement in renal functions of renal allograft recipients while being treated with cyclosporin A and intravenous acyclovir, and by Shepp et al.,[53] who observed a deterioration in the renal functions of BMT patients on cyclosporin A therapy following treatment with intravenous acyclovir.

1.2.3.2   Herpes Zoster in HIV-Infected Patients

VZV infections are among the most frequent viral opportunistic infections in HIV-infected patients.[224] The incidence of herpes zoster among HIV-infected patients is nearly seven times higher as compared to the general population.[225]

The most general presentation of such infection in that population is a multidermatomal zoster with or without dessimination.[226] In addition, some patients may experience recurrent attacks.[227-230] Furthermore, eruptions often occur as an early sign of a compromised immune system, thereby making them an important indicator of HIV infection among younger individuals.

Persistent VZV infections with atypical cutaneous lesions have also been recognized with increasing frequency;[231-238] nodular, pox-like, hyperkerotic or necrotic skin lesions in AIDS patients have been reported.[239-241] Colebunders et al.[238] reported atypical VZV infections in four HIV-positive patients with severe immunodeficiencies. Three of the patients had been treated initially with subtherapeutic doses of acyclovir. However, when oral acyclovir was given four to five times daily at 800 mg, the lesions resolved. In one of the patients, the lesions were clinically resistant to high doses of acyclovir and disappeared only when foscarnet (200 mg/kg IV)–famciclovir (750 mg, t.i.d.) was applied.[238] In another case of atypical VZV infection in an AIDS patient, the lesions persisted despite repeated treatment with oral (800 mg, five times daily for 20 d) and IV (750 mg, t.i.d. for over 10 d) acyclovir, but cleared temporarily when foscarnet (4.0 g, t.i.d. for 2 weeks) was administered intravenously. It has been suggested that prolonged therapy may have allowed for the selection of acyclovir-resistant VZV strains that led to an atypical clinical course.[237]

Hellinger et al.[242] have described a case of VZV-induced retinitis in a patient with AIDS-related complex (ARC). Rousseau et al.[243] have reported three similar cases in HIV-infected patients who in addition have developed cerebral vasculitis which was likely due to VZV. All three patients had ARC when the ophthalmic complications occurred, and five of six episodes of necrotizing retinitis were diagnosed when the patients' CD4 cell counts were below 50 cells/mm^3. Therapy with either acyclovir or foscarnet did not prevent complete destruction of the retina and all patients became blind.

Snoeck et al.[226] described a case of an AIDS patient who developed meningoradiculoneuritis while receiving oral acyclovir prophylactically (400 mg, b.i.d.) for 8 months following recurrent multidermatomal zoster. A thymidine kinase (TK)-deficient, acyclovir-resistant VZV strain has been isolated from the cerebrospinal fluid (CSF). Upon initiation of foscarnet therapy, the virus became undetectable and the CSF was cleared from mononuclear cells (pleiocytosis) and protein overload (proteinorachia). In addition to foscarnet, which does not need to be phosphorylated to act at the viral DNA polymerase level, two acyclic nucleoside phosphonate derivatives, (S)-9-(3-hydroxy-2-phosphonylmethoxypropyl)adenine (HPMPA) and (S)-1-(3-hydroxy-2-phosphonyl-methoxypropyl)cytosine (HPMPC), also do not need the viral TK to be phosphorylated into the active diphosphate form. Like foscarnet, HPMPA and HPMPC were active *in vitro* against the acyclovir-resistant VZV isolates.[226]

1.2.3.3 Congenital Herpes Zoster

Manifestations of intrauterine VZV infections vary roughly according to the gestational week of maternal varicella.[244] Varicella embriopathy,[245-248] varicella of the newborn,[216,249-251] and zoster in early childhood[248,252,253] are the three different manifestations of VZV-associated intrauterine infections. Kusuhara et al.[244] have described the first case of congenital herpes zoster in a 5-d-old infant which may have occurred in the prenatal period. This case supports the hypothesis[254] that varicella embryopathy is the sequela of intrauterine herpes zoster. The patient was treated with intravenous acyclovir administered in four divided doses of 15 mg/kg daily. After healing, eruption occurred twice; however, each recurrent episode was relatively milder, and during the second recurrence, the course of disease was self-limiting and eruption disappeared without treatment.

1.2.3.4 Management of Drug-Resistant Varicella-Zoster Virus Infections

Acyclovir, which is inactive as nucleoside, exerts its antiviral activity after phosphorylation to the nucleotide acyclovir triphosphate.[255] The monophosphorylation of the drug is carried out by a virally encoded enzyme, the thymidine kinase (TK). Viral TK is induced in cells infected with VZV. The acyclovir monophosphate is further phosphorylated to its triphosphate nucleotide form by host cell enzymes. Decreased or absent induction of virus-encoded TK is one mechanism by which VZV becomes resistant to acyclovir.[6,256] One other potential mode to acquire resistance is alterations in substrate specificity of either viral TK or viral DNA polymerase.[5] Acyclovir-resistant VZV infection has been reported exclusively in HIV-seropositive patients, usually in the setting of advanced immunosuppression and previous exposure to acyclovir.[6,257-260] One acyclovir-resistant isolate was obtained from a bone marrow transplant recipient who had received the drug intravenously;[256] five other isolates were recovered from chronic hyperkeratotic skin lesions of AIDS patients who had received multiple courses of acyclovir therapy.[6,258] The mean ED_{50} value of the four isolates from AIDS patients reported by Jacobson et al.[6] was 85 μM, as compared to 3.3 μM for the reference VZV strain Oka.

The vast majority of acyclovir-resistant VZV strains isolated from patients have been either TK-deficient or have reduced TK activity.[6,159,261] Chatis et al.[262] presented evidence that acyclovir-resistant strains (encoding for deficient, truncated TK) have been selected under the pressure of antiviral therapy.

Intravenous foscarnet has been evaluated as an alternative therapy for acyclovir-resistant VZV at dosage regimens of 60 mg/kg twice daily or 40 mg/kg (t.i.d.) for 10 d or until the lesion is completely healed.[5] At daily doses of 120 mg/kg, IV for 10 d, foscarnet produced complete healing in four of five AIDS patients with TK-deficient VZV strains; the remaining patient developed resistance to foscarnet.[159] Smith et al.[160] described a patient with chronic hyperkeratotic VZV lesions and acyclovir resistance who responded well to a 3-week course of foscarnet (120 mg/kg). Adverse effects included nausea, vomiting, bloating, as well as hypokalemia and hyperphosphatemia.

1.2.3.5 Specific Immunoglobulin Therapy

In 1985, Kaufmann[263] described passive immunotherapy in 20 patients with herpes zoster using intravenous hyperimmune globulins. When therapy was initiated early, a rapid and complete resolution of symptoms occurred in all patients. Later, the efficacy of specific anti-VZV hyperimmune globulins was compared with that of acyclovir in both immunocompetent and immunocompromised patients with varicella, herpes zoster, and disseminated zoster.[264] While the response rate of acyclovir and immunoglobulins were 100% and 92%, respectively, the results were difficult to interpret because of the heterogeneity of the patient group. Zaia et al.[265] reported that varicella-zoster immunoglobulin was effective in reducing the likelihood of developing severe illness in a seronegative patient when administered within 48 to 72 h after exposure.

In another study, two groups of 20 patients each were treated respectively with intralesional and intramuscular hyperimmune anti-VZV immunoglobulins, and the results compared with those of a third group given intravenous acyclovir.[266] There was positive response in all patients as demonstrated by the disappearance of fever, local pain, and the improvement of cutaneous lesions 2 d after the onset of treatment.

Although in severely immunocompromised patients, the use of specific immunoglobulin therapy may be beneficial in preventing cutaneous and visceral dissemination by hematogeneous route, two studies[267,268] proved that hyperimmune immunoglobulin therapy did not prevent cutaneous dissemination in immunocompromised patients suffering from herpes zoster.

1.2.3.6 Varicella-Zoster Virus Pneumonitis

It was not until 1992 that VZV-associated pneumonitis was recognized as a separate clinical entity with potentially lethal outcome in even otherwise healthy adults.[269] Currently, VZV-induced pneumonitis is considered to be one of the most serious complications of disseminated VZV infection, especially in immunocompromised individuals.[270] Bone marrow transplant,[211,271,272] renal[273,274] and liver[275] transplant recipients, children with cancer,[276-278] and HIV-positive patients[279] are at the highest risk of developing VZV pneumonitis. Corticosteroid therapy administered to patients with underlying disease, such as renal or collagen-vascular disorders, has also been associated with an increased risk of VZV pneumonitis.[270] In addition, several reports have indicated that conventional "low-dose" corticosteroid therapy (< 2.0 mg/kg daily, or 5.0 to 20 mg daily),[280] topical nasal corticosteroids for chronic sinusitis,[281] and short-course corticosteroid therapy for acute asthma attack when administered during the incubation period of varicella[282] may predispose to disseminated varicella infections.

Intravenous acyclovir is the drug of choice in the therapy of VZV pneumonitis. Thus, in children with cancer and varicella, there was no evidence of VZV pneumonitis after 2 d of acyclovir therapy; by comparison, 30% of vidarabine-treated patients developed pulmonary complications.[277] The overall mortality from VZV pneumonitis in immunocompromised and immunocompetent hosts treated with acyclovir is between 10% and 20%.[283,284]

The recommended daily dose regimens of intravenous acyclovir in the treatment of VZV pneumonitis is 30 mg/kg daily divided every 8 h (1500 mg/m^2 daily divided every 8 h for children less than 12 years old). For intravenous vidarabine, the recommended daily doses are 10 mg/kg infused over 12 h. Intravenous foscarnet, another drug used in the therapy of VZV pneumonitis, is usually given at 40 mg/kg daily, divided every 8 h.[270]

The role of corticosteroids in the therapy of VZV pneumonitis is controversial. In spite of some reports to the contrary, because of their impairment of host immune responses to infection, corticosteroid therapy is contraindicated in most cases of varicella infections with pulmonary involvement.[270]

1.2.3.7 Herpes Zoster Oticus (Ramsay Hunt Syndrome)

Herpes zoster oticus (Ramsay Hunt syndrome)[285] is one of the less common causes of facial paralysis, accounting for 3% to 12% of these patients.[286-289] It is a debilitating disease producing cranial nerve damage, primarily facial nerve paralysis. The otological complications include facial paralysis, tinnitus, hearing loss, hyperacusis (dysacousia), vertigo, and dysgeusia.[290,291] In more severe cases, there was high incidence of complete degeneration.[292] The syndrome is characterized with severe pain and small vesicles in the external ear canal and adjacent concha, and rapidly developing facial paralysis. Frequently, there is also involvement of other cranial nerves (particularly the VIIIth, and to a lesser extent, the Vth, IXth-XIIth).[289]

Treatment of herpes zoster oticus is usually nonspecific and involves high-dose regimens of steroids.[288] Although steroid treatment significantly relieved viral-induced vestibular vertigo[293] and reduced the number of facial nerve degeneration,[288] no conclusion can be made about the effect on hearing loss.[290] Surgical decompression of the facial nerve has been both recommended[286,294] and also contradicted.[295,296]

The use of acyclovir in the therapy of the Ramsay Hunt syndrome has been also reported.[289,297,298] Uri et al.[289] have used intravenous acyclovir at a dose of 5 mg/kg administered every 8 h, for 5 to 8 d. In some cases, parenteral treatment was followed by one more week of oral administration (400 mg, five times daily) with no side effects.

1.2.3.8 Herpes Zoster Ophthalmicus

Herpes zoster ophthalmicus (HZO) affects the first division of the trigeminal nerve and is associated with a high rate of ocular involvement, often leading to serious morbidity.[299-304] In the majority of HZO cases, the eye complications appear shortly after the rash and are assumed to be the result by the presence of replicating VZV.[301,305-308] HZO complications are inflammatory and include conjunctivitis, episcleritis, keratitis, and anterior uveitis. While conjunctivitis and episcleritis tend to be transient and self-limiting, the other inflammatory lesions can become chronic or recurrent.[300] Three types of corneal involvement occur: epithelial keratitis, stromal keratitis, and neurotrophic keratopathy; in addition, corneal edema may develop in association with iritis.[304] The onset of acute ocular complications ranges between 1 and 4 weeks with as many as 93% of the patients experiencing acute pain.[305] Chronic pain occurs in up to 34% of patients, becoming more frequent in older persons.[305,309-312]

Intravenous acyclovir and vidarabine are the mainstay of therapy in patients with VZV retinitis.[313] The recommended dose of acyclovir is 1.5 g/m^2 every 8 h for 7 days; intravenous courses of acyclovir are frequently followed by 1- to 2-week courses of oral acyclovir as the retinitis regresses. The recommended dose for vidarabine is 10 mg/kg daily in a 12-h infusion for 5 d, both in normal and immunocompromised patients.[313]

Recent attention has been centered on the use of acyclovir in both prophylaxis and disease management.[299,300] Current evidence favors the use of topical acyclovir alone in the treatment of established ocular complications.[314] There have also been recommendations for topical use of steroids but the precise relationship between antiviral therapy and steroids is still unclear,[315,316] and the use of topical steroids should be considered only for most severe cases.[314]

When administered orally, acyclovir (800 mg five times daily) has only limited therapeutic benefits because it is only partially absorbed, and its plasma levels remain virtually unchanged at doses over 800 mg.[317] In addition, these plasma levels have been only slightly higher than the mean effective dose (ED$_{50}$) for most strains of VZV.[318,319] However, the aqueous humoral levels have been significantly higher if acyclovir was administered topically to the eye.[299,320]

Aylward et al.[300] have conducted a retrospective, case-control study to evaluate the influence of oral acyclovir on HZO in immunocompetent patients. There was no difference observed in the rate of ocular complications due to HZO between treated and untreated patients.

Netland et al.[321] have described an unusual case of post-traumatic activation of HZO that was associated with HIV-1 infection. The patient, who developed pain, erythema, and vesicles in the distribution of the 1st division of the left 5th cranial nerve one day after being struck in the left eye, was successfully treated with oral acyclovir (800 mg five times daily) and topical corticosteroids. The reported case indicated that VZV may be activated by local trauma, and that HZO in young patients may be associated with underlying HIV infection.[322-324]

Rosencrance[325] has described a case of herpes zoster keratitis involving the right trigeminal nerve and suggested in addition to intravenous acyclovir, the use of trifluridine and sulfacetamide-prednisolone eyedrops. However, Harris[326] strongly questioned the topical use of trifluridine due to its potential side effects, such as superficial punctate keratopathy and epithelial defects. Because of its toxicity trifluridine is indicated only for the treatment of external eye infections caused by herpes simplex virus.

In two studies on the prophylactic use of acyclovir, the beneficial effects have been observed only when the treatment was initiated within 72 h of the onset of rash.[327,328] However, the results were conflicting, since in one study the effect was noticed early,[327] while in the other it occurred late.[328] To study the possibility whether ocular treatment with acyclovir provides better efficacy than oral administration, Neoh et al.[299] used a multicenter, open randomized trial to compare the ocular prophylactic effects of topical and oral acyclovir. The patients received prophylactic treatment within 72 h of the onset of rash consisting of either topical acyclovir ointment or 800 mg of oral acyclovir, both five times daily for 1 week; a follow-up examination was carried out 12 months after completion of treatment. The results have shown that in spite of its better penetration, topical acyclovir apparently did not offer prophylactic value in the management of early HZO.[299]

1.2.3.8.1 Acute retinal necrosis syndrome

The acute retinal necrosis (ARN) syndrome is a potentially devastating ocular disorder which affects otherwise healthy immunocompetent adults of either sex and any age,[329,330] as well as immuno-compromised patients, including those with AIDS.[331-334] Although VZV is believed to be the causative agent in the vast majority of ARN cases, herpes simplex virus[333,335-339] has also been implicated in the ARN etiology.

The clinical symptoms of ARN may be insidious in the onset, with the initial presentation of mild anterior uveitis accompanied by blurred vision. In some cases, severe ocular pain may be present. With the advance of necrotizing retinitis, an increase in vitreous turbidity may also be observed. The active phase of the disease is often associated with acute swelling of the optic nerve head and macular edema.[313]

The recommended therapy for ARN is IV acyclovir at a daily regimen of 1.5 g/m^2 in three divided doses for 1 to 3 weeks, followed by oral acyclovir (400 mg five times daily) for 4 to 6 weeks.[313,331]

The use of corticosteroids in the treatment of ARN syndrome remains controversial. Cytotoxic agents, such as chlorambucil are contraindicated because of their immunosuppressive effects.[340]

1.2.3.8.2 Progressive outer retinal necrosis syndrome in AIDS patients

Progressive outer retinal necrosis syndrome is described as a distinct variant of necrotizing herpetic retinopathy in patients with AIDS.[341-345] VZV is the only agent associated with this syndrome to date. After human cytomegalovirus-induced retinopathy, the progressive outer retinal necrosis is believed to be the second most frequent opportunistic retinal infection in AIDS patients in the U.S.[345] Even though successful treatment of this syndrome with intravenous acyclovir or ganciclovir have been described, the overall prognosis in this population is poor.[341-343,346,347]

One of the most characteristic clinical features of the disease is the development of multiple discrete areas of retinal opacification in the deep layers, measuring from less than 50 μm to several thousand microns in diameter.[345,348] Other features that help differentiate the progressive outer retinal necrosis syndrome from ARN syndrome include distinctive early involvement of the outer retina, the lack of occlusive vasculopathy, and minimal or no intraocular inflammation. Furthermore, while tractional retinal detachment may occur in patients with ARN syndrome, it is not a feature in retinal detachments associated with the progressive outer retinal necrosis syndrome.[345] Kuppermann et al.[349] have observed an additional new feature that comprises the clinical profile of progressive outer retinal necrosis in AIDS patients, namely, the increased risk of these patients to develop life-threatening encephalitis.[350]

Treatment of progressive outer retinal necrosis is based on experience in patients with other forms of VZV infections. Parenteral therapy with acyclovir (10 mg/kg or more, every 8 h) for 10 to 14 d is usually followed by maintenance therapy with oral acyclovir (800 mg five times daily). The latter is necessary to preserve serum drug levels above the ID_{50} for VZV.[351] Johnston et al.[352] have used either of two regimens: combined high-dose intravenous acyclovir (10 to 20 mg/kg every 8 h) and foscarnet (60 mg/kg every 8 h), or combined ganciclovir (5.0 mg/kg every 12 h) and foscarnet (60 mg/kg every 8 h).

Pinnolis et al.[353] described a case of an AIDS patient suffering from progressive outer retinal necrosis who was successfully treated with a combination of intravitreal ganciclovir (200 µg injected twice weekly) and oral sorivudine (40 mg every day). Both high-dose IV acyclovir (10 mg/kg, t.i.d.) and foscarnet (60 mg/kg t.i.d., IV) failed to bring clinical improvement.

1.2.3.9 Syndrome of Inappropriate Antidiuretic Hormone Secretion (SIADH)

The syndrome of inappropriate secretion of diuretic hormone (SIADH) constitutes a common clinical complication in immunosuppressed individuals that may be associated with tumors, drug intake, or viral infections such as varicella-zoster virus infection.[153,354-360] VZV infections associated with SIADH predominate in patients with lymphoma, leukemia, and carcinoma. SIADH has also been associated with the use of vidarabine and pentamidine.[153,361] The effect of vidarabine is more likely related to the large amounts of fluid required for its dilution rather than to the direct effect of the drug itself.[153]

Generally, SIADH is characterized as a disseminated infection of the skin caused by excess of antidiuretic hormone, and presenting with multiple cutaneous dermatoma and occasionally producing ocular and visceral complications, such as encephalitis, hepatitis, pneumonitis, and even peritonitis and Reye's syndrome.[362]

In patients with AIDS, SIADH is the second most common cause of hyponatremia after sodium depletion through the digestive tract.[362,363] The latter is due to the frequent digestive disorders (vomiting, diarrhea) associated with AIDS. However, some AIDS patients experience acute hyponatremic situations, predominantly due to SIADH coinciding with severe opportunistic infections.[363] Arzuaga et al.[362] reported the first case of SIADH associated with VZV infection in an AIDS patient. The patient was successfully treated with saline hypertonic infusion, water restriction, and intravenous administration of acyclovir (750 mg every 8 h) for 8 d.

1.2.3.10 Neurological Complication of Herpes Zoster

Postherpetic neuralgia is the most common neurological complication of herpes zoster. Other less common but still serious complications of herpes zoster include acute herpetic neuralgia, peripheral motor neuropathy, cranial nerve palsies, myelitis, encephalitis, thrombotic cerebral vasculopathy, acute ascending polyradiculitis, aseptic meningitis, and zoster sine herpete.[364]

1.2.3.10.1 Postherpetic neuralgia

Postherpetic neuralgia, a potentially very debilitating neurological complication of herpes zoster, is characterized by pain persisting for more than 1 month after healing of the initial skin eruption.[312,365,366]

There is little direct evidence about the causes and potential mechanism(s) of herpes zoster-associated pain during an attack of shingles, and even less direct evidence on the causes of pain of postherpetic neuralgia.[367] One major mechanism producing pain during an attack of shingles has been linked to the escape of VZV from the sensory nerve fibers into the skin and subcutaneous tissues. This event, in turn, will trigger a massive inflammatory response which is the primary cause of much of the actual tissue damage. Once it occurs, the tissue damage will excite the nociceptors; the latter represent primary afferent neurons that innervate the skin and nearly all subcutaneous tissues, and which respond specifically to real or impending tissue damage.[367] The nociceptor sensitization is characterized by three acquired abnormalities: (1) spontaneous discharge, (2) a lowered activation threshold triggered by normally innocuous stimuli, and (3) an exaggerated response to stimuli that exceed the normal pain threshold. Taken together these abnormalities will produce "spontaneous" or ongoing pain, allodynia (pain to normally innocuous stimulation), and hyperalgesia (pain of exaggerated severity following a normally noxious stimulus).[367] In addition, there is evidence of other mechanisms likely to produce pain, such as activity transmitted to the spinal cord by unmyelinated C-fiber nociceptors resulting in a state of central hyperexcitability in spinal dorsal horn neurons,[368] as well as pain and dysesthesia resulting from an inflammatory response that will excite and sensitize the nociceptors which innervate the sheath surrounding the nerve and ganglion.[369]

Postherpetic neuralgia, a serious complication affecting nearly 45% of patients,[145] is a common sequela of herpes zoster infections, especially in the elderly. It is possible that once sensitized, nociceptors may fail to return to their normal state after the inflammation subsides. There is evidence for human pain due to a persistent, abnormal (i.e., in the absence of ongoing injury or inflammation) sensitization of C-fiber nociceptors.[367] Furthermore, several reports[370-372] have suggested the possibility that abnormalities in CNS function may also contribute to postherpetic neuralgia.

Nociceptor-evoked central hyperexcitability is known to involve activity at spinal glutaminergic synapses of the N-methyl-D-aspartate (NMDA) type resulting in an increase of intracellular calcium, ultimately giving rise to long-term cellular changes.[373,374] Therefore, the use of both competitive and non-competitive NMDA receptor antagonists, such as dextrorphan, dextromethorphan, and memantine, may effectively prevent nociceptor-evoked central hyperexcitability.[90]

Of the many therapies suggested for postherpetic neuralgia, several have been proven ineffective, including the use of conventional analgesics, such as epidurally administered morphine, anticonvulsant monotherapy, somatic and sympathetic nerve blocks, skin infiltration with steroids and other agents, transcutaneous nerve stimulation, vibration, acupuncture, and epidural steroids.[375,376]

1.2.3.10.2   Topical treatment of postherpetic neuralgia

Although postherpetic neuralgia, unlike herpes zoster, is mainly a CNS syndrome, the pain is referred to the body surface, and in many patients local treatment with anesthetics have been proven beneficial. The use of local anesthetics to alleviate the pain in postherpetic neuralgia dates several decades back when Wood reported[377] a complete relief of ophthalmic postherpetic neuralgia after injection of procaine into the supraorbital nerve.

Among the drugs used most often are lidocaine, capsaicin, and the nonsteroidal anti-inflammatory drugs. Over the years, local anesthetics have been administered by various routes, including epidural, skin infiltration, intravenously, as stelate ganglion blocks, and as peripheral nerve and intercostal nerve blocks.[371,378-382] The administration of local anesthetics by either regional nerve block or local infiltration, although providing useful relief of variable duration,[383,384] is associated with substantial discomfort and some risk because of the use of needles.[385] One useful alternative to this route of administration is the topical percutaneous formulations of local anesthetics.[386-388] The barrier presented by the stratum corneum of the intact skin will require special formulations for topical drug delivery.[389,390] These formulations contain the base (i.e., uncharged) form of one or more local anesthetics. When formulations specially designed to penetrate the skin have been used,[391-394] the local anesthetics produced effective cutaneous analgesia, such as in acute herpes zoster.[395-398] In a double-blind, three-session study, 5% lidocaine gel or vehicle was applied simultaneously to both the area of pain and to the contralateral mirror-image unaffected skin of postherpetic neuralgia patients with painfully sensitive skin.[386] In the remote session, lidocaine gel was applied to mirror-image skin; in the placebo session, the vehicle was applied bilaterally. The results showed that in patients with cranial postherpetic neuralgia the pain relief was significant for local drug application at 30 min, 2, 4, and 8 h. For those patients with torso or limb postherpetic neuralgia, local drug application at 8 h was most beneficial. Furthermore, remote lidocaine application to mirror-image skin was no different from placebo. Overall, the study demonstrated that 5% lidocaine gel is capable of relieving pain from postherpetic neuralgia by a direct action on the painful skin.[386]

EMLA (an eutectic mixture of local anesthetics containing 2.5% lidocaine and 2.5% prilocaine in emulsion form) has also been recommended.[387] On balance, however, lidocaine 5% lotion seemed to have the most effective topical activity of the local anesthetics.[388]

Capsaicin, a naturally occurring alkaloid, has been shown to selectively stimulate and then block the unmyelinated C-fiber nociceptive afferents from the skin and mucous membranes containing substance P, as well as other neuropeptide transmitters, such as somatostatin, and the calcitonin gene-related peptide.[399] It is thought that its mode of action involves the ability to enhance the release of substance P from the C-fiber nociceptors and prevent its reaccumulation in these fibers.[400-405] Several open-label[406,407] and double-blind, vehicle-controlled trials[408-409] have indicated that topical capsaicin was effective in relieving the pain in postherpetic neuralgia, and that its efficacy was significantly greater than its vehicle.[408] The drug, which was applied either as 0.025%[410,411] or 0.075%[409] cream, caused only a transient stinging/burning sensation, sometimes appearing with erythema at the application sites.[409] This reaction is thought to be provoked by the release of substance P stores from the peripheral sensory neurons into the skin and is, therefore, related to the pharmacologic action of the drug.[408] To alleviate this effect, it has been recommended[375] that EMLA or lidocaine ointment 5% be applied 20 to 30 min prior to capsaicin in order to obviate the worst of the burning sensation.

Nonsteroidal anti-inflammatory drug creams have also been used extensively to relieve pain in postherpetic neuralgia. Among the most effective of this group of agents, benzydamine[412] and aspirin (acetylsalicylic acid)[413-415] appeared to be most beneficial. It has been suggested that the analgesic action of aspirin (applied as either chloroform or diethyl ether mixtures) in cases of postherpetic neuralgia was related to its membrane-stabilizing property at the superficial sensory receptors rather than its anti-inflammatory activity.[414] However, Bowsher and Gill,[416] in a double-blind crossover trial, found aspirin-in-chloroform to be no more active than placebo.

Indomethacin stupes have also been shown to have some beneficial effects (40% mean pain relief) in an open trial of 18 postherpetic neuralgia cases.[417]

Nicholls[418] used topical piroxicam gel 0.5% in the treatment of 12 patients with postherpetic neuralgia. The results showed excellent response in six patients, good in three, and moderate in one patient; there has been little benefit in the remaining two patients. The interpretation of these results was, however, questioned.[419]

1.2.3.10.3 Systemic treatment of postherpetic neuralgia

In several controlled trials as well as extensive clinical experience, some of the tricyclic antidepressant drugs have been shown to reduce the severity of postherpetic neuralgia.[420] Amitryptiline was the first drug of this class to be used for treatment of postherpetic neuralgia[421] and initially its efficacy was attributed to relief of depression. However, five placebo-controlled trials[422-426] have established that reducing the pain of postherpetic neuralgia was independent of the antidepressant effect. Amitriptiline was effective in 44% to 67% of patients.[422,425] Desipramine, another norepinephrine reuptake blocker, was also found effective (63% of patients).[426] Maprotilene was inferior to amitryptiline (44% vs. 18% response),[425] whereas zimeldine (a specific serotonin reuptake blocker) had no effect on postherpetic neuralgia.[424] Two other selective serotonin reuptake inhibitors, fluoxetine and fluvoxamine, have also been shown to be ineffective. To this end, it has been demonstrated that the efficacy of the tricyclic antidepressants in the treatment of postherpetic neuralgia was related to the degree of their adrenergic activity.[427]

It is generally agreed that for therapy of postherpetic neuralgia, the antidepressants should be initiated at a small dose (10 mg or 25 mg) and increased every week by 10 mg or 25 mg (according to the patient's tolerance) until a dose of 50 mg or 75 mg is reached.[375] Since the tricyclic antidepressants have long biological half-lives they may be taken at any time during the day. However, because of their hypnotic effect it would be advisable for the whole dose to be administered at bedtime. Side effects of the antidepressants are mainly anticholinergic, including dry mouth, urinary retention, and constipation; distigmine bromide (5.0 mg every morning) should be given concomitantly. There is evidence suggesting that distigmine might have analgesic effect itself.[428]

Other systemic therapies of postherpetic neuralgia include the use of oral corticosteroids. Their use remains controversial at best.[429,430] Several double-blind, randomized controlled studies[431-433] have demonstrated no benefit in prevention of postherpetic neuralgia. Other investigators have shown some efficacy when corticosteroids were given at the early eruptive stages of herpes zoster,[429,434-436] especially in immunocompetent patients.[437,438] A combination therapy of acyclovir and methylprednisolone (40 to 80 mg) produced better results than acyclovir alone, particularly in alleviating pain.[439] However, Wood et al.[440] found that acyclovir (800 mg, five times daily for 1 to 3 weeks) with or without prednisolone (40 mg daily tapered over a 3-week period) for treatment of acute herpes zoster proved that no benefit was gained by the corticosteroid. Experience accumulated over the years has demonstrated that systemic corticosteroids should be avoided in the course of cutaneous or visceral herpes zoster, and in general their use in prevention of postherpetic neuralgia or other neurological complications should not be recommended.[154]

Hoffmann et al.[441] treated initially a patient with postherpetic neuralgia with a subanesthetic dose of ketamine: an intramuscular bolus injection of 15 mg (0.2 mg/kg) relieved the pain for about 2 h, then, a continuous subcutaneous infusion of 5 mg/h (0.06 mg/kg/h) in the abdomen was instituted. Oral ketamine medication was also applied. The initial oral dose of 40 mg six times daily (6 × 0.5 mg/kg daily) was increased after pain reappeared to 200 mg five times daily. Both the oral and subcutaneous therapies were comparable in providing relief from pain.

Results from controlled studies investigating the effect of acyclovir on the incidence of postherpetic neuralgia have been inconclusive.[442-444] Trials with oral acyclovir (800 mg five times daily for 7 to 10 d) have indicated a marked reduction in the incidence of postherpetic neuralgia.[80,445,446] While intravenous therapy with acyclovir decreased the incidence of postherpetic neuralgia, no statistically significant differences compared to placebo were observed.[43,447] Malin[448] conducted a retrospective and an observational study showing that the incidence of postherpetic neuralgia can be reduced when acyclovir is administered for 7 to 10 d.

The inconsistency of data as to the effect of oral acyclovir therapy on chronic pain has prompted Huff et al.[449] to reexamine the results of the largest U.S. placebo-controlled trial of 187 immunocompetent patients with herpes zoster[442] by using a method that considered the pain of herpes zoster as a continuum, rather than distinguishing acute pain from an arbitrary definition of postherpetic neuralgia. When a survival analysis was applied to data collected for 7 months beginning on study enrollment, acyclovir was shown to reduce significantly the median duration of pain to 20 d vs. 62 d for the placebo-receiving counterparts ($p = .02$).[449]

Over the last several decades, therapies against intractable postherpetic neuralgia included exclusively neurosurgical procedures, such as the dorsal root entry operation, ganglionectomy, and spinal-cord stimulation.[450] However, the poor efficacy and high morbidity rate have limited the overall usefulness of these procedures.

Recently, chronic opioid therapy was suggested as an alternative treatment for intractable postherpetic neuralgia. Although the chronic use of opioids for cancer pain is no longer controversial, their long-term use for management of chronic non-cancer pain remain controversial.[451-454] It was believed that neuropathic pain syndromes, such as postherpetic neuralgia, were inherently nonresponsive to opioids and that treatment may only lead to drug dependence. Several recent studies,[455-458] however, seem to challenge that assertion directly. Thus, intravenous morphine has been reported to be effective in reducing pain and hyperalgesia in patients with postherpetic neuralgia.[459] Pappagallo and Campbell[460] conducted an open-label study of patients with intractable postherpetic neuralgia to assess the effects on pain and cognition of two long-acting opioids, controlled-release morphine and compounded-slow release oxycodone. The opioid dose was gradually increased until satisfactory pain relief or unmanageable side effects occurred; median duration of upward dose titration was 4 weeks (range, 1 to 8 weeks). The mean daily dose of controlled-release oral morphine was 45 mg (range, 15 to 90 mg) at 2- and 6-month follow-up. At the 6-month follow-up, five patients showed excellent pain relief, nine reported good pain relief, and two patients reported slight to moderate pain relief. Some of the patients, however, experienced severe side effects of morphine (nausea/vomiting, dysphoria, constipation, and depression and drowsiness). Hydroxyzine was used as needed to control opioid-related nausea and vomiting.[460]

In another three-session, double-blind, placebo-controlled study[461] comparing the efficacy of lidocaine and morphine in patients with postherpetic neuralgia, each drug was administered by slow intravenous infusion over 1 h to allow for the drugs to take effect slowly. The patients received average total doses of 19.2 mg of morphine (range, 11 to 25 mg), and 316 mg of lidocaine (range, 180 to 450 mg). There was subjective normalization of sensation in 10 of 11 patients who reported the morphine session as best, and 1 of 4 patients who reported the lidocaine session as best.

1.2.3.10.4   Encephalitis

Symptomatic herpes zoster-associated encephalitis is a relatively less common CNS complication affecting immunocompromised patients with cutaneous zoster.[462] Clinically, the disease is characterized with altered level of consciousness, headache, photophobia, and meningism.[463] Risk factors for development of encephalitis include cranial or mixed cranial and cervical dermatomal involvement, two or more prior episodes of cutaneous zoster, older age, dissemination of cutaneous zoster eruption, and impaired cellular immunity.[462,464,465] The latter two risk factors accounted for about 30% of all cases of encephalitis.[462,464]

VZV-induced focal encephalopathy, although uncommon, has been described.[24,466-468] Immunocompromised patients may have more variable presentation, such as progressive encephalopathy identified with extensive small vessel infarction and thrombosis throughout most of the small- and medium-sized blood vessels in the brain.[364] In AIDS patients, this situation may result in leukoencephalopathy characterized with predominantly white matter demyelination and infiltration of VZV in the brain.[25,465] The encephalopathy may be associated with cerebral vasculopathy and may occur without the presence of cutaneous zoster.[466]

Resolution of encephalitis was achieved with systemic acyclovir therapy.[469,470] Thus, Carmack et al.[468] have described a successful treatment of VZV-induced multifocal leukoencephalopathy in a child with leukemia using intravenous acyclovir, initially at 500 mg/m^2 daily every 8 h (17 mg/kg dose), then increased to 20 mg/kg every 8 h in order to maximize drug concentrations in brain tissue sites.

1.2.3.10.5   Myelitis

Myelitis is a rare neurological complication of herpes zoster.[467,471-476] It is characterized most often with unilateral motor and posterior column dysfunction evolving into paraplegia, with or without sensory features and sphincter problems, after thoracic cutaneous herpes zoster eruptions.[364,477,478] Even less common are reports of progressive, often fatal, myelopathy in immunocompromised patients in which VZV invasion of the spinal cord has occurred.[471,472] Recurrent cases of myelitis have been especially rare.[479-481]

Systemic antiviral therapy of myelitis (acyclovir, vidarabine, steroids, interferon-α) have been used in attempts to halt or reverse the progression of disease.[474-477] In one study, Gilden et al.[477] treated four patients at various times with intravenous (10 to 15 mg/kg every 8 h) and oral (800 mg five times daily) acyclovir and concomitant therapy with steroids (intravenous dexamethasone at 16 to 24 mg daily) but failed to observe a conclusive favorable response.

Nakano et al.[481] used interferon-α to treat a patient with recurrent herpes zoster myelitis after initial methylprednisolone therapy. IFN-α was given intramuscularly in two courses each consisting of 3 million units daily for 4 weeks. There were clinical improvements in the refractory sensory disturbance, natural killer cell activity, the helper T cell/suppressor T cell ratio, as well as an increase in the κ/λ ratio of B cells, all believed to result from the immunomodulating effects of IFN-α. Contrary to previous reports,[474,482] steroid therapy was not sufficiently effective.[481]

1.2.3.10.6   Thrombotic cerebral vasculopathy

Thrombotic cerebral vasculopathy, also known as herpes zoster ophthalmicus with delayed contralateral hemiparesis, is a very rare neurological disorder associated with herpes zoster ophthalmicus eruption.[483-485] The patients usually develop headache and a catastrophic onset of hemiplagia.[364]

Imaging studies reveal infarction in the distribution of the involved vessel, and angiography demonstrates multifocal thrombosis of the proximal branches of the anterior or middle cerebral artery.[486]

High-dose acyclovir has been recommended for management of thrombotic cerebral vasculopathy, which has a mortality rate of at least 20%, with survivors experiencing major neurological morbidity.[364,484]

1.2.3.10.7 Peripheral motor neuropathy

Peripheral motor neuropathy (segmental motor paresis) is a neurological complication occurring in 2.5% to 3.2% of all patients with cutaneous herpes zoster.[487,488] The motor impairment occurs with pain and sensory abnormalities in the dermatomal distribution of the rash.[364] Patients who develop peripheral motor neuropathy also show an increased incidence of an underlying malignancy.[487] Thomas and Howard[487] have reported slow recovery from peripheral motor neuropathy in 75% of patients, with 25% left with residual motor deficit.

1.2.3.10.8 Cranial nerve palsies

While reviewing cases of herpes zoster ophthalmicus, Marsh et al.[489] found that one third of the patients had developed a variety of cranial nerve abnormalities consisting mainly of partial or complete 3rd nerve palsies, followed in descending order by 4th nerve palsies, 6th nerve palsies, and a subgroup of patients with bilateral palsies.[490] Other cranial neuropathies include optic neuritis,[490] which may lead to permanent visual loss and facial paresis accompanying the Ramsey Hunt syndrome.[487,490,491]

1.2.3.10.9 Zoster sine herpete

Zoster sine herpete has been defined generally as pain in a dermatomal distribution without the rash of cutaneous zoster.[492-494] However, reports from the literature suggest that it has a more complex nature, encompassing such neurological disorders as multiple cranial neuropathies and acute polyneuropathy,[495] meningitis,[496,497] meningoencephalitis/meningoradiculitis,[498] encephalitis,[466,495] and myelitis.[499]

1.2.4 REFERENCES

1. Roizman, B., Herpesviridae: a brief introduction, in *Fields Virology*, 2nd ed., Fields, B. N., Knipe, D. M., Chanock, R. M., Hirsch, M. S., Melnick, J. L., Monath, T. P., and Roizman, B., Eds., Raven Press, New York, 1990, 1787.
2. Liesegang, T. J., Diagnosis and therapy of herpes zoster ophthalmicus, *Ophthalmology*, 98, 1216, 1991.
3. Gershon, A. A. and Steinberg, S. P., Antibody response to varicella- zoster virus and the role of antibody in host defense, *Am. J. Med. Sci.*, 282, 12, 1981.
4. Straus, S. E., Ostrove, J. M., Inchauspé, G., Felser, J. M., Freifeld, A., Croen, K. D., and Sawyer, M. H., NIH conference varicella-zoster virus infections. Biology, natural history, treatment, and prevention, *Ann. Intern. Med.*, 108, 221, 1988.
5. Balfour, H. H., Benson, C., Braun, J., Cassens, B., Erice, A., Friedman- Kien, A., Klein, T., Polsky, B., and Safrin, S., Management of acyclovir-resistant herpes simplex and varicella-zoster virus infection, *J. Acquir. Immune Defic. Syndr.*, 7, 254, 1994.
6. Jacobson, M. A., Berger, T. G., Fikrig, S., Becherer, P., Moohr, J. W., Stanat, S. C., and Biron, K. K., Acyclovir-resistant varicella-zoster virus infection after chronic oral acyclovir therapy in patients with the acquired immunodeficiency syndrome (AIDS), *Ann. Intern. Med.*, 112, 187, 1990.
7. Gelb, L. D., Varicella-zoster virus, in *Fields Virology*, 2nd ed., Fields, B. N., Knipe, D. M., Chanock, R. M., Hirsch, M. S., Melnick, J. L., Monath, T. P., and Rozman, B., Eds., Raven Press, New York, 2011, 1990.
8. Gilden, D. H., Vafai, A., Shtram, Y., Becker, Y., Devlin, M., and Wellish, M., Varicella zoster virus DNA in human sensory ganglia, *Nature*, 306, 478, 1983.
9. Mahalingam, R., Wellish, M., Wolf, W., Dueland, A. N., Cohrs, R., Vafai, A., and Gilden, D., Latent varicella-zoster viral DNA in human trigeminal and thoracic ganglia, *N. Engl. J. Med.*, 323, 627, 1990.

10. Hyman, R. W., Ecker, J. R., and Tenser, R. B., Varicella zoster virus RNA in human trigeminal ganglia, *Lancet*, 2, 814, 1983.
11. Arvin, A. M., Koropchak, C. M., and Wittek, A. E., Immunologic evidence of reinfection with varicella-zoster virus, *J. Infect. Dis.*, 148, 200, 1983.
12. Brunell, P. A., Gershon, A. A., Hughes, W. T., Riley, H. D., Jr., and Smith, J., Prevention of varicella in high risk children: a collaborative study, *Pediatrics*, 50, 718, 1972.
13. Gershon, A. A., Steinberg, S. P., Gelb, L., and NIAID Collaborative Varicella Vaccine Study Group, Clinical reinfection with varicella-zoster virus, *J. Infect. Dis.*, 149, 127, 1984.
14. Weigle, K. A. and Grose, C., Molecular dissection of the humoral immune response to individual varicella-zoster viral proteins during chickenpox, quiescence, reinfection, and reactivation, *J. Infect. Dis.*, 149, 741, 1984.
15. Berlin, B. S. and Campbell, T., Hospital acquired herpes zoster following exposure to chickenpox, *JAMA*, 211, 1831, 1970.
16. Hope-Simpson, R. E., Infectiousness of communicable diseases in the household (measles, chickenpox, and mumps), *Lancet*, 2, 549, 1952.
17. Head, H. and Campbell, A. W., The pathology of herpes zoster and its bearing on sensory localization, *Brain*, 23, 353, 1900.
18. Juel-Jensen, B. W. and MacCallum, F. O., *Herpes Simplex, Varicella and Zoster*, J. B. Lippincott, Philadelphia, 1972.
19. Schimpff, S., Serpick, A., Stoler, B., Rumack, B., Mellin, H., Joseph, J. M., and Block, J., Varicella-zoster infection in patients with cancer, *Ann. Intern. Med.*, 76, 241, 1972.
20. Easton, H. G., Zoster sine herpete causing trigeminal neuralgia, *Lancet*, 2, 1065, 1970.
21. Luby, J. P., Ramirez-Ronda, C., Rinner, S., Hull, A., and Vergne-Marini, P., A longitudinal study of varicella zoster infections in renal transplant recipients, *J. Infect. Dis.*, 135, 659, 1977.
22. Merselis, J. G., Kaye, D., and Hook, E. W., Disseminated herpes zoster. A report of 17 cases, *Arch. Intern. Med.*, 113, 679, 1964.
23. Gallagher, J. G. and Merigan, T. C., Prolonged herpes-zoster infection associated with immuno-suppressive therapy, *Ann. Intern. Med.*, 91, 842, 1972.
24. Horten, B., Price, R. W., and Jimenez, D., Multifocal varicella-zoster virus leukoencephalitis temporarily remote from herpes zoster, *Ann. Neurol.*, 9, 251, 1981.
25. Ryder, J. W., Croen, K., Kleinschmidt-DeMasters, B. K., Ostrove, J. M., Straus, S. E., and Cohn, D. L., Progressive encephalitis three months after resolution of cutaneous zoster in a patient with AIDS, *Ann. Neurol.*, 19, 182, 1986.
26. Dolin, R., Reichman, R. C., Masur, M. H., and Whitley, R. J., Herpes zoster-varicella infection in immunocompromised patients, *Ann. Intern. Med.*, 89, 375, 1978.
27. Atkinson, K., Meyers, J. D., Storb, R., Prentice, R. L., and Thomas, E. D., Varicella-zoster virus after marrow transplantation for aplastic anaemia or leukaemia, *Transplantation*, 29, 47, 1980.
28. Rand, K. H., Rasmussen, L. E., Pollard, R. B., Arvin, A., and Merigan, T. C., Cellular immunity and herpes virus infections in cardiac-transplant patient, *N. Engl. J. Med.*, 296, 1372, 1976.
29. Guinee, V. F., Guido, J. J., Pfalzgraf, K. A., Giacco, G. G., Lagarde, C., Durand, M., van der Velden, J. W., Löwenberg, B., Jereb, B., Bretsky, S., Meilof, J., Hamersma, E. A. M., Dische, S., and Anderson, P., The incidence of herpes zoster in patients with Hodgkin's disease: an analysis of prognostic factors, *Cancer*, 56, 642, 1985.
30. Correale, J., Monteverde, D. A., Bueri, J. A., and Reich, E. G., Peripheral nervous system and spinal cord involvement in lymphoma, *Acta Neurol. Scand.*, 83, 45, 1991.
31. Rusthoven, J. J., Ahlgren, P., Elhakim, T., Pinfold, P., Reid, J., Stewart, L., and Feld, R., Varicella zoster infection in adult cancer patients: a population study, *Arch. Intern. Med.*, 148, 1561, 1988.
32. Sokal, J. E. and Firat, D., Varicella-zoster infection in Hodgkin's disease, *Am. J. Med.*, 39, 452, 1965.
33. Norum, J., Bremnes, R. M., and Wist, E., The ChlVPP regimen, a risk factor for herpes zoster virus infection in patients treated for Hodgkin's disease, *Eur. J. Haematol.*, 53, 51, 1994.
34. Feld, R., Evans, W. K., and DeBoer, G., Herpes zoster in patients with carcinoma of the lung, *Am. J. Med.*, 73, 795, 1982.
35. Maiche, A. G., Kajanti, M. J., and Pirhönen, S., Simultaneous disseminated herpes zoster and bacterial infection in cancer patients, *Acta Oncol.*, 31, 681, 1992.

36. Gottlieb, M. S., Wolfe, P. R., Fahey, J. L., Knight, S., Hardy, D., Eppolito, L., Ashida, E., Patel, A., Beall, G. N., and Sun, N., The syndrome of persistent generalized lymphadenopathy: experience with 101 patients, in *AIDS-Associated Syndromes*, Gupta, S., Ed., Plenum Press, New York, 1984, 85.

37. Colebunders, R., Francis, H., Izaley, L., Kakonde, N., Kabasele, K., Ifoto, L., Nzilambi, N., Quinn, T. C., Van der Groen, G., Curran, J. W., Vercauteren, G., and Piot, P., Evaluation of a clinical case-definition of acquired immunodeficiency syndrome in Africa, *Lancet*, 1, 492, 1987.

38. Mandal, B. K., Herpes zoster and the immunocompromised, *J. Infect.*, 14, 1, 1987.

39. King, D. H., History, pharmacokinetics, and pharmacology of acyclovir, *J. Am. Acad. Dermatol.*, 18, 176, 1988.

40. Hopefl, A. W., The clinical use of intravenous acyclovir, *Drug Intell. Clin. Pharm.*, 17, 623, 1983.

41. Whitley, R. J. and Gnann, J. W., Acyclovir: a decade later, *N. Engl. J. Med.*, 327, 782, 1992.

42. Elion, G. B., Furman, P. A., Fyfe, J. A., de Miranda, P., Beauchamp, L., and Schaeffer, H. J., Selectivity of action of an antiherpetic agent, 9-(2-hydroxyethoxymethyl)guanine, *Proc. Natl. Acad. Sci. U.S.A.*, 74, 5716, 1977.

43. Schaeffer, H. J., Beauchamp, L., de Miranda, P., Elion, G. B., Bauer, D. J., and Collins, P., 9-(2-Hydroxyethoxymethyl)guanine activity against viruses of the herpes group, *Nature*, 272, 583, 1978.

44. Bridgen, D. and Whiteman, P., The mechanism of action, pharmacokinetics and toxicity of acyclovir — a review, *J. Infect. Dis.*, 6(Suppl.1), 3, 1983.

45. Fyfe, J. A., Keller, P. M., Furman, P. A., Miller, R. L., and Elion, G. B., Thymidine kinase from herpes simplex virus phosphorylates the new antiviral compound, 9-(2-hydroxyethoxymethyl)guanine, *J. Biol. Chem.*, 253, 8721, 1978.

46. Derse, D., Cheng, Y.-C., Furman, P. A., St. Clair, M. H., and Elion, G. M., Inhibition of purified human and herpes simplex virus-induced DNA polymerases by 9-(2-hydroxyethoxymethyl)guanine triphosphate: effects on primer-template function, *J. Biol. Chem.*, 256, 11447, 1981.

47. Furman, P. A., St. Clair, M. H., and Spector, T., Acyclovir triphosphate is a suicide inactivator of the herpes simplex virus DNA polymerase, *J. Biol. Chem.*, 259, 9575, 1984.

48. Furman, P. A., St. Clair, M. H., Fyfe, J. A., Rideout, J. L., Keller, P. M., and Elion, G. B., Inhibition of herpes simplex virus-induced DNA polymerase activity and viral DNA replication by 9-(2- hydroxyethoxymethyl)guanine and its triphosphate, *J. Virol.*, 32, 72, 1979.

49. Appelboom, T. M. and Flowers, F. P., Acyclovir, *South. Med. J.*, 76, 905, 1983.

50. Davenport, A., Goel, S., and Mackenzie, J. C., Neurotoxicity of acyclovir in patients with end-stage renal failure treated with continuous ambulatory peritoneal dialysis, *Am. J. Kidney Dis.*, 20, 647, 1992.

51. Wingard, J. R., Viral infections in leukemia and bone marrow transplant patients, *Leukemia Lymphoma*, 11(Suppl. 2), 115, 1993.

52. Heidl, M., Scholz, H., and Dörffel, W., Die wirksamkeit von aciclovir und vidarabin bei immun-insuffzienten kindern mit varizellen und zoster — eine kontrollierte klinische studie, *Z. Klin. Med.*, 2107, 1987.

53. Shepp, D. H., Dandliker, P. S., and Meyers, J. D., Treatment of varicella-zoster virus infection in severely immunocompromised patients: a randomized comparison of acyclovir and vidarabine, *N. Engl. J. Med.*, 314, 208, 1986.

54. Guinee, V. F., Guido, J. J., Pfalzgraf, K. A., Giacco, G. G., Lagarde, C., Durand, M., von der Velden, J. W., Löwenberg, B., Jereb, B., Bretsky, S., Meilof, J., Hamersma, E. A. M., Dische, S., and Anderson, P., The incidence of herpes zoster in patients with Hodgkin's disease, *Cancer*, 56, 642, 1985.

55. Heidl, M., Scholz, H., Dörffel, W., and Wutzler, P., Varicella and zoster in children with malignant diseases. II. Prophylaxis and therapy, *Z. Arztl. Fortbild.*, 83, 136, 1989.

56. Biron, K. K., Fyfe, J. A., Noblin, J. E., and Elion, G. B., Selection and preliminary characterization of acyclovir-resistant mutants of varicella-zoster virus, *Am. J. Med.*, 73(Suppl. A), 383, 1982.

57. Wade, J. C. and Meyers, J. D., Neurologic symptoms associated with parenteral acyclovir treatment after marrow transplantation, *Ann. Intern. Med.*, 98, 921, 1983.

58. Keeney, R. E., Kirk, M. S., and Bridgen, D., Acyclovir tolerance in humans, *Am. J. Med.*, 73(Suppl.), 176, 1982.

59. Tomson, C. R. V., Goodship, T. H. J., and Rodger, R. S. C., Psychiatric side-effects of acyclovir in patients with chronic renal failure, *Lancet*, 2, 385, 1985.

60. Wellcome Medical Division, Zovirax in ABPI Data sheet compendium 1991-1992, Datafarm Publishers, London, 1991, 1748.
61. Bataille, P., Devos, P., Noel, J. L., Dautrevaux, C., and Lokiec, F., Psychiatric side-effects with acyclovir, *Lancet*, 2, 724, 1985.
62. Rubin, R., Overdose with acyclovir in a CAPD patient, *Perit. Dial. Bull.*, 7, 42, 1987.
63. Swan, S. K. and Bennett, W. M., Oral acyclovir and neurotoxicity, *Ann. Intern. Med.*, 111, 188, 1989.
64. Krigel, R. L., Reversible neurotoxicity due to acyclovir in a patient with chronic lymphatic leukaemia, *J. Infect. Dis.*, 154, 189, 1986.
65. Beales, P., Almond, M. K., and Kwan, J. T. C., Acyclovir neurotoxicity following oral therapy: prevention and treatment in patients on haemodialysis, *Nephron*, 66, 362, 1994.
66. Blum, M. R., Liao, S. H. T., and de Miranda, P., Overview of acyclovir pharmacokinetic desposition in adults and children, *Am. J. Med.*, 73 (Suppl. 1A), 186, 1982.
67. Laskin, O. L., Longstreth, J. A., Whelton, A., Krasny, H. C., Keeney, R. E., Rocco, L., and Lietman, P. S., Effect of renal failure on the pharmacokinetics of acyclovir, *Am. J. Med.*, 73(Suppl. 1A), 197, 1982.
68. MacDiarmaid-Gordon, A. R., O'Connor, M., Beaman, M., and Ackrill, P., Neurotoxicity associated with oral acyclovir in patients undergoing dialysis, *Nephron*, 62, 280, 1992.
69. Spiegal, D. M. and Lau, K., Acute renal failure and coma secondary to acyclovir therapy, *JAMA*, 255, 1882, 1986.
70. Johnson, R., Douglas, J., Corey, L., and Krasney, H., Adverse effects with acyclovir and meperidine, *Ann. Intern. Med.*, 103, 962, 1985.
71. Gill, M. J. and Burgess, E., Neurotoxicity of acyclovir in end stage disease, *J. Antimicrob. Chemother.*, 25, 300, 1990.
72. Feldman, S., Rodman, J., and Gregory, B., Excessive serum concentrations of acyclovir and neurotoxicity, *J. Infect. Dis.*, 157, 385, 1988.
73. Haefeli, W. E., Schoenenberger, R. A. Z., Weiss, P., and Ritz, R. F., Acyclovir-induced neurotoxicity: concentration-side effect relationship in acyclovir overdose, *Am. J. Med.*, 94, 212, 1993.
74. Selby, P., Blake, S., Mbidde, E. K., Hickmott, E., Powles, R. L., Stolle, K., McElwain, T. J., and Whiteman, P. D., Amino(hydroxyethoxymethyl)purine: a new well-absorbed prodrug of acyclovir, *Lancet*, 2, 1428, 1984.
75. Peterslund, N. A., Esmann, V., Geil, J. P., Munck Petersen, C., and Mogensen, C. E., Open study of 2-amino-9-(hydroxyethoxymethyl)-9*H*-purine (desciclovir) in the treatment of herpes zoster, *J. Antimicrob. Chemother.*, 20, 743, 1987.
76. Purifoy, D. J. M., Beauchamp, L. M., de Miranda, P., Ertl, P., Lacey, S., Roberts, G., Rahim, S. G., Darby, G., Krenitsky, T. A., and Powell, K. L., Review of research leading to new anti-herpesvirus agents in clinical development: valaciclovir hydrochloride (256U, the L-valyl ester of acyclovir) and 882C, a specific agent for varizella zoster virus, *J. Med. Virol. Suppl.*, 1, 139, 1993.
77. Beauchamp, L. M., Orr, G. F., de Miranda, P., Doucette, M., Burnette, T., and Krenitsky, T. A., Amino acid ester prodrugs of acyclovir, *Antiviral Chem. Chemother.*, 3, 157, 1992.
78. Gnann, J. W., New antivirals with activity against varicella-zoster virus, *Ann. Neurol.*, 34, S69, 1994.
79. de Miranda, P., Krasny, H. C., Page, D. A., and Elion, G. B., The disposition of acyclovir in different species, *J. Pharmacol. Exp. Ther.*, 219, 309, 1981.
80. Huff, J. C., Bean, B., Balfour, H. H., Jr., Laskin, O. L., Connor, J. D., Corey, L., Bryson, Y. J., and McGuirt, P., Therapy of herpes zoster with oral acyclovir, *Am. J. Med.*, 85(Suppl. 2A), 84, 1988.
81. Morton, P. and Thompson, A. N., Oral acyclovir in the treatment of herpes zoster in general practice, *N.Z. Med. J.*, 102, 93, 1989.
82. Blum, M. R., Weller, S., de Miranda, P., Lederberg, D., Burnette, T., and Smiley, L., Single and multiple dose pharmacokinetics of a new acyclovir prodrug, 256U, in healthy volunteers, *Proc. 31st Intersci. Conf. Antimicrob. Agents Chemother.*, Chicago, American Society for Microbiology, Washington, D.C., Abstr. 763, 1991.
83. Weller, S., Blum, M. R., Doucette, M., Smiley, M. L., Burnette, T., and de Miranda, P., Multiple-dose pharmacokinetics (PK) of 256U, a new acyclovir (ACV) prodrug in normal volunteers, *Pharm. Res.*, 8(Suppl.), 314, 1991.
84. Jacobson, M. A., Valaciclovir (BW256U87): the L-valyl ester of acyclovir, *J. Med. Virol. Suppl.*, 1, 150, 1993.

85. Feinberg, J., Gallant, J., Weller, S., Coakley, D., Gary, D., Squires, L., Smiley, M. L., Blum, M. R., and Jacobson, M., A phase I evaluation of 256U87, an acyclovir prodrug, in HIV-infected patients, *Proc. 8th Int. Conf. AIDS*, Amsterdam, 1992, Abstr. PoB 3885.

86. Smiley, M. L., and the International Valaciclovir Zoster Study Group, The efficacy and safety of valaciclovir for the treatment of herpes zoster, *Proc. 33rd Intersci. Conf. Antimicrob. Agents Chemother.*, American Society for Microbiology, Washington, D.C., Abstr. 1203, 1993.

87. Editorial, Valaciclovir more effective than acyclovir in reducing pain from shingles, *Infect. Control Hosp. Epidemiol.*, 15, 61, 1991.

88. Darby, G., The acyclovir legacy: its contribution to antiviral drug discovery, *J. Med. Virol. Suppl.*, 1, 134, 1993.

89. Earnshaw, D. L., Bacon, T. H., Darlison, S. J., Edmunds, K., Perkins, R. M., and Vere Hodge, R. A., Mode of antiviral action of penciclovir in MRC-5 cells infected with herpes simplex virus type 1 (HSV-1), HSV-2, and varicella-zoster virus, *Antimicrob. Agents Chemother.*, 36, 2747, 1992.

90. Vere Hodge, R. A. and Cheng, Y.-C., The mode of action of penciclovir, *Antiviral Chem. Chemother.*, 4(Suppl. 1), 13, 1993.

91. Earnshaw, D. L. and Vere Hodge, R. A., Effective inhibition of herpesvirus DNA synthesis by (*S*)-penciclovir-triphosphate, *Proc. 32nd Intersci. Conf. Antimicrob. Agents Chemother.*, American Society for Microbiology, Washington, D.C., Abstr. 1707, 1992.

92. Boyd, M. R., Safrin, S., and Kern, E. R., Penciclovir: a review of spectrum of activity, selectivity, and cross-resistance pattern, *Antiviral Chem. Chemother.*, 4(Suppl. 1), 3, 1993.

93. Boyd, M. R., Bacon, T. H., Sutton, D., and Cole, M., Antiherpes activity of 9-(4-hydroxy-3-hydroxymethylbutyl-1-yl)guanine (BRL 39123) in cell culture, *Antimicrob. Agents Chemother.*, 31, 1238, 1987.

94. Vere Hodge, R. A., Famciclovir and penciclovir: the mode of action of famciclovir including its conversion to penciclovir, *Antiviral Chem. Chemother.*, 42, 67, 1993.

95. Harnden, M. R., Jarvest, R. L., Boyd, M. R., Sutton, D., and Vere Hodge, R. A., Prodrugs of the selective anti-herpes virus agent 9-(4-hydroxyethoxy-3-hydroxymethylbut-1-yl)guanine (BRL 31123) with improved gastrointestinal absorption properties, *J. Med. Chem.*, 32, 1738, 1989.

96. Pue, M. A. and Benet, L. Z., Pharmacokinetics of famciclovir in man, *Antiviral Chem. Chemother.*, 4(Suppl. 1), 47, 1993.

97. Abramowitz, M., Famciclovir for herpes zoster, *Med. Lett. Drugs Ther.*, 36, 97, 1994.

98. Saltzman, R., Jurewicz, R., and Boon, R., Safety of famciclovir in patients with herpes zoster and genital herpes, *Antimicrob. Agents Chemother.*, 38, 2454, 1994.

99. Tyring, S., Nahlik, J., Cunningham, A., and the Collaborative Famciclovir Herpes Zoster Clinical Study Group, Efficacy and safety of famciclovir in the treatment of patients with herpes zoster, *Proc. 33rd Intersci. Conf. Antimicrob. Agents Chemother.*, American Society for Microbiology, Washington, D.C., Abstr. 1540, 1993.

100. Gheeraert, P., and the Famciclovir Herpes Zoster Virus Clinical Study Group, Efficacy and safety of famciclovir in the treatment of uncomplicated herpes zoster, *Proc. 32nd Intersci. Conf. Antimicrob. Agents Chemother.*, American Society for Microbiology, Washington, D.C., Abstr. 1108, 1992.

101. Sacks, S. L., Bishop, A. M., Fox, R., and Lee, G. C. Y., A double-blind, placebo-controlled trial of the effect of chronically administered oral famciclovir on sperm production in men with recurrent genital herpes infection, *Antiviral Res.*, 23(Suppl. 1), 72, 1994.

102. Machida, H. and Nishitani, M., Drug susceptibilities of isolates of varicella zoster virus in a clinical study of oral brovavir, *Microbiol. Immunol.*, 34, 407, 1990.

103. Machida, H., In vitro anti-herpesvirus action of a novel antiviral agent, brovavir (BV-araU), *Chemotherapy*, 58, 256, 1990.

104. Sherman, J., De Vault, A., Natarajan, M. et al., SQ 32756 (BV-araU): characteristics and pharmacokinetics in healthy young and elderly male volunteers, *Proc. 30th Intersci. Conf. Antimicrob. Agents Chemother.*, American Society for Microbiology, Washington, D.C., Abstr. 1103, 1990.

105. Niimura, M., Takahashi, M., Nishikawa, T., Ogawa, H., Asada, Y., and Ishii, J., Multicenter double-blind study of YN-72 (BV-araU, brovavir) in patients with herpes virus, *Jpn. J. Clin. Dermatol.*, 44, 447, 1990.

106. Niimura, M., A double-blind clinical study in patients with herpes zoster to establish YN-72 (brovavir) case, *Adv. Exp. Med. Biol.*, 278, 267, 1990.

107. Hiraoka, A., Masaoka, T., Nagai, K., Horiuchi, A., Kanamaru, A., Niimura, M., Hamada, T., and Takahashi, M., Clinical effect of BV-ara-U on varicella-zoster virus infection in immunocompromised patients with haematological malignancies, *J. Antimicrob. Chemother.*, 27, 361, 1991.

108. Young, C. W., Schneider, R., Leyland-Jones, B., Armstrong, D., Tan, C. T. C., Lopez, C., Watanabe, K. A., Fox, J. J., and Philips, F. S., Phase I evaluation of 2′-fluoro-5-iodo-1-D-arabinofuranosylcytosine in immunosuppressed patients with herpes virus infection, *Cancer Res.*, 43, 5006, 1983.

109. Leyland-Jones, B., Donnelly, H., Groshen, S., Myskowski, P., Donner, A. L., Fannuchi, M., Fox, J., and the Memorial Sloan-Kettering Antiviral Working Group, 2′-Fluoro-5-iodoarabinocytosine, a new potent antiviral agent: efficacy in immunosuppressed individuals with herpes zoster, *J. Infect. Dis.*, 154, 430, 1986.

110. Rahim, S. G., Trivedi, N., Selway, J., Darby, G. K., Collins, P., Powell, K. L., and Purifoy, D. J. M., 5-Alkynyl pyrimidine nucleosides as potent selective inhibitors of varicella-zoster virus, *Antiviral Chem. Chemother.*, 3, 293, 1992.

111. Talarico, C. L., Stanat, S. C., Rahim, S. G., Purifoy, D. J. M., and Biron, K. K., In vitro antiviral activity of 1-(beta-D-arabinofuranosyl)-5-(1-propynyl)uracil against varicella zoster virus, *Antiviral Res.*, 20(Suppl. 1), 128, 1993.

112. Peck, R. W., Posner, J., Weatherley, B., Holditch, T. A., and Whiteman, P. D., Tolerability and pharmacokinetics of 882C87, a novel nucleoside analogue in healthy male volunteers, *Br. J. Clin. Pharmacol.*, 33, 568P, 1992.

113. Peck, R. W., Orme, P., Weatherley, B., and Posner, J., The tolerability and pharmacokinetics of 882C87, a novel nucleoside analogue in healthy elderly volunteers, *Br. J. Clin. Pharmacol.*, 35, 74P, 1993.

114. Wood, M. J., McKendrick, M. W., Bannister, B., Mandal, B. K., Peck, R. W., and Crooks, R. J., Preliminary pharmacokinetics and safety of 882C87 in patients with herpes zoster, *J. Med. Virol. Suppl.*, 1, 154, 1993.

115. Peck, R. W., Crome, P., Weatherly, B. C., and Posner, J., Tolerability and pharmacokinetics of 882C, a novel nucleoside analogue, in healthy elderly volunteers, *Br. J. Clin. Pharmacol.*, 35, 74, 1993.

116. Crooks, R. J., Peck, R. W., and Wood, M. J., An open study to investigate the clinical potential, pharmacokinetics, and safety of 882C in patients with herpes zoster, *Antiviral Res.*, 20(Suppl. 1), 144, 1993.

117. Jones, A. S., Verhelst, G., and Walker, R. T., The synthesis of the potent anti-herpes virus agent, *E*-5-(2-bromovinyl)-2′-deoxyuridine and related compounds, *Tetrahedron Lett.*, 45, 4415, 1979.

118. De Clercq, E., Descamps, J., De Somer, P., Barr, P. J., Jones, A. S., and Walker, R. T., (*E*)-5-(2-bromovinyl)-2′-deoxyuridine: a potent and selective anti-herpes agent, *Proc. Natl. Acad. Sci. U.S.A.*, 76, 2947, 1979.

119. Shigeta, S., Yokota, T., Iwabuchi, T., Baba, M., Konno, K., Ogata, M., and De Clercq, E., Comparative efficacy of antiherpes drugs against various strains of varicella-zoster virus, *J. Infect. Dis.*, 147, 576, 1983.

120. De Clercq, E. and Walker, R. T., Synthesis and antiviral properties of 5- vinyl-pyrimidine nucleoside analogues, *Pharmacol. Ther.*, 26, 1, 1984.

121. De Clercq, E., Biochemical aspects of the selective antiherpes activity of nucleoside analogues, *Biochem. Pharmacol.*, 33, 2159, 1984.

122. Allaudeen, H. S., Chen, M. S., Lee, J. J., De Clercq, E., and Prusoff, W. H., Incorporation of *E*-5-(2-halovinyl)-2′-deoxyuridines into deoxyribonucleic acids of herpes simplex virus type 1-infected cells, *J. Biol. Chem.*, 257, 603, 1982.

123. Allaudeen, H. S., Kozarich, J. W., Bertino, J. R., and De Clercq, E., On the mechanism of selective inhibition of herpes-virus replication by (*E*)-5-(2-bromovinyl)-2′-deoxyuridine, *Proc. Natl. Acad. Sci. U.S.A.*, 78, 2698, 1981.

124. Mancini, W. R., De Clercq, E., and Prusoff, W. H., The relationship between incorporation of *E*-5-(2-bromovinyl)-2′-deoxyuridine into herpes simplex virus type 1 DNA with virus infectivity and DNA integrity, *J. Biol. Chem.*, 258, 792, 1983.

125. Busson, R., Colla, L., Vanderhaeghe, H., and De Clercq, E., Synthesis and antiviral activity of some sugar-modified derivatives of (*E*)-5-(2- bromovinyl)-2′-deoxyuridine, *Nucleic Acids Symp. Ser.*, 9, 49, 1981.

126. De Clercq, E., Balzarini, J., Descamps, J., Huang, G.-F., Torrence, P. F., Bergstrom, D. E., Jones, A. S., Serafinowski, P., Verhelst, G., and Walker, R. T., Antiviral, antimetabolic, and cytotoxic activities of 5-substituted 2'-deoxycytidines, *Mol. Pharmacol.*, 21, 217, 1982.

127. De Clercq, E., Descamps, H., Wildiers, J., De Jonge, G., Drochmans, A., Descamps, J., and De Somer, P., Oral (*E*)-5-(2-bromovinyl)-2'-deoxyuridine in severe herpes zoster, *Br. Med. J.*, 281, 1178, 1980.

128. Baba, M., Shigeta, S., and De Clercq, E., Serum and urine concentrations of oral bromovinyl-deoxyuridine in humans as monitored by a bioassay system based on varicella-zoster virus focus inhibition, *J. Med. Virol.*, 22, 17, 1987.

129. Desgranges, C., Razaka, G., Raubaud, M., Bricaud, H., Balzarini, J., and de Clercq, E., Phosphorolysis of (*E*)-5-(2-bromovinyl)-2'-deoxyuridine (BVDU) and other 5-substituted-2'-deoxyuridines by purified human thymidine phosphorylase and intact blood platelets, *Biochem. Pharmacol.*, 32, 3583, 1983.

130. Wingard, J. R., Hess, A. D., Stuart, R. K., Saral, R., and Burns, W. H., Effect of several antiviral agents on human lymphocyte functions and marrow progenitor cell proliferation, *Antimicrob. Agents Chemother.*, 23, 593, 1983.

131. Wittek, A. E., Cohren, P. S., Arvin, A. M., Smith, S. D., Koropchak, C. M., and De Clercq, E., Effect of (*E*)-5-(2-bromovinyl)-2'-deoxyuridine on proliferation of human fibroblasts, peripheral blood mononuclear cells, and granulocyte-monocyte progenitor cells in vitro, *Antimicrob. Agents Chemother.*, 24, 803, 1983.

132. Tricot, G., De Clercq, E., Boogaerts, M. A., and Verwilghen, R. L., Oral bromovinyldeoxyuridine therapy for herpes simplex and varicella-zoster virus infections in severely immunosuppressed patients: a preliminary clinical trial, *J. Med. Virol.*, 18, 11, 1986.

133. Heidl, M., Scholz, H., Dörffel, W., and Hermann, J., Antiviral therapy of varicella-zoster virus infection in immunocompromised children — a prospective randomized study of aciclovir versus brivudin, *Infection*, 19, 401, 1991.

134. Benoit, Y., Laureys, G., Delbeke, M.-J., and De Clercq, E., Oral BVDU treatment of varicella and zoster in children with cancer, *Eur. J. Pediatr.*, 143, 198, 1985.

135. Wildiers, J. and De Clercq, E., Oral (*E*)-5-(2-bromovinyl)-2'-deoxyuridine treatment of severe herpes zoster in cancer patients, *Eur. J. Cancer Clin. Oncol.*, 20, 471, 1984.

136. Wutzler, P., Wutke, K., Bärwolff, D., and Reefschläger, J., BVDU-therapie von zostererkrankungen bei patienten mit malignem grundleiden, *Z. Gesamte Inn. Med.*, 43, 677, 1988.

137. Dawber, R., Idoxuridine in herpes zoster: further evaluation of intermittent topical therapy, *Br. Med. J.*, 2, 526, 1974.

138. Wildenhoff, K. E., Esmann, V., Ipsen, J., Harving, H., Peterslund, N. A., and Schonheyder, H., Treatment of trigeminal and thoracic zoster with idoxuridine, *Scand. J. Infect. Dis.*, 13, 257, 1981.

139. Jeul-Jensen, B. E., MacCullum, F., and MacKensie, A., Treatment of zoster with idoxuridine in dimethyl sulphoxide. Results of two double-blind trials, *Br. Med. J.*, 4, 776, 1970.

140. Wildenhoff, K. E., Ipsen, J., and Esmann, V., Treatment of herpes zoster with idoxuridine ointment including a multivariate analysis of symptoms and signs, *Scand. J. Infect. Dis.*, 11, 1, 1979.

141. Esmann, V. and Wildenhoff, K. E., Idoxuridine in herpes zoster, *Lancet*, 2, 474, 1980.

142. Aliaga, A., Armijo, M., Camacho, F., Castro, A., Cruces, M., Diaz, J. L., Fernandez, J. M., Iglesias, L., Ledo, A., Mascaró, J. M. et al., Solucion topica de idoxuridina al 40% en dimetilsulfoxido frente a aciclovir oral en el tratamiento del herpes zoster: ensayo clinico multicentrico a doble ciego, *Med. Clin.*, 98, 245, 1992.

143. Senff, H., Engelmann, L., Kunze, J., and Hausen, B. M., Allergic contact dermatitis from idoxuridine, *Contact Dermatitis*, 23, 43, 1990.

144. Whitley, R., Ch'ien, L. T., Dolin, R., Galasso, G. J., Alford, C. A., Jr., Eds., and the Collaborative Study Group, Adenine arabinoside therapy of herpes zoster in the immunosuppressed, *N. Engl. J. Med.*, 294, 1193, 1976.

145. Whitley, R. J., Soong, S.-J., Dolin, R., Betts, R., Linnemann, C., Jr., Alford, C. A., Jr., and the NIAID Collaborative Antiviral Study Group, Early vidarabine therapy to control the complications of herpes zoster in immunosuppressed patients, *N. Engl. J. Med.*, 307, 971, 1982.

146. Whitley, R. J., Gnann, J. W., Jr., Hinthorn, D., Liu, C., Pollard, R. B., Hayden F., Mertz, G. J., Oxman, M., Soong, S.-J., and the NIAID Collaborative Antiviral Study Group, Disseminated herpes zoster in the immunocompromised host: a comparative trial of acyclovir and vidarabine, *J. Infect. Dis.*, 165, 450, 1992.

147. Kunitomi, T., Akazai, A., Ikeda, M., Oda, M., and Kodani, N., Comparison of acyclovir and vidarabine in immunocompromised children with varicella- zoster virus infection, *Acta Pediatr. Jpn.*, 31, 702, 1989.

148. Shepp, D. H., Dandlinker, P. S., and Meyers, J. D., Current therapy of varicella zoster virus infection in immunocompromised patients: a comparison of acyclovir and vidarabine, *Am. J. Med.*, 85, 96, 1988.

149. Vildé, J. L., Bricaire, F., Leport, C., Renaudie, M., and Brun-Vézinet, F., Comparative trial of acyclovir and vidarabine in disseminated varicella-zoster virus infections in immunocompromised patients, *J. Med. Virol.*, 20, 127, 1986.

150. Nagafuchi, S., Moriyama, K., Takamatsu, Y., Hayashi, S., Niho, Y., Takenaka, A., and Mori, R., Treatment of disseminated herpes zoster in six severely immunocompromised patients: acyclovir and vidarabine, *Jpn. J. Med.*, 28, 100, 1989.

151. Moriyama, K., Asano, Y., Fujimoto, K., Okamura, T., Shibuya, T., Harada, M., and Niho, Y., Successful combination therapy with acyclovir and vidarabine for disseminated varicella zoster infection with retinal involvement in a patient with B-cell lymphoma and adult T-cell leukemia, *Am. J. Med.*, 85, 885, 1985.

152. Burdge, D. R., Chow, A. W., and Sacks, S. L., Neurotoxic effects during vidarabine therapy for herpes zoster, *Can. Med. Assoc. J.*, 132, 392, 1985.

153. Semel, J. D. and McNerney, J. J., Jr., AIADH during disseminated herpes varicella-zoster infections: relationship to vidarabine therapy, *Am. J. Med. Sci.*, 291, 115, 1986.

154. Nikkels, A. F. and Piérard, G. E., Recognition and treatment of shingles, *Drugs*, 48, 528, 1994.

155. Stevens, D. A., Jordan, G. W., Waddell, T. F., and Merigan, T. C., Adverse effect of cytosine arabinoside on disseminated zoster in a controlled trial, *N. Engl. J. Med.*, 289, 873, 1973.

156. Sklar, S. H., Blue, W. T., Alexander, E. J., and Bodian, C. A., Herpes zoster: the treatment and prevention of neuralgia with adenosine monophosphate, *JAMA*, 253, 1427, 1985.

157. Sherlock, C. H. and Corey, L., Adenosine monophosphate for the treatment of varicella zoster infections: a large dose of caution, *JAMA*, 253, 1444, 1985.

158. Hengee, U. R., Brockmeyer, N. H., Malessa, R., Ravens, U., and Goos, M., Foscarnet penetrates the blood-brain barrier: rationale for therapy of cytomegalovirus encephalitis, *Antimicrob. Agents Chemother.*, 37, 1010, 1993.

159. Safrin, S., Berger, T. G., Gilson, I., Wolfe, P. R., Wolfsy, C. B., and Biron, K. K., Foscarnet therapy in five patients with AIDS and acyclovir-resistant varicella-zoster virus infection, *Ann. Intern. Med.*, 115, 19, 1991.

160. Smith, K. J., Kahlter, D. C., Davis, C., James, W. D., Skelton, H. G., and Angritt, P., Acyclovir-resistant varicella zoster responsive to foscarnet, *Arch. Dermatol.*, 127, 1069, 1991.

161. Merigan, T. C., Rand, K. H., Pollard, R. B., Abdallah, P. S., Jordan, G. W., and Fried, R. P., Human leukocyte interferon for the treatment of herpes zoster in patients with cancer, *N. Engl. J. Med.*, 298, 981, 1978.

162. Winston, D. J., Eron, L. J., Ho, M., Pazin, G., Kessler, H., Pottage, J. C., Jr., Gallacher, J., Sartiano, G., Ho, W. G., Champlin, R. E., Bernhardt, L., Bigley, J., Kanitra, L., Nadler, P. I., and the Hoffmann-La Roche Herpes Zoster Study Group, Recombinant interferon-alpha-2a for treatment of herpes zoster in immunosuppressed patients with cancer, *Am. J. Med.*, 85, 147, 1988.

163. Emödi, G., Rufli, T., Just, M., and Hernandez, R., Human interferon therapy for herpes zoster in adults, *Scand. J. Infect. Dis.*, 7, 1, 1975.

164. Duschet, P., Schwarz, T., Soyer, P., Henk, A., Hausmaninger, H., and Gschnait, F., Treatment of herpes zoster: recombinant alpha interferon versus acyclovir, *Int. J. Dermatol.*, 27, 193, 1988.

165. Georgiev, V. St., Immunomodulatory activity of small peptides, *Trends Pharmacol. Sci.*, 11, 373, 1990.

166. Georgiev, V. St., Immunomodulating peptides of natural and synthetic origin, *Med. Res. Rev.*, 11, 81, 1991.

167. Schlesinger, D. and Goldstein, G., The amino acid sequence of thymopentin II, *Cell*, 5, 361, 1975.

168. Goldstein, G., Scheid, M. P., Boyse, E. A., Schlesinger, D. H., and Van Wauwe, J., A synthetic pentapeptide with biological activity characteristic of the thymic hormone thymopoietin, *Science*, 204, 1309, 1979.

169. Tischio, J. P., Patrick, J. E., Weintraub, H. S., Chasin, M., and Goldstein, G., Short *in vitro* half-life of thymopoietin$_{32-36}$ pentapeptide in human plasma, *Int. J. Peptide Protein Res.*, 14, 479, 1979.

170. Di Perri, T., Laghi Pasini, F., and Autori, A., Immunokinetics of a single dose of thymopoietin pentapeptide, *J. Immunopharmacol.*, 2, 567, 1980.
171. Sundal, E. and Bertelletti, D., Management of viral infections with thymopentin, *Arzneim.-Forsch.*, 44, 866, 1994.
172. Sapuppo, A., Guaneri, B., Di Prima, T. M., De Pasquale, R., Nier, M. A., Califano, L. et al., *Farmaco*, 14, 35, 1990.
173. Carco, F., Gilli, C., Gobber, M., Bianchi, B., and Guazzotti, G., Indicazioni terapeutiche nell herpes zoster, *Clin. Ter.*, 136, 327, 1991.
174. Kokelj, F., Thymopentin and acyclovir association in the treatment of herpes zoster, *G. Ital. Dermatol. Venereol.*, 126, 453, 1991.
175. Lomuto, M., Zenarola, P., Ditano, G., and Cascavilla, N., Thymopentin in the treatment of herpes zoster, *Curr. Ther. Res.*, 44, 672, 1988.
176. Scarpa, C. and Kokelj, F., Experience with immune stimulation by thymopentin in herpes zoster, *Akt. Dermatol.*, 13, 247, 1987.
177. Wood, M. J., Current experience with antiviral therapy for acute herpes zoster, *Ann. Neurol.*, 35, S65, 1994.
178. Bunta, S. and Peris, E., Immunstimulierende zostertherapie, *Z. Hautkrankheit*, 56, 147, 1981.
179. Editorial, Inosiplex: antiviral, immunomodulator, or neither? *Lancet*, 1, 1052, 1982.
180. Jones, C. E., Dyken, P. R., Huttenlocher, P. R., Jabbow, J. T., and Maxwell, K. W., Inosiplex therapy in subacute sclerosing panencephalitis. A multicentre non-randomized study in 98 patients, *Lancet*, 1, 1034, 1982.
181. Payne, C. M., Menday, A. P., Rogers, T., and Staughton, R. C. D., Isoprinosine does not influence the natural history of herpes zoster or postherpetic neuralgia, *Scand. J. Infect. Dis.*, 21, 15, 1989.
182. Castelli, M., Zanca, A., Giubertoni, G., Zanca, A., and Bertolini, A., Griseofulvin-methisoprinol combination in the treatment of herpes zoster, *Pharmacol. Res. Commun.*, 18, 991, 1986.
183. Bruni, L., Tagliapietra, G., and Innocenti, P., Herpes zoster treatments: results of a clinical trial relative to the use of rifamycin SV versus neuramide, *J. Int. Med. Res.*, 12, 255, 1984.
184. Mavlight, G. M. and Talpaz, M., Cimetidine for herpes zoster, *N. Engl. J. Med.*, 310, 318, 1984.
185. Miller, A., Harel, D., Laor, A., and Lahat, N., Cimetidine as an immunomodulator in the treatment of herpes zoster, *J. Neuroimmunol.*, 22, 69, 1989.
186. Benze, L., Marcusson, J. A., and Ramsten, T., Effect of cimetidine on herpes zoster infection, *Drug Intell. Clin. Pharm.*, 21, 803, 1987.
187. Wood, M. J., Ogan, P. H., McKendrick, M. W., Care, C. D., McGill, J. I., and Webb, E. M., Efficacy of oral acyclovir treatment of acute herpes zoster, *Am. J. Med.*, 85(Suppl. 2A), 79, 1988.
188. Gnann, J. W. and Whitley, R. J., Natural history and treatment of varicella-zoster in high-risk populations, *J. Hosp. Infect.*, 18(Suppl.), 317, 1991.
189. Balfour, H. H., Jr., Current management of varicella zoster virus infections, *J. Med. Virol. Suppl.*, 1, 74, 1993.
190. Wood, M. J., Johnson, R. W., McKendrick, M. W., Taylor, J., Mandal, B. K., and Crooks, J., A randomized trial of acyclovir for 7 days with and without prednisolone for treatment of acute herpes zoster, *N. Engl. J. Med.*, 330, 896, 1994.
191. van den Broek, P. J., Stuyt, P. M. J., van der Meer, J. W. M., Tangeman, J. C., Kuzminski, A. M., Svahn, D. S., Wood, M. J., McKendrick, M. W., and Johnson, R. W., Acyclovir for herpes zoster, *N. Engl. J. Med.*, 331, 481, 1994.
192. Bean, B., Braun, C., and Balfour, H. H., Jr., Acyclovir therapy for acute herpes zoster, *Lancet*, 2, 118, 1982.
193. Peterslund, N. A., Seyer-Hansen, K., Ipsen, J., Esmann, V., Schonheyder, H., and Juhl, H., Acyclovir in herpes zoster, *Lancet*, 2, 827, 1981.
194. McGill, J., MacDonald, D. R., Fall, C., McKendrick, G. D. W., and Copplestone, A., Intravenous acyclovir in acute herpes zoster infection, *J. Infect. Dis.*, 6, 157, 1983.
195. Balfour, H. H., Jr., Bean, B., Laskin, O. L., Ambinder, R. F., Meyers, J. D., Wade, J. C., Zaia, J. A., Aeppli, D., Kirk, L. E., Segretti, A. C., Keeney, R. E., and the Burroughs Wellcome Collaborative Acyclovir Study Group, Acyclovir halts progression of herpes zoster in immunocompromised patients, *N. Engl. J. Med.*, 308, 1448, 1983.

196. Petrozza, J. C., Monga, M., Oshiro, B. T., Graham, J. M., and Blanco, J. D., Disseminated herpes zoster in a pregnant woman positive for human immunodeficiency virus, *Am. J. Perinatol.*, 10, 463, 1993.

197. Sempere, A., Sanz, G. F., Scnent, L., de la Rubia, J., Jarque, I., López, F., Arilla, M. J., Guinot, M., Martin, G., Martinez, J., Marty, M. L., and Sanz, M. A., Long-term acyclovir prophylaxis for prevention of varicella zoster virus infection after autologous blood stem cell transplantation in patients with acute leukemia, *Bone Marrow Transplant.*, 10, 495, 1992.

198. Acyclovir sodium, in *AMA Drug Evaluation*, 6th ed., American Medical Association, Chicago, 1986, 1623.

199. Wood, M. J., McKendrick, M. W., Freris, M. W., Jeal, S. C., Jones, D. A., and Gilbert, A. M., Trough plasma acyclovir concentrations and safety of oral acyclovir, 800 mg five times daily for 7 days in elderly patients with herpes zoster, *J. Antimicrob. Chemother.*, 33, 1245, 1994.

200. Whitley, R. J., Hilty, M., Haynes, R., Bryson, Y., Connor, J. D., Soong, S. J., and Alford, C. A., Vidarabine therapy of varicella in immunosuppressed patients, *J. Pediatr.*, 101, 125, 1982.

201. Ch'ien, L. T., Whitley, R. J., Alford, C. A., Jr., Galasso, G. J., and the Collaborative Antiviral Study Group, Adenine arabinoside for therapy of herpes zoster in immunosuppressed patients: preliminary results of a collaborative study, *J. Infect. Dis.*, 133 (Suppl.), A184, 1976.

202. Whitley, R. J., Ch'ien, L. T., Dolin, R., Galasso, G. J., Alford, C. A., Jr., and the Collaborative Antiviral Study Group, Adenine arabinoside therapy of herpes zoster in the immunosuppressed, *N. Engl. J. Med.*, 294, 1193, 1976.

203. Whitley, R. J., Therapeutic approaches to varicella-zoster virus infections, *J. Infect. Dis.*, 166(Suppl.), S51, 1992.

204. Deray, G., Martinez, F., Katlama, C., Levaltier, B., Beaufils, H., Danis, M., Rosenheim, M., Baumelou, A., Dohin, E., Gentilini, M., and Jacobs, C., Foscarnet nephrotoxicity: mechanism, incidence and prevention, *Am. J. Nephrol.*, 9, 316, 1989.

205. Bendel, A. E., Gross, T. G., Woods, W. G., Edelman, C. K., and Balfour, H. H., Jr., Failure of foscarnet in disseminated herpes zoster, *Lancet*, 341, 1342, 1993.

206. Mallett, R. B. and Staughton, R. C. D., The treatment of herpes zoster with flamazine — a double-blind placebo-controlled trial, *Clin. Exp. Dermatol.*, 18, 196, 1993.

207. Chang, T. W. and Weinstein, L., Prevention of herpes keratoconjunctivitis in rabbits by silver sulphadiazine, *Antimicrob. Agents Chemother.*, 8, 677, 1975.

208. Montes, L. F., Muchnick, G., and Fox, C. L., Response of varicella zoster virus and herpes zoster to silver sulphadiazine, *Cutis*, 38, 363, 1986.

209. Gwiezdzinski, Z. and Protas-Drozo, F., Gryzeofulvina w leczeniu polpasca, *Przegl. Dermatol.*, 76, 45, 1989.

210. Paryani, S. G. and Azuin, A. M., Intrauterine infection with varicella- zoster virus after maternal varicella, *N. Engl. J. Med.*, 314, 1542, 1986.

211. Locksley, R. M., Flournoy, N., Sullivan, K. M., and Mayers, J. D., Infection with varicella-zoster virus after marrow transplantation, *J. Infect. Dis.*, 152, 1172, 1985.

212. Bustamantem, C. I. and Wade, J. C., Herpes zoster virus infection in the immunocompromised cancer patient, *J. Clin. Oncol.*, 9, 1903, 1991.

213. Selby, P. J., Jameson, B., and Watson, J. G., Parenteral acyclovir: therapy for herpes virus infection in man, *Lancet*, 2, 1267, 1979.

214. Gluckman, E., Devergie, A., and Melo, R., Prophylaxis of herpes infections after bone marrow transplantation by oral acyclovir, *Lancet*, 2, 706, 1983.

215. Horowitz, G. M. and Hankins, G. D. V., Early-second-trimester use of acyclovir in treating herpes zoster in a bone marrow transplant patient: a case report, *J. Reprod. Med.*, 37, 280, 1992.

216. Stemmer, S. M., Kinsman K., Tellschow, S., and Jones, R. B., Fatal noncutaneous visceral infection with varicella-zoster virus in a patient with lymphoma after autologous bone marrow transplantation, *Clin. Infect. Dis.*, 16, 497, 1993.

217. Feldman, S., Varicella zoster infections in bone marrow transplants, *Recent Results Cancer Res.*, 132, 177, 1993.

218. Ben, B., Buren, C. T., and Balfour, H. H., Jr., Acyclovir therapy for acute herpes zoster, *Lancet*, 2, 118, 1982.

219. Bridgen, D., Rosling, A. E., and Woods, N. C., Renal function after acyclovir intravenous injection, *Am. J. Med.*, 73(Suppl. 1A), 182, 1982.
220. Stoffel, M., Squifflet, J. P., Pirson, Y., Lamy, M., and Alexandre, G. P. J., Effectiveness of oral acyclovir prophylaxis in renal transplant recipients, *Transplant. Proc.*, 19, 2190, 1987.
221. Meyers, J. D., Wade, J. C., Shepp, D. H., and Newton, B., Acyclovir treatment of varicella-zoster virus infection in the compromised host, *Transplantation*, 37, 571, 1984.
222. Hayes, K., Shakuntala, V., Pingle, A., Dhawan, I. K., and Masri, M. A., Safe use of acyclovir (zovirax) in renal transplant patients on cyclosporine A therapy: case reports, *Transplant. Proc.*, 24, 1926, 1992.
223. Johnson, P. C., Kumor, K., Welsh, M. S., Woo, J., and Kahan, B. D., Effects of coadministration of cyclosporine and acyclovir on renal function of renal allograft recipients, *Transplantation*, 44, 329, 1987.
224. Glesby, M. J., Moore, R. D., Chaisson, R. E., and the Zidovudine Epidemiology Study Group, Herpes zoster in patients with advanced human immunodeficiency virus infection treated with zidovudine, *J. Infect. Dis.*, 168, 1264, 1993.
225. Friedman-Kien, A. E., Lafleur, F. L., Gendler, E., Hennessey, N. P., Montagna, R., Halbert, S., Rubinstein, P., Krasinski, K., Zang, E., and Poiesz, B., Herpes zoster: a possible early sign for development of acquired immunodeficiency syndrome in high-risk individuals, *J. Am. Acad. Dermatol.*, 14, 1023, 1986.
226. Snoeck, R., Gérard, M., Sadzot-Delvaux, C., Andrei, G., Balzarini, J., Reymen, D., Ahadi, N., De Bruyn, J. M., Piette, J., Rentier, B., Clumeck, N., and De Clercq, E., Meningoradiculoneuritis due to acyclovir-resistant varicella zoster in an acquired immune deficiency syndrome patient, *J. Med. Virol.*, 42, 338, 1994.
227. Kaplan, M. H., Sadick, N., McNutt, N. S., Meltzer, M., Sarngadharan, M. G., and Pahwa, S., Dermatologic findings and manifestations of acquired immunodeficiency syndrome (AIDS), *J. Am. Acad. Dermatol.*, 16, 485, 1987.
228. Janier, M., Hillion, B., Baccard, M., Morinet, F., Scieux, C., Perol, Y., and Givatte, J., Chronic varicella-zoster infection in acquired immunodeficiency syndrome, *J. Am. Acad. Dermatol.*, 18, 584, 1988.
229. Colebunders, R., Mann, J. M., Francis, H., Bila, K., Izaley, L., Ilwaya, M., Kakonde, N., Quinn, T. C., Curran, J. W., and Piot, P., Herpes zoster in African patients: a clinical predictor of human immunodeficiency virus infection, *J. Infect. Dis.*, 157, 314, 1988.
230. Acheson, D. W. K., Leen, C. L. S., Tariq, W. U. Z., and Mandal, B. K., Severe and recurrent varicella-zoster virus infection in a patient with the acquired immune deficiency syndrome, *J. Infect.*, 16, 193, 1988.
231. Quinnan, G. V., Jr., Masur, H., Rook, A. H., Armstrong, G., Frederick, W. R., Epstein, J., Manischewitz, J. F., Macher, A. M., Jackson, L., Ames, J., Smith, H. A., Parker, M., Pearson, G. R., Parrillo, J., Mitchell, C., and Straus, S. E., Herpesvirus infection in the acquired immune deficiency syndrome, *JAMA*, 252, 72, 1984.
232. Ryder, J. W., Croen, K., Kleinschmidt-DeMasters, B. K., Ostrove, J. M., Straus, S. E., and Cohn, D. L., Progressive encephalitis three months after resolution of cutaneous zoster in a patient with AIDS, *Ann. Neurol.*, 19, 182, 1986.
233. Cohen, P. R., Beltrani, V. P., and Grossman, M. E., Disseminated herpes zoster in patients with human immunodeficiency virus infection, *JAMA*, 84, 1076, 1988.
234. Nelson, J. A., Ghazal, P., and Wiley, C. A., Role of opportunistic viral infections in AIDS, *AIDS*, 4, 1, 1990.
235. Cockerell, C. J., Human immunodeficiency virus infection and the skin, *Arch. Intern. Med.*, 151, 1295, 1991.
236. Leibovitz, E., Kaul, A., Rigaud, M., Bebenroth, D., Krasinski, K., and Borkowsky, W., Chronic varicella zoster in a child infected with human immunodeficiency virus: case report and review of the literature, *Cutis*, 49, 27, 1992.
237. Lokke Jensen, B., Weismann, K., Mathiesen, L., and Klem Thomsen, H., Atypical varicella-zoster infection in AIDS, *Acta Derm. Venereol. (Stockholm)*, 73, 123, 1993.
238. Colebunders, R., Van Damme, L., Van den Abbeele, K., Fleerackers, Y., Van den Enden, E., and Dockx, P., Atypical varicella zoster infection in persons with HIV infection, *Acta Clin. Belg.*, 49, 104, 1994.
239. Linnemann, C. C., Biron, K. K., Hoppenjans, W. G., and Solinger, A. M., Emergence of acyclovir-resistant varicella-zoster virus in an AIDS patient on prolonged acyclovir therapy, *AIDS*, 4, 577, 1990.

240. Disler, R. S. and Dover, J. S., Chronic localized herpes zoster in AIDS, *Arch. Dermatol.*, 126, 1105, 1990.

241. Hoppenjans, W. B., Bibler, M. R., Orme, R. L., and Solinger, A. M., Prolonged cutaneous herpes zoster in acquired immunodeficiency syndrome, *Arch. Dermatol.*, 126, 1048, 1990.

242. Hellinger, W. C., Bolling, J. P., Smith, T. F., and Campbell, R. J., Varicella-zoster virus retinitis in a patient with AIDS-related complex: case report and brief review of the acute retinal necrosis syndrome, *Clin. Infect. Dis.*, 16, 208, 1993 (comment in *Clin. Infect. Dis.*, 17, 943, 1993).

243. Rousseau, F., Perronne, C., Raguin, G., Thouvenot, D., Vidal, A., Leport, C., and Vildé, J. L., Necrotizing retinitis and cerebral vasculitis due to varicella-zoster virus in patients infected with the human immunodeficiency virus, *Clin. Infect. Dis.*, 17, 943, 1993.

244. Kusuhara, K., Miyazaki, C., Ise, K., Hidaka, Y., Tokugawa, K., and Ueda, K., A case of congenital herpes zoster, *Acta Paediatr. Jpn.*, 35, 141, 1993.

245. Srabstein, J. C., Morris, N., Bryle Larke, R. P., de Sa, D. J., Castelino, B. B., and Sum, E., Is there a congenital varicella syndrome? *J. Pediatr.*, 84, 239, 1974.

246. Brunell, P. A., Fetal and neonatal varicella-zoster infections, *Semin. Perinatol.*, 7, 47, 1986.

247. Alkalay, A. L., Pomerance, J. J., and Rimoin, D. L., Fetal varicella syndrome, *J. Pediatr.*, 111, 320, 1987.

248. Paryani, S. G. and Arvin, A. M., Intrauterine infection with varicella- zoster virus after maternal varicella, *N. Engl. J. Med.*, 314, 1542, 1986.

249. Newman, C. G. H., Perinatal varicella, *Lancet*, 2, 1159, 1965.

250. Meyers, J. D., Congenital varicella in term infants: risk reconsidered, *J. Infect. Dis.*, 129, 215, 1974.

251. Bennet, R., Forsgren, M., and Herin, P., Herpes zoster in a 2 week old premature infant with possible congenital varicella encephalitis, *Acta Pediatr. Scand.*, 75, 979, 1985.

252. Brunell, P. A. and Miller, L. H., Zoster in children, *Am. J. Dis. Child.*, 115, 432, 1968.

253. Brunell, P. A. and Kotchmar, G. S., Zoster in infancy: failure to maintain virus latency following intrauterine infection, *J. Pediatr.*, 98, 71, 1981.

254. Higa, K., Dan, K., and Manabe, H., Varicella-zoster virus infections during pregnancy: hypothesis concerning the mechanisms of congenital malformations, *Obstet. Gynecol.*, 69, 214, 1987.

255. Balfour, H. H., Jr., Acyclovir, in *The Antimicrobial Agents Annual/3*, Peterson, P. K. and Verhoef, J., Eds., Elsevier Science, New York, 1988, 345.

256. Collins, P., Viral sensitivity following the introduction of acyclovir, *Am. J. Med.*, 85, 129, 1988.

257. Janier, M., Hillion, M., Baccard, M., Morinet, F., Scieux, C., Perol, Y., and Civatte, J., Chronic varicella zoster infection in acquired immunodeficiency syndrome, *J. Am. Acad. Dermatol.*, 18, 584, 1988.

258. Pahwa, S., Biron, K., Lim, W., Swenson, P., Kaplan, M. H., Sadick, N., and Pahwa, R., Continuous varicella-zoster infection associated with acyclovir resistance in a child with AIDS, *JAMA*, 260, 2879, 1988.

259. Linneman, C. C., Biron, K. K., Hoppenjans, W. G., and Solinger, A. M., Emergence of acyclovir-resistant varicella zoster virus in an AIDS patient on prolonged acyclovir therapy, *AIDS*, 4, 577, 1990.

260. Hoppenjans, W. B., Bibler, M. R., Ormer, R. L., and Solinger, A. M., Prolonged cutaneous herpes zoster in acquired immunodeficiency syndrome, *Arch. Intern. Med.*, 126, 1048, 1990.

261. Erlich, K. S., Jacobson, M. A., Koehler, J. E., Folansbee, S. E., Drennan, D. P., Gooze, L., Safrin, S., and Mills, J., Foscarnet therapy for severe acyclovir-resistant herpes simplex virus type-2 infections in patients with the acquired immunodeficiency syndrome (AIDS): an uncontrolled trial, *Ann. Intern. Med.*, 110, 710, 1989.

262. Chatis, P. A., Miller, C. H., Schrager, L. E., and Crumpacker, C. S., Successful treatment with foscarnet of an acyclovir-resistant mucocutaneous infection with herpes simplex virus in a patient with acquired immunodeficiency syndrome, *N. Engl. J. Med.*, 320, 297, 1989.

263. Kaufmann, R., Passive immunotherapy in herpes zoster: a pilot study with intravenous hyperimmune globulin, *Z. Hautkr.*, 60, 207, 1985.

264. Senneville, E., Chidiac, C., Brouillard, M., Beuscart, C., Leroy, O., Sivery, B., Beaucaire, G., and Mouton, Y., Aciclovir et immunoglobulines specifiques anti-varicelle-zona dans le traitement des infections par le virus de la varicelle at du zona chez 113 patients, *Pathol. Biol.*, 38, 568, 1990.

265. Zaia, J. A., Levin, M. J., Preblud, S. R., Leszczynski, J., Wright, G. G., Ellis, R. J., Curtis, A. C., Valerio, M. A., and LeGore, J., Evaluation of varicella-zoster immune globulin: protection of immunosuppressed children after household exposure to varicella, *J. Infect. Dis.*, 147, 737, 1983.

266. Agostini, G. and Agostini, S., Le immunoglobuline nel trattamento dell'herpes zoster, *Clin. Ter.*, 141, 11, 1992.

267. Groth, K. E., McCullough, J., Marker, S. C., Howard, R. J., Simmons, R. L., Najarian, J. S., and Balfour, H. H., Jr., Evaluation of zoster immune plasma: treatment of cutaneous disseminated zoster in immunocompromised patients, *JAMA*, 239, 1877, 1978.

268. Stevens, D. A. and Merigan, T. C., Zoster immune globulin prophylaxis of disseminated zoster in compromised hosts, *Arch. Intern. Med.*, 140, 52, 1980.

269. Waring, J. J., Neubuerger, K., and Geever, E. F., Severe forms of chickenpox in adults, *Arch. Intern. Med.*, 69, 384, 1942.

270. Feldman, S., Varicella-zoster virus pneumonitis, *Chest*, 106 (Suppl.), 22S, 1994.

271. Schuchter, L. M., Wingard, J. R., Piantadosi, S., Burns, W. H., Santos, G. W., and Saral, R., Herpes zoster infection after autologous bone marrow transplantation, *Blood*, 74, 1424, 1989.

272. Wacker, P., Hartmann, O., Benhamou, E., Salloum, E., and Lemerle, J., Varicella-zoster virus infections after autologous bone marrow transplantation in children, *Bone Marrow Transplant.*, 4, 191, 1989.

273. Feldhoff, C. M., Balfour, H. H., Jr., Simmons, R. L., Najarian, J. S., and Mauer, S. M., Varicella in children with renal transplants, *J. Pediatr.*, 98, 25, 1981.

274. Lynfield, R., Herrin, J. T., and Rubin, R. H., Varicella in pediatric renal transplant recipients, *Pediatrics*, 90, 216, 1992.

275. McGregor, R. S., Zitelli, B. J., Urbach, A. H., Malatack, J. J., and Gartner, J. C., Jr., Varicella in pediatric orthotopic liver transplant recipients, *Pediatrics*, 83, 256, 1989.

276. Feldman, S., Hughes, W. T., and Daniel, C. B., Varicella in children with cancer: 77 cases, *Pediatrics*, 56, 388, 1975.

277. Feldman, S. and Lott, L., Varicella in children with cancer: impact of antiviral therapy and prophylaxis, *Pediatrics*, 80, 465, 1987.

278. Feldman, S., Hughes, W. T., and Kim, H. Y., Herpes zoster in children with cancer, *Am. J. Dis. Child.*, 126, 178, 1973.

279. Jura, E., Chadwick, E. G., Josephs, S. H., Steinberg, S. P., Yogev, R., Gershon, A. A., Krasinski, K. M., and Borkowsky, W., Varicella-zoster virus infections in children infected with human immunodeficiency virus, *Pediatr. Infect. Dis. J.*, 8, 586, 1989.

280. Dowell, S. F. and Bresee, J. S., Severe varicella associated with steroid use, *Pediatrics*, 92, 223, 1993.

281. Abzug, M. J. and Cotton, M. F., Severe chickenpox after intranasal use of corticosteroids, *J. Pediatr.*, 123, 577, 1993.

282. Kasper, W. J. and Howe, P. M., Fatal varicella after a single course of corticosteroids, *Pediatr. Infect. Dis. J.*, 9, 729, 1990.

283. Haake, D. A., Zakowski, P. C., Haake, D. L., and Bryson, Y. J., Early treatment with acyclovir for varicella pneumonia in otherwise healthy adults: retrospective controlled study and review, *Rev. Infect. Dis.*, 12, 788, 1990.

284. Gogos, C. A., Bassaris, H. P., and Vagenakis, A. G., Varicella pneumonia in adults: a review of pulmonary manifestations, risk factors and treatment, *Respiration*, 59, 339, 1992.

285. Hunt, J. R., On herpetic inflammations of the geniculate ganglion: a new syndrome and its complications, *J. Nerv. Ment. Dis.*, 34, 73, 1907.

286. Crabtree, J. A., Herpes zoster oticus, *Laryngoscope*, 78, 1853, 1968.

287. Mair, I. W. S. and Flugsrud, L. B., Peripheral palsy and herpes zoster infection, *J. Laryngol. Otol.*, 90, 373, 1976.

288. Robillard, R. B., Hilsinger, R. L., Jr., and Adour, K. K., Ramsay Hunt facial paralysis: clinical analyses of 185 patients, *Otolaryngol. Head Neck Surg.*, 95, 292, 1986.

289. Uri, N., Greenberg, E., Meyer, W., and Kitzes-Cohen, R., Herpes zoster oticus: treatment with acyclovir, *Ann. Otol. Rhinol. Laryngol.*, 101, 161, 1992.

290. Adour, K. K., Otological complications of herpes zoster, *Ann. Neurol.*, 35, S62, 1994.

291. Wayman, D. M., Pham, H. N., Byl, F. M., and Adour, K. K., Audiological manifestations of Ramsay Hunt syndrome, *J. Laryngol. Otol.*, 104, 104, 1990.

292. Kanzaki, J., Electrodiagnostic findings in the early stages of Bell's palsy and Ramsay-Hunt's syndrome, *Acta Otolaryngol. Suppl. (Stockholm)*, 446, 42, 1988.

293. Ariyasu, L., Byl, F., Sprague, M. S., and Adour, K., The beneficial effect of methylprednisolone in acute vestibular vertigo, *Arch. Otolaryngol. Head Neck Surg.*, 116, 700, 1990.

294. Fleury, P., Basset, J. M., and Compere, J. F., Idiopathic facial paralysis and facial paralysis due to herpes zoster. Follow-up and therapeutic indications, *Rev. Laryngol. Otol. Rhinol. (Bordeaux)*, 99, 307, 1978.

295. Teverner, D., Electrodiagnosis in facial palsy, *Arch. Otolaryngol.*, 81, 470, 1965.

296. Payten, R. J. and Dawes, J. D. K., Herpes zoster of the head and neck, *J. Laryngol. Otol.*, 86, 1031, 1972.

297. Dickins, J. R. E., Smith, J. T., and Graham, S. S., Herpes zoster oticus: treatment with intravenous acyclovir, *Laryngoscope*, 98, 776, 1988.

298. Stafford, F. W. and Welch, A. R., The use of acyclovir in Ramsay Hunt syndrome, *J. Laryngol. Otol.*, 100, 337, 1986.

299. Neoh, C., Harding, S. P., Saunders, D., Wallis, S., Tullo, A. B., Nylander, A., and Nelson, M. E., Comparison of topical and oral acyclovir in early herpes zoster ophthalmicus, *Eye*, 8, 688, 1994.

300. Aylward, G. W., Claoué, C. M. P., Marsh, R. J., and Yasseem, N., Influence of oral acyclovir on ocular complications of herpes zoster ophthalmicus, *Eye*, 8, 70, 1994.

301. Womack, L. W. and Leisegang, T. J., Complications of herpes zoster ophthalmicus, *Arch. Ophthalmol.*, 101, 42, 1983.

302. Karbassi, M., Raizman, M. B., and Schuman, J. S., Herpes zoster ophthalmicus, *Surv. Ophthalmol.*, 36, 395, 1992.

303. Harding, S. P., Lipton, J. R., and Wells, J. C. D., Natural history of herpes zoster ophthalmicus: predictors of postherpetic neuralgia and ocular involvement, *Br. J. Ophthalmol.*, 71, 353, 1987.

304. Mader, T. H. and Stulting, R. D., Viral keratitis, *Infect. Dis. Clin. North Am.*, 6, 831, 1992.

305. Harding, S. P., Lipton, J. R., and Wells, J. C. D., Natural history of herpes zoster ophthalmicus, predictors of postherpetic neuralgia and ocular involvement, *Br. J. Ophthalmol.*, 71, 353, 1986.

306. Scheie, H. G., Herpes zoster ophthalmicus, *Trans. Ophthalmol. Soc. U.K.*, 90, 899, 1970.

307. Leisegang, T. J., Corneal complications from herpes zoster ophthalmicus, *Ophthalmology*, 92, 316, 1985.

308. Marsh, R. J. and Cooper, M., Ophthalmic herpes zoster, *Eye*, 7, 350, 1993.

309. Hope-Simpson, R. E., Postherpetic neuralgia, *J. R. Coll. Gen. Pract.*, 25, 571, 1975.

310. Burgoon, C. F., Burgoon, J. S., and Baldridge, G. D., The natural history of herpes zoster, *JAMA*, 164, 265, 1957.

311. Brown, G. R., Herpes zoster: correlation of age, sex distribution, neuralgia and associated disorders, *South. Med. J.*, 69, 576, 1976.

312. de Moragas, J. M. and Kierland, R. R., The outcome of patients with herpes zoster ophthalmicus, *Arch. Dermatol.*, 75, 193, 1957.

313. Yoser, S. L., Forster, D. J., and Rao, N. A., Systemic viral infections and their retinal and choroidal manifestations, *Surv. Ophthalmol.*, 37, 313, 1993.

314. Harding, S. P., Management of ophthalmic zoster, *J. Med. Virol. Suppl.*, 1, 97, 1993.

315. McGill, J. and Chapman, C. A., A comparison of topical acyclovir with steroids in the treatment of herpes zoster keratouveitis, *Br. J. Ophthalmol.*, 67, 746, 1983.

316. Marsh, R. J. and Cooper, M., Double-masked trial of topical acyclovir and steroids in the treatment of herpes zoster ocular inflammations, *Br. J. Ophthalmol.*, 75, 542, 1991.

317. Bridgen, D., Foule, A., and Rosling, A., Acyclovir, a new antiherpetic drug: early experience in man with systemically administered drug, in *Developments in Antiviral Therapy*, Collier, L. H. and Oxford, J., Eds., Academic Press, London, 1980, 53.

318. Biron, K. K. and Elion, G. B., *In vitro* susceptibility of varicella zoster virus to acyclovir, *Antimicrob. Agents Chemother.*, 18, 443, 1980.

319. Crumpacker, C. S., Schnipper, L. E., Zaia, J. A., and Levin, H. J., Growth inhibition by acycloguanosine of herpesvirus isolated from human infections, *Antimicrob. Agents Chemother.*, 15, 642, 1979.

320. Poirier, R. H., Kingham, J. D., de Miranda, P., and Annel, M., Intraocular antiviral penetration, *Arch. Ophthalmol.*, 100, 1964, 1982.

321. Netland, P. A., Zicrhut, M., and Raizman, M. B., Posttraumatic herpes zoster ophthalmicus as a presenting sign of human immunodeficiency virus infection, *Ann. Ophthalmol.*, 25, 14, 1993.

322. Sandor, E. V., Millman, A., Croxson, T. S., and Mildvan, D., Herpes zoster ophthalmicus in patients at risk for the acquired immune deficiency syndrome (AIDS), *Am. J. Ophthalmol.*, 101, 153, 1986.

323. Cole, E. L., Meisler, D. M., Calabrese, L. H., Holland, G. N., Mondino, B. J., and Conant, M. A., Herpes zoster ophthalmicus and acquired immune deficiency syndrome, *Arch. Ophthalmol.*, 102, 1027, 1984.

324. Lewallen, S., Herpes zoster ophthalmicus in Malawi, *Ophthalmology*, 101, 1801, 1994.

325. Rosencrance, G., Herpes zoster, *N. Engl. J. Med.*, 330, 906, 1994.

326. Harris, D. J., Jr., Trifluridine for herpes zoster, *N. Engl. J. Med.*, 331, 481, 1994.

327. Cobo, L. M., Foulks, G. N., Leisegang, T., Lass, J., Sutphin, J. E., Wilhelmus, K., Jones, D. B., Chapman, S., Segretti, A. C., and King, D. H., Oral acyclovir in the treatment of acute herpes zoster ophthalmicus, *Ophthalmology*, 93, 763, 1986.

328. Harding, S. P. and Porter, S. M., Oral acyclovir in herpes zoster ophthalmicus, *Curr. Eye Res.*, 10, 177, 1991.

329. Urayama, A., Yamada, N., and Sasaki, T., Unilateral acute uveitis with retinal periarteritis and detachment, *Jpn. J. Clin. Ophthalmol.*, 25, 607, 1971.

330. Duker, J. S. and Blumenkranz, M. S., Diagnosis and management of the acute retinal necrosis (ARN) syndrome, *Surv. Ophthalmol.*, 35, 327, 1991.

331. Blumenkranz, M. S., Culbertson, W. W., Clarkson, J. G., and Dix, R., Treatment of the acute retinal necrosis syndrome with intravenous acyclovir, *Ophthalmology*, 93, 296, 1986.

332. Chess, J. and Marcus, D. M., Zoster-related bilateral acute retinal necrosis syndrome as presenting sign in AIDS, *Ann. Ophthalmol.*, 20, 431, 1988.

333. Freeman, W. R., Thomas, E. L., Rao, N. A., Pepose, J. S., Trousdale, M. D., Howes, E. L., Nadel, A. J., Mines, J. A., and Bowe, B., Demonstration of herpes group virus in acute retinal necrosis syndrome, *Am. J. Ophthalmol.*, 102, 701, 1986.

334. Jabs, D. A., Schachat, A. P., Liss, R., Knox, D. L., and Michels, R. G., Presumed varicella zoster retinitis in immunocompromised patients, *Retina*, 7, 9, 1987.

335. Ludvig, I. H., Zegarra, H., and Zakov, Z. N., The acute retinal necrosis syndrome. Possible herpes simplex retinitis, *Ophthalmology*, 91, 1659, 1984.

336. Matsuo, T., Nakayama, T., Matsuo, N., and Koide, N., Immunological studies of uveitis. I. Immune complex containing herpes virus antigens in four patients with acute retinal necrosis syndrome, *Jpn. J. Ophthalmol.*, 30, 472, 1986.

337. Peyman, G. A., Goldberg, M. F., Uninsky, E., Tessler, H., Pulido, J., and Hendricks, R., Vitrectomy and intravitreal antiviral drug therapy in acute retinal necrosis syndrome: report of two cases, *Arch. Ophthalmol.*, 102, 1618, 1984.

338. Rabinovitch, T., Nozik, R. A., and Verenhorst, M. P., Bilateral acute retinal necrosis syndrome, *Am. J. Ophthalmol.*, 108, 735, 1989.

339. Reese, L., Sheu, M. M., Lee, F., Kaplan, H. J., and Nahmias, A., Intraocular antibody production suggests herpes zoster is only one cause of acute retinal necrosis (ARN), *Invest. Ophthalmol. Vis. Sci.*, 27(Suppl.), 12, 1986.

340. Willerson, D., Jr., Aaberg, T. M., and Reeser, F. H., Necrotizing vaso-occlusive retinitis, *Am. J. Ophthalmol.*, 84, 209, 1977.

341. Johnson, W. H., Holland, G. N., Engstrom, R. E., Jr., and Rimmer, S., Recurrence of presumed varicella-zoster virus retinopathy in patients with acquired immunodeficiency syndrome, *Am. J. Ophthalmol.*, 116, 42, 1993.

342. Forster, D. J., Dugel, P. U., Frangieh, G. T., Liggett, P. E., and Rao, N. A., Rapidly progressive outer necrosis in the acquired immunodeficiency syndrome, *Am. J. Ophthalmol.*, 110, 341, 1990.

343. Margolis, T. P., Lowder, C. Y., Holland, G. N., Spaide, R. F., Logan, A. G., Weissman, S. S., Irvine, A. R., Josephberg, R., Meisler, D. M., and O'Donnell, J. J., Varizella-zoster virus retinitis in patients with the acquired immunodeficiency syndrome, *Am. J. Ophthalmol.*, 112, 119, 1991.

344. Schulman, J. A. and Peyman, G. A., Management of viral retinitis, *Ophthal. Surg.*, 19, 876, 1988.

345. Engstrom, R. E., Holland, G. N., Margolis, T. P., Muccioli, C., Lindley, J. I., Belfort, R., Jr., Holland, S. P., Johnstone, W. H., Wolitz, R. A., and Kreiger, A. E., The progressive outer retinal necrosis syndrome. A variant of necrotizing herpetic retinopathy in patients with AIDS, *Ophthalmology*, 101, 1488, 1994.

346. Morley, M. G., Duker, J. S., and Zacks, C., Successful treatment of rapidly progressive outer retinal necrosis in the acquired immunodeficency syndrome, *Am. J. Ophthalmol.*, 117, 264, 1994.

347. Laby, D. M., Nasrallah, F. P., Butrus, S. I., and Whitmore, P. V., Treatment of outer retinal necrosis in AIDS patients, *Graefes Arch. Clin. Exp. Ophthalmol.*, 231, 271, 1993.

348. Friedman, S. M., Margo, C. E., and Connelly, B. L., Varicella-zoster virus retinitis as the initial manifestation of the acquired immunodeficiency syndrome, *Am. J. Ophthalmol.*, 117, 536, 1994.

349. Kuppermann, B. D., Quiceno, J. I., Wiley, C., Hesselink, J., Hamilton, R., Keefe, K., Garcia, R., and Freeman, W. R., Clinical and histological study of varicella zoster virus retinitis in patients with the acquired immunodeficiency syndrome, *Am. J. Ophthalmol.*, 118, 589, 1994.

350. Gray, F., Mohr, M., Rozenberg, F., Belec, L., Lescs, M. C., Dournon, E., Sinclair, E., and Scaravilli, F., Varicella-zoster virus encephalitis in acquired immunodeficiency syndrome: report of four cases, *Neuropathol. Appl. Neurobiol.*, 18, 502, 1992.

351. Teich, S. A., Cheung, T. W., and Friedman, A. H., Systemic antiviral drugs used in ophthalmology, *Surv. Ophthalol.*, 37, 19, 1992.

352. Johnston W. H., Holland, G. N., Engstrom, R. E., and Rimmer, S., Recurrence of presumed varicella-zoster virus retinopathy in patients with acquired immunodeficiency syndrome, *Am. J. Ophthalmol.*, 116, 42, 1993.

353. Pinnolis, M. K., Foxworthy, D., and Kemp, B., Treatment of progressive outer retinal necrosis with sorivudine, *Am. J. Ophthalmol.*, 119, 516, 1995.

354. Moses, A. M. and Streeten, D. H. P., Disorders of neurohypophysis, in *Harrison's Principles of Internal Medicine*, 12th ed., Wilson, J. D., Braunwald, E., Isselbacher, K. J., Petersdorf, R. G., Martin, J. B., Fauci, A. S., and Root, R. K., Eds., McGraw-Hill, New York, 1991, 1682.

355. Ramos, E., Timmons, R. F., and Schimpff, S. C., Inappropriate antidiuretic hormone following adenine arabinoside administration, *Antimicrob. Agents Chemother.*, 15, 142, 1979.

356. White, T. M., Hoffman, J. H., Holmes, W. H., and Huntly, R. G., Disseminated herpes zoster and the syndrome of inappropriate antidiuretic hormone, *Conn. Med.*, 46, 373, 1982.

357. Maze, S. S., Klaff, L. J., and Yach, D., Syndrome of inappropriate antidiuretic hormone secretion in association with herpes zoster of the chest wall, *S. Afr. Med. J.*, 63, 735, 1983.

358. Ingraham, I. E., Jr., Estes, M. N. A., Bern, M. M., and De Girolami, P. C., Disseminated varicella-zoster virus infection with the syndrome of inappropriate antidiuretic hormone, *Arch. Intern. Med.*, 143, 1270, 1983.

359. Kageyama, Y., Nakamura, M., Sato, A., Sato, M., Nakayama, S., Komatsuzaki, O., and Fukuda, H., Syndrome of inappropriate antidiuretic hormone (SIADH) associated with Ramsay Hunt syndrome: report of a case and review of the literature, *Jpn. J. Med.*, 28, 219, 1989.

360. Gabriele, G. and Raimondi, A., Probabile sindrome da inappropriata secrezione di ADH in varicella, *Pediatr. Med. Chir.*, 12, 57, 1990.

361. Strauss, K. W., Endocrine complications of AIDS, *Arch. Intern. Med.*, 151, 1441, 1991.

362. Arzuaga, J. A., Estirado, E., Roman, F., Perez-Maestu, R., Masa, C., and de Letona, J. M., Syndrome of inappropriate antidiuretic hormone secretion and herpes zoster infection. I. Report of this association in a patient suffering from AIDS, *Nephron*, 68, 262, 1994.

363. Hoen, J. B., Tallot, B., May, Th., Amiel, C., Gérard, A., Dureux, J. B., and Canton, Ph., Hyponatrémie au cours du SIDA. Etiologie et diagnostic, *Presse Med.*, 22, 1028, 1991.

364. Elliott, K. J., Other neurological complications of herpes zoster and their management, *Ann. Neurol.*, 35(Suppl.), S57, 1994.

365. Hope-Simpson, R. E., The nature of herpes zoster: a long term study and a new hypothesis, *Proc. R. Soc. Med.*, 58, 9, 1965.

366. Ragozzino, M. W., Melton, L. J. III, Kurland, L. T., Chu, C. P., and Perry, H. O., Population-based study of herpes zoster and its sequelae, *Medicine (Baltimore)*, 61, 310, 1982.

367. Bennett, G. J., Hypotheses on the pathogenesis of herpes zoster-associated pain, *Ann. Neurol.*, 35, 538, 1994.

368. Woolf, C. J., Recent advances in the pathophysiology of acute pain, *Br. J. Anaesth.*, 63, 139, 1989.

369. Asbury, A. K. and Fields, H. L., Pain due to peripheral nerve damage: a hypothesis, *Neurology*, 34, 1587, 1984.

370. Watson, C. P. N. and Deck, J. H., The neuropathology of herpes zoster with particular reference to postherpetic neuralgia and its pathogenesis, in *Herpes Zoster and Postherpetic Neuralgia. Pain Research and Clinical Management*, Vol. 8, Watson, C. P. N., Ed., Elsevier, Amsterdam, 1993, 139.

371. Rowbotham, M. C. and Fields, H. L., Post-herpetic neuralgia: the relation of pain complaint, sensory disturbance, and skin temperature, *Pain*, 39, 129, 1989.

372. Tal, M. and Bennett, G. J., Extra-territorial pain in rats with a peripheral mononeuropathy: mechano-hyperalgesia and mechano-allodynia in the territory of an uninjured nerve, *Pain*, 57, 375, 1994.

373. Woolf, C. J. and Thompson, S. W. N., The induction and maintenance of central sensitization is dependent on *N*-methyl-D-aspartic acid receptor activation: implication for the treatment of post-injury pain hypersensitivity states, *Pain*, 44, 293, 1991.

374. Bennett, G. J., Evidence from animal models on the pathogenesis of painful peripheral neuropathy: relevance for pharmacotherapy, in *Towards a New Pharmacotherapy of Pain. Report of the Dahlem Workshop, Berlin 1989*, Basbaum, A. I. and Besson, J. M., Eds., John Wiley & Sons, Chichester, 1991, 365.

375. Bowsher, D., Post-herpetic neuralgia in older patients: incidence and optimal treatment, *Drugs Aging*, 5, 411, 1994.

376. Watson, C. N., Postherpetic neuralgia, *Eur. J. Pain*, 15, 3, 1994.

377. Wood, H., Herpes zoster ophthalmicus complicated by persistent neuritis, *Am. J. Ophthalmol.*, 12, 759, 1929.

378. Coldin, A., Treatment of pain. Organization of a pain clinic: treatment of acute herpes zoster, *Proc. R. Soc. Med.*, 66, 541, 1971.

379. Dan, K., Higa, K., and Noda, B., in *Advances in Pain Research and Therapy*, Vol. 9, Fields, H., Dubner, R., and Cervero, F., Eds., Raven Press, New York, 1985, 831.

380. Riopelle, J. M., Naraghi, M., and Grush, K., Chronic neuralgia incidence following local anesthetic therapy for herpes zoster, *Arch. Dermatol.*, 120, 747, 1984.

381. Shanbrom, E., Treatment of herpetic pain and postherpetic neuralgia with intravenous procain, *JAMA*, 176, 1041, 1961.

382. Secunda, L., Wolf, W., and Price, J., Herpes zoster: local anesthesia in the treatment of pain, *N. Engl. J. Med.*, 224, 501, 1961.

383. Riopelle, J. M., Naraghi, M., and Grush, K. P., Chronic neuralgia incidence following local anesthetic therapy for herpes zoster, *Arch. Dermatol.*, 120, 747, 1984.

384. Bonica, J. J., *The Management of Pain*, 2nd ed., Lea and Febiger, Philadelphia, 1990, 257.

385. Swerdlow, M., Complications of local anesthetic neural blockade, in *Neural Blockade in Clinical Anesthesia and Management of Pain*, Cousins, M. J. and Bridenbaugh, P. O., Eds., J. B. Lippincott, Philadelphia, 1980, 526.

386. Rowbotham, M. C., Davies, P. S., and Fields, H. L., Topical lidocaine gel relieves postherpetic neuralgia, *Ann. Neurol.*, 37, 246, 1995.

387. Stow, P. J., Glynn, C. J., and Minor, B., EMLA cream in the treatment of post-herpetic neuralgia: efficacy and pharmacokinetic profile, *Pain*, 39, 301, 1989.

388. Kissin, I., McDanal, J., and Xavier, A. V., Topical lidocaine for relief of post-herpetic neuralgia, *Neurology*, 39, 1132, 1989.

389. Dalili, H. and Adriani, J., The efficacy of local anesthetics in blocking the sensations of itch, burning, and pain in normal and "sunburned" skin, *Clin. Pharmacol. Ther.*, 12, 913, 1971.

390. Niamtu, J. III, Campbell, R. L., and Garrett, M. S., The anesthetic skin patch for topical anesthesia, *J. Oral Maxillofac. Surg.*, 42, 839, 1984.

391. Ehrenstrom, G. M. E. and Reiz, S. L. A., EMLA — a eutectic mixture of local anesthetics for topical anesthesia, *Acta Anaesthesiol. Scand.*, 26, 596, 1982.

392. Evers, H., VonDardel, O., Johlin, L., Ohlsén, L., and Vinnars, E., Dermal effects of compositions based on the eutectic mixture of lignocaine and prilocaine (EMLA), *Br. J. Anaesth.*, 57, 997, 1985.

393. Hallen, B., Olsson, G. L., and Uppfeldt, A., Pain-free venipuncture, *Anaesthesia*, 39, 969, 1984.

394. Lahteenmaki, T., Lillieborg, M., Ohlsén, L., Olenius, M., and Strömbeck, J. O., Topical analgesia for the cutting of split-skin grafts: a multicenter comparison of two doses of a lidocaine/prilocaine cream, *Plast. Reconstr. Surg.*, 82, 458, 1988.

395. Wheeler, J. G., EMLA cream and herpetic neuralgia, *Med. J. Aust.*, 154, 781, 1991.

396. Riopelle, J. M., Naraghi, M., and Lopez-Anaya, A., Treatment of severe skin pain and allodynia in acute herpes zoster using topical 4.5% lidocaine (base) in petrolatum: report of a case, *L.A. Soc. Anesthesiol. Newslett.*, 1, 6, 1992.

397. Riopelle, J. M., Lopez-Anaya, A., Heitler, D., Hood, K. T., McKenzie, G., Dunston, A., Eyrich, J., Heaton, J., and Naraghi, M., Topical percutaneous local anesthesia: a year of experience using lidocaine and tetracaine (amethocaine) ointments, *Reg. Anesth.*, 18(Suppl.), 11, 1993.

398. Riopelle, J., Lopez-Anaya, A., Cork, R. C., Heitler, D., Eyrich, J., Dunston, A., Riopelle, A. J., Johnson, W., Ragan, A., and Naraghi, M., Treatment of the cutaneous pain of acute herpes zoster with 9% lidocaine (base) in petrolatum/paraffin ointment, *J. Am. Acad. Dermatol.*, 30, 757, 1994.

399. Fitzgerald, M., Capsaicin and sensory neurons — a review, *Pain*, 15, 109, 1983.

400. Jessell, T. M., Iversen, L. L., and Cuello, A. C., Capsaicin-induced depletion of substance P from primary sensory neurons, *Brain Res.*, 152, 183, 1978.

401. Yaksh, T. L., Farb, D. H., Leeman, S. E., and Jessell, T. M., Intrathecal capsaicin depletes substance P in the rat spinal cord and produces thermal analgesia, *Science*, 206, 481, 1979.

402. Hökfelt, T., Kellerth, J. O., Nilsson, G., and Pernow, B., Substance P: localization in the central nervous system and in some primary sensory neurons, *Science*, 190, 889, 1975.

403. Hökfelt, T., Johansson, O., Ljundahl, A., Lundberg, J. M., and Schultzberg, M., Peptidergic neurones, *Nature*, 284, 515, 1980.

404. Jessell, T. M., Neurotransmitters and CNS disease. Pain, *Lancet*, 2, 1084, 1982.

405. Theriault, E., Otsuka, M., and Jessell, T., Capsaicin-evoked release of substance P from primary sensory neurons, *Brain Res.*, 170, 209, 1979.

406. Bernstein, J. E., Capsaicin in dermatologic disease, *Semin. Dermatol.*, 17, 304, 1988.

407. Bernstein, J. E., Bickers, D. R., Dahl, M. V., and Roshal, J. Y., Treatment of chronic postherpetic neuralgia with topical capsaicin, *J. Am. Acad. Dermatol.*, 17, 93, 1987.

408. Bernstein, J. E., Korman, N. J., Bickers, D. R., Dahl, M. V., and Millikan, L. E., Topical capsaicin treatment of chronic postherpetic neuralgia, *J. Am. Acad. Dermatol.*, 21, 265, 1989.

409. Watson, C. P. N., Tyler, K. L., Bickers, D. R., Millikan, L. E., Smith, S., and Coleman, E., A randomized vehicle-controlled trial of topical capsaicin in the treatment of postherpetic neuralgia, *Clin. Ther.*, 15, 510, 1993.

410. Watson, C. P. N., Evans, R. J., and Watt, V. R., Postherpetic neuralgia and topical capsaicin, *Pain*, 33, 333, 1988.

411. Peikert, A., Hentrich, M., and Ochs, G., Topical 0.025% capsaicin in postherpetic neuralgia: efficacy, predictors of response and long-term course, *J. Neurol.*, 238, 452, 1991.

412. Coniam, S. W. and Hunton, J., A study of benzydamine cream in post-herpetic neuralgia, *Res. Clin. Forums*, 10, 65, 1988.

413. King, R. B., Concerning the management of pain associated with herpes zoster and postherpetic neuralgia, *Pain*, 33, 73, 1988.

414. King, R. B., Topical aspirin in chloroform and the relief of pain due to herpes zoster and postherpetic neuralgia, *Ann. Neurol.*, 50, 1046, 1993.

415. De Benedittis, G., Besana, F., and Lorenzetti, A., A new topical treatment for acute herpetic neuralgia and post-herpetic neuralgia: the aspirin/diethyl ether mixture. An open-label study plus a double-blind controlled clinical trial, *Pain*, 48, 383, 1992.

416. Bowsher, D. and Gill, H., Aspirin-in-chloroform for the topical treatment of postherpetic neuralgia: a double-blind trial, *J. Pain Soc.*, 9, 16, 1991.

417. Morimoto, M., Inamori, K., and Hyodo, M., The effect of indomethacin stupe for post-herpetic neuralgia — particularly in comparison with chloroform-aspirin solution, *Pain*, 5(Suppl.), S59, 1990.

418. Nicholls, D. S. H., Treatment of postherpetic neuralgia with topical piroxicam gel, *N.Z. Med. J.*, 106, 233, 1993.

419. Jones, D., Post herpetic neuralgia, *N.Z. Med. J.*, 106, 296, 1993.

420. Max, M. B., Treatment of post-herpetic neuralgia: antidepressant, *Ann. Neurol.*, 35, S50, 1994.

421. Woodforde, J. M., Dwyer, B., McEwen, B. W., De Wilde, F.W., Bleasel, K., Connelley, T. J., and Ho, C. Y., The treatment of postherpetic neuralgia, *Med. J. Aust.*, 2, 869, 1965.

422. Watson, C. P., Evans, R. J., Reed, K., Merskey, H., Goldsmith, L., and Warsh, J., Aminotryptiline versus placebo in postherpetic neuralgia, *Neurology*, 32, 671, 1982.

423. Max, M. B., Schafer, S. C., Culnane, M., Smoller, B., Dubner, R., and Gracely, R. H., Aminotryptiline, but not lorazepam, relieves postherpetic neuralgia, *Neurology*, 38, 1427, 1988.

424. Watson, C. P. N. and Evans, R. J., A comparative trial of amitriptyline and zimelidine in post-herpetic neuralgia, *Pain*, 23, 387, 1985.

425. Watson, C. P. N., Chipman, M., Reed, K., Evans, R. J., and Birkett, N., Amitriptyline versus maprotiline in postherpetic neuralgia: a randomized, double-blind, crossover trial, *Pain*, 48, 29, 1992.

426. Kishore-Kumar, R., Max, M. B., Schafer, S. C., Gaughan, A. M., Smoller, B., Gracely, R. H., and Dubner, R., Desipramine relieves postherpetic neuralgia, *Clin. Pharmacol. Ther.*, 47, 305, 1990.
427. Ardid, D. and Guilbaud, G., Antinociceptive effects of acute and "chronic" injections of tricyclic antidepressant drugs in a new model of mononeuropathy in rats, *Pain*, 49, 279, 1992.
428. Hampf, G., Bowsher, D., and Nurmikko, T., Distigmine and amitryptiline in the treatment of chronic pain, *Anesth. Prog.*, 36, 58, 1989.
429. Woolner, E., Oral corticosteroids and postherpetic neuralgia, *Am. Family Phys.*, 48, 1384, 1993.
430. Dickinson, J. A., Should we treat herpes zoster with corticosteroid agents? *Med. J. Aust.*, 144, 378, 1986.
431. Benoldi, D., Mirizzi, S., Zucchi, A., and Allegra, F., Prevention of post-herpetic neuralgia. Evaluation of treatment with oral prednisone, oral acyclovir, and radiotherapy, *Int. J. Dermatol.*, 30, 288, 1991.
432. Esmann, V., Geil, J. P., Kroon, S., Fogh, H., Peterslund, N. A., Petersen, C. S., Petersen, C. S., Ronne-Rasmussen, J. O., and Danielsen, L., Prednisolone does not prevent post-herpetic neuralgia, *Lancet*, 2, 126, 1987.
433. Schmader, K. E. and Studenski, S., Are current therapies useful for the prevention of postherpetic neuralgia? A critical analysis of the literature, *J. Gen. Intern. Med.*, 4, 83, 1989.
434. Keczkes, K. and Basheer, A. M., Do corticosteroids prevent post-herpetic neuralgia? *Br. J. Dermatol.*, 102, 551, 1980.
435. Eaglstein, W. H., Katz, R., and Brown, J. A., The effects of early corticosteroid therapy on the skin eruption and pain of herpes zoster, *JAMA*, 211, 1681, 1970.
436. Elliott, F. A., Treatment of herpes zoster with high doses of prednisone, *Lancet*, 2, 610, 1964.
437. Arnold, H. A., Jr., Odom, R. B., and James, W. D., *Andrews' Diseases of the Skin: Clinical Dermatology*, 8th ed., W. B. Saunders, Philadelphia, 1990.
438. Habif, T. P., *Clinical Dermatology: a Color Guide to Diagnosis and Therapy*, 2nd ed., Mosby, St. Louis, 1990.
439. Soltz-Szots, J., Acyclovir-corticosteroid therapy in herpes zoster, *Hautarzt*, 37, 152, 1986.
440. Wood, M., Johnson, R. W., McKendrick, M. W., Taylor, J., Mandal, B. K., and Crooks, J., A randomized trial of acyclovir for 7 days or 21 days with and without prednisolone for treatment of acute herpes zoster, *N. Engl. J. Med.*, 330, 896, 1994.
441. Hoffmann, V., Coppejans, H., Vercauteren, M., and Adriansen, H., Successful treatment of postherpetic neuralgia with oral ketamine, *Clin. J. Pain*, 10, 240, 1994.
442. McKendrick, M. W., McGill, J. I., and Wood, M. J., Lack of effect of acyclovir on postherpetic neuralgia, *Br. J. Med.*, 298, 431, 1989.
443. Huff, J. C., Oral acyclovir therapy of acute herpes zoster: a multicenter study, *Res. Clin. Forums*, 9, 37, 1987.
444. Wassilew, S. W., Reimlinger, S., Nasemann, T., and Jones, D., Oral acyclovir for herpes zoster: a double blind controlled trial in normal subjects, *Br. J. Dermatol.*, 117, 495, 1987.
445. McKendrick, M. W., McGill, J. I., White, J. E., and Wood, M., Oral acyclovir in acute herpes zoster, *Br. Med. J.*, 293, 1529, 1986.
446. Harding, S. P. and Porter, S. M., Oral acyclovir in herpes zoster ophthalmicus, *Curr. Eye Res.*, 10(Suppl.), 17, 1991.
447. Juel-Jensen, B. E., Khan, J. A., and Pasvol, G., High-dose intravenous acyclovir in the treatment of zoster: a double-blind, placebo controlled trial, *J. Infect.*, 6(Suppl. 1), 31, 1983.
448. Malin, J.-P., A retrospective and an observational study with acyclovir, *J. Med. Virol. Suppl.*, 1, 102, 1993.
449. Huff, J. C., Drucker, J. L., Clemmer, A., Laskin, O. L., Connor, J. D., Bryson, Y. J., and Balfour, H. H., Jr., Effect of oral acyclovir on pain resolution in herpes zoster: a reanalysis, *J. Med. Virol. Suppl.*, 1, 93, 1993.
450. Tasker, R. R., Management of nociceptive, deafferentation and central pain by surgical intervention, in *Pain Syndromes in Neurology*, Fields, H. L., Ed., Butterworth, Stoneham, MA, 1990, 143.
451. Maruta, T., Swanson, D. W., and Finlayson, R. E., Drug abuse and dependency in patients with chronic pain, *Mayo Clin. Proc.*, 54, 241, 1979.
452. Taub, A., Opioid analgesics in the treatment of chronic intractable pain of non-neoplastic origin, in *Narcotic Analgesics in Anesthesiology*, Kitihata, L. M. and Collins, J. D., Eds., Williams and Wilkins, Baltimore, 1982, 199.

453. Porter, J. and Jick, H., Addiction rare in patients treated with narcotics, *N. Engl. J. Med.*, 302, 123, 1980.

454. Turk, D. C. and Brody, M. C., Chronic opioid therapy for persistent noncancer pain: panacea or oxymoron? *Am. Pain Soc. Bull.*, 1, 1, 1991.

455. Portenoy, R. K. and Foley, K. M., Chronic use of opioid analgesics in non-malignant pain: report of 38 cases, *Pain*, 25, 171, 1986.

456. Zenz, M., Strumpf, M., and Tryba, M., Long-term opioid therapy in patients with non-malignant pain, *J. Pain Symptom Manag.*, 7, 68, 1992.

457. Urban, B. J., France, R. D., Steinberger, D. L., Scott, D. L., and Maltbie, A. A., Long-term use of narcotic/antidepressant medication in the management of phantom limb pain, *Pain*, 24, 191, 1986.

458. Watson, C. P. N., Evans, R. J., Watt, V. R., and Birkett, N., Postherpetic neuralgia: 208 cases, *Pain*, 35, 289, 1988.

459. Rowbotham, M. C., Reisner-Keller, L. A., and Fields, H. L., Both intravenous lidocaine and morphine reduce the pain of postherpetic neuralgia, *Neurology*, 41, 1024, 1991.

460. Pappagallo, M. and Campbell, J. N., Chronic opioid therapy as alternative treatment for post-herpetic neuralgia, *Ann. Neurol.*, 35, S54, 1994.

461. Rowbotham, M. C., Managing post-herpetic neuralgia with opioids and local anesthetics, *Ann. Neurol.*, 35, S46, 1994.

462. Masur, M. H. and Dolin, R., Herpes zoster at the NIH: a 20 year experience, *Am. J. Med.*, 65, 738, 1978.

463. Arvin, A. M., Clinical manifestations of varicella and herpes zoster and the immune response to varicella-zoster virus, in *Natural History of Varicella-Zoster Virus*, Hyman, R. W., Ed., CRC Press, Boca Raton, FL, 1987, 67.

464. Jemsek, J., Greenberg, S. B., Taber, L., Harvey, D., Gershon, A., and Couch, R. B., Herpes zoster associated encephalitis: clinicopathologic report of 12 cases and review of the literature, *Medicine (Baltimore)*, 62, 81, 1983.

465. Gilden, D. H., Murray, R. S., Wellish, M., Kleinschmidt-DeMasters, B. K., and Vafai, A., Chronic progressive varicella zoster virus encephalitis in an AIDS patient, *Neurology*, 38, 1150, 1988.

466. Morgello, S., Block, G. A., Price, R. W., and Petito, C. K., Varicella- zoster virus leukocncephalitis and cerebral vasculopathy, *Arch. Pathol. Lab. Med.*, 112, 173, 1988.

467. McCormick, W. F., Rodnitzky, R. L., Schochet, S. S., and McKee, A. P., Varicella-zoster encephalomyelitis, *Arch. Neurol.*, 21, 559, 1969.

468. Carmack, M. A., Twiss, J., Enzmann, D. R., Amylon, M. D., and Arvin, A. M., Multifocal leukoencephalitis caused by varicella-zoster virus in a child with leukemia: successful treatment with acyclovir, *Pediatr. Infect. Dis. J.*, 12, 402, 1993.

469. Steele, R. W., Keeney, R. E., Bradsher, R. W., Moses, E. B., and Soloff, B. L., Treatment of varicella-zoster meningoencephalitis with acyclovir — demonstration of virus in cerebrospinal fluid by electron microscopy, *Am. J. Clin. Pathol.*, 80, 57, 1983.

470. Johns, D. R. and Gress, D. R., Rapid response to acyclovir in herpes zoster-associated encephalitis, *Am. J. Med.*, 82, 560, 1987.

471. Devinsky, O., Cho, E.-S., Petito, C. K., and Price, R. W., Herpes zoster myelitis, *Brain*, 114, 1181, 1991.

472. Hogan, E. L. and Krigman, M. R., Herpes zoster myelitis: evidence for viral invasion of spinal cord, *Arch. Neurol.*, 29, 309, 1973.

473. Muder, R. R., Lumish, R. M., and Corsello, G. R., Myelopathy after herpes zoster, *Arch. Neurol.*, 40, 445, 1983.

474. Baethge, B. A., King, J. W., Husain, F., and Embree, L. J., Case report: herpes zoster myelitis occurring during treatment for systemic lupus erythematosus, *Am. J. Med. Sci.*, 298, 264, 1989.

475. Friedman, D. P., Herpes zoster myelitis: MR appearance, *AJNR Am. J. Neuroradiol.*, 13, 1404, 1992.

476. Corston, R. N., Logsdail, S., and Godwin-Austen, R. B., Herpes-zoster myelitis treated successfully with vidarabine, *Br. Med. J.*, 283, 698, 1981.

477. Gilden, D. H., Beinlich, B. R., Rubinstein, E. M., Stommel, E., Swenson, R., Rubinsterin, D., and Mahalingam, R., Varicella-zoster virus myelitis: an expanding spectrum, *Neurology*, 44, 1818, 1994.

478. Gilden, D. H., Mahalingam, R., Dueland, A. N., and Cohrs, R., Herpes zoster: pathogenesis and latency, in *Progress in Medical Virology*, Vol. 39, Melnick, J. L., Ed., S. Karger, Basel, 1992, 19.

479. McAlpine, D., Kuroiwa, Y., Toyokura, Y., and Araki, S., Acute demyelinating disease complicating herpes zoster, *J. Neurol. Neurosurg. Psychiat.*, 22, 120, 1959.

480. O'Donnell, P. P., Pula, T. P., Sellman, M., and Camenga, L., Recurrent herpes zoster encephalitis. A complication of systemic lupus erythematosus, *Arch. Neurol.*, 38, 49, 1981.

481. Nakano, T., Awaki, E., Araga, S., Takai, H., Inoue, K., and Takahashi, K., Recurrent herpes zoster myelitis treated with human interferon alpha: a case report, *Acta Neurol. Scand.*, 85, 372, 1992.

482. Kanehisa, Y., Hokesu, Y., and Nagamatsu, K., Three cases of herpes zoster myelitis, *Clin. Neurol. (Jpn.)*, 22, 514, 1982.

483. Doyle, P. W., Gibson, G., and Dolman, C. L., Herpes zoster ophthalmicus with contralateral hemiplegia: identification of cause, *Ann. Neurol.*, 14, 84, 1983.

484. Reshef, E., Greenberg, S. B., and Jankovic, J., Herpes zoster ophthalmicus followed by contralateral hemiparesis: report of two cases and review of literature, *Neurol. Neurosurg. Psychiat.*, 48, 122, 1985.

485. Hilt, D. C., Buchholz, D., Krumholz, A., Weiss, H., and Wolinsky, J. S., Herpes zoster ophthalmicus and delayed contralateral hemiparesis caused by cerebral angiitis: diagnosis and management approaches, *Ann. Neurol.*, 14, 543, 1983.

486. Eidelberg, D., Sotrel, A., Horoupian, D. S., Neumann, P. E., Pumarola-Sune, T., and Price, R. W., Thrombotic cerebral vasculopathy associated with herpes zoster, *Ann. Neurol.*, 19, 7, 1986.

487. Thomas, J. E. and Howard, F. M., Segmental zoster paresis — a disease profile, *Neurology*, 22, 459, 1972.

488. Chang, C. M., Woo, E., Yu, Y. L., Huang, C. Y., and Chin, D., Herpes zoster and its neurological complications, *Postgrad. Med. J.*, 63, 85, 1987.

489. Marsh, R. J., Dulley, B., and Kelly, V., External ocular motor palsies in ophthalmic zoster: a review, *Br. J. Ophthalmol.*, 61, 677, 1977.

490. Edgerton, A. E., Herpes zoster ophthalmicus: report of cases and review of literature, *Arch. Ophthalmol.*, 34, 40, 1945.

491. McKendall, R. R. and Klawans, H. L., Nervous system complications of varicella-zoster virus, in *Handbook of Clinical Neurology*, Vol. 34, Vinken, P. J. and Bruyn, G. W., Eds., North Holland, Amsterdam, 1978, 161.

492. Lewis, G. W., Zoster sine herpete, *Br. Med. J.*, 2, 418, 1958.

493. Easton, H. G., Zoster sine herpete causing acute trigeminal neuralgia, *Lancet*, 2, 1065, 1970.

494. Gilden, D. H., Dueland, A. N., Cohrs, R., Martin, J. R., Kleinschmidt-DeMasters, B. K., and Mahalingam, R., Preherpetic neuralgia, *Neurology*, 41, 1215, 1991.

495. Mayo, D. R. and Booss, J., Varicella zoster-associated neurologic disease without skin lesions, *Arch. Neurol.*, 46, 313, 1989.

496. Martinez-Martin, P., Garcia-Saiz, A., Rapun, J. L., and Echevarria, J. M., Intrathecal synthesis of IgG antibodies to varicella-zoster virus in two cases of acute aseptic meningitis syndrome with no cutaneous lesions, *J. Med. Virol.*, 16, 201, 1985.

497. Echevarria, J. M., Martinez-Martin, P., Telléz, A., de Ory, F., Rapun, J. L., Bernal, A., Estévez, E., and Najera, R., Aseptic meningitis due to varicella-zoster virus: serum antibody levels and local synthesis of specific IgG, IgM and IgA, *J. Infect. Dis.*, 155, 959, 1987.

498. Dueland, A. N., Devlin, M., Martin, J. R., Mahalingam, R., Cohrs, R., Manz, H., Trombley, I., and Gilden, D., Fatal vericella-zoster virus meningoradiculitis without skin involvement, *Ann. Neurol.*, 29, 569, 1991.

499. Heller, H. M., Carnevale, N. T., and Steigbigel, R. T., Varicella zoster virus transverse myelitis without cutaneous rash, *Am. J. Med.*, 68, 550, 1990.

1.3 HERPES SIMPLEX VIRUS

1.3.1 INTRODUCTION

The herpesviruses (family Herpesviridae) are highly disseminated in nature. Herpesvirus hominis is the etiologic agent of herpes simplex in humans. Forty years after the isolation of the herpes simplex viruses (HSV), Schneweiss[1] established the existence of two serotypes, HSV-1 and HSV-2, currently designated under ICTV rules as human herpes viruses 1 and 2.[2] Type 1 infections are primarily nongenital (e.g., herpes labialis and ocular herpes), whereas type 2 infections are primarily genital (herpes genitales).

Since their discovery, nearly 100 herpesviruses have been, at least partially, characterized and six of them have been isolated from humans: HSV-1,[3-8] HSV-2,[3-5,8,9] human cytomegalovirus (HCMV),[10] varicella-zoster virus (VZV),[11-13] Epstein-Barr virus (EBV),[14,15] and human herpesvirus 6 (HHV6).[16,17] The virion architecture of a typical herpesvirus consists of: (1) a core containing a linear, double-stranded DNA; (2) an icosadeltahedral capsid, approximately 100 to 110 nm in diameter, and containing 162 capsomers with a hole running down the long axis; (3) an amorphous, sometimes asymmetric material surrounding the capsid and known as the tegument;[18] and (4) an envelope containing viral glycoprotein spikes on its surface.[3,4] The herpesviruses mature in the nucleus of the infected cell, where they induce the formation of a characteristic inclusion body; some also induce the formation of a cytoplasmic inclusion body. The reproductive cycle of host cells infected with herpesviruses undergoes major structural and biochemical changes that will ultimately lead to the destruction of the cells.

Prior to the emergence of the AIDS pandemic, chronic mucocutaneous HSV infections were seen primarily in patients with congenital cellular immune deficiencies, or acquired immune defects associated most often with lymphoproliferative malignancies[19-21] and organ transplantations.[19,21-26] Thus, 80% of marrow transplant recipients with antibody to HSV before transplantation have reactivated virus after the transplantation.[24,27] The absence of specific cellular immune response to HSV during the first month after the transplant significantly contributes to the severe, prolonged, and debilitating course of HSV disease.[27] Frequent reactivation also has been reported in renal transplant recipients,[28,29] and in patients receiving leukemic induction therapy.[30]

Currently, HIV-infected patients represent the major population affected by persistent active HSV infections.[31] Since asymptomatic shedding of HSV can continue despite clinically effective suppression with antiviral chemotherapy, the possibility of person-to-person transmission persists.[32]

Mucocutaneous HSV infections in immunocompromised patients may be much more severe than in normal subjects. The lesions tend to be more invasive, slower to heal, and associated with prolonged viral shedding.[33]

Since seropositivity for HSV is high in HIV-positive patients, it is very likely that clinical HSV disease is associated with reactivation of latent virus.[34] The most common clinical manifestations, usually identified with high morbidity and mortality rate, include orolabial, genital, and anorectal mucocutaneous lesions, esophagitis, and, less often, encephalitis. According to the Centers for Disease Control definition,[35] ulcerative HSV lesions that have been present for more than 1 month in an HIV-positive individual, or in persons with no other apparent cause of immunodeficiency, are considered an AIDS-defining condition.

Chronic perianal HSV lesions causing severe morbidity (pain, itching, and painful defecation), have been considered among the first opportunistic infections associated with AIDS in homosexual men.[36] The clinical manifestations of orolabial and genital HSV disease in HIV-infected patients (mild to severe tissue destructive lesions) are usually similar to that observed in other immuno-suppressed individuals.[34]

Cases of HSV-associated encephalitis in AIDS patients usually occur as complications of orolabial HSV infection. HSV encephalitis is a life-threatening condition with substantial morbidity and mortality despite the use of antiviral therapy.[37,38]

Although HSV disease affects primarily the upper respiratory tract, lower respiratory tract infections have also been reported.[39] In a study by Ramsey et al.,[40] mucocutaneous lesions antedated the pneumonia in 17 of 21 patients with HSV pneumonitis. HSV-associated pneumonitis has been diagnosed in immunocompromised patients,[41-44] alcoholic hepatitis,[45] burn victims,[46,47] and as a consequence of disseminated HSV infection in neonates.[48,49] While the majority of cases affected adults, HSV pneumonitis has also been described in children.[39,41,42,46,47,50-52]

1.3.2 HOST IMMUNE RESPONSE TO HERPES SIMPLEX VIRUS INFECTIONS

Experiments in animal models have provided most of the information with regard to the relationship between host defense and disease pathogenesis. Thus, host genetic background, macrophages, natural killer cells, specific T cell subpopulations, specific antibodies, and lymphokine responses have all been shown to play important roles in the host defense against HSV.[5]

Zweerink and Stanton[53] have demonstrated a direct relationship between the intensity of antibody response and both the severity of primary infection and the frequency of recurrence. Furthermore, the frequency of recurrences has been directly linked to the viability of cell-mediated responses. In numerous lymphocyte blastogenesis studies,[54-63] reactivity was demonstrated within 4 to 6 weeks after the onset of infection and sometimes as early as 2 weeks.

With regard to specific cytotoxic T cell responses, Thong et al.[64] have found that cytotoxic cells were depressed in patients having frequent recurrences. Similar observations have been made for natural killer cells.[5] Torseth et al.[65] have demonstrated that viral envelope glycoproteins may play a role in the establishment of cell-mediated immunity.

Lymphokine production has also been related to the pathogenesis of frequently recurrent genital and orolabial HSV infections — a decrease in the production of interferon-γ as well as natural killer cells during disease prodrome has been observed.[65-68]

Humoral responses to HSV infections involving IgM and IgG antibodies have also been well defined.[5,63,69] Kahlon and Whitley[69] made the interesting observation that antibodies to the gene responsible for initiating viral replication, ICP4, were not only reflective of the extent of viral replication, but also were predictive of long-term neurologic impairment.

Antibodies with complement, and antibodies mixed with killer lymphocytes, monocytes, macrophages, or polymorphonuclear leukocytes have been found to lyse HSV-infected cells *in vitro*.[70] In addition, antibody-dependent cell-mediated cytotoxicity has also been shown to play an important part in the development of host immunity to infection.[71]

1.3.3 EVOLUTION OF THERAPIES AND TREATMENT OF HERPES SIMPLEX VIRUS INFECTIONS

Vidarabine was the first antiviral agent used in the treatment of mucocutaneous HSV infections in immunocompromised hosts.[24,72] However, it proved to be relatively weak and was quickly displaced by acyclovir.

Currently, acyclovir is the most commonly prescribed medication for HSV infections.[73-77] Immunocompromised patients receiving acyclovir showed shorter duration of viral shedding and more rapid healing of lesions than patients given placebo.[76,78,79] The recommended oral dose for mild to moderate mucocutaneous disease is 200 mg, five times daily for 7 d. Higher dose regimens (400 to 800 mg, three to five times daily over a 10-d period) have also proven beneficial in more severe conditions (marrow transplant recipients).[33,74] The therapy should be initiated within 48 h of onset of rash. In more serious settings (bone marrow transplantation, HSV encephalitis, and viscerally disseminated HSV disease in immunocompromised patients)[80] or when absorption of oral drug is doubtful, intravenous acyclovir (5.0 to 10 mg/kg, every 8 h) for 7 to 10 d may be used in patients without renal insufficiency.[33,75]

Intravenous acyclovir (5% solution) is the most effective treatment for a first episode of genital herpes and results in a significant reduction of median duration of viral shedding, pain, and length of time to complete healing.[75,81,82] Treatment of mucocutaneous lesions should be continued until they have all crusted.[33] In a multicenter randomized, double-blind, placebo-controlled trial of 97 immunocompromised patients with mucocutaneous HSV infection conducted by Meyers et al.,[76] intravenous acyclovir significantly shortened the periods of virus shedding ($p < .0002$), lesion pain ($p < .01$), lesion scabbing ($p < .004$), and lesion healing ($p < .04$).

Oral therapy (200 mg, five times daily) is nearly as effective as intravenous infusions for initial episodes of genital herpes infections[83,84] and has become the standard treatment.[33] The use of oral acyclovir has not been associated with any hepatic, renal, or neurologic toxicity.[85]

Topically applied acyclovir (5% ointment) while reducing the duration of viral shedding and the length of time for lesions to crust, is less effective for genital HSV infections than the orally or intravenously administered drug.[86,87] Topical treatment of mucocutaneous HSV infections in normal subjects with vidarabine or other antiviral agents has been largely disappointing.[88-91]

In cases of orolabial herpes, despite promising results in early trials with 5% topical acyclovir,[92] subsequent studies showed no clinical benefit[93,94] because of the poor drug penetration to the site of viral replication. Current data do not support the use of topical acyclovir for orolabial herpes.[33] The recommended treatment is oral acyclovir at 200 mg, five times daily for 5 d. While this regimen did not diminish the pain and the time for complete healing, it still reduced the length of time to the loss of crusts by approximately 1 d (7 vs. 8 d).[95] In another trial, Spruance et al.[96] used increased dosing (400 mg, five times daily for 5 d) and initiated treatment during the prodromal or erythematous stages of infection — the duration of pain was reduced by 36% and the length of time to the loss of crust by 27%. Although, if started early after recurrence, oral acyclovir may be useful, it still cannot be recommended as a routine therapy for treating orolabial herpes.[33]

For HSV-associated encephalitis, administration of acyclovir at doses of 10 mg/kg, t.i.d., for 10 to 14 d reduced mortality at 3 months to 19%, as compared to nearly 50% in patients treated with vidarabine.[37] Moreover, 38% treated with acyclovir regained normal function. The therapy was most beneficial when initiated before the development of coma or semicoma.[33]

Acyclovir prophylaxis of HSV infections should be of clinical benefit in severely immuno-compromised patients, especially those undergoing induction chemotherapy or organ transplantation. Computer modeling has been used to test different dose schedules in order to determine the optimal total intravenous daily dose of acyclovir; dose regimens of 125 mg/m^2 every 6 h, and 62.5 mg/m^2 every 4 h were found to be highly effective as prophylactic therapy.[21] In a randomized, double-blind, controlled trial conducted in bone marrow transplant recipients, acyclovir prophylaxis (250 mg/m^2, IV every 8 h) was carried out for 18 d starting 3 d before transplantation — no patient given acyclovir developed HSV infection. By comparison, 7 of 10 patients receiving placebo developed HSV disease.[97] The recommended oral prophylaxis doses of acyclovir have been 400 mg every 4 to 8 h.[85]

Neither intravenous nor oral antiviral therapy of acute HSV infections reduced the frequency of recurrence.[75,82,84] It has been suggested that virus reactivation and antigen exposure is necessary to restore the specific immune response to HSV after organ transplantation.[27,28] To this end, acyclovir treatment may delay immune reconstitution by limiting the period of antigen exposure. In addition, acyclovir may also be directly immunosuppressive, as found by Levin et al.[98] for lymphocyte transformation responses *in vitro*; however, similar suppression was not found by Steele et al.[99] using higher concentrations of acyclovir.

Management of recurrent HSV disease may be carried out with low-dose suppressive therapy with oral acyclovir.[85,100] Doses of 200 mg, four times daily or 400 mg, b.i.d., appeared to be equally effective; in some patients, however, doses of 400 mg, four times daily (or 800 mg, b.i.d.) may be clinically necessary to control HSV recurrences.[80] Long-term oral administration of acyclovir effectively suppressed the recurrence of genital HSV infections.[101-103]

On average, intravenous or oral acyclovir reduced the incidence of symptomatic HSV infections from about 70% to 5–20%.[85,97,102,104] As demonstrated by Shepp et al.[105] in chronically immuno-compromised bone marrow transplant recipients, a sequential regimen of intravenous followed by oral acyclovir for 3 to 6 months can virtually eliminate symptomatic HSV disease. The two-part regimen included intravenous infusions of acyclovir (250 mg/m^2, b.i.d.) from 5 d before until 30 d after transplantation; on day 31, in a random and double-blind approach patients were assigned to receive either oral acyclovir (800 mg, b.i.d.) or an identical placebo until day 75 after transplantation.

The results demonstrated that the two-part sequential regimen was effective and convenient for extended prophylaxis of HSV infection following marrow transplantation and should be effective in other chronically immunosuppressed patients as well.[105]

Acyclovir treatment should usually be interrupted every 12 months to reassess the need for continued suppression.[106]

Vidarabine when applied intravenously has been shown to affect favorably the course of both HSV encephalitis[107] and neonatal HSV infection.[108] However, against HSV infection in immuno-compromised patients, vidarabine was inferior to acyclovir.[109] One explanation for the observed lack of potency is the need of a modicum of host immune response for efficacy[110] thus rendering the drug largely ineffective in severely immunocompromised patients. In addition, because of its low solubility vidarabine has required administration in large fluid volumes over 12 to 24-h periods, although this should be improved by using the more soluble monophosphate derivative. In several studies vidarabine was found to cause significant CNS toxicity in some patients.[111-114]

Tricot et al.[115] have used bromovinyldeoxyuridine (BVDU), a highly potent and selective anti-herpes agent, to treat an intercurrent mucocutaneous HSV infection in 14 severely immunosup-pressed patients. The drug was administered orally at daily doses of 7.5 mg/kg (divided over 3-4 doses a day) for 5 d. In all but two patients, BVDU arrested progression of the HSV disease within 1 to 2 d after beginning treatment. The results of this uncontrolled trial indicated that BVDU may be safe and effective for oral treatment of HSV type 1 infections.[115] The mechanism of action of BVDU to a large extent is similar to that of acyclovir. Initially, it is specifically phosphorylated by the virus-encoded thymidine kinase, which limits its further action to the virus-infected cell. In its 5′-triphosphate form, BVDU interacted with the DNA polymerase as either an inhibitor to cut off the DNA synthesis, or as a substrate which is incorporated selectively into the DNA of virus-infected cells.[116]

The primary mechanism of acyclovir resistance has been the induction of viral mutants defective or deficient of thymidine kinase, the viral-encoded enzyme, which catalyzes the rate-limiting step of triphosphorylation of acyclovir to its active form, acyclovir triphosphate (see Section 1.3.3.1 below). Foscarnet, a potent inhibitor of HSV DNA polymerases, does not require phosphorylation for its antiviral activity, thereby making it a potentially useful therapeutic agent against acyclovir-resistant HSV infections.

Foscarnet (trisodium phosphonoformate) is a pyrophosphate analog with activity *in vitro* against all human herpesviruses, as well as HIV.[117,118] In several clinical studies in AIDS patients with HSV infections that were refractory to acyclovir therapy, foscarnet proved to be efficacious and well tolerated.[119-128] Since its oral absorption is poor, foscarnet is usually administered intravenously to achieve adequate serum levels.[94]

In a controlled, randomized, dose-comparative trial in AIDS patients with acyclovir-resistant HSV infections, two regimens of foscarnet (40 mg/kg, administered every 8 or 12 h, respectively) have provided evidence supporting its safety and therapeutic efficacy, as well as its usefulness in maintenance therapy to delay recurrence of HSV lesions.[117] The analysis of data from this trial, however, was complicated by the extensive variability in the lesion size at initiation of therapy, making any statistically valid comparison of treatment regimens nearly impossible.

Acyclovir-resistant mucocutaneous HSV infections have been recognized with increasing frequency in AIDS patients. However, alternative therapies in this setting have not been widely studied, with the exception of foscarnet.[119-124] Safrin et al.[119] have conducted a study of 26 consecutive AIDS patients treated with foscarnet for mucocutaneous acyclovir-resistant HSV infections. The drug was administered parenterally over 1 to 2 h through either a peripheral or a central venous catheter. The initial dosage in patients who had normal creatinine clearance ranged from 40 to 60 mg/kg every 8 h and was serially adjusted according to calculated creatinine clearance as described previously.[129] Clinical response was noted in 81% of patients, with complete re-epithelialization of HSV lesions in 73%. Cessation of viral shedding was documented in all of the 11 patients who were recultured. Even though there were frequent adverse reactions to foscarnet (rise in serum creatinine levels to ≥3.0 mg/dl, decrease in the absolute number of polymorphonuclear leukocytes to ≤750 cells/mm^3, abnormal serum calcium and phosphorous levels), in only 3 patients (12%) did the observed toxicities necessitated discontinuation of therapy. Before the initiation of the foscarnet therapy, 14 of the patients who did receive vidarabine (10 to 20 mg/kg daily, for 4 to 21 d) failed to respond and therapy was ceased in 4 patients (29%) due to unwarranted toxicity.[119]

Chatis et al.[120] have described the use of foscarnet in a patient with AIDS and a severe HSV-2 mucocutaneous infection who did not respond to therapy with acyclovir, but healed completely after a 16-d course of intravenous foscarnet medication (50 mg/kg, t.i.d.). Again, the major side effect was the rise of the serum creatinine from 70 to 105 μM/l on day 15 of therapy, making necessary the lowering of the foscarnet dosage to 40 mg/kg, t.i.d. In addition, during the 16-d course of treatment, the serum phosphate level rose gradually from 1.1 to 1.7 mmol/l — this condition was treated with basic aluminum carbonate gel (Basaljel®). While the calcium concentration rose from 2.0 to 2.6 mmol/l, no specific treatment was given for this effect.[120]

In an open-labeled trial, four AIDS patients with severe progressive, ulcerative mucocutaneous lesions of the genitals, perineum, perianal region, or finger due to acyclovir resistant HSV-2, were successfully treated with intravenous foscarnet at 60 mg/kg, t.i.d., for 12 to 50 d (each infusion was given over 2 h).[122] Clinical findings revealed a significant clearing of mucocutaneous lesions and eradication of HSV from the mucosal surface. Two of the patients also received maintenance foscarnet therapy at 42 to 60 mg/kg daily, given for 5 to 7 d weekly.

An allogeneic bone marrow transplant recipient who acquired severe mucocutaneous HSV-1 infection during acyclovir prophylaxis, and subsequently failed to respond to high-dose acyclovir, was completely cured after a 16-d course of intravenous foscarnet at 40 mg/kg, t.i.d.[130]

The therapeutic efficacies of foscarnet and vidarabine have been compared in a randomized trial of 14 patients with AIDS and mucocutaneous HSV lesions that had been unresponsive to intravenous acyclovir therapy for a minimum of 10 d.[128] The patients were randomly assigned to receive intravenously either foscarnet (40 mg/kg, every 8 h) or vidarabine (15 mg/kg daily) for 10 to 42 d. The results have shown foscarnet to have superior efficacy and less frequent toxicity. Once the treatment was stopped, however, there were numerous cases of relapse.

Sall et al.[126] have described the successful treatment of progressive acyclovir-resistant orofacial HSV infection in an AIDS patient using intravenous foscarnet at 40 mg/kg three times daily — improvement was noted within 4 d. The patient completed 3 weeks of therapy without any clinical complications or abnormal laboratory values, and with complete re-epithelialization except for a residual peripheral crust.

The intermittent administration of foscarnet (every 8 h) usually produces peak and trough serum drug concentrations of 530 and 100 μM, respectively.[131] Excretion of the drug occurs solely by renal mechanisms, and with a serum half-life ranging between 0.7 and 4.8 h.[131,132] However, progressive impairment of renal functions can take place after its prolonged use, thereby making dosage adjustments essential in patients with renal dysfunction.[117,132]

1.3.3.1 Acyclovir-Resistant Herpes Simplex Virus

The incidence of acyclovir-resistant HSV in immunocompromised patients, while still relatively low, appears to be on the rise;[75,124,133-142] by one estimate only 4.7% of patients (7 of 148 immunocompromised patients but none in 59 immunocompetent patients).[143] In another study, Nugier et al.[144] detected resistance in 2.5% of HSV strains from more than 800 strains tested. While most acyclovir resistance has been reported among AIDS patients, some cases of lethal disseminated visceral HSV infections caused by acyclovir-resistant mutants have been described in bone marrow transplant recipients[145] and in one case of meningoencephalitis in an AIDS patient.[146] In bone marrow transplant recipients, acyclovir-resistant HSV isolates have been identified more frequently after therapeutic acyclovir administration than during prophylaxis.[134]

Acyclovir resistance is even less frequent in immunocompetent patients.[147-150] Erlich et al.[133]have reported the presence of acyclovir-resistant HSV in patients with AIDS. The major mechanism of resistance appeared to be a deficiency of viral thymidine kinase.[151-155] Contrary to early reports for reduced virulence,[156-157] thymidine kinase-deficient HSV not only maintains its virulence undiminished, but also has been shown capable of establishing latent infections.[133] Acyclovir-resistant isolates with mutation in the DNA polymerase have also been found in immuno-compromised patients.[151,152,158-162]

Treatment of severe, acyclovir-resistant HSV infections include continuous therapy with intravenous acyclovir, vidarabine, and foscarnet.[133,163-165] Foscarnet (trisodium phosphonoformate) is probably the most effective antiviral agent for treatment of acyclovir-resistant HSV infections.[128,166] Neither vidarabine nor foscarnet required activation of its active moiety by viral thymidine kinase.[167] Vidarabine (adenine arabinoside), a nucleoside analog, is phosphorylated by host-cell enzymes, whereas foscarnet is an active inhibitor of HSV DNA polymerase in its native form and does not require phosphorylation for antiviral activity.[167,168]

Since the oral absorption of foscarnet is poor, its intravenous infusion is the preferred route of administration in order to achieve adequate serum levels.[169] Intermittent administration of 60 mg/kg every 8 h (infused over a 2-h period) produced peak and through serum concentrations of 530 μM and 100 μM, respectively.[170] Foscarnet is excreted exclusively through the kidney with a serum half-life between 0.7 and 4.8 h.[132,170] Because a prolonged treatment with foscarnet may cause progressive impairment of renal functions, dosage adjustments would be necessary in patients with renal dysfunction.[132,169]

In an uncontrolled trial of AIDS patients with severe acyclovir-resistant HSV type 2 infection, Erlich et al.[164] administered foscarnet intravenously at 60 mg/kg every 8 h (with reduced dosage for renal impairment) for 12 to 50 d. All patients showed dramatic improvement in their clinical condition with a marked clearing of mucocutaneous lesions and eradication of HSV from mucosal surfaces. Chatis et al.[120] also observed complete healing of mucocutaneous lesions in an AIDS patient with severe HSV type 2 infection, following a 16-d course with intravenous foscarnet (50 mg/kg, t.i.d.). In another uncontrolled trial,[166] 21 of 26 AIDS patients (81%) with acyclovir-resistant HSV infection showed clinical response to foscarnet, with complete re-epithelialization of lesions occurring in 19 of those patients (73%). In the same study, the outcome of vidarabine therapy was also investigated. Even though HSV was found susceptible to vidarabine *in vitro*, there was clinical benefit observed in only 2 of 14 patients who received vidarabine, and toxicity required discontinuation of the drug in 4 patients. Safrin et al.[128] have compared foscarnet (40 mg/kg every 8 h) with vidarabine (15 mg/kg once daily) in 14 randomly selected AIDS patients with acyclovir-resistant HSV infections. Foscarnet was found to be more effective and less toxic; lesions healed in all eight patients receiving foscarnet compared with none of the six patients who received vidarabine. In addition, three of the patients given vidarabine showed neurologic abnormalities. However, HSV disease recurred in all patients following discontinuation of therapy.[128] Vinckier et al.[124] have also reported a beneficial clinical response to intravenous foscarnet in an immunocompromised patient with severe HSV infection.

HSV strains resistant to acyclovir by virtue of alteration in the substrate specificity of the thymidine kinase or the viral DNA polymerase, however, may develop concurrent resistance to either foscarnet or vidarabine.[162,171] Thus, in two studies by Birch et al.,[79,80] HSV strains resistant to both acyclovir and foscarnet have been described.

1.3.4 REFERENCES

1. Schneweiss, K. E., Serologische untersuchungen zur typendifferenzierung des herpesvirus hominis, *Z. Immuno-Forsch.*, 124, 24, 1962.
2. Roizman, B., Carmichael, L. E., Deinhardt, F., de-The, G., Nahmias, A. J., Plowright, W., Rapp, F., Sheldrick, P., Takahashi, M., and Wolf, K., Herpesviridae: definition, provisional nomenclature and taxonomy, *Intervirology*, 16, 201, 1981.

3. Roizman, B., Herpesviridae: a brief introduction, in *Fields Virology*, 2nd ed., Fields, B. N., Knipe, D. M., Chanock, R. M., Hirsch, M. S., Melnick, J. L., Monath, T. P., and Roizman, B., Eds., Raven Press, New York, 1990, 1787.

4. Roizman, B. and Sears, A. E., Herpes simplex viruses and their replication, in *Fields Virology*, 2nd ed., Fields, B. N., Knipe, D. M., Chanock, R. M., Hirsch, M. S., Melnick, J. L., Monath, T. P., and Roizman, B., Eds., Raven Press, New York, 1990, 1795.

5. Whitley, R., Herpes simplex viruses, in *Fields Virology*, 2nd ed., Fields, B. N., Knipe, D. M., Chanock, R. M., Hirsch, M. S., Melnick, J. L., Monath, T. P., and Roizman, B., Eds., Vol. 2, Raven Press, New York, 1990, 1843.

6. Gruter, W., Das herpesvirus, seine aetiologische und klinische bedeutung, *Munch. Med. Wochenschr.*, 71, 1058, 1924.

7. McGeoch, D. J., Dalrymple, M. A., Davison, A. J., Dolan, A., Frame, M. C., McNab, D., Perry, L. J., Scott, J. E., and Taylor, P., The complete DNA sequence of the long unique region of the genome of herpes simplex virus type 1, *J. Gen. Virol.*, 69, 1531, 1988.

8. Roizman, B., The structure and isomerization of herpes simplex virus genomes, *Cell*, 16, 481, 1979.

9. Nahmias, A. J. and Dowdle, W. R., Antigenic and biologic differences in herpesvirus hominis, *Prog. Med. Virol.*, 10, 110, 1968.

10. Smith, M. G., Propagation in tissue cultures of a cytopathogenic virus from human salivary gland virus (SGV) disease, *Proc. Soc. Exp. Biol. Med.*, 92, 424, 1956.

11. Davison, A. J. and Scott, J. E., The complete DNA sequence of varicella-zoster virus, *J. Gen. Virol.*, 67, 1759, 1986.

12. Dumas, A. M., Geelen, J. L. M. C., Maris, W., and Van der Noordas, J., Infectivity and molecular weight of varicella-zoster virus DNA, *J. Gen. Virol.*, 47, 233, 1980.

13. Ludwig, H. O., Biswal, N., and Benyesh-Melnick, M., Studies on the relatedness of herpesviruses through DNA-DNA hybridization, *Virology*, 49, 95, 1972.

14. Baer, R., Bankier, A. T., Biggin, M. D., Deininger, P. L., Farrell, P. J., Gibson, T. J., Hatful, G., Hudson, G. S., Satchwell, S. G., Séguin, C., Tuffnell, P. S., and Barell, B. G., DNA sequence and expression of the B95-8 Epstein-Barr virus genome, *Nature*, 310, 207, 1984.

15. Epstein, M. A., Henle, W., Achong, B. G., and Barr, Y. M., Morphological and biological studies on a virus in cultured lymphoblasts from Burkitt's lymphoma, *J. Exp. Med.*, 121, 761, 1965.

16. Lopez, C., Pellett, P., Stewart, J., Goldsmith, C., Sanderlin, K., Black, J., Warfield, D., and Feorino, P., Characteristics of human herpesvirus-6, *J. Infect. Dis.*, 157, 1271, 1988.

17. Salahuddin, S. Z., Ablashi, D. V., Markham, P. D., Josephs, S. F., Sturzenegger, S., Kaplan, M., Halligan, G., Biberfeld, P., Wong-Stall, F., Kramarsky, B., and Gallo, R. C., Isolation of a new virus, HBLV, in patients with lymphoproliferative disorder, *Science*, 234, 596, 1986.

18. Roizman, B. and Furlong, D., The replication of herpesviruses, in *Comprehensive Virology*, Fraenkel-Conrat, H. and Wagner, R. R., Eds., Plenum Press, New York, 1974, 229.

19. Muller, S. A., Herrmann, E. C., Jr., and Winkelmann, R. K., Herpes simplex infections in hematologic malignancies, *Am. J. Med.*, 52, 102, 1972.

20. Dreizen, S., McCredie, K. B., Bodey, G. P., and Keating, M. J., Mucocutaneous herpetic infections during cancer chemotherapy, *Postgrad. Med. J.*, 84, 181, 1988.

21. Wingard, J. R., Viral infections in leukemia and bone marrow transplant patients, *Leukemia Lymphoma*, 11(Suppl. 2), 115, 1993.

22. Stone, W. J., Scowden, E. B., Spannuth, C. L., Lowry, S. P., and Alford, R. H., Atypical simplex virus hominis type 2 infection in uremic patients receiving immunosuppressive therapy, *Am. J. Med.*, 63, 511, 1977.

23. Schneidman, D. W., Barr, R. J., and Graham, J. H., Chronic cutaneous herpes simplex, *JAMA*, 241, 542, 1979.

24. Straus, S. E., Smith, H. A., Brickmann, C., de Miranda, P., McLaren, C., and Keeney, R. E., Acyclovir for chronic mucocutaneous herpes simplex virus infections in immunosuppressed patients, *Ann. Intern. Med.*, 96, 270, 1982.

25. Armstrong, D., Opportunistic infections in the acquired immune deficiency syndrome, *Semin. Oncol.*, 14(Suppl. 3), 40, 1987.

26. Levin, M. J., Impact of herpesvirus infections in the future, *J. Med. Virol. Suppl.*, 1, 158, 1993.

27. Meyers, J. D., Flornoy, N., and Thomas, E. D., Infection with herpes simplex virus and cell-mediated immunity after marrow transplant, *J. Infect. Dis.*, 142, 338, 1980.

28. Rand, K. H., Rasmussen, L. E., Pollard, R. B., Arvin, A., and Merigan, T. C., Cellular immunity and herpesvirus infections in cardiac transplant patients, *N. Engl. J. Med.*, 296, 1372, 1977.

29. Pass, R. F., Whitley, R. J., Whelchel, J. D., Diethelm, A. G., Reynolds, D. W., and Alford, C. A., Identification of patients with increased risk of infection with herpes simplex virus after renal transplantation, *J. Infect. Dis.*, 140, 487, 1979.

30. Lam, M. T., Pazin, G. J., Armstrong, J. A., and Ho, M., Herpes simplex infection in acute myelogenous leukemia and other hematologic malignancies: a prospective study, *Cancer*, 48, 2168, 1981.

31. Straus, S. E., Treatment of persistent active herpesvirus infections, *J. Virol. Meth.*, 21, 305, 1988.

32. Straus, S. E., Seidlin, M., Takiff, H. E., Rooney, J. F., Felser, J. M., Smith, H. A., Roane, P., Johnson, F., Hallahan, C., Ostrove, J. M., and Nusinoff Lehrman, S., Effect of oral acyclovir treatment on symptomatic and asymptomatic virus shedding in recurrent genital herpes, *Sex. Transm. Dis.*, 16, 107, 1989.

33. Whitley, R. J. and Gnann, J. W., Jr., Acyclovir: a decade later, *N. Engl. J. Med.*, 327, 782, 1992.

34. Fletcher, C. V., Treatment of herpesvirus infections in HIV-infected individuals, *Ann. Pharmacother.*, 26, 955, 1992.

35. Centers for Disease Control, Revision of the CDC surveillance case definition for acquired immunodeficiency syndrome, *Morbid. Mortal. Wkly. Rep.*, 36(Suppl.), S1, 1987.

36. Siegel, F. P., Lopez, C., Hammer, B. S., Brown, A. E., Kornfeld, S. J., Gold, J., Hassett, J., Hirschman, S. Z., Cunningham-Rundles, C., Adelsberg, B. R., Parham, D. M., Siegal, M., Cunningham-Rundles, S., and Armstrong, D., Severe acquired immunodeficiency in male homosexuals, manifested by chronic perianal ulcerative herpes simplex lesions, *N. Engl. J. Med.*, 305, 1439, 1981.

37. Whitley, R. J., Alford, C. A., Hirsch, M. S., Schooley, R. T., Luby, J. P., Aoki, F. Y., Hanley, D., Nahmias, A. J., Soong, S.-J., and the NIAID Collaborative Antiviral Study Group, Vidarabine versus acyclovir therapy in herpes simplex encephalitis, *N. Engl. J. Med.*, 314, 144, 1986.

38. Sköldenberg, B., Forsgren, M., Alestig, K., Bergström, T., Burman, L., Dahlqvist, E., Forkman, A., Frydén, A., Lövgren, K., Norlin, K., Norrby, R., Olding-Stenkvist, E., Stiernstedt, G., Uhnoo, I., and de Vahl, K., Acyclovir versus vidarabin in herpes simplex encephalitis: randomized multicentre study in consecutive Swedish patients, *Lancet*, 2, 707, 1984.

39. Hull, H. F., Blumhagen, J. D., Benjamin, D., and Corey, L., Herpes simplex virus pneumonitis in childhood, *J. Pediatr.*, 104, 211, 1984.

40. Ramsey, P. G., Fife, K. H., Hackman, R. C., Meyers, J. D., and Corey, L., Herpes simplex pneumonia: clinical, virologic and pathologic features in 20 patients, *Ann. Intern. Med.*, 97, 813, 1982.

41. Herout, V., Vortel, V., and Vondrackova, A., Herpes simplex involvement of the lower respiratory tract, *Am. J. Clin. Pathol.*, 46, 411, 1966.

42. Morgan, H. R. and Finland, J., Isolation of herpesvirus from a case of atypical pneumonia and erythema multiforme exudativum, with studies of four additional cases, *Am. J. Med. Sci.*, 217, 91, 1949.

43. Douglas, R. G., Jr., Anderson, M. S., Weg, J. G., Williams, T., Jenkins, D. E., Knight, V., and Beall, A. C., Jr., Herpes simplex virus pneumonia: occurrence in an allotransplanted lung, *JAMA*, 210, 902, 1966.

44. Jordan, S. W., McLaren, L. C., and Crosby, J. H., Herpetic tracheobronchitis: cytologic and virologic detection, *Arch. Intern. Med.*, 135, 784, 1975.

45. Caldwell, J. E. and Porter, D. D., Herpetic pneumonia in alcoholic hepatitis, *JAMA*, 217, 1703, 1971.

46. Nash, G. and Foley, F. D., Herpetic infection of the middle and lower respiratory tract, *Am. J. Clin. Pathol.*, 54, 857, 1970.

47. Nash, G., Necrotizing tracheobronchitis and bronchopneumonitis consistent with herpetic infection, *Human Pathol.*, 3, 283, 1972.

48. Wheeler, C. E., Jr. and Huffines, W. D., Primary disseminated herpes simplex of the newborn, *JAMA*, 191, 455, 1965.

49. Haynes, R. E., Azimi, P. H., and Cramblett, H. G., Fatal herpesvirus hominis (herpes simplex virus) infection in children, *JAMA*, 206, 312, 1968.

50. Bland, J. D. and Lilleyman, J. S., Fatal pneumonia associated with two viruses in a child with lymphoblastic leukemia, *Br. Med. J.*, 284, 82, 1982.

51. Tucker, E. S. and Scofield, G. F., Hepatoadrenal necrosis: fatal systemic herpes simplex infection: review of the literature and report of two cases, *Arch. Pathol.*, 71, 84, 1961.

52. Kipps, A., Becker, W., Wainwright, J., and McKenzie, D., Fatal disseminated primary herpesvirus in children: epidemiology based on 93 non-neonatal cases, *S. Afr. Med. J.*, 41, 647, 1967.

53. Zweerink, H. J. and Stanton, L. W., Immune response to herpes simplex virus infections: virus-specific antibodies in sera from patients with recurrent facial infections, *Infect. Immun.*, 31, 624, 1981.

54. Corey, L., Reeves, W. C., and Holmes, K. K., Cellular immune response in genital herpes simplex virus infection, *N. Engl. J. Med.*, 299, 986, 1978.

55. Pass, R. F., Dworsky, M. E., Whitley, R. J., August, A. M., Stagno, S., and Alford, C. A., Jr., Specific lymphocyte blastogenic responses in children with cytomegalovirus and herpes simplex virus infections acquired early in infancy, *Infect. Immun.*, 34, 166, 1981.

56. Rasmussen, L. E., Jordan, G. W., Stevens, D. A., and Merigan, T. C., Lymphocyte interferon production and transformation after herpes simplex infections in humans, *J. Immunol.*, 112, 728, 1974.

57. Russell, A. S., Cell-mediated immunity to herpes simplex virus in man, *Am. J. Clin. Pathol.*, 60, 826, 1973.

58. Russell, A. S., Cell-mediated immunity to herpes simplex virus in man, *J. Infect. Dis.*, 129, 142, 1974.

59. Russell, A. S., HL-A transplantation antigens in subjects susceptible to recrudescent herpes labialis, *Tissue Antigens*, 6, 257, 1975.

60. Russell, A. S. and Schlaut, J., Association of HLA-AI antigen and susceptibility to recurrent cold sores, *Arch. Dermatol.*, 113, 1721, 1977.

61. Shillitoe, E. J., Wilton, J. M. A., and Lehner, T., Sequential changes in T and B lymphocyte responses to herpes simplex virus in man, *Scand. J. Immunol.*, 7, 357, 1978.

62. Starr, S. E., Kartela, S. A., Shore, S. L., Duffey, A., and Nahmias, A. J., Stimulation of human lymphocytes by herpes simplex virus antigens, *Infect. Immun.*, 11, 109, 1975.

63. Sullender, W. M., Miller, J. L., Yasukawa, L. L., Bradley, J. S., Black, S. B., Yeager, A. S., and Arvin, A. M., Humoral and cell-mediated immunity in neonates with herpes simplex virus infection, *J. Infect. Dis.*, 155, 28, 1987.

64. Thong, Y. H., Vincent, M. M., Hensen, S. A., Fuccello, D. A., Rola-Pleszczynski, M., and Bellanti, J. A., Depressed specific cell-mediated immunity to herpes simplex virus type 1 in patients with recurrent herpes labialis, *Infect. Immun.*, 12, 76, 1975.

65. Torseth, J. W., Cohen, G. H., Elsenberg, R. J., Berman, P. W., Lasky, L. A., Cerini, C. P., Heilman, C. J., Kerwar, S., and Merigan, T. C., Native and recombinant herpes simplex virus type 1 envelope proteins induce human immune T-lymphocyte responses, *J. Virol.*, 61, 1532, 1987.

66. Cunningham, A. L. and Merigan, T. C., Alpha interferon production appears to predict time of recurrence of herpes labialis, *J. Immunol.*, 130, 2397, 1983.

67. Overall, J. C., Jr., Spruance, S. L., and Green, J. A., Viral-induced leukocyte interferon in vesicle fluid from lesions of recurrent herpes labialis, *J. Infect. Dis.*, 143, 543, 1981.

68. Sheridan, J. F., Dounenberg, A. D., Aurelian, L., and Elpern, D. J., Immunity to herpes simplex virus type 2. IV. Impaired lymphokine production during recrudescence correlates with an imbalance in T-lymphocyte subsets, *J. Immunol.*, 129, 326, 1982.

69. Kahlon, J. and Whitley, R. J., Antibody response of the newborn, *J. Infect. Dis.*, 158, 925, 1988.

70. Rouse, B. T., The herpesviruses, in *Immunobiology and Prophylaxis of Human Herpesvirus Infections*, Vol. 4, Roizman, B. and Lopez, C., Eds., Plenum Press, New York, 1985, 103.

71. Kohl, S., Frazier, J. P., Pickering, L. K., and Loo, L. S., Normal function of neonatal polymorphonuclear leukocytes in antibody-dependent cellular cytotoxicity to herpes simplex virus infected cells, *J. Pediatr.*, 98, 783, 1981.

72. Whitley, R. J., Spruance, S., Hayden, F. G., Overall, J., Alford, C. A., Jr., Gwaltney, J. M., Jr., Soong, S.-J., and the NIAID Collaborative Antiviral Study Group, Vidarabine therapy for mucocutaneous herpes simplex virus infections in immunocompromised hosts, *J. Infect. Dis.*, 149, 1, 1984.

73. Conant, M., Current clinical issues in the management of herpes simplex virus infections in patients with HIV, *Dermatology*, 194, 93, 1997.

74. Shepp, D. H., Newton, B. A., Dandliker, P. S., Flornoy, N., and Meyers, J. D., Oral acyclovir therapy for mucocutaneous herpes simplex virus infection in immunocompromised marrow transplant recipients, *Ann. Intern. Med.*, 102, 783, 1985.

75. Wade, J. C., Newton, B., McLaren, C., Flournoy, N., Keeney, R. E., and Meyers, J. D., Intravenous acyclovir to treat mucocutaneous herpes simplex virus infection after marrow transplantation: a double-blind trial, *Ann. Intern. Med.*, 96, 265, 1982.

76. Meyers, J. D., Wade, J. C., Mitchell, C. D., Saral, R., Lietman, P. S., Durack, D. T., Levine, M. J., Segretti, A. C., and Balfour, H. H., Jr., Multicenter collaborative trial of intravenous acyclovir for treatment of mucocutaneous herpes simplex virus infection in the immunocompromised host, *Am. J. Med.*, 73(Suppl. 1A), 229, 1982.

77. Griffiths, P. D., Future management of herpesvirus infections, *J. Med. Virol. Suppl.*, 1, 165, 1993.

78. Mitchell, D., Bean, B., Gentry, S. R., Groth, K. E., Boen, J. R., and Balfour, H. H., Jr., Acyclovir therapy for mucocutaneous herpes simplex virus infections in immune compromised patients, *Lancet*, 1, 1389, 1981.

79. Chou, S., Gallagher, J. G., and Merigan, T. C., Controlled trial of intravenous acyclovir in heart-transplant patients with mucocutaneous herpes simplex infections, *Lancet*, 2, 1392, 1981.

80. Drew, W. L., Buhles, W., Dworkin, R. J., and Erlich, K. S., Management of herpes virus infections (CMV, HSV, VZV), in *The Management of AIDS*, 2nd ed., Sande, M. A. and Volberding, P. A., Eds., 2nd ed., W. B. Saunders, Philadelphia, 1990, 316.

81. Corey, L., Fife, K. H., Benedetti, J. K., Winter, C. A., Fahnlander, A., Connor, J. D., Hintz, M. A., and Holmes, K. K., Intravenous acyclovir for the treatment of primary genital herpes, *Ann. Intern. Med.*, 98, 914, 1983.

82. Peacock, J. E., Jr., Kaplowitz, L. G., Sparling, P. F., Durack, D. T., Gnann, J. W., Jr., Whitley, R. J., Lovett, M., Bryson, Y. J., Klein, R. J., Friedman-Kien, A. E., Knowlton, G. M., and Davis, L. G., Intravenous acyclovir therapy of first episodes of genital herpes: a multicenter double-blind, placebo-controlled trial, *Am. J. Med.*, 85, 301, 1988.

83. Bryson, Y. J., Dillon, M., Lovett, M., Aguna, G., Taylor, S., Cherry, J. D., Johnson, B. L., Wiesmeier, E., Growdon, W., Creagh-Kirk, T., and Keeney, R., Treatment of first episodes of genital herpes simplex virus infection with oral acyclovir: a randomized double-blind controlled trial in normal subjects, *N. Engl. J. Med.*, 308, 916, 1983.

84. Mertz, G. J., Critchlow, C. W., Benedetti, J., Reichman, R. C., Dolin, R., Connor, J., Redfield, D. C., Savoia, M. C., Richman, D. D., Tyrell, D. L., Miedzinski, L., Portnoy, J., Keeney, R. E., and Corey, L., Double-blind placebo-controlled trial of oral acyclovir in first-episode genital herpes simplex virus infection, *JAMA*, 252, 1147, 1984.

85. Wade, J. C., Newton, B., Flournoy, N., and Meyers, J. D., Oral acyclovir for prevention of herpes simplex virus reactivation after marrow transplantation, *Ann. Intern. Med.*, 100, 823, 1984.

86. Corey, L., Nahmias, A. J., Guinan, M. E., Benedetti, J. K., Critchlow, C. W., and Holmes, K. K., A trial of topical acyclovir in genital herpes simplex infections, *N. Engl. J. Med.*, 306, 1313, 1982.

87. Corey, L., Benedetti, J., Critchlow, C., Mertz, G., Douglas, J., Fife, K., Fahnlander, A., Remington, M. L., Winter, C., and Dragovony, J., Treatment of primary first-episode genital herpes simplex virus infections with acyclovir: results of topical, intravenous and oral therapy, *J. Antimicrob. Chemother.*, 12(Suppl. B), 79, 1983.

88. Adams, H. G., Benson, E. A., Alexander, E. R., Vontver, L. A., Remington, M. A., and Holmes, K. A., Genital herpetic infection in men and women: clinical course and effect of topical application of adenine arabinoside, *J. Infect. Dis.*, 133(Suppl. A), 151, 1976.

89. Spruance, S. L., Crumpacker, C. S., Haines, H., Bader, C., Mehr, K., MacCalman, J., Schniffer, L. E., Klauber, M. R., Overall, J. C., and the Collaborative Study Group, Ineffectiveness of topical adenine arabinoside 5'-monophosphate in the treatment of recurrent herpes simplex labialis, *N. Engl. J. Med.*, 300, 1180, 1979.

90. Corey, L., Reeves, W. C., Chiang, W. T., Vontver, L. A., Remington, M., Winter, C., and Holmes, K. K., Ineffectiveness of topical ether for the treatment of genital herpes simplex virus infection, *N. Engl. J. Med.*, 299, 237, 1978.

91. Myers, M. G., Oxman, M. N., Clark, J. E., and Arndt, K. A., Failure of neutral-red photodynamic inactivation in recurrent herpes simplex virus infection, *N. Engl. J. Med.*, 293, 945, 1975.

92. Fiddian, A. P., Yeo, J. M., Stubbings, R., and Dean, D., Successful treatment of herpes labialis with topical acyclovir, *Br. Med. J.*, 286, 1699, 1983.

93. Spruance, S. L., Schnipper, L. E., Overall, J. C., Jr., Kern, E. R., Wester, B., Modlin, J., Wenerstrom, G., Burton, C., Arndt, K. A., Chiu, G. L., and Crumpacker, C. S., Treatment of herpes simplex labialis with topical acyclovir in polyethylene glycol, *J. Infect. Dis.*, 146, 85, 1982.

94. Shaw, M., King, M., Best, J. M., Banatvala, J. E., Gibson, J. R., and Klaber, M. R., Failure of acyclovir cream in treatment of recurrent herpes labialis, *Br. Med. J.*, 291, 7, 1985.

95. Raborn, G. W., McGaw, W. T., Grace, M., Tyrrell, L. D., and Samuels, S. M., Oral acyclovir and herpes labialis: a randomized, double-blind, placebo-controlled study, *J. Am. Dent. Assoc.*, 115, 38, 1987.

96. Spruance, S. L., Stewart, J. C. B., Rowe, N. H., McKeough, M. B., Wenerstrom, G., and Freeman, D. J., Treatment of recurrent herpes simplex labialis with oral acyclovir, *J. Infect. Dis.*, 161, 185, 1990.

97. Saral, R., Burns, W. H., Laskin, O. L., Santos, G. W., and Lietman, P. S., Acyclovir prophylaxis of herpes-simplex-virus infections: a randomized, double-blind, controlled trial in bone-marrow-transplant recipients, *N. Engl. J. Med.*, 305, 63, 1981.

98. Levin, M. J., Leary, P. L., and Arbeit, R. D., Effect of acyclovir on the proliferation of human fibroblasts and peripheral blood mononuclear cells, *Antimicrob. Agents Chemother.*, 17, 947, 1980.

99. Steele, R. W., Marmer, D. J., and Keeney, R. E., Comparative in vitro immunotoxicology of acyclovir and other antiviral agents, *Infect. Immunol.*, 28, 957, 1980.

100. Straus, S. E., Seidlin, M., Takiff, H., Jacobs, D., Bowen, D., and Smith, H. A., Oral acyclovir for suppression of recurrent herpes simplex virus infections in immunodeficient patients, *Ann. Intern. Med.*, 100, 522, 1984.

101. Douglas, J. M., Critchlow, C., Benedetti, J., Mertz, G. J., Connor, J. D., Hintz, M. A., Fahnlander, A., Remington, M., Winter, C., and Corey, L., A double-blind study of oral acyclovir for suppression of recurrences of genital herpes simplex virus infection, *N. Engl. J. Med.*, 310, 1551, 1984.

102. Mertz, G. J., Jones, C. C., Mills, J., Fife, K. H., Lemon, S. M., Stapleton, J. T., Hill, E. L., Davis, L. G., and the Acyclovir Study Group, Long-term acyclovir suppression of frequently recurring genital herpes simplex virus infection: a multicenter double-blind trial, *JAMA*, 260, 201, 1988.

103. Straus, S. E., Takiff, H. E., Seidlin, M., Bachrach, S., Lininger, L., DiGiovanna, J. J., Western, K. A., Smith, H. A., Nusinoff Lehrman, S., Creagh-Kirk, T., and Alling, D. W., Suppression of frequently recurring genital herpes: a placebo-controlled double-blind trial of oral acyclovir, *N. Engl. J. Med.*, 310, 1545, 1984.

104. Kaplowitz, L. G., Baker, D., Gelb, L., Blythe, J., Hale, R., Frost, P., Crumpacker, C., Rabinovich, S., Peacock, J. E., Jr., Herndon, J., Davis, L. G., and the Acyclovir Study Group, Prolonged continuous acyclovir treatment of normal adults with frequently recurring genital herpes simplex virus infection, *JAMA*, 265, 747, 1991.

105. Shepp, D. H., Dandliker, P. S., Flournoy, N., and Meyers, J. D., Sequential intravenous and twice-daily oral acyclovir for extended prophylaxis of herpes simplex virus infection in marrow transplant patients, *Transplantation*, 43, 654, 1987.

106. Straus, S. E., Croen, K. D., Sawyer, M. H., Freifeld, A. G., Felser, J. M., Dale, J. K., Smith, H. A., Hallahan, C., and Nusinoff Lehrman, S., Acyclovir suppression of frequently recurring genital herpes: efficacy and diminishing need during successive years of treatment, *JAMA*, 260, 2227, 1988.

107. Whitley, R. J., Soong, S.-J., Dolin, R., Galasso, G. J., Ch'ien, L. T., Alford, C. A., and the Collaborative Study Group, Adenine arabinoside therapy of biopsy-proven herpes simplex encephalitis, *N. Engl. J. Med.*, 297, 289, 1977.

108. Whitley, R. J., Nahmias, A. J., Soong, S.-J., Gallasso, G. H., Fleming, C. L., and Alford, C. A., Vidarabine therapy of neonatal herpes simplex virus infection, *Pediatrics*, 66, 495, 1980.

109. Ch'ien, L. T., Cannon, N. J., Charamella, L. J., Dismukes, W. E., Whitley, R. J., Buchanan, R. A., and Alford, C. A., Jr., Effect of adenine arabinoside on severe herpesvirus hominis infections in man, *J. Infect. Dis.*, 128, 658, 1973.

110. Steele, R. W., Keeney, R. E., Brown, J., and Young, E. J., Cellular immune responses to herpesviruses during treatment with adenine arabinoside, *J. Infect. Dis.*, 135, 893, 1977.

111. Lauter, C. B., Bailey, E. J., and Lerner, A. M., Microbiologic assays and neurological toxicity during use of adenine arabinoside in humans, *J. Infect. Dis.*, 134, 75, 1976.

112. Sacks, S. L., Smith, J. L., Pollard, R. B., Sawhney, V., Mahol, A. S., Gregory, P., Merigan, T. C., and Robinson, W. S., Toxicity of vidarabine, *JAMA*, 241, 28, 1979.

113. Marker, S. C., Howard, R. J., Groth, K. E., Mastri, A. R., Simmons, R. L., and Balfour, H. H., Jr., A trial of vidarabine for cytomegalovirus infection in renal transplant patients, *Arch. Intern. Med.*, 140, 1441, 1980.

114. Van Etta, L., Brown, J., Mastri, A., and Wilson, T., Fatal vidarabine toxicity in a patient with normal renal function, *JAMA*, 246, 1703, 1981.

115. Tricot, G., De Clercq, E., Boogaerts, M. A., and Verwilghen, R. L., Oral bromovinyldeoxyuridine therapy for herpes simplex and varicella-zoster virus infections in severely immunosuppressed patients: a preliminary clinical trial, *J. Med. Virol.*, 18, 11, 1986.

116. De Clercq, E., Biochemical aspects of the selective antiherpes activity of nucleoside analogues, *Biochem. Pharmacol.*, 33, 2159, 1984.

117. Oberg, B., Antiviral effects of phosphonoformate, *Pharmacol. Ther.*, 19, 387, 1983.

118. Sandstrom, E. G., Byington, R. E., Kaplan, J. C., and Hirsch, M. S., Inhibition of human T cell lymphotropic virus type III in vitro by phosphonoformate, *Lancet*, 2, 1480, 1985.

119. Smith, N. A., Wood, C., Asboe, D., and Bingham, J. S., Topical foscarnet for acyclovir-resistant mucocutaneous herpes infection in AIDS, *AIDS*, 11, 254, 1997.

120. Chatis, P. A., Miller, C. H., Schrager, L. E., and Crumpacker, C. S., Successful treatment with foscarnet of an acyclovir-resistant mucocutaneous infection with herpes simplex virus in a patient with the acquired immunodeficiency syndrome, *N. Engl. J. Med.*, 320, 297, 1989.

121. Causey, D. M., Rarick, M. U., and Melancon, H., Foscarnet treatment of acyclovir-resistant herpes simplex proctitis in an AIDS patient, *Proc. IVth Int. Conf. AIDS*, Stockholm, 1988, Abstr. 3589.

122. Erlich, K. S., Jacobson, M. A., Koehler, J. E., Follansbee, S. E., Drennan, D. P., Goose, L., Safrin, S., and Mills, J., Foscarnet therapy of severe acyclovir-resistant herpes simplex virus infections in patients with the acquired immunodeficiency syndrome, *Ann. Intern. Med.*, 110, 710, 1989.

123. Youle, M. M., Hawkins, D. A., Collins, P., Shanson, D. C., Evans, R., Oliver, N., and Lawrence, A., Acyclovir-resistant herpes in AIDS treated with foscarnet, *Lancet*, 2, 341, 1988.

124. Vinckier, F., Boogaerts, M., De Clercq, D., and De Clercq, E., Chronic herpetic infection in an immunocompromised patient: report of a case, *J. Oral Maxillofac. Surg.*, 45, 723, 1987.

125. Hardy, W. D., Foscarnet treatment of acyclovir-resistant herpes simplex virus infection in patients with acquired immunodeficiency syndrome: preliminary results of a controlled, randomized, regimen-comparative trial, *Am. J. Med.*, 92(Suppl. 2A), 30S, 1992.

126. Sall, R. K., Kauffmann, C. L., and Levy, C. S., Successful treatment of progressive acyclovir-resistant herpes simplex virus using intravenous foscarnet in a patient with the acquired immunodeficiency syndrome, *Arch. Dermatol.*, 125, 1549, 1989.

127. Balfour, H. H., Jr., Benson, C., Braun, J., Cassens, B., Erice, A., Friedman-Kien, A., Klein, T., Polsky, B., and Safrin, S., Management of acyclovir-resistant herpes simplex and varicella-zoster virus infection, *J. Acquir. Immune Defic. Syndr.*, 7, 254, 1994.

128. Safrin, S., Crumpacker, C., Chatis, P., Davis, R., Hafner, R., Rush, J., Kessler, H. A., Landry, B., and Mills, J., A controlled trial comparing foscarnet with vidarabine for acyclovir-resistant mucocutaneous herpes simplex in the acquired immunodeficiency syndrome, *N. Engl. J. Med.*, 325, 551, 1991.

129. Jacobson, M. A., O'Donnell, J. J., and Mills, J., Foscarnet treatment of cytomegalovirus retinitis in patients with the acquired immunodeficiency syndrome, *Antimicrob. Agents Chemother.*, 33, 736, 1989.

130. Verdonck, L. F., Cornelissen, J. J., Smit, J., Lepoutre, J., de Gast, G. C., Dekker, A. W., and Rozenberg-Arska, M., Successful foscarnet therapy for acyclovir-resistant mucocutaneous infection with herpes simplex virus in a recipient of allogeneic BMT, *Bone Marrow Transplant.*, 11, 177, 1993.

131. Aweeka, F., Gambertoglio, J. G., Mills, J., and Jacobson, M. A., Pharmacokinetics of intermittently administered intravenous foscarnet in the treatment of AIDS patients with serious CMV retinitis, *Proc. IVth Int. Conf. AIDS*, Stokholm, 1988, Abstr. 3591.

132. Ringdén, O., Lönnqvist, B., Paulin, T., Ahlmén, J., Klintmalm, G., Wahren, B., and Lernestedt, J.-O., Pharmacokinetics, safety and preliminary clinical experiences using foscarnet in the treatment of cytomegalovirus infections in bone marrow and renal transplant recipients, *J. Antimicrob. Chemother.*, 17, 373, 1986.

133. Erlich, K. S., Mills, J., Chatis, P., Mertz, G. J., Busch, D. F., Follansbee, S. E., Grant, R. M., and Crumpacker, C. S., Acyclovir- resistant herpes simplex virus infections in patients with the acquired immunodeficiency syndrome, *N. Engl. J. Med.*, 320, 293, 1989.

134. Wade, J. C., McLaren, C., and Meyers, J. D., Frequency and significance of acyclovir-resistant herpes simplex virus isolated from marrow transplant patients receiving multiple courses of treatment with acyclovir, *J. Infect. Dis.*, 148, 1077, 1983.

135. Crumpacker, C. S., Schnipper, L. E., Marlowe, S. I., Kowalsky, P. N., Hershey, B. J., and Levin, M. J., Resistance to antiviral drugs of herpes simplex virus isolated from a patient treated with acyclovir, *N. Engl. J. Med.*, 306, 343, 1982.

136. Westheim, A. I., Tenser, R. B., and Marks, J. G., Jr., Acyclovir resistance in a patient with chronic mucocutaneous herpes simplex virus infection, *J. Am. Acad. Dermatol.*, 17, 875, 1982.

137. Collins, P. and Darby, G., Laboratory studies of herpes simplex virus strains resistant to acyclovir, *Rev. Med. Virol.*, 1, 19, 1991.

138. Ljungman, P., Herpes virus infections in immunocompromised patients: problems and therapeutic interventions, *Ann. Med.*, 25, 329, 1993.

139. Burns, W. H., Saral, R., Santos, G. W., Laskin, O. L., Lietman, P. S., McLaren, C., and Barry, D. W., Isolation and characterization of resistant herpes simplex virus after acyclovir therapy, *Lancet*, 1, 421, 1982.

140. Sibrack, C. D., Gutman, L. T., Wilfert, C. M., McLaren, C., St. Clair, M. H., Keller, P. M., and Barry, D. W., Pathogenicity of acyclovir-resistant herpes simplex virus type 1 from an immunodeficient child, *J. Infect. Dis.*, 146, 673, 1982.

141. Schinazi, R. F., del Bene, V., Scott, R. T., and Dudley-Thorpe, J. B., Characterization of acyclovir-resistant and -sensitive herpes simplex viruses isolated from a patient with an acquired immune deficiency, *J. Antimicrob. Chemother.*, 18(Suppl.), 127, 1986.

142. Norris, S. A., Kessler, H. A., and Fife, K. H., Severe, progressive herpetic whitlow caused by an acyclovir-resistant virus in a patient with AIDS, *J. Infect. Dis.*, 157, 209, 1988.

143. Englund, J. A., Zimmerman, M. K., Swierkosz, E. M., Goodman, J. L., Scholl, D. R., and Balfour, H. H., Jr., Herpes simplex virus resistant to acyclovir: a study in a tertiary care center, *Ann. Intern. Med.*, 112, 416, 1990.

144. Nugier, F., Colin, J. N., Aymard, M., and Langlois, M., Occurrence and characterization of acyclovir-resistant herpes simplex virus isolates: report on a two-year sensitivity screening survey, *J. Med. Virol.*, 36, 1, 1992.

145. Ljungman, P., Ellis, M. N., Hackman, R. C., Sheep, D. H., and Meyers, J. D., Acyclovir-resistant herpes simplex virus causing pneumonia after marrow transplantation, *J. Infect. Dis.*, 162, 244, 1990.

146. Gateley, A., Gander, R. M., Johnson, P. C., Kit, S., Otsuka, H., and Kohl, S., Herpes simplex virus type 2 meningoencephalitis resistant to acyclovir in a patient with AIDS, *J. Infect. Dis.*, 161, 711, 1990.

147. Nisinoff Lehrman, S., Douglas, J. M., Corey, L., and Barry, D. W., Recurrent genital herpes and suppressive oral acyclovir therapy: relation between clinical outcome and in-vitro drug sensitivity, *Ann. Intern. Med.*, 134, 786, 1986.

148. Parris, D. S. and Harrington, J. E., Herpes simplex virus variants resistant to high concentrations of acyclovir exist in clinical isolates, *Antimicrob. Agents Chemother.*, 22, 71, 1982.

149. McLaren, C., Corey, L., Dekket, C., and Barry, D. W., In vitro sensitivity to acyclovir in genital herpes simplex virus from acyclovir-treated patients, *J. Infect. Dis.*, 148, 868, 1983.

150. Lehrman, S. N., Douglas, J. M., Corey, L., and Barry, D. W., Recurrent genital herpes and suppressive oral acyclovir therapy: relation between clinical outcome and in-vitro sensitivity, *Ann. Intern. Med.*, 104, 786, 1986.

151. Schnipper, L. E. and Crumpacker, C. S., Resistance of herpes simplex virus to acylguanosine: role of viral thymidine kinase and DNA polymerase, *Proc. Natl. Acad. Sci. U.S.A.*, 77, 2270, 1980.

152. Coen, D. and Schaffer, P. A., Two distinct loci confer resistance to acylguanosine in herpes simplex virus type 1, *Proc. Natl. Acad. Sci. U.S.A.*, 77, 2265, 1980.

153. Darby, G., Field, H. J., and Salisbury, S. A., Altered substrate specificity of herpes simplex virus thymidine kinase confers acyclovir resistance, *Nature*, 289, 81, 1981.

154. Ellis, M. N., Keller, P. M., Fyfe, J. A., Martin, J. L., Rooney, J. F., Straus, S. E., Lehrman, S. N., and Barry, D. W., Clinical isolate of herpes simplex virus type 2 that induces a thymidine kinase with altered substrate specificity, *Antimicrob. Agents Chemother.*, 31, 1117, 1987.

155. Sasadeusz, J. J., Tufaro, F., Safrin, S., Schubert, K., Hubinette, M. M., Cheung, P. K., and Sacks, S. L., Homopolymer mutational hot spots mediate herpes simplex virus resistance to acyclovir, *J. Virol.*, 71, 3872, 1997.

156. Field, H. J. and Darby, G., Pathogenicity in mice of strains of herpes simplex virus which are resistant to acyclovir in vitro and in vivo, *Antimicrob. Agents Chemother.*, 17, 209, 1980.

157. Sibrack, C. D., McLaren, C., and Barry, D. W., Disease and latency characteristics of clinical herpes simplex virus isolates after acyclovir therapy, *Am. J. Med.*, 73(Suppl.), 372, 1982.

158. Collins, P., Larder, B. A., Oliver, N. M., Kemp, S., Smith, I. W., and Darby, G., Characterization of a DNA polymerase mutant of herpes simplex virus from a severely immunocompromised patient receiving acyclovir, *J. Gen. Virol.*, 70, 375, 1989.

159. Knopf, K. W., Kaufman, E. R., and Crumpacker, C., Physical mapping of drug resistance mutations defines an active center on the herpes simplex virus DNA polymerase enzyme, *J. Virol.*, 39, 746, 1981.

160. Sacks, S. L., Wanklin, R. J., Reece, D. E., Hicks, K. A., Tyler, K. L., and Coen, D. M., Progressive esophagitis from acyclovir-resistant herpes simplex: clinical roles for the DNA polymerase mutants and viral heterogeneity? *Ann. Intern. Med.*, 111, 893, 1989.

161. Parker, A. C., Craig, J. I., Collins, Oliver, N., and Smith, I., Acyclovir-resistant herpes simplex virus infection due to altered DNA polymerase, *Lancet*, 2, 1461, 1987.

162. Birch, C., Tachedjian, G., Doherty, R., Hayes, K., and Gust, I., Altered sensitivity to antiviral drugs of herpes simplex virus isolates from a patient with the acquired immunodeficiency syndrome, *J. Infect. Dis.*, 162, 731, 1990.

163. Fletcher, C. V., Englund, J. A., Bean, B., Chinnock, B., Brundage, D. M., and Balfour, H. H., Jr., Continuous infusion high-dose acyclovir for serious herpesvirus infections, *Antimicrob. Agents Chemother.*, 33, 1375, 1989.

164. Erlich, K. S., Jacobson, M. A., Koehler, J. E., Follansbee, S. E., Dreenan, D. P., Gooze, L., Safrin, S., and Mills, J., Foscarnet therapy for severe acyclovir-resistant herpes simplex virus type-2 infections in patients with the acquired immunodeficiency syndrome, *Ann. Intern. Med.*, 110, 710, 1989.

165. Engel, J. P., Englund, J. A., Fletcher, C. V., and Hill, E. L., Treatment of resistant herpes simplex virus with continuous-infusion acyclovir, *JAMA*, 263, 1662, 1990.

166. Safrin, S., Assaykeen, T., Follansbee, S., and Mills, J., Foscarnet therapy for acyclovir-resistant mucocutaneous herpes simplex virus infection in 26 AIDS patients: preliminary data, *J. Infect. Dis.*, 161, 1078, 1990.

167. Crumpacker, C., Resistance of herpes viruses to nucleoside analogues — mechanisms and clinical importance, in *Antiviral Chemotherapy*, Mills, J. and Corey, L., Eds., Elsevier, New York, 1986, 226.

168. Dorsky, D. I. and Crumpacker, C. S., Drugs five years later: acyclovir, *Ann. Intern. Med.*, 107, 859, 1987.

169. Oberg, B., Antiviral effects of phosphonoformate, *Pharmacotherapy*, 19, 387, 1983.

170. Aweeka, F., Gambertoglio, J. G., Mills, J., and Jacobson, M. A., Pharmacokinetics of intermittently administered intravenous foscarnet in the treatment of AIDS patients with serious CMV retinitis, *Proc. IVth Int. Conf. AIDS*, Stockholm, 1988, Abstr. 3591.

171. Birch, C., Tyssen, D., Tachedjian, G., Doherty, R., Hayes, K., Mijch, A., and Lucas, C. R., Clinical effects and *in vitro* studies of trifluorothymidine combined with interferon-alfa for treatment of drug-resistant and -sensitive herpes simplex infections, *J. Infect. Dis.*, 166, 108, 1992.

1.4 EPSTEIN-BARR VIRUS

1.4.1 INTRODUCTION

The impact of acute clinical manifestations in immunocompromised patients induced by the Epstein-Barr virus is less well understood, although there has been suspicion that this virus may be the cause of high morbidity and severe illness in immunosuppressed hosts.

The Epstein-Barr virus (EBV) was discovered during the course of research trying to establish the cause of Burkitt's lymphoma,[1] a tumor commonly affecting children in some parts of East Africa, which was thought to be induced by a virus.[2] In 1964, Epstein and Barr[3] and Pulvertaft[4] simultaneously reported the first successful attempts to establish continuous lymphoblastoid cell lines from explants of Burkitt's lymphoma, which led subsequently to the isolation from thin sections of these cell lines of viral particles that were morphologically similar to herpesviruses.[5] During ensuing studies, such particles were found not to be confined solely to lymphoid cell lines originating from Burkitt's lymphoma tissues but were present also in lymphoid cell lines from patients with various malignancies, infectious mononucleosis, and from apparently normal individuals.[6,7]

EBV is a B-lymphotropic virus ubiquitously found worldwide, which contains a double-stranded DNA core surrounded by an icosahedral nucleocapsid and complex envelope and is morphologically indistinguishable from other herpesviruses.[7,8]

There has been no convincing evidence that strain differences among various EBV isolates account for the wide range of clinical conditions associated with EBV infections.[8]

Primary EBV infections are most frequent in an earlier age among lower socioeconomic groups and in developing countries. Nevertheless, it has been estimated that about 50% of the population in industrialized countries have had a primary EBV infection by adolescence, either clinically inapparent or mild and nonspecific.[8] In adolescence and young adulthood, primary EBV infections account for most cases of infectious mononucleosis, and by adulthood, most individuals are EBV-seropositive.[9]

Although EBV can be transmitted through blood transfusions, the main portal of entry is the oropharynx. It is most commonly transmitted by saliva and the oropharynx is the initial site of replication within many epithelial elements, such as the parotid and other salivary gland ducts, buccal and pharyngeal epithelial cells, and possibly the tongue.[10-12] The virus is shed continously from the oropharynx for up to 18 months after the infection, and thereafter intermittently by all seropositive individuals. The asymptomatic shedding of EBV by healthy people accounts for most of the spread to uninfected members of the population. Immunosuppressed persons shed the virus more frequently.

B lymphocytes are the only cells known to have surface receptors for EBV and replication in the epithelial cells of the oropharynx is thought to provide the source of virus which infects the B lymphoid cells.[9]

In addition to African Burkitt's lymphoma,[13] EBV has been linked epidemiologically with nasopharyngeal carcinoma,[14] and the Epstein-Barr viral genome was detected in a host of lymphoid neoplasms, including lethal midline granuloma,[15] Hodgkin's lymphoma,[16] T cell lymphoma,[17] thymic carcinoma,[18] congenital and acquired immunodeficiency, such as post-transplantation B cell lymphoproliferative disorders,[19-23] and AIDS.[20] Post-transplantation T cell lymphoproliferative disorders have been rare.[24]

1.4.2   Immune Response to Epstein-Barr Virus Infection

The presence of EBV in epithelial and B cells triggers an intense immune response consisting of antibodies to a large host of virally encoded products, a panoply of cell-mediated responses, and secretion of lymphokines.[6]

Although the exact role of the antibodies in controlling the infection is not known, neutralizing antibodies which appear early after infection will persist for life and may act to limit the spread of infection.

In normal individuals, the control of EBV proliferation in B lymphocytes is carried out by a variety of cell-mediated immune responses. The global cellular immune hyporesponsiveness, which is readily demonstrated during primary EBV infection, resolves after resolution of the illness.

Reactivation of EBV is facilitated by conditions that interfere with viability of the cell-mediated immunity. While less intense and of shorter duration than that associated with cytomegalovirus infections, the cellular hyporesponsiveness associated with EBV reactivation may contribute to morbidity observed in immunocompromised patients.[9]

Interferons, which inhibit EBV-induced proliferation and induction of immunoglobulin synthesis, and have been detected in the supernatants of blood lymphocytes exposed to EBV *in vitro*, are considered to be an important component of the immune control of EBV.[25]

1.4.2.1   Epstein-Barr Infection in Immunocompromised Hosts

The combination of cell-mediated and humoral immune responses acts to control the B cell proliferation and most oropharyngeal replication of EBV. In immunocompromised hosts such control has been weakened, thereby resulting in increased numbers of circulating infected B lymphocytes and increased levels of EBV in the saliva of such patients. For example, EBV nucleic sequences have been detected in approximately half of the B cell malignancies encountered in immunosuppressed patients.[9]

Even though EBV may reactivate frequently in immunocompromised patients, it does not usually cause any severe symptoms.[26] However, in patients with global immunodeficiency that is either congenital, such as severe combined immunodeficiency or ataxia telangiectasia, or acquired (organ or tissue transplant recipients, AIDS patients), some oncogenic viruses, such as EBV, may induce even fatal lymphoproliferative disease with the features of frank lymphoma.[6]

In patients with congenital immunodeficiencies, primary EBV infection is often present at the time they develop lymphoproliferative disease. Similarly, Ho et al.[27] made the observation that children who experienced primary EBV infection during organ transplantation appeared to be at increased risk for development of lymphoma.

In many cases, the post-transplantation lymphoproliferative disorders have been attributed to immunosuppressive therapy, especially with OKT3 and cyclosporin A.[19,28-30] Profound immunodeficiency induced by immunosuppressive therapy after organ transplantation has been shown[31] to be occasionally associated with EBV-induced B cell proliferation. In transplant recipients receiving immunosuppressive therapy with cyclosporin A, the lymphoproliferative lesions have occasionally been found to regress upon cessation of therapy.[32] In a related development, Bird et al.[33] have reported that in cell cultures, cyclosporin A enhanced *in vitro* the outgrowth of EBV-induced B lymphoid cell lines from normal EBV-seropositive donors. However, some oncogenic viruses such as EBV may also play a role in the development of B cell lymphoproliferative disorders.[20-22,34,35]

Randhawa et al.[21] reported that all five cases of B-cell post-transplantation lymphoproliferative disorders in 53 heart-lung transplant recipients were associated with primary EBV infection, and Nalesnik et al.[19] found 28 of 43 patients to develop also primary EBV infection. Because most of the reported B cell post-transplantation lymphoproliferative syndromes appeared to represent primary EBV infections, the lack of a previous EBV infection may be a risk factor for these B cell syndromes.

In contrast, chronic EBV infections are presumed to be the cause of EBV-associated T cell lymphomas.[17,36,37] Thus, all 10 cases of EBV-induced T cell lymphomas reported by Su et al.[37] have been past infections, and none of them had elevated IgM class anti-Epstein-Barr viral capsid antigen. However, since the EBV receptor, C3dR (CD21), has not been demonstrated uniformly[37,38] this raises the possibility that the expression of CD21 on these neoplastic cells may be either transient, cell cycle-dependent, or at low level.[37] The exact mechanism by which EBV infiltrates the T cells, and why the majority of the EBV-associated T cells have been of T helper phenotype has not yet been elucidated.[38]

EBV-driven lymphoproliferative disorders may also occur in transplant patients treated with antithymocyte globulin or monoclonal antibodies directed against T cells.

Severe Epstein-Barr viral infections have been infrequently reported in recipients of HLA-matched bone marrow transplants that have not been T cell-depleted.[39-42] However, a high incidence of B cell proliferation has been observed[43] in recipients of bone marrow transplants treated with monoclonal anti-CD3 antibody for severe graft-versus-host disease. These disorders, if left untreated, may frequently and rapidly become fatal.

Recipients of T cell-depleted HLA-matched bone marrow transplants have also been reported to develop potentially lethal B lymphoproliferative disorders.[44] One of the factors predisposing the occurrence of this syndrome has been the introduction of T cell-depleted HLA-mismatched (incompatible) bone marrow transplants.[45,46]

These observations have suggested that deficiency in one or more of the immune effector mechanisms necessary to recognize and eliminate EBV-transformed cells is central to the pathogenesis of progressive lymphoproliferative disease in the immunocompromised patient.[6] Thus, in transplant recipients three factors are thought to contribute to the pathogenesis: (1) the dose, duration, and number of immunosuppressive drugs, particularly cyclosporin A; (2) whether the patient is undergoing primary or reactivated infection; and (3) the use of antibody to T cells in order to maintain the graft or, in case of bone marrow transplantation, to prevent graft-versus-host disease.[6,43]

1.4.2.2 Pathogenesis of EBV-Associated Diseases in AIDS Patients

Three different EBV-associated lesions have been characterized in AIDS patients:[6] (1) diffuse polyclonal lymphomas that are frequently localized in extranodal sites, such as the gut and CNS; (2) lymphocytic interstitial pneumonitis; and (3) oral "hairy" leukoplakia of the tongue.[10] The specific host factors facilitating the development of these lesions are not well known.

EBV-induced lymphomas in AIDS patients may sometimes take the form of classic Burkitt's lymphoma with its associated chromosome abnormality. However, in contrast to cases of Burkitt's lymphoma within endemic regions, it should be emphasized that on many occasions Burkitt's lymphoma (and B cell lymphomas, in general) which occur in globally immunodeficient hosts such as AIDS patients have not always been associated with the Epstein-Barr virus.[47,48]

Lymphocytic interstitial pneumonitis (LIP), which has been diagnosed primarily among infants and children with AIDS, is characterized with significant hypergammaglobulinemia, high antibody levels to EBV replicative antigens, and a poor antibody response to EBV-induced nuclear antigens (EBNAs).[49] LIP is not a progressive lymphoproliferative disorder, but rather chronic and highly variable.

One of the forms of chronic EBV infection is the oral "hairy" leukoplakia.[50] It is a slowly progressive disorder of the tongue and buccal epithelium that is usually associated with AIDS patients.[10] The replicating forms of virus DNA predominate, with mature virions found in the lesions.[6] Even when asymptomatic, HIV-infected patients have presented with increased levels of EBV as evidenced by both bioassays and nucleic acid hybridization in the oropharynx.[51,52]

Katz et al.[53] have found that patients with AIDS may become infected simultaneously with several different genotypes of EBV.

1.4.3 EVOLUTION OF THERAPIES AND TREATMENT OF EPSTEIN-BARR VIRUS INFECTIONS

Several agents that have been shown to inhibit some aspects of EBV replication *in vitro* were not completely efficacious in clinical settings. Thus, leukocyte-derived human interferon-α, which was found to inhibit the stimulation of cellular DNA synthesis and cell growth of fresh lymphocytes inoculated with EBV,[54] when tested in renal transplant recipients prevented EBV excretion in only 38% of patients, compared with 68% in the control group.[55]

Another antiviral agent, acyclovir, was found to inhibit the lytic (but not latent) phase of EBV replication.[6] It is thought that acyclovir is incorporated preferentially into viral DNA through the action of EBV thymidine kinase. While the drug suppressed the viral linear DNA synthesis leading to virion production, it had no effect on the number of latent (circular) genomes.[56] Further studies have revealed that acyclovir suppressed the EBV DNA polymerase but not EBV-induced B cell immortalization. The latter finding suggested that lytic replication of the viral genome is not required for B cell transformation by the virus.[6]

Ernberg and Andersson[57] have used acyclovir to treat patients with acute infectious mono-nucleosis. While the level of oropharyngeal viral replication during the period of administration was efficiently reduced, following cessation of therapy the viral replication returned to its previous high levels. Moreover, since there was little or no reduction in the number of EBV-infected B cells found in the peripheral circulation, the oropharyngeal replication of EBV is not likely to be a major reservoir for B cell immortalization. Overall, the efficacy of acyclovir in the treatment of mono-nucleosis has been minimal.

Acyclovir and its prodrug, 6-deoxyacyclovir, have been reported to induce substantial regression of EBV-associated oral "hairy" leukoplakia in AIDS patients.[58,59]

The occasional reports of beneficial effects of acyclovir in the therapy of EBV-associated post-transplantation lymphoma,[60-62] as well as other lymphomas in immunosuppressed patients, have not been confirmed by controlled clinical trials.

Since Burkitt's lymphoma is a multifocal condition at the time of diagnosis, systemic chemo-therapy has been the treatment of choice.[6] Surgery and radiotherapy have also been used to reduce tumor lesions. In general, chemotherapeutic regimens have been very effective, especially when administered in cyclic fashions. In a typical example, six single doses of 40 mg/kg of cyclo-phosphamide are given at close intervals, usually every 2 to 3 weeks, allowing time for the recovery of the peripheral granulocyte counts to reach 1500 cells/mm³. Other agents that have been used to induce remission of Burkitt's lymphoma include vincristine, methotrexate, and prednisolone. So far, in African Burkitt's lymphomas remission following chemotherapy has been attained in 80% to 90% of the cases. However, outside the endemic regions, the prognosis for Burkitt's lymphomas and for EBV-negative B cell lymphomas has been poor.[6]

Blanche et al.[63] have used a combination of two monoclonal anti-B cell antibodies to treat two patients who had developed severe polyclonal EBV-induced lymphoproliferative syndrome after bone marrow transplantation for congenital (inherited) immunodeficiency. The syndrome, which occurred 50 to 60 d after the bone marrow infusion, was diagnosed by the presence of spontaneously growing B cells containing Epstein-Barr nuclear antigen in the blood and bone marrow. The two mouse monoclonal anti-B cell antibodies were a CD21-specific antibody recognizing the CR2 receptor on B cells (BL13, Ig1) and a CD24-specific antibody binding B cells at all steps of differentiation (ALB9, Ig1). Both antibodies have been injected intravenously daily at 0.2 mg/kg for 10 d. All clinical and biological manifestations resolved in both patients within 3 weeks of treatment, and there has been no recurrence at the 15- and 18-month follow-up examinations, respectively.[63] The reported results suggested that monoclonal anti-B cell antibody therapy may prove to be useful in controlling EBV-induced severe polyclonal lymphoproliferative syndrome in profoundly immunodeficient patients after bone marrow transplantation.

Shiong et al.[24] have described a rare case of fatal EBV-associated T cell lymphoma after renal transplantation and ensuing antirejection chemotherapy with prednisolone (10 mg daily), azathioprine (50 mg daily), and oral cyclosporin A. The presence of the EBV genome in the tissue was demonstrated by *in situ* hybridization and immunofluorescent techniques.

1.4.4 REFERENCES

1. Burkitt, D., A sarcoma involving the jaws in Afrikan children, *Br. J. Surg.*, 46, 218, 1958.
2. Burkitt, D., Determining the climatic limitations of a children's cancer common in Africa, *Br. Med. J.*, 2, 1019, 1962.
3. Epstein, M. A. and Barr, Y. M., Cultivation *in vitro* of human lymphoblasts from Burkitt's malignant lymphoma, *Lancet*, 1, 252, 1964.
4. Pulvertaft, R. J. V., Cytology of Burkitt's tumor (Afrikan lymphoma), *Lancet*, 1, 238, 1964.
5. Epstein, M. A., Achong, B. G., and Barr, Y. M., Virus particles in cultured lymphoblasts from Burkitt's lymphoma, *Lancet*, 1, 702, 1964.

6. Miller, G., Epstein-Barr virus, in *Fields Virology*, 2nd ed., Fields, B. N., Knipe, D. M., Chanock, R. M., Hirsch, M. S., Melnick, J. L., Monath, T. P., and Roizman, B., Eds., Raven Press, New York, 1990, 1921.

7. Miller, G., Human lymphoblastoid cell lines and Epstein-Barr virus (a review of their interrelationships and their relevance to the etiology of leukoproliferative states in man), *Yale J. Biol. Med.*, 43, 358, 1971.

8. Yoser, S. L., Forster, D. J., and Rao, N. A., Systemic viral infections and their retinal and choroidal manifestations, *Surv. Ophthalmol.*, 37, 313, 1993.

9. Schooley, R. T., Epstein-Barr virus infections, including infectious mononucleosis, in *Harrison's Principles of Internal Medicine*, 12th ed., Wilson, J. D., Braunwald, E., Isselbacher, K. J., Petersdorf, R. G., Martin, J. B., Fauci, A. S., and Root, R. K., Eds., McGraw-Hill, New York, 1991, 689.

10. Greenspan, J. S., Greenspan, D., Lennette, E. T., Abrams, D. I., Conant, M. A., Petersen, V., and Freese, U. K., Replication of Epstein-Barr virus within the epithelial cells of oral "hairy" leukoplakia, an AIDS-associated lesion, *N. Engl. J. Med.*, 313, 1564, 1985.

11. Sixbey, J. W., Nedrud, J. G., Raab-Traub, N., Hanes, R. A., and Pagano, J. S., Epstein-Barr virus replication in oropharyngeal epithelial cells, *N. Engl. J. Med.*, 310, 1225, 1984.

12. Wolf, H., Haus, M., and Wilmes, E., Persistence of Epstein-Barr virus in the parotid gland, *J. Virol.*, 51, 795, 1984.

13. de Thé, G., Geser, A., Day, N. E., Tukei, P. M., Williams, E. H., Beri, D. P., Smith, P. G., Dean, A. G., Bornkamm, G. W., Feorino, P., and Henle, W., Epidemiological evidence for casual relationship between Epstein-Barr virus and Burkitt's lymphoma from Ugandan prospective study, *Nature*, 274, 756, 1978.

14. de Thé, G. and Zeng, Y., Population screening for EBV markers: toward improvement of nasopharyngeal carcinoma control, in *The Epstein-Barr Virus: Recent Advances*, Epstein, M. A. and Achong, B. G., Eds., John Wiley & Sons, New York, 1986, 237.

15. Harabuchi, Y., Yamanaka, N., Kitaura, A., Imai, S., Kineshita, T., Mizuno, F., and Osato, T., Epstein-Barr virus in nasal T-cell lymphomas in patients with lethal midline granuloma, *Lancet*, 335, 128, 1990.

16. Weiss, L. M., Movahed, L. A., Warnke, R. A., and Sklar, J., Detection of Epstein-Barr viral genomes in Reed-Sternberg cells of Hodgkin's disease, *N. Engl. J. Med.*, 320, 502, 1989.

17. Jones, J. F., Shurin, S., Abramowsky, C., Tubbs, R. R., Sciotto, C. G., Wahl, R., Sands, J., Gottman, D., Katz, B. Z., and Sklar, J., T-cell lymphomas containing Epstein-Barr viral DNA in patients with chronic Epstein-Barr virus infection, *N. Engl. J. Med.*, 318, 733, 1988.

18. Leyvraz, S., Henle, W., Chahinian, A. P., Perlmann, C., Klein, G., Gordon, R. E., Rosenblum, M., and Holland, J. F., Association of Epstein-Barr virus with thymic carcinoma, *N. Engl. J. Med.*, 312, 1296, 1985.

19. Nalesnik, M. A., Jaffe, R., Starzl, T. E., Demetris, A. J., Porter, K., Burnham, J. A., Makowka, L., Ho, M., and Locker, J., The pathology of posttransplant lymphoproliferative disorders occurring in the setting of cyclosporine A-prednisone immunosuppression, *Am. J. Pathol.*, 133, 173, 1988.

20. Cohen, J. I., Epstein-Barr virus lymphoproliferative disease associated with acquired immunodeficiency, *Medicine (Baltimore)*, 70, 137, 1991.

21. Randhawa, P. S., Yousem, S. A., Paradis, I. L., Dauber, J. A., Griffith, B. P., and Locker, J., The clinical spectrum, pathology, and clonal analysis of Epstein-Barr virus-associated lymphoproliferative disorders in heart-lung transplant recipients, *Am. J. Clin. Pathol.*, 92, 177, 1989.

22. Locker, J. and Nalesnik, M., Molecular genetic analysis of lymphoid tumors arising after organ transplantation, *Am. J. Pathol.*, 135, 977, 1989.

23. Hanto, D. W., Gajl-Peczalska, K. J., Frizzera, G., Arthur, D. C., Balfour, H. H., Jr., McClain, K., Simmons, R. L., and Najarian, J. S., Epstein-Barr virus (EBV) induced polyclonal and monoclonal B-cell lymphoproliferative diseases occurring after renal transplantation, *Ann. Surg.*, 198, 356, 1983.

24. Shiong, Y. S., Lian, J. D., Lin, C. Y., Shu, K. H., Lu, Y. S., and Chou, G., Epstein-Barr virus-associated T-cell lymphoma of the maxillary sinus in a renal transplant recipient, *Transplant. Proc.*, 24, 1929, 1992.

25. Thorley-Lawson, D. A., The transformation of adult but not newborn human lymphocytes by Epstein-Barr virus and phytohemagglutinin is inhibited by interferon: the early suppression by T cells of Epstein-Barr infection is mediated by interferon, *J. Immunol.*, 126, 829, 1981.

26. Ljungman, P., Herpes virus infections in immunocompromised patients: problems and therapeutic interventions, *Ann. Med.*, 25, 329, 1993.

27. Ho, M., Miller, G., Atchison, R. W., Breinig, M. K., Dummer, J. S., Andiman, W., Starzl, T. E., Eastman, R., Grifith, B. P., Hardesty, R. L., Bahnson, H. T., Hakata, T. R., and Rosenthal, J. T., Epstein-Barr virus infections and DNA hybridization studies in posttransplantation lymphoma and lymphoproliferative lesions: the role of primary infections, *J. Infect. Dis.*, 152, 876, 1985.

28. Nalesnik, M. A., Makowka, L., and Starzl, T. E., The diagnosis and treatment of posttransplant lymphoproliferative disorders, *Curr. Probl. Surg.*, 25, 376, 1988.

29. Swinnen, L. J., Costanzo-Nordin, M. R., Fisher, S. G., O'Sullivan, E. J., Johnson, M. R., Heroux, A. L., Dizikes, G. J., Pifarre, R., and Fisher, R. I., Increased incidence of lymphoproliferative disorders after immunosuppression with the monoclonal antibody OKT3 in cardiac-transplant recipients, *N. Engl. J. Med.*, 323, 1723, 1990.

30. Penn, I., Cancer complicating organ transplantation, *N. Engl. J. Med.*, 323, 1767, 1990.

31. Hanto, D. W., Frizzera, G., Gajl-Peczalska, K. J., and Simmons, R. L., Epstein-Barr virus, immuno-deficiency and B-cell lymphoproliferation, *Transplantation*, 39, 461, 1985.

32. Starzl, T. E., Nalesnik, M. A., Porter, K. A., Ho, M., Iwatsuki, S., Griffith, B. P., Rosenthal, J. T., Hakala, T. R., Shaw, B. W., Jr., Hardesty, R. L., Atchison, R. W., Jaffe, R., and Bahnson, H. T., Reversibility of lymphomas and lymphoproliferative lesions developing under cyclosporin-steroid therapy, *Lancet*, 1, 583, 1984.

33. Bird, A. G., McLachlan, S. M., and Britton, S., Cyclosporin A promotes spontaneous outgrowth *in vitro* of Epstein-Barr virus-induced B-cell lines, *Nature*, 289, 300, 1981.

34. Ho, M., Jaffe, R., Miller, G., Breinig, M. K., Dummer, J. S., Makowka, L., Atchison, R. W., Karrer, F., Nalesnik, M. A., and Starzl, T. E., The frequency of Epstein-Barr virus infection and associated lymphoproliferative syndrome after transplantation and its manifestations in children, *Transplantation*, 45, 719, 1988.

35. Talenti, A., Marshall, W. F., and Smith, T. F., Detection of Epstein-Barr virus by polymerase chain reaction, *J. Clin. Microbiol.*, 28, 2187, 1990.

36. Su, I.-J., Chan, H.-L., Kuo, T., Eimoto, T., Maeda, Y., Kikuchi, M., Kuan, Y.-Z., Shih, L.-Y., Chen, M.-J., and Takeshitan, M., Adult T-cell leukemia/lymphoma in Taiwan: a clinicopathologic observation, *Cancer*, 56, 2217, 1985.

37. Su, I.-J., Hsieh, H.-C., Lin, K.-H., Uen, W.-C, Kao, C.-L., Chen, C.-J., Cheng, A.-L., Kadin, M. E., and Chen, J.-Y., Aggressive peripheral T-cell lymphomas containing Epstein-Barr viral DNA: a clinicopathologic and molecular analysis, *Blood*, 77, 799, 1991.

38. Su, I.-J., Shih, L.-Y., Kadin, M. E., Dun, P., and Hsu, S.-M., Pathologic and immunologic characterization of malignant lymphoma in Taiwan, with special reference to retrovirus-associated adult T-cell lymphoma/leukemia, *Am. J. Clin. Pathol.*, 84, 715, 1985.

39. Gossett, T. C., Gale, R. P., Fleischman, H., Austin, G. E., Sparkes, R. S., and Taylor, C. R., Immunoblastic sarcoma in donor cells after bone marrow transplantation, *N. Engl. J. Med.*, 30, 904, 1979.

40. Crawford, D. H., Mulholland, N., Iliescu, V., Hawkins, R., and Powles, R., Epstein-Barr virus infection and immunity in bone marrow transplant recipients, *Transplantation*, 42, 50, 1986.

41. Lange, B., Henle, W., Meyers, J. D., Yang, L. C., August, C., Koch, P., Arbeter, A., and Henle, G., Epstein-Barr virus-related serology in marrow transplant recipients, *Int. J. Cancer*, 26, 151, 1980.

42. Schubach, W. M., Hackman, R., Neiman, P. E., Miller, G., and Thomas, E. D., A monoclonal immunoblastic sarcoma in donor cells bearing Epstein-Barr virus genomes following allogeneic marrow grafting for acute lymphoblastic leukemia, *Blood*, 60, 180, 1982.

43. Martin, P. J., Shulman, H. M., Schubach, W. H., Hansen, J. A., Fefer, A., Miller, G., and Thomas, E. D., Fatal EBV-associated proliferation of donor B cells following treatment of acute graft-versus-host-disease with a murine monoclonal anti-T cell antibody, *Ann. Intern. Med.*, 101, 310, 1984.

44. Bozdech, M. J., Finlay, J. L., Trigg, M. E., Billing, R., Hong, R., Sugden, W., and Sondel, P. M., Monoclonal B-cell lymphoproliferative disorder following monoclonal antibody (CT2) T-cell depleted allogeneic bone marrow transplantation, *Blood*, 62(Suppl. 1A), 218, 1983.

45. Shearer, W. T., Ritz, J., Finegold, M. J., Guerra, I. C., Rosenblatt, H. M., Lewis, D. E., Pollack, M. S., Taber, L. H., Sumaya, C. V., Grumet, F. C., Cleary, M. L., Warnke, R., and Sklar, J., Epstein-Barr-virus-associated B-cell proliferations of diverse clonal origins after bone marrow transplantation in a 12-year-old patient with severe combined immunodeficiency, *N. Engl. J. Med.*, 312, 1151, 1985.

46. Kapoor, N., Jung, L. K., Engelhardt, D., Filler, J., Shalit, I., Landreth, K. S., and Good, R. A, Lymphoma in a patient with severe combined immunodeficiency with adenosine deaminase deficiency following unsustained engraftment of histocompatible T cell-depleted bone marrow, *J. Pediatr.*, 108, 435, 1986.

47. Subar, M., Neri, A., Inghirami, G., Knowles, D. M., and Dalla-Favera, R., Frequent c-*myc* oncogene activation and infrequent presence of Epstein-Barr virus genome in AIDS-associated lymphoma, *Blood*, 72, 667, 1988.

48. Garcia, C. R., Brown, N. A., Schreck, R., Stiehm, E. R., and Hudnall, S. D., B-cell lymphoma in severe combined immunodeficiency not associated with the Epstein-Barr virus, *Cancer*, 60, 2941, 1987.

49. Andiman, W. A., Eastman, R., Martin, K., Katz, B. Z., Rubinstein, A., Pitt, J., Pahwa, S., and Miller, G., Opportunistic lymphoproliferations associated with Epstein-Barr viral DNA in infants and children with AIDS, *Lancet*, 2, 1390, 1985.

50. Straus, S. E., Treatment of persistent active herpesvirus infections, *J. Virol. Meth.*, 21, 305, 1988.

51. Sumaya, C. V., Boswell, R. N., Ench, Y., Kisner, D. L., Hersh, E. M., Reuben, J. M., and Mansell, P. W., Enhanced serological and virological findings of Epstein-Barr virus in patients with AIDS and AIDS-related complex, *J. Infect. Dis.*, 154, 864, 1986.

52. Alsip, G. R., Ench, Y., Sumaya, C. V., and Boswell, R. N., Increased Epstein-Barr virus DNA in oropharyngeal secretions from patients with AIDS, AIDS-related complex, or asymptomatic human immunodeficiency virus infections, *J. Infect. Dis.*, 157, 1072, 1988.

53. Katz, B. Z., Andiman, W. A., Eastman, R., Martin, K., and Miller, G., Infection with two genotypes of Epstein-Barr virus of an infant with AIDS and lymphoma of the central nervous system, *J. Infect. Dis.*, 153, 601, 1986.

54. Garner, J. G., Hirsch, M. S., and Schooley, R. T., Interferon-alpha prevention of Epstein-Barr virus-induced B-cell outgrowth, *Infect. Immun.*, 43, 920, 1984.

55. Cheeseman, S. H., Henle, W., Rubin, R. H., Tolkoff-Rubin, N. E., Cosimi, B., Cantell, K., Winkle, S., Herrin, J. T., Black, P. H., Russell, P. S., and Hirsch, M. S., Epstein-Barr virus infection in renal transplant recipients: effects of antithymocyte globulin and interferon, *Ann. Intern. Med.*, 93, 39, 1980.

56. Colby, B. M., Shaw, J. E., Elion, G. B., and Pagano, J. S., Effect of acyclovir [9-(2-hydroxyethoxy-methyl)guanine] on Epstein-Barr virus replication, *J. Virol.*, 34, 560, 1980.

57. Ernberg, I. and Andersson, J., Acyclovir efficiently inhibits oropharyngeal excretion of Epstein-Barr virus in patients with acute infectious mononucleosis, *J. Gen. Virol.*, 67, 2267, 1986.

58. Resnick, L., Herbst, J. S., Ablashi, D. V., Atherton, S., Frank, B., Rosen, L., and Horwitz, S. N., Regression of oral "hairy" leukoplakia after orally administered acyclovir therapy, *JAMA*, 15, 384, 1988.

59. Shöfer, H., Ochsendorf, F. R., Helm, F., and Milbradt, R., Treatment of oral "hairy" leukoplakia in AIDS patients with vitamin A acid (topically) or acyclovir (systemically), *Dermatologica*, 174, 150, 1987.

60. Hanto, D. W., Frizzera, G., Gajl-Peczalska, K. J., Sakamoto, K., Purtilo, D. T., Balfour, H. H., Jr., Simmons, R. L., and Najarian, J. S., Epstein-Barr virus-induced B-cell lymphoma after renal transplantation: acyclovir therapy and transition from polyclonal to monoclonal B-cell proliferation, *N. Engl. J. Med.*, 306, 913, 1982.

61. Sullivan, J. L., Byron, K. S., Brewster, F. E., Sakamoto, K., Shaw, J. E., and Pagano, J. S., Treatment of life-threatening Epstein-Barr virus infection with acyclovir, *Am. J. Med.*, 73(1A), 262, 1982.

62. Sullivan, J. L., Medveczky, P., Forman, S. J., Baker, S. M., Monroe, J. E., and Mulder, C., Epstein-Barr virus-induced lymphoproliferation: implication for antiviral chemotherapy, *N. Engl. J. Med.*, 311, 1163, 1984.

63. Blanche, S., Le Deist, F., Veber, F., Lenoir, G., Fischer, A. M., Brochier, J., Boucheix, C., Delaage, M., Griscelli, C., and Fischer, A., Treatment of severe Epstein-Barr virus-induced polyclonal B-lymphocyte proliferation by anti-B-cell monoclonal antibodies, *Ann. Intern. Med.*, 108, 199, 1988.

1.5   HUMAN HERPESVIRUS-6, HUMAN HERPESVIRUS-7, AND HUMAN HERPESVIRUS-8

1.5.1   INTRODUCTION

In 1986, Salahuddin et al.[1] described the first isolates of a previously unrecognized human herpesvirus which they designated as human B-lymphotropic virus (HBLV) based on the fact that it was initially discovered in freshly isolated infected B cells from cultures of peripheral blood mononuclear cells derived from AIDS patients with lymphoreticular (leukemia/lymphoma) disorders. Later, similar viral isolates were obtained from AIDS patients in Uganda,[2] Gambia,[3] Zaire,[4] and the Ivory Coast.[5] Genomes from viruses isolated in Uganda, Gambia, Zaire, and the Ivory Coast have been shown to contain fragments homologous to sequences from a U.S. isolate represented in the pZVH14 recombinant clone.[6]

It was initially proposed[1] that HBLV infects exclusively B cells. However, isolates from Uganda, Gambia, and Zaire have been shown to replicate preferentially in T cell populations from peripheral blood or cord blood mononuclear cells.[2-5] Moreover, Lusso et al.,[7,8] after thoroughly evaluating the growth of HBLV in cultures of mononuclear cells from adult peripheral blood, cord blood, and thymic tissues, have found that most cells supporting HBLV replication displayed markers characteristic of immature T cells, i.e., CD2, CD4, CD5, CD7, and CD8. HBLV was also reported capable of infecting and replicating in macrophages,[9] where it could lead to dysregulated production of cytokines that may potentiate any inflammatory process. Therefore, the continuous usage of human B cell lymphotropic virus (HBLV) as a label for this virus has been deemed inappropriate and the name human herpesvirus-6 (HHV-6) was adopted instead.

The viral genome of HHV-6 represents a linear, double-stranded DNA molecule with a mean composition of 43% to 44% (G + C) and a size of 160 to 170 kbp.[10] The existence of genetic heterogeneity among HHV-6 isolates has been reported.[11,12] Lawrence et al.[13] have sequenced approximately 13% of the HHV-6 genome and noted more homology between HHV-6 and regions of the cytomegalovirus DNA than with that of other herpesviruses.

Currently, there is convincing evidence to suggest that infection with HHV-6 is widespread in normal adults.[14-16] A number of studies[17-19] have provided evidence that infection with HHV-6 typically develops in early infancy and is the causative agent of exanthem subitum. It is generally believed that a primary infection with HHV-6 acquired early confers permanent immunity, although reinfection should not be excluded in profoundly immunosuppressed individuals since most adults with the antibody to HHV-6 excrete the virus into saliva.[20-22] It has been suggested that several tissues, such as lungs,[23,24] liver,[25] lymph nodes,[26] kidney,[27] and salivary glands[28] contain HHV-6.

HHV-6 has been implicated in some cases of severe hepatitis, transverse myelitis, meningoencephalitis, and mononucleosis syndromes.[29-33] Sumiyoshi et al.[34] have reported two cases of a severe, infectious, mononucleasosis-like syndrome resulting from a primary HHV-6 infection in immunocompetent adults. In addition, both patients had a skin condition known as erythroderma. Immunohistochemical examination of a skin biopsy specimen revealed the presence of HHV-6-infected lymphocytes. It has been suggested that erythroderma in immunocompetent hosts infected with primary HHV-6 may be provoked by infiltration of infected inflammatory cells or infected neoplastic lymphocytes into the dermis. Jones et al.[35] have described a previously healthy infant who developed status epilepticus with high fever due to acute HHV-6 infection.

Sumiyoshi et al.[36] have analyzed the HHV-6 genomes in patients with lymphoid malignancies, and detected the virus in 50% to 68.8% of all cases. The results suggested that HHV-6 DNA was not related to the lymphoid malignancy but rather was a latent infection of non-neoplastic cells in tumor tissue. In a related study, Fox et al.[37] detected high levels of HHV-6 DNA in a lymphoma of a patient with Sjögren's syndrome.

Similarly to other herpes viruses, HHV-6 seems to remain latent in the body after primary infection and reactivate in immunocompromised hosts.[38] Thus, Okuno et al.[39] and Ward et al.[25] have reported reactivation or activation of HHV-6 after kidney and liver transplantations, respectively. Okuno et al.[39] have suggested that the active infection by HHV-6 in renal transplantations may be due to the immunosuppressive treatment for kidney rejection. In this regard, Jacobs et al.[40] have reported a severe kidney allograft dysfunction following OKT3-induced HHV-6 reactivation.

HHV-6 has also been associated with graft failure and meningoencephalitis after bone marrow transplantation.[41] According to a study by Yoshikawa et al.,[42] HHV-6 was isolated from the blood of 40% of bone marrow transplant recipients studied.

The development of early interstitial pneumonia following bone marrow transplantation has been associated with the isolation of HHV-6.[23]

1.5.2 Role of Herpesvirus-6 in HIV Disease

The occurrence of three events relevant to both HHV-6 and HIV, namely, (1) the common isolation of HHV-6 from HIV-infected patients; (2) the finding that HHV-6 can infect CD4-T cells (also the target cells for HIV); and (3) the observation that human herpesvirus immediate-early proteins can *trans*-activate the HIV long terminal repeat (LTR),[43,44] have suggested the possibility that HHV-6 may be a cofactor in the progression of HIV-positive patients to symptomatic AIDS. The presence of HHV-6 in most patients with AIDS has been ascertained by direct isolation,[1-3] DNA amplification technique,[45] and serological analysis.[46]

In further studies, Lusso et al.[44] have demonstrated that both HHV-6 and HIV-1 can productively coinfect individual human CD4+ T lymphocytes, resulting in accelerated HIV-1 expression and cellular death. This finding and the observed transactivation of the HIV-1 LTR by HHV-6 (using human CD4+ T-line MOLT-3) represent a direct evidence of interaction between HIV-1 and HHV-6.

In another related development, infection of a human neoplastic T cell line with HHV-6 dramatically upregulated the expression of CD4 (the receptor for HIV-1[47-49]).[50] More importantly, HHV-6 induced the *de novo* expression of CD4 messenger RNA and protein in normal mature CD8+ T lymphocytes, rendering them susceptible to infection with HIV-1.[50] The results of this study have demonstrated a novel mechanism, receptor regulation, through which HHV-6 may positively interact with HIV-1 in coinfected patients.

The seroprevalence of HHV-6 infection in HIV-positive patients has been investigated by Roldan et al.[51]

1.5.3 Drug Susceptibility of Human Herpesvirus-6

Bapat et al.[52] have evaluated the inhibitory properties of various deoxynucleoside triphosphate and pyrophosphate analogs on the HHV-6 DNA polymerase activity. Based on the inhibition constant value of acyclovir triphosphate and its ratio to 2-deoxyguanosine-5′-triphosphate, it has been predicted that acyclovir may not be as selective against HHV-6 as well as some of the other herpesviruses, whereas similar data for ganciclovir (DHPG) and bromovinyldeoxyuridine (BVdU) indicated that these two antiviral agents may be more selective against HHV-6. Subsequent studies by Burns and Sandford[53] have shown that HHV-6 was susceptible *in vitro* to ganciclovir and foscarnet but resistant to acyclovir (at 10 μM) and BVdU (at concentrations as high as 100 μM). Russler et al.[54] have also found HHV-6 susceptible to ganciclovir. These results supported the findings of Bapat et al.[52] that ganciclovir may effectively inhibit the HHV-6 DNA synthesis, whereas acyclovir and BVdU were less active. The lack of potency of acyclovir and BVdU suggested that HHV-6 may lack thymidine kinase capable of phosphorylating these two compounds.

Nakagami et al.[55] have examined the antiviral activity of biliverdin, a bile pigment, against HHV-6 *in vitro*. At 10 µg/ml, biliverdin significantly inhibited the replication of HHV-6 in MT-4 cells, when the cells were treated during a virus adsorption period. The activity was weakened when the cells were treated after adsorption, and there was no activity when cells were treated with 40 µg/ml, 3 h after virus infection.

1.5.4 HUMAN HERPESVIRUS-7

Recently, Frenkel et al.[56] have isolated a new herpesvirus, human herpesvirus-7 (HHV-7), which shared some genomic homology with HHV-6. Although HHV-6 and HHV-7 exhibited similar cytopathic effects and virion structure, still there is not sufficient information about the genomic and antigenic properties of HHV-7 and its role as an etiologic agent of infections in immunocompromised hosts.

1.5.5 HUMAN HERPESVIRUS-8

Kaposi's sarcoma and non-Hodgkin's lymphoma are the two most common neoplasms occurring in patients infected with the HIV.[57-60] Approximately 15% to 20% of AIDS patients are expected to develop Kaposi's sarcoma, which otherwise has been rarely seen in immunocompetent individuals.[57,58] In some cohorts of homosexual male AIDS patients, the lifetime risk of Kaposi's sarcoma may approach 50%.[61]

Epidemiologic evidence has suggested that the AIDS-associated Kaposi's sarcoma may have an infectious etiology[57,62-67] since homosexual and bisexual male AIDS patients have been nearly 20 times more likely to develop this neoplasia than hemophiliac AIDS patients.[57,63] In addition, the development of Kaposi's sarcoma may be linked to specific sexual practices among gay men with AIDS.[62,63,68,69] The finding of Friedman-Kien et al.[70] that frequency of Kaposi's sarcoma in HIV-negative homosexual men has been higher than expected supported the hypothesis that its etiologic agent can be sexually transmitted and is also distinct from HIV-1. Moreover, Kaposi's sarcoma has been uncommon among adult AIDS patients infected through heterosexual or parenteral HIV transmission, or among pediatric patients infected through vertical HIV transmission.[71]

Various infectious agents have been suspected to cause Kaposi's sarcoma, including cytomegalovirus, hepatitis B virus, human herpesvirus-6, HIV, and *Mycoplasma penetrans*.[71-78] Extensive follow-up studies, however, failed to demonstrate any etiologic association between these agents and Kaposi's sarcoma in AIDS patients.[79-82] Noninfectious agents, such as nitrite inhalants, have also been suggested as potential causes of Kaposi's sarcoma tumorogenesis.[83]

In addition to Kaposi's sarcoma in AIDS patients, histopathologically similar forms of this neoplasia have been observed in non-HIV-infected individuals. The classic form represents an indolent disease that usually affects the low extremities.[84] It has been observed most often in elderly men of Mediterranean, Middle Eastern, or eastern European ethnic origin.[85,86] Some serologic evidence has suggested that the classic form of Kaposi's sarcoma may be associated with cytomegalovirus infection.[87,88]

Endemic African Kaposi's sarcoma[89,90] and post-transplantation Kaposi's sarcoma[91] are two additional forms of the disease that were diagnosed in immunocompetent and immunocompromised patients, respectively.

In HIV-seronegative homosexual men with Kaposi's sarcoma, there has been no detectable immunodeficiency, and the tumor resembles that of classic Kaposi's sarcoma both in its presentation and clinical course.[92]

In 1994, while studying Kaposi's sarcoma tissues obtained from AIDS patients, Chang et al.[93] discovered distinct herpesvirus-like DNA sequences which were subsequently recognized as a new human herpesvirus, designated as human herpesvirus-8 (HHV-8). The technique used to isolate, identify, and characterize the two unique DNA sequences, known as KS330Bam (330 bp) and KS631Bam (631 bp), involved representational difference analysis. These DNA sequences were either absent or present in low copy number in nondiseased tissue obtained from the same patient.[94]

Both KS330Bam and KS631Bam coded for amino acid sequences with homology to herpesvirus polypeptides, in particular to the minor capsid and tegument protein genes of two gammaherpesviruses, the Epstein-Barr virus and the herpesvirus saimiri. Thus, KS330Bam was 51% identical by amino acid homology to a portion of the ORF26 open reading frame encoding the capsid protein VP23 of herpesvirus saimiri,[95] a gammaherpesvirus that causes fulminant lymphoma in New World monkeys. In addition, this fragment was also 39% identical to the amino acid sequence encoded by the corresponding BDLFI ORF of the Epstein-Barr virus.[96] The amino acid sequence encoded by KS631Bam was homologous to the tegument protein (ORF75) of herpesvirus saimiri and to the tegument protein of the Epstein-Barr virus (ORF BNRFI, p140).

The findings of Chang et al.[93] provided strong evidence that a new human herpesvirus (HHV-8) is the cause of AIDS-associated Kaposi's sarcoma. However, it is also possible that this agent may preferentially colonize preexisting Kaposi's sarcoma in immunosuppressed patients and did not play an etiologic role.[97]

Comparative experiments by Moore and Chang[92] have demonstrated that the same herpesvirus-like DNA sequences (HHV-8) were also present in AIDS-associated Kaposi's sarcoma, classic Kaposi's sarcoma, and the Kaposi's sarcoma that affects HIV-seronegative homosexual men. Ceserman et al.[97] have found the HHV-8 DNA sequences in an unusual subgroup of AIDS-related body-cavity-based B cell lymphomas, but not in any other lymphoid neoplasm studied so far. In spite of the extensive similarity, polymorphism among the herpesvirus-like DNA sequences identified in Kaposi's sarcoma tissues from different populations still existed as shown by both single-strand conformational polymorphism and direct sequencing.[98]

So far, the currently available information clearly indicates that HHV-8 should not be considered solely as the cause of an opportunistic infection in patients with AIDS, but may be involved in the pathogenesis of different forms of Kaposi's sarcoma seen among distinct and unrelated populations.[86,98] The presence of HHV-8 DNA sequences in a very large fraction of Kaposi's sarcomas, both AIDS-related and classic, points to HHV-8 as either a highly preferred colonizing agent or an etiologic agent, and the available information does not permit discrimination between these two alternatives.[99]

1.5.5.1 Treatment of Kaposi's Sarcoma

At present, the treatment of Kaposi's sarcoma involves the use of chemotherapy, interferons, radiation, and different kinds of local treatment that can offer palliation. However, short remission or considerable toxicities have limited the benefits of these therapeutic approaches.

So far, only a few cases of spontaneous resolution of epidemic Kaposi's sarcoma have been reported.[100-102] In one of the patients described, foscarnet was used.[102] Several studies failed to demonstrate any beneficial effect of zidovudine in the treatment of this neoplasia.[103,104]

Morfeldt and Torssander[105] have described a long-term remission of Kaposi's sarcoma in HIV-infected patients (four of the five patients treated suffered from severe immunodeficiency with CD4[+] counts below 30×10^6/l), following treatment with foscarnet. The patients received intravenous foscarnet at 100 mg/kg daily for 10 d. Three of the patients went into long-term remission as seen from observation at 12, 13, and 20 months, respectively.

In another report, Jones et al.[106] have examined data collected on HIV-infected patients in more than 100 medical facilities in ten metropolitan areas in the U.S. Of three antiviral medications used (acyclovir, ganciclovir, and foscarnet), only the latter proved to be associated with a significant reduction in the risk of Kaposi's sarcoma.

1.5.6 REFERENCES

1. Salahuddin, S. Z., Ablashi, D. V., Markham, P. D., Josephs, S. F., Sturenegger, S., Kaplan, M., Halligan, G., Biberfeld, P., Wong-Staal, F., Kramarsky, B., and Gallo, R. C., Isolation of a new virus, HBLV, in patients with lymphoproliferative disorders, *Science*, 234, 596, 1986.
2. Downing, R. G., Sawankambo, N., Serwadda, D., Honess, R., Crawford, D., Jarrett, R., and Griffin, B. E., Isolation of human lymphotropic herpesviruses from Uganda, *Lancet*, 2, 390, 1987.
3. Tedder, R. S., Briggs, M., Cameron, C. H., Honess, R., Robertson, D., and Whittle, H., A novel lymphotropic herpesvirus, *Lancet*, 2, 390, 1987.

4. Lopez, C., Pellett, P., Stewart, J., Goldsmith, C., Sanderlin, K., Black, J., Warfield, D., and Feorino, P., Characteristics of human herpesvirus-6, *J. Infect. Dis.*, 157, 1271, 1988.
5. Agut, H., Guetard, D., and Collandre, H., Concomitant infection by human herpesvirus 6, HTLV-1, and HIV-2, *Lancet*, 1, 712, 1988.
6. Josephs, S. F., Salahuddin, S. A., Ablashi, D. V., Schachter, F., Wong-Staal, F., and Gallo, R. C., Genomic analysis of the human B-lymphotropic virus (HBLV), *Science*, 234, 601, 1986.
7. Lusso, O., Markham, P. D., Tschachler, E., di Marzo Veronese, S., Salahuddin, S. Z., Ablashi, D. V., Pahwa, S., Krohn, K., and Gallo, R. C., *In vitro* cellular tropism of human B-lymphotropic virus (human herpesvirus- 6), *J. Exp. Med.*, 167, 1659, 1988.
8. Lusso, P., Salahuddin, S. Z., Ablashi, D. V., Gallo, R. C., Veronese, F., and Markham, P. D., Diverse tropism of human B-lymphotropic virus (human herpesvirus-6), *Lancet*, 2, 743, 1987.
9. Levy, J. A., Ferro, F., Lennette, E. T., Oshiro, L., and Poulin, L., Characterization of a new strain of HHV-6 (HHV-6$_{SF}$) recovered from the saliva of an HIV-infected individual, *Virology*, 178, 113, 1990.
10. Lopez, C. and Honess, R. W., Human herpesvirus-6, in *Fields Virology*, 2nd ed., Fields, R. M., Knipe, M. S., Chanock, R. M., Hirsch, M. S., Melnick, J. L., Monath, T. P., and Roizman, R., Eds., Raven Press, New York, 1990, 2055.
11. Kikuta, H., Ly, H., Matsumoto, S., Josephs, S. F., and Gallo, R. C., Polymorphism of human herpesvirus 6 DNA from five Japanese patients with exanthem subitum, *J. Infect. Dis.*, 160, 550, 1989.
12. Aubin, J. T., Agut, H., Collandre, H., Yamanishi, K., Chandran, B., Montagnier, L., and Huraux, J. M., Antigenic and genetic differentiation of the two putative types of human herpesvirus-6, *J. Virol. Meth.*, 41, 223, 1993.
13. Lawrence, G. L., Chee, M., Craxton, M. A., Gompels, U. A., Honess, R. W., and Barrell, B. G., Human herpesvirus 6 is closely related to human cytomegalovirus, *J. Virol.*, 64, 287, 1990.
14. Briggs, M., Fox, J., and Tedder, R. S., Age prevalence of antibody to human herpesvirus-6, *Lancet*, 1, 1058, 1988.
15. Brown, H. A., Sumaya, C. V., Liu, C.-R., Ench, Y., Kovacs, A., Coronesi, M., and Kaplan, M. H., Fall in human herpesvirus-6 seropositivity with age, *Lancet*, 2, 396, 1988.
16. Takahashi, K., Sonoda, S., Kawakami, K., Miyata, K., Oki, T., Nagata, T., Okuno, T., and Kamanishi, K., Human herpesvirus 6 and exanthem subitum, *Lancet*, 1, 1463, 1988.
17. Biggar, R., Henle, W., Fleisher, G., Bocker, J., Lennette, E. T., and Henle, G., Primary Epstein-Barr virus infections in African infants. I. Decline of maternal antibodies and time of infection, *Int. J. Cancer*, 22, 239, 1978.
18. Yamanishi, K., Okuno, T., Shiraki, K., Takahashi, M., Kondo, T., Asano, Y., and Kurata, T., Identification of human herpesvirus-6 as a causal agent for exanthem subitum, *Lancet*, 1, 1065, 1988.
19. Pruksananonda, P., Hall, C. B., Insel, R. A., McIntyre, K., Pellett, P. E., Long, C. E., Schnabel, K. C., Pincus, P. H., Stamey, F. R., Dambaugh, T. R., and Stewart, J. A., Primary human herpesvirus 6 infection in young children, *N. Engl. J. Med.*, 326, 1445, 1992.
20. Pietroboni, G. R., Harnett, G. B., Bucens, M. R., and Honess, R. W., Antibody to human herpesvirus 6 in saliva, *Lancet*, 1, 1059, 1988.
21. Harnett, G., Farr, T., Pietroboni, G., and Bucens, M., Frequent shedding of human herpesvirus 6 in saliva, *J. Med. Virol.*, 30, 128, 1990.
22. Levy, J. A., Ferro, F., Greenspan, D., and Lennette, E. T., Frequent isolation of HHV-6 from saliva and high prevalence of the virus in the population, *Lancet*, 335, 1047, 1990.
23. Carrigan, D. R., Drobyski, W. R., Russler, S. K., Tapper, M. A., Knox, K. K., and Ash, R. C., Interstitial pneumonitis associated with human herpes virus-6 infection after marrow transplantation, *Lancet*, 338, 147, 1991.
24. Pitalia, A. K., Liu-Yin, J. A., Freemont, A. J., Morris, D. J., and Fitzmaurice, R. J., Immunohistological detection of human herpesvirus 6 in formalin-fixed, paraffin-embedded lung tissues, *J. Med. Virol.*, 41, 103, 1993.
25. Ward, K. N., Gray, J. J., and Efstathiou, S., Brief report: primary human herpesvirus 6 infection in a patient following liver transplantation from a seropositive donor, *J. Med. Virol.*, 28, 69, 1989.
26. Eizuru, Y., Minamatsu, T., Minamishima, Y., Kikuchi, M., Yamanishi, K., Takahashi, M., and Kurata, T., Human herpesvirus-6 in lymph nodes, *Lancet*, 1, 40, 1990.
27. Asano, Y., Yoshikawa, T., Suga, S., Yazaki, T., Hirabayashi, S., Ono, Y., Tsuzuki, K., and Oshima, S., Human herpesvirus-6 harboring in kidney, *Lancet*, 2, 1391, 1989.

28. Fox, J. D., Briggs, M., Ward, P. A., and Tedder, R. S., Human herpesvirus-6 in salivary glands, *Lancet*, 336, 590, 1990.

29. Niederman, J. C., Kaplan, M. H., Liu, C.-R., and Brown, N. A., Clinical and serological features of human herpesvirus-6 infection in three adults, *Lancet*, 2, 817, 1988.

30. Sobue, R., Miyazaki, H., Okamoto, M., Hirano, M., Yoshikawa, T., Suga, S., and Asano, Y., Fulminant hepatitis in primary human herpesvirus-6 infection, *N. Engl. J. Med.*, 324, 1290, 1991.

31. Buchwald, D., Cheney, P. R., Peterson, D. L., Henry, B., Wormsley, S. B., Geiger, A., Ablashi, D. V., Salahuddin, Z., Saxinger, C., Biddle, R., Kikinis, R., Jolesz, F. A., Folks, T., Balachandran, N., Peter, J. B., Gallo, R. C., and Komaroff, A. L., A chronic illness characterized by fatigue, neurologic and immunologic disorders, and active human herpesvirus type 6 infection, *Ann. Intern. Med.*, 116, 103, 1992.

32. Prezioso, P. J., Cangiarella, J., Lee, M., Nuovo, G. J., Borkowsky, W., Orlow, S. J., and Greco, M. A., Fatal disseminated infection with human herpesvirus-6, *J. Pediatr.*, 120, 921, 1992.

33. Hill, A. E., Hicks, E. M., and Coyle, P. V., Human herpes virus 6 and central nervous system complications, *Dev. Med. Child. Neurol.*, 36, 651, 1994.

34. Sumiyoshi, Y., Akashi, K., and Kikuchi, M., Detection of human herpes virus 6 (HHV 6) in the skin of a patient with primary HHV 6 infection and erythroderma, *J. Clin. Pathol.*, 47, 762, 1994.

35. Jones, C. M., Dunn, H. C., Thomas, E. E., Cone, R. W., and Weber, J. M., Acute encephalopathy and status epilepticus associated with human herpes virus 6 infection, *Dev. Med. Child. Neurol.*, 36, 646, 1994.

36. Sumiyoshi, Y., Kikuchi, M., Ohshima, K., Takeshita, M., Eizuro, Y., and Minamishima, Y., Analysis of human herpesvirus-6 genomes in lymphoid malignancy in Japan, *J. Clin. Pathol.*, 46, 1137, 1993.

37. Fox, R. I., Luppi, M., Kang, H. I., Ablashi, D., and Josephs, S., Detection of high levels of human herpesvirus-6 DNA in a lymphoma of a patient with Sjögren's syndrome, *J. Rheumatol.*, 20, 764, 1993.

38. Ljungman, P., Herpes virus infections in immunocompromised patients: problems and therapeutic interventions, *Ann. Med.*, 25, 329, 1993.

39. Okuno, T., Higashi, K., Shiraki, K., Yamanishi, K., Takahashi, M., Kokado, Y., Ishibashi, M., Takahara, S., Sonoda, T., Tanaka, K., Baba, K., Yabuuchi, H., and Kurata, T., Human herpesvirus 6 infection in renal transplantation, *Transplantation*, 49, 519, 1990.

40. Jacobs, U., Ferber, J., and Klehr, H. U., Severe allograft dysfunction after OKT3-induced human herpes virus-6 reactivation, *Transplant. Proc.*, 26, 3121, 1994.

41. Levin, M. J., Impact of herpesvirus infections in the future, *J. Med. Virol. Suppl.*, 1, 158, 1993.

42. Yoshikawa, T., Suga, S., Asano, Y., Nakashima, T., Yazaki, T., Sobue, R., Hirano, M., Fukuda, M., Kojima, S., and Matsuyama, T., Human herpes virus-6 infection in bone marrow transplantation, *Blood*, 78, 1381, 1981.

43. Rando, R. F., Pellett, P. E., Luciw, P. A., Bohan, C. A., and Srinivasan, A., *Trans*-activation of human immunodeficiency virus by herpesviruses, *Oncogene*, 1, 13, 1987.

44. Lusso, P., Ensoli, B., Markham, P. D., Ablashi, D. V., Salahuddin, S. Z., Tschachler, E., Wong-Staal, F., and Gallo, R. C., Productive dual infection of human CD4+ T lymphocytes by HIV-1 and HHV-6, *Nature*, 337, 370, 1989.

45. Biberfeld, P., Petrén, A.-L., Eklund, A., Lindemalm, C., Barkhem, T., Ekman, M., Ablashi, D., and Salahuddin, S. Z., Human herpesvirus-6 (HHV-6, HBLV) in sarcoidosis and lymphoproliferative disorders, *J. Virol. Meth.*, 21, 49, 1988.

46. Ablashi, D. V., Josephs, S. F., Buchbinder, A., Hellman, K., Nakamura, S., Llana, T., Lusso, P., Kaplan, M., Dahlberg, J., Memon, S., Imam, F., Ablashi, K. L., Markham, P. D., Kramarsky, B., Krueger, G. R. F., Biberfeld, P., Wong-Staal, F., Salahuddin, S. Z., and Gallo, R. C. Human B-lymphotropic virus (human herpesvirus-6), *J. Virol. Meth.*, 21, 29, 1988.

47. Dalgleish, A. G., Beverley, P. C. L., Claphan, P. R., Crawford, D. H., Greaves, M. F., and Weiss, R. A., The CD4 (T4) antigen is an essential component of the receptor for AIDS retrovirus, *Nature*, 312, 763, 1984.

48. Klatzmann, D., Champagne, E., Chamaret, S., Gruest, J., Guetard, D., Hercend, T., Gluckman, J.-C., and Montagnier, L., T-lymphocyte T4 molecule behaves as the receptor for human retrovirus LAV, *Nature*, 312, 767, 1984.

49. McDougal, J. S., Kennedy, M. S., Sligh, J. M., Cort, S. P., Mawle, A., and Nicholson, K. K. A., Binding of HTLV-III/LAV to T4⁺ T cells by a complex of HOK viral protein and the T4 molecule, *Science*, 231, 382, 1986.

50. Lusso, P., De Maria, A., Malnati, M., Lori, F., DeRocco, S. E., Baseler, M., and Gallo, R. C., Induction of CD4 and susceptibility to HIV-1 infection in human CD8⁺ T lymphocytes by human herpesvirus 6, *Nature*, 349, 533, 1991.

51. Roldan, C., Gutierrez, J., Maroto, M. C., and Bernal, M. C., Seroprevalence of infection by human type 6 herpes virus in patients with the human immunodeficiency virus infection, *Med. Clin. (Barcelona)*, 101, 637, 1993.

52. Bapat, A. R., Bodner, A. J., Ting, R. C. Y., and Cheng, Y. C., Identification of some properties of a unique DNA polymerase from cells infected with human B-lymphotropic virus, *J. Virol.*, 63, 1400, 1989.

53. Burns, W. H. and Sandford, G. R., Susceptibility of human herpes virus-6 to antivirals *in vitro*, *J. Infect. Dis.*, 162, 634, 1990.

54. Isakov, V. A., Ermolenko, D. K., Chaika, N. A., Ermolenko, E. I., and Norman, L. L., Epidemiologic aspects of human herpes virus type VI, *Vestn. Ross. Akad. Med. Nauk*, 9, 15, 1994.

55. Nakagami, T., Taji, S., Takahashi, M., and Yamanishi, K., Antiviral activity of a bile pigment, biliverdin, against human herpesvirus 6 (HHV- 6) in vitro, *Microbiol. Immunol.*, 36, 381, 1992.

56. Frenkel, N., Schirmer, E. C., Wyatt, L. S., Katsafanas, G., Roffman, E., Danovich, R. M., and June, C. H., Isolation of a new herpesvirus from human CD4⁺ T cells, *Proc. Natl. Acad. Sci. U.S.A.*, 87, 784, 1990.

57. Beral, V., Peterman, T. A., Berkelman, R. L., and Jaffe, H. W., Kaposi's sarcoma among persons with AIDS: a sexually transmitted infection? *Lancet*, 335, 123, 1990.

58. Beral, V., Bull, D., Jaffe, H., Evans, B., Gill, N., Tillett, H., and Swerdlow, A. J., Is risk of Kaposi's sarcoma in AIDS patients in Britain increased if sexual partners came from the United States or Africa? *Br. Med. J.*, 302, 624, 1991 [correction in *Br. Med. J.*, 302, 752, 1991].

59. Beral, V., Peterman, T., Berkelman, R., and Jaffe, H., AIDS-associated non-Hodgkin lymphoma, *Lancet*, 337, 805, 1991.

60. Levine, A. M., AIDS-related malignancies: the emerging epidemic, *J. Natl. Cancer Inst.*, 85, 1382, 1993.

61. Katz, M. H., Hessol, N. A., Buchbinder, S. P., Hirozawa, A., O'Malley, P., and Holmberg, S. D., Temporal trends of opportunistic infections and malignancies in homosexual men with AIDS, *J. Infect. Dis.*, 170, 198, 1994.

62. Beral, V., Bull, D., Darby, S., Weller, I., Carne, C., Beecham, M., and Jaffe, H., Risk of Kaposi's sarcoma and sexual practices with faecal contact in homosexual or bisexual men with AIDS, *Lancet*, 339, 632, 1992.

63. Archibald, C. P., Schechter, M. T., Le, T. N., Craib, K. J. P., Montaner, J. S. G., and O'Shaughnessy, M. V., Evidence for a sexually transmitted cofactor for AIDS-related Kaposi's sarcoma in a cohort of homosexual men, *Epidemiology*, 3, 203, 1992.

64. Jaffe, H. W., Choi, K., Thomas, P. A., Haverkos, H. W., Auerbach, D. M., Guinan, M. E., Rogers, M. F., Spira, T. J., Darrow, W. W., Kramer, M. A., Friedman, S. M., Monroe, J. M., Friedman-Kien, A. E., Laubenstein, L. J., Marmor, M., Safai, B., Dritz, S. K., Crispi, S. J., Fannin, S. L., Orkwis, J. P., Kelter, A., Rushing, W. R., Thacker, S. B., and Curran, J. W., National case-control study of Kaposi's sarcoma and *Pneumocystis carinii* pneumonia in homosexual men. I. Epidemiologic results, *Ann. Intern. Med.*, 99, 145, 1983.

65. Biggar, R. J., Cancer in acquired immunodeficiency syndrome: an epidemiological assessment, *Semin. Oncol.*, 17, 251, 1990.

66. Lassoued, K., Clauvel, J. P., Fegueux, S., Matheron, S., Gorin, I., and Oksenhendler, E., AIDS-associated Kaposi's sarcoma in female patients, *AIDS*, 5, 877, 1991.

67. Beral, V., Epidemiology of Kaposi's sarcoma, in *Cancer, HIV and AIDS*, Beral, V., Jaffe, H. W., and Weiss, R. A., Eds., Cold Spring Harbor Laboratory, Cold Spring Harbor, NY, 1991, 5.

68. Lifson, A. R., Darrow, J. J., Hessol, N. A., O'Malley, P. M., Barnhart, J. L., Jaffe, H. W., and Rutherford, G. W., Kaposi's sarcoma in a cohort of homosexual and bisexual men: epidemiology and analysis for cofactors, *Am. J. Epidemiol.*, 131, 221, 1990.

69. Schechter, M. T., Marion, S. A., Elmslie, K. D., Ricketts, M. N., Nault, P., and Archibald, C. P., Geographic and birth cohort association of Kaposi's sarcoma among homosexual men in Canada, *Am. J. Epidemiol.*, 134, 485, 1991.

70. Friedman-Kien, A. E., Saltzman, B. R., Cao, Y. Z., Nestor, M. S., Mirabile, M., Li, J. J., and Peterman, T. A., Kaposi's sarcoma in HIV- negative homosexual men, *Lancet*, 335, 168, 1990.

71. Peterman T. A., Jaffe, H. W., Friedman-Kien, A. E., and Weiss, A., The etiology of Kaposi's sarcoma, in *Cancer Survey*, Vol. 10, *Cancer, HIV and AIDS*, Imperial Cancer Research Fund, London, 1991, 23.

72. Drew, W. L., Conant, M. A., Miner, R. C., Huang, E. S., Ziegler, J. L., Groundwater, J. R., Gullett, J. H., Volberding, P., Abrams, D. I., and Mintz, L., Cytomegalovirus and Kaposi's sarcoma in young homosexual men, *Lancet*, 2, 125, 1982.

73. Siddiqui, A., Hepatitis B virus DNA in Kaposi's sarcoma, *Proc. Natl. Acad. Sci. U.S.A.*, 80, 4861, 1983.

74. Bovenzi, P., Mirandola, P., Secchiero, P., Strumia, R., Cassai, E., and Di Luca, D., Human herpesvirus 6 (variant A) in Kaposi's sarcoma, *Lancet*, 341, 1288, 1993.

75. Vogel, J., Hinrichs, S. H., Reynolds, R. K., Luciw, P. A., and Jay, G., The HIV *tat* gene induces dermal lesions resembling Kaposi's sarcoma in transgenic mice, *Nature*, 335, 606, 1968.

76. Wang, R. Y.-H., Shih, J. W.-K., Weiss, S. H., Grandinetti, T., Pierce, P. F., Lange, M., Alter, H. J., Wear, D. J., Davies, C. L., Mayur, R. K., and Lo, S.-C., *Mycoplasma penetrans* infection in male homosexuals with AIDS: high seroprevalence and association with Kaposi's sarcoma, *Clin. Infect. Dis.*, 17, 724, 1993.

77. Giraldo, G., Beth, E., and Buonaguro, F. M., Kaposi's sarcoma: a natural model of relationships between viruses, immunologic responses, genetics and oncogenesis, *Antibiot. Chemother.*, 32, 1, 1983.

78. Bendsöe, N., Dictor, M., Blomberg, J., Agren, S., and Merk, K., Increased incidence of Kaposi's sarcoma in Sweden before the AIDS epidemic, *Eur. J. Cancer*, 26, 699, 1990.

79. van den Berg, F., Shipper, M., Jiwa, M., Rook, R., van de Rijke, F., and Tigges, B., Implausibility of an aetiological association between cytomegalovirus and Kaposi's sarcoma shown by four techniques, *J. Clin. Pathol.*, 42, 128, 1989.

80. Johnston, G. S., Jockusch, J., McMurtry, L. C., and Shandera, W. X., Cytomegalovirus (CMV) titers among acquired immunodeficiency syndrome (AIDS) patients with and without history of Kaposi's sarcoma, *Cancer Detect. Prev.*, 14, 337, 1990.

81. Jahan, N., Razzaque, A., Greenspan, J., Conant, M. A., Josephs, S. F., Nakamura, S., and Rosenthal, L. J., Analysis of human KS biopsies and cloned cell lines for cytomegalovirus, HIV-1, and other selected DNA virus sequences, *AIDS Res. Hum. Retroviruses*, 5, 225, 1989.

82. Holmberg, S. D., Possible cofactors for the development of AIDS-related neoplasms, *Cancer Detect. Prev.*, 14, 331, 1990.

83. Haverkos, H. W., Pinskey, P. F., Drotman, P., and Bregman, D. J., Disease manifestation among homosexual men with acquired immunodeficiency syndrome: a possible role of nitrites in Kaposi's sarcoma, *Sex. Transm. Dis.*, 12, 203, 1985.

84. Friedman-Kien, A. E. and Saltzman, B. R., Clinical manifestations of classical, endemic African, and epidemic AIDS-associated Kaposi's sarcoma, *J. Am. Acad. Dermatol.*, 22, 1237, 1990.

85. DiGiovanna, J. J. and Safai, B., Kaposi's sarcoma: retrospective study of 90 cases with particular emphasis on the familial occurrences, ethnic background and prevalence of other diseases, *Am. J. Med.*, 71, 779, 1981.

86. Dupin, N., Grandadam, M., Calvez, V., Gorin, I., Aubin, J. T., Havard, S., Lamy, F., Leibowitch, M., Huraux, J. M., Escande, J. P., and Agut, H., Herpesvirus-like DNA sequences in patients with Mediterranean Kaposi's sarcoma, *Lancet*, 345, 761, 1995.

87. Giraldo, G., Beth, E., Henle, W., Henle, G., Miké, V., Safai, B., Huraux, J. M., McHardy, J., and de Thé, G., Antibody patterns to herpesvirus in Kaposi's sarcoma. II. Serological association of American Kaposi's sarcoma with cytomegalovirus, *Int. J. Cancer*, 22, 126, 1978.

88. Giraldo, G., Beth, E., Kourilsky, F. M., Henle, W., Henle, G., Miké, V., Huraux, J. M., Andersen, H. K., Gharbi, M. R., Kyalwazi, S. K., and Puissant, A., Antibody patterns to herpesviruses in Kaposis's sarcoma: serological association of European Kaposi's sarcoma with cytomegalovirus, *Int. J. Cancer*, 15, 839, 1975.

89. Ambinder, R. F., Newman, C., Hayward, G. S., Biggar, R., Melbye, M., Kestens, L., Van Marck, E., Piot, P., Gigase, P., Wright, P. B., and Quinn, T. C., Lack of association of cytomegalovirus with endemic African Kaposi's sarcoma, *J. Infect. Dis.*, 156, 193, 1985.

90. Kestens, L., Melbye, M., Biggar, R. J., Stevens, W. J., Piot, P., De Muynck, A., Taelman, H., De Feyter, M., Paluku, L., and Gigase, P. L., Endemic African Kaposi's sarcoma is not associated with immuno-deficiency, *Int. J. Cancer*, 36, 49, 1985.

91. Penn, I., Kaposi's sarcoma in organ transplant recipients: report of 20 cases, *Transplantation*, 27, 8, 1979.

92. Moore, P. S. and Chang, Y., Detection of herpesvirus-like DNA sequences in Kaposi's sarcoma in patients with and those without HIV infection, *N. Engl. J. Med.*, 332, 1181, 1995.

93. Chang, Y., Ceserman, E., Pessin, M. S., Lee, F., Culpepper, J., Knowles, D. M., and Moore, P. S., Identification of herpesvirus-like DNA sequences in AIDS-associated Kaposi's sarcoma, *Science*, 266, 1865, 1994.

94. Lisitsyn, N., Lisitsyn, N., and Wigler, M., Cloning the differences between two complex genomes, *Science*, 259, 946, 1993.

95. Albrecht, J.-C., Nicholas, J., Biller, D., Cameron, K. R., Biesinger, B., Newman, C., Wittmann, S., Craxton, M. A., Coleman, H., Fleckenstein, B., and Honess, R. W, Primary structure of the herpesvirus saimiri genome, *J. Virol.*, 66, 5047, 1992.

96. Baer, R., Bankier, A. T., Biggin, M. D., Deininger, P. L., Farrell, P. J., Gibson, T. J., Hatfull, G., Hudson, G. S., Satchwell, S. C., Séguin, C., Tuffnell, P. S., and Barrell, B. G., DNA sequence and expression of the B95-8 Epstein-Barr virus genome, *Nature*, 310, 207, 1984.

97. Ceserman, E., Chang, Y., Moore, P. S., Daid, J. W., and Knowles, D. M., Kaposi's sarcoma-associated herpesvirus-like DNA sequences in AIDS-related body-cavity-based lymphomas, *N. Engl. J. Med.*, 332, 1186, 1995.

98. Huang, Y. Q., Li, J. J., Kaplan, M. H., Poiesz, B., Katabira, E., Zhang, W. C., Felner, D., and Friedman-Kien, A. E., Human herpesvirus-like nucleic acid in various forms of Kaposi's sarcoma, *Lancet*, 345, 759, 1995.

99. Roizman, B., New viral footprints in Kaposi's sarcoma, *N. Engl. J. Med.*, 223, 1227, 1995.

100. Janier, M., Vignon, M. D., and Cottenot, F., Spontaneously healing Kaposi's sarcoma in AIDS, *N. Engl. J. Med.*, 312, 1638, 1985.

101. Real, F. X. and Krown, S. E., Spontaneous regression of Kaposi's sarcoma in patients with AIDS, *N. Engl. J. Med.*, 313, 1659, 1985.

102. O'Connell, K. A., Resolution of Kaposi's sarcoma, *Lancet*, 343, 741, 1994.

103. Lane, H. C., Falloon, J., Walker, R. E., Deyton, L., Kovacs, J. A., Masur, H., Banks, S., Kirk, L. E., Baseler, M. W., Salzman, N. P., and Fauci, A. S., Zidovudine in patients with human immunodeficiency virus (HIV) infection and Kaposi's sarcoma, *Ann. Intern. Med.*, 111, 41, 1989.

104. de Wit, R., Reiss, P., Bakker, P. J. M., Lange, J. M. A., Danner, S. A., and Veenhof, K. H. N., Lack of activity of zidovudine in AIDS-associated Kaposi's sarcoma, *AIDS*, 3, 847, 1989.

105. Morfeldt, L. and Torssander, J., Long-term remission of Kaposi's sarcoma following foscarnet treatment in HIV-infected patients, *Scand. J. Infect. Dis.*, 26, 749, 1994.

106. Jones, J. L., Hanson, D. L., Chu, S. Y., Ward, J. W., and Jaffe, H. W., AIDS-associated Kaposi's sarcoma, *Science*, 267, 1078, 1995.

2 Papovaviridae

The family Papovaviridae comprises two subfamilies, polyomaviruses and papillomaviruses, based on several common characteristic features, including their small size, nonenveloped virion, icosahedral capsid, superhelical, double-stranded, circular DNA genome, and the nucleus as a site of replication. However, the polyoma-papillomaviruses are not related immunologically and they do not share similar genetic organization. Thus, in contrast to polyomaviruses, which carry approximately one half of the genetic information on each DNA strand, all of the genomic information of the papillomaviruses is held in one DNA strand.

2.1 HUMAN PAPILLOMAVIRUS

2.1.1 Introduction

Human papillomavirus (HPV) infections have been steadily rising for the last 20 years and are now the most commonly diagnosed sexually transmitted disease in the U.S.[1-5] When the subclinical and latent infections are also taken into account, the statistics are even more alarming.

Papillomaviruses are a widespread class of small, nonenveloped viruses that replicate mainly in the nucleus of squamous epithelial cells of higher vertebrates, including humans.[6] They contain the viral genome in a double-stranded DNA in a covalently closed circular pattern, surrounded by a icosahedral (20 faces) capsid. Together with the polyomaviruses, the papillomaviruses form the large papovavirus family. At present, more than 70 distinct human papillomaviruses have been identified.[7,8] They have been identified by the composition of the DNA nucleotide sequence — if the DNA sequence of a given HPV differed by more than 50% from the known strains, it was classified as a new type.[9,10] To a large degree, the intense research on human papillomaviruses during the last 20 years or so has been aroused by the association of some members of this class of viruses with genital cancers — so far, nearly 18 HPVs have been linked to anogenital lesions. Because of the ability of HPVs to exert a marked display of cellular tropism, they have been divided into two large groups, cutaneous and mucosal HPVs. In another classification, HPV infections have been divided into genital-mucosal, nongenital, and epidermodysplasia verruciformis (EV)-specific.[11] The latter infection is a rare skin condition associated with widespread, chronic nongenital cutaneous HPV lesions.[12]

The HPVs infect exclusively the surface epithelia of the skin and the mucous membranes (external and internal genitalia, oral cavity, respiratory tract), forming self-limiting proliferative lesions (papillomas). The oncogenic potential of HPVs is expressed mainly as cancers of the skin (carcinomas and epidermodysplasia verruciformis) and genitalia. The viral infection may occur by either skin abrasions involving the basal cell layer through traumatized epithelium, sexual intercourse, or during passage through an infected birth canal (juvenile-onset laryngeal papilloma).

The incubation period following infection of the epithelium lasts between 6 weeks to 8 months during which the viral genome stabilizes as a provirus. However, in some patients the incubation period may persist for months, years, or even for life.

The active phase of the infection lasts for 3 to 6 months, and is characterized by rapid epithelial and capilary growth resulting in condyloma.[10] The clinical manifestations of human papillomavirus infections[6] include:

1. Cutaneous lesions (warts) which are easily transmitted from one person to another by direct contact with infected tissue or indirectly by contaminated objects; in addition, in infected individuals, transmission from one site to another by self-inoculation is common
2. Epidermodysplasia verruciformis, a rare life-long dermatological disorder where wart virus infections will not resolve and occasionally may progress to malignancy[13,14]
3. Anogenital warts (genital warts, genital papilloma, condyloma)[15-18]
4. HPV-associated cervical intraepithelial neoplasma (CIN) and cancer of the cervix[19-23] (in developing countries, the latter is the most frequent female malignancy, accounting for approximately 24% of all cancers in women)[19]
5. Neoplasia at other lower-anogenital tract sites (the vulva, vagina, penis, perineum, and the anus)[24-27]
6. Respiratory tract infections, such as respiratory papillomatosis (laryngeal papilloma), nasal papillomas, cancers of the respiratory tract
7. Conjunctival papilloma
8. Oral cavity infections, such as focal epithelial hyperplasia,[28,29] squamous papillomas, oral leukoplakias,[30] and oral cancers[6]

HPV types 6, 11, 16, 18, 31, 33, 35, 39, 41–45, 51–56, and 59 have been known to infect genitalia.[10] HPV-6 and HPV-11, two genital-tract viruses, have been identified as the etiologic agents of nearly all respiratory papillomas,[31-33] squamous and inverted papillomas,[34-37] severe dysplasias[38] and cancers,[39,40] childhood conjunctival papillomas, and adult tumors.[41-43]

By light microscopy, histologic evidence of HPV-induced neoplasia included koilocytosis, multinucleation, hyperkeratosis, parakeratosis, dyskeratosis, and papillomatosis.[44] The presence of koilocytes appeared to be the most sensitive index for detecting human HPV infection.[45]

2.1.2   STUDIES ON THERAPEUTICS

2.1.2.1   Interferons

First discovered by Issacs and Lindemann,[46] the interferons (IFNs) represent a group of antiviral proteins (cytokines), endogenously produced by infected eukaryotic cells. Their use for the treatment of condyloma acuminatum was first reported in 1974.[47] After approval by the Food and Drug Administration (FDA) of interferon-α3 (natural interferon-α) and recombinant interferon-α2b for treatment of recurrent condyloma acuminatum,[48] increasingly, the IFNs have been used in the treatment of symptomatic and asymptomatic HPV infections, both as a primary and adjunctive therapy.[49] Structurally related to the glycoproteins, the IFNs are divided into three groups: α-, β-, and γ-IFNs, based on their antigenic specificity and the cell type from which individual IFNs were derived.[50] While pharmacologic amounts of IFNs can be produced by *in vitro* fibroblast or leukocyte stimulation, large quantities of them are generated by recombinant DNA techniques.

Reports from a number of investigators have indicated that all three interferons (α-, β-, and γ-) have been effective against human papillomavirus infections.[51-55] However, the IFN-α was the one most often applied.[56] The biological activities of these glycoproteins are both cell- and interferon-specific. In general, IFNs inhibit the cell proliferation, enhance the natural killer cell activity, T cell cytotoxicity, and macrophage activation.[50,57-59] Minor impairment of the immune system may trigger reactivation of latent HPV infection or keep it clinically active, especially in immunosuppressed patients or those receiving corticosteroids. In those patients, interferon therapy is rarely successful.[49]

Gall et al.[49] have undertaken a study to determine the efficacy of two types of interferon, consensus interferon (r-Met-Hu IFN-Con) and interferon-α-2a, in the treatment of resistant and/or persistent HPV infections of the female genital tract. Consensus interferon is a designer protein molecule produced by a synthetic gene that is most closely related to interferon F, a natural subtype of the interferon-α family of proteins (there are only 10 amino acid positions at which consensus interferon differs from interferon F). The other type, interferon-α-2a was selected because it represents a single interferon-α. Twenty-one of 31 patients with persistent HPV infection (condyloma acuminatum) received consensus interferon (mean 55.2 μU per patient, administered intramuscularly), and 6 patients were given placebo; 19 of those receiving the drug (76%) showed complete or partial clearing of condyloma 10 and 16 weeks after initiation of therapy; in 22 of 24 patients (91%) who were treated with interferon-α-2a (mean 88 μU per patient, intramuscularly), clearing was observed after a similar time period. Both drugs were also effective when administered as adjunctive therapy.[49]

Consensus interferon is a 166-amino acid protein produced by *Escherichia coli* through the expression of a synthetic gene that is carried on a plasmid vector. It differs from interferon-α in that its amino acid sequence reflects the most frequently occurring amino acid residues at each position of the 13 known members of the interferon-α family.

Einhorn et al.[60] compared the efficacy of semipurified (P-IFN) and purified (NK2-IFN) human leukocyte interferon in the treatment of 12 patients with advanced condyloma acuminatum. When applied systemically (3×10^6 IU daily, intramuscularly), both preparations were able to affect the condylomatous growth, resulting in one complete remission, six partial remissions, four minimal responses, and one patient showing progressive disease. Side effects (shivers, fatigue, fever, erythema, and reduced kidney function) were unexpectedly common in this advanced disease stage and therapy had to be stopped on four occasions. P-IFN was derived from blood cells, while the purified preparation, NK2-IFN was made with the help of monoclonal antibodies.[61,62]

The toxic side effects of IFNs appear to be dose-dependent but not route-dependent.[7] The most common adverse reaction is the "flu-like syndrome" (fever, chills, nausea, emesis, headaches, myalgias, and fatigue) which is usually observed at doses exceeding 1.0 MU and becomes more severe at doses above 5.0 MU. In addition, mild to moderate but transient leukopenia, thrombocytopenia, as well as minor elevations in the serum levels of some liver enzymes have also been observed in the 1.0 to 5.0 MU dose range. Antibodies to IFN, although rare, develop in 2% to 3% of patients on systemic IFN medication, and in less than 1% of patients receiving intralesional injections.[63] At present, the significance of these antibodies is not well understood.

2.1.2.2 5-Fluorouracil

Topical application of 5-fluorouracil (5-FU) 5% cream has been used successfully to treat HPV-associated vaginal dysplasia and condyloma acuminata.[64-68] When given as a single dose once weekly for a period of 10 weeks, the drug is well tolerated.[65,67] However, side effects, such as acute inflammatory changes with superficial erosions of the vaginal and/or cervical epithelium, are frequently observed following intravaginal 5-FU therapy; usually the alterations will heal within 4 to 5 weeks after completion of therapy.[68] Continuous application of 5-FU once or twice daily for 5 to 14 d in one or more treatment cycles often produced acute vulvovaginitis with formation of shallow vaginal erosions.[64,66] Even periodic applications of the cream may cause localized erythema and edema in 30% and acute ulceration of the vaginal and/or cervical mucosa in 10% of patients.[67] While the acute toxicities of 5-FU are well recognized, there is little information about long-term vaginal mucosal alterations. In one such study, Krebs and Helmkamp[68] investigated chronic ulcerations caused by topical 5-FU therapy of 220 patients with vaginal lesions. The total amount of 5-FU used and the underlying clinical conditions (e.g., vaginal dysplasia or condyloma acuminatum) did not influence the formation of ulcers. It seemed to be related mainly to the duration of therapy since it was more prominent in women applying 5-FU for longer than 10 weeks than in those who used 5-FU for 10 weeks or less (9.6% vs. 5.7%, $p = .05$). One likely explanation for the ulcer formation is that repeated applications of 5-FU would damage the epithelium, thereby preventing reepithelialization of the denuded area. In a related study, Mansell et al.[69] reported that following its use for cutaneous cancers, 5-FU triggered a delayed hypersensitivity reaction which may be an important factor for the etiology of chronic vaginal ulcers.

Reid et al.[70] used external laser vaporization and adjunctive 5-FU therapy to treat HPV-associated vulvar disease. Two 5-FU regimens were applied: (1) routine once-weekly prophylactic application to prevent postoperative recurrence, and (2) twice-weekly dosing to avoid further laser surgery among patients with early but diffused failures.

2.1.2.3 Podophyllin Derivatives

Podophyllum resin is an extract derived from the May apple perennial plant, mainly *Podophyllum peltatum* and *P. emodi*. It contains a number of biologically active lignins which have the ability to bind to microtubules and induce tissue necrosis by blocking the cell mitosis.[71] Depending on the plant species, different extracts will consist of different lignins in different ratios; however, their therapeutic efficacy was not determined by the total lignin concentrations.[72]

Podophylotoxin is one of the active lignin ingredients of the podophyllum resin that has the advantages over the crude resin of having higher purity, stable shelf life, negligible systemic absorption, and lesser local toxicity when applied topically.[73] At present, podophyllotoxin is not approved by the FDA for treatment of genital warts.

2.1.2.4 Retinoic Acid Derivatives

Several retinoid derivatives (13-*cis*-retinoic acid, β-all-*trans*-retinoic acid) have proven effective in reversing premalignant lesions of squamous epithelium, such as leukoplakia of the oral cavity and cervical dysplasia.[74-78] In a randomized, double-blind, placebo-controlled clinical study, 13-*cis*-retinoic acid, when given at daily doses of 1.0 to 2.0 mg/kg for 3 months, significantly decreased the size of lesions in 63% of the patients; 54% had their dysplasia reversed.[75] Adverse side effects included cheilitis, facial erythema, dryness and peeling of the skin, conjunctivitis, and hyper-triglyceridemia; the toxicity was reversed by reducing the dose or discontinuing the therapy.

Markowska et al.[79] used a topical combination of 13-*cis*-retinoic acid and IFN-β to treat HPV infection of the uterine cervix. The cure response was 94.2%, as compared to an 88% rate when IFN-β was applied alone. Similar synergistic effects between various retinoids (9-*cis*-retinoic acid, all-*trans*-retinoic acid, and 13-*cis*-retinoic acid) and IFN-α were found by Majewski et al.[80] in the treatment of tumor-induced angiogenesis caused by HPV-16- and HPV-18-harboring tumor cell lines.

Graham et al.[76] conducted a phase II clinical trial using β-all-*trans*-retinoic acid for treatment of cervical intraepithelial neoplasia delivered by a collagen sponge and cervical cap. A dose of 1.0 ml (0.372%) of the drug was applied in a cream-based vehicle that contained polyethylene 400, butylated hydroxytoluene, and 55% ethyl alcohol. A complete response with total regression of disease was obtained in 50% of the patients.[76]

2.1.2.5 Phosphorothioate Oligonucleotides

Antisense oligonucleotides have been found to act as specific inhibitors of gene expression,[81] as well as to be effective agents against a number of viruses, including Rous sarcoma virus,[82] vesicular stomatitis virus,[83] herpes simplex virus type 1,[84] influenza virus,[85] and HIV.[86]

Using the similarities of gene structure and function of bovine papillomavirus type 1 (BPV-1) and HPV-6 and HPV-16, Cowsert et al.[87] tested the hypothesis that the viral E2 gene may represent a rational therapeutic target. It is known,[88,89] that the E2 open reading frame of papillomaviruses encodes a family of sequence-specific DNA-binding proteins that regulate the transcription of papillomavirus early genes. First observed in BPV-1,[90] the role of E2 was later confirmed in several human papillomaviruses (HPV-11,[91] HPV-16,[92] and HPV-18[93]), where E2 was found to regulate the expression of viral genes responsible for transformation, replication,[94,95] and transcriptional regulation. A number of phosphorothioate oligonucleotides complementary to E2 mRNAs have been synthesized and tested *in vitro* in BPV and HPV models for their ability to inhibit E2 transactivation and virus-induced focus formation.[87] Based on these observations, Cowsert et al.[87] synthesized ISIS 2105, a 20-residue phosphorothioate oligonucleotide derivative targeted to hybridize to the AUG region of the HPV-11 E2 transactivator mRNA covering nts 2713 to 2732. ISIS 2105 was found to suppress HPV-11 E2-dependent transactivation in a concentration-dependent, sequence-specific manner, with an IC_{50} between 5.0 and 7.0 μM.

Although the precise mechanism by which ISIS 2105 and other active oligonucleotides modulate the E2 transactivation is not very clear, one potential mechanism is a hybridization arrest in which the protein synthesis is inhibited as a result of the binding of the oligonucleotide to the RNA, causing disruption of the protein translation process.[96] Such a mechanism seems to be in agreement with the finding that many potent oligonucleotides are targeted to sites associated with the initiation of translation.[87] Another potential mechanism is cleavage of the oligonucleotide:RNA complex by RNase H, leading to degradation of the RNA.[81] While ISIS 2105 was demonstrated to support RNase H cleavage of E2 mRNA *in vitro*, there was no conclusive evidence that this process is responsible for the observed activity in cells.[87] The overall data from these experiments strongly suggested that the E2 transactivator protein of papillomaviruses is a sensitive target for antisense oligonucleotides. ISIS 2105 is being evaluated in phase 1 clinical trials for the treatment of genital warts.[87]

2.1.2.6   9-(2-Phosphonylmethoxy)ethylguanidine

The effectiveness of 9-(2-phosphonylmethoxy)ethylguanidine (PMEG), an acyclic nucleotide, was evaluated against Shope papillomavirus infection in rabbits, and HPV-11 infections of human foreskin xenografts in athymic mice.[97] The drug was found active against both conditions. When PMEG was started in the latent period and continued for the duration of the experiment, it inhibited the HPV-11 infection of human skin, including condyloma growth, and synthesis of viral DNA and capsid antigen. The PMEG toxicity paralled its therapeutic effects in rabbits, but was much less toxic in athymic mice.[97]

2.1.3   Evolution of Therapies and Treatment of Papillomavirus Infections

It is estimated that human papillomavirus infections are widespread, with about 20% of women carrying HPV. At least 14 of the known human papillomaviruses have been associated with anogenital infections. Clinical manifestations of such infection can range from subclinical to benign warts, abnormal genital cytology and dysplastic lesions to carcinomas. The HPV DNA has been found in the majority of squamous cancers of the female genital tract,[98-102] and genital warts (condyloma acuminatum) are considered to be the most prevalent sexually transmitted disease in the U.S.[103] Furthermore, there is also increasing frequency in the incidence of HPV-related anogenital infections in HIV-infected patients.

HPV-associated anogenital infections can involve the cervix, vagina, vulva, perianal area and anal canal, penis, and the urethra. Bouchaud et al.[104] have diagnosed HPV in the esophagus of HIV-positive patients. In the latter study, since HPV was found both in esophagus with and without lesion, it is likely that it is not an etiologic agent of esophagitis but probably a cofactor.

Consensus about the appropriate management of HPV disease is yet to emerge, especially of subclinical infections. A variety of treatment regimens are available for treatment of HPV infections.[71] In general, several criteria are taken into consideration in determining the most appropriate therapy: the histologic grade of the lesion (i.e., benign vs. neoplastic), the size and number of lesions, the history of previous therapy, the clinical appearance and anatomic site of the growth (flat vs. exophytic), and the immune status of the patient.[7] However, it is the patient tolerance that could be the most important factor in selecting a particular modality.

Therapies for HPV disease include carbon dioxide laser vaporization,[105] cryotherapy, electrocautery, excision and surgery, radiation, and systemic chemotherapy. While therapeutic options for neoplasia include surgery, radiotherapy, and chemotherapy, laser treatment and cryotherapy are also commonly used for dysplastic lesions.[7] Systemic interferon-α has been approved for use in condyloma acuminatum. Local chemotherapy for benign tumors (i.e., warts) with cytotoxic agents, such as dichloro- and trichloroacetic acids, podophyllin resin, podophyllotoxin, and 5-fluorouracil (5-FU), have been reported, as well as ablative techniques (excisional surgery, electrocautery, laser vaporization, and cryotherapy). Other anti-infective agents that have been investigated include isotretinoin and hypericin. The primary disadvantage of surgical interventions is that such treatment, while removing the clinically apparent lesions, will have no direct effect on the HPV infection itself. The presence of subclinical disease is one major factor for the high rates of recurrence due to latent HPV in clinically normal-appearing skin.[106] Therefore, in order to achieve rapid clearance of lesions with reduced recurrence rate, one logical choice of treatment would be to combine cytodestructive techniques or surgical excision with antiviral therapy.[7]

One common such strategy is to apply a combination of IFN-α or IFN-γ with surgery.[107-110] For example, recurrence of infection was significantly less likely to occur when laser surgery was followed by IFN-α treatment, than surgery alone.[111-115] In another study, Tiedemann and Ernst[116] found the recurrence rate to be only 9% (2 of 22 patients) when electrocautery was followed by rIFN-α2b therapy, as compared to 45% recurrence of infection (5 of 11 patients) with electrocautery alone. Similarly, Piccoli et al.[117] reported 25% recurrence of condyloma acuminatum at 6 to 12 months after combination of electrocautery and rIFN-β, vs. 67% for electrocautery alone. However, it is important to note that even after IFN therapy, HPV DNA can still persist during periods of complete clinical remission.[118]

In two studies by Handley et al.[119] and Eron et al.,[120] however, cryotherapy combined with IFN-α did not prove superior to cryotherapy alone. Thus, subcutaneous administration of IFN-α2a followed by cryotherapy led to 50% recurrence rate at 3 months in contrast to 38% for cryotherapy alone,[119] and in the reverse case when initial cryotherapy was followed by subcutaneous rIFN-α2a, the corresponding values at 6 months were 69% and 73% (for cryotherapy alone).[120]

Another combination therapy studied was podophyllin with intralesional administration of rIFN-α2b. The results, however, showed no difference with those achieved with podophyllin alone (67% and 65% recurrence rates at 40 and 31 d, respectively).[121] Self-treatment with podophyllotoxin (podofilox 0.5%) solution with local (subcutaneous) administration of IFN-α (e.g., in the suprabubic area/inguinal folds) has also been recommended for patients with moderate number/size of refractory or recurrent condyloma acuminatum.[7]

Some recommended strategies for external treatment of HPV-associated lesions are listed in Table 2.1.[122,123] However, caution should be used with several of these treatments. Thus, podofilox and podophyllin solutions are not recommended for use in pregnant women. In addition, warts that remain after four podofilox or six podophyllin treatments should be considered for another therapy. Trichloroacetic acid should be applied to wart tissue only, and talc or sodium bicarbonate may be used to remove unreacted acid. Furthermore, warts that persist after six treatments should be evaluated for another therapy. Depending on the circumstances, oral warts may be treated with either cryotherapy, liquid nitrogen, electrodesiccation, electrocautery, or surgical excision.

Studies of topical IFN applications have involved randomized, double-blinded, and placebo-controlled trials of human leukocyte IFN-α preparations,[124-127] as well as recombinant IFN-α which was used in an open trial[107] (Table 2.1). The vaginal and cervical application of rIFN-α was by a vaginal cream applicator and diaphragm, respectively.[107] The reported 100% therapeutic efficacy

TABLE 2.1
Treatment Strategies of Human Papillomavirus Exophytic Genital Infections

Indication	Treatment[a]
External Genital/Perianal Warts	
Cryotherapy	Liquid nitrogen or cryoprobe
Podofilox (0.5% solution)	Self-treatment (genital warts only) applied twice daily for 3 days, followed by 4 days of no therapy[b]
Podophyllin (10–25% in compound tincture of benzoin)	0.5 ml (or less) or 10 cm² per session (repeat weekly if necessary)[c]
Trichloroacetic acid (60–90%)	Applied to warts only[d]
Electrodessication or electrocautery	Local anesthesia is required[e]
Cervical Warts	
Cryotherapy	Liquid nitrogen[f]
Trichloroacetic acid (80–90%)	Applied only to warts[d]
Podophyllin (10–25% in compound tincture of benzoin)	Treatment area 2 cm² (or less) must be dry before removing the speculum[g]
Urethral Meatus Warts	
Cryotherapy	Liquid nitrogen
Podophyllin (10–25% in compound tincture of benzoin)	Treatment area must be dry before contact with normal mucosa[c,g]
Anal Warts	
Cryotherapy	Liquid nitrogen
Trichloroacetic acid (80–90%)	Applied only to warts[d]
Surgical Removal	
Oral Warts	
Cryotherapy	Liquid nitrogen
Electrodesiccation or electrocautery	
Surgical Removal	

[a] Treatment of human papillomavirus genital warts should be guided by the preference of the patient. A specific treatment regimen should be chosen with consideration given to anatomic site, size, and number of warts as well as the expense, efficacy, convenience, and potential for adverse effects. Carbon dioxide and conventional surgery are considered useful in the management of extensive warts (but not limited lesions), particularly in patients who have not responded to other regimens. Interferon therapy is not recommended because of its cost and its association with a high frequency of adverse side effects; in addition, the interferon efficacy has been no greater than that of other available therapies. Treatment with 5-FU cream has not been evaluated in controlled studies; in addition, it often may cause local irritation, and has not been recommended for the treatment of genital warts.[122]

(continues)

TABLE 2.1 (continued)

b This cycle may be repeated as necessary for a total of four cycles. The total wart area treated should not exceed 10 cm^2, and total volume of podofilox should not exceed 0.5 ml per day. Its use is contraindicated during pregnancy.[122]

c Because of problems with systemic absorption and toxicity, the recommended treatment should not be exceeded, with the treated area being thoroughly washed off in 1–4 hours. The use of podophyllin is contraindicated during pregnancy.[122]

d Powder with talc or sodium bicarbonate (baking soda) should be used to remove unreacted acid. The treatment may be repeated if necessary; however, if warts persist after six applications, other therapies should be considered.[122]

e Both therapies are contraindicated for patients with cardiac pacemakers or for lesions proximal to the anal verge.[122]

f The use of cryoprobe in the vagina is not recommended because of the risk of vaginal perforation and fistula formation.[122]

g The treatment may be repeated at weekly intervals; however, because of potential systemic absorption caution should be applied in vaginal application. The use of podophyllin is contraindicated during pregnancy.[122]

(10 of 10 patients) of the first randomized, double-blinded, placebo-controlled trial[124] using human leukocyte IFN-α was not confirmed in two subsequent similar studies where the reported complete clearance rates of genital warts were 38% (3 of 8 patients)[125,126] and 33% (10 of 30 patients).[127]

In general, HIV-positive patients with HPV disease may not respond well to genital wart therapy.

2.1.3.1   Administration of Interferons

Several factors regarding the most appropriate route of administration of IFNs should be considered. Intra- or perilesional injections of IFN, although more effective for the treatment of individual lesions and cases of refractory condyloma acuminatum than systemic IFN administration, because of pain and discomfort, are often less acceptable to patients. On the other hand, systemic IFN (subcutaneous or intramuscular) in most instances would produce only mild to moderate rates of complete response. To this end, various IFN preparations, dose regimens, and the schedules and sites (whether the area is closer to or away from lesions) of administration may also influence the outcome of a systemic therapy.[128,129] In several studies, immunocompromised hosts, such as AIDS patients,[121] organ transplant recipients,[130] and patients with certain autoimmune diseases[131] have been found to be less responsive to even low-dose IFN therapy.

In several reports,[107,124,125,127] a topical application of IFN cream was described. Such a procedure has the advantage of being painless and with minimal or no toxicity. However, currently there is no topical IFN preparation available for general clinical use. Imiquimod, a topical inducer of IFNs, is also being tested as a cream in patients with genital and perianal warts.[132]

2.1.3.2   Condyloma Acuminatum

Condyloma acuminatum (condylomata acuminata) are HPV-associated benign lesions (genital warts) found among sexually active individuals (both females and males), and lately found with increased frequency in HIV-positive patients.[133-136] HIV-positive patients are difficult to treat because of recurrence of infection.[137] Most condylomata lesions contain the low-risk HPV types 6 or 11; however, the high-risk HPV-16 and HPV-18 have been occasionally detected.[138-140] Various detection methods, including *in situ* hybridization, polymerase chain reaction, and Southern blot, have shown that more than one HPV type is present in up to 32% of condylomata lesions.[141-146] Recently, a new detection technique, the hybrid capture method, has also been used successfully to determine the number of HPV types in condyloma lesions.[140,147] Most of the lesions containing multiple HPV types have been found in immunocompromised patients having either impaired cell-mediated immunity, such as HIV-positive individuals or organ transplant recipients receiving immunosuppressive medication.[147] Furthermore, it was found that in immunosuppressed patients with genital lesions, the predominant HPV type may not remain constant but rather change dramatically in a short period of time, and that this change may coincide with changes in histopathology.[147] There have been cases, however, where multiple HPV types were isolated from patients with no known immune defects.

In earlier studies,[47,124] topical application of IFN-α was found to produce complete response between 90% (36 of 40 patients) and 100% (10 of 10 patients) of patients with vulvar and vaginal warts. By comparison, topical IFN-β for therapy of condylomata acuminata was not only less effective (7 of 13 patients; 38%), but also resulted in 100% recurrence rate at 1 to 2 months.[125]

In a number of placebo- and non-placebo-controlled clinical trials, various IFN preparations have been used intralesionally to treat condyloma acuminatum.[54,121,128,148-153] In general, intralesional injections were applied 2 to 3 times weekly for 3 to 8 weeks, with the number of genital warts treated varying from a single lesion to all of a patient's genital warts. The usual IFN dose injected into each lesion was 10^6 U. In placebo-controlled trials where patients received 10^5 U of rIFN-α for 3 weeks, the interferon-treated genital wart cleared completely in 19% of patients,[153] and in 36%[154] and 53%,[153] respectively, of patients who received 10^6 U of the drug for 3 weeks. In those patients who received 10^6 U of IFN-α for 4 weeks complete clearance was observed in 47%;[128] and in 62% of patients whose dose was determined by surface area and who received injections for up to 8 weeks.[150] In the largest study involving intralesionally applied IFN-α, 41 of 66 patients (62%) had a complete response, as compared to 21% (14 of 66 patients) treated with placebo; the recurrence rates were 25% (at 4 months) and 23% (at 2 months) for IFN-α and placebo, respectively.[150] In a comparative study involving intralesional treatment of condyloma acuminatum with recombinant IFN-α2b, IFN-α, and IFN-β, Reichman et al.[128] observed complete responses in 48%, 45%, and 50% of patients, respectively, vs. 22% in the placebo group.

Systemic treatment of condyloma acuminatum with IFNs has been the subject of numerous clinical trials.[53,89,129,154-162] When used systemically, IFNs may be administered either subcutaneously or intramuscularly away from the lesion. Following intramuscular administration of IFN-α against condyloma acuminatum, Gall et al.[156] described complete response in 43% (6 of 14 patients), 57% (17 of 30 patients), and 69% (11 of 16 patients) at 1.0 MU (million units per treatment), 3.0 MU, and 5.0 MU, respectively. In several other reports,[157,158] the observed complete response was somewhat lower, varying between 21% to 25% and 25% to 33% for 1.0 and 3.0 MU of IFN-α, respectively; recurrence of infection has been reported to be 5% at 4 months[158] and 44% at 1 month.[157] Results from a double-blind, placebo-controlled, comparative study[129] showed that subcutaneous administration of IFN-α, IFN-β, and IFN-α2b (at 2.0 MU each) for condyloma acuminatum elicited a similar complete response: 17% (22 of 133 patients) vs. 10% (4 of 42 patients) in the placebo group. Recombinant IFN-α2a when used subcutaneously at 3.0 and 9.0 MU produced a similar low efficacy rate (21% complete response vs. 18% in placebo-treated patients); at 9 months, the 9.0-MU group had a 36% (5 of 14 patients) recurrence of infection.[159] Gross et al.[160,161] studied the efficacy of low- and high-dose (from 1.5 to 18.0 MU; subcutaneously) regimens of two recombinant IFN-α preparations, INF-α2b and IFN-α2c; while the complete response ranged between 43% and 71%, the low-dose regimens were considered to be superior. Gall et al.[162] compared the efficacies of recombinant IFN-α2 (3.0 MU; intramuscularly) with consensus IFN (2.5 or 5.0 MU; intramuscularly) for treatment of persistent papillomavirus disease, and found complete responses of 50% (12 of 24 patients) and 36% (9 of 25 patients), respectively. Adverse side effects have been observed in nearly all trials; in several cases the adverse symptoms necessitated discontinuance of therapy or dose reduction in 45 of 157 patients (29%),[71] and concurrent administration of ibuprofen (600 mg b.i.d.) did not significantly reduce toxicity of a 5.2×10^6 U dose regimen of IFN given five times weekly for 6 weeks.[71] In one study where the adverse side effects did not require a dose reduction, the IFN regimen was 1.7×10^6 U.[53]

Panici et al.[163] did not observe any therapeutic difference between subcutaneous and intramuscular administration of 3.0 MU of recombinant IFN-α2b.

The systemic use of IFN-γ for treatment of condyloma acuminatum has also been investigated, with variable outcomes.[109,164-167] Thus, Zouboulis et al.[166] observed no response to short-term treatment with recombinant IFN-γ (1.5 MU; subcutaneously), whereas Kirby et al.[167] found only 7% complete response in patients (2 of 28) receiving 0.2 MU IFN-γ. In an earlier study, Kirby et al.[164] described a complete response rate between 9% (0.2 to 2.0 MU) and 20% (0.2 to 0.5 MU). Fierlbeck and Rassner[109] reported more optimistic results (29% complete response) following subcutaneous injections of 1.5 to 3.0 MU of recombinant IFN-γ, while Gross et al.[165] observed the highest rate at 56% (34 of 64 patients receiving 0.75 to 6.0 MU of recombinant IFN-γ; subcutaneously), and no recurrence of infection at 7 to 16 months.

In several open trials,[66,67,168-171] topical 5-fluorouracil (5-FU) cream was used to treat condyloma acuminatum. The results showed complete clearance of warts in 10% to 73% of patients with lesions on the external genitalia; in 25% to 95% of men with urethral lesions; and in 83% to 85% of women with vaginal lesions; the recurrence rate for vaginal warts was in the 10% to 12% range.[71] Various adverse side effects (local irritation of skin and mucosal membranes, vaginal discharge, vulvitis, and ulcerative balanitis and urethral meatitis in men) caused by 5-FU, have been reported. It should be noted that the FDA has not approved 5-FU cream for treatment of genital warts.

Even though the reported cure rates have been relatively low, podophyllin and podophylotoxin have been used often in various regimens to treat genital warts mainly because of their convenience and low costs.[72,172-180] The observed local toxicities included erythema, tenderness, itching, burning, pain, swelling, and superficial erosions.[71] Because of the potential of their systemic absorption, and related toxicity and damage to the fetus, the use of podophyllin derivatives in pregnant women has been contraindicated. In order to avoid serious systemic side effects, it has been recommended that the maximal volume to be used in one session should not exceed 1.0 ml of podophyllin resin derived from *P. peltatum*, and 0.5 ml of that made from *P. emodi*.[179] The reported cure rates for genital warts in clinical trials using podophyllin were in the 22% to 77% range, with recurrence rates as high as 74%.[72,173-178] In a placebo-controlled trial of patient-applied podophyllotoxin, the observed efficacy was similar to that of podophyllin.[177]

There is limited information on the efficacies of di- and trichloroacetic acids to treat condylomas. In one randomized clinical trial,[180] the efficacy and frequency of side effects of trichloroacetic acid were similar to that of cryotherapy. Another randomized trial did not demonstrate any advantages of a combination of trichloroacetic acid and podophyllin over podophyllin alone.[181]

In CO_2 laser treatment of genital warts, the high-intensity light emitted is absorbed by the tissues it collides with. Inside the cells, the light energy is converted into heat energy with the resulting high temperatures vaporizing the tissue and sealing the blood vessels during the process.[71] Tissue destruction occurs from both immediate vaporization and delayed tissue necrosis; the latter can be controlled by keeping the power density over 750 W/cm³. The area and depth of tissue destruction are usually controlled with the laser's adjustable power density and port size. Genital warts on or in the vulva, vagina, cervix, urethra, anus, rectum, penis, and the scrotum are treated with different laser techniques. The procedure is commonly performed under general anesthesia, and recurrence rates, which vary between 3% and 95%, will decrease if the laser treatment is extended to include normal-appearing skin or mucosa surrounding the wart.[71] In one study, however, histologic evidence for persistent subclinical HPV was found in 88% of the patients.[182] Laser vaporization is not appropriate as initial therapy in cases where the disease is still in the proliferative stage, characterized by rapid epithelial and papillary growth formation. Rather, it should be used in patients with resistant, thick keratotic lesions that will not respond to local chemotherapy; if used in this fashion, it could lead to remission rates of about 85%.[5]

Happonen et al.[183] treated 40 heterosexual men with treatment-resistant penile warts of long duration (mean 12.9 months) with CO_2 laser therapy immediately followed by topical application (b.i.d.) of 0.5% idoxuridine cream for 2 weeks. After 2 weeks of treatment, 32 patients (87.5%) showed complete response; no controls were used in the study. All patients had been previously treated with a combination of CO_2 laser therapy and topical podophyllotoxin 0.5% solution with no success.

Cryotherapy of genital warts has been used more often than the standard surgical or electro-surgical procedures.[71,175,176,178,180,184-186] It involves freezing of the wart and small parts of surrounding tissue with one or more freeze-thaw cycles with liquid nitrogen applied either as a fine spray or with a cotton swab. The procedure is associated with pain which usually subsides within 10 to 15 min. Complete clearance of genital warts following cryotherapy has been demonstrated in 63% to 88% of patients,[175,180,184-186] with recurrence rates ranging between 21% and 39%.[176,178,180] Complete clearance in electrodessication and standard surgical excision have been observed in 94% and 93% of patients, respectively, with corresponding recurrence rates of 22% and 29%.[178]

2.1.3.3 Cervical Intraepithelial Neoplasia (CIN)

There is a close association of genital neoplasia with initial HPV infection.[11] Therefore, the differences in the morphology, HPV type, and histologic appearance of condyloma lesions and a true cervical intraepithelial neoplasia are important clinically relevant factors that should be considered in deciding the course and nature of HPV disease management.[5,187-191] Based on the existing relationship between HPV infection and the development of precursor lesions in the cervix, the cervical intraepithelial neoplasia has been defined as mild (CIN 1), moderate (CIN 2), and severe (CIN 3). In patients with squamous intraepithelial lesions (SIL), the low-grade lesions have been defined as CIN 1, and the high-grade lesions as CIN 2 and CIN 3.[11] The highest incidence of cervical cancer seems to occur in women over 35 years of age.[192]

Hartvejt et al.[193] investigated the occurrence of CIN in women with glomerulonephritis and its possible association with immunosuppressive treatment. The results showed that CIN was more prevalent in these patients as compared to controls (24% and 4%, respectively). While the increased occurrence of CIN was found to be independent of the use of immunosuppressive therapy, individual lesions tended to be more advanced when such therapy had been used.

When IFN-α was used topically in the treatment of CIN, the complete response varied between 50% and 54% in two trials[194,195] and in the 23% to 44% range in two placebo-controlled trials.[196,197] However, in the cases of patients treated with placebo, the relapse rate at 16 months was 29%, as compared to 0% for complete responders treated with IFN-α. In CIN infections treated with topical recombinant IFN-α2c, complete response was observed in 6 of 9 patients (67%).[107] Marcovici et al.[198] reported complete cure in all 25 patients (100%) when using topical plus intralesional IFN-β.

Topical application of IFN-α for cervical cancer produced complete response in 33% of patients (2 of 6); combination of topical IFN-α and intramuscular IFN-α resulted in only 11% complete response. No recurrences have been observed during the following 11 to 34 months.[7]

The intralesional use of IFNs for cervical intraepithelial neoplasia has also been the subject of numerous investigations.[199-209] The results have been promising. In some of the non-placebo-controlled trials, complete response for IFN-β was observed from 59% (19 of 32 patients)[209] to 100% (2 of 2 patients);[199] for IFN-α, the complete response was 29% (36 of 125 patients)[204] and 100% (3 of 3 patients);[202] and for recombinant IFN-α2b, 11% (1 of 11 patients)[205] and 33% (8 of 24 patients).[208] In a comparative study conducted by Choo et al.,[203] the complete responses to intralesional treatment of CIN with IFN-α and IFN-β were 86% (6 of 7 patients) and 40% (2 of 5 patients), respectively. In one trial using intralesional IFN-γ for therapy of CIN, the complete response was 68% (5 of 8 patients) vs. 13% (1 of 8 patients) with placebo.[207] However, in a double-blind study, Frost et al.[210] found no beneficial effect of intralesional IFN-α2b (intron a) in women with histologically confirmed CIN 2 lesions. Because of pronounced side effects the treatment was ceased in all patients.

Systemic IFN-α has also been used for the treatment of CIN.[7] In one such study, Schneider et al.[107] reported 20% (1 of 5 patients) complete response with a combination of topical and systemic (subcutaneous) administration of recombinant IFN-α2c, and 71% response (5 of 7 patients) when rIFN-α2c was used only subcutaneously; none of the patients had a recurrence at 7.5 months. However, Yliskoski et al.[108] found no statistical difference between subcutaneously administered IFN-α and placebo.

Several reports[64,65,68] describe the use of topical 5-fluorouracil 5% cream alone or in combination with laser treatment for therapy of CIN.

2.1.3.4 Vulvar Intraepithelial Neoplasia (VIN)

Vulvar intraepithelial neoplasia (VIN) is a condition manifested by epithelial abnormalities characterized by a broad spectrum of cellular atypia, such as Bowen's disease, bowenoid papulosis, bowenoid dysplasia, and bowenoid atypia.[211] Bowen's disease is assumed to be the precursor of invasive squamous cell carcinoma, while bowenoid atypia, and the more or less synonymous bowenoid dysplasia and bowenoid papulosis are considered benign. By and large, both groups of lesions represent a continuous spectrum of atypical vulvar squamous lesions.[211] Zachow et al.[212] have identified HPV DNA in both the premalignant and benign types of VIN.

In several other studies,[211,213-219] intraepithelial neoplasia and invasive vulvar cancer have also been associated with HPV infection. Of the various types of HPV, HPV-16 was found in as many as 81% of patients with VIN, 61% in those with invasive vulvar cancer, and only 12% of patients with condyloma acuminata.[213]

Various treatments of vulvar HPV infections without histologic evidence of VIN have included symptomatic therapy (topical antipruritics, such as 1% hydrocortisone), CO_2 laser vaporization, 85% trichloroacetic acid, and topical 5-fluorouracil ointment. In patients with HPV infection and VIN, CO_2 laser vaporization was the preferred therapy.[214]

2.1.3.5 Human Papillomavirus-Associated Buschke-Löwenstein Carcinoma (Giant Condyloma Acuminatum)

The Buschke-Löwenstein carcinoma (giant condyloma acuminatum) is a destructive malignancy clinically resembling squamous cell carcinoma. Microscopically, it represents a form of condyloma acuminatum usually occurring on the uncircumcised penis but also diagnosed elsewhere in the anogenital area, especially the anus and vulva. Clinically, it presents as a large verrucous to fungating, cauliflower-like mass that erodes the involved skin and progresses to penetrate and destroy the deeper tissues.

Piepkorn et al.[215] described a case of a patient who developed a Buschke-Löwenstein giant penile condyloma following 4 years of intermittent cyclosporine therapy for generalized pustular psoriasis. The condition was clearly associated with several HPV genotypes, including HPV-16. Treatment was successful and included biopsies of the penile skin lesions followed by debulking with CO_2 laser; no lymphadenopathy was observed at the 6-month follow-up examination. This case signifies the enhanced risk of cutaneous carcinogenesis from either HPV infection or chronic actinic damage that has become evident in patients with organ allografts and cyclosporine therapy.[216-221] In most reports, this association occurred against a background of chronic actinic damage[217,218,220] or HPV infection.[220,222]

Recently, the diagnosis made by Piepkorn et al.[215] has been challenged by Noel and de Dobbeleer.[223] In the opinion of the latter, the patient probably had two simultaneous tumors: a verrucous carcinoma containing HPV-6, and a squamous cell carcinoma harboring HPV-16. Among findings presented in support of their hypothesis, Noel and de Dobbeleer cited studies suggesting HPV-6 as the major causative agent of the Buschke-Löwenstein carcinoma in contrast to HPV-16 which (together with HPV-18) is mostly associated with epidermoid carcinoma or condylomatous (warty) carcinomas.[224,225] In addition, Noel and de Dobbeleer cited evidence[226] that condyloma acuminatum and/or squamous cell carcinoma may also occur adjacent to verrucous carcinomas, particularly on the vulva, as well as the fact that Buschke-Löwenstein tumors are typically diploid, whereas classic squamous cell carcinomas are aneuploid.[227] Noel and de Dobbeleer suggested digital cell analysis as one methodology that can prove their hypothesis.[223]

2.1.3.6 Human Papillomavirus-Associated Squamous Cell Carcinoma

Squamous cell carcinoma (SCC) is a rare complication found in patients with cutaneous lupus erythematosus, especially those with chronic cutaneous lesions of discoid lupus erythematosus, and has been attributed to chronic scarring.[228,229] The incidence of multiple verrucae and cutaneous SCC is high in organ transplant recipients, and the risk will increase with the length of graft survival.[230,231] It is believed that this phenomenon results from an altered immunity, not only from the immunosuppressive medication but also from the presence of the non-native transplanted tissue.

So far, there have been no reports associating SCC with nonscarring cutaneous lupus erythematosus lesions (subacute cutaneous lupus erythematosus). However, in a highly unusual case, Cohen et al.[232] described a patient with subacute cutaneous lupus erythematosus who was treated for his condition with azathioprine and prednisone, and who developed SCC that was found to harbor HPV-11.

2.1.3.7 Role of Human Papillomavirus in Human Cancers

There is a close relationship between genital HPV infections and genital malignancies.[11] It has been estimated that cervical cancer is the second leading cause of death in women worldwide.[233] Data from molecular diagnosis of HPV suggested that advanced HIV-related clinical disease or immunosuppression predispose to higher rates of cervical intraepithelial neoplasia.[234-238] However, there have been other reports[239,240] describing no such association.

In several reports,[241-243] evidence for the role of HPV in human cancers has been derived from studies of patients with epidermodysplasia verruciformis and organ transplant recipients where viral examination has revealed the presence of HPV-5 and HPV-8 in these patients. HPV-6 and HPV-11 most frequently infect external genitalia, causing formation of warts (condyloma acuminatum); they are very rarely isolated from cervical cancers, although malignant cutaneous neoplasms harboring HPV-11 have been reported.[232] HPV-16 and HPV-18 are the types most often associated with cervical cancers, with HPV-16 being found in 40% to 60% of cervical tumors and HPV-18 present in another 10% to 20%; about 10% of cervical cancers lack detectable HPV DNA.[244-247] The majority of the remaining tumors contained DNA from HPV-31, HPV-33, and HPV-45.[11]

The overwhelming evidence about the etiologic relationship between HPV infection and cervical malignancies has been derived from molecular biology[248,249] and epidemiologic studies. It is also believed that patients on immunosuppressive drug therapy will have impaired immune systems that are unable to clear viral infections, or in the case of epidermodysplasia verruciformis, a defective cell-mediated immunity that will increase the propensity for HPV infection and the malignant transformation of otherwise benign warts.[250,251] Other experimental studies have also shown that during carcinogenesis there is concurrence of action between a protein encoded by HPV and the activated *ras* oncogene.[252-254]

The prevalence of anorectal cancer among homosexual men is increasing.[255] Several studies have indicated the HPVs as a possible cause of these malignancies.[256,257] In addition, the T cell depletion associated with AIDS may also be a contributing factor for the transformation of benign HPV-induced condylomata lesions to a malignant state.[258-261] Although the natural history of HPV infections in men is less well understood, there is a strong correlation between CIN and male genital HPV infections in their regular partners.[24,262] However, the incidence of penile cancer is much lower than that of cervical cancer and the involvement of HPV is identified in only 20% to 50% of cases.[27,263,264]

Anal cancers, which are relatively uncommon in both men and women, seem to be more strongly associated with HPV infection. Thus, in two recent studies,[263,265] HPV DNA was detected in nearly 70% of patients. Furthermore, Ampel et al.[74] have demonstrated that a persistent rectal ulcer in a homosexual AIDS patient was associated with severe cellular atypia and the presence of HPV type 33 within the koilocytotic nuclei; the latter genotype has previously been isolated from cervical intraepithelial neoplasia in women,[266,267] but not from condyloma lesions in homosexual men or AIDS patients. According to Rudlinger et al.[268] anal condylomas in homosexual men are caused mainly by HPV types 6 and 11, which have not been associated with severe dysplasia or carcinoma in immunocompetent hosts. Finally, results from a study conducted by Frazer et al.[260] have clearly demonstrated a link between dysplastic changes in the anal epithelium of homosexual men and the presence of HPV.

2.1.3.8   Human Papillomavirus Infections in Immunosuppressed Patients

HPV infections in immunosuppressed patients with compromised cell-mediated immunity are more likely to occur, and often such patients do not respond well to conventional treatment.[269-271] For example, lower genital neoplasia was diagnosed more frequently in immunosuppressed women than in the general population.[272-274] An abnormal immunological status was indicated in 80% of these patients by an altered T helper/T suppressor cell ratio, a deficient response to mitogenic stimulation,[275] or both.[276] In a study conducted by Carson et al.[277] when compared to controls, immunosuppressed patients with genital neoplasia-papilloma syndrome had a significantly higher percentage of OKT8-positive T suppressor cells (mean 33% vs. 18%), and a lower proportion of OKT4-positive T helper cells (mean 35% vs. 50%); the mean T helper/T suppressor cell ratio of these patients was 1.72 as compared to 3.21 in the control group.

Schneider et al.[278] presented data collected over a 17-year period which demonstrated an increased incidence of cervical dysplasia among female renal transplant recipients mainly due to iatrogenic immunosuppression; all transplant recipients had been maintained on a regimen of immunosuppressive drugs (imuran and prednisone at average daily doses of 150 mg and 15 mg, respectively).

2.1.3.9   Human Papillomavirus Infections in HIV-Positive and AIDS Patients

Asymptomatic and immunosuppressed HIV-positive women are at significantly higher risk of developing HPV infection and CIN than HIV-seronegative women.[279,280] In this context, HIV-positive women and AIDS patients are more likely to present intraepithelial neoplasia, not only with high-grade lesions,[281,282] but also disease at more than one site (cervix, vagina, vulva, and perianal region).[235] Thus, Klein et al.[283] found that HIV-positive women have a higher rate of squamous intraepithelial lesions on PAP smear than HIV-negative women (25% and 10%, respectively). Vermund et al.[234] also reported a high risk of HPV infection and cervical squamous intraepithelial lesions among women with symptomatic HIV infection. According to Vernon et al.,[284] asymptomatic HIV-positive women are at significantly higher risk to develop HPV-associated CIN than HIV-negative women. Furthermore, HIV-positive women with CD4 counts below 500/mm^3 and evidence of HPV infection are more likely to develop neoplastic changes in the cervix.[285] CIN in HIV-infected women may be recalcitrant and more likely to recur,[286,287] especially with advancing immunosuppression.

Using data from 21 studies, 5 of which included comparison groups and contained sufficient information for inclusion in the analysis, Mandelblatt et al.[288] studied the association between HIV infection and cervical neoplasia, and its implications for the clinical care of women at risk for both conditions. The data consistently supported the close association between HIV disease and cervical neoplasia across individual studies, geographic locations (U.S., Europe, and Australia) and populations, and stressed the importance of Pap smear screening of women with HIV infection.

The presence of a strong link in homosexual men engaging in unprotected receptive anal intercourse between HPV infection, HIV, and the development of anal dysplasia[255-259,289,290] suggests a common HIV-induced immunosuppression-mediated mechanism of HPV-related neoplastic changes in selected genital epithelial tissues in both males and females.[234] Thus, Croxson et al.[258] reported epithelial carcinoma that developed from rectal condylomata in seven homosexual men; four of these patients later developed AIDS. In another study, Howard et al.[259] described two immunosuppressed homosexual men with T lymphocyte depletion who developed squamous cell carcinoma within perianal warts. Similarly, evidence of HPV infection in anal squamous proliferative lesions was found in five of eight homosexual men.[256]

Ampel et al.[74] successfully treated a persistent rectal ulcer of a homosexual man with AIDS with 60 mg daily of oral 13-*cis*-retinoic acid (isotretinoin) for 2 months; a follow-up sigmoidoscopic examination at 2 months after treatment showed resolution of the ulcer.

In summary, there has been compelling evidence presented about the interactions between HPV and HIV infections and their potential role in the development of intraepithelial neoplasia. Undoubtedly, the HIV-induced immunosuppression will accelerate the intensity and duration of anogenital warts, as well as increase their infectiousness and diminish the treatment efficacy.[282]

2.1.3.9.1   Localization of HIV-1 in HPV-induced cervical lesions

It has been discovered that the human immunodeficiency virus frequently colocalizes with HPV in CIN lesions, and that this colocalization is independent of both the clinical status and CD4 counts.[291] Relative to the clinical course of CIN, the progression to cervical cancer, as well as the risk of HIV transmission, would be greater if HIV and HPV are colocalized in CIN lesions. Using polymerase chain reaction for HIV and HPV, HIV-1 was detected in 52% (17 of 33) of cervical biopsy samples from HIV-infected women.[291] This finding corroborated a previous study[292] showing that the HIV-1 *tat* protein enhanced the E2-dependent HPV-16 transcription. The importance of such interaction between HIV-1 and HPV is not to be underestimated because of the possibility that it may adversely affect the HPV pathogenicity. Furthermore, the colocalization of the two viruses in HPV-associated lesions also raises the concern that such an increased concentration of HIV in those lesions may also increase the risk of HIV transmission during and after surgical removal of the lesions.[291]

2.1.3.10   Human Papillomavirus Infections During Pregnancy

Pregnancy may be a predisposing factor for HPV infections in women. It could be that the disease is acquired more readily during pregnacy or that reactivation of infection may occur at a higher rate than in nonpregnant women. Such findings are compatible with the concept of a permissive immune status during pregnancy.[10,293] In addition, clinically evident lesions have often been observed to grow more rapidly during pregnancy. Thus, Schneider et al.,[294] while studying cervical samples of women without prior history of cervical dysplasia or abnormal Pap smears, detected HPV DNA in 9% of samples during the first trimester, in 28% during the second trimester, and in 33% during the third trimester; by comparison, 28% is the prevalence rate in nonpregnant women. In addition, infected pregnant women had greater amounts of HPV DNA in their cells than infected nonpregnant women. Similar increase in HPV DNA prevalence in pregnant women (20.9% and 46% for the first and third trimesters, respectively) was also reported by Rando et al.[295]

The hormonal ambience during pregnancy would favor HPV replication. HPV growth is stimulated by estrogen, glucocorticoids, and other cellular factors.[295] In addition, the ratio of T helper to T suppressor cells decreases as gestational age progresses. Such a shift in the T cell population would also favor viral replication.[293]

Management of HPV infections in pregnant women is directed primarily at attainment and maintenance of a lesion-free state and reducing the risk of intrapartum maternal morbidity and exposure of the fetus to a large inoculum of HPV. Destruction of lower genital tract lesions may also reduce the risk of perinatal infection during labor and delivery.[10] Several of the available drugs for treating genital condylomas (podophyllin, 5-FU, and IFN-α) have been contraindicated in pregnant women (Table 2.1). Thus, podophyllin has been linked to both maternal and fetal toxicity (and even death), and 5-FU and IFN-α have shown systemic effects following local application. In one report by Stephens et al.,[296] 5-FU was suggested as the cause of multiple congenital abnormalities in a fetus exposed to the drug during the first trimester. Previously, Stadler and Knowles[297] described a case of neonatal intoxication following intrauterine exposure to 5-FU at approximately 22 to 23 weeks of gestation. In the context of these two reports, Odom et al.[298] found no teratogenic effects in two patients after exposure to topical vaginal 5-FU for HPV-induced lesions during the period of conception. However, caution should be applied since much more information is needed to assess the potential risks of human developmental toxicity associated with the use of vaginal topical 5-FU.[299]

The therapies most often used for HPV lesions in pregnancy include laser vaporization, cryocautery, and dichloro- and trichloroacetic acids.[10] In laser vaporization, the procedure is usually guided by colposcopy to allow for accurate treatment of all gross and visible condylomas and avoid unnecessary tissue destruction. When performed by experienced surgeons, laser vaporization is associated with minimal morbidity.

Cryotherapy is applied with local anesthesia; however, if patients require multiple treatments, there may be the possibility of profuse discharge produced by the sloughing of tissue. Electrocautery may also be applied, but will require general or regional conduction anesthesia.

One advantage of trichloroacetic acid is that it denatures on contact with tissue and, therefore, is not absorbed systemically. Although no anesthesia is required, treatment of large areas in one sitting is not practical. Trichloroacetic acid is also useful in treating small lesions on the vagina and cervix, and in combination with laser vaporization in cases of recurrent infection.[10]

2.1.3.10.1   Laryngeal papillomatosis

Even though fetal contamination with HPV during delivery is unavoidable, the factors that contribute to vertical transmission of HPV are still not well understood. Although transplacental or hematogenous routes of infection are likely to occur in some cases, transvaginal contamination is by far the most frequent.[10] Some pediatric infections, such as those of the anogenital, respiratory, and digestive tracts may have longer latency periods between the infection and clinically apparent disease, extending for as long as 5 years, as in the case of laryngeal papillomas.[300] Sedlacek et al.[301] found that nasopharyngeal aspirates of infants born to HPV-infected mothers tested positive for HPV DNA in 47.8% of the cases. Since HPV-6 and HPV-11, the two most prevalent HPV types of laryngeal papillomatosis, have also been commonly identified in mothers with genital condylomas, the association between genital and laryngeal HPV disease should be considered a distinct possibility.

The histopathologic features of laryngeal papilloma lesions include abnormal squamous maturation with parakeratosis, retardation of superficial cell maturation, and basal hyperplasia.[302] There was no correlation observed between the HPV type, histologic appearance, and clinical pattern.[303]

Early diagnosis of laryngeal papillomas are important, since it is the most dangerous manifestation of perinatal HPV infection, and in many cases, its complications can be severe (hoarseness, airway obstruction) and even fatal. The prolonged latency period makes it more difficult to estimate the true incidence of the disease.[304] Weiss and Kashima[305] studied the tracheal involvement in laryngeal papillomatosis and found extension of the papillomatous growth into the tracheostomy site. The incidence of subglottic and tracheal extension occurs in 2% to 63% of the cases. Although rare (in less than 1% of patients), papillomata may spread even into the lung parenchyma causing extensive destruction and restrictive lung disease.[10] Malignant transformation of laryngeal papillomatosis to a fatal metastatic squamous lung cancer has also been reported.[10]

Although over the years many different treatment modalities have been applied, there has been only limited success in the management of laryngeal papillomatosis. The various therapies for treatment of laryngeal papillomas included ultrasound and cryosurgery, hormones, steroids, antibiotics, chemotherapy, as well as an autogenous vaccine, transfer factor, and interferon.[304] Currently, the most commonly used procedures for treatment include endolaryngeal forceps removal, or carbon dioxide laser vaporization. However, recurrence of infection even after removal of papillomata lesions remains a serious problem. One explanation for the observed multiple recurrence of laryngeal HPV infections is the existence of latent HPV-6 and HPV-11 in morphologically normal tissues surrounding the papillomas.[302]

Interferon therapy for recurrent respiratory papillomatosis (RRP) has been discussed in several reports.[306-308] In an uncontrolled study of seven patients, Haglund et al.[309] have found human leukocyte IFN to be beneficial in the treatment of juvenile laryngeal papillomatosis. Later, in several other reports[310-312] involving small numbers of patients, IFN was shown to possess various degrees of efficacy in laryngeal papillomatosis. Kashima et al.[306] evaluated the effect of IFN-α-n1 (wellferon; a mixture of IFNs prepared by stimulation of human Burkitt's lymphoma cell line by the Sendai virus) as an adjuvant to CO_2 laser surgical excision in a 1-year randomized, cross-over study of severe juvenile-onset RRP. Patients received either 6 months of IFN-α-n1 followed by 6 months of surgery only (observation group), or 6 months of surgery only followed by 6 months of IFN-α-n1 (same dose as above) (wellferon group). IFN-α-n1 was administered intramuscularly at 5 MU/m^2 body surface area daily for 28 days and three times weekly for 5 months. The results, which showed a statistically significant improvement in the wellferon group, indicated that IFN-α-n1 may be a useful adjuvant to surgical management of RRP.[306] Mullooly et al.[307] have investigated the clinical effects of IFN-α dose variation on laryngeal papillomas. The results showed that achieving optimal clinical control of RRP with prolonged treatment of human leukocyte IFN-α appeared to be dose-dependent and often required individualized dosage elevation (six of eight patients needed a maximum dose of 18×10^6 IU per week for part of the therapy period in order to achieve better disease control). The observed strong correlation between dosage and drug response lends credence to the notion that to a large degree it is IFN causing the effect on disease expression, not just the unpredictable nature of the illness.[307]

The erratic natural history of RRP and the lack of properly controlled trials have hampered efforts to determine the efficacy of IFN treatment. Furthermore, there is also a concern whether previous studies had properly distinguished between spontaneous remission and IFN-related response.[308] Addressing these concerns, in a randomized, multicenter, controlled trial, Healy et al.[308] found no efficacy of human leukocyte IFN either as curative or as an adjunctive agent in the treatment of RRP. They treated 123 patients who were randomly assigned to receive therapy with either surgery plus IFN, or surgery alone. IFN (2×10^6 IU/m^2 of body surface area) was given daily for 1 week, then three times weekly for 1 year. During the first 6 months of the IFN-treated group, the growth of papillomas was significantly lower than in the control group ($p = .0007$); however, the difference diminished during the following 6 months, and was no longer statistically significant ($p = .68$).

Ogura et al.[313] found that one particular subtype, HPV-6e, was persistently present in multiple laryngeal papilloma and in the counterpart false cord of an IFN-α-treated adult patient.

Although the concept to apply a photosensitive dye activated by light to selectively destroy malignant cells is not new and has been previously applied to treat cancer,[314-316] photodynamic therapy (PDT) is the newest modality to be used in the therapy of laryngeal papillomatosis.[317-319] The procedure utilizes dihematoporphyrin ether (DHPE), a purified photosensitive agent, to selectively destroy papillomata lesions. When activated by light of appropriate wavelength (630 nm), DHPE, which is selectively localized and retained in virally induced lesions, will destroy them.[320-322] Studying the biodistribution of DHPE, Shikowitz et al.[323] were first to demonstrate its increased localization in papillomas, as compared with normal surrounding body tissues. Abramson et al.[324] established the safety parameters for photodynamic therapy to the larynx.

Abramson et al.[317] described two cases of adults with recurrent laryngeal papillomas treated with PDT. The hematoporphyrin dye (6.0 mg/kg) was injected intravenously 72 h prior to endoscopic surgery, at which time 32 J/cm^2 was delivered to the endolarynx by an argon pump dye laser with a red light output of 630 nm. Although at a follow-up examination 3 years later no visible evidence was present, Southern blot hybridization analysis revealed the presence of latent HPV DNA. The infusion of DHPE, 72 h prior to photoactivation was found to be the upper limit of the time interval needed for localization and retention of DHPE in the papillomas.[322] However, Abramson et al.[319] have recommended that this time interval be shortened to 48 h if no adverse effects are observed. Shikowitz[325] compared the efficacy of a pulsed light emission from a gold vapor laser, and that of continuous wave light emitted from an argon pumped-dye laser. Molecular and histologic analyses of the treated tissues showed similar results when either of the two activating light sources was used.

The antiviral agent ribavirin was used as an adjunct therapy to laser surgery of laryngeal papillomatous lesions.[326] Ribavirin was started in three adult patients at oral daily doses of 23 mg/kg prior to laser vaporization and continued for the next 6 months; one infant received oral ribavirin for 2 months. Two of the adult patients achieved complete remission for at least 2 consecutive months, but developed recurrent disease (although only minimal) in 4 months of follow-up; the other adult patient and the infant showed only a partial response and an increased interval between the required surgeries. In another study by the same group of investigators,[327] intradermally injected ribavirin successfully inhibited in a dose-dependent manner, cottontail rabbit papillomavirus-induced warts; at 30 mg/kg daily, the average reduction in the number of warts was 52% as compared to controls.

2.1.3.11   Vulvar Vestibulitis Syndrome

Vulvar vestibulitis syndrome (VVS), one of the leading causes of chronic vulvar pain,[328] is a condition characterized with severe pain on vestibular touch or attempted vaginal entry, tenderness to pressure within the vulvar vestibule, and various degrees of vulvar erythema.[329] While the etiology of VVS is still poorly understood, Turner and Marinoff[330] have discovered the presence of HPV DNA in the vulvar tissue of several patients with VVS who were lacking clinical evidence of condyloma acuminatum. These and other similar findings[331-333] implied the involvement of subclinical HPV infection, although a direct cause-and-effect relationship was not proven.[334]

Initially, the only successful therapy for VVS was the surgical removal of the vestibule with vaginal advancement (perineoplasty).[335] Later, laser vulvectomy was introduced to treat VVS, but the results were inconsistent and improvement was observed in no more than 60% of patients.[336]

In an attempt to introduce a less aggressive, nonsurgical alternative to perineoplasty, Marinoff et al.[334] have evaluated the response of 55 patients with VVS to intralesional recombinant IFN-α. Evidence of subclinical HPV infection was found in 46 patients. Substantial or partial improvement was observed in 49% of patients (27 of 55). Of the remaining 25 patients (51%) who did not improve following IFN-α therapy, 19 elected to have surgery. The latter resulted in substantial improvement in 84% and partial improvement in 11% of the patients.

2.1.3.12 Human Papillomavirus-Associated Balanoposthitis

Balanoposthitis is a condition involving inflammation of the glans penis and prepuce. Birley et al.,[337] who followed the features and clinical course of five patients with chronic balanitis, found upon histologic examination of cutaneous biopsy samples the presence of HPV-6 DNA. This finding was also confirmed by polymerase chain reaction and Southern blot analysis. Although the HPV infection did not clearly identify HPV as the causative agent, the histological evidence and the failure of topical steroids to clear the infection strongly suggest an association of HPV with this condition. Treatment with oral isotretinoin elicited positive response in one of the patients.[337]

2.1.4 References

1. de Villiers, E.-M., Wagner, D., Schneider, A., Wesch, H., Miklaw, H., Wahrendorf, J., Papendick, U., and zur Hausen, H., Human papillomavirus infections in women without and with abnormal cervical cytology, *Lancet*, 2, 703, 1987.
2. Kjaer, S. K., Engholm, G., Teisen, C., Haugaard, B. J., Lynge, E., Christensen, R. B., Moller, K. A., Jensen, H., Poll, P., Vestergaard, B. F., de Villiers, E.-M., and Jensen, O. M., Risk factors for cervical human papillomavirus and herpes simplex virus infections in Greenland and Denmark: a population-based study, *Am. J. Epidemiol.*, 131, 669, 1990.
3. Toon, P. G., Arrand, J. R., Wilson, L. P., and Sharp, D. S., Human papillomavirus infection of the uterine cervix of women without cytological signs of neoplasia, *Br. Med. J. Clin. Res.*, 293, 1261, 1986.
4. Becker, T. M., Stone, K. M., and Alexander, E. R., Genital human papillomavirus infection: a growing concern, *Obstet. Gynecol. Clin. North Am.*, 14, 389, 1987.
5. Hatch, K. D., Vulvovaginal human papillomavirus infections: clinical implications and management, *Am. J. Obstet. Gynecol.*, 165, 1183, 1991.
6. Shah, K. V. and Howley, P. M., Papillomaviruses, in *Fields Virology*, 2nd ed., Fields, B. N., Knipe, D. M., Chanock, R. M., Hirsch, M. S., Melnick, J. L., Monath, T. P., and Roizman, B., Eds., Raven Press, New York, 1990, 1651.
7. Cirelli, R. and Tyring, S. K., Interferons in human papillomavirus infections, *Antiviral Res.*, 24, 191, 1994.
8. de Villiers, E.-M., Heterogeneity of the human papillomavirus group, *J. Virol.*, 63, 4896, 1989.
9. Howley, P. M., Papillomavirinae and their replication, in *Fields Virology*, 2nd ed., Fields, B. N., Knipe, D. M., Chanock, R. M., Hirsch, M. S., Melnick, J. L., Monath, T. P., and Roizman, B., Eds., Raven Press, New York, 1990, 1625.
10. Osborne, N. G. and Adelson, M. D., Herpes simplex virus and human papillomavirus genital infections: controversy over obstetric management, *Clin. Obstet. Gynecol.*, 33, 801, 1990.
11. Lowy, D. R., Kirnbauer, R., and Schiller, J. T., Genital human papillomavirus infection, *Proc. Natl. Acad. Sci. U.S.A.*, 91, 2436, 1994.
12. Orth, G., Epidermodysplasia verruciformis, in *The Papovaviridae: The Papilloviruses*, Vol. 2, Salzman, N. P. and Howley, P. M., Eds., Plenum Press, New York, 1987, 199.
13. Jablonska, S., Dabrowski, J., and Jakubowicz, K., Epidermodysplasia verruciformis as a model in studies on the role of papovaviruses in oncogenesis, *Cancer Res.*, 32, 485, 1961.
14. Orth, G., Epidermodysplasia verruciformis, in *The Papovaviridae: The Papilloviruses*, Vol. 2, Salzman, N. P. and Howley, P. M., Eds., Plenum Press, New York, 1987, 199.
15. Meisels, A. and Fortin, R., Condylomatous lesions of the cervix and vagina. I. Cytologic patterns, *Acta Cytol.*, 20, 505, 1976.
16. Meisels, A., Fortin, R., and Roy, M., Condylomatous lesions of the cervix. II. Cytologic, colposcopic and histopathologic study, *Acta Cytol.*, 21, 379, 1977.
17. Meisels, A., Morin, C., and Casas-Cordero, M., Human papillomavirus infection of the uterine cervix, *Int. J. Gynecol. Pathol.*, 1, 75, 1982.
18. Reid, R., Laverty, C., Coppleson, M., Isarangkul, W., and Hills, E., Non-condylomatous cervical wart virus infection, *Obstet. Gynecol.*, 55, 476, 1980.
19. Peto, R., Introduction: geographic patterns and trends, in *Viral Etiology Cervical Cancer*, Peto, R. and zur Hausen, H., Eds., Banbury Report 21. Cold Spring Harbor Laboratory, Cold Spring Harbor, New York, 1986, 3.

20. Ferenczy, A. and Winkler, B., Cervical intraepithelial neoplasia and condyloma, in *Blaustein's Pathology of the Female Genital Tract*, 3rd ed., Kurman, R. J., Ed., Springer-Verlag, New York, 1987, 177.
21. Ferenczy, A. and Winkler, B., Carcinoma and metastatic tumors of the cervix, in *Blaustein's Pathology of the Female Genital Tract*, 3rd ed., Kurman, R. J., Ed., Springer-Verlag, New York, 1978, 218.
22. Reid, R., Crum, C. P., Herschman, B. R., Fu, Y. S., Braun, L., Shah, K. V., Agronow, S. J., and Stanhope, C. R., Genital warts and cervical cancer. III. Subclinical papillomaviral infection and cervical neoplasia are linked by a spectrum of continuous morphologic and biologic change, *Cancer*, 53, 943, 1984.
23. Saito, K., Saito, A., Fu, Y. S., Smotkin, D., Gupta, J., and Shah, K. V., Topographical study of cervical condyloma and intraepithelial neoplasia, *Cancer*, 59, 2064, 1987.
24. Barasso, R., De Brux, J., Croissant, O., and Orth, G., High prevalence of papillomavirus-associated penile intraepithelial neoplasia in sexual partners of women with cervical intraepithelial neoplasia, *N. Engl. J. Med.*, 317, 916, 1987.
25. Gupta, J., Pilotti, S., Rilke, F., and Shah, K., Association of human papillomavirus type 16 with neoplastic lesions of the vulva and other genital sites by *in situ* hybridization, *Am. J. Pathol.*, 127, 206, 1987.
26. Henderson, B. R., Thompson, C. H., Rose, B. R., Cossart, Y. E., and Morris, B. J., Detection of specific types of human papillomavirus in cervical scrapes, anal scrapes, and anogenital biopsies by DNA hybridization, *J. Med. Virol.*, 21, 381, 1987.
27. McCance, D. J., Kalache, A., Ashdown, K., Andrade, L., Menezes, F., Smith, P., and Doll, R., Human papillomavirus type 16 and 18 in carcinomas of the penis in Brasil, *Int. J. Cancer*, 37, 55, 1986.
28. Praetorius-Clausen, F., Rare oral viral disorder (molluscum contagiosum, localized keratoacanthoma, verrucae, condyloma acuminatum, and focal epithelial hyperplasia), *Oral Surg. Oral Med. Oral Pathol.*, 34, 604, 1972.
29. Syrjanen, S. M., Human papillomavirus infections in the oral cavity, in *Papillomaviruses and Human Disease*, Syrjanen, K., Gissmann, L., and Koss, L. G., Eds., Springer-Verlag, New York, 1987, 104.
30. Shklar, G., Oral leukoplakia, *N. Engl. J. Med.*, 315, 1544, 1986.
31. Gissmann, L., Diehl, V., Schultz-Loulon, H. J., and zur Hausen, H., Molecular cloning and characterization of human papillomavirus DNA derived from laryngeal papilloma, *J. Virol.*, 44, 393, 1982.
32. Kashima, H. and Mounts, P., Tumors of the head and neck, larynx, lung and esophagus and their possible relation to HPV, in *Papillomaviruses and Human Disease*, Syrjanen, K., Gissmann, L., and Koss, L. G., Eds., Springer-Verlag, New York, 1987, 138.
33. Mounts, P. and Shah, K., Respiratory papillomatosis: etiological relation to genital tract papillomaviruses, *Prog. Med. Virol.*, 29, 90, 1984.
34. Brandsma, J., Abramson, A., Sciubba, J., Shah, K., Barrezuetta, N., and Galli, R., Papillomavirus infection of the nose, in *Cancer Cells 5: Papillomaviruses*, Steinberg, B. M., Brandsma, J. L., and Taichman, L. B., Eds., Cold Spring Harbor Laboratory, Cold Spring Harbor, New York, 1987, 301.
35. Respler, D. S., Jahn, A., Pater, A., and Pater, M. M., Isolation and characterization of papillomavirus DNA from nasal inverting (Schneiderian) papillomas, *Ann. Otol. Rhinol. Laryngol.*, 96, 170, 1987.
36. Syrjanen, S., Happonen, R. P., Virolainen, E., Silvonen, L., and Syrjanen, K., Detection of human papillomavirus (HPV) structural antigens and DNA types in inverted papillomas and squamous cell carcinomas of the nasal cavities and paranasal sinuses, *Acta Otolaryngol. (Stockholm)*, 104, 334, 1987.
37. Weber, R. S., Schillitoe, E. J., Robbins, K. T., Luna, M. A., Batsakis, J. G., Donovan, D. T., and Adler-Storthz, K., Prevalence of human papillomavirus in inverted nasal papillomas, *Arch. Otolaryngol. Head Neck Surg.*, 114, 23, 1988.
38. Crissman, J. D., Kessis, T., Shah, K. V., Fu, Y. S., Stoler, M. H., Zarbo, R. J., and Wei, M. A., Squamous papillary neoplasia of the adult upper aerodigestive tract, *Hum. Pathol.*, 19, 1387, 1988.
39. Byrne, J. C., Tsao, M. S., Fraser, R. S., and Howley, P. M., Human papillomavirus-11 DNA in a patient with chronic laryngotracheobronchial papillomatosis and metastatic squamous-cell carcinoma of the lung, *N. Engl. J. Med.*, 317, 873, 1987.
40. Kashima, H., Wu, T.-C., Mounts, P., Heffner, D., Cachay, A., and Hyams, V., Carcinoma ex-papilloma histologic and virologic studies in whole-organ sections of the larynx, *Laryngoscope*, 98, 619, 1988.
41. Lass, J. H., Jenson, A. B., Papale, J. J., and Albert, D. M., Papillomavirus in human conjuctival papillomas, *Am. J. Ophthalmol.*, 95, 364, 1983.

42. McDonnell, P. J., McDonnell, J. M., Kessis, T., Green, W. R., and Shah, K. V., Detection of human papillomavirus type 6/11 DNA in conjuctival papillomas by *in situ* hybridization with radioactive probes, *Hum. Pathol.*, 18, 1115, 1987.

43. Pfister, H., Fuchs, P. G., and Volcler, H. E., Human papillomavirus DNA in conjuctival papilloma, *Graefes Arch. Clin. Exp. Ophthalmol.*, 223, 164, 1985.

44. Meisels, A., Roy, M., Fortier, M., Morin, C., Casas-Cordero, M., Shah, K. V., and Turgeon, H., Human papillomavirus infection of the cervix. The atypical condylomata, *Acta Cytol.*, 25, 7, 1981.

45. Grunebaum, A., Sedlis, A., Sillman, F., Fruchter, R., Stanek, A., and Boyce, J., Association of human papillomavirus infection with cervical intraepithelial neoplasia, *Obstet. Gynecol.*, 62, 448, 1983.

46. Isaacs, A. and Lindemann, J. J., Virus interference: the interferon, *Proc. R. Soc. London Biol.*, 147, 258, 1957.

47. Ikic, D., Orescanin, M., Krusic, J., Cestar, Z., Alac, Z., Soos, E., Jusic, D., and Smerdel, S., Preliminary study of the effect of human leukocyte interferon on condyloma acuminata in women, in *Proc. Symp. Clin. Use Interferon*, Ikic, D., Ed., Yugoslav Academy of Science and the Arts, Zagreb, 1975, 223.

48. Food and Drug Administration, Alpha interferon for venereal warts, *FRD Drug Bull.*, 18, 19, 1988.

49. Gall, S. A., Constantine, L., and Koukol, D., Therapy of persistent human papillomavirus disease with two different interferon species, *Am. J. Obstet. Gynecol.*, 164, 130, 1991.

50. Georgiev, V. St., Immunomodulating peptides of natural and synthetic origin, *Med. Res. Rev.*, 11, 81, 1991.

51. Einhorn, N., Ling, P., and Strander, H., Systemic interferon alpha treatment of human condylomata acuminata, *Acta Obstet. Gynaecol. Scand.*, 62, 285, 1983.

52. Gall, S. A., Hughes, C. E., Mounts, P., Segriti, A., Weck, P. K., and Whisnant, J. K., Efficacy of human lymphoblastoid interferon in the therapy of resistant condyloma acuminata, *Obstet. Gynecol.*, 67, 643, 1986.

53. Gall, S. A., Hughes, C. E., and Trofatter, K., Interferon for the therapy of condyloma acuminatum, *Am. J. Obstet. Gynecol.*, 153, 157, 1985.

54. Eron, L. F., Judson, F., Tucker, S., Prawer, S., Mills, J., Murphy, K., Hickey, M., Rogers, M., Flannigan, S., Hien, N., Katz, H. I., Goldman, S., Gottlieb, A., Adams, K., Burton, P., Tanner, D., Taylor, E., and Peets, E., Interferon therapy for condyloma acuminata, *N. Engl. J. Med.*, 315, 1059, 1986.

55. Horowitz, B. J., Interferon therapy for condylomatous vulvitis, *Obstet. Gynecol.*, 73, 446, 1989.

56. Pestka, S., Interferon: a decade of accomplishments, in *Foundations of the Future in Antiviral Chemotherapy*, Mills, J. and Corey, L., Eds., Elsevier, New York, 1986, 9.

57. Preble, O. T. and Friedman, R. M., Interferon-induced alterations in cells: relevance to viral and nonviral diseases, *Lab. Invest.*, 49, 4, 1983.

58. Santoli, D., Trinchieri, G., and Koprowski, H., Cell-mediated cytotoxicity against virus-infected target cells in humans. II. Interferon induction and activation of natural killer cells, *J. Immunol.*, 121, 532, 1978.

59. Jones, C. M., Varesio, L., Herberman, R. B., and Pestka, S., Interferon activates macrophages to produce plasminogen activator, *J. Interferon Res.*, 2, 377, 1982.

60. Einhorn, N., Ling, P., Secher, D., and Strander, H., Treatment of advanced condylomata acuminata with semi-purified and purified human leukocyte interferon, *Acta Oncol.*, 30, 343, 1991.

61. Secher, D. S. and Burke, D. C., A monoclonal antibody for large-scale purification of human leukocyte interferon, *Nature*, 285, 446, 1980.

62. Scott, G., Secher, D., Flowers, D., Bate, J., Cantell, K., and Tyrell, D., Toxicity of interferon, *Br. Med. J.*, 282, 1345, 1981.

63. Spiegel, R. J., Spicehandler, J. R., Jacobs, S. L., and Oden, E. M., Low incidence of serum neutralizing factors in patients receiving recombinant alfa-2b interferon (intron A), *Am. J. Med.*, 80, 223, 1986.

64. Ballon, S. C., Roberts, J. A., and Lagasse, L. D., Topical 5-fluorouracil in the treatment of intraepithelial neoplasia of the vagina, *Obstet. Gynecol.*, 54, 163, 1979.

65. Krebs, H.-B., Treatment of vaginal intraepithelial neoplasias with laser and topical 5-fluorouracil, *Obstet. Gynecol.*, 73, 657, 1989.

66. Ferenczy, A., Comparison of 5-fluorouracil and CO_2 laser for treatment of vaginal condylomata, *Obstet. Gynecol.*, 64, 773, 1984.

67. Krebs, H.-B., Treatment of vaginal condylomata acuminata by weekly topical application of 5-fluorouracil, *Obstet. Gynecol.*, 70, 68, 1987.

68. Krebs, H.-B. and Helmkamp, B. F., Chronic ulcerations following topical therapy with 5-fluorouracil for vaginal human papillomavirus-associated lesions, *Obstet. Gynecol.*, 78, 205, 1991.

69. Mansell, P. W. A., Litwin, M. S., Ichinose, H., and Krementz, E. T., Delayed hypersensitivity to 5-fluorouracil following topical chemotherapy of cutaneous cancers, *Cancer Res.*, 35, 1288, 1975.

70. Reid, R., Greenberg, M. D., Lörincz, A. T., Daoud, Y., Pizzuti, and Stoler, M., Superficial laser vulvectomy. IV. Extended laser vaporization and adjunctive 5-fluorouracil therapy of human papillomavirus-associated vulvar disease, *Obstet. Gynecol.*, 76, 439, 1990.

71. Kraus, S. J. and Sone, K. M., Management of genital infection caused by human papillomavirus, *Rev. Infect. Dis.*, 12(suppl. 6), S620, 1990.

72. von Krogh, G., Topical treatment of penile condylomata acuminata with podophyllin, podophyllotoxin and colchicine, *Acta Derm. Venereol. (Stockholm)*, 58, 163, 1978.

73. Beutner, K. R., Podophyllotoxin in the treatment of genital human papillomavirus infection: a review, *Semin. Dermatol.*, 6, 10, 1987.

74. Ampel, N. M., Stout, M. L., Garewal, H. S., and Davis, J. R., Persistent rectal ulcer associated with human papillomavirus type 33 in a patient with AIDS: successful treatment with isotretinoin, *Rev. Infect. Dis.*, 12, 1004, 1990.

75. Hong, W. K., Endicott, J., Itri, L. M., Doos, W., Batsakis, J. G., Bell, R., Fofonoff, S., Byers, R., Atkinson, E. N., Vaughan, C., Toth, B. B., Kramer, A., Dimery, I. W., Skipper, P., and Strong, S., 13-*cis*-Retinoic acid in the treatment of oral leukoplakia, *N. Engl. J. Med.*, 315, 1501, 1986.

76. Graham, V., Surwit, E. S., Weiner, S., and Meyskens, F. L., Jr., Phase II trial of beta-all-*trans*-retinoic acid for cervical intraepithelial neoplasia delivered via a collagen sponge and cervical cap, *West. J. Med.*, 145, 192, 1986.

77. Cordero, A. A., Allevato, M. A. J., Barclay, C. A., Traballi, C. A., and Donatti, L. B., Treatment of lichen planus and leukoplakia with the oral retinoid Ro 10-039, in *Retinoids*, Orfanos , C. E., Braun-Falco, O., Farber, E. M., Grupper, Ch., Polano, M. K., and Schuppli, R., Eds., Springer-Verlag, Basel, 1981, 273.

78. Shah, J. P., Strong, E. W., DeCosse, J. J., Itri, L., and Sellers, P., Effects on retinoids in oral leukoplakia, *Am. J. Surg.*, 146, 466, 1983.

79. Markowska, J., Nowak, M., Niecewicz, R., Breborowicz, J., Wiese, E., and Zengteler, G., Results of topical treatment of HPV infection in the uterine cervix using interferon beta, 13-*cis*-retinoic acid and TFX, *Eur. J. Gynaecol. Oncol.*, 15, 65, 1994.

80. Majewski, S., Szmurlo, A., Marczak, M., Jablonska, S., and Bollag, W., Synergistic effect of retinoids and interferon alpha on tumor-induced angiogenesis: anti-angiogenic effect on HPV-harboring tumor-cell lines, *Int. J. Cancer*, 57, 81, 1994.

81. Helene, C. and Toulme, J.-J., Specific regulation of gene expression by antisense, sense, and antigene nucleic acids, *Biochim. Biophys. Acta*, 1049, 99, 1990.

82. Zamecnik, P. C. and Stephenson, M. L., Inhibition of Rous sarcoma virus replication and cell transformation by a specific oligonucleotide, *Proc. Natl. Acad. Sci. U.S.A.*, 75, 280, 1978.

83. Agris, C. H., Blake, K. R., Miller, P. S., Reddy, M. P., and Ts'o, P. O. P., Inhibition of vesicular stomatitis virus protein synthesis and infection by sequence-specific oligodeoxyribonucleoside methylphosphonates, *Biochemistry*, 25, 6268, 1986.

84. Smith, C. C., Aurelian, L., Reddy, M., Miller, P. S., and Ts'o, P. O. P., Antiviral effect of an oligo(nucleotide methylphosphonate) complementary to the splice-junction of herpes simplex virus type 1 immediate early pre-mRNAs 4 and 5, *Biochemistry*, 83, 2787, 1986.

85. Zerial, A., Thuong, N. T., and Helene, C., Selective inhibition of the cytopathic effect of type A influenza viruses by oligonucleotides covalently linked to an intercalating agent, *Nucleic Acids Res.*, 15, 9909, 1987.

86. Zamecnik, P. C., Goodchild, J., Taguchi, Y., and Sarin, P. S., Inhibition of replication and expression of human T-cell lymphotropic virus type II in cultured cells by exogenous synthetic oligonucleotides complementary to viral RNA, *Proc. Natl. Acad. Sci. U.S.A.*, 83, 4143, 1986.

87. Cowsert, L. M., Fox, M. C., Zon, G., and Mirabelli, C. K., In vitro evaluation of phosphorothioate oligonucleotides targeted to the E2 mRNA of papillomavirus: potential treatment for genital warts, *Antimicrob. Agents Chemother.*, 37, 171, 1993.

88. McBride, A. A., Romanczuk, H., and Howley, P. M., The papillomavirus E2 regulatory proteins, *J. Biol. Chem.*, 266, 18411, 1991.

89. Sousa, R., Dostatni, N., and Yanive, M., Control of papillomavirus gene expression, *Biochim. Biophys. Acta*, 1032, 19, 1990.

90. Spalholz, B. A., Yang, Y.-C., and Howley, P. M., Transactivation of a bovine papillomavirus transcriptional regulatory element by the E2 gene product, *Cell*, 42, 183, 1985.

91. Hirochika, H., Broker, T. R., and Chow, L. T., Enhancers and *trans*-acting E2 transcriptional factors of papillomaviruses, *J. Virol.*, 61, 2599, 1987.

92. Phelps, W. C. and Howley, P. M., Transcriptional transactivation by the human papillomavirus type-16 E2 gene product, *J. Virol.*, 61, 1630, 1987.

93. Guis, D., Grossman, S., Bedell, M. A., and Laimons, L. A., Inducible and constitutive enhancer domains in the noncoding region of human papillomavirus type 18, *J. Virol.*, 62, 665, 1988.

94. del Vecchio, A. M., Romanczuk, H., Howley, P. M., and Baker, C. C., Transient replication of human papillomavirus DNAs, *J. Virol.*, 66, 5949, 1992.

95. Mohr, I., Clark, R., Sun, S., Androphy, E., MacPherson, P., and Botchan, M., Targeting the E1 replication protein to the papillomavirus origin of replication by complex formation with the E2 transactivator, *Science*, 250, 1694, 1990.

96. Liebhaber, S. A., Russel, J. E., Cash, F. E., and Eshleman, S. S., Inhibition of mRNA translation by antisense sequences, in *Gene Regulation: Biology of Antisense RNA and DNA*, Erickson, R. P. and Izant, J. G., Eds., Raven Press, New York, 1992, 163.

97. Kreider, J. W., Balogh, K., Olson, R. O., and Martin, J. C., Treatment of latent rabbit and human papillomavirus infections with 9-(2-phosphonylmethoxy)ethylguanidine (PMEG), *Antiviral Res.*, 14, 51, 1990.

98. Wickenden, C., Malcolm, A. D. B., Steele, A., and Coleman, D. V., Screening for wart virus infection in normal and abnormal cervices by DNA hybridization of cervical scrapes, *Lancet*, 1, 65, 1985.

99. Reid, R., Stanhope, C. R., Herschman, B. R., Booth, E., Phibbs, G. D., and Smith, J. P., Genital warts and cervical cancer. I. Evidence of an association between subclinical papillomaviral infection and cervical malignancy, *Cancer*, 50, 377, 1982.

100. zur Hausen, H., Human papillomaviruses and their possible role in squamous cell carcinoma, *Curr. Top. Microbiol. Immunol.*, 78, 1, 1977.

101. Zachow, K. R., Ostrow, R. S., Bender, M., Watts, S., Okagaki, T., Pass, F., and Faras, A. J., Detection of human papillomavirus DNA in anogenital neoplasias, *Nature*, 300, 771, 1982.

102. Smotkin, D., Berek, J. S., Fu, Y. S., Hacker, N. F., Major, F. J., and Wettstein, F. O., Human papillomavirus deoxyribonucleic acid in adenocarcinoma and adenosquamous carcinoma of the uterine cervix, *Obstet. Gynecol.*, 68, 241, 1986.

103. Koutsky, L. A., Galloway, D. A., and Holmes, K. K., Epidemiology of genital human papillomavirus infection, *Epidemiol. Rev.*, 10, 122, 1988.

104. Bouchaud, O., Marche, C., Cadiot, G., Longuet, P., René, E., and Coulaud, J. P., Human papillomavirus in the esophagus in HIV patients, *Proc. Xth Int. Conf. AIDS*, Yokohama, 1994, Abstr. PB0171.

105. Baggish, M., Carbon dioxide laser treatment for condylomata acuminata venereal infections, *Obstet. Gynecol.*, 55, 711, 1980.

106. Ferenczy, A., Mitao, M., Nagai, N., Silverstein, S. J., and Crum, C. P., Latent papillomavirus and recurring genital warts, *N. Engl. J. Med.*, 313, 784, 1985.

107. Schneider, A., Papendick, U., Gissmann, I., and De Villiers, E. M., Interferon treatment of human genital papillomavirus infection: importance of viral type, *Int. J. Cancer*, 40, 610, 1987.

108. Yliskoski, M., Syrjanen, K., Syrjanen, S., Saarikoski, S., and Nethersell, A., Systemic alpha-interferon (wellferon) treatment of genital human papillomavirus (HPV) type 6, 11, 16 and 18 infections: double-blind, placebo-controlled trial, *Gynecol. Oncol.*, 43, 55, 1991.

109. Fierlbeck, G. and Rassner, G., Treatment of condylomata acuminata with systemically administered recombinant gamma interferon, *Z. Hautkr.*, 62, 1280, 1987.

110. Erpenbach, K., Derschum, W., and Vietsch, H. V., Adjuvant-systemische interferon-α2b-behandlung bei therapieresistenten anogenitalen condyloma acuminata, *Urologie*, 29, 43, 1990.

111. Vance, J. C. and Davis, D., Interferon alpha-2b injections used as an adjuvant therapy to carbon dioxide laser vaporization of recalcitrant ano-genital condylomata acuminata, *J. Invest. Dermatol.*, 95, 146S, 1990.

112. Hohenleutner, U., Landthaler, M., and Braun-Falco, O., Post-operative adjuvante therapie mit interferon-alfa-2b nach laserchirurgie von condylomata acuminata, *Hautarzt*, 41, 545, 1990.

113. Peterson, C. S., Bjerring, P., Larsen, J., Blaakaer, J., Hagdrup, H., From, E., and Obergarrd, L., Systemic interferon alpha-2b increases the cure rate in laser treated patients with multiple persistent genital warts: a placebo-controlled study, *Genitourin. Med.*, 67, 99, 1991.

114. Davis, B. E. and Noble, M. J., Initial experience with combined interferon alpha-2b and carbon dioxide laser for the treatment of condyloma acuminata, *J. Virol.*, 147, 627, 1992.

115. Reid, R., Greenberg, M. D., Pizzuti, D. J., Omoto, K. H., Rutledge, L. H., and Soo, W., Superficial laser vulvectomy. V. Surgical debulking is enhanced by adjuvant systemic interferon, *Am. J. Obstet. Gynecol.*, 166, 815, 1992.

116. Tiedemann, K. H. and Ernst, T. M., Combination therapy of recurrent condylomata acuminata with electrocautery and alpha-2-interferon, *AKT Dermatol.*, 14, 200, 1988.

117. Piccoli, R., Santoro, M. G., Nappi, C., Capodanno, M., De Santis, V., La Torre, P. C., Costa, S., and Montemagno, U., Vulvo-vaginal condylomatosis and relapse: combined treatment with electrocauterization and beta-interferon, *Clin. Exp. Obstet. Gynecol.*, 16, 30, 1989.

118. Macnab, J. C. M., Walkinshaw, S. A., Cordiner, J. W., and Clements, J. B., Human papillomavirus in clinically and histologically normal tissue of patients with genital cancer, *N. Engl. J. Med.*, 315, 1052, 1986.

119. Handley, J. M., Horner, T., Maw, R. D., Lawther, H., and Dinsmore, W. W., Subcutaneous interferon alpha 2a combined with cryotherapy vs. cryotherapy alone in the treatment of primary anogenital warts: a randomized observer blind placebo-controlled study, *Genitourin. Med.*, 67, 297, 1991.

120. Eron, L. J., Alder, M. B., O'Rourke, J. M., Rittweger, K., DePamphilis, J., and Pizzuti, D. J., Recurrence of condylomata acuminata following cryotherapy is not prevented by systemically administered interferon, *Genitourin. Med.*, 69, 91, 1993.

121. Douglas, J. M., Rogers, M., and Judson, F. N., The effect of asymptomatic infection with HTLV-III on the response of anogenital warts to intralesional treatment with recombinant α2 interferon, *J. Infect. Dis.*, 154, 331, 1986.

122. Centers for Disease Control and Prevention. 1993 Sexually transmitted diseases treatment guidelines, *Morbid. Mortal. Wkly Rep.*, 42(No. RR-14), 1, 1993.

123. Buntin, D. M., The 1993 sexually transmitted disease treatment guidelines, *Semin. Dermatol.*, 13, 269, 1994.

124. Ikic, D., Bosnic, N., Smerdel, S., Jusic, D., Soos, E., and Delimar, N., Double blind clinical study with human leukocyte interferon in the therapy of condylomata acuminata, in *Proc. Symp. Clin. Use Interferon*, Ikic, D., Ed., Yugoslav Academy of Science and the Arts, Zagreb, 1975, 229.

125. Vesterinen, E., Meyer, B., Purola, E., and Cantell, K., Treatment of vaginal flat condyloma with interferon cream, *Lancet*, 1, 157, 1984.

126. Vesterinen, E., Meyer, B., Cantell, K., and Purola, E., Topical treatment of flat vaginal condyloma with human leukocyte interferon, *Obstet. Gynecol.*, 64, 535, 1984.

127. Keay, S., Teng, N., Eisenberg, M., Story, B., Sellers, P. W., and Merigan, T. C., Topical interferon for treating condyloma acuminata in women, *J. Infect. Dis.*, 158, 934, 1988.

128. Reichman, R. C., Oakes, D., Bonnez, W., Greisberger, C., Tyring, S., Miller, L., Whitley, R., Carveth, H., Wiedner, M., Krueger, G., Yorkey, L., Roberts, N. J., Jr., and Dolin, R., Treatment of condyloma acuminatum with three different interferons administered intralesionally: a double-blind, placebo-controlled trial, *Ann. Intern. Med.*, 108, 675, 1988.

129. Reichman, R. C., Oakes, D., Bonnez, W., Brown, D., Mattison, H. R., Bailey-Farchione, A., Stoler, M. H., Demeter, L. M., Tyring, S. K., Miller, L., Whitley, R., Carveth, H., Weidner, M., Krueger, G., and Choi, A., Treatment of condyloma acuminatum with three different interferon-α preparations administered parenterally: a double-blind, placebo-controlled trial, *J. Infect. Dis.*, 162, 1270, 1990.

130. Kovarik, J., Mayer, G., Pohanka, E., Schwarz, M., Traindl, O., Graf, H., and Smolen, J., Adverse effect of low-dose prophylactic human recombinant leukocyte interferon alpha treatment in renal transplant recipients, *Transplantation*, 45, 402, 1988.

131. Rohnblom, L. E., Alm, G. V., and Oberg, K. E., Autoimmunity after alpha-interferon therapy for malignant carcinoid tumors, *Ann. Intern. Med.*, 115, 178, 1991.

132. Spruance, S., Douglas, J., Hougham, A., Fox, T., and Beutner, K., Multicenter trial of 5% imiquimod (IQ) cream for the treatment of genital and perianal warts, *Proc. 33rd Intersci. Conf. Antimicrob. Agents Chemother.*, American Society for Microbiology, Washington, D.C., Abstr. 1432, 1993.

133. Oriel, J. D., Natural history of genital warts, *Br. J. Vener. Dis.*, 47, 1, 1971.

134. Simmons, P. O., Genital warts, *Int. J. Dermatol.*, 22, 410, 1983.

135. Lutzner, M. A., The human papillomaviruses — a review, *Arch. Dermatol.*, 119, 631, 1983.

136. Howley, P. M. and Broker, T. R., *Papillomaviruses — Molecular and Clinical Aspects*, Alan R. Liss, New York, 1985.

137. Margolis, S., Therapy for condyloma acuminatum: a review, *Rev. Infect. Dis.*, 4(Suppl.), 829, 1982.

138. Gissmann, L., Wolnik, L., Ikenberg, H., Koldovsky, U., Schnurch, H. G., and zur Hausen, H., Human papillomavirus types 6 and 11 DNA sequences in genital and laryngeal papillomas and in some cervical cancers, *Proc. Natl. Acad. Sci. U.S.A.*, 80, 560, 1983.

139. Brown, D. R., Bryan, J. T., Cramer, H., and Fife, K. H., Analysis of human papillomavirus types in exophytic condylomata acuminata by hybrid capture and Southern blot techniques, *J. Clin. Microbiol.*, 31, 2667, 1993.

140. Pfister, H., Human papillomaviruses and genital cancer, *Adv. Cancer Res.*, 48, 113, 1987.

141. Reid, R., Greenberg, M., Jenson, A. B., Husain, M., Willett, J., Daoud, Y., Temple, G., Stanhope, C. R., Sherman, A. I., Phibbs, G. D., and Lörincz, A. T., Sexually transmitted papillomaviral infections, *Am. J. Obstet. Gynecol.*, 156, 212, 1987.

142. Bergeron, C., Ferenczy, A., Shah, K. V., and Naghashfar, Z., Multicenter human papillomavirus infections of the female genital tract: correlation of viral types with abnormal mitotic figures, colposcopic presentation and location, *Obstet. Gynecol.*, 69, 736, 1987.

143. Wilbur, D. C., Reichman, R. C., and Stoler, M. H., Detection of infection by human papillomavirus in genital condylomata. A comparison study using immunocytochemistry and in situ nucleic acid hybridization, *Am. J. Clin. Pathol.*, 89, 505, 1988.

144. Beckmann, A. M., Sherman, K. J., Myerson, D., Daling, J. R., McDougall, J. K., and Galloway, D. A., Comparative virologic studies of condylomata acuminata reveal a lack of dual infections with human papillomavirus, *J. Infect. Dis.*, 163, 393, 1991.

145. Yang, G. C. H., Demopoulos, R. I., Chan, W., and Mittal, K. R., Superficial nuclear enlargement without koilocytosis as an expression of human papillomavirus infection of the uterine cervix: an in situ hybridization study, *Int. J. Gynecol. Pathol.*, 11, 283, 1992.

146. Langenberg, A., Cone, R., McDougall, J., Kiviat, N., and Corey, L., Dual infection with human papillomavirus in a population with overt genital condylomas, *J. Am. Acad. Dermatol.*, 28, 434, 1993.

147. Brown, D. R., Bryan, J. T., Cramer, H., Katz, B. P., Handy, V., and Fife, K. H., Detection of multiple human papillomavirus types in condylomata acuminata from immunosuppressed patients, *J. Infect. Dis.*, 170, 759, 1994.

148. Geffen, J. R., Klein, R. J., and Friedman-Kien, A. E., Intralesional administration of large doses of human leukocyte interferon for the treatment of condyloma acuminata, *J. Infect. Dis.*, 150, 612, 1986.

149. Vance, J. C., Bart, B. J., Bart, B., Welander, C. E., Smiles, K. A., and Tanner, D. J., Effectiveness of intralesional human recombinant alpha-2b interferon (intron-A) for the treatment of patients with condyloma acuminatum, *Clin. Res.*, 34, 993A, 1986.

150. Friedman-Kien, A. E., Eron, L. J., Conant, M., Growdon, W., Badiak, H., Bradstreet, P. W., Fedorczyk, D., Trout, R., and Plasse, T. F., Natural interferon alpha for treatment of condylomata acuminata, *JAMA*, 259, 533, 1988.

151. Boot, J. M., Blog, B., and Stolz, E., Intralesional interferon alpha-2b treatment of condylomata acuminata previously resistant to podophyllum resin application, *Genitourin. Med.*, 65, 50, 1989.

152. Scott, G. M. and Csonka, G. W., Effect of injections of small doses of human fibroblast interferon into genital warts: a pilot study, *Br. J. Vener. Dis.*, 55, 442, 1979.

153. Vance, J. C., Bart, B. J., Hansen, R. C., Reichman, R. C., McEwen, C., Hatch, K. D., Berman, B., and Tanner, D. J., Intralesional recombinant alpha-2 interferon for the treatment of patients with condyloma acuminatum or vertica plantaris, *Arch. Dermatol.*, 122, 272, 1986.

154. Gross, G., Ikenberg, H., Roussaki, A., Kunze, B., and Drees, N., Does the papillomavirus DNA persist in the epithelium after successful treatment of genital warts with subcutaneous injections of recombinant interferon alpha? *J. Invest. Dermatol.*, 90, 242, 1988.

155. Schonfeld, A., Nitke, S., Schattner, A., Wallach, D., Crespi, M., Hahn, T., Levavi, H., Yarden, O., Shoham, J., Doerner, T., and Revel, M., Intramuscular human interferon-β injections in treatment of condylomata acuminata, *Lancet*, 1, 1038, 1984.

156. Gall, S. A., Hughes, C. E., and Trofatter, K., Interferon for the therapy of condyloma acuminata, *Am. J. Obstet. Gynecol.*, 153, 157, 1985.

157. Olsen, E. A., Trofatter, K. F., Gall, S. A., Medoff, J. R., Hughes, C. E., Weiner, M. S., and Kelly, F. F., Human lymphoblastoid alpha-interferon in the treatment of refractory condyloma acuminata, *Clin. Res.*, 33, 673A, 1985.

158. Reichman, R. C., Micha, J. P., Weck, P. K., Bonnez, W., Wold, D., Whisnant, J. K., Mounts, P., Trofatter, K. F., Kucera, P., and Gall, S. A., Interferon alpha-nl (wellferon) for refractory genital warts: efficacy and tolerance of low dose systemic therapy, *Antiviral Res.*, 10, 41, 1988.

159. Condylomata International Collaborative Study Group. Randomized placebo-controlled double-blind combined therapy with laser surgery and systemic IFN-α2a in the treatment of anogenital condylomata acuminatum, *J. Infect. Dis.*, 176, 824, 1993.

160. Gross, G., Ikenberg, H., Roussaki, A., Dress, N., and Schopf, E., Systemic treatment of condylomata acuminata with recombinant interferon-alpha-2a: low-dose superior to high-dose regimen, *Chemotherapy*, 32, 537, 1986.

161. Gross, G., Roussaki, A., Schopf, E., deVilliers, E.-M., and Papendick, U., Successful treatment of condyloma acuminata and bowenoid papulosis with subcutaneous injections of low-dosage recombinant interferon-α, *Arch. Dermatol.*, 122, 749, 1986.

162. Gall, S. A., Constantine, L., and Koukol, D., Therapy of persistent human papillomavirus disease with two different interferon species, *Am. J. Obstet. Gynecol.*, 164, 130, 1991.

163. Panici, P. B., Scambia, G., Baiocchi, G., Perrone, L., Pintus, C., and Mancuso, S., Randomized clinical trial comparing systemic IFN with diathermocoagulation in primary multiple and widespread anogenital condyloma, *Obstet. Gynecol.*, 74, 393, 1989.

164. Kirby, P., Wells, D., Kiviat, N., and Corey, L., A phase I trial of intramuscular recombinant human gamma interferon for refractory genital warts, *J. Infect. Dis.*, 86, 485, 1986.

165. Gross, G., Roussaki, A., and Brzoska, J., Low doses of systemically administered recombinant interferon-gamma effective in the treatment of genital warts, *J. Invest. Dermatol.*, 90, 242, 1988.

166. Zouboulis, C., Stadler, R., Ikenberg, H., and Orfanos, C. E., Short-term systemic recombinant interferon-γ treatment is ineffective in recalcitrant condyloma acuminata, *J. Am. Acad. Dermatol.*, 24, 302, 1991.

167. Kirby, P. K., Kiviat, N., Beckman, A., Wells, D., Sherwin, S., and Corey, L., Tolerance and efficacy of recombinant human interferon gamma in the treatment of refractory genital warts, *Am. J. Med.*, 85, 183, 1988.

168. Nel, W. S. and Fourie, E. D., Immunotherapy and 5% topical 5-fluorouracil ointment in the treatment of condylomata acuminata, *S. Afr. Med. J.*, 47, 45, 1973.

169. Haye, K. R., Treatment of condyloma acuminata with 5 per cent 5-fluorouracil (5-FU) cream, *Br. J. Vener. Dis.*, 50, 466, 1974.

170. Dretler, S. P. and Klein, L. A., The eradication of intraurethral condyloma acuminata with 5 per cent 5-fluorouracil cream, *J. Urol.*, 113, 195, 1975.

171. von Krogh, G., The beneficial effect of 1% 5-fluorouracil in 70% ethanol on therapeutically refractory condylomas in the preputial cavity, *Sex. Transm. Dis.*, 5, 137, 1978.

172. Simmons, P. D., Podophyllin 10% and 25% in the treatment of anogenital warts: a comparative double-blind study, *Br. J. Vener. Dis.*, 57, 208, 1981.

173. von Krogh, G., Penile condylomata acuminata: an experimental model for evaluation of topical self-treatment with 0.5%-1.0% ethanolic preparation of podophyllotoxin for three days, *Sex. Transm. Dis.*, 8, 179, 1981.

174. Lassus, A., Haukka, K., and Forsstrom, S., Podophyllotoxin for treatment of genital warts in males: a comparison with conventional podophyllin therapy, *Eur. J. Sex. Transm. Dis.*, 2, 31, 1984.

175. Bashi, S. A., Cryotherapy versus podophyllin in the treatment of genital warts, *Int. J. Dermatol.*, 24, 535, 1985.

176. Jensen, S. L., Comparison of podophyllin application with simple surgical excision in clearance and recurrence of perianal condylomata acuminata, *Lancet*, 2, 1146, 1985.

177. Beutner, K. R., Conant, M. A., Friedman-Kien, A. E., Illeman, M., Artman, N. N., Thisted, R. A., and King, D. H., Patient-applied podofilox for treatment of genital warts, *Lancet*, 1, 831, 1989.

178. Stone, K., Becker, T., Hadgu, A., and Kraus, S., Treatment of external genital warts: a randomized clinical trial comparing podophyllin, cryotherapy, and electrodessication, *Genitourin. Med.*, 66, 16, 1990.

179. von Krogh, G., Condylomata acuminata 1983: an updated review, *Semin. Dermatol.*, 2, 109, 1983.

180. Godley, M. J., Bradbeer, C. S., Gellan, M., and Thin, R. N. T., Cryotherapy compared with trichloro-acetic acid in treating genital warts, *Genitourin. Med.*, 63, 390, 1987.

181. Gabriel, G. and Thin, R. N. T., Treatment of anogenital warts: comparison of trichloroacetic acid and podophyllin versus podophyllin alone, *Br. J. Vener. Dis.*, 59, 124, 1983.

182. Riva, J. M., Sedlacek, T. V., Cunnane, M. F., and Mangan, C. E., Extended carbon dioxide laser vaporization in the treatment of subclinical papillomavirus infection of the lower genital tract, *Obstet. Gynecol.*, 73, 25, 1989.

183. Happonen, H. P., Lassus, A., Santalahti, J., Forsstrom, S., and Lassus, J., Combination of laser-therapy with 0.5% idoxuridine cream in the treatment of therapy-resistant genital warts in male patients: an open study, *Sex. Transm. Dis.*, 17, 127, 1990.

184. Balsdon, M. J., Cryosurgery of genital warts, *Br. J. Vener. Dis.*, 54, 352, 1978.

185. Ghosh, A. K., Cryosurgery of genital warts in cases in which podophyllin treatment failed or was contraindicated, *Br. J. Vener. Dis.*, 53, 49, 1977.

186. Simmons, P. D., Langler, F., and Thin, R. N. T., Cryotherapy versus electrocautery in the treatment of genital warts, *Br. J. Vener. Dis.*, 57, 273, 1981.

187. Willett, G. D., Kurman, R. J., Reid, R., Greenberg, M., Jenson, A. B., and Lörincz, A. T., Correlation of the histologic appearance of intraepithelial neoplasia of the cervix with human papillomavirus types, *Int. J. Gynecol. Pathol.*, 8, 15, 1989.

188. The 1988 Bethesda system for reporting cervical/vaginal cytological diagnosis, *JAMA*, 262, 931, 1989.

189. Wilcynski, S. P., Bergen, S., Walker, J., Liao, S.-Y., and Pearlman, L. F., Human papillomavirus and cervical cancer: analysis of the histopathologic features associated with different viral types, *Hum. Pathol.*, 19, 697, 1988.

190. Barnes, W., Delgado, G., Kurman, R. J., Petrilli, E. S., Smith, D. M., Ahmed, S., Lörincz, A. T., Temple, G. F., Jenson, A. B., and Lancaster, W. D., Possible prognostic significance of human papillomavirus type in cervical cancer, *Gynecol. Oncol.*, 29, 267, 1988.

191. Kurman, R. J., Schiffman, M. H., Lancaster, W. D., Reid, R., Jenson, A. B., Temple, G. F., and Lörincz, A. T., Analysis of individual human papillomavirus types in cervical neoplasia: a possible role for type 18 in rapid progression, *Am. J. Obstet. Gynecol.*, 159, 293, 1988.

192. Schiffman, M. H., Recent progress in defining the epidemiology of human papillomavirus infection and cervical neoplasia, *J. Natl. Cancer Inst.*, 84, 394, 1992.

193. Hartvejt, F., Bertelsen, B., Thunold, S., Maehle, B. O., Skaarland, E., and Christensen, J., Risk of cervical intraepithelial neoplasia in women with glomerulonephritis, *Br. Med. J.*, 302, 375, 1991.

194. Moller, B. R., Jahannesen, P., Osther, K., Ulmsteen, U., Hastrup, J., and Berg, K., Treatment of dysplasia of the cervical epithelium with an interferon gel, *Obstet. Gynecol.*, 62, 625, 1983.

195. Ikic, D., Singer, Z., Beck, M., Soos, E., Sips, D. J., and Jasic, D., Interferon treatment of uterine cervical precancerosis, *J. Cancer Res. Clin. Oncol.*, 101, 303, 1981.

196. Byrne, M. A., Moller, B. R., Taylor-Robinson, D., Harris, J. R. W., Wickenden, C., Malcolm, A. D. B., Anderson, M. C., and Coleman, D. V., The effect of interferon on human papillomaviruses associated with cervical intraepithelial neoplasia, *Br. J. Obstet. Gynaecol.*, 93, 1136, 1986.

197. Yliskoski, M., Cantell, K., Syrjanen, K., and Syrjanen, S., Topical treatment with human leukocyte interferon of HPV 16 infections associated with cervical and vaginal intraepithelial neoplasias, *Gynecol. Oncol.*, 36, 353, 1990.

198. Marcovici, R., Peretz, B. A., and Paldi, E., Human fibroblast interferon therapy in patients with condylomata acuminata, *Isr. J. Med. Sci.*, 19, 104, 1983.

199. Uyeno, K. and Ohtsu, A., Interferon treatment of viral warts and some skin diseases, in *The Clinical Potential of Interferons*, Kono, R. and Vilcek, J., Eds., University of Tokyo Press, Tokyo, 1982.

200. Stefanon, D., Activity of interferon-beta in small condylomatous lesions of the uterine cervix, *Cervix*, 1, 23, 1983.

201. De Palo, G., Stefanon, B., Rilke, E., Pilotti, S., and Ghione, M., Human fibroblast interferon in cervical and vulvar intraepithelial neoplasia associated with papilloma virus infection, *Int. J. Tissue React.*, 6, 523, 1984.

202. Hsu, C., Choo, Y. C., Seto, W. H., Pang, S. W., Tan, C. Y. H., Merigan, T. C., and Ng, M. H., Exfoliative cytology in the evaluation of interferon treatment of cervical intraepithelial neoplasia, *Acta Cytol.*, 28, 111, 1984.

203. Choo, Y. C., Seto, W. H., Hsu, C., Merigan, T. C., Tan, Y. H., Ma, H. K., and Ng, M. H., Cervical intraepithelial neoplasia treated by perilesional injection of interferon, *Br. J. Obstet. Gynaecol.*, 93, 372, 1986.

204. Vasilyev, R. V., Bokhman, J. V., Smorodintsev, A. A., Chepik, O. F., Novik, V. I., Garmanova, N. V., Stepanov, A. M., and Iovlev, V. I., An experience with application of human leucocyte interferon for cervical cancer treatment, *Eur. J. Gynaecol. Oncol.*, 11, 313, 1990.

205. Frost, L., Skajaa, K., Hvidman, L. E., Fay, S. J., and Larsen, P. M., No effect of intralesional injection of interferon on moderate cervical intraepithelial neoplasia, *Br. J. Obstet. Gynaecol.*, 97, 626, 1990.

206. Dunham, A. M., McCartney, J. C., McCance, D. J., and Taylor, R. W., Effect of perilesional injection of alpha-interferon on cervical intraepithelial neoplasia and associated human papillomavirus infection, *J. R. Soc. Med.*, 83, 490, 1990.

207. Iwasaka, T., Hayashi, Y., Yokoyama, M., Hachisuga, T., and Sugimori, H., Interferon-γ treatment for cervical intraepithelial neoplasia, *Gynecol. Oncol.*, 37, 96, 1990.

208. Stellato, G., Intralesional recombinant alpha 2b interferon in the treatment of human papillomavirus-associated cervical intraepithelial neoplasia, *Sex. Transm. Dis.*, 19, 124, 1992.

209. Micheletti, L., Barbero, M., Preti, M., Zanotto-Valentino, M. C., Nicolaci, P., Corbella, L., and Borgno, G., Il beta-interferone intralesionale nel trattamento delle CIN associate ad infezione da HPV, *Minerva Ginecol.*, 44, 329, 1992.

210. Frost, L., Skajaa, K., Hvidman, L. E., and Larsen, P. M., No effect of intralesional injection of interferon on moderate cervical intraepithelial neoplasia, *Br. J. Obstet. Gynaecol.*, 97, 626, 1990.

211. Twiggs, L. B., Okagaki, T., Clark, B., Fukushima, M., Ostrow, R., and Faras, A., A clinical, histo-pathologic, and molecular biologic investigation of vulvar intraepithelial neoplasia, *Int. J. Gynaecol. Pathol.*, 7, 48, 1988.

212. Zachow, K. R., Ostrow, R. S., Bender, M., Okagaki, T., Pass, F., and Faras, T., Detection of human papillomavirus DNA in anogenital neoplasias, *Nature*, 300, 771, 1981.

213. Buscema, J., Naghashfar, Z., Swada, E., Daniel, R., Woodruff, J. D., and Shah, K., The predominance of human papilomavirus type 16 in vulvar neoplasia, *Obstet. Gynecol.*, 71, 601, 1988.

214. Planner, R. S. and Hobbs, J. B., Intraepithelial and invasive neoplasia of the vulva in association with human papillomavirus infection, *J. Reprod. Med.*, 33, 503, 1988.

215. Piepkorn, M., Kumasaka, B., Krieger, J. N., and Burmer, G. C., Development of human papillomavirus-associated Buschke-Löwenstein penile carcinoma during cyclosporine therapy for generalized pustular psoriasis, *J. Am. Acad. Dermatol.*, 29, 321, 1993.

216. Thompson, J. F., Allen, R., Morris, P. J., and Wood, R., Skin cancer in renal transplant patients treated with cyclosporine, *Lancet*, 1, 158, 1985.

217. Bencini, P. L., Montagnino, G., Crosti, C., and Sala, F., Squamous-cell epitheliomata and cyclosporine treatment, *Br. J. Dermatol.*, 113, 373, 1985.

218. Price, M. L., Tidman, M. J., Ogg, C. S., and McDonald, D. M., Skin cancer and cyclosporine therapy, *N. Engl. J. Med.*, 313, 1420, 1985.

219. Chapman, J. R., Taylor, H. M., Thompson, J. F., Wood, R. F., and Morris, P. J., The problems associated with conversion from azathioprine and prednisolone to cyclosporine, *Uremia Invest.*, 9, 19, 1986.

220. McLelland, J., Rees, A., Williams, G., and Chu, T., The incidence of immunosuppression-related skin disease in long-term transplant patients, *Transplantation*, 46, 871, 1988.

221. Abel, E. A., Cutaneous manifestations of immunosuppression in organ transplant recipients, *J. Am. Acad. Dermatol.*, 21, 167, 1989.

222. Couetil, J.-P., McGoldrick, J. P., Wallwork, J., and English, T. A. H., Malignant tumors after heart transplantation, *J. Heart Transplant.*, 9, 622, 1990.

223. Noel, J. C. and de Dobbeleer, G., Development of human papillomavirus-associated Buschke-Löwenstein penile carcinoma during cyclosporine therapy for generalized pustular psoriasis, *J. Am. Acad. Dermatol.*, 31, 299, 1994.

224. Noel, J. C., Vandenbossche M., Peny, M. O., Sassine, A., de Dobbeleer, G., Schulman, C. C., and Verhest, A., Verrucous carcinoma of the penis: importance of human papillomavirus typing for diagnosis and therapeutic decision, *Eur. Urol.*, 22, 83, 1992.

225. Boshart, M. and zur Hausen, H., Human papillomavirus in Buschke- Löwenstein tumors: physical state of the DNA and identification of a tandem duplication in the noncoding region of a human papillomavirus 6 subtype, *J. Virol.*, 58, 963, 1986.

226. Dihn, T. V., Powell, L. G., Hannigan, E. V., Yang, H. L., Wirt, D. P., and Yandel, R. B., Simultaneously occurring condylomata acuminatum carcinoma in situ and verrucous carcinoma of the vulva and carcinoma in situ of the cervix in a young woman, *J. Reprod. Med.*, 33, 510, 1988.

227. Kurman, R. J., Norris, H. J., and Wilkinson, E., Verrucous carcinoma, in *Tumors of the Cervix, Vagina and Vulva (Atlas of Tumor Pathology; 3rd Series, Fascicle 4)*, Armed Forces Institute of Pathology, Washington, D.C., 1992, 200.

228. Millard, L. G. and Barker, D. J., Development of squamous cell carcinoma in chronic discoid lupus erythematosus, *Clin. Exp. Dermatol.*, 3, 161, 1978.

229. Caruso, W. P., Stewart, M. L., Nanda, V. K., and Quismorio, F. P., Squamous cell carcinoma of the skin in black patients with discoid lupus erythematosus, *J. Rheumatol.*, 14, 156, 1987.

230. Gupta, A. K., Cardella, C. J., and Haberman, H. F., Cutaneous malignant neoplasms in patients with renal transplants, *Arch. Dermatol.*, 122, 1288, 1986.

231. Liddington, M., Richardson, A. J., Higgins, R. M., Endre, Z. H., Murie, J. A., and Morris, P. J., Skin cancer in renal transplant recipients, *Br. J. Surg.*, 76, 1002, 1989.

232. Cohen, L. M., Tyring, S. K., Rady, P., and Callen, J. P., Human papillomavirus type 11 in multiple squamous cell carcinomas in a patient with subacute lupus erythematosus, *J. Am. Acad. Dermatol.*, 26, 840, 1992.

233. Parkin, D. M., Stjernward, J., and Muir, C. S., Estimates of the worldwide frequency of twelve major cancers, *Bull. WHO*, 62, 163, 1984.

234. Vermund, S. H., Kelley, K. F., Klein, R. S., Feingold, A. R., Schreiber, K., Munk, G., and Burk, R. D., High risk of human papillomavirus infection and cervical squamous intraepithelial lesions among women with symptomatic human immunodeficiency virus infection, *Am. J. Obstet. Gynecol.*, 165, 392, 1991.

235. Byrne, M. A., Taylor-Robinson, D., Munday, P. E., and Harris, J. R. W., The common occurrence of human papillomavirus infection and intraepithelial neoplasia in women infected by HIV, *AIDS*, 3, 379, 1989.

236. Caubel, P., Foulques, H., Blondon, J., and LeFranc, J. P., Lesions cervico-vaginales et vulvaires a papillomavirus: epidemiologie chez les femmes seropositives pour le HIV. Etude preliminaire sur une serie continue, *Presse Med.*, 18, 1239, 1989.

237. Feingold, A. R., Vermund, S. H., Burk, R. D., Keley, K. F., Schrager, L. K., Schreiber, K., Munk, G., Friedland, G. H., and Klein, R. S., Cervical cytologic abnormalities and papillomavirus in women infected with human immunodeficiency virus, *J. Acquir. Immune Defic. Syndr.*, 3, 896, 1990.

238. Schafer, A., Wolfgang, F., Mielke, M., Schwartlander, B., and Koch, M. A., Increased frequency of cervical dysplasia/neoplasia in HIV-infected women is related to the extent of immunosuppression, in *Proc. VIth Int. Conf. AIDS*, San Francisco, 1990, 215 (Abstr. 519).

239. Kreiss, J., Kiviat, N., Plummer, F., Ngugi, E., Waiaki, P., and Holmes, K., HIV, human papillomavirus, and cervical dysplasia in Nairobi prostitutes, in *Proc. Vth Int. Conf. AIDS*, Montreal, 1989, 1, 230 (Abstr. 53).

240. Hiller, K. F., Baur, S., Lutz, R., Stauber, M., and Jacobs, U., Human papilloma virus infection and cervical intraepithelial neoplasia (CIN) in HIV-infected female patients, in *Proc. VIth Int. Conf. AIDS*, San Francisco, 1990, 380 (Abstr. 2104).

241. Ostrow, R. S., Bender, M., Niimura, M., Seki, T., Kawashima, M., Pass, F., and Faras, A. J., Human papillomavirus DNA in cutaneous primary and metastasized squamous cell carcinomas from patients with epidermodysplasia verruciformis, *Proc. Natl. Acad. Sci. U.S.A.*, 79, 1634, 1982.

242. Blessing, K., McLaren, K. M., Morris, R., Barr, B. B. B., Benton, E. C., Alloub, M., Bunney, M. H., Smith, I. W., Smart, G. E., and Bird, C. C., Detection of human papillomavirus in skin and genital lesions of renal allograft recipients by in situ hybridization, *Histopathology*, 16, 181, 1990.

243. Lutzner, M. A., Croissant, O., Ducasse, M.-F., Kreis, H., Crosnier, J., and Orth, G., A potentially oncogenic human papillomavirus (HPV-5) found in two renal allograft recipients, *J. Invest. Dermatol.*, 75, 353, 1980.

244. Van den Brule, A. J., Walboomers, J. M. M., du Maine, M., Kenemans, P., and Meijer, C. J. L. M., Difference in prevalence of human papillomavirus genotypes in cytomorphologically normal cervical intraepithelial neoplasia, *Int. J. Cancer*, 48, 404, 1991.

245. Riou, G., Favre, M., Jeannel, D., Bourhis, J., Le Doussal, V., and Orth, G., Association between poor prognosis in early-stage invasive cervical carcinomas and non-detection of HPV DNA, *Lancet*, 335, 1171, 1990.
246. Lorincz, A. T., Reid, R., Jenson, A. B., Greenberg, M. D., Lancaster, W., and Kurman, R. J., Human papillomavirus infection of the cervix: relative risk association of 15 common anogenital types, *Obstet. Gynecol.*, 79, 328, 1992.
247. Higgins, G. D., Davy, M., Roder, D., Uzelin, D. M., Phillips, G. E., and Burrell, C. J., Increased age and mortality associated with cervical carcinomas negative for human papillomavirus RNA, *Lancet*, 338, 910, 1991.
248. Boshart, M., Gissmann, L., Ikenberg, H., Kleinheinz, A., Scheurlen, W., and zur Hausen, H., A new type of papillomavirus DNA, its presence in genital cancer biopsies and in cell lines derived from cervical cancer, *EMBO J.*, 3, 1151, 1984.
249. Dürst, M., Gissmann, L., Ikenberg, H., and zur Hansen, H., A papillomavirus DNA from a cervical carcinoma and its prevalence in cancer biopsy samples from different geographic regions, *Proc. Natl. Acad. Sci. U.S.A.*, 80, 3812, 1983.
250. Vardy, D. A., Baadsgaard, O., Hansen, E. R., Lisby, S., and Vejlsgaart, G. L., The cellular immune response to human papillomavirus infection, *Int. J. Dermatol.*, 29, 603, 1990.
251. Pfister, H., Human papillomaviruses and impaired immunity vs. epidermodysplasia verruciformis, *Arch. Dermatol.*, 123, 1469, 1987.
252. Matlashewski, G., Schneider, J., Banks, L., Jones, N., Murray, A., and Crawford, L. V., Human papillomavirus type 16 DNA cooperates with activated *ras* in transforming primary cells, *EMBO J.*, 6, 1741, 1987.
253. Crook, T., Storey, A., Almond, N., Osborn, K., and Crawford, L., Human papillomavirus type 16 cooperates with activated *ras* and *fos* oncogenes in the hormone-dependent transformation of primary mouse cells, *Proc. Natl. Acad. Sci. U.S.A.*, 85, 8820, 1988.
254. DiPaolo, J. A., Woodworth, C. D., Popescu, N. C., Notario, V., and Doniger, J., Induction of human cervical squamous cell carcinoma by sequential transfection with human papillomavirus 16 DNA and viral Harvey *ras*, *Oncogene*, 4, 395, 1989.
255. Daling, J. R., Weiss, N. S., Klopfenstein, L. L., Cochran, L. E., Chow, W. H., and Daifuku, R., Correlates of homosexual behavior and the incidence of anal cancer, *JAMA*, 247, 1988, 1982.
256. Gal, A. A., Meyer, P. R., and Taylor, C. R., Papillomavirus antigens in anorectal condyloma and carcinoma in homosexual men, *JAMA*, 257, 337, 1987.
257. Hill, S. A. and Coghill, S. B., Human papillomavirus in sqamous carcinoma of anus, *Lancet*, 2, 1333, 1986.
258. Croxson, T., Chabon, A. B., Rorat, E., and Barash, I. M., Intraepithelial carcinoma of the anus in homosexual men, *Dis. Colon Rectum*, 27, 325, 1984.
259. Howard, L. C., Paterson-Brown, S., Weber, J. N., Chan, S. T. F., Harris, J. R. W., and Glazer, G., Squamous carcinoma of the anus in young homosexual men with T helper cell depletion, *Genitourin. Med.*, 62, 393, 1986.
260. Frazer, I. H., Crapper, R. M., Medley, G., Brown, T. C., and Mackay, I. R., Association between anorectal dysplasia, human papillomavirus, and human immunodeficiency virus infection in homosexual men, *Lancet*, 2, 657, 1986.
261. Milburn, P. B., Brandsma, J. L., Goldsman, C. I., Teplitz, E. D., and Heilman, E. I., Disseminated warts and evolving squamous cell carcinoma in a patient with acquired immunodeficiency syndrome, *J. Am. Acad. Dermatol.*, 19, 401, 1988.
262. Schneider, A., Sawada, E., Gissmann, L., and Shah, K., Human papillomaviruses in women with a history of abnormal Papanicolaou smears and in their male partners, *Obstet. Gynecol.*, 69, 554, 1987.
263. Daling, J. R., Sherman, K. J., Hislop, T. G., Maden, C., Mandelson, M. T., Beckman, A. M., and Weiss, N. S., Cigarette smoking and the risk of anogenital cancer, *Am. J. Epidemiol.*, 135, 180, 1992.
264. Maden, C., Sherman, K. J., Beckman, A. M., Hislop, T. G., Teh, C. Z., Ashley, R. L., and Daling, J. R., History of circumcision, medical conditions, and sexual activity and risk of penile cancer, *J. Natl. Cancer Inst.*, 85, 19, 1993.
265. Crook, T., Wrede, D., Tidy, J., Sholefield, J., Crawford, L., and Vousden, K. H., Status of c-*ras*, p53, and retinoblastoma genes in human papillomavirus positive and negative squamous cell carcinomas in the anus, *Oncogene*, 6, 1251, 1991.

266. Pfister, H., Relationship of papillomaviruses to anogenital cancer, *Obstet. Gynecol. Clin. North Am.*, 14, 349, 1987.
267. Howley, P. M., On human papillomaviruses, *N. Engl. J. Med.*, 315, 1089, 1986.
268. Rudlinger, R., Grob, R., Buchmann, P., Christen, D., and Steiner, R., Anogenital warts of the condyloma acuminatum type in HIV-positive patients, *Dermatologica*, 176, 277, 1988.
269. Morison, W. L., Viral warts, herpes simplex and herpes zoster in patients with secondary immune deficiencies and neoplasms, *Br. J. Dermatol.*, 92, 625, 1975.
270. Halpert, R., Fruchter, R. G., Sedlis, A., Butt, K., Boyce, J. G., and Sillman, F. H., Human papillomavirus and lower genital neoplasia in renal transplant recipients, *Obstet. Gynecol.*, 68, 251, 1986.
271. Sillman, F., Stanek, A., Sedlis, A., Rosenthal, J., Lanks, K. W., Buchhagen, D., Nicastri, A., and Boyce, J., The relationship between human papillomavirus and lower genital intraepithelial neoplasia in immunosuppressed women, *Am. J. Obstet. Gynecol.*, 150, 300, 1984.
272. Porrero, R., Penn, I., Droegmueller, W., Greer, B., and Makowski, E., Gynecologic malignancies in immunosuppressed organ homograft recipients, *Obstet. Gynecol.*, 45, 359, 1975.
273. Penn, I., Malignancies associated with immunosuppressive or cytotoxic therapy, *Surgery*, 83, 492, 1978.
274. Sillman, F. H., Boyce, J. G., Macasaet, M. A., and Nicastri, A. D., 5-Fluorouracil/chemosurgery for intraepithelial neoplasia of the lower genital tract, *Obstet. Gynecol.*, 58, 356, 1981.
275. Seski, J. C., Reinhalter, E. R., and Silva, J., Jr., Abnormalities of lymphocyte transformation in women with condylomata acuminata, *Obstet. Gynecol.*, 51, 188, 1978.
276. Sillman, F., Stanek, A., Sedlis, A., Rosenthal, J., Lanks, K. W., Buchhagen, D., Nicastri, A., and Boyce, J., The relationship between human papillomavirus and lower genital intraepithelial neoplasia in immunosuppressive women, *Am. J. Obstet. Gynecol.*, 150, 300, 1984.
277. Carson, L. F., Twiggs, L. B., Fukushima, M., Ostrow, R. S., Faras, A. J., and Okagaki, T., Human genital papilloma infections: an evaluation of immunologic competence in the genital neoplasia-papilloma syndrome, *Am. J. Obstet. Gynecol.*, 155, 784, 1986.
278. Schneider, V., Kay, S., and Lee, H. M., Immunosuppression as a high-risk factor in the development of condyloma acuminatum and squamous neoplasia of the cervix, *Acta Cytol.*, 27, 220, 1983.
279. Laga, M., Icenogle, J. P., Marsella, R., Manoka, A. T., Nzila, N., Ryder, R. W., Vermund, S. H., Heyward, W. L., Nelson, A., and Reeves, W. C., Genital papillomavirus infection and cervical dysplasia: opportunistic complications of HIV infection, *Int. J. Cancer*, 50, 45, 1992.
280. Vernon, S. D., Reeves, W. C., Clancy, K. A., Laga, M., St. Louis, M., Gary, H. E., Jr., Ryder, R. W., Manoka, A. T., and Icenogle, J. P., A longitudinal study of human papillomavirus DNA detection in HIV-1 seropositive and seronegative women, *J. Infect. Dis.*, 169, 1108, 1994.
281. American Foundation For AIDS Research, *AIDS/HIV Treatment Directory*, 4(4), 91, 1995.
282. Judson, F. N., Interaction between human papillomavirus and human immunodeficiency virus infections, in *The Epidemiology of Human Papillomavirus and Cervical Cancer*, Munoz, N., Bosch, F. X., Shah, K. V., and Meheus, A., Eds., International Agency of Cancer, Lyon, 1992, 199.
283. Klein, R. S., Adachi, A., Fleming, I., Ho, G. Y. F., and Burk, R., A prospective study of genital neoplasia and human papillomavirus (HPV) in HIV-infected women, *Proc. VIIIth Int. Conf. AIDS*, Amsterdam, 1992, Abstr. Tub0527.
284. Vernon, S. D., Zaki, S. R., and Reeves, W. C., Localization of HIV-1 to human papillomavirus associated cervical lesions, *Lancet*, 344, 54, 1994.
285. Regcvik, N., Sen, P., Raska, K., Jr., Raskova, J., Middleton, J., Nilsson, S., Jiminez, G., and Jensson, A. B., Cervical human papillomavirus (HPV) in correlation with immune status and Pappanicolaou smear abnormalities, *Proc. VIIIth Int. Conf. AIDS*, Amsterdam, 1992, Abstr. Tub0528.
286. Maiman, M., Fruchter, R. G., Guy, L., Cuthill, S., Levine, P., and Serur, E., Human immunodeficiency virus infection and invasive cervical carcinoma, *Cancer*, 71, 402, 1993.
287. Maiman, M., Fruchter, R. G., Serur, E., Levine, P. A., Arrastia, C. D., and Sedlis, A., Recurrent cervical intraepithelial neoplasia in human immunodeficiency virus-seropositive women, *Obstet. Gynecol.*, 82, 170, 1993.
288. Mandelblatt, J. S., Fahs, M., Garibaldi, K., Senie, R. T., and Peterson, H. B., Association between HIV infection and cervical neoplasia: implications for clinical care of women at risk for both conditions, *AIDS*, 6, 173, 1992.

289. Palefsky, J. M., Gonzales, J., Greenbelt, R. M., Ahn, D. K., and Hollander, H., Anal intraepithelial neoplasia and anal papillomavirus infection among homosexual males with group IV HIV disease, *JAMA*, 263, 2911, 1990.

290. Caussy, D., Goedert, J. J., Palefsky, J., Gonzales, J., Rabkin, C. S., DiGiola, R. A., Sanchez, W. C., Grossman, R. J., Colclough, G., Wiktor, S. Z., and Blattner, W. A., Infection of human immunodeficiency and papilloma viruses: association with anal epithelial abnormality in homosexual men, *Int. J. Cancer*, 46, 214, 1990.

291. Vernon, S. D., Zaki, S. R., and Reeves, W. C., Localization of HIV-1 to human papillomavirus associated cervical lesions, *Lancet*, 344, 954, 1994.

292. Vernon, S. D., Hart, C. E., Reeves, W. C., and Icenogle, J. P., The HIV-1 *tat* protein enhances E2-dependent human papillomavirus 16 transcription, *Virus Res.*, 27, 133, 1993.

293. Sridama, V., Pacini, F., Yang, S.-L., Moawad, A., Reilly, M., and DeGroot, L. J., Decreased levels of helper T cells a possible of immunodeficiency in pregnancy, *N. Engl. J. Med.*, 307, 352, 1982.

294. Schneider, A., Hotz, M., and Gissmann, L., Increased prevalence of human papillomaviruses in the lower genital tract of pregnant women, *Int. J. Cancer*, 40, 198, 1987.

295. Rando, R. F., Lindeim, S., Hasty, L., Sedlacek, T. V., Woodland, M., and Eder, C., Increased frequency of detection of human papillomavirus deoxyribonucleic acid in exfoliated cervical cells during pregnancy, *Am. J. Obstet. Gynecol.*, 161, 50, 1989.

296. Stephens, J. D., Golbus, M. S., Miller, T. R., Wiber, R. R., and Epstein, C. J., Multiple congenital anomalies in a fetus exposed to 5-fluorouracil during the first trimester, *Am. J. Obstet. Gynecol.*, 137, 747, 1980.

297. Stadler, H. E. and Knowles, J., Fluorouracil in pregnancy: effect on the neonate, *JAMA*, 217, 214, 1971.

298. Odom, L. D., Plouffe, L., Jr., and Butler, W. J., 5-Fluorouracil exposure during the period of conception: report on two cases, *Am. J. Obstet. Gynecol.*, 163, 76, 1990.

299. Otaño, L., Amestoy, G., Paz, J., and Gadow, E. C., Periconceptional exposure to topical 5-fluorouracil, *Am. J. Obstet. Gynecol.*, 166, 263, 1992.

300. Davis, A. J. and Emans, S. J., Human papilloma virus infection in the pediatric and adolescent patient, *J. Pediatr.*, 115, 1, 1989.

301. Sedlacek, T. V., Lindheim, S., Eder, C., Hasty, L., Woodland, M., Ludomirsky, A., and Rando, R. F., Mechanism for human papillomavirus transmission at birth, *Am. J. Obstet. Gynecol.*, 161, 55, 1989.

302. Steinberg, B. M., Topp, W., Schneider, P. S., and Abramson, A. L., Laryngeal papillomavirus infection during clinical remission, *N. Engl. J. Med.*, 308, 1261, 1983.

303. Abramson, A. L., Steinberg, B. M., and Winkler, B., Laryngeal papillomatosis: clinical, histopathologic and molecular studies, *Laryngoscope*, 97, 678, 1987.

304. Steinberg, B. M. and Abramson, A. L., Laryngeal papillomas, *Clin. Dermatol.*, 3, 130, 1985.

305. Weiss, M. D. and Kashima, H. K., Tracheal involvement in laryngeal papillomatosis, *Laryngoscope*, 93, 45, 1983.

306. Kashima, H., Leventhal, B., Clark, K., Cohen, S., Dedo, H., Donovan, D., Fearon, B., Gardiner, L., Goepfert, H., Lusk, R., McCabe, B. F., Mounts, P., Muntz, H., Richardson, M., Singleton, G., Weck, P., Whisnant, J., Wold, D., and Yonkers, A., Interferon alfa-n1 in juvenile onset recurrent respiratory papillomatosis: results of a randomized study in twelve collaborative institutions, *Laryngoscope*, 98, 334, 1988.

307. Mullooly, V. M., Abramson, A. L., Steinberg, B. M., and Horowitz, M., Clinical effects of alpha-interferon dose variation on laryngeal papillomas, *Laryngoscope*, 98, 1324, 1988.

308. Healy, G. B., Gelber, R. D., Trowbridge, A. L., Grundfast, K. M., Ruben, R. J., and Price, K. N., Treatment of recurrent respiratory papillomatosis with human leukocyte interferon, *N. Engl. J. Med.*, 319, 401, 1988.

309. Haglund, S., Lundqvist, P.-G., Cantell, K., and Strander, H., Interferon therapy in juvenile laryngeal papillomatosis, *Arch. Otolaryngol.*, 107, 327, 1981.

310. Goepfert, H., Sessions, R. B., Gutterman, J., Cangir, A., Dichtel, W. J., and Sulek, M., Leukocyte interferon in patients with juvenile laryngeal papillomas, *Ann. Otol. Rhinol. Laryngol.*, 91, 431, 1982.

311. McCabe, B. F. and Clark, K. F., Interferon and laryngeal papillomatosis: the Iowa experience, *Ann. Otol. Rhinol. Laryngol.*, 92, 2, 1983.

312. Göbel, U., Arnold, W., Wahn, V., Treuner, J., Jürgens, H., and Cantell, K., Comparison of human fibroblast and leukocyte interferon in the treatment of severe laryngeal papillomatosis in children, *Eur. J. Pediatr.*, 137, 175, 1981.

313. Ogura, H., Watanabe, S., Fukushima, K., Baba, Y., Masuda, Y., Fujiwara, T., and Yabe, Y., Persistence of human pappilomavirus type 6e in adult multiple laryngeal pappiloma and the counterpart false corde of an interferon-treated patient, *Jpn. J. Clin. Oncol.*, 23, 130, 1993.

314. Dahlman, A., Wile, A. G., Burns, R. G., Mason, G. R., Johnson, F. M., and Berns, M. N., Laser photoradiation therapy of cancer, *Cancer Res.*, 43, 430, 1983.

315. Jesionek, A. and Tappeiner, V. H., Zur behandlung der hautcarcinomemet fluorescendent stoffen, *MMW*, 47, 2042, 1903.

316. Henderson, R. W., Christie, G. S., Clezy, P. S., and Lineman, J., Hematoporphyrin diacetate: a probe to distinguish malignant from normal tissue by selective fluorescence, *Br. J. Exp. Pathol.*, 61, 345, 1980.

317. Abramson, A. L., Waner, M., and Brandsma, J., The clinical treatment of laryngeal papillomas with hematoporphyrin therapy, *Arch. Otolaryngol. Head Neck Surg.*, 114, 795, 1988.

318. Kavaru, M. S., Mehta, A. C., and Eliachar, I., Effect of photodynamic therapy and external beam radiation therapy on juvenile laryngotracheobronchial papillomatosis, *Am. Rev. Respir. Dis.*, 141, 509, 1990.

319. Abramson, A. L., Shikowitz, M. J., Mullooly, V. M., Steinberg, B. M., Amella, C. A., and Rothstein, H. R., Clinical effects of photodynamic therapy on recurrent laryngeal papillomas, *Arch. Otolaryngol. Head Neck Surg.*, 118, 25, 1992.

320. Dougherty, T. J., Photoradiation therapy for cutaneous and subcutaneous malignancies, *J. Invest. Dermatol.*, 77, 122, 1981.

321. Dougherty, T. J., Photodynamic therapy: new approaches, *Semin. Surg. Oncol.*, 5, 6, 1989.

322. Shikowitz, M. J., Steinberg, B. M., and Abramson, A. L., Hematoporphyrin derivative therapy of papillomas, *Arch. Otolaryngol. Head Neck Surg.*, 112, 42, 1986.

323. Shikowitz, M. J., Galli, R., Bandyopadhyay, D., and Hoory, S., Biodistribution of indium 111-labeled dihematoporphyrin ether in papillomas and body tissues, *Arch. Otolaryngol. Head Neck Surg.*, 115, 845, 1989.

324. Abramson, A. L., Barrezueta, N. X., and Shikowitz, M. J., Thermal effects of photodynamic therapy on the larynx, *Arch. Otolaryngol. Head Neck Surg.*, 113, 854, 1987.

325. Shikowitz, M. J., Comparison of pulsed and continuous wave light in photodynamic therapy of papillomas: an experimental study, *Laryngoscope*, 102, 300, 1992.

326. McGlennen, R. C., Adams, G. L., Lewis, C. M., Faras, A. J., and Ostrow, R. S., Pilot trial of ribavirin for the treatment of laryngeal papillomatosis, *Head Neck*, 15, 504, 1993.

327. Ostrow, R. S., Forslund, K. M., McGlennen, R. C., Shaw, D. P., Schlievert, P. M., Ussery, M. A., Higgins, J. W., and Faras, A. J., Ribavirin mitigates wart growth in rabbits at early stages of infection with cottontail rabbit papillomavirus, *Antiviral Res.*, 17, 99, 1992.

328. McKay, M., Frankman, O., Horowitz, B. J., Lecart, C., Micheletti, L., Ridley, C. M., Chanco Turner, C. M., and Woodruff, J. D., Vulvar vestibulitis and vestibular papillomatosis: report of the ISSVD Committee on Vulvodynia, *J. Reprod. Med.*, 36, 413, 1991.

329. Friedrich, E. G., Vulvar vestibulitis syndrome, *J. Reprod. Surg.*, 32, 110, 1987.

330. Turner, M. L. and Marinoff, S. C., Association of human papillomavirus with vulvodynia and the vulvar vestibulitis syndrome, *J. Reprod. Med.*, 33, 533, 1988.

331. Boden, E., Rylander, E., Evander, M., Wadel, G., and von Schoultz, B., Papilloma virus infection of the vulva, *Acta Obstet. Gynaecol. Scand.*, 68, 179, 1989.

332. Umpierre, S. A., Kaufman, R. H., Adam, E., Woods, K. V., and Adler-Storthz, K., Human papillomavirus DNA in tissue biopsy of vulvar vestibulitis patients treated with interferon, *Obstet. Gynecol.*, 78, 693, 1991.

333. Pyka, R. E., Wilkinson, E. J., Friedrich, E. G., Jr., and Croker, B. P., The histopathology of vulvar vestibulitis syndrome, *Int. J. Gynecol. Pathol.*, 7, 249, 1988.

334. Marinoff, S. C., Turner, M. L., Hirsch, R. P., and Richard, G., Intralesional alpha interferon. Cost-effective therapy for vulvar vestibulitis syndrome, *J. Reprod. Med.*, 38, 19, 1993.

335. Woodruff, J. D. and Parmley, T. H., Infection of the major vestibular gland, *Obstet. Gynecol.*, 62, 609, 1983.

336. Davis, G. D., The management of vulvar vestibulitis syndrome with the carbon dioxide laser, *J. Gynecol. Surg.*, 5, 87, 1989.

337. Birley, H. D., Luzzi, G. A., Walker, M. M., Ryait, B., Taylor-Robinson, D., and Renton, H., The association of human papillomavirus infection with balanoposthitis: a description of five cases with proposals for treatment, *Int. J. STD AIDS*, 5, 139, 1994.

2.2 POLYOMAVIRUSES

Polyomavirus infections in humans have been recognized recently.[1] One major event related to polyomavirus human disease has been the exposure of millions of people to simian virus 40 (SV40), an oncogenic polyomavirus of Asian macaques, as a result of immunization in the U.S. with poliovirus vaccines unintentionally prepared in SV40-contaminated monkey kidney culture.[2,3]

The polyomaviruses are ubiquitous in nature and have been isolated from humans and a wide variety of mammals (monkeys, cattle, rabbits, mice, hamsters, rats), and parakeets. By and large, the polyomaviruses are species-specific and have been known to infect either only one species or a few closely related species.

In addition to SV40, two other viruses, the JC virus and the BK virus, have been associated with human disease. The JC virus has been identified as the etiologic agent of progressive multifocal leukoencephalopathy and was isolated from infected brain tissue. The BK virus has been cultivated from the urine of a renal transplant recipient.[4,5] In addition, the BK virus has been associated with human brain and pancreatic tumors,[6,7] as well as hemorragic cystitis, urethral stenosis, and some of the urinary tract illnesses.[1]

There has been indirect evidence for human infection with another polyomavirus when antibodies that reacted with a lymphotropic polyomavirus of African green monkeys were identified in human sera.[8,9] However, the lymphotropic polyomavirus has not yet been isolated from humans.[1]

2.2.1 PROGRESSIVE MULTIFOCAL LEUKOENCEPHALOPATHY (JC VIRUS INFECTION)

2.2.1.1 Introduction

Progressive multifocal leukoencephalopathy (PML) has been the first human disease associated with polyomavirus. It is a rare, fatal disorder of the central nervous system which occurs in patients with immune deficiencies, and was first related to a viral infection by Richardson.[10] The key pathogenic event of PML is the infection of oligodendrocytes in the brain by the JC virus.

In the vast majority of cases of PML, the JC virus (JCV) is the etiologic agent. Simian virus 40 (SV40), a polyomavirus closely associated with JCV, has also been implicated in several cases of PML.[11] In several studies,[12,13] varicella-zoster virus was determined to be the causative agent of multifocal leukoencephalopathy.

PML is a demyelinating disease affecting the brain of patients with impaired cell-mediated immunity and decreased immune competence,[11-19] such as AIDS patients[15,20-25] and allograft recipients with severely suppressed cellular immunity.[26] Over the last several decades, an association of PML with an underlying disease of the reticuloendothelial system (leukemia, lymphoma, and sarcoidosis) has been observed.[27-30] On rare occasions, PML can affect individuals without underlying disease or compromised immune state.[31]

First described in 1958,[27] PML is manifested with mental aberration, blindness, aphasias, hemiparesis, ataxia, glial reaction, and other focal deficits which slowly progress until death. Even though partial recovery and prolonged survival have been documented,[32,33] PML is almost invariably relentlessly progressive with a life expectancy between 3 and 18 months.[24,28]

Exposure to JCV usually occurs early in life and results in the persistence of an archtypic virus in a large percentage of the human population.[34,35] The prevalence of antibody to the virus is 76% of individuals by late adult life.[36] However, primary infection with JC virus does not usually result in disease in an immunocompetent host. Most likely the virus will establish a benign latent infection.[37] Reactivation of the latent virus, especially in immunosuppressed patients, can lead to infection and cytolytic destruction of the myelin-producing oligodendrocytes of the CNS, resulting in severe demyelination.[14] Demyelination is usually found in the white matter[38] but, although rarely, it can also be seen in the brain stem and cerebellum. One unusual feature of PML is the absence of inflammation and the presence of astrocyte cells and enlarged oligodendrocytes containing intranuclear inclusions surrounding the areas of demyelination.[39] Viral isolates from infected brain tissues,[40] such as the prototypic JC viral strain MAD-1,[41] exhibit marked specificity for glial cells.[42,43] The tissue tropism of JCV is determined at transcription level and is conferred by the hypervariable noncoding region which controls DNA replication[44,45] and promotes both the early regulatory and late capsid genes.[42]

2.2.1.2 Host Factors in the Development of Progressive Multifocal Leukoencephalopathy

In general, an overwhelming majority of patients with PML will have some degree of underlying cellular immunodeficiency.[14] Initially, Hodgkin's disease and chronic lymphocytic leukemia were the underlying conditions most frequently associated with PML.[15,46] Other disorders included autoimmune diseases, granulomatous processes, myeloproliferative disorders, soft tissue malignancies, and immunosuppression acquired during organ transplantation or secondary to chemotherapy.[14] With the spread of the AIDS epidemic, the incidence of PML increased dramatically, with 55% to 85% of all recent cases of PML having the profound immune suppression associated with AIDS as the underlying pathology leading to reactivation of the JC virus.[23,47,48] In addition, there has been evidence of a possible direct interaction between HIV-1 and JCV proteins.[49,50]

In a study of seven patients with PML, Willoughby et al.[51] found that in vitro lymphocyte proliferation in response to mitogen stimulation has been less sensitive. The production of leukocyte migration factor from lymphocytes in response to JCV antigens has been used to measure the cellular immunity directed specifically against JCV. Usually, the production of this factor was normal in non-PML patients. However, in PML patients with cellular immunodeficiencies this factor was absent, suggesting that in such patients, in addition to the general immunodeficiency, there was a selective deficiency in the cellular immune response to JCV antigens. Other studies have also indicated that loss of immunocompetence would likely predispose patients to reactivation of a latent JCV infection.[52] Attempts to identify brain cells as the cell type harboring latent JCV failed to produce convincing evidence.[53-56] Apparently, the virus remained latent outside the CNS and during reactivation gained passage into the nervous system sometime during the immunosuppression. Since JCV latency is most likely established during primary infection, identifying the sites of viral persistence would provide the minimum number of cell types affected by the primary infection.[14] To this end, Grinnell et al.[57] have found JCV DNA in the lung, liver, lymph node, and spleen cells in non-PML-affected patients, some of whom were children with combined immunodeficiency syndromes; however, none of the organs studied expressed viral antigens that would have indicated a productive phase of infection. Greenlee and Keeney[58] also failed to observe expression of viral antigens by extraneural tissues of patients with PML. All of these findings unequivocally suggested the presence of widespread dissemination of JCV in cases of severe immunodeficiency.

There is evidence indicating JCV latent infection of two extraneural sites, the kidney and the B lymphocytes. The virus has been isolated from urine of immunosuppressed patients with and without PML,[59,60] and viral DNA has been detected in kidney cells by in situ hybridization.[14] Houff et al.[59] have found that B cells from the spleen and bone marrow of patients with PML were capable of expressing JCV antigens. Further experiments have revealed that JCV-infected B cells were present in a perivascular location and in the Virchow-Robins space of the brain parenchyma of

PML patients.[60] It is evident from these results that JCV infects B cells, which then may remain latent in the marrow.

Since the long-lived B lymphocyte memory cells provide a stable cell type for maintenence of JCV latency, studying the biology of their growth and development[61-63] may provide insights into the mechanism of JCV latency and reactivation. For their growth and development, which is controlled by immunoregulatory T lymphocytes, the B cells will require synthesis of nuclear transcription factors not present in resting memory cells.[14] Even though T cell immune deficiency (such as in AIDS) may seriously damage the immunoregulatory functions of T lymphocytes, B cells can still become activated, leading to synthesis of nuclear transcription factors and to their growth and differentiation.[60] The JC virus which has remained latent because of the absence of the required transcription factors could be reactivated as an unintended consequence of B lymphocyte activation.[14]

Wegner et al.[64] presented evidence that the glial transcription factor Tst-1, a member of the POU-domain family, stimulated transcription of both early and late viral genes. This stimulation was dependent on site-specific binding of Tst-1 to the JC viral regulatory region, and on the presence of an intact amino-terminal transactivation domain within the Tst-1. Because of its ability to increase the expression of viral large tumor antigen, Tst-1 stimulated the viral DNA replication without participating directly in the replication event, and might thus be one of the factors which determines the specificity of JCV for the myelin-producing oligodendrocytes.[64]

Following the loss of an integrated cellular immunity in cases of cellular immunodeficiency, the B cell population may polyclonally expand as evidenced in HIV infections when the CD4+ counts decrease. The activated B cells, now in the active phase of viral application and transcription, will cross the blood-brain barrier and invade the CNS. The JC virus can enter the brain in activated B cells.[59] Furthermore, JCV-infected B cells may gain access to glial cells since activated lymphocytes will not require antigen-specific recognition to cross the blood-brain barrier.[61,63] This hematogenous spread to the CNS is supported by the multifocal nature of the demyelinating lesions as well as their location near the gray-white junction where the end arterioles of the cerebrospinal tree are found.[14] Although the macrophages are the primary cellular immune response to JCV neuroglial infection, the mechanism of their recruitment into demyelinating lesions is still unknown.

Results from JCV-specific cellular immune studies in a small number of patients have shown that T cell cytotoxicity is still being displayed in spite of the presence of immunodeficiency. However, the failure of cytotoxic T lymphocytes to clear the JCV infection may be associated with the inability of JCV-infected glial cells to express viral antigens with the major histocompatibility complex class I and II antigens. While these antigens are not constitutively expressed in the CNS, they can be induced by viral infection.[14]

2.2.1.3   Evolution of Therapies and Treatment of Progressive Multifocal Leukoencephalopathy

Prior to the AIDS epidemic, cases of PML were relatively rare. However, with the growth of the HIV-infected population,[24] the need for effective therapies against PML has become evident. So far, treatments for PML, either directed specifically at JCV, or to bolster the cellular immunity of patients, have not been satisfactory. Furthermore, even with the increased incidence of PML in AIDS patients, there have not been randomized, double-blind studies involving large groups of patients.

So far, there is no effective therapy for PML. Attempts using cytosine arabinoside,[16,21,47] adenine arabinoside,[16] and acyclovir[20] have been largely disappointing. Other antimicrobial agents, such as zidovudine, vidarabine, dideoxycytidine, ganciclovir, and dideoxyinosine, were also found ineffective to alter the rapid progression of PML.[65] However, data from several reports,[65-70] describing potential therapies for PML, although involving small numbers of patients, have suggested that the disease may remain stable for longer periods and occasionally even remit. Proposed therapies for PML include the use of nucleoside analogs (cytosine arabinoside, adenine arabinoside, iododeoxyuridine, AZT), heparin, transfer factor, recombinant interferon-2α, interferon-β, and corticosteroids.

2.2.1.3.1 Nucleoside congeners

Early reports on the therapeutic efficacy of cytosine arabinoside (ARA-C, cytarabine), one of several nucleoside agents used in the therapy of PML, were not conclusive[71-80] — one patient with underlying chronic lymphocytic leukemia (CCL) died after receiving daily doses of 40 mg/m^2 of ARA-C,[71] while in another case,[72] the patient (also with underlying CCL) improved within 48 h after IV infusion of 60 mg/m^2 daily for 6 d, followed by intrathecal administration of 10 mg/m^2 for 2 d. In a third case, Marriott et al.[74] described a patient with underlying sarcoidosis, showing significant improvement within 6 weeks and continued improvement over 18 months after treatment with 2.0 mg/kg daily of ARA-C for 5 d every 3 weeks for 18 months. Several other regimens involving initially intravenous ARA-C (10 mg/m^2 daily for 5 to 6[75,76] or 18 d[77]), followed by intrathecal ARA-C (10 mg/m^2 for 2 d[75,76]) or intravenous ARA-C (100 mg/m^2 for 8 d[77]), were also not conclusive, leading to either improvement followed by deterioration over a 20-month period,[75] gradual improvement over 3 weeks,[76] or deterioration.[77] However, Buckman and Wiltshaw[81] observed resolution of neurological symptoms in a patient with Hodgkin's disease and suspected PML (not proven by biopsy) after therapy with intravenous and intrathecal ARA-C.

Adenine arabinoside (ARA-A) proved to be not beneficial.[82-84] Thus, after a 14-d course of ARA-A at 20 mg/kg daily for 2 weeks, two patients with PML failed to improve and showed continued deterioration.[82]

The combination of prednisone and intrathecal iododeoxyuridine (2.0 mg/kg/12 h) was also unsuccessful when given for 7 weeks; the patient (with PML complicating sarcoidosis) failed to improve until interferon-β was initiated.[85] Another combination consisting of corticosteroid, transfer factor, adrenocorticotropin, and ARA-C also failed to treat PML.[79]

Selhorst et al.[86] reported stabilization in neurological damage in a renal transplant recipient with PML after receiving tilorone (an immune enhancer); the initial therapy with azathioprine was ineffective. However, cessation of immunosuppressive therapy alone failed to improve the condition of a patient with PML and myasthenia gravis.[87]

2.2.1.3.2 Interferons

The antiviral activity of interferons (IFNs) has been linked directly to their ability to activate the natural killer cells.[88] IFN-α has been found effective against various papovaviruses, especially the human papillomavirus (HPV).[89] While the genetic homology between HPV and JCV is small, IFN-α has also shown activity against simian virus 40 (SV40). Colosimo et al.[90] have treated a patient with PML with IFN-α starting with 5^6 U (intramuscularly every other day) and increasing the dose to 10^6 after 3 weeks. The neurological state and magnetic resonance imaging (MRI) findings gradually improve and, 18 months after the onset of therapy, the patient showed significant recovery from both aphasia and motor impairment. IFN-α has also been used in the treatment of PML associated with AIDS.[14]

Steiger et al.[91] treated a patient with PML associated with sarcoidosis with IFN-α (3^6 U daily, subcutaneously) for 19 d, followed by a regime of daily injections 5 d weekly. In addition, intermittent cytarabine (2.0 mg/kg daily) in 5-d courses at 10-d intervals was also administered; a total of seven cytarabine courses were given. The patient made significant improvent by regaining full functional independence. The rationale for using IFN-α was to stimulate the immune system and, at the same time, prevent viral replication; cytarabine when given alone will further depress the patient's immunity in an attempt to prevent viral replication.[91]

IFN-β combined with ARA-A has been applied but failed in the therapy of PML complicating sarcoidosis.[85] An ensuing 7-d course of intravenous ARA-A (90 mg daily) supplemented with 2 d of intrathecal ARA-A (10 mg daily) also failed to elicit a beneficial response. However, when the patient received intrathecal IFN-β at 10^6 U weekly for 19 weeks and monthly thereafter, a modest improvement in the clinical conditions and MRI was observed.[85]

2.2.1.3.3   Treatment of progressive multifocal leukoencephalopathy in AIDS patients

The recent increase in the incidence of PML among the AIDS population[15,92] is not surprising because of the growing number of patients with compromised cell-mediated immunity.[17-19,27,93] It has been suggested that currently PML occurs more frequently in AIDS patients than in any other immunodeficiency disorders,[94] affecting between 0.5% and 3.8%,[15,21,24,25,47,48] and as high as 4.2%[75] of the AIDS population.

At present, since there is no known therapy effective for PML, survival of AIDS patients is uniformly poor.[24,65,95] One potentially useful approach, as suggested by Karahalios et al.,[65] is to diagnose early PML by stereotactic brain biopsy and allow for swift initiation of antiviral therapy.

Fong et al.[96] have studied the correlation between the natural history of PML in HIV-infected patients and the CD4+ counts, as well as the effect of systemic cyclical ARA-C (2.0 mg/kg daily for 5 d each month) on the disease course. The results have shown that although there was a trend for slightly greater survival time in patients with higher CD4+ counts, there was no direct linear correlation, and a high CD4+ cell count did not translate into a longer survival time. In addition, no benefit from systemic ARA-C was observed.[96]

Since the JC virus enters the brain through the bloodstream, in particular the mononuclear cells, systemic antiviral therapy with ARA-C would be most appropriate. However, it seems rational that locally (intrathecally) administered ARA-C may increase the response. Thus, Lidman et al.[22] treated an AIDS patient with PML with cytarabine as a bolus infusion (2.0 mg/kg) given daily over a 5-d period, then repeated at intervals of 15 d between each 5-d treatment period; intrathecal cytarabine (50 mg/m²) was started concomitantly on day 1, and then adminstered once a week. At 5-month follow-up examination, the patient showed significant improvement. In another clinical trial,[97] AIDS patients with PML and CD4+ cell counts ranging from 7/mm³ to 690/mm³ (mean 106/mm³) received ARA-C intrathecally. Eight of the 13 patients treated have stabilized and improved, including 60% of patients with CD4+ cell counts of less than 50/mm³. Four of the patients had sustained improvement for up to 2 years, and four had transient improvement up to 6 months. O'Riordan et al.[78] also observed rapid improvement and complete remission of PML when intrathecal administration of ARA-C (50 mg/m²) was added to intravenous ARA-C (2.0 mg/kg daily for 5 d, repeated every 3 weeks). Portegies et al.[80] have treated three AIDS patients with PML (not confirmed by brain biopsy) with intravenous ARA-C at doses of 2.0 mg/kg for 5 d every 4 weeks. Both the clinical and MRI improvement observed at the end of treatment have been attributed to the longer period of therapy. Nicoli et al.[98] also reported the benefit of long-term cytarabine therapy in AIDS patients with PML.

However, results from several studies[99-102] did not confirm any previously reported therapeutic efficacy of ARA-C in AIDS patients with PML. In contrast to results by Portegies et al.[80] and Nicoli et al.,[98] long-term cytarabine therapy was also found to be ineffective.[101] Moreover, in spite of contemporary intravenous and intrathecal administration of ARA-C, an increased JCV burden was observed in the cerebrospinal fluid of patients.[102] Thus, according to Urtizberea et al.,[99] seven patients were treated monthly with ARA-C intravenously (2.0 mg/kg for 5 d) and intrathecally (50 mg; five patients with three or more courses, and two patients with one and two courses). While clinical symptoms were transiently reduced in three of seven patients, after 2 to 3 months worsening was observed in all but one patient; in six patients death occurred in 3 to 11 months (mean 4.5 months) after therapy.[99] Asbill et al.[100] also reported failure of intravenous and intrathecal cytarabine to improve the neurological deterioration in two AIDS patients with PML.

Therapy of PML with zidovudine (AZT, azidothymidine, 3′-azido-3′-deoxythymidine) in HIV-infected patients was also studied.[23,103-105] In one report,[103] after doses of 200 mg given every 4 h, the patient continued to deteriorate until death. However, in a recent study,[104] the clinical condition of an HIV-positive patient with PML improved significantly after the administration of AZT at doses of 200 mg every 4 h, but worsened when the dose was reduced to 200 mg every 8 h because of the development of granulocytopenia. After the initial higher-dose regimen was restored, the patient remained neurologically stable. Lortholary et al.[23] described a case of prolonged survival (>5 years) of an AIDS patient with PML after treatment with azidothymidine. Initially, the drug was given at daily doses of 1.2 mg, but the treatment was stopped for 3 months because of cytopenia; it was restarted at a lower dosage (600 mg daily). Singer et al.[106] also reported positive response to a high-dose AZT treatment (1.2 mg daily) in an AIDS (CD4+ count of 162 cells/mm^3) patient with JCV-associated PML.

Vago et al.,[107] who have studied the relations between neurologic findings, duration of treatment, and the cumulative AZT dose, found that the greatest reduction in frequency of multinucleated giant cells (their presence indicates the degree of HIV infection of the CNS) occurred after 6 to 12 months of treatment, while the frequency of HIV-induced cytopathic lesions increased in patients treated for more than 12 months. A cumulative zidovudine dose greater than 200 g has been associated with the lowest frequency of multinucleated giant cells.

The mechanism by which zidovudine might exert its therapeutic efficacy in the treatment of PML is still not clear. It is unlikely that zidovudine will have a direct effect on the JCV replication since polyomaviruses use a host-cell DNA polymerase, whereas zidovudine inhibits the retroviral RNA-dependent DNA polymerase. Since HIV itself may also cause encephalopathy, it is possible that the observed clinical response of patients with PML to zidovudine may be due to its effects on the HIV replication in the CNS,[108] rather than its effects on JCV replication. In addition, there is also evidence for a stimulatory effect of the HIV-1 *tat* protein on the expression of JCV late genes encoding JCV capsid proteins.[102] Consequently, any reduction of the HIV load in the CNS due to zidovudine might diminish the stimulus for JCV replication and thereby allow the host immune responses to control the JCV replication.[109]

Data collected by Major et al.[14] on HIV-infected patients with PML did not corroborate any beneficial neurological effect of zidovudine at various dose regimens used. Allegre et al.[110] also failed to confirm any efficacy of zidovudine administered intrathecally (by bolus injections 100 mg daily for 3 months) to two AIDS patients with PML.

The clinical efficacy of IFN-α in the treatment of AIDS patients with PML has been evaluated, in spite of the previously observed[111] selective defect in its production in HIV-1-infected monocytes. In an open label trial,[14] 19 HIV-1-seropositive patients with PML (confirmed by brain biopsies) were treated subcutaneously with 3×10^6 U of recombinant IFN-2α daily, with a gradual increment (typically, by 3×10^6 U every third day). A daily dose of rIFN-2α of 18×10^6 U was maintained following initiation. AZT, at 100 mg every 4 h, was also administered, and if not tolerated, the AZT was substituted with dideoxyinosine (ddI). In spite of the short period of treatment, modest improvement was observed in several patients, and none of the patients who responded to therapy showed any reversal in neurological functions. At least three patients remained clinically stable for a period of 6 months, and one patient exhibited significant improvement as seen by MRI; four patients did not respond to therapy.[14]

2.2.1.3.4 Heparin sulfate

The use of low-dose heparin sulfate in the therapy of PML as an adjunct to other drugs is based on the hypothesis by Houff et al.[59] that PML is the consequence of activated JCV-infected B cells crossing the blood-brain barrier and initiating new areas of neurological infection during the course of the disease. Since in animal models heparin sulfate prevented activated B lymphocytes from crossing the blood-brain barrier by stripping the lymphocyte glycoprotein cell surface receptors for cerebrovascular endothelial cells,[61] it has been postulated that such activity in humans may prevent the formation of new demyelinating lesions.[14] To examine this hypothesis, four HIV-1-infected patients with PML manifested by single demyelinating lesions, CD4+ lymphocyte counts below 200 cells/m³, and no prior history of opportunistic infections have been treated with 5000 U of heparin sulfate administered subcutaneously every 12 h. The results have been encouraging in three of four patients; PML did not progress after heparin sulfate administration for periods of 15, 18, and 27 months, respectively. The fourth patient had neurological disease progression that resulted in death 4 months after initiation of therapy.[14]

2.2.1.3.5 Progressive multifocal leukoencephalopathy in children

In general, children with HIV infection as underlying disease are less likely to develop neurological disorders as a result of opportunistic infection as compared with adults.[112] Thus, in adults with AIDS the likelihood of a neurological disorder following opportunistic infection is between 26% and 72%.[15,21,113] Rather, the overwhelming majority of children will develop neurological disorders as a direct consequence of HIV-1 infection of the CNS,[114] with only a small percentage of them developing a CNS opportunistic infection.[112,115,116] Although seroepidemiologic evidence suggests a high prevalence of antibodies to JCV in children (40% to 60% of children between the ages of 10 and 14 years carry JCV antibodies),[34,117,118] PML is rarely diagnosed in children with any form of immune deficiency.[112,119-121] Therapy for PML in children remains largely unsatisfactory. In one report,[112] treatment with zidovudine (200 mg, four times daily) and incrementally increasing doses of subcutaneous recombinant IFN-α2a (a total dose of 18^6 U) was found ineffective.

Redfearn et al.[122] have described a highly unusual case of a child with immunodeficiency and hyperimmunoglobulinemia M (dysgammaglobulinemia type I) who died of JCV-induced PML. In addition to JCV, the patient also had a BK virus infection. Pediatric cases of PML are very rare, and only once previously has a case of immunodeficiency with hyperglobulinemia M with BK virus infection been described.[123,124] The BK virus is the only other member of the papovaviridae to cause disease in immunocompromised patients.[125] What makes such cases very unusual is that PML, in general, is observed in patients with cell-mediated immune defects, such as HIV infection or severe combined immunodeficiency.[119] Immunodeficiency with hyperimmunoglobulinemia M is an antibody deficiency syndrome often characterized by other hematologic or lymphoreticular abnormalities.[126,127]

2.2.1.3.6 Leukoencephalopathy and immunosuppressive therapy

Leukoencephalopathy is a well-recognized complication resulting from immunosuppressive therapy, especially cancer chemotherapy (e.g., acute lymphocytic leukemia). Methotrexate is, by far, the most common drug associated with this neurologic disease.[128-132] Cytosine arabinoside-associated leukoencephalopathy is usually produced by intrathecal administration of high doses of ARA-C in combination with methotrexate.[133-138] Systemic ARA-C has not been linked to this complication.[135] Other immunosuppressive agents associated with leukoencephalopathy include 5-fluorouracil,[139-141] carmofur (1-hexylcarbamoyl-5-fluorouracil),[142-144] tegafur (a 5-fluorouracil derivative),[145] BCNU (carmustine, 1,3-bis(2-chloroethyl)-1-nitrosourea),[146-148] cyclophosphamide,[66,149] levamisole,[140,141] corticosteroids,[149] cyclosporin A,[150,151] azathioprine,[66] cisplatin,[152] lomustine (combined with irradiation),[153] and thiotepa.

Intrathecal methotrexate is used extensively in the therapy to or prevent meningeal leukemia and lymphoma[154,155] as well as against meningeal carcinomatosis, especially in cases of breast carcinoma.[156-158] Treatment is usually combined with cranial or craniospinal radiotherapy and occasionally with systemic methotrexate. The neurological complications of intrathecal methotrexate can be either acute or late effects.[159] The most serious delayed neurologic complication is disseminated necrotizing leukoencephalopathy. It is diagnosed usually 3 to 15 months after treatment and is clinically manifested by an insiduous onset of personality changes, lethargy, and dementia, usually followed by hemiplagia or quadriparesis and coma.[160,161] Cohen et al.[162] reported a case of methotrexate-induced leukoencephalopathy which was successfully treated with high-dose folinic acid; the neurologic disorder was cleared after 2.35 mg of folinic acid (leucovorin) was given in addition to the 135 mg administered as part of the initial therapy.

Multifocal inflammatory leukoencephalopathy secondary to treatment with levamisole alone or in combination with 5-fluorouracil has also been reported.[139,140,163] Results from stereotactic biopsies revealed reactive gliosis and infiltration of macrophages strongly positive for class II antigens, and interleukins 6 and 1α.[140] Concomitant administration of glucocorticoids has been recommended for more rapid resolution of clinical and radiographic symptoms of this neurologic disorder.[141]

PML has been reported in patients with Wegener's granulomatosis receiving immunosuppressive therapy of either cyclophosphamide and corticosteroids[149] or cyclosporin A.[150] Embrey et al.[66] reported a case of long-term survival of a renal transplant recipient who suffered late development of invasive bladder cancer and who developed PML following therapy of azathioprine (later substituted with cyclophosphamide because of hepatotoxicity) and prednisone; PML had been in remission for 56 after its diagnosis.

2.2.1.4 References

1. Shah, K. V., Polyomaviruses, in *Fields Virology*, 2nd ed., Fields, B. N., Knipe, D. M., Chanock, R. M., Hirsch, M., S., Melnick, J. L., Monath, T. P., and Roizman, B., Eds., Raven Press, New York, 1990, 1609.

2. Fraumeni, J. F., Jr., Stark, C. R., Gold, E., and Lepow, M. L., Simian virus 40 in polio vaccine: follow-up of newborn recipients, *Science*, 167, 59, 1970.

3. Shah, K. and Nathanson, N., Human exposure to SV40: review and comment, *Am. J. Epidemiol.*, 103, 1, 1976.

4. Gardner, S., The new human papovaviruses: their nature and significance, in *Recent Advances in Clinical Virology*, Waterson, A. P., Ed., Churchill Livingstone, New York, 1977, 93.

5. Padgettt, B. and Walker, D., Natural history of human polyomavirus infections, in *Persistent Viruses*, Stevens, J. G., Todaro, G. J., and Fox, C. F., Eds., Academic Press, New York, 1978, 751.

6. Corallini, A., Pagnani, M., Viadana, P., Silini, E., Mottes, M., Milanesi, G., Gerna, G., Vettor, R., Trapella, G., Silvani, V., Gaist, G., and Barbanti-Brodano, G., Association of BK virus with human brain tumors and tumors of pancreatic islets, *Int. J. Cancer*, 39, 60, 1987.

7. Dorries, K., Loeber, G., and Meixensberger, J., Association of polyomaviruses JC, SV-40, and BK with human brain tumors, *Virology*, 160, 268, 1987.

8. Takemoto, K., Furuno, A., Kata, K., and Yoshike, K., Biological and biochemical studies of African green monkey lymphotropic papovavirus, *J. Virol.*, 42, 502, 1982.

9. zur Hausen, H., Gissman, L., Mincheva, A., and Bocker, J., Characterization of lymphotropic papovaviruses, in *Viruses in Naturally Occurring Cancers*, Cold Spring Harbor Conferences on Cell Proliferation, Vol. 7, Cold Spring Harbor Laboratory, Essex, M., Todaro, G., and zur Hausen, H., Eds., Cold Spring Harbor, NY, 1980, 365.

10. Richardson, E., Progressive multifocal leukoencephalopathy, *N. Engl. J. Med.*, 265, 815, 1961.

11. Weiner, L. P., Herndon, R. M., Navayan, O., Johnson, R. T., Shah, K., Rubinstein, L. J., Prefiosi, T. J., and Conley, F. K., Isolation of virus related to SV40 from patients with progressive multifocal leukoencephalopathy, *N. Engl. J. Med.*, 288, 1103, 1972.

12. Morgello, S., Block, G. A., Price, R. W., and Petito, C. K., Varicella-zoster virus leukoencephalitis and cerebral vasculopathy, *Arch. Pathol. Lab. Med.*, 112, 173, 1988.

13. Carmack, M. A., Twiss, J., Enzmann, D. R., Amylon, M. D., and Arvin, A. M., Multifocal leukoencephalitis caused by varicella-zoster virus in a child with leukemia: successful treatment with acyclovir, *Pediatr. Infect. Dis. J.*, 12, 402, 1993.

14. Major, E. O., Amemiya, K., Tornatore, C. S., Houff, S. A., and Berger, J. R., Pathogenesis and molecular biology of progressive multifocal leukoencephalopathy, the JC virus-induced demyelinating disease of the human brain, *Clin. Microbiol. Rev.*, 5, 49, 1992.

15. Levy, R. M., Bredesen, D. E., and Rosenblum, M. L., Neurological manifestations of the acquired immunodeficiency syndrome (AIDS): experience at UCSF and review of the literature, *J. Neurosurg.*, 62, 475, 1985.

16. Miller, J. R., Barrett, R. E., Britton, C. B., Tapper, M. L., Bahr, G. S., Bruno, P. J., Marquardt, M. D., Hays, A. P., McMurtry, J. G. III, Weissman, J. B., and Bruno, M. S., Progressive multifocal leukoencephalopathy in a male homosexual with T-cell immune deficiency, *N. Engl. J. Med.*, 307, 1436, 1982.

17. Richardson, E. P., Progressive multifocal leukoencephalopathy 30 years later, *N. Engl. J. Med.*, 318, 315, 1988.

18. Padgett, B. L., Walker, D. L., Zu Rhein, G. M., and Eckroade, R. J., Cultivation of popova-like virus from human brain with progressive multifocal leukoencephalopathy, *Lancet*, 1, 1257, 1971.

19. Narayan, O., Penney, J. B., Jr., Johnson, R. T., Herndon, R. M., and Weiner, L. P., Etiology of progressive multifocal leukoencephalopathy, *N. Engl. J. Med.*, 289, 1278, 1973.

20. Bedri, J., Weinstein, W., DeGregorio, P., and Verity, M. A., Progressive multifocal leukoencephalopathy in acquired immunodeficiency syndrome, *N. Engl. J. Med.*, 309, 492, 1983.

21. Snider, W. D., Simpson, D. M., Nielsen, S., Gold, J. W. M., Metroka, C. E., and Posner, J. B., Neurological complications of the acquired immune deficiency syndrome: analysis of 50 patients, *Ann. Neurol.*, 14, 403, 1983.

22. Lidman, C., Lindqvist, L., Mathiesen, T., and Grane, P., Progressive multifocal leukoencephalopathy in AIDS, *AIDS*, 5, 1039, 1991.

23. Lortholary, O., Pialoux, G., Dupont, B., Trotot, P., Vazeux, R., Mikol, J., Thiebaut, J. B., and Gonzalez-Canali, G., Prolonged survival of a patient with AIDS and progressive multifocal leukoencephalopathy, *Clin. Infect. Dis.*, 18, 826, 1994.

24. Berger, J. R., Kaszovitz, B., Donovan-Post, M. J., and Dickinson, G., Progressive multifocal leukoencephalopathy associated with human immunodeficiency virus: a review of the literature with report of sixteen cases, *Ann. Intern. Med.*, 107, 78, 1987.

25. Trotot, P. M., Vazeux, R., Yamashita, H. K., Sandoz-Tronca, C., Mikol, J., Vedrenne, C., Thiébaux, J. B., Gray, F., Cikurel, M., Pialoux, G., and Levillain, R., MRI pattern of progressive multifocal leukoencephalopathy (PML) in AIDS, *J. Neuroradiol.*, 17, 233, 1990.

26. Brooks, B. R. and Walker, D. L., Progressive multifocal leukoencephalopathy, *Neurol. Clin.*, 2, 299, 1984.

27. Aström, K. E., Mancall, E. L., and Richardson, E. P., Jr., Progressive multifocal leuko-encephalopathy: a hitherto unrecognized complication of chronic lymphatic leukaemia and Hodgkin's disease, *Brain*, 81, 93, 1958.

28. Davies, J. A., Hughes, J. T., and Oppenheimer, D. R., Richardson's disease (progressive multifocal leucoencephalopathy), *Q. J. Med.*, 167, 481, 1973.

29. Marriott, P. J., O'Brien, M. D., Mackenzie, C. K., and Janota, I., Progressive multifocal leuko-encephalopathy: remission with cytarabine, *J. Neurol. Neurosurg. Psychiatry*, 38, 205, 1975.

30. Walker, D. L., Progressive multifocal leukoencephalopathy: an opportunistic viral infection of the central nervous system, in *Handbook of Clinical Neurology*, Vol. 47, Vinken, P. J., Bruyn, G. W., and Klawans, H. L., Eds., Elsevier Science Publishers, Amsterdam, 1985, 503.

31. Ast, D. and Cunha, B. A., Chronic encephalitis caused by leukoencephalopathy, *Heart Lung*, 19, 678, 1990.

32. Price, R. W., Nielsen, S., Horten, B., Rubino, M., Padgett, E., and Walker, D., Progressive multifocal leukoencephalopathy: a burnt-out case, *Ann. Neurol.*, 13, 485, 1983.

33. Brun, A., Nordenfeldt, E., and Kjellén, L., Aspects on the variability of progressive multifocal leuko-encephalopathy, *Acta Neuropathol. (Berlin)*, 24, 232, 1973.

34. Padgett, B. L. and Walker, D. L., Prevalence of antibodies in human sera against JC virus, an isolate from a case of progressive multifocal leukoencephalopathy, *J. Infect. Dis.*, 127, 467, 1973.

35. Yogo, Y., Kitamura, T., Sugimoto, C., Ueki, T., Aso, Y., Hara, K., and Taguchi, F., Isolation of a possible archtypal JC virus DNA sequence from nonimmunocompromised individuals, *J. Virol.*, 64, 3139, 1990.

36. Greenlee, J. E., Progressive multifocal leukoencephalopathy, *Curr. Clin. Top. Infect. Dis.*, 10, 140, 1989.

37. Price, R. W., Progressive multifocal leukoencephalopathy, in *Cecil Textbook of Medicine*, Plum, F., Ed., W. B. Saunders, Philadelphia, 1988, 2207.

38. Atlas, S. W., Grossman, R. I., Packer, R. J., Goldberg, H. I., Hackney, D. B., Zimmerman, R. A., and Bilaniuk, L. T., Magnetic resonance imaging diagnosis of disseminated necrotizing leuko-encephalopathy, *J. Computed Tomography*, 11, 39, 1987.

39. Zu Rhein, G. M., Association of popova-virions with a human demyelinating disease (progressive multifocal leukoencephalopathy), *Prog. Med. Virol.*, 11, 185, 1969.

40. Iida, T., Kitamura, T., Guo, J., Taguchi, F., Aso, Y., Nagashima, K., and Yogo, Y., Origin of JC polyomavirus variants associated with progressive multifocal leukoencephalopathy, *Proc. Natl. Acad. Sci. U.S.A.*, 90, 5062, 1992.

41. Frisque, R., Bream, G., and Cannella, M., Human polyomavirus JC virus genome, *J. Virol.*, 51, 458, 1984.

42. Kenney, S., Natarajan, V., Strike, D., Khoury, G., and Salzman, N. P., JC virus enhancer-promoter active in human brain cells, *Science*, 226, 1337, 1984.

43. Assouline, J. G. and Major, E. O., Human fetal Schwann cells support JC virus multiplication, *J. Virol.*, 65, 1002, 1991.

44. Lynch, K. J. and Frisque, R. J., Identification of critical elements within the JC virus DNA replication origin, *J. Virol.*, 64, 5812, 1990.

45. Sock, E., Wegner, M., and Grummt, F., DNA replication of human polyomavirus JC is stimulated by NF-I *in vivo*, *Virology*, 182, 298, 1991.

46. Richardson, E. P., Jr. and Johnson, P. C., Atypical progressive multifocal leukoencephalopathy with plasma-cell infiltrates, *Acta Neuropathol.*, 6(Suppl.), 247, 1975.

47. Krupp, L. B., Lipton, R. B., Swerdlow, M. L., Leeds, N. E., and Llena, J., Progressive multifocal encephalopathy: clinical and radiographic features, *Ann. Neurol.*, 17, 344, 1985.

48. Stoner, G., Ryschkewitsch, C., Walker, D., Stoffer, D., and Webster, H. deF., A monoclonal antibody to SV40 large T-antigen labels a nuclear antigen in JC virus-transformed cells and in progressive multifocal leukoencephalopathy (PML) brain infected with JC virus, *J. Neuroimmunol.*, 17, 331, 1988.

49. Gendelman, H., Phelps, W., Feigenbaum, L., Ostrove, J., Adachi, A., Howley, P., Khoury, G., Ginsberg, H., and Martin, M., Trans-activation of the human immunodeficiency virus long terminal repeat by DNA viruses, *Proc. Natl. Acad. Sci. U.S.A.*, 83, 9759, 1986.

50. Krupp, L. B., Lipton, R. B., Swerdlow, M. L., Leeds, N. E., and Llena, J., Progressive multifocal leukoencephalopathy: clinical and radiographic features, *Ann. Neurol.*, 17, 344, 1985.

51. Willoughby, E., Price, R. W., Padgett, B. L., Walker, D. L., and Dupont, B., Progressive multifocal encephalopathy (PML): in vitro cell-mediated immune responses to mitogens and JC virus, *Neurology*, 30, 256, 1980.

52. Gardner, S., Mackenzie, E., Smith, C., and Porter, A., Prospective study of the human polyomavirus BK and JC and cytomegalovirus in renal transplant recipients, *J. Clin. Pathol.*, 37, 578, 1984.

53. Hogan, T. F., Padgett, B. L., Walker, D. L., Bordon, E. C., and McBain, J. A., Rapid detection and identification of JC virus and BK virus in human urine by using immunofluorescence microscopy, *J. Clin. Microbiol.*, 11, 178, 1980.

54. Arthur, R. R., Dagostin, S., and Shah, K., Detection of BK virus and JC virus in urine and brain tissue by the polymerase chain reaction, *J. Clin. Microbiol.*, 27, 1174, 1989.

55. Telenti, A., Aksamit, A. J., Proper, J., and Smith, T. F., Detection of JC virus DNA by polymerase chain reaction in patients with progressive multifocal leukoencephalopathy, *J. Infect. Dis.*, 162, 858, 1990.

56. Henson, J., Rosenblum, M., and Furneaux, H., A potential diagnostic test for PML: PCR analysis of JC virus DNA, *Neurology*, 41(Suppl.), 338, 1991.

57. Grinnell, B. W., Padgett, B. L., and Walker, D. L., Distribution of nonintegrated DNA from JC papovavirus in organs of patients with progressive multifocal leukoencephalopathy, *J. Infect. Dis.*, 147, 669, 1983.

58. Greenlee, J. and Keeney, P. M., Immunoenzymatic labeling of JC papovavirus T antigen in brains of patients with progressive multifocal leukoencephalopathy, *Acta Neuropathol.*, 71, 150, 1986.

59. Houff, S. A., Major, E. O., Katz, D., Kufta, C., Sever, J., Pittaluga, S., Roberts, J., Gitt, J., Saini, N., and Lux, W., Involvement of JC virus-infected mononuclear cells from the bone marrow and spleen in the pathogenesis of progressive multifocal leukoencephalopathy, *N. Engl. J. Med.*, 318, 301, 1988.

60. Major, E. O., Amemiya, K., Elder, G., and Houff, S. A., Glial cells of the human developing brain and B cells of the immune system share a common DNA binding factor for recognition of the regulatory sequences of the human polyomavirus, JCV, *J. Neurosci. Res.*, 27, 461, 1990.
61. Brenan, M. and Parish, C. R., Modification of lymphocyte migration by sulphated polysaccharides, *Eur. J. Immunol.*, 16, 423, 1986.
62. Cooper, M., B lymphocytes: new development and function, *N. Engl. J. Med.*, 317, 1452, 1987.
63. Wekerle, Z. H., Linington, H., Lassman, H., and Meyerman, R., Cellular immune reactivity within the central nervous system, *Trends Neurosci.*, 9, 271, 1986.
64. Wegner, M., Drolet, D. W., and Rosenfeld, M. G., Regulation of JC virus by the POU-domain transcription factor Tst-1: implication for progressive multifocal leukoencephalopathy, *Proc. Natl. Acad. Sci. U.S.A.*, 90, 4743, 1993.
65. Karahalios, D., Breit, R., Dal Canto, M. C., and Levy, R. M., Progressive multifocal encephalopathy in patients with HIV infection: lack of impact of early diagnosis by stereotactic brain biopsy, *J. Acquir. Immune Defic. Syndr.*, 5, 1030, 1992.
66. Embrey, J. R., Silva, F. G., Helderman, J. H., Peters, P., and Sagalowsky, A. I., Long term survival and late development of bladder cancer in renal transplant patient with progressive multifocal leukoencephalopathy, *J. Urol.*, 139, 580, 1988.
67. Berger, J. R. and Mucke, L., Prolonged survival and partial recovery in AIDS-associated progressive multifocal leukoencephalopathy, *Neurology*, 38, 1060, 1988.
68. Padgett, B. L. and Walker, D. L., Virologic and serologic studies of progressive multifocal leukoencephalopathy, *Prog. Clin. Biol. Res.*, 105, 107, 1983.
69. Price, R. W., Nielsen, S., Horten, B., Rubino, M., Padgett, B., and Walker, D., Progressive multifocal leukoencephalopathy: a burnt-out case, *Ann. Neurol.*, 13, 485, 1983.
70. Sima, A. A. F., Finkelstein, S. D., and McLachlan, D. R., Multiple malignant astrocytomas in a patient with spontaneous progressive multifocal leukoencephalopathy, *Ann. Neurol.*, 14, 183, 1983.
71. Castleman, B., Scully, R. E., and McNeely, B. J., Weekly clinicopathological exercise, case 1901972, *N. Engl. J. Med.*, 286, 1047, 1972.
72. Bauer, W. R., Turci, A. P., Jr., and Johnson, K. P., Progressive multifocal leukoencephalopathy and cytarabine, *JAMA*, 226, 174, 1973.
73. Conomy, J. P., Beard, N. S., Matsumoto, H., and Roessmann, U., Cytarabine treatment of progressive multifocal leukoencephalopathy, *JAMA*, 229, 1313, 1974.
74. Marriott, P. J., O'Brian, M. D., Mackenzie, I. C., and Janota, I., Progressive multifocal leukoencephalopathy: remission with cytarabine, *J. Neurol. Neurosurg. Psychiatry*, 38, 205, 1975.
75. Rockwell, D., Ruben, F. L., Winkelstein, A., and Mendelow, H., Absence of immune deficiencies in a case of progressive multifocal leukoencephalopathy, *Am. J. Med.*, 61, 433, 1976.
76. Peters, A. C. B., Veersteeg, J., Bots, G. T. A., Boogerd, W., and Vielvoye, G. J., Progressive multifocal leukoencephalopathy: immunofluorescent demonstration of SV40 antigen in CSF cells and response to cytarabine therapy, *Arch. Neurol.*, 37, 497, 1980.
77. Smith, C. R., Sima, A. A. F., Salit, I. E., and Gentili, F., Progressive multifocal leukoencephalopathy: failure of cytarabine therapy, *Neurology*, 32, 200, 1982.
78. O'Riordan, T., Daly, P. A., Hutchinson, M., Shattock, A. G., and Gardner, S. D., Progressive multifocal leukoencephalopathy — remission with cytarabine, *J. Infect.*, 20, 51, 1990.
79. Van Horn, G., Bastien, F. O., and Moake, J. L., Progressive multifocal leukoencephalopathy: failure of response to transfer factor and cytarabine, *Neurology*, 28, 794, 1978.
80. Portegies, P., Algra, P. R., Hollak, C. E. M., Prins, J. M., Reiss, P., Valk, J., and Lange, J., Response to cytarabine in progressive multifocal leukoencephalopathy in AIDS, *Lancet*, 337, 680, 1991.
81. Buckman, R. and Wiltshaw, E., Progressive multifocal leukoencephalopathy successfully treated with cytosine arabinoside, *Br. J. Haematol.*, 34, 153, 1976.
82. Wolinsky, J. S., Johnson, K. P., Rand, K., and Merigan, T. C., Progressive multifocal leukoencephalopathy: clinical pathological correlates and failure of a drug trial in two patients, *Trans. Am. Neurol. Assoc.*, 101, 81, 1976.
83. Rand, K. H., Johnson, K. P., Rubenstein, L. J., Wolinsky, J., Penney, J., Walker, D., Padgett, B., and Merigan, T., Adenine arabinoside in the treatment of progressive multifocal leukoencephalopathy: use of virus containing cells in the urine to assess response to therapy, *Ann. Neurol.*, 1, 458, 1977.

84. Walker, D. L., Progressive multifocal leukoencephalopathy: an opportunistic viral infection of the central nervous system, in *Handbook of Clinical Neurology*, Vol. 34, Bruyn, G. W., Ed., Elsevier/North-Holland, New York, 1978, 307.

85. Tashiro, K., Doi, S., Moriwaka, F., Maruo, Y., and Nomura, M., Progressive multifocal leukoencephalopathy with magnetic resonance imaging verification and therapeutic trials with interferon, *J. Neurol.*, 234, 427, 1987.

86. Selhorst, J. B., Ducy, K. F., Thomas, J. M., and Reggelson, W., Remission and immunologic reversals, *Neurology*, 28, 337, 1978.

87. Dawson, D. M., Progressive multifocal leukoencephalopathy, *Ann. Neurol.*, 11, 218, 1982.

88. Tyring, S. K., Cauda, R., Ghanta, V., and Hiramoto, R., Activation of natural killer cell function during interferon-alpha treatment of patients with condyloma acuminatum is predictive of clinical response, *J. Biol. Regul. Homeo Agents*, 2, 63, 1988.

89. Weck, P. K., Buddin, D. A., and Whinant, J. K., Interferons in the treatment of genital human papillomavirus infections, *Am. J. Med.*, 85, 159, 1988.

90. Colosimo, C., Lebon, P., Martelli, M., Tumminelli, F., and Mandelli, F., Alpha-interferon therapy in a case of probable progressive multifocal leukoencephalopathy, *Acta Neurol. Belg.*, 92, 24, 1992.

91. Steiger, M. J., Tarnesby, G., Gabe, S., McLaughlin, J., and Schapira, A. H. V., Successful outcome of progressive multifocal leukoencephalopathy with cytarabine and interferon, *Ann. Neurol.*, 33, 407, 1993.

92. Levy, R. M., Janssen, R., Bush, T., and Rosenblum, M., Neuroepidemiology of AIDS in the United States, *J. Acquir. Immune Defic. Syndr.*, 1, 31, 1988.

93. McCormick, W. F., Schochet, S. S., Sarles, H. E., and Calverley, J. R., Progressive multifocal leukoencephalopathy in renal transplant recipients, *Arch. Intern. Med.*, 136, 829, 1976.

94. Weiss, S. H., Goedert, J. J., Sangadharan, M. G., Bodner, A. J., Gallo, R. C., and Blattner, W. A., Screening test for HTLV-III (AIDS agent) antibodies, *JAMA*, 253, 221, 1985.

95. Levy, R. M. and Bredesen, D. E., Central nervous system dysfunction in acquired immunodeficiency syndrome, *J. Acquir. Immune Defic. Syndr.*, 1, 41, 1988.

96. Fong, I. W., Toma, E., Cameron, W., Genereaux, M., Gill, J., and Ostrowski, M., The natural history of progressive multifocal leukoencephalopathy (PML) in HIV patients, *Proc. IXth Int. Conf. AIDS*, Berlin, 1993, Abstr. PO-B01-0864.

97. Britton, C. B., Romagnoli, M., Sisti, M., and Powers, J. M., Progressive multifocal leukoencephalopathy: disease progression, stabilization and response to intrathecal ARA-C in 26 patients, *Proc. VIIIth Int. Conf. AIDS*, Amsterdam, 1992, Abstr. ThB 1512.

98. Nicoli, F., Chave, B., Peragut, J. C., and Gastaut, J. L., Efficacy of cytarabine in progressive multifocal leukoencephalopathy in AIDS, *Lancet*, 339, 306, 1992.

99. Urtizberea, J. A., Flament-Saillour, M., Clair, B., and de Truchis, P., Cytarabine for progressive multifocal leucoencephalopathy (PML) in AIDS patients, *Proc. IXth Int. Conf. AIDS*, Berlin, 1993, Abstr. PO-B16-1717.

100. Asbill, M. C., Marmarelis, P. Z., and Brownstone, P. K., Two gay patients with demyelinating disorders, *Hosp. Pract.*, 21(5A), 54, 1986.

101. de Truchis, P., Flament-Saillour, M., Urtizberea, J.-A., Hassine, D., and Clair, B., Inefficacy of cytarabine in progressive multifocal leukoencephalopathy in AIDS, *Lancet*, 342, 622, 1993.

102. Antinori, A., De Luca, A., Ammassari, A., Cingolani, A., Murri, R., Colosimo, G., Roselli, R., Scerrati, M., and Tamburrini, E., Failure of cytarabine and increased JC virus-DNA burden in the cerebrospinal fluid of patients with AIDS-related progressive multifocal leukoencephalopathy, *AIDS*, 8, 1022, 1994.

103. Tarsy, D., Holden, E. M., Segarra, J. M., and Feldman, R. G., 5-Iodo-2'- deoxyuridine (IUDR): (NSC-39661) given intraventricularly in the treatment of progressive multifocal leukoencephalopathy, *Cancer Chemother. Rep.*, 57, 73, 1973.

104. Conway, B., Halliday, W. C., and Brunham, R. C., Human immunodeficiency virus-associated progressive multifocal leukoencephalopathy: apparent response to 3'-azido-3'-deoxythymidine, *Rev. Infect. Dis.*, 12, 479, 1990.

105. Fiala, M., Cone, L. A., Cohen, N., Patel, D., Williams, K., Casareale, D., Shapshak, P., and Tourtelotte, W., Responses of neurologic complications of AIDS to 3'-azido-3'-deoxythymidine and 9-(1,3-dihydroxy-2-propoxymethyl)guanine. I. Clinical features, *Rev. Infect. Dis.*, 10, 250, 1988.

106. Singer, E. J., Stoner, G. L., Singer, P., Tomiyasu, U., Licht, E., Fahy- Chandon, B., and Tourtellotte, W. W., AIDS presenting as progressive multifocal leukoencephalopathy with clinical response to zidovudine, *Acta Neurol. Scand.*, 90, 443, 1994.

107. Vago, L., Castagna, A., Lazzarin, A., Cinque, P., Trabattoni, G., and Costanzi, G., Zidovudine and frequency of HIV-induced diffuse leukoencephalopathy, *Lancet*, 337, 1488, 1991.

108. Geleziunas, R., Schipper, H. M., and Wainberg, M. A., Pathogenesis and therapy of HIV-1 infection of the central nervous system, *AIDS*, 6, 1411, 1992.

109. Tada, H., Rappaport, J., Lashgari, M., Amini, S., Wong-Staal, F., and Khalili, K., Trans-activation of the JC virus late promoter by the tat protein to type 1 human immunodeficiency virus in glial cells, *Proc. Natl. Acad. Sci. U.S.A.*, 87, 3479, 1990.

110. Allegre, Th., Routy, J. P., Cailleres, S., Blanc, A. P., Toma, E., and Beaulieu, Intrathecal zidovudine (IT-AZT) treatment of patients with HIV associated progressive multifocal leukoencephalitis (PML), *Proc. IXth Int. Conf. AIDS*, Berlin, 1993, Abstr. PO-B16-1727.

111. Gendelman, H. E., Friedman, R. M., Joe, S., Baca, L., Turpin, I., Dveksler, G., Meltzer, M., and Dieffenbach, C., A selective defect of interferon alpha production in human immunodeficiency virus-infected monocytes, *J. Exp. Med.*, 172, 1433, 1990.

112. Berger, J. R., Scott, G., Albrecht, J., Belman, A. L., Tornatore, C., and Major, E. O., Progressive multifocal leukoencephalopathy in HIV-1-infected children, *AIDS*, 6, 837, 1992.

113. Berger, J. R., Moskowitz, L., Fischl, M., and Kelley, R. E., Neurologic disease as the presenting manifestation of acquired immunodeficiency syndrome, *South. Med. J.*, 80, 685, 1987.

114. Epstein, L. G., Sharer, L. R., Oleske, J. M., Connor, E. M., Goulsmit, J., Bagdon, L., Robert-Guroff, M., and Koenigsberger, M. R., Neurologic manifestations of human immunodeficiency virus infection in children, *Pediatrics*, 78, 678, 1986.

115. Belman, A. L., Diamond, G., Dickson, D., Horoupian, D., Llena, J., Lantos, G., and Rubinstein, A., Pediatric acquired immunodeficiency syndrome: neurologic syndromes, *Am. J. Dis. Child.*, 142, 29, 1988.

116. Dickson, D. W., Belman, A. L., Park, Y. D., Wiley, C., Horoupian, D. S., Llena, J., Kure, K., Lyman, W. D., Morecki, R., Mitsudo, S., and Cho, S., Central nervous system pathology in pediatric AIDS: an autopsy study, *APMIS*, S8, 40, 1989.

117. Padgett, B. L. and Walker, D. L., Virologic and serologic studies of progressive multifocal leukoencephalopathy, in *Polyomaviruses and Human Neurological Diseases*, Sever, J. L. and Madden, D. L., Eds., Alan R. Liss, New York, 1983, 107.

118. Taguchi, F., Kajioka, J., and Miyamura, T., Prevalence rate and age of acquisition of antibodies against JC virus and BK virus in human sera, *Microbiol. Immunol.*, 26, 1057, 1982.

119. Stoner, G. L., Walker, D. L., and Webster, H. D., Age distribution of progressive multifocal leuko-encephalopathy, *Acta Neurol. Scand.*, 78, 307, 1988.

120. Krasinski, K., Borkowsky, W., and Holzman, R. S., Prognosis of human immunodeficiency virus infection in children and adolescents, *Pediatr. Infect. Dis. J.*, 8, 216, 1989.

121. Vandersteenhoven, J. J., Dbaibo, G., Boyko, O. B., Huletta, C. M., Anthony, D. C., and Wilfert, C., Progressive multifocal leukoencephalopathy in pediatric acquired immunodeficiency syndrome, *Pediatr. Infect. Dis. J.*, 11, 232, 1992.

122. Redfearn, A., Pennie, R. A., Mahony, J. B., and Dent, P. B., Progressive multifocal leukoencephalopathy in a child with immunodeficiency and hyperimmunoglobulinemia M, *Pediatr. Infect. Dis. J.*, 12, 399, 1993.

123. Zu Rhein, G. M., Padgett, B. L., Walker, D. L., Chun, R. W. M., Horowitz, S. D., and Hong, R., Progressive multifocal leukoencephalopathy in a child with severe combined immunodeficiency, *N. Engl. J. Med.*, 299, 256, 1978.

124. Rosen, S., Harmon, W., Krensky, A. M., Edelson, P. J., Padgett, B. L., Grinell, B. W., Rubino, M. J., and Walker, D. L., Tubulo-interstitial nephritis associated with polyomavirus (BK type) infection, *N. Engl. J. Med.*, 308, 1192, 1983.

125. Padgett, B. and Walker, D. L., New human papovaviruses, in *Comprehensive Virology*, Vol. 18, Frankel-Conrat, H. and Wagner, R. R., Eds., Plenum Press, New York, 1983, 161.

126. Stiehm, E. R. and Fudenberg, H. H., Clinical and immunologic features of dysgammaglobulinemia type I, *Am. J. Med.*, 40, 805, 1966.

127. Goldstein, G. W., Krivit, W. J., and Hong, R., Hypoimmunoglobulin G, hyperimmunoglobulin M, intestinal nodular lymphoid hyperplasia and thrombocytopenia: an unusual association, *Arch. Dis. Child.*, 44, 621, 1969.

128. Kaplan, R. S. and Wiernik, P. H., Neurotoxicity of antineoplastic drugs, *Semin. Oncol.*, 9, 103, 1982.

129. Bleyer, W. A. and Griffin, T. W., White matter necrosis, mineralizing microangiopathy and intellectual abilities in survivors of childhood leukemia: association with central nervous system irradiation and methotrexate therapy, in *Radiation Damage to the Nervous System*, Gilbert, H. A. and Kagen, A. R., Eds., Raven Press, New York, 1980, 155.

130. Young, D. F. and Posner, J. B., Nervous system toxicity of the chemotherapeutic agents, in *Handbook of Clinical Neurology*, Vol. 39, Vinken, P. J. and Bruyn, G. W., Eds., Elsevier North-Holland, Amsterdam, 91. 1980,

131. Shapiro, W. R., Allen, J. C., and Horten, B. C., Chronic methotrexate toxicity to the central nervous system, *Clin. Bull.*, 10, 49, 1980.

132. Allen, J. C., Rosen, G., Mehta, B. M., and Horten, B., Leukoencephalopathy following high-dose IV methotrexate chemotherapy with leucovorin rescue, *Cancer Treat. Rep.*, 64, 1261, 1980.

133. Fusner, J. E., Poplack, D. G., Pizzo, P. A., and Di Chiro, G., Leukoencephalopathy following chemotherapy for rhabdomyosarcoma: reversibility of cerebral changes demonstrated by computed tomography, *J. Pediatr.*, 91, 77, 1977.

134. Rubinstein, L. J., Herman, M. M., Long, T. F., and Wilbur, J. R., Disseminated necrotizing leukoencephalopathy: a complication of treated central nervous system leukemia and lymphoma, *Cancer*, 35, 291, 1975.

135. Hwang, T.-L., Yung, W. K. A., Lee, Y.-Y., Borit, A., and Fields, W. S., High dose Ara-C related leukoencephalopathy, *J. Neuro-Oncology*, 3, 335, 1986.

136. Tsukada, T., Morita, N., Ikeda, T., Katayama, N., Nishikawa, M., Kobayashi, T., Deguchi, K., and Shirakawa, S., An adult case of acute lymphoblastic leukemia with necrotizing leukoencephalopathy, *Jpn. J. Med.*, 29, 56, 1990.

137. Hayashi, Y., Hanada, R., Yamamoto, K., Taguchi, N., and Shikano, T., Leukoencephalopathy in children with t(1;19) acute lymphoblastic leukaemia, *Lancet*, 340, 316, 1992.

138. Gay, C. T., Bodensteiner, J. B., Nitschke, R., Sexauer, C., and Wilson, D., Reversible treatment-related leukoencephalopathy, *J. Child. Neurol.*, 4, 208, 1989.

139. Aoki, N., Reversible leukoencephalopathy caused by 5-fluorouracil derivatives, presenting as akinetic mutism, *Surg. Neurol.*, 25, 279, 1986.

140. Chen, T. C., Hinton, D. R., Leichman, L., Atkinson, R. D., Apuzzo, M. L. J., and Couldwell, W. T., Multifocal inflammatory leukoencephalopathy associated with levamisole and 5-fluorouracil: case report, *Neurosurgery*, 35, 1138, 1994.

141. Kimmel, D. W. and Schutt, A. J., Multifocal leukoencephalopathy: occurrence during 5-fluorouracil and levamisole therapy and resolution after discontinuation of chemotherapy, *Mayo Clin. Proc.*, 68, 363, 1993.

142. Kuzihara, S., Ohkoshi, N., Kanazawa, K., Hashimoto, H., Nakanishi, T., and Toyokura, Y., Subacute leukoencephalopathy induced by carmofur, a 5-fluorouracil derivative, *J. Neurol.*, 234, 365, 1987.

143. Yamada, T., Okamura, S., Okazaki, T., Ushiroyama, T., Yanagawa, Y., Ueki, M., Sugimoto, O., Yamazaki, H., Sugino, M., and Masui, Y., Leukoencephalopathy following treatment with carmofur: a case and review of Japanese literature, *Asia-Oceania J. Obstet. Gynaecol.*, 15, 161, 1989.

144. Suzuki, T., Koizumi, J., Uchida, K., Shiraishi, H., and Hori, M., Carmofur-induced organic mental disorders, *Jpn. J. Psychiatry Neurol.*, 44, 723, 1990.

145. Hayashi, R., Hanyu, N., and Kitahara, A., Leukoencephalopathy induced by tegafur: serial studies of somatosensory evoked potentials and cerebrospinal fluid, *J. Intern. Med.*, 31, 828, 1992.

146. Burger, P. C., Kamenar, E., Schold, S. C., Fay, J. W., Phillips, G. L., and Herzig, G. P., Encephalopathy following high-dose BCNU therapy, *Cancer*, 48, 1318, 1981.

147. Kleinschmidt-Demasters, B. K., Intracarotid BCNU leukoencephalopathy, *Cancer*, 57, 1276, 1986.

148. Watne, K., Nome, O., Hager, B., and Hirschberg, H., Combined intra-arterial chemotherapy and irradiation of malignant gliomas, *Acta Oncol.*, 30, 835, 1991.

149. Choy, D. S. J., Weiss, A., and Lin, P. T., Progressive multifocal encephalopathy following treatment for Wegener's granulomatosis, *JAMA*, 268, 600, 1992.

150. Ettinger, J., Feiden, W., Hubner, G., and Shreiner, M., Progressive multifokale leukoenzephakopathie bei Wegener'scher graunulomatose unter therapie mit cyclosporin A, *Klin. Wochenschr.*, 67, 260, 1989.

151. Shimizu, C., Kimura, S., Yoshida, Y., Nezu, A., Saitoh, K., Osaka, H., Aihara, Y., and Nagasaka, Y., Acute leucoencephalopathy during cyclosporin A therapy in a patient with nephrotic syndrome, *Pediatr. Nephrol.*, 8, 483, 1994.

152. Brück, W., Heise, E., and Friede, R. L., Leukoencephalopathy after cisplatin therapy, *Clin. Neuropathol.*, 8, 263, 1989.

153. Frytak, S., Shaw, J. N., O'Neill, B. P., Lee, R. E., Eagan, R. T., Shaw, E. G., Richardson, R. L., Coles, D. T., and Jett, J. R., Leukoencephalopathy in small cell lung cancer patients receiving prophylactic cranial irradiation, *Am. J. Clin. Oncol.*, 12, 27, 1989.

154. Bleyer, W. A. and Poplack, D. G., Prophylaxis and treatment of leukemia in the central nervous system and other sanctuaries, *Semin. Oncol.*, 12, 131, 1985.

155. MacKintosh, F. R., Colby, T. V., Podolsky, W. J., Burke, J. S., Hoppe, R. T., Rosenfelt, F. P., Rosenberg, S. A., and Kaplan, H. S., Central nervous system involvement in non-Hodgkin's lymphoma, *Cancer*, 49, 586, 1982.

156. Wasserstrom, W. R., Glass, J. P., and Posner, J. B., Diagnosis and treatment of leptomeningeal metastasis from solid tumors, *Cancer*, 49, 759, 1982.

157. Yap, H. Y., Yap, B. S., Rasmussen, S., Levens, M. E., Hortobagui, G. N., and Blumenschein, G. R., Treatment for meningeal carcinomas in breast cancer, *Cancer*, 49, 219, 1982.

158. Ongerboer de Visser, B. W., Somers, R., Nooyen, W. H., van Heerde, P., Hart, A. A. M., and McVie, J. G., Intraventricular methotrexate therapy of leptomeningeal metastasis from breast carcinoma, *Neurology*, 33, 1565, 1983.

159. Boogerd, W., Sande, J. J. vd, and Moffie, D., Acute fever and delayed leukoencephalopathy following low dose intraventricular methotrexate, *J. Neurol. Neurosurg. Psychiatry*, 51, 1277, 1988.

160. Bleyer, W. A., Neurologic sequelae of methotrexate and ionizing radiation: a new classification, *Cancer Treat. Rep.*, 65, 89, 1981.

161. Jellinger, K., Pathologic effects of chemotherapy, in *Oncology of the Nervous System*, Walker, M. D., Ed., Martinus Nijhoff, Boston, 1983, 185

162. Cohen, I. J., Stark, B., Kaplinsky, C., Weitz, R., Matz, S., Lerman, P., Rakowsky, E., Vogel, R., and Zaizov, R., Methotrexate-induced leukoencephalopathy is treatable with high-dose folinic acid: a case report and analysis of the literature, *Pediatr. Hematol. Oncol.*, 7, 79, 1990.

163. Hook, C. C., Kimmel, D. W., Kvols, L. K., Scheithauer, B. W., Forsyth, P. A., Rubin, J., Moertel, C. G., and Rodriguez, M., Multifocal inflammatory leukoencephalopathy with 5-fluorouracil and levamisole, *Ann. Neurol.*, 31, 262, 1992.

3 Adenoviridae

The adenoviruses is a group of viruses found in all regions of the world and known to cause disease of the upper respiratory tract and conjunctivae and also present in latent infection in normal persons. In addition to human adenovirus types, there are simian, bovine, avian, canine, and murine types, and many of them have induced malignancy in certain species.

Currently, some 31 distinct adenovirus serotypes have been identified and given numbers. Types 1, 2, and 5 have been recovered from tonsils and adenoids of both persons not ill with respiratory disease and patients with febrile respiratory infections. On the other hand, types 3, 4, 7, 14, and 21 have been isolated only from patients with acute respiratory disease. Adenovirus type 3 is considered to be the specific etiologic agent of pharyngoconjunctival fever, whereas adenovirus type 8 is though to be the causative agent of the epidemic keratoconjunctivitis.

3.1 ADENOVIRUSES

3.1.1 INTRODUCTION

Adenoviruses were first cultured and reported as a distinct viral taxonomic group by Rowe et al.[1] in 1953. They are classified into two genera *Mastadenovirus* and *Aviadenovirus*.[2] The genus *Mastadenovirus* includes human, simian, bovine, equine, porcine, ovine, canine, and oppossum viruses.[3] Morphologically, the adenoviruses represent nonenveloped, regular icosahedrons that are 65 to 80 nm in diameter.[4] Multiple numbers of structures known as "fibers" project from each of the viral vertices. Their length varies depending on the viral serotype.[5,6] The subclassification of the human adenoviruses is based on the hemagglutination patterns (the hemagglutinin is a determinant of the fiber polypeptide) with red blood cells of rat, rhesus monkeys, and other species.[7,8] The patterns defined four hemagglutination groups (I to IV). In addition, each of the latter comprises subgroups, namely: I (subgenus B), II (subgenus D), III (subgenera C, E, and F), and IV (subgenus A).[2,9,10] The subgenus B has been further subdivided into two subgroups B1 and B2 based on DNA and protein homology.[11] Each of the A to F subgroups consists of different serotypes designated with Arabic numbers.

Although adenoviruses of different groups do not recombine, there are polypeptides capable of functioning in complementation reactions between unrelated serotypes. However, within a group, viruses can recombine very efficiently.[12]

The antigenic relatedness of adenovirus tumor (T) antigens has been the basis of another classification scheme.[13] Members of each group will have at least one T-antigenic determinant in common.

Although, in general, viruses produce toxins on rare occasions, one of the adenovirus structural proteins, the penton, has been shown to be directly toxic to cells other than those intrinsically infected with replicating adenoviruses.[14,15] Ladisch et al.[16] have found penton in the blood of several fatal cases of adenovirus pneumonia.

The family of more than 42 serotypes of human adenoviruses has been associated with a wide variety of infections, including respiratory infections, conjunctivitis, hemorrhagic cystitis, and gastroenteritis.[17] Primary adenovirus infections with serotypes 1, 2, and 5 (parts of subgenus C) are common in infancy.[17] The infection is usually restricted to the upper respiratory tract, and the adenovirus may persist after infancy in tonsilar, adenoidal, and other lymphoid tissues. Not very common, but still described, have been infections of the central nervous system, such as meningo-encephalitis complicating infection of the respiratory tract.[18] While many adenovirus infections are subclinical, they result in antibody formation, and the adenovirus itself may be grown, especially from the gastrointestinal[19] and respiratory[20] tracts for months after the initial infection and immune response. The occurrence of oral ulcerations associated with adenovirus infection has also been documented.[21]

Nosocomial hospital outbreaks of adenovirus infections has been reported in both pediatric and adult units.[22-33] In addition, acute respiratory disease associated with adenovirus in military recruits is well known.[34,35]

The adenoviral serotype may be an important factor in determining whether a specific illness is associated with overwhelming infection. Thus, it has been determined that serotypes 1 to 3 and 5 to 7 were the major types responsible for respiratory infections in children.[32,36-40] For serotypes 3, 4, 7, 14, and 17, which predominate in cases of acute respiratory illness[32,35,37-40] and in the majority of reported hospital nosocomial outbreaks,[22-32] the presence of virulence factor may be possible.[33] Adenoviruses of subgenus B1, serotypes 3, 7 (especially 7h, a new genome type isolated in South America[38,41-43]), 16, and 21, have been associated with clinical manifestations of considerable severity.[27,38,44-46] Other virulent serotype 7 genome types are 7b (in Australia, Europe, and the U.S.), 7c (in Africa), and 7d (in China).[38,47] B2 adenovirus types 11, 34, and 35 are primarily isolated from urine.[48]

The association of adenoviruses with gastroenteritis is well established for serotypes 40 and 41 (subgenus F),[49] 12, 18, and 31 (subgenus A), and 1, 2, 5, and 6 (subgenus C).[37]

The role of adenovirus as a cause of hemorrhagic cystitis in children was first described by Numazaki et al.;[50] serotypes 11 and 35 appeared to be mostly involved.[51] In bone marrow transplant recipients, the risk of developing hemorrhagic cystitis is greatest from 2 weeks to 3 months after the transplantation.[52] While the precise mechanism of viral spread to the bladder is not known, it appeared that the initial viremia was followed by viruria and the travel of viral particles from the kidney to the bladder via the urine.[53]

3.1.2 ADENOVIRUS MODULATION OF IMMUNE RESPONSES

Several interesting *in vitro* studies have revealed the ability of some adenovirus early proteins to modulate host immune responses by interference with the expression of major histocompatibility complex (MHC) class I antigens.[54] As reported by Vaessen et al.,[55] in cells transformed by adenovirus type 12 (subgenus A), a serotype that is highly oncogenic to rodents, the adenovirus early region E1A was shown to specifically inhibit the post-transcriptional processing of class I mRNA. In another mechanism for reducing MHC antigen expression, in serotype 2 (subgenus C)-infected cells and in cells transfected with the serotype 2 early region 3 (E3), the E3-19K glycoprotein bound to class I antigens in the endoplasmic reticulum.[56,57]

In addition, Paabo et al.[58] demonstrated that antibody to MHC class I antigens co-immunoprecipitated the adenovirus early glycoproteins in cells infected with other subgenus B serotypes, as well as with serotypes of subgenera D and E. Furthermore, the fact that cell surface expression of class I MHC antigens was inhibited in cells infected with all of these serotypes appears to suggest this to be a general trait of the adenovirus family, including types 7 (a virulent serotype associated with severe lower respiratory tract disease), 35 (a serotype isolated primarily from immunocompromised hosts[59]), and 2 (a serotype commonly associated with upper respiratory tract infections in children).[54]

Taken into account, these protein–protein interactions indicate that inhibition of the normal processing and transport of the MHC antigens would result in their reduced expression on the cell surface *in vivo*. Since class I MHC antigen are necessary for cytotoxic T lymphocyte recognition of virus-infected cells, a reduction in the level of cell surface MHC antigens may not only modulate acute adenovirus pathogenicity,[60] but also play a role in the establishment of viral persistence and latency.[54]

3.1.2.1 Adenovirus Infections in Immunocompromised Hosts

Adenovirus infections in immunocompromised patients are manifested by high morbidity and mortality.[61-70] Patients (renal transplant recipients,[62,71] hematologic malignancies,[72] and AIDS[63,73]) have shown increased incidence of infections involving serotypes 11, 34, 35 (subgenus B1), and 43 (subgenus D).[48,54,62,66,73-81] Other studies have revealed serotype 5 (subgenus C) as the frequent cause of serious infections in patients undergoing chemotherapy,[74,82,83] in severe combined immuno-deficiency (SCID),[84] and in children receiving liver transplants.[85]

Adenoviruses of subgenus C have been implicated in cases of disseminated infections in immunocompromised host disease.[61,72,74,86-91] Krilov et al.[86] have described disseminated adenovirus infection with fatal hepatic necrosis in 16 patients (median age 4.7 years), 15 of whom had immunocompromised conditions most commonly due to HIV; serotypes 1, 2, 3, and 5 were the most prevalent.

Serotype 31 (subgenus A) has been the cause of considerable mortality in children with SCID,[92] and other immunocompromised patients.[64,73,74,93] Increasingly, type 31 has been associated with gastroenteritis.[37,49,94-98] Horoupian et al.[64] have described a case of an AIDS patient in whom a terminal dementing process and signs of upper motor neuron dysfunction were associated with symmetrical multiple tract degeneration involving frontopontine, corticospinal, and pontocerebellar fibers; adenovirus type 31 was isolated once from his cerebrospinal fluid.

Serotypes 40 and 41 (subgenus F) are only second in importance to rotaviruses as the etiologic agents of gastroenteritis in infants and young children.[49,99-101] Gastroenteritis due to adenovirus type 41 was also diagnosed in adult patients with AIDS[102] and chronic lymphocytic leukemia.[99]

Although cell-mediated immune deficiency appears to be a major predisposing factor to severe adenovirus disease, overwhelming infection cannot be limited to a particular immune defect, and the diagnosis should be considered in a broad range of immunocompromised hosts.[33]

Adenovirus infections can also be a consequence of reactivation of a persistent infection[72,74,86,91] acquired during childhood. However, primary adenovirus infections have not been excluded.[72,87,103] Renal transplantation has been suggested as a route of transmission for adenoviruses.[71] Patients with isolated defects in the humoral immunity (agammaglobulinemia),[75] hematologic malig-nancies,[61] bone marrow,[66,72,88] and liver[85] transplant recipients, have been reported to be also at risk.

Clinical manifestations of adenovirus infections include pharyngitis, pneumonitis, hematuria, diarrhea, liver dysfunction, disseminated intravascular coagulation, hepatitis, and multiorgan involvement.[34,104] Fulminant hepatitis has been diagnosed in association with the acquired immuno-deficiency syndrome, inherited immunodeficiency syndromes, and following liver or bone marrow transplantation.[86] Frequent coinfections with herpes simplex virus, cytomegalovirus, or both have been recognized.[65]

Morris et al.[103] and others[65,87] have reported fatal disseminated adenovirus subgenus C (serotype 2) infections following bone marrow transplantation. Major factors predisposing to adeno-virus infections in bone marrow transplant recipients may have included graft-vs.-host disease (GVHD),[65,74] pretransplant disease, or irregularities with the conditioning drug regimens.[91] To this end, minimizing immunosuppression by avoiding intensive pretransplant conditioning regimens and prevention of post-transplant GVHD would be beneficial.

Johansson et al.[82] have described adenovirus type 5 as the possible cause of severe gastroenteritis in an immunocompromised child undergoing cytostatic therapy (vincristine, adriamycin, predniso-lone, and methotrexate) for acute lymphatic leukemia. In addition, adenovirus infection has been associated with gastroenteritis in bone marrow transplant recipients; four of nine patients died as a result.[105] Adenovirus has also been suggested as the cause of colitis in an AIDS patient.[83] Elevated liver enzymes have been described in 8 of 11 (78%) immunocompromised patients with severe adenovirus infection.[106]

In conclusion, while immunocompromised hosts are no more at risk to adenovirus infections than immunocompetent persons, they have higher morbidity and mortality rates.[61,62,75,89]

3.1.3 TREATMENT OF ADENOVIRUS INFECTIONS

At present, antiviral therapy against adenovirus infection is not very efficacious. Although ribavirin showed *in vitro* antiviral activity, it has not been fully assessed *in vivo*.[86]

Several cases of hemorrhagic cystitis due to adenovirus have been described in immunocompromised patients.[53,76] In one of the studies, Londergan and Walzak[53] used intravenous ribavirin at 25 mg/kg, t.i.d. for 2 weeks to treat the infection (caused by serotype 11) in two bone marrow transplant recipients; the therapy had no effect in one of the patients, and possible beneficial effect in the other. Two other reports[107,108] described the use of ribavirin in the treatment of children with hemorrhagic cystitis secondary to bone marrow transplantation. In one of the studies,[108] the young patient (who weighed 30 kg) received 333 mg of intravenous ribavirin every 8 h for 3 doses, then 166 mg every 8 h for 24 doses, for a total course of 9 d; there was rapid resolution of symptoms and virus-negative urine cultures, with no adverse side effects being observed. Another case of successful therapy with intravenous ribavirin has been reported by McCarthy et al.[109] The patient, an infant with disseminated adenovirus infection with persistent high fever, received a loading dose of 30 mg/kg daily in three doses, followed by a maintenance dose of 15 mg/kg daily. The medication was well tolerated and daily blood counts remained normal throughout the period of ribavirin therapy. Prior administration of ganciclovir (5.0 mg/kg, b.i.d.) for 2 weeks at full dosage failed to bring any improvement,[109] even though ganciclovir has been shown to reduce adenovirus titers *in vitro*.[110,111]

Despite therapy with intravenous broad-spectrum antibiotics, amphotericin B, and acyclovir, a case of disseminated adenovirus type 2 infection secondary to bone marrow transplantation was fatal in an infant.[103]

3.1.4 REFERENCES

1. Rowe, W. P., Huebner, R. J., Gilmore, L. K., Parrott, R. H., and Ward, T. G., Isolation of a cytopathogenic agent from human adenoids undergoing spontaneous degeneration in tissue culture, *Proc. Soc. Exp. Biol. Med.*, 84, 570, 1953.
2. Norrby, E., Bartha, A., Boulanger, P., Dreizin, R. S., Ginsberg, H. S., Kalter, S. S., Kawamura, H., Rowe, W. P., Russell, W. C., Schlesinger, R. W., and Wigand, R., Adenoviridae, *Intervirology*, 7, 117, 1976.
3. Horwitz, M. S., Adenoviridae and their replication, in *Fields Virology*, 2nd ed., Fields, B. N., Knipe, D. M., Chanock, R. M., Hirsch, M. S., Melnick, J. L., Monath, T. P., and Roizman, B., Eds., Raven Press, New York, 1990, 1679.
4. Horne, R. W., Bonner, S., Waterson, A. P., and Wildy, P., The icosahedral form of an adenovirus, *J. Mol. Biol.*, 1, 84, 1959.
5. Norrby, E., The relationship between soluble antigens and the virion of adenovirus type 3. I. Morphological characteristics, *Virology*, 28, 236, 1966.
6. Norrby, E., The relationship between soluble antigens and the virion of adenovirus type 3. III. Immunologic characteristics, *Virology*, 37, 565, 1969.
7. Rosen, I., A hemagglutination-inhibition technique for typing adenoviruses, *Am. J. Hyg.*, 71, 120, 1960.
8. Hierholzer, J. C., Further subgrouping of the human adenoviruses by differential hemagglutination, *J. Infect. Dis.*, 128, 541, 1973.
9. Baum, S. G., Adenoviridae, in *Principles and Practice of Infectious Diseases*, 2nd ed., Mandel, G. L., Douglas, R. G., and Bennet, J. E., Eds., John Wiley & Sons, New York, 1984, 1353.
10. Wadell, G., Molecular epidemiology of human adenoviruses, *Curr. Top. Microbiol. Immunol.*, 110, 191, 1984.

11. Wadell, G., Hammarskjöld, M.-L., Winberg, G., Varsanyi, T. M., and Sundell, G., Genetic variability of adenoviruses, *Ann. NY Acad. Sci.*, 354, 16, 1980.

12. Sambrook, J., Williams, J. F., Sharp, P. A., and Grodzicker, T., Physical mapping of temperature sensitive mutations of adenoviruses, *J. Mol. Biol.*, 97, 369, 1975.

13. McAllister, R. M., Nicholson, M. O., Reed, G., Kern, J., Gilden, R. V., and Huebner, R. J., Transformation of rodent cells by adenovirus 19 and other group D adenoviruses, *J. Natl. Cancer Inst.*, 43, 917, 1969.

14. Pettersson, U. and Hoglund, S., Structural proteins of adenoviruses, *Virology*, 39, 90, 1969.

15. Valentine, R. C. and Periera, H. G., Antigens and structure of the adenovirus, *J. Mol. Biol.*, 13, 13, 1965.

16. Ladisch, S., Lovejoy, F. H., Hierholzer, J. C., Oxman, M. N., Strieder, D., Vawter, G. F., Finer, N., and Moore, M., Extrapulmonary manifestations of adenovirus type 7 pneumonia simulating Reye syndrome and the possible role of an adenovirus toxin, *J. Pediatr.*, 95, 348, 1979.

17. Horwitz, M. S., Adenovirus, in *Fields Virology*, 2nd ed., Fields, B. N., Knipe, D. M., Chanock, R. M., Hirsch, M. S., Melnick, J. L., Monath, T. P., and Roizman, B., Eds., Raven Press, New York, 1990, 1723.

18. Kelsey, D. S., Adenovirus meningoencephalitis, *Pediatrics*, 61, 291, 1978.

19. Fox, J. P., Brandt, C. D., Wassermann, F. E., Hall, C. E., Spigland, I., Kogon, A., and Elveback, L. R., The Virus Watch Program: a continuing surveillance of viral infections in metropolitan New York families. VI. Observation of adenovirus infections: virus excretion patterns, antibody response, efficiency of surveillance, patterns of infection and relations to illness, *Am. J. Epidemiol.*, 89, 25, 1969.

20. Evans, A. S., Latent adenovirus infections of the human respiratory tract, *Am. J. Hyg.*, 67, 256, 1958.

21. Sallay, K., Kulcsar, G., Nasz, I., Dan, P., and Geck, P., Adenovirus isolation from recurrent oral ulcers, *J. Periodontol.*, 44, 712, 1973.

22. Barr, J., Kjellén, L., and Svedmyr, A., Hospital outbreaks of adenovirus type 3 infections: a clinical and virological study on 38 patients partly involved in a nosocomial outbreak, *Acta Paediatr.*, 47, 365, 1958.

23. Flewett, T. H., Bryden, A. S., Davies, H., and Morris, C. A., Epidemic viral enteritis in a long-stay children's ward, *Lancet*, 1, 4, 1975.

24. Herbert, F. A., Wilkinson, D., Burchak, E., and Morgante, O., Adenovirus type 3 pneumonia causing lung damage in childhood, *Can. Med. Assoc. J.*, 116, 274, 1977.

25. Harrison, H. R., Howe, P., Minnich, L., and Ray, C. G., A cluster of adenovirus 19 infection with multiple clinical infections, *J. Pediatr.*, 94, 917, 1979.

26. Centers for Desease Control, Nosocomial outbreak of pharyngoconjunctivitis fever due to adenovirus, type 4 — New York, *Morbid. Mortal. Wkly Rep.*, 27, 49, 1978.

27. Straube, R. C., Thompson, M. A., Van Dyke, R. B., Wadell, G., Connor, J. D., Wingard, D., and Spector, S. A., Adenovirus type 7b in a children's hospital, *J. Infect. Dis.*, 147, 814, 1983.

28. Pingleton, S. K., Pingleton, E. W., Hill, R. H., Dixon, A., Sobonya, R. E., and Gertzen, J., Type 3 adenoviral pneumonia occurring in a respiratory intensive care unit, *Chest*, 73, 554, 1978.

29. Levandowski, R. A. and Rubenis, M., Nosocomial conjunctivitis caused by adenovirus type 4, *J. Infect. Dis.*, 143, 28, 1981.

30. Larsen, R. A., Jacobson, J. T., Jacobson, J. A., Strikas, R. A., and Hierholzer, J. C., Hospital-associated epidemic of pharyngitis and conjunctivitis caused by adenovirus (21/H21 + 35), *J. Infect. Dis.*, 154, 706, 1986.

31. Alpert, G., Charney, E., Fee, M., and Plotkin, S. A., Outbreak of fatal adenoviral type 7a respiratory disease in a children's long-term care inpatient facility, *Am. J. Infect. Control*, 14, 188, 1986.

32. Chany, C., Lépine, P., Lelong, M., Vihn, L.-T., Satge, P., and Virat, J., Severe and fatal pneumonia in infants and young children associated with adenovirus infections, *Am. J. Hyg.*, 67, 367, 1958.

33. Brummitt, C. F., Cherrington, J. M., Katzenstein, D. A., Juni, B. A., Van Drunen, N., Edelman, C., Rhame, F. S., and Jordan, M. C., Nosocomial adenovirus infections: molecular epidemiology of an outbreak due to adenovirus 3a, *J. Infect. Dis.*, 158, 423, 1988.

34. Dudding, B. A., Wagner, S. C., Zeller, J. A., Gmelich, J. T., French, G. R., and Top, F. H., Jr., Fatal pneumonia associated with adenovirus type 7 in three military trainees, *N. Engl. J. Med.*, 286, 1289, 1972.

35. Dudding, B. A., Top, F. H., Jr., Winter, P. E., Buescher, E. L., Lamson, T. H., and Liebovitz, A., Acute respiratory disease in military trainees: the adenovirus surveillance program, 1966-1971, *Am. J. Epidemiol.*, 97, 187, 1973.

36. Brandt, C. D., Kim, H. W., Vargosko, A. J., Jeffries, B. C., Arrobio, J. O., Rindge, B., Parrott, R. H., and Chanock, R. M., Infections in 18,000 infants and children in a controlled study of respiratory tract disease. I. Adenovirus pathogenicity in relation to serologic type and illness syndrome, *Am. J. Epidemiol.*, 90, 484, 1969.

37. Schmitz, H., Wigand, R., and Heinrich, W., Worldwide epidemiology of human adenovirus infections, *Am. J. Epidemiol.*, 117, 455, 1983.

38. Murtagh, P., Cerqueiro, C., Halac, A., Avila, M., and Kajon, A., Adenovirus type 7h respiratory infections: a report of 29 cases of acute lower respiratory disease, *Acta Pediatr.*, 82, 557, 1993.

39. Steen-Johnsen, J., Orstavik, J., and Attramadal, A., Severe illness due to adenovirus type 7 in children, *Acta Paediatr. Scand.*, 58, 157, 1969.

40. Becroft, D. M. O., Bronchiolitis obliterans, bronchiectasis and other sequelae of adenovirus type 21 infection in young children, *J. Clin. Pathol.*, 24, 72, 1971.

41. Kajon, A. E. and Wadell, G., Characterization of adenovirus genome type 7h: analysis of its relationship to other members of serotype 7, *Intervirology*, 33, 86, 1992.

42. Kajon, A. E. and Vicente Suarez, M., Molecular epidemiology of adenoviruses isolated from hospitalized children with severe lower acute respiratory infection in Santiago, Chile, *J. Med. Virol.*, 30, 294, 1990.

43. Kajon, A. E. and Wadell, G., Molecular epidemiology of adenoviruses associated with acute lower respiratory disease of children in Buenos Aires, Argentina (1984-1988), *J. Med. Virol.*, 36, 292, 1992.

44. Nahmias, A. J., Griffith, D., and Snitzer, J., Fatal pneumonia associated with adenovirus type 7, *Am. J. Dis. Child.*, 114, 36, 1967.

45. Wadell, G., Varsanyi, T. M., Lord, A., and Sutton, R. N. P., Epidemic outbreaks of adenovirus 7 with special reference to the pathogenicity of adenovirus genome type 7b, *Am. J. Epidemiol.*, 112, 619, 1980.

46. Simila, S., Linna, O., Lanning, P., Heikkinen, E., and Ala-Houhala, M., Chronic lung damage caused by adenovirus type 7: a ten-year follow-up study, *Chest*, 80, 127, 1981.

47. Wadell, G., Cooney, M. K., da Costa Linhares, A., de Silva, L., Kenett, M. L., Kono, R., Gui-Fang, R., Lindman, K., Nascimento, J. P., Schoub, B. D., and Smith, C. D., Molecular epidemiology of adenoviruses: global distribution of adenovirus 7 genome types, *J. Clin. Microbiol.*, 21, 403, 1985.

48. Flomenberg, P. R., Chen, M., Munk, G., and Horwitz, M. S., Molecular epidemiology of adenovirus type 35 infections in immunocompromised hosts, *J. Infect. Dis.*, 155, 1127, 1987.

49. Uhnoo, I., Wadell, G., Svensson, L., and Johansson, M. E., Importance of enteric adenoviruses 40 and 41 in acute gastroenteritis in infants and young children, *J. Clin. Microbiol.*, 20, 365, 1984.

50. Numazaki, Y., Shigeta, S., Kumasaka, T., Miyazura, T., Yamanaka, M., Yano, N., Takai, S., and Ishida, N., Acute hemorrhagic cystitis in children: isolation of adenovirus type 11, *N. Engl. J. Med.*, 278, 700, 1968.

51. Mufson, M. A., Belshe, R. B., Horrigan, T. J., and Zollar, L. M., Cause of acute hemorrhagic cystitis in children, *Am. J. Dis. Child.*, 126, 605, 1973.

52. Miyamura, K., Takeyama, K., Kojima, S., Minami, S., Matsuyama, K., Morishima, Y., and Kodera, Y., Hemorrhagic cystitis associated with urinary excretion of adenovirus type 11 following allogeneic bone transplantation, *Bone Marrow Transplant.*, 4, 533, 1989.

53. Londergan, T. A. and Walzak, M. P., Hemorrhagic cystitis due to adenovirus infection following bone marrow transplantation, *J. Urol.*, 151, 1013, 1994.

54. Flomenberg, P. R., Chen, M., and Horwitz, M. S., Characterization of a major histocompatibility complex class I antigen-binding glycoprotein from adenovirus type 35, a type associated with immunocompromised hosts, *J. Virol.*, 61, 3665, 1987.

55. Vaessen, R. T. M. J., Houweling, A., and Van Der Eb, A. J., Post-transcriptional control of class I MHC mRNA expression in adenovirus 12-transfected cells, *Science*, 235, 1486, 1987.

56. Andersson, M., Paabo, S., Nilsson, T., and Peterson, P. A., Impaired intracellular transport of class I MHC antigens as a possible means for adenoviruses to evade immune surveillance, *Cell*, 43, 215, 1985.

57. Burgert, H. and Kvist, S., An adenovirus type 2 glycoprotein blocks cell surface expression of human histocompatibility class I antigens, *Cell*, 41, 987, 1985.

58. Paabo, S., Nilsson, T., and Peterson, P. A., Adenoviruses of subgenera B, D, and E modulate cell-surface expression of major histocompatibility complex class I antigens, *Proc. Natl. Acad. Sci. U.S.A.*, 83, 9665, 1986.
59. Valderrama-Leon, G., Flomenberg, P., and Horwitz, M. S., Restriction endonuclease mapping of adenovirus 35, a type isolated from immunocompromised hosts, *J. Virol.*, 56, 647, 1985.
60. Doherty, P. C. and Zinkernagel, R. M., H-2 compatibility is required for T-cell-mediated lysis of target cell infected with lymphocytic choriomeningitis virus, *J. Exp. Med.*, 141, 502, 1975.
61. Zahradnik, J. M., Spenser, M. J., and Porter, D. D., Adenovirus infection in the immunocompromised patient, *Am. J. Med.*, 68, 725, 1980.
62. Stadler, H., Hierholzer, J. C., and Oxman, M. N., New human adenovirus (candidate adenovirus type 35) causing a fatal disseminated infection in a renal transplant recipient, *J. Clin. Microbiol.*, 6, 257, 1977.
63. De Jong, P. J., Valderrama, G., Spigland, I., and Horwitz, M. S., Adenovirus isolates from the urines of patients with acquired immunodeficiency syndrome, *Lancet*, 1, 1293, 1983.
64. Horoupian, D. S., Pick, P., Spigland, I., Smith, P., Portenoy, R., Katzman, R., and Cho, S., Acquired immune deficiency syndrome and multiple tract degeneration in a homosexual man, *Ann. Neurol.*, 15, 502, 1984.
65. Landry, M. L., Fong, C. K. Y., Neddermann, K., Solomon, L., and Hsiung, G. D., Disseminated adenovirus infection in an immunocompromised host: pitfalls in diagnosis, *Am. J. Med.*, 83, 555, 1987.
66. Ambinder, R. H., Burns, W. H., Forman, M., Santos, M., Santos, G. W., and Saral, R., Adenovirus infections in bone marrow transplant recipients, *Clin. Res.*, 32, 363A, 1984.
67. Akhter, J., Qadri, S. M. H., and Myint, S. H., Adenovirus infections in compromised and other patients at a tertiary referral centre in Saudi Arabia, *J. Infect.*, 31, 85, 1995.
68. Teague, M. W., Glick, A. D., and Fogo, A. B., Adenovirus infection of the kidney: mass formation in a patient with Hodgkin's desease, *Am. J. Kidney Dis.*, 18, 499, 1991.
69. Ljungman, P., Ehrnst, A., Bjorkstrand, B., Hellström, E., Ingelman- Sundberg, H., Juliusson, G., and Lönnqvist, B., Lethal disseminated adenovirus type 1 infection in a patient with chronic lymphocytic leukemia, *Scand. J. Infect. Dis.*, 22, 601, 1990.
70. Zahradnik, J. M., Adenovirus pneumonia, *Semin. Respir. Infect.*, 2, 104, 1987.
71. Myerowitz, R. L., Stadler, J., Oxman, M. N., Levin, M. J., Moore, M., Leith, J. D., Gantz, N. M., Pellegrini, J., and Hierholzer, J. C., Fatal disseminated adenovirus infection in a renal transplant recipients, *Am. J. Med.*, 59, 591, 1975.
72. Shields, A. F., Hackman, R. C., Meyers, J. D., Fife, K. H., and Corey, L., Fulminant liver failure induced by adenovirus after bone marrow transplantation, *N. Engl. J. Med.*, 312, 1708, 1985.
73. Hierholzer, J. C., Wigand, R., Anderson, L., Adrian, T., and Gold, J., Adenoviruses from patients with AIDS: a plethora of serotypes and a description of five new serotypes of subgenus D (types 43-47), *J. Infect. Dis.*, 158, 804, 1988.
74. Shields, A. F., Hackman, R. C., Fife, K. H., Corey, L., and Meyers, J. D., Adenovirus infection in patients undergoing bone marrow transplantation, *N. Engl. J. Med.*, 312, 529, 1985.
75. Siegal, F. P., Dikman, S. H., Arayata, R. B., and Bottone, E. J., Fatal disseminated adenovirus 11 pneumonia in an agammaglobulinemic patient, *Am. J. Med.*, 71, 1062, 1981.
76. Fiala, M., Payne, J. E., Berne, T. V., Poosawat, S., Schieble, J., and Guze, L., Role of adenovirus type 11 in hemorrhagic cystitis secondary to immunosuppression, *J. Urol.*, 112, 595, 1974.
77. Johansson, M. E., Brown, M., Hierholzer, J. C., Thörner, A., Ushijima, H., and Wadell, G., Genome analysis of adenovirus type 31 strains from immunocompromised and immunocompetent patients, *J. Infect. Dis.*, 163, 293, 1991.
78. Keller, E. W., Rubin, R. H., Black, P. H., Hirsch, M. S., and Hierholzer, J. C., Isolation of adenovirus type 34 from a renal transplant recipient with interstitial pneumonia, *Transplantation*, 23, 188, 1977.
79. Hammond, G. W., Mauthe, G., Joshua, J., and Hannan, C. K., Examination of uncommon clinical isolates of human adenoviruses by restriction endonuclease analysis, *J. Clin. Microbiol.*, 21, 611, 1985.
80. Ljungman, P., Gleaves, C. A., and Meyers, J. D., Respiratory virus infection in immunocompromised patients, *Bone Marrow Transplant.*, 4, 35, 1989.
81. Harnett, G. B., Bucens, M. R., Clay, S. J., and Saker, B. M., Acute hemorrhagic cystitis caused by adenovirus type 11 in a recipient of a transplanted kidney, *Med. J. Aust.*, 1, 565, 1982.

82. Johansson, M. E., Zweygberg Wirgart, B., Grillner, L., and Björk, O., Severe gastroenteritis in an immunocompromised child caused by adenovirus type 5, *Pediatr. Infect. Dis. J.*, 9, 449, 1990.

83. Carmichael, G. P., Zahradnik, J. M., Moyer, G. H., and Porter, D., Adenovirus hepatitis in an immunocompromised adult patient, *Am. J. Clin. Pathol.*, 71, 352, 1979.

84. South, M. A., Dolen, J., Beach, D. K., and Mirkovic, R. R., Fatal adenovirus hepatic necrosis in severe combined immune deficiency, *Pediatr. Infect. Dis. J.*, 1, 416, 1982.

85. Koneru, B., Jaffe, R., Esquivel, C. O., Kunz, R., Todo, S., Iwatsuki, S., and Starzl, T. E., Adenoviral infections in pediatric liver transplant recipients, *JAMA*, 258, 489, 1987.

86. Krilov, L. R., Rubin, L. G., Frogel, M., Gloster, E., Ni, K., Kaplan, M., and Lipson, S. M., Disseminated adenovirus infection with hepatic necrosis in patients with human immunodeficiency virus infection and other immunodeficiency states, *Rev. Infect. Dis.*, 12, 303, 1990.

87. Purtilo, D. T., White, R., Filipovich, A., Kersey, J., and Zelkowitz, L., Fulminant liver failure induced by adenovirus after bone marrow transplantation, *N. Engl. J. Med.*, 312, 1707, 1985.

88. Webb, D. H., Shields, A. F., and Fife, K. H., Genomic variation of adenovirus type 5 isolates recovered from bone marrow transplant recipients, *J. Clin. Microbiol.*, 25, 305, 1985.

89. Wigger, H. J. and Blanc, W. A., Fatal hepatic and bronchial necrosis in adenovirus infection with thymic alymphoplasia, *N. Engl. J. Med.*, 275, 870, 1966.

90. Ohbu, M., Sasaki, K., Okudaira, M., Iidaka, K., and Aouama, Y., Adenovirus hepatitis in a patient with severe combined immunodeficiency, *Acta Pathol. Jpn.*, 37, 655, 1987.

91. Wasserman, R., August, C. S., and Plotkin, S. A., Viral infections in paediatric bone marrow transplant patients, *Pediatr. Infect. Dis. J.*, 7, 109, 1988.

92. Gold, J. W. M., Yu, B., Brigati, D., Bernard, E. M., Brown, A. E., O'Reilly, R. J., Hierholzer, J., and Armstrong, D., Disseminated adenovirus infection in marrow transplant unit patients, *Clin. Res.*, 29, 385A, 1981.

93. Rodriguez, F. H., Liuzza, G. E., and Gohd, R. H., Disseminated adenovirus 31 infection in an immunocompromised host, *Am. J. Clin. Pathol.*, 82, 615, 1984.

94. Brown, M., Laboratory identification of adenoviruses associated with gastroenteritis in Canada from 1983 to 1986, *Clin. Microbiol.*, 28, 1525, 1990.

95. Johansson, M. E., Brundin, M., Adamson, L., Grillner, L., Landqvist, M., Thörner, A., and Zweygbert Wirgart, B., Characterization of two genome types of adenovirus type 31 isolated in Stockholm during 1987, *J. Med. Virol.*, 28, 63, 1989.

96. Ushijima, H. J., Eshita, Y., Araki, K., Shinozaki, T., Togo, T., and Matsunaga, Y., A study of adenovirus gastroenteritis in the Tokyo area, *Eur. J. Pediatr.*, 147, 90, 1988.

97. Adrian, T. and Wigand, R., Genome type analysis of adenovirus 31, a potential causative agent of infant's enteritis, *Arch. Virol.*, 105, 81, 1989.

98. Johansson, M. E., Uhnoo, I., Kidd, A. H., Madeley, C. R., and Wadell, G., Direct identification of enteric adenovirus, a candidate new serotype, associated with infantile gastroenteritis, *J. Clin. Microbiol.*, 12, 95, 1980.

99. Bates, P. R., Bailey, A. S., Wood, D. J., Morris, D. J., and Couriel, J. M., Comparative epidemiology of rotavirus, subgenus F (types 40 and 41) adenovirus and astrovirus gastroenteritis in children, *J. Med. Virol.*, 39, 224, 1993.

100. Morris, D. J., Virus infections in children with cancer, *Rev. Med. Microbiol.*, 1, 49, 1990.

101. de Jong, J. C., Bijlsma, K., Wermenbol, A. G., Verweij-Uijterwaal, M. W., van der Avoort, H. G. A. M., Wood, D. J., Bailey, A. S., and Osterhaus, A. D. M. E., Detection, typing, and subtyping of enteric adenoviruses 40 and 41 from fecal samples and observation of changing incidences of infections with these types and subtypes, *J. Clin. Microbiol.*, 31, 1562, 1993.

102. Cunningham, A. L., Grohman, G. S., Harkness, J., Law, C., Marriott, D., Tindall, B., and Cooper, D. A., Gastrointestinal viral infections in homosexual men who were symptomatic and seropositive for human immunodeficiency virus, *J. Infect. Dis.*, 158, 386, 1988.

103. Morris, D. J., Corbitt, G., Bailey, A. S., Newbould, M., Smith, E., Picton, S., and Stevens, R. F., Fatal disseminated adenovirus type 2 infection following bone marrow transplantation for Hurler's syndrome: a primary infection, *J. Infect.*, 26, 181, 1993.

104. Odio, C., McCracken, G. H., Jr., and Nelson, J. D., Disseminated adenovirus infection: a case report and review of the literature, *Pediatr. Infect. Dis. J.*, 3, 46, 1984.

105. Yolken, R. H., Bishop, C. A., Townsend, T. R., Bolyard, E. A., Bartlett, J., Santos, G. W., and Saral, R., Infectious gastroenteritis in bone- marrow-transplant recipients, *N. Engl. J. Med.*, 306, 1010, 1982.

106. Andiman, W. A., Jacobson, R. I., and Tucker, G., Leukocyte-associated viremia with adenovirus type 2 in an infant with lower-respiratory-tract disease, *N. Engl. J. Med.*, 297, 100, 1977.

107. Murphy, G. F., Wood, D. P., Jr., McRoberts, J. W., and Henslee-Downey, P. J., Adenovirus-associated hemorrhagic cystitis treated with intravenous ribavarin, *J. Urol.*, 149, 565, 1993.

108. Cassano, W. F., Intravenous ribavirin treatment for adenovirus cystitis after allogeneic bone marrow transplantation, *Bone Marrow Transplant.*, 7, 247, 1991.

109. McCarthy, A. J., Bergin, M., De Silva, L. M., and Stevens, M., Intravenous ribavirin therapy for disseminated adenovirus infection, *Pediatr. Infect. Dis. J.*, 14, 1003, 1995.

110. Taylor, D. L., Jeffries, D. J., Taylor-Robinson, D., Parkin, J. M., and Tyms, A. S., The susceptibility of adenovirus infection to the anti-cytomegalovirus drug, ganciclovir (DHPG), *FEMS Microbiol. Lett.*, 49, 337, 1988.

111. Wreghitt, T. G., Gray, J. J., Ward, K. N., Salt, A., Taylor, D. L., Alp, N. J., and Tyms, A. S., Disseminated adenovirus infection after liver transplantation and its possible treatment with ganciclovir, *J. Infect.*, 19, 88, 1989.

4 Parvoviridae

The parvovirus (also called picodnavirus) is a genus of viruses that belongs to the family Parvoviridae, which comprises three genera: *Parvovirus, Densovirus* (densonucleosis virus), and *Dependovirus,* which includes the adeno-associated satellite virus (AAV). Parvoviridae are the smallest known DNA viruses (18 to 25 nm; 1.39 to 1.45 g/ml density), comprised entirely of protein and DNA. They lack envelopes and are composed of a 5.5-kb length single-strand DNA, either positive or negative sense, each type of which is fully capable of infection and replication.[1,2] The viral capsid is of cubic symmetry with 32 capsomeres. Molecular analysis has demonstrated that both viral replication and assembly occur in the nucleus of the infected cells.[3,4]

The parvoviruses and dependoviruses are widespread among warm-blooded animals and humans. The adeno-associated viruses are unique among the animal viruses because (except for special conditions) they require coinfection with an unrelated virus, either adenovirus or herpesvirus, for productive infection in cell culture. The densonucleosis viruses have so far been isolated only from *Lepidoptera* and *Orthoptera* species.

Possibly because of their simplicity, the parvoviruses are extremely resistant to inactivation — they were found to be stable at pH ranging between 3 and 9, and at 60°C for 60 min. However, the virus still can be inactivated with formalin, β-propiolactone, hydroxylamine, and oxidizing agents.

4.1 HUMAN PARVOVIRUS B19

4.1.1 INTRODUCTION

The B19 strain is the only strain of human parvovirus that has been consistently demonstrated and studied. It was identified initially[5] during screening of blood for hepatitis B antigen in serum samples that tested negative for hepatitis B, and later confirmed as parvovirus by electron microscopy.[6,7] A comparison of 17 B19 isolates has revealed the existence of several restriction endonuclease variants within B19 isolates.[8] The parvovirus B19 strain has been found resistant at temperatures below 100°C.[9-12] Transmission of human parvovirus B19 by blood transfusion as a source of infection, although not firmly established, has been suspected in a patient with chronic myelomonocytic leukemia who received multiple erythrocyte transfusions.[13] Both seroconversion[11,14] and clinical infection with seroconversion[10] have been observed after administration of heat-treated factor concentrates to patients with hemophilia. However, the possibility that a solvent-detergent and terminally dry-heated factor VIII concentrate may transmit human parvovirus B19 infection in previously untreated hemophilia patients[15,16] is still the subject of debate.[17,18]

A second parvovirus strain, RA-1, which is antigenically distinct from B19, has been reported in association with rheumatoid arthritis.[19,20]

In humans, the B19 strain of parvovirus can directly infect hematopoietic cells, causing several distinct clinical diseases:[21] aplastic crisis in patients with chronic hemolytic anemia,[22-26] persistent bone marrow depression (chronic marrow hypoplasia) in immunocompromised hosts, and non-immune hydrops fetalis and fetal wastage.[27-29] While neutropenia and thrombocytopenia with decreased myeloid and megakaryocytic cells may occur in B19 infections, the erythroid cell line is the one most frequently susceptible to inhibition by parvovirus.[30-33] Giant pronormoblasts in the bone marrow are characteristic of human parvovirus B19 infections. The degree of hematologic expression of parvovirus B19 may also be related to bone marrow proliferation. It is well known that the replication of autonomous parvoviruses required that the host cell pass through an S-phase.[34]

Erythema infectiosum, arthritis, and purpuric vasculitis are postinfectious manifestations of B19 parvovirus infections.[1,35,36] Well over 50% of the adult human population has been found to carry anti-B19 antibodies,[37] an indication of earlier infection and likely lifelong immunity to the virus.[1]

Patients with congenital or acquired immunodeficiencies are susceptible to chronic parvovirus B19 infection and bone marrow suppression affecting all cell lines.[38-40] Thus, patients with congenital immunodeficiencies, such as Nazelof's syndrome, bone marrow transplant recipients,[41] malignancies (acute lymphoblastic leukemia,[38,40,42-50] Burkitt's lymphosarcoma,[6] rabdomyosarcoma[44,51]), or AIDS[52-54] have been reported to develop persistent B19 infection.[35,37,39] Such patients failed to develop neutralizing antibodies to the minor capsid protein, VP1.[37,55] Azzi et al.[43] reported aplastic crisis caused by B19 parvovirus in an immunosuppressed child during induction of therapy for acute lymphoblastic leukemia. In another report, persistent B19 infection leading to chronic bone marrow failure was described in a subject with combined immunodeficiency.[39]

In a study by Naides et al.,[56] some patients with AIDS who developed severe anemia while receiving zidovudine therapy also had persistent B19 parvovirus viremia. The authors suggested that the possibility of B19 infection exists whenever cytopenias occur, particularly in the setting of severe anemia. However, data from a study[57] which included all HIV-infected patients with anemia (and not only those receiving zidovudine) indicated that B19 infections may not be a common cause of anemia in patients on concomitant zidovudine therapy, and that anemia in HIV-infected patients may, in fact, be multifactorial in origin.[58,59] Taken together, the aforementioned results[56,57] indicated that AIDS patients with lower CD4+ cell counts are at greater risk of B19 viremia and B19-related anemia than HIV-positive patients without symptoms or those in the early stage of the disease when the CD4+ cell counts were still relatively normal. Whether the increased risk in late HIV infection represents B19 reactivation of latent infection or a higher infection rate on exposure remains to be determined.[56]

Graeve et al.[42] have reported several cases of cancer patients who developed human parvovirus infection while receiving myelosuppressive or immunosuppressive chemotherapy. In addition to aplastic crisis, the patients presented with some atypical manifestations (prolonged myelosuppression, and absent or prolonged cutaneous eruption) associated with parvovirus B19 infection.

The relationship between parvovirus B19 infection and classic rheumatoid arthritis remains to be determined. Although rheumatoid factor as a marker of classic rheumatoid arthritis has been reported only rarely in association with human parvovirus B19 arthropathy,[60-65] reports of a rheumatoid-like arthritis of variable duration following acute human parvovirus B19 infection have suggested HPV as the etiologic candidate for at least a subset of rheumatoid arthritis.[36,60-62,65,66] Naides and Field[36] described two cases of adult erythema infectiosum (fifth disease) associated with transiently elevated levels of rheumatoid factor.

Human parvovirus B19 has also been associated with various neuropathies and vasculitises.[67] Thus, the B19 virus was serologically confirmed in nonthrombocytic purpura, such as the Henoch-Schönlein purpura.[67,68] In addition, the presence of positive parvovirus B19 IgM immunoglobulins with subsequent conversion to IgG immunoglobulins has been established in association with temporal arteritis, polyarteritis nodosa, and Wegener's granulomatosis.[69,70] The development of disease symptoms was believed to be related to postinfectious, immune-mediated mechanisms.[67] In a study of patients with immune-mediated inner ear disease, Cotter et al.[71] found 14 of 17 patients to have parvovirus B19 IgM and/or IgG antibodies, and to respond to immunosuppressive therapy. Because of the association of parvovirus B19 with systemic immune disorders known to have otologic manifestations, these authors suggested that B19 virus may be a possible etiology of the immune-mediated inner ear disease.[71]

4.1.2. Aplastic Crisis and Chronic Bone Marrow Suppression

In normal individuals, this syndrome is characterized mainly with transient inhibition of erythropoiesis with reticulocytopenia,[30,72] although to a lesser extent other blood cells may also be affected. The bone marrow depression commonly appears 1 week after infection and usually lasts for another week. In persons with a normal life span of circulating red blood cells (120 d) these changes usually go unnoticed. However, in patients with chronic hemolytic anemias the life span of circulating red blood cells is shortened (10 to 15 d), and parvovirus B19 infections in these individuals may result in aplastic crisis manifested by a precipitous fall in hemoglobin without reticulocyte response.[1] During aplastic crisis reticulocytes are absent from the blood, and erythroid precursors are significantly diminished in the bone marrow for a period of 5 to 10 d. Bone marrow depression (very few erythroid line precursors)[72] is especially frequent in patients with sickle cell anemia,[22,23,73-75] with hereditary spherocytosis,[76] pyruvate kinase deficiency,[77] heterozygous beta-thalassemia,[78] dyserythropoietic anemia,[79] autoimmune hemolytic anemia,[80] and G6PD deficiency.[1] However, it has been reported that in some patients with aplastic crisis there has been no evidence of recent human parvovirus infection,[81] probably due to false-negative testing or because of different pathogens that can cause this syndrome.

4.1.3 Bone Marrow Necrosis

Defined as extensive necrosis of the myelogenous tissue, bone marrow necrosis is a rare syndrome with unknown pathogenesis, but generally related to an underlying disorder, such as sickle cell disease and acute leukemia.[82-87] So far, several hypotheses have been proposed to explain the pathophysiology of bone marrow necrosis, including microcirculatory failure, vascular occlusion, compression by tumoral process, bacterial endotoxins, a drop of regional oxygen tension, tumor necrosis factor, and viral agents.[85] Petrella et al.[88] have described a case of bone marrow necrosis associated with serologically documented recent parvovirus B19 infection preceding the development of a Ph1+ acute lymphoblastic leukemia. This finding may suggest the possibility of B19 virus being a cofactor of bone marrow necrosis induction in conjunction with an underlying disorder.

4.1.4 Erythema Infectiosum (Fifth Disease)

Erythema infectiosum was the fifth of the original childhood exanthematous diseases, which now has been firmly established to be caused by human parvovirus infection.[24,89-91] The illness is manifested with a lacy rash, most frequently on the face (known as the "slapped-cheek" facial rash). In general, erythema infectiosum is a benign disease except in patients with chronic hemolytic anemia, immunocompromised individuals, and during pregnancy.[1]

Erythema infectiosum may be associated with arthralgia with or without arthritis.[36] Thus, Ager et al.[92] found arthralgia in 7.8% of 307 patients with fifth disease and under 20 years of age, and in 77.2% of 57 adult patients.

4.1.5 Evolution of Therapies and Treatment of Human Parvovirus B19 Infections

The greatest risk of parvovirus B19 infection is to immunocompromised hosts, such as patients with acquired or congenital immune deficiency,[35,38,39,41,53] those with leukemia, and the fetus.

In general, the management of pure red cell aplasia (PRCA)[93-95] is difficult because of its different and poorly understood pathophysiology.[96] However, high-dose intravenous immunoglobulin therapy has been found effective in PRCA associated with human parvovirus B19 infection and impaired IgG-antibody response.[97-100] Normally, the B19 infection is terminated with the development of specific antibodies which neutralize the activity of the virus.[35,48,51,101]

In immunocompromised and possibly also in immunocompetent patients[102] the B19 parvovirus persists because of the impaired ability of the host to produce neutralizing antibodies.[96]

The most often recommended treatment regimen consists of intravenous gammaglobulin at 400 mg/kg daily for 5 to 10 d; maintenance therapy or retreatment may be needed.[48,52,53,96] The role of immunoglobulins in the treatment of PRCA is thought to involve blockade of the Fc-receptors and neutralization of host antibodies with anti-idiotype IgG.[103-105]

In two studies by Frickhofen et al.[52] and Griffin et al.,[53] HIV-infected patients with chronic human parvovirus B19-induced erythroid hypoplasia were treated with intravenous gammaglobulin at 400 mg/kg daily for 5 to 10 days. Prompt reticulocytosis and rise in hemoglobin levels followed the treatment. However, all patients with CD4$^+$ cell counts of <100 cells/mm^3 had relapses of erythroid hypoplasia requiring retreatment; by comparison, patients with CD4$^+$ cell counts of >100 cells/mm^3 had remissions lasting 7 to 13 months after a single course of gammaglobulin therapy.[52] Maintenance therapy with monthly infusion of gammaglobulin (400 mg/kg) was necessary in patients with severely depressed CD4$^+$ cell counts.[52,53]

Symptomatic aplastic crisis is usually treated with transfusion of red blood cells; recurrence is unlikely.[1] In immunocompromised patients, chronic bone marrow depression has been treated with intravenous gammaglobulin and/or withdrawal chemotherapy.[106] However, this therapy has not been systematically studied. Kurtzman and Young[107] have successfully treated with immunoglobulin an adult immunodeficient patient with chronic parvovirus B19 infection and pure red blood cell aplasia.

Treatment of another chronically anemic and transfusion-dependent patient with plasma containing anti-B19 antibodies produced a decrease in the serum virus levels, as well as improvement in the reticulocyte count and development of the fifth disease.[50]

In several AIDS patients with concurrent B19 infection and chronic anemia, intravenous administration of commercial immunoglobulin has corrected chronic anemia secondary to persistent B19 infection, presumably because of passive immunization with B19 neutralizing antibodies.[52] In addition to intravenous infusion, intramuscular administration of immune serum globulin (ISG) also prevented the B19 viremia and presumably the viral shedding; ISG increased the reticulocyte counts and hemoglobin.[56] Furthermore, treatment with ISG may have also reduced the risk of inadvertent transmission of parvovirus B19 to other immunocompromised patients or women of childbearing age.

Atypical exanthema manifestations (nonspecific itching, macular eruption) have been associated with parvovirus B19 infections.[108,109] To this end, Lobkowitz et al.[110] described a case of a patient with acute parvovirus B19 infection who developed erythema multiforme after oral administration of methylprednisolone; the case resolved during gradual tapering and withdrawal of steroid therapy.

4.1.6 REFERENCES

1. Rotbart, H. A., Human parvovirus infections, *Annu. Rev. Med.*, 41, 25, 1990.
2. Summers, J., Jones, S. E., and Anderson, M. E., Characterization of the genome of the agent of erythrocyte aplasia permits its classification as a human parvovirus, *J. Gen. Virol.*, 64, 2527, 1983.
3. Young, N., Harrison, M., Moore, J., Mortimer, P., and Humphries, P. K., Direct demonstration of the human parvovirus in erythroid progenitor cells infected in vitro, *J. Clin. Invest.*, 74, 2024, 1984.
4. Kurtzman, G. J., Gascon, P., Caras, M., Cohen, B., and Young, N. S., B19 parvovirus replicates in circulating cells of acutely infected patients, *Blood*, 71, 1448, 1988.
5. Cossart, Y. E., Field, A. M., Cant, B., and Widdows, D., Parvovirus-like particles in human sera, *Lancet*, 1, 72, 1975.
6. Courouce, A.-M., Ferchal, F., Morinet, F., Muller, A., Drouet, J., Soulier, J. P., and Perol, Y., Human parvovirus infection in France, *Lancet*, 1, 160, 1984.
7. Okochi, K., Mori, R., Miyazaki, M., Cohen, B. J., and Mortimer, P. P., Nakatani antigen and human parvovirus (B19), *Lancet*, 1, 160, 1984.

8. Morinet, F., Tratschin, J.-D., Perol, Y., and Siegl, G., Comparison of 17 isolates of the human parvovirus B19 by restriction enzyme analysis, *Arch. Virol.*, 90, 165, 1986.

9. Azzi, A., Ciappi, S., Zakrzewska, K., Morfini, M., Mariani, G., and Marcucci, P. M., Human parvovirus B19 infection in hemophiliacs first infused with two high-purity, virally attenuated factor VIII concentrates, *J. Haematol.*, 39, 228, 1992.

10. Lyon, D. G., Chapman, C. S., Martin, C., Brown, K. E., Clewley, J. P., Flower, A. J. E., and Mitchell, V. E., Symptomatic parvovirus B19 infection and heat-treated factor IX concentrate, *Lancet*, 1, 1085, 1989.

11. Corsi, O. B., Azzi, A., Morfini, M., Fauci, R., and Ferrini, P. R., Human parvovirus infection in haemophiliacs first infused with treated clotting factor concentrate, *J. Med. Virol.*, 25, 165, 1988.

12. Rubinstein, A., Rubinstein, D. B., and Coughlin, J., Combined solvent detergent and 100°C (boiling) sterilizing dry-heat treatment of factor VIII concentrates to assure sterility, *Vox Sang.*, 60, 60, 1991.

13. Malarme, M., Vandervelde, D., and Brasseur, M., Parvovirus infection, leukaemia and immunodeficiency, *Lancet*, 1, 1457, 1989.

14. Mortimer, P. P., Luban, N. L. C., Kelleher, J. F., and Cohen, B. J., Transmission of serum parvovirus-like virus by clotting factor concentrates, *Lancet*, 2, 482, 1983,

15. Santagostino, E., Mannucci, P. M., Gringeri, A., Azzi, A., and Morfini, M., Eliminating parvovirus B19 from blood products, *Lancet*, 343, 798, 1994.

16. Guillaume, T., Parvovirus B19 and blood products, *Lancet*, 343, 1101, 1994.

17. Di Napoli, G. and Bucci, E., Human parvovirus B19 after concentrates for haemophilia, *Lancet*, 343, 1566, 1994.

18. Prowse, C. V., Parvovirus B19 and blood products, *Lancet*, 343, 1101, 1994.

19. Simpson, R. W., McGinty, L., Simon, L., Smith, C. A., Godzeski, C. W., and Boyd, R. J., Association of parvoviruses with rheumatoid arthritis of humans, *Science*, 223, 1425, 1983.

20. Stierle, G., Brown, K. A., Rainsford, S. G., Smith, C. A., Hamermann, D., Stierle, H, E., and Dumonde, D. C., Parvovirus associated antigen in the synovial membrane of patients with rheumatoid arthritis, *Ann. Rheum. Dis.*, 46, 219, 1987.

21. Anderson, L. J., Role of parvovirus B19 in human disease, *Pediatr. Infect. Dis. J.*, 6, 711, 1987.

22. Pattison, J. R., Jones, S. E., Hodgson, J., Davis, L. R., White, J. M., Stroud, C. E., and Murtaza, L., Parvovirus infections and hypoplastic crisis in sickle-cell anaemia, *Lancet*, 1, 664, 1981.

23. Serjeant, G. R., Mason, K., Topley, J. M., Serjeant, B. E., Pattison, J. R., Jones, S. E., and Mohamed, R., Outbreak of aplastic crisis in sickle cell anaemia associated with parvovirus-like agent, *Lancet*, 2, 595, 1981.

24. Chorba, T., Coccia, P., Holman, R. C., Tattersall, P., Anderson, L. J., Sudman, J., Young, N. S., Kurczynski, E., Saarinen, U. M., Moir, R., Lawrence, D. N., Jason, J. M., and Evatt, B., The role of parvovirus B19 in aplastic crisis and erythema infectiosum (fifth disease), *J. Infect. Dis.*, 154, 383, 1986.

25. Anderson, M. J., Davis, L. R., Hodgson, J., Jones, S. E., Murtaza, L., Pattison, J. R., Stroud, C. E., and White, J. M., Occurrence of infection with a parvovirus-like agent in children with sickle cell anemia during a two year period, *J. Clin. Pathol.*, 35, 744, 1982.

26. Rao, K. R. P., Patel, A. R., Anderson, M. J., Hodgson, J., Jones, S. E., and Pattison, J. R., Infection with parvovirus-like virus and aplastic crisis in chronic hemolytic anemia, *Ann. Intern. Med.*, 98, 930, 1983.

27. Anand, A., Gray, E., Brown, T., Clewley, J. P., and Cohen, B. J., Human parvovirus infection in pregnancy and hydrops fetalis, *N. Engl. J. Med.*, 316, 183, 1987.

28. Woernle, C. H., Anderson, L. J., Tattersall, P., and Davison, J. M., Human parvovirus B19 infection during pregnancy, *J. Infect. Dis.*, 156, 17, 1987.

29. Clarke, H. C., Erythema infectiosum: an epidemic with a probable posterythema phase, *Can. Med. Assoc. J.*, 130, 603, 1984.

30. Anderson, M. J., Higgins, P. G., Davis, L. R., Willman, J. S., Jones, S. E., Kidd, I. M., Pattison, J. R., and Tyrrell, D. A., Experimental parvovirus infection in humans, *J. Infect. Dis.*, 152, 257, 1985.

31. Saunders, P. W. G., Reid, M. M., and Cohen, B. J., Human parvovirus induced cytopenias, *Br. J. Haematol.*, 63, 407, 1986.

32. Frickhofen, N., Raghavachar, A., Heit, W., and Heimpel, H., Human parvovirus infection, *N. Engl. J. Med.*, 314, 646, 1986.

33. Mortimer, P. P., Humphries, R. K., Moore, J. G., Purcell, R. H., and Young, N. S., A human parvovirus-like virus inhibits haematopoietic colony formation in vitro, *Nature*, 302, 426, 1983.

34. Siegl, G., Biology and pathogenicity of autonomous parvoviruses, in *The Parvoviruses*, Berns, K. I., Ed., Plenum Press, New York, 1984, 297.

35. Naides, S. J., Parvoviruses, in *Clinical Virology Manual*, 2nd ed., Specter, S. and Lancz, G., Eds., Elsevier Science Publishers, Cambridge, UK, 1992, 547.

36. Naides, S. J. and Field, E. H., Transient rheumatoid factor positivity in acute human parvovirus B19 infection, *Arch. Intern. Med.*, 148, 2587, 1988.

37. Kurtzman, G. J., Cohen, B. J., Field, A. M., Oseas, R., Blaese, R. M., and Young, N. S., Immune response to B19 parvovirus and an antibody defect in persistent viral infection, *J. Clin. Invest.*, 84, 1114, 1989.

38. Van Horn, D. K., Mortimer, P. P., Young, N., and Hanson, G. R., Human parvovirus-associated red cell aplasia in the absence of underlying hemolytic anemia, *Am. J. Pediatr. Hematol./Oncol.*, 8, 235, 1986.

39. Kurtzman, G. J., Ozawa, K., Cohen, B., Hanson, G., Oseas, R., and Young, N. S., Chronic bone marrow failure due to persistent B19 parvovirus infection, *N. Engl. J. Med.*, 317, 287, 1987.

40. Smith, M. A., Shah, N. R., Lobel, J. S., Cera, P. J., Gary, G. W., and Anderson, L. J., Severe anemia caused by human parvovirus in a leukemia patient on maintenance chemotherapy, *Clin. Pediatr.*, 27, 383, 1988.

41. Weiland, H. T., Salimans, M. M. M., Fibbe, W. E., Kluin, P. M., and Cohen, B. J., Prolonged parvovirus B19 infection with severe anaemia in a bone marrow transplant recipient, *Br. J. Haematol.*, 71, 300, 1989.

42. Graeve, J. L. A., de Alarcon, P. A., and Naides, S. J., Parvovirus B19 infection in patients receiving cancer chemotherapy: the expanding spectrum of disease, *Am. J. Pediatr. Hematol./Oncol.*, 11, 441, 1989.

43. Azzi, A., Macchia, P. A., Favre, C., Nardi, M., Zakrzewska, K., and Corsi, O. B., Aplastic crisis caused by B19 virus in a child during induction therapy for acute lymphoblastic leukemia, *Haematologica*, 74, 191, 1989.

44. Rao, S. P., Miller, S. T., and Cohen, B. J., Severe anemia due to B19 parvovirus infection in children with acute leukemia in remission, *Am. J. Pediatr. Hematol./Oncol.*, 12, 194, 1990.

45. Sallan, S. and Buchanan, G., Selective erythroid aplasia during therapy for lymphoblastic leukemia, *Pediatrics*, 59, 895, 1977.

46. Coulombel, L., Morinet, F., Mielot, F., and Tchernia, G., Parvovirus infection: leukaemia and immuno-deficiency, *Lancet*, 1, 101, 1989.

47. Carstensen, H., Ornvold, K., and Cohen, B. J., Human parvovirus B19 infection associated with prolonged erythroblastopenia in a leukemic child, *Pediatr. Infect. Dis. J.*, 8, 56, 1989.

48. Koch, W. C., Massey, G., Russell, C. E., and Adler, S. P., Manifestations and treatment of human parvovirus B19 infection in immunocompromised patients, *J. Pediatr.*, 116, 355, 1990.

49. Takahashi, M., Moriyama, Y., Shibata, A., Takai, K., and Sanada, M., Anemia caused by parvovirus in an adult patient with acute lymphoblastic leukemia in complete remission, *Eur. J. Haematol.*, 46, 47, 1991.

50. Kurtzman, G. J., Meyers, P., Cohen, B., Amunullah, A., and Young, N. S., Persistent B19 parvovirus infection as a cause of severe chronic anaemia in children with acute lymphocytic leukaemia, *Lancet*, 2, 1159, 1988.

51. Shaw, P. J., Eden, T., and Cohen, B. J., Parvovirus B19 as a cause of chronic anemia in rhabdo-myosarcoma, *Cancer*, 72, 945, 1993.

52. Frickhofen, N., Abkowitz, J. L., Safford, M., Berry, J. M., Antunez-de-Mayolo, J., Astrow, A., Cohen, R., Halperin, I., King, L., Mintzer, D., Cohen, B., and Young, N. S., Persistent B19 parvovirus infection in patients infected with human immunodeficiency virus type 1 (HIV-1): a treatable cause of anemia in AIDS, *Ann. Intern. Med.*, 113, 926, 1990.

53. Griffin, T. C., Squires, J. E., Timmons, C. F., and Buchanan, G. R., Chronic human parvovirus B19-induced erythroid hypoplasia as the initial manifestation of human immunodeficiency virus infection, *J. Pediatr.*, 118, 899, 1991.

54. Naides, S. J., Howard, E. J., Swack, N. S., True, C. A., and Stapleton, J. T., Parvovirus B19 as a cause of anemia in human immunodeficiency virus-infected patients, *J. Infect. Dis.*, 169, 939, 1994.

55. Rosenfeld, S. J., Yoshimoto, K., Kajigaya, S., Anderson, S., Young, N. S., Field, A., Warrener, P., Bansal, G., and Collett, M. S., Unique region of the minor capsid protein of human parvovirus B19 is exposed on the virion surface, *J. Clin. Invest.*, 89, 2023, 1992.

56. Naides, S. J., Howard, E. J., Swack, N. S., True, C. A., and Stapleton, J. T., Parvovirus B19 infection in human immunodeficiency virus type 1-infected persons failing or intolerant to zidovudine therapy, *J. Infect. Dis.*, 168, 101, 1993.

57. Bremner, J. A. G. and Cohen, B. J., Parvovirus B19 as a cause of anemia in human immunodeficiency virus-infected patients, *J. Infect. Dis.*, 169, 938, 1994.

58. Spivak, J. L., Bender, B. S., and Quinn, T. C., Hematologic abnormalities in the acquired immune deficiency syndrome, *Am. J. Med.*, 77, 224, 1984.

59. Zon, L. I. and Groopman, J. E., Hematologic manifestations of the human immune deficiency virus (HIV), *Semin. Hematol.*, 25, 208, 1988.

60. White, D. G., Woolf, A. D., Mortimer, P. P., Cohen, B. J., Blake, D. R., and Bacon, P. A., Human parvovirus arthropathy, *Lancet*, 1, 419, 1985.

61. Reid, D. M., Reid, T. M. S., Brown, T., Rennie, J. A. N., and Eastmond, C. J., Human parvovirus-associated arthritis: a clinical and laboratory description, *Lancet*, 1, 422, 1985.

62. Smith, C. A., Woolf, A. D., and Lenci, M., Parvoviruses: infections and arthropathies, *Rheum. Dis. Clin. North Am.*, 13, 249, 1987.

63. Luzzi, G. A., Kurtz, J. B., and Chapel, H., Human parvovirus arthropathy and rheumatoid factor, *Lancet*, 2, 1218, 1985.

64. Semble, E. L., Agudelo, C. A., and Pegram, P. S., Human parvovirus B19 arthropathy in two adults after contact with childhood erythema infectiosum, *Am. J. Med.*, 83, 560, 1987.

65. Cohen, B. J., Buckley, M. M., Clewley, J. P., Jones, V. E., Puttick, A. H., and Jacoby, R. K., Human parvovirus infection in early rheumatoid arthritis and inflammatory arthritis, *Ann. Rheum. Dis.*, 45, 832, 1986.

66. Schwarz, T. F., Roggendorf, M., Suschke, H., and Deinhard, F., Human parvovirus B19 infection and juvenile chronic polyarthritis, *Infection*, 15, 264, 1987.

67. Torok, T. J., Parvovirus B19 and human disease, *Adv. Intern. Med.*, 37, 431, 1992.

68. Thurn, J., Human parvovirus B19: historical and clinical review, *Rev. Infect. Dis.*, 10, 1005, 1988.

69. Corman, L. C. and Dolson, D. J., Polyarteritis nodosa and parvovirus B19 infection, *Lancet*, 339, 491, 1992.

70. Corman, L. C. and Dolson, D. J., Parvovirus B19 and necrotizing vasculitis, *Arthritis Rheum.*, 35(Suppl.), 5165, 1992.

71. Cotter, C. S., Singleton, G. T., and Corman, L. C., Immune-mediated inner ear disease and parvovirus B19, *Laryngoscope*, 104, 1235, 1994.

72. Potter, C. G., Potter, A. C., Hatton, C. S. R., Chapel, H. M., Anderson, M. J., Pattison, J. R., Tyrrell, D. A., Higgins, P. G., Willman, J. S., Parry, H. F., and Cotes, P. M., Variation of erythroid and myeloid precursors in the marrow and peripheral blood of volunteer subjects infected with human parvovirus (B19), *J. Clin. Invest.*, 79, 1486, 1987.

73. Anderson, M. J., Davis, L. R., Hodgson, J., Jones, S. E., Murtaza, L., Pattison, J. R., Stroud, C. E., and White, J. M., Occurrence of infection with a parvovirus-like agent in children with sickle cell anaemia during a two-year period, *J. Clin. Pathol.*, 35, 744, 1982.

74. Kelleher, J. F., Luban, N. L. C., Cohen, B. J., and Mortimer, P. P., Human serum parvovirus as the cause of aplastic crisis in sickle cell disease, *Am. J. Dis. Child.*, 138, 401, 1984.

75. Gowda, N., Rao, S. P., Cohen, B., Miller, S. T., Clewley, J. P., and Brown, A., Human parvovirus infection in patients with sickle cell disease with and without hypoplastic crisis, *J. Pediatr.*, 110, 81, 1987.

76. Kelleher, J. F., Luban, N. L. C., Mortimer, P. P., and Kamimura, T., Human serum "Parvovirus": a specific cause of aplastic crisis in children with hereditary spherocytosis, *J. Pediatr.*, 102, 720, 1983.

77. Duncan, J. R., Cappellini, M. D., Anderson, M. J., Potter, C. G., Kurtz, J. B., and Weatherall, D. J., Aplastic crisis due to parvovirus infection in pyruvate kinase deficiency, *Lancet*, 2, 14, 1983.

78. Lefrere, J.-J., Courouce, A.-M., Girot, R., and Cornu, P., Human parvovirus and thalassaemia, *J. Infect.*, 13, 45, 1986.

79. West, N. C., Meigh, R. E., Mackie, M., and Anderson, M. J., Parvovirus infection associated with aplastic crisis in a patient with HEMPAS, *J. Clin. Pathol.*, 39, 1019, 1986.

80. Tomiyama, J., Adachi, Y., Hanada, T., and Matsunaga, Y., Human parvovirus B19-induced aplastic crisis in autoimmune haemolytic anaemia, *Br. J. Haematol.*, 69, 288, 1988.
81. Lefrere, J.-J., Courouce, A.-M., and Bertrand, Y., Aplastic crisis in haemolytic anaemias not associated with human parvovirus infection, *J. Clin. Pathol.*, 40, 700, 1987.
82. Bernard, C., Sick, H., Boilletot, A., and Oberling, F., Bone marrow necrosis: acute microcirculation failure in myelomonocytic leukemia, *Arch. Intern. Med.*, 138, 1569, 1978.
83. Brown, C., Bone marrow necrosis: study of 70 cases, *Johns Hopkins Med. J.*, 131, 189, 1972.
84. Charache, S. and Page, D. L., Infarction of bone marrow in the sickle cell disorders, *Ann. Intern. Med.*, 67, 1195, 1967.
85. Kiraly, J. F. and Wheby, M. S., Bone marrow necrosis, *Am. J. Med.*, 60, 361, 1976.
86. Pardoll, D. M., Rodeheffer, R. J., Smith, R. L., and Charache, S., Aplastic crisis due to extensive bone marrow necrosis in sickle cell disease, *Arch. Intern. Med.*, 142, 2223, 1982.
87. Conrad, M. E., Studdard, H., and Anderson, L. J., Aplastic crisis in sickle cell disorders: bone marrow necrosis and human parvovirus infection, *Am. J. Med. Sci.*, 295, 212, 1988.
88. Petrella, T., Bailly, F., Mugneret, F., Caillot, D., Chavanet, P., Guy, H., Solary, E., Waldner, A., Devilliers, E., Carli, P.-M., and Michiels, R., Bone marrow necrosis and human parvovirus associated infection preceding an Ph1+ acute lymphoblastic leukemia, *Leukemia Lymphoma*, 8, 415, 1992.
89. Anderson, M. J., Lewis, E., Kidd, I. M., Hall, S. M., and Cohen, B. J., An outbreak of erythema infectiosum associated with human parvovirus infection, *J. Hyg.*, 93, 85, 1984.
90. Plummer, F. A., Hammond, G. W., Forward, K., Sekla, L., Thompson, L. M., Jones, S. E., Kidd, I. M., and Anderson, M. J., An erythema infectiosum- like illness caused by human parvovirus infection, *N. Engl. J. Med.*, 313, 74, 1985.
91. Anderson, M. J., Jones, S. E., Fisher-Hoch, S. P., Lewis, E., Hall, S. M., Bartlett, C. L. R., Cohen, B. J., Mortimer, P. P., and Pereira, M. S., Human parvovirus, the cause of erythema infectiosum (fifth disease?), *Lancet*, 1, 1378, 1983.
92. Ager, E. A., Chin, T. D. Y., and Poland, J. D., Epidemic erythema infectiosum, *N. Engl. J. Med.*, 275, 1326, 1966.
93. Dessypris, E. N., *Pure Red Cell Aplasia*, The Johns Hopkins University Press, Baltimore, 1988.
94. Sieff, C., Pure red cell aplasia, *Br. J. Haematol.*, 54, 331, 1983.
95. Tohda, S., Nara, N., Tanikawa, S., Imai, Y., Murakami, N., and Aoki, N., Pure red cell aplasia following autoimmune haemolytic anaemia: cell-mediated suppression of erythropoiesis as a possible pathogenesis of pure red cell aplasia, *Acta Haematol.*, 87, 98, 1992.
96. Raghavachar, A., Pure red cell aplasia: review of treatment and proposal for a treatment strategy, *Blut*, 61, 47, 1990.
97. Frickhofen, N., Abkowitz, J., King, L., Astrow, A., Halperin, I., and Young, N., Red cell aplasia due to persistent B19 parvovirus infection in HIV-infected patients and its treatment with immunoglobulin, *Blood*, 74(Suppl. 1), 44a, 1989.
98. Kurtzman, G., Frickhofen, N., Kimball, J., Jenkins, D. W., Nienhuis, A. W., and Young, N. S., Pure red cell aplasia of 10 years' duration due to persistent parvovirus B19 infection and its cure with immunoglobulin therapy, *N. Engl. J. Med.*, 321, 519, 1989.
99. Mintzer, D. and Reilly, R., Pure red blood cell aplasia associated with human immunodeficiency virus infection: response to intravenous gammaglobulin, *Blood*, 70(Suppl. 1), 124a, 1987.
100. Needleman, S. W., Durable remission of pure red cell aplasia after treatment with high-dose intravenous gammaglobulin and prednisone, *Am. J. Hematol.*, 32, 150, 1989.
101. Schwarz, T. F., Roggendorf, M., Hottenträger, B., Modrow, S., Deinhardt, F., and Middeldorp, J., Immunoglobulins in the prophylaxis of parvovirus B19 infection, *J. Infect. Dis.*, 162, 1214, 1990.
102. Belloy, M., Morinet, F., Blondin, G., Courouce, A. M., Peyrol, Y., and Vilmer, E., Erythroid hypoplasia due to chronic infection with parvovirus B19, *N. Engl. J. Med.*, 322, 633, 1990.
103. Berkman, S. A., Lee, M. L., and Gale, R. P., Clinical use of intravenous immunoglobulins, *Semin. Hematol.*, 25, 140, 1988.
104. Clauvel, J. P., Vainchenker, W., Herrera, A., Dellagi, K., Vinci, G., Tabilio, A., and Lacombe, C., Treatment of pure red cell aplasia by high dose intravenous immunoglobulins, *Br. J. Haematol.*, 55, 380, 1983.

105. McGuire, W. A., Yank, H. H., Bruno, E., Brandt, J., Briddell, R., Coates, T. D., and Hoffman, R., Treatment of antibody-mediated pure red cell aplasia with high-dose intravenous gammaglobulin, *N. Engl. J. Med.*, 317, 1004, 1987.

106. Koch, W. C., Adler, S. P., and Massey, G., Manifestations and therapy of chronic human parvovirus B19 (B19) infections, *Pediatr. Res.*, 25 (Abstr.), 182A, 1989.

107. Kurtzman, G. and Young, N., Clinical spectrum of bone marrow failure due to chronic B19 parvovirus infection and the immunologic mechanism responsible for persistence, *Blood*, 72, 45a, 1988.

108. Shirley, J. A., Revill, S., Cohen, B. J., and Buckley, M. M., Serological study of rubella-like illnesses, *J. Med. Virol.*, 21, 369, 1987.

109. Schwarz, T. F., Roggendorf, M., and Deinhard, F., Human parvovirus infections in Germany, *Lancet*, 1, 739, 1987.

110. Lobkowicz, F., Ring, J., Schwarz, T. F., and Roggendorf, M., Erythema multiforme in a patient with acute human parvovirus B19 infection, *J. Am. Acad. Dermatol.*, 20 (5 Part 1), 849, 1989.

5   Paramyxoviridae

Based on morphological and biologic criteria, the Paramyxoviridae family of viruses is classified in three genera: *Paramyxovirus*, *Morbillivirus*, and *Pneumovirus*. The paramyxoviruses have been found only in warm-blooded animals.

One common structural characteristic of paramyxoviruses is the lipoprotein envelope enclosing the helically symmetrical nucleocapsids. In addition, the paramyxoviruses have similar features with the rhabdoviruses and myxoviruses, two other families of negative-stranded RNA viruses. Thus, the paramyxoviruses and rhabdoviruses are the only negative-strand RNA viruses that possess nonsegmented genomes coupled with striking similarities in genome organization and expression.

Among the three genera of Paramyxoviridae, major distinctions include the ability of the *Paramyxovirus* genus to agglutinate mammalian and avian erythrocytes together with an easily demonstrable neuraminidase activity; by comparison, members of the [*Morbillivirus*] genus hemagglutinate but lack neuraminidase. The members of the genus *Pneumovirus*, which comprises the human and bovine respiratory syncytial viruses, have been known to be morphologically different from the other two genera by having narrower nucleocapsids.

5.1   RESPIRATORY SYNCYTIAL VIRUS

5.1.1   INTRODUCTION

The respiratory syncytial virus (RSV) remains the most common cause of viral lower airway disease in infants and children.[1-3] It is a medium-sized membrane-coated RNA virus which was first isolated by Morris et al.[4] Because of its morphologic similarity (size and shape) to other members, RSV was initially classified into the genus *Paramyxovirus*. Although the nucleocapsid of RSV represents a symmetrical helix closely related to that of paramyxoviruses, RSV is still different in several respects. The main difference is that of the diameter of the RSV helix, which in negatively stained preparations was 12 to 15 nm rather than 18 nm of the paramyxoviruses.[5-8] Together with animal strains of RSV and the pneumonia virus of mice, which shared the same nucleocapsid diameter, human RSV was classified into the separate genus *Pneumovirus*.[3]

For many years RSV, which has shown evidence of antigenic heterogeneity when assessed by neutralization kinetics of animal sera, epidemiologically behaved as a single serotype.[9] Not until monoclonal antibodies were used have at least two distinct subtypes (A and B) been identified.[10-12] While these two RSV strains were able to co-circulate,[11,13] subtype A was more prevalent during most epidemics and appeared to cause the more severe illness.[13] In general, immunity in response to natural infection has been poor and reinfections occur regularly throughout life.[14-18] The latter phenomenon is still poorly understood.[2]

The precise role of immunity in RSV infection is still not clear.[3] There is increasing evidence that neutrophils and alveolar macrophages may play an important role in the acute and long-term pathology within the respiratory tract, as well as being central factors in defense against the pathogen.[19-21] There is little doubt that RSV can exert significant immunosuppressive effect, thus preventing the development of effective immunity.[2]

5.1.2 RESPIRATORY SYNCYTIAL VIRUS INFECTIONS IN IMMUNOCOMPROMISED PATIENTS

It has been estimated that half of all infants will be infected by RSV in the first year of life, and about half of those infected will develop lower respiratory tract illness.[1]

Compared to immunocompetent hosts, immunocompromised patients, either children[22-27] or adults,[28] are at greater risk of developing much more severe lower respiratory tract infection due to RSV.[29] Thus, the mortality rate in hospitalized infants with underlying diseases has been strikingly higher (15% to 40%) than that of infants who were previously normal (less than 1%).[23,27,30-32] Risk factors for serious RSV infection in children include congenital heart disease, chronic lung disease (particularly bronchopulmonary dysplasia), organ and bone marrow transplant recipients, and either inherited or acquired immunodeficiencies.[22-31,33,34]

Milner et al.[27] have reported a fatal outcome of RSV infection in two infants with severe combined immunodeficiency syndrome (SCIDS) presenting with interstitial giant cell pneumonitis and thymic dysplasia. Patients with SCIDS have been noted to have frequent and multiple viral infections, such as RSV disease.[23,26,27,32,35-40]

Pohl et al.[22] have reviewed the course of RSV infection in 17 children who underwent liver transplantation. Thirteen of the patients developed nosocomial infection resulting in two deaths. In the latter two cases, the fatal outcome was associated with progressive pulmonary disease and occurred in children who developed the infection early in the postoperative period (when the immunosuppression tended to be greatest) and were intubated before the onset of symptoms. Overall, the severity of illness was greater in children with early onset of infection (<20 d) after transplantation. A preexisting lung disease (pneumonia, atelectasis due to increased abdominal girth, respiratory insufficiency requiring mechanical ventilation, and asthma) has also predisposed to more severe disease.[22] Intubation itself may be a risk factor by providing a direct pathway to the lower respiratory tract and by impairing normal host mechanisms of defense, such as cough.[41]

Another important factor contributing to more severe course of RSV infection in children may be age. Both fatal cases described by Pohl et al.[22] occurred in patients less than 15 months old. Infants less than 3 months old were observed to experience increased morbidity,[42] perhaps reflecting both immunologic immaturity and a higher risk of primary infections.[43]

Although symptomatic RSV-induced disease is most often associated with the very young, the virus may be found in respiratory secretion of infected persons at any age.[44] Thus, outbreaks among the elderly have been associated with serious and even fatal illness,[45,46] and RSV infections in immunocompromised adults have been reported with increasing incidence.[28,35,36,47-51] Underlying conditions included solid organ (kidney, pancreas) and bone marrow transplantation, and hematologic malignancies (T cell lymphoma).[28] While patients receiving corticosteroids alone did not appear to be at the same level of increased risk as other patient populations (as described above), corticosteroid therapy seemed to increase the quantity of viral shedding.[23] In gnotobiotic calves infected with bovine RSV, the administration of dexamethasone for 10 d has been shown to result not only in increased viral shedding but also in enhancement of pulmonary lesions and suppression of the specific IgM antibody response.[52]

Results from several studies have suggested that some of the clinical and pathologic findings observed in patients with RSV-associated wheezing may be immunomodulated, possibly secondary to the development of virus-specific IgE, and other homocytotropic (IgG4) antibody activity and the subsequent release of histamine, leukotrienes, and other cellular mediators of bronchospasm.[53,54] In one study by Welliver et al.,[55] anti-RSV-specific IgE antibody was undetectable in the acute phase of the disease in non-wheezing children with only upper respiratory tract illness or pneumonia. However, RSV-specific IgE antibody has been detected in 30% of patients with pneumonia and wheezing, and in 40% of patients with bronchiolitis and wheezing. In a related investigation, McIntosh et al.[56,57] have found that in the majority of infants younger than 6 months, anti-RSV IgA antibody developed to RSV infection, and this capacity improved with age; in addition, there has been a marked discrepancy between the secretory antibody and secretory neutralizing activity against RSV. Nevertheless, the development of IgA antibody to RSV correlated in time with the disappearance of virus from the respiratory tract.[56,57] However, the role of IgA in the elimination of RSV has been questioned based on the observation that patients with IgA deficiency have no increase in the incidence and/or severity of respiratory tract viral infections.[58,59]

In HIV-related immunodeficiency in children, the RSV infection frequently resulted in pneumonia, while bronchiolitis with wheezing occurred rarely.[24] In addition, bacterial infections in HIV-infected children occurred more frequently (20%) than in immunocompetent children hospitalized with RSV infection (2.9%).[60] It may well be that the RSV infection has predisposed the children to superinfection by other pathogens.[24,61]

It is likely that the defective cell-mediated immunity in HIV-positive patients may be responsible for the prolonged viral shedding.[23,26,38]

5.1.3 EVOLUTION OF THERAPIES AND TREATMENT OF RESPIRATORY SYNCYTIAL VIRUS INFECTIONS

The use of aerosolized ribavirin in the treatment of RSV-induced infections, particulary in severe disease, has been well established.[2,62,63]

Ribavirin (1β-D-ribofuranosyl-1,2,4-triazole-3-carboxamide) is a synthetic nucleoside analog, structurally similar to guanosine and inosine. It appeared to have activity against a number of DNA and RNA viruses, including RSV.[64,65] Although its exact mechanism of action is still being investigated, it is thought that ribavirin acts on several stages of viral replication.[66]

During administration, ribavirin is nebulized into an oxyhood, tent, or mask from a solution containing 20 mg of the drug per milliliter of water with the help of a small-particle aerosol generator supplied by the manufacturer (mass median aerosol diameter, 1 to 2 μm). The aerosol is administered for 12 to 18 h daily for 3 to 7 days.[62]

Ribavirin when administered orally has mild hepatic and bone marrow toxicity. Furthermore, when ribavirin is being delivered almost continuously (i.e., 18 to 20 h daily) as small-particle aerosol, its systemic toxicity is nearly nonexistent.[3] Daily oral administration of ribavirin to adults in doses of up to 1.0 g for more than 1 week has resulted in as much as 20% of transient decrease in hematocrit value.[67] By comparison, adult volunteers receiving ribavirin aerosol by mask for 12 h daily for 3 d showed no toxic side effects.[68]

The use of aerosolized ribavirin in experimental RSV infection in adult volunteers and naturally occurring RSV lower respiratory tract disease in infants has suggested a modest but consistent beneficial effect on both viral shedding and clinical illness.[67,69-71] However, even though ribavirin decreased the degree of viral shedding and increased the level of oxidation, there has been no convincing evidence that this drug actually decreased the duration of hospitalization or lessened the need for supportive therapies.[3]

Clinical studies of hospitalized infants with RSV lower respiratory tract diseases have involved both normal patients and those with underlying diseases.[25,69-74]

Rosner et al.[75] have found that ribavirin markedly impaired the development of virus-specific serum IgG, secretory IgA, and specific IgE mucosal antibody responses. While such immunologic alterations seemed not to have any deleterious effect on the outcome of primary infection or reinfection in otherwise normal children, their role in immunity against reinfection in immunocompromised patients is still not fully understood. It is possible that suppression of the IgE response may be beneficial in reducing mucosal inflammation by inhibiting the release of inflammatory products of mast cell activation, as well as other mediators of bronchospasm, such as histamine and leukotrienes.[29]

The use of ribavirin in the management of RSV-induced acute bronchiolitis in infants has been controversial since results from early trials.[69-72,76,77] There was the opinion that since the therapeutic benefits of ribavirin have been firmly established, any further studies with the drug would be unethical,[77] even though the early studies demonstrated no more than a trend towards more rapid improvement in treated patients.[2] The major drawbacks of the early trials, namely the limited number of patients as well as concerns regarding their design, led to renewed calls for larger double-blind prospective studies to establish the efficacy of ribavirin in resolving such issues as reducing mortality, the need for ventilation, and duration of hospitalization, particularly in high-risk patients (infants with chronic lung disease or cardiac disease).[78-80]

The American Academy of Pediatrics concluded that ribavirin should be "considered" in infants at high risk of severe RSV illness, such as those with congenital cardiac disease,[30,81,82] chronic lung disease, cystic fibrosis, or immunodeficiencies, as well as in cases where the severity of RSV infection would preclude a prolonged treatment course.[62] The recommended duration of treatment was for at least 3, and preferably 5 d.[70] However, in the absence of convincing evidence obtained from larger trials to demonstrate that the use of ribavirin in cases such as those advocated by the American Academy of Pediatrics would reduce the incidence of subsequent recurrent respiratory symptoms, it is still unclear whether its use would produce the intended results.[2] To this end, results from a large prospective study[83] in which ribavirin was used early in the course of RSV infections in patients considered to be at high risk of severe disease, suggested that such early treatment may help reduce morbidity. The fact that none of the patients on active treatment or the placebo-receiving group had required ventilation or died (a situation which was very different from that reported in historical studies[30]), has been attributed to the early and aggressive medical support and meticulous attention to oxygenation.[83]

McIntosh et al.[25] successfully used aerosolized ribavirin to treat pneumonitis and combined infection of RSV and parainfluenza virus type 3 in an infant with SCIDS secondary to adenosine deaminase deficiency. The drug was administered as a small-particle aerosol in four separate courses. Neither virus returned during profound immunosuppression for bone marrow transplantation.

Englund et al.[28] have treated bone marrow transplant recipients who developed RSV infections with aerosolized ribavirin (6.0 g daily, diluted in 300 ml distilled water and delivered over 18- to 24-h time periods) either by mask or assisted ventilation for 7 to 25 d (mean duration, 16 d). Two patients also received ribavirin intravenously for 4 and 5 d. Three of the six patients treated initially by mask subsequently required assisted ventilation but died. The fatal outcomes were associated with RSV infection that developed early after transplantation (within 5 to 32 d; median, 12 d), whereas the bone marrow transplant recipients who survived had RSV diagnosed at median of 82 d after transplantation (range, 7 to 157 days). All recipients of renal transplants survived the RSV infection.[28]

Results from recent studies of experimental RSV infection in animal models[84-87] have suggested that immunotherapy may prove useful in the treatment of serious RSV-induced lower respiratory tract illness in infants and young children. Thus, when purified human intravenous IgG was inoculated parenterally at the height of RSV infection, it elicited a $10^{-1.7}$ to $10^{-2.7}$ reduction in the level of pulmonary virus without evidence of potentiation of pulmonary pathology.[88,89] IgG was also shown to be beneficial when instilled directly into the airways of cotton rats at the height of RSV infection.[88]

In a clinical trial conducted by Hemming et al.,[90] the therapeutic efficacy of intravenous IgG (at 2.0 g/kg daily) against RSV pneumonia or bronchiolitis in infants and children was found to be similar to that of aerosolized ribavirin in producing a more rapid improvement in oxygenation (within 24 h) and a decrease in viral shedding (within 48 h), but the treatment did not reduce the mean duration of hospitalization. The prophylactic efficacy of IgG is being currently evaluated in infants and children at high risk for RSV infection.[3]

Since RSV is a poor inducer of IFN-α, it was postulated that its administration would be therapeutically useful in infants with RSV bronchiolitis. However, a study by Portnoy et al.[91] demonstrated no discernible beneficial effects even though the IFN-α aerosol was well tolerated.

5.1.4 REFERENCES

1. Stark, J. M., Lung infections in children, *Curr. Opin. Pediatr.*, 5, 273, 1993.
2. Everard, M. L. and Milner, A. D., The respiratory syncitial virus and its role in acute bronchiolitis, *Eur. J. Paediatr.*, 151, 638, 1992.
3. McIntosh, K. and Chanock, R. M., Respiratory syncytial virus, in *Fields Virology*, 2nd ed., Fields, B. N., Knipe, D. M., Chanock, R. M., Hirsch, M. S., Melnick, J. L., Monath, T. P., and Roizman, B., Eds., Raven Press, New York, 1990, 1045.
4. Morris, J. A., Blount, R. E., and Savage, R. E., Recovery of cytopathogenic agent from chimpanzees with coryza, *Proc. Soc. Exp. Biol. Med.*, 92, 544, 1956.
5. Kalica, A. R., Wright, P. F., Hetrick, F. M., and Chanock, R. M., Electron microscopic studies of respiratory syncytial temperature-sensitive mutants, *Arch. Ges. Virusforsch.*, 41, 248, 1973.
6. Berthiaume, L., Joncas, J., and Pavilanis, V., Comparative structure, morphogenesis and biological characteristics of the respiratory synsytial (RS) virus and the pneumonia virus in mice, *Arch. Ges. Virusforsch.*, 45, 39, 1974.
7. Joncas, J., Berthiaume, L., and Pavilanis, L., The structure of the respiratory syncytial virus, *Virology*, 38, 493, 1969.
8. Zakstelskaya, L. Y. and Shendervoch, S. F., On mechanisms of interference of respiratory syncytial virus by influenza A2 virus, *Vopr. Virusol.*, 15, 552, 1970.
9. McIntosh, K. and Fishaut, J. M., Immunopathologic mechanisms in lower respiratory tract disease of infants due to respiratory syncytial virus, *Prog. Med. Virol.*, 26, 94, 1980.
10. Anderson, L. J., Hierholzer, J. C., Tsou, C., Hendry, R. M., Fernie, B. F., Stone, Y., and McIntosh, K., Antigenic characteristics of respiratory syncytial virus strains with monoclonal antibodies, *J. Infect. Dis.*, 151, 626, 1985.
11. Hendry, R. M., Talis, A. L., Goodfrey, E., Anderson, L. J., Fernie, B. F., and McIntosh, K., Concurrent circulation of antigenically distinct strains of respiratory syncytial virus during community outbreaks, *J. Infect. Dis.*, 153, 291, 1986.
12. Mufson, M. A., Orvell, C., Rafnar, B., and Norbby, E., Two distinct subtypes of human respiratory syncytial virus, *J. Gen. Virol.*, 66, 2111, 1985.
13. Taylor, C. E., Morrow, S., Scott, M., Young, B., and Toms, G. L., Comparative virulence of respiratory syncytial virus subgroups A and B, *Lancet*, 1, 777, 1989.
14. Glezen, W. P., Taber, L. H., Frank, A. L., and Kasel, J. A., Risk of primary infection and re-infection with respiratory syncytial virus, *Am. J. Dis. Child.*, 140, 543, 1986.
15. Hall, C. B., Geiman, J. M., Biggar, R., Kotok, D. I., Hogan, P. M., and Douglas, R. G., Respiratory syncytial virus infections within families, *N. Engl. J. Med.*, 294, 414, 1976.
16. Hall, J. W., Hall, C. B., and Speers, D. M., Respiratory syncytial virus infections in adults, *Ann. Intern. Med.*, 88, 203, 1978.
17. Mufson, M. A., Belshe, R. B., Orvell, C., and Norbby, E., Subgroup characteristics of respiratory syncytial virus strains recovered from children with two consecutive infections, *J. Clin. Microbiol.*, 25, 1535, 1987.
18. Parrott, R. H., Kim, H. W., Arrobio, J. O., Hodes, D. S., Murphy, B. R., Brandt, C. D., Camargo, E., and Chanock, R. M., Epidemiology of respiratory syncytial virus infections in Washington DC. II. Infection and disease with respect to age, immunological status, race and sex, *Am. J. Epidemiol.*, 98, 289, 1973.
19. Fantone, J. C., Feltner, D. E., Brieland, K. K., and Ward, P. A., Phagocytic cell-derived inflammatory mediators and lung disease, *Chest*, 91, 428, 1987.
20. Sibille, Y. and Reynolds, H. Y., State of the art: macrophages and polymorphonuclear neutrophils in lung defense and injury, *Am. Rev. Respir. Dis.*, 141, 471, 1990.
21. Faden, H. S., Kaul, T. N., Lin, T. Y., and Ogra, P. L., Activation and mucosal migration of polymorphonuclear leukocytes during respiratory syncytial virus infection, *Pediatr. Res.*, 18, 274A, 1984.
22. Pohl, C., Green, M., Wald, E. R., and Ledesma-Medina, J., Respiratory syncytial virus infections in pediatric liver transplant recipients, *J. Infect. Dis.*, 165, 166, 1992.
23. Hall, C. B., Powell, K. R., MacDonald, N. E., Gala, C. L., Menegus, M. E., Suffin, S. C., and Cohen, H. J., Respiratory syncytial viral infection in children with compromised immune function, *N. Engl. J. Med.*, 315, 77, 1986.

24. Chandwani, S., Borkowsky, W., Krasinski, K., Lawrence, R., and Welliver, R., Respiratory syncytial virus infection in human immunodeficiency virus-infected children, *J. Pediatr.*, 117, 251, 1990.

25. McIntosh, K., Kurachek, S. C., Cairns, I. M., Burns, J. C., and Goodspeed, B., Treatment of respiratory viral infection in an immunodeficient infant with ribavirin aerosol, *Am. J. Dis. Child.*, 238, 305, 1984.

26. Jarvis, W. R., Middleton, R. J., and Gelfond, E. W., Significance of viral infections in severe combined immunodeficiency disease, *Pediatr. Infect. Dis. J.*, 2, 187, 1983.

27. Milner, M. E., de la Monte, S. M., and Hutchins, G. M., Fatal respiratory syncytial virus infection in severe combined immunodeficiency syndrome, *Am. J. Dis. Child.*, 139, 1111, 1985.

28. Englund, J. A., Sullivan, C. J., Jordan, M. C., Dehner, L. P., Vercillotti, G. M., and Balfour, H. H., Jr., Respiratory syncytial virus infection in immunocompromised adults, *Ann. Intern. Med.*, 109, 203, 1988.

29. Ogra, P. L. and Patel, J., Respiratory syncytial virus infection and the immunocompromised host, *Pediatr. Infect. Dis. J.*, 7, 246, 1988.

30. MacDonald, N. E., Hall, C. B., Suffin, S. C., Alexson, C., Starris, P. J., and Manning, J. A., Respiratory syncytial viral infection in infants with congenital heart disease, *N. Engl. J. Med.*, 307, 397, 1982.

31. Aherne, W., Bird, T., Court, S. D. M., Gardner, P. S., and McQuillin, J., Pathological changes in virus infections of the lower respiratory tract in children, *J. Clin. Pathol.*, 23, 7, 1970.

32. Craft, A. W., Reid, M. M., Gardner, P. S., Jackson, E., Kernahan, J., McQuillin, J., Noble, T. C., and Walker, W., Virus infection in children with acute lymphoblastic leukemia, *Arch. Dis. Child.*, 54, 755, 1979.

33. Plotkin, S. A., Peter, G., Daum, R. S., Giebink, G. S., Hall, C. B., Halsey, N. A., Lepow, M. L., Marcuse, E. K., Marks, M. I., McCracken, G. H. et al., Ribavarin therapy of respiratory syncytial virus, in *Report of the Committee on Infectious Diseases*, 22nd ed., Peter, G., Ed., American Academy of Pediatrics, Elk Grove, IL, 1991, 581.

34. Harrington, R. D., Hooton, T. M., Hackman, R. C., Storch, G. A., Osborne, B., Gleaves, C. A., Benson, A., and Meyers, J. D., An outbreak of respiratory syncytial virus in a bone marrow transplant center, *J. Infect. Dis.*, 165, 987, 1992.

35. Crane, L. R., Kish, J. A., Ratanatharathora, V., Merline, J. R., and Raval, M. F., Fatal syncytial virus pneumonia in a laminar airflow room, *JAMA*, 246, 366, 1987.

36. Milder, J. E., McDearmon, S. C., and Walzer, P. D., Presumed respiratory syncytial virus pneumonia in an adolescent compromised host, *South. Med. J.*, 72, 1195, 1979.

37. Delage, G., Brochu, P., Pelletier, M., Tasmin, G., and Lapointe, N., Giant-cell pneumonia caused by parainfluenza virus, *J. Pediatr.*, 94, 426, 1979.

38. Fishaut, M., Tubergen, B., and McIntosh, K., Cellular response to respiratory viruses with particular reference to children with disorders of cell-mediated immunity, *J. Pediatr.*, 96, 179, 1980.

39. Bruce, E., Reid, M. M., Craft, A. W., Kernahan, J., and Gardner, P. S., Multiple virus isolations in children with acute lymphoblastic leukaemia, *J. Infect.*, 1, 243, 1979.

40. Brugman, S. and Hutter, J., Jr., Respiratory syncytial virus (RSV) pneumonitis in acute leukemia, *Am. J. Pediatr. Hematol. Oncol.*, 2, 371, 1980.

41. Krasinsky, K., Severe respiratory syncytial virus infection: clinical features, nosocomial acquisition and outcome, *Pediatr. Infect. Dis. J.*, 4, 250, 1985.

42. Green, M., Brayer, A., Shenkman, K., and Wald, E. R., Duration of hospitalization in previously well infants with respiratory syncytial virus infection, *Pediatr. Infect. Dis. J.*, 8, 601, 1989.

43. Gree, M. and Michaels, M., Infectious complications of solid-organ transplantation in children, *Adv. Pediatr. Infect. Dis.*, 7, 181, 1992.

44. Cooney, M. K., Fox, J. P., and Hall, C. E., The Seattle virus watch. VI. Observation of infections with and illness due to parainfluenza, mumps, and respiratory syncytial viruses and mycoplasma pneumoniae, *Am. J. Epidemiol.*, 101, 532, 1975.

45. Public Health Laboratory Service Communicable Disease Surveillance Centre, Respiratory syncytial virus infection in the elderly, 1976-1982, *Br. Med. J.*, 287, 1618, 1983.

46. Mathur, U. S., Bentley, D. W., and Hall, C. B., Concurrent respiratory syncytial virus and influenza A infections in the institutionalized elderly and chronically ill, *Ann. Intern. Med.*, 93, 49, 1980.

47. Solomon, L. R., Raftery, A. T., Mallick, N. P., Johnson, R. W., and Longson, M., Respiratory syncytial virus infection following renal transplantation, *J. Infect.*, 3, 280, 1981.

48. Spelman, D. W. and Stanley, P. A., Respiratory syncytial virus pneumonitis in adults, *Med. J. Aust.*, 1, 430, 1983.

49. Kasupski, G. J. and Leers, W. D., Presumed respiratory syncytial virus pneumonia in three immuno-compromised adults, *Am. J. Med. Sci.*, 285, 28, 1983.

50. Levenson, R. M. and Kantor, O. S., Fatal pneumonia in an adult due to respiratory syncytial virus, *Arch. Intern. Med.*, 147, 791, 1987.

51. Chandra, R. S., Giant cell pneumonia, *Pediatr. Pathol.*, 2, 226, 1984.

52. Thomas, L. H., Stott, E. J., Collins, A. P., Crouch, S., and Jebbett, J., Infection of gnotobiotic calves with a bovine and human isolate of respiratory syncytial virus: modification of the response by dexamethasone, *Arch. Virol.*, 79, 67, 1984.

53. Welliver, R. C., Kaul, T. N., and Ogra, P. L., The appearance of cell-bound IgE in respiratory-tract epithelium after respiratory syncytial virus infection, *N. Engl. J. Med.*, 303, 1198, 1980.

54. Bui, R. H., Molinaro, G. A., Kettering, J. D., Heiner, D. C., Imagawa, D. T., and St. Geme, J. W., Jr., Virus-specific IgE and IgG4 antibodies in serum of children infected with respiratory syncytial virus, *J. Pediatr.*, 110, 87, 1987.

55. Welliver, R. C., Wong, D. T., Sun, M., Middleton, E., Vaughan, R. S., and Ogra, P. L., The development of respiratory syncytial virus specific IgE and the release of histamine in nasopharyngeal secretions after infection, *N. Engl. J. Med.*, 305, 841, 1981.

56. McIntosh, K., Masters, H. B., Orr, I., Chao, R. K., and Barkin, R. M., The immunologic response to infection with respiratory syncytial virus in infants, *J. Infect. Dis.*, 138, 24, 1978.

57. McIntosh, K., Masters, H. B., Orr, I., Chao, R. K., and Barkin, R. M., Secretory antibody following respiratory syncytial virus infection in infants, *Pediatr. Res.*, 10, 389 (Abstr. No. 530), 1976.

58. Ogra, P. L., Coppola, M. R., MacGillivray, M. H., and Dzierba, J. L., Mechanism of mucosal immunity to viral infections in IgA deficiency syndromes, *Proc. Soc. Exp. Biol. Med.*, 145, 811, 1974.

59. Aho, K., Pyhälä, R., and Koistinen, J., IgA deficiency in influenza infection, *Scand. J. Immunol.*, 5, 1089, 1976.

60. Hall, C. B., Powell, K. R., Schnabel, K. C., Gala, C. L., and Pincus, P. H., Risk of secondary bacterial infection in infants hospitalized with respiratory syncytial virus infection, *J. Pediatr.*, 113, 266, 1988.

61. Korppi, M., Leinonen, M., Koskela, M., Makela, H., and Launiala, K., Bacterial co-infection in children hospitalized with respiratory syncytial virus infections, *Pediatr. Infect. Dis. J.*, 8, 687, 1989.

62. Brunell, P. S., Daum, R. S., Giebink, G. S., Hall, C. B., Lepow, M. L., McCracken, G. H., Jr., Nahmias, A. J., Phillips, C. F., Plotkin, S. A., and Wright, H. T., Jr. for the Committee on Infectious Diseases, Ribavirin therapy of respiratory syncytial virus, *Pediatrics*, 79, 475, 1987.

63. Hall, C. B. and Douglas, R. G., Modes of transmission of respiratory syncytial virus, *J. Pediatr.*, 99, 100, 1981.

64. Hruska, J. F., Bernstein, J. M., Douglas, R. G., and Hall, C. B., Effects of ribavirin on RSV *in vitro*, *Antimicrob. Agents Chemother.*, 17, 770, 1980.

65. Hruska, J. F., Morrow, P. E., Suffin, S. C., and Douglas, R. G., *In vitro* inhibition of respiratory syncytial virus by ribavirin, *Antimicrob. Agents Chemother.*, 21, 125, 1982.

66. Patterson, J. L. and Fernandez-Larsson, R., Molecular mechanisms of action of ribavirin, *Rev. Infect. Dis.*, 12, 1139, 1990.

67. Hall, C. B., Walsh, E. E., Hruska, J. F., Betts, R. F., and Hall, W. J., Ribavirin treatment of experimental respiratory syncytial virus infection, *JAMA*, 249, 2666, 1983.

68. McCormick, J. B., King, I. J., Webb, P. A., Scribner, C. L., Craven, R. B., Johnson, K. M., Elliott, L. H., and Belmont-Williams, R., Lassa fever: effective therapy with ribavirin, *N. Engl. J. Med.*, 314, 20, 1986.

69. Hall, C. B., McBride, J. T., Walsh, E. E., Bell, D. M., Gala, C. L., Hildereth, S., Ten Eyck, L. G., and Hall, W. J., Aerosolized ribavirin treatment of infants with respiratory syncytial viral infection: a randomized double-blind study, *N. Engl. J. Med.*, 308, 1443, 1983.

70. Hall, C. B., McBride, J. T., Gala, C. L., Hildreth, S. W., and Schnabel, K. C., Ribavirin treatment of respiratory syncytial viral infection in infants with underlying cardiopulmonary disease, *JAMA*, 254, 3047, 1985.

71. Taber, L. H., Knight, V., Gilbert, B. E., McClung, H. W., Wilson, S. Z., Norton, H. J., Thurson, J. M., Gordon, W. H., Atmar, R. L., and Schlaudt, W. R., Ribavirin aerosol treatment of bronchiolitis associated with respiratory syncytial virus infection in infants, *Pediatrics*, 72, 613, 1983.

72. Rodriguez, W. J., Kim, H. W., Brandt, C. D., Fink, R. J., Getson, P. R., Arrobio, J., Murphy, T. M., McCarthy, V., and Parrott, R. H., Aerosolized ribavirin in the treatment of patients with respiratory, syncytial virus disease, *Pediatr. Infect. Dis. J.*, 6, 159, 1987.

73. Gelfand, E. W., McCurdy, D., Rao, C. P., and Middleton, P. J., Ribavirin treatment of viral pneumonitis in severe combined immunodeficiency disease, *Lancet*, 2, 732, 1983.

74. Connor, J. D., Hintz, M., Van Dyke, R., McCormick, J. B., and McIntosh, K., Ribavirin pharmaco-kinetics in children and adults during the therapeutic trials, in *Clinical Applications of Ribavirin*, Smith, R. A., Knight, V., and Smith, J. A. D., Eds., Academic Press, Orlando, FL, 1984, 107.

75. Rosner, I. K., Welliver, R. C., Edelson, P. J., Geraci-Ciardullo, K., and Sun, M., Effect of ribavirin therapy on respiratory syncytial virus-specific IgE and IgA responses after infection, *J. Infect. Dis.*, 155, 1043, 1987.

76. Barry, W., Cockburn, F., Cornall, R., Price, J. F., Sutherland, G., and Vardag, A., Ribavirin aerosol for acute bronchiolitis, *Arch. Dis. Child.*, 61, 593, 1986.

77. Conrad, D. A., Christenson, J. C., Waner, J. L., and Marks, M. I., Aerosolized ribavirin treatment of respiratory syncytial virus infection in infants hospitalized during an epidemic, *Pediatr. Infect. Dis. J.*, 6, 152, 1987.

78. Isaacs, D., Moxon, E. R., Harvey, D., Kovar, I., Madeley, C. R., Richardson, R. J., Levin, M., Whitelaw, A., and Modi, N., Ribavirin in respiratory syncytial virus infection: a double blind placebo controlled trial is needed, *Arch. Dis. Child.*, 63, 986, 1988.

79. Ray, C. G., Ribavirin: ambivalence about an antiviral agent, *Am. J. Dis. Child.*, 142, 488, 1988.

80. Wald, E. R., Dashefsky, B., and Green, M., In re ribavirin: a case of premature abjudication? *J. Pediatr.*, 112, 154, 1988.

81. Gardner, P. S., Turk, D. C., Aherne, W. A., Bird, T., Holdaway, M. D., and Court, S. D. M., Deaths associated with respiratory tract infection in childhood, *Br. Med. J.*, 4, 316, 1967.

82. Downham, M. A. P. S., Gardner, P. S., McQuillin, J., and Ferris, J. A. J., Role of respiratory viruses in childhood mortality, *Br. Med. J.*, 1, 235, 1975.

83. Groothius, J. R., Woodin, K. A., Katz, R., Robertson, A. D., McBride, J. T., Hall, C. B., McWilliams, B. C., and Lauer, B. A., Early ribavirin treatment of respiratory syncytial viral infection in high-risk children, *J. Pediatr.*, 117, 792, 1990.

84. Walsh, E. E., Schlesinger, J. J., and Brandriss, M. W., Protection from respiratory syncytial virus infection in cotton rats by passive transfer of monoclonal antibodies, *Infect. Immun.*, 43, 756, 1984.

85. Prince, G. A., Horswood, R. L., and Chanock, R. M., Quantitative aspects of passive immunity to respiratory syncytial virus infection in infant cotton rats, *J. Virol.*, 55, 517, 1985.

86. Hemming, V. G., Prince, G. A., Horswood, R. L., London, W. J., Murphy, B. R., Walsh, K. E., Fischer, G. W., Weisman, L. E., Baron, P. A., and Chanock, R. M., Studies of passive immunotherapy for infections of respiratory syncytial virus in the respiratory tract of a primate model, *J. Infect. Dis.*, 152, 1083, 1985.

87. Suffin, S. C., Prince, G. A., Muck, K. B., and Porter, D. D., Immunoprophylaxis of respiratory syncytial virus infection in the infant ferret, *J. Immunol.*, 123, 10, 1979.

88. Prince, G. A., Hemming, V. G., Horswood, R. L., and Chanock, R. M., Immunoprophylaxis and immunotherapy of respiratory syncytial virus infection in the cotton rat, *Virus Res.*, 3, 193, 1985.

89. Prince, G. A., Hemming, V. G., Horswood, R. L., Baron, P. A., and Chanock, R. M., Effectiveness of topically administered neutralizing antibodies in experimental immunotherapy of respiratory syncytial virus infection in cotton rats, *J. Virol.*, 61, 1851, 1987.

90. Hemming, V. G., Rodriguez, W., Kim, H. W., Brandt, C. D., Parrott, R. H., Burch, B., Prince, G. A., Baron, P. A., Fink, R. J., and Reaman, G., Intravenous immunoglobulin treatment of respiratory syncytial virus infections in infants and young children, *Antimicrob. Agents Chemother.*, 31, 1882, 1987.

91. Portnoy, J., Hicks, R., Pacheco, F., and Olson, L., Pilot study of recombinant interferon alpha-2a for treatment of infants with bronchiolitis induced by respiratory syncytial virus, *Antimicrob. Agents Chemother.*, 32, 589, 1988.

6 Poxviridae

Poxviridae represent a large family of complex DNA viruses capable of infecting a wide array of vertebrate and invertebrate hosts. Since long ago, the best recognized member of this family has been the variola virus, the causative agent of smallpox.

Structurally, the poxviruses are characterized by a large and complex virion containing enzymes associated with mRNA synthesis, and a genome comprising a single linear double-stranded DNA molecule (130 to 300 kbp). The poxviruses have the ability to replicate within the cytoplasmic compartment of the host cell.

In their most recent classification, the Poxviridae family is divided into two subfamilies, Chordopoxviridae and Entemopoxviridae. The Chordopoxviridae (vertebrate poxviruses) has been further subdivided into six genera: *Orthopoxvirus, Parapoxvirus, Avipoxvirus, Capripoxvirus, Leporipoxvirus,* and *Suipoxvirus.* The establishment of two additional genera of vertebrate poxviruses, *Molluscipoxvirus* and *Yatapoxvirus*, is currently being considered. The Entemopoxviridae (insect poxviruses) subfamily consists of two members, *Amsacta moori* and *Chironimus luridus.*

Nine different poxviruses can cause human disease, namely four members of *Orthopoxvirus* (the variola virus, monkeypox virus, cowpox virus, and the vaccinia virus), two *Parapoxviruses* (the orf virus and the paravaccinia virus), and three unclassified viruses: the tanapoxvirus, the yabapoxvirus, and *Poxvirus mollusci.*

6.1 MOLLUSCUM CONTAGIOSUM

6.1.1 Introduction

Molluscum contagiosum is a superficial infection of the skin caused by *Poxvirus mollusci,* a double-stranded DNA virus that is morphologically similar to vaccinia virus.

Poxvirus mollusci has been isolated from humans, primates, and marsupials and has a worldwide distribution. It is estimated that molluscum contagiosum affects between 2% to 5% of the general population.[1] In general, the disease afflicts mostly children less than 5 years of age, but recent evidence suggests that adolescents and young adults could also be affected.[2] Molluscum contagiosum has also been reported to occur in AIDS patients.[3-11]

The viral transmission is usually by direct contact and possibly by fomites.[12] Autoinoculation, especially among young children and infants, is also common. Transmission of molluscum contagiosum by skin contact associated with sexual intercourse has also been reported among adults, and has been recently linked to the 11-fold increase in incidence in adolescents and young adults.[2]

The incubation period of the infection is between 2 and 7 weeks. The infection is manifested by the appearance of pinhead-sized discrete, flesh-colored, dome-shaped umbilicated papules. In cases of nonsexually transmitted infections, the lesions are most commonly found on the trunk, the extremities, and occasionally, the face. Although usually 2 to 4 mm, the lesions may become extremely large on the eyelids.[13-16] By contrast, the primary lesions of sexually transmitted disease occur on the lower abdomen and the genital region.[2,12] Even though unique in appearance, lesions by the molluscum virus may occasionally by confused with other skin diseases, such as fungal infections (histoplasmosis, cryptococcosis) which may elicit similar umbilicated papules.[17-19]

Naert and Lachapelle[20] have described an unusual case of a patient with systemic lupus erythematosus receiving therapy of azathioprine and methylprednisolone who developed molluscum contagiosum lesions associated with metaplastic ossification. The latter consisted of primary bone tissue located in the upper dermis in close relation to the epidermal molluscum lesions.

6.1.2 TREATMENT OF MOLLUSCUM CONTAGIOSUM

Usually lesions of molluscum contagiosum will resolve spontaneously and without scarring within 6 to 12 weeks. When secondary infections or eczematoid dermatitis is involved, patients should receive systemic treatment with antimicrobial drugs or a topical corticosteroid, respectively.[12] Removal of molluscum lesions by surgical excision, curettage, cryotherapy, carbon dioxide laser vaporization, or electrodissection has also been recommended in cases where there is no spontaneous resolution or recurrent infection.[13,21,22]

Disseminated molluscum contagiosum has been observed in patients with immune deficiencies,[23-27] such as those receiving immunosuppressive chemotherapy (methotrexate),[23] corticosteroids (prednisone),[21,23] patients with sarcoidosis,[25] eczema,[21,26-28] congenital IgM deficiency,[29] and AIDS.[3-11] The development of lesions has been associated with depletion of T helper cells and occasionally will precede worsening of clinical and immunologic status.[8] In AIDS patients, lesions of molluscum contagiosum are multiple and will usually appear on the face, scalp, and the neck.[7]

Mayumi et al.[29] have reported a case of severe selective IgM immunodeficiency (as evidenced by significantly lower serum levels of IgM) associated with disseminated molluscum contagiosum; at the same time, the levels of IgG, IgA, and especially IgE were elevated. Selective IgM deficiency is a disorder presenting with heterogeneous immunologic abnormalities typified with normal B cell counts[30-33] but impaired T lymphocyte functions,[30] including IgM-specific T suppressor cells.[34] While it is known that patients with selective T cell deficiency have been highly susceptible to bacterial and/or viral infections,[30,35-41] the case reported by Mayumi et al. was the first to describe dysgammaglobulinemia in a patient with persistent disseminated molluscum contagiosum. The latter was treated with intravenous interferon-α (10^6 U daily for 7 d, followed by 2×10^6 U three times weekly for 5 weeks). Contrary to a previous report,[42] no improvement in the clinical manifestations of molluscum contagiosum was observed.[29]

Betlloch et al.[8] have described a case of molluscum contagiosum in an AIDS patient who responded well to treatment with zidovudine (200 mg every 4 h). Since a decrease of T helper and Langerhans cells of the skin is the first immunologic event that predisposes to cutaneous viral infections, zidovudine has been thought to act by reestablishing the cellular immune response, thus stopping the rapid replication of the molluscum virus.[8]

Topical treatment with cantharidin (in a collodion-type of vehicle) has been recommended to treat molluscum contagiosum; usually five to six applications are needed to eradicate the lesions.[43-45]

Ohkuma[46] has reported a new topical procedure for molluscum lesion removal using 10% propridine iodine solution and 50% salicylic acid plaster application.

Podophyllotoxin (as 0.5% solution) has also been applied topically to treat molluscum contagiosum.[47] Syed et al.[48] conducted a multicenter, double-blind, placebo-controlled trial to evaluate the clinical efficacy and tolerance of 0.3% and 0.5% podophyllotoxin cream preparations. The latter, in general, have been found more convenient and easy to use than solution forms. The results from the study indicated that 0.5% podophyllotoxin cream when applied twice daily for three consecutive days cured molluscum lesions, thus making prolonged repetitive applications unnecessary.

Trichloroacetic acid was also used successfully for topical treatment of molluscum papules.[21]

Gross et al.[49] introduced inosiplex as a systemic therapy of molluscum contagiosum in children. The drug, which is devoid of major toxic side effects,[50,51] was given orally at daily doses of 50 mg/kg; seven of nine patients showed lesion regression. Inosiplex seemed to act indirectly by mediating the host immunologic responses. It has immunomodulating properties by stimulating the host cellular immune response, thus increasing the overall number of lymphocytes (and T helper cells, in particular[50,52]), and the activity of the natural killer cells. In a double-blind, placebo-controlled trial, inosiplex helped restore the cellular immunity in moderately immunosuppressed patients suffering from chronic lymphadenopathy.[49]

6.1.3 REFERENCES

1. Felman, Y. and Nikitis, J. D., Genital molluscum contagiosum, *Cutis*, 26, 28, 1980.
2. Becker, T. M., Blount, J. H., Douglas, J., and Judson, F. N., Trends in molluscum contagiosum in the United States, 1966-1983, *Sex. Trans. Dis.*, 13, 88, 1986.
3. Fischer, B. and Warner, L., Cutaneous manifestations of the acquired immune deficiency syndrome, *Int. J. Dermatol.*, 26, 615, 1987.
4. Redfield, R. R., Severe molluscum contagiosum infection in a patient with human T cell lymphotropic (HTLV-III) disease, *J. Am. Acad. Dermatol.*, 13, 821, 1985.
5. Sarma, D. P. and Weilbaedheer, T. G., Molluscum contagiosum in the acquired immunodeficiency syndrome, *J. Am. Acad. Dermatol.*, 13,, 682, 1985.
6. Katzman, M., Carey, J. T., Elmets, C. A., Jacobs, G. H., and Lederman, M. M., Molluscum contagiosum and the acquired immunodeficiency syndrome: clinical and immunological details of two cases, *Br. J. Dermatol.*, 116, 131, 1987.
7. Lombardo, P. C., Molluscum contagiosum and the acquired immunodeficiency syndrome, *Arch. Dermatol.*, 121, 834, 1985.
8. Betlloch, I., Pinazo, I., Mestre, F., Altés, J., and Villalonga, C., Molluscum contagiosum in human immunodeficiency virus infection: response to zidovudine, *Int. J. Dermatol.*, 28, 351, 1989.
9. Sindrup, J. H., Lisby, G., Weismann, K., and Wantzin, G. L., Skin manifestations in AIDS, HIV infection and AIDS-related complex, *Int. J. Dermatol.*, 26, 267, 1987.
10. Reichert, C. M., O'Leary, T. J., Levens, D. L., Simrell, C. R., and Macher, A. M., Autopsy pathology in the acquired immune deficiency syndrome, *Am. J. Pathol.* 112, 357, 1983.
11. Penneys, N. S. and Hicks, B., Unusual cutaneous lesions associated with acquired immunodeficiency syndrome, *J. Am. Acad. Dermatol.*, 13, 845, 1985.
12. Ginsburg, C. M., Management of selected skin and soft tissue infections, *Pediatr. Infect. Dis. J.*, 5, 735, 1986.
13. Gonnering, R. S., Treatment of periorbital *Molluscum contagiosum* by incision and curettage, *Ophthalmol. Surg.*, 19, 325, 1988.
14. Van der Meer Maastricht, B. C. J. and Gomperts, C. E., Molluscum contagiosum giganteum, *Am. J. Ophthalmol.*, 33, 965, 1950.
15. Einaugler, R. B. and Henkind, P., Molluscum contagiosum of the eyelids: an interesting case, *J. Pediatr. Ophthalmol. Strabismus*, 5, 201, 1968.
16. Rao, V. A., Baskaran, R. K., and Krishnan, M. M., Unusual cases of molluscum contagiosum of eye, *Indian J. Ophthalmol.*, 33, 263, 1985.
17. Feuillade de Chauvin, M., Revuz, J., and Deniau, M., Histoplasmose a histoplasma duboisii, *Ann. Dermatol. Venereol.*, 110, 716, 1983.
18. Rico, M. J. and Penneys, N. S., Cutaneous cryptococcosis resembling molluscum contagiosum in a patient with AIDS, *Arch. Dermatol.*, 121, 901, 1985.
19. Picon, L., Vaillant, L., Duong, T., Lorette, G., Bacq, Y., Besnier, J. M., and Choutet, P., Cutaneous cryptococcosis resembling molluscum contagiosum: a first manifestation of AIDS, *Acta Derm. (Stockholm)*, 69, 365, 1989.
20. Naert, F. and Lachapelle, J. M., Multiple lesions of molluscum contagiosum with multiple ossification, *Am. J. Dermatol.*, 11, 238, 1989.
21. Hellier, F. F., Profuse mollusca contagiosa of the face induced by corticosteroids, *Br. J. Dermatol.*, 85, 398, 1970.
22. Friedman, M. and Gal, D., Keloid scars as a result of carbon dioxide laser for molluscum contagiosum, *Obstet. Gynecol.*, 70, 394, 1987.

23. Rosenberg, E. G. and Yusk, J. W., Molluscum contagiosum: eruption following treatment with prednisone and methotrexate, *Arch. Dermatol.*, 101, 439, 1970.

24. Vilmer, C., Molluscum contagiosum profus chez un enfant immunodeprime, *Ann. Dermatol. Venereol.*, 110, 781, 1983.

25. Ganpule, M. and Garretts, M., Molluscum contagiosum and sarcoidosis: report of a case, *Br. J. Dermatol.*, 85, 587, 1971.

26. Peachey, R. D. G., Severe molluscum contagiosum infection with T cell deficiency, *Br. J. Dermatol.*, 97(Suppl. 15), 49, 1977.

27. Pauly, C. R., Artis, W. M., and Jones, H. E., Atopic dermatitis, impaired cellular immunity, and molluscum contagiosum, *Arch. Dermatol.*, 114, 391, 1978.

28. Solomon, L. M. and Telner, P., Eruptive molluscum contagiosum in atopic dermatitis, *Can. Med. Assoc. J.*, 95, 978, 1966.

29. Mayumi, M., Yamaoka, K., Tsutsui, T., Mizue, H., Doi, A., Matsuyama, M., Ito, S., Shinomyiya, K., and Mikawa, H., Selective immunoglobulin M deficiency associated with disseminated molluscum contagiosum, *Eur. J. Paediatr.*, 145, 99, 1986.

30. De La Concha, E. G., Garcia-Rodriguez, M. C., Zabay, J. M., Laso, M. T., Alonso, F., Bootello, A., and Fontan, G., Functional assessment of T and B lymphocytes in patients with selective IgM deficiency, *Clin. Exp. Immunol.*, 49, 670, 1982.

31. Yocum, M. W., Strong, D. M., Chusid, M. J., and Lakin, J. D., Selective immunoglobulin M (IgM) deficiency in two immunodeficient adults with recurrent staphylococcal pyoderma, *Am. J. Med.*, 60, 486, 1976.

32. Endoh, M., Kaneshige, H., Tomino, Y., Nomoto, Y., Sakai, H., and Arimori, S., Selective IgM deficiency: a case study, *Tokai J. Exp. Clin. Med.*, 6, 327, 1981.

33. Ross, I. N. and Thompson, R. A., Severe selective IgM deficiency, *J. Clin. Pathol.*, 29, 773, 1976.

34. Cooper, M. D., Lawton, A. R., Preud'homme, J. L., and Seligmann, M., Primary antibody deficiencies, in *Immune Deficiency*, Cooper, M. D., Miescher, P. A., and Mueller-Eberhand, H. J., Eds., Springer-Verlag, Berlin, 1979, 31.

35. Chandra, R. K., Kaveramma, B., and Soothill, J. F., Generalized non-progressive vaccinia associated with IgM deficiency, *Lancet*, 1, 687, 1969.

36. Faulk, W. P., Kiyasu, W. S., Cooper, M. D., and Fudenberg, H. H., Deficiency of IgM, *Pediatrics*, 47, 399, 1971.

37. Gilbert, C. and Hong, R., Qualitative and quantitative immunoglobulin deficiency, *Am. J. Med.*, 37, 602, 1964.

38. Hobbs, J. R., Milner, R. D. G., and Watt, P. J., Gamma-M deficiency predisposing to meningococcal septicemia, *Br. Med. J.*, 4, 583, 1967.

39. Jones, D. M., Tobin, B. M., and Butterworth, A., Three cases of meningococcal infection in a family, associated with a deficient immune response, *Arch. Dis. Child.*, 48, 742, 1973.

40. Silber, H. K. B., Shuster, J., Gold, P., and Freedman, S. O., Leukopenia, leukoagglutinins, and low IgM in a family with severe febrile illnesses, *Clin. Immunol. Immunopathol.*, 1, 220, 1973.

41. Stoelinga, G. B. A., van Munster, P. J. J., and Slooff, J. P., Antibody deficiency syndrome and autoimmune haemolytic anaemia in a boy with isolated IgM deficiency dysimmunoglobulinaemia type 5, *Acta Paediatr. Scand.*, 58, 352, 1969.

42. Uyeno, K. and Ohtsu, A., Interferon treatment of viral warts and some skin diseases, in *The Clinical Potential of Interferons*, Kono, R. and Vicek, J., Eds., Publication No. 15, Japan Medical Research Foundation, 1982, 149.

43. Funt, T. R., Cantharidin treatment of molluscum contagiosum, *Arch. Dermatol.*, 83, 504, 1961.

44. Funt, T. R. and Mehr, K. A., Cantharidin: a valuable office treatment of molluscum contagiosum, *South. Med. J.*, 72, 1019, 1979.

45. Epstein, E., Cantharidin treatment of molluscum contagiosum, *Acta Derm. Venereol. (Stockholm)*, 69, 91, 1989.

46. Ohkuma, M., Molluscum contagiosum treated with iodine solution and salicylic acid plaster, *Int. J. Dermatol.*, 29, 443, 1990.

47. Deleixhe, M., Piérard-Franchimont, C., and Piérard, G. E., Podophyllotoxin in the treatment of molluscum contagiosum, *J. Dermatol. Treat.*, 2, 99, 1991.

48. Syed, T. A., Lundin, S., and Ahmad, M., Topical 0.3% and 0.5% podophyllotoxin cream for self-treatment of molluscum contagiosum in males, *Dermatology*, 189, 65, 1994.
49. Gross, G., Jogerst, C., and Schöpf, E., Systemic treatment of mollusca contagiosa with inosiplex, *Acta Derm. Venereol. (Stockholm)*, 66, 76, 1986.
50. Editorial, Inosiplex: antiviral, immunomodulator, or neither? *Lancet*, 1, 1052, 1982.
51. Gross, G., Treatment of viral warts with inosiplex, *Akt. Dermatol.*, 10, 197, 1984.
52. Jones, C. E., Dyken, P. R., Huttenlocher, P. R., Jabbow, J. T., and Maxwell, K. W., Inosiplex therapy in subacute sclerosing panencephalitis. A multicentre non-randomized study in 98 patients, *Lancet*, 1, 1034, 1984.

7 Hepadnaviridae

Although the development of acute hepatitis following percutaneous exposure to human serum or blood had been known for over a century, not until the 1960s was the actual etiologic agent of hepatitis identified, when the hepatitis B surface antigen (HBsAg) was discovered and recognized as a viral antigen associated with acute hepatitis B.

Structural features that are commonly shared by the hepadnaviruses include the size and ultrastructure of the virion, with an envelope surrounding an electron-dense spherical nucleocapsid or core; a characteristic polypeptide and antigenic composition; common virion DNA size, structure, and genetic organization; and a unique mechanism of viral DNA replication which involves reverse transcription of a greater-than-genome-length viral RNA transcript utilizing a viral encoded protein primer in forming the first synthesized viral DNA strand.

Because of distinct differences in the genome nucleotide sequences, the gene number and organization, the virion ultrastructure and polypeptide size and organization, the absence of antigenic cross-reaction, and the host-range differences, the mammalian and avian hepadnaviruses appear to represent two groups (or genera) within the Hepadnaviridae family.

7.1 HEPATITIS

7.1.1 INTRODUCTION

Viral hepatitis, a general term that has been reserved for liver infections caused by one of at least five distinct hepatitic agents, continues to be one of the major health problems worldwide. The causative agents of hepatitis are nonopportunistic hepatotropic viruses, known as hepadnaviruses (family Hepadnaviridae),[1-3] including hepatitis A virus, hepatitis B virus, hepatitis D virus, hepatitis C virus, and the non-A non-B hepatitis virus.

Currently, viral hepatitis is ranked third among all reportable diseases behind venereal infections and chickenpox.[4] Although not directly opportunistic, some hepadnaviruses, such as hepatitis B virus, have been implicated as potential cofactors in the development and progression of HIV infection. There is, however, much more to be understood about the complex relationship between HIV infection and the hepadnaviruses.

7.1.2 HEPATITIS A

In most cases, the hepatitis A virus (HAV) causes a subclinical disease. HAV, which has no known carrier state and plays no role in the production of chronic active hepatitis or cirrhosis, disappears following acute infection. Transmission of the disease has been primarily through oral-fecal contact.

7.1.3 HEPATITIS B

Hepatitis B virus (HBV) is the prototype virus of the Hepadnaviridae family that exhibits striking tropism for hepatocytes but may also be detected in peripheral blood mononuclear cell and tissues.[4]

Studies in recent years have renewed interest in the hepatitis B virus as a possible cofactor in HIV disease progression to AIDS. Thus, HBV is also a lymphotropic virus,[5-7] and infections caused by HBV have been common among HIV-infected persons,[8-10] as evidenced by HBV DNA being recovered from lymphoid cells of patients coinfected with HBV and HIV.[11] Furthermore, the HBV protein X was shown to activate the long terminal repeat (LTR) of HIV and thus to enhance its replication *in vitro*.[12,13]

Some extrachromosomal sequences of HBV DNA in peripheral mononuclear cells have been reported to be more prevalent among AIDS patients than among asymptomatic HIV carriers.[14] In addition, results from two reports[15,16] have indicated a possible reactivation of HBV infection in HIV-seropositive patients. All of these findings have strongly suggested the presence of a complex interaction between HIV and HBV on a cellular level.

It has been estimated that over 84% of HIV-infected patients have presented with HBV blood markers. The observed frequency of superinfection has been consistent with the similar transmission pathways of HBV and HIV. Thus, HBV has often been transmitted parenterally through contaminated blood or blood products, as well as by sexual and perinatal routes.

In a prospective study of HIV-positive patients from HIV diagnosis to diagnosis of AIDS, or to the end of the follow-up period (mean follow-up time, 62 months), Eskild et al.[17] have found that the presence of antibodies to HBV core antigen (HBcAb) in HIV-infected persons will facilitate a more rapid clinical progression to AIDS. The association between progression to AIDS and the presence of HBcAb was strengthened in the multivariate analysis as compared with the univariate. The adjusted relative risk of progression to AIDS for the 48 subjects who were HBV-antibody-positive at study entry was 3.6 (95% confidence interval, 1.3–10.1).

However, other studies such as the Multicenter AIDS Cohort Study[18] and the Vancouver Lymphadenopathy-AIDS Study[19] have not found previous or present HBV infection to be associated with progression to AIDS. Also, recent data from a retrospective study by Stevenson et al.[20] have suggested that in HIV-positive patients, coinfection with HBV made no difference in the clinical outcome of HIV disease. The rate of decline in CD4+ counts in those HIV-infected patients with hepatitis B markers was compared with that of patients without the HBV markers. Split-plot analysis of variance showed that there was no significant difference between the two groups in terms of CD4+ percentages ($p = .3371$).

The immunologic dysfunction (predominantly in cell-mediated immunity) caused by HIV could be expected to modify the course of HBV infection since viable cell-mediated immunity is important for resolution of HBV infection and inflammation in HBV-induced chronic liver disease.[21-26] Thus, Taylor et al.[27] have shown that when HIV-1 infection preceded HBV infection, the risk of becoming an HBV carrier increased threefold.[27] Furthermore, in those patients with chronic hepatitis B, patients with HIV-1 infection have increased HBV replication and decreased liver inflammation as compared with HIV-1-negative individuals.[8,28,29] Other studies have demonstrated a diminished response to hepatitis B vaccine, a potential for reactivation of quiescent HBV infection, and the loss of detectable HBV antibodies in those infected with HIV-1.[16,30-32] Hadler et al.[33] have studied the outcome of HBV infection and its relation to prior HIV infection. The results of their study, which were consistent with those obtained by Taylor et al.,[27] have shown that when adjusted for prior hepatitis B vaccination status, patients with HIV-1 infection preceding HBV infection had a substantially higher risk of developing HBV carriage, viremia, prolonged alanine aminotransferase (ALT) elevation, and clinical illness. T helper functions, the primary defect of HIV infection, seemed to be directly involved in the resolution of acute HBV disease since the latter may be dependent on such components of cell-mediated immunity as cytotoxic T lymphocytes,[34-38] which in turn, are dependent on normally functioning T helper cells.[33]

Chronic HBV infection when accompanied by HIV infection has been shown to be associated with less severe liver histology.[39-41] Also some studies,[28,39] but not others, have demonstrated lower serum transaminase levels. Furthermore, concurrent HIV infection has been linked with increased

HBcAg and HBeAg (hepatitis B "e" antigen) expression on hepatocyte nuclei.[42] In order to clarify the relationship between HIV and HBV infections, Bodsworth et al.[29] have examined serum markers of HBV replication and the severity of liver disease, as determined by ALT levels in 150 male homosexual chronic hepatitis B surface antigen (HBsAg) carriers, about half of whom were also infected with HIV. The results of the study revealed a higher prevalence of both HBeAg ($p = .001$) and HBV DNA ($p < .0005$) in serum of chronic HBV carriers with concurrent HIV infection. Furthermore, there was an apparent protective effect on the liver of concurrent HIV infection when there was detectable HBeAg in the serum. (This finding was in agreement with necropsy and biopsy studies of AIDS patients that showed milder liver damage due to chronic hepatitis B than in patients without AIDS.)[8] In addition, in patients with HBeAg and HIV infection, the immune suppression correlated with lower serum transaminase levels, which provided further evidence implicating the host's immune response in the pathogensis of chronic HBV infection.[29] This conclusion was consistent with evidence[37,38] suggesting that cytotoxic T cells sensitized to HBeAg have played a major role in the lysis of hepatocytes in chronic HBV infection. Overall, the study of Bodsworth et al.[29] did not show a trend towards greater immunosuppression in HIV-positive subjects who expressed serum markers of HBV replication (HBeAg, HBV DNA) than in those without such markers.

Based on their examination of the relationship between serologic evidence of HBV infection and the presence of AIDS, Scharschmidt et al.[43] concluded that patients with the more advanced immunosuppression characteristic of AIDS may be less likely to clear HBV infection after exposure or more likely to reactivate latent HBV infection, or both.

7.1.3.1 Treatment of Hepatitis B Infection

The morbidity and mortality of hepatitis B-related cirrhosis and hepatocellular carcinoma have been considerable. Several promising clinical trials for treatment of chronic hepatitis B using interferon-α (IFN-α) have been carried out.[9-11,44-46] IFN-α can enhance the immune response to the virus while inhibiting the viral replication in the liver. The drug is typically administered by injection for 16 weeks. Overall, therapy-associated remission of 25% or more has been reported. Since the results of most studies were based on only 1 year of follow-up examination, this period may be too short to determine whether the suppression of viral replication and the associated decrease in hepatic inflammation will be sustained and whether patients subsequently will lose markers of HBV infection. For these reasons, Korenman et al.[47] have assessed the long-term benefit in a cohort of patients with chronic hepatitis B 3 to 7 years after the therapy was completed. Apparently the patients responded favorably to IFN-α treatment, with only 3 of 23 patients relapsing (reappearance of both HBeAg and abnormal serum aminotransferase within 1 year of therapy).[47]

In HIV-infected patients, the combined administration of IFN-α and zidovudine has shown only limited response rates, with high relapse rates for responders who discontinued treatment. Common side effects included flu-like symptoms that, though rarely severe, can make long-term administration difficult.

Currently, the nucleoside analog 3TC is under investigation for the treatment of chronic hepatitis B. At oral daily doses of 100 mg or 300 mg, 3TC reduced the viral levels after 3 months of treatment.

Reactivation of chronic HBV infection by corticosteroid chemotherapy is a well documented complication — development of fulminant hepatitis accompanied with high mortality may follow the withdrawal of these drugs.[48]

7.1.4 Hepatitis C

In 1974, Prince et al.[49] made the observation that 25% of 204 cardiovascular surgery patients followed prospectively had developed post-transfusion hepatitis. Since of those 25%, 71% presented with hepatitis that was not caused by HBV, it was suggested that the disease was caused by a new virus which the investigators tentatively designated as hepatitis C virus. Similarly, neither HBV nor HAV were the etiologic agents for the post-transfusion hepatitis in a group of cardiac surgery patients monitored prospectively at the U.S. National Institutes of Health,[50] and the term non-A, non-B (NANB) hepatitis was coined[51] to account for those cases.

In 1989 this new virus, which was responsible for most of the post-transfusion hepatitis, and a large proportion of sporadic or community-acquired non-A, non-B hepatitis,[52,53] was finally cloned by using a recombinant immunoscreening approach,[54,55] and identified as hepatitis C virus (HCV).[56]

As with chronic hepatitis B infection, evidence is emerging that liver damage may be mediated by the immune reaction to infected hepatocytes, rather than by HCV itself.[48,57] Nevertheless, there have also been reports suggesting direct HCV cytopathic effect on liver cells.[58-61]

Antibodies to hepatitis C virus (anti-HCV), which are detectable with both enzyme-linked immunosorbent assay (ELISA) and the recombinant immunoblot assay (RIBA), should reveal either a past resolved infection or chronic persistent condition. HCV viremia has been frequently associated with liver histologic lesions even in patients with normal serum ALT levels. Usually, RIBA positivity is associated with chronic infection as assessed by polymerase chain reaction.[62,63] After evaluating HCV viremia in HIV-seronegative and -seropositive patients by using the indeterminate HCV recombinant immunoblot assay (RIBA2), Marcellin et al.[64] have suggested that in anti-HIV-positive persons, the antibody response to HCV infection may be impaired by concurrent HIV infection, and therefore, serologic tests must be interpreted with caution.

One of the major routes of transmission of HCV and hepatitis C infection has been through infected blood and blood products. Before anti-HCV screening was implemented, as much as 80% to 90% of post-transfusion hepatitis in the U.S.,[52,65,66] Europe,[67-69] and Asia[70,71] was caused by HCV. Based on various reports, other risk factors included injection drug use,[52,72,73] tattooing,[72-74] needlestick accidents,[75,76] blood exchanges during ritual ceremonies,[77] and use of folk remedies.[78] Transplantation with organs from HCV-infected donors may also transmit the virus,[79-81] although not on all occasions.[82] Vertical transmission of HCV has been uncommon but well documented.[83-87]

Although hepatitis C is generally considered to be a parenterally transmitted disease,[88,89] data from a nationwide surveillance study in the U.S. have shown that parenterally transmitted non-A, non-B hepatitis accounted for less than half of the reported acute cases.[90] In a case-control study, patients with non-A, non-B hepatitis were significantly more likely to have had either sexual or household contact with a person who had previously had hepatitis, or to have had several heterosexual partners.[91] Combined, these exposures accounted for 11% of all non-A, non-B infections, indicating that heterosexual transmission may play an important role in the etiology of the disease.[92] In contrast, the results of two small studies evaluating the heterosexual partners of anti-HCV-positive intravenous drug users,[93] and the heterosexual partners of patients with transfusion-associated non-A, non-B hepatitis, have failed to demonstrate statistically significant heterosexual transmission of HCV. Similarly, Bresters et al.[94] have reported that, since none of 50 heterosexual partners of hepatitis C viremic patients had detectable anti-HCV or HCV RNA by second-generation antibody assay and polymerase chain reaction assay, the risk of sexual transmission of HCV may be absent or low. However, data by Kao et al.[95] and Benezra[96] have provided direct evidence for sexual transmission of HCV infection.

Eyster et al.[92] have compared the frequency of heterosexual co-transmission of HCV and HIV and found that HCV transmission to sexual partners was five times higher when HIV was also transmitted, suggesting that HIV may be a cofactor for the sexual transmission of HCV.

Since 1989, when serologic testing for HCV first became available,[97] cirrhosis secondary to HCV has been recognized as one of the most common indications for orthotopic liver transplantation. It has also been well documented[98-100] that HCV will recur in virtually all patients infected with this virus prior to orthotopic liver transplantation, and cause histologic hepatitis within the allograft of the infected patients.[101,102]

A significant proportion of hemophiliac patients who have been given transfusion with non-heat-treated clotting factor concentrates have also been infected with HCV,[103-107] with the majority remaining chronically infected.[108] Moreover, most of them have also become infected with HIV.[109]

Eyster et al.[110] have found that liver failure occurred more frequently in HCV-seropositive hemophiliacs coinfected with HIV than those who were HCV-seropositive but without HIV infection. In addition, hemophiliac patients with lower CD4 lymphocyte counts or lymphocytopenia have had increased probability to experience liver failure. These findings suggested that HIV or its associated immune deficiency may accelerate the development of liver failure, perhaps by enhancing HCV replication.

In further studies, Eyster et al.[111] quantitated HCV RNA levels in serial samples from HIV-positive and HIV-negative hemophiliac patients before and after HIV seroconversion, and examined the relationships of HCV RNA levels to CD4 cell counts and to hepatic dysfunction over time. Over the entire period of the study, HCV RNA levels increased almost threefold in those patients who remained HIV-seronegative (mean 9.47×10^5 to 2.81×10^6/ml; $p = .02$). Among those hemophiliacs who become HIV-seropositive, the HCV RNA levels increased 58-fold (mean 2.85×10^5 to 1.66×10^7 eq/ml; $p = .0001$). The rate of increase in HCV RNA levels was eightfold faster for the HIV-positive patients than for those who remained HIV-seronegative ($p = .009$). Furthermore, the HCV RNA levels correlated significantly with the CD4 counts ($p = .01$) and serum aspartate aminotransferase ($p = .007$) levels. Overall, the HCV RNA levels were significantly higher in HIV-positive than HIV-negative multitransfusion hemophiliac patients — the HCV load increased over time, in correlation with the progress of immune deficiency, and was enhanced by HIV. Furthermore, the HCV RNA levels were directly associated with high aminotransferase levels. Sherman et al.[112] have also found that in patients with hepatitis C and concurrent HIV infection, the HCV RNA levels measured by the same methodology were higher in HIV-positive than in HIV-negative individuals.

These findings have strongly indicated that the HIV-induced immune deficiency may promote increased HCV replication.[111] Indeed, chronic hepatitis C was reported to be more severe in patients with HIV infection than in those without the disease and can lead to cirrhosis with fatal complication.[113] However, in a recent study by Roger et al.,[114] no evidence was found from liver biopsies in HCV-infected patients with and without HIV infection, to indicate that HIV had influenced chronic HCV disease, although liver tests were commonly abnormal in the HIV-infected group.

Idiopathic cryoglobulinemia is a disorder known to cause clinical manifestations, such as purpura, arthralgia, neuralgia, glomerulonephritis, and/or vasculitis.[115] The pathogenesis of cryoglobulinemia has been often associated with infectious pathogens, including the Epstein-Barr virus, cytomegalovirus, and the hepatitis virus. In several reports, HCV has been implicated as the most likely of the hepatitis viruses to be the causative agent of cryoglobulinemia,[116-119] but few have confirmed the existence of HCV RNA in cryoglobulin.[118,119] Matsuda et al.[120] have studied the role of HCV and HIV in cryoglobulinemia of hemophiliac patients with HIV and/or HCV infection. Since it is well known that circulating immune complex is present in patients infected with HIV-1,[121,122] the possibility exists that HIV-1 may also be associated with the formation of cryoglobulin in HIV-infected hemophiliac patients. The studies of Matsuda et al.[120] have shown that HCV RNA was present in the sera of all 52 hemophiliacs, and cryoglobulin was detected in 48 (92%) of these patients; the remaining 4 hemophiliacs were HIV-infected. The discovery of HCV RNA in the cryoglobulin of these hemophiliac patients has confirmed the close association between HCV and cryoglobulinemia. With regard to p24 antigen, it was detected in the sera of 12 (46%) of 26 hemophiliacs who were infected with HIV-1 and who had cryoglobulinemia; however, p24 antigen was not detected in the cryoglobulin of these 12 or in that of the remaining 14 patients who did not have p24 antigen. The fact that p24 antigen was not detected in any cryoglobulin suggested one of three possibilities: that either HIV-1 is not associated with formation of cryoglobulin, the test applied for p24 antigen has been less sensitive than the ELISA for HCV RNA, or because an HIV-1 protein(s) other than p24 has a role in the formation of cryoglobulin.[120]

7.1.4.1 Treatment of Hepatitis C Infection

Recombinant IFN-α has been the recommended therapy for chronic hepatitis C,[56] based on clinical trials showing sustained normalization of aminotransferase levels in approximately 25% of patients treated with 3×10^6 U three times weekly for 24 weeks.[123,124] Increasing the duration of treatment to 48 or 60 weeks resulted in an increase in the sustained response rates to IFN-α.[125-128] An alternative treatment regimen consisting of 10×10^6 U of IFN-α six times weekly for 2 weeks, followed by three times weekly for 12 weeks led to sustained responses in 48% (14 of 29) of patients.[129]

By several accounts,[130-135] serum HCV RNA became undetectable or titers decreased in patients responding to IFN-α; however, during the relapse, serum HCV RNA once again become elevated. Nevertheless, there have been exceptions to these observations, with patients achieving sustained normalization of hepatic aminotransferase levels despite the re-emergence or persistence of serum HCV RNA,[128,136,137] or relapsing despite continued loss of serum HCV RNA.[138]

Boyer et al.[139] have assessed the response to and tolerance of recombinant IFN-α in 12 patients with chronic hepatitis C and HIV infection. The patients received either 1, 2, or 5 million units three times weekly, for 4 or 6 months. The results have shown a complete response (normal serum alanine aminotransferase activity) in four patients, three had a near-complete response (serum ALT less than one and one half times the upper limit of normal), and five had no response at the end of treatment. The overall conclusion was that the response to and tolerance of rIFN-α were not different from those usually observed in HIV-seronegative patients with chronic hepatitis C infection. In chronic hepatitis C, the effect of IFN-α seemed to be related more to an antiviral mechanism than to an immunomodulatory mechanism.[140]

The therapeutic efficacy of intravenous human IFN-β against hepatitis C and non-A, non-B hepatitis has been tested in a short-course 4-week therapy.[141,142] In one early pilot study,[141] five of five patients with chronic post-transfusion non-A, non-B hepatitis responded initially with decreases in aminotransferase levels, but no sustained effect. In the second study,[142] 10 of 11 randomized patients with non-A, non-B hepatitis had detectable HCV RNA. At 4 weeks of therapy, seven patients responded with sustained normalization of aminotransferase levels, and three of four patients who initially were nonresponders, have been retreated after 1 year and also responded.[142]

Randomized studies have also been conducted to evaluate the therapeutic efficacy of IFN-α in acute post-transfusion hepatitis C.[143,144] After 3 months of therapy, the aminotransferase levels returned to normal in a mean 66% of patients from both trials, compared to only 38% of controls.

In two studies,[145,146] although therapy with ribavirin decreased the HCV RNA titers and normalized serum aminotransferase levels, the response was not sustained. When ribavirin was applied in combination with IFN-β there was no significant improvement.[147]

In another preliminary study,[148] a combination of IFN-α with oral N-acetylcysteine improved the aminotransferase levels in patients who were previously unresponsive to IFN-α alone, despite the persistence of HCV RNA in most patients.

In contrast to HBV, HCV has rarely been the cause of fulminant hepatitis.[149] Vento et al.[150] have described fulminant hepatitis on withdrawal of chemotherapy for malignant lymphoma in two patients with chronic HCV infection — the ALT concentrations were markedly elevated (6030 and 3870 IU/l, respectively) while the serum HCV RNA levels were low in both patients when the severe disease had developed. One of the patients died after massive liver necrosis.

7.1.5 HEPATITIS D (DELTA)

The hepatitis delta virus (HDV) is a unique RNA virus, discovered in 1977 by Rizzetto et al.,[151] that requires for its replication a helper function provided by HBV,[152-154] during which the HBsAg will actually envelope the infectious HDV RNA.

Consequently, HDV may only replicate in patients who have already been infected with HBV.[155]

The clinical course of HDV infection, which may present as either acute or chronic disease,[155,156] has been variable but is usually more severe than that of other forms of hepatitis.[157] The acute HDV infection may be manifested as fulminant hepatitis,[158] a rare sequela of the acute hepatitis caused by other hepatitis viruses. The chronic form of HDV infection is a serious and rapidly progressive liver disease.[159,160]

7.1.5.1   Treatment of Hepatitis Delta Infection

Currently, there is no effective therapy for hepatitis delta. Because of its wide spectrum of antiviral activity,[161,162] IFN-α is being investigated as a possible treatment for hepatitis delta.[163]

Preliminary studies[164-166] have indicated that a 3- to 4-month course of IFN-α did suppress the replication of HDV, resulting in clinical improvement in some patients, but not in all cases; discontinuation of therapy has been followed by a relapse. The results of longer courses of IFN-α,[167-172] although more promising, were difficult to interpret because of too many variables, including enrolment criteria (inadequate control groups), large variations in drug doses, duration of treatment, and the characteristics of the patients.[173] In addition, the criteria (i.e., decrease in serum ALT, histologic findings, and HDV replication) used to evaluate the response to therapy have not been uniform in all studies, and were rarely taken together in assessing the overall effectiveness of IFN-α.[174]

In a randomized, controlled trial, Farci et al.[163] have evaluated the activity of IFN-α_{2a} in patients with chronic HDV disease, all of them recruited from the region of Sardinia, Italy, where infection with HDV is endemic.[174] The efficacy of high (9 million units) vs. low (3 million units) doses of IFN-α_{2a} (three times weekly for 48 weeks) was compared in the long-term treatment of chronic HDV, and patients were followed for up to 4 years after termination of therapy. Multiple factors were analyzed simultaneously to evaluate the response to treatment. By the end of therapy, the serum ALT values had become normal in 10 of 14 patients (71%) receiving the high IFN-α_{2a} dose, as compared with 4 of 14 patients (29%, $p = .029$) treated with the low IFN-α_{2a} dose and 1 of 13 untreated (8%) controls ($p = .001$). Furthermore, complete response (normal serum ALT levels and no detectable serum HDV RNA) was achieved in seven patients treated with the high dose (50%) as compared to only three of those receiving the low dose (21%, $p = .118$) and none of the controls ($p = .004$). However, relapse became common after treatment was stopped.[163]

7.1.6   References

1. Gust, I. D., Burrell, C. J., Couplis, A. G., Robinson, W. S., and Zuckerman, A. J., Taxonomic classification of human hepatitis B virus, *Intervirology*, 25, 14, 1986.
2. Robinson, W. S., Genetic variation among hepatitis B and related viruses, *Ann. NY Acad. Sci.*, 354, 371, 1980.
3. Robinson, W. S., Marion, P. L., Feitelson, M., and Siddiqui, A., in *Viral Hepatitis: 1981 International Symposium*, Szmuness, W., Alter, H. J., and Maynard, J. E., Eds., Franklin Institute Press, Philadelphia, 1982, 57.
4. Hollinger, F. B., Hepatitis B virus, in *Fields Virology*, 2nd ed., Fields, B. N., Knipe, D. M., Chanock, R. M., Hirsch, M. S., Melnick, J. L., Monath, T. P., and Roizman, B., Eds., Raven Press, New York, 1990, 2171.
5. Pontisso, P., Poon, M. C., Tiollais, P., and Brechot, O., Detection of hepatitis B virus in DNA in mononuclear cells, *Br. Med. J.*, 288, 1563, 1984.
6. Yoffe, B., Noonan, C. A., Melnick, J. L., and Hollinger, F. B., Hepatitis B virus in DNA in mononuclear cells and analysis of cell subsets for the presence of replicative intermediates of viral DNA, *J. Infect. Dis.*, 153, 471, 1986.
7. Laure, F., Zagury, D., Saimont, A. G., Gallo, R. C., Hahn, B. H., and Brechot, C., Hepatitis B virus sequences in lymphoid cells from patients with AIDS and AIDS-related complex, *Science*, 229, 561, 1985.

8. Perrillo, R. P., Regenstein, F. G., and Roodman, S. T., Chronic hepatitis B in asymptomatic homosexual men with antibody to human immunodeficiency virus, *Ann. Intern. Med.*, 105, 382, 1986.

9. Dooley, J. S., Davis, G. L., Peters, M., Waggoner, J. G., Goodman, Z., and Hoofnagle, J. H., Pilot study of recombinant human alpha-interferon for chronic type B hepatitis, *Gastroenterology*, 90, 150, 1986.

10. Hoofnagle, J. H., Peters, M. G., Mullen, K. D., Jones, D. B., Rustgi, V., Di Bisceglie, A., Hallahan, C., Park, Y., Meschievitz, C., and Jones, E. A., Randomized, controlled trial of recombinant human alpha-interferon in patients with chronic hepatitis B, *Gastroenterology*, 95, 1318, 1988.

11. Alexander, G. J., Brahm, J., Fagan, E. A., Smith, H. M., Daniels, H. M., Eddleston, A. L., and Williams, R., Loss of HBsAg with interferon therapy in chronic hepatitis B virus infection, *Lancet*, 2, 66, 1987.

12. Seto, E., Yen, T. S., Peterlin, B. M., and Ou, J. H., Transactivation of the human immunodeficiency virus long terminal repeat by the hepatitis B virus X protein, *Proc. Natl. Acad. Sci. U.S.A.*, 85, 8286, 1988.

13. Twu, J.-S., Chu, K., and Robinson, W. S., Hepatitis B virus X gene activates KB-like enhancer sequences in the long terminal repeat of the human immunodeficiency virus 1, *Proc. Natl. Acad. Sci. U.S.A.*, 86, 5168, 1989.

14. Noonan, C., Yoffe, B., Mansell, P. E. A., Melnick, J. L., and Hollinger, F. B., Extrachromosomal sequences of hepatitis B virus DNA in peripheral blood mononuclear cells of acquired immune deficiency syndrome patients, *Proc. Natl. Acad. Sci. U.S.A.*, 83, 5698, 1986.

15. Waite, J., Gilson, R. J. C., Weller, I. V. D., Lacey, C. J., Hambling, M. H., Hawkins, A., Briggs, M., and Tedder, R. S., Hepatitis B virus reactivation or reinfection associated with HIV-1 infection, *AIDS*, 2, 443, 1988.

16. Lazizi, Y., Grangeot-Keros, L., Delfraissy, J.-E., Bone, F., Debrenil, P., Badur, S., and Pillot, J., Reappearance of hepatitis B virus in patients infected with the human immunodeficiency virus type-1, *J. Infect. Dis.*, 158, 666, 1988.

17. Eskild, A., Magnus, P., Petersen, G., Sohlberg, C., Jensen, F., Kittelsen, P., and Skaug, K., Hepatitis B antibodies in HIV infected homosexual men are associated with more rapid progression to AIDS, *AIDS*, 6, 571, 1992.

18. Solomon, R. E., VanRaden, M., Kaslow, R. A., Lyter, D., Vissher, B., Farzadegan, H., and Phair, J., Association of hepatitis B surface antigen and core antibody with aquisition and manifestation of human immunodeficiency virus type 1 (HIV-1) infection, *Am. J. Public Health*, 80, 1475, 1990.

19. Schechter, M. T., Craib, K. J. P., Le, T. N., Willoughby, B., Douglas, B., Sestak, P., Montaner, J. S., Weaver, M. S., Elmslie, K. D., and O'Shaughnessy, M. V., Progression to AIDS and predictors of AIDS in seroprevalent and seroincident cohorts of homosexual men, *AIDS*, 3, 347, 1989.

20. Stevenson, M., Natin, D., Fernando, R., and Shahmanesh, M., Hepatitis B markers do not predict decline in CD4 counts, *Proc. IVth Int. Conf. AIDS,* Berlin, 1993, Abstr. PO-B02-0947.

21. Thomas, H. C., Montano, L., Goodall, A., de Koning, R., Oladapo, J., and Wiedman, K. H., Immunological mechanisms in chronic hepatitis B virus infection, *Hepatology*, 2(Suppl.), 116S, 1982.

22. Dienstag, J. L., Immunological mechanisms in chronic viral hepatitis, in *Viral Hepatitis and Liver Disease*, Vyas, G. N., Dienstag, J. L., and Hoofnagle, J. H., Eds., Grune & Stratton, Orlando, FL, 1984, 135.

23. Mondelli, M. and Eddleston, A. L. W. F., Mechanisms of liver cell injury in acute and chronic hepatitis B, *Semin. Liver Dis.*, 4, 47, 1984.

24. Ganem, D., Persistent infection of humans with hepatitis B virus: mechanisms and consequences, *Rev. Infect. Dis.*, 4, 1026, 1982.

25. Ferrari, C., Penna, A., DegliAntoni, A., and Fiaccadori, F., Cellular immune response to hepatitis B virus antigens: an overview, *J. Hepatol.*, 7, 21, 1988.

26. Thomas, H. C., Jacyna, M., Waters, J., and Main, J., Virus-host interaction in chronic hepatitis B virus infection, *Semin. Liver Dis.*, 8, 342, 1988.

27. Taylor, P. E., Stevens, C. E., Rodriguez de Cordoba, S., and Rubenstein, P., Hepatitis B virus and human immunodeficiency virus: possible interactions, in *Viral Hepatitis and Liver Disease*, Zuckerman, A. J., Ed., Alan R. Liss, New York, 1988, 198.

28. Krogsgaard, K., Lindhardt, B. O., Nielson, J. O., Andersson, P., Kryger, P., Aldershvile, J., Gerstoft, J., and Pedersen, C., The influence of HTLV-III infection on the natural history of hepatitis B virus infection in male homosexual HBsAg carriers, *Hepatology*, 7, 37, 1987.

29. Bodsworth, N., Donovan, B., and Nightingale, B. N., The effect of concurrent human immuno-deficiency virus on chronic hepatitis B: a study of 150 homosexual men, *J. Infect. Dis.*, 160, 577, 1989.

30. Collier, A. C., Corey, L., Murphy, V. L., and Handsfield, H. H., Antibody to human immunodeficiency virus and suboptimal response to hepatitis B vaccination, *Ann. Intern. Med.*, 109, 101, 1988.

31. Davis, G. L. and Hoofnagle, J. H., Reactivation of chronic hepatitis B virus infection, *Gastroenterology*, 92, 2028, 1987.

32. Biggar, R. J., Goedert, J. J., and Hoffnagle, J. H., Accelerated loss of antibody to hepatitis B surface antigen among immunodeficient homosexual men infected with HIV, *N. Engl. J. Med.*, 316, 630, 1987.

33. Hadler, S. C., Judson, F. N., O'Malley, P. M., Altman, N. L., Penley, K., Buchbinder, S., Schable, C. A., Coleman, P. J., Ostrow, D. N., and Francis, D. P., Outcome of hepatitis B virus infection in homosexual men and its relation to prior human immunodeficiency virus infection, *J. Infect. Dis.*, 163, 454, 1991.

34. Naumov, N. V., Mondelli, M., Alexander, G. J. M., Tedder, R. S., Eddleston, A. L. W. F., and Williams, R., Relationship between expression of hepatitis B virus antigens in isolated hepatocytes and autologous lymphocyte cytotoxicity in patients with chronic hepatitis B virus infection, *Hepatology*, 4, 63, 1984.

35. Eddleston, A. L. W. F., Mondelli, M., Mieli-Vergani, G., and Williams, R., Lymphocyte cytotoxicity to autologous hepatocytes in chronic HBV infection, *Hepatology*, 2, 122, 1982.

36. Kakumi, S., Yata, K., and Kashio, T., Immunoregulatory T-cell function in acute and chronic liver disease, *Gastroenterology*, 79, 613, 1980.

37. McDonald, J. A., Harris, S., Waters, J. A., and Thomas, H. C., Effect of human immunodeficiency virus (HIV) infection on chronic hepatitis B hepatic viral antigen display, *J. Hepatol.*, 4, 337, 1987.

38. Pignatelli, M., Waters, J., Lever, A., Iwarson, S., Gerety, R., and Thomas, H. C., Cytotoxic T-cell responses to the nucleocapsid proteins of HBV in chronic hepatitis: evidence that antibody modulation may cause protracted infection, *J. Hepatol.*, 4, 15, 1987.

39. McDonald, J. A., Caruso, L., Karayiannis, P., Scully, L. J., Harris, J. R. W., Forster, G. E., and Thomas, H. C., Diminished responsiveness of male homosexual chronic hepatitis B virus carriers with HTLV-III antibodies to recombinant alpha-interferon, *Hepatology*, 7, 719, 1987.

40. Gordon, S. C., Reddy, K. R., Gould, E. E., Mcfadden, R., O'Brien, C., DeMedina, M., Jeffers, L. J., and Schiff, E. R., The spectrum of liver disease in the acquired immune deficiency syndrome, *J. Hepatol.*, 2, 475, 1986.

41. Lebovics, E., Thung, S. N., Schaffner, F., and Radensky, P. W., The liver in the acquired immuno-deficiency syndrome: a clinical and histologic study, *Hepatology*, 5, 293, 1985.

42. Rector, W. G., Jr., Govindarajan, S., Horsburgh, C. R., Jr., Penley, K. A., Cohn, D. L., and Judson, F. N., Hepatic inflammation, hepatitis B replication, and cellular immune function in homosexual males with chronic hepatitis B and antibody to human immunodeficiency virus, *Am. J. Gastroenterol.*, 83, 262, 1988.

43. Scharschmidt, B. F., Held, M. J., Hollander, H. H., Read, A. E., Lavine, J. E., Veereman, G., McGuire, R. F., and Thaler, M. M., Hepatitis B in patients with HIV infection: relationship to AIDS and patient survival, *Ann. Intern. Med.*, 117, 837, 1992.

44. Brook, M. G., McDonald, J. A., Karayinnis, P., Caruso, L., Forster, G., Harris, J. R., and Thomas, H. C., Randomized controlled trial of interferon alfa 2a (rbe) (Roferon-A) for the treatment of chronic hepatitis B virus (HBV) infection: factors that influence response, *Gut*, 30, 1116, 1989.

45. Saracco, G., Mazzella, G., Rosina, F., Cancellieri, C., Lattore, V., Raise, E., Rocca, G., Giorda, L., Verme, G., Gasbarrini, G., Barbara, L., Bonino, F., Rizzetto, M., and Roda, E., A controlled trial of human lymphoblastoid interferon in chronic hepatitis B in Italy, *Hepatology*, 10, 336, 1989.

46. American Foundation for AIDS Research, Hepatitis, *AIDS/HIV Treatment Directory*, 7(4), 88, 1995.

47. Korenman, J., Baker, B., Waggoner, J., Everhart, J. E., Di Bisceglie, A. M., and Hoofnagle, J. H., Long-term remission of chronic hepatitis B after alpha-interferon therapy, *Ann. Intern. Med.*, 114, 629, 1991.

48. Bird, G. L. A., Smith, H., Portmann, B., Alexander, G. J. M., and Williams, R., Acute liver decompensation on withdrawal of cytotoxic chemotherapy and immunosuppressive therapy in hepatitis B carriers, *Q. J. Med.*, 73, 895, 1989.

49. Prince, A. M., Brotman, B., Grady, G. F., Kuhns, W. J., Hazzi, C., Levine, R. W., and Millian, S. J., Long-incubated post-transfusion hepatitis without serological evidence of exposure to hepatitis-B virus, *Lancet*, 2, 241, 1974.

50. Feinstone, S. M., Kapikian, A. Z., Purcell, R. H., Alter, H. J., and Holland, P. V., Transfusion-associated hepatitis not due to viral hepatitis type A or B, *N. Engl. J. Med.*, 292, 767, 1975.

51. Anonymous, Non-A, non-B? *Lancet*, 2, 64, 1975.

52. Alter, M. J., Margolis, H. S., Krawczynski, K., Judson, F. N., Maree, A., Alexander, W. J., Hu, P. Y., Miller, J. K., Gerber, M. A., Sampliner, R. E., Meeks, E. L., and Beach, M. J., The natural history of community- acquired hepatitis C in the United States, *N. Engl. J. Med.*, 327, 1899, 1992.

53. Seeff, L. B., Buskell-Bales, Z., Wright, E. C., Durako, S. J., Alter, H. J., Iber, F. L., Hollinger, F. B., Gitnick, G., Knodell, R. G., Perillo, R. P., Stevens, C. E., Hollingsworth, C. G., and the National Heart, Lung and Blood Institute Study Group, Long-term mortality after transfusion- associated non-A, non-B hepatitis, *N. Engl. J. Med.*, 327, 1906, 1992.

54. Choo, Q.-L., Kuo, G., Weiner, A. J., Overby, L. R., Bradley, D. W., and Houghton, M., Isolation of a cDNA clone derived from a blood-borne non-A, non-B viral hepatitis genome, *Science*, 244, 359, 1989.

55. Kuo, G., Choo, Q.-L., Alter, H. J., Gitnick, G. L., Redeker, A. G., Purcell, R. H., Miyamura, T., Dienstag, J. L., Alter, M. J., Stevens, C. E., Tegmeier, G. E., Bonino, F., Colombo, M., Lee, W.-S., Kuo, C., Berger, K., Shuster, J. R., Overby, L. R., Bradley, D. W., and Houghton, M., An assay for circulating antibodies to a major etiologic virus of human non-A, non-B hepatitis, *Science*, 244, 362, 1989.

56. Cuthbert, J. A., Hepatitis C: progress and problems, *Clin. Microbiol. Rev.*, 7, 505, 1994.

57. Koziel, M. J., Dudley, D., Wong, J. T., Dienstag, J., Houghton, M., Ralston, R., and Walker, B. D., Intrahepatic cytotoxic T lymphocytes specific for hepatitis C virus in persons with chronic hepatitis, *J. Immunol.*, 149, 3339, 1992.

58. Lau, J. Y. N., Davis, G. L., Kniffen, J., Qian, K. P., Urdea, M. S., Chan, C. S., Mizokami, M., Neuwald, P. D., and Wilber, J. C., Significance of serum hepatitis C virus RNA levels in chronic hepatitis C, *Lancet*, 341, 1501, 1993.

59. Yuki, N., Hayashi, N., and Kamada, T., HCV viraemia and liver injury in symptom-free blood donors, *Lancet*, 342, 444, 1993.

60. Krawczynski, K., Beach, M. J., Bradley, D. W., Kuo, G., Di Bisceglie, A. M., Houghton, M., Reyes, G. R., Kim, J. P., Choo, Q. L., and Alter, M. J., Hepatitis C virus antigen in hepatocytes: immuno-morphologic detection and identification, *Gastroenterology*, 103, 622, 1992.

61. Fong, T. L., Valinluck, B., Govindarajan, S., Charboneau, F., Adkins, R. H., and Redeker, A. G., Short-term prednisone therapy affects aminotransferase activity and hepatitis C virus RNA levels in chronic hepatitis C, *Gastroenterology*, 107, 196, 1994.

62. van der Poel, C. L., Cuypers, H. T. M., Reesink, H. W., Weiner, A. J., Quan, S., Di Nello, R., Van Boven, J. J., Winkel, I., Mulder-Folkerts, D., Exel-Oehlers, P. J., Schaasberg, W., Leentvaar-Kuypers, A., Polito, A., Houghton, M., and Lelie, P. N., Confirmation of hepatitis C virus infection by new four-antigen recombinant immunoblot assay, *Lancet*, 337, 317, 1991.

63. Follett, E. A. C., Dow, B. C., McOmish, F., Lee Yap, P., Hughes, W., Mitchell, R., and Simmonds, P., HCV confirmatory testing of blood donors, *Lancet*, 338, 1024, 1991.

64. Marcellin, P., Martinot-Peignoux, M., Elias, A., Branger, M., Courtois, F., Level, R., Erlinger, S., and Benhamou, J. P., Hepatitis C virus (HCV) viremia in human immunodeficiency virus-seronegative and -seropositive patients with indeterminate HCV recombinant immunoblot assay, *J. Infect. Dis.*, 170, 433, 1994.

65. Aach, R. D., Stevens, C. E., Hollinger, F. B., Mosley, J. W., Peterson, D. A., Taylor, P. E., Johnson, R. G., Barbosa, L. H., and Nemo, G. J., Hepatitis C virus infection in post-transfusion hepatitis: an analysis with first- and second-generation assays, *N. Engl. J. Med.*, 325, 1325, 1991.

66. Koretz, R. L., Abbey, H., Coleman, E., and Gitnick, G., Non-A, non-B post-transfusion hepatitis: looking back in the 2nd decade, *Ann. Intern. Med.*, 119, 110, 1993.

67. Giuberti, T., Ferrari, C., Marchelli, S., Degli, A. A. M., Schianchi, C., Pizzaferri, P., and Fiaccadori, F., Long-term follow-up of anti-hepatitis C virus antibodies in patients with acute nonA nonB hepatitis and different outcome of liver disease, *Liver*, 12, 94, 1992.

68. Mattsson, L., Grilner, L., and Weiland, O., Seroconversion to hepatitis C virus antibodies in patients with acute posttransfusion non-A, non-B hepatitis in Sweden with a second generation test, *Scand. J. Infect. Dis.*, 24, 15, 1992.

69. Tremolada, F., Casarin, C., Alberti, A., Drago, C., Tagger, A., Ribero, M. L., and Realdi, G., Long-term follow-up of non-A, non-B (type C) post-transfusion hepatitis, *J. Hepatol.*, 16, 273, 1992.

70. Luo, K. X., Liang, Z. S., Yang, S. C., Zhou, R., Meng, Q. H., Zhu, Y. W., He, H. T., and Jiang, S., Etiological investigation of acute post-transfusion non-A, non-B hepatitis in China, *J. Med. Virol.*, 39, 219, 1993.

71. Wang, J. T., Wang, T. H., Sheu, J. C., Lin, J. T., Wang, C. Y., and Chen, D. S., Posttransfusion hepatitis revisited by hepatitis C antibody assays and polymerase chain reaction, *Gastroenterology*, 103, 609, 1992.

72. Kaldor, J. M., Archer, G. T., Buring, M. L., Ismay, S. L., Kenrick, K. G., Lien, A. S. M., Purusothaman, K., Tulloch, R., Bolton, W. V., and Wylie, B. R., Risk factors for hepatitis C virus infection in blood donors — a case control study, *Med. J. Aust.*, 157, 227, 1992.

73. McCaughan, G. W., McGuinness, P. H., Bishop, G. A., Painter, D. M., Lien, A. S. M., Tulloch, R., Wylie, B. R., and Archer, G. T., Clinical assessment and incidence of hepatitis C RNA in 50 consecutive RIBA-positive volunteer blood donors, *Med. J. Aust.*, 157, 231, 1992.

74. Ko, Y. C., Ho, M. S., Chiang, T. A., Chang, S. J., and Chang, P. Y., Tattooing as a risk of hepatitis C virus infection, *J. Med. Virol.*, 38, 288, 1992.

75. Kiyosawa, K., Sodeyama, T., Tanaka, E., Nakano, Y., Furuta, S., Nishioka, K., Purcell, R. H., and Alter, H. J., Hepatitis C in hospital employees with needlestick injuries, *Ann. Intern. Med.*, 115, 367, 1991.

76. Mitsui, T., Iwano, K., Masuko, K., Yamazaki, C., Okamoto, H., Tsuda, F., Tanaka, T., and Mishiro, S., Hepatitis C virus infection in medical personnel after needlestick accident, *Hepatology*, 16, 1109, 1992.

77. Atrah, H. I., Ala, F. A., and Gough, D., Blood exchanged in ritual ceremonies as a possible route for infection with hepatitis C virus, *J. Clin. Pathol.*, 47, 87, 1994.

78. Kiyosawa, K., Tanaka, E., Sodeyama, T., Yoshizawa, K., Yabu, K., Furuta, K., Imai, H., Nakano, Y., Usuda, S., Uemura, K., Furuta, S., Watanabe, Y., Watanabe, J., Fukuda, Y., Takeyama, T., Urushibara, A., Matsumoto, A., Mori, H., Kobayashi, M., Suzuki, T., Yamada, S., Seki, T., Shimizu, S., Nakamura, M., Sone, H., Hara, K., Ichijo, T., Ohike, Y., Gibo, Y., Nakatsuji, Y., Yoda, H., Tsuchiya, K., Hayata, T., Imai, Y., Kobayashi, M., and Hara, N., Transmission of hepatitis C in an isolated area of Japan: community-acquired infection, *Gastroenterology*, 106, 1596, 1994.

79. Pereira, B. J. G., Milford, E. L., Kirkman, R. L., and Levey, A. S., Transmission of hepatitis C virus by organ transplantation, *N. Engl. J. Med.*, 325, 454, 1991.

80. Pereira, B. J. G., Milford, E. L., Kirkman, R. L., Quan, S., Sayre, K. R., Johnson, P. J., Wilber, J. C., and Levey, A. S., Prevalence of hepatitis C virus RNA in organ donors positive for hepatitis C antibody and in the recipients of their organs, *N. Engl. J. Med.*, 327, 910, 1992.

81. Roth, D., Fernandez, J. A., Babischkin, S., Demattos, A., Buck, B. E., Quan, S., Olson, L., Burke, G. W., Nery, J. R., Esquenazi, V., Schiff, E. R., and Miller, J., Detection of hepatitis C virus infection among cadaver organ donors — evidence for low transmission of disease, *Ann. Intern. Med.*, 117, 470, 1992.

82. Vincenti, F., Lake, J., Wright, T., Kuo, G., Weber, P., and Stempel, C., Nontransmission of hepatitis C from cadaver kidney donors to transplant recipients, *Transplantation*, 55, 674, 1993.

83. Inoue, Y., Takeuchi, K., Chou, W. H., Unayama, T., Takahashi, K., Saito, I., and Miyamura, T., Silent mother-to-child transmission of hepatitis C virus through two generations determined by comparative nucleotide sequence analysis of the viral cDNA, *J. Infect. Dis.*, 166, 1425, 1992.

84. Novati, R., Thiers, V., Monforte, A. D., Maisonneuve, P., Principi, N. R., Conti, M., Lazzarin, A., and Bréchot, C., Mother-to-child transmission of hepatitis C virus detected by nested polymerase chain reaction, *J. Infect. Dis.*, 165, 720, 1992.

85. Ohto, H., Terazawa, S., Sasaki, N., Sasaki, N., Hino, K., Ishiwata, C., Kako, M., Ujiie, N., Endo, C., Matsui, A., Okamoto, H., Mishiro, S., Kojima, M., Aikawa, T., Shimoda, K., Sakamoto, M., Akahane, Y., Yoshizawa, H., Tanaka, T., Tokita, H., and Tsuda, F., Transmission of hepatitis C virus from mothers to infants, *N. Engl. J. Med.*, 330, 744, 1994.

86. Thaler, M. M., Park, C. K., Landers, D. V., Wara, D. W., Houghton, M., Veereman-Wauters, G., Sweet, R. L., and Han, J. H., Vertical transmission of hepatitis C virus, *Lancet*, 338, 17, 1991.

87. Weiner, A. J., Thaler, M. M., Crawford, K., Ching, K., Kansopon, J., Chien, D. Y., Hall, J. E., Hu, F., and Houghton, M., A unique, predominant hepatitis C virus variant found in an infant born to a mother with multiple variants, *J. Virol.*, 67, 4365, 1993.

88. Alter, H. J., Holland, P. V., Morrow, A. G., Purcell, R. H., Feinstone, S. M., and Moritsugi, Y., Clinical and serological analysis of transfusion-associated hepatitis, *Lancet*, 2, 838, 1975.

89. Dienstag, J. L., Non-A, non-B hepatitis. I. Recognition, epidemiology, and clinical features, *Gastroenterology*, 85, 439, 1983.

90. U.S. Department of Health and Human Services, Hepatitis Surveillance Report 51, Centers for Disease Control, Atlanta, GA, 1987, 19.

91. Alter, M. J., Coleman, P. J., Alexander, W. J., Kramer, E., Miller, J. K., Mandel, E., Hadler, S. C., and Margolis, H. S., Importance of heterosexual activity in the transmission of hepatitis B and non-A, non-B hepatitis, *JAMA*, 262, 1201, 1989.

92. Eyster, M. E., Alter, H. J., Aledorf, L. M., Quan, S., Hatzakis, A., and Goedert, J. J., Heterosexual co-transmission of hepatitis C virus (HCV) and human immunodeficiency virus (HIV), *Ann. Intern. Med.*, 115, 764, 1991.

93. Esteban, J. I., Esteban, R., Viladomiu, L., Lopez-Talavera, J. C., Gonzalez, A., Hernandez, J. M., Roget, M., Vargas, V., Genesca, J., Buti, M., Giardia, J., Houghton, M., Choo, Q.-L., and Kuo, G., Hepatitis C virus antibodies among risk groups in Spain, *Lancet*, 2, 294, 1989.

94. Bresters, D., Mauser-Bunschoten, E. P., Reesink, H. W., Roosendaal, G., van der Poel, C. L., Chamuleau, R. A. F. M., Jansen, P. L. M., Weegink, C. J., Cuypers, H. T. M., Lelie, P. N., and van den Berg, H. M., Sexual transmission of hepatitis C virus, *Lancet*, 342, 210, 1993.

95. Kao, J.-H., Chen, P.-J., Lei, M.-Y., Wang, T.-H., and Chen, D.-S., Sexual transmission of HCV, *Lancet*, 342, 626, 1993.

96. Benezra, J., Sexual transmission of HCV, *Lancet*, 342, 626, 1993.

97. Kuo, G., Choo, Q. L., Alter, H. J., Gitnick, G. L., Redeker, A. G., Purcell, R. H., Miyamura, T., Dienstag, J. L., Alter, M. J., Stevens, C. E., Tegtmeier, G. E., Bonino, F., Colombo, M., Lee, W.-S., Kuo, C., Berger, K., Shuster, J. R., Overby, L. R., Bradley, D. W., and Houghton, M., An assay for circulating antibodies to a major etiologic virus of human non-A, non-B hepatitis, *Science*, 244, 362, 1989.

98. Shiffman, M. L., Contos, M. J., Luketic, V. A., Sanyal, A. J., Purdum, P. P. III, Mills, A. S., Fisher, R. A., and Posner, M. P., Biochemical and histological evaluation of recurrent hepatitis C following orthotopic liver transplantation, *Transplantation*, 57, 526, 1994.

99. Martin, P., Munoz, S. J., Di Bisceglie, A. M., Rubin, R., Waggoner, J. G., Armenti, V. T., Moritz, M. J., Jarrell, B. E., and Maddrey, W. C., Recurrence of hepatitis C infection following orthotopic liver transplantation, *Hepatology*, 13, 719, 1991.

100. Wright, T. L., Donegan, E., Hsu, H. H., Ferrell, L., Lake, J. R., Kim, M., Combs, C., Fennessy, S., Roberts, J. P., Ascher, N. L., and Greenberg, H. B., Recurrent and acquired hepatitis C viral infection in liver transplant recipients, *Gastroenterology*, 103, 317, 1992.

101. Thung, S. W., Shim, K. S., Shieh, Y. S. C., Schwartz, M., Thiese, N., Bercich, A., Katz, E., Miller, C., and Gerber, M. A., Hepatitis C in liver allografts, *Arch. Pathol. Lab. Med.*, 117, 145, 1993.

102. Ferrel, L., Wright, T. L., Lake, J., Roberts, J., and Ascher, N., Pathology of hepatitis C virus infection in liver transplant recipients, *Lab. Invest.*, 66, 96A, 1992.

103. Schramm, W., Roggendorf, M., Rommel, F., Kammerer, R., Pohlmann, H., Rasshofer, R., Gürtler, L., and Deinhardt, F., Prevalence of antibodies to hepatitis C virus (HCV) in haemophiliacs, *Blut*, 59, 390, 1989.

104. Makris, M., Preston, F. E., Triger, D. R., Underwood, J. C. E., Choo, Q. L., Kuo, G., and Houghton, M., Hepatitis C antibody and chronic liver disease in haemophilia, *Lancet*, 335, 1117, 1990.

105. Brettler, D. B., Alter, H. J., Dienstag, J. L., Forsberg, A. D., and Levine, P. H., Prevalence of hepatitis C virus antibody in a cohort of hemophilia patients, *Blood*, 76, 254, 1990.

106. Blanchette, V. S., Vorstman, E., Shore, A., Wang, E., Petric, M., Jett, B. W., and Alter, H. J., Hepatitis C infection in children with hemophilia A and B, *Blood*, 78, 285, 1991.

107. Rumi, G. M., Colombo, M., Gringeri, A., and Mannucci, P. M., High prevalence of antibody to hepatitis C virus in multitransfused hemophiliacs with normal transaminase levels, *Ann. Intern. Med.*, 112, 379, 1990.

108. Allain, J. P., Dailey, S. H., Laurian, Y., Vallari, D. S., Rafawicz, A., Desai, S. M., and Devare, S. G., Evidence for persistent hepatitis C virus (HCV) infection in hemophiliacs, *J. Clin. Invest.*, 88, 1672, 1991.

109. Goedert, J. J., Kessler, C. M., Aledorf, L. M., Biggar, R. J., Andes, W. A., White, G. C., Drummond, J. E., Vaidya, K., Mann, D. L., Eyster, M. E., Ragni, M. V., Lederman, M. M., Cohen, A. R., Bray, G. L., Rosenberg, P. S., Friedman, R. M., Hilgartner, M. W., Blattner, W. A., Kroner, B., and Gail, M. H., A prospective study of human immunodeficiency virus type 1 infection and the development of AIDS in subjects with hemophilia, *N. Engl. J. Med.*, 321, 1141, 1989.

110. Eyster, M. E., Diamondstone, L. S., Lien, J. M., Ehmann, W. C., Quan, S., and Goedert, J. J., The natural history of hepatitis C virus (HCV) infection in multitransfused hemophiliacs: effect of coin-fection with human immunodeficiency virus (HIV), *J. AIDS*, 6, 602, 1993.

111. Eyster, M. E., Fried, M. W., Di Bisceglie, A. M., Goedert, J. J., and the Multicenter Hemophilia Cohort Study, Increasing hepatitis C virus RNA levels in hemophiliacs: relationship to human immunodefi-ciency virus infection and liver disease, *Blood*, 84, 1020, 1994.

112. Sherman, K. E., O'Brien, J., Gutierrez, A. G., Harrison, S., Urdea, M., Neuwald, P., and Wilber, J., Quantitative evaluation of hepatitis C virus RNA in patients with concurrent immunodeficiency virus infections, *J. Clin. Microbiol.*, 31, 2679, 1993.

113. Martin, P., Di Bisceglie, A. M., Kassianides, C., Lisker-Melman, M., and Hoofnagle, J. H., Rapidly progressive non-A non-B hepatitis in patients with human immunodeficiency virus infection, *Gastro-enterology*, 97, 1559, 1989.

114. Roger, P. M., Tran, A., Saint Paul, M. C., Fuzibet, J. G., Benzaken, S., Michiels, J. F., Rampal, P., and Dellamonica, P., Influence of HIV infection in chronic C hepatitis: a case-control study, *Proc. 36th Intersci. Conf. Antimicrob. Agents Chemother.*, American Society for Microbiology, Washington, D.C., Abstr. H-68, 1996.

115. Brouet, J. C., Clauvel, J. P., Danon, F., Klein, M., and Seligmann, M., Biologic and clinical significance of cryoglobulins: a report of 86 cases, *Am. J. Med.*, 57, 775, 1974.

116. Pechere-Bertschi, A., Perrin, L., De Saussure, P., Wildmann, J. J., Giostra, E., and Schifferli, J. A., Hepatitis C: a possible etiology for cryoglobulinemia type II, *Clin. Exp. Immunol.*, 89, 419, 1992.

117. Ferri, C., Greco, F., Longobardo, G., Palla, P., Marzo, E., and Moretti, A., Antibodies to hepatitis C virus in patients with mixed cryoglobulinemia, *Arthritis Rheum.*, 34, 1606, 1991.

118. Angello, V., Chung, R. T., and Kaplan, L. M., A role for hepatitis C virus infection in type II cryoglobulinemia, *N. Engl. J. Med.*, 327, 1490, 1992.

119. Werner, C., Joller-Jemelka, H. I., and Fontana, A., Hepatitis C virus and cryoglobulinemia, *N. Engl. J. Med.*, 328, 1122, 1993.

120. Matsuda, J., Tsakamoto, M., Gonchi, K., Saitoh, N., and Gotoh, M., Hepatitis C virus (HCV) RNA and human immunodeficiency virus (HIV) p24 antigen in the cryoglobulin of hemophiliacs with HIV and/or HCV infection, *Clin. Infect. Dis.*, 18, 832, 1994.

121. Ellaurie, M., Calvelli, T. A., and Rubinstein, A., Human immunodeficiency virus (HIV) circulating immune complexes in infected children, *AIDS Res. Hum. Retrovir.*, 6, 1437, 1990.

122. Simon, F., Rahimy, C., Krivine, A., Levine, M., Pepin, J. M., Lapierro, D., Denamur, E., Vernoux, L., De Crepy, A., Blot, P., Vilmer, E., and Brun-Vezinet, F., Antibody avidity measurement and immune complex dissociation for serological diagnosis of vertically acquired HIV-1 infection, *J. Acquir. Immune Defic. Syndr.*, 6, 201, 1993.

123. Davis, G. L., Balart, L. A., Schiff, E. R., Lindsay, K., Bodenheimer, H. C., Perrillo, R. P., Carey, W., Jacobson, I. M., Payne, J., Dienstag, J. L., Van Thiel, D. H., Tamburro, C., Lefkovitch, J., Albrecht, J., Meschievitz, C., Ortego, T. J., Gibas, A., and the Hepatitis Interventional Therapy Group, Treatment of chronic hepatitis C with recombinant interferon alpha: a multicenter randomized, controlled trial, *N. Engl. J. Med.*, 321, 1501, 1989.

124. Di Bisceglie, A. M., Martin, P., Kassianides, C., Lisker-Melman, M., Murray, L., Waggoner, J., Goodman, Z., Banks, S. M., and Hoofnagle, J. H., Recombinant interferon alfa therapy for chronic hepatitis C: a randomized, double-blind, placebo-controlled trial, *N. Engl. J. Med.*, 321, 1506, 1989.

125. Jouet, P., Rudet-Thoraval, F., Dhumeaux, D., Métreau, J.-M., and Le Groupe Francais pour l'Etude du Traitement des Hépatities Chroniques NANB/C, Comparative efficacy of interferon alfa in cirrhotic and noncirrhotic patients with non-A, non-B, C hepatitis, *Gastroenterology*, 106, 686, 1994.

126. Lindsay, K. L., Davis, G. L., Schiff, E., Bodenheimer, H., Balart, L., Dienstag, J., Perrillo, R., Tamburro, C., Silva, M., Goff, C., Everson, G., Sanghvi, B., and Albrecht, J., Long-term response to higher doses of interferon alfa-2b treatment of patients with chronic hepatitis C: a randomized multicenter trial, *Hepatology*, 18, 106A, 1993.

127. Reichard, O., Foberg, U., Frydén, A., Mattsson, L., Norkrans, G., Sönnenborg, A., Westjal, R., Yun, Z.-B., and Weiland, O., High sustained response rate and clearance of viremia in chronic hepatitis C after treatment with interferon-α_{2b} for 60 weeks, *Hepatology*, 19, 280, 1994.

128. Saracco, G., Rosina, F., Abate, M. L., Chiandussi, L., Gallo, V., Cerutti, E., Dinapoli, A., Solinas, A., Deplano, A., Tocco, A., Cossu, P., Chien, D., Kuo, G., Polito, A., Weiner, A. J., Houghton, M., Verme, G., Bonino, F., and Rizzetto, M., Long-term follow-up of patients with chronic hepatitis C treated with different doses of interferon-α_{2b}, *Hepatology*, 18, 1300, 1993.

129. Iino, S., Hino, K., Kuroki, T., Suzuki, H., and Yamamoto, S., Treatment of chronic hepatitis C with high-dose interferon α-2b: a multicenter study, *Dig. Dis. Sci.*, 38, 612, 1993.

130. Brillanti, S., Garson, J. A., Tuke, P. W., Ring, C., Briggs, M., Masci, C., Miglioli, M., Barbara, L., and Tedder, R. S., Effect of alpha-interferon therapy on hepatitis C viraemia in community-acquired chronic non-A, non-B hepatitis: a quantitative polymerase chain reaction study, *J. Med. Virol.*, 34, 136, 1991.

131. Chayama, K., Saitoh, S., Arase, Y., Ikeda, K., Matsumoto, T., Sakai, Y., Kobayashi, M., Unakami, M., Morinaga, T., and Kumada, H., Effect of interferon administration on serum hepatitis C virus RNA in patients with chronic hepatitis C, *Hepatology*, 13, 1040, 1991.

132. Hagiwara, H., Hayashi, N. R., Mita, E., Ueda, K., Takehara, T., Kasahara, A., Fusamoto, H., and Kamada, T., Detection of hepatitis C virus RNA in serum of patients with chronic hepatitis C treated with interferon-alpha, *Hepatology*, 15, 37, 1992.

133. Magrin, S., Craxi, A., Fabiano, C., Fiorentino, G., Marino, L., Almasio, P., Pinzello, G. B., Palazzo, U., Vitale, M., Maggio, A., Bucca, G., Gianguzza, F., Shyamala, V., Han, J. H., and Pagliaro, L., Serum hepatitis C virus (HCV)-RNA and response to alpha-interferon in anti-HCV positive chronic hepatitis, *J. Med. Virol.*, 38, 200, 1992.

134. Shindo, M., Di Bisceglie, A. M., Cheung, L., Shih, J. W., Cristiano, K., Feinstone, S. M., and Hoofnagle, J. H., Decrease in serum hepatitis C viral RNA during alpha-interferon therapy for chronic hepatitis C, *Ann. Intern. Med.*, 115, 700, 1991.

135. Shindo, M., Di Bisceglie, M., and Hoofnagle, J. H., Long-term follow-up of patients with chronic hepatitis C treated with alpha-interferon, *Hepatology*, 15, 1013, 1992.

136. Kakumi, S., Yoshika, K., Tanaka, K., Higashi, Y., Kurokawa, S., Hirofuji, H., and Kusakabe, A., Long-term carriage of hepatitis C virus with normal aminotransferase after interferon treatment in patients with chronic hepatitis C, *J. Med. Virol.*, 41, 65, 1993.

137. Lau, J. Y. N., Mizokami, M., Ohno, T., Diamond, D. A., Kniffen, J., and Davis, G. L., Discrepancy between biochemical and virological responses to interferon-α in chronic hepatitis C, *Lancet*, 342, 1208, 1993.

138. Kobayashi, Y., Watanabe, S., Konishi, M., Yokoi, M., Ikoma, J., Kakehashi, R., Kojima, Y., and Suzuki, S., Detection of hepatitis C virus RNA by nested polymerase chain reaction in sera of patients with chronic non-A, non-B hepatitis treated with interferon, *J. Hepatol.*, 16, 138, 1992.

139. Boyer, N., Marcellin, P., Degott, C., Degos, F., Saimot, A. G., Erlinger, S., Benhamou, J. P., and the Comité des Anti-Viraux, Recombinant interferon-α for chronic hepatitis C in patients positive for antibody to human immunodeficiency virus, *J. Infect. Dis.*, 165, 723, 1992.

140. Hoofnagle, J. H., Mullen, K. D., Jones, D. R., Rustgi, V., Di Bisceglie, A., Peters, M., Waggoner, J. G., Park, Y., and Jones, E. A., Treatment of chronic non-A, non-B hepatitis with recombinant human alpha interferon: a preliminary report, *N. Engl. J. Med.*, 315, 1575, 1986.

141. Ohnishi, K., Nomura, F., and Iida, S., Treatment of post-transfusion non-A, non-B acute and chronic hepatitis with human fibroblast beta-interferon: a preliminary report, *Am. J. Gastroenterol.*, 84, 596, 1989.

142. Omata, M., Yokosuka, O., Takano, S., Kato, N. R., Hosoda, K., Imazeki, F., Tada, M., Ito, Y., and Ohto, M., Resolution of acute hepatitis C after therapy with natural beta interferon, *Lancet*, 338, 914, 1991.

143. Lampertico, P., Rumi, M., Romeo, R., Craxi, A., Soffredini, R., Biassoni, D., and Colombo, M., A multicenter randomized controlled trial of recombinant interferon-α_{2b} in patients with acute transfusion-associated hepatitis C, *Hepatology*, 19, 19, 1994.

144. Viladomiu, L., Genesca, J., Esteban, J. I., Allende, H., Gonzalez, A., Lopez-Talavera, J. C., Esteban, R., and Guardia, J., Interferon-alpha in acute posttransfusion hepatitis C: a randomized, controlled study, *Hepatology*, 15, 767, 1992.

145. Di Bisceglie, A. M., Shindo, M., Fong, T.-L., Fried, M. W., Swain, M. G., Bergasa, N. V., Axiotis, C. A., Waggoner, J. G., Park, Y., and Hoofnagle, J. H., A pilot study of ribavirin therapy for chronic hepatitis C, *Hepatology*, 16, 649, 1992.

146. Reichard, O., Yun, Z. B., Sonnenborg, A., and Weiland, O., Hepatitis C viral RNA titers in serum prior to, during, and after oral treatment with ribavirin for chronic hepatitis C, *J. Med. Virol.*, 41, 99, 1993.

147. Kakumi, S., Yoshioka, K., Wakita, T., Ishikawa, T., Takayanagi, M., and Higashi, Y., A pilot study of ribavirin and interferon beta for the treatment of chronic hepatitis C, *Gastroenterology*, 105, 507, 1993.

148. Beloqui, O., Prieto, J., Suarez, M., Gil, B., Qian, C. H., Garcia, N., and Civeira, M. P., *N*-Acetyl cysteine enhances the response to interferon-alpha in chronic hepatitis C: a pilot study, *J. Interferon Res.*, 13, 279, 1993.

149. Wright, T. L., Hsu, H., Donegan, E., Feinstone, S., Greenberg, H., Read, A., Ascher, N. L., Roberts, J. P., and Lake, J. R., Hepatitis C virus not found in fulminant non-A, non-B hepatitis, *Ann. Intern. Med.*, 115, 111, 1991.

150. Vento, S., Cainelli, F., Mirandola, F., Cosco, L., Di Perri, G., Solbiati, M., Ferraro, T., and Concia, E., Fulminant hepatitis on withdrawal of chemotherapy in carriers of hepatitis C virus, *Lancet*, 347, 92, 1996.

151. Rizzetto, M., Canese, M. G., Arico, S., Crivelli, O., Trepo, C., Bonino, F., and Verme, G., Immuno-fluorescence detection of a new antibody-antibody system (δ/anti-δ) associated to hepatitis B virus in liver and in serum of HBsAg carriers, *Gut*, 18, 997, 1977.

152. Rizzetto, M. and Verme, G., Delta hepatitis — present status, *J. Hepatol.*, 1, 187, 1985.

153. Taylor, J., Structure and replication of hepatitis delta virus, *Semin. Virol.*, 1, 135, 1990.

154. Purcell, R. H. and Gerin, J. L., Hepatitis delta virus, in *Fields Virology*, 2nd ed., Fields, B. N., Knipe, D. M., Chanock, R. M., Melnick, J. L., Monath, T. P., and Roizman, B., Eds., Raven Press, New York, 1990, 2275.

155. Rizzetto, M., Verme, G., Gerin, J. L., and Purcell, R. H., Hepatitis delta virus disease, in *Progress in Liver Disease*, Vol. 8, Popper, H. and Schaffner, F., Eds., Grune and Stratton, Orlando, FL, 1986, 417.

156. Hoofnagle, J. H., Type D (delta) hepatitis, *JAMA*, 261, 1321, 1989 (correction in *JAMA*, 261, 3552, 1989).

157. Bonino, F., Negro, F., Baldi, M., Brunetto, M. R., Chiaberge, E., Capalbo, M., Maran, E., Lavarini, C., Tocca, N., and Rocca, G., The natural history of chronic delta hepatitis, in *The Hepatitis Delta Virus and Its Infection*, Progress in Clinical and Biological Research, Vol. 234, Rizzetto, M., Gerin, J. L., and Purcell, R. H., Eds., Alan R. Liss, New York, 1987, 145.

158. Smedile, A., Farci, P., Verme, G., Carreda, F., Cargnel, A., Caporaso, N., Dentico, P., Trepo, C., Opolon, P., Gimson, A., Vergani, D., Williams, R., and Rizzetto, M., Influence of delta infection on severity of hepatitis B, *Lancet*, 2, 945, 1982.

159. Rizzetto, M., Verme, G., Recchia, S., Bonino, F., Farci, P., Arico, S., Calzia, R., Picciotto, A., Colombo, M., and Popper, H., Chronic hepatitis in carriers of hepatitis B surface antigen, with intrahepatic expression of delta antigen: an active and progressive disease unresponsive to immuno-suppressive treatment, *Ann. Intern. Med.*, 98, 437, 1983.

160. Saracco, G., Rosina, F., Brunetto, M. R., Amoroso, P., Caredda, F., Farci, P., Piantino, P., Bonino, F., and Rizzetto, M., Rapidly progressive HBsAg-positive hepatitis in Italy: the role of hepatitis delta virus infection, *J. Hepatol.*, 5, 274, 1987.

161. Peters, M., Mechanisms of action of interferons, *Semin. Liver Dis.*, 9, 235, 1989.

162. Baron, S., Tyring, S. K., Fleischmann, W. R., Jr., Coppenhaver, D. H., Niesel, D. W., Klimpel, G. R., Stanton, G. J., and Hughes, T. K., The interferons: mechanisms of action and clinical applications, *JAMA*, 266, 1375, 1991.

163. Farci, P., Mandas, A., Coiana, A., Lai, E. M., Desmet, V., Van Eyken, P., Gibo, Y., Caruso, L., Scaccabarozzi, S., Criscuolo, D., Ryff, J.-C., and Balestrieri, A., Treatment of chronic hepatitis D with interferon alpha-2a, *N. Engl. J. Med.*, 330, 88, 1994.

164. Thomas, H. C., Farci, P., Shein, R., Karayiannis, P., Smedile, A., Caruso, L., and Gerin, J., Inhibition of hepatitis delta virus (HDV) replication by lymphoblastoid human alpha interferon, in *The Hepatitis Delta Virus and Its Infection* [Progress in Clinical and Biological Research, Vol. 234], Rizzetto, M., Gerin, J. L., and Purcell, R. H., Eds., Alan R. Liss, New York, 1987, 277.

165. Hoofnagle, J., Mullen, K., Peters, M., Avigan, M., Park, Y., Waggoner, J., Gerin, J., Hoyer, B., and Smedile, A., Treatment of chronic delta hepatitis with recombinant human alpha interferon, in *The Hepatitis and Its Infection*, Rizzetto, M., Gerin, J. L., and Purcell, R. H., Eds. [Progress in Clinical and Biological Research, vol. 234], Alan R. Liss, New York, 291, 1987.

166. Rosina, F., Saracco, G., Lattore, V., Quartarone, V., Rizzetto, M., Verme, G., Trinchero, P., Sansalvadore, F., and Smedile, A., Alpha 2 recombinant interferon in the treatment of chronic hepatitis delta virus (HDV) hepatitis, in *The Hepatitis and Its Infection* [Progress in Clinical and Biological Research, Vol. 234], Rizzetto, M., Gerin, J. L., and Purcell, R. H., Eds., Alan R. Liss, New York, 1987, 299.

167. Hoofnagle, J. H. and Di Bisceglie, A. M., Therapy of chronic viral hepatitis: chronic hepatitis D and non-A, non-B hepatitis, in *Viral Hepatitis and Liver Disease*, Zuckerman, A. J., Ed., Alan R. Liss, New York, 1988, 823.

168. Farci, P., Karayiannis, P., Brook, M. G., Smedile, A., Lai, M. E., Balestriere, A., Saldanha, J. A., Monjardino, J., Gerin, J., and Thomas, H. C., Treatment of chronic hepatitis delta virus (HDV) infection with human lymphoblastoid alpha interferon, *Q. J. Med.*, 73, 1045, 1989.

169. Di Bisceglie, A. M., Martin, P., Lisker-Melman, M., Kassianides, C., Korenman, J., Bergasa, N. V., Baker, B., and Hoofnagle, J. H., Therapy of chronic delta hepatitis with interferon alfa-2b, *J. Hepatol.*, 11(Suppl. 1), S151, 1990.

170. Porres, J. C., Carreno, V., Bartolome, J., Moreno, A., Galiana, F., and Quiroga, J. A., Treatment of chronic delta infection with recombinant human interferon alpha 2c at high doses, *J. Hepatol.*, 9, 338, 1989.

171. Marinucci, G., Hassan, G., Di Giacomo, C., Barlattani, A., Costa, F., Rasshofer, R., and Roggendorf, M., Long term treatment of chronic delta hepatitis with alpha recombinant interferon, in *The Hepatitis Delta Virus* [Progress in Clinical and Biological Research, Vol. 364], Gerin J. L., Purcell, R. H., and Rizzetto, M., Eds., Wiley-Liss, New York, 1991, 405.

172. Rosina, F., Pintus, C., Meschievitz, C., and Rizzetto, M., A randomized controlled trial of a 12-month course of recombinant human interferon- alpha in chronic delta (type D) hepatitis: a multicenter Italian study, *Hepatology*, 13, 1052, 1991.

173. Hadziyannis, S. J., Use of α-interferon in the treatment of chronic delta hepatitis, *J. Hepatol.*, 13(Suppl. 1), S21, 1991.

174. Farci, P., Orgiana, G., Coiana, A., Peddis, G., Mandas, A., Lai, E., Farci, A. M. G., Chessa, L., Balestrieri, A., Arnone, M., Casula, P., Montis, S., Bolasco, F., Deiana, E., De Virgilis, S., Podda, R., Targhetta, R., Biddau, P. F., Faa, G., and Pilleri, G., Epidemiology of HDV infection in Sardinia, an island with a high epidemiology for HBV: a multicenter study, in *The Hepatitis Delta Virus* [Progress in Clinical and Biological Research, Vol. 364], Gerin, J. L., Purcell, R. H., and Rizzetto, M., Eds., Wiley-Liss, New York, 1991, 41.

Section II

Bacterial Infections

8 Actinomycetes

The term aerobic actinomycetes is being used informally to designate a class of bacteria that has been classified to the order *Actinomycetales*.[1] Initially, the actinomycetes were considered fungi because of the presence of true aerial hyphae, which is considered to be a fungal attribute. However, based on the composition of their cell wall components, and in particular the cell envelope lipids and peptidoglycans, the actinomycetes are currently considered to represent true aerobic bacteria.

In general, the actinomycetes are Gram-positive, filamentous, partially acid-fast, branched bacteria which have some common characteristics with species of the genera *Mycobacterium* and *Corynebacterium*.

Medically important aerobic actinomycetes include such genera as *Nocardia*, *Rhodococcus*, *Actinomadura*, *Gordona*, and *Dermatophilus congolensis*.[1]

Clinically, even though not frequently associated with human disease, some actinomycetes have the potential to become opportunistic, causing serious human infections, especially in immuno-compromised hosts.

8.1 *NOCARDIA* SPP.

8.1.1 INTRODUCTION

The genus *Nocardia* comprises aerobic bacteria which are widespread worldwide in soil and organic matter.[2] They are considered to be sporophytic and primarily responsible for the decomposition of organic plant material.[2-4] Most of the pathogenic *Nocardia* spp. (*N. asteroides*, *N. brasiliensis*, and *N. caviae*) are acid-resistant, especially when material is examined directly or from glycerol-containing media.[5,6]

In a recent taxonomic revision of the *N. asteroides* taxon (*N. asteroides* complex), two new species, *N. nova* and *N. farcinica*, were separated from it.[7-10] The latter has been further reestablished as a separate species[9] because of its distinct antimicrobial resistance pattern.[10]

The heterogeneity within the species *N. asteroides*, which has been well established by numerous taxonomic,[3,11-15] genetic,[16,17] and immunologic[4,18,19] studies, resulted in the formation of several *N. asteroides* subgroups. One of these subgroups, containing the *N. farcinica* taxon, was found to be biochemically, genetically, and immunologically distinct from other isolates identified as *N. asteroides*, which led to the establishment of a separate species status for *N. farcinica*. Studies by Wallace et al.[10] have shown that *N. farcinica* had a specific drug resistance pattern that has confirmed the previously described concept that the drug resistance patterns of *N. asteroides* may be associated with specific taxonomic groups. In a subsequent study, Wallace et al.[9] demonstrated that another drug resistance pattern was specific for *N. nova*, another subgroup of *N. asteroides*.

One constant morphologic feature of *Nocardia* spp. is the proclivity of both aerial and substrate hyphae to fragment into bacillary and coccoid elements.[20] Currently, the chemotaxonomic criteria applied for the assignment of new species to the genus *Nocardia* include the presence of *meso*-2,6-diaminopimelic acid and the whole-cell sugars arabinose and galactose (cell wall type IV);[21] intermediate-chain (C_{46-60}) mycolic acids;[22-27] a fatty acid profile showing major amounts of straight-chain, unsaturated, and tuberculostearic acids;[28] and a menaquinone fraction containing a tetrahydrogenated menaquinone moiety with eight isoprene units [MK-8(H$_4$)] as the predominant isoprenoic quinone.[29-32]

Several *Nocardia* species have been known to be pathogenic to humans and animals, among them, *N. asteroides, N. brasiliensis, N. otitidiscaviarum* (formerly known as *N. caviae*), *N. farcinica, N. nova,* and *N. transvalensis*.[1] Nocardial infection is usually transmitted through inhalation or by traumatic inoculation of the skin.[33,34]

The first report of an aerobic *Nocardia*-associated clinical disease was published in 1888 by Nocard,[35] who described a bovine farcy in cattle. Shortly thereafter, the etiologic agent isolated by Nocard was characterized as *N. farcinica*.[36] In humans, a disease caused by *Nocardia* was first reported in 1890 by Eppinger,[37] who described a patient with pneumonia and brain abscess due to *N. asteroides*.

In immunocompetent hosts, primary nocardiosis has been associated most frequently with cutaneous and ocular infections.[1] A fatal case of a generalized (lungs, subcutaneous tissue, and brain) nocardiosis with meningoencephalitis has also been described.[38] Rosendale et al.[39] reported a case of *N. asteroides*-induced cervical osteomyelitis.

Primary cutaneous and subcutaneous *Nocardia* infections, which will usually result from traumatic inoculations (e.g., from insect bites,[40] pet scratches[41]), may present as mycetoma,[42-48] lymphocutaneous infection,[41,49,50] and superficial skin infections (abscess or cellulitis). Secondary cutaneous involvement with disseminated disease in AIDS patients has also been described.[51,52] Of the three mostly pathogenic species (*N. asteroides, N. brasiliensis,* and *N. otitidiscaviarum*), *N. brasiliensis* seemed to predominate as the etiologic agent of primary cutaneous infections in the Americas and Australia, and *N. somaliensis* in Africa;[53-57] sporadic cases have been caused by *N. asteroides*[58] and *N. otitidiscaviarum*.[32,59-75] Cutaneous infections due to *N. transvalensis*[43] and *N. farcinica*[76] have also been reported.

Nocardial ocular disease, although rare, has been reported to develop in both immunocompetent and immunocompromised patients as the result of exogenous inoculation with *Nocardia* spp. or secondary to a traumatic corneal injury.[77-81] In immunocompromised hosts, endogenous ocular nocardiosis may develop following bloodstream dissemination from a distant pulmonary or other infective focus.[1]

Septic arthritis due to *N. asteroides* has been reported in both adult immunocompromised patients with disseminated infection,[82-84] as well as in an immunocompetent child.[85]

Even though invasive pulmonary and disseminated nocardiosis can occur in immunocompetent hosts, these two forms have been increasingly recognized as opportunistic infections associated with immunocompromised patients.[1,33,86-97]

Inhalation of infectious airborn *Nocardia* spores or mycelia is considered the major route of invasive pulmonary infection. In addition, there has been evidence that the prevalence of respiratory tract colonization may be much higher in defined populations of severely immunocompromised patients, such as cardiac transplant recipients — according to Simpson et al.,[90] 44% to 51% of them may be colonized with *Nocardia* spp.

N. asteroides, which has been the major cause of primary pulmonary nocardiosis, was implicated in as many as 80% of all cases.[87] However, *N. brasiliensis*,[53] *N. otitidiscaviarum*,[59] and *N. transvalensis*[98] have also been related to pulmonary disease in both immunocompromised and immunocompetent hosts. Patients with impaired local pulmonary defenses, such as those with chronic obstructive pulmonary conditions (chronic bronchitis and emphysema), asthma, and bronchiectasis,[60,91] have been at higher risk of developing pulmonary nocardiosis. In addition, *Nocardia* spp. was also reported to cause infections in solid organ (renal,[99-108] liver,[109-112] cardiac[113-115]) and bone marrow transplant[116-119] recipients.[120] Seggev[121] has described a fatal case of overwhelming pulmonary nocardiosis (10 months after an apparent cure) complicating chronic mucocutaneous candidiasis.

There have been several reports[92,122-126] in which a coexistence between pulmonary nocardiosis and alveolar proteinosis was described. In view of the well-established association between pulmonary alveolar proteinosis and hematologic malignancies, it is still unclear whether the connection between pulmonary nocardiosis and alveolar proteinosis represents a true independent association, or it merely reflects the independent correlation of each of these two conditions with an underlying hematologic malignancy.[123]

Systemic immunosuppression from prolonged treatment with corticosteroids and/or cytotoxic drugs has been a major predisposing factor for the development of invasive pulmonary nocardiosis.[1,127,128] In particular, renal[99-106] and cardiac[113,114,129] transplant recipients, patients with lymphoma,[130-134] malignant neoplasms,[87,135,136] sarcoidosis,[137] collagen vascular disease (e.g., systemic lupus erythemathosus),[138-141] dysgammaglobulinemia,[92] chronic granulomatous disease,[142-146] chronic alcoholism,[147] diabetes mellitus,[60,148] trauma or surgery,[92] patients undergoing continuous ambulatory peritoneal analysis (CAPD),[141] and patients infected with HIV,[60,149-158] all have been reported to develop invasive pulmonary nocardiosis. Another group at risk has been the intravenous drug abusers, mostly because of bacterial contamination of needles.[159-162]

In immunocompromised patients, one complication related to invasive pulmonary nocardiosis has been the development of suppurative and/or chronic pericarditis.[163-168]

Furthermore, in severely immunocompromised patients invasive pulmonary nocardial infections have the tendency to progress rapidly and disseminate through the bloodstream, although in some patients it may follow a gradually progressive indolent course, very often mimicking pulmonary involvement associated with tuberculosis, fungal disease, sarcoidosis, and neoplasia.[1]

Disseminated nocardiosis is frequently a late-presenting and potentially life-threatening infection having originated endogenously (i.e., secondary to hematogenous spread from the lungs),[169,170] but occasionally, also from a primary nonpulmonary (cutaneous) infection.[53,171] Most often, dissemination results in brain and skin lesions with mortality rates reaching 7% to 44%[87,92] or even higher (85%) as was the case in severely immunocompromised hosts.[172] Nocardial metastatic lesions may occur in nearly every part of the body.

Borget et al.[173] have reported the development of a primary nocardial muscle abscess in an immunosuppressed patient receiving corticosteroid therapy for Horton disease.

In addition to N. asteroides[92] and N. brasiliensis,[53,174,175] other species, such as N. otitidiscaviarum,[59,176,177] N. transvalensis,[43,98,178,179] N. farcinica,[10,76,127,129,180-186] and N. nova[9,187] have been implicated in disseminated and occasionally fatal human nocardiosis. While initially recognized as a cause of mycetoma,[188] N. transvalensis has been known to elicit life-threatening invasive and disseminated infections in severely immunocompromised patients.[98,178,179]

Patients at higher risk for developing disseminated disease include those who are severely immunocompromised, such as renal,[80,89,104,189-192] cardiac,[90,113] and liver[109,193] transplant recipients, HIV-infected patients,[51,194-196] and patients with carcinomatosis,[135] and sarcoidosis.[197]

In addition to the brain, which is the most frequent nonpulmonary site involved in disseminated disease (25% to 40% of all cases of nocardiosis),[170,198-208] other organs involved include the kidneys,[209,210] spleen,[209] liver,[209,211] and less often bone,[212-220] eyes,[22,221] skin,[169,222-225] and the joints.[82,169,226-228]

In a retrospective analysis by Barnicoat et al.,[229] patients with primary cerebral nocardiosis (that is, cerebral abscess without concurrent pulmonary involvement) and an underlying immunosuppressive disorder had an increased rate of mortality, reaching as high as 95%.

Even though nocardiosis has been most often a late-presenting, community-acquired infection, nosocomial outbreaks have also been reported.[88,90,100,103,230]

Despite the high degree of cellular immunodeficiency characteristic for patients infected with HIV, opportunistic Nocardia spp. infections in this particular population has been relatively uncommon.[51,149,152,154,155,162,194,195,231-241] In advanced HIV disease (lymphocyte counts below 266 cells/mm^3), however, nocardiosis can be a fatal complication.[162] By one estimate,[232] only 0.19%

to 0.3% of AIDS patients reported to the Centers for Disease Control had been found to develop nocardiosis complicating AIDS. However, this assessment may have underestimated the frequency of infection due to the fact that AIDS surveillance techniques rarely take into consideration follow-up information on infections that such patients may acquire after the diagnosis of AIDS. Findings from postmortem case series on AIDS patients seemed to support the apparent low incidence of opportunistic nocardiosis in HIV-infected patients.[242,243] In this regard, one factor that should be taken into consideration is the widespread prophylactic use of trimethoprim-sulfamethox-azole (TMP-SMX) against *Pneumocystis carinii*, which may account for the low incidence of nocardiosis in HIV-infected patients since it is known that TMP-SMX also has a protective effect against *Nocardia* spp.[162,232] Nevertheless, this has not always been the case. Thus, in bone marrow recipients with graft-vs.-host disease, TMP-SMX prophylaxis for *P. carinii* failed to consistently prevent nocardial infection although it may have prevented or delayed dissemination.[116,117]

Of all *Nocardia* spp., *N. asteroides* was the most common species involved as the causative agent of opportunistic nocardiosis in AIDS patients.[194,239] Reports of infections by other *Nocardia* spp. were rare and included *N. brasiliensis*,[51,233,244,245] *N. farcinica*,[238,241] and *N. nova*.[239]

There have been several reports about simultaneous infections of *N. asteroides* with *Mycobacterium tuberculosis*[51,237,246-249] and nontuberculous mycobacteria (as many as 6% of all cases of nocardiosis).[250] To this end, a statistically significant association has been observed between primary pulmonary nocardial disease and the subsequent development of nontuberculous pulmonary myco-bacteriosis caused by *Mycobacterium kansasii* and the *M. avium-intracellulare–M. scrofulaceum* complex in cardiac transplant recipients.[251] It should be noted that currently there is no clear evidence that such coinfections represent a true association that may indicate some interrelationship between these microbial agents.[1]

Concomitant pulmonary infections by *N. asteroides* and *Pneumocystis carinii* have also been described in patients undergoing immunosuppressive therapy for organ transplantations and cancer.[252,253]

8.1.2 Evolution of Therapies and Treatment of Nocardiosis

The treatment of nocardiosis remains problematic since there have been no large controlled clinical trials, and the available empiric recommendations for specific antimicrobial agents have been based on a limited number of patients.[1,254] As with other infections in which cell-mediated immunity plays a large defensive role, nocardiosis in immunocompromised patients can relapse after an apparent cure and occasionally remote from the original infection.[255]

In some patients treatment with antimicrobial drugs for primary infection may result in failure, thus leading to metastatic spread of the disease or late relapse.[256] To improve the clinical outcome of nocardiosis, surgical intervention in addition to antimicrobial therapy has often been recom-mended.[42,185,257-263] For example, the successful management of suppurative and/or chronic constric-tive pericarditis (often observed in immunocompromised patients) required an agressive approach that combined appropriate antimicrobial therapy and pericardiectomy,[164-166] and in HIV-infected individuals, nocardiosis has been treated with antimicrobial regimens often coupled with surgical drainage.[51,152,200,233,234]

The spectrum of nocardiosis may also be changing from a predominantly *N. asteroides*-induced infection to increasing incidence of illness due to *N. farcinica*.[238] According to published statistics, *N. farcinica* constituted the prevailing pathogenic actinomycete in Germany from 1979 to 1991,[63] and in France one quarter of all *Nocardia* isolates were *N. farcinica*.[264] The changing etiologic pattern of nocardiosis may also affect the way initial therapy is administered.[238] Though *N. aster-oides* remains sensitive to most antimicrobial agents,[10,265] *N. farcinica*, which is almost indistin-guishable from *N. asteroides* by regular laboratory methods, has been resistant to cephalosporins.[10] It is important that because of the rising incidence of *N. farcinica* and its drug resistance, third-generation cephalosporins were not to be used in the initial management of *Nocardia* infections.[238]

Currently, there is no known therapy of choice against *N. transvalensis*. Furthermore, clinical isolates of this species have demonstrated a high degree of drug resistance, and therapy with TMP-SMX has not always been successful.[98]

Treatment with sulfonamides (sulfisoxazole,[90,162] sulfadiazine,[94,162] sulfadimidine[266]) alone[90,92,267] or in combination with trimethoprim has been the mainstay of antimicrobial therapy for human nocardiosis.[1,110,162,185,252,268-280] While the combination of sulfamethoxazole with trimethoprim (co-trimoxazole) is frequently used either orally or intravenously,[83,170,229,254,281-283] its beneficial therapeutic effect may come not as much from the synergistic relationship between these two drugs but from an improved penetration into the cerebrospinal fluid and generally favorable pharmacokinetics.[284]

Sulfonamide dose regimens should be adjusted to achieve the recommended blood levels of 100 to 150 µg/ml approximately 2 h after an oral dose. For effective treatment, generally high doses of sulfonamides (3 to 6 g daily) should be given for extended periods (6 to 12 months).[1,274] While primary cutaneous disease may be cured within 1 to 3 months and uncomplicated pulmonary nocardiosis may respond to therapy for 6 months or less, the therapy in immunocompromised hosts and for disseminated nocardiosis may have to be carried out for prolonged periods of time (12 months or more).[254,285]

One of the unwarranted side effects of the sulfonamides (e.g., sulfadiazine[286]) has been the development of drug-induced lithiasis due to their poor solubility in urine.[287] The result may be an obstructive uropathy leading to acute renal failure. Rapid improvement can be achieved by drug discontinuation or decrease of dosage, systemic administration of fluid, and urine alkalinization.[156]

Some problems posed by sulfonamide-trimethoprim combinations[288-291] included patient's intolerance[76] (acute pancreatitis[177,292]) and drug incompatiblity with cyclosporine, which is used as an antirejection agent in organ transplant recipients. The latter may result in reversible cyclosporine-induced nephrotoxicity.[93,293-296] Furthermore, when the concentration of the sulfonamide component has been high relative to that of trimethoprim, *in vitro* antagonism has been demonstrated.[33,297]

It is also important to note that 50% of HIV-infected patients will still experience adverse reactions (fever, severe hypersensitivity reactions, and prolonged myelosuppression) due to TMP-SMX, which could be of sufficient severity to cause discontinuation.[238,298]

Single sulfonamide drugs used most frequently in the treatment of nocardiosis included sulfisoxazole (4 to 8 g daily) and sulfadiazine (4 to 6 g daily).[162,286,299,300]

Miralles[238] has described an AIDS patient presenting with disseminated *N. farcinica* infection diagnosed by percutaneous kidney biopsy. Intravenous therapy with TMP-SMX (350 mg/1750 mg) given four times daily (at a dose of 5.0 mg/kg TMP) over 4 weeks led to significant clinical improvement.

Several reports have indicated that sulfonamide resistance could be overcome by treatment with minocycline,[301,302] amikacin, or erythromycin in combination with ampicillin.[76,106,274,303,304] Stella et al.[305] have described a complete cure of a systemic infection due to *N. asteroides* with a 2-month course of erythromycin (500 mg, four times daily) and amoxicillin/clavulanic acid (500 mg/125 mg, once daily), combined with ultrasound-guided transcutaneous aspiration of multiple subcutaneous metastatic abscesses. In another example, a 15-month course consisting of minocycline (400 to 600 mg daily), cefotaxime (1.2 to 3.0 g daily), and probenicide cured *N. asteroides*-induced pneumonia and brain abscess persisting after therapy with sulfonamides, minocycline, and cefotaxime.[199]

Reports of other antibiotics used in the therapy of nocardiosis included cefuroxime (2.25 to 4.5 g daily), ceftriaxone (2.0 g daily), cefotaxime, amikacin (1.0 g daily), minocycline (200 mg daily), imipenem, and meropenem.[162,299,301,306-308] Drug combinations, such as imipenem–amikacin, ceftriaxone–amikacin, imipenem–rifampicin, imipenem–cilastatin, imipenem–ciprofloxacin, ciprofloxacin–doxacycline, cefotaxime–amikacin, and amoxicillin–clavulanic acid–amikacin, have shown evidence of synergy *in vitro*[309] as well as in clinical setting,[197,310-317] Metronidazole–flucloxacillin has been used successfully in several cases in Europe.[190,318]

Intravenous amikacin and imipenem at doses of 250 mg and 1.5 g, respectively, four times daily cured endocarditis of a prosthetic aortic valve due to *N. asteroides*.[319]

After failure to achieve cure with co-trimoxazole, Overkamp et al.[197] effectively treated disseminated nocardiosis in an immunosuppressed patient with a combination of oral rifampicin and intravenous imipenem, followed by oral rifampicin and ampicillin–clavulanic acid.

Bauwens et al.[320] described two cases of nocardiosis in immunocompromised renal transplant recipients successfully treated with amoxicillin (500 mg, four times daily for 10 d), and TMP-SMX/cefotaxime (for 6 months, then followed by TMP-SMX alone for 1 year), respectively. In another report, a renal transplant recipient with an unusual case of nocardial psoas and perinephric abscess responded to treatment with ciprofloxacin and cefuroxime combined with surgical drainage.[321]

Several cases of concomitant pulmonary nocardiosis and aspergillosis in immunocompromised patients have also been described.[115,322,323] In one study, one such patient who also had renal vasculitis was treated successfully with a combination of imipenem, co-trimoxazole and a prolonged course of itraconazole.[323]

In general, the apparent response to nonsulfonamide agents seemed to have supported published data regarding their *in vitro* efficacy against *Nocardia* spp.[324-326]

A rare case of pleuropulmonary nocardiosis in an immunosuppressed patient with systemic lupus erythematosus and receiving chronic treatment with corticosteroids and immunosuppressive drugs was successfully treated with intravenous imipenem (500 mg, b.i.d.); following hospital discharge, the patient continued therapy with oral ciprofloxacin at 500 mg daily.[140]

Other unusual cases of *Nocardia* pulmonary involvement may present with endobronchial lesions[275,327,328] that could mimic a bronchogenic tumor.[275,327]

Intravenous imipenem (1.0 g, t.i.d.) combined with oral erythromycin (500 mg, four times daily) and roxithromycin (300 mg, b.i.d.) successfully resolved a case of sphenoidal sinusitis due to *N. asteroides*.[266]

Among the various forms of ocular nocardiosis, there have been case reports of *Nocardia*-associated keratitis,[78,280,329-332] conjunctivitis,[333] corneal ulcer,[79,334,335] episcleral granuloma,[336] dacryocystitis,[337] subretinal abscess,[338] and endogenous nocardial endophthalmitis.[335,339-354] The majority of cases involving endogenous intraocular nocardiosis followed some form of debilitating disease, including immunosuppression after renal or heart transplantation or illnesses related to immunodeficiency. Several cases occurred as a result of presumed metastatic involvement from the lungs. In addition, there have also been reports of exogenous *Nocardia* endophthalmitis following either intracapsular cataract extraction,[344,355] trabeculectomy,[356] or corneal laceration/injuries.[357-359]

Delayed chronic intraocular *Nocardia* infection has been known to complicate extracapsular cataract extraction[339] and intraocular lens (IOL) implantation.[342] Zimmerman et al.[339] have described a case of chronic *N. asteroides* endophthalmitis following extracapsular cataract extraction that was treated with a combination of antibiotics, including intravitreal (200 μg, done twice) and intra-cameral (200 μg, b.i.d. for 4 weeks) injections of amikacin sulfate, and topical amikacin sulfate (33 g/l, every 4 h); intravenous imipenem (500 mg, t.i.d. for 6 weeks) was also administered after the surgery in addition to oral TMP-SMX, minocycline hydrochloride (100 mg, b.i.d.), and 1% prednisolone (four times daily). In spite of the therapy, the patient's clinical course continued to deteriorate, leading to enucleation of the globe.[339] The use of intravenous imipenem was also considered after a report[360] has shown that its aqueous humor concentrations were sufficiently high after intravenous administration.

Srinivasan and Sundar[341] reported eight cases of nocardial endophthalmitis following posterior chamber IOL implantation, which all responded to various topical antibiotic agents (10% ampicillin sodium, 0.2% trimethoprim sulfate, 30% sulfacetamide sodium, 0.3% norfloxacin, and 0.3% ciprofloxacin hydrochloride) administered according to the sensitivity of the isolates.

Although rarely, testicular nocardiosis in immunocompromised patients has also been diagnosed.[95,257,259-261] The mortality in such cases was high (three of five reported patients, 60%), and the two survivors required long-term sulfonamide treatment combined with orchiectomy.[257,261]

Lopez et al.[257] have reported a case of epididymo-orchitis due to *N. asteroides* in an immunocompromised liver transplant recipient receiving immunosuppressive therapy. Treatment with co-trimoxazole (20 mg/kg trimethoprim daily) for 5 months, followed by orchiectomy and additional 4 months of TMP-SMX therapy led to clinical resolution of nocardiosis.[257]

Treatment of primary cutaneous nocardiosis included the use of intravenous (TMP: 240 mg/SMX: 1.2 g, daily)[58] or oral (TMP: 480 mg/SMX: 2.4 g, b.i.d.)[62] trimethoprim-sulfamethoxazole, and various antibiotic combinations,[61] namely, rifampin (600 mg daily)–clofazimine (300 mg daily)–minocycline (1.0 g daily),[61] cefalexine 500 (1.0 g daily)–gentamicin (1.0 g daily for 5 d),[61] and enoxacin (600 mg daily)–minocycline (200 mg daily)–doxycycline (100 mg daily).[32] Rees et al.[129] have reported the successful treatment of primary cutaneous *N. farcinica* nocardiosis in an immunosuppressed heart transplant recipient with oral doxycycline (100 mg daily) — prior treatment with imipenem (1.0 g daily, IV) and amikacin (1.0 g daily, IV) had failed to bring clinical improvement.

Trimethoprim–sulfamethoxazole alone or in combination with diaminodiphenylsulfone has been the treatment of choice for actinomycetoma. Amikacin has been used in severe cases that were unresponsive to previous treatment and in danger of dissemination to adjacent organs.[277] Gomez et al.[46] have treated *N. brasiliensis*-induced mycetoma with bone involvement with oral amoxicillin–clavulanic acid (500 mg and 125 mg, respectively, given three times daily for 5 to 6 months).

8.1.2.1 *In Vitro* Susceptibility Testing of *Nocardia* spp.

The *in vitro* antimicrobial sensitivity testing of *Nocardia* spp. remains problematic because of the typically slow growth of the aerobic actinomycetes.[5,360] Consequently, the slow growth may eventually facilitate spontaneous drug decomposition compromising the testing results. The most common techniques used so far include a modified[361,362] disk diffusion assay, and the agar dilution and broth microdilution assays.[264,265,363-365] The degree of success in each of these methods has depended upon achievement of adequate initial suspension of microorganisms from which a standard inoculum is made.[1]

Results from a number of studies on the *in vitro* antimicrobial susceptibility of clinical isolates of *Nocardia* spp. have shown a variable degree of drug resistance among the various species.[98,363,366-368] Thus, while all clinical isolates of *N. asteroides*, *N. farcinica*, and *N. otitidiscaviarum* displayed 100% resistance to erythromycin,[363,366] only 50% of *N. transvalensis* were resistant,[98] and none of *N. brasiliensis*[367] and *N. nova*.[366] Resistance against sulfamethoxazole (part of the trimethoprim–sulfamethoxazole combination) was 100% and 10%, respectively, among the *N. otitidiscaviarum* and *N. transvalensis* isolates tested; by comparison, the *N. asteroides*,[366] *N. brasiliensis*,[367] *N. farcinica*,[366] and *N. nova*[366] isolates were all susceptible. There has been a great degree of resistance towards ciprofloxacin (87/100%, 100%, 70%, and 40%, respectively for *N. asteroides*,[366] *N. nova*,[366] *N. brasiliensis*,[367] and *N. transvalensis*,[98] but none for *N. farcinica* isolates[366]) and ampicilin (100%, 100%, 100%, 90%, and 86%, respectively for *N. asteroides*,[366] *N. farcinica*,[366] *N. otitidiscaviarum*,[363] *N. transvalensis*,[98] and *N. brasiliensis*[367] but none for *N. nova*[366]).

Results for cefotaxime (100%, 83%, 50%, and 25% resistance, respectively, for *N. farcinica*,[366] *N. otitidiscaviarum*,[363] *N. transvalensis*,[98] and *N. brasiliensis*[367] but 0% for *N. asteroides* and *N. nova*[366]), imipenem (70%, 25/0%, 18%, and 10% resistance, respectively, for *N. brasiliensis*,[367] *N. asteroides*,[366] *N. farcinica*,[366] and *N. transvalensis*,[98] but 0% for *N. nova*[366]), and amoxicillin–clavulanic acid (100%, 97%, 53.3%, and 35%, respectively, for *N. otitidiscaviarum*,[363] *N. nova*,[366] *N. farcinica*,[366] and *N. brasiliensis*[367]) were variable.

With the exception of *N. transvalensis* (18% resistance),[363] all clinical isolates of *N. asteroides*,[366] *N. brasiliensis*,[367] *N. farcinica*,[366] *N. nova*,[366] and *N. otitidiscaviarum*[363] were completely susceptible to amikacin.

In general, *N. asteroides* isolates were usually sensitive to all aminoglycosides, third-generation cephalosporins, sulfonamides, and tetracyclines.[10,369] By comparison, isolates of *N. farcinica* have been resistant to gentamicin, tobramycin, tetracyclines, and the third-generation of cephalosporins.[10]

N. otitidiscaviarum isolates were resistant to β-lactams, amoxicillin–clavulanic acid, cefamandole, and cefotaxime,[363,370] as well as quinolones (enoxacin, norfloxacin, ofloxacin, and ciprofloxacin),[265,324,369] but most strains remained susceptible to chloramphenicol, minocycline, erythromycin, and clindamycin;[363] susceptibility to aminoglycosides has been variable.[363,366,370] Some of the newer quinolones (tosufloxacin, PD-117596, PD-127391, PD-117558) appeared to have good *in vitro* activity against *N. otitidiscaviarum*.[265,324,369]

8.1.2.2 Acquired Drug Resistance of *Nocardia* spp.

Joshi and Hamory[371] have reported the development of a multiple drug-resistant strain of *N. asteroides* in a patient with AIDS and concomitant disseminated histoplasmosis. The pattern of resistance, known as type 5, has been specific for broad-spectrum cephalosporins, ciprofloxacin, and all aminoglycosides (except amikacin). In another case, a patient with *N. asteroides*-associated brain abscess and ventriculitis developed resistance to sulfonamides but was susceptible to β-lactams.[372]

An acquired resistance to clavulanic acid (as part of a combination with amoxicillin) by *N. brasiliensis* has been attributed to mutational change in the inhibitor and active site(s) in the β-lactamase.[373]

8.1.3 BIOLOGICAL RESPONSE MODIFIERS FROM *NOCARDIA* SPP.

Several biologically active fractions isolated from cell walls of *Nocardia* spp. have shown effective immunomodulating activity, namely, inducing interferon-γ production, activating natural killer cells, and exerting antitumor activity.[374,375]

8.1.3.1 *Nocardia rubra* Cell Wall Skeleton

Mice, when immunized with either crude cell extract antigens of *N. asteroides* or its purified fraction F1, showed increased levels of humoral and cellular immune responses.[376] When challenged with 50% lethal dose of *N. asteroides*, two weeks after complete immunization the animals exhibited significant protection against systemic nocardiosis as seen by the decreased mortality and viable counts as compared to those of nonimmunized controls.[376]

However, it is the immunomodulating properties of the *Nocardia rubra* cell wall skeleton (N-CWS) that have shown most promising activities, as demonstrated extensively in both studies in animal models[377,378] and clinical settings.

The protective effect of the *N. rubra* N-CWS on experimental infections was investigated both in normal and immunosuppressed mice.[379,380] In normal mice, pretreatment with N-CWS provided protection against acute systemic infections due to *Pseudomonas aeruginosa*, *Escherichia coli*, *Klebsiella pneumoniae*, and herpes simplex virus. In addition, in cyclophosphamide-, hydrocortisone-, or X-ray-immunosuppressed mice, treatment with N-CWS markedly restored host defense ability against pseudomonal infection.[379]

The antitumor activity of N-CWS was investigated using syngeneically transplanted P388 leukemia cells in a solid form.[381] Systemically administered N-CWS significantly suppressed the subcutaneous growth of P388 tumors in DBA/2 mice in a dose-dependent manner. While the antitumor effect of N-CWS was not affected in T cell- or natural killer (NK) cell-deficient mice, it was partially but statistically significantly abrogated in splenectomized mice. Moreover, the splenic cytostatic activity resided neither in the T cells nor NK cells, but in the macrophages. The macrophages acted as the major effector cells in the suppression of P388 tumor growth in DBA/2 mice, and tumor necrosis factor produced by these cells may have been involved in the macrophage-mediated cytostatic effect induced by N-CWS.[381] In an earlier study, analysis of surface markers of cells after intratumor injection of N-CWS has shown gradually increasing percentage of macrophage, Pan T and BoCD4+ cells.[382] The tumorigenic effect of *N. rubra* N-CWS was further evaluated on Meth A fibrosarcoma (Meth A) in BALB/a mice,[383] and by its ability to prevent Friend leukemia virus-induced splenomegaly in C3H/HeN mice.[384] N-CWS suppressed or regressed the intradermal growth of syngeneic Meth A cells in both normal and athymic mice. However, pre-treatment of normal mice with immunosuppressive drugs markedly reduced the antitumor effect of N-CWS. Again, the macrophages acted as the main effector cells in the early stage of tumor rejection.[383]

In a series of experiments in BALB/c-Meth A and C3H-MH 134 systems, the immuno-modulating activity of N-CWS was compared with that of another immunomodulatory agent, OK-432.[385] Peritoneal exudate cells obtained from mice injected intraperitoneally with OK-432 or N-CWS showed stronger *in vitro* cytotoxicity against Meth A and YAC-1 cells than did those from untreated mice. Overall, there have been no significant differences in the direct tumor-inhibiting activities of OK-432 and N-CWS *in vitro*. However, while administration of N-CWS had no therapeutic effect against intraperitoneally inoculated tumor cells, OK-432 showed a strong therapeutic effect by the same treatment schedule.

Studies by Kawase et al.[386] and Miyasaki et al.[387] have demonstrated the presence of a synergistic effect between *N. rubra* N-CWS and recombinant interleukin-2 (rIL-2) in the *in vivo* induction of murine lymphokine-activated killer cell activity. Thus, combination of an intraperitoneal injection of N-CWS and three daily injections of human rIL-2 into C3H/HeN mice resulted not only in a significant increase in the number of peritoneal cells but also in a potent induction of their lymphokine-activated killer (LAK) activity compared with results obtained with N-CWS or rIL-2 alone.[386] The augmented LAK activity was mediated by nonadherent, nonphagocytic, Thy-1.2+(−) and asialo GM-1+ cells. In the suggested mode of action, N-CWS potentiated the accumulation of LAK precursors (CD3+CD4−CD8− T cells and asialo GM-1+ natural killer cells) and elevated their responsiveness to rIL-2 at the injection site.[386,387]

The clinical usefulness of *N. rubra* N-CWS has been investigated in several studies.[388-398] For example, the continuous treatment with N-CWS of eight patients with erythromycin-resistant diffuse panbronchiolitis who had repeated intractable airway infections led to reduction of subjective symptoms and decreased antibiotic dose regimens.[388]

The effect of immunotherapy with N-CWS on the remission duration and survival of adult patients with acute myelogenous leukemia was examined by Ohno et al.[395,396] in a prospective, randomized, controlled study. The results of the trial demonstrated that after being induced into complete remission, patients who received maintenance chemotherapy plus immunotherapy with N-CWS and irradiated allogeneic acute myelogeneous leukemia cells, had their 50% remission periods prolonged by 120 d. However, this treatment did not change in any significant way the survival time ($p = .306$) of patients.

In a comparative study, children with acute lymphoblastic leukemia, who had been in continuous remission for 3 years on chemotherapy, received treatment with N-CWS, as well as other biological response modifiers (bestatin, OK-432, and/or PSK), in order to prevent relapses after treatment suspension.[390] Only 8 of 57 patients who were treated with N-CWS or OK-432 relapsed; by comparison, 6 of 20 patients who received PSK relapsed within 13 months, which was similar to the rate observed with those patients who were off chemotherapy (4 relapses in 17 patients within 13 months). Best results were achieved with bestatin, where only 3 of 31 patients ($p < .05$) relapsed.[390]

In a randomized controlled study, the postoperative survival rates of patients with gastric carcinoma receiving either chemotherapy with tagafur (400 to 800 mg daily) or adjuvant immunotherapy with N-CWS (400 µg, daily within the second postoperative week, then weekly during the first month and subsequently monthly for as long as practicable), were compared.[393] No statistical difference was detected between the two groups in terms of age, sex, surgical curability, or stage of carcinoma. However, the overall survival rate for all patients was markedly higher in the N-CWS-receiving group than those treated with tagafur (p <.05). The side effects of N-CWS were limited to transient skin lesions in the injected sites and fever.[393]

When given as a cancer-preventive measure, N-CWS showed a statistically significant reduction in the incidence of lung cancer in a high-risk group of retired chemical weapons factory workers.[389] In addition, patients receiving N-CWS have shown markedly elevated production of IL-2 and lymphocyte proliferation as well.[391,394] By comparison, normal controls not receiving N-CWS had a substantial decrease in their lymphocyte proliferation, but only slight and not statistically significant reduction in IL-2 production.[394]

After considering the results of experimental and clinical studies, it was concluded that immunostimulant therapy with N-CWS when employed as a nonspecific adjuvant after cancer chemotherapy, may play an important role, not only in eradicating tumor cells which have escaped from chemotherapy, but also in preventing infectious complication by activating host defense mechanisms common to cancer and infection.[399]

8.1.3.2   *Nocardia opaca* Cell Wall Fractions

A water-soluble mitogen, NWSM, isolated from *Nocardia opaca*, was shown to be a very potent antitumor agent. Intratumoral administration of NWSM into Lewis lung carcinoma (LLC) in mice resulted in a massive accumulation of inflammatory cells around the tumor. The thick rim of infiltrating cells consisted of macrophages and lymphocytes, which were directly implicated in the antitumor activity of NWSM; by comparison, untreated tumors provoked only a sparse lymphocyte infiltration.[374]

The involvement of macrophages and lymphocytes in the activity of the *Nocardia* delipidated cell mitogen (NDCM)-induced tumor-inhibiting effect was also investigated.[400-402] Macrophages activated by NDMC exerted a cytotoxic effect on LLC cells *in vitro*. This finding was found to correlate with previous data showing local accumulation of macrophages (and lymphocytes) at the tumor site in NDCM-treated mice. Furthermore, in tumor-bearing mice (both treated and untreated with NDCM), a splenomegaly due to a pronounced extramedullary hematopoiesis was observed. Concomitant with the gradual evolution of the extramedullary hematopoiesis in the red pulp, a depletion in white pulp component has been noticed — the effect was more pronounced in the control LLC-bearing mice than in the LLC-inoculated NDCM-treated animals. It has been postulated that the disappearance of the lymphatic follicles in LLC-bearing mice might have been responsible for the failure to cope with the tumor. If so, it would appear possible that the tumor-inhibiting activity of NDCM may be related to its ability to delay white pulp depletion, thereby potentiating a better host defense response against the tumor.[401]

In a separate study,[402] NDCM when injected parenterally in an oil/water emulsion to F6 rhabdomyosarcoma-bearing rats, has inhibited the development of pulmonary metastases. Next, repeated intraperitoneal administration of emulsified NDCM, NWSM, and purified cell walls (CW; an insoluble macromolecular *N. opaca* fraction) in LLC-bearing mice resulted in a significant reduction of lung metastases. The efficiency of these three fractions was enhanced by association with monokines. Thus, a combination regimen of NDCM, NWSM, and CW (100 µg/0.1 ml) and monokines (0.1 ml), when injected intraperitoneally in LLC-bearing mice, produced greater anti-metastatic effect than either therapy alone. Further experiments have suggested that activated peritoneal macrophages may have played a role in mediating the antimetastatic effect of both soluble and insoluble *N. opaca* fractions, and the monokines.[402]

When tested in BALB/c mice, *Nocardia* lysozyme digest (NLD), a particulate fraction from *N. opaca*, was able to suppress the tumor growth in SaL-1 tumor cells (lung sarcoma).[403] Macrophages isolated from peritoneal cavity and stimulated with NLD have released arachidonic acid metabolites (mostly PGE_2). In addition, macrophages recovered from tumor-bearing mice were found more sensitive to *Nocardia* antigens compared to normal macrophages.

Ehrenfeld and Haas[404] have applied immunotherapy with a *N. opaca* cell wall extract in a male patient who was in the final stage of recurring lung metastases by infiltrating breast carcinoma (T2NOMO). The treatment resulted in a complete remission without serious side effects.

8.1.3.3   Antitumor *Nocardia* spp. Antibiotics

A number of novel antibiotics produced by *Nocardia* spp. have also been shown to elicit useful biological activities. Rasmussen et al.[405] have isolated from the fermentation broth of *Nocardia lurida* benzanthrins A and B two representatives of a new class of quinone antibiotics. Structurally, benzanthrins A and B were diglycosides of a trihydroxy benz[*a*]anthraquinone chromophore in which one of the sugar moieties was linked through a carbon atom and the other through a nitrogen. The two compounds differed in the stereochemistry of the *O*-glycosidic sugar. When tested for activity, both antibiotics inhibited the growth of Gram-positive bacteria and 9KB, 9PS, and 0ASK tumor cells in tissue cultures.[405]

The mycelium of the actinomycete strain C-38,383, which closely resembled strains of *N. aerocolonigenes* (recently renamed *Saccharothrix aerocolonigenes*), was found to produce rebeccamycin, a novel antibiotic with activity against P388 leukemia, L1210 leukemia, and B16 melanoma implanted in mice.[406] In addition, rebeccamycin inhibited the growth of human lung adenocarcinoma cells (A549) as well as effected single-strand breaks in the DNA of these cells. It is worth noting that a strain selection isolate without aerial mycelium, C-38,383-RK-1, failed to produce rebeccamycin, while a strain with aerial mycelium, C-38,383-RK-2, did so.

PC-766B, a new macrolide antibiotic, was isolated from *N. brasiliensis* (Lindenberg) Pinoy.[407] While PC-766B showed activity against Gram-positive bacteria, and some fungi and yeasts, it was inactive against Gram-negative bacteria. The compound showed antitumor activity against murine tumor cells *in vitro* and *in vivo*, but weak inhibitory effect against Na^+ and K^+-ATPases *in vitro*.

SO-75R1 is another antibiotic produced by *N. brasiliensis* which belongs to a new anthracycline group of antibiotics structurally related to mutactimycin.[408] SO-75R1 was found active against Gram-positive bacteria but inactive against Gram-negative bacteria and fungi. All tested *N. brasiliensis* strains as well as the producer itself were resistant to SO-75R1; however, four other pathogenic *Nocardia* (*N. asteroides*, *N. nova*, *N. farcinica*, and *N. otitidoscaviarum*) were found to be sensitive.[408]

8.1.4   REFERENCES

1. McNeil, M. M. and Brown, J. M., The medically important aerobic Actinomycetes: epidemiology and microbiology, *Clin. Microbiol. Rev.*, 7, 357, 1994.
2. Goodfellow, M., Ecology of actinomycetes, *Annu. Rev. Microbiol.*, 37, 189, 1983.
3. Orchard, V. A. and Goodfellow, M., Numerical classification of some named strains of *Nocardia asteroides* and related isolates from soil, *J. Gen. Microbiol.*, 118, 295, 1980.
4. Pier, A. C. and Fichtner, R. E., Distribution of serotypes of *Nocardia asteroides* from animal, human, and environmental sources, *J. Clin. Microbiol.*, 13, 548, 1981.
5. Lerner, P. I., Nocardia species, in *Infectious Diseases*, 3rd ed., Mandell, G. L., Douglas, R. G., and Bennett, J. E., Eds., Churchill Livingston, New York, 1990, 1926.
6. Causey, W. A. and Sieger, B., Systemic nocardiosis caused by *Nocardia brasiliensis*, *Am. Rev. Respir. Dis.*, 109, 134, 1974.

7. Lechevalier, H. A., Nocardioforms, in *Bergey's Manual of Systematic Bacteriology*, Vol. 4, Williams, S. T., Sharpe, M. E., and Holt, J. G., Eds., Williams & Wilkins, Baltimore, 1989, 2348.

8. Tsukamura, M., Numerical analysis of the taxonomy of nocardiae and rhodococci. Division of *Nocardia asteroides* sensu stricto into two species and descriptions of *Nocardia paratuberculosis* sp. nov. Tsukamura (formerly the Kyoto-I-group of Tsukamura), *Nocardia nova* sp. nov. Tsukamura, *Rhodococcus aichiensis* sp. nov. Tsukamura, *Rhodococcus chubuensis* sp. nov. Tsukamura, and *Rhodococcus obuensis* sp. nov. Tsukamura, *Microbiol. Immunol.*, 26, 1101, 1982.

9. Wallace, R. J., Jr., Brown, B. A., Tsukamura, M., Brown, J. M., and Onyi, G. O., Clinical and laboratory features of *Nocardia nova*, *J. Clin. Microbiol.*, 29, 2407, 1991.

10. Wallace, R. J., Jr., Tsukamura, M., Brown, B. A., Brown, J., Steingrube, V. A., Zhang, Y. S., and Nash, D. R., Cefotaxime-resistant *Nocardia asteroides* strains are isolates of the controversial species *Nocardia farcinica*, *J. Clin. Microbiol.*, 28, 2726, 1990.

11. Goodfellow, M., Numerical taxonomy of some nocardioform bacteria, *J. Gen. Microbiol.*, 69, 33, 1971.

12. Goodfellow, M. and Orchard, V. A., Antibiotic sensitivity of some nocardioform bacteria and its value as a criterion for taxonomy, *J. Gen. Microbiol.*, 83, 375, 1974.

13. Schaal, K. P. and Reutersberg, H., Numerical taxonomy of *Nocardia asteroides*, *Zentralbl. Bakteriol. Mikrobiol. Hyg. Abt. 1 Orig. Reihe A*, 6, 53, 1978.

14. Tsukamura, M., Numerical taxonomy of the genus *Nocardia*, *J. Gen. Microbiol.*, 56, 265, 1969.

15. Tsukamura, M., Extended numerical taxonomy study of *Nocardia*, *Int. J. Syst. Bacteriol.*, 27, 311, 1977.

16. Franklin, A. A., Jr. and McClung, N. M., Heterogeneity among *Nocardia asteroides* strains, *J. Gen. Appl. Microbiol.*, 22, 151, 1976.

17. Mordarski, M., Schaal, K. P., Tkacz, A., Pulverer, G., Szyba, K., and Goodfellow, M., Deoxyribonucleic acid base composition and homology studies on *Nocardia*, *Zentralbl. Bakteriol. Mikrobiol. Hyg. Abt. 1 Orig. Reihe A*, 6, 91, 1978.

18. Magnusson, M. and Mariat, F., Delineation of *Nocardia farcinica* by delayed type skin reactions on guinea pigs, *J. Gen. Microbiol.*, 51, 151, 1968.

19. Ridell, M., Immunodiffusion studies of some *Nocardia* strains, *J. Gen. Microbiol.*, 123, 69, 1980.

20. Locci, R., Developmental micromorphology of actinomycetes, in *Actinomycetes: The Boundary Microorganisms*, Arai, T., Ed., University Park Press, London, 1976, 249.

21. Lechevalier, H. A. and Lechevalier, M. P., A critical evaluation of the genera of *Actinomycetales*, in *The Actinomycetales*, Prauser, H., Ed., Gustav Fischer Verlag, Jena, 1970, 393.

22. Alshamaony, L., Goodfellow, M., and Minnikin, D. E., Free mycolic acids as a criterion in the classification of *Nocardia* and the rhodochrous complex, *J. Gen. Microbiol.*, 92, 188, 1976.

23. Butler, W. R., Ahearn, D. G., and Kilburn, J. O., High-performance liquid chromatography of mycolic acids as a tool in the identification of *Corynebacterium*, *Nocardia*, *Rhodococcus*, and *Mycobacterium* species, *J. Clin. Microbiol.*, 23, 182, 1986.

24. Butler, W. R., Kilburn, J. O., and Kubica, G. P., High-performance liquid chromatography analysis of mycolic acids as an aid in laboratory identification of *Rhodococcus* and *Nocardia* species, *J. Clin. Microbiol.*, 25, 2126, 1987.

25. Goodfellow, M. and Cross, T., Classification, in *The Biology of the Actinomycetes*, Goodfellow, M., Mordarski, M., and Williams, S. T., Eds., Academic Press, London, 1984, 7.

26. Goodfellow, M. and Minnikin, D. E., The genera *Nocardia* and *Rhodococcus*, in *The Procaryotes: a Handbook on Habitats, Isolation, and Identification of Bacteria*, Starr, M. P., Stolp, H., Trüper, H. G., Balows, A., and Schlegel, H. G., Eds., Springer-Verlag, Berlin, 1981, 2016,

27. Lechevalier, M. P., The taxonomy of the genus *Nocardia*: some light in the end of the tunnel? in *The Biology of the Nocardiae*, Goodfellow, M., Brownell, G. H., and Serrano, J. A., Eds., Academic Press, New York, 1976, 1.

28. Lechevalier, M. P., Lipids in bacterial taxonomy — a taxonomist's view, *Crit. Rev. Microbiol.*, 5, 109, 1977.

29. Collins, M. D., Goodfellow, M., Minnikin, D. E., and Alderson, G., The menaquinone composition of mycolic acid-containing actinomycetes and some sporoactinomycetes, *J. Appl. Bacteriol.*, 58, 77, 1985.

30. Yamada, Y., Inouye, G., Tahara, Y., and Kondo, K., The menaquinone system in the classification of coryneform and nocardioform bacteria and related organisms, *J. Gen. Appl. Microbiol.*, 22, 203, 1976.

31. Yamada, Y., Yishikawa, T., Tahara, Y., and Kondo, K., The menaquinone system in the classification of the genus *Nocardia, J. Gen. Appl. Microbiol.*, 23, 207, 1977.

32. Suzuki, Y., Toyama, K., Utsugi, K., Yazawa, K., Mikami, Y., Fujita, M., and Shinkai, H., Primary lymphocutaneous nocardiosis due to *Nocardia otitidiscaviarum*: the first case report from Japan, *J. Dermatol.*, 22, 344, 1995.

33. Curry, W. A., Human nocardiosis: a clinical review with selected case reports, *Arch. Intern. Med.*, 140, 818, 1980.

34. Kahn, F. W., Gornick, C. C., and Tofte, R. W., Primary cutaneous *Nocardia asteroides* infection with dissemination, *Am. J. Med.*, 70, 859, 1981.

35. Nocard, M. E., Note sur la maladie des boeufs de la Guadeloupe connue sous le nom de farcin, *Ann. Inst. Pasteur*, 2, 293, 1888.

36. Trevisan, V., I generi e le specie delle battieriacee, Milano: Zanabon and Gabuzzi, *Int. Bull. Bacteriol. Nomencl. Taxon.*, 2, 13, 1889.

37. Eppinger, H., Über eine neue pathogene *Cladothrix* und eine durch sie hervorgerufene pseudotuberculosis (cladothricia), *Beitr. Pathol. Anat. Allg. Pathol.*, 9, 287, 1980.

38. Hanneman, J., Dalitz, M., Hell, W., Lebeau, A., Busch, D., and Dalhoff, K., Generalized nocardiosis with meningoencephalitis in a nonimmunosuppressed female patient, *Dtsch. Med. Wochenschr.*, 118, 1281, 1993.

39. Rosendale, D. E., Myers, C., Boyko, E. J., and Jafek, B., *Nocardia asteroides* cervical osteomyelitis in an immunocompetent host, *Otolaryngol. Head Neck Surg.*, 99, 334, 1988.

40. O'Connor, P. T. and Dire, D. J., Cutaneous nocardiosis associated with insect bites, *Cutis*, 50, 301, 1992.

41. Sachs, M. K., Lymphocutaneous *Nocardia brasiliensis* infection acquired from a cat scratch: case report and review, *Clin. Infect. Dis.*, 15, 710, 1992.

42. Madiba, T. E., Hoosen, A. A., Madaree, A., and Abdool Carrim, A. T. O., Surgical excision of scalp mycetoma due to *Nocardia, Trop. Geogr. Med.*, 46, 185, 1994.

43. Mirza, S. H. and Campbell, C., Mycetoma caused by *Nocardia transvalensis, J. Clin. Pathol.*, 47, 85, 1994.

44. Saraca, G. D., Towersey, L., Hay, R. J., Londero, A. T., Martins, E. de C., Amora, A. T., Reis, K. M., Mendonca, A. M., and Estrella, R. R., Mycetoma by *Nocardia asteroides*: a 9 year follow-up, *Rev. Inst. Trop. Med. Sao Paolo*, 35, 199, 1993.

45. Wortman, P. D., Treatment of a *Nocardia brasiliensis* mycetoma with sulfamethoxazole and trimethoprim, amikacin, and amoxicillin and clavulinate, *Arch. Dermatol.*, 129, 564, 1993.

46. Gomez, A., Saul, A., Bonifaz, A., and Lopez, M., Amocillin and clavulanic acid in the treatment of actinomycetoma, *Int. J. Dermatol.*, 32, 218, 1993.

47. Martinez, R. E., Couchel, S., Swartz, W. M., and Smith, M. B., Mycetoma of the hand, *J. Hand Surg. (Am.)*, 14, 909, 1989.

48. Orellano Ocampo, F., Arellano Huacuja, A., and Leon Valle, C., Surgical treatment of mycetoma located in the face, *Med. Cutan. Ibero Lat. Am.*, 17, 9, 1989.

49. Schwartz, J. G., McGough, D. A., Thorner, R. E., Fetchick, R. J., Tio, F. O., and Rinaldi, M. G., Primary lymphocutaneous *Nocardia brasiliensis* infection: three case reports and a review of the literature, *Diagn. Microbiol. Infect. Dis.*, 10, 113, 1988.

50. Moeller, C. A. and Burton, C. S. III, Primary lymphocutaneous *Nocardia brasiliensis* infection, *Arch. Dermatol.*, 122, 1180, 1986.

51. Kim, J., Minamoto, G. Y., and Grieco, M. H., Nocardial infection as a complication of AIDS: report of six cases and a review, *Rev. Infect. Dis.*, 13, 624, 1991.

52. Seidel, J. F., Younce, D. C., Hupp, J. R., and Kaminski, Z. C., Cervicofacial nocardiosis: report of case, *J. Oral Maxillofac. Surg.*, 52, 188, 1994.

53. Smego, R. A., Jr. and Gallis, H. A., The clinical spectrum of *Nocardia brasiliensis* infection in the United States, *Rev. Infect. Dis.*, 6, 164, 1984.

54. Beaman, B. L., Boiron, P., Beaman, L., Brownell, G. H., Schaal, K., and Gombert, M. E., *Nocardia* and nocardiosis, *J. Med. Vet. Mycol.*, 30, 317, 1992.

55. Neubert, U. and Schaal, K. P., Sporotrichoid infection caused by *Nocardia brasiliensis, Hautarzt*, 33, 548, 1982.

56. Spehn, J., Grosser, S., Jessel, A., von Essen, J., and Klose, G., High-dosage cotrimoxazole therapy of disseminated *Nocardia brasiliensis* infection, *Dtsch. Med. Wochenschr.*, 111, 215, 1986.

57. Shifren, J. D. and Milliken, R. G., An acute *Nocardia brasiliensis* infection of the hand: a case report, *J. Hand Surg. (Am.)*, 21, 309, 1996.
58. Marck, Y., Meunier, L., Perez, C., and Meynadier, J., Nocardiose cutanée primitive a *Nocardia asteroides* chez un malade immunodéprimé, *Ann. Dermatol. Venereol.*, 122, 675, 1995.
59. Causey, W. A., *Nocardia caviae*: a report of 13 new isolations with clinical correlation, *Appl. Environ. Microbiol.*, 28, 193, 1974.
60. Georghiou, P. R. and Blacklock, Z. M., Infection with *Nocardia* species in Queensland: a review of 102 clinical isolates, *Med. J. Aust.*, 156, 692, 1992.
61. Freland, C., Fur, J. L., Nemirovsky-Trebucq, B., Lelong, P., and Boiron, P., Primary cutaneous nocardiosis caused by *Nocardia otitidiscaviarum*: two cases and a review of the literature, *J. Trop. Med. Hyg.*, 98, 395, 1995.
62. Clark, N. M., Braun, D. K., Pasternak, A., and Chenoweth, C. E., Primary cutaneous *Nocardia otitidiscaviarum* infection: case report and review, *Clin. Infect. Dis.*, 20, 1266, 1995.
63. Schaal, K. P. and Lee, H. J., Actinomycetes infections in humans — a review, *Gene*, 115, 201, 1992.
64. Mariat, F., Étude comparative de souches de *Nocardia* isolées de mycétomes, *Ann. Inst. Pasteur*, 109, 90, 1965.
65. Juminer, B., Khalfat, A., Heldt, N., and Mariat, F., Deuxième cas tunisien de mycétome a *Nocardia*, *Bull. Soc. Pathol. Exot.*, 58, 177, 1965.
66. Fukushiro, R. and Mariat, F., Note sur un mycétome a *Nocardia caviae* observé au Japon, *Bull. Soc. Pathol. Exot.*, 58, 185, 1965.
67. Thammayya, A., Basu, N., Sur-Roy-Chowdhury, D., Banerjee, A. K., and Sanyal, M., Actinomycetoma pedis caused by *Nocardia caviae* in India, *Sabouraudia*, 10, 19, 1972.
68. Sandhu, D. K., Mishra, S. K., Damodaran, V. N., Sandhu, R. S., and Randhawa, H. S., Mycetoma of the knee due to *Nocardia caviae*, *Sabouraudia*, 13, 170, 1975.
69. Alteras, I., Feuerman, E. J., and Dayan, I., Mycetoma due to *Nocardia caviae*: the first Israeli patient, *Int. J. Dermatol.*, 19, 260, 1980.
70. Lampe, R. M., Baker, C. J., Septimus, E. J., and Wallace, R. J., Jr., Cervicofacial nocardiosis in children, *J. Pediatr.*, 99, 593, 1981.
71. Alteras, I. and Feuerman, E. J., The second case of mycetoma due to *Nocardia caviae* in Israel, *Mycopathologia*, 93, 185, 1986.
72. Saul, A., Bonifaz, A., Messina, M., and Andrade, R., Mycetoma due to *Nocardia caviae*, *Int. J. Dermatol.*, 26, 174, 1987.
73. Girouard, Y., Albert, G., Thivierge, B., and Lorange-Rodrigues, M., Primary cutaneous nocardiosis due to *Nocardia caviae*, *Can. Med. Assoc. J.*, 136, 844, 1987.
74. Hachisuka, H., Ichiki, M., Yoshida, N., Nakano, S., and Sasai, Y., Primary subcutaneous abscess caused by *Nocardia otitidiscaviarum*, *J. Am. Acad. Dermatol.*, 21, 137, 1989.
75. Yang, L.-J., Chan, H.-L., Chen, W.-J., and Kuo, T.-T., Lymphocutaneous nocardiosis caused by *Nocardia caviae*: the first case report from Asia, *J. Am. Acad. Dermatol.*, 29, 639, 1993.
76. Schiff, T. A., McNeil, M. M., and Brown, J. M., Cutaneous *Nocardia farcinica* infection in a nonimmunocompromised patient: case report and review, *Clin. Infect. Dis.*, 16, 756, 1993.
77. Chiemchaisri, Y. W., Imwidthaya, S., and Parichatikanond, P., Exogenous intraocular nocardiosis, *J. Med. Assoc. Thailand*, 68, 29, 1985.
78. Climenhaga, D. B., Tokarewicz, A. C., and Willis, N. R., Nocardia keratitis, *Can. J. Ophthalmol.*, 19, 284, 1984.
79. Douglas, R. M., Grove, D. I., Elliott, J., Looke, D. F., and Jordan, A. S., Corneal ulceration due to *Nocardia asteroides*, *Aust. NZ J. Ophthalmol.*, 19, 317, 1991.
80. Heathcote, J. G., McCartney, A. C., Rice, N. S., Peacock, J., and Seal, D. V., Endophthalmitis caused by exogenous nocardial infection in a patient with Sjogren's syndrome, *Can. J. Ophthalmol.*, 25, 29, 1990.
81. King, L. P., Furlong, W. B., Gilbert, W. S., and Levy, C., *Nocardia asteroides* infection following scleral buckling, *Ophthalm. Surg.*, 22, 150, 1991.
82. Clague, H. W., Harth, M., Hellyer, D., and Morgan, W. K., Septic arthritis due to *Nocardia asteroides* in association with pulmonary alveolar proteinosis, *J. Rheumatol.*, 9, 469, 1982.
83. Baikie, A. G., Macdonald, C. B., and Mundy, G. R., Systemic nocardiosis treated with trimethoprim and sulfamethoxazole, *Lancet*, 2, 261, 1970.

84. Rao, K. V., O'Brien, T. J., and Anderson, R. C., Septic arthritis due to *Nocardia asteroides* after successful kidney transplantation, *Arthritis Rheum.*, 24, 99, 1981

85. Asmar, B. I. and Bashour, B. N., Septic arthritis due to *Nocardia asteroides*, *South. Med. J.*, 84, 933, 1991.

86. Beaman, B. L. and Beaman, L., *Nocardia* species: host-parasite relationships, *Clin. Microbiol. Rev.*, 7, 213, 1994.

87. Beaman, B. L., Burnside, J., Edwards, B., and Causey, W., Nocardial infections in the United States, 1972-1974, *J. Med. Vet. Dis.*, 134, 286, 1976.

88. Cox, F. and Hughes, W. T., Contagious and other aspects of nocardiosis in the compromised host, *Pediatrics*, 55, 135, 1975.

89. Wilson, J. P., Turner, H. R., Kirchner, K. A., and Chapman, S. W., Nocardial infections in renal transplant recipients, *Medicine (Baltimore)*, 68, 38, 1989.

90. Simpson, G. L., Stinson, E. B., Egger, M. J., and Remington, J. S., Nocardial infections in the immunocompromised host: a detailed study in a defined population, *Rev. Infect. Dis.*, 3, 492, 1981.

91. Murray, J. F., Finegold, S. M., Froman, S., and Will, D. W., The changing spectrum of nocardiosis: a review and presentation of nine cases, *Am. Rev. Respir. Dis.*, 83, 315, 1961.

92. Palmer, D. L., Harvey, R. L., and Wheeler, J. K., Diagnostic and therapeutic considerations in *Nocardia asteroides* infection, *Medicine (Baltimore)*, 53, 391, 1974.

93. Arduino, R. C., Johnson, P. C., and Miranda, A. G., Nocardiosis in renal transplant recipients undergoing immunosuppression with cyclosporine, *Clin. Infect. Dis.*, 16, 505, 1993.

94. Frazier, A. R., Rosenow, E. C. III, and Roberts, G. D., Nocardiosis: a review of 25 cases occurring during 24 months, *Mayo Clin. Proc.*, 50, 657, 1975.

95. Young, L. S., Armstrong, D., Blevins, A., and Lieberman, P., *Nocardia asteroides* infection complicating neoplastic disease, *Am. J. Med.*, 50, 356, 1971.

96. Bani-Sadr, F., Hamidou, M., Raffi, F., Chamoux, C., Caillon, J., and Freland, C., Aspects cliniques et bactériologiques des nocardioses: 9 observations, *Presse Med.*, 24, 1062, 1995.

97. Ledesma Castano, F., Hernandez Hernandez, J. L., Echevarria Viema, S., and Conde Yague, R., Immunosuppression and pulmonary nocardiosis, *Ann. Med. Intern.*, 13, 50, 1996.

98. McNeil, M. M., Brown, J. M., Georghiou, P. R., Allworth, A. M., and Blacklock, Z. M., Infections due to *Nocardia transvalensis*: clinical spectrum and antimicrobial therapy, *Clin. Infect. Dis.*, 15, 453, 1992.

99. Anonymous, Cavitary lung disease following renal transplantation, *Am. J. Med.*, 72, 145, 1982.

100. Baddour, L. M., Baselski, V. S., Herr, M. J., Christensen, G. D., and Bisno, A. L., Nocardiosis in recipients of renal transplants: evidence for nosocomial acquisition, *Am. J. Infect. Control*, 14, 214, 1986.

101. Barmeir, E., Mann, J. H., and Marcus, R. H., Cerebral nocardiosis in renal transplant patients, *Br. J. Radiol.*, 54, 1107, 1981.

102. Carter, J. M., Green, W. R., Callender, C. O., and Peters, B., Pulmonary cavitation with *Nocardia* and *Aspergillus* in a renal transplant patient, *J. Natl. Med. Assoc.*, 82, 527, 1990.

103. Hellyar, A. G., Experience with *Nocardia asteroides* in renal transplant recipients, *J. Hosp. Infect.*, 12, 13, 1988.

104. Leaker, B., Hellyar, A., Neild, G. H., Rudge, C., Mansell, M., and Thompson, F. D., *Nocardia* infection in a renal transplant unit, *Transplant. Proc.*, 21, 2103, 1989.

105. Lovett, I. S., Houang, E. T., Burge, S., Turner-Warwick, M., Thompson, F. D., Harrison, A. R., Joekes, A. M., and Parkinson, M. C., An outbreak of *Nocardia asteroides* infection in a renal transplant unit, *Q. J. Med.*, 50, 123, 1981.

106. Avram, M. M., Ramachandran Nair, S., Lipner, H. I., and Cherubin, C. E., Persistent nocardemia following renal transplantation: association with pulmonary nocardiosis, *JAMA*, 239, 2779, 1978.

107. Wilson, J. P., Turner, H. R., Kirchner, K. A., and Chapman, S. W., Nocardial infections in renal transplant recipients, *Medicine (Baltimore)*, 68, 38, 1989.

108. Santamaria Saber, L. T., Figueiredo, J. F., Santos, S. B., Levy, C. E. et al., *Nocardia* infection in renal transplant recipient: diagnostic and therapeutic considerations, *Rev. Inst. Med. Trop. Sao Paolo*, 35, 417, 1993.

109. Forbes, G. M., Harvey, F. A., Philpott-Howard, J. N., O'Grady, J. G., Jensen, R. D., Sahathevan, M., Casewell, M. W., and Williams, R., Nocardiosis in liver transplantation: variation in presentation, diagnosis and therapy, *J. Infect.*, 20, 11, 1990.

110. Weinberger, M., Eid, A., Schreiber, L., Shapiro, M., Ilan, Y., Libson, E., Sacks, T., and Tur-Kaspa, R., Disseminated *Nocardia transvalensis* resembling pulmonary infection in a liver transplant patient, *Eur. J. Clin. Microbiol. Infect. Dis.*, 14, 337, 1995.

111. Lumbreras, C., Lizasoian, M., Moreno, E., Aguado, J. M., Gomez, R., Garcia, I., Gonzalez, I., Loinaz, C., Cisneros, C., and Noriega, A. R., Major bacterial infections following liver transplantation: a prospective study, *Hepato-Gastroenterology*, 39, 362, 1992.

112. Schroter, G. P. J., Hoelscher, M., Putnam, C. W., Porter, K. A., Hansbrough, J. F., and Starzl, T. E., Infections complicating orthotopic liver transplantation: a study emphasizing graft-related septicemia, *Arch. Surg.*, 111, 1337, 1976.

113. Krick, J. A., Stinson, E. B., and Remington, J. S., *Nocardia* infection in heart transplant patients, *Ann. Intern. Med.*, 82, 18, 1975.

114. Mahgoub, E. S., Medical management of mycetoma, *Bull. WHO*, 54, 303, 1976.

115. Monteforte, J. S. and Wood, C. A., Pneumonia caused by *Nocardia nova* and *Aspergillus fumigatus* after cardiac transplantation, *Eur. J. Clin. Microbiol. Infect. Dis.*, 12, 112, 1993.

116. Shearer, C., Chandrasekar, P. H., and the Bone Marrow Transplantation Group, *Bone Marrow Transplant.*, 15, 479, 1995.

117. Freites, V., Sumoza, A., Bisotti, R., Mujica, M., Cabrera, A., Costa, M., Anguilo, R., and Rolston, K., Subcutaneous *Nocardia asteroides* in a bone marrow transplant recipient, *Bone Marrow Transplant.*, 15, 135, 1995.

118. Petersen, D. L., Hudson, L. D., and Sullivan, K., Disseminated *Nocardia caviae* with positive blood cultures, *Arch. Intern. Med.*, 138, 1164, 1978.

119. Hodohara, K., Fujiyama, Y., Hiramita, Y., Sumiyoshi, K., Kotoh, K., Hosada, S., and Sugiura, H., Disseminated subcutaneous *Nocardia asteroides* abscesses in a patient after bone marrow transplantation, *Bone Marrow Transplant.*, 11, 341, 1993.

120. Chapman, S. W. and Wilson, J. P., Nocardiosis in transplant recipients, *Semin. Respir. Infect.*, 5, 74, 1990.

121. Seggev, J. S., Fatal pulmonary nocardiosis in a patient with chronic mucocutaneous candidiasis, *J. Allergy Clin. Immunol.*, 94, 259, 1994.

122. Andriole, V. T., Baldas, M., and Wilson, G. L., The association of nocardiosis and pulmonary alveolar proteinosis, *Ann. Intern. Med.*, 60, 266, 1964.

123. Anonymous, Case records of the Massachusetts General Hospital. Weekly clinicopathological exercises: case 18 - 1988. A 30-year-old man with bilateral pulmonary consolidation and cavitation, *N. Engl. J. Med.*, 318, 1186, 1988.

124. Burbank, B., Morrione, T. G., and Cutler, S. S., Pulmonary alveolar proteinosis and nocardiosis, *Am. J. Med.*, 28, 1002, 1960.

125. Teleghani-Far, M., Barber, J. B., Sampson, C., and Marsden, K. A., Cerebral nocardiosis and pulmonary alveolar proteinosis, *Am. Rev. Respir. Dis.*, 89, 561, 1964.

126. Pascual, J., Sureda, A., Gomez Aguinaga, M. A., and Vidal, R., Alveolar proteinosis: a report of a case treated by total bronchopulmonary lavage, *An. Med. Intern.*, 7, 276, 1990.

127. Debieuvre, D., Dalphin, J. C., Jacoulet, P., Breton, J. L., Boiron, P., and Depierre, A., Disseminated infection due to an unusual strain of *Nocardia farcinica*, *Rev. Mal. Respir.*, 10, 356, 1993.

128. Borges, A. A., Krasnow, S. H., Wadleigh, R. G., and Cohen, M. H., Nocardiosis after corticosteroid therapy for malignant thymoma, *Cancer*, 71, 1746, 1993.

129. Rees, W., Schuler, S., Hummel, M., and Hetzer, R., Primary cutaneous *Nocardia farcinica* infection following heart transplantation, *Dtsch. Med. Wochenschr.*, 119, 1276, 1994 (correction in *Dtsch. Med. Wochenschr.*, 119, 1276, 1994).

130. Abdi, E. A., Ding, J. C., and Cooper, I. A., *Nocardia* in splenectomized patients: case reports and review of the literature, *Postgrad. Med. J.*, 63, 455, 1987.

131. Noto, N., Sugaya, N., Wakabayashi, Y., and Hirose, S., A case of pulmonary nocardiosis in malignant lymphoma under VEMP therapy, *Rinsho Ketsueki*, 26, 1140, 1985.

132. Pinkhas, J., Oliver, I., de Vries, A., Spitzer, S. A., and Henig, E., Pulmonary nocardiosis complicating malignant lymphoma successfully treated with chemotherapy, *Chest*, 63, 367, 1973.

133. Shelkovitz-Shilo, L., Feinstein, A., Trau, H., Kaplan, B., Sofer, E., and Schewach-Millet, M., Lymphocutaneous nocardiosis due to *Nocardia asteroides* in a patient with intestinal lymphoma, *Int. J. Dermatol.*, 31, 178, 1992.

134. Taylor, G. D. and Turner, A. R., Cutaneous abscess due to *Nocardia* after "alternative" therapy for lymphoma, *Can. Med. Assoc. J.*, 133, 767, 1985.

135. Berkey, P. and Bodey, G. P., Nocardial infection in patients with neoplastic disease, *Rev. Infect. Dis.*, 11, 407, 1989.

136. Tang, L. M. and Hsi, M. S., Nocardial cerebral abscess: report of a case, *J. Formos. Med. Assoc.*, 88, 186, 1989.

137. Ziza, J. M., Mayaud, C., and Carnot, F., Anatomo-clinical conference. Pitie-Salpetriere Hospital: case n. 1-1988. Degradation of the respiratory function in a patient followed for severe sarcoidosis, *Ann. Med. Intern. (Paris)*, 139, 41, 1988.

138. Garty, B. Z., Stark, H., Yaniv, I., Varsano, I., and Danon, Y. I., Pulmonary nocardiosis in a child with systemic lupus erythematosus, *Pediatr. Infect. Dis. J.*, 4, 66, 1985.

139. Gorevic, P. D., Katler, E. I., and Agus, B., Pulmonary nocardiosis: occurrence in men with systemic lupus erythematosus, *Arch. Intern. Med.*, 140, 361, 1980.

140. Nzeusseu Toukap, A., Hainaut, P., Moreau, M., Pieters, T., Noirhomme, P., and Gigi, J., Nocardiosis: a rare cause of pleuropulmonary disease in the immunocompromised host, *Acta Clin. Belg.*, 51, 161, 1996.

141. Lopes, J. O., Alves, S. H., Benevenga, J. P., Salla, A., and Tatsch, I., *Nocardia asteroides* peritonitis during continuous ambulatory peritoneal dialysis, *Rev. Inst. Med. Trop. Sao Paolo*, 35, 377, 1993.

142. Tirapu, J. M., Alvarez, M., Crespo, J. A., Rojo, P., Gonzalez-Igual, J., Arriaga, I., and Cisterna, R., Chronic granulomatous disease and pulmonary nocardiosis, *Med. Clin. (Barcelona)*, 99, 27, 1992.

143. Casale, T. B., Macher, A. M., and Fauci, A. S., Concomitant pulmonary aspergillosis and nocardiosis in a patient with chronic granulomatous disease of childhood, *South. Med. J.*, 77, 274, 1984.

144. Fernandez-Funez, V. A., Solera, J., Castro, C., Beato, J. L., Medrano, F., and Camino, E., Chronic granulomatous disease and infection by *Nocardia*, *Enferm. Infecc. Microbiol. Clin.*, 7, 564, 1989.

145. Johnston, H. C., Shigeoka, A. O., Hurley, D. C., and Pysher, T. J., *Nocardia* pneumonia in a neonate with chronic granulomatous disease, *Pediatr. Infect. Dis. J.*, 8, 526, 1989.

146. Jonsson, S., Wallace, R. J., Jr., Hull, S. I., and Musher, D. M., Reccurent *Nocardia* pneumonia in an adult with chronic granulomatous disease, *Am. Rev. Respir. Dis.*, 133, 932, 1986.

147. Valencia, M. E., Lavilla, P., Lopez Dupla, J. M., and Gil Aguado, A., Disseminated nocardiosis in a patient with chronic alcoholism, *Rev. Clin. Esp.*, 186, 146, 1990.

148. Sahl, B., Fegan, C., Hussain, A., Jaulim, A., Whale, K., and Webb, A., Pulmonary infection with *Nocardia caviae* in a patient with diabetes mellitus and liver cirrhosis, *Thorax*, 43, 933, 1988.

149. Kramer, M. R. and Uttamchandani, R. B., The radiographic appearance of pulmonary nocardiosis associated with AIDS, *Chest*, 98, 382, 1990.

150. Marin Casanova, P., Garcia-Martos, P., Fernandez Gutierez del Alamo, C., Garcia Herruzo, J., Escribano Moriana, J. C., and Aznar Martin, A., Nocardiosis in a patient with AIDS, *Rev. Clin. Esp.*, 188, 83, 1991.

151. Perez Perez, M., Garcia-Martos, P., Escribano Moriana, J. C., and Marin Casanova, P., *Nocardia caviae* meningitis in a patient with HIV infection, *Rev. Clin. Esp.*, 187, 374, 1990.

152. Rodriguez, J. L., Barrio, J. L., and Pitchenik, A. E., Pulmonary nocardiosis in the acquired immuno-deficiency syndrome: diagnosis with bronchoalveolar lavage and treatment with non-sulphur containing drugs, *Chest*, 90, 912, 1986.

153. Allworth, A. M. and Bowden, F. J., Managing HIV. V. Treating secondary outcomes: HIV and bacterial infections, *Med. J. Aust.*, 164, 546, 1996.

154. Sanchez Munoz-Torrero, J. F., Yniguez, T. R., Garcia-Onieva, E., Pascua, F. J., Crespo, L., Bacaicoa, A., and Martin, C., Nocardiosis in patients with human immunodeficiency virus infection in Spain, *Rev. Clin. Esp.*, 195, 468, 1995.

155. Meyer, C. N., Nocardiosis in HIV patients, *Ugeskr. Laeger*, 157, 4358, 1995.

156. Farina, L. A., Palou Redorta, J., and Chechile Toniolo, G., Reversible acute renal failure due to sulfonamide-induced lithiasis in an AIDS patient, *Arch. Esp. Urol.*, 48, 418, 1995.

157. Khorrami, P. and Heffeman, E. J., Pneumonia and meningitis due to *Nocardia asteroides* in a patient with AIDS, *Clin. Infect. Dis.*, 17, 1084, 1993.

158. Weiss, D., Bodmer, T., Mathieu, R., and Malinverni, R., Systemic *Nocardia* infection in an AIDS patient, *Schweiz. Med. Wochenschr.*, 122, 1057, 1992.

159. Garcia-Martos, P., Diaz, J., Perez, M., Alvarez, M. M., and Rubin, J., Meningeal syndrome in a patient addicted to parenteral drugs, *Enferm. Infecc. Microbiol. Clin.*, 8, 313, 1990.
160. Hershewe, G. L., Davis, L. E., and Bicknell, J. M., Primary cerebellar brain abscess from nocardiosis in a heroin addict, *Neurology*, 38, 1655, 1988.
161. Vanderstigel, M., Leclercq, R., Brun-Buisson, C., Schaeffer, A., and Duval, J., Blood-borne pulmonary infection with *Nocardia asteroides* in a heroin addict, *J. Clin. Microbiol.*, 23, 175, 1986.
162. Uttamchandani, R. B., Daikos, G. L., Reyes, R. R., Fischl, M. A., Dickinson, G. M., Yamaguchi, E., and Kramer, M. R., Nocardiosis in 30 patients with advanced human immunodeficiency virus infection: clinical features and outcome, *Clin. Infect. Dis.*, 18, 348, 1994.
163. Anonymous, *Nocardia asteroides* pericarditis, *Mayo Clin. Proc.*, 65, 1276, 1990.
164. Kessler, R., Follis, F., Daube, D., and Wernly, J., Constrictive pericarditis from *Nocardia asteroides* infection, *Ann. Thorac. Surg.*, 52, 861, 1991.
165. Leung, W. H., Wong, K. L., Lau, C. P., and Wong, C. K., Purulent pericarditis and cardiac tamponade caused by *Nocardia asteroides* in mixed connective tissue disease, *J. Rheumatol.*, 17, 1237, 1990.
166. Poland, G. A., Jorgensen, C. R., and Sarosi, G. A., *Nocardia asteroides* pericarditis: report of a case and review of the literature, *Mayo Clin. Proc.*, 65, 819, 1990.
167. Hornick, P., Harris, P., and Smith, P., *Nocardia asteroides* purulent pericarditis, *Eur. J. Cardiothorac. Surg.*, 9, 468, 1995.
168. Susens, G. P., Al-Shamma, A., Rowe, J. C., Herbert, C. C., Bassis, M., and Coggs, G. C., Purulent constrictive pericarditis caused by *Nocardia asteroides*, *Ann. Intern. Med.*, 67, 1021, 1967.
169. Boudoulas, O. and Camisa, C., *Nocardia asteroides* infection with dissemination to skin and joints, *Arch. Dermatol.*, 121, 898, 1985.
170. Naguib, M. T. and Fine, D. P., Brain abscess due to *Nocardia brasiliensis* hematogenously spread from a pulmonary infection, *Clin. Infect. Dis.*, 21, 459, 1995.
171. Welsh Lozano, O. and Lopez Lopez, J. R., Mycetomas with pulmonary dissemination, *Med. Cutan. Ibero Lat. Am.*, 13, 517, 1985.
172. Presant, C. A., Wiernik, P. H., and Serpick, A. A., Factors affecting survival in nocardiosis, *Am. Rev. Respir. Dis.*, 108, 1444, 1973.
173. Borget, C., Gepner, P., Piette, A. M., and Chapman, A., Primary *Nocardia asteroides* deltoid abscess in treated Horton disease, *Rev. Rhum. Mal. Osteoartic.*, 59, 149, 1992.
174. Klein-Gitelman, M. S. and Szer, I. S., Disseminated *Nocardia brasiliensis* infection: an unusual complication of immunosuppressive treatment for childhood dermatomyositis, *J. Rheumatol.*, 18, 1243, 1991.
175. Zufferey, P., Wenger, A., Bille, J., and Hofstetter, J. R., Disseminated nocardiosis due to *Nocardia brasiliensis* in an ambulatory patient, *Schweiz. Rundsch. Med. Prax.*, 78, 718, 1989.
176. Bradsher, R. W., Monson, T. P., and Steele, R. W., Brain abscess due to *Nocardia caviae*: report of a fatal outcome associated with abnormal phagocyte function, *Am. J. Clin. Pathol.*, 78, 124, 1982.
177. Simmons, B. P., Gelfand, M. S., and Roberts, G. D., *Nocardia otitidiscaviarum* (*caviae*) infection in a heart transplant patient presented as having a thigh abscess (Madura thigh), *J. Heart Lung Transplant.*, 11, 824, 1992.
178. Baghdadlian, H., Sorger, S., Knowles, K., McNeil, M., and Brown, J., *Nocardia transvalensis* pneumonia in a child, *Pediatr. Infect. Dis. J.*, 8, 470, 1989.
179. McNeil, M. M., Brown, J. M., Magruder, C. H., Shearlock, K. T., Saul, R. A., Allred, D. P., and Ajello, L., Disseminated *Nocardia transvalensis* infection: an unusual opportunistic pathogen in severely immunocompromised patients, *J. Infect. Dis.*, 165, 175, 1992.
180. Dietlein, E., Firsching, R., and Peters, G., Therapy of brain abscess caused by *Nocardia farcinica*, *Med. Klin.*, 83, 613, 1988.
181. Miksits, K., Stoltenburg, G., Neumayer, H. H., Spiegel, H., Schaal, K. P., Cervos-Navarro, J., Distler, A., Stein, H., and Hahn, H., Disseminated infection of the central nervous system caused by *Nocardia farcinica*, *Nephrol. Dial. Transplant.*, 6, 209, 1991.
182. Tsukamura, M., Nocardiae that recently caused lung infection in Japan — *Nocardia asteroides* and *Nocardia farcinica*, *Microbiol. Immunol.*, 26, 341, 1982.
183. Tsukamura, M. and Ohta, M., *Nocardia farcinica* as a pathogen of lung infection, *Microbiol. Immunol.*, 24, 237, 1980.

184. Tsukamura, M., Shimoide, H., Kaneda, K., Sakai, R., and Seino, A., A case of lung infection caused by an unusual strain of *Nocardia farcinica*, *Microbiol. Immunol.*, 32, 541, 1988.

185. Granier, F., Kahla-Clemenceau, N., Richardin, F., Leclerc, V., Bourgeois- Droin, C., Bérardi-Grassias, L., and Trémolières, F., *Nocardia farcinica* infection: cutaneous form in an immunodepressed patient, *Presse Med.*, 23, 329, 1994.

186. Liassine, N. and Rahal, K., Peritonitis caused by *Nocardia farcinica* in a patient undergoing continuous ambulatory peritoneal analysis, *Arch. Inst. Pasteur Alger.*, 58, 95, 1992.

187. Schiff, T. A., Sanchez, M., Moy, J., Klirsfeld, D., McNeil, M. M., and Brown, J. M., Cutaneous nocardiosis caused by *Nocardia nova* occurring in an HIV-infected individual: a case report and review of the literature, *J. Acquir. Immune Defic. Syndr.*, 6, 849, 1993.

188. Pijper, A. and Pullinger, B. D., South African nocardiases, *J. Trop. Med. Hyg.*, 30, 153, 1927

189. Kong, N. C., Morad, Z., Suleiman, A. B., Cheong, I. K., and Lajin, I., Spectrum of nocardiosis in renal patients, *Ann. Acad. Med. Singapore*, 19, 375, 1990.

190. King, C. T., Chapman, S. W., and Butkus, D. E., Recurrent nocardiosis in a renal transplant recipient, *South. Med. J.*, 86, 225, 1993.

191. Carpintero, Y., Mendaza, P., Portero, F., Sanchez, B. et al., *Nocardia asteroides* pneumonia in a patient undergoing a kidney transplant, *Enferm. Infecc. Microbiol. Clin.*, 14, 65, 1996.

192. Gutierrez, H., Salgado, O., Garcia, R., Henriquez, C., Herrera, J., and Rodriguez-Iturbe, B., Nocardiosis in renal transplant patients, *Transplant. Proc.*, 26, 341, 1994.

193. Raby, N., Forbes, G., and Williams, R., *Nocardia* infection in patients with liver transplants or chronic liver disease: radiologic findings, *Radiology*, 174, 713, 1990.

194. Javaly, K., Horowitz, H. W., and Wormser, G. P., Nocardiosis in patients with human immunodeficiency virus infection: report of 2 cases and review of the literature, *Medicine (Baltimore)*, 71, 128, 1992.

195. Aguilar, P. H., Pahl, F. H., Uip, D. E., Vellutini, E. A. et al., Cerebellar abscess by *Nocardia*: a case report, *Arq. Neurosiquiatr.*, 53, 307, 1995.

196. Desfemmes, T., Cadranel, J., Delisle, F., Akoun, G., and Mayaud, C., Pulmonary and cerebral nocardiosis in a patient infected with HIV, *Rev. Mal. Respir.*, 10, 262, 1993.

197. Overkamp, D., Waldmann, B., Lins, T., Lingenfelser, T., Petersen, D., and Eggstein, M., Successful treatment of brain abscess caused by *Nocardia* in an immunocompromised patient after failure of co-trimoxazole, *Infection*, 20, 365, 1992.

198. Findley, J. C., Arafah, B. M., Silverman, P., and Aron, D. C., Cushing's syndrome with cranial and pulmonary lesions: necessity for tissue diagnosis, *South. Med. J.*, 85, 204, 1992.

199. Fried, J., Hinthorn, D., Ralstin, J., Gerjarusak, P., and Liu, C., Cure of brain abscess caused by *Nocardia asteroides* resistant to multiple antibiotics, *South. Med. J.*, 81, 412, 1988.

200. Idemyor, V. and Cherubin, C. E., Pleurocerebral *Nocardia* in a patient with human immunodeficiency virus, *Ann. Pharmacother.*, 26, 188, 1992.

201. Ohguni, S., Yamamoto, D., Furuya, H., Masaki, Y., Oka, N., Kamura, T., and Kato, Y., A case of adult T-cell leukemia (ATL) complicated with multiple nocardial abscesses, *Kansenshogaku Zasshi*, 65, 1459, 1991.

202. Tanaka, M., Sato, Y., Ito, H., Ichikawa, Y., Oizumi, K., and Shigemori, M., A case of Cushing's syndrome associated with *Nocardia* cerebral abscess, *Kansenshogaku Zasshi*, 65, 243, 1991.

203. Buxton, N. and McIntosh, J., Multiple nocardial brain abscesses: report of two patients, *Br. J. Neurosurg.*, 8, 501, 1994.

204. Coutant-Perronne, V., Lutz, V., Mainardi, J. L., Acar, J. F., Kugelstadt, P., and Goldstein, F., Méningite a *Nocardia* sans abscès cérébral a la scanographie, *Presse Med.*, 24, 1271, 1995.

205. Hall, W. A., Martinez, A. J., Dunne, J. S., and Linsford, L. D., Nocardial brain abscess: diagnostic and therapeutic use of stereotactic aspiration, *Surg. Neurol.*, 28, 114, 1987.

206. Kruege, E. G., Norson, L., Kenney, M., and Price, P. A., Nocardiosis of the central nervous system, *J. Neurosurg.*, 11, 226, 1954.

207. Turner, E. and Whiting, J. L., Nocardial cerebral abscesses with systemic involvement successfully treated by aspiration and sulphonamides, *J. Neurosurg.*, 31, 227, 1969.

208. Philit, F., Boibieux, A., Coppere, B., Reverdy, M. E., Peyramond, D., and Bertrand, J. L., *Nocardia asteroides* meningitis without brain abscess in a nonimmunodepressed adult, *Presse Med.*, 23, 346, 1994.

209. Kulkarni, S. A. and Kulkarni, A. G., Disseminated nocardiosis, *J. Assoc. Physicians India*, 39, 779, 1991.

210. Raghavan, R., Date, A., and Bhaktaviziam, A., Fungal and nocardial infections of the kidney, *Histopathology*, 11, 9, 1987.

211. Roman, H. O., Vilar, J. H., Corrales, J. L., and Lanari Zubiaur, F. J., Liver abscess caused by *Nocardia*: report of a case, *Rev. Esp. Enferm. Apar. Dig.*, 80, 282, 1991.

212. Almekinders, L. C. and Lechiewicz, P. F., *Nocardia* osteomyelitis: case report and review of the literature, *Orthopedics*, 12, 1583, 1989.

213. Awad, I., Bay, J. W., and Petersen, J. M., Nocardial osteomyelitis of the spine with epidural spinal cord compression — a case report, *Neurosurgery*, 15, 254, 1984.

214. De Luca, J., Walsh, B., Robbins, W., and Visconti, E. B., *Nocardia asteroides* osteomyelitis, *Postgrad. Med. J.*, 62, 673, 1986.

215. Guiral, J., Refolio, C., Carrero, P., and Carbajosa, S., Sacral osteomyelitis due to *Nocardia asteroides*: a case report, *Acta Orthop. Scand.*, 62, 389, 1991.

216. Laurin, J. M., Resnik, C. S., Wheeler, D., and Needleman, B. W., Vertebral osteomyelitis caused by *Nocardia asteroides*: report and review of the literature, *J. Rheumatol.*, 18, 455, 1991.

217. Masters, D. L., and Lentino, J. R., Cervical osteomyelitis related to *Nocardia asteroides*, *J. Infect. Dis.*, 149, 824, 1984.

218. Petersen, J. M., Awad, I., Ahmad, M., Bay, J. W., and McHenry, M. C., *Nocardia* osteomyelitis and epidural abscess in the nonimmunocompromised host, *Cleve. Clin. Q.*, 50, 453, 1983.

219. Law, B. J. and Marks, M. I., Pediatric nocardiosis, *Pediatrics*, 70, 560, 1982.

220. Schwartz, J. G. and Tio, F. O., Nocardial osteomyelitis: a case report and review of the literature, *Diagn. Microbiol. Infect. Dis.*, 8, 37, 1987.

221. Price, N. C., Frith, P. A., and Awdry, P. N., Intraocular nocardiosis: a further case and review, *Int. Ophthalmol.*, 13, 177, 1989.

222. Curley, R. K., Hayward, T., and Holden, C. A., Cutaneous abscesses due to systemic nocardiosis — a case report, *Clin. Exp. Dermatol.*, 15, 459, 1990.

223. Kalb, R. E., Kaplan, M. H., and Grossman, M. E., Cutaneous nocardiosis: case reports and review, *J. Am. Acad. Dermatol.*, 13, 125, 1985.

224. Nishimoto, K. and Ohno, M., Subcutaneous abscesses caused by *Nocardia brasiliensis* complicated by malignant lymphoma: a survey of cutaneous nocardiosis reported in Japan, *Int. J. Dermatol.*, 24, 437, 1985.

225. Yu, C. T., Tsai, Y. H., Leu, H. S., and Shieh, W. B., Pulmonary nocardiosis with skin and subcutaneous dissemination: an imitator mimicking tuberculosis, *Chang Keng I Hsueh*, 15, 54, 1992.

226. Cons, F., Trevino, A., and Lavalle, C., Septic arthritis due to *Nocardia brasiliensis*, *J. Rheumatol.*, 12, 1019, 1985.

227. Di Vittorio, G., Carpenter, J. T., Jr., and Bennett, J. C., Arthritis in systemic nocardiosis, *South. Med. J.*, 75, 507, 1982.

228. Koll, B. S., Brown, A. E., Kiehn, T. E., and Armstrong, D., Disseminated *Nocardia brasiliensis* infection with septic arthritis, *Clin. Infect. Dis.*, 15, 469, 1992.

229. Barnicoat, M. J., Wierzbicki, A. S., and Norman, P. M., Cerebral nocardiosis in immunosuppressed patients: five cases, *Q. J. Med.*, 72, 689, 1989.

230. Houang, E. T., Lovett, I. S., Thompson, F. D., Harrison, A. R., Joekes, A. M., and Goodfellow, M., *Nocardia asteroides* infection — a transmissible disease, *J. Hosp. Infect.*, 1, 31, 1980.

231. Macher, A. M., De Vinatea, M. L., and Daly, M. J., AIDS case for diagnosis, *Milit. Med.*, 151, M73, 1986.

232. Holtz, H. A., Lavery, D. P., and Kapila, R., *Actinomycetales* infection in the acquired immunodeficiency syndrome, *Ann. Intern. Med.*, 102, 203, 1992.

233. Bonacini, M. and Walden, J. M., *Nocardia brasiliensis* peritonitis in a patient with AIDS, *Am. J. Gastroenterol.*, 85, 1432, 1990.

234. Adair, J. C., Beck, A. C., Apfelbaum, R. I., and Baringer, J. R., Nocardial cerebral abscess in the acquired immunodeficiency syndrome, *Arch. Neurol.*, 44, 548, 1987.

235. Telzak, E. E., Hii, J., Polsky, B., Kiehn, T. E., and Armstrong, D., Nocardia infection in the acquired immunodeficiency syndrome, *Diagn. Microbiol. Infect. Dis.*, 12, 517, 1989.

236. Struillou, L. and Raffi, F., Cerebro-meningeal infections in patients with human immunodeficiency virus infections, *Rev. Prat.*, 44, 2187, 1994.
237. Lynn, W., Whyte, M., and Weber, J., Nocardia, mycobacteria and AIDS, *AIDS*, 3, 766, 1989.
238. Miralles, G. D., Disseminated *Nocardia farcinica* infection in an AIDS patient, *Eur. J. Clin. Microbiol. Infect. Dis.*, 13, 497, 1994.
239. Long, P. F., A retrospective study of *Nocardia* infections associated with the acquired immune deficiency syndrome (AIDS), *Infection*, 22, 362, 1994.
240. Cherubin, C. E., Nocardiosis in patients with AIDS, *Clin. Infect. Dis.*, 15, 370, 1992.
241. Parmentier, L., Salmon-Ceron, D., and Boiron, P., Pneumonopathy and kidney abscess due to *Nocardia farcinica* in an HIV-infected patient, *AIDS*, 6, 891, 1992.
242. Niedt, G. W., and Schinella, R. A., Acquired immunodeficiency syndrome: clinicopathologic study of 56 autopsies, *Arch. Pathol. Lab. Med.*, 109, 727, 1985.
243. Schinella, R., Chaitin, B., and Gross, E., The AIDS autopsy: comparison of intravenous drug abusers with non-intravenous drug abusers, in *Progress in AIDS Pathology*, Rotterdam, H. and Sommers, S. C., Eds., Field and Wood, New York, 1989, 219.
244. Sieratzki, H. J., *Nocardia brasiliensis* infection in patients with AIDS, *Clin. Infect. Dis.*, 14, 977, 1992.
245. Sieratzki, H. J., Nocardiosis in patients with AIDS, *Clin. Infect. Dis.*, 15, 370, 1992.
246. Hathway, B. M. and Mason, K. N., Nocardiosis: study of fourteen cases, *Am. J. Med.*, 32, 903, 1962.
247. Lerner, P. I., Pneumonia due to *Actinomycetes*, *Arachnia*, and *Nocardia*, in *Respiratory Infections: Diagnosis and Management*, Pennington, J. E., Ed., Raven Press, New York, 1983, 387.
248. Weed, L. A., Andersen, H. A., Good, A., and Baggenstoss, A. H., Nocardiosis: clinical, bacteriologic and pathological aspects, *N. Engl. J. Med.*, 253, 1137, 1955.
249. Aisu, T. O., Eriki, P. P., Morrisey, A. B., Ellner, J. J., and Daniel, T. M., Nocardiosis mimicking pulmonary tuberculosis in Ugandan AIDS patients, *Chest*, 100, 888, 1991.
250. Georg, L. K., Ajello, L., McDurmont, C., and Hosty, T. S., The identification of *Nocardia asteroides* and *Nocardia brasiliensis*, *Am. Rev. Respir. Dis.*, 84, 337, 1961.
251. Simpson, G. L., Raffin, T. A., and Remington, J. S., Association of prior nocardiosis and subsequent occurrence of nontuberculous mycobacteriosis in a defined, immunosuppressed population, *J. Infect. Dis.*, 146, 211, 1982.
252. Ruiz, L. M., Montejo, M., Benito, J. R., Aguirrebengoa, K. et al., Simultaneous pulmonary infection by *Nocardia asteroides* and *Pneumocystis carinii* in a renal transplant patient, *Nephrol. Dial. Transplant.*, 11, 711, 1996.
253. Perschak, H., Gubler, J., Speich, R., and Russi, E., Pulmonary nocardiosis concurrent with *Pneumocystis carinii* pneumonia in two patients undergoing immunosuppressive therapy, *J. Infect.*, 23, 183, 1991.
254. Filice, G. A. and Simpson, G. L., Management of *Nocardia* infections, in *Current Clinical Topics in Infectious Diseases*, Vol. 5, Remington, J. S. and Swartz, M. N., Eds., McGraw-Hill, New York, 1984, 49.
255. King, C. T., Chapman, S. W., and Butkus, D. E., Recurrent nocardiosis in renal transplant recipient, *South. Med. J.*, 86, 225, 1993.
256. Byrne, E., Brophy, B. P., and Perrett, L. V., Nocardia cerebral abscess: new concepts in diagnosis, management, and prognosis, *J. Neurol. Neurosurg. Psychiatry*, 42, 1038, 1979.
257. Lopez, E., Ferrero, M., Lumbreras, C., Gimeno, C., Gonzalez-Pinto, I., and Palengue, E., A case of transient nocardiosis and literature review, *Eur. J. Clin. Microbiol. Infect. Dis.*, 13, 310, 1994.
258. Hall, W. A., Martinez, A. J., Dummer, J. S., and Linsford, L. D., Nocardial abscess: diagnostic and therapeutic use of stereotactic aspiration, *Surg. Neurol.*, 28, 114, 1987.
259. Wheeler, J. S., Culkin, D. J., O'Connell, J., and Winters, G., Nocardia epididymo-orchitis in an immunosuppressed patient, *J. Urol.*, 136, 1314, 1986.
260. Geelhoed, G. W. and Myers, G. H., Nocardiosis of the testis, *J. Urol.*, 111, 791, 1974.
261. Strong, D. W. and Hodges, C. V., Disseminated nocardiosis presenting as testicular abscess, *Urology*, 1, 57, 1976.
262. Hadley, M. N., Spetzler, R. F., Martin, N. A., and Johnson, P. C., Middle cerebral artery aneurysm due to *Nocardia asteroides*: case report of aneurysm excision and extracranial-intracranial bypass, *Neurosurgery*, 22, 923, 1988.

263. Meier, B., Metzger, U., Muller, F., Siegenthaler, W., and Luthy, R., Successful treatment of a pancreatic *Nocardia asteroides* abscess with amikacin and surgical drainage, *Antimicrob. Agents Chemother.*, 29, 150, 1986.

264. Boiron, P., Provost, F., Chevrier, G., and Dupont, B., Review of nocardial infections in France 1987 to 1990, *Eur. J. Clin. Microbiol. Infect. Dis.*, 11, 709, 1992.

265. Yazawa, K., Mikami, Y., and Uno, J., *In vitro* susceptibility of *Nocardia* spp. to a new fluoroquinolone, tosufloxacin (T-3262), *Antimicrob. Agents Chemother.*, 33, 2140, 1989.

266. Roberts, S. A., Bartley, J., Braatvedt, G., and Ellis-Pegler, R. B., *Nocardia asteroides* as a cause of sphenoidal sinusitis: case report, *Clin. Infect. Dis.*, 21, 1041, 1995.

267. Geisler, P. J. and Andersen, B. R., Results of therapy in systemic nocardiosis, *Am. J. Med. Sci.*, 278, 188, 1979.

268. Chosidow, O., Wolkenstein, P., Bagot, M., Girard-Pipau, F., Brun-Buisson, C., Fraitag, S., Roujeau, J. C., and Revuz, J., *Nocardia asteroides* septicemia in a pemphigus patient: successful treatment with trimethoprim-sulfamethoxazole and amikacin association, *Dermatologica*, 181, 311, 1990.

269. Smego, R. A., Jr., Mueller, M. B., and Gallis, H. A., Trimethoprim-sulfamethoxazole therapy for *Nocardia* infections, *Arch. Intern. Med.*, 143, 711, 1983.

270. Bach, M. C., Sabath, L. D., and Finland, M., Susceptibility of *Nocardia asteroides* to 45 antimicrobial agents *in vitro*, *Antimicrob. Agents Chemother.*, 3, 1, 1973.

271. Petersen, E. A., Nash, M. L., Mammana, R. B., and Copeland, J. G., Minocycline treatment of pulmonary nocardiosis, *JAMA*, 250, 930, 1983.

272. Balikian, J. P., Herman, P. G., and Kopit, S., Pulmonary nocardiosis, *Radiology*, 126, 569, 1978.

273. Rice, S. A., Barton, L. L., and Gartner, G. S., Fever and skin lesions in a five-year-old boy, *Pediatr. Infect. Dis. J.*, 12, 887, 1993.

274. Mamelak, A. N., Obana, W. G., Flaherty, J. F., and Rosenblum, M. L., Nocardial brain abscess: treatment strategies and factors influencing outcome, *Neurosurgery*, 35, 622, 1994.

275. Casty, F. E. and Wencel, M., Endobronchial nocardiosis, *Eur. Respir. J.*, 7, 1903, 1994.

276. Adams, H. G., Beeler, B. A., Wann, L. S., Chin, C. K., and Brooks, G. F., Synergistic action of trimethoprim and sulfamethoxazole for *Nocardia asteroides*: efficacious therapy in five patients, *Am. J. Med.*, 287, 8, 1984.

277. Welsh, O., Salinas, M. C., and Rodriguez, M. A., Treatment of eumycetoma and actinomycetoma, *Curr. Top. Med. Mycol.*, 6, 47, 1995.

278. Lyos, A. T., Tuchler, R. E., Malpica, A., and Spira, M., Primary soft-tissue nocardiosis, *Ann. Plast. Surg.*, 34, 212, 1995.

279. Huang, C. C., Lee, C. C., and Chu, N. S., A case of cerebral nocardiosis successfully treated with trimethoprim-sulfamethoxazole, *J. Formos. Med. Assoc.*, 90, 407, 1991.

280. Donnenfeld, E. D., Cohen, E. J., Barza, M., and Baum, J., Treatment of *Nocardia* keratitis with topical trimethoprim-sulfamethoxazole, *Am. J. Ophthalmol.*, 99, 601, 1985.

281. Pourmand, G., Jazaeri, S. A., Mehrsai, A., Kalhori, S., and Afshar, K., Nocardiosis: report of four cases in renal transplant recipients, *Transplant. Proc.*, 27, 2731, 1995.

282. Maderazo, E. G. and Quintiliani, R., Treatment of nocardial infection with trimethoprim and sulfamethoxazole, *Am. J. Med.*, 57, 671, 1974.

283. Wallace, R. J., Jr., Septimus, E. J., Williams, T. W., Conklin, R. H., Satterwhite, T. K., Bushby, M. B., and Hollowell, D. C., Use of trimethoprim-sulfamethoxazole for treatment of infections due to nocardia, *Rev. Infect. Dis.*, 4, 315, 1982.

284. Stevens, D. A., Clinical and clinical laboratory aspects of nocardial infection, *J. Hyg.*, 91, 377, 1983.

285. Geiseler, P. J. and Andersen, B. R., Results of therapy in systemic nocardiosis, *Am. J. Med. Sci.*, 278, 188, 1979.

286. de la Hoz Caballer, B., Fernandez-Rivas, M., Fraj Lazaro, J., Quirce Gancedo, S., Davilla Ruiz, I., Puyana Ruiz, J., Cuesta Herranz, J., Alvarez Cuesta, E., Cuevas, M., and Perez Elias, M. J., Management of sulfadiazine allergy in patients with acquired immunodeficiency syndrome, *J. Allergy Clin. Immunol.*, 88, 137, 1991.

287. Portoles, J., Torralbo, A., Prats, D., Blanco, J., and Barrientos, A., Acute renal failure and sulphadiazine crystalluria in kidney transplant, *Nephrol. Dial. Transplant.*, 9, 180, 1994.

288. Burman, L. G., Significance of the sulfonamide component for the clinical efficacy of trimethoprim-sulfonamide combinations, *Scand. J. Infect. Dis.*, 18, 89, 1986.

289. Burman, L. G., The antimicrobial activities of trimethoprim and sulfonamides, *Scand. J. Infect. Dis.*, 18, 3, 1986.

290. Cockerill, F. R. III and Edson, R. S., Trimethoprim-sulfamethoxazole, *Mayo Clin. Proc.*, 62, 921, 1987.

291. Spehn, J., Grosser, S., Jessel, A., von Essen, J., and Klose, G., High- dosage cotrimoxazole therapy of disseminated *Nocardia brasiliensis* infection, *Dtsch. Med. Wochenschr.*, 111, 215, 1986.

292. Antonow, D. R., Acute pancreatitis associated with trimethoprim-sulfamethoxazole, *Ann. Intern. Med.*, 104, 363, 1986.

293. Nyberg, G., Gabel, H., Althoff, P., Bjork, S., Herlitz, H., and Brynger, H., Adverse effect of trimethoprim on kidney function in renal transplant patients, *Lancet*, 1, 394, 1984.

294. Ringdén, O., Myrenfors, P., Klintmalm, G., Tyden, G., and Ost, L., Nephrotoxicity by cotrimazole and cyclosporine in transplanted patients, *Lancet*, 1, 1016, 1984.

295. Sands, M. and Brown, R. B., Interactions of cyclosporine with antimicrobial agents, *Rev. Infect. Dis.*, 11, 691, 1989.

296. Thompson, J. F., Chalmers, D. H. K., Hunnisett, A. G. W., Wood, R. F. M., and Morris, P. J., Nephrotoxicity of trimethoprim and cotrimoxazole in renal allograft recipients treated with cyclosporine, *Transplantation*, 36, 204, 1983.

297. Bennett, J. E. and Jennings, A. E., Factors influencing susceptibility of *Nocardia* species to trimethoprim sulfamethoxazole, *Antimicrob. Agents Chemother.*, 13, 624, 1978.

298. Gordin, F. M., Simon, G. L., Wofsy, C. B., and Mills, J., Adverse reactions to trimethoprim-sulfamethoxazole in patients with the acquired immunodeficiency syndrome, *Ann. Intern. Med.*, 100, 495, 1984.

299. Jansen, C., Frenay, H. M., Vandertop, W. P., and Visser, M. R., Intracerebral *Nocardia asteroides* abscess treated by neurosurgical aspiration and combined therapy with sulfadiazine and cefotaxime, *Clin. Neurol. Neurosurg.*, 93, 253, 1991.

300. Fraj Lazaro, J., de la Hoz Caballer, B., Davilla Gonzalez, I., Puyana Ruiz, J., and Alvarez Cuesta, E., Desensitization to sulfadiazine in patients with AIDS and opportunistic infection, *Rev. Clin. Esp.*, 185, 167, 1989.

301. Kim, J., Minamoto, G. Y., Hoy, C. D., and Grieco, M. H., Presumptive cerebral *Nocardia asteroides* infection in AIDS: treatment with ceftriaxone and minocycline, *Am. J. Med.*, 90, 656, 1991.

302. Wren, M. V., Savage, A. M., and Alford, R. H., Apparent cure of intracranial *Nocardia asteroides* infection by minocycline, *Arch. Intern. Med.*, 139, 249, 1979.

303. Bach, M. C., Monaco, A. P., and Finland, M., Pulmonary nocardiosis: therapy with minocycline and with erythromycin plus ampicillin, *JAMA*, 224, 1378, 1973.

304. Yogev, R., Greenslade, T., Firlit, C. F., and Lewy, P., Successful treatment of *Nocardia asteroides* infection with amikacin, *J. Paediatr.*, 96, 771, 1980.

305. Stella, P. R., Vermeulen, E. J., Roggeveen, Ch., Overbosch, E. H., and van Dorp, W. T., Systemic infection with *Nocardia asteroides* cured with amoxicillin/clavulanic acid, erythromycin and ultrasound-guided transcutaneous aspiration, *Neth. J. Med.*, 44, 178, 1994.

306. Velasco, N., Farrington, K., Greenwood, R., and Rahman, A. F., Atypical presentation of systemic nocardiosis and successful treatment with meropenem, *Nephrol. Dial. Transplant.*, 11, 709, 1996.

307. Garcia del Palacio, J. I. and Martin Perez, I., Response of pulmonary nocardiosis to ceftriaxone in a patient with AIDS, *Chest*, 103, 1925, 1993.

308. Lo, W. and Rolston, K. V., Use of imipenem in the treatment of pulmonary nocardiosis, *Chest*, 103, 951, 1993.

309. Gombert, M. E. and Aulicino, T. M., Synergism of imipenem and amikacin in combination with other antibiotics against *Nocardia asteroides*, *Antimicrob. Agents Chemother.*, 24, 810, 1983.

310. Gombert, M. E., Aulicino, T. M., duBouchet, L., Silverman, G. E., and Sheinbaum, W. M., Therapy of experimental cerebral nocardiosis with imipenem, amikacin, trimethoprim-sulfamethoxazole, and minocycline, *Antimicrob. Agents Chemother.*, 30, 270, 1986.

311. Garlando, F., Bodmer, T., Lee, C., Zimmerli, W., and Pirovino, M., Successful treatment of disseminated nocardiosis complicated by cerebral abscess with ceftriaxone and amikacin: case report, *Clin. Infect. Dis.*, 15, 1039, 1992.

312. Bartels, R. H., van der Spek, J. A., and Oosten, H. R., Acute pancreatitis due to sulfamethoxazole-trimethoprim, *South. Med. J.*, 85, 1006, 1992.

313. Thaler, F., Gotainer, B., Teodori, G., Dubois, C., and Loirat, P., Mediastinitis due to *Nocardia asteroides* after cardiac transplantation, *Intensive Care Med.*, 18, 127, 1992.

314. Krone, A., Schaal, K. P., Brawanski, A., and Schuknecht, B., Nocardial cerebral abscess cured with imipenem/amikacin and enucleation, *Neurosurg. Rev.*, 12, 333, 1989.

315. Bath, P. M., Pettingale, K. W., and Wade, J., Treatment of multiple subcutaneous *Nocardia asteroides* abscesses with ciprofloxacin and doxycycline, *Postgrad. Med. J.*, 65, 190, 1989.

316. Ruppert, S., Reinold, H. M., Jipp, P., Schroter, G., Egner, E., and Schaal, K. P., Successful antibiotic treatment of a pulmonary infection with *Nocardia asteroides* (biovariety A3), *Dtsch. Med. Wochenschr.*, 113, 1801, 1988.

317. Stasiecki, P., Diehl, V., Vlaho, M., Krueger, G. R., and Schaal, K. P., New effective therapy of systemic infection with *Nocardia asteroides*, *Dtsch. Med. Wochenschr.*, 110, 1733, 1985.

318. Buggy, B. P., *Nocardia asteroides* meningitis without brain abscess, *Rev. Infect. Dis.*, 9, 228, 1987.

319. Ertl, G., Schaal, K. P., and Kochsiek, K., Nocardial endocarditis of an aortic valve prosthesis, *Br. Heart J.*, 57, 384, 1987.

320. Bauwens, M., Hauet, T., Crevel, J., Goujon, J., Patte, D., and Touchard, G., Nocardiosis in recipients of renal transplants: two case reports, *Transplant. Proc.*, 27, 2430, 1995.

321. Shohaib, S., Nocardial psoas and perinephric abscess in a renal transplant treated by surgery and antibiotics, *Nephrol. Dial. Transplant.*, 9, 1209, 1994.

322. Varma, P. P., Church, S., Gupta, K. L., Sakhuja, V., and Chugh, K. S., Invasive pulmonary aspergillosis and nocardiosis in an immunocompromised host, *J. Assoc. Physicians India*, 41, 237, 1993.

323. Holt, R. I., Kwan, J. T., Sefton, A. M., and Cunningham, J., Successful treatment of concomitant pulmonary nocardiosis and aspergillosis in an immunocompromised renal patient, *Eur. J. Clin. Microbiol. Infect. Dis.*, 12, 110, 1993.

324. Berkey, P., Moore, D., and Rolston, K., *In vitro* susceptibilities of *Nocardia* species to newer antimicrobial agents, *Antimicrob. Agents Chemother.*, 32, 1078, 1988.

325. Gombert, M. E., Susceptibility of *Nocardia asteroides* to various antibiotics, including newer beta-lactams, trimethoprim-sulfamethoxazole, amikacin, and *N*-formimidoyl thienamycin, *Antimicrob. Agents Chemother.*, 21, 1011, 1982.

326. Wallace, R. J., Jr., Steele, L. C., Sumter, G., and Smith, J. M., Antimicrobial susceptibility patterns of *Nocardia asteroides*, *Antimicrob. Agents Chemother.*, 32, 1776, 1988.

327. Brown, A., Geyer, S., Arbitman, M., and Pestic, B., Pulmonary nocardiosis presenting as a bronchogenic tumor, *South. Med. J.*, 73, 660, 1980.

328. Henkle, J. Q. and Nair, S. V., Endobronchial pulmonary nocardiosis, *JAMA*, 256, 1331, 1986.

329. Newmark, E., Polack, F. M., and Ellison, A. C., Report of a case of *Nocardia asteroides* keratitis, *Am. J. Ophthalmol.*, 72, 813, 1971.

330. Srinivasan, M. and Sharma, S., *Nocardia asteroides* as a cause of corneal ulcer, *Arch. Ophthalmol.*, 105, 464, 1987.

331. Parsons, M. R., Holland, E. J., and Agapitos, P. J., *Nocardia asteroides* keratitis associated with extended-wear soft contact lenses, *Can. J. Ophthalmol.*, 24, 120, 1989.

332. Perry, H. D., Nauheim, J. S., and Donnenfeld, S. D., *Nocardia asteroides* keratitis presenting as a persistent epithelial defect, *Cornea*, 8, 41, 1898.

333. Benedict, W. L. and Iverson, H. A., Chronic keratoconjunctivitis associated with *Nocardia*, *Arch. Ophthalmol.*, 32, 84, 1944.

334. Schardt, W. M., Unsworth, A. C., and Hayes, C. V., Corneal ulcer due to *Nocardia asteroides*, *Am. J. Ophthalmol.*, 42, 303, 1956.

335. Davidson, S. and Foerster, H. C., Intraocular nocardia abscess, endogenous, *Trans. Am. Acad. Ophthalmol. Otolaryngol.*, 71, 847, 1967.

336. Gregor, R. J., Chong, C. A., Augsburger, J. J., Eagle, R. C., Jr., Carlson, K. M., Jessup, M., Wong, S., and Naids, R., Endogenous *Nocardia asteroides* subretinal abscess diagnosed by transvitreal fine-needle aspiration biopsy, *Retina*, 9, 118, 1989.

337. Peniket, E. J. K. and Rees, D. L., *Nocardia asteroides* infection, *Am. J. Ophthalmol.*, 53, 1006, 1962.

338. Henderson, J. W., Wellman, W. E., and Weed, L. A., Nocardiosis of the eye: report of a case, *Mayo Clin. Proc.*, 35, 614, 1960.

339. Zimmerman, P. L., Mamalis, N., Alder, J. B., Teske, M. P., Tamura, M., and Jones, G. R., Chronic *Nocardia asteroides* endophthalmitis after extracapsular cataract extraction, *Arch. Ophthalmol.*, 111, 837, 1993.

340. Zimmerman, P. L., Mamalis, N., and Teske, M. P., Nocardial endophthalmitis, *Arch. Ophthalmol.*, 112, 871, 1994.

341. Srinivasan, M. and Sundar, K., Nocardial endophthalmitis, *Arch. Ophthalmol.*, 112, 871, 1994.

342. Srinivasan, M., Channa, P., Gopal Raju, C. V., and George, C., Nocardial endophthalmitis following IOL surgery, *J. Tamil Nadu Ophthalmol. Assoc.*, 30, 29, 1992.

343. Bullock, J. D., Endogenous ocular nocardiosis: a clinical and experimental study, *Trans. Am. Ophthalmol. Soc.*, 81, 451, 1983.

344. Meyer, S. L., Font, R. L., and Shaver, R. P., Intraocular nocardiosis, *Arch. Ophthalmol.*, 83, 536, 1970.

345. Burpee, J. C. and Starke, W. R., Bilateral metastatic intraocular nocardiosis, *Arch. Ophthalmol.*, 86, 666, 1971.

346. Panijayanond, P., Olsson, C. A., Spivack, M. L., Schmitt, G. W., Idelson, B. A., Sachs, B. J., and Nahseth, D. C., Intraocular nocardiosis in a renal transplant patient, *Arch. Surg.*, 104, 845, 1972.

347. Jampol, L. M., Strauch, B. S., and Albert, D. M., Intraocular nocardiosis, *Am. J. Ophthalmol.*, 76, 568, 1973.

348. Sher, N. A., Hill, C. W., and Elfrig, D. E., Bilateral intraocular *Nocardia asteroides* infection, *Arch. Ophthalmol.*, 95, 1415, 1977.

349. Rogers, S. J. and Johnson, B. L., Endogenous *Nocardia* endophthalmitis: report of a case in a patient treated for lymphocytic lymphoma, *Ann. Ophthalmol.*, 9, 1123, 1977.

350. Lissner, G. S., O'Grady, R., and Choromokos, E., Endogenous intraocular *Nocardia asteroides* in Hodgkin's disease, *Am. J. Ophthalmol.*, 86, 388, 1978.

351. Mamalis, N., Daily, M. J., and Ross, D., Presumed intraocular nocardiosis in a cardiac-transplant patient, *Ann. Ophthalmol.*, 20, 271, 1988.

352. Ferry, A. P., Font, R. L., Weinberg, R. S., Boniuk, M., and Schaffer, C. L., *Nocardia* endophthalmitis: report of two cases studied histopathologically, *Br. J. Ophthalmol.*, 72, 55, 1988.

353. Price, N. C., Frith, P. A., and Awdry, P. N., Intraocular nocardiosis: a further case and review, *Int. Ophthalmol.*, 13, 177, 1989.

354. Ishibashi, Y., Watanabe, R., Hommura, S., Koyama, A., Ishikawa, T., and Mikami, Y., Endogenous *Nocardia asteroides* endophthalmitis in a patient with systemic lupus erythematosus, *Br. J. Ophthalmol.*, 74, 433, 1990.

355. Atkinson, P. L., Jackson, H., Philpot-Howard, J., Patel, B. C., and Aclimandos, W., Exogenous *Nocardia asteroides* endophthalmitis following cataract surgery, *J. Infect.*, 26, 305, 1993.

356. Chiemchaisri, Y. W., Imwidthaya, S., and Parichatikanond, P., Exogenous intraocular nocardiosis, *J. Med. Assoc. Thailand*, 68, 29, 1985.

357. Batchon, B. A., Brosius, O. C., and Snyder, J. C., A case report of *Nocardia asteroides* of the eye, *Mycologia*, 63, 459, 1971.

358. Lass, J. H., Thoft, R. A., Bellows, A. R., and Slansky, H. H., Exogenous *Nocardia asteroides* endophthalmitis associated with malignant glaucoma, *Ann. Ophthalmol.*, 13, 317, 1981.

359. Chen, C. J., *Nocardia asteroides* endophthalmitis, *Ophthalm. Surg.*, 14, 502, 1983.

360. Denis, F., Adenis, J. P., and Mounier, M., Intraocular passage of imipenem in man, *Pathol. Biol. (Paris)*, 37, 415, 1989.

361. Federal Register, Antibiotic susceptibility disks, *Fed. Regist.*, 37, 20525, 1072.

362. National Committee for Clinical Laboratory Standards, *Methods For Dilution Antimicrobial Susceptibility Tests For Bacteria That Grow Aerobically*, National Committee for Clinical Laboratory Standards, Villanova, Pennsylvania, 1985.

363. Boiron, P. and Provost, F., In-vitro susceptibility testing of *Nocardia* spp. and its taxonomic implication, *J. Antimicrob. Chemother.*, 22, 623, 1988.

364. Carroll, G. F., Brown, J. M., and Haley, L. D., A method for determining in-vitro susceptibilities of some Nocardiae and Actinomadurae, *Am. J. Clin. Pathol.*, 68, 279, 1977.

365. Wallace, R. J., Jr., Septimus, E. J., Musher, D. M., and Martin, M. M., Disk diffusion susceptibility testing of *Nocardia* species, *J. Infect. Dis.*, 35, 568, 1977.

366. Wallace, R. J., Jr. and Steele, L. C., Susceptibility testing of *Nocardia* species for the clinical laboratory, *Diagn. Microbiol. Infect. Dis.*, 9, 155, 1988.

367. McNeil, M. M., Brown, J. M., Jarvis, W. R., and Ajello, L., Comparison of species distribution and antimicrobial susceptibility of aerobic actinomycetes from clinical specimens, *Rev. Infect. Dis.*, 12, 778, 1990.
368. Dewsnup, S. H. and Wright, D. B., *In vitro* susceptibility of *Nocardia asteroides* to 25 antimicrobial agents, *Antimicrob. Agents Chemother.*, 25, 165, 1984.
369. Khardori, N., Shawar, R., Gupta, R., Rosenbaum, B., and Rolston, K., *In vitro* antimicrobial susceptibilities of *Nocardia* species, *Antimicrob. Agents Chemother.*, 37, 882, 1993.
370. Wallace, R. J., Jr., Wiss, K., Curvey, R., Vance, P. H., and Steadham, J., Differences among *Nocardia* spp. in susceptibility to aminoglycosides and β-lactam antibiotics and their potential use in taxonomy, *Antimicrob. Agents Chemother.*, 23, 19, 1983.
371. Joshi, N. and Hamory, B. H., Drug-resistant *Nocardia asteroides* infection in a patient with acquired immunodeficiency syndrome, *South. Med. J.*, 84, 1155, 1991.
372. Oda, Y., Kamijyo, Y., and Kang, Y., *Nocardia* brain abscess and ventriculitis — resistance of *Nocardia* to sulfonamides and susceptibilities to beta-lactams, *No Shinkei Geka*, 14(3 Suppl.), 340, 1986.
373. Steingrube, V. A., Wallace, R. J., Jr., Brown, B. A., Pang, Y., Zeluff, B., Steele, L. C., and Zhang, Y., Acquired resistance of *Nocardia brasiliensis* to clavulanic acid related to change in beta-lactamase following therapy with amoxicillin-clavulanic acid, *Antimicrob. Agents Chemother.*, 35, 524, 1991.
374. Leibovici, J., Hoenig, S., Pinchassov, A., and Barot-Ciobaru, R., Antitumoral activity of an immuno-modulatory fraction of *Nocardia opaca*: mechanism of action, *Int. J. Immunopharmacol.*, 16, 475, 1994.
375. Azuma, I., Review: inducer of cytokines *in vivo*: over of field and romurtide experience, *Int. J. Immunopharmacol.*, 14, 487, 1992.
376. Gupta, R., Pancholi, V., Vinayak, V. K., and Khuller, G. K., Protective immunity to systemic nocardiosis in mice immunized with cell extract antigens of *Nocardia asteroides*, *Med. Microbiol. Immunol. (Berlin)*, 174, 157, 1985.
377. Ogiu, T., Furita, K., Matsuoka, C., Maekawa, A., and Azuma, I., Effect of *Nocardia rubra* cell wall skeleton and/or cyclophosphamide on leukogenesis induced by *N*-ethyl-*N*-nitrosourea in Donryu rats, *J. Cancer Res. Clin. Oncol.*, 109, 173, 1985.
378. Haraguchi, S., Kurakata, S., Matsuo, T., and Yoshida, T. O., Strain differences in the antitumor activity of an immunopotentiator, *Nocardia rubra* cell-wall skeleton, in B10 congenic and recombinant mice, *Jpn. J. Cancer Res.*, 76, 400, 1985.
379. Mine, Y., Yokota, Y., Nonoyama, S., and Kikuchi, H., Protective effect of *Nocardia rubra* cell wall skeleton on experimental infection in normal and immunosuppressed mice, *Arzneim.-Forsch.*, 36, 1489, 1986.
380. Ogura, T., Hara, H., Yokota, S., Hosoe, S., Kawase, I., Kishimoto, S., and Yamamura, Y., Effector mechanism in concomitant immunity potentiated by intratumoral injection of *Nocardia rubra* cell wall skeleton, *Cancer Res.*, 45, 6371, 1985.
381. Izumi, S., Ogawa, T., Miyauchi, M., Fujie, K., Okuhara, M., and Kohsaka, M., Antitumor effect of *Nocardia rubra* cell wall skeleton on syngeneically transplanted P388 tumors, *Cancer Res.*, 51, 4038, 1991.
382. Yasutomi, Y., Onuma, M., Davis, W. C., and Kawakami, Y., Properties of tumor infiltrated cells induced by N-CWS, *Nippon Juigaku Zasshi*, 52, 1205, 1990.
383. Hirai, C., Fujitsu, T., Oku, R., Satoh, H. et al., Host mediated anti-tumor effect of *Nocardia rubra* cell wall skeleton on syngeneic tumor in mice, *Nippon Yakurigaku Zasshi*, 89, 307, 1987.
384. Mine, Y., Yokota, Y., and Kikuchi, H., Inhibitory effect of *Nocardia rubra* cell wall skeleton on splenomegaly induced by Friend leukemia virus in mice, *Arzneim.-Forsch.*, 35, 1563, 1985.
385. Mizushima, Y., Iwata, M., Sato, M., Hirata, H., Takashima, A., and Yano, S., Differences in the immunostimulatory activity and antitumor therapeutic effect of OK-432 and N-CWS, *Gan To Kagaku Ryoho*, 13, 2404, 1986.
386. Kawase, I., Komuta, K., Shirasaka, T., Hara, H., Tanio, Y., Watanabe, M., Saito, S., Ikeda, T., Masuno, T., Kishimoto, Y. et al., Synergy of *Nocardia rubra* cell wall skeleton and interleukin 2 in the *in vivo* induction of murine lymphokine-activated killer cell activity, *Jpn. J. Cancer Res.*, 80, 1089, 1989.
387. Miyazaki, K., Yasumoto, K., Yano, T., Matsuzaki, G., Sugimachi, K., and Nomoto, K., Synergistic effect of *Nocardia rubra* cell wall skeleton and recombinant interleukin 2 for *in vivo* induction of lymphokine-activated killer cells, *Cancer Res.*, 51, 5261, 1991.

388. Ishioka, S., Hozawa, S., Hasegawa, K., Saito, T., Takaishi, M., and Yamakido, M., Clinical usefulness of continuous administration of *Nocardia rubra* cell wall skeleton (N-CWS) in diffuse panbronchiolitis (DPB), *Biotherapy*, 6, 19, 1993.

389. Yamakido, M., Ishioka, S., Hozawa, S., Matsuzaka, S., Yanegida, J., Shigenoba, T., Otake, M., and Nishimoto, Y., Effect of *Nocardia rubra* cell-wall skeleton on cancer prevention in humans, *Cancer Immunol. Immunother.*, 34, 389, 1992.

390. Kawa, K., Konishi, S., Tsujino, G., and Mabuchi, S., Effects of biological response modifiers on childhood ALL being in remission after chemotherapy, *Biomed. Pharmacother.*, 45, 113, 1991.

391. Hozawa, S., Ishioka, S., Yaniguda, J., Takaishi, M., Matsuzaka, S., Ohsaki, M., and Yamakido, M., Effects of periodic adminstration of *Nocardia rubra* cell-wall skeleton on immunoglobulin production and B-cell-stimulatory factor activity *in vitro* in workers at a poison gas factory, *Cancer Immunol. Immunother.*, 30, 190, 1989.

392. Tsubura, E., Intratumoral injections of *Nocardia rubra* cell-wall skeleton for hilar type lung cancer in humans and Lewis lung carcinoma in mice, *Jpn. J. Med.*, 24, 84, 1985.

393. Koyama, S., Ozaki, A., Iwasaki, Y., Sakita, T., Osuga, T., Watanabe, A., Suzuki, M., Kawasaki, T., Soma, T., Tabuchi, T., Nakayama, M., Koizumi, S., Yokoyama, K., Uchida, T., Orii, K., and Tanaka, T., Randomized controlled study of postoperative adjuvant immunotherapy with *Nocardia rubra* cell wall skeleton (N-CWS) and tegafur for gastric carcinoma, *Cancer Immunol. Immunother.*, 22, 148, 1986.

394. Yamakido, M., Yanagida, J., Ishioka, S., Matsuzaka, S., Hozawa, S., Takaishi, M., Inamizo, T., Akiyama, M., and Nishimoto, Y., Effect of *Nocardia rubra* cell wall skeleton on interleukin 2 production and lymphocyte proliferation in former poison gas factory workers, *Jpn. J. Cancer Res.*, 77, 406, 1986.

395. Ohno, R., Nakamura, H., Kodera, Y., Masaoka, T., and Yamada, K., Immunotherapy of acute myelogenous leukemia (AML) in adults with the *Nocardia rubra* cell wall skeleton, *Gan To Kagaku Ryoho*, 13, 1264, 1986.

396. Ohno, R., Nakamura, H., Kodera, Y., Ezaki, K., Yokomaku, S., Oguma, S., Kubota, Y., Shibata, H., Ogawa, N., Masaoka, T., and Yamada, K., Randomized controlled study of chemoimmunotherapy of acute myelogenous leukemia (AML) in adults with *Nocardia rubra* cell-wall skeleton and irradiated allogeneic AML mice, *Cancer*, 57, 1483, 1986.

397. Ogura, T. and Sakatani, M., Randomized controlled study on adjuvant immunotherapy for unresectable lung cancer with *Nocardia rubra* cell wall skeleton, *Nippon Kyobu Shikkan Gakkai Zasshi*, 23, 62, 1985.

398. Sakai, S., Itoh, M., Matsunaga, T., Yoshida, J., Sato, T., Miyahara, Y., Matsunaga, T., Hyoh, Y., Ohyama, K., Katsuta, K. et al., A randomized controlled study of adjuvant immunotherapy with N-CWS for head and neck malignancies, *Gan No Rinsho*, 31, 1353, 1985.

399. Ogura, T., Bases on timing of combined modality of chemotherapy and immunotherapy, *Gan To Kagaku Ryoho*, 17, 1414, 1990.

400. Mandel, L., Trebichavsky, I., Tlaskalova, H., Sinkora, J., Splichal, I., and Barot-Ciorbaru, R., Treatment of radiation disease by *Nocardia* fraction: possible effect of inflammatory cytokines, *Int. J. Immunopharmacol.*, 16, 481, 1994.

401. Leibovici, J., Hoenig, S., Pinchassov, A., and Barot-Ciobaru, R., Macrophage involvement in the antitumoral effect of *Nocardia*-delipidated cell mitogen (NDCM), *In Vivo*, 5, 365, 1991.

402. Barot-Ciorbaru, R., Cornil, I., Grand-Perret, T., and Poupon, M. F., Antimetastatic effect of immuno-modulators from *Nocardia opaca* in mice and rats: activation of peritoneal macrophages by these fractions, *Cancer Immunol. Immunother.*, 25, 111, 1987.

403. Tomecki, J. K., Cieslik, K., Kordowiak, A. M., and Barot, R., Immunomodulatory activities of *Nocardia opaca*, *Acta Microbiol. Pol.*, 42, 151, 1993.

404. Ehrenfeld, U. and Haas, R., Complete remission of metastatic breast cancer by non-specific immuno-stimulation with *Nocardia opaca* cell-wall extract after failure of conventional therapy, *Sb. Led.*, 95, 1, 1994.

405. Rasmussen, R. R., Nuss, M. E., Scherr, M. H., Mueller, S. L., McAlpine, J. B., and Mitscher, L. A., Benzanthrins A and B, a new class of quinone antibiotics, *J. Antibiot.*, 39, 1515, 1986.

406. Bush, J. A., Long, B. H., Catino, J. J., Bradner, W. T., and Tomita, K., Production and biological activity of rebeccamycin, a novel antitumor agent, *J. Antibiot.*, 40, 668, 1987.

407. Kumagai, K., Taya, K., Fukui, A., Fukasawa, M., Fukui, M., and Nabeshima, S., PC-766B, a new macrolide antibiotic produced by *Nocardia brasiliensis*. I. Taxonomy, fermentation and biological activity, *J. Antibiot.*, 46, 972, 1993.

408. Maeda, A., Yazawa, K., Mikami, Y., Ishibashi, M., and Kobayashi, J., The producer and biological activities of SO-75R1, a new mutactimycin group antibiotic, *J. Antibiot.*, 45, 1848, 1992 (corrected: *J. Antibiot.*, 46, C-1, 1993).

8.2 RHODOCOCCUS EQUI

8.2.1 INTRODUCTION

Rhodoccocus equi is a well-recognized bacterial pathogen in veterinary medicine.[1] It was first isolated in 1932 from foals and described initially as *Corynebacterium equi*.[2] In addition to foals, where *R. equi* is the etiologic agent of a serious and often fatal chronic granulomatous pneumonia, these bacteria have also been isolated from the cervical lymph nodes of swine as well as other mammals, often following immunosuppression by various causes.[3] Infections by *R. equi* in animals is often presented by granulomatous pneumonia and lung abscesses, lymphadenitis of the mesenteric, bronchial, or cervical lymph nodes, wound infections, and abscesses of different parts of the body.[1,4-6]

Inhalation or ingestion appears to be the major route of infection in foals, and the primary source of infection is believed to be the soil.[4]

In humans, *R. equi* infections are relatively rare, with the first case reported in 1963.[7] Before 1983, only 12 human infections were described.[8] However, with the spread of the AIDS epidemic, *R. equi* is increasingly emerging as an opportunistic pathogen in patients with underlying immuno-suppression, and in most cases who have history of contact with farm animals, contaminated soil, and manure.[9] The first description of *R. equi* infection in a patient with AIDS was reported in 1986.[10]

The taxonomic history of *R. equi* has been rather confusing. Currently, this pathogen is being described[11] as either *Rhodococcus equi* or *Corynebacterium equi*. However, with the generally resolved classification of the nocardioform actinomycetes,[12] the taxonomic status of *Rhodococcus* has been determined as a distinct genus belonging to the phylogenetic group of nocardioform actinomycetes. In general, the nocardioform actinomycetes represent Gram-positive, aerobic, catalase-positive bacteria, best characterized by biochemical criteria.[13-18] In addition to *Rhodococcus*, other genera classified as nocardioform actinomycetes include *Caseobacter*, *Corynebacterium*, *Mycobacterium*, *Nocardia*, and the "*aurantiaca*" taxon.[13,15] Subsequently, the "*aurantiaca*" taxon has been classified as the genus *Tsukamurella*.[19]

Morphologically, the genus *Rhodococcus* has been characterized by variations in its growth cycle typified by the presence of: diphosphatidylglycerol, phosphatidylethanolamine, and phosphatidylinositol mannosides; C_{34-64} mycolic acids containing up to four double bonds; dihydrogenated menaquinones with either eight or nine isoprene units as their major building blocks; large amounts of straight-chain, unsaturated fatty acids; and tuberculostearic acid.[1] The genus *Rhodococcus* is heterogeneous and has been divided into two groups, *Gordona* and *Rhodococcus*.[15] All three species originally classified in the genus *Gordona* (*R. bronchialis*, *R. rubropectinis*, and *R. terrae*) contain C_{48-66} mycolic acids and nine isoprene dihydrogenated menaquinones, and produce mycobactins. The species of the genus *Rhodococcus* contain C_{34-52} mycolic acids with up to two double bonds and eight isoprene dihydrogenated menaquinones, but no mycobactins.[15,20,21] Based on these structural differences, Stackebrandt et al.[22] have proposed that the three species comprising *Gordona* be reinstated as a separate genus, while keeping the genus *Rhodococcus* the second group. The redefined genus *Rhodococcus* comprises 12 recognized species that are widely distributed in nature, particularly in soil and herbivore manure.[14,22-24] In addition, some unidentified *Rhodococcus* species have been isolated from a variety of noncaseating granulomatous lesions in the lungs, lymph nodes, pleura, meninges, pericardium, and skin of human patients, often associated with immunosuppressive disease or drug treatments.[25]

Structurally, *R. equi* is a mucoid bacterium with a distinct lamellar polysaccharide capsule and pili,[26,27] which produces soluble factors (*equi* factors) that can interact with the phospholipase C of *Corynebacterium pseudotuberculosis* to generate complete hemolysis of mammalian crythrocytes.[28] It has been long recognized that variations in the outcome of experimental infections of foals were related to differences in bacterial virulence.[29-31]

Attempts have been made to determine the virulence of *R. equi*, and evidence has been presented about difference in the virulence in mouse models of equine lung isolates and soil isolates and its correlation with the ability of the pathogen to resist phagocytosis and intracellular killing by murine macrophages.[32,33] While both the bacterial capsule[34,35] and *equi* factors (cholesterol oxidase and phospholipase C exoenzymes)[28,36-40] were thought to be of potential value as virulence determinants, in general, they seem not to play any important role in the bacterial pathogenesis, and little is known about markers and/or factors associated with the virulence of *R. equi*. Takai et al.[41] have analyzed antigens of *R. equi* by immunoblotting with naturally infected foal sera. Their data have shown that major 15- to 17-kDa diffuse protein bands were present in all clinical isolates tested and in all isolates virulent for mice, but not in ATCC 6939, a type strain of *R. equi* that was avirulent for mice. Immunoblotting experiments by Mastroianni et al.[42] of sera from AIDS patients who had recovered from *R. equi* infection have shown only a well-defined narrow 15-kDa protein band; however, no seroactivity was found in AIDS patients with severe *R. equi* disease.

In recent studies, Tan et al.[43] have corroborated the findings of Takai et al.[41] They demonstrated by sodium dodecyl sulfate-polyacrylamide gel electrophoresis the presence of three antigenically related virulence-associated proteins: a diffuse 18- to 22-kDa, a 17.5-kDa, and a 15-kDa protein, all expressed from a single gene (designated as VapA). Opsonization of virulent *R. equi* with an IgG1 mouse monoclonal antibody (Mab103) to the VapA protein significantly enhanced uptake in the murine macrophage cell line IC-20. Intraperitoneal injection of mice with Mab103 increased the initial clearance from the liver of mice challenged intravenously with *R. equi*.

8.2.2 IMMUNOLOGIC RESPONSE TO *RHODOCOCCUS EQUI* INFECTION

Studies on the mechanism of acquired immunity to *R. equi* in a murine model have revealed that protective immunity may be induced by live but not killed bacteria.[44] Furthermore, adoptive transfer of resistance was obtained with spleen cells but not immune serum from mice immunized intravenously 30 d earlier with live bacteria. Finally, *in vivo* depletion with monoclonal antibodies showed that both CD4+ and CD8+ T cell subsets participated in the clearance of bacteria and that CD8+ T lymphocytes play a major role in the mechanism of acquired immunity to *R. equi*.[44]

In general, impairment of cell-mediated immunity is considered to be the major predisposing factor in humans to *R. equi* infections. In many renal and bone marrow transplant recipients, and in patients with lymphatic leukemias, treatment with imunosuppressive drugs (cyclosporin A, corticosteroids, antimetabolites) can be inhibitory to mitogen-induced production of interferon-γ by CD4+ lymphocytes.[1]

The ability of *R. equi* to remain in and to destroy the macrophages has been the basic feature of its pathogenicity. For example, foal alveolar macrophages cultured *in vitro* rapidly ingested opsonized *R. equi*; however, 75% of the ingested organisms remained viable after 4 h of incubation.[45] As evidenced by electron microscopic examination, *R. equi* within cultured foal and adult horse macrophages was able to evade killing by preventing phagosome-lysosome fusion, then multiplying in and eventually killing the phagocytes.[46,47] Foal neutrophils were most efficient in ingesting and killing cells when opsonized with a specific antibody.[46] To this end, a heat-stable surface component of *R. equi*, possibly a capsular polysaccharide, has been shown to inhibit the oxygen-dependent cytotoxic mechanisms of adult horse neutrophils against *Streptococcus aureus*.[48] Even though the inhibition against *S. aureus* did not appear to be sufficient to damage the overall bactericidal activity of equine neutrophils against opsonized *R. equi in vitro*,[49-51] this impairment may be significant *in vivo*, perhaps in the absence of a specific antibody.[1]

Mastroianni et al.[42] have studied in AIDS patients the antibody response to *R. equi* infection and its correlation with the clinical outcome of the disease. The results indicated that patients who recovered from *R. equi* pneumonia showed a pronounced antibody response to all major bacterial protein antigens; by comparison, the clinical course was more severe in patients who exhibited a negligible humoral response. The findings of Mastroianni et al.[42] may prove important by suggesting that a specific antibody production in AIDS patients infected with *R. equi* might be a needed function in the protection against and recovery from *R. equi* pneumonia, possibly by enhancing the uptake and killing the bacteria by alveolar macrophages and neutrophils.

8.2.3 EVOLUTION OF THERAPIES AND TREATMENT OF *RHODOCOCCUS EQUI* INFECTION

The increased number of human *R. equi* infections has been primarily associated with underlying immunosuppressive disorder,[5,7,12,52-57] immunosuppressive chemotherapy (organ transplant recipients,[55,56,58-62] sarcoidosis[63]), and with the spread of AIDS.[7,10,41,64-99]

Clinically, the *R. equi* infection is most often manifested as cavitary pneumonia, which is characterized by a high mortality rate despite prolonged antibiotic chemotherapy.[1,42,45,79,82,93,97,100] In several reports, *R. equi* infections were associated with penetrating eye injuries,[101,102] inflammatory mass in the pelvis,[65] bloody diarrhea and cachexia,[67] pleural effusion,[103] osteomyelitis secondary to a pneumonic episode,[59] paraspinal abscess,[55] psoas abscess,[65] lung abscess,[5] and cervical lymphadenitis.[104]

Cases of pulmonary malacoplakia secondary to *R. equi*-associated pneumonia in AIDS patients have also been described.[80,89] The occurrence of these two conditions was apparently due to deficiency in cellular immunity and macrophage cellular activity as well as failure of the intracellular bactericidal and phagolysosomal functions.[80]

R. equi infections in children, although rare, have been described, but with no pediatric death so far reported.[105] Treatment with multiple antibiotics seemed to be successful.

The usual manifestations of *R. equi* pneumonia include gradually developing fever (several days to several weeks in duration), malaise, dyspnea, and nonproductive cough; hemoptysis has also been noticed.[1]

Treatment of *R. equi* infection in non-HIV-infected patients has been comprised of either multiple antibiotics alone or combination of antibiotics and surgery.[71,88,106] Relapses have been common, requiring a second course of antibiotics. Dissemination of infection (subcutaneous abscesses,[7,53] multiple brain abscesses,[8,100,107] lung, kidneys, brain, bloodstream,[98] and osteomyelitis[59]) following discontinuation of antimicrobial therapy have been reported on several occasions. By one account,[71] the overall mortality from *R. equi* infection in non-HIV-infected patients may reach 20%.

A review of the treatment of *R. equi* disease in HIV-infected patients showed that patients had received multiple antibiotic treatments comprising, on average, 4.1 antibiotics during the course of their illness.[71] Relapses were frequent after discontinuation of therapy.[99,108] Mortality rates for patients undergoing surgery was 50% — a value similar to the 57% for those receiving antibiotics alone.[71]

The selection of lipid-soluble antibiotics capable of intracellular penetration has been considered to be critical for the successful treatment of *R. equi* disease. Antibiotic susceptibilities of 24 *R. equi* isolates tested showed the following values (in %): vancomycin (100), rifampin (100), tobramycin (100), streptomycin (100), erythromycin (95), chloramphenicol (92), gentamicin (95), kanamycin (86), trimethoprim-sulfamethoxazole (80), tetracycline (53), and carbenicillin (50); there was little sensitivity towards ampicillin (25), clindamycin (22), oxacillin (14), cephalothin (13), and penicillin (9).[71] In general, there were no differences in the susceptibility patterns between isolates from HIV-infected individuals and those from non-HIV-infected patients.

According to Colebunders et al.,[109] in three cases of AIDS complicated by *R. equi* infection, despite the fact that the pathogen was susceptible to tetracycline, erythromycin, amikacin, co-trimoxazole, rifampicin, and vancomycin, these antibiotics were not clinically successful. Clinical improvement was noticed only in one patient following teicoplanin and imipenem-cilastatin therapy. In the experience of Mascellino et al.,[110] the combinations of erythromycin–rifampin and imipenem–teicoplanin were the most effective treatments of *R. equi* infections. However, resistance to imipenem,[75] rifampicin,[94] and rifampin–fluoroquinolone[111] has been reported.

Combination antibiotic treatments that included clarithromycin,[83] imipenem–vancomycin,[84,95] imipenem–teicoplanin,[96] and erythromycin–rifampin,[106,112,113] have also been recommended.[113] Frequent relapses (as high as 87.5%) necessitated longer duration of treatment.[113]

In addition to using antimicrobial drugs, surgical treatment of human *R. equi* infections included drainage of suppurative lesions, and resection of granulomatous tissue. Control of predisposing factors by decreasing the dosage of concurrent immunosuppressive therapy, or controlling underlying malignancies, have also been recommended to prevent *R. equi* infections.[1,71]

Spark et al.[114] have stressed the importance of using biochemical profiles of known non-*equi* strains and ribosomal DNA analysis to unequivocally identify the *Rhodococcus* species.

8.2.4 REFERENCES

1. Prescott, J. F., *Rhodococcus equi*: an animal and human pathogen, *Clin. Microbiol. Rev.*, 4, 20, 1991.
2. Magnusson, H., Spezifische infecktioese pneumonie beim fohlen: eine neuer eitererreger beim pferd, *Arch. Wiss. Prakt. Tierheilkd.*, 50, 22, 1923.
3. Carman, M. G. and Hodges, R. T., Distribution of *Rhodococcus equi* in animals, birds and from the environment, *NZ Vet. J.*, 35, 114, 1987.
4. Barton, M. D. and Hughes, K. L., *Corynebacterium equi*: a review, *Vet. Bull.*, 50, 65, 1980.
5. Elissalde, G. S. and Renshaw, H. W., *Corynebacterium equi*: an interhost review with emphasis on the foal, *Comp. Immunol. Microbiol. Infect. Dis.*, 3, 433, 1980.
6. Ellenberger, M. A. and Ganetzky, R. P., *Rhodococcus equi* infections: literature review, *Comp. Cont. Educ. Pract. Vet.*, 8, S414, 1986.
7. Golub, B., Falk, G., and Spink, W. W., Lung abscess due to *Corynebacterium equi*: report of first human infection, *Ann. Intern. Med.*, 66, 1174, 1967.
8. Van Etta, L. L., Filice, G. A., Ferguson, R. M., and Gerding, D. N., *Corynebacterium equi*: a review of 12 cases of human infection, *Rev. Infect. Dis.*, 5, 1012, 1983.
9. Verville, T. D., Huycke, M. M., Greenfield, R. A., Fine, D. P., Kuhls, T. L., and Slater, L. N., *Rhodococcus equi* infections in humans: 12 cases and a review of the literature, *Medicine (Baltimore)*, 73, 119, 1994.
10. Sane, D. C. and Durack, D. T., Infection with *Rhodococcus equi* in AIDS, *N. Engl. J. Med.*, 314, 56, 1986.
11. Skerman, V. D. B., McGowan, V., and Sneath, P. H. A., Approved list of bacterial names, *Int. J. Syst. Bacteriol.*, 30, 225, 1980.
12. Borleffs, J. C., Petersen, E. J., Kaasjager, K., Teding van Berkhout, F., and Rozenberg-Arska, M., *Rhodococcus equi* pneumonia in patients with immunodeficiency, *Ned. Tijdschr. Geneeskd.*, 138, 2587, 1994.
13. Goodfellow, M., The taxonomic status of *Rhodococcus equi*, *Vet. Microbiol.*, 14, 205, 1987.
14. Goodfellow, M., Beckman, A. R., and Barton, M. D., Numerical classification of *Rhodococcus equi* and related actinomycetes, *J. Appl. Bacteriol.*, 53, 199, 1982.
15. Goodfellow, M., Genus *Rhodococcus*, in *Bergey's Manual of Systematic Bacteriology*, Vol. 2, Sneath, P. H. A., Mair, N. S., Sharpe, M. E., and Holt, J. G., Eds., Williams and Wilkins, Baltimore, 1986, 1472.
16. Butler, W. R., Ahearn, D. G., and Kilburn, J. O., High-performance liquid chromatography of mycolic acids as a tool in the identification of *Corynebacterium*, *Nocardia*, *Rhodococcus*, and *Mycobacterium* species, *J. Clin. Microbiol.*, 23, 182, 1986.
17. Goodfellow, M. and Cross, T., Classification, in *The Biology of the Actinomycetes*, Goodfellow, M., Mordaski, M., and Williams, S. T., Eds., Academic Press, London, 1984, 7.

18. Lipsky, B. A., Goldberger, A. C., Tompkins, L. S., and Plorde, J. J., Infections caused by nondiphtheria corynebacteria, *Rev. Infect. Dis.*, 4, 1220, 1982.
19. Collins, M. D., Smida, J., Dorsch, M., and Stackebrandt, E., *Tsukamurella* gen. nov. harboring *Corynobacterium paurometabolum* and *Rhodococcus auranticus*, *Int. J. Syst. Bacteriol.*, 38, 385, 1988.
20. Hall, R. M. and Ratledge, C., Distribution and application of mycobactins for the characterization of species within the genus *Rhodococcus*, *J. Gen. Microbiol.*, 132, 853, 1986.
21. Tsukamura, M., Proposal of a new genus, *Gordona*, for slightly acid-fast organisms occurring in the sputa of patients with pulmonary disease and in soil, *J. Gen. Microbiol.*, 68, 15, 1971.
22. Stackebrandt, E., Smida, J., and Collins, M. D., Evidence of phylogenetic heterogeneity within the genus *Rhodococcus*: revival of the genus *Gordona* (Tsukamura), *J. Gen. Appl. Microbiol.*, 34, 341, 1988.
23. Zakrzewska-Czerwinska, J., Mordarski, M., and Goodfellow, M., DNA base composition and homology values in the classification of some *Rhodococcus* species, *J. Gen. Microbiol.*, 134, 2807, 1988.
24. Apajalahti, J. H. A., Karpanoja, P., and Salkinoja-Salonen, M. S., *Rhodococcus chlorophenolicus* sp. nov., a chlorophenol-mineralizing actinomycete, *Int. J. Syst. Bacteriol.*, 36, 246, 1986.
25. Tsukamura, M., Genus *Rhodococcus* and *Rhodococcus* infection, *Kekkaku*, 63, 779, 1988.
26. Woolcock, J. B. and Mutimer, M. D., Capsules of *Corynebacterium equi* and *Streptococcus equi*, *J. Gen. Microbiol.*, 109, 127, 1978.
27. Yanagawa, Y. and Honda, E., Presence of pili in species of human and animal parasites and pathogens of the genus *Corynebacterium*, *Infect. Immun.*, 13, 1293, 1976.
28. Bernheimer, A. W., Linder, R., and Avigad, L. S., Stepwise degradation of membrane sphingomyelin by corynebacterial phospholipases, *Infect. Immun.*, 29, 123, 1980.
29. Flatla, J. L., Infeksjion med *Corynebacterium equi* hos foll, *Nor. Vet. Tidsskr.*, 54, 249, 1942.
30. Martens, R. J., Fiske, R. A., and Renshaw, H. W., Experimental subacute foal pneumonia induced by aerosol administration of *Corynebacterium equi*, *Equine Vet. J.*, 14, 111, 1982.
31. Takai, S., Kawasu, S., and Tsubaki, S., Humoral immune response of foals to experimental infection with *Rhodococcus equi*, *Vet. Microbiol.*, 14, 321, 1987.
32. Nakazawa, M., Haritani, M., Sugimoto, C., and Isayama, Y., Virulence of *Rhodococcus equi* for mice, *Jpn. J. Vet. Sci.*, 45, 679, 1983.
33. Takai, S., Michizoe, T., Matsumura, K., Nagai, M., Sato, H., and Tsubaki, S., Correlation of *in vitro* properties of *Rhodococcus* (*Corynebacterium*) *equi* with virulence for mice, *Microbiol. Immunol.*, 29, 1175, 1985.
34. Nakazawa, M., Kubo, M., Sugimoto, C., and Isayama, Y., Serogrouping of *Rhodococcus equi*, *Microbiol. Immunol.*, 27, 837, 1983.
35. Prescott, J. F., Capsular serotypes of *Corynebacterium equi*, *Can. J. Comp. Med.*, 45, 130, 1981.
36. Prescott, J. F., Lastra, M., and Barksdale, L., *Equi* factors in the identification of *Corynebacterium equi* Magnusson, *J. Clin. Microbiol.*, 16, 988, 1982.
37. Skalka, B. and Svastova, A., Serodiagnostics of *Corynebacterium* (*Rhodococcus*) *equi*, *Zentralbl. Veterinaermed. Reihe B*, 32, 137, 1985.
38. Fraser, G., The effect on animal erythrocytes of combinations of diffusable substances produced by bacteria, *J. Pathol. Bacteriol.*, 88, 43, 1964.
39. Linder, R. and Bernheimer, A. W., Enzymatic oxidation of membrane cholesterol oxidase in relation to lysis of sheep erythrocytes by corynebacterial enzymes, *Arch. Biochem. Biophys.*, 213, 395, 1982.
40. Machang'u, R. S. and Prescott, J. F., Role of antibody to extracellular proteins of *Rhodococcus equi* in protection against *R. equi* pneumonia in foals, *Vet. Microbiol.*, 26, 323, 1991.
41. Takai, S., Koike, K., Ohbushi, S., Izumi, C., and Tsubaki, S., Identification of 15- to 17-kilodalton antigens associated with virulent *Rhodococcus equi*, *J. Clin. Microbiol.*, 29, 439, 1991.
42. Mastroianni, C. M., Lichtner, M., Vullo, V., and Delia, S., Humoral immune response to *Rhodococcus equi* in AIDS patients with *R. equi* pneumonia, *J. Infect. Dis.*, 169, 1179, 1994.
43. Tan, C., Prescott, J. F., Patterson, M. C., and Nicholson, V. M., Molecular characterization of a lipid-modified virulence-associated protein of *Rhodococcus equi* and its potential in protective immunity, *Can. J. Vet. Res.*, 59, 51, 1995.
44. Nordman, P., Ronco, E., and Nauciel, C., Role of T-lymphocyte subsets in *Rhodococcus equi* infection, *Infect. Immun.*, 60, 2748, 1992.

45. Zink, M. C., Yager, J. A., Prescott, J. F., and Wilkie, B. N., *In vitro* phagocytosis and killing of *Corynebacterium equi* by alveolar macrophages of foals, *Am. J. Vet. Res.*, 46, 2171, 1985.

46. Hietala, S. K. and Ardans, A. A., Interaction of *Rhodococcus equi* with phagocytic cells from *R. equi*-exposed and non-exposed foals, *Vet. Microbiol.*, 14, 307, 1987,

47. Zink, M. C., Yager, J. A., Prescott, J. F., and Fernando, M. A., Electron microscopic investigation of intracellular events after ingestion of *Rhodococcus equi* by foal alveolar macrophages, *Vet. Microbiol.*, 14, 295, 1987.

48. Ellenberger, M. A., Kabaerle, M. L., and Roth, J. A., Effect of *Rhodococcus equi* on equine poly-morphonuclear leucocyte function, *Vet. Immunol. Immunopathol.*, 7, 315, 1984.

49. Hietala, S. K. and Ardans, A. A., Neutrophil phagocytic and serum opsonic response of the foal to *Corynebacterium equi*, *Vet. Immunol. Immunopathol.*, 14, 279, 1987.

50. Martens, J. G., Martens, R. J., and Renshaw, H. W., *Rhodococcus (Corynebacterium) equi*: bactericidal capacity of neutrophils from neonatal and adult horses, *Am. J. Vet. Res.*, 49, 295, 1988.

51. Yager, J. A., Foster, S. F., Zink, M. C., Prescott, J. F., and Lumsden, J. H., *In vitro* bactericidal efficacy of equine polymorphonuclear leukocytes against *Corynebacterium equi*, *Am. J. Vet. Med.*, 47, 348, 1986.

52. Marsch, J. C. and von Graevenitz, A., Recurrent *Corynebacterium equi* infection with lymphoma, *Cancer*, 32, 147, 1973.

53. Berg, R., Chmel, H., Mayo, J., and Armstrong, D., *Corynebacterium equi* infection complicating neoplastic disease, *Am. J. Clin. Pathol.*, 68, 73, 1977.

54. Gardner, S. E., Pearson, T., and Hughes, W. T., Pneumonitis due to *Corynebacterium equi*, *Chest*, 70, 92, 1976.

55. Jones, M. R., Say, P. J., Neale, T. J., and Horne, J. G., *Rhodococcus equi*: an emerging opportunistic pathogen? *Aust. NZ J. Med.*, 19, 103, 1989.

56. Williams, G. D., Flanigan, W. J., and Campbell, G. S., Surgical management of localized thoracic infections in immunosuppressed patients, *Ann. Thor. Surg.*, 12, 471, 1971.

57. Carpenter, J. L. and Blom, J., *Corynebacterium equi* pneumonia in a patient with Hodgkin's disease, *Am. Rev. Respir. Dis.*, 114, 235, 1987.

58. Gainsford, S. A. and Frater, E., Two cases of infection involving *Rhodococcus equi*, *NZ J. Med. Lab. Technol.*, 40, 100, 1986.

59. Novak, R. M., Polisky, E. L., Janda, W. M., and Libertin, C. R., Osteomyelitis caused by *Rhodococcus equi* in a renal transplant recipient, *Infection*, 16, 186, 1988.

60. Rubin, R. H., Pneumonia in the compromised host, in *Update: Pulmonary Disease and Disorders*, Fishman, A. P., Ed., McGraw-Hill, New York, 1982, 1.

61. Savdie, E., Pigott, P., and Jennis, F., Lung abscess due to *Corynebacterium equi* in a renal transplant recipient, *Med. J. Aust.*, 1, 817, 1977.

62. Segovia, J., Pulpón, L. A., Crespo, M. G., Daza, R., Rodriguez, J. C., Rubio, A., Serrano, S., Carreno, M. C., Varela, A., Aranguena, R., and Yebra, M., *Rhodococcus equi*: first case in a heart transplant recipient, *J. Heart Lung Transplant.*, 13, 332, 1994.

63. Hillerdal, G., Riesenfeldt-örn, I., Pedersen, A., and Ivanicova, E., Infection with *Rhodococcus equi* in a patient with sarcoidosis treated with corticosteroids, *Scand. J. Infect. Dis.*, 20, 673, 1988.

64. Bishopric, G. A., d'Agay, M. F., Schlemmer, B., Sarfati, E., and Brocheriou, C., Pulmonary pseudot-umour due to *Corynebacterium equi* in a patient with the acquired immunodeficiency syndrome, *Thorax*, 43, 486, 1988.

65. Fierer, J., Wolf, P., Seed, L., Gay, T., Noonan, K., and Haghighi, P., Non-pulmonary *Rhodococcus equi* infections in patients with acquired immune deficiency syndrome (AIDS), *Clin. Pathol.*, 40, 556, 1987.

66. Kunke, P. J., Serious infection in an AIDS patient due to *Rhodococcus equi*, *Clin. Microbiol. Newslett.* 9, 163, 1987.

67. Samies, J. H., Hathaway, B. N., Echols, R. M., Veazey, J. M., Jr., and Pilon, V. A., Lung abscess due to *Corynebacterium equi*: report of the first case in a patient with acquired immune deficiency syndrome, *Am. J. Med.*, 80, 685, 1986.

68. Sonnet, J., Wauters, G., Zech, F., and Gigi, J., Opportunistic *Rhodococcus equi* infection in an African AIDS case (1976-1981), *Acta Clin. Belg.*, 42, 215, 1987.

69. Wang, H. H., Tollerud, D., Danar, D., Hanff, P., Gottesdiener, K., and Rosen, S., Another Whipple-like disease in AIDS? *N. Engl. J. Med.*, 314, 1577, 1986.

70. Weingarten, J. S., Huang, D. Y., and Jackman, J. D., Jr., *Rhodococcus equi* pneumonia: an unusual early manifestation of the acquired immunodeficiency syndrome (AIDS), *Chest*, 94, 195, 1988.

71. Harvey, R. L. and Sunstrom, J. C., *Rhodococcus equi* infection in patients with and without human immunodeficiency virus infection, *Rev. Infect. Dis.*, 13, 139, 1991.

72. Haglund, L. A., Trotter, J. A., Slater, L. N., Harris, S. L., Rettig, P. J., and Harkess, J. R., Case 9-1989: AIDS and a cavitary pulmonary lesion, *N. Engl. J. Med.*, 321, 395, 1989.

73. MacGregor, J. H., Samuelson, W. M., Sane, D. C., and Godwin, J. D., Opportunistic lung infection caused by *Rhodococcus* (*Corynebacterium*) *equi*, *Radiology*, 160, 83, 1986.

74. Marco, M. L., Remacha, A., and Echevarri, B., *Rhodococcus equi* pneumonia in patients with AIDS, *Arch. Bronconeumol.*, 30, 519, 1994.

75. Fernandez, A., Santos, J., Sanchez, M. A., and Alfaro, C., *Rhodococcus equi* pneumonia in a patient with AIDS, *Enferm. Infecc. Microbiol. Clin.*, 12, 471, 1994.

76. Legras, A., Lemmens, B., Dequin, P. F., Cattier, B., and Besnier, J. M., Tamponade due to *Rhodococcus equi* in acquired immunodeficiency syndrome, *Chest*, 106, 1278, 1994.

77. Figueras Villalba, M. P., Martinez Alvarez, R. M., and Munoz Marco, J. J., Pneumonia by *Rhodococcus equi* in patients with HIV infection, *Ann. Med. Intern.*, 11, 238, 1994.

78. Heudier, P., Taillan, B., Garnier, G., Vialla, I., Diaine, B., Elbaze, P., Fuzibet, J. G., and Dujardin, P., L'infection a *Rhodococcus equi* au cours du sida: un cas avec abcès pulmonaire. Revue de la littérature, *Rev. Med. Intern.*, 15, 268, 1994.

79. Nzerue, C., *Rhodococcus equi* infection: a cause of cavitary pulmonary disease in immuno-compromised patients, *Cent. Afr. J. Med.*, 39, 262, 1993.

80. Lemmens, B., Besnier, J. M., Diot, P., Fetissof, F., Anthonioz, P., Cattier, B., and Choutet, P., Malacoplasie pulmonaire et pneumonie a *Rhodococcus equi* chez un patients infecté par le virus de l'immunodépression humaine: a propos d'un cas avec revue de la littérature, *Rev. Mal. Respir.*, 11, 301, 1994.

81. Fiaccadori, F., Emergent pathologies: *Rhodococcus equi* infection in the acquired immunodeficiency syndrome, *Ann. Ital. Med. Int.*, 9, 10, 1994.

82. Frame, B. C. and Petcus, A. F., *Rhodococcus equi* pneumonia: case report and literature review, *Ann. Pharmacother.*, 27, 1340, 1993.

83. Pialoux, G., Goldstein, F., Dupont, B., Gonzalez Canali, G., and Sansonetti, P., Combination antibiotic treatment with clarithromycin for human immunodeficiency virus-associated *Rhodococcus equi* infection, *Clin. Infect. Dis.*, 17, 513, 1993.

84. Javaloyas, M., Garcia, D., and Ruffi, G., Recurrent abscess of the lung caused by *Rhodococcus equi* in an HIV-positive patient: response to a combination imipenem/vancomycin, *Med. Clin. (Barcelona)*, 100, 759, 1993.

85. Gazquez, I., Garcia Gonzalez, M., Pena, J. M., Rubio, M., and Nogues, A., A pulmonary abscess due to *Rhodococcus equi* in an AIDS patient, *Rev. Clin. Esp.*, 192, 152, 1993.

86. Clotet, B., Sirera, G., and Erice, A., *Rhodococcus equi* infection in HIV-infected patients, *J. Acquir. Immune Defic. Syndr.*, 6, 429, 1993.

87. Piersantelli, N., Casini-Lemmi, M., Cavanna, E., Cassola, G., Crisalli, M. P., Guida, B., Paladino, M., Penco, G., Piscopo, R., and Torresin, A., *Rhodococcus equi* infections in AIDS: personal cases, *Pathologica*, 84, 517, 1992.

88. Curry, J. D., Harrington, P. T., and Hosein, I. K., Successful medical therapy of *Rhodococcus equi* pneumonia in a patient with HIV infection, *Chest*, 102, 1619, 1992.

89. Rouveix, E., Dupont, C., Ichai, P., Nicolas, M. H., Julie, C., Lesur, G., and Dorra, M., Two particular aspects of *Rhodococcus equi* infection: malacoplakia and acquisition of resistance to antibiotics, *Presse Med.*, 21, 1086, 1992.

90. Pialoux, G. and Dupont, B., Lung abscess caused by *Rhodococcus equi* in HIV infection: two cases, *Presse Med.*, 21, 1086, 1992.

91. Pialoux, G., Fournier, S., Dupont, B., Fleury, J., Sansonetti, Ph., Goldstein, F., and Trotot, P., Lung abscess caused by *Rhodococcus* (*Corynebacterium*) *equi* in HIV infection: two cases, *Presse Med.*, 21, 417, 1992.

92. Gray, B. M., Case report: *Rhodococcus equi* pneumonia in a patient infected by the human immunodeficiency virus, *Am. J. Med. Sci.*, 303, 180, 1992.

93. Drancourt, M., Bonnet, E., Gallais, H., Peloux, Y., and Raoult, D., *Rhodococcus equi* infection in patients with AIDS, *J. Infect.*, 24, 123, 1992.

94. Nordman, P., Chavanet, P., Caillon, J., Duez, J. M., and Portier, H., Recurrent pneumonia due to rifampicin-resistant *Rhodococcus equi* in a patient infected with HIV, *J. Infect.*, 24, 104, 1992.

95. Rouquet, R. M., Clave, D., Massip, P., Moatti, N., and Leophonte, P., Imipenem/vancomycin for *Rhodococcus equi* pulmonary infection in HIV-positive patient, *Lancet*, 337, 375, 1991.

96. Chavanet, P., Bonnotte, B., Caillot, D., and Portier, H., Imipenem/teicoplanin for *Rhodococcus equi* pulmonary infection in AIDS patient, *Lancet*, 337, 794, 1991.

97. Roca, V., Vinuelas, J., Perez-Cecilia, E., Picardo, A., Rabadan, P. M., Ortega, L., Torres, A., and Picazo, J. J., Bacteremic pneumonia caused by *Rhodococcus equi* and HIV infection: report of a new case and review of the literature, *Enferm. Infecc. Microbiol. Clin.*, 9, 627, 1991.

98. Sirera, G., Romeu, J., Clotet, B., Velasco, P., Arnal, J., Rius, F., and Foz, M., Relapsing systemic infection due to *Rhodococcus equi* in a drug abuser seropositive for human immunodeficiency virus, *Rev. Infect. Dis.*, 13, 509, 1991.

99. Flepp, M., Luthy, R., Wust, J., Steinke, W., and Greminger, P., *Rhodococcus equi* infection in HIV disease, *Schweiz. Med. Wochenschr.*, 119, 566, 1989.

100. Daley, C. L., Bacterial pneumonia in HIV-infected patients, *Semin. Respir. Dis.*, 8, 104, 1993.

101. Ebersole, L. L. and Paturzo, J. L., Endophthalmitis caused by *Rhodococcus equi* Prescott serotype 4, *J. Clin. Microbiol.*, 26, 1221, 1988.

102. Hillman, D., Garretson, B., and Fiscella, R., *Rhodococcus equi* endophthalmitis, *Arch. Ophthalmol.*, 107, 20, 1989.

103. LeBar, W. D. and Pensler, M. I., Pleural effusion due to *Rhodococcus equi*, *J. Infect. Dis.*, 154, 919, 1986.

104. Thomsen, V. F., Henriques, U., and Magnusson, M., *Corynebacterium equi* Magnusson isolated from a tuberculoid lesion in a child with adenitis coli, *Dan. Med. Bull.*, 15, 135, 1968.

105. McGowan, K. L. and Mangano, M. F., Infections with *Rhodococcus equi* in children, *Diagn. Microbiol. Infect. Dis.*, 14, 347, 1991.

106. Sladek, G. G. and Frame, J. N., *Rhodococcus equi* causing bacteremia in an adult with acute leukemia, *South. Med. J.*, 86, 244, 1993.

107. Obana, W. G., Scannell, K. A., Jacobs, R., Greco, C., and Rosenblum, M. L., A case of *Rhodococcus equi* brain abscess, *Surg. Neurol.*, 35, 321, 1991.

108. Jablonowski, H., Armbrecht, C., Mauss, S., Szelényi, H., Manegold, C., Borchard, F., and Niederau, C., *Rhodococcus equi* pneumonia in an HIV- infected patient, *Bildgebung*, 61, 206, 1994.

109. Colebunders, R., De Roo, A., Verstraeten, T., van den Abbeele, K., Levens, M., Hauben, E., Van Marck, E., Schaal, K., and Portaels, F., *Rhodococcus equi* infection in 3 AIDS patients, *Acta Clin. Belg.*, 51, 101, 1996.

110. Mascellino, M. T., Iona, E., Ponzo, R., Mastroianni, C. M., and Delia, S., Infections due to *Rhodococcus equi* in three HIV-infected patients: microbiological findings and antibiotic susceptibility, *Int. J. Clin. Pharmacol. Res.*, 14, 157, 1994.

111. Nordman, P., Rouveix, E., Guenounou, M., and Nicolas, M. H., Pulmonary abscess due to a rifampin and fluoroquinolone resistant *Rhodococcus equi* strain in a HIV infected patient, *Eur. J. Clin. Microbiol. Infect. Dis.*, 11, 557, 1992.

112. Hillidge, C. J., Use of erythromycin-rifampin combination in treatment of *Rhodococcus equi* pneumonia, *Vet. Microbiol.*, 14, 337, 1987.

113. Arrizabalaga, J., Hernandez, J., Iribarren, J. A., Uriz, J., Rodriguez Arrondo, F., Agud, J. M., von Wichmann, M. A., and Arrieta, J., *Rhodococcus equi* infection in immunocompromised host: 11 cases, *Proc. 36th Intersci. Conf. Antimicrob. Agents Chemother.*, American Society for Microbiology, Washington, D.C., Abstr. I24, 1996.

114. Spark, R. P., McNeil, M. M., Brown, J. M., Lasker, B. A., Montano, M. A., and Garfield, M. D., *Rhodococcus* species fatal infection in an immunocompetent host, *Arch. Pathol. Lab. Med.*, 117, 515, 1993.

8.3 TSUKAMURELLA PAUROMETABOLUM

8.3.1 INTRODUCTION

Tsukamurella paurometabolum is a Gram-positive, weakly or variably acid-fast, non-motile, non-sporoforming, rod-shaped obligate aerobic actinomycete. Morphologically, it is characterized by the absence of aerial hyphae. The composition of its cell wall is notable for the presence of unusually very long-chain (68 to 76 carbon atoms) and highly unsaturated (two to six double bonds) mycolic acids,[1] as well as other novel glycolipids and menaquinones with unsaturated multiprenyl side chains.[1-6]

The natural habitat of *T. paurometabolum* is soil, sludge, and arthropods. It is a psychrophilic bacterium that grows best at temperatures cooler than that of a human body.

There is some controversy surrounding the taxonomic placement of *T. paurometabolum*.[10,13] *T. paurometabolum* was first isolated in 1941 by Steinhaus[7] from mycetomas and ovaries of bedbugs (*Cimex lectularius*), and was originally classified as *Corynebacterium paurometabolum*. Until 1988, *T. paurometabolum* was also referred to as either *Rhodococcus aurantiacus* or *Gordona aurantiaca*.[8,9]

Subsequently, the placement of *T. paurometabolum* in the genus *Corynebacterium* has been questioned by several investigators.[1,10,11,13] At present, there is a general agreement that *Tsukamurella* (*Corynebacterium*) *paurometabolum* is more closely associated with the rhodococci, and quite distinct from authentic corynebacteria.

It is generally accepted that the genus *Corynebacterium* should be restricted to species that are characterized by the presence of: *meso*-diaminopimelic acid and arabinogalactan in their cell wall (wall chemotype IV[23]); relatively short-chain C_{22-36} mycolic acids, and dihydrogenated menaquinones with eight isoprene units, or both; and have a deoxyribonucleic acid (DNA) base composition within the approximate range of 51 to 67 mol%.[10,24] While *Tsukamurella* (*Corynebacterium*) *paurometabolum* resembles authentic corynebacteria by containing a directly cross-linked murein based on *meso*-diaminopimelic acid and an arabinogalactan polymer,[25,26] it can be distinguished from them because it contains an unusual series of very long (C_{68-76}) and highly unsaturated (two to six double bonds) acids.[1,13]

A similar series of very long and highly unsaturated mycolic acids has been found in *Rhodococcus aurantiacus*[6,27] (first described as *Gordona aurantiaca*[12]). The generic position of *R. aurantiacus*, which has now been firmly established, comprises strains previously classified in the genus *Gordona* and members of the "rhodochrous" complex;[2,6,10,14] Tsukamura[8,15,16] subsequently assigned *Gordona aurantiaca* to the genus *Rhodococcus*.

Extensive studies on the reverse transcriptase sequencing of long regions of 16S ribosomal ribonucleic acids of *Corynebacterium paurometabolum* and *Rhodococcus aurantiacus* conducted by Collins et al.[13] have demonstrated that not only were these two species highly related to each other (over 99% sequence homology in a large stretch of 1184 nucleotides, and the presence of menaquinones with unsaturated multiprenyl side chains[1,6]) but they were also distinct from the genera *Corynebacterium*, *Nocardia*, *Mycobacterium*, and *Rhodococcus* (invariably containing menaquinones with partially saturated side chains). In addition to their unusual colony morphology, the absence of aerial hyphae, and a negative 3-d arylsulfatase test have been helpful to distinguish *T. paurometabolum* from the other rapidly growing *Mycobacterium* and *Nocardia* species with which it is most often confused.[28]

Tsukamurella organisms may be further differentiated from *Rhodococcus* species by their β-galactosidase activity, resistance to mitomycin C (5.0 µg/ml), inability to reduce nitrate to nitrite, and the use of galactose as a sole carbon source.[8,18]

On the basis of their own as well as other findings,[6,8,14-16] Collins et al.[13] proposed that *C. paurometabolum* and *R. aurantiacus* be reduced to a single species and reclassified in a new genus, *Tsukamurella*, with *T. paurometabolum* comb. nov. representing the type species (new type strain W4779).[13]

T. paurometabolum infection was first described in humans in 1971 by Tsukamura and Mizuno,[12] who isolated the bacterium from sputum of patients with tuberculosis.

Although rarely, it is an opportunistic pathogen for humans, specifically in patients with predisposing conditions, such as immunosuppression, chronic pathology, and foreign bodies.[17] So far, only several cases of human disease caused by *T. paurometabolum* have been described: pneumonia in a patient with tuberculosis,[18] meningitis in a patient with hairy cell leukemia,[19] necrotizing fasciitis in a previously healthy patient,[20] and peritonitis in a patient undergoing peritoneal dialysis with an indwelling catheter.[21] In addition, central venous catheter-related infections due to *Gordona rubropertincta* and *G. terrae* in two immunocompetent patients who had been receiving total parenteral nutrition in their homes have also been reported.[29] Auerbach at al.[22] have described a hospital outbreak of pseudoinfection with *T. paurometabolum* which was traced to laboratory contamination.

Shapiro et al.[28] and Lai[30] have described central venous catheter-related sepsis due to *T. paurometabolum* in immunocompromised cancer patients.

In a recent report, Rey et al.[17] reported what appeared to be the first described case of *T. paurometabolum* infection in an HIV-infected individual.

8.3.2 EVOLUTION OF THERAPIES AND TREATMENT OF *T. PAUROMETABOLUM* INFECTION

T. paurometabolum appears to be pathogenic to humans only in specific conditions, such as immunosuppression, presence of an indwelling foreign body, and a chronic infection, such as pulmonary tuberculosis.

Shapiro et al.[28] have tested *in vitro* the susceptibilities of an ATCC type strain 25938 of *T. paurometabolum* and three clinical isolates and found them highly susceptible to sulfamethoxazole, imipenem, third generation of cephalosporins (three of four isolates), amikacin, and ciprofloxacin, but resistant to the penicillins and second generation of cephalosporins. However, the results of *in vitro* testing may not always correlate with the outcome *in vivo*, as evidenced by a case of a patient with subcutaneous abscesses and necrotizing tenosynovitis who despite amputation and treatment with a four-drug regimen (to which *T. paurometabolum* was susceptible *in vitro*), did not improve.[20]

Lai[30] successfully used a combination of erythromycin and gentamicin (IV administration for 4 weeks) to treat an immunosuppressed cancer patient with central venous catheter-associated sepsis caused by *T. paurometabolum*. However, in this as well as other similar cases,[28] because of prolonged bacteremia, removal of the catheter was essential for cure.

Jones et al.[31] effectively treated a patient with persistent *T. paurometabolum* bacteremia with a 6-week course of vancomycin (1.0 g/week).

Therapeutic regimens used by Shapiro et al.[28] to treat three cases of *T. paurometabolum* bacteremia included: a 2-week intravenous therapy with trimethoprim–sulfamethoxazole (TMX-SMZ), followed by 2 weeks with oral TMP-SMZ; a 4-week course of intravenous erythromycin and gentamicin; and intravenous vancomycin and ceftazidime for 4 d, followed by intravenous ceftriaxone for 10 d.

8.3.3 REFERENCES

1. Collins, M. D. and Jones, D., Lipid composition of *Corynebacterium paurometabolum* (Steinhaus), *FEMS Microbiol. Lett.*, 13, 13, 1982.
2. Goodfellow, M., Genus *Rhodococcus*, in *Bergey's Manual of Systematic Bacteriol.*, Vol. 2, Sneath, P. H. A., Mair, N. S., Sharpe, M. E., and Holt, J. G., Eds., Williams and Wilkins, Baltimore, 1986, 1472.
3. Tomiyasu, I. and Yano, I., Separation and analysis of novel polyunsaturated mycolic acids from a psychrophylic, acid-fast bacterium, *Gordona aurantiaca*, *Eur. J. Biochem.*, 139, 173, 1984.

4. Rastogi, N., David, H. L., and Frehel, C., Ultrastructure of "*Gordona aurantiaca*" Tsukamura 1981, *Curr. Microbiol.*, 13, 51, 1986.
5. Tomiyasu, I., Yoshinaga, J., Kurano, F., Kato, Y., Kaneda, K., Imaizumi, S., and Yano, I., Occurrence of a novel glycolipid trehalose 2,3,6′- trimycolate in a psychrophylic, acid-fast bacterium, *Rhodococcus aurantiacus* (*Gordona aurantiaca*), *FEBS Lett.*, 203, 239, 1986.
6. Goodfellow, M. P., Orlean, P. A. B., Collins, M. D., Alshamaony, L., and Minnikin, D. E., Chemical and numerical taxonomy of strains received as *Gordona aurantiaca*, *J. Gen. Microbiol.*, 109, 57, 1978.
7. Steinhaus, E. A., A study of the bacteria associated with thirty species of insects, *J. Bacteriol.*, 42, 757, 1941.
8. Tsukamura, M. and Yano, I., *Rhodococcus sputi* sp. nov., nom. rev., and *Rhodococcus aurantiacus* sp. nov., nom. rev., *Int. J. Syst. Bacteriol.*, 35, 364, 1985.
9. Stackebrandt, E., Smida, J., and Collins, M. D., Evidence of phylogenetic heterogeneity within the genus *Rhodococcus:* revival of the genus *Gordona* (Tsukamura), *J. Gen. Appl. Microbiol.*, 34, 341, 1988.
10. Collins, M. D. and Cummins, C. S., Genus *Corynebacterium*, in *Bergey's Manual of Systematic Bacteriology*, Vol. 2, Sneath, P. H. A., Mair, N. S., Sharpe, M. E., and Holt, J. G., Eds., Williams and Wilkins, Baltimore, 1986, 1266.
11. Jones, D., A numerical taxonomic study of coryneform and related bacteria, *J. Gen. Microbiol.*, 87, 52, 1975.
12. Tsukamura, M. and Mizuno, S., A new species, *Gordona aurantiaca*, occurring in sputa of patients with pulmonary disease, *Kekkaku*, 46, 93, 1971.
13. Collins, M. D., Smida, J., Dorsch, M., and Stackebrandt, E., *Tsukamurella* gen. nov. harboring *Corynebacterium paurometabolum* and *Rhodococcus aurantiacus*, *Int. J. Syst. Bacteriol.*, 38, 385, 1988.
14. Goodfellow, M. and Alderson, G., The actinomycete genus *Rhodococcus*: a home for the "rhodochrous" complex, *J. Gen. Microbiol.*, 100, 99, 1977.
15. Tsukamura, M., A further taxonomic study of the rhodochrous group, *Jpn. J. Microbiol.*, 18, 37, 1974.
16. Tsukamura, M., Numerical classification of *Rhodococcus* (formerly *Gordona*) organisms recently isolated from sputa of patients: description of *Rhodococcus sputi* Tsukamura sp. nov., *Int. J. Syst. Bacteriol.*, 28, 169, 1978.
17. Rey, D., De Briel, D., Heller, R., Fraisse, Ph., Partisani, M., Leiva-Mena, M., and Lang, J. M., Tsukamurella and HIV infection, *AIDS*, 9, 1379, 1995.
18. Tsukamura, M. and Kawakami, K., Lung infection caused by *Gordona aurantiaca* (*Rhodococcus auranticus*), *J. Clin. Microbiol.*, 16, 604, 1982.
19. Prinz, G., Ban, E., Fekete, S., and Szabo, Z., Meningitis caused by *Gordona aurantiaca* (*Rhodococcus aurantiacus*), *J. Clin. Microbiol.*, 22, 472, 1985.
20. Tsukamura, M., Hikosaka, K., Nishimura, K., and Hara, S., Severe progressive subcutaneous abscesses and necrotizing tenosynovitis caused by *Rhodococcus aurantiacus*, *J. Clin. Microbiol.*, 26, 201, 1987.
21. Casella, P., Tommasi, A., and Tortorano, A. M., Peritonie da *Gordona aurantiaca* (*Rhodococcus aurantiacus*) in dialisi peritoneale ambulatorie continua, *Microbiol. Med.*, 2, 47, 1987.
22. Auerbach, S. B., McNeil, M. M., Brown, J. M., Lasker, B. A., and Jarvis, W. R., Outbreak of pseudoinfection with *Tsukamurella paurometabolum* traced to laboratory contamination: efficacy of joint epidemiological and laboratory investigation, *Clin. Infect. Dis.*, 14, 1015, 1992.
23. Lechevalier, M. P. and Lechevalier, H. A., Chemical composition as a criterion in the classification of aerobic actinomycetes, *Int. J. Syst. Bacteriol.*, 20, 435, 1970.
24. Pitcher, D. G., Deoxyribonucleic acid base composition of *Corynebacterium diphtheriae* and other corynebacteria with cell wall type IV, *FEMS Microbiol. Lett.*, 16, 291, 1983.
25. Cummins, C. S., Cell wall composition in *Corynebacterium bovis* and some other corynebacteria, *J. Bacteriol.*, 105, 1227, 1971.
26. Schleifer, K. H. and Kandler, O., Peptidoglycan types of bacterial cell wall and their taxonomic implications, *Bacteriol. Rev.*, 36, 407, 1972.
27. Tomoyasu, I. and Yano, I., Separation and analysis of novel polyunsaturated mycolic acids from a psychrophilic, acid-fast bacterium, *Gordona aurantiaca*, *Eur. J. Biochem.*, 139, 173, 1984.

28. Shapiro, C. L., Haft, R. F., Gantz, N. M., Doern, G. V., Christenson, J. C., O'Brien, R., Overall, J. C., Brown, B. A., and Wallace, R. J., Jr., *Tsukamurella paurometabolum*: a novel pathogen causing catheter-related bacteremia in patients with cancer, *Clin. Infect. Dis.*, 14, 200, 1992.

29. Buchman, A. L., McNeil, M. M., Brown, J. M., Lasker, B. A., and Ament, M. E., Central venous catheter sepsis caused by unusual *Gordona* (*Rhodococcus*) species: identification with a digoxigenin-labeled rDNA probe, *Clin. Infect. Dis.*, 15, 694, 1992.

30. Lai, K. K., A cancer patient with central venous catheter-related sepsis caused by *Tsukamurella paurometabolum* (*Gordona aurantiaca*), *Clin. Infect. Dis.*, 17, 285, 1993.

31. Jones, R. S., Fekete, T., Truant, A. L., and Satishchandran, V., Persistent bacteremia due to *Tsukamurella paurometabolum* in a patient undergoing hemodialysis: case report and review, *Clin. Infect. Dis.*, 18, 830, 1994.

8.4   *MYCOBACTERIUM TUBERCULOSIS*

8.4.1   INTRODUCTION

Pulmonary tuberculosis (consumption, phthisis) is considered to be one of the most devastating human diseases, causing death and prolonged disability among people over many centuries. The incidence of tuberculosis increased dramatically during the Industrial Revolution, probably as a result of the serious social consequences that characterized that period. The causative agent of the disease, the human tubercle bacillus, was discovered by Robert Koch in 1882, and since then tuberculosis has become one of the most intensely studied infectious diseases. Following a decline in prevalence during the latter part of this century, the incidence of tuberculosis has substantially risen in recent years.[1,2]

The pattern of tuberculosis has also changed and in recent years the incidence of extrapulmonary tuberculosis has become more common.[3] Among the various contributing factors responsible for this disturbing trend, special attention has been given to the continuously increasing population of immunocompromised patients, such as organ transplant recipients,[4-9] patients on immuno-suppressive therapy,[10] patients with idiopathic CD4[+]-lymphocytopenia,[11] severe combined immuno-deficiency,[12] and especially patients who are HIV-positive or already have AIDS,[13-17] as well as patients with chronic renal failure undergoing continuous ambulatory peritoneal dialysis.[18] Cases of extrapulmonary involvement, most often cerebral tuberculosis, have also been described.[19]

Outbreaks of multiple drug-resistant tuberculosis among HIV-infected and AIDS patients, which have been reported to occur in hospitals and prisons, were characterized by high mortality rates, disease transmission within the institutions, and high transmission rates to health care workers.[20-23] Data reported by Pearson et al.[24] have also underscored the possibility that nosocomial transmission of multiple drug-resistant tuberculosis may occur both from patient to patient, and from patient to health care worker.

In the context of HIV infection, tuberculosis has been the only bacterial infection to which HIV-positive subjects are prone that can be readily transmitted to non-HIV-infected individuals. Githui et al.[25] have examined various aspects associated with HIV-related tuberculosis in a cohort study of HIV-positive and HIV-negative patients from Kenya. The 2-year incidence of tuberculosis in cohorts of HIV-infected and uninfected urban Rwandan women has shown the rate ratio for development of tuberculosis among HIV-positive patients to be 22%.[26]

A small, but statistically significant, increase of tuberculosis in intravenous drug users has recently also been observed.

In contrast to most pathogenic bacteria, which are either facultative aerobes or anaerobes, the human tuberculous bacillus (*Mycobacterium tuberculosis*) is an obligate aerobe. In man, the bacilli are observed as slightly bent or curved, slender rods, approximately 2 to 4 μm long and 0.2 to 0.5 μm wide. In culture media, the cells may vary from coccoid to filamentous. Most of the virulent tubercle strains form rough colonies, whereas many avirulent laboratory strains produce less rough colonies. An interesting feature of the virulent strains is their ability to grow as intertwining "serpentine cords" in which the bacilli aggregate with their long axes parallel.

The well known "Bacille Calmette Guérin" (BCG), is an attenuated mutant of *M. bovis* which has been carried through several hundred serial cultures on unfavorable, bile-containing media. As a result, it multiplies in the host to a limited extent, causing at most only minor and transient lesions. BCG has been used to immunize humans against tuberculosis, and has remained avirulent for over 40 years.[27]

One of the most characteristic features of mycobacteria has been their unusually high lipid content (20% to 40% of the dry weight). The mycobacteria, which replicate slowly and may remain dormant for prolonged periods of time, can be eradicated by drugs only when the organisms are replicating.

In humans, *M. tuberculosis* can be found in open cavities, closed caseous lesions, and within macrophages. Unlike *Mycobacterium leprae*, *M. tuberculosis* is not found inside cells other than macrophages and polymorphonuclear cells. *In vitro*, however, the microorganisms readily penetrated all cell lines tested. In cultured human macrophages, the organisms multiply within membrane-enclosed vesicles which are generally thought to be acidic. Immunochemical experiments by Crawle et al.[28] demonstrated that any observed acidity has been associated with killed and not living mycobacteria, and that the macrophage vesicles containing mycobacteria were not acidic. Chloroquine, a lysomotropic base which can be used to raise the phagolysosomal pH, was found effective when used alone or in combination with other antimycobacterial agents in inhibiting intracellular mycobacteria residing in the vacuoles.[29]

Within macrophages, *M. tuberculosis* produces large amounts of lipoarabinomannan, a highly immunogenic, cell wall-associated glycolipid.[30] Lipoarabinomannan is a potent inhibitor of interferon (IFN)-γ-mediated activation of murine macrophages by scavenging cytotoxic oxygen-free radicals. In addition, lipoarabinomannan inhibits the protein kinase C activity and blocks the transcriptional activation of IFN-γ-inducible genes in human macrophage-like cells. The adverse activity of lipoarabinomannan may contribute to the observed persistence of mycobacteria within mononuclear phagocytes.

8.4.2 DIAGNOSTIC AND DIFFERENTIATION PROCEDURES FOR *M. TUBERCULOSIS*

New diagnostic and differentiation procedures are being developed based on the presence of antigens exclusive to *M. tuberculosis*.[31] These antigens were initially identified by Western blots using sera from patients with active pulmonary tuberculosis against sonic extracts from *M. tuberculosis* and *M. bovis* BCG.

Among the several proteins present in *M. tuberculosis* but absent in the *M. bovis* BCG sonic extracts and currently under investigation, the denoted MTP40 antigen has been extensively studied. In addition to having the nucleotide sequence of the *mtp*40 gene being elucidated, hybridization studies have shown that this DNA fragment is also exclusive to *M. tuberculosis*.[31] Based on this genomic fragment, a polymerase chain reaction (PCR)-based diagnostic test which allowed the specific identification of a minimum of 10 fragments of *M. tuberculosis* DNA has been developed and tested on uncultured clinical samples in order to determine its usefulness in routine diagnosis.

Clinico-immunogenetic correlations based on HLA-typing of both patients with infiltrative tuberculosis and healthy controls, have provided evidence for significantly higher incidence of antigens A11, B12, Cw2, DR2, DR5 in patients with infiltrative tuberculosis as compared with the healthy subjects.[32] Furthermore, antigens Cw2 and DR2 were observed to occur more frequently in progressive disease, while in disseminated disease, antigens HLA-DR2 were more prevalent.

A radiometric method using the BACTEC 460-TB apparatus has been developed to differentiate between various clinical mycobacterial isolates belonging either to *Mycobacterium tuberculosis* complex (comprised of *M. tuberculosis*, *M. bovis*, *M. bovis* BCG, and *M. africanum*) or nontuberculous mycobacteria.[33]

A number of PCR-based assays have been developed for detection of mycobacteria.[34-38] In a related study, a rapid thin-layer chromatographic method for detection of 2,3,6,6'-tetraacyltrehalose-2'-sulfate (sulfolipid I) from *M. tuberculosis* was found to be a simple and rapid procedure for the identification of mycobacteria in a clinical setting.[39] Evans et al.[40] used acridinium ester-labeled DNA probes to identify *M. tuberculosis* directly from primary BACTEC cultures. A coagglutination technique using lipoarabinomannan as a diagnostic test for tuberculosis was also developed.[41] Measurement of IgG antibody response to A60 antigen as a means for serological diagnosis of pulmonary tuberculosis has also been investigated.[42,43]

DNA amplification of three *M. tuberculosis*-specific DNA sequences, IS6110, the 65-kDa antigen, and the MPB64, by PCR have been used for rapid diagnosis of tuberculous meningitis.[44] The DNA sequences amplified were a 123-bp region of the IS6110 insertion elements which occur in multiple copies in the mycobacterial genome, a 240-bp region (nts 460–700) from the MPB64 protein coding gene, and the 383–bp region of the 65–kDa heat shock protein (HSP) antigen. The main drawback of the proposed DNA amplification procedure has been its extreme sensitivity, giving rise to false positive results, especially the repeat copy sequences generated from IS6110 and the 65-kDa HSP (62% and 33%, respectively).

Sugita et al.[45] have combined PCR technique with dot-blot hybridization to diagnose tuberculous lymphadenitis that had developed following treatment with systemic prednisolone.

The clinical efficiency of the amplified *M. tuberculosis* direct test for the diagnosis of pulmonary tuberculosis has been examined by Bradley et al.[46] The test, which is based on a nucleic acid amplification technique, when used directly on processed clinical specimens and in conjunction with routine smear and culture, may become a useful rapid diagnostic tool for suspected pulmonary tuberculosis.

Nelson and Taber[47] have used a fluorochrome stain, and Bertolaccini et al.[48] suggested a [67]-gallium-citrate scan for early diagnosis of pericarditis.[49]

Choy et al.[50] proposed an assay measuring the synovial fluid lymphocyte proliferation to tuberculin protein antigens as a diagnostic tool in patients with tuberculous and reactive arthritis.

8.4.3 *Mycobacterium tuberculosis* Infections in AIDS Patients

It has been well documented that HIV-infected persons are at particular risk of infections with *M. tuberculosis*, and the course of the disease in such patients is accelerated.[51] It is believed that tuberculosis may be the most common opportunistic infection and the leading cause of death among patients infected with HIV worldwide, even though a number of retrospective and prospective studies have shown that the disease may be treatable and often preventable.[52]

While the disease affects predominantly the alveoli of the lung,[53] extrapulmonary involvement is not unusual in HIV-positive patients, especially those with low $CD4^+$ counts where the extrapulmonary manifestations may occur in as many as half of the cases.[54,55] In this regard, the lymphatic system has been frequently involved.[56] Disseminated cutaneous tuberculosis with concurrent pulmonary infection in AIDS patients has been rare and may present as a febrile illness and an abnormal chest radiograph, as well as with the development of widespread cutaneous tuberculous pustules.[57]

Berenguer et al.[58] have found that while the incidence of tuberculous meningitis has been higher among HIV-infected persons, the clinical outcome of the disease has been similar to that in non-HIV-infected patients. However, Fortun et al.[59] reported a fatal outcome following treatment failure for tuberculous meningitis of two HIV-positive patients.

In a retrospective clinical review of all cases of tuberculous meningitis identified among adults over a 12-year period, Yechoor et al.[60] have determined that the majority of patients (65%) were HIV-seropositive — fever and abnormal mental status were commonly observed (83% and 71%, respectively). In another case of neurologic involvement due to *M. tuberculosis*, an AIDS patient has developed a yellow-white chorioretinal infiltrate with indistinct borders and mild vitreitis of the eye most likely caused by mycobacteria.[61]

Martinez-Vazquez et al.[62] have conducted a comparative study to determine the clinical characteristics of cerebral tuberculoma in patients with and without HIV infection. Thus, while disease-associated seizures were observed in HIV-negative individuals, in HIV-positive patients this finding was absent. Instead, all patients studied (n = 4) had headache and fever and their CSF specimens showed the presence of lymphocytic meningitis. HIV-infected persons, in which the cerebral tuberculoma was the result of dissemination, presented with spontaneous hypodense cerebral lesions; in contrast, the HIV-negative patients showed hyperdense cerebral lesions.

Two cases of splenic abscess due to *M. tuberculosis* in AIDS patients have been described by Salazar et al.[63] The patients presented with peripheral polyadenopathies and enhancement of hiliary and paratracheal lymph nodes, and multiple hypoechenogenic and hypodense splenic lesions.

While most of the clinical symptoms of tuberculosis (cough, weight loss, fever, night sweats, fatigue)[64,65] may be present, they are not always indicative of tuberculosis in patients with AIDS. Calpe et al.[66] have used routine fibrobronchoscopy to determine the frequency of endobronchial tuberculosis in HIV-positive patients.

Recurrence of HIV-related tuberculosis may be due to either relapse to the original infection, subtherapeutic concentrations of antituberculosis agents, or reinfection with a different strain of *M. tuberculosis*.[67-69]

One serious problem confronting clinicians treating HIV-positive patients with tuberculosis has been the high incidence of multiple drug-resistant strains of *M. tuberculosis* compounding the mortality rate, which can reach 80%. In addition, such cases usually progress very rapidly.

Inadequate treatment has been thought to be one major reason for the development of multidrug-resistant tuberculosis, especially likely to occur when single drugs have been added to a failing regimen.[70] To avoid potential pitfalls, when initiating treatment in patients with confirmed multiple drug-resistant tuberculosis, both the treatment history and the *in vitro* susceptibilities of the patient's tuberculous strains should be thoroughly evaluated — the selected regimen should include between four and seven antimycobacterial agents, including such drugs as pyrazinamide, ethambutol, streptomycin, ofloxacin, ciprofloxacin, ethionamide, cycloserine, capreomycin, and *p*-aminosalicylic acid (PAS).[71]

8.4.4   HOST DEFENSE AGAINST *MYCOBACTERIUM TUBERCULOSIS*

The spread of the AIDS epidemic, coupled with the reemergence of tuberculosis, has presented the scientific and medical communities with an enormous public health challenge that rekindled the interest in the mechanisms by which the immune system may control mycobacterial infections.

There is a sequence of events that follows intracellular penetration of *M. tuberculosis* into phagocytic cells. This sequence includes the activation of accessory cells to trigger the host immune response, the activation of various effector cells and cytotoxic lymphocytes, and the enhanced production of cytokines. Wallis et al.[72] have identified two fractions of mycobacterial proteins (molecular weight of 20,000 and 46,000, respectively) which have consistently stimulated the production of interleukin-1 and the tumor necrosis factor-α (TNF-α) by monocytes. The increased levels of these two cytokines may cause fever and cachexia that have been readily associated with tuberculosis.

Although the relationship between host and mycobacteria is still not very well understood, recent evidence has shown that in the presence of antimycobacterial drugs and normal host defense mechanisms, the tubercle bacilli are converted into metabolically inactive, non-acid fast (NAF) granular forms. The latter represent cell wall-deficient variants which remain dormant but may also revert back to the parent, acid-fast bacilli in the case of immunocompromised patients, thus causing the disease to persist in spite of chemotherapy.[73] Experimental evidence has suggested that humoral (B cell) responses in tuberculosis will precede the protective cell-mediated immunity. In the majority of patients, the humoral response is characterized by an initial rise of specific IgM immunoglobulins, followed by an increase in the IgG production during the subclinical infection stage. Eventually, the B cell responses are suppressed as protective cell-mediated immunity is established during the protracted subclinical phase of infection.[74] In addition to the well-known immunologic role of T cells bearing the conventional $\alpha\beta$ T cell receptor, recent studies by Janis et al.[75] have indicated that $\gamma\delta$ T cells may also play a distinct role in generating the primary immune response to mycobacteria. Hubbard et al.[76] have studied the memory T cell-mediated resistance to *M. tuberculosis* infection in innately susceptible and resistant mice.

The growth of *M. tuberculosis* in human macrophages was investigated at both ambient oxygen concentrations (5% CO_2 and 95% air, corresponding to 20% O_2 or 140 mmHg PO_2) and concentrations corresponding to tissue levels (5% CO_2 and 5% CO_2 in nitrogen balance, corresponding to 36 mmHg PO_2).[77] When cultivated at lower PO_2 concentrations, macrophages had an increased glycolytic (but decreased oxidative) metabolism. Upon stimulation, such macrophages had a better preserved ability to respond with an increased production of superoxide anion. Following infection with *M. tuberculosis*, macrophages cultivated at lower PO_2 concentrations permitted significantly less growth of the pathogen than macrophages cultured at higher PO_2 levels. Crude lymphokines, recombinant IFN-γ, or recombinant TNF-α have not consistently affected the growth of mycobacteria in macrophages cultured at either high or low oxygen pressure. The observed reduced growth of mycobacteria cultivated in macrophages at physiologic PO_2 levels may explain the preferential localization of tuberculous lesions in body areas, such as the lung apex, where the tissue levels of PO_2 are high.

Results from a related study by Chan et al.[78] have demonstrated that murine macrophages activated by IFN-γ and lipopolysaccharide or TNF-α inhibited the growth and also killed *M. tuberculosis*. The observed effect was independent of the capacity of macrophages to produce reactive oxygen intermediates. The latter finding was later confirmed by experiments showing that various oxygen radical scavengers (superoxide dismutase, catalase, mannitol, and diazabicyclooctane) did not affect the antimycobacterial activity of macrophages. Similarly, O'Brien et al.[79] have also demonstrated that guinea pig alveolar macrophages eradicated *M. tuberculosis in vitro* independently of susceptibility to hydrogen peroxide or triggering of the respiratory burst. Based on such findings, it would be unlikely that reactive oxygen intermediates play any substantial role in killing mycobacteria.

In contrast, the antimycobacterial activity of these macrophages strongly correlated with the induction of L-arginine-dependent generation of reactive nitrogen intermediates (NO, NO_2, and HNO_2). The action of such nitrogen-containing species may be one major effector mechanism by which activated murine macrophages inhibit the growth and kill virulent *M. tuberculosis*. Data by Denis[80] also indicated that IFN-γ-treated murine macrophages restricted the growth of *M. tuberculosis* by promoting the release of reactive inorganic nitrogen species. Involvement of reactive nitrogen intermediates in the antimicrobial activity of human macrophages, however, has not yet been clearly demonstrated.

Studying the macrophage cell line J-774, Rastogi and Blom-Potar[81] have demonstrated that addition of IFN-γ, 1,25-dihydroxyvitamin D_3 and lipopeptide RP-56142 to macrophages increased their ability to kill intracellularly multiplying *M. tuberculosis* and *M. avium*.

Jones et al.[82] found that the mechanism by which neutrophils exert their bactericidal effect against *M. tuberculosis* is independent of the oxygen metabolic burst.

When tested on monocytes, sulfatide, a lipid from *M. tuberculosis*, blocked the priming for enhanced release of superoxide anion (O_2^-) by such macrophage-activating factors as lipopolysaccharide (LPS), IFN-γ, IL-1β, TNF-α, and muramyl dipeptide.[83] In the presence of LPS, sulfatide also caused an increased secretion of IL-1β and TNF-α into the monocyte culture medium. Furthermore, sulfatide altered the pattern of phosphorylation of monocyte proteins; consequently, the monocytes showed a decreased protein kinase C activity, implicating this enzyme as a part of the mechanism of priming. By the scope of its activity (increasing the levels of both IL-1β and TNF-α, which are known to promote formation of granulomata, and blocking the priming for enhanced release of O_2^-), it is possible that sulfatide has a role in the pathogenesis of *M. tuberculosis*.

Invoking delayed hypersensitivity reaction by *M. tuberculosis* has been an important element in the diagnosis of the disease. Yet, many patients with tuberculosis remain anergic. Fibronectin, a protein secreted by activated T cells, was closely associated with the initiation of delayed-type hypersensitivity reactions. Addressing the specific lack of immune response in anergic patients, Godfrey et al.[84] presented evidence indicating that mycobacterial antigen 85 (Ag85) proteins were capable of strongly binding plasma fibronectin, thereby inhibiting its ability to potentiate delayed hypersensitivity reaction during mycobacterial infections. Using culture filtrate antigens of *M. tuberculosis*, Espitia et al.[85] have demonstrated strong fibronectin binding (in 55.9% of tuberculosis sera) by a 30- to 31-kDa protein (Fn 30-31) that was also found present in *M. leprae*. To this end, Thole et al.[86] have performed molecular and immunologic analyses of Fn 30-31.

In the context of host immune responses against mycobacteria, the lymphocyte response has been an essential part of the human defense against these organisms. Thus, in human pulmonary tuberculosis, CD4[+] lymphocytes were found in substantially increased numbers in the pleural fluid, but relatively depleted in the blood. In the bronchoalveolar lavage fluid their numbers varied widely in localized pulmonary and miliary tuberculosis but were highest in lavage fluid from patients with miliary tuberculosis. In the latter case, the increase was the result of an increase in CD8[+] lymphocytes, which were also increased in the blood.[87]

The virulence of mycobacteria appears to be inversely related to the organisms' ability to provoke the production of cytokines in infected hosts. Consequently, the presence of TNF-α and IFN-γ has been of great importance, and mycobacterial polysaccharides seemed to be the major constituents responsible for stimulation of these cytokines.[88] Barnes et al.[89] examined the patterns of cytokine production by *Mycobacterium*-reactive human T cell clones in order to evaluate their functional capacity as part of the immune response towards the pathogen. Nine of the 11 T cell clones bearing α, β or γ/δ receptors produced both Th1 and Th2 cytokines, a pattern resembling that of murine Th0 clones. The most frequent was the secretion of IFN-γ, TNF-α, and IL-1, in combination with IL-2, IL-5, or both. Although IL-4 was not observed in cell culture supernatants, IL-4 mRNA was detected by polymerase chain reaction amplification in two of six clones. These markedly elevated concentrations of TNF-α in clone supernatants, independent of other cytokines produced, was a rather striking finding. Further experiments have also suggested that TNF-α produced by T cells may be an important co-stimulus for the granulomatous host response to mycobacteria. Although studies in experimental animal models have indicated that γ/δ T cells may have taken part in the immune response against mycobacteria, evidence of their participation during the course of the disease is still fragmentary.[90]

Friedland et al.[91] have investigated the plasma concentrations of TNF-α, IL-6, and IL-8 before and after maximal lipopolysaccharide stimulation *ex vivo* of whole blood leukocytes from Zambian patients. Thirty-two patients with nonfatal tuberculosis (25 of whom were seropositive for HIV) were followed for 9 months. Concurrent HIV infection resulted in persistently decreased IL-6 secretions *ex vivo*, although the erythrocyte sedimentation rate remained high. Overall, after antibiotic therapy *in vivo*, the IL-8 secretion *ex vivo* increased, thus lending credence to the hypothesis that IL-8 may play a role in immunity to tuberculosis.[91]

In an overall assessment, the effects of various T cell-produced cytokines may be not only immunoregulatory but also immunopathologic, thus mediating some of the clinical manifestations of the disease.

Parronchi et al.[92] have found that IL-4 and IFN (both -α and -γ) exerted opposite regulatory effects on the development of the cytolytic potential by Th1 or Th2 human T cell clones. IL-4 when added in bulk culture before cloning suppressed not only the differentiation of T cells specific for the purified protein derivative (PPD) from *M. tuberculosis* into Th1-like cell lines and clones, but also the development of their cytolytic potential. The observed inhibitory effect of IL-4 on the development of PPD-specific T cell lines with both Th1 cytokine profile and cytolytic potential was dependent on early addition of IL-4 to the bulk cultures. In contrast, the addition to bulk cultures of IFN-γ enhanced both the cytolytic activity of PPD-specific T cell lines and the proportion of PPD-specific T cell clones with cytolytic activity. These and other results suggested that the majority of human T cell clones that produce IFN-γ but not IL-4 (Th1-like), as well as T cell clones that produce IFN-γ in combination with IL-4 (Th0-like), are cytolytic. Furthermore, the results strongly indicated that addition of either IFN-α or IFN-γ, or IL-4 to bulk cultures before cloning may influence not only the cytokine profile of human CD4+ T cell clones but also their cytolytic potential. Kawamura et al.[93] have presented experimental data showing an increased ability of protective CD4+ T cells to produce IFN-γ upon stimulation with mycobacterial antigen.

Incubation of human monocytes with crude lymphokines in combination with calcitriol (1,25-dihydroxyvitamin D_3) led to total stasis of the growth of *M. tuberculosis*.[94] Similarly, a combination of recombinant cytokines (IFN-γ, TNF-α) and calcitriol have induced a significant amount of intramonocyte killing of the mycobacteria. While calcitriol alone at doses of 10^{-7} to 10^{-9} M promoted significantly the ability of human monocytes to suppress intracellular growth, various crude lymphokines and recombinant cytokines (IFN-γ, CSF-1, IL-1, IL-3, and IL-6) alone, failed to stimulate antimycobacterial properties.

Another cytokine, the granulocyte-macrophage colony-stimulating factor (GM-CSF), suppressed the intracellular growth of *M. tuberculosis in vitro* in human monocyte-derived macrophages.[95] However, TNF-α, alone, was the most effective cytokine in potentiating intracellular growth suppression of the pathogen in human macrophages.[96]

IFN-γ and clofazimine had a synergistic effect on phagocyte functions.[97,98] At concentrations of 25 U/ml and 0.3 µg/ml, respectively, IFN-γ and clofazimine restored the phagocytic functions inhibited by a 25-kDa glycolipoprotein from *M. tuberculosis*; when used alone, the two agents were ineffective.

IL-8 was found to be a chemoattractant for activated human lymphocytes in mononuclear cell cultures with anti-CD3 or purified protein derivative of *M. tuberculosis*.[99] The reported data were in agreement with *in vivo* observations that lymphocytes that migrate selectively into inflammatory sites have been activated.

Studies have been carried out to examine the effects of supernatants derived from CD8+ lymphocytes treated with high-molecular-weight components of *M. tuberculosis* on cytokine production.[100] The supernatants increased the production of IL-4 and IL-6, but inhibited the production of IL-1β, TNF-α, IL-2, and IFN-γ by monocytes and lymphocytes. The suppression of IL-1β and TNF-α was due to increased levels of IL-6 in the supernatants of nonadherent lymphocytes incubated with mycobacterial components. Such findings strongly supported the possibility that mycobacterial components may inhibit host cellular responses by manipulating the host's cytokine network. Theisen-Popp et al.[101] reported that heat-killed *M. tuberculosis* was a strong inducer of IL-6 production by spleen cells *in vitro*.

It has been shown that normal human cells of types that were likely to be involved in tuberculosis lesions have become much more sensitive to the cytotoxic effect of TNF-α after exposure to *M. tuberculosis*.[102] For example, fibroblasts, after taking up live (but not killed) *M. tuberculosis* strain H37Rv, have developed greatly increased sensitivity to the toxic effect of TNF-α, regardless of whether the cell line was inherently sensitive to TNF-α or not.[103] The possibility has been raised that some virulent mycobacterial strains may acquire the capacity to produce a factor(s) capable of distorting the normal protective function of TNF-α, thus rendering it toxic to host tissues and leading to the classical immunopathology of tuberculous lesions.

In continuing studies to elucidate the role of host immune defenses against mycobacteria, the intracellular growth of *M. tuberculosis* strain H37Rv was compared in human peripheral blood monocytes and in cultured macrophages.[104] The cells were treated with 300 U of human rIFN-γ either 48 h prior to phagocytosis or after infection; in some cases, indomethacin (a potent inhibitor of prostaglandin E_2 synthesis) was added immediately after the infection of macrophages. IFN-γ pretreatment of monocytes resulted in approximately 50% decrease in mycobacterial uptake, but had no effect on macrophages, suggesting that the latter cells may have been more efficient in controlling the intracellular growth of *M. tuberculosis*. The overall effect of IFN-γ was to endow both monocytes and macrophages with significant bacteriostatic activity that was further potentiated by the addition of indomethacin.

The effect of HIV on the mycobacterial antibody production was investigated by Barrera et al.[105] A decreased responsiveness of humoral immune mechanisms to *M. tuberculosis* was observed during the progression of HIV infections to AIDS.

Geluk et al.[106] have conducted functional analysis of DR17(DR3)-restricted mycobacterial T cell epitopes that revealed the presence of a DR17-binding motif which may encourage the design of allele-specific competitor peptides for use as potential immunotherapeutics.

The addition of hydrocortisone has impaired the enhanced antimycobacterial activity of macrophages activated with the BCG-purified derivative (BCG-PPD).[107] While the release of H_2O_2 was not affected by BCG-PPD, the production of NO_2^- was inhibited.

Table 8.1 is an illustration of cells and mediators involved in the host immune responses to tuberculosis.

TABLE 8.1
Cells and Cytokines Involved in the Host Immune Responses in Tuberculosis

Cells	Cytokines
Macrophages	Interferon (IFN)-γ
Neutrophils	Tumor necrosis factor (TNF)-α
	Interleukin (IL)-1
	IL-4
	Granulocyte-macrophage colony-stimulating factor (GM-CSF)

8.4.5 STUDIES ON THERAPEUTICS

In vivo studies by Gangadharam et al.[108,109] have demonstrated that a single implant of polylactic-co-glycolic acid (PLGA) copolymer containing isoniazid provided a sustained release of the drug for up to 6 weeks with drug levels being comparable to those obtained by daily medication with free isoniazid. The implant caused no local or systemic toxicity.

The effect of pyrazinamide has been mostly bacteriostatic with little bactericidal activity against *M. tuberculosis* which has been grown in broth medium at pH 5.6.[110] However, when the organisms are cultured in 7H12 broth at pH 4.8 to 5.0, they usually convert into a semidormant state that is especially vulnerable to pyrazinamide; thus, at concentrations of 50 µg/ml, the drug decreased the number of viable bacteria by 1000-fold.[111]

It has been known that strains susceptible to pyrazinamide transformed the drug into pyrazinoic acid with the help of a bacterial enzyme, pyrazinamidase. In contrast, drug-resistant strains lack this enzyme. To examine the activity of pyrazinoic acid, comparative studies with pyrazinamidase-positive or -negative strains were conducted in cultured human macrophages and in broth BACTEC system with 7H12 medium at pH 6.0.[112,113] It has been found that while the addition of pyrazinoic acid did not inhibit mycobacteria in cultured macrophages, at very high concentrations, pyrazinoic acid suppressed the pathogen in the BACTEC broth. In another effort to elucidate the mechanism of action of pyrazinoic acid, Heifets et al.[114] studied its ability to lower the pH of the medium in conjunction with the observed inhibition of mycobacterial growth. Depending on its concentration, pyrazinoic acid did lower the pH of 7H12 broth medium to 5.8 and 4.5, at 120 and 960 µg/ml, respectively. At an adjusted pH of 5.6, the pyrazinoic acid also elicited a specific antimicrobial effect, suggesting that its antimycobacterial activity may be a combined effect of specific activity and the ability to lower the acidity of the environment below the limits of tolerance of the mycobacteria.

Gangadharam et al.[115] examined the effects of exposure time, drug concentration, and temperature on the activity of ethambutol against *M. tuberculosis* in a series of dynamic *in vitro* studies. The maximal bactericidal activity of ethambutol was observed at 37°C, at a drug concentration of 10 μg/ml, and with constant contact with the pathogen.

Yamori et al.[116] have found differences in the bacteriostatic and bactericidal activities of rifampicin, isoniazid, streptomycin, enviomycin, and ethambutol against various mycobacteria in different growth phases. For example, while isoniazid, streptomycin, and rifampicin were all bactericidal against *M. tuberculosis*, the activity of isoniazid was most potent in the log phase.

Studies of antimycobacterial drugs in Middlebrook 7H10 (a susceptibility testing medium) have shown acceptable stability when stored at 3 to 7°C for 1 month. However, during incubation at 37°C, approximately 50% of the activities of isoniazid, ethionamide, ethambutol, cycloserine, and rifampin were lost after periods ranging from 2 to 4 d (e.g., ethambutol) to 2 weeks (e.g., rifampin).[117]

8.4.5.1 Antimycobacterial Antibiotics

Dhillon et al.[118] investigated the therapeutic efficacy of two long-acting rifamycins, rifapentine and FCE 22807, in a mouse model of experimental tuberculosis caused by *M. tuberculosis* strain H37Rv, by counting viable bacilli in the spleen. Two weeks after infection, a daily treatment comprising isoniazid (25 mg/kg), rifampicin (10 mg/kg), and pyrazinamide (150 mg/kg) was commenced for a period of 6 weeks. Next, the mice were divided into groups given rifapentine and FCE 22807 at intervals of 1, 2, or 3 weeks with spleen counts following 18 and 24 weeks of chemotherapy. Experimental results have demonstrated that rifapentine when administered once a week at doses of 16 mg/kg, elicited a rapid sterilization, but was less effective at 10 mg/kg, and completely inactive at 6.25 mg/kg. Regimens of rifapentine given every 2 or 3 weeks were less effective.

In other experiments, the activities of rifapentine and FCE 22807 were compared; each drug was administered at doses of 12 and 8.0 mg/kg. Although the effects of both drugs were similar, at doses of 8.0 mg/kg given every 2 or 3 weeks, FCE 22807 was slightly more effective than rifapentine. Dhillon and Mitchison[119] have also determined the activities of rifabutin, FCE 22807, rifapentine, and rifampin against *M. tuberculosis in vitro* in 7H-9 medium containing no Tween 80. The same investigators have also examined the *in vitro* activities of FCE 22807 and another long-acting rifampicin analog, CGP 40/469A (SPA-S-565) against *M. tuberculosis*.[120] While their minimal inhibitory concentration (MIC) values were four times lower when compared with rifampicin, neither drug was particularly active against rifampicin-resistant strains of the pathogen.

The therapeutic efficacies of three combinations, isoniazid, rifampin, and pyrazinamide; isoniazid and rifampin; and rifampin and pyrazinamide, have been evaluated in mice inoculated with the H37Rv strain of *M. tuberculosis*.[121] At the end of the initial 6-month period of chemotherapy, all three combinations were highly effective in reducing the number of colony-forming units (CFU) in the spleen. While the bactericidal activities of isoniazid/rifampin/pyrazinamide and isoniazid/rifampin were similar, that of rifampin/pyrazinamide was significantly greater (2 $\log_{10}$ more killing during the initial phase and a 30% lower relapse rate). The overall results from the initial and the follow-up periods of treatment indicated the presence of antagonism between isoniazid and the combination rifampin/pyrazinamide. As a result, the activity of the combination isoniazid/rifampin/pyrazinamide was reduced to the same level as that of isoniazid/rifampin, thus compromising the benefit conferred by the addition of pyrazinamide to the combination. Preliminary pharmacokinetic experiments have indicated that the mechanism of the antagonism very likely involved a pharmacological interaction between isoniazid and rifampin, although a microbiological interaction might have also been possible.

The antituberculosis activity of rifampin was substantially increased after it was encapsulated in egg phosphatidylcholine liposomes.[122] A further increase in the therapeutic potency has been observed when tuftsin, a macrophage activator tetrapeptide, was grafted on the surface of the drug-loaded liposomes. Moreover, intermittent treatment with this formulation proved to be significantly more beneficial than continuous medication — when given twice weekly for 2 weeks, this regimen was at least 2000 times more effective than the free drug in lowering the load of lung bacilli in infected animals.

Kuze[123] has reviewed the synthesis and antimycobacterial activities of a number of novel 3′-hydroxy-5′-alkylpiperazinylbenzoxazinorifamycins (KRMs), namely KRM-1648, KRM-1657, KRM-1668, KRM-1674, and KRM-2312. The MIC_{90} values of these five KRMs against 20 clinical isolates of *M. tuberculosis* were between 0.035 and 0.07 μg/ml. By comparison, the MIC_{90} of rifampicin was 1.25 μg/ml.[124] Hirata et al.[125] compared KRM-1648 with rifampin and rifabutin against 30 fresh isolates of *M. tuberculosis* and reported MIC_{90} and MIC_{50} values of 2.0 and 0.016 μg/ml, >128 and 4.0 μg/ml, and 8.0 and 0.125 μg/ml, respectively. However, a correlational analysis of the MICs showed the presence of cross-resistance of the clinical isolates to KRM-1648 and either rifampin or rifabutin. KRM-1648 and rifampin at concentrations of 1.0 to 10 μg/ml almost completely inhibited the bacterial growth of rifampin-susceptible strains (H37Rv, Kurono, and Fujii) of *M. tuberculosis* phagocytized in macrophage-derived J774.1 cells.

The *in vivo* activity of KRM-1648 has also been the subject of several studies.[125-128] When KRM-1648 was given to *M. tuberculosis*-infected mice at 5.0 to 20 mg/kg by gavage once daily, 6 d per week from day 1 after infection, it was much more effective than rifampin against infections induced in mice by the rifampin-sensitive Kurono strain.

Reddy et al.[126] have examined the activity of KRM-1648 against *M. tuberculosis* in C57BL/6 mice infected with either a drug-susceptible but virulent strain (H37Rv) or a multidrug-resistant strain (2230), and the results obtained were compared to those of rifabutin and rifampin tested under the same conditions. Treatment started 1 d postinfection or after 2 weeks following infection (i.e., established infection) with 20 mg/kg of each of the three drugs. All compounds tested prevented mortality for up to 28 weeks of observation compared to untreated control mice which died by week 4. Analysis of the CFU counts revealed that KRM-1648 and rifabutin were superior to rifampin against the drug-susceptible strain of *M. tuberculosis,* which was completely eradicated from the lungs after 12 weeks of treatment. However, residual organisms started to appear in the spleens 6 weeks after cessation of therapy with rifabutin and 16 weeks after KRM-1648 treatment. In mice infected with the multidrug-resistant strain of *M. tuberculosis,* which was susceptible to KRM-1648 *in vitro,* all three drugs appeared not to have any activity.[126] In a separate study,[127] KRM-1648 at 20 mg/kg was found superior to rifampin and rifabutin (both given at 20 mg/kg) in *M. tuberculosis*-infected mice. The combinations of KRM-1648 and pyrazinamide, and KRM-1648 and isoniazid, proved to be the most active ones when tested in the same model.

A new rifamycin derivative, the 3-(4-cinnamylpiperazinyl iminomethyl)rifamycin SV (T9) has been tested against 20 susceptible and drug-resistant strains of *M. tuberculosis.*[129] The rifampin-susceptible strains were inhibited at $MIC_{90} = 0.25$ μg/ml or less; the corresponding value for rifampin was 0.5 μg/ml. The MICs of T9 against rifampin-resistant strains were also lower. Furthermore, when tested *in vivo* T9 showed excellent activity in both the lungs and spleens of C57BL/6 mice infected with strain H37Rv of *M. tuberculosis*; again, rifampin was less active.

The activities of meropenem and imipenem, two carbapenem antibiotics, against *M. tuberculosis* were evaluated *in vitro* by using a BACTEC 460 radiometric apparatus.[130] One problem that has been confronted while studying the therapeutic effect of these antibiotics is their potential instability over the prolonged incubation period which is required for the slow-growing mycobacteria. It was found that both meropenem and imipenem lost activity in the test medium in time. This was circumvented by daily dosing of the antibiotic vials with calculated amounts of the test compounds that led to a considerable increase in the observed activity.

Two patients with multidrug-resistant tuberculosis were successfully treated with the addition of amoxicillin–clavulanic acid combination to a second-line antimycobacterial drugs.[131] Apparently, the presence of clavulanic acid, a β-lactamase inhibitor, acted by neutralizing the β-lactamase which is produced by *M. tuberculosis* and may contribute to the development of resistance against β-lactam antibiotics. That conclusion has been corroborated by Zhang et al.,[132] who have found that in

10 clinical isolates of *M. tuberculosis* strain H3Rv, β-lactamase was produced intracellularly. Furthermore, when exposed to BRL 42715, a new β-lactamase inhibitor, mycobacterial β-lactamase enzyme preparations have been highly susceptible, with $I_{50} = 0.0001$ µg/ml. The preparations were also susceptible to both clavulanic acid ($I_{50} = 0.05$ µg/ml) and a synergistic clavulanic acid–amoxicillin combination.[132]

When tested in two different mouse experiments, a 6-week course of clarithromycin at 200 mg/kg given six times weekly did not produce any bactericidal or bacteriostatic effects against *M. tuberculosis;* the antiobiotic inhibited 12 mycobacterial strains *in vitro* ($MIC_{50} = 64$ µg/ml and $MIC_{90} \geq 128$ µg/ml).[133] In a separate study, Luna-Herrera et al.[134] investigated the antituberculosis activity of clarithromycin *in vitro*, in macrophages, and in C57BL/6 mice. While the MIC values were high (4.0 to >16 µg/ml), inside J774A.1 macrophages, clarithromycin exerted potent activity and was synergistic with rifampin against some strains of *M. tuberculosis* susceptible or resistant to isoniazid and rifampin. In the mouse experiments, CFU data for lungs and spleens revealed that clarithromycin was inferior to both isoniazid and streptomicin, even though it showed activity against the drug-sensitive H37Rv strain by reducing the mortality rate for up to 8 weeks of observation.[134]

Addition of clarithromycin[133,134] and its biologically active 14-hydroxy metabolite (at fixed concentrations of 2.0 and 0.5 µg/ml, respectively) to various combinations comprised of isoniazid, rifampin, and ethambutol resulted in 4- to 32-fold reductions in the value of MICs of the latter three drugs, and made resistant strains susceptible. The fractional inhibitory concentrations for all strains were in the 0.23 to 0.50 range, suggesting a synergistic interaction between the isoniazid/rifampin/ethambutol combination and clarithromycin/14-hydroxyclarithromycin.[135]

The *in vivo* activity of paromomycin against susceptible and multidrug-resistant strains of *M. tuberculosis* has been investigated in C57BL/6 and beige mice.[136] Against drug-susceptible strains, paromomycin when given at 100 and 200 mg/kg was significantly less active than isoniazid (25 mg/kg; $p < .0005$) in reducing the mean log CFU in the lungs, livers, and spleens of infected mice. When evaluated against multidrug-resistant strains, paromomycin at 200 mg/kg was effective in reducing the mean log CFU of an isolate resistant to isoniazid, rifampin, and streptomycin.

The antimycobacterial activity of tuberactinomycin against 114 clinical isolates of *M. tuberculosis* was tested *in vitro* in Lowenstein-Jensen medium.[137] At concentrations of 25 mg/l and 50 mg/l, respectively, 83.3% and 13.2% of the strains were susceptible. There was a cross-resistance in 53.6% of the strains between tuberactinomycin and kanamycin.

Bleomycin, a known antitumor antibiotic, was reported to be also effective *in vitro* and *in vivo* (guinea pigs) against *M. tuberculosis;* the MIC value of the drug was 0.1 mg/l.[138]

Capreomycin, a cyclic peptide antibiotic with tuberculostatic properties, is usually injected intramuscularly at doses of 15 mg/kg, five times weekly. The dose and/or frequency of administration may be lowered if renal insuffiency is observed.[139]

8.4.5.2 Fluoroquinolone Derivatives

The anti-infective activity of nalidixic acid, the prototype drug of the first generation of quinolone antimicrobials, is somewhat limited in scope and confined exclusively to aerobic and Gram-negative microorganisms. Introduction of a fluorine atom at the 6-position resulted in the development of a second generation of quinolone derivatives having an improved antibacterial spectrum that also included activity against Gram-positive and aerobic bacteria.[140-142]

The *in vitro* activities of ofloxacin and ciprofloxacin against 50 strains of *M. tuberculosis* were evaluated in Lowenstein-Jensen medium — the corresponding MIC_{90} values were 1.0 and 4.0 mg/l, respectively.[143] Previously, Yew et al.[144] tested the activity of ofloxacin against 159 clinical isolates of *M. tuberculosis* and determined MIC values of 0.63 to 1.25 mg/l against 147 (92%) of these isolates.

The MIC values of ciprofloxacin, ofloxacin, and lomefloxacin were determined against 90 strains of *M. tuberculosis* isolated from both AIDS and non-AIDS patients.[145] The MIC_{90} of ofloxacin against *M. tuberculosis* (2.0 mg/l) was three dilutions lower than that of pefloxacin, and well within the range of that drug concentration achievable in man.[146]

Enoxacin showed a moderate *in vitro* activity against *M. tuberculosis* when tested in either modified Saunton or modified Lowenstein-Jensen media with MICs ranging between 1.0 and 8.0 µg/ml.[147] In the same experiments, ofloxacin was superior to enoxacin with MIC values of 0.5 to 2.0 µg/ml. Furthermore, enoxacin when given to mice at doses of 3.0 mg (about 150 mg/kg) daily, or 6.0 mg (about 300 mg/kg) intermittently, was inactive ($p > .05$) against *M. tuberculosis*; by comparison, ofloxacin at the same doses was significantly more effective ($p < .01$).

In a mouse model, pefloxacin at daily doses of up to 150 mg/kg was inactive against *M. tuberculosis*.[146] By comparison, the minimal effective dose of ofloxacin (given either by gavage or with food) to achieve survival was 150 mg/kg daily. Furthermore, the therapeutic efficacy of ofloxacin was also dose-dependent; thus, 300 mg/kg daily by gavage, or 0.4% in the mouse diet, produced a much better therapeutic effect than several lower dose regimens.[146]

The effect of ofloxacin and ciprofloxacin on the intracellular growth of *M. tuberculosis* in the J-774 macrophage cell line has also been examined.[148] The two drugs were highly bactericidal.

The *in vitro* and *in vivo* antimycobacterial efficacy of sparfloxacin (AT-4140) was evaluated by Ji et al.[149] Against 18 clinical isolates of *M. tuberculosis*, the drug showed MIC_{50} and MIC_{90} values of 0.25 and 0.5 mg/l, respectively; these values were one and two dilutions, respectively, lower than the corresponding values of ciprofloxacin and ofloxacin.

In mice infected with the H37Rv strain of *M. tuberculosis*, the minimum effective dose of sparfloxacin was 12.5 mg/kg. Tomioka et al.[150] and Rastogi and Goh[151] have reported similar MICs for sparfloxacin against *M. tuberculosis*.

The antimycobacterial activity of fleroxacin [6,8-difluoro-1-(2-fluoroethyl)-1,4-dihydro-7-(4-methyl-1-piperazinyl)-4-oxo-3-quinolinecarboxylic acid] was evaluated *in vitro* in 7H11 agar medium, and compared to that of ofloxacin; against *M. tuberculosis*, the MIC_{90} of fleroxacin (6.25 mg/l) was comparable to that of ofloxacin.[152] Kawahara et al.[153] have also conducted *in vitro* studies comparing the efficacy of fleroxacin against clinical isolates of *M. tuberculosis* with those of lomefloxacin, spafloxacin, and ofloxacin.

In tests against 18 drug-susceptible strains of *M. tuberculosis*, the MIC_{90} of levofloxacin and ofloxacin were similar.[154] In mice infected with the H37Rv strain, levofloxacin (300 mg/kg) was compared to other antituberculosis drugs, all given six times weekly for 4 weeks. It was equipotent with sparfloxacin (100 mg/kg), but superior to sparfloxacin (50 mg/kg), isoniazid, and ofloxacin (300 mg/kg and 150 mg/kg).[154] When tested in a murine model of tuberculosis, levofloxacin at 100, 200, and 300 mg/kg was less effective than isoniazid and rifampin, but equipotent to ethambutol and pyrazinamide in reducing the number of organisms in the spleens.[155]

Another fluoroquinolone derivative, the 1-cyclopropyl-7-(2,6-dimethyl-4-pyridinyl)-6-fluoro-1,4-dihydro-4-oxo-3-quinolonecarboxylic acid (WIN 57273) was tested for *in vitro* activity against *M. tuberculosis*.[156] The broth-determined MIC values ranged between 1.0 to 4.0 µg/ml. One distinct feature of WIN 57273, as compared to ofloxacin and ciprofloxacin, was its substantially greater activity at lower pH values of the medium.

Y-26611, a fluoroquinolone derivative containing a morpholine moiety at the 7-position, was examined *in vitro* for antimycobacterial activity using the agar dilution method in 7H11 medium.[157] Against 25 strains of *M. tuberculosis*, Y-26611 was more potent than ofloxacin with a MIC_{90} value of 0.4 µg/ml. However, against *M. tuberculosis* phagocytosed in cultured murine peritoneal macrophages, Y-26611 was less potent than ofloxacin.

8.4.5.3 Miscellaneous Compounds

p-Aminosalicylic acid (PAS) conjugated to maleylated bovine serum albumin (MBSA) was taken up efficiently through high-affinity MBSA-binding sites on cultured mouse peritoneal macrophages infected with *M. tuberculosis*.[158] The drug conjugate was nearly 100 times more effective in killing the intracellular mycobacteria than free PAS. Evidently, a lysosomal hydrolysis of the internalized conjugate resulted in the intracellular release of PAS.

Some new pyrazinoic acid esters when tested *in vitro* for activity against susceptible isolates of *M. tuberculosis* were more potent than pyrazinamide.[159] A number of new *N*-pyrazinylthioureas were synthesized and found active *in vitro*.[160]

A series of N^1-aryliden-2-pyridinecarboxyamidrazone derivatives were also synthesized and shown to elicit activity against some clinical isolates of *M. tuberculosis*.[161]

Mir et al.[162] have reported the synthesis of the α-[5-(5-nitro-2-furyl)-1,3,4-oxadiazol-2-ylthio]acethydrazide and some related derivatives and studied their activity against *M. tuberculosis*. Some *N*-(2-naphthyl)glycine hydrazide analogs were found to exert potent inhibitory activity against *M. tuberculosis* H37Rv in Youman's medium at concentrations of 0.5 to 10.0 µg/ml.[163]

The DL-*S*-*n*-[3-(4-acetyl)-2-oxo-5-oxazolidinylmethyl]acetamide (DuP-721) is an orally active oxazolidinone which at concentrations ranging from 1.5 to 4 µg/ml inhibited several susceptible and resistant strains of *M. tuberculosis*.[164] *In vitro*, the activity of DuP-721 was not affected by changes in the pH of the medium (from 6.8 to 5.5). The ED_{50} value of DuP-721 in mice was 13.2 mg/kg, following its daily administration starting 4 h postinfection and continuing for 17 d.

Broth-determined MIC values for thiacetazone against 14 wild strains of *M. tuberculosis* ranged between 0.08 and 1.2 µg/ml.[165]

Trifluoperazine, a calmodulin antagonist, was found to completely abolish mycobacterial growth.[166] When measured in shake cultures in a synthetic medium containing 0.2% Tween 80 against the human pathogenic strain H37Rv and a strain of *M. tuberculosis* resistant to isoniazid, the corresponding MICs of trifluoperazine were 5.0 and 8.0 µg/ml, respectively.

The activity of fusidic acid was tested against 40 strains of *M. tuberculosis* (20 of the strains studied were either mono- or multiresistant to conventional antimycobacterial agents).[167] MICs, which were determined by using the radiometric (BACTEC) broth method, ranged between 8.0 mg/l and 32 mg/l (MIC_{90} = 16 mg/l). The minimal bactericidal concentration (MBC), defined as the lowest concentration at which the drug kills 99% or more of the pathogen, varied between 32 and 500 mg/l (MBC_{90} = 250 mg/l). There has been no cross-resistance observed between strains resistant to one or more standard antimycobacterial agents. In addition, the combination of fusidic acid (64 mg/l) and ethambutol (4.0 mg/l) was synergistic.[168]

The observed antimycobacterial activity of auramine in 7H12 Middlebrook liquid medium has been thought to result from its dual interaction with mycobacterial DNA and mycolic acid.[169]

A series of novel imidazo[4,5-b]pyridine analogs were synthesized and found to exert antimyco-bacterial activity.[170-172] Among a number of phenoxymethylbenzimidazole and 2-benzylbenzi-midazole derivatives, the 2-chloro-2-phenoxymethylbenzimidazole was the most active analog (MIC = 125 µg/ml). Overall, the 2-benzylbenzimidazoles had the more potent *in vitro* activity.[173]

Dannhardt et al.[174] have reported the presence of a significant inhibitory effect in a number of 2-hydroxyquinolizin-4-ones against the *M. tuberculosis* strain H37Ra.

Various antihistaminic compounds were found to exert antimycobacterial activity at concentrations of 8 to 32 µg/ml.[175]

Immunomodulatory polysaccharides isolated from *Acanthopanax senticosus* were reported active against mycobacteria when tested in mice and guinea pigs.[176] The tuberculostatic activity of henna (*Lawsonia inermis* Linn.) has also been tested *in vitro* and *in vivo*.[177] The growth of the *M. tuberculosis* strain H37Rv was inhibited by 6.0 µg/ml. In guinea pigs and mice, a dose of 5.0 mg/kg caused a significant resolution of experimental infection caused by strain H37Rv.

A number of metal ligands have been studied and found to demonstrate antimycobacterial activities. Chohan and Rauf[178] have studied the antimycobacterial activity of a series of complexes of cobalt(II) and nickel(II) with dithiooxamide-derived ligands. Also, several new chromium(III) and titanium(III) complexes with isonicotinic acid hydrazide have shown significant tuberculostatic activity.[179] The synthesis and antimycobacterial activity of oxovanadium(IV) complexes with two aromatic acid hydrazides have been described.[180]

The antimycobacterial effect of the DS6A mycobacteriophage was examined in guinea pigs with disseminated tuberculous infection.[181] Although the mycophage was found active, its activity was less than that of isoniazid. The tissue changes caused by the mycophage included incomplete phagocytosis and development of granulomatous processes characterized by a gradual loss of the morphological signs of tuberculous inflammation and evolution of typical sarcoidosis features.

A poloxamer surfactant, CRL8131, has been evaluated for activity against *M. tuberculosis* (Erdman) in broth culture, by a macrophage cell line, and in a mouse model.[182] In the broth culture, CRL8131 inhibited mycobacterial growth and produced synergistic effect on intracellular killing of *M. tuberculosis* (including against two drug-resistant isolates) when applied in combination with isoniazid, rifampin, streptomycin, pyrazinamide, thiacetazone, D-cycloserine, ethionamide, amikacin, clindamycin, and p-aminosalicylic acid. When tested in C57BL/6 mice infected with *M. tuberculosis*, CRL8131 in combination with either thiacetazone or pyrazinamide significantly reduced the number of mycobacteria in both the lungs and spleens of mice and produced 100% survival at 40 d; thiacetazone or pyrazinamide alone elicited only 33% survival, whereas CRL8131 alone was inactive (0% survival).

8.4.5.4 Development of Drug Testing Methodologies

An *ex vivo* human macrophage model has been used to evaluate activity of drugs against intracellular virulent mycobacteria. Sbarbaro et al.[183] have found an enhanced bacteriostatic effect when low, nonbactericidal levels of rifampin were applied with clinically achievable levels of pyrazinamide, but not with higher bactericidal levels of rifampin. Adding pyrazinamide 2 d after the introduction of rifampin has clearly enhanced the combined killing effect. However, reversing the order and adding rifampin 2 d after the introduction of pyrazinamide produced a result weaker than introducing the agents simultaneously. The latter finding underscored the importance of timing in the administration of these two agents in order to achieve a maximal effect. In previous studies using the human macrophage model, rifampin when applied alone was found bactericidal, whereas pyrazinamide even when applied at clinically unachievable levels was only bacteriostatic.

A plasmapheresis model to be used in chronic rabbit experiments has been developed to evaluate the effect of plasmapheresis on the course of experimental tuberculosis, as well as the tolerance of chemotherapy by patients with renal tuberculosis.[184] Rabbits subjected to plasmapheresis have developed a more benign course of the disease, with the activities of isoniazid and rifampicin being significantly decreased. Clinical studies of patients with renal tuberculosis and poor tuberculostatic tolerance have shown that plasmapheresis promoted both the improvement of renal functions and the restoration of drug tolerance by decreasing the side effects of antituberculosis drugs.

Smith et al.[185] have developed a guinea pig model of experimental airborne tuberculosis capable of assessing the activity of chemotherapeutic regimens against virulent mycobacterial strains during the initial phase of drug treatment.

Jacobs et al.[186] and Cooksey et al.[187] have reported an efficient assay aimed at assessing drug susceptibility of *M. tuberculosis* by using luciferase reporter phages. The proposed methodology is based on the ability of viable mycobacteria to emit photons when infected with specific reporter phages expressing the firefly luciferase gene. The latter catalyzes the reaction of luciferin with ATP to generate photons with a quantum yield of 0.85 photons per molecule of substrate reacted. When delivered into *M. tuberculosis*, the luciferase reporter gene will facilitate the measurement of bacterial growth or inhibition by drugs. The light production, which is dependent on the phage infection, expression of luciferase genes, and the level of cellular ATP, may be detected shortly after infecting mycobacteria with the reporter phages. The assay, which usually requires small amounts of test compounds, has been designed to screen large numbers of antimycobacterial drugs and be able to distinguish drug-resistant from drug-susceptible mycobacteria.

Schaberg et al.[188] have proposed a rapid susceptibility testing procedure suitable for isoniazid, rifampin, ethambutol, streptomycin, and pyrazinamide based on agar-dilution technique (Middlebrook 7H11 agar solid medium and microcolony detection).

8.4.6 EVOLUTION OF THERAPIES AND TREATMENT OF *MYCOBACTERIUM TUBERCULOSIS* INFECTIONS

Specific chemotherapy for tuberculosis was started in the early 1940s. Soon after its discovery as an antituberculosis agent, isoniazid became an essential part of any antimycobacterial therapy. Next, the introduction of rifampicin antibiotics, streptomycin, pyrazinamide, and the fluoroquinolones, not only made it possible that such therapy could be relatively short in duration, but also to be given intermittently, thus allowing for closer supervision and monitoring.

The mechanisms of action of various antimycobacterial drugs are different, as are their primary sites of action.[189] Thus, isoniazid and rifampin exert bactericidal activity against all populations of mycobacteria. By comparison, streptomycin is most effective against bacilli found in open cavities, whereas the bactericidal activity of pyrazinamide is most pronounced against pathogens within the macrophages.

In therapeutic doses, isoniazid, rifampin, and pyrazinamide usually achieve adequate tissue and body fluid concentrations to kill *M. tuberculosis* in all body sites. Ethambutol, ethionamide, and *p*-aminosalicylic acid (PAS) are all bacteriostatic.

Resistance against drugs is very common in mycobacteria, and the number of drug-resistant mutants is usually proportional to the size of the mycobacterial population. The main rationale for antituberculosis treatment is to give a regimen combining drug(s) with bactericidal activity with bacteriostatic agent(s) that suppress the emergence of drug-resistant mutants. Microbiologic cure usually requires between 18 and 24 months of therapy. It is generally accepted that using at least two bactericidal drugs against susceptible isolates is likely to provide a cure in 6 to 9 months.[190]

One of the recommended chemotherapeutic regimens for newly diagnosed patients (both children and adults) involves a 6-month daily course of isoniazid and rifampicin, supplemented with pyrazinamide for the first 2 months.[191,192] At least nine studies of 6-month (short-course) antituberculosis chemotherapy have demonstrated promising results in children.[193-201] However, variation from a standard 6-month treatment may become necessary when there has been a high level of initial drug resistance, particularly against isoniazid. After taking into account results from recent clinical trials, recommendations have also been made on antituberculosis chemotherapy in infants and children.[190]

The optimal treatment of tuberculosis in HIV-positive patients is still being defined. Small et al.[202] have conducted a retrospective study of 132 patients listed in both the AIDS and tuberculosis case registries in San Francisco from 1981 through 1988. In HIV-infected patients who complied with conventional multidrug therapy, the results indicated a rapid sterilization of sputum, radiographic improvement, and low rates of relapse. In contrast, in patients with advanced HIV infection, the disease caused significantly high mortality. It has been reported that prophylactic medication with isoniazid, by far, is more beneficial to both HIV-infected, tuberculin-positive patients and anergic HIV-infected patients than the risks of potential isoniazid side effects.[203]

Since 1986, powerful short-course regimens have also been commonly used.[204] One preferred combination has been isoniazid, rifampin, and pyrazinamide administered on a daily basis for 2 months, followed by isoniazid and rifampin for 4 more months. Also, a 9-month regimen of isoniazid and rifampin has been found equally effective. However, supplementation (in case of drug resistance) or extension (when immunosuppression has been present) of short-course regimens has been strongly recommended.

Table 8.2 contains a list of drugs currently used in the chemotherapy of tuberculosis. Column A of the table lists the more effective and less toxic first-line antimycobacterials which have usually been applied in multidrug combinations; the less effective and more toxic second-line of drugs are presented in column B.

Some of the more promising antimycobacterial agents currently in development are given in Table 8.3.

TABLE 8.2
Antimycobacterial Agents Currently Used in the Chemotherapy of Tuberculosis

Isoniazid	Ethionamide
Rifampin	p-Aminosalicylic acid (PAS)
Pyrazinamide	Cycloserine
Ethambutol	Kanamycin
Streptomycin	Amikacin
	Capreomycin
	Ciprofloxacin

TABLE 8.3
Experimental Antimycobacterial Agents Currently in Development

Antibiotics	Quinolones	Aminophenazines
Rifapentine	Ofloxacin	Clofazimine
Enviomycin	Lomefloxacin	
FCE 22807	Sparfloxacin (AT-4140)	
CGP 40/469A	Fleroxacin	

The incidence of hypersensitivity reactions to antimycobacterial agents has been relatively uncommon. However, when such reactions occur they may result in cessation of therapy. Matz et al.[205] have described a procedure for rapid oral desensitization to ethambutol and rifampin based on a desensitization protocol for penicillin and increased dosing intervals to account for the different kinetics of these two drugs.

Corticosteroid therapy in conjunction with conventional antimycobacterial treatment was initiated in 120 patients with active pulmonary tuberculosis.[206] The corticosteroids were administered in the morning every other day. Daily doses of 20 mg corticosteroids when given for at least 2 months increased treatment efficacy to 83.3%; when used for over 3 months, the observed efficacy was even higher (89.5%). However, the issue of using corticosteroids in treatment of tuberculosis still remains controversial because of the prevailing notion that a decrease in cell-mediated immunity associated with steroids would diminish the efficacy of treatment.

A rapid resolution of tuberculous pericardial effusion was achieved after treatment with prednisone at 120 mg daily — dramatic clinical improvement was observed within 1 week of therapy.[207]

Levamisole, a widely used anthelminthic drug, has been shown to restore cutaneous hypersensitivity in anergic patients with cancer and to amplify the activation of T lymphocyte by mitogens *in vitro*. Taki and Schwartz[208] described a patient who presented with fulminant, disseminated mycobacterial infection of the joints secondary to a cell-mediated immune deficiency associated immunosuppressive chemotherapy for a T cell leukemia. Treatment with levamisole led to restoration of T cell functions and resolution of mycobacterial infection. The effect of adding once-weekly levamisole to an antituberculosis regimen lasting for 4 or 8 weeks to 6 months, has been studied in a double-blind, placebo-controlled clinical trial.[209] There has been no evidence of clinical and/or bacteriologic improvement from adding levamisole to the standard chemotherapy regimen.

8.4.6.1 Pulmonary Tuberculosis

In a prospective comparative study of 124 patients with pulmonary tuberculosis, the combined efficacy of ofloxacin, rifampicin, and isoniazid was compared to that of a regimen comprising ethambutol, rifampicin, and isoniazid.[210] All drugs were administered orally on a daily basis for 9 months. Culture conversion rates determined 3 months after commencing therapy were 98% in the ofloxacin group and 94% in the ethambutol group; by the end of six months, all patients from both groups were culture-negative. From the reported findings, it appears that in combination with isoniazid and rifampicin, ofloxacin is as useful as ethambutol in the treatment of pulmonary tuberculosis.

Information from several large clinical trials conducted in Southeast Asia and East Africa is now available. These trials, which involved short-course chemotherapy, were performed under the auspices of the British Medical Research Council (BMRC). In one of the studies conducted in Hong Kong, 1386 patients with pulmonary tuberculosis were randomly divided to receive four 6-month regimens, all given three times weekly and containing isoniazid and rifampin throughout.[211] Three of the regimens contained streptomycin for the first 4 months and pyrazinamide for 2, 4, or 6 months. The fourth regimen contained pyrazinamide for 6 months but no streptomycin. In another of the BMRC-sponsored trials conducted in Singapore,[212] 310 patients with pulmonary tuberculosis were randomly selected to receive daily regimens comprising streptomycin, isoniazid, rifampin, and pyrazinamide for 1 or 2 months; a third group was given a 2-month regimen consisting of isoniazid, rifampin, and pyrazinamide. After completion of their respective courses, all patients were treated three times weekly with isoniazid and rifampin for a total duration of 6 months. The results showed no therapeutic benefit from continuing streptomycin/isoniazid/rifampin/pyrazinamide medication beyond 1 month of treatment, or from adding streptomycin to isoniazid/rifampin/pyrazinamide.

Data from the aforementioned and some earlier trials conducted by BMRC and their colleagues have been critically reviewed by Iseman and Sbarbaro.[213]

A controlled study of three short-course (one 3- and two 5-month) regimens was carried out in South Indian patients with newly diagnosed, sputum-positive pulmonary tuberculosis.[214] The patients were randomly allocated to receive one of three regimens: (1) rifampicin/streptomycin/isoniazid/pyrazinamide (daily for 3 months); (2) the same regimen as in (1) but followed by streptomycin/isoniazid/pyrazinamide (twice weekly for an additional 2 months); and (3) the same regimen as in (2) but without rifampicin. The results of the trial demonstrated that a bacteriologic relapse requiring treatment occurred by 5 years in 16.8% of 113 patients receiving regimen (1), in 5.2% of 97 patients receiving regimen (2), and in 20% of 115 patinets given regimen (3), with organisms sensitive to streptomycin and isoniazid initially. Furthermore, the observed differences in the relapse rates between the (1) and (2) and between the (2) and (3) regimens were statistically significant. Considering patients with organisms initially resistant to streptomycin or isoniazid, or both, 7 of 52 patients had a bacteriologic relapse that required retreatment.

Wolde et al.[215] have compared the therapeutic benefits of a short-term (6 and 8 months) vs. standard long-term (12 months) treatment of pulmonary tuberculosis with a fixed-dose combination of isoniazid, rifampicin, and pyrazinamide. Based on their experience, the investigators concluded that short-course regimens with these drugs, when applied either alone or in combination, were more effective than the standard long-term regimens.

Studying the time course of smear and culture conversion in 50 previously untreated patients with cavitary pulmonary tuberculosis, Novak et al.[216] have found that in 76% of patients who were treated with isoniazid, rifampicin, and pyrazinamide, the cultural conversion preceded microscopic conversion. While examination of smears can still be a good indicator of the presence of bacilli, the cultural conversion is currently the recognized means to determine an effective response to a drug treatment.

Clinical and laboratory data by Starostenko et al.[217] have raised the possibility of lowering the doses of antimycobacterial drugs in patients with pulmonary tuberculosis by giving them in combination with two antioxidants, α-tocopherol and sodium thiosulfate. While the addition of the two antioxidants have increased the efficacy of the antimycobacterial drugs, as evidenced by the shorter periods to achieve sputum negativity, their mechanism of action was unclear.

A controlled study was undertaken to evaluate the therapeutic effect of rifabutin (LM 427, ansamycin)[218] in the retreatment of 22 patients from Hong Kong with chronic pulmonary tuberculosis who were resistant to isoniazid, streptomycin, and rifampicin.[219] The patients were divided into pairs showing similar drug resistance patterns. Randomly, one member of the pair was given rifabutin only, while the other received rifampicin only; both members of the pair were also given the same or similar second drug chosen on the basis of susceptibility testing results and the history of previous antituberculosis chemotherapy. There was no bacteriological evidence to show sustained benefits in any patient. A total of 17 patients (including 7 not in the paired comparison) were subsequently retreated with ofloxacin; 10 patients showed a response with the disease becoming and remaining quiescent in 3 of them.

In a multicenter, randomized, comparative study to assess the efficacy, tolerability, and toxicity of two regimens containing different daily dosages of rifabutin in comparison with rifampicin, 520 patients received either 150 mg daily of rifampicin (n = 175) (or rifabutin [n = 174]), or 300 mg daily of rifabutin (n = 171) for 6 months.[220] In addition, each group of patients received concurrent medication with isoniazid (for the entire 6-month period), and pyrazinamide and ethambutol (both for only the first 2 months). The success rates at the last valid observation for each patient were 89%, 94%, and 92% in the rifampicin (150 mg), rifabutin (150 mg), and rifabutin (300 mg) groups, respectively. While all three regimens proved effective and well tolerated, rifabutin at 150 mg daily showed the best risk-to-benefit ratio (the highest number of patients completing the treatment), the highest bacteriologic conversion rates, and the lowest incidence of adverse reactions.[220]

Chan et al.[221] have conducted a study in Hong Kong in which previously untreated patients with smear-positive pulmonary tuberculosis were randomly allocated to receive in addition to rifabutin (600-mg, 300-mg, 150-mg, or 75-mg doses), also rifampicin (600-mg, 300-mg, or 150-mg doses) and 300 mg of isoniazid (or no drug at all) daily for 2 d. The early bactericidal activity (EBA) of rifabutin was measured by the fall in the number of viable counts of *M. tuberculosis* in sputum collections during the 2 d of combined therapy; EBA was estimated from counts of colony-forming units on selective 7H11 agar medium. When compared with rifampicin, the EBA value of rifabutin was lower, suggesting that rifabutin was inactive or less active than rifampicin against extracellular pathogens in the pulmonary cavities. The lower EBA of rifabutin was probably the result of its low plasma concentrations (seven times lower than those after the same dose size of rifampicin).

In another study, Pretet et al.[222] conducted a prospective multicenter open trial to evaluate the efficacy and tolerability of rifabutin as part of a multiple-drug regimen given to patients with pulmonary tuberculosis who showed resistance to isoniazid and rifampicin. The patients received rifabutin (450 to 600 mg) on a daily basis concomitantly with other drugs (preferably, a fluoroquinolone) to which the pathogen was still susceptible. Of the 39 patients enrolled in the trial, 23 received treatment for at least 12 months. Twenty-one of them experienced adverse side effects, and in four, the therapy had to be discontinued.

The therapeutic efficacy and tolerability of rifabutin as a salvage therapy for cases of chronic multiple drug-resistant pulmonary tuberculosis was assessed in patients with tuberculosis who had become progressively resistant to isoniazid, rifampin, and other conventional antimycobacterial drugs.[223] Rifabutin was administered at 300 mg or 450 mg daily in conjunction with available antituberculosis agents for a mean 353 d (range, 42 to 678 d). Forty-seven percent of all evaluable patients (n = 36) achieved a sustained conversion to a negative sputum culture in a mean 47.7 d (range, 14 to 120 d), and clinical and radiologic cure and significant improvement in more than half of treated cases.[223]

A single-blind, randomized study conducted in Ugandan patients with HIV-1 infection and pulmonary tuberculosis was carried out to evaluate the feasibility of a larger phase III trial utilizing rifabutin as a substitute for rifampin in short-course therapy.[224] In addition to either rifabutin or rifampin, the treatment regimens contained isoniazid, ethambutol, and pyrazinamide. While the overall results have shown that both rifabutin- and rifampin-containing regimens were safe, well-tolerated, and with comparable efficiency, the rifabutin-receiving patients had significantly more rapid clearance of acid-fast bacilli from sputum at 2 months ($p < .05$, Fisher exact test) and over the entire period ($p < .05$, logrank test) than rifampin-treated patients. One surprising result of the study was the isolation of *Mycobacterium africanum* from 49% of the sputum cultures, demonstrating a high prevalence of this mycobacterial species in human tuberculosis in Uganda.

A patient with pulmonary tuberculosis had suffered a severe skin eruption, prominent esinophilia, and liver dysfunction after taking 750 mg of streptomycin given daily in combination with rifampicin (450 mg daily) and isoniazid (400 mg daily). Ceasing the streptomycin medication led to gradual improvement of symptoms.[225]

The fluoroquinolone drug ofloxacin was also used in the treatment of intractable pulmonary tuberculosis.[226] It was administered orally to 118 patients at daily doses of 300 to 600 mg for periods of over 3 months. Within 5 months, 19.5% of the patients showed negative sputum cultures and remained culture-negative for at least 6 months. Side effects were rare and included arthralgia (one patient) and abdominal fullness (one patient). However, the development of a significant resistance against ofloxacin has been a serious drawback.

In another clinical trial, 22 patients with multidrug-resistant pulmonary tuberculosis were treated for 8 to 12 months with ofloxacin (300 mg or 800 mg, once daily) together with second-line antimycobacterial agents.[144] In the 300-mg group, the peak serum concentrations of the ofloxacin were 3.71 to 8.08 mg/l; in the 800-mg group, the corresponding values were 10.0 to 18.7 mg/l. Concomitant medication with second-line antimycobacterial drugs led to a more rapid sputum culture conversion.

Ziegler et al.[227] have described an unusual case of a patient with advanced HIV infection (CD4+ count of 90 cells/µl, and CD4+/CD8+ ratio of 0.2) and pulmonary tuberculosis who failed to respond to standard antituberculosis therapy consisting of isoniazid, rifampin, ethambutol, and amikacin despite an initial clinical improvement. However, upon cessation of therapy, extrapulmonary spread (severe arthritis of the elbow) and recurrence of pulmonary tuberculosis have been observed. Renewed and lasting control of the infection was achieved only by continuous administration of corticosteroids (prednisolone at 10 mg, b.i.d.) in conjunction with an unconventional antibiotic regimen consisting of amikacin, protionamide, terizidone, clarithromycin, and sparfloxacin for 5 months.[227]

8.4.6.2 Extrapulmonary Tuberculosis

The influence of dosage (10 and 20 mg/kg) and acetylation status on the concentration levels of isoniazid in cerebrospinal fluid (CSF) and plasma of children with tuberculous meningitis was studied by Donald et al.[228] While maximum drug levels in CSF were reached 2 to 4 h after dosing, they did not differ significantly from those in the plasma. The CSF levels after 10-mg/kg dosing were markedly lower than those following a dosage of 20 mg/kg. However, 14 to 16 h after the administration of both dosing regimens, the isoniazid concentrations in CSF were in excess of its MIC value for *M. tuberculosis*.

The activity of ofloxacin in the treatment of urogenital tuberculosis was assessed and compared to that of other antimycobacterial drugs.[229] The preliminary data indicated that at doses of 200 mg given every 12 h for 6 months, the therapeutic efficacy of ofloxacin was comparable to that of rifampicin (600 mg, every 24 h for 3 months) and isoniazid (300 mg, every 24 h for 3 months).

With the increased incidence of extrapulmonary tuberculosis, ocular infections have become more prevalent. The predominant route by which tubercle bacilli can reach the eye is through the bloodstream, after infecting the lungs, even though the pulmonary loci may not be initially evident clinically or radiographically.[230] The most common ocular involvement in patients with pulmonary tuberculosis has been choroiditis. Retinal periphlebitis has been rarely induced by a direct invasion of the retina by tubercle bacilli. Usually (but not always) retinal tuberculosis has been secondary to an underlying choroiditis.

A case of posterior uveitis and choroiditis in an AIDS patient was treated successfully with isoniazid, rifampin, and ethambutol.[61] The increased risk of development of severe ocular tuberculosis in immunocompromised patients was further demonstrated by Anders and Wollensak,[10] who described a patient with systemic lupus eruthematosus and on immunosuppressive therapy — fundoscopy revealed severe subretinal exudation with overlying serious retinal detachment progressing to panuveitis with spontaneous perforation and the presence of acid-fast bacilli in orbital lesions.

Tuberculous dacryocystitis, an acute infection and inflammation of the nasolacrymal sac may complicate congenital obstruction of the nasolacrimal duct. Cotton et al.[231] have described a pediatric patient with acute left dacryocystitis with fever and cervical adenitis. Although the involvement of both the lacrymal and lymph node persisted despite antibiotic and corticosteroid therapy, the patient was eventually cured with izoniazid and rifampin for 9 months, and pyrazinamide for 2 months. Drainage of the sac area was also performed after 1 month of therapy, followed by dacryocystorhinostomy.

Sais et al.[232] have described a patient with cervical lymphadenitis due to *M. tuberculosis* infection who also developed cutaneous vasculitis. Clinical resolution was achieved with conventional antituberculosis therapy. The association between leukocytoclastic vasculitis and tuberculous infection has been uncommon and rarely reported. Cutaneous leukocytoclasic vasculitis is an inflammatory vascular disorder resulting from the deposition of immune complexes in dermal vessels, and a direct or indirect role of infectious agents in the pathogenesis of this condition has been postulated.[232] Cases of cervical lymphadenitis in children, although uncommon, have also been reported.[233]

Another rare example of extrapulmonary tuberculous involvement was reported in a patient with skeletal tuberculosis with extravertebral location.[234] The tuberculous osteomyelitis, which had affected simultaneously two right ribs and the left ulna, was treated with a multidrug regimen incliding rifampin and streptomycin. Kreder and Davey[235] have described a case of tuberculous infection complicating total hip arthroplasty which had been performed 4 years earlier for degenerative arthritis — the patient had no prior history of exposure to tuberculosis and no evidence of skeletal or nonskeletal tuberculous infection.

Delayed prosthetic joint infection due to *M. tuberculosis*, although uncommon, may result from either local reactivation of initial infection (as far back as 40 years) or from hematogenous spread. Treatment usually consisted of removal of the prosthesis in addition to administration of antituberculosis drugs.[236]

Chen et al.[237] have described an AIDS patient with a nonspinal psoas abscess due to *M. tuberculosis* without pulmonary involvement. The characteristic hypodense lesion within the right psoas muscle, which was noted by a computerized tomographic (CT) scanning, responded rapidly to antituberculosis therapy.

A fatal case was reported of a patient with dermatomyositis associated with carcinoma, despite therapy with steroids and antimycobacterial antibiotics.[238] Autopsy revealed the overwhelming presence of diffuse nongranulomatous infection by *M. tuberculosis* of only the skeletal muscles and one inguinal lymph node. This rare localization was probably due to steroid immunosuppression and the humoral immune attack on muscle blood vessels that is part of dermatomyositis.[238]

Duodenal tuberculosis due to *M. tuberculosis* in an elderly patient has been identified as the cause of a covered perforation of the duodenal bulb.[239] Daily antimycobacterial treatment with isoniazid (300 mg), rifampicin (450 mg), ethambutol (800 mg), and pyrazinamide (1.5 g), in addition to 50 mg prednisolone to prevent stricture, resulted in a marked reduction in the size of the tuberculous ulcer within 2 weeks, followed by nearly complete healing without stricture after 6 months of therapy.

Primary tuberculosis in the oral cavity is yet another rare entity which was described in a patient who had suffered an exodontia 20 d before. Usually the microorganisms will need a disruption of the oral mucosa to become pathogenic.[240]

Shafik[241] has compared the results of treating patients with tuberculous epididymitis by rifampin injection into the tunica vaginalis sac (600 mg every 4 to 6 d) with those following daily oral antituberculosis therapy consisting of rifampin (600 mg), isoniazid (300 mg), and ethambutol (25 mg/kg). Treatment in both groups continued for 6 months, with 3-month follow-up thereafter. While in the intratunical injection group (n = 4) the epididymal swellings disappeared in 3 to 6 months and the semen and hydrocele fluid became sterile in 4 months, in the orally treated group (n = 4), semen remained positive for tubercle bacilli and only one patient showed partial diminution of the epididymal mass, whereas one patient had developed scrotal fistula. Another potential advantage of intratunical rifampin injections has been the use of a single drug as compared to the multidrug oral medication which may enhance the incidence of side effects.[241]

An unusual case of tuberculous paronychia with skin infection of the big toe and complicated by inguinal lymphadenitis and tuberculous abscess formation, was successfully treated with surgery and chemotherapy with ethambutol, rifampin, and isoniazid.[242]

8.4.6.3   Drug Resistance in Tuberculosis

With the emergence of drug-resistant strains of *M. tuberculosis*, the effective chemotherapy of the disease will require rapid assessment of drug resistance. The currently available methodology will not allow determination of drug susceptibility for 2 to 18 weeks because of the 20- to 24-h doubling time of *M. tuberculosis*. However, some new techniques (e.g., firefly luciferase-based assay) in development may remedy this situation by significantly shortening the ascertainment times.

Table 8.4 lists the results of a drug susceptibility test of 10 drugs from a study conducted by the Centers for Disease Control in collaboration with 31 health departments that surveyed the frequency of both primary and acquired drug resistance in 464 *M. tuberculosis* isolates from previously treated patients (but not during the last 3 months prior to specimen collection) and 3760 isolates from never-treated patients.[243,244]

Worldwide, the incidence rate of drug-resistant tuberculosis, while variable, has often been seen as influenced by the overall economic strength of the region.[245,246] However, it should be noted that the level of drug resistance may still remain relatively low in poor nations where antituberculosis medication is inadequate and drugs are scarce, while in some developed regions the higher level of drug resistance has been attributed to a combination of poor quality of treatment in the past, the uncontrolled use of antituberculosis agents in the private sector, noncompliance with tuberculosis treatment,[247] as well as poverty, alcoholism, intravenous substance abuse, and HIV infection.[248-250] In general, areas with high frequency of active disease are also very likely to have high rates of drug resistance (Table 8.5).[139,251-254] Data on the incidence of multidrug-resistant (that is, two drugs or more) tuberculosis, although more difficult to obtain, have shown case fatality rates in several countries already ranging from 40 to 60% in immunocompetent patients, to over 80% in immuno-compromised patients.

TABLE 8.4

Proportion of Patients with Resistance to Antituberculosis Drugs

Drugs	% Resistance	
	Never treated	Previously treated
Isoniazid	5.3	19.4
Streptomycin	4.8	10.3
Rifampin	0.6	3.2
Ethambutol	0.6	2.2
Pyrazinamide[a]	0.5	1.5
Ethionamide	1.5	3.7
PAS	1.0	3.5
Kanamycin	0.03	0.4
Capreomycin	0.08	0.2
Cycloserine	0.00	0.03
Any drug	9.0	22.8

[a] Excludes isolates with unknown pyrazinamide results (31%).

TABLE 8.5

Regions of High Prevalence of Multiple Drug-Resistant Tuberculosis[a]

Country	Population	Annual incidence rate per 100,000 population	Initial drug resistance (in %)
China	1.1 billion	300–500	20
India	700 million	200–300	20
Pakistan	100 million	500	30
Philippines	80 million	500	33

[a] Data taken from Ref. 139.

With the dramatic increase of the HIV-infected population, the frequency of multiple drug-resistant *M. tuberculosis* is also on the rise. While reviewing the clinical course of 171 patients (median age, 46 years) with pulmonary tuberculosis, Goble et al.[255] have found significant resistance to isoniazid and rifampin. The patients were treated between 1973 and 1983 with multidrug combinations and their regimens, while determined individually, have included preferably three medications that had not been used previously and against which the mycobacterial strain was fully susceptible in immunocompetent persons.

Based on tuberculosis susceptibility patterns, predictors of multidrug resistance, and implications for initial therapeutic regimens, a theoretically effective antituberculosis regimen was assumed to contain at least two drugs to which an *M. tuberculosis* isolate was susceptible.[256]

In a study by Frieden et al.,[257] 44% of 239 patients receiving antituberculosis multiple drug therapy had isolates which were resistant to one or more drugs, and 30% had isolates resistant to both isoniazid and rifampin. Patients who had never been treated and were HIV-positive were more likely to present with resistant isolates than non-HIV-infected individuals.[257] However, as reported in a number of studies,[258,259] there has been no significant difference in the overall frequency of resistance between patients at risk for HIV infection and those without the risk. This trend, however, may have already started to change with the additional cases of multidrug-resistant *M. tuberculosis* infection being described in HIV-positive patients.

To investigate the relationship between isoniazid resistance and HIV infection in patients with tuberculosis, Asch ct al.[260] have evaluated data in the Los Angeles County tuberculosis registry encompassing 1506 patients for whom drug susceptibility results were available. The conclusion was that in a setting where there has been no ongoing outbreak of drug-resistant tuberculosis, isoniazid-resistant tuberculosis was no more commonly detected in HIV-infected patients.[260]

Salomon et al.[261] have identified early predictors of multiple drug-resistant tuberculosis and described improved clinical outcomes, including survival, for HIV-infected patients under a direct drug-treatment observation. Thus, analysis using the Cox proportional hazards model revealed that failure to defervesce while receiving a standard four-drug antituberculosis regimen was independently associated with multidrug resistance ($p = .004$). In a specific example, patients with HIV-related multidrug-resistant tuberculosis were prospectively identified and treated with at least two agents that were active *in vitro*; 100% bacteriologic conversion and improved survival (4 months and over for 88% of patients, and 1 year or more for 59% of patients) has been observed.[261] In a parallel study, Turett et al.[262] have also found by bivariate analysis that HIV-infected patients with multidrug-resistant tuberculosis responded better and had increased survival rates after receiving for 2 or more consecutive weeks appropriate therapy consisting of at least two drugs to which the isolate was susceptible *in vitro*; starting appropriate therapy within 4 weeks of the diagnosis; and having tuberculosis that was limited to the lungs.

Rastogi et al.[263] have cultured serial isolates of *M. tuberculosis* from a patient who failed to respond to standard antituberculosis chemotherapy. Each successive isolate was found to be resistant to a wider range of drugs than the preceding one. Evidence from bacteriophage typing profiles and DNA restriction fragment patterns confirmed that the patient had been infected with a single mycobacterial strain that developed resistance to a number of drugs but did not significantly change its typing patterns.

Comparison of protein spectra of taxonomically different mycobacteria with spectra of isoniazid-, streptomycin-, and rifampicin-resistant strains have shown distinct differences in the protein complexes.[264]

While the resistance mechanisms for rifampicin and streptomycin are associated and similar to those found in other bacteria, the isoniazid susceptibility and resistance was found to be unique to *M. tuberculosis*.[265,266]

So far, mutations in two chromosomal loci, *kat*G and *inh*A, have been found to be involved in the isoniazid resistance in tuberculosis.[266] Zhang et al.[267] studied the role of *kat*G, a catalase-peroxidase gene, in the isoniazid resistance of *M. tuberculosis*. Usually in a guinea pig model, clinical isolates of isoniazid-resistant mycobacteria have been shown to reduce the catalase activity. The *kat*G gene, which encodes for both catalase and peroxidase, restored sensitivity to isoniazid in a resistant mutant of *M. smegmatis*. In further experiments, the deletion of the gene from the chromosome was associated with isoniazid resistance in two clinical isolates of *M. tuberculosis*.

Zhang et al.[268] have also performed genetic analysis of six *M. tuberculosis* strains differing in their virulence towards guinea pigs. The results demonstrated the presence of an altered restriction enzyme fragmentation pattern associated with the superoxide dismutase gene in one low-virulence and isoniazid-resistant strain. Moreover, the superoxide dismutase enzyme produced by this isoniazid-resistant strain differed in its electrophoretic mobility from the superoxide dismutase of the other mycobacterial strains studied. Such genetic changes may be related to the strain-dependent differences in virulence observed in *M. tuberculosis*.

Biochemical variations in the cell wall and membrane structures associated with ethambutol resistance have been observed in a single-step mutant of *M. tuberculosis* strain H37Ra.[269] The drug-resistant strain had a reduced phospholipid content, particularly in the cell membrane fraction. Additional significant alterations were found in the individual phospholipid content and the phospholipid fatty acid acyl group composition of whole cells and subcellular fractions. Structural changes on the cell surface were also present.

Historically, the majority of multiple-drug antituberculosis regimens contained isoniazid and rifampin as part of the same regimen. As a consequence of this combined therapy, acquired rifampin resistance without preexisting isoniazid resistance[270] is highly unusual in patients with tuberculosis,[271] and strains resistant only to rifampin have been rarely recovered. However, there has been an increased incidence of HIV-positive patients infected with mono-rifampin-resistant *M. tuberculosis* strains.[272] Nolan et al.[271] have described an unusual pattern of acquired rifampin resistance in three HIV-infected patients who initially had *M. tuberculosis* strains susceptible to both rifampin and isoniazid. During treatment in two patients and after completion of therapy in the remaining one, each patient developed active, rifampin-resistant but isoniazid-susceptible tuberculosis (one patient subsequently developed isoniazid resistance also).

To test the hypothesis that acquired rifampin resistance is the result of dissemination of a single clone, Lutfey et al.[272] performed IS6110 DNA fingerprinting[273] and automated DNA sequencing on a region of the RNA polymerase β-subunit structural gene (*rpo*B) containing mutations that confer rifampin resistance. The results indicated that all organisms independently acquired the mono-rifampin-resistant phenotype. Furthermore, the data obtained ruled out the possibility of person-to-person strain transmission among patients, and instead suggested that host factors, such as poor compliance with antituberculosis medication or decreased absorption of rifampin may have been the driving force in the origin of resistance in these strains.[272] Using similar techniques, Nolan et al.[271] have also reached the conclusion that acquired rifampin resistance was the result of *rpo*B gene mutation in the original *M. tuberculosis* isolate.

Jarallah et al.[274] have noticed a higher incidence of resistance towards streptomycin (16%) and rifampicin (15%) in patients from the Taif region of Saudi Arabia. A rapid procedure for determination of rifampin resistance in clinical isolates of *M. tuberculosis* was developed by using PCR technique to amplify a known region around a cluster of mutations in the *rpo*B gene, and an optimized single-stranded conformational polymorphism analysis to screen for mutations in the amplified region.[275] The procedure was sensitive for 95% of rifampin-resistant isolates.

Experimental results by Tsukamura[276] strongly suggested that prior antimycobacterial therapy with aminoglycoside antibiotics, such as streptomycin or kanamycin, led to an increase in the bacterial populations more resistant to rifampicin. It was also shown that the ratio of streptomycin-resistant mutants increased after pretreatment with kanamycin, and the ratio of kanamycin-resistant mutants expanded after pretreatment with streptomycin.[276,277]

Mutations in the *rps*L and *rrs* genes have been associated with streptomycin resistance.[266]

A strain of *M. tuberculosis* resistant to ofloxacin has produced a mutation in the *gyr*A gene which was hypothesized to be responsible for the acquired resistance.[278] The chromosomal DNA was amplified by PCR using two oligonucleotide primers highly homologous to DNA sequences flanking the quinolone resistance-determining region in the *gyr*A of the mycobacteria. Comparison of the nucleotide sequences of the 150-bp fragments obtained by PCR revealed a point mutation in the ofloxacin-resistant strain, leading to the substitution of histidine for aspartic acid at a position corresponding to residues involved in quinolone resistance in *Escherichia coli* (Asp87), *Staphylococcus aureus* (Glu88), and *Campylobacter jejuni* (Asp90).[268]

Bibergal and Palian[279] applied a radiometric procedure to determine resistance against pyrazinamide. The use of a gas chromatographic technique to detect drug resistance by *Mycobacterium* was also reported.[280]

Plikaytis et al.[281] have proposed a procedure for the rapid identification of a multidrug-resistant strain of *M. tuberculosis*, designated as strain W (IS6110 restriction fragment length polymorphism type 212071), and which was resistant to isoniazid, rifampin, ethambutol, streptomycin, kanamycin, ethionamide, and rifabutin, using a multiplex PCR assay to target a direct repeat of IS6110 with a 556-bp intervening sequence (NTF-1). The amplification generated two amplicons from strain W, which indicated the presence and orientation of the NTF-1 sequence between the direct repeat of

IS6110, and a third amplicon, which served as an internal PCR control. The sensitivity of the procedure was 100% — all 48 strain W isolates among 193 isolates studied were correctly identified.

Changes in the degree of drug susceptibility of the bacterial population in patients with tuberculosis during chemotherapy can be monitored quantitatively by testing *M. tuberculosis* isolates against various concentrations of the drugs in 7H12 broth to determine radiometrically the minimum inhibitory concentrations.[282]

Acknowledging the seriousness of multiple drug-resistance in the U.S., a task force comprising representatives from various federal agencies proposed a National Action Plan to combat this problem.[283]

8.4.6.4 Adoptive Immunotherapy

Kitsukawa et al.[284] have reported the use of adoptive immunotherapy to treat a case of pulmonary tuberculosis caused by multidrug-resistant mycobacteria. The patient was treated with adoptively transferred autologous peripheral blood leukocytes (PBL) sensitized with killed *M. tuberculosis in vitro*. The PBL were obtained by leukapheresis and separated with Ficoll-Hypaque solution, then cultured with the killed mycobacteria in media containing rIL-2. Although the patient did not show roentgenologic improvement, there was weight gain, alleviation of fever, and the number of organisms in the sputum was temporarily decreased.

8.4.6.5 Prophylaxis of Tuberculosis in HIV-Infected Patients

In a recent report,[285] the Advisory Council for the Elimination of Tuberculosis has recommended a model for tuberculosis control programs to be implemented in the U.S., including three priority strategies for prevention and control: identifying and treating persons with active tuberculosis; finding and screening persons who had contact with patients with tuberculosis to determine whether they have been infected with *M. tuberculosis* or have active disease, and providing appropriate treatment if necessary; and screening populations at high risk for tuberculosis and providing therapy to prevent progression of active disease.

Preventive therapy of patients exposed to multiple drug-resistant *M. tuberculosis* is still somewhat controversial and of unknown efficacy.[2]

In general, while prophylaxis with isoniazid for 6 to 12 months has been very important, it is often a neglected preventive measure for patients latently infected but still without active disease.[204] Daily therapy with 300 mg of isoniazid for at least 9 months has been recommended for patients at high risk for tuberculosis.[286]

In a prospective observational cohort study conducted among 2960 community-based injecting drug users (including 942 HIV-seropositive persons) during 1988 to 1994, Graham et al.[287] have evaluated the expanded access to isoniazid chemoprophylaxis on the tuberculosis incidence. Directly observed chemoprophylaxis with twice-weekly isoniazid (10 to 15 mg/kg) was offered to purified protein derivative (PPD) tuberculin-positive individuals, but not to those with cutaneous anergy; disease incidence was monitored by using Poisson regression. Following preventive therapy, there has been a dramatic decrease in incidence from a peak of 6 per 1000 person-years in 1991 to only one case in 1992 and 0 cases for 24 months thereafter (mid-1992 to mid-1994), for an overall 83% drop in tuberculosis incidence. The results obtained were consistent with those observed in clinical trials of isoniazid prophylaxis and were obtained without offering chemoprophylaxis to HIV-infected patients with cutaneous anergy.

8.4.7 References

1. Fry, D. E., The reemergence of mycobacterial infections, *Arch. Surg.*, 131, 14, 1996.
2. Peloquin, C. A. and Berning, S. E., Infection caused by *Mycobacterium tuberculosis, Ann. Pharmacother.*, 28, 72, 1994.

3. Huebner, R. E. and Castro, K. G., The changing face of tuberculosis, *Annu. Rev. Med.*, 46, 47, 1995.
4. Park, S. B., Joo, I., Park, Y. I., Suk, J., Cho, W. H., Park, C. H., and Kim, H. C., Clinical manifestations of tuberculosis in renal transplant patients, *Transplant. Proc.*, 28, 1520, 1996.
5. Munoz, P., Palomo, J., Munoz, R., Rodriguez-Creixems, M., Pelaez, T., and Bouza, E., Tuberculosis in heart transplant recipients, *Clin. Infect. Dis.*, 21, 398, 1995.
6. Ahsan, N., Blanchard, R. L., and Mai, M. L., Gastrointestinal tuberculosis in renal transplantation, *Clin. Transplant.*, 9, 349, 1995.
7. Miller, R. A., Lanza, L. A., Kline, J. N., and Geist, L. J., *Mycobacterium tuberculosis* in lung transplant recipients, *Am. J. Respir. Crit. Care Med.*, 152, 374, 1995.
8. Tantawichien, T., Suwangool, P., and Suvanapha, R., Tuberculosis in renal transplant recipients, *Transplant. Proc.*, 26, 2187, 1994.
9. Chen, C. H., Hsieh, H., and Lai, M. K., Pulmonary tuberculosis or MOTT infection in kidney transplant recipients, *Transplant. Proc.*, 26, 2136, 1994.
10. Anders, N. and Wollensak, G., Ocular tuberculosis in systemic lupus erythematosus and immunosuppressive therapy, *Klin. Monatsbl. Augenheilkd.*, 207, 368, 1995.
11. Neukirch, B. and Kremer, G. J., Disseminated extrapulmonary tuberculosis in idiopathic CD4-lymphocytopenia, *Dtsch. Med. Wochenschr.*, 120, 23, 1995.
12. Nagasawa, M., Maeda, H., Okawa, H., and Yata, J., Pulmonary miliary tuberculosis and T-cell abnormalities in a severe combined immunodeficient patient reconstituted with haploidentical bone marrow transplantation, *Int. J. Hematol.*, 59, 303, 1994.
13. Phair, J. P., Gross, P. A., Kaplan, J. E., Masur, H., Holmes, K. K., Wilfert, C. M., Martone, W. J., and Castro, K. G., Quality standard for the identification and treatment of persons coinfected with human immunodeficiency virus and *Mycobacterium tuberculosis*, *Clin. Infect. Dis.*, 21(Suppl. 1), S130, 1995.
14. Molina-Gamboa, J. D., Ponce-de-Leon, S., Sifuentes-Osornio, J., Bobadilla del Valle, M., and Ruiz-Palacios, G. M., Mycobacterial infection in Mexican AIDS patients, *J. Acquir. Immune Defic. Syndr. Hum. Retrovirol.*, 11, 53, 1996.
15. Drobniewski, F. A., Pozniak, A. L., and Uttley, A. H., Tuberculosis and AIDS, *J. Med. Microbiol.*, 43, 85, 1995.
16. Kritski, A., Dalcolmo, M., del Bianco, R., del Melo, F. F., Pinto, W. P., Schechther, M., and Castelo, A., Association of tuberculosis and HIV infection in Brasil, *Bol. Oficina Sanit. Panam.*, 118, 542, 1995.
17. Waxman, S., Gang, M., and Goldfrank, L., Tuberculosis in the HIV-infected patient, *Emerg. Med. Clin. North Am.*, 13, 179, 1995.
18. Yalcinkaya, F., Tumer, N., Akar, N., Ekim, M., and Bildirici, Y., Tuberculous osteomyelitis: an unusual case of tuberculous infection in a child undergoing continuous ambulatory peritoneal dialysis, *Pediatr. Nephrol.*, 9, 485, 1995.
19. Labhard, N., Nicod, L., and Zellweger, J. P., Cerebral tuberculosis in the immunocompetent host: 8 cases observed in Switzerland, *Tuber. Lung Dis.*, 75, 454, 1994.
20. Farley, T. A., AIDS and multidrug-resistant tuberculosis: an epidemic transforms an old disease, *J. La. State Med. Soc.*, 144, 357, 1992.
21. Bagg, J., Tuberculosis: a re-emerging problem for health care workers, *Br. Dent. J.*, 180, 376, 1996.
22. Moroni, M., Gori, A., Rusconi, S., Franzetti, F., and Antinori, S., Mycobacterial infections in AIDS: an overview of epidemiology, clinical manifestations, therapy and prophylaxis, *Monaldi Arch. Chest Dis.*, 49, 432, 1994.
23. Fraser, V. J., Kilo, C. M., Bailey, T. C., Medoff, G., and Dunagan, W. C., Screening of physicians for tuberculosis, *Infect. Control Hosp. Epidemiol.*, 15, 95, 1994.
24. Pearson, M. L., Jereb, J. A., Frieden, T. R., Crawford, J. T., Davis, B. J., Dooley, S. W., and Jarvis, W. R., Nosocomial transmission of multidrug-resistant *Mycobacterium tuberculosis*: a risk to patients and health care workers, *Ann. Intern. Med.*, 117, 191, 1992.
25. Githui, W., Nunn, P., Juma, E., Karimi, F., Bridle, R., Kamunyi, R., Gathua, S., Gicheha, C., Morris, J., and Omwega, M., Cohort study of HIV-positive and HIV-negative tuberculosis, Nairobi, Kenya: comparison of bacteriological results, *Tuber. Lung Dis.*, 73, 203, 1992.
26. Allen, S., Batungwanayo, J., Kerlikowske, K., Lifson, A. R., Wolf, W., Granich, R., Taelman, H., Van de Perre, P., Serufilira, A., Bogaerts, J., Slutkin, G., and Hopewell, P. C., Two-year incidence of tuberculosis in cohorts of HIV-infected and uninfected urban Rwandan women, *Am. Rev. Respir. Dis.*, 146, 1439, 1992.

27. Davis, B. D., Dulbecco, R., Eisen, H. N., Ginsberg, H. S., Wood, W. B., and McCarty, M., *Microbiology*, 2nd ed., Harper and Row, New York, 1973.

28. Crowle, A. J., Dahl, R., Ross, E., and May, M. H., Evidence that vesicles containing living, virulent *Mycobacterium tuberculosis* or *Mycobacterium avium* in cultured human macrophages are not acidic, *Infect. Immun.*, 59, 1823, 1991.

29. Crawle, A. J. and May, M. H., Inhibition of tubercle bacilli in cultured human macrophages by chloroquine used alone and in combination with streptomycin, isoniazid, pyrazinamide, and two metabolites of vitamin D_3, *Antimicrob. Agents Chemother.*, 34, 2217, 1990.

30. Chan, J., Fan, X. D., Hunter, S. W., Brennan, P. J., and Bloom, B. R., Lipoarabinomannan, a possible virulence factor involved in persistence of *Mycobacterium tuberculosis* within macrophages, *Infect. Immun.*, 59, 1755, 1991.

31. Leao, S. C., Tuberculosis: new strategies for the development of diagnostic tests and vaccines, *Braz. J. Med. Biol. Res.*, 26, 827, 1993.

32. Pospelov, L. E. and Mikhailova, I. V., Effect of HLA genotype on bacterial colonization and antigenemia in patients with infiltrative pulmonary tuberculosis, *Probl. Tuberk.*, (5), 35, 1993.

33. Goh, K. S. and Rastogi, N., Rapid preliminary differentiation of species within the *Mycobacterium tuberculosis* complex: proposition of a radiometric method, *Res. Microbiol.*, 142, 659, 1991.

34. Fauville-Dufaux, M., Vanfleteren, B., De Wit, L., Vincke, J. P., Van Vooren, J. P., Yates, M. D., Serruys, E., and Content, J., Rapid detection of tuberculous and nontuberculous mycobacteria by polymerase chain reaction amplification of a 162 bp DNA fragment from antigen 85, *Eur. J. Clin. Microbiol. Infect. Dis.*, 11, 197, 1992.

35. Bollet, C., De Lamballerie, X., Zandotti, C., Vignoli, C., Gevaudan, M. J., and De Micco, P., Detection and identification of *Mycobacterium tuberculosis*, *M. bovis*/BCG, and *M. avium* by two-step polymerase chain reaction: comparison with ELISA using A60 antigen, *Microbiologica*, 15, 345, 1992.

36. Narita, M., Shibata, M., Togashi, T., and Kobayashi, H., Polymerase chain reaction for detection of *Mycobacterium tuberculosis*, *Acta Paediatr.*, 81, 141, 1992.

37. Bocart, D., Lecossier, D., De Lassence, A., Valeyre, D., Battesti, J. P., and Hence, A. J., A search for mycobacterial DNA in granulomatous tissues from patients with sarcoidosis using the polymerase chain reaction, *Am. Rev. Respir. Dis.*, 145, 1142, 1992.

38. de Lassence, A., Lecossier, D., Pierre, C., Cadranel, J., Stern, M., and Hence, A. J., Detection of mycobacterial DNA in pleural fluid from patients with tuberculous pleurisy by means of the polymerase chain reaction: comparison of two protocols, *Thorax*, 47, 265, 1992.

39. Luquin, M., Papa, F., and David, H. L., Identification of sulpholipid I by thin-layer chromatography in the rapid identification of *Mycobacterium tuberculosis*, *Res. Microbiol.*, 143, 225, 1992.

40. Evans, K. D., Nakasone, A. S., Sutherland, P. A., de la Maza, L. M., and Peterson, E. M., Identification of *Mycobacterium tuberculosis* and *Mycobacterium avium-M. intracellulare* directly from primary BACTEC cultures by using acridinium-ester-labeled DNA probes, *J. Clin. Microbiol.*, 30, 2427, 1992.

41. Sada, E., Aguilar, D., Torres, M., and Herrera, T., Detection of lipoarabinomannan as a diagnostic test for tuberculosis, *J. Clin. Microbiol.*, 30, 2415, 1992.

42. Ladron de Guevara, M. C., Beltran, M., Gutierrez, A., and Saz, J. V., Effect of chemotherapy on the antibody response to A60 antigen, *Enferm. Infecc. Microbiol. Clin.*, 10, 26, 1992.

43. Ladron de Guevara, M. C., Gonzalez, A., Ortega, A., and Saz, V., Serological diagnosis of pulmonary tuberculosis using ELISA and the A60 antigen, *Enferm. Infecc. Microbiol. Clin.*, 10, 17, 1992.

44. Lee, B. W., Tan, J. A., Wong, S. C., Tan, C. B., Yap, H. K., Low, P. S., Chia, J. N., and Tay, J. S., DNA amplification by the polymerase chain reaction for the rapid diagnosis of tuberculous meningitis: comparison of protocols involving three mycobacterial DNA sequences, IS6110, 65 kDa antigen, and MPB64, *J. Neurol. Sci.*, 123, 173, 1994.

45. Sugita, Y., Sasaki, T., Okuda, K., and Nakajima, H., Practical use of polymerase chain reaction for the diagnosis of steroid induced tuberculous lymphadenitis, *J. Trop. Med. Hyg.*, 97, 65, 1994.

46. Bradley, S. P., Reed, S. L., and Catanzaro, A., Clinical efficacy of the amplified *Mycobacterium tuberculosis* direct test for the diagnosis of pulmonary tuberculosis, *Am. J. Respir. Crit. Care Med.*, 153, 1606, 1996.

47. Nelson, C. T. and Taber, L. H., Diagnosis of tuberculous pericarditis with a fluorochrome stain, *Pediatr. Infect. Dis. J.*, 14, 1004, 1995.

48. Bertolaccini, P., Chimenti, M., Bianchi, S., Manfredini, G., Berattini, G., and Maneschi, A., Gallium-67 scintography in an AIDS patient presenting tuberculous pericarditis, *J. Nucl. Biol. Med.*, 37, 245, 1993.

49. Hugo-Hamman, C. T., Scher, H., and De Moor, M. M., Tuberculous pericarditis in children: a review of 44 cases, *Pediatr. Infect. Dis. J.*, 13, 13, 1994.

50. Choy, E. H., Chieco-Bianchi, F., Panayi, G. S., and Kingsley, G. H., Synovial fluid lymphocyte proliferation to tuberculin protein product derivative: a novel way of diagnosing tuberculous arthritis, *Clin. Exp. Rheumatol.*, 12, 187, 1994.

51. Daley, C. L., Small, P. M., Schecter, G. F., Schoolnik, G. K., McAdam, R. A., Jacobs, W. R., Jr., and Hopewell, P. C., An outbreak of tuberculosis with accelerated progression among persons infected with HIV, *N. Engl. J. Med.*, 326, 231, 1992.

52. Shafer, R. W. and Edlin, B. R., Tuberculosis in patients infected with human immunodeficiency virus: perspective on the past decade, *Clin. Infect. Dis.*, 22, 683, 1996.

53. Wada, M., Yamamoto, S., Ogata, H., Sugita, N., Kino, T., and Hayashi, A., Two pulmonary tuberculosis cases with HIV infection, *Kekkaku*, 69, 367, 1994.

54. Jones, E., Young, S. M. M., Antoniskis, D., Davidson, P. T., Kramer, F., and Barnes, P. F., Relationship of the manifestations of tuberculosis to CD4 cell counts in patients with human immunodeficiency virus infections, *Am. Rev. Respir. Dis.*, 148, 1292, 1993.

55. Dupon, M., Texier-Maugein, J., Leroy, V., Sentilhes, A., Pellegrin, J.-L., Morlat, P., Ragnaud, J.-M., Chene, G., Dabis, F., and Groupe d'Epidémiologie Clinique du SIDA en Aquitaine, Tuberculosis and HIV infection: a cohort study of incidence and susceptibility to antituberculous drugs, Bordeaux, 1985-1993, *AIDS*, 9, 577, 1995.

56. Greten, T., Hautmann, H., Trauner, A., and Huber, R. M., Esophagomediastinal fistulae as a rare complication of tuberculosis in an HIV-infected patient, *Dtsch. Med. Wochenschr.*, 119, 1613, 1994.

57. Corbett, E. L., Crossley, I., De Cock, K. M., and Miller, R. F., Disseminated cutaneous *Mycobacterium tuberculosis* infection in a patient with AIDS, *Genitourin. Med.*, 71, 308, 1995.

58. Berenguer, J., Moreno, S., Laguna, F., Vicente, T., Adrados, M., Ortega, A., Gonzalez-Lattoz, J., and Bouza, E., Tuberculous meningitis in patients infected with the human immunodeficiency virus, *N. Engl. J. Med.*, 326, 668, 1992.

59. Fortun, J., Gomez-Mampaso, E., Navas, E., Hermida, C. M., Antela, A., and Guerrero, A., Tuberculous meningitis caused by resistant microorganisms, *Enferm. Infecc. Microbiol. Clin.*, 12, 150, 1994.

60. Yechoor, V. K., Shandera, W. X., Rodriguez, P., and Cate, T. R., Tuberculous meningitis among adults with and without HIV infection: experience in an urban public hospital, *Arch. Intern. Med.*, 156, 1710, 1996.

61. Muccioli, C. and Belfort, R., Jr., Presumed ocular and central nervous system tuberculosis in a patient with the acquired immunodeficiency syndrome, *Am. J. Ophthalmol.*, 121, 217, 1996.

62. Martinez-Vazquez, C., Bordon, J., Rodriguez-Gonzalez, A., de la Fuente-Aguado, J., Sopena, B., Gallego-Rivera, A., and Martinez-Cueto, P., Cerebral tuberculoma — a comparative study in patients with and without HIV infection, *Infection*, 23, 149, 1995.

63. Salazar, A., Carratala, J., Santin, M., Meco, F., and Rufi, G., Splenic abscesses caused by *Mycobacterium tuberculosis* in AIDS, *Enfer. Infecc. Microbiol. Clin.*, 12, 146, 1994.

64. Moreno, S., Baraia, J., Parras, F., Solera, J., Bernacer, B., Meana, A., and Bouza, E., Fever evolution after treatment in patients with tuberculosis and HIV infection, *Rev. Clin. Esp.*, 195, 150, 1995.

65. Albrecht, H., Stelbrink, H. J., Eggers, C., Rusch-Gerdes, S., and Greten, H., A case of disseminated *Mycobacterium bovis* infection in an AIDS patient, *Eur. J. Clin. Microbiol. Infect. Dis.*, 14, 226, 1995.

66. Calpe, J. L., Chiner, E., and Larramendi, C. H., Endobronchial tuberculosis in HIV-infected patients, *AIDS*, 9, 1159, 1995.

67. Dronda, F., Fernandez-Martin, I., Chaves, F., and Gonzalez-Lopez, M., Recurrent *Mycobacterium tuberculosis* bacteremia in AIDS: subtherapeutic concentrations of antitubercular agents? *Med. Clin. (Barcelona)*, 103, 478, 1994.

68. Godfrey-Faussett, P., Githui, W., Batchelor, B., Brindle, R., Paul, J., Hawken, M., Gathua, S., Odhiambo, J., Ojoo, S., Nunn, P., Gilks, C., McAdam, K., and Stoker, N., Recurrence of HIV-related tuberculosis in an endemic area may be due to relapse or reinfection, *Tuber. Lung Dis.*, 75, 199, 1994.

69. Small, P. M., Shafer, R. W., Hopewell, P. C., Singh, S. P., Murphy, M. J., Desmond, E., Sierra, M. F., and Schoolnik, G. K., Exogenous reinfection with multidrug-resistant *Mycobacterium tuberculosis* in patients with advanced HIV infection, *N. Engl. J. Med.*, 328, 1137, 1993 (see also comments in *N. Engl. J. Med.*, 329, 811 & 812, 1993).

70. Mahmoudi, A. and Iseman, D., Pitfalls in the care of patients with tuberculosis: common errors and their association with the acquisition of drug resistance, *JAMA*, 270, 65, 1993.

71. Iseman, M. D., Treatment of multidrug-resistant tuberculosis, *N. Engl. J. Med.*, 329, 784, 1993.

72. Wallis, R. S., Amir-Tahmasseb, M., and Ellner, J. J., Induction of interleukin 1 and tumor necrosis factor by mycobacterial proteins: the monocyte western blot, *Proc. Natl. Acad. Sci. U.S.A.*, 87, 3348, 1990.

73. Chandrasekhar, S. and Ratnam, S., Studies on cell-wall deficient non-acid fast variants of *Mycobacterium tuberculosis*, *Tuber. Lung Dis.*, 73, 273, 1992.

74. David, H. L., Papa, F., Cruaud, P., Berlie, H. C., Moroja, M. F., Salem, J. I., and Costa, M. F., Relationships between titers of antibodies immunoreacting against glycolipid antigens from *Mycobacterium leprae* and *M. tuberculosis*, the Mitsuda and Mantoux reactions, and bacteriological loads: implications in the pathogenesis, epidemiology and serodiagnosis of leprosy and tuberculosis, *Int. J. Lepr. Other Mycobact. Dis.*, 60, 208, 1992.

75. Janis, E. M., Kaufmann, S. H., Schwartz, R. H., and Pardoll, D. M., Activation of gamma delta T cells in the primary immune response to *Mycobacterium tuberculosis*, *Science*, 244, 713, 1989.

76. Hubbard, R. D., Flory, C. M., and Collins, F. M., Memory T cell-mediated resistance to *Mycobacteria tuberculosis* infection in innately susceptible and resistant mice, *Infect. Immun.*, 59, 2012, 1991.

77. Meylan, P. R., Richman, D. D., and Kornbluth, R. S., Reduced intracellular growth in human macrophages cultivated at physiologic oxygen pressure, *Am. Rev. Respir. Dis.*, 145, 947, 1992.

78. Chan, J., Xing, Y., Magliozzo, R. S., and Bloom, B. R., Killing of virulent *Mycobacterium* tuberculosis by reactive nitrogen intermediates produced by activated murine macrophages, *J. Exp. Med.*, 175, 1111, 1992.

79. O'Brien, S., Jackett, P. S., Lowrie, D. B., and Andrew, P. W., Guinea-pig alveolar macrophages kill *Mycobacterium tuberculosis in vitro*, but killing is independent of susceptibility to hydrogen peroxide or triggering of the respiratory burst, *Microb. Pathol.*, 10, 199, 1991.

80. Denis, M., Interferon-gamma-treated macrophages inhibit growth of tubercle bacilli via the generation of reactive nitrogen intermediates, *Cell Immunol.*, 132, 150, 1990.

81. Rastogi, N. and Blom-Potar, M. C., A comparative study on the activation of J-774 macrophage-like cells by gamma-interferon, 1,25-dihydroxyvitamin D_3 and lipopeptide RP-56142: ability to kill intracellularly multiplying *Mycobacterium tuberculosis* and *Mycobacterium avium*, *Int. J. Med. Microbiol.*, 273, 344, 1990.

82. Jones, G. S., Amirault, H. J., and Andersen, B. R., Killing of *Mycobacterium tuberculosis* by neutrophils: a nonoxidative process, *J. Infect. Dis.*, 162, 700, 1990.

83. Brozna, J. P., Horan, M., Rademacher, J. M., Pabst, K. M., and Pabst, M. J., Monocyte responses to sulfatide from *Mycobacterium tuberculosis*: inhibition of priming for enhanced release of superoxide, associated with increased secretion of interleukin-1 and tumor necrosis factor alpha, and altered protein phosphorylation, *Infect. Immun.*, 59, 2542, 1991.

84. Godfrey, H. P., Feng, Z., Mandy, S., Mandy, K., Huygen, K., De Bruyn, J., Abou-Zeid, C., Wiker, H. G., Nagai, S., and Tasaka, H., Modulation of expression of delayed hypersensitivity by mycobacterial antigen 85 fibronectin-binding proteins, *Infect. Immun.*, 60, 2522, 1992.

85. Espitia, C., Sciutto, E., Bottasso, O., Gonzalez-Amaro, R., Hernandez Pando, R., and Mancilla, R., High antibody levels to the mycobacterial fibronectin-binding antigen of 30-31 kD in tuberculosis and lepromatous leprosy, *Clin. Exp. Immunol.*, 87, 362, 1992.

86. Thole, J. E., Schöningh, R., Janson, A. A., Garbe, T., Cornelisse, Y. E., Clark-Curtiss, J. E., Kolk, A. H., Ottenhoff, T. H., De Vries, R. R., and Abou-Zeid, C., Molecular and immunological analysis of a fibronectin-binding protein antigen secreted by *Mycobacterium leprae*, *Mol. Microbiol.*, 6, 153, 1992.

87. Ainslie, G. M., Solomon, J. A., and Bateman, E. D., Lymphocyte and lymphocyte subset numbers in blood and in bronchoalveolar lavage and pleural fluid in various forms of human pulmonary tuberculosis at presentation and during recovery, *Thorax*, 47, 513, 1992.

88. Wallis, R. S., Ellner, J. J., and Shiratsuchi, H., Macrophages, mycobacteria and HIV: the role of cytokines in determining mycobacterial virulence and regulating viral replication, *Res. Microbiol.*, 143, 398, 1992.

89. Barnes, P. F., Abrams, J. S., Lu, S., Sieling, P. A., Rea, T. H., and Modlin, R. L., Patterns of cytokine production by mycobacterium-reactive human T-cell clones, *Infect. Immun.*, 61, 197, 1993.

90. Tazi, A., Bouchonnet, F., Valeyre, D., Cadranel, J., Battesti, J. P., and Hance, A. J., Characterization of gamma/delta T-lymphocytes in the peripheral blood of patients with active tuberculosis: a comparison with normal subjects and patients with sarcoidosis, *Am. Rev. Respir. Dis.*, 146, 1216, 1992.

91. Friedland, J. S., Hartley, J. C., Hartley, C. G., Shattock, R. J., and Griffin, G. E., Cytokine secretion *in vivo* and ex vivo following chemotherapy of *Mycobacterium tuberculosis* infection, *Trans. R. Soc. Trop. Med. Hyg.*, 90, 199, 1996.

92. Parronchi, P., De Carli, M., Manetti, R., Simonelli, C., Piccinni, M. P., Macchia, D., Maggi, E., Del Prete, G., Ricci, M., and Romagnani, S., IL-4 and IFN (alpha and gamma) exert opposite regulatory effects on the development of cytolytic potential by Th1 or Th2 human T cell clones, *J. Immunol.*, 149, 2977, 1992.

93. Kawamura, I., Tsukada, H., Yoshikawa, H., Fujita, M., Nomoto, K., and Mitsuyama, M., IFN-gamma-producing ability as a possible marker for the protective T cells against *Mycobacterium bovis* BCG in mice, *J. Immunol.*, 148, 2887, 1992.

94. Denis, M., Killing of *Mycobacterium tuberculosis* within human monocytes: activation by cytokines and calcitriol, *Clin. Exp. Immunol.*, 84, 200, 1991.

95. Denis, M. and Ghadirian, E., Granulocyte-macrophages colony-stimulating factor restricts growth of tubercle bacilli in human macrophages, *Immunol. Lett.*, 24, 203, 1990.

96. Denis, M., Gregg, E. O., and Ghandirian, E., Cytokine modulation of *Mycobacterium tuberculosis* growth in human macrophages, *Int. J. Immunopharmacol.*, 12, 721, 1990.

97. Wadee, A. A., A 25-kDa fraction from *Mycobacterium tuberculosis* that inhibits leukocyte bactericidal activity: reversal by gamma interferon and clofazimine, *Res. Microbiol.*, 141, 249, 1990.

98. Parak, R. B. and Wadee, A. A., The synergistic effects of gamma interferon and clofazimine on phagocyte function: restoration of inhibition due to a 25 kilodalton fraction from *Mycobacterium tuberculosis*, *Biotherapy*, 3, 265, 1991.

99. Wilkinson, P. C. and Newman, I., Identification of IL-8 as a locomotor attractant for activated human lymphocytes in mononuclear cell cultures with anti-CD3 or purified protein derivative of *Mycobacterium tuberculosis*, *J. Immunol.*, 149, 2689, 1992.

100. Sussman, G. and Wadee, A. A., Supernatants derived from CD8+ lymphocytes activated by mycobacterial fractions inhibit cytokine production: the role of interleukin-6, *Biotherapy*, 4, 87, 1992.

101. Theisen-Popp, P., Pape, H., and Muller-Peddinghaus, R., Interleukin-6 (IL-6) in adjuvant arthritis of rats and its pharmacological modulation, *Int. J. Immunopharmacol.*, 14, 565, 1992.

102. Filley, E. A., Bull, H. A., and Dowd, P. M., The effect of *Mycobacterium tuberculosis* on the susceptibility of human cells to the stumulatory and toxic effects of tumour necrosis factor, *Immunology*, 77, 505, 1992.

103. Filley, E. A. and Rook, G. A., Effect of mycobacteria on sensitivity to the cytotoxic effects of tumor necrosis factor, *Infect. Immun.*, 59, 2567, 1991.

104. Carvalho de Sousa, J. P. and Rastogi, N., Comparative ability of human monocytes and macrophages to control the intracellular growth of *Mycobacterium avium* and *Mycobacterium tuberculosis*: effect of interferon-gamma and indomethacin, *FEMS Microbiol. Immunol.*, 4, 329, 1992.

105. Barrera, L., de Kantor, I., Ritacco, V., Reniero, A., Lopez, B., Benetucci, J., Beltran, M., Libonatti, O., Padula, E., Castagnino, J., and Gonzalez Montaner, L., Humoral response to *Mycobacterium tuberculosis* in patients with human immunodeficiency virus infection, *Tuber. Lung Dis.*, 73, 187, 1992.

106. Geluk, A., Van Meijgaarden, K. E., Janson, A. A., Drijfhoot, J. W., Meloen, R. H., De Vries, R. R., and Ottenhoff, T. H., Functional analysis of DR17(DR3)-restricted mycobacterial T cell epitopes reveals DR17- binding motif and enables the design of allele-specific competitor peptides, *J. Immunol.*, 149, 2864, 1992.

107. Stokvis, H., Langermans, J. A., de Backer Vledder, E., van der Hulst, M. E., and van Furth, R., Hydrocortisone treatment of BCG-infected mice impairs the activation and enhancement of antimicrobial activity of peritoneal macrophages, *Scand. J. Immunol.*, 36, 299, 1992.

108. Gangadharam, P. R., Ashtekar, D. R., Farhi, D. C., and Wise, D. L., Sustained release of isoniazid *in vivo* from a single implant of a biodegradable polymer, *Tubercle*, 72, 115, 1991.

109. Gangadharam, P. R., Kailasam, S., Srinivasan, S., and Wise, D. L., Experimental chemotherapy of tuberculosis using single dose treatment with isoniazid in biodegradable polymers, *J. Antimicrob. Chemother.*, 33, 265, 1994.

110. Heifets, L. B. and Lindholm-Levy, P. J., Is pyrazinamide bactericidal against *Mycobacterium tuberculosis*? *Am. Rev. Respir. Dis.*, 141, 250, 1990.

111. Cynamon, M. H., Klemens, S. P., Chou, T. S., Gimi, R. H., and Welch, J. T., Antimycobacterial activity of a series of pyrazinoic acid esters, *J. Med. Chem.*, 35, 1212, 1992.

112. Salfinger, M., Reller, L. B., Demchuk, B., and Johnson, Z. T., Rapid radiometric method for pyrazinamide susceptibility testing of *Mycobacterium tuberculosis*, *Res. Microbiol.*, 140, 301, 1989.

113. Salfinger, M., Crowle, A. J., and Reller, L. B., Pyrazinamide and pyrazinoic acid activity against tubercle bacilli in cultured human macrophages and in the BACTEC system, *J. Infect. Dis.*, 162, 201, 1990.

114. Heifets, L. B., Flory, M. A., and Lindholm-Levy, P. J., Does pyrazinoic acid as an active moiety of pyrazinamide have specific activity against *Mycobacterium tuberculosis*? *Antimicrob. Agents Chemother.*, 33, 1252, 1989.

115. Gangadharam, P. R., Pratt, P. F., Perumal, V. K., and Iseman, M. D., The effects of exposure time, drug concentration, and temperature on the activity of ethambutol versus *Mycobacterium tuberculosis*, *Am. Rev. Respir. Dis.*, 141, 1478, 1990.

116. Yamori, S., Ichiyama, S., Shimokata, K., and Tsukamura, M., Bacteriostatic and bactericidal activities of antituberculosis drugs against *Mycobacterium tuberculosis*, *Mycobacterium avium-Mycobacterium intracellulare* complex and *Mycobacterium kansasii* in different growth phases, *Microbiol. Immunol.*, 36, 361, 1992.

117. Griffith, M. E. and Bodily, H. L., Stability of antimycobacterial drugs in susceptibility testing, *Antimicrob. Agents Chemother.*, 36, 2398, 1992.

118. Dhillon, J., Dickinson, J. M., Guy, J. A., Ng, T. K., and Mitchison, D. A., Activity of two long-acting rifamycins, rifapentin and FCE 22807, in experimental murine tuberculosis, *Tuber. Lung Dis.*, 73, 116, 1992.

119. Dhillon, J. and Mitchison, D. A., Activity *in vitro* of rifabutin, FCE 22807, rifapentine, and rifampin against *Mycobacterium microti* and *Mycobacterium tuberculosis* and their penetration into mouse peritoneal macrophages, *Am. Rev. Respir. Dis.*, 145, 212, 1992.

120. Dickinson, J. M. and Mitchison, D. A., *In vitro* activities against mycobacteria of two long-acting rifamycins, FCE 22807 and CGP 40/496A (SPA-S-565), *Tubercle*, 71, 109, 1990.

121. Grosset, J., Truffot-Pernot, C., Lacroix, C., and Ji, B., Antagonism between isoniazid and the combination pyrazinamide-rifampin against tuberculosis infection in mice, *Antimicrob. Agents Chemother.*, 36, 548, 1992.

122. Agarwal, A., Kandpal, H., Gupta, H. P., Singh, N. B., and Gupta, C. M., Tuftsin-bearing liposomes as rifampin vehicles in treatment of tuberculosis in mice, *Antimicrob. Agents Chemother.*, 38, 588, 1994.

123. Kuze, F., Antimycobacterial activities of rifamycin derivatives, *Kekkaku*, 66, 679, 1991.

124. Yamamoto, T., Amitani, R., Kuze, F., and Suzuki, K., *In vitro* activities of new rifamycin derivatives against *Mycobacterium tuberculosis* and *M. avium* complex, *Kekkaku*, 65, 805, 1990.

125. Hirata, T., Saito, H., Tomioka, H., Sato, K. et al., *In vitro* and *in vivo* activities of the benzoxazinorifamycin KRM-1648 against *Mycobacterium tuberculosis*, *Antimicrob. Agents Chemother.*, 39, 2295, 1995.

126. Reddy, M. V., Luna-Herrera, J., Daneluzzi, D., and Gangadharam, P. R., Chemotherapeutic activity of benzoxazinorifamycin, KRM-1648, against *Mycobacterium tuberculosis* in C57BL/6 mice, *Tuber. Lung Dis.*, 77, 154, 1996.

127. Klemens, S. P., Grossi, M. A., and Cynamon, M. H., Activity of KRM-1648, a new benzoxazinorifamycin, against *Mycobacterium tuberculosis* in a murine model, *Antimicrob. Agents Chemother.*, 38, 2245, 1994.

128. Tomioka, H. and Saito, H., Studies on therapeutic efficacy of a new anti-tuberculous drug, benzoxazinorifamycin, against murine experimental mycobacterial infections: attempt at various regimens and protocols, *Kekkaku*, 69, 703, 1994.

129. Reddy, V. M., Nadadhur, G., Daneluzzi, D., Dimova, V., and Gangadharam, P. R., Antimycobacterial activity of a new rifamycin derivatives, 3-(4-cinnamylpiperazinyl iminomethyl) rifamycin SV (T9), *Antimicrob. Agents Chemother.*, 39, 2320, 1995.

130. Watt, B., Edwards, J. R., Rayner, A., Grindey, A. J., and Harris, G., *In vitro* activity of two carbapenem antibiotics, meropenem and imipenem, against mycobacteria: development of a daily antibiotic dosing schedule, *Tuber. Lung Dis.*, 73, 134, 1992.

131. Nadler, J. P., Berger, J., Nord, J. A., Cofsky, R., and Saxena, M., Amoxicillin-clavulanic acid for treating drug-resistant *Mycobacterium tuberculosis*, *Chest*, 99, 1025, 1991.

132. Zhang, Y., Steingrube, V. A., and Wallace, R. J., Jr., Beta-lactamase inhibitors and the inducibility of the beta-lactamase of *Mycobacterium tuberculosis*, *Am. Rev. Respir. Dis.*, 145, 657, 1992.

133. Truffot-Pernot, C., Lounis, N., Grosset, J. H., and Ji, B., Clarithromycin is inactive against *Mycobacterium tuberculosis*, *Antimicrob. Agents Chemother.*, 39, 2827, 1995.

134. Luna-Herrera, J., Reddy, Y. M., Daneluzzi, D., and Gangadharam, P. R., Antituberculosis activity of clarithromycin, *Antimicrob. Agents Chemother.*, 39, 2692, 1995.

135. Cavalieri, S. J., Biehle, J. R., and Sanders, W. E., Jr., Synergistic activities of clarithromycin and antituberculous drugs against multidrug-resistant *Mycobacterium tuberculosis*, *Antimicrob. Agents Chemother.*, 39, 1542, 1995.

136. Kanyok, T. P., Reddy, M. V., Chinnaswamy, J., Danziger, L. H., and Gangadharam, P. R., *In vivo* activity of paromomycin against susceptible and multidrug-resistant *Mycobacterium tuberculosis* and *M. avium* complex strains, *Antimicrob. Agents Chemother.*, 38, 170, 1994.

137. Selvakumar, N., Kumar, V., Acharyulu, G. S., Rehman, F., Paramasivan, C. N., and Prabhakar, R., Susceptibility of south Indian strains of *Mycobacterium tuberculosis* to tuberactinomycin, *Indian J. Med. Res.*, 101, 1992.

138. Ertem, E., Yüce, K., Karakartal, G., Onal, O., and Yücem G., The antituberculous effect of bleomycin, *J. Antimicrob. Chemother.*, 26, 862, 1990.

139. Iseman, M. D. and Madsen, L. A., Drug-resistant tuberculosis, *Clin. Chest Med.*, 10, 341, 1989.

140. Nakanishi, N., Kojima, T., Fujimoto, T., and Mitsuhashi, S., *In vitro* properties of newer quinolones, *Prog. Drug Res.*, 38, 19, 1992.

141. Klopman G., Fercu, D., Li, J. Y., Rosenkranz, H. S., and Jacobs, M. R., Antimycobacterial quinolones: a comparative analysis of structure-activity and structure-toxicity relationships, *Res. Microbiol.*, 147, 86, 1996.

142. Jacobs, M. R., Activity of quinolones against mycobacteria, *Drugs*, 49(Suppl.), 67, 1995.

143. Aysev, D., *In vitro* activity of ofloxacin and ciprofloxacin against *Mycobacterium tuberculosis* strains, *Microbiol. Bul.*, 27, 31, 1993.

144. Yew, W. W., Kwan, S. Y., Ma, W. K., Khin, M. A., and Chau, P, Y., *In vitro* activity of ofloxacin against *Mycobacterium tuberculosis* and its clinical efficacy in multiple resistant tuberculosis, *Antimicrob. Agents Chemother.*, 261, 227, 1990.

145. Piersimoni, C., Morbiducci, V., Bornigia, S., De Sio, G., and Scalise, G., *In vitro* activity of the new quinolone lomefloxacin against *Mycobacterium tuberculosis*, *Am. Rev. Respir. Dis.*, 146, 1445, 1992.

146. Truffot-Pernot, C., Ji, B., and Grosset, J., Activities of pefloxacin and ofloxacin against mycobacteria: *in vitro* and mouse experiments, *Tubercle*, 72, 57, 1991.

147. Xu, G., Li, H., and Liu, S., Comparison of in-vitro and in-vivo activities of enoxacin and ofloxacin against *Mycobacterium tuberculosis*, *Chung Hua Chieh Ho Ho Hu Hsi Tsa Chih*, 18, 175, 1995.

148. Rastogi, N. and Blom-Potar, M. C., Intracellular bactericidal activity of ciprofloxacin and ofloxacin against *Mycobacterium tuberculosis* H37Rv multiplying in the J-774 macrophage cell line, *Int. J. Med. Microbiol.*, 273, 195, 1990.

149. Ji, B., Truffot-Pernot, C., and Grosset, J., *In vitro* and *in vivo* activities of sparfloxacin (AT-4140) against *M. tuberculosis*, *Tubercle*, 72, 181, 1991.

150. Tomioka, H., Sato, K., and Saito, H., Antimycobacterial activities of a new quinolone, sparfloxacin, *Kekkaku*, 66, 643, 1991.

151. Rastogi, N. and Goh, K. S., *In vitro* activity of the new difluorinated quinolone sparfloxacin (AT-4140) against *Mycobacterium tuberculosis* compared with activities of ofloxacin and ciprofloxacin, *Antimicrob. Agents Chemother.*, 35, 1933, 1991.

152. Tomioka, H., Sato, K., and Saito, H., Comparative *in vitro* and *in vivo* activity of fleroxacin and ofloxacin against various mycobacteria, *Tubercle*, 72, 176, 1991.

153. Kawahara, S., Kamisaka, K., Tada, A., Nakada, H., Mishima, Y., Yoshimoto, S., Matsuyama, T., Kibata, M., and Nagare, J., *In vitro* activities of newly developed quinolones, fleroxacin, lomefloxacin and sparfloxacin against *Mycobacterium tuberculosis*, *Kekkaku*, 66, 429, 1991.

154. Ji, B., Lounis, N., Truffot-Pernot, C., and Grosset, J., *In vitro* and *in vivo* activities of levofloxacin against *Mycobacterium tuberculosis*, *Antimicrob. Agents Chemother.*, 39, 1341, 1995.

155. Klemens, S. P., Sharpe, C. A., Rogge, M. C., and Cynamon, M. H., Activity of levofloxacin in a murine model of tuberculosis, *Antimicrob. Agents Chemother.*, 38, 1476, 1994.

156. Heifets, L. B. and Lindholm-Levy, P. J., MICs and MBCs of WIN 57273 against *Mycobacterium avium* and *M. tuberculosis*, *Antimicrob. Agents Chemother.*, 34, 770, 1990.

157. Tomioka, H., Sato, K., Saito, H., and Ikeda, Y., Antimycobacterial activity of a newly synthesized fluoroquinolone, Y-26611, *Kekkaku*, 67, 515, 1992.

158. Majumdar, S. and Basu, S. K., Killing of intracellular *Mycobacterium tuberculosis* by receptor-mediated drug delivery, *Antimicrob. Agents Chemother.*, 35, 135, 1991.

159. Heifets, L. and Lindholm-Levy, P., Pyrazinamide sterilizing activity *in vitro* against semidormant *Mycobacterium tuberculosis* bacterial populations, *Am. Rev. Respir. Dis.*, 145, 1223, 1992.

160. Wisterowicz, K., Foks, H., Janowiec, M., and Zwolska-Kwiek, Z., Studies on pyrazine derivatives. XXVI. Synthesis and tuberculostatic activity of *N*-pyrazinylthiourea, *Acta Pol. Pharm.*, 46, 101, 1989.

161. Mamolo, M. G., Vio, L., Banfi, E., Predominato, M., Fabris, C., and Asaro, F., Synthesis and antimycobacterial activity of some 2-pyridinecarboxyamidrazone derivatives, *Farmaco*, 47, 1055, 1992.

162. Mir, I., Siddiqui, M.T., and Comrie, A. M., Alpha-[5-(5-nitro-2-furyl)-1,3,4-oxadiazol-2-ylthio]acethy-drazide and related compounds, *J. Pharm. Sci.*, 80, 548, 1991.

163. Ramamurthy, B. and Bhatt, M. V., Synthesis and antitubercular activity of *N*-(2-naphthyl)glycine hydrazide analogs, *J. Med. Chem.*, 32, 2421, 1989.

164. Ashtekar, D. R., Costa-Periera, R., Shrinivasan, T., Iyyer, R., Vishvanathan, N., and Rittel, W., Oxazolidinones, a new class of synthetic antituberculosis agents: *in vitro* and *in vivo* activities of DuP-721 against *Mycobacterium tuberculosis*, *Diagn. Microbiol. Infect. Dis.*, 14, 465, 1991.

165. Heifets, L. B., Lindholm-Levy, P. J., and Flory, M., Thiacetazone: *in vitro* activity against *Mycobacterium avium* and *M. tuberculosis*, *Tubercle*, 71, 287, 1990.

166. Ratnakar, P. and Murthy, P. S., Antitubercular activity of trifluoperazine, a calmodulin antagonist, *FEMS Microbiol. Lett.*, 76, 73, 1992.

167. Fuursted, K., Askgaard, D., and Faber, V., Susceptibility of strains of the *Mycobacterium tuberculosis* complex to fusidic acid, *APMIS*, 100, 663, 1992.

168. Hoffner, S. E., Olsson-Liljequist, B., Rydgard, K. J., Svenson, S. B., and Källenius, G., Susceptibility of mycobacteria to fusidic acid, *Eur. J. Clin. Microbiol. Infect. Dis.*, 9, 294, 1990.

169. Botis, S., Koemoth, P. P., Correa de Brito, J. M., and Brock, M., Growth of some mycobacterial strains in 7H12 Middlebrook liquid medium in the presence of auramine, *Rev. Ig. (Pneumoftiziol.)*, 38, 137, 1989.

170. Bukowski, L. and Janowiec, M., Synthesis and some reactions of 1-methyl-1*H*-2-cyanomethy-limidazo[4,5-*b*]pyridine: tuberculostatic activity of obtained compounds, *Pharmazie*, 45, 904, 1990.

171. Bukowski, L. and Kaliszan, R., Imidazo[4,5-*b*]pyridine derivatives of potential tuberculostatic activity. I. Synthesis and quantitative structure-activity relationships, *Arch. Pharm. (Weinheim)*, 324, 121, 1991.

172. Bukowski, L. and Kaliszan, R., Imidazo[4,5-*b*]pyridine derivatives of potential tuberculostatic activity. II. Synthesis and bioactivity of designed and some other 2-cyanomethylimidazo[4,5-*b*]pyridine derivatives, *Arch. Pharm. (Weinheim)*, 324, 537, 1991.

173. Gümüs, F., Altuntas, T. G., Saygun, N., Ozden, T., and Ozden, S., *In vitro* tuberculostatic activities of some 2-benzylbenzimidazole and 2-phenoxymethylbenzimidazole derivatives, *J. Pharm. Belg.*, 44, 398, 1989.

174. Dannhardt, G., Kappe, T., Meindle, W., and Schober, B., Antimycobacterial acting 2-hydroxy-quinolizin-4-ones, *Arch. Pharm. (Weinheim)*, 323, 375, 1990.

175. Meindl, W., Antimycobacterial antihistaminics, *Arch. Pharm. (Weinheim)*, 322, 493, 1989.

176. Shen, M. L., Zhai, S. K., Chen, H. L., Luo, Y. D., Tu, G. R., and Ou, D. W., Immunopharmacological effects of polysaccharides from *Acanthopanax senticosus* on experimental animals, *Int. J. Immuno-pharmacol.*, 13, 549, 1991.

177. Sharma, V. K., Tuberculostatic activity of henna (*Lawsonia inermis* Linn.), *Tubercle*, 71, 293, 1990.

178. Chohan, Z. H. and Rauf, A., Studies on biologically active complexes of cobalt(II) and nickel(II) with dithiooxamide-derived ligands, *J. Inorg. Biochem.*, 46, 41, 1992.

179. Pin, Y. and Zhang, X. P., Synthesis and characterization of new chromium(III), vanadium(IV), and titanium(III) complexes with biologically active isonicotinic acid hydrazide, *J. Inorg. Biochem.*, 37, 61, 1989.

180. Maiti, A. and Ghosh, S., Synthesis and reactivity of the oxovanadium(IV) complexes of two N-O donors and potentiation of the antituberculosis activity of one of them on chelation to metal ions. IV, *J. Inorg. Biochem.*, 36, 131, 1989.

181. Zemskova, Z. S. and Dorozhkova, I. R., Pathomorphological assessment of the therapeutic effect of mycobacteriophages in tuberculosis, *Probl. Tuberk.*, 63, 1991.

182. Jagannath, C., Allaudeen, H. S., and Hunter, R. L., Activities of poloxamer CRL8131 against *Mycobacterium tuberculosis in vitro* and *in vivo*, *Antimicrob. Agents Chemother.*, 39, 1349, 1995.

183. Sbarbaro, J. A., Iseman, M. D., and Crowle, A. J., The combined effect of rifampin and pyrazinamide within the human macrophage, *Am. Rev. Respir. Dis.*, 146, 1448, 1992.

184. Bispen, A. V., Aleksandrova, A. E., Vakhmistrova, T. I., and Vinogradova, T. I., Effect of plasmapheresis on the course of experimental tuberculosis and the tolerance of chemotherapy by patients with renal tuberculosis, *Probl. Tuberk.*, 53, 1992.

185. Smith, D. W., Balasubramanian, V., and Wiegeshaus, E., A guinea pig model of experimental airborne tuberculosis for evaluation of the response to chemotherapy: the effect on bacilli in the initial phase of treatment, *Tubercle*, 72, 223, 1991.

186. Jacobs, W. R., Jr., Barletta, R. G., Udani, R., Chan, J., Kalkut, G., Sosne, G., Kieser, T., Sarkis, G. J., Hatfull, G. F., and Bloom, B. R., Rapid assessment of drug susceptibility of *M. tuberculosis* by means of luciferase reporter phages, *Science*, 260, 819, 1993.

187. Cooksey, R. C., Crawford, J. T., Jacobs, W. R., Jr., and Shinnick, T. M., A rapid method for screening agents for activity against a strain of *M. tuberculosis* expressing firefly luciferase, *Antimicrob. Agents Chemother.*, 37, 1348, 1993.

188. Schaberg, T., Reichert, B., Schulin, T., Lode, H., and Mauch, H., Rapid drug susceptibility testing of *Mycobacterium tuberculosis* using conventional solid media, *Eur. Respir. J.*, 8, 1688, 1995.

189. Georgiev, V. St., Treatment and developmental therapeutics of *Mycobacterium tuberculosis* infections, *Int. J. Antimicrob. Agents*, 4, 157, 1994.

190. Committee on Infectious Diseases, Chemotherapy for tuberculosis in infants and children, *Pediatrics*, 89, 161, 1992.

191. Blom-Bülow, B., Dosing regimens in the treatment of tuberculosis, *Scand. J. Infect. Dis. Suppl.*, 74, 258, 1990.

192. Doganay, M., Calangu, S., Turgut, H., Bakir, M., and Aygen, B., Treatment of tuberculous meningitis in Turkey, *Scand. J. Infect. Dis.*, 27, 135, 1995.

193. Ibanez, S. and Ross, G., Quimioterapia abreviada de 6 meses en tuberculosis pulmonar infantil, *Rev. Chil. Pediatr.*, 51, 249, 1980.

194. Anane, T., Cernay, J., and Bensenovci, A., Resultats compares des regimens et des regimens long dans la chimiotherapie de la tuberculose de l'enfant en Algerie, *African Regional Meeting of International Union Against Tuberculosis*, Tunis, Tunisia, 1984.

195. Varudkar, B. L., Short-course chemotherapy for tuberculosis in children, *Indian J. Pediatr.*, 52, 593, 1985.

196. Pelosi, F., Budani, H., Rubinstein, C., Diaz Vélez, H., Bonavena, B., Beltran, O. P., and Gonzalez Montaner, J., Isoniazid, rifampin and pyrazinamide in the treatment of childhood tuberculosis with duration adjusted to the clinical status, *Am. Rev. Respir. Dis.*, 131(Suppl.), A229, 1985.

197. Starke, J. R. and Taylor-Watts, K. T., Six-month chemotherapy of intrathoracic tuberculosis in children, *Am. Rev. Respir. Dis.*, 139(Suppl.), A314, 1989.

198. Medical Research Council Tuberculosis and Chest Disease Unit, Management and outcome of chemotherapy for childhood tuberculosis, *Arch. Dis. Child.*, 64, 1004, 1989.

199. Biddulph, J., Short-course chemotherapy for childhood tuberculosis, *Pediatr. Infect. Dis. J.*, 9, 794, 1990.

200. Khubchandani, R. P., Kumta, N. B., Bharucha, N. B., and Ramakantan, R., Short-course chemotherapy in childhood pulmonary tuberculosis, *Am. Rev. Resp. Dis.*, 141(Suppl.), A338, 1990.

201. Kumar, L., Dhand, R., Singhi, P. D., Rao, K. L., and Katariya, S., A randomized trial of fully intermittent vs. daily followed by intermittent short-course chemotherapy for childhood tuberculosis, *Pediatr. Infect. Dis. J.*, 9, 802, 1990.

202. Small, P. M., Schecter, G. F., Goodman, P. C., Sande, M. A., Chaisson, R. E., and Hopewell, P. C., Treatment of tuberculosis in patients with advanced human immunodeficiency virus infection, *N. Engl. J. Med.*, 324, 289, 1991.

203. Rose, D. N., Schechter, C. B., and Sacks, H. S., Preventive medicine for HIV-infected patients: an analysis of isoniazid prophylaxis for tuberculin reactors and for anergic patients, *J. Gen. Intern. Med.*, 7, 589, 1992.

204. Pust, R. E., Tuberculosis in the 1990's: resurgence, regimens, and resources, *South. Med. J.*, 85, 584, 1992.

205. Matz, J., Borish, L. C., Routes, J. M., and Rosenwasser, L. J., Oral desensitization to rifampin and ethambutol in mycobacterial disease, *Am. J. Respir. Crit. Care Med.*, 149, 815, 1994.

206. Iareshko, A. G., The optimization of the corticosteroid therapy of patients with destructive pulmonary tuberculosis, *Vrach. Delo*, 39, 1989.

207. Strang, J. I., Rapid resolution of tuberculous pericardial effusion with high dose prednisone and anti-tuberculous drugs, *J. Infect.*, 28, 251, 1994.

208. Taki, H. N. and Schwartz, S. A., Levamisole as an immunopotentiator for T cell deficiency, *Immunopharmacol. Immunotoxicol.*, 16, 129, 1994.

209. Kenian/Zambian/British Medical Research Council Collaborative Study, Controlled clinical trial of levamisole in short-course chemotherapy for pulmonary tuberculosis, *Am. Rev. Respir. Dis.*, 140, 990, 1989.

210. Kohno, S., Koga, H., Kaku, M., Maesaki, S., and Hara, K., Prospective comparative study of ofloxacin or ethambutol for the treatment of pulmonary tuberculosis, *Chest*, 102, 1815, 1992.

211. Hong Kong Chest Service/British Medical Research Council, Controlled trial of 2, 4, and 6 months of pyrazinamide in 6-month, three-times-weekly regimens for smear-positive pulmonary tuberculosis, including an assessment of a combined preparation of isoniazid, rifampin, and pyrazinamide: results at 30 months, *Am. Rev. Respir. Dis.*, 143, 700, 1991.

212. Singapore Tuberculosis Service/British Medical Research Council, Assessment of daily combined preparation of isoniazid, rifampin, and pyrazinamide in a controlled trial of three 6-month regimens for smear-positive pulmonary tuberculosis, *Am. Rev. Respir. Dis.*, 143, 707, 1991.

213. Iseman, M.D. and Sbarbaro, J. A., Short-course chemotherapy of tuberculosis, *Am. Rev. Respir. Dis.*, 143, 697, 1991.

214. Balasubramanian, R., Sivasubramanian, S., Vijayan, V. K., Ramachandran, R., Jawahar, M. S., Paramasivan, C. N., Selvakumar, N., and Somasusundaram, P. R., Five year results of a 3-month and two 5-month regimens for the treatment of sputum-positive pulmonary tuberculosis in South India, *Tubercle*, 71, 253, 1990.

215. Wolde, K., Lema, E., Roscigno, G., and Abdi, A., Fixed dose combination short course chemotherapy in the treatment of pulmonary tuberculosis, *Ethiop. Med. J.*, 30, 63, 1992.

216. Novak, D., Radenbach, D., and Magnussen, H., In 76% of patients with active tuberculosis treated with triple therapy (isoniazid-rifampicin-pyrazinamide) cultural conversion precedes microscopic conversion, *Pneumologie*, 44(Suppl.), 497, 1990.

217. Starostenko, E. V., Dolzhanskii, B. M., Salpagarov, A. M., and Levchenko, T. N., The use of antioxidants in the complex therapy of patients with infiltrating pulmonary tuberculosis, *Probl. Tuberk.*, 9, 1991.

218. Brogden, R. N. and Fitton, A., Rifabutin: a review of its antimicrobial activity, pharmacokinetic properties and therapeutic efficacy, *Drugs*, 47, 983, 1994.

219. Hong Kong Chest Service/British Medical Research Council, A controlled study of rifabutin and an uncontrolled study of ofloxacin in the retreatment of patients with pulmonary tuberculosis resistant to isoniazid, streptomycin and rifampicin, *Tuber. Lung Dis.*, 73, 59, 1992.

220. Gonzalez-Montaner, L. J., Natal, S., Yongchaiyud, P., and Olliaro, P., Rifabutin for the treatment of newly-diagnosed pulmonary tuberculosis: a multinational, randomized, comparative study versus rifampicin. Rifabutin Study Group, *Tuber. Lung Dis.*, 75, 341, 1994 (see also comment in *Tuber. Lung Dis.*, 76, 582, 1995).

221. Chan, S. L., Yew, W. W., Ma, W. K., Girling, D. J., Aber, V. R., Felmingham, D., Allen, B. W., and Mitchison, D. A., The early bactericidal activity of rifabutin measured by sputum viable counts in Hong Kong patients with pulmonary tuberculosis, *Tuber. Lung Dis.*, 73, 33, 1992.

222. Pretet, S., Lebeaut, A., Parrot, R., Truffot, C., Grosset, J., and Dinh-Xuan, A. T., Combined chemotherapy including rifabutin for rifampicin and isoniazid resistant pulmonary tuberculosis. G.E.T.I.M. (Group for the Study and Treatment of Resistant Mycobacterial Infection), *Eur. Respir. J.*, 5, 680, 1992.

223. Lee, C. N., Lin, T. P., Chang, M. F., Jimenez, M. V., Dolfi, L., and Olliaro, P., Rifabutin as salvage therapy for cases of chronic multidrug-resistant pulmonary tuberculosis in Taiwan, *J. Chemother.*, 8, 137, 1996.

224. Schwander, S., Rusch-Gerdes, S., Mateega, A., Lutalo, T. et al., A pilot of antituberculosis combinations comparing rifabutin with rifampicin in the treatment of HIV-1 associated tuberculosis: a single-blind randomized evaluation in Ugandan patients with HIV-1 infection and pulmonary tuberculosis, *Tuber. Lung Dis.*, 76, 210, 1995.

225. Matsuzawa, Y., Nakamura, Y., Nakagawa, S., Fujimoto, K., Honda, T., Kubo, K., Kobayashi, T., and Sekiguchi, M., A case of pulmonary tuberculosis associated with severe skin eruption, prominent eosinophilia, and liver dysfunction induced by streptomycin, *Kekkaku*, 67, 413, 1992.

226. Nakae, I., Nakatani, K., Inoue, S., Takahashi, K., Ikeda, N., Matsumoto, T., Ozawa, S., Sakatani, M., Kita, N., and Tanaka, S., Therapeutic effect of ofloxacin on intractable pulmonary tuberculosis and ofloxacin resistance of tubercle bacilli isolated from the patients. Chest Disease Cooperative Study Unit of National Sanatoriums in Kinki District, *Kekkaku*, 66, 299, 1991.

227. Ziegler, D., Lode, H., Raffenberg, M., Schaberg, T., Mauch, H., and Grassot, A., Incompatibility of tuberculosis therapy in a patient with AIDS, *Dtsch. Med. Wochenschr.*, 119, 1728, 1994.

228. Donald, P. R., Gent, W. L., Seifart, H. I., Lamprecht, J. H., and Parkin, D. P., Cerebrospinal fluid isoniazid concentrations in children with tuberculous meningitis: the influence of dosage and acetylation status, *Pediatrics*, 89, 247, 1992.

229. Estebanez Zarranz, M. J., Martinez Sagarra, J. M., Alberte, A., Amon Sesmero, J., and Rodriguez Toves, A., Treatment of urogenital tuberculosis with ofloxacin: preliminary study, *Actas Urol. Esp.*, 16, 64, 1992.

230. Helm, C. J. and Holland, C. N., Ocular tuberculosis, *Surv. Ophthalmol.*, 38, 229, 1993.

231. Cotton, J. B., Ligeon-Ligeonnet, P., Durra, A., Sartre, J., Bureau, E., Chetail, N., and Grenier, J. L., Tuberculous dacryocistis, *Arch. Pediatr.*, 2, 147, 1995.

232. Sais, G., Vidaller, A., Jucgla, A., and Peyri, J., Tuberculous lymphadenitis presenting with cutaneous leukocytoclastic vasculitis, *Clin. Exp. Dermatol.*, 21, 65, 1996.

233. Dabrowski, M. T. and Keith, A. O., Three cases of mycobacterial cervical lymphadenitis, *J. Laryngol. Otol.*, 108, 514, 1994.

234. Di Natale, M., Fiusti, R., Lai, F., and Corradi, F., Extrapulmonary tuberculosis: an unusual case, *Minerva Med.*, 86, 555, 1995.

235. Kreder, H. J. and Davey, J. R., Total hip arthroplasty complicated by tuberculous infection, *J. Arthroplasty*, 11, 111, 1996.

236. Tokumoto, J. I., Follansbee, S. E., and Jacobs, R. A., Prosthetic joint infection due to *Mycobacterium tuberculosis*: report of three cases, *Clin. Infect. Dis.*, 21, 134, 1995.

237. Chen, Y. C., Chang, S. C., Hsieh, W. C., Luh, K. T., and Shen, M. C., Non-spinal psoas abscess due to *Mycobacterium tuberculosis* in a patient with acquired immunodeficiency syndrome: report of a case, *J. Formos. Med. Assoc.*, 93, 433, 1994.

238. Davidson, G. S., Voorneveld, C. R., and Krishnan, N., Tuberculous infection of skeletal muscle in a case of dermatomyositis, *Muscle Nerve*, 17, 730, 1994.

239. Nowak, B., Lautenschlager, G., Hennermann, K. H., Hubner, K., and Teschke, R., Duodenal tuberculosis: a rare cause of a covered perforation in the duodenal bulb, *Dtsch. Med. Wochenschr.*, 119, 141, 1994.

240. Junquera Gutierrez, L. M., Alonso Vaquero, D., Albertos Castro, J. M., Palacios Gutierrez, J. J., and Vicente Rodriguez, J. C., Primary tuberculosis of the oral cavity, *Rev. Stomatol. Chir. Maxilofac.*, 97, 3, 1996.

241. Shafik, A., Treatment of tuberculous epididymitis by intratunical rifampicin injection, *Arch. Androl.*, 36, 239, 1996.

242. Goh, S. H., Ravintharan, T., Sim, C. S., and Chung, H. C., Nodular skin tuberculosis with lymphatic spread — a case report, *Singapore Med. J.*, 36, 99, 1995.

243. Centers for Disease Control, Nosocomial transmission of multidrug- resistant tuberculosis among HIV-infected persons — Florida and New York, 1988-1991, *Morbid. Mortal. Wkly. Rep.*, 40, 585, 1991.

244. Snider, D. E., Jr., Cauthen, G. M., Farer, L. S., Kelly, G. D., Kilbern, J. O., Good, R. C., and Dooley, S. W., Drug-resistant tuberculosis, *Am. Rev. Respir. Dis.*, 144, 732, 1991.

245. Cole, S. T. and Telenti, A., Drug resistance in *Mycobacterium tuberculosis*, *Eur. Respir. J. Suppl.*, 20, 701s, 1995.

246. Nunn, P. and Felten, M., Surveillance of resistance to antituberculosis drugs in developing countries, *Tuber. Lung Dis.*, 75, 163, 1994.

247. Olle-Goig, J. E., Non-compliance with tuberculosis treatment: patients and physicians, *Tuber. Lung Dis.*, 76, 277, 1995.

248. Kochi, A., The global tuberculosis situation and the new control strategy of the World Health Organization, *Tubercle*, 72, 1, 1991.

249. Lambregts-van Weezenbeek, C. S. and Veen, J., Control of drug-resistant tuberculosis, *Tuber. Lung Dis.*, 76, 455, 1995.

250. Yew, W. W. and Chau, C. H., Drug-resistant tuberculosis in the 1990s, *Eur. Respir. J.*, 8, 1184, 1995.

251. Kleeberg, H. and Olivier, M., *A World Atlas of Initial Drug Resistance*, 2nd ed., Tuberculosis Research Institute of the South African Medical Resarch Council, Pretoria, South Africa, 1984.

252. Borchardt, J., Kirsten, D., Jorres, R., Kroeger, C., and Magnussen, H., Incidence of resistance and risk factors for resistance in *Mycobacterium tuberculosis*: a retrospective study of 1,055 patients of a specialty hospital 1984 to 1993, *Pneumologie*, 50, 28, 1996.

253. Schaberg, T., Gloger, G., Reichert, B., Mauch, H., and Lode, H., Resistant lung tuberculosis in Berlin 1987-1993, *Pneumologie*, 50, 21, 1996.

254. Ausina, V., Multidrug-resistant tuberculosis: remarks and reflections on a controversial subject of current utmost importance, *Med. Clin. (Barcelona)*, 106, 15, 1996.

255. Goble, M., Iseman, M. D., Madsen, L. A., Waite, D., Ackerson, L., and Horsburgh, C. R., Jr., Treatment of 171 patients with pulmonary tuberculosis resistant to isoniazid and rifampin, *N. Engl. J. Med.*, 328, 527, 1993.

256. Weltman, A. C. and Rose, D. N., Tuberculosis susceptibility patterns, predictors of multidrug resistance, and implication for initial therapeutic regimens at a New York City hospital, *Arch. Intern. Med.*, 154, 2161, 1994.

257. Frieden, T. R., Sterling, T., Pablos-Mendez, A., Kilburn, J. O., Cauthen, G. M., and Dooley, S. W., The emergence of drug-resistant tuberculosis in New York City, *N. Engl. J. Med.*, 328, 521, 1993.

258. Chawla, K., Klapper, P. J., Kamholz, S. L., Pollack, A. H., and Heurich, A. E., Drug-resistant tuberculosis in an urban population including patients at risk for human immunodeficiency virus infection, *Am. Rev. Respir. Dis.*, 146, 280, 1992.

259. Braun, M. M., Kilburn, J. O., Smithwick, R. W., Coulibaly, I. M., Coulibaly, D., Silcox, V. A., Gnaore, E., Adjorlolo, G., and De Cock, K. M., HIV infection and primary resistance to antituberculosis drugs in Abidjan, Cote d'Ivoire, *AIDS*, 6, 1327, 1992.

260. Asch, S., Knowles, L., Rai, A., Jones, B. E. et al., Relationship of isoniazid resistance to human immunodeficiency virus infection in patients with tuberculosis, *Am. J. Respir. Crit. Care Med.*, 153, 1708, 1996 (see also comment in *Am. J. Respir. Crit. Care Med.*, 153, 1472, 1996).

261. Salomon, N., Perlman, D. C., Friedmann, P., Buchstein, S., Kreiswirth, B. N., and Mildvan, D., Predictors and outcome of multidrug-resistant tuberculosis, *Clin. Infect. Dis.*, 21, 1245, 1995.

262. Turett, G. S., Telzak, E. E., Torian, L. V., Blum, S., Alland, D., Weisfuse, I., and Fazal, B. A., Improved outcomes for patients with multidrug-resistant tuberculosis, *Clin. Infect. Dis.*, 21, 1238, 1995.

263. Rastogi, N., Ross, B. C., Dwyer, B., Goh, K. S., Clavel-Sérès, S., Jeantils, V., and Cruaud, P., Emergence during unsuccessful chemotherapy of multiple drug resistance in a strain of *Mycobacterium tuberculosis*, *Eur. J. Clin. Microbiol. Infect. Dis.*, 11, 901, 1992.

264. Fadeeva, N.I., Golyshevskaya, V. I., Bibergal, E. A., and Safonova, S. G., Protein spectrum of mycobacteria in relation to their taxonomy and resistance to antitubercular drugs, *Probl. Tuberk.*, 65, 1991.

265. Zhang, Y. and Young, D., Molecular genetics of drug resistance in *Mycobacterium tuberculosis*, *J. Antimicrob. Chemother.*, 34, 313, 1994.

266. Heym, B., Honore, N., Truffot-Pernot, C., Banerjee, A., Schurra, C., Jacobs, W. R., Jr., van Embden, J. D. A., Grosset, J. H., and Cole, S. T., Implications of multidrug resistance for the future of short-course chemotherapy of tuberculosis: a molecular study, *Lancet*, 344, 293, 1994 (see also comment in *Lancet*, 344, 277, 1994).

267. Zhang, Y., Heym, B., Allen, B., Young, D., and Cole, S., The catalase- peroxidase gene and isoniazid resistance of *Mycobacterium tuberculosis*, *Nature*, 358, 591, 1992.

268. Zhang, Y., Garcia, M. J., Lathigra, R., Allen, B., Moreno, C., van Embden, J. D., and Young, D., Alterations in the superoxide dismutase gene of an isoniazid-resistant strain of *Mycobacterium tuberculosis*, *Infect. Immun.*, 60, 2160, 1992.

269. Sareen, M. and Khuller, G. K., Cell wall and membrane changes associated with ethambutol resistance in *Mycobacterium tuberculosis* H37Ra, *Antimicrob. Agents Chemother.*, 34, 1773, 1990.

270. Ausina, V., Riutort, N., Vinado, B., Manterola, J. M., Ruiz Manzano, J., Rodrigo, C., Matas, L., Giménez, M., Tor, J., and Roca, J., Prospective study of drug-resistant tuberculosis in a Spanish urban population including patients at risk for HIV infection, *Eur. J. Clin. Microbiol. Infect. Dis.*, 14, 105, 1995.

271. Nolan, C. M., Williams, D. L., Cave, M. D., Eisenach, K. D., El-Hajj, H., Hooton, T. M., Thompson, R. L., and Goldberg, S. V., Evolution of rifampin resistance in human immunodeficiency virus-associated tuberculosis, *Am. J. Respir. Crit. Care Med.*, 152, 1067, 1995.

272. Lutfey, M., Della-Latta, P., Kapur, V., Palumbo, L. A., Gurner, D., Stotzky, G., Brudney, K., Dobkin, J., Moss, A., Musser, J. M., and Kreiswirth, B. N., Independent origin of mono-rifampin-resistant *Mycobacterium tuberculosis* in patients with AIDS, *Am. J. Respir. Crit. Care Med.*, 153, 837, 1996.

273. Huh, Y. J., Ahn, D. I., and Kim, S. J., Limited variation of DNA fingerprints (IS6110 and IS1081) in Korean strains of *Mycobacterium tuberculosis*, *Tuber. Lung Dis.*, 76, 324, 1995.

274. Jarallah, J. S., Elias, A. K., al-Hajjaj, M. S., Bukhari, M. S., al-Shareef, A. H., and al-Shammari, S. A., High rate of rifampicin resistance of *Mycobacterium tuberculosis* in the Taif region of Saudi Arabia, *Tuber. Lung Dis.*, 73, 113, 1992.

275. Pretorius, G. S., Sirgel, F. A., Schaaf, H. S., van Helden, P. D., and Victor, T. C., Rifampicin resistance in *Mycobacterium tuberculosis* — rapid detection and implications in chemotherapy, *S. Afr. Med. J.*, 86, 50, 1996.

276. Tsukamura, M., *In vitro* experiment showing that chemotherapy of tuberculosis by aminoglycoside antibiotics may influence successive chemotherapy with rifampicin, *Kekkaku*, 66, 13, 1991.

277. Tsukamura, M., Cross-resistance relationship between streptomycin and kanamycin resistances in *Mycobacterium smegmatis* (strain Jucho) — comparison of the development patterns of resistance to streptomycin and kanamycin among *Mycobacterium tuberculosis*, *Mycobacterium avium* complex, and *Mycobacterium smegmatis*, *Kekkaku*, 65, 785, 1990.

278. Cambau, E., Sougakoff, W., Besson, M., Truffot-Pernot, C., Grosset, J., and Jarlier, V., Selection of a gyrA mutant of *Mycobacterium tuberculosis* resistant to fluoroquinolones during treatment with ofloxacin, *J. Infect. Dis.*, 170, 479, 1994 (correction in *J. Infect. Dis.*, 170, 1351, 1994).

279. Bibergal, E. A. and Palian, A. B., Determination of resistance of *Mycobacterium tuberculosis* to pyrazinamide by radiometric method, *Probl. Tuberk.*, 7, 1991.

280. He, Z., Li, J., Zhao, S., Ding, S., Wu, L., and Zhao, Q., Studies of rapid detection of drug-resistance of *Mycobacterium* by gas chromatography, *Hua Hsi I Ko Ta Hsueh Pao*, 21, 301, 1990.

281. Plikaytis, B. B., Marden, J. L., Crawford, J. T., Woodley, C. L., Butler, W. R., and Shinnick, T. M., Multiplex PCR assay specific for the multidrug resistant strain W of *Mycobacterium tuberculosis*, *J. Clin. Microbiol.*, 32, 1542, 1994.

282. Chen, C. H., Suo, J., Goble, M., and Heifets, L., Quantitative measurement of drug susceptibility of *Mycobacterium tuberculosis* for monitoring chemotherapy response, *J. Formos. Med. Assoc.*, 93, 35, 1994.

283. Task Force. National action plan to combat multidrug-resistant tuberculosis, *Morbid. Mortal. Wkly. Rep.*, 41(RR-11), 5, 1992.

284. Kitsukawa, K., Higa, F., Takushi, Y., Miyagi, H., Kakazu, T., Fukuhara, H., Nakamura, H., Kaneshima, H., Irabu, Y., Shimoji, K. et al., Adoptive immunotherapy for pulmonary tuberculosis caused by multi-resistant bacteria using autologous peripheral blood leucocytes sensitized with killed *Mycobacteria tuberculosis* bacteria, *Kekkaku*, 66, 563, 1991.

285. Essential components of a tuberculosis prevention and control program. Recommendation of the Advisory Council for the Elimination of Tuberculosis, *Morbid. Mortal. Wkly. Rep.*, 44(RR-11), 1, 1995.

286. Stearn, B. F. and Polis, M. A., Prophylaxis of opportunistic infections in persons with HIV infection, *Cleve. Clin. J. Med.*, 61, 187, 1994.

287. Graham, N. M., Galai, N., Nelson, K. E., Astemborski, J., Bonds, M., Rizzo, R. T., Sheeley, L., and Vlahov, D., Effect of isoniazid chemoprophylaxis on HIV-related mycobacterial disease, *Arch. Intern. Dis.*, 156, 889, 1996.

8.5 *MYCOBACTERIUM BOVIS*

8.5.1 INTRODUCTION

Mycobacterium bovis is a virulent organism, which was first isolated from cattle infected with tuberculous tubercles. *M. bovis* was found together with *M. tuberculosis* and *M. africanum* to cause tuberculosis in humans and lower animals. Most of the cases reported in the literature were effected by the Bacille Calmette-Guérin (BCG), a live attenuated strain of *M. bovis* which has been used to prepare the BCG vaccine since 1921.

In recent years, human tuberculosis caused by *M. bovis* has been rare in the developed countries, and when it occurs such infections are most likely the result of either reactivation of a latent infection,[1-3] or acquired in developing countries or regions where the pathogen is still endemic.[4-6] Although in humans the disease is usually seen in children, acquired mainly through infected milk, an increase in the incidence among adult patients has also been seen.[7] Dankner et al.[8] have described 73 mostly Hispanic patients with *M. bovis* infection who were identified in the San Diego, California area during a 12-year period between 1980 and 1991. Of these, 13 were HIV-positive, with 1 patient having pulmonary disease, 4 with mesenteric adenitis, and 8 patients with disseminated disease; there was no case of meningitis. Of the 60 HIV-negative patients, only 1 presented with disseminated disease, and 3 of the patients had meningitis as documented by positive CSF cultures.

With the spread of the AIDS epidemic, *M. bovis*-associated tuberculosis in this population has grown steadily.[4,9-16] The majority of reported cases have been on disseminated infections.[9,10,17] While the BCG strain was the most commonly isolated,[9-11] AIDS patients with *M. bovis* infections not due to the BCG strain have also been reported.[4,12] Bouvet et al.[16] described a nosocomial outbreak of multidrug-resistant *M. bovis* tuberculosis among HIV-infected patients in what appeared to be a single-strain source.

Because of the possibility of developing progressive disease, the BCG vaccination of asymptomatic HIV-positive patients[18] and infants born of HIV-seropositive mothers[17,19] is still controversial[9,20-22] and should be considered with caution.[11,22] Cases of immunocompetent and previously healthy children who had developed infections due to *M. bovis*-BCG inoculation have also been reported.[23-25]

Rovatti et al.[26] have evaluated a Western blot serum test for the diagnosis of *M. bovis* infection using the BCG A60 antigen complex in both purified protein derivative (PPD)-negative and PPD-positive individuals as well as subjects undergoing BCG vaccination and HIV-infected patients. The discriminant score identified 100% of the PPD-positives and none (0%) of the PPD-negatives. In the BCG-vaccinated subjects, 1.4% tested positive before vaccination and 90% after vaccination, and in the HIV-infected patients, 90% of the PPD-positive and 5% of the PPD-negative individuals had a positive score. The data obtained suggested the Western blot discriminant score as a viable and accurate test to survey for tuberculosis infection in serum samples.[26]

Cerebral tuberculosis, a rare but severe and often fatal form of extrapulmonary disease caused by both *M. tuberculosis* and *M. bovis,* has been diagnosed in several immunocompetent hosts, all of whom also showed radiological or bacteriological signs of pulmonary tuberculosis or miliary tuberculosis.[27]

Leach and Halpin[28] described a case of *M. bovis* infection of a total hip arthroplasty. Other nonpulmonary involvement of *M. bovis* included lymphadenitis, pleural effusion, and peritoneal infection.[7] There have been at least two fatal cases, one from ovarian neoplasia with abdominal dissemination,[7] and the other from a disseminated BCG disease.[29]

8.5.2 HOST IMMUNE RESPONSE TO *MYCOBACTERIUM BOVIS* INFECTION

In a study aimed at investigating the role of IFN-γ in host defense against *M. bovis*, IFN-γ mRNA was induced in murine lungs prior to mycobacterial infection.[30] Treatment with anti-IFN-γ monoclonal antibodies (mAb) prevented the activation of pulmonary intraparenchymal macrophages by *M. bovis*-BCG. In addition, these mAb also inhibited the activation by BCG of Mac1$^+$CD4$^-$CD8$^-$ T cells bearing α/β antigen receptor. The population of these T cells, which are found in murine lungs and thought to play a role in host defense mechanisms against mycobacterial infection, has been significantly increased by the administration of IFN-γ. *In vivo* studies in mice by Kawakami et al.[31] have shown that anti-IFN-γ mAb suppressed the enhanced expression of MHC class II and ICAM-1 on pulmonary parenchymal macrophages induced by intravenous injection of *M. bovis*-BCG.

In another immunologic investigation, Denis[32] has examined the contribution of transforming growth factor-β1 (TGF-β1) in the inflammatory response and fibrotic reaction using a mouse model of immune-induced lung fibrosis caused by repeated intranasal exposure to heat-killed bacillus Calmette-Guérin. The mice were treated with 200 μg of BCG 3 d weekly for 4 weeks, and simultaneous intraperitoneal injections of a nonspecific rabbit antiserum against mouse TFG-β1 or a preimmune serum (normal rabbit globulin). BCG instillations generated a copious release of antigenic TFG-β1 in the lungs at 1, 2, 3, and 4 weeks (up to 15 ng/lungs/mouse). Next, treatment with anti-TFG-β1 antiserum markedly decreased the number of free lung cells recovered by bronchoalveolar lavage without affecting the latter's cellular profile. Furthermore, the anti-TFG-β1 treatment of challenged mice diminished in a very substantial manner the total levels of IL-1β and TNF-α in the lungs of mice challenged with BCG. Overall, histologic examination has demonstrated a significant decrease in lung fibrosis and granulomatous response of challenged mice given anti-TFG-β1, thereby suggesting a role for TFG-β1 in inducing inflammation and lung fibrosis in response to an immune stimulus.[32]

8.5.3 TREATMENT OF *MYCOBACTERIUM BOVIS* INFECTIONS

A BCG-induced sepsis in mice was treated with combination antibiotic and corticosteroid therapy consisting of isoniazid, rifampin, and prednisolone.[33] The 53% survival rate observed, as compared with 25% survival in controls ($p = .0209$), and even worse 10.5% in mice receiving prednisolone alone, suggested that BCG-induced sepsis probably has components of both a hypersensitivity reaction and bacterial sepsis, thereby lending support to the current use of combination antibiotic and steroid therapies for treatment of BCG sepsis in clinical settings.[33]

Combination therapy with isoniazid and dihydromycoplanecin A (a cyclic peptide antibiotic) was successfully carried out in experimental tuberculosis in mice infected with *M. bovis* Ravanel.[34] In another *in vivo* study, Tsukamura[35] examined the therapeutic effect of ofloxacin on mice challenged by ofloxacin-resistant *M. bovis* strains.

An HIV-positive intravenous drug user with a non-BCG *M. bovis* infection was successfully treated with a daily regimen consisting of isoniazid (300 mg) and rifampin (450 mg) given over a 12-week period.[4]

In the first case of disseminated *M. bovis* (non-BCG) infection with meningitis in AIDS, the patient presented with fever, weight loss, inappetence, fatigue, and malaise. A five-drug antituberculosis therapy consisting of isoniazid (300 mg daily), rifampin (600 mg daily), ethambutol (400 mg, t.i.d.), streptomycin (1.0 g daily for a total of 20 g), and pyrazinamide (1.0 g daily) plus prednisone (50 mg daily) resulted in complete recovery.[12]

M. bovis sepsis in a HIV-positive infant was treated with intravenous isoniazid (20 mg/kg daily) and rifampin (20 mg/kg daily).[11] After steady clinical improvement from the therapy, which was given for 1 year, and despite a prophylactic treatment with trimethoprim-sulfamethoxazole, the patient's condition worsened dramatically, resulting in death from what was interpreted as a relapse of *Pneumocystis* pneumonia.

Noah et al.[36] have evaluated in a randomized, placebo-controlled prospective trial the efficacy of oral erythromycin and local isoniazid instillation therapy in infants with BCG lymphadenitis and abscesses. When patients who developed subsequent regional abscesses were excluded, erythromycin caused significantly earlier resolution of lymphadenitis compared with placebo (5.1 months vs. 5.7 months for placebo; $p < .01$). There was no marked difference in the percentage of patients who developed subsequent regional abscesses between the two groups (47% for erythromycin vs. 60% for placebo; $p = .14$). Local isoniazid instillation caused significantly earlier resolution of abscesses compared with erythromycin therapy (3.9 months for isoniazid vs. 5.2 months for erythromycin; $p < .001$).[36]

Lin et al.[37] have treated an immunodeficient infant with progressive BCG infection with thymostimulin, a specific bovine thymic extract.

A short-course chemotherapy for pulmonary infection due to *M. bovis* was effective in three alcoholic patients suffering from malnutrition.[3]

The therapeutic efficacy of erythromycin in the treatment of BCG infections was examined by Singh.[38]

8.5.3.1 BCG Vector-Based Vaccines in Immunotherapy Against HIV Infection

A recombinant *M. bovis* bacillus Calmette-Guérin vector-based vaccine capable of secreting the V3 principal neutralizing epitope of HIV was shown to induce immune response to the epitope and prevent HIV infection in guinea pigs.[39] Furthermore, immunization of mice with the rBCG resulted in induction of cytotoxic T lymphocytes. Administration of serum IgG from vaccinated guinea pigs was found effective in completely blocking the HIV infection in thymus/liver transplanted severe combined immunodeficiency (SCID)/hu or SCID/PBL mice. In addition, the immune serum IgG was shown to neutralize primary field isolates of HIV that match the neutralizing sequence motif by a peripheral blood mononuclear cell-based virus neutralization assay. The information obtained has supported the concept that the antigen-secreting rBCG system may be used as a tool for the development of HIV vaccines.[39]

In a study conducted in rhesus monkeys, Yasutomi et al.[40] have demonstrated that a vaccine-elicited, single viral epitope-specific cytotoxic T lymphocyte response did not protect against intravenous, cell-free simian immunodeficiency virus challenge.

8.5.3.2 BCG in the Treatment of Bladder Cancer and Carcinoma *in Situ*

The intravesical application of BCG has proven to be an effective therapy for some superficial cancers of the bladder and carcinoma *in situ*.[41-56]

During intravesical BCG treatment, patients typically show a local inflammatory response involving mainly T lymphocytes having the helper-induced phenotype (CD4+) (CD4+/CD8+ ratio >1).[49] To evaluate whether this immunophenotypic profile of the lymphocytes persisted after completion of immunotherapy, Boccafoschi et al.[49] examined bladder biopsy specimens of patients previously submitted to a 2-year BCG administration. A reversal to the pretreatment CD4+/CD8+ ratio of <1 occurred in the majority of patients, including those with histologically confirmed tumor recurrence. Based on these findings, it appeared that the long-term host response to BCG did not depend exclusively on an intense, long-lasting local mononuclear immune reaction.

Nakamura et al.[57] have investigated the role of monocytes in conjunction with BCG in the cell-mediated cytolysis of bladder-cancer cells. Human peripheral monocytes released a cytolytic factor which lysed T24 bladder-cancer cells and a number of human tumor cells, but not normal lymphocytes or fibroblasts. After *in vitro* incubation of monocytes with BCG for 48 h, cytolysis of T24 cells increased up to 56.7 ± 4.1%. Furthermore, treatment of monocytes with actinomycin D (an inhibitor of RNA transcription) reduced the release of cytolytic factor from 27.3 ± 5.7% cytolysis to 4.5 ± 1.4% (p <.05). The reported findings may be associated with the antitumor activity of BCG in intravesical therapy of bladder cancer.

Schneider et al.[58] have studied the cellular immune mechanism of the BCG anticancer activity by using an *in vitro* adhesion assay to investigate the interaction of radiolabeled BCG with urothelial bladder-tumor cells. A BCG dose-dependent binding to bladder-tumor cell lines derived from tumors of different gradings was observed to occur by electron microscope technique in less than 30 min of incubation. Furthermore, the binding was apparently specific since competition experiments showed an inhibition by nonradioactive BCG, but not by *Escherichia coli*. In addition, the role of fibronectin as an adhesion molecule that is also present in the bladder wall has been investigated. It was demonstrated that BCG was capable of binding to fibronectin-coated surfaces in a dose-dependent manner, but competitive binding assays failed to show inhibition of BCG binding to bladder-tumor cells by anti-fibronectin. The conclusion was made that the *in vitro* attachment of BCG to bladder-tumor cells appeared not to be mediated by fibronectin.[58]

An extract from the Tice substrain BCG, used clinically in the immunotherapy of superficial bladder cancer, has shown antitumor activity against murine S180 sarcoma model.[48,59] Using Sephadex LH-20 chromatography, Wang et al.[48] have further fractionated the extract into fractions A, B, and C. An antitumor glucan, PS1A1 (65 to 97 kDa), was isolated from fraction PS1A and shown to consist structurally of 1→6-α-linked glucose units.

MY-1, a DNA fraction, was isolated and purified from *M. bovis*-BCG.[60,61] Comprised of water-soluble and heat-denatured nucleic acid, MY-1, when tested in animal models, showed host-mediated antitumor activity against various cancers combined with low toxicity. In human phase I clinical studies, MY-1 was used as a single subcutaneous injection at doses of 0.25 to 20 mg, or at 3.0 to 12.5 mg given subcutaneously three times weekly.[60]

Infrequent, but still serious complications of intravesical treatment have become apparent as its use grew more widespread.[62] Thus, infected aortic aneurysm,[41,47,63,64] vertebral osteomyelitis,[63,65,66] mycobacteremia/sepsis,[33,47,67,68] pulmonary infection,[69-71] miliary tuberculosis,[72,73] granulomatous hepatitis,[68] tuberculous spondylitis,[74] a generalized BCG infection,[75] psoas abscess,[66,69,76] arthritis,[77,78] endophthalmitis,[79] and prosthetic total knee infection[80] have been reported as complications after intravesical BCG therapy. Stone et al.[81] have reported the development of meningitis in two immunocompromised children due to iatrogenic BCG infection, and Ribera et al.[82] have described a case of *M. bovis*-BCG infection of the glans penis.

Maes et al.[45] have compared the antitumor activity of BCG and a thermostable macromolecular antigen complex of BCG known as A60.When used as preventive therapies (in conjunction with or without tumor antigens) against growth and dissemination of the EMT6 tumor cell line, it has been demonstrated that tumor antigens alone did not significantly alter the oncological indexes, although a slight increase in both T lymphocyte and macrophage activation was observed. It has been further demonstrated that not only A60 induced a protective activity that was as much as 40% greater than that of live BCG, but also its effect was not accompanied by any of the adverse toxicity observed during BCG immunotherapy. Stimulation of T lymphocytes by A60 was the key step which led to activation of the immunocompetent cells involved in the tumor rejection.[46,83]

8.5.4 REFERENCES

1. Hardie, R. M. and Watson, J. M., *Mycobacterium bovis* in England and Wales: past, present and future, *Epidemiol. Infect.*, 109, 23, 1992.
2. Stoller, J. K., Late recurrence of *Mycobacterium bovis* genitourinary tuberculosis: case report and review of literature, *J. Urol.*, 134, 565, 1985.

3. O'Donohue, W. J., Jr., Bedi, S., Bittner, M. J., and Preheim, L. C., Short-course chemotherapy for pulmonary infection due to *Mycobacterium bovis*, *Arch. Intern. Med.*, 145, 703, 1985.

4. Cornuz, J., Fitting, J. W., Beer, V., and Chave, J. P., *Mycobacterium bovis* and AIDS, *AIDS*, 5, 1038, 1991.

5. Collins, C. H. and Grange, J. M., A review: the bovine tubercle bacillus, *J. Appl. Bacteriol.*, 55, 13, 1983.

6. Moda, G., Daborn, C. J., Grange, J. M., and Cosivi, O., The zoonotic importance of *Mycobacterium bovis*, *Tuber. Lung Dis.*, 77, 103, 1996.

7. Sauret, J., Jolis, R., Ausina, V., Castro, E., and Cornudella, R., Human tuberculosis due to *Mycobacterium bovis*: report of 10 cases, *Tuber. Lung Dis.*, 73, 388, 1992.

8. Dankner, W. M., Waecker, N. J., Essey, M. A., Moser, K., Thompson, M., and Davis, C. E., *Mycobacterium bovis* infections in San Diego: a clinicoepidemiologic study of 73 patients and a historical review of a forgotten pathogen, *Medicine (Baltimore)*, 72, 11, 1993.

9. Boudes, P., Sobel, A., Deforges, L., and Leblic, E., Disseminated *Mycobacterium bovis* infection from BCG vaccination and HIV infection, *JAMA*, 262, 2386, 1989.

10. Centers for Disease Control, Disseminated *Mycobacterium bovis* infection from BCG vaccination of a patient with acquired immunodeficiency syndrome, *Morbid. Mortal. Wkly. Rep.*, 234, 227, 1985.

11. Houde, C. and Dery, P., *Mycobacterium bovis* species in an infant with human immunodeficiency virus infection, *Pediatr. Infect. Dis. J.*, 7, 810, 1988.

12. Albrecht, H., Stellbrink, H. J., Eggers, C., Rusch-Gerdes, S., and Greten, H., A case of disseminated *Mycobacterium bovis* infection in an AIDS patient, *Eur. J. Clin. Microbiol. Infect. Dis.*, 14, 226, 1995.

13. Grange, J. M., Daborn, C., and Cosivi, O., HIV-related tuberculosis due to *Mycobacterium bovis*, *Eur. Respir. J.*, 7, 1564, 1994.

14. Daborn, C. J. and Grange, J. M., HIV/AIDS and its implications for the control of animal tuberculosis, *Br. Vet. J.*, 149, 405, 1993.

15. Kitching, R. P., Tuberculosis and AIDS — a deadly combination, *Br. Vet. J.*, 149, 405, 1993.

16. Bouvet, E., Casalino, E., Mendoza-Sassi, G., Lariven, S., Valée, E., Pernet, M., Gottot, S., and Vachon, F., A nosocomial outbreak of multidrug-resistant *Mycobacterium bovis* among HIV-infected patients: a case-control study, *AIDS*, 7, 1453, 1993.

17. Ninane, J., Grymonprez, A., Burtonboy, G., Francois, A., and Cornu, G., Disseminated BCG in HIV infection, *Arch. Dis. Child.*, 63, 1268, 1988.

18. Lumb, R. and Shaw, D., *Mycobacterium bovis* (BCG) vaccination: progressive disease in a patient asymptomatically infected with the human immunodeficiency virus, *Med. J. Aust.*, 156, 286, 1992.

19. Anonymous, BCG vaccination and pediatric HIV infection — Rwanda, 1988-1990, *Morbid. Mortal. Wkly. Rep.*, 40, 833, 1991.

20. TenDam, H. G. and Hitze, K. L., Does BCG vaccination protect the newborn and young infants? *Bull. WHO*, 58(part 1), 37, 1980.

21. Reichman, L. B., Why hasn't BCG proved dangerous in HIV-infected patients? *JAMA*, 261, 3246, 1989.

22. Streeton, J. A., *Mycobacterium bovis* (BCG) vaccination, *Med. J. Aust.*, 156, 812, 1992.

23. Tardieu, M., Truffot-Pernot, C., Carriere, J. P., Dupic, Y., and Landrieu, P., Tuberculous meningitis due to BCG in two previously healthy children, *Lancet*, 1, 440, 1988.

24. Murugasu, B., Quah, T. C., Quak, S. H., Low, P. S., and Wong, H. B., Disseminated BCG infection: a case report, *J. Singapore Paediatr. Soc.*, 30, 139, 1988.

25. Marik, I., Kubat, R., Filipsky, J., and Galliova, J., Osteitis caused by BCG vaccination, *J. Pediatr. Orthop.*, 8, 333, 1988.

26. Rovatti, E., Corradi, M. P., Amicosante, M., Tartoni, P. L. et al., Evaluation of a Western blot serum test for the diagnosis of *Mycobacterium tuberculosis*, *Eur. Respir. J.*, 9, 288, 1996.

27. Labhard, N., Nicod, L., and Zellweger, J. P., Cerebral tuberculosis in the immunocompetent host: 8 cases observed in Switzerland, *Tuber. Lung Dis.*, 75, 459, 1994.

28. Leach, W. J. and Halpin, D. S., *Mycobacterium bovis* infection of a total hip arthroplasty: a case report, *J. Bone Joint Surg. Br.*, 75, 661, 1993.

29. de la Monte, S. M. and Hutchins, G. M., Fatal disseminated bacillus Calmette-Guérin infection and arrested growth of cutaneous malignant melanoma following intralesional immunotherapy, *Am. J. Dermatopathol.*, 8, 331, 1986.

30. Kawakami, K., Analysis of host defense mechanism against mycobacterial infection and its application to therapy with biological response modifiers, *Kekkaku*, 69, 719, 1994.

31. Kawakami, K., Teruya, K., Tohyama, M., Kudeken, N., and Saito, A., A therapeutic trial of experimental tuberculosis with gamma-interferon in an immunocompromised mouse model, *Kekkaku*, 69, 607, 1994.

32. Denis, M., Neutralization of transforming growth factor-beta 1 in a mouse model of immune-induced lung fibrosis, *Immunology*, 82, 584, 1994.

33. Koukol, S. C., DeHaven, J. I., Riggs, D. R., and Lamm, D. L., Drug therapy of bacillus Calmette-Guérin sepsis, *Urol. Res.*, 22, 373, 1995.

34. Haneishi, T., Nakajima, M., Shiraishi, A., Katayama, T., Torikata, A., Kawahara, Y., Kurihara, K., Arai, M., Arai, T., Aoyagi, T., Koseki, Y., Kondo, E., and Tokunaga, T., Antimycobacterial activities *in vitro* and *in vivo* and pharmacokinetics of dihydromycoplanecin A, *Antimicrob. Agents Chemother.*, 32, 110, 1988.

35. Tsukamura, M., Therapeutic effect of ofloxacin on mice challenged by ofloxacin-resistant *Mycobacterium bovis* strains, *Kekkaku*, 62, 235, 1987.

36. Noah, P. K., Pande, D., Johnson, B., and Ashley, D., Evaluation of oral erythromycin and local isoniazid instillation therapy in infants with Bacillus Calmette-Guérin lymphadenitis and abscesses, *Pediatr. Infect. Dis. J.*, 12, 136, 1993.

37. Lin, C. Y., Hau, H. C., and Hsieh, H. C., Treatment of progressive Bacillus Calmette-Guérin infection in an immunodeficient infant with a specific bovine thymic extract (thymostimulin), *Pediatr. Infect. Dis. J.*, 4, 402, 1985.

38. Singh, G., Erythromycin for BCG infections, *Clin. Pediatr. (Philadelphia)*, 24, 470, 1985.

39. Honda, M., Matsuo, K., Nakasone, T., Okamoto, Y., Yoshizaki, H., Kitamura, K., Sugiura, W., Watanabe, K., Fukushima, Y., Haga, S., Katsura, Y., Tasaka, H., Komuro, K., Yamada, T., Asano, T., Yamazaki, A., and Yamazaki, S., Protective immune responses induced by secretion of a chimeric soluble protein from a recombinant *Mycobacterium bovis* bacillus Calmette-Guérin vector candidate vaccine for human immunodeficiency virus type 1 in small animals, *Proc. Natl. Acad. Sci. U.S.A.*, 92, 10693, 1995.

40. Yasutomi, Y., Koenig, S., Woods, R. M., Madsen, J., Wassef, N. M., Alving, C. R., Klein, H. J., Nolan, T. E., Boots, L. J., Kessler, J. A., Emini, E. A., Conley, A. J., and Letvin, N. L., A vaccine-elicited, single viral epitope-specific cytotoxic T lymphocyte response does not protect against intravenous, cell-free simian immunodeficiency virus challenge, *J. Virol.*, 69, 2279, 1995.

41. Wolf, Y. G., Wolf, D. G., Higginbottom, P. A., and Dilley, R. B., Infection of a ruptured aortic aneurysm and an aortic graft with bacille Calmette-Guérin after intravesical administration for bladder cancer, *J. Vasc. Surg.*, 22, 80, 1995.

42. Cheng, C., Consigliere, D., Foo, K. T. et al., Bacillus Calmette-Guérin (BCG) in the treatment of superficial bladder cancer, *Ann. Acad. Med. Singapore*, 24, 562, 1995.

43. Malekos, M. D., Zarakovitis, I. E., Fokaefs, E. D., Dandinis, K. et al., Intravesical bacillus Calmette-Guérin versus epirubicin in the prophylaxis of recurrent and/or multiple superficial bladder tumours, *Oncology*, 53, 281, 1996.

44. Bohle, A., Rusch-Gerdes, S., Ulmer, A. J., Braasch, H., and Jocham, D., The effect of lubricants on viability of bacillus Calmette-Guérin for intravesical immunotherapy against bladder carcinoma, *J. Urol.*, 155, 1892, 1996.

45. Maes, H., Taper, H., and Cocito, C., Comparison between bacillus Calmette-Guérin and the A60 mycobacterial antigen complex used as cancer-preventive immunotherapies, *J. Cancer Res. Clin. Oncol.*, 122, 296, 1996.

46. Maes, H. and Cocito, C., Cancer prevention by adoptive transfer of antigen 60-activated immunocompetent cells, *Scand. J. Immunol.*, 43, 283, 1996.

47. Hellinger, W. C., Oldenburg, W. A., and Alvarez, S., Vascular and other serious infections with *Mycobacterium bovis* after bacillus Calmette-Guérin therapy for bladder cancer, *South. Med. J.*, 88, 1212, 1995.

48. Wang, R., Klegerman, M. E., Marsden, I., Sinnott, M., and Groves, M. J., An anti-neoplastic glycan synthesis isolated from *Mycobacterium bovis* (BCG vaccine), *Biochem. J.*, 311, 867, 1995.

49. Boccafoschi, C., Montefiore, F., Pavesi, M., Pastormerlo, M., and Betta, P. G., Late effects of intravesical bacillus Calmette-Guérin immunotherapy on bladder mucosa infiltrating lymphocytes: an immunohistochemical study, *Eur. Urol.*, 27, 334, 1995.

50. Bowyer, L., Hall, R. R., Reading, J., and Marsh, M. M., The persistence of bacille Calmette-Guérin in the bladder after intravesical treatment for bladder cancer, *Br. J. Urol.*, 75, 188, 1995.

51. Uekado, Y., Hirano, A., Shinka, T., and Ohkawa, T., The effects of intravesical chemoimmunotherapy with epirubicin and bacillus Calmette-Guérin for prophylaxis of recurrence of superficial bladder cancer: a preliminary report, *Cancer Chemother. Pharmacol.*, 35(Suppl.), S65, 1994.

52. Stassar, M. J., Vegt, P. D., Steerenberg, P. A., van der Mejden, A. P., Meiring, H. D., Dessens-Kroon, M., Geertzen, H. G., and den Otter, W., Effects of isoniazid (INH) on the BCG-induced local immune response after intravesical BCG therapy for superficial bladder cancer, *Urol. Res.*, 22, 177, 1994.

53. Ratliff, T. L., Mechanisms of action of BCG in superficial bladder cancer, *Prog. Clin. Biol. Res.*, 378, 103, 1992.

54. Pagano, F., Bassi, P., Milani, C., Piazza, N., Meneghini, A., and Garbeglio, A., BCG in superficial bladder cancer: a review of phase III European trials, *Eur. Urol.*, 21(Suppl. 2), 7, 1992.

55. Lamm, D. L., Blumenstein, B. A., Crawford, E. D., Montie, J. E., Scardino, P., Grossman, H. B., Stamisic, T. H., Smith, J. A., Jr., Sullivan, J., Sarosdy, M. F., Crissman, J. D., and Coltman, C. A., A randomized trial of intravesical doxorubicin and immunotherapy with bacille Calmette-Guérin for transitional-cell carcinoma of the bladder, *N. Engl. J. Med.*, 325, 1205, 1991.

56. van der Meijden, A. P., Steerenberg, P. A., de Jong, W. H., and Debruyne, F. M., Intravesical bacillus Calmette-Guérin treatment for superficial bladder cancer: results after 15 years of experience, *Anti-cancer Res.*, 11, 1253, 1991.

57. Nakamura, K., Chiao, J. W., Nagamatsu, G. R., and Addonizio, J. C., Monocyte cytolytic factor in promoting monocyte-mediated lysis of bladder cancer cell by bacillus Calmette-Guérin, *J. Urol.*, 138, 867, 138.

58. Schneider, B., Thanhäuser, A., Jocham, D., Loppnow, H., Vollmer, E., Galle, J., Flad, H. D., Ulmer, A. J., and Böhle, A., Specific binding of bacillus Calmette-Guérin to urothelial tumor cells *in vitro*, *World J. Urol.*, 12, 337, 1994.

59. Lou, Y., Klegerman, M. E., Muhamad, A., Dai, X., and Greves, M. J., Initial characterization of an antineoplastic, polysaccharide-rich extract of *Mycobacterium bovis* BCG, Tice substrain, *Anticancer Res.*, 14, 1469, 1994.

60. Majima, H. and Nomura, K., Phase I clinical study of MY-1, a new biological response modifier, *Gan To Kagaku Ryoho*, 13, 109, 1986.

61. Shimada, S., Yano, O., Inoue, H., Kuramoto, E., Fukuda, T., Yamamoto, H., Kataoka, T., and Tokunaga, T., Antitumor activity of the DNA fraction from *Mycobacterium bovis* BCG. II. Effects on various syngeneic mouse tumors, *J. Natl. Cancer Inst.*, 74, 681, 1985.

62. Steg, A., Adjiman, S., and Debre, B., BCG therapy in superficial bladder tumours — complications and precautions, *Eur. Urol.*, 21(Suppl. 2), 35, 1992.

63. Rozenblit, A., Wasserman, E., Marin, M. L., Veith, F. J., Cynamon, J., and Rozenblit, G., Infected aortic aneurysm and vertebral osteomyelitis after intravesical bacillus Calmette-Guérin therapy, *Am. J. Roentgenol.*, 167, 711, 1996.

64. Woods, J. M. IV, Schellack, J., Stewart, M. T., Murray, D. R., and Schwartzman, S. W., Mycotic abdominal aortic aneurysm induced by immunotherapy, *J. Vasc. Surg.*, 7, 808, 1988.

65. Morgan, M. B. and Iseman, M. D., *Mycobacterium bovis* vertebral osteomyelitis as complication of intravesical administration of bacillus Calmette-Guérin, *Am. J. Med.*, 100, 372, 1996.

66. Katz, D. S., Wogalter, H., D'Esposito, R. F., and Cunha, B. A., *Mycobacterium bovis* vertebral osteomyelitis and psoas abscess after intravesical BCG therapy for bladder carcinoma, *Urology*, 40, 63, 1992.

67. Izes, J. K., Bihrle, W. III, and Thomas, C. B., Corticosteroid-associated fatal mycobacterial sepsis occurring 3 years after instillation of intravesical bacillus Calmette-Guérin, *J. Urol.*, 150, 1498, 1993.

68. Proctor, D. D., Chopra, S., Rubenstein, S. C., Jokela, J. A., and Uhl, L., Mycobacteremia and granulomatous hepatitis following initial intravesical bacillus Calmette-Guérin instillation for bladder carcinoma, *Am. J. Gastroenterol.*, 88, 1112, 1993.

69. Kristjansson, M., Green, P., Manning, H. L., Slutsky, A. M., Brecher, S. M., von Reyn, C. F., Arbeit, R. D., and Maslow, J. N., Molecular confirmation of bacillus Calmette-Guérin as the cause of pulmonary infection following urinary tract instillation, *Clin. Infect. Dis.*, 17, 228, 1993.

70. Hoffler, D., Niemeyer, R., Strack, G., and Zieschang, M., Sputum-positive lung tuberculosis after instillation of BCG for bladder cancer, *Clin. Nephrol.*, 36, 307, 1991.

71. Kesten, S., Title, L., Mullen, B., and Grossman, R., Pulmonary disease following intravesical BCG treatment, *Thorax*, 45, 709, 1990.
72. Reparaz, J., Uriz, J., Castiello, J., and Sola, J., Miliary tuberculosis after bacillus Calmette-Guérin administration, *Enferm. Infecc. Microbiol. Clin.*, 11, 570, 1993.
73. McParland, C., Cotton, D. J., Gowda, K. S., Hoeppner, V. H., Martin, W. T., and Weckworth, P. F., Miliary *Mycobacterium bovis* induced by intravesical bacille Calmette-Guérin immunotherapy, *Am. Rev. Respir. Dis.*, 146, 1330, 1992.
74. Fishman, J. R., Walton, D. T., Flynn, N. M., Benson, D. R., and deVere White, R. W., Tuberculous spondylitis as a complication of intravesical bacillus Calmette-Guérin therapy, *J. Urol.*, 149, 584, 1993.
75. de Saint Martin, L., Boiron, C., Poveda, J. D., and Herreman, G., Generalized BCG infection after intravesical instillations of Calmette-Guérin bacillus, *Presse Med.*, 22, 1352, 1993.
76. Hakim, S., Heaney, J. A., Heinz, T., and Zwolak, R. W., Psoas abscess following intravesical bacillus Calmette-Guérin for bladder cancer: a case report, *J. Urol.*, 150, 188, 1993.
77. Ochsenkuhn, T., Weber, M. M., and Caselman, W. H., Arthritis after *Mycobacterium bovis* immunotherapy for bladder cancer, *Ann. Intern. Med.*, 111, 581, 1989.
78. Yu, D. T. Y., Choo, S. Y., and Schaack, T., Molecular mimicry in HLA-B27- related arthritis, *Ann. Intern. Med.*, 111, 581, 1989.
79. Lester, H., Erdey, R. A., Fastenberg, D. M., Schwartz, P. L., and Rosenhaus, J. B., Bacillus Calmette-Guérin (BCG) endophthalmitis, *Retina*, 8, 182, 1988.
80. Chazerain, P., Desplaces, N., Mamoudy, P., Leonard, P., and Ziza, J. M., Prosthetic total knee infection with a bacillus Calmette-Guérin (BCG) strain after BCG therapy for bladder cancer, *J. Rheumatol.*, 20, 2171, 1993.
81. Stone, M. M., Vannier, A. M., Storch, S. K., Peterson, C., Nitta, A. T., and Zhang, Y., Brief report: meningitis due to iatrogenic BCG infection in two immunocompromised children, *N. Engl. J. Med.*, 333, 651, 1995.
82. Ribera, M., Bielsa, J., Manterola, J. M., Fernandez, M. T., and Ferrandiz, C., *Mycobacterium bovis*-BCG infection of the glans penis: a complication of intravesical administration of bacillus Calmette-Guérin, *Br. J. Dermatol.*, 132, 309, 1995.
83. Maes, H., Taper, H., and Cocito, C., Alteration of the immune response during cancer development and prevention by administration of a mycobacterial antigen, *Scand. J. Immunol.*, 41, 53, 1995.

8.6 NONTUBERCULOUS MYCOBACTERIAL INFECTIONS

8.6.1 INTRODUCTION

The incidence of infections caused by mycobacteria other than *Mycobacterium tuberculosis* (MOTT) have increased dramatically over the last decade or so.[1-23] In some areas and patient populations, the isolation of nontuberculous (also referred to as "atypical" or "anonymous")[24,25] mycobacteria, such as *Mycobacterium avium-intracellulare* complex (MAI) has even surpassed that of *M. tuberculosis*. In addition to MAI, other nontuberculous mycobacteria (NTM) species that have been implicated in human disease include, among others, *M. haemophilium*, *M. kansasii*, *M. fortuitum*, *M. chelonae*, *M. bovis*, *M. malmoense*, *M. neoaurum*, *M. gordonae*, *M. terrae-triviale*, and *M. scrofulaceum*.

Because of antigenic similarities between *M. scrofulaceum* and MAI, occasional isolates identified biochemically as *M. scrofulaceum* have been serotyped as MAI and vice versa. For this reason some investigators have classified MAI and *M. scrofulaceum* together as a new pathogenic entity, the *M. avium-intracellulare scrofulaceum* complex (MAC).[1,27,28]

According to one of the earliest methods used to classify nontuberculous mycobacteria, suggested by Runyon,[26] they have been divided into four groups: (1) photochromogenes; (2) scotochromogenes; (3) nonphotochromogenes; and (4) rapid growers (on the basis of colony pigmentation and growth rate). However, there have been several exceptions to this classification. For example, *M. kansasii*, which for the most part is photochromogenic, has some of its strains being nonpigmented or scotochromogenic. Furthermore, often *M. avium-intracellulare* can be slightly pigmented, thereby leading to the erroneous misinterpretaion of them as being scotochromogenic. In another example, while *M. szulgai* is scotochromogenic at 37°C, it is also photochromogenic at 25°C.

Woods and Washington[1] have proposed that the nontuberculous mycobacteria be classified into two groups according to the degree of their pathogenicity to humans. The first group includes NTM that are potentially pathogenic in humans: *M. avium-intracellulare*, *M. kansasii*, *M. fortuitum-chelonae* complex, *M. scrofulaceum*, *M. xenopi*, *M. szulgai*, *M. malmoense*, *M. simiae*, *M. marinum*, *M. ulcerans*, *M. bovis*, *M. genavense*, and *M. haemophilium*. The second group of NTM, which consists of saprophitic mycobacterium species that rarely cause disease in humans, has been further divided into three subgroups based on their growth rates. The slow-growing subgroup includes *M. gordonae*, *M. asiaticum*, *M. terrae-triviale*, *M. gastri*, *M. nonchromogenicum*, and possibly *M. paratuberculosis*. The intermediate-growth subgroup contains currently only one species, *M. flavescens*. The third subgroup of rapid growers comprises *M. thermoresistibile*, *M. smegmatus*, *M. vaccae*, *M. parafortium* complex, *M. neoaurum*, and *M. phlei*.

The nontuberculous mycobacteria are rather ubiquitous in nature, and their pathogenic potential for humans varies.[1,29] As compared with *M. tuberculosis*, there is generally a lack of person-to-person transmission with nontuberculous mycobacteria. Furthermore, NTM may colonize an individual without causing invasive disease, which very often will require the presence of a predisposing factor. Patients with malignancies[30] and immunosuppression, such as those with AIDS,[10,31] and organ transplant recipients,[7] and patients on continuous ambulatory peritoneal dialysis (CAPD),[32] have been particularly vulnerable to NTM infections.

Infections caused by NTM include chronic pulmonary disease, lymphadenitis, skin and soft-tissue involvement,[11] and infections of the skeletal system.[33] Since the 1980s, disseminated NTM disease has become not only common, especially in association with opportunistic infections in AIDS patients,[34] but also in an increasingly growing immunocompromised population of patients with malignancies, organ transplant recipients, and those receiving immunosuppressive (e.g., corticosteroid[35]) therapy.[36]

Patients with NTM infections have been usually started on conventional multiple-drug antituberculosis therapy once acid-fast bacilli (AFB) have been detected, and before the exact type of mycobacteria has been identified.[11,37,38] In general, combinations containing rifampicin and ethambutol have been effective.[39] Dautzenberg et al.[13] have treated AIDS patients with fever and AFB on microscopic examination of bacteriologic samples or mycobacteria isolated by culture with a daily four-drug combination consisting of rifabutin (7 to 10 mg/kg), isoniazid (5.0 mg/kg), ethambutol (20 mg/kg), and clofazimine (100 mg).

Based on *in vitro* susceptibility testing, Tsukamura and Yamori[40] have recommended the following drug regimens for the treatment of various atypical mycobacteria: rifampicin–enviomycin–ethambutol for *M. avium-intracellulare*; ofloxacin–enviomycin–rifampicin for *M. kansasii*; enviomycin–ethambutol–isoniazid for *M. szulgai*; and ofloxacin for *M. fortuitum*.

However, the therapy of NTM infections may often be difficult in patients with severe underlying conditions and the natural resistance of most of the NTM to currently available antituberculosis drugs. In addition, as opposed to *M. tuberculosis*, the NTM, while sharing generally reduced sensitivity to antimycobacterial agents, may also differ in terms of drug specificity.[41]

In general, in order to avoid the development of resistant strains,[42] and based on the frequently found synergism *in vitro*, nearly all NTM infections may have to be treated by combined chemotherapy.[43] The latter, coupled with surgical debridement,[44,45] has been found especially beneficial in the therapy of difficult to treat infections due to *M. ulcerans*, *M. scrofulaceum*, and *M. fortuitum/chelonae*.[41]

8.6.2   *In Vitro* and *in Vivo* Activities of Anti-Nontuberculous Mycobacterial Agents

Rastogi et al.[46] have examined the *in vitro* activity of 13 drugs against 552 clinical isolates of atypical mycobacteria representing 12 species using the 1% proportion method with 7H11 agar medium. All the species tested were resistant to isoniazid and pyrazinamide. With the exception of *M. fortuitum* and *M. chelonae*, which were resistant to both drugs, clofazimine and D-cycloserine have displayed the broadest spectrum of activity; *M. szulgai* and *M. terrae* complex were resistant to D-cycloserine. The next broad-spectrum was ethionamide, followed by ansamycin, rifampin, capreomycin, kanamycin, streptomycin, and ethambutol. Among the fluoroquinolones, both ciprofloxacin and ofloxacin were active against *M. xenopi*, *M. gordonae,* and *M. fortuitum*, whereas *M. kansasii* and *M. gastri* were sensitive to ofloxacin only. The results of this study have demonstrated that critical drug concentrations established for *M. tuberculosis* may not be appropriate for atypical mycobacteria.[46]

The therapeutic potential of sparfloxacin against NTM infection was evaluated *in vitro* using the actual count method on Ogawa egg medium.[47] The reported MIC values were as follows: ofloxacin-sensitive *M. tuberculosis*, 0.16 to 0.32 µg/ml; ofloxacin-resistant *M. tuberculosis*, 0.63 to 2.5 µg/ml; *M. avium*, 0.63 to 10.0 µg/ml (MICs were equal to or less than 1.25 µg/ml in 7 of 11 strains); *M. intracellulare*, 2.5 to 10.0 µg/ml (MICs were equal to or more than 10.0 µg/ml in 17 of 23 strains); *M. kansasii*, ≤0.08 to 0.16 µg/ml; *M. fortuitum*, ≤0.08 µg/ml; *M. chelonae* subsp. *abscessus*, >10.0 µg/ml; *M. chelonae* subsp. *chelonae*, 0.63 µg/ml; *M. scrofulaceum*, ≤0.08 µg/ml; *M. nonchromogenicum*, 1.25 µg/ml; *M. xenopi*, ≤0.08 µg/ml; and *M. gordonae*, ≤0.08 µg/ml. Based on the average serum concentrations of sparfloxacin during the period of multiple oral administration (200 mg daily) (0.67 ± 0.32, 1.13 ± 0.21, 1.27 ± 0.32, and 1.31 ± 0.34 µg/ml after 1, 2, 4, and 6 h, respectively), its therapeutic potential against *M. tuberculosis*, *M. kansasii*, *M. fortuitum*, *M. chelonae* subsp. *chelonae*, *M. scrofulaceum*, *M. xenopi*, and *M. gordonae* is expected to be strong.[47] In a previous study by Tomioka et al.,[48] although still more potent than ofloxacin, sparfloxacin showed more variable MIC_{90} values against *M. tuberculosis*, *M. kansasii*, and *M. fortuitum* (0.2, 6.25, and 1.6 µg/ml, respectively). Furthermore, sparfloxacin inhibited the growth of *M. intracellulare* in 7H9 broth when added at a concentration of 0.2 µg/ml and rapidly killed the pathogen at 1.0 µg/ml, but exhibited only weak therapeutic activity against *M. intracellulare*-induced infection in mice.[48]

The susceptibilities to ciprofloxacin and ofloxacin of 548 clinical isolates of 8 subgroups or species of rapidly growing mycobacteria have been determined with demonstration of acquired resistance following single-drug therapy.[49] With regard to ciprofloxacin, the 170 isolates of *M. fortuitum* biovar. *fortuitum* were most sensitive (MIC_{90} = 0.125 µg/ml). The other biovariants of *M. fortuitum*, *M. smegmatis*, and the *M. chelonae*-like organisms have been less susceptible; the modal MIC value has been 0.5 µg/ml, and that of MIC_{90} was 1.0 µg/ml. Isolates of the two subspecies of *M. chelonae* have been generally resistant to ciprofloxacin, with only 8% of 206 isolates considered to be moderately susceptible (MIC = 2.0 µg/ml) and only 2% being susceptible (MIC ≤ 1.0 µg/ml). By comparison, the MIC values of ofloxacin averaged 1 to 2 dilutions higher than those of ciprofloxacin for all subgroups tested.[49]

Tomioka et al.[50] have compared the *in vitro* and *in vivo* efficacies of fleroxacin and ofloxacin against various nontuberculous mycobacteria. In the agar dilution assay with 7H11 medium, fleroxacin has shown MIC_{90} values of 3.13, 6.25, and 6.25 µg/ml against *M. kansasii*, *M. fortuitum*, and *M. tuberculosis*, respectively; *M. marinum*, *M. scrofulaceum*, *M. chelonae*, and *M. avium-intracellulare* were highly resistant to the drug. Overall, the activity of fleroxacin was comparable to that of ofloxacin. *In vivo*, fleroxacin was superior to ofloxacin against *M. fortuitum*-induced infection in mice. Neither drug, however, was efficacious against *M. intracellulare*-induced infection.[50]

Comparative studies evaluating the *in vitro* and *in vivo* activities of pefloxacin and ofloxacin against *M. xenopi* and *M. tuberculosis* have shown the MIC_{90} values for ofloxacin to be 2.0 mg/l, which was three dilutions lower than that of pefloxacin, and well within the range of drug concentrations achievable in man.[51] *M. avium-intracellulare* was resistant to both drugs.

A new fluoroquinolone, DU-6859a, was studied for its *in vitro* and *in vivo* antimycobacterial activity.[52] MIC_{90} determination in the agar dilution assay with 7H11 medium has shown values of 0.78, 1.56, 1.56, 0.39, 6.25, 1.56, and 12.5 µg/ml for *M. kansasii*, *M. marinum*, *M. scrofulaceum*, *M. fortuitum*, *M. chelonae* subsp. *abscessus*, *M. chelonae* subsp. *chelonae*, and MAI, respectively; the corresponding MIC_{90} value for *M. tuberculosis* was 0.2 µg/ml. Compared to sparfloxacin and ofloxacin, DU-6859a was more potent against most atypical mycobacterium species.[52]

Tsukamura[53] has compared the minimal inhibitory concentrations (MICs) of isoniazid and ethambutol against various nontuberculous mycobacteria and clinical strains of *M. tuberculosis* recovered from patients untreated previously by any antituberculosis drugs. The MICs for isoniazid against *M. tuberculosis*, *M. xenopi*, *M. szulgai*, and *M. kansasii* were 0.03 to 0.1, 0.1 to 0.4, 0.2 to 0.8, and 0.8 to 1.6 µg/ml, whereas the MIC value for ethambutol against *M. tuberculosis* ranged from 0.8 to 3.13 µg/ml. The percentage of strains of various mycobacteria which were susceptible to 3.13 µg/ml of ethambutol were 100%, 100%, 90%, 88%, 77%, 46%, and 30% for *M. szulgai*, *M. nonchromogenicum*, *M. gordonae*, *M. marinum*, *M. kansasii*, *M. malmoense*, and *M. scrofulaceum*, respectively; in contrast, the percentage of susceptible *M. avium* complex strains remained only 19%. Based on these findings, it has been suggested that isoniazid may be effective in the therapy of infections due to *M. xenopi*, *M. szulgai*, and *M. kansasii*, whereas ethambutol may be useful in the treatment of diseases caused by *M. szulgai*, *M. marinum*, and *M. kansasii*.[53]

The *in vitro* and *in vivo* activities of DuP-721, a new orally active oxazolidinone agent were studied by Ashtekar et al.[54] At concentrations ranging from 1.5 to 4.0 µg/ml, DuP-721 inhibited equally strains of *M. tuberculosis* both susceptible and resistant to conventional antituberculosis drugs. Furthermore, it inhibited strains of *M. kansasii*, *M. gordonae*, *M. fortuitum*, and *M. scrofulaceum* at 1.95, 3.9, 3.9, and 15.6 µg/ml, respectively, but was completely inactive against *M. avium-intracellulare* (≤ 250 µg/ml).

Tsukamura[55] has determined the *in vitro* efficacy of rifampicin against 295 nontuberculous and *M. tuberculosis* strains using the Ogawa egg medium. The MIC values were determined after incubation at 37°C. Overall, the drug was most active against *M. kansasii* and least potent against *M. fortuitum*. Against different strains of *M. tuberculosis*, the MIC values ranged between 3.13 and 12.5 µg/ml. The latter value was foreseen to be the critical concentration at which a clinical efficacy of rifampicin could be expected.

Klemens and Cynamon[56] have investigated the activities of azithromycin and clarithromycin against a number of nontuberculous mycobacteria (*M. kansasii*, *M. xenopi*, *M. simiae*, and *M. malmoense*) in beige C57BL/6J bgj/bgj mice with disseminated infection. Treatment with azithromycin (200 mg/kg), clarithromycin (200 mg/kg), ethambutol (125 mg/kg), rifampin (20 mg/kg), and clofazimine (20 mg/kg) was started 7 d postinfection, and the drugs were administered 5 d per week for 4 weeks. Overall, both azithromycin and clarithromycin showed activities comparable to or better than that of rifampin, ethambutol, or clofazimine against all mycobacterial strains tested. Azithromycin (200 mg/kg) was more active than clarithromycin (200 mg/kg) against organisms in the spleen for *M. xenopi* and *M. malmoense*; the corresponding activities against *M. kansasii* and *M. simiae* were comparable for both drugs. Against organisms in the lungs, the activities of azithromycin and clarithromycin were comparable for all four species.[56] Previously, Rapp et al.[57] also compared the pharmacology, *in vitro* activity, and the clinical potential of azithromycin and clarithromycin in the treatment of nontuberculous mycobacteria. Clarithromycin has been recommended as a component of the combination therapy for *M. avium* complex infection in patients with AIDS.

Haifets[58] has reviewed extensively the *in vitro* activity and general principles in selecting antimicrobial agents for different treatment regimens.

8.6.3   VIRULENCE ANTIGENS OF NONTUBERCULOUS MYCOBACTERIA

The nature of the virulence antigens associated with nontuberculous mycobacteria is yet to be fully understood.[59,60] It has been postulated that such antigens have been responsible for the observed persistence of the more virulent nontuberculous species within the lymphoreticular organs of the hosts.[61]

In general, nontuberculous mycobacteria are considered to be less pathogenic than *M. tuberculosis* even though some of the species (*M. kansasii*, *M. avium*, and *M. ulcerans*) have been capable of inducing progressive disease in normal immunocompetent adults.[62,63]

Schaefer[64] has demonstrated that first-time tissue isolates of *M. avium,* when cultured on Lowenstein-Jensen egg medium or Middlebrook 7H10 agar, produced thin and translucent virulent colonies. However, when these strains were cultivated on laboratory media, the colonies they formed were domed and opaque in appearance with attenuated virulence; eventually, rough and avirulent variants may also develop.

This type of colonial variation has been correlated with a progressive loss of mouse virulence,[60,65] as well as differences in susceptibility to antituberculous drugs and mycobacteriophages, to the plasmid content of these organisms.[66-68] Thus, when environmental isolates of *M. intracellulare* lack plasmids, they generally produced domed colonies which were avirulent to mice.[69] In contrast, isolates from AIDS patients tended to produce thin and translucent colonies that usually carry a number of plasmids.[70] These differences may result in selective pressure being exerted on MAI strains when they reach the gut-associated lymphoid tissue organs of pre-AIDS patients.[59] In such case, the mucosal macrophages as part of the host immune defense may select any translucent variants which happen to be present, and these more virulent organisms will then multiply within the immunodepleted host. This phenomenon has been demonstrated experimentally in mice infected with a mixture of translucent and opaque colony variants of *M. intracellulare* which yielded nearly pure cultures of the translucent colony form as the infection developed and the host defense eliminated the opaque variant.[60] It has been assumed that a similar type of selection process may occur within AIDS-related complex (ARC) patients who had ingested environmental mycobacteria, a small proportion of which were of the translucent colony types.[59]

8.6.4   NONTUBERCULOUS MYCOBACTERIAL INFECTIONS AND AIDS

Although less pathogenic than *M. tuberculosis*, in AIDS patients a number of nontuberculous mycobacteria have caused unexpectedly severe mycobacteriosis similar to that seen previously in a few cancer patients and transplant recipients. In general, during the time of their illness as many as 50% of AIDS patients may be infected with acid-fast bacilli,[71] with an estimated 5% of them developing life-threatening disseminated disease as a result of infection with *M. avium*-complex (MAC) serovars 4 and 8.[72] The virtual absence in the U.S. AIDS population of some of the other virulent MAC serotypes (types 2, 6, 9, 12, 14, and 16), given that they are known to exist in other patients living within the same communities, has been surprising.[73-75] Furthermore, about 10% of the mycobacterial isolates have been identified as *M. kansasii* (mostly coming from AIDS patients living in the midwestern U.S.), with another 6% to 9% being attributed to *M. chelonae, M. scrofulaceum, M. gordonae,* and *M. fortuitum.*[74]

In contrast to the U.S. and Europe, there has been no detailed epidemiological data on nontuberculous mycobacteriosis in African AIDS patients.[76,77] Most of the information currently available, which has been accumulated from African AIDS patients treated in Europe,[78] shows a preponderance of *M. tuberculosis* in these patients.[79] In European AIDS patients, there has been an increasing incidence of MAC serotypes 4 and 8,[80] especially during the development of clinical AIDS.[77]

8.6.5 *Mycobacterium avium* Complex (MAC)

8.6.5.1 Introduction

M. avium, M. intracellulare, and *M. scrofulaceum* are the three major pathogens comprising the *Mycobacterium avium* complex (MAC). *M. avium* and *M. intracellulare* are the most commonly isolated nontuberculous mycobacteria and are often referred to as *M. avium-intracellulare* (MAI).

Studies conducted in the U.S. show that members of the MAC family grow well in natural waters, particularly in the southeast region of the country.[28] It was also observed[81] that MAC strains containing virulent plasmids may be aerosolized, thus providing an airborne mechanism for spreading the disease. In general, natural waters are considered to be the primary environmental source for most human infections caused by MAC,[82,83] but also barnyards, where *M. avium* is a common pathogen infecting poultry and pigs.

In 1982, for the first time disseminated MAC disease was described in AIDS patients.[84,85] Presently the disease, which may start as gastrointestinal infection,[86,87] affects approximately one third of these patients.[88,89] In the U.S., *M. avium* is recognized as one of the most common opportunistic infections in HIV-positive patients.[90-93] The frequency of disseminated MAC infections in AIDS patients has risen significantly with diagnosis rates ranging from 18% to 56%.[94] Compared to *M. tuberculosis,* infections with MAC tend to occur later in the course of AIDS, when immuno-suppression is more advanced.[94] Autopsy studies[95] have indicated that between 30% and 50% of AIDS patients have evidence of disseminated MAC infection at their death.

One striking feature of *M. avium* infections in AIDS patients is the fact that the majority of isolates belong to serotype 4, and over 95% belong to one of three serotypes (1, 4, and 8).[96] The latter finding suggests not only that serotypes 1, 4, and 8 may have a more virulent nature, but also that in the context of HIV disease, *M. avium* isolates are more virulent than those of *M. intracellulare.* Other unusual features of serotypes 1, 4, and 8 include the observation that most strains are pigmented,[96] and that nearly all of them contain one or more small plasmids showing some degree of homology in their DNA content.[97]

Sato et al.[98] studied the differential susceptibilities of *M. avium* and *M. intracellulare* to sodium nitrite. While 67 of 72 strains (93.1%) of *M. avium* were found resistant to sodium nitrite at a concentration of 3 mg/ml in 7H11 agar medium, 57 of 59 strains (96.6%) of *M. intracellulare* were susceptible to the agent. The observed difference in susceptibilities may prove useful in differentiating between these two species. The presence of epidemiological and genetic markers, virulence factors, and intracellular growth of *M. avium* in AIDS patients have been reviewed extensively.[99]

In a retrospective study conducted in a cohort of 702 HIV-infected patients, Flegg et al.[100] have analyzed 46 cases of disseminated MAC infection. While concomitant colonization of the respiratory and gastrointestinal tracts was common (61% and 48%, respectively), dissemination was diagnosed antemortem in 18% of AIDS patients, and was the AIDS-defining diagnosis in 6% of all AIDS cases. Even though the overall survival from AIDS was not significantly different between patients who did or did not develop disseminated MAC disease, the latter markedly contributed to AIDS morbidity, and its incidence increased with prolonged AIDS survival.[100]

In disseminated disease, it is most likely for mycobacteria to be found in macrophages within the liver and spleen.[101] However, during the course of infection MAC was also found to invade fibroblasts, thus triggering a natural killer (NK) cell-mediated cytotoxicity against the infected cells.[101] *In vivo* studies by Harshan and Gangadharam[102] provided direct evidence that depletion of NK cell activity enhanced the multiplication of *M. avium* complex in mice.

Torriani et al.[103] have studied the relationship between the levels of MAC in blood and tissues by histopathologic examination and quantitation of MAC cultures on blood and tissue samples of seven organs at autopsy of 10 AIDS patients who had been treated for MAC bacteremia. The numbers of MAC colony-forming units (CFUs) in the blood and tissues were highly correlated.

Furthermore, the highest concentrations of MAC were observed in the reticuloendothelial organs, with a maximum of 6.9 $\log_{10}$ CFU/g in mesenteric lymph nodes and 6.9 $\log_{10}$ CFU/g in the spleen. The histopathologic findings paralleled quantitative cultures and were consistent with entry of MAC via the lymphatics through the gastrointestinal tract, followed by hematologic dissemination.[103]

Assessing the relative risks associated with a history of prior opportunistic infections, changes in the CD4+ levels, and baseline prognostic factors, Finkelstein et al.[104] have found that the occurrence of each opportunistic infection has increased the risk of subsequent opportunistic infection, even after adjusting for the CD4+ count. Specifically, the occurrence of *Pneumocystis carinii* pneumonia significantly increased the risk of MAC and cytomegalovirus infections, and to a certain degree the risk of systemic mycoses. Thus, diagnosis of MAC was associated with an increased risk of subsequent cytomegalovirus infection, where the occurrence of the latter increased the risk of a MAC infection.[104]

Claass et al.[105] have described a case of opportunistic disseminated MAC disease in a pediatric patient following chemotherapy for acute myeloid leukemia. The patient's cellular immunity was severely compromised, with a marked depression of the CD4+ counts.

In another report, a fatal case of maxillary sinusitis caused by *M. avium-intracellulare* was described in a pediatric patient with AIDS.[106]

8.6.5.2 Studies on Therapeutics

One of the drawbacks of antimycobacterial chemotherapy is that, although various agents may show appreciable bactericidal activity in the early phase (2 to 4 weeks after infection) of MAC disease, hardly any drug is known to continue to exert growth-inhibiting activity at the site of infection during the progressed stage. Using a mouse model, Sato et al.[107] have investigated the mechanism of bacterial regrowth, which usually starts about 2 to 4 weeks postinfection. Changes in the levels of tumor necrosis factor-α (TNF-α), interferon-γ (IFN-γ), and interleukins IL-6 and -10 in the lungs and spleen, have shown increased concentrations of TNF-α and IL-10 around weeks 2 to 4, a rapid decrease thereafter, and a return to normal levels by week 8; the levels of IFN-γ and IL-6 remained very low throughout the observation period. In this experiment, the bacterial CFU counts rapidly diminished during the first 2 weeks of treatment with the rifamycin derivative, KRM-1648; then a bacterial regrowth took place even in mice treated continuously with KRM-1648, although at a much lower rate than untreated controls. In another set of experiments, anti-transforming growth factor-β (anti-TGF-β) and anti-IL-10 antibodies potently reduced the intracellular growth of MAC in human monocytes cultured *in vitro* in the medium with or without the addition of TNF-α or IFN-γ. The effects of TNF-α and IFN-γ in decreasing mycobacterial growth were potentiated by the addition of either anti-TGF-β or anti-IL-10 antibodies. In addition, the anti-IL-10 antibody augmented to some extent the therapeutic efficacy of KRM-1648 against MAC infection, when the drug was given to mice 2 to 4 weeks postinfection. The overall results of these experiments strongly indicated that IL-10 derived from MAC-infected macrophages in response to stimulation by bacterial components, such as lipoarabinomannan, may have downregulated the antimicrobial function of the host macrophages against MAC.[107]

Tomioka et al.[108] have studied differences in the *in vitro* susceptibilities of *M. avium* and *M. intracellulare* clinical isolates to various antimycobacterial drugs. Test strains of *M. avium* were more resistant to rifampicin, rifabutin, kanamycin, streptomycin, amikacin, ethambutol, and clofazimine than test strains of *M. intracellulare*. Conversely, the *M. avium* strains were more susceptible to ofloxacin, ciprofloxacin, and cycloserine than *M. intracellulare* strains. There was no statistically significant difference between the two species in their susceptibility towards isoniazid.

The ability of various *in vitro* methods of antimycobacterial susceptibility testing to predict the therapeutic outcome in patients infected with *M. avium* complex has been evaluated by Sison et al.[109] Pretreatment bloodstream MAC isolates from AIDS patients, previously treated in a randomized fashion with either ethambutol, rifampin, or clofazimine, were tested by three conventional assays using broth or agar, as well as by co-cultivation with macrophages, and the obtained results were compared with the quantitatively determined bacteriologic response to the administration of the single agent in humans. None of the conventional *in vitro* susceptibility assays was predictive of the therapeutic outcome. The results of co-cultivation with macrophages were of moderate predictive value — the positive predictive value of a response in humans based on the response in macrophages (as defined by ≥1.0 log reduction in baseline colony counts after 5 d of treatment) was 74%, while the negative predictive value was 82%.

8.6.5.2.1   Fluoroquinolone derivatives

The fluoroquinolones have been shown to be highly active *in vitro* against various mycobacterial species, including *M. avium-intracellulare*.[110] Ciprofloxacin, ofloxacin, and sparfloxacin have been the best studied and among the most effective fluoroquinolone derivatives. The most important structural features determining the activity against MAI include the cyclopropyl ring at the N'–position, the fluorine atoms at C-6 and C-8, and a C-7 heterocyclic substituent.[110]

The activity of sparfloxacin (CI-978, AT 4140) was tested against 30 strains of MAC.[111,112] The observed MIC values (≤0.06 to 4 µg/ml) were lower than those of ciprofloxacin for all 30 strains; the MBC values for acid-fast bacteria were lower for 28 of 30 strains tested.[111] The combination of sparfloxacin and ethambutol was synergistic against 9 strains, whereas the combination of sparfloxacin, ethambutol, and rifampin was synergistic against all 30 strains. Sparfloxacin given in association with only rifampin was antagonistic against three of the MAC strains.[111]

Results by Rastogi et al.[113] have shown satisfactory correlations between extracellular and intracellular drug activity data. The *in vitro* activity of ciprofloxacin against 31 clinical isolates of MAC was studied by microdilution technique and compared to that of two other DNA gyrase inhibitors, coumermycin and novobiocin.[114] The broth-determined mean MIC values for ciprofloxacin, coumermycin, and novobiocin were 4.1 µg/ml, 17.4 µg/ml, and 54.7 µg/ml, respectively. The corresponding MBC values (determined by subculturing to Middlebrook 7H10 agar) were, in general, more than two dilution steps higher than MICs.

Oh et al.[115] have studied different methods to prepare liposome encapsulated ciprofloxacin, and were able to produce over 90% efficiency regardless of the content of negatively charged lipids by using a remote-loading technique that utilized both pH and potential gradients to drive the drug into preformed liposomes. Furthermore, both the cellular accumulation and the anti-*M. avium* activity of ciprofloxacin increased in proportion to the liposome negative charge — the maximal enhancement of potency was 43-fold in liposomes consisting of distearoylphosphatidylglycerol and cholesterol in a 10:5 ratio.

Against *M. avium-intracellulare* isolated from non-AIDS patients, two quinolone derivatives, difloxacin and A-56620, each inhibited 50% of the strains at a concentration of 2.0 µg/ml.[116]

Lomefloxacin (SC47111) is a difluorinated quinolone derivative with a relatively long half-life and high serum concentration. When tested *in vitro* against MAC isolated from AIDS patients, the majority of strains studied showed resistance to lomefloxacin (MIC_{90} > 8.0 µg/ml).[117]

A new quinolone derivative, WIN 57273 [1-cyclopropyl-7-(2,6-dimethyl-4-pyridinyl)-6-fluoro-1,4-dihydro-4-oxo-3-quinolinecarboxylic acid] was tested *in vitro* against *M. avium* and *M. tuberculosis*.[118] The broth-determined MIC values against *M. avium* ranged between 0.25 and 8.0 µg/ml; the corresponding concentrations against *M. tuberculosis* were 1.0 to 4.0 µg/ml. When compared with ofloxacin and ciprofloxacin, WIN 57273 had a significantly greater activity at low pH values; for example, against *M. avium*, MIC values of 2.0 µg/ml or less were observed for 54.5% of the strains at pH 6.8, while 85.5% of the strains were inhibited at pH 5.0. Since the predominant location of mycobacteria in the host is within the phagosomes and phagolysosomes of macrophages, i.e., in an acidic environment (that is, pH 5.0 or lower), the antimycobacterial activity of WIN 57273 seemed promising, especially against *M. avium*. The observed bactericidal activity of WIN 57273 against *M. avium* strains (MBC = 4.0 to 16.0 µg/ml) was equipotent to that of ciprofloxacin.[118] Cohen et al.[119] studied the activities of WIN 57273, minocycline, and 14-hydroxyclarithromycin (a human metabolite of clarithromycin) against two virulent strains of MAC in a model of intracellular infection, and compared them with that of clarithromycin. The concentrations used (equal to the serum peak levels) were 3.0, 4.0, 4.0, and 4.0 µg/ml for WIN 57273, 14-hydroxyclarithromycin, minocycline, and clarithromycin, respectively. On day 7 postinfection, compared with controls, WIN 57273, minocycline, clarithromycin, or different combinations of clarithromycin and the other drugs had slowed the intracellular replication of strain MO-1. 14-Hydroxyclarithromycin, clarithromycin, and the combinations of clarithromycin/minocycline, clarithromycin/14-hydroxy-clarithromycin, and clarithromycin/minocycline/14-hydroxyclarithromycin also slowed the intracellular replication of strain LV-2. The overall results showed that while WIN 57273 was less effective than clarithromycin against strain MO-1, the combination of clarithromycin, minocycline, and 14-hydroxyclarithromycin was more effective than clarithromycin alone against strain LV-2.[119]

Using a 7H9 broth microdilution technique, Barrett et al.[120] tested the activities of sparfloxacin, WIN 57273, CI-960, and isepamicin against 35 clinical isolates of *M. avium-intracellulare*, and compared them with those of other antimycobacterial drugs. While sparfloxacin ($MIC_{90} = 0.5$ µg/ml) was the most active fluoroquinolone, isepamicin (MIC_{90} = 4.0 µg/ml) was the most potent aminoglycoside.

The *in vitro* potency and *in vivo* activity of DU-6859a, a new fluoroquinolone derivative, against *M. avium* complex have been investigated by Saito et al.[52] The MIC_{90} value determined by the agar dilution method in 7H11 medium was 12.5 µg/ml and comparable to that of sparfloxacin, but lower than that of ofloxacin. When given at approximately 50 mg/kg to mice infected with MAC, DU-6859a reduced the frequency of occurrence and the degree of gross pulmonary or renal lesions, and the bacterial loads in the lungs, spleens, and kidneys.

Patil et al.[121] studied *in vitro* the effect of quinolones on the mycolic acid metabolism of mycobacteria. At concentrations of 6.0 µg/ml, norfloxacin exerted the maximum inhibitory activity on mycolic acids in *M. intracellulare*. The effect appeared to be direct and secondary to DNA gyrase.

8.6.5.2.2   Antimycobacterial antibiotics

Presently, the exclusive use of multiple drug combinations represents the fundamental principle of conventional therapy against MAC infections. Alongside such established antimycobacterial agents as isoniazid, ethambutol, and ethionamide, a number of antimycobacterial antibiotics (streptomycin, rifampin) have been used in various combinations for treatment of *M. avium-intracellulare* disease.

Furthermore, in addition to semisynthetic rifamycin analogs, some aminoglycoside antibiotics and novel macrolide antibiotics (azithromycin, clarithromycin, and roxithromycin), have been shown to possess promising antimycobacterial activity. Some recent data on their therapeutic efficacy when given alone or in combinations with other antimycobacterial agents is presented in this section.

8.6.5.2.2.1   Rifamycin and congeners — A number of semisynthetic rifamycin analogs have been tested for activity against *M. avium-intracellulare*. The most active compounds include rifampin (a derivative of rifamycin B), rifapentine (MDL 473, a cyclopentyl derivative of rifampin), rifabutin (ansamycin, a spiropiperidyl derivative of rifamycin S), and CGP 7040 (a rifamycin analog containing a trimethylbenzylpiperazinyl side chain at C-3).

The MIC and MBC values of rifampin, rifabutin, rifapentine, CGP-7040, and P-DEA were determined against 50 *M. avium* strains in 7H12 liquid medium under various pH conditions, and the results were compared to the corresponding values for *M. tuberculosis*.[122] One half of the strains were clinical isolates from AIDS patients, while the remaining were recovered from non-AIDS patients but with pulmonary disease. The bactericidal activity of all rifamycin derivatives against

M. avium was substantially lower than that against *M. tuberculosis*; rifapentine, P-DEA, and CGP-7040 were the most active compounds.

Treatment of MAC-infected thymectomized C57BL/6 mice with rifabutin at doses of 40 mg/kg for a period of 120 d sterilized the infection.[123] The activity of rifabutin in combination with clofazimine, kanamycin, and ethambutol was also investigated.[124,125] Against *M. intracellulare* strain N-260 infection in mice, the combinations of rifabutin/ethambutol, rifabutin/clofazimine, rifabutin/kanamycin, rifabutin/ethambutol/clofazimine, rifabutin/ethambutol/kanamycin, and rifabutin/clofazimine/kanamycin enhanced the elimination of mycobacteria from the lungs, liver, and spleen; the combinations containing clofazimine were especially active.[124]

The antimycobacterial activity of rifapentine was evaluated in a beige mouse (C57BL/6-bgj-bgj) model of disseminated *M. avium* infection.[126] Treatment commenced at day 7 postinfection with a dose of 20 mg/kg given intraperitoneally or orally. The antibiotic was given once daily for 5 d, followed by twice weekly administration for 3 weeks. The drug acted in a dose-dependent manner and reduced organisms in the spleen, liver, and lungs.

Studying the efficacy of various rifampin combinations against cavitary lung disease caused by MAC and untreated previously, Tsukamura et al.[127] have found that regimens comprising rifampin, isoniazid, and enviomycin, and rifampin, isoniazid, and streptomycin were superior to rifampin, isoniazid, and ethambutol. In MAI strains not exposed to antituberculosis drugs prior to testing, resistance to rifampin, minocycline, and kitasamycin, as well as to streptomycin and kanamycin, appeared frequently in the same strains.[128]

A combination consisting of rifampicin, thiacetazone, and isonicotinic acid hydrazide (or ethambutol) was reported to be highly effective in the treatment of patients (including HIV-positive) infected with multiple drug-resistant MAC.[129] A similar, highly synergistic combination comprising rifampicin, thiacetazone, isoniazid, and/or ethambutol was also reported to be effective in the treatment of patients with MAC disease.[130]

The susceptibility of *M. avium-intracellulare* to rifampicin and streptomycin was augmented by the addition of Tween 80 into 7H10 agar medium with OADC; by comparison, the susceptibility to ethambutol was either unchanged or reduced by the addition of Tween 80.[131] In 7H10 agar medium without OADC, however, susceptibilities to both rifampicin and sulfadimethoxine were reduced by the addition of Tween 80 to the medium.

A number of 3'-hydroxy-5'-alkylpiperazinyl-benzoxazinorifamycins (KRMs), a new class of synthetic rifamycin analogs, were reported to exert potent *in vitro* and *in vivo* activities against *M. tuberculosis, M. intracellulare,* and *M. avium* comparable to those of rifampicin and rifabutin.[132-134] Five derivatives (KRM-1648, KRM-1657, KRM-1668, KRM-1674, and KRM-2312) have elicited 100% inhibition of 20 clinical isolates of *M. avium* complex at 1.25 µg/ml, while only 35% and 10% of the strains were suppressed by the same concentration of rifabutin and rifampicin, respectively. The observed MIC_{90} values of the five KRMs were 0.07 to 0.3 µg/ml, and 5.0 and 40 to 50 µg/ml for rifabutin and rifampicin, respectively.[135]

The *in vivo* activity of KRMs was evaluated in mouse and rabbit models with experimentally induced tuberculosis and/or *M. avium-intracellulare* infections.[136-143] Female beige mice were inoculated with the *M. avium-intracellulare* mouse-virulent strain 31F093T. The treatment with KRM drugs was started at 24 h postinfection at daily oral doses of 20 mg/kg and continued for 12 weeks. In the case of experimental tuberculosis, the treatment by daily oral administration of 10 mg/kg of the drugs was commenced at 24 h after infection and continued until day 40. All controls died within a 20- to 22-d period, while all of the KRM-treated animals survived.[136] In a continuing study Tomioka et al.[144] have examined the therapeutic efficacy of KRM-1648 against *M. intracellulare* strain N-260 (virulent) and N-478 (nonvirulent) in mice. KRM-1648 exerted potent activity against *M. intracellulare* infection induced in NK cell-deficient beige mice. The latter is a plausible model for AIDS-associated MAC infections in which a much more progressed state of gross lesions and bacterial loads at the sites of infection are observed. One drawback of the therapeutic efficacy of KRM-1648 has been its inability to suppress the progression of pulmonary lesions and the increase in bacterial loads at the sites of infection (including lungs and spleen) at the late phase of infection.[144]

The antimycobacterial activity of a new rifampin derivative, the 3-(4-cinnamylpiperazinyl iminomethyl) rifampicin SV (T9) against 20 strains of *M. avium* complex was investigated by Reddy et al.[145] Against MAC strains, the MIC_{90} values were 0.125 µg/ml or less; the corresponding values of rifampin were 2.0 µg/ml or less.

8.6.5.2.2.2 Aminoglycoside antibiotics — The anti-MAC activity of free and liposome-encapsulated streptomycin inside peritoneal macrophages has recently been examined.[146-148] In beige mice, free streptomycin at 100 mg/kg (given intramuscularly 5 d a week for 4 weeks) caused a significant reduction of the CFU counts of MAC from spleen, lungs, and liver.[148] In the same experiment, streptomycin encapsulated in multilamellar liposomes at 15 mg/kg in two intravenous injections elicited greater reduction of CFU in all three tissues.[146,147] The therapeutic efficacies of both unilamellar and multilamellar liposome preparations were similar.[147]

Majumdar et al.[149] also examined the effects of liposome-encapsulated streptomycin and ciprofloxacin against growth of MAC infection inside human peripheral blood monocyte/macrophages. The treatment was commenced 24 h postinfection and lasted for 20 h, then the cells were incubated for another 7 d. Throughout the concentration range studied (10 to 50 µg/ml), the liposome-encapsulated streptomycin reduced the CFU count about threefold more than the free antibiotic. At concentrations of 5.0 µg/ml, the liposome-encapsulated ciprofloxacin was about 50 times more effective than its free counterpart, and at the end of the 7-day incubation period, the CFUs were reduced 1000-fold compared with the untreated controls. Streptomycin encapsulated in sterically stabilized liposomes was bactericidal against MAC strain 101 in the spleen and liver, but not lungs, of beige mice.[150]

The bactericidal activity of injectable streptomycin against *M. avium* and *M. tuberculosis* was tested and compared to that of amikacin, kanamycin, and capreomycin.[151] All four agents were found to be highly bactericidal against *M. tuberculosis* with low MBC/MIC ratios and MBC values that were markedly lower than the maximum achievable concentrations in the serum (C_{max}). However, all four antibiotics possessed very low bactericidal activities against *M. avium*, with the broth-determined MBC values being considerably higher than the C_{max}. Overall, one third of the 100 strains of *M. avium* tested have been tentatively considered as susceptible to streptomycin, amikacin, and kanamycin, but not to capreomycin. In general, streptomycin and kanamycin were equipotent in activity and substantially less costly than amikacin.[151,152]

Yamori et al.[153] have found that the bactericidal activity of streptomycin and enviomycin against *M. avium-intracellulare* was most pronounced in the lag growth phase of mycobacteria.

The therapeutic efficacy of liposome-encapsulated kanamycin was examined against experimental infection of *M. intracellulare* in mice.[154] Injections of liposomal kanamycin were given once weekly for up to 8 weeks. When compared to the free antibiotic administered either alone or in combination with empty liposomal vesicles, the liposomal kanamycin elicited greater reduction in the degree of gross pulmonary lesions as well as in the growth of pathogen in the lungs, liver, spleen, and the kidneys. Furthermore, the effect of the liposomal drug was dose-dependent within the range of 50 to 200 µg/mouse/injection. It also markedly changed the tissue distribution of kanamycin in the serum and lungs, as well as in the reticuloendothelial organs (liver and spleen) where accumulation and retention of the liposome-encapsulated drug was significantly enhanced as compared with free kanamycin.[154]

The MIC values of amikacin against 50% and 90% of *M. avium* isolates were 4.8 and 13.4 µg/ml, respectively.[155] Similar values of 2.65 and 6.75 µg/ml, respectively, have been reported by other investigators.[151,152]

Treatment of a disseminated MAC (strain 101) infection in beige mice with amikacin prevented mortality and decreased the infection in the blood, liver, and spleen.[156] In other studies, liposome-encapsulated amikacin showed significantly greater inhibitory activity against MAC inside mouse peritoneal macrophages than the free drug.[157] In beige mice, liposome-encapsulated amikacin and gentamicin markedly reduced the bacterial counts in the blood, liver, and spleen (98.5%, 92.7%, and 92.8%, respectively, for 1.0-mg dose of amikacin, and 92.8%, 99.7%, and 99.4%, respectively, for gentamicin) as compared with placebo liposomes and buffer.[158]

Unlike rifapentine, amikacin showed a long post-treatment effect against *M. avium*.[159] This finding suggested that amikacin may still be active therapeutically even though its serum levels may have exceeded the MIC value for only a few hours.

Haifets et al.[160] have found that the inhibitory activity of gentamicin against *M. avium* depended on the pH of the medium. For example, the broth-determined MIC values for 90% of the strains studied were 5.0 µg/ml at pH 7.4, 9.5 µg/ml at pH 6.8, and greater than 16 µg/ml at pH 5.0. The MBC values were two- to eightfold higher than the MIC values. The combined effect of gentamicin and clarithromycin was additive, and the corresponding MICs and MBCs for each antibiotic were either the same as measured in single-drug tests or reduced twofold.[160]

The activity of TLC G-65, a liposomal gentamicin preparation, given alone or in combinations with rifapentine, clarithromycin, clofazimine, and ethambutol, was evaluated in a beige mouse (C57BL/6J-bgj/bgj) model of disseminated *M. avium* infection.[161] While the combination of TLC G-65 and rifapentine was more potent than either drug alone, the combination of TLC G-65 with clarithromycin showed activity similar to that of the individual antibiotics. Clofazimine and etham- butol improved the activity of TLC G-65 in the spleen and liver, respectively; both drugs enhanced the antimycobacterial potency of TLC G-65 in the lungs.[161]

Kanyok et al.[162] examined the *in vivo* activity of paromomycin against susceptible and multi- drug-resistant MAC strains in C57BL/6 mice and their beige counterparts. When given at 200 mg/kg, paromomycin was as effective as amikacin (50 mg/kg) in reducing the mean log CFU in the lungs, livers, and spleens of infected mice.

The efficacies of various antimycobacterial aminoglycosides against either colonizing *M. intracellulare* isolates from patients with underlying pulmonary disease, or infectious *M. intracellulare* (pathogens) isolated from patients with atypical mycobacterial disease, were investigated by Maesaki et al.[163] The results reported have demonstrated that aminoglycosides, in general, were more effective against the colonizing organisms than against the pathogens. Among the other drugs tested under the same conditions, isoniazid, ethambutol, and rifampicin were less potent against both colonizing organisms and pathogens, whereas the activity of cyclosporine was equipotent against both colonizing organisms and pathogens.

8.6.5.2.2.3 Macrolide antibiotics

— In recent years, several macrolide antibiotics, such as clarithromycin (CP 62,993), azithromycin (A-56268, TE-031), and roxithromycin (RU 28965) have shown promising activities against *M. avium-intracellulare* complex.[164]

Clarithromycin is a semisynthetic macrolide antibiotic which differs from erythromycin by an *O*-methyl substituent at C-6 of the 14-membered lactate ring. It appears to have a selective activity against MAC infections.[165] Compared with erythromycin, clarithromycin was twofold more active against most aerobic bacteria, and also achieved higher levels in serum and tissues.[166] When tested *in vitro* by the BACTEC method, the antibiotic inhibited 90% of 28 strains of MAC isolated from AIDS patients (MIC = 4.0 µg/ml); under the same conditions, roxithromycin and erythromy- cylamine inhibited 90% of strains at 16 µg/ml.[167]

Rastogi and Labrousse[168] have determined the MIC and MBC values of clarithromycin alone and in combinations with ethambutol and rifampin at sublethal concentrations (1.0 µg/ml) against 10 strains of *M. avium*. When given alone the antibiotic was bactericidal against all 10 strains. Its potency was augmented by ethambutol (in 8 of 9 strains) and rifampin (in 3 of 9 strains). In 7 of 9 strains, the combination of all three drugs elicited higher bactericidal effect than any individual drug or two-drug combination.

The bactericidal effect of clarithromycin (alone or in combinations, and at concentrations obtainable in human serum) was also evaluated against strain ATCC 15769 in 7H9 broth and BACTEC radiometry (extracellular action), and in the J-774 macrophage cell line (intracellular action).[168] The results showed a good correlation between extracellular and intracellular activities. As evidenced by electron microscopy, clarithromycin disorganized the outer cell wall layer and the cytoplasmic membrane of the mycobacterial cell envelope, which led to formation of large vacuoles inside the cytoplasm, solubilization of ribosomal structures, and ensuing plasmolysis.[168]

In other studies, the MIC and MBC values of clarithromycin were determined against 49 *M. avium* strains isolated from patients with AIDS.[169] As with other antibiotics, the pH of the medium affected the inhibitory effect of clarithromycin.[169,170] The antibiotic was more effective at physiologic (7.4) than acidic (5.0) pH.[170] For most strains tested in broth and pH 7.4, the MIC values ranged between 0.25 and 0.5 μg/ml; by comparison, the agar-determined MIC values were 1.0 to 4.0 μg/ml. The MBC values of clarithromycin were 8- to 64-fold higher than the corresponding MICs. The latter finding may indicate that the antimycobacterial efficacy of clarithromycin is determined more by its inhibitory rather than bactericidal activity.[169]

Yajko et al.[171] have evaluated the intracellular activities of clarithromycin and erythromycin, alone or in combinations with other antimicrobial agents, against MAC strains inside the mouse J-774 cell line and inside alveolar macrophages obtained from HIV-1-infected individuals. Clarithromycin alone was superior to erythromycin, and combinations that included clarithromycin were generally more effective than combinations that included erythromycin.

The activity of clarithromycin in combination with ethambutol and rifampicin was tested at concentrations achievable in serum against 20 strains of MAC.[172] The combination of clarithromycin and rifampicin was inhibitory against 11 strains, and bactericidal synergism was observed against 7 of them. When ethambutol was added, the bactericidal effect increased to include 16 strains.

The potency of clarithromycin, sulfisoxazole, and rifabutin against three virulent clinical isolates of *M. avium* from AIDS patients were evaluated in infected human monocyte-derived macrophages.[173] The MIC values against the three strains were as follows: for clarithromycin — 4.0, 4.0, and 4.0 μg/ml; for sulfisoxazole — 50, 25, and 25 μg/ml; and for rifabutin — 2.0, 0.5, and 0.5 μg/ml. At the concentrations applied (4.0 μg/ml for clarithromycin, 50 μg/ml for sulfisoxazole, and 0.5 μg/ml for rifabutin), clarithromycin and rifabutin were equipotent in reducing the intracellular replication of all strains, while sulfisoxazole was ineffective. The combinations of clarithromycin with either rifabutin or sulfisoxazole were as effective as clarithromycin alone.

Combinations of clarithromycin with amikacin, rifampicin, rifabutin, clofazimine, and ciprofloxacin were assessed for activity by agar dilution and radiometric technique in broth against 11 *M. avium-intracellulare* strains isolated from AIDS patients.[174] Clear synergistic activity was observed only with clarithromycin/rifampicin. The combination of clarithromycin, rifampicin, and amikacin was partially synergistic, while that of clarithromycin with rifabutin and clofazimine showed only an additive effect.

Daily treatment of C57BL/6 mice challenged with *M. avium* complex with clarithromycin (50 mg/kg, subcutaneously) and low- (15 μg/kg, intraperitoneally) or high-dose (300 μg/kg, intraperitoneally) of granulocyte colony-stimulating factor (G-CSF) reduced the CFU counts in both lung and spleen tissue.[175]

Starting on day 6 postinfection, beige mice infected with *M. avium* ATCC 25291 were treated with clarithromycin twice daily at 8-h intervals for 9 d.[166] At doses of 25 mg/kg, the antibiotic reduced the viable bacterial counts in the spleen when administered subcutaneously or orally. Other antimycobacterial drugs (erythromycin, difloxacin, temafloxacin, ciprofloxacin, rifampin, amikacin, and ethambutol) were also tested under the same conditions; only amikacin showed *in vivo* activity.[166]

Bermudez et al.[176] used a C57BL/6 beige mouse model to evaluate the oral activity of clarithromycin (200 mg/kg daily), dapsone (15 mg/kg daily), and combination of both against disseminated

MAC (serovar 1) infection. While clarithromycin alone markedly reduced bacteremia and the CFU counts in the liver and spleen, dapsone itself and in combination with clarithromycin had no beneficial effect. Clarithromycin (200 mg/kg daily) in combination with the rifamycin analog KRM-1648 (40 mg/kg daily) has decreased significantly the number of bacteria in the blood and spleen of beige mice as compared to untreated controls ($p < .001$).[139]

Drug therapy with clarithromycin, alone or in combinations, may also lead to resistance.[177-180] Thus, Ji et al.[177] have reported the isolation of clarithromycin-resistant mutants of *M. avium* from beige mice treated with 200 mg/kg of the antibiotic, six times weekly for 8 weeks. The frequency of drug-resistant mutants was estimated to be between 10^{-8} and 10^{-9}, and the MIC value of clarithromycin against the resistant organisms was ≥ 512 µg/ml.[177] Furthermore, the clarithromycin-resistant strains of MAC isolated from AIDS patients and beige mice as well as derivatives selected *in vitro* have shown a unique pattern of acquired cross-resistance to other macrolides and other antibiotics.[181] In contrast, the resistance pattern to non-macrolide antibiotics remained unchanged in clarithromycin-resistant strains. In addition, a dramatic decrease in ribosome affinity for clarithromycin and erythromycin was found in clarithromycin-resistant strains, but no mutation was present in the peptidyl domain of the 23S rRNA, indicating that another ribosomal modification has been involved.[181]

The acquired resistance to clarithromycin and combined therapy for *M. avium-intracellulare* infections has also been the subject of research.[182-184] Meier et al.[184] have investigated the peptidyl-transferase region of the 23S rRNA gene (the probable target site of the macrolide antibiotics) in blood isolates of *M. avium* recovered from 38 patients before and after the development of clarithromycin resistance. Point mutations were identified in 100% of the 74 resistant relapse blood isolates, but in none of 69 susceptible pretreatment isolates. Furthermore, multiple mutations have been identified in isolates from 23 of 38 patients (61%), and of the 63 identified mutations, 95% involved adenine at bp 2058. Single-colony clones from cultures that were mixtures of more than one mutation revealed a single mutation within each clone, and pulsed field gel electrophoresis of genomic DNA restriction fragments showed that 13 of 16 multiple mutations (81%) identified in the same patient were derived from a single infection strain.[184]

Azithromycin and roxithromycin, two of the newer macrolide antibiotics, were also examined for activity against *M. avium* and *M. xenopi in vitro*.[185,186] The two drugs were evaluated alone or in combinations with two other antibiotics, amikacin and rifabutin, and 1,25-dihydroxyvitamin D_3. After treating macrophage monolayers with the four antibiotics alone or in combination for 4 consecutive days, intracellular killing of mycobacteria did take place, with the combinations being markedly superior to the individual antibiotics. The effect was enhanced when 1,25-dihydroxy-vitamin D_3 was added to the culture.[185] Inderlied et al.[187] have also studied the *in vitro* potency and *in vivo* efficacy of azithromycin administered alone against MAC.

Cynamon et al.[188-190] have examined, in beige mice infected with *M. avium-intracellulare*, the comparative activities of azithromycin and clarithromycin and the activities of azithromycin alone and in combination with other antimycobacterial agents. The investigators found azithromycin and clarithromycin to be comparable in activity. Combination of azithromycin, clofazimine, and ethambutol reduced the number of organisms in the spleen more than azithromycin alone; however, the same combination was less potent than azithromycin alone in reducing mycobacteria in the lungs. Further testing showed that while rifabutin and azithromycin had similar activity for organisms in the spleen and lungs, in combination they were more efficacious than either drug alone for MAI in the spleen, and comparable to rifabutin for organisms in the lungs. All three drugs showed little correlation between *in vitro* and *in vivo* activities.[188]

Liposome-encapsulated azithromycin, prepared as a freeze-dried formulation to avoid chemical instability during storage, has shown enhanced anti-*M. avium* activity — the potency increased in parallel to the percentage of moles of negatively charged lipids.[115] Thus, in liposomes consisting of distearoylphosphatidylglycerol and cholesterol (10:5 ratio), azitrhromycin inhibited the intracellular *M. avium* growth 41-fold more effectively than did conventional azithromycin.

Roxithromycin alone reduced the level of bacteremia caused by *M. avium* complex liver and splenic infection (in CFU per gram) in beige mice and mortality compared with untreated controls ($p < .05$).[191] When combined with ethambutol, roxithromycin significantly reduced the number of bacteria in splenic tissue compared with those in control splenic tissues of mice and mice treated with roxithromycin alone and ethambutol alone. However, the *in vivo* efficacy of the combination of roxithromycin with levofloxacin was not better than roxithromycin alone.[191]

In vitro studies on the sensitivity of *M. avium* to roxithromycin, erythromycin, and doxycycline showed the pathogen to be highly and uniformly resistant to doxycycline ($MIC_{50} = 64$ mg/l). However, for roxithromycin some strains were moderately susceptible: MIC_{50} and MIC_{90} were, respectively, 8.0 and 16 mg/l; the corresponding values for erythromycin were 16 and 64 mg/l.[192]

The activity of roxithromycin against three clinical isolates of *M. avium* has been compared with that of clarithromycin both in a model of infection of human monocyte-derived macrophages and in a model of established infection of C57BL/6 mice.[193] In the cell culture model, roxithromycin and clarithromycin were bactericidal for strains MO-1 and N-92159 and bacteriostatic for strain N-93043. In the mice model, both drugs were given by gavage at a dosage of 200 mg/kg 6 d weekly for 16 weeks starting 5 weeks postinfection. At the end of treatment, clarithromycin was superior to roxithromycin in the lungs, while the two antibiotics were equipotent in the spleens.[193]

The activities of azithromycin, sparfloxacin, temafloxacin, and rifapentine against intracellular replication of two virulent strains of MAC in human macrophages isolated from AIDS patients were evaluated and compared to that of clarithromycin.[194] Compared to controls, clarithromycin, sparfloxacin, and azithromycin slowed the intracellular replication of both strains while rifapentine and temafloxacin were effective against only one strain.

When tested against *M. avium-M. intracellulare* strains, streptomycin and enviomycin were bactericidal; by comparison, the bactericidal activities of rifampicin and ethambutol were weak or absent even against the most susceptible strains 13008 (serotype 20) and 13016 (serotype 4).[195,196] It should be noted, however, that the susceptibilities of *M. avium-intracellulare* may be influenced by the size of the inoculum used in the determination, and the extent to such an inoculum effect may vary considerably with various drugs.[197]

Yet in another study,[198] the efficacy of various antibiotics (amikacin, rifampicin, rifabutin, ciprofloxacin, temafloxacin, erythromycin, and clarithromycin) was evaluated against pigmented and unpigmented variants of *M. avium-intracellulare*[199] isolated from AIDS patients. It was found that in intracellularly growing bacteria, the unpigmented variants were more resistant to antibiotics. The combinations of temafloxacin or ciprofloxacin with rifabutin and amikacin were the most effective against unpigmented variants.

The activities of amikacin, roxithromycin, rifampicin, rifapentine, and clofazimine, used alone or in combinations, were evaluated *in vitro* against *M. avium-intracellulare*. With all established combinations, the MIC values observed for each drug alone was appreciably reduced. Clofazimine, amikacin, and rifapentine were shown to be the most active.[200]

Some of the more serious side effects of various antimycobacterial antibiotics are presented in Table 8.6.

8.6.5.2.3 Folate antagonists

Various synergistic combinations containing folate antagonists (trimethoprim, sulfonamides) have often been used for treating MAC infections. The mode of action of sulfonamides involves suppression of the conversion of bacterial *p*-aminobenzoic acid to dihydrofolic acid. Trimethoprim, a 3,4,5-trimethoxybenzylpyrimidine analog, acts by blocking the activity of hydrofolate reductase, a bacterial enzyme that catalyzes the next step of the folate metabolism. When applied in combination, sulfamethoxazole (the most commonly used sulfonamide derivative) and trimethoprim act synergistically to block sequential stages of the folic acid biosynthesis. Trimethoprim is usually used together with sulfamethoxazole in a 1:5 ratio.

TABLE 8.6
Toxic Side Effects of Antimycobacterial Antibiotics

Antibiotic	Toxicities
Streptomycin, amikacin	Vestibulary/auditory disturbancy (dizziness, vertigo, ataxia, tinnitus, hearing loss), nephrotoxicity (tubular necrosis, nonoliguric azotemia, neuromuscular blockade, hypersensitivity (streptomycin: rash, fever, eosinophilia)
Rifampin	Gastrointestinal intolerance (nausea, vomiting), rash, fever, hepatitis, "flulike" syndrome, thrombocytopenia, renal failure associated with intermittent therapy, discoloration of secretion and urine, increased hepatic metabolism of drugs administered concomitantly (contraceptives, ketoconazole, oral hypoglycemics, prednisolone, quinidine, warfarin, methadone)
Rifabutin	Hepatitis, hemolytic anemia, leukopenia, thrombocytopenia

When tested *in vitro* against 11 isolates of MAC, sulfamethoxazole inhibited 3 of the isolates at a concentration of 32 μg/ml.[201] The latter is below the mean peak serum level obtained after a single 800-mg oral dose of sulfamethoxazole. Under the same conditions, trimethoprim was not active against any of the isolates tested, and in combination with sulfamethoxazole, it was not better than sulfamethoxazole alone.[202] Results by Raszka et al.[203] have corroborated these findings. The response of *M. avium-intracellulare* infections to treatment with trimethoprim–sulfamethoxazole was discussed by Chang and Goetz.[204]

Tsukamura[205,206] has found sulfadimethoxine to be the most effective sulfonamide derivative against *M. avium* complex strains. The activity was bacteriostatic and the MIC values of the drug when measured in Ogawa egg medium were influenced by the number of viable bacteria (expressed as CFU) used in the susceptibility testing.[207] Thus, when small inocula (50 to 100 CFU) were used, the MIC values ranged between 0.8 and 3.13 μg/ml; with large inocula, however, the MIC values were 6.25 to 25 μg/ml. Furthermore, prolongation of the incubation times resulted in higher MIC values.[207]

The antimycobacterial activity of sulfisoxazole against *M. avium-intracellulare* was also evaluated. The drug inhibited 12 of 20 isolates at 10 μg/ml.[208] However, other experiments have shown that sulfisoxazole was more effective — at concentrations of 0.2 μg/ml, it suppressed 24 of 25 isolates studied.[209]

Trimetrexate and piritrexim, two folate antagonists structurally related to methotrexate, were found active against MAC at concentrations of 8.0 μg/ml and 36 μg/ml, respectively.[210]

8.6.5.2.4 Inhibitors of cell wall synthesis

One of the strategies to circumvent multiple-drug resistance in antimycobacterial therapy is to enhance the *M. avium* susceptibility to drugs by inhibiting the synthesis of the outermost layer of its envelope, which appears to function as an exclusionary lipophilic barrier for drugs. The cell wall of various *Mycobacterium* species was found to contain a chemotype IV peptidoglycan to which an arabinogalactan moiety is covalently attached.[211] This arabinogalactan moiety is further modified by esterification with mycolic acid residues.[212,213] In addition, small amounts of highly immunogenic proteins are also present.[214] The mycolylarabinogalactan moiety of the mycobacterial cell wall has been implicated in a number of biological responses associated with human and experimental mycobacterioses, including the high titer of IgG antibodies in tuberculosis and leprosy sera,[215,216] and the state of T cell-mediated immunological anergy present in the multibacillary form of the disease.[217]

The integrity of the mycobacterial cell envelope in general, and the mycolylarabinogalactan moiety, in particular, have long been recognized as critical for the survival of the pathogen in the hostile host environment, and therefore, as important targets for antimycobacterial drugs.[218] Studies in recent years have resulted in the detailed chemical characterization of the mycobacterial cell wall, including a full definition of the glycopeptidolipids which comprise the typing antigens of the *M. avium* complex.[211,219-223] Of particular interest has been the recognition of a pentaarabino-furanosyl motif equating the nonreducing termini of the arabinan segment of arabinogalactan with the dominant antigenic determinant of arabinogalactan.[211] These and other findings have provided the necessary knowledge of those structural details required to facilitate the design of compounds capable of inhibiting the attachment of mycolic acids to arabinogalactan. Such information coupled with the increased ability to prepare derivatives inhibiting various carbohydrate-recognizing enzymes[224] will expand the opportunities for design and synthesis of antimycobacterial drugs acting on cell wall biosynthesis.

One such strategy used by Rastogi et al.[225] has included the simultaneous use of conventional antimycobacterial agents with drugs known for their ability to inhibit the *M. avium* cell envelope formation, such as *m*-fluorophenylalanine (an inhibitor of mycoside-C biosynthesis), DL-norleucine (an inhibitor of transmethylation reactions), ethambutol (an inhibitor of arabinogalactan synthesis), EDTA (a divalent-ion chelator), and colistin (an inducer of the membrane flux of divalent cations). All these drugs were used in low concentrations not to cause potential damage to the host. The testing results against seven strains of *M. avium* complex showed that both *m*-fluorophenylalanine and ethambutol were effective in significantly enhancing MAC susceptibility.[225]

David et al.[226] found that radioactivity from [^3H]-methylmethionine was rapidly incorporated into the surface lipids of *M. avium*. This transmethylation reaction was efficiently inhibited by DL-ethionine, D-norleucine, and DL-norleucine. Of the three amino acids, DL-norleucine profoundly altered the structure of the envelope outer layer of the mycobacteria.

8.6.5.2.5 *Miscellaneous antimycobacterial compounds*

In addition to the major classes of known antimycobacterial drugs, a number of other agents have shown various degrees of anti-*M. avium* complex activity. Heifets et al.[227] compared the bacterio-static and bactericidal activities (MICs and MBCs, respectively) of isoniazid and ethionamide against 68 strains of *M. avium* and 14 wild drug-susceptible strains of *M. tuberculosis*. The MIC values of isoniazid ranged between 0.025 and 0.05 µg/ml for *M. tuberculosis*, and from 0.6 µg/ml to greater than 10.0 µg/ml for *M. avium*. The corresponding values of ethionamide for *M. tuber-culosis* were from 0.3 to 1.25 µg/ml; values for 42.7% of the *M. avium* strains were within the same range. While both drugs have been highly bactericidal against *M. tuberculosis*, their bacteri-cidal activity against *M. avium* was markedly less potent.[227]

Using strains which were isolated from sputum specimens of patients previously not treated with antimycobacterial drugs, Tsukamura[228] investigated drug cross-resistance patterns in MAC infections. Among the various agents studied, cross-resistance was observed only between ethionamide and isoniazid. The *in vitro* susceptibility of *M. avium-intracellulare* to low concentrations (as measured in the blood) of isoniazid (0.2 µg/ml) and ethionamide (5.0 µg/ml) has also been investigated.[229]

Gangadharam et al.[230] have studied the activity of compound B746, a derivative of clofazimine, against MAC. When applied alone against experimental *M. avium-intracellulare* infections in beige mice at the required optimal dose of 20 mg/kg, B746 was inferior to clofazimine but slightly superior to streptomycin when given intramuscularly at 150 mg/kg. Combinations of B746 with either clofazimine or streptomycin were inferior to any of the three drugs administered alone.

Kaufman et al.[231] successfully treated a localized MAC-induced granuloma in a cat with clofazimine and doxycycline.

Peterson et al.[232] reported the synthesis and anti-*M. intracellulare* activity of several ring A- and B-substituted sampangine (a group of copyrine alkaloids) analogs. Structure-activity relation-ship studies demonstrated more potent activity for compounds containing a C-3 substituent or a 4,5-benzene ring. In Mueller-Hinton broth, the most active derivatives exhibited MIC values of 0.39 and 0.78 µg/ml; by comparison, the MIC of rifampin was 0.78 µg/ml.

A combination, known as CQQ or gangamicin, and comprising of vitamin K and coenzyme Q, was found active against *M. tuberculosis* and *M. avium*.[233,234] All of the 40 isolates of *M. avium* studied were inhibited by CQQ at concentrations of 16 µg/ml.[234]

Peripheral blood mononuclear cells (PBMC) of healthy subjects preincubated with 100 to 1000 ng/ml of diethyldithiocarbamate (DTC), and then infected with *M. tuberculosis* H37Rv or *M. avium-intracellulare* exhibited increased antimycobacterial activity.[235] When tested *ex vivo* in monocytes derived from healthy volunteers, the beneficial effect of DTC (5.0 mg/mL) was most evident at 24 h postinfection.

Wright and Barrow[236] have found that 2-deoxy-D-glucose inhibited in a dose-dependent manner the glycopeptidolipid biosynthesis of cultures of *M. avium* complex serovar 4.

The bacteriostatic and bactericidal activity of thiacetazone was determined against 68 clinical isolates of *M. avium* and 14 wild drug-susceptible strains of *M. tuberculosis*.[237] The bactericidal activity of thiacetazone was equally low against both mycobacterial species. Its bacteriostatic activity was greater against *M. avium*; measured in broth, the MIC values against *M. avium* and *M. tuberculosis* were 0.02 to 0.15 µg/ml and 0.08 to 1.2 µg/ml, respectively.

Dihydromycoplanecin A, a semisynthetic cyclic peptide antibiotic derived from mycoplanecin A, was reported to be active against MAC *in vitro*.[238,239] Studies in a murine model of tuberculosis showed dihydromycoplanecin A to be synergistic with isoniazid.[238]

When tested *in vitro* against 17 strains of *M. avium* complex, fusidic acid, at concentrations of up to 64 mg/l, was found inactive against all but one strain. However, synergistic effects were observed in 11 of the 17 strains when fusidic acid was applied in combination with ethambutol.[240]

The efficacy of dapsone against *M. avium*, *M. intracellulare*, *M. tuberculosis*, *M. kansasii*, and *M. fortuitum* was determined by disc elution in agar.[241] The MIC_{90} values were 8.0 mg/l for *M. avium*, *M. intracellulare*, and *M. kansasii*, and ≥32 mg/l for *M. tuberculosis* and *M. fortuitum*. However, the use of potentiators, such as 4-amino-*N*-(4,6-dimethyl-2-pyrimidinyl)benzenesulfonamide (sulfamethazine, BN 2409) and 1-(4-chlorophenyl)-1,6-dihydro-6,6-dimethyl-1,3,5-triazine-2,4-diamine·HCl (cycloquanil chloride, BN 2410), reduced the MIC_{90} values from 8.0 mg/l to 2.0 mg/l.

Forty-six derivatives of 6-acylamido-2-alkylthiobenzothiazole were tested *in vitro* for activity against *M. avium* and several structure-activity relationship correlations reported.[242]

When screened for activity against MAC isolates, two β-lactam antibiotics, meropenem and imipenem, were for the most part inactive; the serotypes of the strains studied were characteristic for patients with disseminated infection.[243]

A number of lipophilic *N*-acylpyrazimine derivatives were prepared and tested for activity against *M. avium-intracellulare*.[244] One liposome-encapsulated preparation containing the *N*-palmitoylpyrazinamide derivative was active at 12.5-25 µg/ml.

JTP3309, a newly synthesized lipid A-subunit analog, was examined for *in vitro* and *in vivo* antimycobacterial activity.[245] In BALB mice, JTP3309 when given at doses of 10 and 20 µg/mouse 4 and 1 d prior to infection with *M. avium*, reduced the number of CFUs recovered from the spleen of infected mice.

8.6.5.3 Evolution of Therapies and Treatment of *M. avium-intracellulare* Infections

The present status of chemotherapy of *M. avium-intracellulare* infections, especially in immunocompromised patients, is still far from being solved. Although in recent years some progress in treating such infections has been made, there is still no viable drug and/or combinations of drugs effective against them. The chemotherapy of these infections still remains a formidable challenge because of the resistance of MAI isolates to the majority of conventional antimycobacterial agents. Results from controlled clinical trials are scarce, and a significant part of the published reports provide recommendations for therapies that are limited in scope, often anecdotal, and based mainly on empirical data.[246]

In general, because of drug resistance, all *M. avium-intracellulare* infections should be treated using combined chemotherapy. The first-line antimycobacterial agents currently in clinical use against *M. tuberculosis* are 10 to 100 times less active *in vitro* against MAC isolates. Such a marked decline in therapeutic potency is considered to result from the highly lipophilic nature of the *M. avium* cell wall which would prevent adequate drug penetration.[247] Antimycobacterial agents that have a better *in vitro* activity against MAC isolates (cycloserine, ethionamide) are usually considered second-line chemotherapeutics because of their more pronounced toxicity.

Thoracic infection caused by MAC typically occurs in patients with underlying lung disease or immunologic abnormality. However, immunocompetent hosts have also been diagnosed with the disease.[248,249]

Current therapies for pulmonary *M. avium-intracellulare* infections include the use of multiple drug combinations.[250-252] Such regimens, however, because of their multiple-drug involvement may create a relatively high risk of toxic side effects. The U.S. Public Health Service has provided some guidelines for treatment of MAC infection in both adults and children. It has been recommended that active disseminated MAC infections be treated with regimens that include at least two drugs, one of which is either clarithromycin or azithromycin; ethambutol may be considered as the second drug. Other potentially useful drugs include clofazimine, rifabutin, rifampin, amikacin, and ciprofloxacin. While clinical response may be observed within 4 to 6 weeks, sterilization of blood cultures usually takes longer.

The development of two new macrolide antibiotics, clarithromycin and azithromycin, may have signaled the turning point in the treatment of *M. avium* infection.[253-270] Results from controlled clinical trials have indicated the high efficiency of clarithromycin in both AIDS patients with disseminated disease and non-AIDS patients having localized pulmonary infection.[266,271,272] Either when given alone or as part of antimycobacterial combinations, clarithromycin at doses of 0.5 to 2.0 g (typically 1.0 g) administered twice daily was found effective in controlling MAC bacteremia in AIDS patients.[273]

In a randomized, double-blind, dose-ranging study,[266] 154 AIDS patients with symptomatic MAC disease were treated for 12 weeks with clarithromycin at dosages of 500 mg, 1.0 g, or 2.0 g, given twice daily. Clarithromycin decreased the mycobacterial CFU counts from 2.7 to 2.8 $\log_{10}$/ml of blood at baseline to less than 0 $\log_{10}$/ml during the follow-up examination ($p < .0001$), and at 6 weeks, the median CFU counts per milliliter of blood was 0 or 1 for all three dose regimens. While clarithromycin-resistant isolates of MAC developed in 46% of patients at a median of 16 weeks, the median survival rate was longer in patients receiving the 500-mg dose (249 d) than in patients given 1.0 g or 2.0 g dosages. Overall, the 500-mg dose of clarithromycin was well tolerated and associated with better survival.[266]

However, even though monotherapy with clarithromycin may result in the elimination of bacteremia in nearly all patients, relapse of disease inevitably occurred in patients who survived long enough to reach this event.

In addition, short-term monotherapy may lead to bacterial resistance (within 12 to 16 weeks), underscoring the importance of long-term treatment with a combination of antimycobacterial drugs.[266,268,273] As reported by Heifets,[274] clinical isolates which were susceptible to clarithromycin before the treatment contained 10^{-8} or 10^{-9} resistant mutants, and the relapses of bacteremia were caused by multiplication of these preexisting mutants. The resistance to clarithromycin was associated with a mutation in the 23S rRNA gene. Cross-resistance between clarithromycin and azithromycin has also been confirmed with both laboratory mutants and clinical isolates.[274] The selection of companion drugs to be used with clarithromycin and azithromycin to preclude the emergence of macrolide resistance has remained largely unsolved and the subject of clinical trials currently in progress.

Dautzenberg et al.[275] studied the therapeutic efficacy of clarithromycin in a randomized, double-blind, placebo-controlled trial involving 15 male AIDS (late-stage) patients with disseminated *M. avium* infection. The patients were divided into two groups. The first one received clarithromycin alone for 6 weeks, then placebo plus rifampin, isoniazid, ethambutol, and clofazimine for 6 weeks; the second group was treated with placebo alone, then clarithromycin plus the other four drugs. The MIC value of clarithromycin for 90% of the strains isolated from patients at baseline (as measured on 7H11 agar at pH 6.6) was 8.0 μg/ml. Eight eligible patients from the first group with initial positive culture responded with a marked decline in the number of *M. avium* CFU; in six cases, CFUs decreased to zero. When seven of the patients were switched to placebo plus the other four drugs, the CFU counts rose in four patients and remained undetectable in three. The five eligible patients from the second group initially treated with placebo had progressive increase in the CFU counts; when three were switched to clarithromycin plus the other four drugs, their CFU counts declined.

Wallace et al.[253] have reviewed the intermediate results of 50 HIV-negative patients treated with clarithromycin regimen for MAI lung disease; pretreatment isolates were all susceptible to the antibiotic. The patients, who received clarithromycin at 500 mg, b.i.d., ethambutol, rifampin, or rifabutin, and initial streptomycin, were treated until they became culture-negative for 1 year. Of the 39 evaluable patients, 36 (92%) converted their sputa to negative, and 32 (82%) have remained culture-negative to date; isolates from 6 of 39 patients (15%) became clarithromycin-resistant.

The side effects of clarithromycin were generaly mild and included a transient hypoacusis. Elevation of the serum glutamic-pyruvic transaminase and/or alkaline phosphatase levels was observed in two patients, one on clarithromycin medication and the other one receiving placebo.[275] Price and Tuazon[276] have reported the existence of clarithromycin-induced thrombocytopenia. Nightingale et al.[277] have observed acute psychosis in two AIDS patients with disseminated MAC infection after therapy with clarithromycin. The psychosis resolved when the treatment was discontinued and recurred when it was resumed. Clarithromycin has also been associated with a case of corneal opacity in an AIDS patient.[278]

In another randomized and double-blind study,[279] nine HIV-positive patients with disseminated MAC disease received clarithromycin or placebo in addition to a basic regimen that included isoniazid, ethambutol, and clofazimine. Blood culture conversion and clinical response were observed in all four patients receiving clarithromycin. Of the five patients not on clarithromycin medication, two showed resolution of mycobacteremia and clinical response, while another two died without showing a response. After 6 weeks of intensive treatment, clarithromycin was administered in an open maintenance phase to all patients, initially in combination with rifabutin for 24 weeks and then alone. One patient had a relapse of MAC infection when treated with clarithromycin alone.[279]

Using a combination of clarithromycin and rifabutin for 8 months, Malessa et al.[280] have described the first case of a successful treatment of MAC-induced meningoencephalitis in an AIDS patient.

The effect of a combination of clarithromycin, ciprofloxacin, and amikacin was evaluated in 12 AIDS patients with *M. avium-intracellulare* infection.[281] Mycobacteremia was cleared and symptoms were resolved in all patients after 2 to 8 weeks of therapy. Although four of the patients died, disseminated *M. avium-intracellulare* disease was not considered the primary cause of their death.

Since rifampin and rifabutin have been known to induce the hepatic cytochrome P450 system,[282] Wallace et al.[283] examined their impact on the metabolism of clarithromycin. The serum levels of clarithromycin and its major metabolite, 14-hydroxyclarithromycin, were measured in the sera of patients receiving 500 mg twice daily before and after the addition of other antimycobacterial drugs, including 600 mg daily of either rifampin or rifabutin. The mean serum levels of clarithromycin when given as a single drug (5.4 ± 2.1 μg/ml) decreased to 0.7 ± 0.6 and 2.0 ± 1.5 μg/ml in patients receiving rifampin and rifabutin, respectively. However, the mean serum levels of 14-hydroxyclarithromycin were not influenced and remained similar in all three groups (1.8 to 1.9 μg/ml). Overall, rifampin and to a lesser extent rifabutin appeared to induce the metabolism of clarithromycin and reduce its serum concentrations when applied as part of the same regimen.

Clinical studies conducted in AIDS patients have shown that azithromycin was active against disseminated MAC infection at daily doses of 600 mg.[257] Wallace at al.[284] have reported senso-rineural ototoxicity associated with azithromycin during treatment of MAC infection.

An initial therapy of pulmonary MAC diseases, which has been recommended by the American Thoracic Society (ATS),[86] consisted of daily administration of isoniazid (300 mg), rifampin (600 mg), and ethambutol (25 mg/kg for the first 2 months, then 15 mg/kg), with streptomycin also given during the initial 3 to 6 months of therapy.[86,285,286] Although the optimal dose or duration of streptomycin medication is still not well defined, daily treatment for 5 d weekly is preferred for patients younger than 70 years of age and with normal renal function; after 6 months of treatment, the streptomycin therapy should become intermittent. The length of the ATS-recommended treat-ment is also not well defined. It has been suggested[86] that patients who failed to convert their sputum cultures after 12 months of treatment should be reassessed, although earlier changes in the course of therapy may still be necessary. Subsequent therapies of such patients are difficult to manage because of the higher risk of drug toxicity.

With regard to the ATS four-drug regimen, Heifets and Iseman[287] objected to the inclusion of isoniazid because of its toxicity and negligible *in vitro* efficacy against *M. avium-intracellulare*. To this end, Tsukamura[288] has studied the bacteriostatic and bactericidal activity of isoniazid against various MAC strains. At concentrations of 0.1 to 25 μg/ml, the drug was bactericidal for several relatively susceptible strains. Overall, *M. avium* strains were more resistant to isoniazid than *M. intracellulare* strains. Although frequently used in various drug combinations, because isoniazid is essentially inactive against MAC at achievable serum concentrations, its usefulness in combined treatment of MAC infections has been seriously questioned.[287,289,290]

Shafran et al.[291] reported results of the Canadian HIV Trial Network Protocol 010, in which two regimens were compared in the treatment of *M. avium* complex bacteremia. Two hundred twenty-nine AIDS patients were randomly assigned to receive either rifampin (600 mg daily), ethambutol (approximately 15 mg/kg daily), clofazimine (100 mg daily), and ciprofloxacin (750 mg, b.i.d.) (regimen A); or rifabutin (600 mg daily), ethambutol (same as above), and clarithromycin (1.0 g, b.i.d.) (regimen B). In the regimen B group, the dose of rifabutin was reduced by half after 125 patients were randomized because 24 of 63 patients developed uveitis. Overall, among the 187 evaluable patients, the three-drug regimen B (rifabutin–ethambutol–clarithromycin) was superior to its four-drug counterpart (regimen A) in several evaluation criteria: blood cultures became negative more often in the regimen B group than in the regimen A group (69% and 29%, respec-tively; $p <.001$); in patients treated at least 4 weeks, the bacteremia resolved more frequently in the regimen B group (78% vs. 40%; $p <.001$); in the regimen B group, bacteremia resolved more often with the 600-mg dose of rifabutin than with the 300-mg dose ($p = .025$), but the latter regimen was still more effective than regimen A ($p <.05$); and the median survival time was 8.6 months and 5.2 months for regimens B and A, respectively ($p = .001$). The incidence rate of mild uveitis that developed in 3 of 53 patients receiving the 300-mg dose of rifabutin was about one quarter that observed with the 600-mg dose ($p <.001$).[291]

The individual effects of clofazimine, ethambutol, and rifampin on MAC bacteremia in AIDS patients were investigated by Kemper et al.[292] Patients were randomized to receive daily doses of either 200 mg clofazimine, 15 mg/kg ethambutol, or 600 mg rifampin for 4 weeks. Only ethambutol resulted in a statistically significant reduction in the level of mycobacteremia — the median range in individual baseline colony counts was $-0.60 \log_{10}$ CFU/ml after 4 weeks of treatment ($p = .046$). By comparison, the median changes in individual baseline colony counts were $-0.2 \log_{10}$ CFU/ml and $+0.2 \log_{10}$ CFU/ml for clofazimine and rifampin, respectively (both, $p >.4$).

Jorup-Ronstrom et al.[293] evaluated the clinical efficacy of ethambutol (15 mg/kg), rifabutin (6.0 mg/kg), and amikacin (15 mg/kg, IV for 2 to 4 weeks) in 31 HIV-infected patients with severe immunodeficiency and MAC infection. Clinical response was observed in 22 of 31 patients after a median time of 14 d; 5 patients had a relapse which was successfully treated with another course of amikacin.

Another recommended multiple-drug regimen involved cycloserine (250 mg, b.i.d.), ethionamide (250 mg twice daily, then increased to three times daily if tolerated), and prolonged use of streptomycin (three to five times weekly).[86] The use of clofazimine and ciprofloxacin has also been reported.[294]

The disseminated form of *M. avium-intracellulare* disease is more likely to affect immunocompromised patients.[295-297] The severity of infection usually depends on the degree of immunosuppression, extent of mycobacterial involvement, and the therapeutic regimen, and recurrence is not unusual.[298] While in non-AIDS patients the four-drug regimen recommended for pulmonary infections appears to be beneficial,[86] in patients with a severely suppressed immune system during the late stages of AIDS, the response and long-term prognosis are generally poor.[90,299] In several reports, multiple-drug therapy that included ethambutol, rifampin (or rifabutin), clofazimine, and an injectable aminoglycoside (streptomycin, amikacin) has provided symptomatic and clinical improvement to some[289,300,301] but not all[302] patients. Thus, using a combination of rifabutin (150 or 300 mg daily) and clofazimine (100 mg daily), Mazur et al.[302] have described a rather insignificant response to long-term therapy: a sustained clearing of mycobacteremia was observed in only 4 of 13 patients with MAC infection. Similarly, Hawkins et al.[90] have reported that treatment of mycobacteremia with a three-drug combination of rifabutin/clofazimine/ethionamide or ethambutol was successful in only 2 of 26 patients.

In a small retrospective study involving long-term therapy of seven patients with AIDS and MAC disease, Agins et al.[289] have found that the response to a combination of rifabutin (150 mg daily), clofazimine (100 mg daily), isoniazid (300 mg daily), and ethambutol (15 mg daily) was positive in six patients. Based on susceptibility data, these investigators recommended that isoniazid be deleted from the combination, and ciprofloxacin be used with ethambutol, ansamycin, and clofazimine.[289] Dautzenberg et al.[303] also conducted a clinical trial assessing the efficacy of rifabutin, ethambutol, clofazimine, and isoniazid in the treatment of disseminated MAC disease (see Section 8.6.9 on *M. xenopi*).

In a clinical trial involving 25 HIV-positive patients with MAC infection, a combination of rifabutin (300 to 600 mg daily), clofazimine (100 mg daily), isoniazid (300 mg daily), and ethambutol (15 mg daily) was administered for 6 to 74 weeks (average of 38 weeks).[304] The results have been encouraging: mycobacteremia was cleared in 22 of 25 patients. On the negative side, however, 6 of the 22 patients involved eventually had a recurrence, most often in the group receiving 300 mg daily of rifabutin. Some of the adverse side effects associated with high-dose rifabutin in macrolide-containing regimens for the treatment of *M. avium* complex lung disease have been discussed by Berning and Peloquin.[305]

In one study, *M. avium* infection was treated with a combination of ethambutol, rifabutin, clofazimine, and protionamide (or cycloserine) in relatively large doses — the median range survival of treated patients was 15.5 (4 to 22) months.[306] Data from clinical trials have indicated that blood cultures from 46% to 92% of patients become sterile after therapy with rifabutin combined with ethambutol, clofazimine, or amikacin.[307]

Rifabutin, a macrophage-penetrating lipophilic rifamycin derivative with long half-life, although showing dose-limiting toxic side effects (mainly arthralgia/arthritis and uveitis),[308-316] can reduce the incidence of MAC infection when given either alone or in combination with other drugs.[317] Compared to those of its structural analog rifampicin, the clinical pharmacokinetics of rifabutin showed important differences. Thus, rifabutin has relatively low oral bioavailability — about 20% after a single dose administration. While its elimination half-life is long (45 h), because of the very large volume of distribution (over 9.0 l/kg), the average plasma concentrations remained relatively low after repeated administration of conventional doses.[318]

In a prospective study conducted by Sullam et al.,[319] rifabutin (600 mg daily) or placebo was evaluated, each in combination with clofazimine and ethambutol, in AIDS patients with MAC bacteremia. The patients in the rifabutin group had a significantly higher rate of microbiological response, as defined by either sterilization of the blood, or at least a 2-$\log_{10}$ reduction in mycobacterial titers.

Griffith et al.[320] have conducted a multiple-drug trial that included high-dose rifabutin for the treatment of MAC disease. Twenty-six patients received 600 mg daily of rifabutin in combination with ethambutol, streptomycin, and either clarithromycin (500 mg, b.i.d.; 15 patients) or azithromycin (600 mg daily; 11 patients). Rifabutin-related adverse side effects occurred in 77% of patients, with 58% requiring either dosage adjustment or discontinuation of rifabutin therapy. The most common toxicity was the reduction of the mean total white blood cell count, which decreased from 8600 ± 2800 cells/mm^3 before treatment to 4500 ± 2100 cells/mm^3 during treatment ($p = .0001$), followed by diffuse polyarthralgia syndrome and anterior uveitis; other adverse side effects included gastrointestinal symptoms (nausea, vomiting, or diarrhea) and abnormal liver enzyme levels. A recommended dose of 300 mg daily is considered to be safe in multidrug regimens containing a macrolide component for the treatment of MAC lung disease.[320] Results from two double-blind, randomized, placebo-controlled trials involving 1100 patients with AIDS and AIDS-related complex have confirmed the safety and efficacy of rifabutin when given at low doses — the therapy decreased in half the rate of MAC bacteremia and significantly reduced symptoms associated with disseminated MAC disease.[321]

The results of several European trials of rifabutin alone or in multiple-drug combinations for treatment of infections due to *M. avium* complex in patients with AIDS have been discussed by Dautzenberg.[322] Thus, in a prospective open study in France involving 50 patients, treatment with rifabutin, isoniazid, ethambutol, and clofazimine was well tolerated, and the rate of conversion of cultures from positive to negative reached 70% at 6 months. Another randomized, double-blind, placebo-controlled, prospective trial (the NTMT01 trial) has assessed the role of rifabutin in treatment with a combination containing clofazimine, isoniazid, and ethambutol — the culture conversion rate was 74% for the rifabutin group and 53% for the patients given placebo, at the last valid observation for evaluable patients. In the ongoing Curavium study, patients receive clarithromycin in addition to either clofazimine or both rifabutin and ethambutol. Overall results have indicated that the best treatment for MAC infection in AIDS patients will require multiple-drug regimens, and rifabutin can be used safely as part of such combinations.[322]

Microcalorimetric studies of the initial interaction between *M. avium* and ethambutol suggested that the latter may potentiate the effect of other antimycobacterial drugs on MAI by increasing the permeability of the bacterial cell wall.[323] For example, in a case report involving a 57-year-old female patient with recurring tenosynovitis due to MAI infection, treatment with a combination of ethambutol and rifabutin proved successful.[324] Hoffner et al.[325] have found combinations of ethambutol with fluorinated quinolones, such as ciprofloxacin, ofloxacin, and norfloxacin, to be synergistic because of the enhanced penetration of quinolones caused by ethambutol.

The potentiating effect of ethambutol, which is thought to be mediated through a specific ethambutol receptor(s) located in the outer cell envelope of MAC,[325] may be the result of interference with the cell wall-permeability barrier of MAC to other drugs.[325,326]

Sullam[307] has observed a markedly enhanced efficacy of ethambutol–clofazimine combination after rifabutin had been added to the regimen. However, in combination with clarithromycin, rifabutin at daily dosages of 450 mg or more has been associated with a high incidence of uveitis, thus prompting the recommendation that only 300 mg of the drug be given daily with this macrolide.

Another four-drug combination consisting of rifampin (600 mg daily, orally), ethambutol (15 mg/kg daily), clofazimine (100 to 200 mg daily), and ciprofloxacin (750 mg, b.i.d., orally) was tried for 12 weeks in 31 patients; in addition, 6 of the patients also received amikacin.[327] At the end of the treatment period, the majority of patients showed improved clinical signs.

Peloquin[328] has found that in some non-AIDS patients infected with MAC, rifampin at 600 mg daily and ciprofloxacin at 750 mg b.i.d. failed to produce serum drug concentrations (SDCs) that would have exceeded the pathogen's MIC, and therefore, may require doubling of these dosages to attain SDCs similar to those observed in patients without the absorption problem.

Ciprofloxacin-induced acute renal dysfunction has also been observed 8 to 10 d after commencement of therapy — the patients recovered spontaneously following cessation of therapy for 2 to 8 weeks, and toxicity did not recur when treatment was restarted with regimens that did not contain ciprofloxacin.[329] In another study,[330] a possible interaction between foscarnet and ciprofloxacin in two patients with AIDS, cytomegalovirus retinitis, and MAC infection has been examined. The incidence of seizures with foscarnet infusion is high, ranging from 13% to 15%, and predisposing factors, such as renal impairment, electrolyte and metabolic abnormalities, and underlying neurologic disorders have been associated with seizures during foscarnet therapy. The two patients developed generalized tonic-clonic seizures while receiving both drugs, with neither of them having any of the aforementioned risk factors.

TLC G-65, a liposome-encapsulated gentamicin, was administered intravenously twice weekly for 4 weeks to AIDS patients with MAC bacteremia at dosages of 1.7 mg/kg/infusion, 3.4 mg/kg/infusion, and 5.1 mg/kg/infusion.[331] The MAC colonies in the blood fell by 75% or more in all three groups ($p < .005$). There has been no drug resistance, and adverse side effects included only a transient renal insufficiency in one patient.

Wormser et al.[332] have recommended the use of a low-dose dexamethasone (typically 2.0 mg daily) as adjunctive therapy for disseminated MAC infections in AIDS patients. All patients experienced substantial and sustained weight gain (12% to 50% of pre-steroid treatment weight; $p < .03$), reduction of fever, and increased serum albumin; the serum alkaline phosphatase level, however, fell from 368 ± 247 U/l to 128 ± 43.6 U/l ($p < .04$).

Osteomyelitis in immunocompetent patients due to dissemination of *M. avium* complex has been reported on several occasions.[93,265,333,334] Jones et al.[333] have described a case of MAC-associated osteomyelitis and septic arthritis in an immunocompetent patient. The infection, which was derived from an injury sustained 13 years earlier and had spread through the bone, joint, and soft tissue emerging at the medial aspect, was treated successfully with surgical debridement, drainage, arthrodesis, and 18 months of chemotherapy consisting of clarithromycin, rifampin, ethambutol, and ciprofloxacin, with an initial 2 weeks of amikacin. However, in another case of MAI-induced osteomyelitis involving the patella, distal femur, and the proximal tibia, the patient failed to respond to arthroscopic synovectomy and combination therapy. The need for aggressive surgical intervention has been stressed.[265] Pirofsky et al.[271] described a case of spinal osteomyelitis due to *M. avium-intracellulare* in an immunocompromised elderly patient undergoing corticosteroid therapy.

A localized MAC-associated mastitis in an immunocompetent patient with silicone breast implants was cured with implant removal and a 6-month course of clarithromycin.[335]

While cutaneous involvement with *M. avium-intracellulare* has been commonly observed in disseminated disease, cutaneous infections alone without bacteremia are unusual and probably associated with traumatic percutaneous inoculation, frequently in immunocompromised patients. Philippot et al.[336] have reported one such case of MAI-induced subcutaneous abscess in a patient with lymphoma. The lesion, which was treated with drainage, excision, and antimycobacterial therapy, was most likely the result of inoculation secondary to IFN-α injections. Another case of severe disseminated MAI infection with unusual cutaneous features was described by Bachelez et al.[337] in a HIV-infected patient who presented with disseminated pustular lesions, which showed necrosis and which led to varioliform scarring. The patient was successfully treated with a multiple-agent antimycobacterial regimen including clarithromycin, which appeared to be the most effective drug.

Mattila et al.[338] have evaluated MAI and other mycobacteria as a possible cause of prurigo nodularis, a chronic skin disorder with unknown etiology. Histopathologic examination of skin specimens revealed 12% of the samples positive for acid-fast bacilli, including *M. avium-intracellulare* and *M. malmoense*, suggesting a mycobacterial cause.

It is important to note that therapy of HIV-positive patients with zidovudine during treatment of MAC infections may result in bone marrow depression and high risk of toxicity. Protionamide (also prothionamide), although effective, often caused nausea. A low maintenance dose of corticosteroids was instituted in order to suppress fever and malaise.[339] Table 8.7 lists some of the toxic side effects caused by drugs currently used to treat MAC infections.

TABLE 8.7
Toxic Side Effects of Drugs Used to Treat MAC Infections

Drug	Toxicities
Isoniazid	Fever, rash, hepatitis, central nervous system disorders, peripheral neuropathy
Ethionamide	Gastrointestinal intolerances (vomiting, abdominal pain, nausea), hepatitis, CNS disorders (depression, seizures, hallucinations), peripheral neuritis
Ethambutol	CNS disorders (optic neuritis, peripheral neuritis, dizziness, disorientation, hallucinations)
Clofazimine	Discoloration of tissue and body fluids, gastrointestinal toxicity (abdominal pain, diarrhea, malabsorption)
Cycloserine	Peripheral neuropathy (dizziness, insomnia, nervousness)
Ciprofloxacin	Gastrointesinal disorders (nausea, vomiting, diarrhea), CNS toxicity (headache, insomnia), hypersensitivity (fever, rash), acute renal dysfunction
Tetracyclines (doxycycline, minocycline)	Gastrointestinal toxicity (nausea, vomiting, diarrhea), CNS disorders (minocycline: dizziness, vertigo), hypersensitivity (rash, photosensitivity, hyperpigmentation), hematologic disturbancies (anemia, leukopenia)
Sulfonamides (trimethoprim/sulfamethoxazole	Gastrointestinal intolerance (nausea, vomiting, diarrhea), leukopenia, anemia, thrombocytopenia, hypersensitivity (rash, fever, Stevens-Johnsone syndrome)
Cefoxitin	Hypersensitivity (fever, rash, eosinophilia), anemia, leukopenia
Rifabutin	Arthralgia, arthritis, uveitis, transient rash, jaundice, pseudojaundice
Clarithromycin	Transient hypoacusis, thrombocytopenia, acute psychosis, elevated glutamic-pyruvic transferase and/or alkaline phosphatase levels, corneal opacity
Azithromycin	Sensorineural ototoxicity

8.6.5.3.1   Immunotherapy of MAC infections

Recently, it has been shown that human alveolar macrophages can be selectively activated without systemic effect by the use of aerosolized IFN-γ, a cytokine capable of enhancing the oxidative and antimicrobial activities of macrophages. In this context, Chatte et al.[340] have used IFN-γ to treat an HIV-negative patient with silicosis and advanced MAI cavitary lung disease with three courses of aerosolized IFN-γ (500 μg 3 d weekly for 5 weeks in two courses, and 200 μg 3 d weekly for 5 weeks after a short single trial of subcutaneous IFN-γ). The numbers of MAI decreased in the sputum during therapy, but cultures remained positive (at the same levels) for the first two treatment periods. However, the patient's sputum became AFB smear negative and the number of colonies decreased significantly after the third course of IFN-γ therapy. Cessation of IFN-γ treatment led to a rapid increase in the number of MAI in the sputum.[340] Previously, Holland et al.[341] treated a refractory MAC infection with a combination of subcutaneous IFN-γ (administered two to three times weekly at 25 to 50 μg/m^2 of body-surface area) and antimycobacterial medication. All patients showed marked clinical and radiologic improvement, abatement of fever, clearing of lesions, and reduced need for paracentesis.[341]

Tsukada et al.[295] have reported a case of an opportunistic disseminated MAI infection in an immunosuppressed patient with myelodysplastic syndrome (refractory anemia) on a long-term corticosteroid therapy. Although the patient responded initially to a combination of antimycobacterial drugs and recombinant human GM-CSF, spike fever recurred and the pantocytopenia progressed. Furthermore, the presence of hepatosplenomegaly and marked retroperitoneal lymphadenopathy indicated further dissemination of MAI. Additional treatment with human rGM-CSF and a very low dose of cytosine arabinoside failed to bring any improvement.

8.6.5.3.2 Prophylaxis of M. avium-intracellulare infections in AIDS patients

According to guidelines established by the U.S. Public Health Service for the prophylactic treatment of MAC infections in HIV-positive patients, AIDS patients with CD4+ cell counts below 100 cells/mm³ should receive 300 mg daily of rifabutin. The proposed dose regimen has been based on results from two clinical trials showing the beneficial effect of prophylactic rifabutin in delaying or preventing MAC bacteremia in AIDS patients with low CD4+ counts.[321,342-347] In both studies, rifabutin was given at 300 mg daily. The first trial involved 590 patients with mean baseline CD4+ cell counts of 65.9 (rifabutin group) and 56.5 (placebo). Only 9% (26 of 292 patients) of the rifabutin recipients developed M. avium-intracellulare bacteremia compared to 16% (47 of 298 patients) for the placebo group. In the second trial, which enrolled 556 patients, the mean baseline CD4+ cell counts were 61.8 for rifabutin recipients and 52.8 for the placebo group; 30 of 274 patients (11%) of the rifabutin-treated patients and 53 of 282 (19%) of the placebo-receiving patients developed MAI bacteremia. Adverse side effects (urine discoloration), although similar in both groups, have been more frequent in the rifabutin-treated recipients. There was no difference in the survival rates of the rifabutin and placebo groups, and MAI isolated from breakthrough bacteremia cases was not rifabutin-resistant. While the overall results of both trials demonstrated that prophylaxis with rifabutin was effective in reducing M. avium-intracellulare bacteremia, the probability of AIDS patients (especially those with CD4+ cell counts below 100 cell/mm³) to develop MAI bacteremia 2 years thereafter was still greater than 20%. Special concerns about rifabutin prophylaxis include its interactions with methadone, ketoconazole, zidovudine, and hepatically metabolized drugs. Although a less potent inducer than rifampin, rifabutin was found to induce hepatic cytochrome P450 that may enhance the clearance of some types of drugs.[348]

The prophylactic efficacies of clarithromycin and azithromycin (alone or in combinations with other drugs) in preventing M. avium-intracellulare bacteremia have also been investigated.[257] In one randomized study, 108 patients received either 500, 1000, or 2000 mg of clarithromycin twice daily.[349] Interim results for the first 72 patients have shown a 2.6 to 2.8 log decline in CFUs of MAI in the blood over a 3-month period. The median sterilization times were 55, 43, and 27 d for 500, 1000, and 2000 mg dosage regimens, respectively. However, a substantial drug intolerance was observed in patients receiving 2000 mg of the drug.

Similarly to azithromycin, one significant drawback of clarithromycin as a single-drug prophylactic therapy has been the emergence of resistance. Hewitt et al.[350] have conducted a nonrandomized retrospective chart review of all patients at their center who had CD4+ counts below 200 cells/mm³. Ninety of 148 patients treated had received for at least 4 weeks, clarithromycin (500 mg daily), rifabutin (300 mg/daily), dapsone (50 mg or 100 mg three times weekly), or clarithromycin and dapsone in combination. While MAI bacteremia was not evident in 22, 11, and 11 patients receiving clarithromycin, dapsone, and dapsone/clarithromycin combination, respectively, 1 of 18 patients receiving rifabutin and 14 of 58 patients who did not receive treatment have showed bacteremia.[350]

Abrams et al.[351] investigated the efficacy of clofazimine as prophylaxis for disseminated M. avium-intracellulare disease. A trial was conducted involving 109 patients randomized to receive either clofazimine at 50 mg daily or no treatment. After a mean follow-up of 299 d, 7 of 53 clofazimine recipients, and 6 of 46 no-treatment patients had developed disseminated MAI infection

($p = .76$). The size of the trial was too small to allow for any definitive conclusions about the prophylactic efficacy of clofazimine.

Some of the prophylaxis studies currently in progress involve a randomized, double-blind study (ACTG 196) comparing rifabutin, clarithromycin, and their combination, as well as a randomized, double-blind placebo-controlled study of clarithromycin.

8.6.5.4   Host Immune Response to MAC Infections

In recent years, the increased realization of how important the host's cell-mediated immune defense in resisting opportunistic infections (especially in immunocompromised patients) has been to the outcome of therapy has led to an intensive investigation of the role of cytokines in enhancing immune responses.

Macrophages play an important role in host defense against intracellular pathogens such as MAC. In cultured human macrophages, both *M. avium* and *M. intracellulare* replicate within membrane-enclosed vesicles, which have been generally thought to be acidic. Crowle et al.,[352] however, presented evidence that vesicle acidity may be associated with killed but not living mycobacteria.

Maylan et al.[353] have reported reduced intracellular growth of *M. avium* and *M. tuberculosis* in human macrophages cultivated at ambient concentration of oxygen (5% CO_2 and 95% air, corresponding to 20% O_2 or 140 mmHg PO_2) and at concentrations corresponding to tissue levels (5% O_2 and 5% CO_2 in nitrogen balance, corresponding to 36 mmHg PO_2). These results may explain the preferential localization of tuberculous lesions in body areas with high tissue PO_2, such as the lung apex. It was also found that crude lymphokines, rIFN-γ and rTNF-α were not consistent in affecting the mycobacterial growth in macrophages at either high or low oxygen conditions.[353]

Rastogi and Blom-Potar[354] conducted a comparative study on the activation of J-774 macrophage-like cells by IFN-γ, 1,25-dihydroxyvitamin D_3 (calcitriol), and lipopeptide RP-56142 in killing intracellularly multiplying *M. tuberculosis* and *M. avium*. The macrophage-like J-774 cell line which serves as a model for intracellular multiplication of pathogenic mycobacteria was used to assess the intracellular bactericidal action of macrophages after the addition of drugs and immunomodulators. The reported data have shown that although all immunomodulators studied significantly changed the morphology of the treated macrophages, they did not affect the release of toxic oxygen radicals.[354] In a study by Yajko et al.,[355] it has been demonstrated that in mouse macrophage J-774 cells, several combinations of antimicrobial agents killed MAC inside the macrophage and suggested that this cell line may be useful for screening of intracellular activity against *M. avium* complex.

Interleukin 12 (IL-12), which is produced mainly by macrophages, plays a critical role in the development of cell-mediated immunity. In a mouse model of disseminated *M. avium* infection, genetically susceptible BALB/c mice had increased mycobacterial growth and decreased IL-12 expression leading to the development of large and numerous granulomas.[356] In contrast, resistant DBA/2 mice exhibited reduced mycobacterial burden with increased IL-12 expression resulting in the development of fewer and smaller granulomas. In susceptible mice with established *M. avium* infection, IL-12 replacement therapy led to persistent reduction of mycobacterial burdens. Although IL-12 itself was unable to inhibit mycobacterial growth *in vitro*, by enhancing the host defenses *in vivo*, IL-12 replacement therapy may prove potentially useful against *M. avium* in susceptible hosts.[356,357]

TNF-α and granulocyte-macrophage colony-stimulating factor (GM-CSF) stimulated human macrophages to restrict the growth of virulent *M. avium* and to kill avirulent *M. avium*.[358,359] Thus, application of 100 U/ml of TNF-α significantly increased the ability of macrophages to restrict the growth of virulent *M. avium* 7497 (10-fold decrease in 7 d). Treatment with GM-CSF (100 to 10,000 U/ml) led macrophages to become as mycobacteriostatic for the virulent strain as

TNF-α-treated cells.[358] Inhibition or killing was observed when GM-CSF was given either before or after the establishment of infection.[359] Treatment of macrophages with both TNF-α and GM-CSF had an additive effect on their bacteriostatic activity against *M. avium*. Experiments by Bermudez et al.[360] suggested that the anti-MAC activity of 1,25-dihydroxyvitamin D_3 in human macrophages was related to increased concentrations of TNF and GM-CSF produced by the vitamin.

The effect of pentoxifyline, a TNF-α inhibitor, on the growth of *M. avium* complex in exogenously infected macrophages was studied by Sathe et al.[361,362] Pentoxifyline when applied at a concentration that decreased MAC-induced TNF-α by 48.1%, enhanced MAC growth by 1.9- to 19.6-fold and by 1.82- to 4.46-fold in macrophages from normal and HIV-infected patients, respectively. Pentoxifyline also induced IL-6 in infected macrophages, which correlated with the increase in MAC growth. Dexamethasone in an equivalent TNF-α-suppressing concentration also augmented MAC growth, but was less effective. However, unlike pentoxifyline, dexamethasone suppressed IL-6 and the suppression correlated with MAC growth.[361]

Blanchard[363] found that large autologous granular lymphocytes (LGLs) were also able to lyse monocytes that contained an established intracellular parasitic stage of *M. avium-intracellulare*. If activated with IL-2, LGLs have shown an even higher degree of lysis of infected monocytes. Experimental data have indicated that a direct interaction between *M. avium* and LGLs may induce the expression of both IL-2 receptor α-protein and mRNA, a process that involved signal transduction mechanisms mediated by tyrosine kinase activity.[364]

Further experiments by Blanchard et al.[365] have also demonstrated that treatment of monocytes with rGM-CSF augmented their activity against MAC complex. Moreover, *M. avium-intracellulare* was found to induce the production of this hemopoietic growth factor in both monocytes and large granular lymphocytes, but not T lymphocytes. Bermudez et al.[366] have examined the effect of GM-CSF on MAC infection *in vivo* using a C57BL/6 beige mouse model, as well as the ability of a combination of GM-CSF with amikacin (or azithromycin) to influence survival of MAC within macrophages *in vitro* and in mouse model of disseminated infection. At 25 mg/kg, GM-CSF induced mycobactericidal and mycobacteriostatic activity in macrophages *in vitro* and *in vivo*, and its combination with amikacin (50 mg/kg) or azithromycin (250 mg/kg) has elicited a marked increase in the killing of MAC both within cultured macrophages and in the beige mouse model.

The mechanism by which macrophages kill avirulent *M. avium* has been shown to be dependent on the generation of reactive nitrogen intermediates. Moreover, there was a correlation between the generation of such intermediates and the mycobactericial activity of macrophages. Addition of superoxide dismutase reversed the killing of avirulent *M. avium* by untreated or TNF-α-treated macrophages.[358] Suzuki et al.[367] reported that following preincubation with either TNF-α or IFN-γ, human alveolar macrophages (PAM) released significantly more superoxide anion (O_2^-) as compared with controls. Pretreatment of PAM with IL-2 or GM-CSF also resulted in the release of higher amounts of O_2^-.

While studying the effects of various cytokines on the production of O_2^- and nitrogen intermediates from normal and BCG-induced alveolar macrophages, Suga et al.[368] found that the intracellular growth of MAC was inhibited by PAM stimulated by TNF-α, but not IFN-γ. As expected, the enhanced O_2^- production by PAM stimulated by cytokines was essential for the intracellular killing of MAC. However, when the production of nitrogen intermediates by PAM was enhanced by stimulation with IFN-γ (or IFN-γ plus TNF-α) in the presence of L-arginine in the culture medium, their defense activity against *M. avium* complex was decreased.[368] To this end, ethanol was shown to impair not only the capacity of PAM to produce O_2^- and TNF-α, but also to reduce their ability to respond to stimulation with TNF-α and GM-CSF and kill *M. avium*.[369,370] Ethanol also inhibited the release of TNF-α and GM-CSF and membrane expression of TNF receptors in human monocyte-derived macrophages.[369]

Appelberg et al.[371,372] have investigated the ability of IL-4 and IFN-γ to influence the effector mechanisms of mouse macrophages. Thus, *in vitro* cultured bone marrow-derived macrophages from C57BL/6 mice were treated with IFN-γ, IL-4, or a combination of both cytokines, and the secretion of superoxide or nitrite and growth restriction of *M. avium* have been evaluated. While IL-4 did not influence the IFN-γ-induced enhanced production of nitrogen reactive intermediates by macrophages, it did inhibit the priming of macrophages for enhanced IFN-γ-induced superoxide production. The observed effect of IL-4 on the IFN-γ-primed superoxide production was also dose-dependent.

The *in vitro* effects of stress-related hormones on macrophage activation in response to TNF-α have also been investigated.[373] Somatostatin, ACTH, angiotensin, insulin, epinephrine, and glucagon were applied at physiologic concentrations to human monocyte-derived macrophages, and the [^{125}I]-TNF-α binding and the ability of TNF-α to activate macrophages to kill *M. avium* were measured. Epinephrine, insulin, glucagon, somatostatin, ACTH, and angiotensin reduced the number of TNF-α receptors by 81% ± 6%, 83% ± 6%, 15% ± 5%, 83% ± 4%, 17% ± 4%, and 21% ± 4%, respectively; rIFN-γ, by comparison, increased the number of receptors by 53% ± 8%. Treatment with insulin, epinephrine, and somatostatin also decreased the killing capacity of the macrophages by 30% ± 1%, 20% ± 6%, and 51% ± 2%, respectively.

When tested alone, neither recombinant IFN-γ nor recombinant M-CSF induced PAM to inhibit the growth of a clinical strain of *M. avium-intracellulare* serovar 4.[374] However, a combination of both cytokines (1 to 50 ng M-CSF plus 10^3 U IFN-γ per well) was remarkably effective in decreasing the replication of mycobacteria, even in the presence of anti-TNF-α antibody. The effect appeared to involve activation of intrinsic macrophage mechanisms for restricting MAC growth.[374] A combination of rIFN-γ and GM-CSF resulted in a significant decrease in intracellular inhibition of growth or killing (13.3% ± 2%) compared with 57.7% ± 5% observed with GM-CSF alone.[359]

The ability of soluble factors to modulate the growth of a virulent strain of *M. avium* in murine peritoneal macrophages was also studied. Experiments with recombinant interleukins showed that while treatment with IL-4 alone will enhance the bacteriostatic activity of murine macrophages against *M. avium*, its combination with IFN-γ rendered the macrophages almost fully bacteriostatic against *M. avium*. The inclusion of scavengers of reactive oxygen species did not modify the beneficial effect of IFN-γ and IL-4.[375]

Murine macrophages coinfected with *Toxoplasma gondii* and *M. avium-intracellulare* complex responded differently to stimulation by IFN-γ and TNF-α than cells infected with either organism alone.[376] This finding may suggest that in AIDS patients, who often suffer infections by multiple intracellular pathogens, including *T. gondii* and *M. avium-intracellulare*, the ability of cytokines to stimulate microbicidal or microbistatic activity in mononuclear phagocytes may be impaired or inadequate.

Treatment of BALB/c mice infected with *M. avium* with IL-2 or IL-4 (in hydrophobic gel delivery systems) led to no significant increase in resistance; by comparison, infusion of muramyl dipeptide (MDP) in hypromellose resulted in a marked enhancement of resistance as ascertained by the significant reduction of CFU in the spleens of infected mice.[377] A similar decrease in the CFU counts in organs of mice was achieved by infusion of IL-1β in hypromellose. Studies on the mechanism(s) of this enhanced resistance revealed that infected mice developed a profound immunosuppression. Mice given MDP/hypromellose developed similar immunosuppression, suggesting that adjuvant immunotherapy with MDP did not act by stimulating the T cell response or by abrogating a putative suppressive phenomenon. These, and other findings suggested that, overall, an adjuvant immunotherapy may be beneficial in MAC infections.[377]

The ability of human peripheral blood monocytes to phagocytize and kill *M. avium* was examined *in vitro*.[378,379] The intracellular growth inhibition of *M. avium* at day 7 after infection was comparable in patients with AIDS and healthy donors for all strains tested. Pretreatment of monocytes with IFN-γ prior to infection decreased monocyte phagocytosis. However, continuous coculturing of monocytes with IFN-γ after the infection enhanced their ability to kill the mycobacteria in both AIDS patients and healthy controls for three of the four strains tested.[379] Using a rapid radiolabeled assay, Blanchard et al.[380] have found peripheral blood monocytes derived from healthy donors capable of killing 40% to 92% of inoculated *M. avium-intracellulare* complex. The addition of IFN-γ inhibited the bactericidal activity of fresh monocytes but not of culture-derived macrophages.[380]

Studying the mechanism of antimycobacterial activation of human monocytes, Zerlauth et al.[381] found that TNF-α is essential in triggering the initial activation signal.

Denis[382] has reported that murine rIFN-β enhanced the resistance of BALB/c mice infected with *M. avium* TMC 702; the mycobacterial growth was reduced in the liver and spleen at 2 months postinfection. These results were corroborated by *in vitro* experiments showing that resident peritoneal macrophages became more bacteriostatic when treated with IFN-β as compared to untreated cells.

A number of recombinant and highly purified human cytokines were tested *in vitro* to evaluate their ability to influence the growth of *M. avium-intracellulare* within human monocytes.[383] Monocytes were infected with two strains of *M. avium*, one AIDS-associated and relatively avirulent, and the other a non-AIDS-associated isolate showing a consistent and rapid growth in cultured human monocytes. The infected monocytes were cultured in medium alone or continuously in the presence of IL-1α, IL-1β, IL-2, IL-3, IL-4, IL-6, IFN-γ, GM-CSF, or M-CSF; in some cases, indomethacin was also added to the cultures.[383,384] IFN-γ, alone or in combination with indomethacin, decreased the mycobacterial growth within the monocytes. None of the other cytokines, alone or in combination with indomethacin, were able to reduce intracellular growth. Rather, IL-1α increased intracellular growth in both strains while IL-3, IL-6, and M-CSF increased the growth in one strain. In addition, IL-1α and IL-6 enhanced the mycobacterial growth in tissue culture medium without monocytes.

Cytokines were also reported to stimulate parasitic and microbial growth.[5,386] Thus, Denis[387] has found that IL-6 was a potent growth factor for four virulent strains of *M. avium* binding to a specific receptor site. Treatment of human macrophages with IL-6 and IFN-γ or IL-4 did not modify the growth-promoting effect of IL-6.[388] These findings strongly indicated that by promoting mycobacterial growth, IL-6 may contribute significantly to the pathogenesis of MAC infection.

Treatment of MAC-infected macrophage monolayers with rIL-6 decreased the ability of TNF-α to activate cultured macrophages, and to inhibit growth of or kill intracellular *M. avium* (a 68% ± 14% decrease compared to untreated controls).[389] The effect of rIL-6 was the result of a downregulation of membrane receptors to TNF-α and was reversible. These and other findings suggested that cytokines may have bidirectional effects on intracellular growth that may influence the outcome of *M. avium* infection.[383]

Denis[390] has reported that inclusion of IFN-γ in the presence of indomethacin or calcitriol significantly reduced mycobacterial growth in human monocytes. Conversely, treatment of monocytes with IL-1, M-CSF, or IL-3 led to an increased permissiveness of these cells for *M. avium*.[390]

Data obtained by Rastogi et al.[391,392] have suggested that the immunosuppression induced in human adherent peripheral blood monocyte-derived macrophages infected with *M. avium* may result, in part, from an increased production of prostaglandin E_2 (PGE_2) and the inhibition of phagosome-lysosome fusions, occurring soon after the infection. Therefore, the addition of indomethacin, a potent inhibitor of PGE_2 biosynthesis, may be beneficial in reducing the intracellular growth of MAC in the macrophages.

Denis and Ghadirian[393] have investigated the *in vitro* and *in vivo* effects of transforming growth factor-β (TGF-β1) on the progression of experimental MAC infections. Control BALB/c mice were injected intravenously with inoculum of *M. avium* TMC 702, and the growth monitored in the spleen. Other infected mice were given weekly doses of 1.0 μg/ml of TGF-β1 or weekly doses of 2.0 mg of rabbit antiserum against mouse TGF-β1 and then evaluated for their resistance to *M. avium* TMC 702. Results from both *in vivo* and *in vitro* experiments suggested that, although by an unclear mechanism, overall, TGF-β1 reduced the progression of experimental MAC infections.

Results by Orme et al.[394] have demonstrated that recombinant migration inhibitory factor (MIF), a 12-kDa protein isolated by COS-1 cell expression screening of cDNA from a human T cell hybridoma, possessed potent inhibitory activity on the growth of a number of clinical isolates of *M. avium* in bone marrow-derived murine macrophages and cultured human blood monocytes.

Ogata et al.[395] have investigated the role of defensins derived from human neutrophilic granulocytes against *M. avium-intracellulare*. One such molecule, the human neutrophil peptide (HNP-1) at 5.0 μg/ml was strongly bactericidal (96.3% to 97.7%), and its activity was independent of the colonial morphology of MAC. Two other defensins, HNP-2 and HNP-3, were as effective as HNP-1 in killing mycobacteria.

Ultraviolet irradiation enhanced the intrinsic antimycobacterial activity of monocytes against MAI in a dose-dependent manner.[396] For example, UV irradiation of ≥25 J/m² resulted in a 50- to 100-fold reduction in mycobacterial growth 7 d after initiation of culture.

Recent studies have indicated that some cytokines may augment the activity of antimycobacterial antibiotics. Thus, stimulation of macrophages with human rIFN-γ or human rTNF-α led to an increase in the intracelullar concentration of azithromycin by approximately 200% within 3 h.[397] The infection of macrophages with MAC had the opposite effect — a decrease in the uptake of [^{14}C]-azithromycin by infected cells, as compared with uninfected controls. Overall, however, the stimulatory effect of IFN-γ and TNF-α overcame the inhibitory effect caused by the infection.

8.6.6 MYCOBACTERIUM SCROFULACEUM

8.6.6.1 Introduction

The name *Mycobacterium scrofulaceum* originated from the original report of Prissick and Masson[398] describing tuberculous cervical lymphadenitis (scrofula) in children caused by this species. *M. scrofulaceum* has been isolated from raw milk and other dairy products, pooled oysters, soil, and water.[399] It grows at 21°C, 31°C, and 37°C in 4 to 6 weeks, forming colonies that are buttery in consistency, smooth, and globoid.

The condition most commonly associated with *M. scrofulaceum* is cervical lymphadenitis in children.[400-408] The disease, which most often is observed in young children, usually affects cervical lymph nodes located near the mandible and high in the neck (submandibular, jugulodigastric); however, other nodes may also be affected.[409] Extranodal manifestations include pulmonary disease,[410,411] disseminated disease,[412,413] and on rare occasions, conjunctivitis, osteomyelitis,[400] meningitis,[414] and granulomatous hepatitis.[415]

In addition to children, *M. scrofulaceum* infections have also been described in adult patients.[2,416-420] Disseminated *M. scrofulaceum* infection, although rare, has been reported.[420,421] Katoh et al.[419] have recounted a case of massive hemoptysis due to *M. scrofulaceum*.

8.6.6.2 Evolution of Therapies and Treatment of *M. scrofulaceum* Infections

Treatment of *M. scrofulaceum* depended on the clinical syndrome.[1,404] Due to the fact that, with the exception of cervical lymphadenitis, other forms of *M. scrofulaceum* disease have been rare, no large-scale clinical trials have been undertaken to evaluate optimal drug therapy.

In the case of cervical lymphadenitis, the recommended treatment has been surgical excision of the involved lymph nodes whenever possible without administration of antimycobacterial agents.[402,409,422,423] For other forms of *M. scrofulaceum* disease, however, surgery has not been a viable option, and antimycobacterial therapy should be implemented.

Sanders et al.[421] have described the first case of disseminated disease in an AIDS patient that presented as chronic ulcerative and nodular skin lesions with probable cavitary lung involvement. Although the patient died before susceptibility testing was completed, the *M. scrofulaceum* isolate was found susceptible to clarithromycin, ethambutol, and clofazimine.

In another case of an immunocompromised patient, a 32-year-old male with systemic lupus erythematosus controlled by corticosteroid therapy developed multifocal cutaneous abscesses due to *M. scrofulaceum*.[420] The distribution and evolution of the lesions suggested hematogenous dissemination without pulmonary or other visceral manifestations of systemic mycobacterial disease. The disease was successfully treated after a 9-month course of isoniazid and rifampin.[420]

In a case of a patient with granulomatous hepatitis due to *M. scrofulaceum*, clinical improvement was noted after therapy with isoniazid, streptomycin, and cycloserine.[415]

In general, *M. scrofulaceum* has shown *in vitro* resistance to isoniazid, streptomycin, ethambutol, and *p*-aminosalicylic acid (PAS). While its susceptibility to rifampin has been variable, the pathogen was reported to be sensitive to cycloserine and erythromycin.[1]

8.6.7 MYCOBACTERIUM KANSASII

8.6.7.1 Introduction

Buhler and Pollack[424] were the first to describe a *M. kansasii* infection in 1953. Initially characterized as the "yellow bacillus," *M. kansasii* is a photochromogenic mycobacterium, with nearly all of its strains being yellow-orange; only occasionally, strains may become nonpigmented or scotochromogenic.

In photochromogenic microorganisms, pigmentation will develop only as a result of exposure to light. When grown in the dark, these bacteria are almost colorless. Induction of color will usually take place within several minutes in the shorter wavelength of visible light, then pigmentation occurs within 24 h if conditions permit continuing growth.

M. kansasii produces rough colonies which, after prolonged exposure to light, will display characteristic red β-carotene crystal precipitates.[425] Acid-fast smears of *M. kansasii* usually demonstrate large cross-barred bacilli.[1]

According to one estimate,[73] *M. kansasii* accounted for 3% of mycobacterial isolates in the U.S. in 1980, with California, Texas, Louisiana, Illinois, and Florida being the states with the most reported isolates. In another retrospective study,[426] *M. kansasii* isolates represented 3.7% of the total significant isolations of mycobacteria in respiratory samples over a 6-year period, and affecting predominantly middle-aged males.

Although *M. kansasii* has been cultured from water and soil samples in various parts of the world, its natural habitat is not known.[5,427]

The most common *M. kansasii* infection has been chronic pulmonary disease, which may resemble that caused by MAI (e.g., caseating granulomas[399]) except that fewer patients had preexisting lung disease and the response to chemotherapy was stronger.[428-433] Chronic pulmonary disease caused by *M. kansasii* can range from mild, self-limiting disease to severe progressive and sometimes fatal illness with extensive cavitation.[24] Pleural effusions and lymphadenopathy have been rare.[1]

Using direct smear, it is nearly impossible to distinguish between *M. tuberculosis*, the bacillus causing tuberculosis, and *M. kansasii* (a nontuberculosis bacillus). Only when culture results become available (three or more weeks after specimens have been taken), it would be possible to differentiate between these two pathogens.[24]

Zvetina et al.[30] have found that structural changes induced by either chemotherapy or radiation therapy may predispose patients to reactivation of latent *M. kansasii* infection, and Gettler and El-Sadr[434] reported a case in which a patient with a history of asthma and non-insulin-dependent diabetes mellitus presented *de novo* with concurrent *M. kansasii* pulmonary infection and a small-cell lung carcinoma. Although several reports have documented the association between *M. kansasii* pulmonary infection and bronchogenic carcinoma,[433,435] what made the latter case unusual was the previously unreported simultaneous occurrence of these two conditions. Although the exact mechanism(s) of *M. kansasii* reactivation by particular malignant conditions still remains speculative, based on similar cases of latent reactivation of *M. tuberculosis*,[436] it has been proposed that disruption of granulomas by either cancer cells or tumor antigens and the effects of general malnutrition and wasting which often accompany solid tumors may have been involved.[434]

Extrapulmonary involvement of *M. kansasii* has been rather diverse, including cervical lymphadenitis (seen most often in children);[399,437] cutaneous disease[438-440] that may resemble pyogenic abscess,[441,442] cellulitis,[443] or sporotrichosis;[444] musculoskeletal involvement presenting as carpal tunnel syndrome,[445] synovitis (characterized by noncaseating granulomas),[446-448] arthritis,[449,450] tendonitis and fasciitis,[451] or osteomyelitis.[452,453] Klotch et al.[454] have described an unusual *M. kansasii* infection presenting as rhinophyma (a manifestation of severe rosacea involving the lower half of the nose and sometimes spreading to adjacent cheek areas, resulting from thickened, lobulated overgrowth of the sebaceous glands and epithelial connective tissue).

Disseminated *M. kansasii* usually involves immunosuppressed patients with impaired cellular immunity.[35,433,455,456] Characteristic manifestations, such as fever, constitutional symptoms, pulmonary symptoms, hepatosplenomegaly, and hematologic abnormalities (leukopenia, pancytopenia) have been common, with lymphadenopathy, diffuse bone involvement, skin lesions,[440] genitourinary involvement,[457,458] pericarditis,[459,460] and gastrointestinal involvement being observed less frequently.[1]

The first incidence of *M. kansasii* infection in AIDS patients was reported by Woods and Washington.[1] Later, more cases of both pulmonary and disseminated disease followed to parallel the rise of the AIDS epidemic.[10,438,442,448,450,453,461-470]

In patients with advanced HIV-related immunosuppression, *M. kansasii* may cause serious and potentially life-threatening pulmonary disease.[467,469,471] Boudon et al.[461] have conducted a retrospective study of 12 HIV-positive patients (10 of them with AIDS) who had developed *M. kansasii* pulmonary infections characterized by nodular, interstitial, or diffuse parenchymal infiltrates, and mediastinal and hilar adenopathies, but no cavitary lung disease. Valainis et al.[470] also did not observe cavitary formation at the time of initial presentation. In contrast, based on chest radiographs, Levine and Chaisson[467] and Bamberger et al.[463] have reported the presence of pulmonary cavitation in AIDS patients with *M. kansasii* mycobacteriosis. In fact, the latter group has found radiographic evidence of either pulmonary cavitation or predominantly upper-lobe disease in 8 of 22 patients with *M. kansasii* pulmonary disease.[463] To explain these discrepancies, it has been suggested that pulmonary cavitations in patients with *M. kansasii* infection may instead be the result of zidovudine medication, which is known to lead to partial reconstitution of the cellular immune responses, thereby increasing the hypersensitivity reaction (e.g., exudative reaction) and resulting in tissue necrosis and cavitation.[468] In the experience of Chaisson and Levine,[471] however, the higher prevalence of pulmonary cavities in AIDS patients with *M. kansasii* disease cannot be explained by zidovudine therapy since in their study only 2 of 8 patients receiving zidovudine at the time of the diagnosis had pulmonary cavitation, compared with 5 of 11 patients not receiving zidovudine therapy.

Singh[472] and Friedman and Ike[450] have presented cases of patients who developed septic arthritis due to *M. kansasii*.

In a retrospective study involving 49 AIDS patients, *M. kansasii* was isolated at a mean CD4+ cell count of 62 cells/mm³ and at a mean interval of 17 months after the diagnosis of AIDS; 17 patients had disseminated disease.[462] In contrast, Urkijo et al.[464] have reported that in all but 2 of 13 AIDS cases, the CD4+ cell counts were lower than 200 cells/mm³ when *M. kansasii* was diagnosed.

8.6.7.2   Evolution of Therapies and Treatment of *M. kansasii* Infections

Most strains of *M. kansasii* were found susceptible *in vitro* to rifampin, cyclosporine, rifabutin, davercin, and ofloxacin, and only slightly resistant to isoniazid, ethambutol, augmentin, and streptomycin.[1,473]

In clinical settings, most patients with *M. kansasii* infections (both pulmonary and extrapulmonary) have been responsive to combinations of two or more antimycobacterial drugs, one of which was rifampin.[28,429,432,433,474] However, Wallace et al.[475] have identified 36 rifampin-resistant *M. kansasii* isolates, with 32% of them being recovered from HIV-positive patients. Previously, Dautzenberg et al.[465] reported on acquired rifampicin resistance during *M. kansasii* infection in an AIDS patient — the minimal inhibitory concentrations of rifampicin against the *M. kansasii* strain were respectively 0.2 μg/ml at the onset and 128 μg/ml after the treatment.

While pulmonary infections have responded well to therapy,[3,426,476] relapses have occurred,[426,475] and although rarely, fatal outcomes due to progression of disease have also been reported.[463,469] Surgical treatment of pulmonary *M. kansasii* infections was reported beneficial in certain specific cases, including localized disease with persistent cavitation in which the organism has not been eradicated from sputum after a 6-month follow-up period; acquired drug resistance resulting from poor compliance; and severe drug intolerance.[415]

With the exception of disseminated disease where despite adequate therapy[456] the outcome may be uncertain (and even fatal[477]), the prognosis of extrapulmonary disease when treated appropriately has been generally favorable.[1] In this respect, reducing the dose of corticosteroids may be a beneficial adjunct to the therapy.[439] Thus, when *M. kansasii* has been confined to the skin, the disease was usually indolent, and chemotherapy with traditional antituberculosis agents as well as erythromycin, minocycline, and doxycycline has been successful.[439] However, Delaporte et al.[440] have found treatment with minocycline followed by ciprofloxacin to be ineffective in a case of an immunocompetent patient with cutaneous infection due to *M. kansasii*. Because erythromycin was well tolerated and showed adequate tissue penetration with excellent activity against *M. kansasii*, its use in the therapy of cutaneous infections has been recommended.[478]

Patel et al.[7] have described *M. kansasii* infections in solid transplant recipients presenting as a cutaneous lesion and a pulmonary nodule which responded well to surgery, reduction in doses of immunosuppressive medication, and/or therapy with antimycobacterial drugs.

Treatment with conventional antituberculosis drugs (including isoniazid and pyridoxine at 300 and 150 mg daily, respectively) of *M. kansasii*-induced cavitating pneumonia in a patient with rheumatoid arthritis had to be stopped because of exacerbation of isoniazid-induced peripheral neuropathy; clinical improvement was observed only after both isoniazid and pyridoxine were withdrawn.[479]

A fatal outcome due to *M. kansasii* pneumonia was reported in a case of a HIV-positive patient despite treatment with isoniazid, rifampin, ethambutol, and clofazimine.[469]

Sauret et al.[480] have evaluated the therapeutic response of *M. kansasii* pulmonary disease to 12- and 18-month courses of daily chemotherapy consisting of rifampicin–isoniazid–ethambutol (ethambutol only for the first 6 months). Since patients from both groups showed essentially the same degree of clinical improvement based on radiographic examination and sputum conversion, the 12-month course (with ethambutol given only during the first 6 months of therapy) has been recommended as adequate.[480] Campbell[31] has disagreed with the role of isoniazid as presented by Sauret et al.[480] and concurred with the finding of the prospective study by the British Thoracic Society[481] that isoniazid may be of no benefit whatsoever in the treatment of *M. kansasii* pulmonary infection.

In a retrospective multicenter study conducted by the British Thoracic Society, the optimal duration of treatment of *M. kansasii* pulmonary infections with rifampicin and ethambutol, and whether isoniazid should also be given, have been found uncertain.[463] The results have shown that while, overall, a 9-month course of treatment with rifampicin and ethambutol appeared to be adequate, patients who contracted *M. kansasii* pulmonary infections had nevertheless a high mortality rate resulting from other causes. In addition, it seemed that isoniazid (which had been recommended at a potentially harmful daily dose of 600 mg[482]) did not appear to be necessary as part of a drug regimen for *M. kansasii* infection, especially when most strains have been resistant to isoniazid and pyrazinamide.[24,481]

Umeda et al.[483] have described a case of *M. kansasii* lung infection associated with myelofibrosis that was refractory to treatment with conventional antituberculosis drugs, and leading to hilar and mediastinal lymph node enlargement and finally their calcification.

Ahn et al.[484] have tested 14 wild strains and 14 relapse or treatment failure isolates of *M. kansasii*, and found them to be highly susceptible to sulfamethoxazole, with 26 of 28 isolates having MICs of less than or equal to 4.0 μg/ml in a broth microdilution assay. In addition, treatment failure isolates frequently exhibited acquired resistance to rifampin (MIC >2.0 μg/ml), isoniazid (MIC >4.0 μg/ml), and ethambutol (MIC >4.0 μg/ml) not seen among the wild isolates. Eight patients with cavitary disease induced by rifampin-resistant *M. kansasii* were treated successfully with a 4- to 10-week course of sulfamethoxazole-containing regimens that also included high-dose isoniazid (900 mg), ethambutol (25 mg/kg), and an aminoglycoside (either streptomycin or amikacin).

In another report,[485] a patient with *M. kansasii* pulmonary infection developed severe aplastic anemia (hypoplastic marrow and pancytopenia) after treatment with a conventional regimen of antituberculosis drugs. Changing to ofloxacin, to which the pathogen was sensitive, did not bring any clinical improvement because of complete resistance after several months of treatment. The disease was cured by lobectomy and postoperative administration of sparfloxacin.

Matthiessen et al.[486] have cultured *M. kansasii* from the sputum of a patient with the Swyer-James syndrome. The lung infection, which responded well to daily administration of rifampicin (600 mg), ethambutol (1.6 g), and protionamide (0.5 g), recurred after 2 years. The recurrence again responded well to the same drug regimen with additional sulfamethoxazole (1.6 g).

Kramers et al.[487] have grown *M. kansasii* from blood samples of a patient with Sweet's syndrome and leukopenia related to hairy cell leukemia. The patient recovered after treatment with recombinant IFN-α and tuberculostatic drugs. Remarkably, the skin lesions completely regressed within 1 week after the start of rIFN-α therapy. Previously, Bennett et al.[488] had reported the development of disseminated atypical mycobacteriosis (*M. kansasii*, *M. avium-intracellulare*, and *M. chelonae*) in 9 of 186 patients with hairy cell leukemia.

According to Kurasawa et al.[489] the use of isoniazid, rifampicin, ethambutol, and/or streptomycin (or kanamycin) was highly effective in the treatment of *M. kansasii* and *M. szulgai* infections.

8.6.8   MYCOBACTERIUM FORTUITUM-CHELONAE COMPLEX

8.6.8.1   Introduction

Two human pathogens have been included in this group: *M. fortuitum* and *M. chelonae*. *M. fortuitum* (also known as *M. ranae*) was first described and named in 1938, but its name did not become official until 1972.[490] Several different names synonymous for *M. chelonae* have also appeared in the literature (*M. friedmannii*, *M. abscessus*, *M. runyonii*, and *M. borstelense*).[1]

In addition, there have been three biovariants of *M. fortuitum*: *fortuitum*, *peregrinum*, and an unnamed biovariant designated as the "third group."[491] There are also three subspecies of *M. chelonae*: *chelonae*, *abscessus*, and an unnamed subspecies known as *M. chelonae*-like organisms.[491]

Both mycobacterial species, which grow on various media (conventional or specific for mycobacteria) in 7 d or less at temperatures of 25 to 40°C, are nonphotochromogenic and produce colonies that may be smooth, rough, or a mixture of both.

In nature, *M. fortuitum* has been isolated from water, soil, and dust. By comparison, the distribution of *M. chelonae* may not be so diverse, and its habitat is still uncertain.[492,493]

The observed clinical manifestations of infection induced by the *M. fortuitum-chelonae* complex include cutaneous lesions, pulmonary disease, postsurgical infections, and a range of miscellaneous infections.[1,491,494]

Disseminated disease has also been observed, with patients having no apparent primary source of infection.[1] The usual presentations of disseminated infections, which most frequently affect immunocompromised patients, include multiple, recurrent abscesses of the skin and soft tissue, most commonly located on the extremities.[495,496] Furthermore, patients with disseminated disease may or may not become systemically ill, and in those who are ill, organisms can be collected from many sources, including blood.[1]

Primary cutaneous disease induced by the *M. fortuitum-chelonae* complex may present with localized cellulitis (frequently with draining abscesses) or individual nodules that are minimally tender.[495,497-499] Osteomyelitis has occasionally complicated cutaneous disease, particularly when puncture wounds to the feet have been present.[495]

Although in one report[495] cavitation was observed in only 3 of 27 patients, in many other cases pulmonary manifestations due to *M. fortuitum-chelonae* complex have been nearly identical to those caused by MAI or *M. kansasii*.[435,500] Burke and Ullian[501] have noticed an association between achalasia (failure to relax of the smooth muscle fibers of the gastrointestinal tract at any point of junction of one part with another; in particular, the thoracic esophagus loosing its normal peristaltic activity and becoming dilated, i.e., megaesophagus) and pulmonary disease induced by *M. fortuitum-chelonae* complex.

Endocarditis with prosthetic valve involvement, which usually will manifest 4 to 12 weeks after surgery, has been fatal despite valve replacement.[495]

Other reported infections associated with *M. fortuitum-chelonae* include keratitis and corneal ulceration secondary to traumatic injury,[502,503] scleral buckle infections,[504] cervical lymphadenitis,[495] mycobacteriosis in continuous ambulatory peritoneal dialysis (CAPD) patients,[505-507] and patients with indwelling catheters.[508,509] Hepatitis, meningitis, synovitis, and epidural abscess, although rarely, have also been observed.[495,498]

8.6.8.2 Evolution of Therapies and Treatment of *M. fortuitum-chelonae* Complex Infections

Using the Etest procedure (an alternative susceptibility-testing method for difficult-to-assess organisms, such as fast-growing mycobacteria), Koontz et al.[510] have determined the sensitivity of *M. chelonae* and *M. fortuitum* isolates to various antituberculosis agents. *M. chelonae* was generally more resistant to all drugs (e.g., amikacin had $MIC_{90} = 32$ µg/ml); by comparison, the MIC_{50} values of amikacin, ciprofloxacin, doxycycline, and trimethoprim–sulfamethoxazole against *M. fortuitum* were 1.0, 0.032, 0.125, and 0.032 µg/ml, respectively.

With the exception of prosthetic valve endocarditis, which has been uniformly fatal, the clinical outcome of *M. fortuitum-chelonae* infections following antimycobacterial therapy has been generally good.[1,511] While cutaneous disease, including both community-acquired infections and nosocomial diseases, such as augmentation mammoplasty, wound infections and sternal wound infections, have been relatively easily diagnosed and treated successfully by combination of surgical debridement and antimycobacterial therapy (amikacin, sulfonamides), pulmonary infections (which can also be readily diagnosed) were more difficult to treat, and in many patients the therapy consisted only of intermittent medical intervention during excerbation of the disease.[16,512] Consequently, if infections persist for longer periods their morbidity will rise and chemotherapy should be given in earnest.[513] Fatal outcomes of *M. fortuitum-chelonae* infections, however, have been rare.

In general, *M. fortuitum* and *M. chelonae* have been resistant to conventional antituberculosis agents but responded to other antimicrobial drugs. One recommended therapy for serious infections included a combination of amikacin and cefoxitin for a minimum of 2 to 4 weeks, followed by the administration of one of the active oral agents — sulfonamides, tetracycline, or erythromycin — depending on the results of *in vitro* susceptibility testing.[1] Some of the newer β-lactams (imipenem),[514,515] cephamycins,[516] and clarithromycin have demonstrated promising *in vitro* activity.[491]

Three patients with *M. fortuitum* cutaneous disease relapsed after an initial response to therapy with ciprofloxacin, and their isolates have shown the presence of acquired drug resistance.[49] Subsequently, the mutational frequencies for *M. fortuitum* with ciprofloxacin were found to be relatively high (10^{-5} to 10^{-7}), whereas the MICs for single-step mutants were similar to those for the clinically resistant strains. It has been postulated that despite the generally excellent activity of ciprofloxacin against *M. fortuitum* and other rapidly growing mycobacterial species (except *M. chelonae*[49]), a single-drug therapy should be viewed with caution because of the potential risk of developing mutational resistance.[49]

Yew et al.[515] successfully treated two patients with *M. fortuitum* (secondary to bronchiectasis and inactive pulmonary tuberculosis) and *M. chelonae* (complicating bronchiectasis and silicosis) lung infections using ofloxacin and imipenem, respectively.

Opie et al.[517] have described a successful permanent endobronchial closure of a serious post-pneumonectomy bronchopleural fistula in a patient with a delayed diagnosis of *M. fortuitum-chelonae* complex infection.

In patients with indwelling catheters, the *M. fortuitum-chelonae* disease presented either as bacteremia or catheter-site infection.[509] For treatment of bacteremia, clinical improvement was achieved only after removal of the catheter and antibiotic therapy. Successful treatment of local catheter infections was accomplished by catheter removal alone or in combination with antibiotic therapy. Patients with infection in the catheter tunnel (tunnel infection) responded only after surgical excision of the tissue surrounding the infected tunnel.[509]

Woods et al.[506] have reported the successful treatment of *M. fortuitum*-induced peritonitis in a CAPD patient with ciprofloxacin. A case of *M. chelonae*-induced peritonitis in a CAPD patient was resolved by therapy with doxycycline.[507]

M. fortuitum and *M. chelonae*, which have been the two most common causes of nontuberculous mycobacterial keratitis, are usually difficult to differentiate at diagnosis. To circumvent that, Lin et al.[518] have suggested using their different sensitivities to ciprofloxacin in an animal model of keratitis. When applied topically, ciprofloxacin (3.0 mg/ml) was more active against *M. fortuitum* than *M. chelonae* ($p = .01$).

A bacterial immunopotentiator, LC 9018 (heat-killed *Lactobacillus casei*) was studied for its protective and therapeutic efficacies against *M. fortuitum* and *M. chelonae* infections in mice.[519] When administered intramuscularly six times weekly (0.1 mg dry weight per injection, one injection on each day of treatment) starting 1 week before and 2 weeks after the infection, LC 9018 reduced the incidence of spinning disease and gross renal lesions and enhanced the elimination of organisms at the site of elimination in the host mice. In addition, LC 9018 elicited a marked increase in the phagocytic functions, oxygen- and IL-1-producing capabilities, and chemiluminescence of the host peritoneal macrophages.[519]

8.6.9 MYCOBACTERIUM XENOPI

8.6.9.1 Introduction

Although it was first isolated in 1957[520], *M. xenopi* was not recognized as a human pathogen until 1965.[399] It is a scotochromogenic organism producing a yellow pigment that varies in intensity.

At optimal temperatures of 42 to 43°C (but also at 43°C after prolonged incubation[521]), *M. xenopi* produces smooth colonies, which on corneal agar may propagate filamentous extensions.[425] Acid-fast stained smears have shown long, slender cells, tapered at both ends with a palisading arrangement.

Little is known about the natural habitat of *M. xenopi*. Birds have been considered a possible natural reservoir — in a peculiar finding in Great Britain, the organism has been found more often in birds from coastal than from inland areas. This finding, coupled with the clustering of *M. xenopi* isolates from humans living in coastal areas,[522] led to the hypothesis that these mycobacteria may be transmitted by seabirds and/or seawater. However, there have been numerous reports describing *M. xenopi* infections in inland areas,[523] and the organisms have not yet been isolated from naturally occurring bodies of fresh or salt water.[28,524]

In some western European laboratories, *M. xenopi* has been the most commonly isolated nontuberculous mycobacteria.[523,525,526]

Since *M. xenopi* has been cultured frequently from both hot- and cold-water taps,[520,527] hospital hot-water generators and storage tanks[528,529] may become potential sources of nosocomial infections.[530,531] In a study examining mycobacteria cultured from tonsils, Stewart et al.[532] found *M. xenopi* to account for more than 60% of isolates.

Human infections by *M. xenopi* have been associated mainly with pulmonary disease, with adult males being more frequently affected than females.[5,14,530,532-543] Most patients had either preexisting lung disease[188] or another predisposing factor, such as immunosuppression due to extrapulmonary malignancies, alcoholism, diabetes mellitus,[1] solid organ[544] and bone marrow[545] transplatations, or AIDS.[546]

The *M. xenopi* infection may be chronic, subacute, or acute. Clinical symptoms, which for the most part have been nearly indistinguishable from pulmonary tuberculosis[17,531,538,542] or illness caused by MAI or *M. kansasii*, included nodular or mass lesions, single or multiple cavities, multifocal nodular densities, apical shadowing, consolidation, and fibrosis.[1]

Extrapulmonary infections induced by *M. xenopi* have been rare and involved bone and joints,[521,536,547-550] lymph node, epididymis, a sinus tract, and a prosthetic temporomandibular joint.[399]

Disseminated disease has been reported on several occasions,[551-554] including in patients with AIDS,[303,553,555,556] in an immunocompromised patient with myelogenous leukemia and diabetes mellitus,[551] and in a patient who was not known to be immunosuppressed.[557]

8.6.9.2   Evolution of Therapies and Treatment of *M. xenopi* Infections

Results from *in vitro* susceptibility testing and clinical management of *M. xenopi* disease have been inconsistent.[1,6] There have been reports in which *in vitro* sensitivities against antimycobacterial agents such as isoniazid, ethambutol, streptomycin, and rifampin correlated well with their clinical efficacy when applied in combinations (such as rifampin–ethambutol[531]).[39,540] However, in other studies,[534] while resistance to the aforementioned drugs has been observed, there was uniform susceptibility to cycloserine and ethionamide. Even so, relapses were not infrequent,[39] and response to retreatment was poor.[534] Baugnee et al.[558] found little evidence of correlation between *in vitro* sensitivity to antimycobacterial drugs and their therapeutic efficacies.

Because of frequent unreability of antimycobacterial drug therapy against *M. xenopi* infections, complications of treatment, and the risk of recurrence after treatment, in most cases, surgical debridement has been beneficial.[559,543]

In a double-blind, randomized, placebo-controlled, 12-week trial involving AIDS patients with disseminated disease due to either *M. avium* or *M. xenopi*, Dautzenberg et al.[303] have evaluated the therapeutic efficacy of rifabutin (450 or 600 mg daily). Companion drugs used in both the infection and placebo arms, included ethambutol, clofazimine, and isoniazid. While no significant difference was observed in clinical improvement, mortality, or toxicity between the two treatment arms, it has been suggested that the addition of rifabutin to a triple-drug combination may contribute to the clearance of disseminated mycobacterial infection in AIDS patients without causing additional toxicity. In a previously conducted French study on mycobacterial infections resistant to rifampin, a treatment protocol for *M. xenopi* infection was proposed.[560] The suggested daily regimen consisted of 5.0 to 7.0 mg/kg rifabutin, 20 mg/kg ethambutol, 3.0 to 5.0 mg/kg isoniazid, and 400 mg of ofloxacin (or 800 mg of pefloxacin). Seventy-seven percent (10 out of 13) of *M. xenopi* cultures were negative, 3 months after commencing therapy.

Huber et al.[546] have described a case of an AIDS patient with *M. xenopi* pneumonia who was successfully treated with an antituberculosis drug regimen consisting of daily administration of isoniazid (300 mg), rifampicin (600 mg), streptomycin (900 mg), and pyrizinamide (2.0 g).

Relapsing peritonitis due to *M. xenopi* in a patient undergoing continuous peritoneal dialysis was treated with oral antibiotics in combination with intraperitoneal streptomycin, permitting peritoneal dialysis to be continued with satisfactory clearance and ultrafiltration capacity. The streptomycin pharmacokinetics revealed that 75% of the intraperitoneally administered dose was absorbed from the dialysate.[541]

Miller et al.[521] have linked a case of Pott's disease with *M. xenopi* infection. Also known as "tuberculosis of the spine," the Pott's disease (osteitis or caries of the vertebrae) usually occurs as a complication of tuberculosis of the lungs.[561] Previously, two reports by Prosser[547] and Rahman et al.[548] described vertebral (lumbar spine) infection due to *M. xenopi*.

Kiehl et al.[562] have described a rare lupus vulgaris-like infection caused by *M. xenopi* in an immunocompetent female patient, which responded well to treatment with isoniazid.

A case of fulminant hepatic encephalopathy and renal failure in a patient with *M. xenopi* infection resulted in death despite combination therapy with isoniazid, rifampin, and prothionamide.[563] This fatal outcome may not be so unusual since there has been a widespread recognition that isoniazid can cause fulminant hepatis failure,[564,565] as well as previous fatalities from hepatic failure after its administration (bilirubin levels exceeding 340 μmol/l).[566] Consideration should be given to regular clinical monitoring of the liver function, especially when patients continue to take isoniazid during the prodromal phase (usually lasting for 1 to 4 weeks and often characterized by vague and nonspecific symptoms) of their illness when the severity of hepatitis correlates with continued drug use during this phase.[567]

8.6.10   MYCOBACTERIUM HAEMOPHILUM

8.6.10.1   Introduction

First described in 1978,[568] *Mycobacterium haemophilum* is the etiologic agent of a rare but rapidly emerging infection[569] associated mainly with the development of ulcerating cutaneous lesions.[569-587] *M. haemophilum* is a short, slightly curved rod existing either singly or in a cord-like formation. The organism is strongly acid-fast by Ziel-Nielsen staining.[568]

Initially, *M. haemophilum* disease was observed in patients receiving immunosuppressive therapy, such as renal transplant recipients.[570,572,576,586] However, in the last several years, the infection has been diagnosed with increased frequency in patients with AIDS.[569,571,575,577-579,581,584] In addition, *M. haemophilum* has also been identified in immunocompetent children with cervical and perihilar lymphadenitis,[574,583,584,587] as well as in patients with lymphoma.[568,586]

The ecology of the pathogen and the mode of its transmission are not well understood.[569] It appears that the infection is sporadic since there was no common source suggested by the case control studies, although atypical mycobacteria have been known to be widespread, particularly in water reservoirs[588,589] and soil.[590] Potential routes of transmission include percutaneous inoculation, inhalation, or ingestion.[569] *M. haemophilum* is a nutritionally fastidious and slow-growing bacterium. Compared to other mycobacteria it requires a lower incubation temperature for growth, and an iron-rich medium.[568,587] Because of the strict growth conditions needed for its isolation, cases of *M. haemophilum*-induced infection and its frequency may be much higher.

M. haemophilum is known to cause disseminated cutaneous lesions, bacteremia, and disease of the bones, joints, lymphatics, and the lungs. Cutaneous lesions are found most often on the extremities (frequently overlying joints), and less commonly on the trunk and face. Patients with severe immune deficiencies caused by AIDS, immunosuppressive therapy (such as organ transplant recipients), and lymphoma are at increased risk of infection. In these patients, in addition to skin lesions, the pathogen has been isolated from vitreous fluid, synovial fluid, bronchoalveolar lavage fluid, lung tissue, blood, lymph nodes, wound specimens, bone marrow, and sputum, which suggests hematogenous spread of the organism.[578,579,581,585,591]

8.6.10.2 Evolution of Therapies and Treatment of *M. haemophilum* Infections

M. haemophilum appears to be an emerging opportunistic pathogen in AIDS patients and should be considered in the differential diagnosis of suspected mycobacterial infections in HIV-positive patients. There are a number of cases described, where the initial response to therapy was favorable, to be followed only by a recurrence of infection.[575]

Careful surgical drainage of lesions and antimycobacterial therapy have been used to treat *M. haemophilum* infections.

Most studies have demonstrated *in vitro* susceptibility of *M. haemophilum* to rifampin and *p*-aminosalicylic acid.[568,572,579,580,582,592] When tested for susceptibility, *M. haemophilum* isolates have been found variously susceptible to amikacin, streptomycin, kanamycin, ethionamide, cycloserine, capreomycin, cefotaxin, minocycline, doxycycline, ciprofloxacin, rifabutin, and trimethoprim-sulfamethoxazole,[569,593] whereas the majority of isolates were resistant to ethambutol, isoniazid, and pyrazinamide.[568,569,579,580,585] However, the correlation between data from *in vitro* susceptibility tests and results from antimycobacterial therapy is not very clear. In one case described by Dever et al.[575] a patient responded dramatically to a regimen of isoniazid, rifampin, ethambutol, and ciprofloxacin. Yet, the infection still recurred to respond markedly to a subsequent treatment with izoniazid, rifampin, ethambutol, ciprofloxacin, amikacin, and clofazimine.

Various treatment regimens have been used, including combinations of antimycobacterial drugs, such as isoniazid, rifampin, and ethambutol,[568] isoniazid and rifampin,[573] trimethoprim-sulfamethoxazole,[580] minocycline,[572,576] erythromycin,[576,594] rifampine and minocycline,[572] rifampin and *p*-aminosalicylic acid,[578] rifampin and erythromycin,[577] as well as doxycycline, clarithromycin, ciprofloxacin,[587] amikacin, clofazimine, streptomycin, and pyrazinamide.[569]

Minocycline administered as either adjunctive therapy with surgery or combined with rifampin has produced some response.[572,576] Improvement has been observed also by using sulfamethoxazole alone.[580] Thus, treatment with sulfamethoxazole at a dose of 1.0 g given twice daily resulted in slow but steady regression of lesions in a patient with *M. haemophilum* infection.[580]

McBride et al.[587] reported a case of a postoperative (coronary artery bypass surgery) *M. haemophilum* infection in an immunocompetent patient who responded with nearly complete resolution of skin lesions to ciprofloxacin given at 500 mg twice daily, for 5 months.

Branger et al.[572] have described a case involving a renal transplant recipient who developed *M. haemophilum* infection associated with *M. xenopi* infection. Initial therapy with isoniazid and rifampin had no clinical effect. After surgical drainage of the lesion and administration of minocycline, the patient recovered. In another case involving an immunosuppressed renal transplant recipient,[582] treatment with rifampin (450 mg daily), isoniazid (300 mg daily), and ethambutol (400 mg daily), as well as reduction of immunosuppressive prednisolone therapy to a maintenance level (20 mg daily) did not bring any regression of lesions; eventually the lesions began to regress and had fully resolved later.

An AIDS patient who developed tenosynovitis caused by *M. haemophilum* was the first documented case in AIDS.[579] Of the several antimycobacterial drugs tested for susceptibility, only rifampin exhibited significant activity against the isolate of the patient. In another report,[581] two AIDS patients failed to respond to any of the applied antimycobacterial therapy (isoniazid, rifampin) against *M. haemophilum* lesions; there was also evidence of hematogenous dissemination of disease (positive blood cultures and distant sites of involvement). Thibert et al.[585] have also reported similar hematogenous dissemination in an AIDS patient.

8.6.11 MYCOBACTERIUM SZULGAI

8.6.11.1 Introduction

In 1972, Marks et al.[595] first recognized *M. szulgai* as a human pathogen. It is a slow-growing mycobacterium which produces colonies after approximately 2 weeks of incubation. *M. szulgai* has unique pigmentation; it is scotochromogenic when grown at 37°C and photochromogenic at 25°C. Although the organism has worldwide distribution, its natural habitat is not known.

In humans, *M. szulgai* most often affects middle-aged men causing usually chronic pulmonary disease with cavitary lesions.[596-600] Clinically, the symptoms of *M. szulgai* have been almost indistinguishable from those of *M. tuberculosis*,[600] MAI, and *M. kansasii*.[1]

Extrapulmonary involvement of *M. szulgai* has been uncommon. Among several reports, two patients presented with infection of the olecranon bursa (one after repeated trauma, and the other after cortisone injection),[399] and another two patients suffered extensive cutaneous lesions while receiving corticosteroid therapy.[601,602] There have been cases of tenosynovitis with carpal tunnel syndrome,[603] cervical lymphadenitis in a child, and disseminated disease where the organism was isolated from bone, skin lesions, and sputum.[604] Disseminated *M. szulgai* infection in AIDS patients has also been reported.[605,606] Zamboni et al.[606] diagnosed the first case in a hemophiliac patient with AIDS. Roig et al.[605] have isolated the organism from bone and kidney of an HIV-positive patient.

8.6.11.2 Treatment of *M. szulgai* Infections

Although *M. szulgai* has been found *in vitro* to be slightly more resistant than *M. tuberculosis* to most antituberculosis agents, in many cases the disease responded well to a multiple-drug regimen consisting of rifampin, isoniazid, and ethambutol, with streptomycin, capreomycin, or viomycin serving as a fourth or substitute drug.[1,489] Thus, Mori et al.[598] used a combination of rifampicin, isoniazid, and streptomycin to treat successfully a patient with pulmonary infection associated with multiple bullous disease of the lung.

Based on *in vitro* susceptibility test results, Tsukamura and Yamori[40] have recommended a combination of enviomycin, ethambutol (100% strain sensitivity to 3.13 µg/ml[53]), and isoniazid for the treatment of *M. szulgai* infections.

While surgical excision appears unnecessary in pulmonary disease, it may be warranted in cases of olecranon bursitis (inflammation and enlargement of the bursa over the olecranon; called also "miners' elbow").[600]

8.6.12 MYCOBACTERIUM MALMOENSE

8.6.12.1 Introduction

In 1977, Schröder and Juhlin[607] described *M. malmoense* as a new species. It is a slow-growing, nonphotochromogenic mycobacterium associated with pulmonary disease in humans.

M. malmoense grows as dysgonic, smooth, colorless colonies at temperatures ranging from 22°C to 37°C. At the latter temperature, growth is usually slow — about 18 d, and incubation may eventually be required for up to 12 weeks.[1] It has the ability to hydrolyze Tween 80, a property which might help to distinguish *M. malmoense* from MAI.[608] Another reliable method to differentiate this organism is thin-layer chromatography of its surface lipids — the pattern of spots which will develop using this method is unique for *M. malmoense*.[609]

While the natural habitat of these organisms is not known, the majority of cases have come from Great Britain[609-611] and Scandinavia,[612] but also from the U.S.[613] and Switzerland.[614-616]

Human *M. malmoense*-associated mycobacteriosis usually presents with chronic pulmonary disease.[1,617] In most instances, the infection has been diagnosed in middle-aged men with previously documented pneumoconiosis, and organisms were isolated from sputum, gastric lavage, bronchial secretions, and lung tissue.[609,613] In addition, cases of cervical lymphadenopathy in children have also been described.[404,618] Recently, Mattila et al.[619] have described *M. malmoense* involvement in prurigo nodularis, a chronic skin disorder with unknown cause.

Immunodeficiencies due to hairy cell leukemia,[620,621] diabetes mellitus, and corticosteroid therapy have been recognized as predisposing factors for *M. malmoense* infections.[622,623]

Cases of disseminated disease caused by *M. malmoense* have also been described,[614,621] including in patients infected with HIV.[608,614,624,225]

8.6.12.2 Treatment of *M. malmoense* Infections

The *in vitro* susceptibility patterns of different *M. malmoense* isolates have varied.[1] While most of the original isolates studied have been uniformly susceptible to ethionamide, ethambutol (46% strain sensitivity to 3.13 μg/ml[53]), kanamycin, and cycloserine, and resistant to isoniazid, streptomycin, rifampin, *p*-aminosalicylic acid, and capreomycin,[1,611] the isolate recovered by Warren et al.[613] has shown susceptibility to rifampin, streptomycin, and capreomycin, as well as to ethionamide and ethambutol. It should be noted that because of the slow growth of *M. malmoense* on conventional, egg-based bacteriologic media, the incubation time of these organisms should be over 6 weeks; special solid and liquid media have been recommended.[614]

The clinical relevance of *in vitro* susceptibilities has been unclear and infections due to *M. malmoense* have been generally difficult to manage, leaving optimum treatment as yet to be established. While some patients have shown clinical improvement (including those with cervical adenitis), in others, the outcome has been either fatal,[608] or patients have developed progressive disease, and those who remained clinically stable still showed positive cultures.[1] The antimycobacterial drugs associated with the most favorable susceptibility patterns were rifampin and ethambutol.[614,615]

The response to conventional antimycobacterial therapy (rifampicin, isoniazid, and ethambutol, with or without pyrazinamide) seemed to have been more favorable when administration of ethambutol was included for at least 9 months.[610,626] Surgical excision (lobectomy) combined with antimycobacterial therapy has also been recommended.[616]

Treatment of *M. malmoense* disease in an alcoholic AIDS patient with rifampin, isoniazid, pyrazinamide, and pyridoxine failed to cure the infection. Ethambutol was added to the regimen and the patient, who responded markedly to therapy, died shortly after jaundice and hepatic encephalopathy had developed.[608] The fatal outcome may well have been the result of isoniazid hepatotoxicity.[566]

Klemens and Cynamon[56] have evaluated the activities of azithromycin and clarithromycin against *M. malmoense* disseminated infection in beige C57BL/6J bgj/bgj mice, and found both antibiotics when administered with other antimycobacterial agents to be useful against the disease (see the discussion on *in vitro* and *in vivo* activities on page 309).

Schafer et al.[622] have described a bronchopulmonary infection caused by *M. malmoense* in a patient with severe immunosuppression due to insulin-dependent diabetes mellitus, humoral immunodeficiency after thymoma (Good's disease), and prolonged immunosuppressive therapy after myasthenic crisis. *In vitro* susceptibility testing revealed sensitivity to ethambutol, rifampin, clarithromycin, and prothionamide. While antimycobacterial multiple-drug treatment for 12 months resulted in stable remission and considerable suppression of mycobacterial load, the pathogen was not completely eradicated.

Zaugg et al.[614] used a combination of rifabutin (ansamycin), clofazimine, and isoniazid to treat successfully a disseminated pulmonary and gastrointestinal *M. malmoense* infection in an AIDS patient.

In another case of disseminated *M. malmoense* infection, an immunosuppressed patient with hairy cell leukemia and fever responded to treatment with doxycycline, ethambutol, and cycloserine given over a 16-month period.[621]

Data from a retrospective study conducted by Katila et al.[612] seemed to suggest that the incidence of childhood cervical adenitis caused by *M. malmoense*, *M. tuberculosis*, and MAC was lower in children given neonatal BCG vaccination.

8.6.13 MYCOBACTERIUM GENAVENSE

M. genavense is a newly recognized, fastidious, acid-fast mycobacterium which did not grow on conventional solid media,[627,628] although some limited growth has been observed in liquid Middle-brook 13A culture.[629] The mycolic acid pattern of *M. genavense* (α-, α'-, and keto-mycolates) as determined by thin-layer chromatography was similar to that of *M. simiae* and *M. malmoense*, and gas chromatography revealed tuberculostearic and hexadecanoic acids.[629] However, amplification and sequencing of the 16S ribosomal RNA gene showed phylogenetically different characteristics, prompting the name *M. genavense*.[630,631]

The natural habitat of *M. genavense* remains to be established. In humans, the striking gastro-intestinal symptoms and signs observed may suggested the gut as the reservoir from which these mycobacteria invade other organs.[631]

In 1992, Hirschel et al.[629] have described the first *M. genavense* infection in a severely immuno-compromised AIDS patient. The patient, who died from the infection, presented with fever, hepatosplenomegaly, and gastrointestinal symptoms. The pathogen was present in massive quanti-ties in nearly all tissues examined (duodenum, feces, urine, and bone marrow).

In a study of 18 AIDS patients with disseminated *M. genavense* disease, Böttger et al.[631] described the main clinical features in the majority of patients as relentless loss of weight, fever, and diarrhea resulting from massive infection of the intestine and liver, as well as lungs, bone marrow, and lymph nodes.

The pathogenicity of *M. genavense* in AIDS patients was described as similar to that of disseminated infection caused by *M. avium-intracellulare*.[631-634] In a study conducted by Pechère et al.,[633] the median CD4+ count of infected patients was $0.016 \times 10^9/l$ (16 cells/mm³).

During the period 1990 to 1992, 12.8% of disseminated mycobacterial infections in AIDS patients from Switzerland were attributed to *M. genavense*.[633] Because of such high incidence, it has been suggested that this mycobacterial species should be considered seriously in the differential diagnosis of patients with AIDS with CD4+ counts below 100 cells/mm³, and presenting with diarrhea, weight loss, and fever.[61,631,633,635] In addition, biopsies of liver, duodenum, bone marrow, or lymph nodes should reveal acid-fast rods that cannot be cultured on solid media, although blood cultures in Middlebrook 13A liquid medium may show some growth.

Berman et al.[636] have described a rather unusual case of *M. genavense* infection in an AIDS patient who presented with grand mal seizures and a brain lesion, with evidence of dissemination.

The optimum treatment of *M. genavense* is yet to be determined, although by analogy with *M. avium-intracellulare* and antibiotic sensitivity tests,[637] amikacin, clofazimine, ethambutol, rifab-utin, clarithromycin, azithromycin, and ciprofloxacin (as well as other fluoroquinolones) may be considered.[631] According to Bessesen et al.,[634] the best clinical response and clearance of bacteremia were associated with clarithromycin therapy. Among patients who had been treated with at least two antimycobacterial drugs for 1 month or more, the median survival was 263 d (95% confidence interval, 144 to 382 d), compared with 81 d (95% confidence interval, 73 to 89 d) for those not treated ($p = .0009$).[633]

8.6.14 MYCOBACTERIUM SIMIAE

8.6.14.1 Introduction

Karassova et al.[638] first isolated these organisms from monkeys in 1965. In 1969, Weiszfeiler[639] named them *Mycobacterium simiae*. In 1971, Valdivia et al.[640] isolated from the sputum of patients with either pulmonary tuberculosis or other respiratory disorders a niacin-positive mycobacterial strain belonging to the Runyon group III for which the name *Mycobacterium habana* was proposed. Later studies have determined that *M. simiae* and *M. habana* were identical species.[641,642]

M. simiae is a photochromogenic mycobacterium which requires prolonged exposure to light in order for pigmentation to occur.[1] In addition to monkeys and humans, it has been isolated from tap water in hospitals, thus raising the possibility of nosocomial infections.

Clinical manifestations of *M. simiae* disease include chronic pulmonary infections,[643-645] osteomyelitis,[646,647] and disseminated disease with renal and bone marrow involvement.[646]

8.6.14.2   Treatment of *M. simiae* Infections

With the exception of ethionamide and cycloserine, *in vitro* susceptibility studies have consistently demonstrated resistance to most antimycobacterial drugs.[1] Because of that and the relatively limited cases described, there has not been any recommendation for optimal approach to therapy of *M. simiae* infections.[40] Nevertheless, the disease has been stabilized following treatment with isoniazid, ethambutol, and rifampine, even though excretion of organisms continued.[1]

Valero et al.[648] have examined the therapeutic activities of clarithromycin, ofloxacin, and clarithromycin–ethambutol combination against experimental *M. simiae* infection in mice. While overall all three modalities have decreased the level of infection in both the lungs and spleen, ofloxacin and clarithromycin–ethambutol were superior to clarithromycin alone in reducing the mycobacterial counts in the spleen. In another *in vivo* study,[56] clarithromycin and azithromycin showed similar activity against spleen infection in beige mice due to *M. simiae*.

Despite multiple-drug resistance *in vitro*, Heap[649] has treated successfully with combination chemotherapy a patient with intra-abdominal disease caused by *M. simiae*.

It has been established in several studies that some proteins from the cell wall (33 kDa), cell membrane (38 kDa), and the cytosol (22 kDa) of *M. simiae* were recognized only by leprosy or tuberculosis antisera.[650] This phenomenon has made these immunoreactive antigens of *M. simiae* useful for the development of diagnostic agents for mycobacteria, and a viable vaccine candidate for mycobacterial infections.[650,651]

8.6.15   *Mycobacterium marinum*

8.6.15.1   Introduction

The first report describing *M. marinum* appeared in 1926, after its isolation from salt-water fish.[652] It was not until 1951 that Norden and Linell[653] identified *M. marinum* as a human pathogen. Over the years, two other synonyms (*M. platypoecilus* and *M. balnei*) have been used to describe the same species.[1,654]

M. marinum is a photochromogenic species, which within 8 to 14 d at optimal temperatures of 31 to 33°C produces slightly wrinkled and shiny, but also smooth and hemispheric, colonies. On rare occasions, the colonies may appear rough and dry.

The most characteristic clinical involvement has been cutaneous disease.[8,655-657] It is usually acquired as the result of trauma to skin while in contact with contaminated nonchlorinated fresh or salt water.[12,658-667] However, *M. marinum* cutaneous lesions may also develop after trauma unassociated with water contact, or after contact with water in the absence of preceding trauma.[1,668,669] The typical presentation has been a single papulonodular lesion confined to one extremity, most commonly involving the elbow, knee, foot, toe, or finger.[670-675] Another presentation of cutaneous *M. marinum* infection may resemble cutaneous sporotrichosis, where there is an abscess formation at the inoculation site, followed by the development of a series of secondary nodules that may progress centrally along the lymphatics.[1,676-680]

Extracutaneous involvement of *M. marinum* has included synovitis, infections of the deep structures of the hands, septic bursitis (mainly in the olecranon bursa),[681] septic arthritis and osteomyelitis,[682-688] sclerokeratitis,[689] and laryngeal lesions.[690]

In immunocompromised patients, the occurrence of disseminated cutaneous lesions has been described.[691-695] Parent et al.[693] have reported a case of disseminated dermatitis, osteomyelitis, and bacteremia due to *M. marinum* in an immunocompromised pediatric patient with severe combined immunodeficiency. An unusual *M. marinum* disseminated infection in an immunocompetent patient has also been reported.[696]

Patients with AIDS have also been affected by *M. marinum*-associated mycobacteriosis.[676,679,697] Because of the risk of relapse, such patients may require prolonged treatment.

8.6.15.2   Treatment of *M. marinum* Infections

When tested *in vitro* for susceptibility to antimycobacterial agents, most *M. marinum* strains were sensitive to rifampin and ethambutol, but resistant to isoniazid, sparfloxacin, and fleroxacin, and moderately susceptible to streptomycin.[1,48,50] In a study by Tsukamura,[53] 88% of *M. marinum* strains were susceptible to 3.13 µg/ml of ethambutol, and Boos at al.[698] have found oral rifampicin effective in the treatment of *M. marinum* in two specis of tropical fish.

The MIC values of dihydromycoplanecin A, amikacin, ofloxacin, norfloxacin, enoxacin, minocycline, sulfamethoxazole, trimethoprim–sulfamethoxazole, trimethoprim, oxytetracycline, and pipemidic acid against 16 *M. marinum* strains were 0.19 to 0.39, 0.78 to 1.56, 1.56 to 3.13, 1.56 to 3.13, 1.56 to 3.13, 1.56 to 6.25, 1.56 to 25, 1.56 to 25, 25 to 200, 3.13 to 12.5, and 50 to 200 µg/ml, respectively.[699]

DU-6859a, a new fluoroquinolone derivative was found active *in vitro* against *M. marinum* with a MIC value of 1.56 µg/ml.[52]

The *in vitro* and *in vivo* activities of KRM-1648, a new synthetic benzoxazinorifamycin analog against *M. marinum* were compared to those of rifampin.[700] The MIC values of KRM-1648, determined by the agar dilution method on 7H11 medium against 10 mycobacterial strains, were 32 to 128 times lower than those of rifampin. *In vivo*, KRM-1648 was again superior to rifampin in markedly reducing the skin lesions and the number of CFUs in the lungs and spleens.

Selection of the approach to treatment of *M. marinum* infections will depend on the presentation of disease. While single cutaneous lesions often resolve spontaneously (even though it may take between 3 months to 3 years), the sporotrichoid form may persist for prolonged periods. Occasionally, the discomfort is serious enough to warrant therapy. In such cases, various methods for localized treatment have been applied, including curettage, electrodesiccation, freezing, excision followed by skin grafting, local heat, intralesional steroid injections, irradiation, and incision and drainage.

While chemotherapy alone may be adequate, surgical intervention, alone or in combination with chemotherapy, has also been used in cases of aggressive *M. marinum* infection,[701] or persistent pain, a discharging sinus, or previous local injection of corticosteroids.[702-704] For unresponsive or disseminated skin disease, or deep infections, systemic therapy with antimycobacterial agents is recommended.[1] Suggested therapeutic modalities consisted of rifampin–ethambutol for advanced disease and infections invading the deeper structures of the hand and wrist, and one of either tetracyclines[705,706] or trimethoprim–sulfamethoxazole (co-trimoxazole) for early or less serious disease.[707] Among other drugs, amikacin and kanamycin, and to a lesser extent tetracycline and minocycline, have demonstrated therapeutic efficacy.[708,709] Doxycycline failed to elicit favorable response in two patients with aquarium-acquired cutaneous *M. marinum* infection.[710]

A case of bilateral, symmetric, sporotrichoid *M. marinum* granulomas involving the dorsa of fingers and wrists was successfully cured by co-trimoxazole.[677] In several previous studies,[657,659,661,662,702,710,711] co-trimoxazole was also found to be the most appropriate drug for treatment of *M. marinum* of less advanced cutaneous infections.

Ries et al.[712] have identifed *M. marinum* complex as the causative agent of multiple sub-cutaneous necrotizing nodules on the chest, extremities, and face of an HIV-infected patient. Therapy with isoniazid, rifampin, and ethambutol led to resolution of lesions.

Treatment of cutaneous infections with ethambutol–rifampin[702,711,713] appeared to be more successful (effective in 5 of 5 cases) than minocycline alone (10 of 14 cases) ($p = .28$).[656] Four culture-positive cases of flexor tenosynovitis of the hand were cured by a combination of flexor tenosynovectomy and therapy with rifampin–ethambutol.[714]

Therapy with rifampin alone was credited for the complete healing of a sporotrichoid skin infection due to *M. marinum*.[680]

Another antimicrobial agent, rifabutin, was also found effective in the treatment of cutaneous disease caused by *M. marinum*.[715]

Clarithromycin has been used by Bonnet et al.[697] to treat connective tissue infection. In a recent report, Kuhn et al.[716] have described its use in the treatment of *M. marinum*-induced facial abscess. The antimicrobial activity of clarithromycin seemed to be enhanced by the formation *in vivo* of the 14-hydroxy metabolite, which appeared to be also microbiologically active.[717]

Hanau et al.[676] have reported one case of an AIDS patient with lymphoma and sporotrichoid *M. marinum* infection. The patient responded completely to antimycobacterial therapy, but relapsed when the medication was discontinued 6 months into its course. Another immunocompromised patient with systemic lupus erythematosus and a protracted *M. marinum* skin infection responded poorly to multiple antimycobacterial regimens.[694]

For the treatment of *M. marinum* arthritis (most often seen in patients with monarticular synovitis of the hands and wrists), Alloway et al.[684] recommended therapy consisting of at least two antimycobacterial agents for a minimum of 6 months. Clark et al.[686] used minocycline, rifampin, and ethambutol in combination with surgical intervention to cure osteomyelitis and synovitis produced by *M. marinum*.

Multiplication of *M. marinum* in mice was prevented by vaccination with lymphoid cells prepared from the popliteal lymph nodes of mice in which the organisms were multiplying logarithmically.[718]

Upon recovery from the immediate effects of total lymphoid irradiation (increasingly used in clinic as an immunosuppressive adjunct in transplantation), mice were found capable of mounting an effective immune response to experimental infection with *M. marinum*.[719]

8.6.16 *Mycobacterium gordonae*

8.6.16.1 Introduction

M. gordonae has been the most frequently isolated saprophyte from water and soil, and one of the most common mycobacteria encountered in the laboratory. It has also been referred to as *Mycobacterium aquae* or the tap-water bacillus. Because of its presence in water sources, *M. gordonae* has often been involved in nosocomial pseudoinfections and pseudoepidemics.[720-725] In addition, *M. gordonae* has been routinely isolated from gastric washings and bronchial secretions.

M. gordonae organisms are chromogenic, and form smooth orange-colored colonies after 4 to 8 weeks of incubation at either 25°C or 37°C.

In most cases, *M. gordonae* is considered nonpathogenic to humans. However, with increasing incidence, this mycobacterium has been identified as a causative agent of disease, including meningitis,[726] keratitis,[727,728] hepatoperitoneal disease (including in CAPD patients),[729-731] prosthetic aortic valve[732] and genitourinary[733] infections, and cutaneous lesions.[734-736] Pulmonary involvement has also been reported.[29,737-746]

In seriously ill patients, such as those with severe underlying disease (HIV-positive individuals with CD4+ cell counts of 180 cells/mm^3 or less,[747-749] organ transplant recipients,[750] or history of pulmonary tuberculosis[751]), *M. gordonae* disease may become opportunistic[59,749] and present with destructive lesions and prolonged morbidity if not properly treated.[738]

M. gordonae has also been implicated in causing clinically significant disseminating disease[726,732,750,752] in both immunosuppressed (HIV-positive,[748] renal failure requiring hemodialysis[753]) and immunocompetent[751] patients.

Failure of high-level disinfection of bronchoscopes has caused several outbreaks of nosocomial infection or pseudoinfection due to *M. gordonae*.[754]

M. gordonae may produce caseating or noncaseating granulomas, and skin lesions showing acute and chronic inflammation with scattered histiocytes and giant cells have been seen.[1]

8.6.16.2   Treatment of *M. gordonae* Infections

In vitro susceptibility testing of *M. gordonae* has demonstrated resistance to isoniazid, streptomycin, and *p*-aminosalicylic acid (PAS), but sensitivity to rifampin and ethambutol.[753] Thus, Tsukamura[53] found 90% of *M. gordonae* strains studied susceptible to 3.13 μg/ml of ethambutol. Among the fluoroquinolone antibiotics, ciprofloxacin and ofloxacin were both active against 6 of 13 strains of *M. gordonae*,[46] and in Ogawa egg medium, the MIC value of sparfloxacin was 0.0 μg/ml or less.[47]

DuP-721, a new oxazolidinone analog was found effective *in vitro* (3.9 μg/ml) in inhibiting *M. gordonae*.[54]

Successful treatment with antimycobacterial agents has included the use of a long-term regimen of isoniazid and ethambutol in a patient with *M. gordonae*-induced meningitis;[726] streptomycin, isoniazid, rifampin, ethambutol, and pyrazinamide in HIV-infected patients;[749] and isoniazid, rifampin, and ethambutol in patients with hepatoperitoneal[729] and prosthetic aortic valve[732] involvement. Daily administration of rifampin at 300 mg for 6 months cured cutaneous ulcers on the hand. However, noncompliance with antimycobacterial medication may lead to relapses.[733]

Weinberger et al.[753] have described a pediatric patient with disseminated *M. gordonae* infection whose course was complicated by renal failure requiring hemodialysis, but who recovered after 15 months of chemotherapy consisting of daily administration of isoniazid (300 mg), rifampin (600 mg), amikacin (300 mg), and ethambutol (1.2 g); ciprofloxacin (500 mg daily) was added on day 28 of hospitalization.

A pulmonary infection in an otherwise healthy patient was successfully treated with daily administration of rifampicin (450 mg), isoniazid (400 mg), and ethambutol (1.0 g) over a 9-month period.[739]

Progressive pulmonary disease, however, may be more difficult to treat. Thus, Guarderas et al.[740] reported a case where the patient failed to improve after multiple-drug antimycobacterial therapy given over a period of 8 years.

Nathan et al.[738] have studied the efficacy of rifabutin in the treatment of a progressive cavitary lung disease due to *M. gordonae*, which failed to show any clinical improvement after 9 months of intensive therapy with a conventional four-drug antimycobacterial regimen. After rifabutin was included, the disease was cured. In another study, daily administration of rifabutin (7 to 10 mg/kg) in combination with clofazimine (100 mg), isoniazid (5.0 mg/kg), and ethambutol (20 mg/kg) was used to treat AIDS patients with *M. gordonae* infection.[13]

Liquid chemical sterilization with glutaraldehyde, iodophor, and peracetic acid have been used to eradicate *M. gordonae* from bronchoscope processing.[754,755]

8.6.17   *Mycobacterium ulcerans*

8.6.17.1   Introduction

The pathogenic nature of *M. ulcerans* in humans was first recognized in Australia in the 1930s.[756] In addition, other regions identified as having endemic *M. ulcerans* disease include Central and

East Africa (Zaire, Uganda, Nigeria, Ghana, Cameroon, Benin, Ivory Coast),[757,758] Central and South America (Mexico, Guyana), Malaysia, and the Pacific (New Guinea, Kiribati).

Neither the natural habitat of these organisms nor the usual route of transmission to humans has been fully elucidated. In general, areas situated in latitudes 25° north to 38° south in both tropical and temperate climates are considered as likely foci for *M. ulcerans* disease to occur.[1] Surveying the incidence of atypical cutaneous mycobacterial diseases in France, Bonafe et al.[12] have reported the occurrence, although very rare, of *M. ulcerans* infections.

Similarly to *M. tuberculosis*, *M. ulcerans* produces rough, hydrophobic, nonpigmented colonies, which have the ability to form cords. The organism has a very slow growth rate even at the optimal temperature (33°C). At 27°C and 37°C, it grows poorly or not at all.[1]

At various times, *M. ulcerans* disease has been referred to as Bairnsdale ulcer (from the area where it was first recognized in Australia) or the Buruli disease (after the area of Uganda reporting the most cases).[759]

Clinically, the disease begins initially as a "boil" or subcutaneous lump, which appears on an exposed area (most often the lower extremities). After several weeks the lump, which may itch but is usually painless, breaks down, revealing a shallow ulcer with a necrotic base and edges that resemble and have the consistency of an orange peel. The condition becomes indolent over a period of weeks to months, with prominent involvement of the subcutaneous tissue.[1,760]

According to Muelder and Nourou,[757] *M. ulcerans* can regress as well as progress, resulting in the simultaneous presence of lesions at different stages of development. A system of disease staging was introduced as follows: stage I (subcutaneous nodule), stage II (cellulitis), stage III (ulceration), and stage IV (scar formation). However, Hayman[761] disagreed with this classification, pointing to some differences in the pathology of disease observed in cases in Australia where the discrete subcutaneous nodule first described in Uganda[762] has only rarely been identified.[763]

8.6.17.2 Treatment of *M. ulcerans* Infections

The most common approach for treating *M. ulcerans* disease is surgical debridement.[1,764-768] For early lesions, excision and primary closure have been recommended, whereas large ulcerated areas have usually been treated by radical excision followed by skin grafting. Less extensive surgery combined with antimycobacterial treatment has been reported.[756]

The most appropriate drug regimen appeared to be streptomycin and dapsone with or without ethambutol for at least 2 weeks after completion of healing.[1] Darie et al.[764] reported a good success rate following treatment of *M. ulcerans* ulcers by streptomycin combined with islet-skin grafting.

In a recent report, co-trimoxazole has also been used for therapy of a leg ulcer due to *M. ulcerans*,[669] and earlier, Song et al.[770] applied antibiotics and dextrans to cure successfully a cutaneous infection on the foot.

8.6.18 MYCOBACTERIUM TERRAE-TRIVIALE COMPLEX

The *Mycobacterium terrae-triviale* complex includes *M. terrae* and *M. triviale*. First isolated in 1950 by Richmond and Cummings[771] from washings of radish, *M. terrae* has also been known as the "radish bacillus."[1] Consequently, it has been cultured from soil and other vegetables.

Both *M. terrae* and *M. triviale* are nonphotochromogenic organisms that grow slowly at 25°C and 37°C, with *M. triviale* forming rough colonies, whereas those of *M. terrae* are intermediate in roughness.

While pathogenicity in humans has been rare,[772,773] *M. terrae* was described as one of the causative agents of atypical cutaneous mycobacteriosis of the upper extremities.[8] Other cases involved *M. triviale*-induced septic arthritis in an infant,[774] and synovitis and osteomyelitis due to *M. terrae* in a young patient with Fanconi's syndrome (a rare recessive disorder characterized by pancytopenia and hypoplasia of the bone marrow, and associated with congenital anomalies of the musculoskeletal and genitourinary systems).[775] A possible case of disseminated *M. terrae* disease in a young patient with a history of miliary tuberculosis has also been reported.[776] Katz[777] has reported a case of *M. terrae*-induced tenosynovitis of the hand, which underscored the possibility of delayed and difficult diagnosis.

8.6.18.1 Treatment of M. terrae-triviale Complex Infections

M. terrae is considered to be less pathogenic than *M. marinum* and has responded to either surgical treatment alone or surgery combined with antimycobacterial therapy.[1,8]

8.6.19 MYCOBACTERIUM ASIATICUM

M. asiaticum is a photochromogenic mycobacterium which was first isolated from healthy monkey in 1965 by Karassova et al.[638] and was described and named by Weiszfeiler et al.[778] in 1971. The organisms grow well at 25°C and 37°C but not at 45°C.[1] The natural habitat of *M. asiaticum* is still unknown.

In humans, *M. asiaticum* infections have been associated with pulmonary mycobacteriosis often presenting with cavitary lesions.[29,779,780] Preexisting lung disease may be a predisposing factor.[779] One case of olecranon bursitis was also described.[781]

8.6.19.1 Treatment of M. asiaticum Infections

In vitro susceptibility testing of clinical isolates of *M. asiaticum* has shown sensitivity to cycloserine and ethionamide, but resistance to isoniazid, rifampin, and *p*-aminosalicylic acid; susceptibility to streptomycin and ethambutol has varied.[779]

Describing two cases of pulmonary involvement, Blacklock et al.[779] were not able to prevent the disease from progressing by treating one of the patients with rifampin and ethambutol for 2 years; sputum cultures remained positive. In the second case, the disease remained stabilized for 32 months after the patient received only a short-term therapy with rifampin, ethambutol, capreomycin, and pyrazinamide. In another report of pulmonary infection due to *M. asiaticum*, treatment with conventional antimycobacterial drugs resulted in a bacteriologic conversion.[780]

In a case of olecranon bursitis, the patient did not receive antimycobacterial therapy since the infection responded to drainage, regular dressing, and immobilization.

8.6.20 MYCOBACTERIUM THERMORESISTIBILE

M. thermoresistibile is a rapidly growing mycobacterium (7 d) which produces either smooth or rough yellowish-orange colonies that become brown with age. The optimal temperatures for growth are 37°C and 45°C. However, these organisms can also grow at 25°C, and have the unique ability to produce colonies even at 52°C. In nature, *M. thermoresistibile* has been isolated from soil.

The first human infection caused by *M. thermoresistibile* was reported by Weitzman et al.[782] in 1981. The organisms were recovered repeatedly from the sputum, a bronchoscopy specimen, and from lung tissue of an immunocompetent patient presenting with cough, fever, weight loss, and cavitary lesions on chest radiography. Lung tissue revealed the presence of microabscesses and granulomas with Langhans' giant cells.[782]

In another first case, Wolfe and Moore[783] reported a *M. thermoresistibile* surgical wound infection following augmentation mammoplasty.

A cutaneous infection due to these organisms occurred 3 months after cardiac transplantation near the surgical scar in a diabetic patient.[784]

8.6.20.1   Treatment of M. thermoresistibile Infections

In vitro sensitivity testing of a clinical isolate of *M. thermoresistibile* has shown resistance to isoniazid, *p*-aminosalicylic acid, and ethionamide, but susceptibility to ethambutol and rifampin, and moderate susceptibility to streptomycin.[782]

Treatment of a pulmonary infection with a combination of rifampin, ethambutol, and streptomycin led to clinical and radiologic improvement.[782]

Neeley and Denning[784] treated cutaneous lesions due to *M. thermoresistibile* with oral rifampin, ethambutol, and isoniazid. Even though the pathogen was isoniazid-resistant, the recovery was complete but slow.

8.6.21   MYCOBACTERIUM NEOAURUM

M. neoaurum is a scotochromogenic species which belongs to the group of rapidly growing mycobacteria. It was first isolated from soil in 1972,[785] but can also be recovered from other environmental sources, such as dust and water. When cultured on horse blood agar, *M. neoaurum* formed small, Gram-variable, acid-fast, smooth yellow colonies. The organisms grew at 25°C and 35°C, but not at 45°C.[786]

Human infections caused by *M. neoaurum* have been reported on at least two occasions and in both cases involved immunocompromised patients with Hickman catheters which seemed to be predisposing factors.[786,787]

8.6.21.1   Treatment of M. neoaurum Infections

In vitro susceptibility testing carried out by a disk diffusion assay on Mueller-Hinton agar (enriched with 10% oleic acid–albumin–dextrose–cathalase) has shown zones of inhibition of >30 mm in diameter by ticarcillin–clavulanic acid (85 μg disk), amikacin (30 μg), tetracycline (30 μg), cefoxitin (30 μg), imipenem (10 μg), ciprofloxacin (5 μg), erythromycin (15 μg), clarithromycin (15 μg), roxithromycin (15 μg), and azithromycin (15 μg). Tobramycin (10 μg) produced an inhibition zone of 25 mm, and trimethoprim-sulfamethoxazole (25 μg) a zone of less than 20 mm in diameter.[786]

Davison et al.[787] were the first to describe an *M. neoaurum* infection in an immunocompromised patient with a Hickman catheter *in situ*. The patient successfully recovered after a 7-week course of cefoxitin and gentamicin and without removal of the catheter.

In the second reported case of *M. neoaurum* infection, the Hickman catheter was removed and the patient, who was neutropenic after a bone marrow transplantation, was treated with ticarcillin–clavulanic acid (18 g daily) and tobramycin (18 mg, t.i.d.).[786]

8.6.22   MYCOBACTERIUM NONCHROMOGENICUM

M. nonchromogenicum is a slow-growing nonphotochromogenic mycobacterium found in soil, which has been rarely implicated as a human pathogen.[1] Several cases of pulmonary disease have been reported, all occurring in men 26 to 57 years old who had been involved in occupations predisposing to lung disease.[788] All clinical isolates from the patients were resistant *in vitro* to streptomycin, isoniazid, *p*-aminosalicylic acid (PAS), ethionamide, rifampin, and cycloserine, but susceptible to ethambutol. One of the patients died from cor pulmonale despite chemotherapy with ethambutol, isoniazid, and kanamycin. The patients who survived had their cavitary lesions resolved and sputum samples culture-negative after receiving treatment with rifampin, streptomycin, and isoniazid.[788]

Christensson et al.[789] have described an extrapulmonary involvement of *M. nonchromogenicum* in agricultural workers, presenting as subcutaneous infection of the hand.

Kawahara et al.[47] have studied the therapeutic potential of sparfloxacin against *M. nonchromogenicum*. The drug, when tested *in vitro* in Ogawa egg medium, showed a MIC value of 1.25 μg/ml.

8.6.23 MYCOBACTERIUM FLAVESCENS

M. flavescens, a scotochromogenic bacterium isolated from drug-treated tuberculous guinea pigs, has been considered nonpathogenic to humans. However, Casimir et al.[790] have reported a patient with metastatic melanoma who presented with dyspnea, cough, weight loss, and night sweats, as well as lung cavitation due to *M. flavescens*. A clinical isolate obtained from bronchial washings was sensitive to rifampin and resistant to streptomycin, PAS, ethambutol, and isoniazid. While treatment with ethambutol, rifampin, and isoniazid resulted in clinical improvement and negative sputum cultures, chest roentgenograms remained unchanged after 6 months of treatment.

8.6.24 MYCOBACTERIUM PARATUBERCULOSIS

8.6.24.1 Introduction

M. paratuberculosis is a Gram-positive, facultative acid-fast bacillus (AFB), measuring 0.5 μm by 1.5 μm. It is dependent on exogenous mycobactin, an iron-chelating agent produced by all mycobacteria, for *in vitro* growth. The colonies of *M. paratuberculosis*, which develop in 4 to 8 weeks, are small, white, glistening, and rough-smooth. However, occasional strains may produce yellow-to-orange pigments.[1]

Mycobacterium paratuberculosis is the causative agent of Johne's disease, a chronic, wasting enteritis widespread throughout the world and affecting most frequently cattle, sheep, goats, but also other ruminants (deer, rabbits).[791-793]

Although *M. paratuberculosis* has been considered nonpathogenic to humans, there has been evidence of its association with Crohn's disease.[794-799] As far back as 80 years ago, a Scottish surgeon, Dalziel, clearly described Crohn's disease and suggested that it might be caused by mycobacteria, but it was not until 1978 and 1984 that mycobacteria were isolated from tissue of patients with Crohn's disease.[800] Thus, Chiodini et al.[794] have isolated from resected terminal-ileum samples of patients with Crohn's disease an acid-fast bacillus, which developed primary colonies after 3 to 18 months of incubation. The organisms, which after optimal growth at 37°C measured 0.5 to 1.0 mm, were white, irregularly shaped, mucoid and rough. In addition, their growth was significantly enhanced when the medium was supplemented with mycobactin J (the mycobactin extracted from *M. paratuberculosis*). The biochemical profiles of all strains studied were identical, and while they did not conform to any of the presently known *Mycobacterium* species, they most closely resembled *M. paratuberculosis*.[794]

Further immunologic and *in vivo* studies have suggested a potential role for this *Mycobacterium* species in some cases of Crohn's disease. Thus, oral inoculation of a 7-d-old goat with one of these *Mycobacterium* strains (strain Linda), while not producing clinical disease during a 5-month observation, did allow for the development of both humoral and cell-mediated immunologic responses in 2 to 3 weeks; autopsy examination revealed the presence of granulomatous disease of the distal small intestine and regional lymph nodes.[795] Moreover, culture of one of the lymph nodes grew a *Mycobacterium* species with properties identical to those of the inoculum. In human experiments, Thayer et al.[796] examined sera of patients with Crohn's disease and found a statistically significant increase in the antibody titer to *M. paratuberculosis* as compared to healthy controls.

Recently, Molina et al.[801] studied the immune response of goats vaccinated with a live strain of *M. paratuberculosis* using a lymphocyte transformation assay and a counterimmunoelectrophoresis test. While proliferative response of blood lymphocyte to specific antigen did occur over a year postvaccination, there has been no humoral response.

Using serological assays highly specific for Crohn's disease (an immunoblot assay and an enzyme-linked immunosorbent assay utilizing the 45/48 kDa doublet antigen of *M. paratuberculosis*), Kreuzpaintner at al.[802] investigated the effect of intestinal resection on serum antibodies specific for Crohn's disease. Both the high specificity of the assays for Crohn's disease and the diminished antibody response after intestinal resection in parallel with a decreased Crohn's disease activity index (CDAI) value, supported a mycobacterial etiology of Crohn's disease. In another experiment, Lisby et al.[799] applied a nested primer polymerase chain reaction to detect the presence of an insertional element (IS900) specific for *M. paratuberculosis* in DNA extracted from fresh and from paraffin-embedded intestinal tissue obtained from patients undergoing surgery.

8.6.24.2 Treatment of *M. paratuberculosis* Infections

Mondal et al.[804] have elicited a marked clinical response in rabbits infected with *M. paratuberculosis* with streptomycin, rifampin, and levamisole given for 2 months. When treatment was extended to 4 weeks, a highly significant inhibition of leukocyte migration was also observed.

In vivo administration of a monoclonal antibody against type I IL-1 receptor inhibited the ability of mice to eliminate *M. paratuberculosis*, indicating a significant role for endogenous IL-1 in host defense against these organisms.[803] In another study aimed at evaluating the host defense against experimental paratuberculosis, purified anti-CD4+ or anti-CD8+ monoclonal antibodies were given to mice before intragastric challenge with *M. paratuberculosis* and on a biweekly basis for 6 months.[805] While the applied treatment resulted in a sustained depletion of CD4+ and CD8+ cells as measured by flow cytometry analysis of spleen cells from infected mice, the reduced titers of these cells did not enhance fecal shedding of mycobacteria, bacillary multiplication in the liver and ceca, nor histopathologic damage to the intestinal tract, mesenteric lymph nodes, spleen, and liver. The results suggested that cells other than CD4+ and CD8+ cells may be involved in the host defense against experimental paratuberculosis.[805]

Monensin sodium (0, 15, or 30 mg/kg of complete feed) was fed prophylactically *ad libitum* for 1 week to female C57BL6/J mice (genetically susceptible to infection with *M. paratuberculosis*). The mice were then inoculated intraperitoneally with *M. paratuberculosis* and 50 d later euthanatized. The results showed that while infected mice given the 50-mg/kg dose of monensin had higher body weight and fewer hepatic granulomas than mice not treated with monensin, acid-fast organisms were still present.[806]

BALB/c mice infected intraperitoneally with *M. paratuberculosis* were treated 30 d postinfection with rifabutin at daily doses of 0, 12.5, 25, and 50 mg/kg.[807] The entire dose was delivered by gavage within a 1-h period. Infection, as assessed by bacterial counts, was reduced only in animals receiving the 50-mg/kg dose.

Rutgeerts et al.[808] have treated resected ileocolonic Crohn's disease patients who had early evidence of recurrence with ethambutol and rifabutin. Since the patients failed to show improvement in the condition of intestinal lesions, the conclusion was made that antimycobacterial therapy had no effect on Crohn's disease. However, in view of the small number of patients involved, short treatment duration, and the little or no activity of ethambutol against *M. paratuberculosis*, some investigators have questioned the validity of this conclusion.[808]

Prantera et al.[809] have reported that two of five patients with Crohn's disease and high antimycobacterial antibody levels were cured with dapsone at 100 mg daily. Clinical improvement was evident after 1 month of therapy, with one of the patients showing complete healing of all cutaneous and rectal lesions.

8.6.25 *MYCOBACTERIUM SHIMOIDEI*

Heller et al.[810] have described a new, well-documented case of a tuberculosis-like cavity in the lung due to *M. shimoidei* infection in a patient with preexisting pulmonary lesions. The identification of the strain was accomplished by 16S ribosomal (rDNA) direct sequencing after *in vitro* amplification, and later confirmed by specific phenotypical tests and by chromatographic methods.

So far, the isolation of less than 10 not epidemiologically related strains of *M. shimoidei* (all originating from human pulmonary samples) has been reported worldwide.

8.6.26 MYCOBACTERIUM CELATUM

A disseminated infection caused by a new, slow-growing atypical mycobacteria, *M. celatum,* has been reported in an AIDS patient hospitalized with fever, cough, and weight loss.[811] The mycobacterial cultures from the sputum, blood, and the bronchoalveolar lavage became positive after 3 weeks of incubation. The organisms were identified as *M. celatum* by sequencing of the 16S rDNA gene.

8.6.27 PHYLOGENY OF FAST-GROWING MYCOBACTERIA

Using the dideoxynucleotide-terminated, primer extension method with cDNA generated by reverse transcriptase, Pitulle et al.[812] were able to partially sequence the 16S ribosomal RNAs (rRNAs) from nine rapidly growing *Mycobacteria*. Next, the sequences were aligned with 47 16S rRNA or DNA sequences which represented 30 previously known and 5 undescribed species of the genus *Mycobacterium*, and a dendrogram was constructed by utilizing equally weighted distance values. The data obtained confirmed the phylogenetic separation of the fast- and slow-growing mycobacteria and showed that the majority of the slowly growing members of the genus represent the most recently evolved organisms.

Furthermore, the 24 strains which represented 21 rapidly growing species constituted several sublines, which were defined by the following taxa: (1) *M. neoaurum* and *M. diernhoferi*; (2) *M. gadium*; (3) *M. kommossense*; (4) *M. sphagni*; (5) *M. fallax* and *M. chitae*; (6) *M. aurum* and *M. vaccae*; (7) the *M. flavescens* cluster; and (8) *M. chelonae* subsp. *abscessus*.[812]

Based on its metabolic and chemotaxonomic properties (unique fatty acid pattern, distinct physiologic properties, and unique primary structure of its ribosomal DNA), a new mycobacterial strain isolated from a fluoranthrene-polluted soil was characterized as *Mycobacterium hodleri*.[813] Phylogenetically, *M. hodleri* clustered with the fast-growing mycobacteria and has been closely related to *M. neoaurum* and *M. diernhoferi*.

8.6.28 REFERENCES

1. Woods, G. L. and Washington, J. A. II, Mycobacteria other than *Mycobacterium tuberculosis*: review of microbiologic and clinical aspects, *Rev. Infect. Dis.*, 9, 275, 1987.
2. Xia, X. X., Clinical analysis of 41 cases of pulmonary atypical mycobacteriosis, *Chung Hua Chieh Ho Ho Hsi Tsa Chih*, 15, 200, 1992.
3. Boggs, D. S., The changing spectrum of pulmonary infections due to nontuberculous mycobacteria, *J. Okla. State Med. Assoc.*, 88, 373, 1995.
4. Choudhri, S., Manfreda, J., Wolfe, J., Parker, S., and Long, R., Clinical significance of nontuberculous mycobacteria isolates in a Canadian tertiary care center, *Clin. Infect. Dis.*, 21, 128, 1995.
5. Hoffner, S. E., Pulmonary infections caused by less frequently encountered slow-growing environmental mycobacteria, *Eur. J. Clin. Microbiol. Infect. Dis.*, 13, 937, 1994.
6. Dautzenberg, B. and Mercat, A., Atypical mycobacterial infections, *Presse Med.*, 23, 1483, 1994.
7. Patel, R., Roberts, G. D., Keating, M. R., and Paya, C. V., Infections due to nontuberculous mycobacteria in kidney, heart, and liver transplant recipients, *Clin. Infect Dis.*, 19, 263, 1994.
8. Kozin, S. H. and Bishop, A. T., Atypical *Mycobacterium* infections of the upper extremity, *J. Hand Surg. (Am.)*, 19, 480, 1994.
9. Kennedy, T. P. and Weber, D. J., Nontuberculous mycobacteria: an underappreciated cause of geriatric lung disease, *Am. J. Respir. Dis.*, 149, 1654, 1994.

10. Idigbe, E. O., Nasidi, A., Anyiwo, C. E., Onubogu, C., Alabi, S., Okeye, R., Ugwu, O., and John, E. K., Prevalence of human immunodeficiency virus (HIV) antibodies in tuberculosis patients in Lagos, Nigeria, *J. Trop. Med. Hyg.*, 97, 91, 1994.

11. Georgiev, V. St., Treatment and developmental therapeutics of *Mycobacterium avium* complex (MAC) infections, *Int. J. Antimicrob. Agents*, 4, 247, 1994.

12. Bonafe, J. L., Grigorieff-Larrue, N., and Bauriaud, R., Atypical cutaneous mycobacterium diseases: results of a national survey, *Ann. Dermatol. Venereol.*, 119, 463, 1992.

13. Dautzenberg, B., Truffot, C., Mignon, A., Rozenbaum, W., Katlama, C., Perronne, C., Parrot, C., and Grosset, J., Rifabutin in combination with clofazimine, isoniazid and ethambutol in the treatment of AIDS patients with infections due to opportunistic mycobacteria, *Tubercle*, 72, 168, 1991.

14. Clague, H. W., el-Ansary, E. H., Hopkins, C. A., and Roberts, C., Pulmonary infection with opportunist mycobacteria on Merseyside 1974-1983, *Postgrad. Med. J.*, 62, 363, 1986.

15. Griffith, D. E., Girard, W. M., and Wallace, R. J., Jr., Clinical features of pulmonary disease caused by rapidly growing mycobacteria: an analysis of 154 patients, *Am. Rev. Respir. Dis.*, 147, 1271, 1993.

16. Wallace, R. J., Jr., The clinical presentation, diagnosis, and therapy of cutaneous and pulmonary infections due to the rapidly growing mycobacteria, *M. fortuitum* and *M. chelonae*, *Clin. Chest Med.*, 10, 419, 1989.

17. Contreras, M. A., Cheung, O. T., Sanders, D. E., and Goldstein, R. S., Pulmonary infection with nontuberculous mycobacteria, *Am. Rev. Respir. Dis.*, 137, 149, 1988.

18. Martinez Moragon, E., Menendez, R., Santos, M., Lorente, R., and Marco, V., Lung diseases due to opportunistic environmental mycobacteria in patients uninfected with human immunodeficiency virus, *Arch. Bronconeumol.*, 32, 170, 1996.

19. Kurasawa, T., Ikeda, N., Sato, A., Nakatani, K. et al., A clinical study of non-tuberculous pulmonary mycobacteriosis, *Kekkaku*, 70, 621, 1995.

20. Skogberg, K., Ruutu, P., Tukiainen, P., and Valtonen, V. V., Nontuberculous mycobacterial infection in HIV-negative patients receiving immunosuppressive therapy, *Eur. J. Clin. Microbiol. Infect. Dis.*, 14, 755, 1995.

21. Molina-Gamboa, J. D., Ponce-de-Leon, S., Sifuentes-Osornio, J., Bobadilla del Valle, M., and Ruiz-Palacios, G. M., Mycobacterial infection in Mexican AIDS patients, *J. Acquir. Immune Defic. Syndr. Hum. Retrovirol.*, 11, 53, 1996.

22. Raszka, W. V., Jr., Skillman, L. P., McEvoy, P. L., and Robb, M. L., Isolation of nontuberculous, non-*avium* mycobacteria from patients infected with human immunodeficiency virus, *Clin. Infect. Dis.*, 20, 73, 1995.

23. Furrer, H., Bodmer, T., and von Overbeck, J., Disseminated nontuberculous mycobacterial infections in AIDS patients, *Schweiz. Med. Wochenschr.*, 124, 89, 1994.

24. Davies, P. D., Infection with *Mycobacterium kansasii*, *Thorax*, 49, 435, 1994.

25. Grange, J. M. and Yates, M. D., Infections caused by opportunistic mycobacteria: a review, *J. R. Soc. Med.*, 79, 226, 1986.

26. Runyon, E. H., Anonymous mycobacteria in pulmonary disease, *Med. Clin. North Am.*, 43, 273, 1959.

27. Noel, S. B., Ray, M. C., and Greer, D. L., Cutaneous infection with *Mycobacterium avium-intracellulare scrofulaceum* intermediate: a new pathogenic entity, *J. Am. Acad. Dermatol.*, 19, 492, 1988.

28. Gruft, H., Falkinham, J. O. III, and Parker, B. C., Recent experience in the epidemiology of disease caused by atypical mycobacteria, *Rev. Infect. Dis.*, 3, 990, 1981.

29. Wongwatana, S. and Sriyabhaya, N., Nontuberculous mycobacterial infection of the lung in a chest hospital in Thailand, *J. Med. Assoc. Thai.*, 75, 1, 1992.

30. Zvetina, J. R., Maliwan, N., Frederick, W. E., and Reyes, C., *Mycobacterium kansasii* infection following primary pulmonary malignancy, *Chest*, 102, 1460, 1992.

31. Campbell, I. A., Treatment of pulmonary disease caused by *Mycobacterium kansasii*, results of 18 vs. 12 months' chemotherapy (comment), *Tuber. Lung Dis.*, 76, 583, 1995.

32. White, R., Abreo, K., Flanagan, R., Gadallah, M., Krane, K., el-Shahawy, M., Shakamuri, S., and McKoy, R., Nontuberculous mycobacterial infections in continuous ambulatory peritoneal dialysis patients, *Am. J. Kidney Dis.*, 22, 581, 1993.

33. O'Brien, R. J., Geiter, L. J., and Snider, D. E., Jr., The epidemiology of nontuberculous mycobacterial diseases in the United States: results from a national survey, *Am. Rev. Respir. Dis.*, 135, 1007, 1987.

34. Joint Position Paper of the American Thoracic Society and the Centers for Disease Control. Myco-bacteriosis and the acquired immunodeficiency syndrome, *Am. Rev. Respir. Dis.*, 136, 492, 1987.

35. Veale, D., Fishwick, D., White, J. E., Gascoigne, A. D., Gould, K., and Corris, P. A., Culture of *Mycobacterium kansasii* in the blood of an HIV-negative patient, *Thorax*, 48, 672, 1993.

36. Wolinsky, E., Mycobacterial diseases other than tuberculosis, *Clin. Infect. Dis.*, 15, 1, 1992.

37. Heurlin, N. and Petrini, B., Treatment of non-tuberculous mycobacterial infections in patients without AIDS, *Scand. J. Infect. Dis.*, 25, 619, 1993.

38. Hornick, D. B., Dayton, C. S., Bedell, G. N., and Fick, R. B., Jr., Nontuberculous mycobacterial lung disease: substantiation of a less aggressive approach, *Chest*, 93, 550, 1988.

39. Al Jarad, N., Demertzis, P., Jones, D. J., Barnes, N. C., Rudd, R. M., Gaya, H., Wedzicha, J. A., Hughes, D. T., and Empey, D. W., Comparison of characteristics of patients and treatment outcome for pulmonary non-tuberculous mycobacterial infection and pulmonary tuberculosis, *Thorax*, 51, 137, 1996.

40. Tsukamura, M. and Yamori, S., Chemotherapeutic regimens for nontuberculous mycobacterial infec-tion based on in-vitro susceptibility test results, *Kekkaku*, 65, 349, 1990.

41. Brodt, H. R., Current therapy of atypical mycobacterial infections, *Immun. Infekt.*, 20, 39, 1992.

42. Neubert, R., Resistant behavior of atypical mycobacteria to antibiotics and sulfonamides, *Z. Erkr. Atmungsorgane*, 167, 47, 1986.

43. Vandiviere, H. M., Dillon, M., and Melvin, I. G., Atypical mycobacteria causing pulmonary disease: rapid diagnosis using skin test profiles, *South. Med. J.*, 80, 5, 1987.

44. Inagaki, K., Arai, T., Yano, M., Komatsu, H., Murakami, K., Koyama, A., Anno, H., Yamamoto, H., and Imura, Y., Role of surgical treatment in atypical mycobacteriosis of the lung, *Kekkaku*, 66, 769, 1991.

45. Plaus, W. J. and Hermann, G., The surgical management of superficial infections caused by atypical mycobacteria, *Surgery*, 110, 99, 1991.

46. Rastogi, N., Goh, K. S., Guillou, N., and Labrousse, V., Spectrum of drugs against atypical mycobac-teria: how valid is the current practice of drug susceptibility testing and the choice of drugs? *Int. J. Med. Microbiol. Virol. Parasitol. Infect. Dis.*, 277, 474, 1992.

47. Kawahara, S., Tada, A., Takeuchi, M., Kamisaka, K., Okada, C., Mishima, Y., Soda, R., Takahashi, K., Kibata, M., Nagare, H. et al., Therapeutic potential of sparfloxacin for preventing mycobacterial infections, *Kekkaku*, 69, 351, 1994.

48. Tomioka, H., Sato, K., and Saito, H., Antimycobacterial activities of a new quinolone, sparfloxacin, *Kekkaku*, 66, 643, 1991.

49. Wallace, R. J., Jr., Bedsole, G., Sumter, G., Sanders, C. V., Steele, L. C., Brown, B. A., Smith, J., and Graham, D. R., Activities of ciprofloxacin and ofloxacin against rapidly growing mycobacteria with demonstration of acquired resistance following single-drug therapy, *Antimicrob. Agents Chemother.*, 34, 65, 1990.

50. Tomioka, H., Sato, K., and Saito, H., Comparative *in vitro* and *in vivo* activity of fleroxacin and ofloxacin in various mycobacteria, *Tubercle*, 72, 176, 1991.

51. Truffot-Pernot, C., Ji, B., and Grosset, J., Activities of perfloxacin and ofloxacin against mycobacteria: *in vitro* and mouse experiments, *Tubercle*, 72, 57, 1991.

52. Saito, H., Tomioka, H., Sato, K., and Dekio, S., *In vitro* and *in vivo* antimycobacterial activities of a new quinolone, DU-6859a, *Antimicrob. Agents Chemother.*, 38, 2877, 1994.

53. Tsukamura, M., Evalution of clinical efficacy of isoniazid and ethambutol in the treatment of nontuberculous mycobacteriosis based on *in vitro* susceptibility testing, *Kekkaku*, 64, 511, 1989.

54. Ashtekar, D. R., Costa-Periera, R., Shrinivasan, T., Iyyer, R., Vishvanathan, N., and Rittel, W., Oxazo-lidinones, a new class of synthetic antituberculosis agent: *in vitro* and *in vivo* activities of DuP-721 against *Mycobacterium tuberculosis*, *Diagn. Microbiol. Infect. Dis.*, 14, 465, 1991.

55. Tsukamura, M., Evaluation of clinical efficacy of rifampicin in the treatment of nontuberculous mycobacteriosis from *in vitro* susceptibility testing, *Kekkaku*, 64, 453, 1989.

56. Klemens, S. P. and Cynamon, M. H., Activities of azithromycin and clarithromycin against nontuber-culous mycobacteria in beige mice, *Antimicrob. Agents Chemother.*, 38, 1455, 1994.

57. Rapp, R. P., McCraney, S. A., Goodman, N. L., and Shadduck, D. J., New macrolide antibiotics: usefulness in infections caused by mycobacteria other than *Mycobacteria tuberculosis*, *Ann. Pharmacother.*, 28, 1255, 1994.

58. Heifets, L. B., Antimycobacterial drugs, *Semin. Respir. Infect.*, 9, 84, 1994 (correction in *Semin. Respir. Infect.*, 10, 121, 1995).

59. Collins, F. M., Mycobacterial disease, immunosuppression, and acquired immunodeficiency syndrome, *Clin. Microbiol. Rev.*, 2, 360, 1989.

60. Collins, F. M., *M. avium*-complex infections and immunodeficiency, in *Mycobacterium tuberculosis — Interactions with the Immune System*, Freedman, H. and Bendinelli, M., Eds., Plenum Press, New York, 1988, 389.

61. Collins, F. M., Morrison, N. E., and Montalbine, V., Immune response to persistent mycobacterial infection in mice, *Infect. Immun.*, 19, 430, 1978.

62. Farhi, D. C., Mason, U. G., and Horsburgh, C. R., Pathologic findings in disseminated *M. avium-intracellulare* infection, *Am. J. Clin. Pathol.*, 85, 67, 1986.

63. Horsburgh, C. R., Mason, V. G., Farhi, D. C., and Iseman, M. D., Disseminated infection with *M. avium-intracellulare*: a report of 13 cases and a review of the literature, *Medicine (Baltimore)*, 64, 36, 1985.

64. Schaefer, W. B., Incidence of serotypes of *M. avium* and atypical mycobacteria in human and animal disease, *Am. Rev. Respir. Dis.*, 97, 18, 1968.

65. Schaefer, W. B., Davis, C. L., and Cohn, M. L., Pathogenicity of translucent, opaque, and rough variants of *M. avium* in chickens and mice, *Am. Rev. Respir. Dis.*, 102, 499, 1970.

66. Crawford, J. T. and Bates, J. H., Phage typing of the *M. avium-intracellulare-scrofulaceum* complex: a study of strains of diverse geographic and host origin, *Am. Rev. Respir. Dis.*, 132, 386, 1985.

67. Meissner, P. S. and Falkinham, J. O., Plasmid DNA profiles as epidemiological markers for clinical and environmental isolates of *M. avium*, *M. intracellulare* and *M. scrofulaceum*, *J. Infect. Dis.*, 153, 325, 1986.

68. Moulding, T., The relative drug-susceptibility of opaque colonial forms of *M. intracellulare-avium*: does it affect therapeutic results? *Am. Rev. Respir. Dis.*, 117, 1142, 1978.

69. Gangadharam, P. R. J., Perumal, V. K., Crawford, J. T., and Bates, J. H., Association of plasmids and virulence of *M. avium*-complex, *Am. Rev. Respir. Dis.*, 137, 212, 1988.

70. Crawford, J. T. and Bates, J. H., Analysis of plasmids in *M. avium-intracellulare* isolates from persons with acquired immunodeficiency syndrome, *Am. Rev. Respir. Dis.*, 134, 659, 1986.

71. Collins, F. M., *M. avium*-complex infections and development of the acquired immunodeficiency syndrome: casual opportunist or casual cofactor, *Int. J. Leprosy*, 54, 458, 1986.

72. Horsburgh, C. R. and Selik, R. M., The epidemiology of disseminated tuberculous mycobacterial infection in the acquired immunodeficiency syndrome (AIDS), *Am. Rev. Respir. Dis.*, 139, 4, 1989.

73. Good, R. C. and Snider, D. E., Jr., Isolation of nontuberculous mycobacteria in the United Sates, 1980, *J. Infect. Dis.*, 146, 829, 19982.

74. Good, R. C., Opportunistic pathogens in the genus *Mycobacterium*, *Annu. Rev. Microbiol.*, 39, 347, 1986.

75. McClatchy, J. K., The seroagglutination test in the study of nontuberculous mycobacteria, *Rev. Infect. Dis.*, 3, 867, 1981.

76. Quinn, T. C., Mann, J. M., Curran, J. W., and Piot, P., AIDS in Africa: an epidimiological paradigm, *Science*, 234, 955, 1986.

77. Lamoureux, G., Davignon, L., Turcotte, R., Leverdier, M., Mankiewicz, E., and Walker, M. C., Is prior mycobacterial infection a common predisposing factor to AIDS in Haitians and Africans? *Ann. Inst. Pasteur*, 138, 521, 1987.

78. Anonymous, Clinical features of AIDS in Europe, *Eur. J. Cancer Clin. Oncol.*, 20, 165, 1984.

79. Pinching, A. J., Acquired immune deficiency syndrome: with special reference to tuberculosis, *Tubercle*, 68, 65, 1987.

80. Goldman, K. P., AIDS and tuberculosis, *Tubercle*, 69, 71, 1988.

81. Meissner, P.S. and Falkinham, J. O., Plasmid DNA profiles as epidemiologic markers for clinical and environmental isolates of *Mycobacterium avium*, *Mycobacterium intracellulare*, and *Mycobacterium scrofulaceum*, *J. Infect. Dis.*, 153, 325, 1986.

82. Perronne, C., Mycobacterial infections in AIDS, *Rev. Prat.*, 45, 729, 1995.

83. Meissner, G. and Anz, W., Sources of *Mycobacterium avium*-complex infection resulting in human disease, *Am. Rev. Respir. Dis.*, 116, 1057, 1977.

84. Macher, A.M., Kovacs, J. A., Gill, V., Roberts, G. D., Ames, J., Park, C. H., Straus, S., Lane, H. C., Parrillo, J. E., Fauci, A. S., and Masur, H., Bacteremia due to *Mycobacterium avium-intracellulare* in the acquired immunodeficiency syndrome, *Ann. Intern. Med.*, 99, 782, 1983.

85. Greene, J. B., Sidhu, G. S., Lewin, S., Levine, J. F., Masur, H., Simberkoff, M. S., Nicholas, P., Good, R. C., Zolla-Pazner, S. B., Pollock, A. A., Tapper, M. L., and Holzman, R. S., *Mycobacterium avium-intracellulare*: a cause of disseminated life-threatening infection in homosexuals and drug abusers, *Ann. Intern. Med.*, 97, 539, 1982.

86. Wallace, R. J., Jr., O'Brien, R., Glassroth, J., Raleigh, J., and Dutt, A., Diagnosis and treatment of disease caused by nontuberculosis mycobacteria, *Am. Rev. Respir. Dis.*, 142, 940, 1990.

87. Damsker, B. and Bottone, E. J., *Mycobacterium avium-Mycobacterium intracellulare* from the intestinal tracts of patients with acquired immunodeficiency syndrome: concepts regarding acquisition and pathogenesis, *J. Infect. Dis.*, 151, 179, 1985.

88. Lerner, C. W. and Tapper, M. L., Opportunistic infection complicating acquired immunodeficiency syndrome, *Medicine (Baltimore)*, 63, 155, 1984.

89. Fauci, A. S., Masur, H., Gelmann, E. P., Markham, P. B., Hahn, B. H., and Lane, H. C., The acquired immunodeficiency syndrome: an update, *Ann. Intern. Med.* 102, 800, 1985.

90. Hawkins, C. C., Gold, J. W. M., Whimbey, E., Kiehn, T. E., Brannon, P., Cammarata, R., Brown, A. E., and Armstrong, D., *Mycobacterium avium*-complex infections in patients with acquired immunodeficiency syndrome, *Ann. Intern. Med.*, 105, 184, 1986.

91. Snider, D. E., Hopewell, P. C., Mills, J., and Reichman, L. B., Mycobacteriosis and the acquired immunodeficiency syndrome, *Am. Rev. Respir. Dis.*, 136, 492, 1987.

92. Moroni, M., Gori, A., Rusconi, S., Franzetti, F., and Antinori, S., Mycobacterial infections in AIDS: an overview of epidemiology, clinical manifestations, therapy and prophylaxis, *Monaldi Arch. Chest Dis.*, 49, 432, 1994.

93. Benson, C., Disseminated *Mycobacterium avium* complex disease in patients with AIDS, *AIDS Res. Hum. Retroviruses*, 10, 913, 1994.

94. Mehta, J. B. and Morris, F., Impact of HIV infection on mycobacterial disease, *Am. Fam. Physician*, 45, 2203, 1992.

95. Wallace, J. M. and Hannah, J. B., *Mycobacterium avium* complex infection in patients with the acquired immunodeficiency syndrome, *Chest*, 93, 926, 1988.

96. Kiehn, T. E., Edwards, F. F., Brannon, P., Tsang, A. Y., Maio, M., Gold, J. W. M., Whimbey, E., Wong, B., McClatchy, J. K., and Armstrong, D., Infections caused by *Mycobacterium avium* complex in immunocompromised patients: diagnosis by blood culture and fecal examination, antimicrobial susceptibility tests, and morphological and seroagglutination characteristics, *J. Clin. Microbiol.*, 21, 168, 1985.

97. Crawford, J. T. and Bates, J. H., Analysis of plasmids in *Mycobacterium avium-intracellulare* isolates from persons with acquired immunodeficiency syndrome, *Am. Rev. Respir. Dis.*, 134, 659, 1986.

98. Sato, K., Tomioka, H., and Saito, H., Differential susceptibilities of *Mycobacterium avium* and *Mycobacterium intracellulare* to sodium nitrite, *J. Clin. Microbiol.*, 30, 2994, 1992.

99. McFadden, J. J., Kunze, Z. M., Portaels, F., Labrousse, V., and Rastogi, N., Epidemiological and genetic markers, virulence factors and intracellular growth of *Mycobacterium avium* in AIDS, *Res. Microbiol.*, 143, 423, 1992.

100. Flegg, P. J., Laing, R. B., Lee, C., Harris, G. et al., Disseminated disease due to *Mycobacterium avium* complex in AIDS, *Q. J. Med.*, 88, 617, 1995.

101. Bermudez, L. E., Infection of "nonprofessional phagocytes" with *Mycobacterium avium* complex, *Clin. Immunol. Immunopathol.*, 61, 225, 1991.

102. Harshan, K. V. and Gangadharam, P. R., *In vivo* depletion of natural killer cell activity leads to enhanced multiplication of *Mycobacterium avium* complex in mice, *Infect. Immun.*, 59, 2818, 1991.

103. Torriani, F. J., Behling, C. A., McCutchan, J. A., Haubrich, R. H., and Havlir, D. V., Disseminated *Mycobacterium avium* complex: correlation between blood and tissue burden, *J. Infect. Dis.*, 173, 942, 1996.

104. Finkelstein, D. M., Williams, P. L., Molenberghs, G., Feinberg, J., Powderly, W. G., Kahn, J., Dolin, R., and Cotton, D., Patterns of opportunistic infections in patients with HIV infection, *J. Acquir. Immune Defic. Syndr. Hum. Retrovirol.*, 12, 38, 1996.

105. Claass, A., Claviez, A., Westphal, E., Rusch-Gerdes, S., and Schneppenheim, R., First case of disseminated *Mycobacterium avium* infection, *Infection*, 23, 301, 1995.

106. Sussman, S. J., Sinusitis caused by *Mycobacterium avium-intracellulare* in a patient with human immunodeficiency virus, *Pediatr. Infect. Dis. J.*, 14, 726, 1995.

107. Sato, K., Tomioka, H., Maw, W. W., and Saito, H., Mechanism of bacterial regrowth at the sites of infection in *Mycobacterium avium* complex-infected mice during treatment with chemotherapeutic agents, *Kekkaku*, 70, 673, 1995.

108. Tomioka, H., Sato, K., and Saito, H., *In vitro* susceptibilities of *Mycobacterium avium* and *Mycobacterium intracellulare* to various drugs, *Kekkaku*, 66, 489, 1991.

109. Sison, J. P., Yao, Y., Kemper, C. A., Hamilton, J. R., Brummer, E., Stevens, D. A., and Deresinski, S. C., Treatment of *Mycobacterium avium* complex infection: do the results of *in vitro* susceptibility tests predict therapeutic outcome in humans? *J. Infect. Dis.*, 173, 677, 1996.

110. Jacobs, M. R., Activity of quinolones against mycobacteria, *Drugs*, 49(Suppl. 2), 67, 1995.

111. Yajko, D. M., Sanders, C. A., Nassos, P. S., and Hadley, W. K., *In vitro* susceptibility of *Mycobacterium avium* complex to the new fluoroquinolone sparfloxacin (CI-978; AT-4140) and comparison with ciprofloxacin, *Antimicrob. Agents Chemother.*, 34, 2442, 1990.

112. Gevaudan, M. J., Bollet, C., Mallet, M. N., de Lamballerie, X., Sambuc, R., and de Micco, P., Extracellular and intracellular activity of sparfloxacin against *Mycobacterium avium* complex and *Mycobacterium xenopi*, *Pathol. Biol. (Paris)*, 40, 443, 1992.

113. Rastogi, N., Labrousse, V., Goh, K. S., and De Sousa, J. P., Antimycobacterial spectrum of sparfloxacin and its activities alone and in association with other drugs against *Mycobacterium avium* complex growing extracellularly and intracellularly in murine and human macrophages, *Antimicrob. Agents Chemother.*, 35, 2473, 1991.

114. Babinchak, T. J. and Fass, R. J., *In vitro* activity of DNA gyrase inhibitors, singly and in combination, against *Mycobacterium avium* complex, *Diagn. Microbiol. Infect. Dis.*, 15, 367, 1992.

115. Oh, Y. K., Nix, D. E., and Straubinger, R. M., Formulation and efficacy of liposome-encapsulated antibiotics for therapy of intracellular *Mycobacterium avium* infection, *Antimicrob. Agents Chemother.*, 39, 2104, 1995.

116. Byrne, S. K., Geddes, G. L., Isaac-Renton, J. L., and Black, W. A., Comparison of *in vitro* antimicrobial susceptibilities of *Mycobacterium avium–M. intracellulare* strains from patients with acquired immunodeficiency syndrome (AIDS), patients without AIDS, and animal sources, *Antimicrob. Agents Chemother.*, 34, 1390, 1990.

117. Inderlied, C. B., Lancero, M. G., Bermudez, L. M., and Young, L. S., *In vitro* activity of lomefloxacin as compared with ciprofloxacin, *Diagn. Microbiol. Infect. Dis.*, 12(Suppl. 3), 17S, 1989.

118. Heifets, L. B. and Lindholm-Levy, P. J., MICs and MBCs of Win 57273 against *Mycobacterium avium* and *M. tuberculosis*, *Antimicrob. Agents Chemother.*, 34, 770, 1990.

119. Cohen, Y., Perronne, C., Truffot-Pernot, C., Grosset, J., Vildé, J. L., and Pocidalo, J. J., Activities of WIN-57273, minocycline, clarithromycin, and 14-hydroxyclarithromycin against *Mycobacterium avium* complex in human macrophages, *Antimicrob. Agents Chemother.*, 36, 2104, 1992.

120. Barrett, M. S., Jones, R. N., Erwin, M. E., and Koontz, F. P., CI-960 (PD 127391 or AM-1091), sparfloxacin, WIN 57273, and isepamicin activity against clinical isolates of *Mycobacterium avium-intracellulare* complex, *M. chelonae*, and *M. fortuitum*, *Diagn. Microbiol. Infect. Dis.*, 15, 169, 1992.

121. Patil, M. A., Katoch, V. M., Venkatesan, K., Sharma, V. D., Shivannar, C. T., Kanaujia, G. V., and Agrawal, B. M., Correlation between inhibitory effect of quinolones and mycolic acid metabolism in mycobacteria, *Indian J. Lepr.*, 64, 331, 1992.

122. Heifets, L. B., Lindholm-Levy, P. J., and Flory, M. A., Bactericidal activity *in vitro* of various rifamycins against *Mycobacterium avium* and *Mycobacterium tuberculosis*, *Am. Rev. Respir. Dis.*, 141, 626, 1990.

123. Furney, S. K., Roberts, A. D., and Orme, I. M., Effect of rifabutin on disseminated *Mycobacterium avium* infections in thymectomized, CD4 T-cell- deficient mice, *Antimicrob. Agents Chemother.*, 34, 1629, 1990.

124. Saito, H. and Sato, K., Activity of rifabutin alone and in combination with clofazimine, kanamycin and ethambutol against *Mycobacterium intracellulare* infections in mice, *Tubercle*, 70, 201, 1989.

125. Gevaudan, M. J., Mallet, M. N., Bollet, C., Gulian, C., and de Micco, P., Bacteriostatic and bactericidal study of rifabutin and clofazimine in combination against *Mycobacterium avium-intracellulare* and *Mycobacterium xenopi*, *Pathol. Biol. (Paris)*, 37, 585, 1989.

126. Klemens, S. P. and Cynamon, M. H., Activity of rifapentine against *Mycobacterium avium* infection in beige mice, *J. Antimicrob. Chemother.*, 29, 555, 1992.

127. Tsukamura, M., Ichiyama, S., and Miyachi, T., Superiority of enviomycin or streptomycin over ethambutol in initial treatment of lung disease caused by *Mycobacterium avium* complex, *Chest*, 95, 1056, 1989.

128. Tsukamura, M. and Miyachi, T., Correlations among naturally occurring resistance to antituberculosis drugs in *Mycobacterium avium* complex strains, *Am. Rev. Respir. Dis.*, 139, 1033, 1989.

129. Seydel, J. K., Schaper, K. J., and Rüsch-Gerdes, S., Development of effective drug combinations for the inhibition of multiply resistant mycobacteria, especially of the *Mycobacterium avium* complex, *Chemotherapy*, 38, 159, 1992.

130. Seydel, J. K. and Schaper, K. J., A new, highly synergistic drug combination for the treatment of infections with multiresistant mycobacteria, especially the *Mycobacterium avium* complex, *Immun. Infekt.*, 20, 46, 1992.

131. Yamori, S. and Tsukamura, M., Paradoxical effect of Tween 80 between the susceptibility to rifampicin and streptomycin and the susceptibility to ethambutol and sulfadimethoxine in the *Mycobacterium avium–Mycobacterium intracellulare* complex, *Microbiol. Immunol.*, 35, 921, 1991.

132. Kuze, F., Antimycobacterial activities of rifamycin derivatives, *Kekkaku*, 66, 679, 1991.

133. Tomioka, H. and Saito, H., Studies on therapeutic efficacy of a new anti-tuberculous drug, benzoxazinorifamycin, against murine experimental mycobacterial infections: attempt at various regimens and protocols, *Kekkaku*, 69, 703, 1994.

134. Yamane, T., Hashizume, T., Yamashita, K., Konishi, E., Hosoe, K., Hidaka, T., Watanabe, K., Kawahadara, H., Yamamoto, T., and Kuze, F., Synthesis and biological activity of 3'-hydroxy-5'-aminobenzoxazinorifamycin derivatives, *Chem. Pharm. Bull.*, 41, 148, 1993.

135. Yamamoto, T., Amitani, R., Kuze, F., and Suzuki, K., *In vitro* activities of new rifamycin derivatives against *Mycobacterium tuberculosis* and *M. avium* complex, *Kekkaku*, 65, 805, 1990.

136. Kuze, F., Yamamoto, T., Amitani, R., and Suzuki, K., *In vivo* activity of new rifamycin derivatives against mycobacteria, *Kekkaku*, 66, 7, 1991.

137. Emori, M., Saito, H., Sato, K., Tomioka, H., Setogawa, T., and Hidaka, T., Therapeutic efficacy of the benzoxazinorifamycin KRM-1648 against experimental *Mycobacterium avium* infection induced in rabbits, *Antimicrob. Agents Chemother,*, 37, 722, 1993.

138. Saito, H., Tomioka, H., Sato, K., Kawahara, S., Hidaka, T., and Dekio, S., Therapeutic effect of KRM-1648 with various antimicrobials against *Mycobacterium avium* complex infection in mice, *Tuber. Lung Dis.*, 76, 51, 1995.

139. Bermudez, L. E., Kolonoski, P., Young, L. S., and Inderlied, C. B., Activity of KRM 1648 alone or in combination with ethambutol or clarithromycin against *Mycobacterium avium* in beige mouse model of disseminated infection, *Antimicrob. Agents Chemother.*, 38, 1844, 1994.

140. Saito, H., Tomioka, H., Sato, K., and Hidaka, T., Therapeutic efficacy of a benzoxazinorifamycin, KRM-1648, in *Mycobacterium intracellulare* infection induced in mice, *Kekkaku*, 69, 59, 1994.

141. Tomioka, H., Sato, K., Saito, H., and Hidaka, T., Therapeutic efficacy of a benzoxazinorifamycin, KRM-1648, combined with an immunopotentiator, LC9018, in *Mycobacterium intracellulare* infection induced in beige mice, *Kekkaku*, 68, 751, 1993.

142. Tomioka, H., Sato, K., Saito, H., Dekio, S., and Hidaka, T., Therapeutic efficacy of a benzoxazinorifamycin, KRM-1648, administered in various frequencies per week in *Mycobacterium intracellulare*-infected mice, *Kekkaku*, 68, 683, 1993.

143. Tomioka, H., Sato, K., Saito, H., and Hidaka, T., Therapeutic efficacy of a benzoxazinorifamycin, KRM-1648, administered at the different periods of infection in *Mycobacterium intracellulare*-infected mice, *Kekkaku*, 68, 631, 1993.

144. Tomioka, H., Saito, H., Sato, K., Yamane, T., Yamashita, K., Hosoe, K., Fujii, K., and Hidaka, T., Chemotherapeutic efficacy of a newly synthesized benzoxazinorifamycin, KRM-1648, against *Mycobacterium avium* complex infection in mice, *Antimicrob. Agents Chemother.*, 36, 387, 1992.

145. Reddy, V. M., Nadadhur, G., Daneluzzi, D., Dimova, V., and Gangadharam, P. R., Antimycobacterial activity of a new rifamycin derivative, 3-(4- cinnamylpiperazinyl iminomethyl) rifamycin SV (T9), *Antimicrob. Agents Chemother.*, 39, 2320, 1995.

146. Ashtekar, D., Düzgünes, N., and Gangadharam, P. R., Activity of free and liposome encapsulated streptomycin against *Mycobacterium avium* complex (MAC) inside peritoneal macrophages, *J. Antimicrob. Chemother.*, 28, 615, 1991.

147. Düzgünes, N., Ashtekar, D. R., Flasher, D. L., Ghori, N., Debs, R. J., Friend, D. S., and Gangadharam, P. R., Treatment of *Mycobacterium avium-intracellulare* complex infection in beige mice with free and liposome-encapsulated streptomycin: role of liposome type and duration of treatment, *J. Infect. Dis.*, 164, 143, 1991.

148. Gangadharam, P. R., Ashtekar, D. A., Ghori, N., Goldstein, J. A., Debs, R. J., and Düzgünes, N., Chemotherapeutic potential of free and liposome encapsulated streptomycin against experimental *Mycobacterium avium* complex infections in beige mice, *J. Antimicrob. Chemother.*, 28, 425, 1991.

149. Majumdar, S., Flasher, D., Friend, D. S., Nassos, P., Yajko, D., Hadley, W. K., and Düzgünes, N., Efficacies of liposome-encapsulated streptomycin and ciprofloxacin against *Mycobacterium avium-intracellulare* complex infections in human peripheral blood monocyte/macrophages, *Antimicrob. Agents Chemother.*, 36, 2808, 1992.

150. Gangadharam, P. R., Ashtekar, D. R., Flasher, D. L., and Düsgünes, N., Therapy of *Mycobacterium avium* complex infections in beige mice with streptomycin encapsulated in sterically stabilized liposomes, *Antimicrob. Agents Chemother.*, 39, 725, 1995.

151. Heifets, L. and Lindholm-Levy, P., Comparison of bactericidal activities of streptomycin, amikacin, kanamycin, and capreomycin against *Mycobacterium avium* and *M. tuberculosis*, *Antimicrob. Agents Chemother.*, 33, 1298, 1989.

152. Inderlied, C. B., *In vitro* activity of amikacin against *Mycobacterium avium*, *Antimicrob. Agents Chemother.*, 34, 378, 1990.

153. Yamori, S., Ichiyama, S., Shimokata, K., and Tsukamura, M., Bacteriostatic and bactericidal activity of antituberculosis drugs against *Mycobacterium tuberculosis*, *Mycobacterium avium-Mycobacterium intracellulare* complex and *Mycobacterium kansasii* in different growth phases, *Microbiol. Immunol.*, 36, 361, 1992.

154. Tomioka, H., Saito, H., Sato, K., and Yoneyama, T., Therapeutic efficacy of liposome-encapsulated kanamycin against *Mycobacterium intracellulare* infection induced in mice, *Am. Rev. Respir. Dis.*, 144, 575, 1991.

155. Inderlied, C. B., Young, L. S., and Yamada, J. K., Determination of *in vitro* susceptibility of *Mycobacterium avium* complex isolates to antimycobacterial agents by various methods, *Antimicrob. Agents Chemother.*, 31, 1697, 1987.

156. Inderlied, C. B., Kolonoski, P. T., Wu, M., and Young, L. S., Amikacin, ciprofloxacin, and imipenem treatment for disseminated *Mycobacterium avium* complex infection of beige mice, *Antimicrob. Agents Chemother.*, 33, 176, 1989.

157. Kesavalu, L., Goldstein, J. A., Debs, R. J., Düzgünes, N., and Gangadharam, P. R., Differential effects of free and liposome encapsulated amikacin on the survival of *Mycobacterium avium* complex in mouse peritoneal macrophages, *Tubercle*, 71, 215, 1990.

158. Bermudez, L. E., Yau-Young, A. O., Lin, J. P., Cogger, J., and Young, L. S., Treatment of disseminated *Mycobacterium avium* complex infection of beige mice with liposome-encapsulated aminoglycosides, *J. Infect. Dis.*, 161, 1262, 1990.

159. Bermudez, L. E., Wu, M., Young, L. S., and Inderlied, C. B., Postantibiotic effect of amikacin and rifapentine against *Mycobacterium avium* complex, *J. Infect. Dis.*, 166, 923, 1992.

160. Heifets, L. B., Lindholm-Levy, P. J., and Comstock, R. D., Bacteriostatic and bactericidal activities of gentamicin alone and in combination with clarithromycin against *Mycobacterium avium*, *Antimicrob. Agents Chemother.*, 36, 1695, 1992.

161. Cynamon, M. H., Klemens, S. P., and Swenson, C. E., TLC G-65 in combination with other agents in the therapy of *Mycobacterium avium* infection in beige mice, *J. Antimicrob. Chemother.*, 29, 693, 1992.

162. Kanyok, T. P., Reddy, M. V., Chinnaswamy, J., Danziger, L. H., and Gangadharam, P. R., *In vivo* activity of paromomycin against susceptible and multidrug-resistant *Mycobacterium tuberculosis* and *M. avium* complex strains, *Antimicrob. Agents Chemother.*, 38, 170, 1994.

163. Maesaki, S., Higashiyama, Y., Mitsutake, K., Matsuda, H., Yamada, H., Sugiyama, H., Kaku, M., Koga, H., Kohno, S., and Hara, K., The comparison of drug susceptibility of antituberculous agents against colonizing *M. intracellulare* and infectious *M. intracellulare*, *Kekkaku*, 66, 503, 1991.

164. Bryskier, A. and Labro, M. T., Macrolides: new therapeutic prospects, *Presse Med.*, 23, 1762, 1994.

165. Tomono, K., Therapeutic efficacy of macrolide in pulmonary nontuberculous mycobacteriosis, *Kekkaku*, 69, 725, 1994.

166. Fernandes, P. B., Hardy, D. J., McDaniel, D., Hanson, C. W., and Swanson, R. N., *In vitro* and *in vivo* activities of clarithromycin against *Mycobacterium avium*, *Antimicrob. Agents Chemother.*, 33, 1531, 1989.

167. Naik, S. and Ruck, R., *In vitro* activities of several new macrolide antibiotics against *Mycobacterium avium* complex, *Antimicrob. Agents Chemother.*, 33, 1614, 1989.

168. Rastogi, N. and Labrousse, V., Extracellular and intracellular activities of clarithromycin used alone and in association with ethambutol and rifampin against *Mycobacterium avium* complex, *Antimicrob. Agents Chemother.*, 35, 462, 1991.

169. Heifets, L. B., Lindholm-Levy, P. J., and Comstock, R. D., Clarithromycin minimal inhibitory and bactericidal concentrations against *Mycobacterium avium*, *Am. Rev. Respir. Dis.*, 145, 856, 1992.

170. Truffot-Pernot, C., Ji, B., and Grosset, J., Effect of pH on the *in vitro* potency of clarithromycin against *Mycobacterium avium* complex, *Antimicrob. Agents Chemother.*, 35, 1677, 1991.

171. Yajko, D. M., Nassos, P. S., Sanders, C. A., Gonzalez, P. C., and Hadley, W. K., Comparison of the intracellular activities of clarithromycin and erythromycin against *Mycobacterium avium* complex strains in J774 cells and in alveolar macrophages from human immunodeficiency virus type 1- infected individuals, *Antimicrob. Agents Chemother.*, 36, 1163, 1992.

172. Stauffer, F., Dortbudak, O., and Lahonik, E., *In vitro* testing of clarithromycin in combination with ethambutol and rifampicin against *Mycobacterium avium* complex, *Infection*, 19, 343, 1991.

173. Perronne, C., Gikas, A., Truffot-Pernot, C., Grosset, J., Pocidalo, J. J., and Vildé, J. L., Activities of clarithromycin, sulfisoxazole, and rifabutin against *Mycobacterium avium* complex multiplication within human macrophages, *Antimicrob. Agents Chemother.*, 34, 1508, 1990.

174. Mascellino, M. T., Iona, E., Fattorini, L., De Gregoris, P., Hu, C. Q., Santoro, C., and Orefici, G., *In vitro* activity of clarithromycin alone or in combination with other antimicrobial agents against *Mycobacterium avium-intracellulare* complex strains isolated from AIDS patients, *J. Chemother.*, 3, 357, 1991.

175. Lazard, T., Perronne, C., Cohen, Y., Grosset, J., Vildé, J.-L., and Pocidalo, J.-J., Efficacy of granulocyte colony-stimulating factor and RU-40555 in combination with clarithromycin against *Mycobacterium avium* complex infection in C57BL/6 mice, *Antimicrob. Agents Chemother.*, 37, 692, 1993.

176. Bermudez, L. E., Inderlied, C. B., Kolonoski, P., Petrofsky, M., and Young, L. S., Clarithromycin, dapsone, and a combination of both used to treat or prevent disseminated *Mycobacterium avium* infection in beige mice, *Antimicrob. Agents Chemother.*, 38, 2717, 1994.

177. Ji, B., Lounis, N., Treuffot-Pernot, C., and Grosset, J., Selection of resistant mutants of *Mycobacterium avium* in beige mice by clarithromycin monotherapy, *Antimicrob. Agents Chemother.*, 36, 2839, 1992.

178. Lounis, N., Ji, B., Truffot-Pernot, C., and Grosset, J., Selection of clarithromycin-resistant *Mycobacterium avium* complex during combined therapy using the beige mouse model, *Antimicrob. Agents Chemother.*, 39, 608, 1995.

179. De Wit, S., D'Abbraccio, M., De Mol, P., Clumeck, N., and D'Abraccio, M., Acquired resistance to clarithromycin as combined therapy in *Mycobacterium avium intracellulare* infection, *Lancet*, 341, 53, 1993 (correction in *Lancet*, 341, 704, 1993).

180. Heifets, L., Mor, N., and Vanderkolk, J., *Mycobacterium avium* strains resistant to clarithromycin and azithromycin, *Antimicrob. Agents Chemother.*, 37, 2364, 1993.

181. Doucet-Populaire, F., Truffot-Pernot, C., Grosset, J., and Jarlier, V., Acquired resistance in *Mycobacterium avium* complex strains isolated from AIDS patients and beige mice during treatment with clarithromycin, *J. Antimicrob. Chemother.*, 36, 129, 1995.

182. De Wit, S., D'Abraccio, M., De Mol, P., and Clumeck, N., Acquired resistance to clarithromycin as combined therapy in *Mycobacterium avium intracellulare* infection, *Lancet*, 341, 53, 1993.

183. Ruf, B., Schürman, D., and Mauch, H., Acquired resistance of MAI to clarithromycin, *Am. Rev. Respir. Dis.*, 145, 1241, 1992.

184. Meier, A., Heifets, L., Wallace, R. J., Jr., Zhang, Y., Brown, B. A., Sander, P., and Böttger, E. C., Molecular mechanisms of clarithromycin resistance in *Mycobacterium avium*: observation of multiple 23S rDNA mutations in a clonal population, *J. Infect. Dis.*, 174, 354, 1996.

185. Gevaudan, M. J., Bollet, C., Mallet, M. N., Gulian, G., Tissot-Dupont, H., and de Micco P., Activity of azithromycin and roxithromycin alone or in combination against *Mycobacterium avium* and *Mycobacterium xenopi*, *Pathol. Biol. (Paris)*, 38, 413, 1990.

186. Lagrange, P. H., Azithromycin, pharmacodynamic evaluation in animal models, *Pathol. Biol. (Paris)*, 43, 515, 1995.

187. Inderlied, C. B., Kolonoski, P. T., Wu, M., and Young, L. S., *In vitro* and *in vivo* activity of azithromycin (CP 62,993) against *Mycobacterium avium* complex, *J. Infect. Dis.*, 159, 994, 1989 (correction in *J. Infect. Dis.*, 160, 1095, 1989).

188. Cynamon, M. H. and Klemens, S. P., Activity of azithromycin against *Mycobacterium avium* infection in beige mice, *Antimicrob. Agents Chemother.*, 36, 1611, 1992.

189. Klemens, S. P. and Cynamon, M. H., Intermittent azithromycin for treatment of *Mycobacterium avium* infection in beige mice, *Antimicrob. Agents Chemother.*, 38, 1721, 1994.

190. Cynamon, M. H., Klemens, S. P., and Grossi, M. A., Comparative activities of azithromycin and clarithromycin against *Mycobacterium avium* infection in beige mice, *Antimicrob. Agents Chemother.*, 38, 1452, 1994.

191. Bermudez, L. E., Kolonoski, P., and Young, L. S., Roxithromycin alone and in combination with either ethambutol or levofloxacin for disseminated *Mycobacterium avium* infections in beige mice, *Antimicrob. Agents Chemother.*, 40, 1033, 1996.

192. Maugein, J., Fourche, J., Mormede, M., and Pellegrin, J. L., *In vitro* sensitivity of *Mycobacterium avium* and *Mycobacterium xenopi* to erythromycin, roxithromycin and doxycycline, *Pathol. Biol. (Paris)*, 37, 565, 1989.

193. Struillou, L., Cohen, Y., Lounis, N., Bertrand, G., Grosset, J., Vildé, J.-L., Pocidalo, J. J., and Perronne, C., Activities of roxithromycin against *Mycobacterium avium* infections in human macrophages and C57BL/6 mice, *Antimicrob. Agents Chemother.*, 39, 878, 1995.

194. Perronne, C., Gikas, A., Truffot-Pernot, C., Grosset, J., Vildé, J. L., and Pocidalo, J. J., Activities of sparfloxacin, azithromycin, temafloxacin, and rifapentine compared with that of clarithromycin against multiplication of *Mycobacterium avium* complex within human macrophages, *Antimicrob. Agents Chemother.*, 35, 1356, 1991.

195. Tsukamura, M. and Yamori, S., Bactericidal activities of rifampicin, ethambutol, enviomycin and streptomycin on *Mycobacterium avium–Mycobacterium intracellulare* complex strains, *Kekkaku*, 65, 519, 1990.

196. Tsukamura, M., Bactericidal activity of antituberculosis drugs against *Mycobacterium avium* complex, *Kekkaku*, 65, 9, 1990.

197. Tsukamura, M., Determination of the susceptibilities to antituberculosis agents in *Mycobacterium avium–Mycobacterium intracellulare* complex, *Kekkaku*, 65, 471, 1990.

198. Gevaudan, M. J., Bollet, C., Mallet, M. N., and de Micco, P., Activity of antibiotics against pigmented and unpigmented variants of *Mycobacterium avium-intracellulare*, *Pathol. Biol. (Paris)*, 39, 429, 1991.

199. Stormer, R. S. and Falkinham, J. O. III, Differences in antimicrobial susceptibility of pigmented and unpigmented colonial variants of *Mycobacterium avium*, *J. Clin. Microbiol.*, 27, 2459, 1989.

200. Casal Romn, M., Rodriguez López, F., Villalba Montoro, R., and Gonzalez Requero, A. I., *In vitro* activity of clofazimine alone and in combination with amikacin, roxithromycin, rifampicin and rifapentine against *Mycobacterium avium-intracellulare*, *Enferm. Infecc. Microbiol. Clin.*, 7, 432, 1989.

201. Wallace, R. J., Jr., Wiss, K., Bushby, M. B., and Hollowell, D. C., *In vitro* activity of trimethoprim and sulfamethoxazole against the nontuberculous mycobacteria, *Rev. Infect. Dis.*, 4, 326, 1982.

202. Cynamon, M. H. and Klemens, S. P., New antimycobacterial agents, *Clin. Chest Med.*, 10, 355, 1989.

203. Raszka, W. V., Jr., Skillman, L. P., and McEvoy, P. L., *In vitro* susceptibility of clinical isolates of *Mycobacterium avium* and *M. intracellulare* to folate antagonists, *Diagn. Microbiol. Infect. Dis.*, 18, 201, 1994.

204. Chang, W. J. and Goetz, M. B., Response to treatment of infection due to *Mycobacterium avium* complex with trimethoprim-sulfamethoxazole, *Clin. Infect. Dis.*, 14, 1267, 1992.

205. Tsukamura, M., Bacteriostatic effects of sulfadimethoxine and kitamycin on *Mycobacterium avium–M. intracellulare* complex, *Kekkaku*, 58, 247, 1983.

206. Tsukamura, M., Chemotherapy of lung disease due to *Mycobacterium avium–Mycobacterium intracellulare* complex by a combination of sulfadimethoxine, minocycline and kitasamycin, *Kekkaku*, 59, 33, 1984.

207. Tsukamura, M., A supplement study on the *in vitro* activity of sulfadimethoxine on *Mycobacterium avium* complex — combined effect with other antituberculosis drugs, *Kekkaku*, 64, 379, 1989.

208. Berlin, O. G. W., Clancy, M. N., and Bruckner, D. A., *In vitro* susceptibility of sulfisoxazole against *Mycobacterium avium* complex, *Proc. 28th Intersci. Conf. Antimicrob. Agents Chemother.*, Abstr. 1227, American Society for Microbiology, Washington, D.C., 1988, 328.

209. Davis, C. E., Jr., Carpenter, J. L., Trevino, S., Koch, J., and Ognibene, A. J., *In vitro* susceptibility of *Mycobacterium avium* complex to antibacterial agents, *Diagn. Microbiol. Infect. Dis.*, 8, 149, 1987.

210. Wu, M., Kolonoski, P. T., Yamada, J. K. et al., Susceptibility of *Mycobacterium avium* complex (MAC) to new antimicrobial agents, *Proc. 27th Intersci. Conf. Antimicrob. Agents Chemother.*, Abstr. 277, American Society for Microbiology, Washington, D.C., 1987, 145.

211. Daffe, M., Brennan, P. J., and McNeil, M., Predominant structural features of the cell wall arabinogalactan of *Mycobacterium tuberculosis* as revealed through characterization of oligoglycosyl alditol fragments by gas chromatography/mass spectrometry and by ^{1}H and ^{13}C NMR analyses, *J. Biol. Chem.*, 265, 6734, 1990.

212. Azuma, I., Yamamura, Y., and Fukushi, K., Fractionation of mycobacterial cell wall: isolation of arabinose mycolate and arabinogalactan from cell wall fraction of *Mycobacterium tuberculosis* strain Aoyama 3, *J. Bacteriol.*, 96, 1885, 1968.

213. Amar-Nacasch, C. and Vilkas, E., Walls of *Mycobacterium tuberculosis*. II. Demonstration of a mycolate of arabinobiose and a glucan in the walls of *M. tuberculosis*, *Bull. Soc. Chim. Biol.*, 52, 145, 1970.

214. Melancon-Kaplan, J., Hunter, S. W., McNeil, M., Stewart, C., Modlin, R. L., Rea, T. H., Convit, J., Salgame, P., Mehra, V., Bloom, B. R., and Brennan, P. J., Immunological significance of *Mycobacterium leprae* cell walls, *Proc. Natl. Acad. Sci. U.S.A.*, 85, 1917, 1988.

215. Misaki, A., Seto, N., and Azuma, I., Structure and immunological properties of D-arabino-D-galactans isolated from cell walls of *Mycobacterium* species, *J. Biochem. (Tokyo)*, 76, 15, 1974.

216. Miller, R. A., Harnisch, J. P., and Buchanan, T. M., Antibodies to mycobacterial arabinomannan in leprosy: correlation with reactional states and variation during therapy, *Int. J. Lepr.*, 52, 133, 1984.

217. Kleinhenz, M. E., Ellner, J. J., Spagnuolo, P. J., and Daniel, T. M., Suppression of lymphocyte responses by tuberculous plasma and mycobacterial arabinogalactan: monocyte dependence and indomethacin reversibility, *J. Clin. Invest.*, 68, 153, 1981.

218. Draper, P., Wall biosynthesis: a possible site of action for new antimycobacterial drugs, *Int. J. Lepr.*, 52, 527, 1984.

219. McNeil, M., Daffe, M., and Brennan, P. J., Location of the mycolyl ester substituents in the cell wall of mycobacteria, *J. Biol. Chem.*, 266, 13217, 1991.

220. McNeil, M., Daffe, M., and Brennan, P. J., Predominant structural features of the cell wall arabinogalactan of *Mycobacterium tuberculosis* as revealed through characterization of oligoglycosyl alditol fragments by gas chromatography/mass spectrometry and by ^{1}H and ^{13}NMR analysis, *J. Biol. Chem.*, 265, 18200, 1990.

221. Hunter, S. W., McNeil, M., Modlin, R. L., Mehra, V., Bloom, B. R., and Brennan, P. J., Isolation and characterization of the highly immunogenic cell wall-associated protein of *Mycobacterium leprae*, *J. Immunol.*, 142, 2864, 1989.

222. Hirschfield, G. R., McNeil, M., and Brennan, P. J., Peptidoglycan-associated polypeptides of *Mycobacterium tuberculosis*, *J. Bacteriol.*, 172, 1005, 1990.

223. Chatterjee, D., Lowell, K., Rivoire, B., McNeil, M. R., and Brennan, P. J., Lipoarabinomannan of *Mycobacterium tuberculosis*: capping with mannosyl residues in some strains, *J. Biol. Chem.*, 267, 6234, 1992.

224. Higgins, C., Synthesizing designer drugs, *Nature*, 327, 655, 1987.

225. Rastogi, N., Goh, K. S., and David, H. L., Enhancement of drug susceptibility of *Mycobacterium avium* by inhibitors of cell envelope synthesis, *Antimicrob. Agents Chemother.*, 34, 759, 1990.

226. David, H. L., Clavel-Seres, S., Clément, F., Lazlo, A., and Rastogi, N., Methionine as methyl group donor in the synthesis of *Mycobacterium avium* envelope lipids, and its inhibition by DL-ethionine, D-norleucine and DL-norleucine, *Acta Leprol.*, 7(Suppl. 1), 77, 1989.

227. Heifets, L. B., Lindholm-Levy, P. J., and Flory, M., Comparison of bacteriostatic and bactericidal activity of isoniazid and ethionamide against *Mycobacterium avium* and *Mycobacterium tuberculosis*, *Am. Rev. Respir. Dis.*, 143, 268, 1991.

228. Tsukamura, M., Cross-resistance relationships of antituberculosis drugs in *Mycobacterium avium* complex, *Kekkaku*, 64, 1, 1989.

229. Tsukamura, M. and Yamori, S., In-vitro susceptibility of *Mycobacterium avium* complex to isoniazid and ethionamide, *Kekkaku*, 65, 243, 1990.

230. Gangadharam, P. R., Ashtekar, D., and O'Sullivan, J. F., *In vitro, in vivo*, and intracellular chemotherapeutic activity of B746, a clofazimine analog against *Mycobacterium avium* complex, *Tuberc. Lung Dis.*, 73, 192, 1992.

231. Kaufman, A. C., Greene, C. E., Rakich, P. M., and Weigner, D. D., Treatment of localized *Mycobacterium avium* complex infection with clofazimine and doxycycline in a cat, *J. Am. Vet. Med. Assoc.*, 207, 457, 1995.

232. Peterson, J. R., Zjawiony, J. K., Liu, S., Hufford, C. D., Clark, A. M., and Rogers, R. D., Copyrine alkaloids: synthesis, spectroscopic characterization, and antimycotic/antimycobacterial activity of A- and B-ring-functionalized sampangines, *J. Med. Chem.*, 35, 4069, 1992.

233. Chakraboty, A., Gangadharam, P. R., Damle, P., Pratt, P., Wright, P., and Davidson, P. T., Antituberculous activity of 6-cyclooctylamino-5,8-quinolinequinone (CQQ), *Tubercle*, 62, 37, 1981.

234. Gangadharam, P. R., Pratt, P. F., Damle, P. B., Davidson, P. T., Porter, T. H., and Folkers, K., Inhibition of *Mycobacterium intracellulare* by some vitamin K and coenzyme Q analogs, *Am. Rev. Respir. Med.*, 118, 467, 1987.

235. Hübner, L., Ernst, M., von Laer, D., Schwander, S., and Flad, H. D., Enhancement of monocyte antimycobacterial activity by diethyldithiocarbamate (DTC), *Int. J. Immunopharmacol.*, 13, 1067, 1991.

236. Wright, E. L. and Barrow, W. W., Inhibition of glycopeptidolipid synthesis resulting from treatment of *Mycobacterium avium* with 2-deoxy-D-glucose, *Res. Microbiol.*, 142, 597, 1991.

237. Heifets, L. B., Lindholm-Levy, P. J., and Flory, M., Thiacetazone: *in vitro* activity against *Mycobacterium avium* and *M. tuberculosis*, *Tubercle*, 71, 287, 1990.

238. Haneishi, T., Nakajima, M., Shiraishi, A., Katayama, T., Torikata, A., Kawahara, Y., Kurihara, K., Arai, M., Arai, T., Aoyagi, T., Koseki, Y., Kondo, E., and Tokunaga, T., Antimycobacterial activities *in vitro* and *in vivo* and pharmacokinetics of dihydromycoplanecin A, *Antimicrob. Agents Chemother.*, 32, 110, 1988.

239. Wu, M., Kolonoski, P. T., Yadegar, S. et al. *In vitro* susceptibility of *Mycobacterium avium* complex (MAC) to novel antimycobacterial drugs, *Proc. 26th Intersci. Conf. Antimicrob. Agents Chemother.*, Abstr. 1102, American Society for Microbiology, Washington, D.C., 1986, 298.

240. Hoffner, S. E., Olsson-Liljequist, B., Rydgård, K. J., Svenson, S, B., and Källenius, G., Susceptibility of mycobacteria to fusidic acid, *Eur. J. Clin. Microbiol. Infect. Dis.*, 9, 294, 1990.

241. Gonzalez, A. H., Berlin, O. G., and Bruckner, D. A., In-vitro activity of dapsone and two potentiators against *Mycobacterium avium* complex, *J. Antimicrob. Chemother.*, 24, 19, 1989.

242. Machacek, M., Kunes, J., Sidorova, E., Odlerova, Z., and Waisser, K., Relation between the chemical structure of substances and their antimicrobial action against atypical strains. II. 6-Acylamido-2-alkylthiobenzothiazoles, quantitative relation to their effectiveness spectrum, *Cesk. Farm.*, 38, 9, 1989.

243. Inderlied, C. B., Lancero, M. G., and Young, L. S., Bacteriostatic and bactericidal *in vitro* activity of meropenem against clinical isolates, including *Mycobacterium avium* complex, *J. Antimicrob. Chemother.*, 24(Suppl. A), 85, 1989.

244. Liu, Z. Z., Guo, X. D., Straub, L. E., Erdos, G., Prankerd, R. J., Gonzalez-Rothi, R. J., and Schreier, H., Lipophilic *N*-acylpyrizinamide derivatives: synthesis, physicochemical characterization, liposome incorporation, and *in vitro* activity against *Mycobacterium avium-intracellulare*, *Drug Res. Discov.*, 8, 57, 1991.

245. Suzuki, H., Saito, H., Sato, K., and Tomioka, H., *In vitro* and *in vivo* activities of chemically synthesized lipid A-subunit analog, JTP3309, against mycobacterial infections in mice and in mouse peritoneal macrophages, *Kekkaku*, 70, 285, 1995.

246. Horsburgh, C. R., Jr., Advances in the prevention and treatment of *Mycobacterium avium* disease, *N. Engl. J. Med.*, 335, 428, 1996.

247. Rastogi, N., Frehel, C., Ryter, A., Ohayon, H., Lesourd, M., and David, H.L., Multiple drug resistance in *Mycobacterium avium*: is the wall architecture responsible for the exclusion of antimicrobial agents? *Antimicrob. Agents Chemother.*, 20, 666, 1981.

248. Sanchez Munoz, M. C., Barrio Gomez de Aguero, M. I., Martinez Carrasco, M. C., and Antelo Landeira, M. C., Primary *Mycobacterium avium* respiratory infection in nonimmunocompromised children, *Arch. Bronconeumol.*, 31, 246, 1995.

249. Patz, E. F., Jr., Swensen, S. J., and Erasmus, J., Pulmonary manifestations of nontuberculous *Mycobacterium*, *Radiol. Clin. North Am.*, 33, 719, 1995.

250. Kalayjian, R. C., Toossi, Z., Tomashefski, J. F., Jr., Carey, J. T., Ross, J. A., Tomford, J. W., and Blinkhorn, R. J., Jr., Pulmonary disease due to infection by *Mycobacterium avium* complex in patients with AIDS, *Clin. Infect. Dis.*, 20, 1186, 1995.

251. Kissinger, P., Clark, R., Morse, A., and Brandon, W., Comparison of multiple drug therapy regimens for HIV-related disseminated *Mycobacterium avium* complex disease, *J. Acquir. Immune Defic. Syndr. Hum. Retrovirol.*, 9, 133, 1995.

252. Calzetti, C., Magnani, G., Elia, G., Avanzi, M., Pasetti, G., and Fiaccadori, F., Retrospective study of *Mycobacterium avium* complex infection in the acquired immunodeficiency syndrome, *Ann. Ital. Med. Int.*, 8, 166, 1993.

253. Wallace, R. J., Jr., Brown, B. A., Griffith, D. E., Girard, W. M., and Murphy, D. T., Clarithromycin regimens for pulmonary *Mycobacterium avium* complex: the first 50 patients, *Am. J. Respir. Crit. Care Med.*, 153, 1766, 1996.

254. Frothingham, R., Clarithromycin treatment for *Mycobacterium avium-intracellulare* complex lung disease, *Am. J. Respir. Crit. Care Med.*, 153, 1990, 1996.

255. Bates, J. H., *Mycobacterium avium* disease: progress at last, *Am. J. Respir. Crit. Care Med.*, 153, 1737, 1996.

256. Young, L. S., Treatment and prophylaxis of *Mycobacterium avium* complex, *Int. J. STD AIDS*, 7(Suppl. 1), 23, 1996.

257. Perronne, C., Azithromycin and *Mycobacterium avium* infection, *Pathol. Biol. (Paris)*, 43, 565, 1995.

258. Coulaud, J. P., Azithromycin: new orientation, *Pathol. Biol. (Paris)*, 43, 547, 1995.

259. Singh, N. and Yu, V. L., Clarithromycin therapy for *Mycobacterium avium* complex bacteremia, *Ann. Intern. Med.*, 123, 154, 1995 (see also *Ann. Intern. Med.*, 121, 905, 1994).

260. van der Meer, J. T. and Danner, S. A., Clarithromycin therapy for *Mycobacterium avium* complex bacteremia, *Ann. Intern. Med.*, 123, 154, 1995.

261. Musher, D. M., Clarithromycin therapy for *Mycobacterium avium* complex bacteremia, *Ann. Intern. Med.*, 123, 154, 1995.

262. Ives, D. V., Davis, R. B., and Currier, J. S., Impact of clarithromycin and azithromycin on patterns of treatment and survival among AIDS patients with disseminated *Mycobacterium avium* complex, *AIDS*, 9, 261, 1995.

263. Dautzenberg, B., Piperno, D., Diot, P., Truffot-Pernot, C., and Chauvin, J. P., Clarithromycin in the treatment of *Mycobacterium avium* lung infections in patients without AIDS. Clarithromycin Study Group of France, *Chest*, 107, 1035, 1995.

264. Havlir, D. V., *Mycobacterium avium* complex: advances in therapy, *Eur. J. Clin. Microbiol. Infect. Dis.*, 13, 915, 1994.

265. Rapp, R. P., McCraney, S. A., Goodman, N. L., and Shaddick, D. J., New macrolide antibiotics: usefulness in infections caused by mycobacteria other than *Mycobacterium tuberculosis*, *Ann. Pharmacother.*, 28, 1255, 1994.

266. Chaisson, R. E., Benson, C. A., Dube, M. P., Heifets, L. B., Korvick, J. A., Elkin, S., Smith, T., Craft, J. C., Sattler, F. R., and the AIDS Clinical Trials Group Protocol 157 Study Team, Clarithromycin therapy for bacteremic *Mycobacterium avium* complex disease: a randomized, double-blind, dose-ranging study in patients with AIDS, *Ann. Intern. Med.*, 121, 905, 1994.

267. Dautzenberg, B., Saint-Marc, T., Durant, J., Reynes, J., Meyohas, M. C., Legrand, M. F., Truffot, C., and Chavin, J. P., Treatment with clarithromycin of 173 HIV+ patients with disseminated *Mycobacterium avium intracellulare* infection, *Rev. Mal. Respir.*, 11, 271, 1994.

268. Husson, R. N., Ross, L. A., Sandelli, S., Inderlied, C. B., Lewis, L. L., Woods, L., Conville, P. S., Witebsky, F. G., and Pizzo, P. A., Orally administered clarithromycin for the treatment of systemic *Mycobacterium avium* complex infection in children with acquired immunodeficiency syndrome, *J. Pediatr.*, 124, 807, 1994.

269. Wallace, R. J., Jr., Brown, B. A., Griffith, D. E., Girard, W. M., Murphy, D. T., Onyi, G. O., Steingrube, V. A., and Mazurek., G. H., Initial clarithromycin monotherapy for *Mycobacterium avium-intracellulare* complex lung disease, *Am. J. Respir. Crit. Care Med.*, 149, 1335, 1994.

270. Dautzenberg, B., Saint Marc, T., Meyohas, M. C., Eliaszewitch, M., Haniez, F., Rogues, A. M., De Wit, S., Cotte, L., Chauvin, J. P., and Grosset, J., Clarithromycin and other antimicrobial agents in the treatment of disseminated *Mycobacterium avium* infections in patients with acquired immuno-deficiency syndrome, *Arch. Intern. Med.*, 153, 368, 1993.

271. Pirofsky, J. G., Huang, C. T., and Waites, K. B., Spinal osteomyelitis due to *Mycobacterium avium-intracellulare* in an elderly man with steroid-induced osteoporosis, *Spine*, 18, 1926, 1993.

272. Goldberger, M. and Masur, H., Clarithromycin therapy for *Mycobacterium avium* complex disease in patients with AIDS: potential and problems, *Ann. Intern. Med.*, 121, 974, 1994.

273. Barradell, L. B., Plosker, G. L., and McTavish, D., Clarithromycin: a review of its pharmacological properties and therapeutic use in *Mycobacterium avium-intracellulare* complex infection in patients with acquired immune deficiency syndrome, *Drugs*, 46, 289, 1993.

274. Heifets, L. B., Clarithromycin against *Mycobacterium avium* complex infections, *Tuberc. Lung Dis.*, 77, 19, 1996.

275. Dautzenberg, B., Truffot, C., Legris, S., Meyohas, M. C., Berlie, H. C., Mercat, A., Chevret, S., and Grosset, J., Activity of clarithromycin against *Mycobacterium avium* infection in patients with the acquired immune deficiency syndrome: a controlled clinical trial, *Am. Rev. Respir. Dis.*, 144, 564, 1991.

276. Price, T. A. and Tuazon, C. U., Clarithromycin-induced thrombocytopenia, *Clin. Infect. Dis.*, 15, 563, 1992.

277. Nightingale, S. D., Koster, F. T., Mertz, G. J., and Loss, S. D., Clarithromycin-induced mania in two patients with AIDS, *Clin. Infect. Dis.*, 20, 1563, 1995.

278. Dorrell, L., Ellerton, C., Cottrell, D. G., and Snow, M. H., Toxicity of clarithromycin in the treatment of *Mycobacterium avium* complex infection in a patient with AIDS, *J. Antimicrob. Chemother.*, 34, 605, 1994.

279. Ruf, B., Schürmann, D., Mauch, H., Jautzke, G., Fehrenbach, F. J., and Pohle, H. D., Effectiveness of microlide clarithromycin in the treatment of *Mycobacterium avium* complex function in HIV-infected patients, *Infection*, 20, 267, 1992.

280. Malessa, R., Diener, H. C., Olbricht, T., Bohmer, B., and Brockmeyer, N. H., Successful treatment of meningoencephalitis caused by *Mycobacterium avium intracellulare* in AIDS, *Clin. Invest.*, 72, 850, 1994.

281. de Lalla, F., Maserati, R., Scarpellini, P., Marone, P., Nicolin, R., Caccamo, F., and Rigoli, R., Clarithromycin-ciprofloxacin-amikacin for therapy of *Mycobacterium avium–Mycobacterium intra-cellulare* bacteremia in patients with AIDS, *Antimicrob. Agents Chemother.*, 36, 1567, 1992.

282. Grange, J. M., Winstanley, P. A., and Davies, P. D., Clinically significant drug interactions with antituberculosis agents, *Drug Saf.*, 11, 242, 1994.

283. Wallace, R. J., Jr., Brown, B. A., Griffith, D. E., Girard, W., and Tanaka, K., Reduced serum levels of clarithromycin in patients treated with multidrug regimens including rifampin or rifabutin for *Mycobacterium avium–M. intracellulare* infection, *J. Infect. Dis.*, 171, 747, 1995.

284. Wallace, M. R., Miller, L. K., Nguyen, M. T., and Shields, A. R., Ototoxicity with azithromycin, *Lancet*, 343, 241, 1994.

285. Ahn, C. H., Ahn, S. S., Anderson, R. A., Murphy, D. T., and Mammo, A., A four-drug regimen for initial treatment of cavitary disease caused by *M. avium* complex, *Am. Rev. Respir. Dis.*, 134, 438, 1986.

286. Seibert, A. F. and Base, J. B., Four drug therapy of pulmonary disease caused by *Mycobacterium avium* complex, *Am. Rev. Respir. Dis.*, 139, A399, 1989.

287. Heifets, L. B. and Iseman, M. D., Individualized therapy versus standard regimens in the treatment of *Mycobacterium avium* infections, *Am. Rev. Respir. Dis.*, 144, 1, 1991.

288. Tsukamura, M., In-vitro bacteriostatic and bactericidal activity of isoniazid on the *Mycobacterium avium–Mycobacterium intracellulare* complex, *Tubercle*, 71, 199, 1990.

289. Agins, B. D., Berman, D. S., Spicehandler, D., Al-Sadr, W., Simberkoff, M. S., and Rahal, J. J., Effect of combined therapy with ansamycin, clofazimine, ethambutol, and isoniazid for *Mycobacterium avium* infection in patients with AIDS, *J. Infect. Dis.*, 159, 784, 1989.

290. Heifets, L. B. and Iseman, M. D., Choice of antimicrobial agents of *M. avium* disease based on quantitative tests of drug susceptibility, *N. Engl. J. Med.*, 323, 419, 1990.

291. Shafran, S. D., Singer, J., Zarowny, D. B., Phillips, B. et al., A comparison of two regimens for the treatment of *Mycobacterium avium* complex bacteremia in AIDS: rifabutin, ethambutol, and clarithromycin versus rifampin, ethambutol, clofazimine, and ciprofloxacin. Canadian HIV Trials Network Protocol 010, *N. Engl. J. Med.*, 335, 377, 1996.

292. Kemper, C. A., Havlir, D., Haghighat, D., Dubé, M., Bartok, A. E., Sison, J. P., Yao, Y., Yangco, B., Leedom, J. M., Tilles, J. G., McCutchan, J. A., and Deresinski, S. C., The individual microbiologic effect of three antimycobacterial agents, clofazimine, ethambutol, and rifampin, on *Mycobacterium avium* complex bacteremia in patients with AIDS, *J. Infect. Dis.*, 170, 157, 1994.

293. Jorup-Ronstrom, C., Julander, I., and Petrini, B., Efficacy of triple drug regimen of amikacin, ethambutol and rifabutin in AIDS patients with symptomatic *Mycobacterium avium* complex infection, *J. Infect.*, 26, 67, 1993.

294. Davidson, P. T., Khanijo, V., Goble, M., and Moulding, T. S., Treatment of disease due to *Mycobacterium intracellulare*, *Rev. Infect. Dis.*, 3, 1052, 1981.

295. Tsukada, H., Chou, T., Ishizuka, Y., Ogawa, O., Saeki, T., Ito, S., Wakabayashi, M., Hayashi, N., and Arakawa, M., Disseminated *Mycobacterium avium-intracellulare* infection in a patient with myelo-dysplastic syndrome (refractory anemia), *Am. J. Hematol.*, 45, 325, 1994.

296. Schelonka, R. L., Ascher, D. P., McMahon, D. P., Drehner, D. M., and Kuskie, M. R., Catheter-related sepsis caused by *Mycobacterium avium* complex, *Pediatr. Infect. Dis. J.*, 13, 236, 1994.

297. Clark, D., Lambert, C. M., Palmer, K., Strachan, R., and Nuki, G., Monoarthritis caused by *Mycobacterium avium* complex in a liver transplant recipient, *Br. J. Rheumatol.*, 32, 1099, 1993.

298. Darouiche, R. O., Koff, A., Rosen, T., Darnule, T. V., Lidsky, M. D., and El-Zaatari, A. K., Recurrent disseminated infection with *Mycobacterium avium* complex identified in tissues by molecular analysis, *Clin. Infect. Dis.*, 22, 714, 1996.

299. Rathbun, R. C., Martin, E. S. III, Eaton, V. E., and Matthew, E.B., Current and investigational therapies for AIDS-associated *Mycobacterium avium* complex disease, *Ther. Rev.*, 10, 280, 1991.

300. Baron, E. J. and Young, L. S., Amikacin, ethambutol and rifampin for treatment of disseminated *Mycobacterium avium-intracellulare* infections in patients with acquired immune deficiency syndrome, *Diagn. Microbiol. Infect. Dis.*, 5, 215, 1986.

301. Bach, M. C., Treating disseminated *Mycobacterium avium-intracellulare* infection, *Ann. Intern. Med.*, 110, 169, 1989.

302. Masur, H., Tuazon C., Gill, V., Grimes, G., Baird, B., Fauci, A. S., and Lane, H. C., Effect of combined clofazimine and ansamycin therapy on *Mycobacterium avium-intracellulare* bacteremia in patients with AIDS, *J. Infect. Dis.*, 155, 127, 1987.

303. Dautzenberg, B., Olliaro, P., Ruf, B., Esposito, R., Opravil, M., Hoy, J. F., Rozenbaum, W., Carosi, G. P., Micoud, M., L'Age, M., Pirotta, N., Sassella, D., and the NTMT001 Study Group, Rifabutin versus placebo in combination with three drugs in the treatment of nontuberculous mycobacterial infection in patients with AIDS, *Clin. Infect. Dis.*, 22, 705, 1996.

304. Hoy, J., Mijch, A., Sandland, M., Grayson, L., Lucas, R., and Dwyer, B., Quadruple-drug therapy for *Mycobacterium avium-intracellulare* bacteremia in AIDS patients, *J. Infect. Dis.*, 161, 801, 1990.

305. Berning, S. E. and Peloquin, C. A., Adverse events associated with high-dose rifabutin in macrolide-containing regimens for the treatment of *Mycobacterium avium* complex lung disease, *Clin. Infect. Dis.*, 22, 885, 1996.

306. Denis, M. and Gregg, E. O., Recombinant interleukin-6 increases the intracellular and extracellular growth of *Mycobacterium avium*, *Can. J. Microbiol.*, 37, 479, 1991.

307. Sullam, P. M., Rifabutin therapy for disseminated *Mycobacterium avium* complex infection, *Clin. Infect. Dis.*, 22(Suppl. 1), S37, 1996.

308. Lowe, S. H., Kroon, F. P., Bollemeyer, J. G., Stricker, B. H., and van't Wout, J. W., Uveitis during treatment of disseminated *Mycobacterium avium-intracellulare* complex infection with the combination of rifabutin, clarithromycin and ethambutol, *Neth. J. Med.*, 48, 211, 1996.

309. Tseng, A. L. and Walmsley, S. L., Rifabutin-associated uveitis, *Ann. Pharmacother.*, 29, 1149, 1995.

310. Frau, E., Gregoire-Cassoux, N., Hannouche, D., Lautier-Frau, M. et al., Uveitis with hypopyon in patients with acquired immunodeficiency syndrome, treated with rifabutin, *J. Fr. Ophthalmol.*, 18, 435, 1995.

311. Chevalley, G. F., Kaiser, L., Bouchenaki, N., Baglivo, E., and Kress, O., Uveitis associated with rifabutin treatment: apropos of 3 patients, *Klin. Monatsbl. Augenheilkd.*, 206, 388, 1995.

312. Rifai, A., Peyman, G. A., Daun, M., and Wafapoor, H., Rifabutin- associated uveitis during prophylaxis for *Mycobacterium avium* complex infection, *Arch. Ophthalmol.*, 113, 707, 1995.

313. Dunn, A. M., Tizer, K., and Cervia, J. S., Rifabutin-associated uveitis in a pediatric patient, *Pediatr. Infect. Dis. J.*, 14, 246, 1995.

314. Jacobs, D. S., Piliero, P. J., Kuperwaser, M. G., Smith, J. A., Harris, S. D., Flanigan, T. P., Goldberg, J. H., and Ives, D. V., Acute uveitis associated with rifabutin use in patients with human immuno-deficiency virus infection, *Am. J. Ophthalmol.*, 118, 716, 1994.

315. Saran, B. R., Maguire, A. M., Nichols, C., Frank, I., Hertle, R. W., Brucker, A. J., Goldman, S., Brown, M., and Van Uitert, B., Hypopyon uveitis in patients with acquired immunodeficiency syndrome treated for systemic *Mycobacterium avium* complex infection with rifabutin, *Arch. Ophthalmol.*, 112, 1159, 1994.

316. Frank, M. O., Graham, M. B., and Wispelway, B., Rifabutin and uveitis, *N. Engl. J. Med.*, 330, 868, 1994.

317. Brogden, R. N. and Fitton, A., Rifabutin: a review of its antimicrobial activity, pharmacokinetic properties and therapeutic efficacy, *Drugs*, 47, 983, 1994.

318. Skinner, M. H. and Blaschke, T. F., Clinical pharmacokinetics of rifabutin, *Clin. Pharmacokinet.*, 28, 115, 1995.

319. Sullam, P. M., Gordin, F. M., and Wynne, B. A., Efficacy of rifabutin in the treatment of disseminated infection due to *Mycobacterium avium* complex. The Rifabutin Treatment Group, *Clin. Infect. Dis.*, 19, 84, 1994.

320. Griffith, D. E., Brown, B. A., Girard, W. M., and Wallace, R. J., Jr., Adverse events associated with high-dose rifabutin in macrolide-containing regimens for the treatment of *Mycobacterium avium* complex lung disease, *Clin. Infect. Dis.*, 21, 594, 1995.

321. Siegal, F. P., Rifabutin prophylaxis for *Mycobacterium avium* complex infection in patient with AIDS, *Clin. Infect. Dis.*, 22(Suppl. 1), S23, 1996.

322. Dautzenberg, B., Rifabutin in the treatment of *Mycobacterium avium* complex infection: experience in Europe, *Clin. Infect. Dis.*, 22(Suppl. 1), S33, 1996.

323. Hoffner, S. E., Svenson, S. B., and Beezer, A. E., Microcalorimetric studies of the initial interaction between antimycobacterial drugs and *Mycobacterium avium*, *J. Antimicrob. Chemother.*, 25, 353, 1990.

324. Eggelmeijer, F., Kroon, F. P., Zeeman, R. J., Dijkmans, B. A., and van't Wout, J. W., Tenosynovitis due to *Mycobacterium avium-intracellulare:* case report and a review of the literature, *Clin. Exp. Rheumatol.* 10, 169, 1992.

325. Hoffner, S. E., Kratz, M., Olsson-Liljequist, B., Svenson, S. B., and Källenius, G., *In vitro* synergistic activity between ethambutol and fluorinated quinolones against *Mycobacterium avium* complex, *J. Antimicrob. Chemother.*, 24, 317, 1989.

326. Källenius, G., Svenson, S. B., and Hoffner, S. E., Ethambutol: a key for *Mycobacterium avium* complex chemotherapy? *Am. Rev. Respir. Dis.,* 140, 264, 1989.

327. Kemper, C. A., Chiu, J., Meng, T. C. et al., Microbiologic and clinical response of patients with AIDS and MAC bacteremia to a four oral drug regimen, *Proc. 30th Intersci. Conf. Antimicrob. Agents Chemother.*, Abstr. 1267, American Society for Microbiology, Washington, D.C., 1990.

328. Peloquin, C. A., Dosage of antimycobacterial agents, *Clin. Pharm.*, 10, 664, 1991.

329. Yew, W. W., Chau, C. H., Wong, P. C., and Choi, H. Y., Ciprofloxacin-induced renal dysfunction in patients with mycobacterial lung infection, *Tuberc. Lung. Dis.*, 76, 173, 1995.

330. Fan-Harvard, P., Sanchorawala, V., Oh, J., Moser, E. M., and Smith, S. P., Concurrent use of foscarnet and ciprofloxacin may increase the propensity for seizures, *Ann. Pharmacother.*, 28, 869, 1994.

331. Nightingale, S. D., Saletan, S. L., Swenson, C. E., Lawrence, A. J., Watson, D. A., Pilkiewicz, F. G., and Cal, S. X., Liposome-encapsulated gentamicin treatment of *Mycobacterium avium–Mycobacterium intracellulare* complex bacteremia in AIDS patients, *Antimicrob. Agents Chemother.*, 37, 1869, 1993.

332. Wormser, G. P., Horowitz, H., and Dworkin, B., Low-dose dexamethasone as adjunctive therapy in AIDS patients, *Antimicrob. Agents Chemother.*, 38, 2215, 1994.

333. Jones, A. R., Bartlett, J., and McCormack, J. G., *Mycobacterium avium* complex (MAC) osteomyelitis and septic arthritis in an immunocompetent host, *J. Infect.*, 30, 59, 1995.

334. King, B. F., Disseminated *Mycobacterium avium* complex in an immunocompetent previously healthy woman, *J. Am. Board Fam. Pract.*, 7, 145, 1994.

335. Lee, D., Goldstein, E. J., and Zarem, H. A., Localized *Mycobacterium avium-intracellulare* mastitis in an immunocompetent woman with silicone breast implants, *Plast. Reconstr. Surg.*, 95, 142, 1995.

336. Philippot, V., Yassir, F., Balme, B., and Perrot, H., *Mycobacterium avium-intracellulare* subcutaneous abscess after injections of interferon alpha in a patient treated for lymphoma, *Ann. Dermatol. Venereol.*, 123, 103, 1996.

337. Bachelez, H., Ducloy, G., Pinquier, L., Rouveau, M., Sibilla, J., and Dubertret, L., Disseminated varioliform pustular eruption due to *Mycobacterium avium intracellulare* in an HIV-infected patient, *Br. J. Dermatol.*, 134, 801, 1996.

338. Mattila, J. O., Vornanen, M., Vaara, J., and Katila, M. L., Mycobacteria in prurigo nodularis: the cause or a consequence? *J. Am. Acad. Dermatol.*, 34, 224, 1996.

339. Weits, J., Sprenger, H. G., Ilic, P., van Klingeren, B., Elema, J. D., and Steensma, J. T., *Mycobacterium avium* disease in AIDS patients; diagnosis and therapy, *Ned. Tijdschr. Geneeskd.*, 135, 2485, 1991.

340. Chatte, G., Panteix, G., Perrin-Fayolle, M., and Pacheco, Y., Aerosolized interferon gamma for *Mycobacterium avium*-complex lung disease, *Am. J. Respir. Crit. Care Med.*, 152, 1094, 1995.

341. Holland, S. M., Eisenstein, E. M., Kuhns, D. B., Turner, M. L., Fleisher, T. A., Strober, W., and Gallin, J. I., Treatment of refractory disseminated nontuberculous mycobacterial infection with interferon gamma: a preliminary report, *N. Engl. J. Med.*, 330, 1348, 1994.

342. Nichols, C. W., *Mycobacterium avium* complex infection, rifabutin, and uveitis — is there a connection? *Clin. Infect. Dis.*, 22(Suppl. 1), S43, 1996.

343. American Foundation for AIDS Research, MAC (*Mycobacterium avium* complex), *AIDS/HIV Treatment Directory*, 6(4), 88, 1993.

344. Wynne, B. et al., The development of *Mycobacterium avium* complex (MAC) bacteremia in AIDS patients in the placebo (PLAC)-controlled MAC prophylaxis studies (087023 and 087027), *Proc. 32nd Intersci. Conf. Antimicrob. Agents Chemother.*, American Society for Microbiology, Washington, D.C., Abstr. 890, 1992.

345. Eccles, E. and Ptak, J., *Mycobacterium avium* complex infection in AIDS: clinical features, treatment, and prevention, *J. Assoc. Nurses AIDS Care*, 6, 37, 1995.

346. Hoy, J. F., Marriott, D., and Gottlieb, T., Managing HIV. V. Treating secondary outcomes: 15 HIV and non-tuberculous mycobacterial infections, *Med. J. Aust.*, 164, 543, 1996.

347. Stearn, B. F. and Polis, M. A., Prophylaxis of opportunistic infections in persons with HIV infection, *Cleve. Clin. J. Med.*, 61, 187, 1994.

348. Chaisson, R. E., McCutchan, J. A., Nightingale, S., and Young, L. S., Managing *Mycobacterium avium* complex infection, *AIDS Clin. Care*, 5, 1, 1993.

349. Chaisson, R. E. et al., Clarithromycin therapy for disseminated *Mycobacterium avium* complex (MAC) in AIDS, *Proc. 32nd Intersci. Conf. Antimicrob. Agents Chemother.*, Abstr. 891, American Society for Microbiology, Washington, D.C., 1992.

350. Hewitt, R. G., Maliszewski, M., Goldberg, M., and Harmon, B., Prevention of *M. avium* complex (MAC) bacteremia in patients with CD4+ <200 by rifabutin, clarithromycin or dapsone, *Proc. IXth Int. Conf. AIDS*, Berlin, 1993, Abstr. PO-B07-1184.

351. Abrams, D. I., Mitchell, T. F., Child, C. C., Shiboski, S. C., Brosgart, C. L., Mass, M. M., and the Community Consortium, Clofazimine as prophylaxis for disseminated *Mycobacterium avium* complex infection in AIDS, *J. Infect. Dis.*, 167, 1459, 1993.

352. Crowle, A. J., Dahl, R., Ross, E., and May, M. H., Evidence that vesicles containing living, virulent *Mycobacterium tuberculosis* or *Mycobacterium avium* in cultured human macrophages are not acidic, *Infect. Immun.*, 59, 1823, 1991.

353. Meylan, P. R., Richman, D. D., and Kornbluth, R. S., Reduced intracellular growth of mycobacteria in human macrophages cultivated at physiological oxygen pressure, *Am. Rev. Respir. Dis.*, 145, 947, 1992.

354. Rastogi, N. and Blom-Potar, M. C., A comparative study on the activation of J-774 macrophage-like cells by gamma-interferon, 1,25- dihydroxyvitamin D_3 and lipopeptide RP-56142: ability to kill intracellularly multiplying *Mycobacterium tuberculosis* and *Mycobacterium avium*, *Int. J. Med. Microbiol.*, 273, 344, 1990.

355. Yajko, D. M., Nassos, P. S., Sanders, C. A., and Hadley, W. K., Killing by antimycobacterial agents of AIDS-derived strains of *Mycobacterium avium* complex inside cells of the mouse macrophage cell line J774, *Am. Rev. Respir. Dis.*, 140, 1198, 1989.

356. Kobayashi, K., Yamazaki, J., Kasama, T., Katsura, T., Kasahara, K., Wolf, S. F., and Shimamura, T., Interleukin (IL)-12 deficiency in susceptible mice infected with *Mycobacterium avium* and amelioration of established infection by IL-12 replacement therapy, *J. Infect. Dis.*, 174, 1996.

357. Kobayashi, K., Kasama, T., Yamazaki, J., Hosaka, M. et al., Protection of mice from *Mycobacterium avium* infection by recombinant interleukin-12, *Antimicrob. Agents Chemother.*, 39, 1369, 1995.

358. Denis, M., Tumor necrosis factor and granulocyte macrophage-colony stimulating factor stimulate human macrophages to restrict growth of virulent *Mycobacterium avium* to kill avirulent *M. avium*: killing effector mechanism depends on the generation of reactive nitrogen intermediates, *J. Leukoc. Biol.*, 49, 380, 1991.

359. Bermudez, L. E. and Young, L. S., Recombinant granulocyte-macrophage colony-stimulating factor activates human macrophages to inhibit growth or kill *Mycobacterium avium* complex, *J. Leukoc. Biol.*, 48, 67, 1990.

360. Bermudez, L. E., Young, L. S., and Gupta, S., 1,25-Dihydroxyvitamin D_3-dependent inhibition of growth or killing of *Mycobacterium avium* complex in human macrophages is mediated by TNF and GM-CSF, *Cell. Immunol.*, 127, 432, 1990.

361. Sathe, S. S., Tsigler, D., Sarai, A., and Kumar, P., Pentoxifylline impairs macrophage defense against *Mycobacterium avium* complex, *J. Infect. Dis.*, 172, 863, 1995.

362. Sathe, S. S., Sarai, A., Tsigler, D., and Nedunchezian, D., Pentoxifylline aggravates impairment in tumor necrosis factor-alpha secretion and increases mycobacterial load in macrophages from AIDS patients with disseminated *Mycobacterium avium-intracellulare* complex infection, *J. Infect. Dis.*, 170, 484, 1994.

363. Blanchard, D. K., Cytokine activation of killer cells in mycobacterial immunity, *Adv. Exp. Med. Biol.*, 319, 105, 1992.

364. Blanchard, D. K., McMillen, S., Hoffman, S. L., and Djeu, J. Y., Mycobacterial induction of activated killer cells: possible role of tyrosine kinase activity in interleukin-2 receptor alpha expression, *Infect. Immun.*, 60, 2843, 1992.

365. Blanchard, D. K., Michelini-Norris, M. B., Pearson, C. A., McMillen, S., and Djeu, J. Y., Production of granulocyte-macrophage colony-stimulating factor (GM-CSF) by monocytes and large granular lymphocytes stimulated with *Mycobacterium avium–M. intracellulare*: activation of bactericidal activity by GM-CSF, *Infect. Immun.*, 59, 2396, 1991.

366. Bermudez, L. E., Martinelli, J., Petrofsky, M., Kolonoski, P., and Young, L. S., Recombinant granulocyte-macrophage colony-stimulating factor enhances the effects of antibiotics against *Mycobacterium avium* complex infection in the beige mouse model, *J. Infect. Dis.*, 169, 575, 1994.

367. Suzuki, K., Yamamoto, T., Yuba, Y., Sato, A., Kubo, Y., Murayama, T., and Kuze, F., Effect of cytokines on anti-*Mycobacterium avium* complex (MAC) activities of human alveolar macrophages, *Kekkaku*, 67, 63, 1992.

368. Suga, M., Doi, T., Akaike, T., and Ando, M., Intracellular killing mechanisms of alveolar macrophages against *Mycobacterium avium* complex, *Kekkaku*, 67, 55, 1992.

369. Bermudez, L. E., Wu, M., Martinelli, J., and Young, L. S., Ethanol affects release of TNF and GM-CSF and membrane expression of TNF receptors by human macrophages, *Lymphokine Cytokine Res.*, 10, 413, 1991.

370. Bermudez, L. E. and Young, L. S., Ethanol augments intracellular survival of *Mycobacterium avium* complex and impairs macrophage responses to cytokines, *J. Infect. Dis.*, 163, 1286, 1991.

371. Appelberg, R., Orme, I. M., Pinto de Sousa, M. I., and Silva, M. T., *In vitro* effects of interleukin-4 on interferon-gamma-induced macrophage activation, *Immunology*, 76, 553, 1992.

372. Appelberg, R. and Orme, I. M., Effector mechanisms involved in cytokine-mediated bacteriostasis of *Mycobacterium avium* infections in murine macrophages, *Immunology*, 80, 352, 1993.

373. Bermudez, L.E., Wu, M., and Young, L.S., Effect of stress-related hormones on macrophage receptors and response to tumor necrosis factor, *Lymphokine Res.*, 9, 137, 1990.

374. Rose, R. M., Fuglestad, J. M., and Remington, L., Growth inhibition of *Mycobacterium avium* complex in human alveolar macrophages by the combination of recombinant macrophage colony-stimulating factor and interferon-gamma, *Am. J. Respir. Cell Mol. Biol.*, 4, 248, 1991.

376 Infectious Diseases in Immunocompromised Hosts

375. Denis, M. and Gregg, E. O., Modulation of *Mycobacterium avium* growth in murine macrophages: reversal of unresponsiveness to interferon-gamma by indomethacin or interleukin-4, *J. Leukoc. Biol.*, 49, 65, 1991.

376. Black, C. M., Bermudez, L. E., Young, L. S., and Remington, J. S., Co-infection of macrophages modulates interferon gamma and tumor necrosis factor-induced activation against intracellular pathogens, *J. Exp. Med.*, 172, 977, 1990.

377. Denis, M., *In vivo* modulation of atypical mycobacterial intervention: adjuvant therapy increases resistance to *Mycobacterium avium* by enhancing macrophage effector functions, *Cell. Immunol.*, 134, 42, 1991.

378. Johnson, J. L., Shiratsuchi, H., Toba, H., and Ellner, J. J., Preservation of monocyte effector functions against *Mycobacterium avium–M. intracellulare* in patients with AIDS, *Infect. Immun.*, 59, 3639, 1991.

379. Toba, H., Crawford, J. T., and Ellner, J. J., Pathogenicity of *Mycobacterium avium* for human monocytes: absence of macrophage-activating factor activity of gamma interferon, *Infect. Immun.*, 57, 239, 1989.

380. Blanchard, D. K., Michelini-Norris, M. B., and Djeu, J. Y., Interferon decreases the growth inhibition of *Mycobacterium avium-intracellulare* complex by fresh human monocytes but not by culture-derived macrophages, *J. Infect. Dis.*, 164, 152, 1991.

381. Zerlauth, G., Eibl, M. M., and Mannhalter, J. W., Induction of anti-mycobacterial and anti-listerial activity of human monocyte requires different activation signals, *Clin. Exp. Immunol.*, 85, 90, 1991.

382. Denis, M., Recombinant murine beta interferon enhances resistance of mice to systemic *Mycobacterium avium* infection, *Infect. Immun.*, 59, 1857, 1991.

383. Shiratsuchi, H., Johnson, J. L., and Ellner, J. J., Bidirectional effects of cytokines on the growth of *Mycobacterium avium* within human monocytes, *J. Immunol.*, 146, 3165, 1991.

384. Carvalho de Sousa, J. P. and Rastogi, N., Comparative ability of human monocytes and macrophages to control the intracellular growth of *Mycobacterium avium* and *Mycobacterium tuberculosis:* effect of interferon-gamma and indomethacin, *FEMS Microbiol. Immunol.*, 4, 329, 1992.

385. Denis, M., Campbell, D., and Gregg, E. O., Cytokine stimulation of parasitic and microbial growth, *Res. Microbiol.*, 142, 979, 1991.

386. Georgiev, V. St. and Albright, J. F., Cytokines and their role as growth factors and in regulation of immune responses, *Ann. NY Acad. Sci.*, 685, 584, 1993.

387. Denis, M., Interleukin-6 is used as a growth factor by virulent *Mycobacterium avium*: presence of specific receptors, *Cell. Immunol.*, 141, 182, 1992.

388. Denis, M. and Gregg, E. O., Recombinant interleukin-6 increases the intracellular and extracellular growth of *Mycobacterium avium*, *Can. J. Microbiol.*, 37, 479, 1991.

389. Bermudez, L. E., Wu, M., Petrofsky, M., and Young, L. S., Interleukin-6 antagonizes tumor necrosis factor-mediated mycobacteriostatic and mycobactericidal activities in macrophages, *Infect. Immun.*, 60, 4245, 1992.

390. Denis, M., Growth of *Mycobacterium avium* in human monocytes: identification of cytokines which reduce and enhance intracellular microbial growth, *Eur. J. Immunol.*, 21, 391, 1991.

391. Rastogi, N., Bachelet, M., and Carvalho de Sousa, J. P., Intracellular growth of *Mycobacterium avium* in human macrophages is linked to the increased synthesis of prostaglandin E_2 and inhibition of the phagosome-lysosome fusions, *FEMS Microbiol. Immunol.*, 4, 273, 1992.

392. Carvalho de Sousa, J. P., Bachelet, M., and Rastogi, N., Effect of indomethacin on the modulation of *Mycobacterium avium* growth in human macrophages by interferon gamma, retinoic acid and 1,25-dihydroxyvitamin D_3, *FEMS Microbiol. Immunol.*, 4, 281, 1992.

393. Denis, M. and Ghadirian, E., Transforming growth factor beta (TGF-b1) plays a detrimental role in the progression of experimental *Mycobacterium avium* infection: *in vivo* and *in vitro* evidence, *Microb. Pathol.*, 11, 367, 1991.

394. Orme, I.M., Furney, S. K., Skinner, P. S., Roberts, A. D., Brennan, P. J., Russell, D. G., Shiratsuchi, H., Ellner, J. J., and Weiser, W. Y., Inhibition of growth of *Mycobacterium avium* in murine and human mononuclear phagocytes by migration inhibitory factor, *Infect. Immun.*, 61, 338, 1993.

395. Ogata, K., Linzer, B. A., Zuberi, R. I., Ganz, T., Lehrer, R. I., and Catanzaro, A., Activity of defensins from human neutrophilic granulocytes against *Mycobacterium avium–Mycobacterium intracellulare*, *Infect. Immun.*, 60, 4720, 1992.

396. Mirando, W. S., Shiratsuchi, H., Tubesing, K., Toba, H., Ellner, J. J., and Elmets, C. A., Ultraviolet-irradiated monocytes efficiently inhibit the intracellular replication of *Mycobacterium avium intracellulare*, *J. Clin. Invest.*, 89, 1282, 1992.

397. Bermudez, L. E., Inderlied, C., and Young, L. S., Stimulation with cytokines enhances penetration of azithromycin into human macrophages, *Antimicrob. Agents Chemother.*, 35, 2625, 1991.

398. Prissick, F. H. and Mason, A. M., Cervical lymphadenitis in children caused by chromogenic mycobacteria, *Can. Med. Assoc. J.*, 75, 798, 1956.

399. Wolinsky, E., Nontuberculous mycobacteria and associated diseases, *Am. Rev. Respir. Dis.*, 119, 107, 1979.

400. Lincoln, E. M. and Gilbert, L. A., Disease in children due to mycobacteria other than *Mycobacterium tuberculosis*, *Am. Rev. Respir. Dis.*, 105, 683, 1972.

401. Hsu, K. H. K., Atypical mycobacterial infections in children, *Rev. Infect. Dis.*, 3, 1075, 1981.

402. Taha, A. M., Davidson, P. T., and Bailey, W. C., Surgical treatment of atypical mycobacterial lymphadenitis in children, *Pediatr. Infect. Dis. J.*, 4, 664, 1985.

403. Edwards, F. G. B., Disease caused by "atypical" (opportunist) mycobacteria: a whole population review, *Tubercle*, 51, 285, 1970.

404. Cox, R. J., Brightwell, A. P., and Riordan, T., Non-tuberculous mycobacterial infections presenting as salivary gland masses in children: investigation and conservative management, *J. Laryngol. Otol.*, 109, 525, 1995.

405. Wolinsky, E., Mycobacterial lymphadenitis in children: a prospective study of 105 nontuberculous cases with long-term follow-up, *Clin. Infect. Dis.*, 20, 954, 1995.

406. Dabrowski, M. T. and Keith, A. O., Three cases of mycobacterial cervical lymphadenitis, *J. Laryngol. Otol.*, 108, 514, 1994.

407. Pang, S. C., Mycobacterial lymphadenitis in Western Australia (1962–1987), *Tuberc. Lung Dis.*, 73, 362, 1992.

408. Gill, M. J., Fanning, E. A., and Chomyc, S., Childhood lymphadenitis in a harsh northern climate due to atypical mycobacteria, *Scand. J. Infect. Dis.*, 19, 77, 1987.

409. Wright, J. E., Non-tuberculous mycobacterial lymphadenitis, *Aust. NZ J. Surg.*, 66, 225, 1996.

410. Gracey, D. R. and Byrd, R. B., Five years experience at a pulmonary disease center with report of a case: scotochromogens and pulmonary disease, *Am. Rev. Respir. Dis.*, 101, 959, 1970.

411. Aiken, K. R. and Johnston, R. F., Tuberculous-like disease produced by *M. scrofulaceum*, *Pennsylvania Medicine*, 81, 38, 1978.

412. Dustin, P., Demol, P., Derks-Jacobovitz, D., Cremer, N., and Vis, H., Generalized fatal chronic infection by *Mycobacterium scrofulaceum* with severe amyloidosis in a child, *Pathol. Res. Pract.*, 168, 237, 1980.

413. McNutt, D. R. and Fudenberg, H. H., Disseminated scotochromogen infection and unusual myeloproliferative disorder: report of a case and review of the literature, *Ann. Intern. Med.*, 75, 737, 1971.

414. Yamamoto, M., Sudo, K., Taga, M., and Hibino, S., A study of diseases caused by atypical mycobacteria in Japan, *Am. Rev. Respir. Dis.*, 96, 779, 1967.

415. Patel, K. M., Granulomatous hepatitis due to *Mycobacterium scrofulaceum*: report of a case, *Gastroenterology*, 81, 156, 1981.

416. Kraus, M., Fliss, D. M., Leiberman, A., Barki, Y., and Hertzanu, Y., Mycobacterial cervical adenitis, *Ann. Otol. Rhinol. Laryngol.*, 104, 409, 1995.

417. Nunez Gonzalez, L. C., Egues Cuenca, C., Silvera Carcashe, E., Perra Salazar, C., and Jimenez Misas, C., Mycobacteriosis caused by *Mycobacterium scrofulaceum*: report of 1 case, *Rev. Cubana Med. Trop.*, 43, 124, 1991.

418. Lindberg, M. C. and Thomas, G. G., Lymphadenitis due to atypical mycobacteria, *Ala. Med.*, 59, 19, 1989.

419. Katoh, O., Yamada, H., Yamaguchi, T., Katoh, H., Itoh, T., and Watanabe, T., A resected case with massive hemoptysis due to *Mycobactrium scrofulaceum* lung infection, *Kekkaku*, 62, 349, 1987.

420. Murray-Leisure, K. A., Egan, N., and Weitekamp, M. R., Skin lesions caused by *Mycobacterium scrofulaceum*, *Arch. Dermatol.*, 123, 369, 1987.

421. Sanders, J. W., Walsh, A. D., Snider, R. L., and Sahn, E. E., Disseminated *Mycobacterium scrofulaceum* infection: a potentially treatable complication of AIDS, *Clin. Infect. Dis.*, 20, 549, 1995.

422. Margileth, A. M., The use of purified protein derivative mycobacterial skin test antigens in children and adolescents: purified protein derivative skin test results correlated with mycobacterial isolates, *Pediatr. Infect. Dis. J.*, 2, 225, 1983.

423. Margileth, A. M., Management of nontuberculous (atypical) mycobacterial infections in children and adolescents, *Pediatr. Infect. Dis. J.*, 4, 119, 1985.

424. Buhler, V. B. and Pollack, A., Human infection with atypical acid-fast organisms, *Am. J. Clin. Pathol.*, 23, 363, 1953.

425. Runyon, E. H., Identification of mycobacterial pathogens utilizing colony characteristics, *Am. J. Clin. Pathol.*, 54, 578, 1970.

426. Echevarria, M. P., Martin, G., Perez, J., and Urkijo, J. C., Pulmonary infection by *Mycobacterium kansasii*: presentation of 27 cases, *Enferm. Infecc. Microbiol. Clin.*, 12, 280, 1994.

427. Arnold, J. H., Scott, A. V., and Spitznagel, J. K., Specificity of PPD skin tests in childhood tuberculin converts: comparison with mycobacterial species from tissues and secretions, *J. Pediatr.*, 76, 512, 1970.

428. Ahn, C. H., McLarty, J. W., Ahn, S. S., Ahn, S. I., and Hurst, G. A., Diagnostic criteria for pulmonary disease caused by *Mycobacterium kansasii* and *Mycobacterium intracellulare*, *Am. Rev. Respir. Dis.*, 125, 388, 1982.

429. Kin, T. C., Arora, N. S., Aldrich, T. K., and Rochester, D. F., Atypical mycobacterial infections: a clinical study of 92 patients, *South. Med. J.*, 74, 1304, 1981.

430. Christensen, E. E., Dietz, G. W., Ahn, C. H., Chapman, J. S., Murry, R. C., and Hurst, G. A., Radiographic manifestations of pulmonary *Mycobacterium kansasii* infections, *Am. J. Radiol.*, 131, 985, 1978.

431. Banks, J., Hunter, A. M., Campbell, I. A., Jenkins, P. A., and Smith, A. P., Pulmonary infection with *Mycobacterium kansasii* in Wales, 1970-9: review of treatment and response, *Thorax*, 38, 271, 1983.

432. Johanson, W. G., Jr. and Nicholson, D. P., Pulmonary disease due to *Mycobacterium kansasii*: an analysis of some factors affecting prognosis, *Am. Rev. Respir. Dis.*, 99, 73, 1989.

433. Lillo, M., Orengo, S., Cernoch, P., and Harris, R. L., Pulmonary and disseminated infection due to *Mycobacterium kansasii*: a decade of experience, *Rev. Infect. Dis.*, 12, 760, 1990.

434. Gettler, J. F. and El-Sadr, W., *Mycobacterium kansasii* infection following primary pulmonary malignancy, *Chest*, 105, 325, 1994.

435. Feld, R., Bodey, G. P., and Gröschel, D., Mycobacteriosis in patients with malignant disease, *Arch. Intern. Dis.*, 136, 67, 1976.

436. Kaplan, M. H., Armstrong, D., and Rosen, P., Tuberculosis complicating neoplastic disease: a review of 201 cases, *Cancer*, 33, 850, 1974.

437. Black, B. G. and Chapman, J. S., Cervical adenitis in children due to human and unclassified mycobacteria, *Pediatrics*, 33, 887, 1964.

438. Nandwani, R., Shanson, D. C., Fisher, M., Nelson, M. R., and Gazzard, B. G., *Mycobacterium kansasii* scalp abscesses in an AIDS patient, *J. Infect. Dis.*, 31, 79, 1995.

439. Breathnach, A., Levell, N., Munro, C., Natarajan, S., and Pedler, S., Cutaneous *Mycobacterium kansasii* infection: case report and review, *Clin. Infect. Dis.*, 20, 812, 1995.

440. Delaporte, E., Savage, C., Alfandari, S., Piette, F., Leclerc, H., and Bergoend, H., *Mycobacterium kansasii* cutaneous infection, *Ann. Dermatol. Venereol.*, 120, 289, 1993.

441. Bolivar, R., Satterwhite, T. K., and Floyd, M., Cutaneous lesions due to *Mycobacterium kansasii*, *Arch. Dermatol.*, 116, 207, 1980.

442. Mandal, D., Curless, E., and Ostick, D. G., Pyogenic abscess caused by *Mycobacterium kansasii* in advanced AIDS, *Int. J. STD AIDS*, 3, 362, 1992.

443. Rosen, T., Cutaneous *Mycobacterium kansasii* infection presenting as cellulitis, *Cutis*, 31, 87, 1983.

444. Dore, N., Collins, J.-P., and Mankiewicz, E., A sporotrichoid-like *Mycobacterium kansasii* infection of the skin treated with minocycline hydrochloride, *Br. J. Dermatol.*, 101, 75, 1979.

445. Kelly, P. J., Karlson, A. G., Weed, L. A., and Lipscomb, P. R., Infection of synovial tissues by mycobacteria other than *Mycobacterium tuberculosis*, *J. Bone Joint Surg. (Am.)*, 49A, 1521, 1967.

446. Sutker, W. L., Lankford, L. L., and Tompsett, R., Granulomatous synovitis: the role of atypical mycobacteria, *Rev. Infect. Dis.*, 1, 729, 1979.

447. Leader, M., Revell, P., and Clarke, G., Synovial infection with *Mycobacterium kansasii*, *Ann. Rheum. Dis.*, 43, 80, 1984.

448. Naguib, M. T., Byers, J. M., and Slater, L. N., Paranasal sinus infection due to atypical mycobacteria in two patients with AIDS, *Clin. Infect. Dis.*, 19, 789, 1994.

449. Demerieux, P., Keystone, E. C., Hutcheon, M., and Laskin, C., Polyarthritis due to *Mycobacterium kansasii* in a patient with rheumatoid arthritis, *Ann. Rheum. Dis.*, 39, 90, 1980.

450. Friedman, A. W. and Ike, R. W., *Mycobacterium kansasii* septic arthritis in a patient with acquired immune deficiency syndrome, *Arthritis Rheum.*, 36, 1631, 1993.

451. Parker, M. D. and Irwin, R. S., *Mycobacterium kansasii* tendonitis and fasciitis: report of a case treated successfully with drug therapy alone, *J. Bone Joint Surg. (Am.)*, 57, 557, 1975.

452. Watanakunatorn, C. and Trott, A., Vertebral osteomyelitis due to *Mycobacterium kansasii*, *Am. Rev. Respir. Dis.*, 107, 846, 1973.

453. Weinroth, S. E., Pincetl, P., and Tuazon, C. U., Disseminated *Mycobacterium kansasii* infection presenting as pneumonia and osteomyelitis of the skull in a patient with AIDS, *Clin. Infect. Dis.*, 18, 261, 1994.

454. Klotch, D. W., Owens, M. H., and Wild, L. M., *Mycobacterium kansasii* presenting as an unusual type of rhinophyma, *Otolaryngol. Head Neck Surg.*, 107, 792, 1992.

455. Mead, G. M., Dance, D. A. B., and Smith, A. G., Lymphadenopathy complicating hairy cell leukemia: a case of disseminated *Mycobacterium kansasii* infection, *Acta Haematol. (Basel)*, 70, 335, 1983.

456. McGeady, S. J. and Murphey, S. A., Disseminated *Mycobacterium kansasii* infection, *Clin. Immunol. Immunopathol.*, 20, 87, 1981.

457. Stewart, C. and Jackson, L., Spleno-hepatic tuberculosis due to *Mycobacterium kansasii*, *Med. J. Aust.*, 2, 99, 1976.

458. Hepper, N. G. G., Karlson, A. G., Leary, F. J., and Soule, E. H., Genitourinary infection due to *Mycobacterium kansasii*, *Mayo Clin. Proc.*, 46, 387, 1971.

459. Palmer, J. A. and Watanakunakorn, C., *Mycobacterium kansasii* pericarditis, *Thorax*, 39, 876, 1984.

460. Bacon, M. E., Whelan, T. V., Mahoney, M. D., Patel, T. G., and Judson, P. L., Pericarditis due to *Mycobacterium kansasii* in a patient undergoing dialysis for chronic renal failure, *J. Infect. Dis.*, 152, 846, 1985.

461. Boudon, P., Le Pennec, M. P., Malbec, D., Mathieu, M. et al., *Mycobacterium kansasii* infection in patients with human immunodeficiency virus infection, *Rev. Med. Intern.*, 16, 747, 1995.

462. Witzig, R. S., Fazal, B. A., Mera, R. M., Mushatt, D. M., Dejace, P. M. J. T., Greer, D. L., and Hyslop, N. E., Jr., Clinical manifestations and implications of coinfection with *Mycobacterium kansasii* and human immunodeficiency virus type 1, *Clin. Infect. Dis.*, 21, 77, 1995.

463. Bamberger, D. M., Driks, M. R., Gupta, M. R., O'Connor, M. C., Jost, P. M., Neihart, R. E., McKinsey, D. S., and Moore, L. A., *Mycobacterium kansasii* among patients infected with human immunodeficiency virus in Kansas City. Kansas City AIDS Research Consortium, *Clin. Infect. Dis.*, 18, 395, 1994.

464. Urkijo, J. C., Montejo, M., Aguirrebengoa, K., Urra, E., and Aguirre, C., Disease caused by *Mycobacterium kansasii* in patients with HIV infection, *Enferm. Infecc. Microbiol. Clin.*, 11, 120, 1993.

465. Dautzenberg, B., Antoun, F., and Truffot, C., Acquired rifampicin resistance during *M. kansasii* infection in a patient with AIDS, *Rev. Mal. Respir.*, 9, 464, 1992.

466. Naher, R. and Peters, B., *Mycobacterium kansasii* seroma of the skin in HIV infection, *Hautarzt*, 43, 361, 1992.

467. Levine, B. and Chaisson, R. E., *Mycobacterium kansasii*: a cause of treatable pulmonary disease associated with advanced human immunodeficiency virus (HIV) infection, *Ann. Intern. Med.*, 114, 861, 1991.

468. Valainis, G. T., *Mycobacterium kansasii* infection, *Ann. Intern. Dis.*, 115, 496, 1991.

469. Jost, P. M. and Hodges, G. R., *Mycobacterium kansasii* infection in a patient with AIDS, *South. Med. J.*, 84, 1501, 1991.

470. Valainis, G. T., Cardona, L. M., and Greer, D. L., The spectrum of *Mycobacterium kansasii* disease associated with HIV-1 infected patients, *J. Acquir. Immune Defic. Syndr.*, 4, 516, 1991.

471. Chaisson, R. E. and Levine, B., *Mycobacterium kansasii* infection: a reply, *Ann. Intern. Med.*, 115, 496, 1991.

472. Singh, G., Treatment of septic arthritis due to *Mycobacterium kansasii*, *Br. Med. J. (Clin. Res. Ed.)*, 290, 857, 1985.

473. Zwolska-Kwiek, Z., Augustynowicz-Kopec, E., and Zalewska-Schontaler, N., Drug sensitivity of bacillus strains *M. avium-intracellulare* (MAIC), *M. kansasii* cultured from patients with mycobacteriosis before treatment, *Pneumonol. Alergol. Pol.*, 61, 248, 1993.

474. Hopewell, P., Cynamon, M., Starke, J., Iseman, M., and O'Brien, R., Evaluation of new anti-infective drugs for the treatment of disease caused by *Mycobacterium kansasii* and other mycobacteria, *Clin. Infect. Dis.*, 15(Suppl. 1), S307, 1992.

475. Wallace, R. J., Jr., Dunbar, D., Brown, B. A., Onyi, G., Dunlap, R., Ahn, C. H., and Murphy, D. T., Rifampin-resistant *Mycobacterium kansasii*, *Clin. Infect. Dis.*, 18, 736, 1994.

476. Nakazono, T., Sugie, T., Ogata, H., Mizutani, S., Sugita, H., Kino, T., and Wada, M., Investigation on the treatment of infection due to *Mycobacterium kansasii*, *Kekkaku*, 69, 587, 1994.

477. Delclaux, C., Laederich, J., Adotti, F., and Kleinknecht, D., Fatal disseminated *Mycobacterium kansasii* infection in a hemodialysis patient, *Nephron*, 64, 155, 1993.

478. Groves, R. W., Newton, J. A., and Hay, R. J., Cutaneous *Mycobacterium kansasii* infection — treatment with erythromycin, *Clin. Exp. Dermatol.*, 16, 300, 1991.

479. Nisar, M., Watkin, S. W., Bucknall, R. C., and Agnew, R. A., Exacerbation of isoniazid induced peripheral neuropathy by pyridoxine, *Thorax*, 45, 419, 1990.

480. Sauret, J., Hernandez-Flix, S., Castro, E., Hernandez, L., Ausina, V., and Coll, P., Treatment of pulmonary disease caused by *Mycobacterium kansasii*: results of 18 vs. 12 months' chemotherapy, *Tuberc. Lung Dis.*, 76, 104, 1995.

481. Research Committee, British Thoracic Society, *Mycobacterium kansasii* pulmonary infection: a prospective study of the results of nine months of treatment with rifampicin and ethambutol, *Thorax*, 49, 442, 1994.

482. Ahn, C. H., Lowell, J. R., Ahn, S. I., and Hurst, G. A., Short-course chemotherapy for pulmonary disease caused by *Mycobacterium kansasii*, *Am. Rev. Respir. Dis.*, 128, 1048, 1983.

483. Umeda, A., Asano, K., Kawai, A., Nakamura, H., Fujita, H., Mori, M., Yamaguchi, K., and Kanazawa, M., *Mycobacterium kansasii* lung infection associated with myelofibrosis — a case refractory to treatment with antitubercular agents, *Nippon Kyobu Shikkan Gakkai Zasshi*, 32, 1170, 1994.

484. Ahn, C. H., Wallace, R. J., Jr., Steele, L. C., and Murphy, D. T., Sulfonamide-containing regimens for disease caused by rifampin-resistant *Mycobacterium kansasii*, *Am. Rev. Respir. Dis.*, 135, 10, 1987.

485. Yoshimoto, S., Konishi, H., Kawahara, S., Tada, A., Shiomi, K., Takeuchi, M., Kamisaka, K., Mishima, Y., Matsuyama, T., and Kibata, M., A case of pulmonary atypical mycobacteriosis complicated with aplastic anemia, treated with surgical resection and postoperative sparfloxacin, *Nippon Kyobu Shikkan Gakkai Zasshi*, 30, 1345, 1992.

486. Matthiessen, W., Schonfeld, N., Mauch, H., Wahn, U., and Grassot, A., Nontuberculous mycobacteriosis as a complication of the Swyer-James syndrome, *Dtsch. Med. Wochenschr.*, 118, 139, 1993.

487. Kramers, C., Raemaekers, J. M., van Baar, H. M., de Pauw, B. E., and Horrevorts, A. M., Sweet's syndrome as the presenting symptom of hairy cell leukemia with concomitant infection by *Mycobacterium kansasii*, *Ann. Hematol.*, 65, 55, 1992.

488. Bennett, C., Vardiman, J., and Golomb, H., Disseminated atypical mycobacterial infection in patients with hairy cell leukemia, *Am. J. Med.*, 80, 891, 1986.

489. Kurasawa, T., Ikeda, N., Sato, A., Nakatani, K. et al., A clinical study of non-tuberculous pulmonary mycobacteriosis, *Kekkaku*, 70, 621, 1995.

490. Runyon, E. H., Conservation of the specific epithet *fortuitum* in the name of the organism known as *Mycobacterium fortuitum* da Costa Cruz, *Int. J. Syst. Bacteriol.*, 22, 50, 1972.

491. Wallace, R. J., Jr., Recent changes in taxonomy and disease manifestations of the rapidly growing mycobacteria, *Eur. J. Clin. Microbiol. Infect. Dis.*, 13, 953, 1994.

492. Wolinsky, E. and Rynearson, T. K., Mycobacteria in soil and their relation to disease-associated strains, *Am. Rev. Respir. Dis.*, 97, 1032, 1968.

493. Goslee, S. and Wolinsky, E., Water as a source of potentially pathogenic mycobacteria, *Am. Rev. Respir. Dis.*, 113, 287, 1976.

494. Tsukamura, M., Kita, N., Shimoide, H., Yoshimoto, K., Wada, T., and Mitani, Y., Lung infections due to *Mycobacterium fortuitum* and *Mycobacterium chelonae*: report of nine cases of *M. fortuitum* infection and four cases of *M. chelonae* infection, *Kekkaku*, 60, 429, 1985.

495. Wallace, R. J., Jr., Swenson, J. M., Silcox, V. A., Good, R. C., Tschen, J. A., and Stone, M. S., Spectrum of disease due to rapidly growing mycobacteria, *Rev. Infect. Dis.*, 5, 657, 1983.

496. Tice, A. D. and Solomon, R. J., Disseminated *Mycobacterium chelonei* infection: response to sulfona-mides, *Am. Rev. Respir. Dis.*, 120, 197, 1979.

497. Hand, W. L. and Sanford, J. P., *Mycobacterium fortuitum* — a human pathogen, *Ann. Intern. Med.*, 73, 971, 1970.

498. Heironimus, J. D., Winn, R. E., and Collins, C. B., Cutaneous nonpulmonary *Mycobacterium chelonae* infection: successful treatment with sulfonamides in an immunosuppressed patient, *Arch. Dermatol.*, 120, 1061, 1984.

499. Damsker, B. and Bottone, E. J., Nontuberculous mycobacteria as unsuspected agents of dermatological infections: diagnosis through microbiological parameters, *J. Clin. Microbiol.*, 11, 569, 1980.

500. Dross, I. C., Abbatiello, A. A., Jenney, F. S., and Cohen, A. C., Pulmonary infection due to *M. fortuitum*, *Am. Rev. Respir. Dis.*, 89, 923, 1964.

501. Burke, D. S. and Ullian, R. B., Megaesophagus and pneumonia associated with *Mycobacterium chelonei*: a case report and a literature review, *Am. Rev. Respir. Dis.*, 116, 1101, 1977.

502. Lauring, L. M., Wergeland, F. L., and Sack, G. E., Anonymous mycobacterium keratitis, *Am. J. Ophthalmol.*, 67, 130, 1969.

503. Turner, L. and Stinson, I., *Mycobacterium fortuitum* as a cause of corneal ulcer, *Am. J. Ophthalmol.*, 60, 329, 1965.

504. Smiddy, W. E., Miller, D., and Flynn, H. W., Jr., Scleral buckle infections due to atypical mycobacteria, *Retina*, 11, 394, 1991.

505. Band, J. D., Ward, J. I., Fraser, D. W., Peterson, N. J., Silcox, V. A., Good, R. C., Ostroy, P. R., and Kennedy, J., Peritonitis due to a *Mycobacterium chelonei*-like organism associated with intermittent chronic peritoneal dialysis, *J. Infect. Dis.*, 145, 9, 1982.

506. Woods, G. L., Hall, G. S., and Schreiber, M. J., *Mycobacterium fortuitum* peritonitis associated with continuous ambulatory dialysis, *J. Clin. Microbiol.*, 23, 786, 1986.

507. Merlin, T. L. and Tzamaloukas, A. H., *Mycobacterium chelonae* peritonitis associated with continuous ambulatory peritoneal dialysis, *Am. J. Clin. Pathol.*, 91, 717, 1989.

508. Bolan, G., Reingold, A. L., Carson, L. A., Silcox, V. A., Woodley, C. L., Hayes, P. S., Hightower, A. W., McFarland, L., Brown, J. W. III, Peterson, N. J., Favero, M. S., Good, R. C., and Broome, C. V., Infections with *Mycobacterium chelonei* in patients receiving dialysis and using processed hemo-dialysers, *J. Infect. Dis.*, 152, 1013, 1985.

509. Raad, I. I., Vartivarian, S., Khan, A., and Bodey, G. P., Catheter-related infections caused by *Mycobacterium fortuitum* complex: 15 cases and review, *Rev. Infect. Dis.*, 13, 1120, 1991.

510. Koontz, F. P., Erwin, M. E., Barrett, M. S., and Jones, R. N., Etest for routine clinical antimicrobial susceptibility testing of rapid-growing mycobacteria isolates, *Diagn. Microbiol. Infect. Dis.*, 19, 183, 1994.

511. McFarland, E. J. and Kuritzkes, D. R., Clinical features of infection due to *Mycobacterium fortuitum/chelonae* complex, *Curr. Clin. Top. Infect. Dis.*, 13, 188, 1993.

512. Wallace, R. J., Jr., Diagnostic and therapeutic consideration in patients with pulmonary disease due to the rapidly growing mycobacteria, *Semin. Respir. Infect. Dis.*, 1, 230, 1986.

513. Wallace, R. J., Jr., Swenson, J. M., Silcox, V. A., and Bullen, M. G., Treatment of nonpulmonary infections due to *Mycobacterium fortuitum* and *Mycobacterium chelonei* on the basis of *in vitro* susceptibilities, *J. Infect. Dis.*, 152, 500, 1985.

514. Yew, W. W., Lau, K. S., Tse, W. K., and Wong, C. F., Imipenem in the treatment of lung infections due to *Mycobacterium fortuitum* and *Mycobacterium chelonae*: further experience, *Clin. Infect. Dis.*, 15, 1046, 1992.

515. Yew, W. W., Kwan, S. Y., Wong, P. C., and Lee, J., Ofloxacin and imipenem in the treatment of *Mycobacterium fortuitum* and *Mycobacterium chelonae* lung infections, *Tubercle*, 71, 131, 1990.

516. Cynamon, M. H. and Palmer, G. S., *In vitro* susceptibility of *Mycobacterium fortuitum* to *N*-formamidoyl thienamycin and several cephamycins, *Antimicrob. Agents Chemother.*, 22, 1079, 1982.

517. Opie, J. C., Vaughn, C. C., Comp, R. A., Radford, J. M., Lowell, P., and Finch, C., Endobronchial closure of a postpneumonectomy bronchial fistula, *Ann. Thorac. Surg.*, 53, 686, 1992.

518. Lin, R., Holland, G. N., Helm, C. J., Elias, S. J., Berlin, O. G., and Bruckner, D. A., Comparative efficacy of topical ciprofloxacin for treating *Mycobacterium fortuitum* and *Mycobacterium chelonae* keratitis in an animal model, *Am. J. Ophthalmol.*, 117, 657, 1994.

519. Saito, H., Tomioka, H., and Nagashima, K., Protective and therapeutic efficacy of *Lactobacillus casei* against experimental murine infections due to *Mycobacterium fortuitum* complex, *J. Gen. Microbiol.*, 133, 2843, 1987.

520. Bullin, C. H., Tanner, E. I., and Collins, C. H., Isolation of *Mycobacterium xenopi* from water taps, *J. Hyg. (Cambridge)*, 68, 97, 1970.

521. Miller, W. C., Perkins, M. D., Richardson, W. J., and Sexton, D. J., Pott's disease case by *Mycobacterium xenopi*: case report and review, *Clin. Infect. Dis.*, 19, 1024, 1994.

522. Marks, J. and Schwabacher, H., Infection due to *Mycobacterium xenopi*, *Br. Med. J.*, 1, 32, 1965.

523. Tortoli, E., Simonetti, M. T., Labardi, C., Lopes Pegna, A., Meli, E., Stanflin, N., and Susini, S., *Mycobacterium xenopi* isolation from clinical specimens in the Florence area: review of 46 cases, *Eur. J. Epidemiol.*, 7, 677, 1991.

524. Collins, C. H., Grange, J. M., and Yates, M. D., Mycobacteria in water, *J. Appl. Bacteriol.*, 57, 193, 1984,

525. Koemoth, P. P., Fraselle, R., Correa de Brito, J. M., and Brock, M., Presumptive identification of *Mycobacterium xenopi* with radiometric Bactec system, *Eur. J. Clin. Microbiol. Infect. Dis.*, 10, 694, 1991.

526. Yates, M. D., Grange, J. M., and Collins, C. H., The nature of mycobacterial disease in south east England, 1977-1984, *J. Epidemiol. Community Health*, 40, 295, 1986.

527. Gross, W., Hawkins, J. E., and Murphy, D. B., *Mycobacterium xenopi* in clinical specimens: water as a source of contamination, *Am. Rev. Respir. Dis.*, 113(Suppl.), 78, 1976.

528. McSwiggan, D. A. and Collins, C. H., The isolation of *M. kansasii* and *M. xenopi* from water systems, *Tubercle*, 55, 291, 1974.

529. Levy, A., Rusu, R., and Mates, A., *Mycobacterium xenopi*, a potent human pathogen, *Isr. J. Med. Sci.*, 28, 772, 1992.

530. Costrini, A. M., Mahler, D. A., Gross, W. M., Hawkins, J. E., Yesner, R., and D'Esopo, N. D., Clinical and roentgenographic features of nosocomial pulmonary disease due to *Mycobacterium xenopi*, *Am. Rev. Respir. Dis.*, 123, 104, 1981.

531. Sniadack, D. H., Ostroff, S. M., Karlix, M. A., Smithwick, R. W., Schwartz, B., Sprauer, M. A., Silcox, V. A., and Good, R. C., A nosocomial pseudo-outbreak of *Mycobacterium xenopi* due to a contaminated potable water supply: lessons in prevention, *Infect. Control Hosp. Epidemiol.*, 14, 636, 1993.

532. Stewart, C. J., Dixon, J. M. S., and Curtis, B. A., Isolation of mycobacteria from tonsils, naso-pharyngeal secretions and lymph nodes in East Anglia, *Tubercle*, 51, 178, 1970.

533. Engbaek, H. C., Vergmann, B., Baess, I., and Will, D. W., *M. xenopi*: a bacteriological study of *M. xenopi* including case reports of Danish patients, *Acta Pathol. Microbiol. Scand.*, 69, 576, 1967.

534. Banks, J., Hunter, A. M., Campbell, I. A., Jenkins, P. A., and Smith, A. P., Pulmonary infection with *Mycobacterium xenopi*: review of treatment and response, *Thorax*, 39, 376, 1984.

535. Galblum, L. I. and Abraham, A. A., *Mycobacterium xenopi* mycobacteriosis, *South. Med. J.*, 74, 1026, 1981.

536. Simor, A. E., Salit, I. E., and Vellend, H., The role of *Mycobacterium xenopi* in human disease, *Am. Rev. Respir. Dis.*, 129, 435, 1984.

537. Platia, E. V. and Vosti, K. L., *Mycobacterium xenopi* pulmonary disease, *West. J. Med.*, 138, 102, 1983.

538. Smith, M. J. and Citron, K. M., Clinical review of pulmonary disease caused by *Mycobacterium xenopi*, *Thorax*, 38, 373, 1983.

539. Koizumi, J. H. and Sommers, H. M., *Mycobacterium xenopi* and pulmonary disease, *Am. J. Clin. Pathol.*, 73, 826, 1980.

540. Terashima, T., Sakamaki, F., Hasegawa, N., Kanazawa, M., and Kawashiro, T., Pulmonary infection due to *Mycobacterium xenopi*, *Intern. Med.*, 33, 536, 1994.

541. Sennesael, J. J., Maes, V. A., Pierard, D., Debeukelaer, S. H., and Verbeelen, D. L., Streptomycin pharmacokinetics in relapsing *Mycobacterium xenopi* peritonitis, *Am. J. Nephrol.*, 10, 422, 1990.

542. Thomas, P., Liu, F., and Weiser, W., Characteristics of *Mycobacterium xenopi* disease, *Bull. Int. Union Tuberc. Lung Dis.*, 63, 12, 1988.

543. Parrot, R. G. and Grosset, J. H., Post-surgical outcome of 57 patients with *Mycobacterium xenopi* pulmonary infection, *Tubercle*, 69, 47, 1988.

544. Branger, B., Gouby, A., Oulès, R., Balducchi, J. P., Mourad, G., Fourcade, J., Mion, C., Duntz, F., and Ramiz, M., *Mycobacterium haemophilum* and *Mycobacterium xenopi* associated infection in a renal transplant patient, *Clin. Nephrol.*, 23, 46, 1985.

545. Busch, F. W., Bautz, W., Dierkesmann, R., Toomes, H., Schalk, K. P., Rüsch-Gerdes, S., and Ehninger, G., Lung changes caused by *Mycobacterium xenopi* infection in a patient with bone marrow transplantation: problems in differential diagnosis, *Pneumologie*, 45, 340, 1991.

546. Huber, W., Bautz, W., Holzmann, B., Classen, M., and Schepp, W., Pneumonia due to a rare atypical *Mycobacterium* in AIDS, *Dtsch. Med. Wochenschr.*, 118, 1636, 1993.

547. Prosser, A. J., Spinal infection with *Mycobacterium xenopi*, *Tubercle*, 67, 229, 1986.

548. Rahman, M. A. A., Phongsathorn, V., Hughes, T., and Bielawska, C., Spinal infection by *Mycobacterium xenopi* in a non-immunosuppressed patient, *Tuberc. Lung Dis.*, 73, 392, 1992.

549. Feyen, J., Martens, M., and Mulier, J. C., Infection of the knee joint with *Mycobacterium xenopi*, *Clin. Orthop.*, 179, 189, 1983.

550. Marks, J., Cook, J., and Pringle, J. A. S., Bone abscess due to *Mycobacterium xenopi*, *Tubercle*, 56, 157, 1975.

551. Damsker, B., Bottone, E. J., and Deligdisch, L., *Mycobacterium xenopi*: infection in an immunocompromised host, *Human Pathol.*, 13, 866, 1982.

552. Eng, R. H. K., Forrester, C., Smith, S. M., and Sobel, H., *Mycobacterium xenopi* infection in a patient with acquired immunodeficiency syndrome, *Chest*, 86, 145, 1984.

553. Tecson-Tumang, F. T. and Bright, J. L., *Mycobacterium xenopi*, and the acquired immunodeficiency syndrome, *Ann. Intern. Med.*, 100, 461, 1984.

554. Price, A. B., Owen, R., Sowter, G., Einberg, J., and Smith, H., Disseminated *Mycobacterium xenopi* infection, *Lancet*, 2, 383, 1985.

555. Ausina, V., Barrio, J., Luquin, M., Sambeat, M. A., Gurgui, M., Verger, G., and Prats, G., *Mycobacterium xenopi* infections in the acquired immunodeficiency syndrome, *Ann. Intern. Med.*, 109, 927, 1988.

556. Shafer, R. W. and Sierra, M. F., *Mycobacterium xenopi*, *Mycobacterium fortuitum*, *Mycobacterium kansasii*, and other nontuberculous mycobacteria in an area of endemicity for AIDS, *Clin. Infect. Dis.*, 15, 161, 1992.

557. Weinberg, J. R., Dootson, G., Gertner, D., Chambers, S. T., and Smith, H., Disseminated *Mycobacterium xenopi* infection, *Lancet*, 1, 1033, 1985.

558. Baugnee, P. E., Pouthier, F., and Dalaunois, L., Pulmonary mycobacteriosis due to *Mycobacterium xenopi*: in-vitro sensitivity to classical antitubercular agents and clinical development, *Acta Clin. Belg.*, 51, 19, 1996.

559. Bellamy, J., Leroy-Terquem, E., Duhamel, J. P., Choffel, C., Fraboulet, G., Tobelem, G., and Verdoux, P., *Mycobacterium xenopi* infection in emphysematous bulla: apropos of 4 cases operated on, *Rev. Mal. Respir.*, 4, 261, 1987.

560. Group for the Study and Treatment of Resistant Mycobacterial Infections (GETIM), Rifabutin in the treatment of mycobacterial infections resistant to rifampicin: preliminary results, *Rev. Mal. Respir.*, 6, 335, 1989.

561. Jones, P. G., Schrager, M. A., and Zabransky, R. J., Pott's disease caused by *Mycobacterium xenopi*, *Clin. Infect. Dis.*, 21, 1352, 1995.

562. Kiehl, P., Eicher, U., and Vakilzaden, F., A lupus-vulgaris-like atypical mycobacteriosis caused by *Mycobacterium xenopi* (lupus xenopi), *Hautarzt*, 43, 569, 1992.

563. Crantock, L., Crawford, D., and Powell, L., Fulminant hepatic failure complicating the treatment of *Mycobacterium xenopi*, *Med. J. Aust.*, 155, 723, 1991.

564. Thompson, J. E., Fulminant hepatic failure complicating the treatment of *Mycobacterium xenopi*, *Med. J. Aust.*, 156, 811, 1992.

565. Garibaldi, R. A., Kaplan, H. S., and Brittingham, T. E., Jaundice and death from isoniazid, *J. Tenn. Med. Assoc.*, 63, 23, 1970.

566. Black, M., Mitchell, J., Zimmermann, H., Ishak, K. G., and Epler, G. R., Isoniazid associated hepatitis in 114 patients, *Gastroenterology*, 69, 289, 1975.

567. Powell, L. W. and Crawford, D. H. G., Fulminant hepatic failure complicating the treatment of *Mycobacterium xenopi*: a reply, *Med. J. Aust.*, 156, 812, 1992.

568. Sompolinsky, D., Lagziel, A., Naveh, D., and Yankilevitz, T., *Mycobacterium haemophilum* sp. nov., a new pathogen of humans, *Int. J. Syst. Bacteriol.*, 28, 67, 1978.

569. Strauss, W. L., Ostroff, S. M., Jernigan, D. B., Kiehn, T. E., Sordillo, E. M., Armstrong, D., Boone, N., Schneider, N., Kilburn, J. O., Silcox, V. A., LaBombardi, V., and Good, R. C., Clinical and epidemiologic characteristics of *Mycobacterium haemophilum*, an emerging pathogen in immuno-compromised patients, *Ann. Intern. Med.*, 120, 118, 1994.

570. Walder, B. K., Jeremy, D., Charlesworth, J. A., MacDonald, G. J., Pussell, B. A., and Robertson, M. R., The skin and immunosuppression, *Australas. J. Dermatol.*, 17, 94, 1976.

571. Becherer, P. and Hopfer, R. L., Infection with *Mycobacterium haemophilum*, *Clin. Infect. Dis.*, 14, 793, 1992.

572. Branger, B., Gouby, A., Oules, R., Balducci, J. P., Mourad, G., Fourcade, J., Mion, C., Duntz, F., and Ramuz, M., *Mycobacterium haemophilum* and *Mycobacterium xenopi* associated infection in a renal transplant recipient, *Clin. Nephrol.*, 23, 46, 1985.

573. Davis, B. R., Brumbach, J., Sanders, W. J., and Wolinsky, E., Skin lesions caused by *Mycobacterium haemophilum*, *Ann. Intern. Med.*, 97, 723, 1982.

574. Dawson, D. J., Blacklock, Z. M., and Kane, D. W., *Mycobacterium haemophilum* causing lymphadenitis in an otherwise healthy child, *Med. J. Aust.*, 2, 289, 1981.

575. Dever, L. L., Martin, J. W., Seaworth, B., and Joegensen, J. H., Varied presentations and responses to treatment of infections caused by *Mycobacterium haemophilum* in patients with AIDS, *Clin. Infect. Dis.*, 14, 1195, 1992.

576. Gouby, A., Branger, B., Oules, R., and Ramuz, M., Two cases of *Mycobacterium haemophilum* infection in a renal-dialysis unit, *J. Med. Microbiol.*, 25, 299, 1988.

577. Holton, J., Nye, P., and Miller, R., *Mycobacterium haemophilum* infection in a patient with AIDS, *J. Infect. Dis.*, 23, 303, 1991.

578. Kristjansson, M., Bieluch, V. M., and Byeff, P. D., *Mycobacterium haemophilum* infection in immunocompromised patients: case report and review of the literature, *Rev. Infect. Dis.*, 13, 906, 1991.

579. Males, B. M., West, T. E., and Bartholomew, W. R., *Mycobacterium haemophilum* infection in a patient with acquired immune deficiency syndrome, *J. Clin. Microbiol.*, 25, 186, 1987.

580. Moulsdale, M. T., Harper, J. M., Thatcher, G. N., and Dunn, B. L., Infection by *Mycobacterium haemophilum*, a metabolically fastidious acid-fast bacillus, *Tubercle*, 64, 29, 1983.

581. Rogers, P. L., Walker, R. E., Lane, H. C., Witebsky, F. G., Kovacs, J. A., Parrillo, J. E., and Masur, H., Disseminated *Mycobacterium haemophilum* infection in two patients with the acquired immuno-deficiency syndrome, *Am. J. Med.*, 84, 640, 1988.

582. Ryan, C. G. and Dwyer, B. W., New characteristics of *Mycobacterium haemophilum*, *J. Clin. Microbiol.*, 18, 976, 1983.

583. Saubolle, M. A., Rudinsky, M., Merritt, E. S., Williams, J., Raines, J. M., and Dinler, M., *Mycobacterium haemophilum* infection in two otherwise normal pediatric patients, *Proc. 91st Annu. Meet. Am. Soc. Microbiol.*, American Society for Microbiology, Washington, D.C.,1991, 391.

584. Thilbert, L., Lebel, F., Martineau, B., and Chicoine, L., *Mycobacterium haemophilum* in Quebec, *Can. Dis. Wkly. Rep.*, 14, 196, 1988.

585. Thibert, L., Lebel, F., and Martineau, B., Two cases of *Mycobacterium haemophilum* infection in Canada, *J. Clin. Microbiol.*, 28, 621, 1990.

586. Mezo, A., Jennis, F., McCarthy, S. W., and Dawson, D. J., Unusual mycobacteria in 5 cases of opportunistic infections, *Pathology*, 11, 377, 1979.

587. McBride, J. A., McBride, M. E., and Wolf, J. E., Jr., Evaluation of commercial blood-containing media for cultivation of *Mycobacterium haemophilum*, *Am. J. Clin. Pathol.*, 98, 282, 1992.

588. Goslee, S. and Wolinsky, E., Water as a source of potentially pathogenic mycobacteria, *Am. Rev. Respir. Dis.*, 113, 287, 1985.

589. Bingaman, C., Water treatment procedures and formaldehyde resistant mycobacteria challenge two Baton Rouge dialysis facilities, *Contemp. Dial.*, 4, 34, 1983.

590. Wolinsky, E. and Rynearson, T. K., Mycobacteria in soil and their relation to disease-associated strains, *Am. Rev. Respir. Dis.*, 97, 1032, 1968.

591. Armstrong, D., Kiehn, T., Boone, N., White, M., Pursell, K., Lewin, S., Sordillo, E. M., Schneider, N., Grieco, M. H., LaBombardi, V., Yarish, R., Larone, D., Tapper, M., Ong, K. R., Morse, D. L., Kocher, J., and Spitalny, K. C., *Mycobacterium haemophilum* infections — New York City metropolitan area, 1990-1991, *Morb. Mortal. Wkly. Rep.*, 40, 636, 1991.

592. Dawson, D. J. and Jennis, F., Mycobacteria with a growth requirement for ferric ammonium citrate identified as *Mycobacterium haemophilum*, *J. Clin. Microbiol.*, 11, 190, 1980.

593. McBride, M. E., Rudolph, A. H., Tschen, J. A., Cernoch, P., Davis, J., Brown, B. A., and Wallace, R. J., Jr.., Diagnostic and therapeutic considerations for cutaneous *Mycobacterium haemophilum* infections, *Arch. Dermatol.*, 127, 276, 1991.

594. Armstrong, K. L., James, R. W., Dawson, D. J., Francis, P. W., and Masters, B., *Mycobacterium haemophilum* causing perihilar or cervical lymphadenitis in healthy children, *J. Pediatr.*, 121, 202, 1992.

595. Marks, J., Jenkins, P. A., and Tsukamura, M., *Mycobacterium szulgai* — a new pathogen, *Tubercle*, 53, 210, 1972.

596. Medinger, A. E. and Spagnolo, S. V., *Mycobacterium szulgai* pulmonary infection: the importance of knowing, *South. Med. J.*, 74, 85, 1981.

597. Davidson, P. T., *Mycobacterium szulgai*: a new pathogen causing infection of the lung, *Chest*, 69, 799, 1976.

598. Mori, K., Yoshikawa, M., Nakamura, T., Tomoda, K. et al., Pulmonary infection due to *Mycobacterium szulgai* associated with multiple bullous disease of the lung, *Kekkaku*, 70, 511, 1995.

599. Olmos, J. M., Peralta, F. G., Mellado, A., and Gonzalez-Macias, J., Infection by *Mycobacterium szulgai* in a patient with pulmonary tuberculosis, *Eur. J. Clin. Microbiol. Infect. Dis.*, 13, 689, 1994.

600. Maloney, J. M., Gregg, C. R., Stephens, D. S., Manian, F. A., and Rimland, D., Infections caused by *Mycobacterium szulgai* in humans, *Rev. Infect. Dis.*, 9, 1120, 1987.

601. Sybert, A., Tsou, E., and Garagusi, V. F., Cutaneous infection due to *Mycobacterium szulgai*, *Am. Rev. Respir. Dis.*, 115, 695, 1977.

602. Cross, G. M., Guill, M. A., and Aton, J. K., Cutaneous *Mycobacterium szulgai*, *Arch. Dermatol.*, 121, 247, 1985.

603. Stratton, C. W., Phelps, D. B., and Reller, L. B., Tuberculoid tenosynovitis and carpal tunnel syndrome caused by *Mycobacterium szulgai*, *Arch. Intern. Med.*, 144, 1861, 1984.

604. Gur, H., Porat, S., Haas, H., Naparstek, Y., and Eliakim, M., Disseminated mycobacterial disease caused by *Mycobacterium szulgai*, *Arch. Intern. Med.*, 144, 1861, 1984.

605. Roig, P., Nieto, A., Navarro, V., Bernacer, B., and Borras, R., Mycobacteriosis from *Mycobacterium szulgai* in a patient with human immunodeficiency virus infection, *Ann. Med. Intern.*, 10, 182, 1993.

606. Zamboni, M., Igreja, R. P., Bonecker, C., and Torres Filho, H. M., *Mycobacterium szulgai* infection in a patient with hemophilia and AIDS, *Rev. Assoc. Med. Bras.*, 38, 150, 1992.

607. Schröder, K. H. and Juhlin, I., *Mycobacterium malmoense* sp. nov., *Int. J. Syst. Bacteriol.*, 27, 241, 1977.

608. Claydon, E. J., Coker, R. J., and Harris, J. R., *Mycobacterium malmoense* infection in HIV-positive patients, *J. Infect.*, 23, 191, 1991.

609. Jenkins, P. A. and Tsukamura, M., Infections with *Mycobacterium malmoense* in England and Wales, *Tubercle*, 60, 71, 1979.

610. France, A. J., Mcleod, D. T., Calder, M. A., and Seaton, A., *Mycobacterium malmoense* infections in Scotland: an increasing problem, *Thorax*, 42, 593, 1987.

611. Connolly, M. J., Magee, J. G., Hendrick, D. J., and Jenkins, P. A., *Mycobacterium malmoense* in the northeast of England, *Tubercle*, 66, 211, 1985.

612. Katila, M. L., Brander, E., and Beckman, A., Neonatal BCG vaccination and mycobacterial cervical adenitis in childhood, *Tubercle*, 68, 291, 1987.

613. Warren, N. G., Body, B. A., Silcox, V. A., and Matthews, J. H., Pulmonary disease due to *Mycobacterium malmoense*, *J. Clin. Microbiol.*, 20, 245, 1984.

614. Zaugg, M., Salfinger, M., Opravil, M., and Luthy, R., Extrapulmonary and disseminated infections due to *Mycobacterium malmoense*: case report and review, *Clin. Infect. Dis.*, 16, 540, 1993.

615. Osterwalder, C., Salfinger, M., and Sulser, H., *Mycobacterium malmoense* infection of the flexor tendon sheath, *Handchir. Mikrochir. Plast. Chir.*, 24, 210, 1992.

616. Leuenberger, P., Aubert, J. D., and Beer, V., *Mycobacterium malmoense* — report of a case in Switzerland, *Respiration*, 51, 285, 1987.
617. Heurlin, N. and Petrini, B., Treatment of non-tuberculous mycobacterial infections in patients without AIDS, *Scand. J. Infect. Dis.*, 25, 619, 1993.
618. Fabbri, J., Welge-Lussen, A., Frei, R., and Zimmerli, W., Cervical lymphadenitis due to *Mycobacterium malmoense* in a child: case report and differential diagnosis of cervical lymphadenitis and lymphadenopathies, *Schweiz. Med. Wochenschr.*, 123, 1756, 1993.
619. Mattila, J. O., Vornanen, M., Vaara, J., and Katila, M. L., Mycobacteria in prurigo nodularis: the cause or a consequence? *J. Am. Acad. Dermatol.*, 34, 224, 1996.
620. Dave, J., Williams, A. T., and Jenkins, P. A., *Mycobacterium malmoense* infection in an immuno-compromised patient, *J. Infect.*, 26, 223, 1993.
621. Brinch, L., Rostad, H., Mehl, A., Blichfeldt, P., and Eng, J., Hairy cell leukemia and *Mycobacterium malmoense* infection, *Tidsskr. Nor. Laegeforen*, 110, 835, 1990.
622. Schafer, H., Ewig, S., Hasper, E., Pakos, E., Wilhelm, K., and Lüderitz, B., Bronchopulmonary infection with *Mycobacterium malmoense* presenting as a bronchoesophageal fistula, *Tuberc. Lung Dis.*, 77, 287, 1996.
623. Smeenk, F. M., Klinkhamer, P. J., Breed, W., Jansz, A. R., and Jansveld, C. A., Opportunistic lung infections in patients with chronic obstructive lung disease: a side effect of inhalation corticosteroids? *Ned. Tijdschr. Geneeskd.*, 140, 94, 1996.
624. Chocarro, A., Gonzalez Lopez, A., Breznes, M. F., Canut, A., Rodriguez, J., and Diego, J. M., Disseminated infection due to *Mycobacterium malmoense* in a patient infected with human immuno-deficiency virus, *Clin. Infect. Dis.*, 19, 203, 1994.
625. Willocks, L., Leen, C. L. S., Brettle, R. P., Rayner, A., Harris, G., and Watt, B., Isolation of *Mycobacterium malmoense* from HIV-positive patients, *J. Infect.*, 26, 345, 1993.
626. Banks, J., Jenkins, P. A., and Smith, A. P., Pulmonary infection with *Mycobacterium malmoense* — a review of treatment and response, *Tubercle*, 66, 197, 1985.
627. Böttger, E. C., Hirschel, B., and Coyle, M. B., *Mycobacterium genavense* sp. nov., *Int. J. Syst. Bacteriol.*, 43, 841, 1993.
628. Coyle, M. B., Carlson, L. C., Wallis, C. K. et al., Laboratory aspects of "*Mycobacterium genavense*," a proposed species isolated from AIDS patients, *J. Clin. Microbiol.*, 30, 3206, 1992.
629. Hirschel, B., Chang, H. R., Mach, N., Piguet, P.-F., Cox, J., Piguet, J.-D., Silva, M. T., Larsson, L., Klatser, P. R., Thole, J. E. R., and Rigouts, L., Fatal infection with a novel unidentified mycobacterium in a man with the acquired immunodeficiency syndrome, *N. Engl. J. Med.*, 323, 109, 1990.
630. Rogall, T., Wolters, J., Flohr, T., and Böttger, E. C., Towards a phylogeny and definition of species at the molecular level within the genus *Mycobacterium*, *Int. J. Syst. Bacteriol.*, 40, 323, 1990.
631. Böttger, E. C., Teske, A., Kirschner, P., Bost, S., Chang, H. R., Beer, V., and Hirschel, B., Disseminated "*Mycobacterium genavense*" infection in patients with AIDS, *Lancet*, 340, 76, 1992.
632. Pechère, M. and Hirschel, B., Infections a *Mycobacterium genavense* fréquence et présentation clinique, *Presse Med.*, 24, 239, 1995.
633. Pechère, M., Opravil, M., Wald, A., Chave, J.-P., Bessesen M., Sievers, A., Hein, R., von Overbeck, J., Clark, R. A., Tortoli, E., Emler, S., Kirschner, P., Gabriel, V., Böttger, E. C., Hirschel, B., and the Swiss HIV Cohort Study, Clinical and epidemiological features of infection with *Mycobacterium genavense*, *Arch. Intern. Med.*, 155, 400, 1995.
634. Bessesen, M. T., Shlay, J., Stone-Venohr, B., Cohn, D. L., and Reves, R. R., Disseminated *Mycobacterium genavense* infection: clinical and microbiological features and response to therapy, *AIDS*, 7, 1357, 1993.
635. Heiken, H., Kirschner, P., Stoll, M., Böttger, E. C., and Schmidt, R. E., *Mycobacterium genavense* infection in AIDS, *Dtsch. Med. Wochenschr.*, 118, 296, 1993.
636. Berman, S. M., Kim, R. C., Haghighat, D., Mulligan, M. E., Fierer, J., and Wyle, F. C., *Mycobacterium genavense* infection presenting as a solitary brain mass in a patient with AIDS: case report and review, *Clin. Infect. Dis.*, 19, 1152, 1994.
637. Dionisio, D., Tortoli, E., Simonetti, M. T., di Lollo, S., Meli, M., Farese, A., Fontana, R., Sterrantino, G., and Leoncini, F., Intestinal mycobacterial infections in AIDS: clinical course and treatment of infections caused by *Mycobacterium avium*, *Mycobacterium kansasii*, *Mycobacterium genavense*, *Recenti Prog. Med.*, 85, 526, 1994.

638. Karassova, V., Weiszfeiler, J., and Krasznay, E., Occurrence of atypical mycobacteria in macacus rhesus, *Acta Microbiol. Acad. Sci. Hung.*, 12, 275, 1965.

639. Weiszfeiler, J. G., Die atypischen mycobakterien und das *Mycobacterium simiae*, in *Die Biologie und Variabilitat des Tuberkelbakteriums und die Atypischen Mycobakterien*, Akadémiai Kiado, Budapest, 1969, 227.

640. Valdivia, A., Mendez, J. S., and Font, M. E., *Mycobacterium habana*: probable nueva especie dentro dellas microbacterias no classificadas, *Boll. Hig. Epidemiol. (Habana)*, 9, 65, 1971.

641. Meissner, G. and Schröder, K.-H., Relationship between *Mycobacterium simiae* and *Mycobacterium habana*, *Am. Rev. Respir. Dis.*, 111, 196, 1975.

642. Weiszfeiler, J. G. and Karczag, E., Synonymy of *Mycobacterium simiae* Karasseva et al. 1965 and *Mycobacterium habana* Valdivia et al. 1971, *Int. J. Syst. Bacteriol.*, 26, 474, 1976.

643. Bell, R. C., Higuchi, J. H., Donovan, W. N., Krasnow, I., and Johanson, W. G., Jr., *Mycobacterium simiae*: clinical features and follow-up of twenty-four patients, *Am. Rev. Respir. Dis.*, 127, 35, 1983.

644. Krasnow, I. and Gross, W., *Mycobacterium simiae* infection in the United States: a case report and discussion of the organism, *Am. Rev. Respir. Dis.*, 111, 357, 1973.

645. Menard, O., Tanguy, B., Ahmed, Z., Caligaris, P., and Desnanot, J., Severe pulmonary mycobacteriosis caused by *Mycobacterium simiae*, *Rev. Mal. Respir.*, 4, 327, 1987.

646. Rose, H. D., Dorff, G. J., Lauwasser, M., and Sheth, N. K., Pulmonary and disseminated *Mycobacterium simiae* infection in humans, *Am. Rev. Respir. Dis.*, 126, 1110, 1982.

647. Kuipers, E. J., Hazenberg, H. J., Ploeger, B., Smit, F. W., and de Jong, A., Nontuberculous mycobacterial sternal osteomyelitis in a patient without predisposing condition, *Neth. J. Med.*, 38, 122, 1991.

648. Valero, G., Moreno, F., and Graybill, J. R., Activities of clarithromycin, ofloxacin, and clarithromycin plus ethambutol against *Mycobacterium simiae* in murine model of disseminated infection, *Antimicrob. Agents Chemother.*, 38, 2676, 1994.

649. Heap, B. J., *Mycobacterium simiae* as a cause of intra-abdominal disease: a case report, *Tubercle*, 70, 217, 1989.

650. Chaturvedi, V., Singh, N. B., and Sinha, S., Immunoreactive antigens of a candidate leprosy vaccine: *Mycobacterium habana*, *Lepr. Rev.*, 66, 31, 1995.

651. Singh, N. B., Lowe, A. C., Rees, R. J., and Colston, M. J., Vaccination of mice against *Mycobacterium leprae* infection, *Infect. Immun.*, 57, 653, 1989.

652. Aronson, J. D., Spontaneous tuberculosis in salt water fish, *J. Infect. Dis.*, 39, 315, 1926.

653. Norden, A. and Linell, F., A new type of pathogenic *Mycobacterium*, *Nature*, 168, 826, 1951.

654. Linnel, F. and Norden, A., *Mycobacterium balnei*: a new acid-fast bacillus occurring in swimming pools and capable of producing skin lesions in humans, *Acta Tuberc. Scand.*, 33(Suppl.), 1, 1954.

655. Gluckman, S. J., *Mycobacterium marinum*, *Clin. Dermatol.*, 13, 273, 1995.

656. Edelstein, H., *Mycobacterium marinum* skin infections: report of 31 cases and review of the literature, *Arch. Intern. Med.*, 154, 1359, 1994.

657. Kullavanijaya, P., Sirimachan, S., and Bhuddhavudhikrai, P., *Mycobacterium marinum* cutaneous infections acquired from occupations and hobbies, *Int. J. Dermatol.*, 32, 504, 1993.

658. Joe, L. and Hall, E., *Mycobacterium marinum* disease in Anne Arundel County: 1995 update, *Md. State Med. J.*, 44, 1043, 1995.

659. Jensen, P., Gabrielsen, T. O., Hovig, B., Engh, V., and Eng, J., Aquarium-borne *Mycobacterium marinum* infection, *Tidsskr. Nor. Laegeforen*, 113, 1569, 1993.

660. Paul, D. and Gulick, P., *Mycobacterium marinum* skin infections: two case reports, *J. Fam. Pract.*, 36, 336, 1993.

661. Kariniemi, A. L., Brander, E., and Huttunen, R., Swimming pools granuloma: hand infection caused by *Mycobacterium marinum*, *Duodecim*, 107, 1437, 1991.

662. Guarda, R., Gubelin, W., Gajardo, J., Rohmann, I., and Valenzuela, M. T., Cutaneous infection by *Mycobacterium marinum*: case report, *Rev. Med. Chil.*, 120, 1027, 1992 (correction in *Rev. Med. Chil.*, 121, 125, 1993).

663. Hoyt, R. E., Bryant, J. E., Glessner, S. F., Littleton, F. C., Jr., Sawyer, R. W., Newman, R. J., Nichols, D. B., Franco, A. P., Jr., and Tingle, N. R., Jr., *M. marinum* infection in a Chesapeake Bay community, *Va. Med.*, 116, 467, 1989.

664. McLain, E. H., Case study: mariner's TB, *AAOHN J.*, 37, 329, 1989.

665. Tsukamura, M., *Mycobacterium marinum* infections in humans. II. Infections caused by *M. marinum*, *Kekkaku*, 63, 577, 1988.
666. Brown, J. W. III and Sanders, C. V., *Mycobacterium marinum* infections: a problem of recognition, not therapy? *Arch. Intern. Med.*, 147, 817, 1987.
667. Collins, C. H., Grange, J. M., Noble, W. C., and Yates, M. D., *Mycobacterium marinum*, *J. Hyg. (London)*, 94, 135, 1985.
668. Fragoso, M. A. and Murray, D. L., *Mycobacterium marinum* infection in a 4-year-old child, *Clin. Pediatr. (Philadelphia)*, 24, 288, 1985.
669. Eriksson, B. and Petrini, B., *Mycobacterium marinum* infection in the hand after a visit to the tropics, *Lakartidningen*, 86, 3054, 1989.
670. Sommer, A. F., Williams, R. M., and Mandel, A. D., *Mycobacterium balnei* infection: report of two cases, *Arch. Dermatol.*, 86, 106, 1962.
671. Jolly, H. W., Jr. and Seabury, J. H., Infections with *Mycobacterium marinum*, *Arch. Dermatol.*, 106, 32, 1972.
672. Cott, R. E., Carter, D. M., and Sall, T., Cutaneous disease caused by atypical mycobacteria: report of two chromogen infections and review of the subject, *Arch. Dermatol.*, 95, 259, 1967.
673. Phillips, S. A., Marya, S. K., Dryden, M. S., and Samuel, A. W., *Mycobacterium marinum* infection of the finger, *J. Hand Surg. (Br.)*, 20, 801, 1995.
674. Goldhagen, M., Nunberg, S., and Freeman, A. M., Right hand and arm rash *Mycobacterium marinum* infection, *Acad. Emerg. Med.*, 2, 919, 1995.
675. Harth, M., Ralph, E. D., and Faraawi, R., Septic arthritis due to *Mycobacterium marinum*, *J. Rheumatol.*, 21, 957, 1994.
676. Hanau, L. H., Leaf, A., Soeiro, R., Weiss, L. M., and Pollack, S. S., *Mycobacterium marinum* infection in a patient with the acquired immunodeficiency syndrome, *Cutis*, 54, 103, 1994.
677. Alinovi, A., Vecchini, F., and Bassissi, P., Sporothricoid mycobacterial infection: a case report, *Acta Derm. Venereol.*, 73, 146, 1993.
678. Borradori, L., Baudraz-Rosselet, F., Beer, V., Monnier, M., and Frenk, E., *Mycobacterium marinum* granuloma in a fish fancier: apropos of a case with sporotrichoid lesions, *Schweiz. Med. Wochenschr.*, 121, 1340, 1991.
679. Zukervar, P., Canillot, S., Gayrard, L., and Perrot, H., Sporotrichoid *Mycobacterium marinum* infection in a patient infected with human immunodeficiency virus, *Ann. Dermatol. Venereol.*, 118, 111, 1991.
680. Puiatti, P., Alberico, G., Cotilli, G., Salvai, M., and Goitre, M., Sporotrichoid infection: two cases, *G. Ital. Dermatol. Venereol.*, 125, 349, 1990.
681. Pien, F. D., Ching, D., and Kim, E., Septic bursitis: experience in a community practice, *Orthopedics*, 14, 981, 1991.
682. Travis, W. D., Travis, L. B., Roberts, G. D., Su, D. W., and Weiland, L. W., The histopathologic spectrum in *Mycobacterium marinum* infection, *Arch. Pathol. Lab. Med.*, 109, 1109, 1985.
683. Patel, S., Duke, O., and Harland, C., Septic arthritis due to *Mycobacterium marinum*, *J. Rheumatol.*, 22, 1607, 1995.
684. Alloway, J. A., Evangelisti, S. M., and Sartin, J. S., *Mycobacterium marinum* arthritis, *Semin. Arthritis Rheum.*, 24, 382, 1995.
685. Harth, M., Ralph, E. D., and Faraawi, R., Septic arthritis due to *Mycobacterium marinum*, *J. Rheumatol.*, 21, 957, 1994.
686. Clark, R. B., Spector, R. B., Friedman, D. M., Oldrati, K. J., Young, C. L., and Nelson, S. C., Osteomyelitis and synovitis produced by *Mycobacterium marinum* in a fisherman, *J. Clin. Microbiol.*, 28, 2570, 1990.
687. Jones, M. W. and Wahid, I. A., *Mycobacterium marinum* infections of the hand and wrist, *J. Bone Joint Surg. (Am.)*, 70, 631, 1988.
688. Aubrey, M. and Fam, A. G., A case of clinically unsuspected *Mycobacterium marinum* infection, *Arthritis Rheum.*, 30, 1317, 1987.
689. Schonherr, U., Naumann, G. O., Lang, G. K., and Bialasiewicz, A. A., Sclerokeratitis caused by *Mycobacterium marinum*, *Am. J. Ophthalmol.*, 108, 607, 1989.
690. Gould, W. M., McMeekin, D. R., and Bright, R. D., *Mycobacterium marinum* (*balnei*) infection: report of a case with cutaneous and laryngeal lesions, *Arch. Dermatol.*, 97, 159, 1968.

691. Gombert, M. E., Goldstein, E. J. C., Corrado, M. L., Shin, A. J., and Butt, K. H., Disseminated *Mycobacterium marinum* infection after renal transplantation, *Ann. Intern. Med.*, 94, 486, 1981.

692. Sage, R. E. and Derrington, A. W., Opportunistic cutaneous *Mycobacterium marinum* infection mimicking *Mycobacterium ulcerans* in lymphosarcoma, *Med. J. Aust.*, 2,434, 1973.

693. Parent, L. J., Salam, M. M., Appelbaum, P. C., and Dossett, J. H., Disseminated *Mycobacterium marinum* infection and bacteremia in a child with severe combined immunodeficiency, *Clin. Infect. Dis.*, 21, 1325, 1995.

694. Enzenauer, R. J., McKoy, J., Vincent, D., and Gates, R., Disseminated cutaneous and synovial *Mycobacterium marinum* infection in a patient with systemic lupus erythematosus, *South. Med. J.*, 83, 471, 1990.

695. Bodemer, C., Durand, C., Blanche, S., Teillac, D., and De Prost, Y., Disseminated *Mycobacterium marinum* infection, *Ann. Dermatol. Venereol.*, 116, 842, 1989.

696. Vazquez, J. A. and Sobel, J. D., A case of disseminated *Mycobacterium marinum* infection in an immunocompetent patient, *Eur. J. Clin. Microbiol. Infect. Dis.*, 11, 908, 1992.

697. Bonnet, E., Debat-Zoguereh, D., Petit, N., Ravaux, I., and Gallais, H., Clarithromycin: a potent agent against infections due to *Mycobacterium marinum*, *Clin. Infect. Dis.*, 18, 664, 1994.

698. Boos, S., Schmidt, H., Ritter, G., and Manz, D., Effectiveness of oral rifampicin against mycobacteriosis in tropical fish, *Berl. Munch. Tierarztl. Wochenschr.*, 108, 253, 1995.

699. Arai, H., Nakajima, H., and Kaminaga, Y., *In vitro* susceptibility of *Mycobacterium marinum* to dihydromycoplanecin A and ten other antimicrobial agents, *J. Dermatol.*, 17, 370, 1990.

700. Yamamoto, Y., Saito, H., Tomioka, H., Sato, K., Yamane, T., Yamashita, K., Hosoe, K., and Hidaka, T., *In vitro* and *in vivo* activities of KRM-1648, a newly synthesized benzoxazinorifamycin, against *Mycobacterium marinum*, *Int. J. Med. Microbiol. Virol. Parasitol. Infect. Dis.*, 277, 204, 1992.

701. Wendt, J. R., Lamm, R. C., Altman, D. I., Cruz, II. G., and Achauer, B. M., An unusually aggressive *Mycobacterium marinum* hand infection, *J. Hand Surg (Am.)*, 11, 753, 1986.

702. Iredell, J., Whitby, M., and Blacklock, Z., *Mycobacterium marinum* infection: epidemiology and presentation in Queensland 1971-1990, *Med. J. Aust.*, 157, 596, 1992.

703. Amrani, M., Renoitre, P., Pieron, P., and Six, C., Skin lesions due to *Mycobacterium marinum*: surgical ablation. Apropos of a case of false paronychia, *Acta Chir. Belg.*, 91, 265, 1991.

704. Chow, S. P., Ip, F. K., Lau, J. H., Collins, R. J., Luk, K. D., So, Y. C., and Pun, W. K., *Mycobacterium marinum* infection of the hand and wrist: results of conservative treatment in twenty-four cases, *J. Bone Joint Surg. (Am.)*, 69, 1161, 1987.

705. Donta, S. T., Levitz, R. E., Quintiliani, R., and Smith, P. W., Tetracyclines in therapy of *Mycobacterium marinum* infections, *Arch. Intern. Med.*, 147, 2054, 1987.

706. Hurst, L. C., Amadio, P. C., Badalamente, M. A., Ellstein, J. L., and Dattwyler, R. J., *Mycobacterium marinum* infections of the hand, *J. Hand Surg. (Am.)*, 12, 428, 1987.

707. Harris, L. F., Striplin, W. H., and Burnside, R. C., Aquatic hazard *Mycobacterium marinum* infection, *Ala. Med.*, 61, 8, 1991.

708. Sanders, W. J. and Wolinsky, E., *In vitro* susceptibility of *Mycobacterium marinum* to eight antimicrobial agents, *Antimicrob. Agents Chemother.*, 18, 529, 1980.

709. Arai, H., Nakajima, H., Naito, S., Kaminaga, Y., and Nagai, R., Amikacin treatment for *Mycobacterium marinum* infection, *J. Dermatol.*, 13, 385, 1986.

710. Ljungberg, B., Christensson, B., and Grubb, R., Failure of doxycycline treatment in aquarium-associated *Mycobacterium marinum* infections, *Scand. J. Infect. Dis.*, 19, 539, 1987.

711. Huminer, D., Pitlik, S. D., Block, C., Kaufman, L., Amit, S., and Rosenfeld, J. B., Aquarium-borne *Mycobacterium marinum* skin infection: report of a case and review of the literature, *Arch. Dermatol.*, 122, 698, 1986.

712. Ries, K. M., White, G. L., Jr., and Murdock, R. T., Atypical mycobacterial infection caused by *Mycobacterium marinum*, *N. Engl. J. Med.*, 322, 633, 1990.

713. Donta, S. T., Smith, P. W., Levitz, R. E., and Quintiliani, R., Therapy of *Mycobacterium marinum* infections: use of tetracyclines vs. rifampin, *Arch. Intern. Med.*, 146, 902, 1986.

714. Lacy, J. N., Viegas, S. F., Calhoun, J., and Mader, J. T., *Mycobacterium marinum* flexor tenosynovitis, *Clin. Orthop.*, 238, 288, 1989.

715. Laing, R. B., Wynn, R. F., and Leen, C. L., New antimicrobials against *Mycobacterium marinum* infection, *Br. J. Dermatol.*, 131, 914, 1994.

716. Kuhn, S. M., Rosen, W., Wong, A., and Jadavji, T., Treatment of *Mycobacterium marinum* facial abscess using clarithromycin, *Pediatr. Infect. Dis. J.*, 14, 631, 1995.

717. Peters, D. H. and Clissold, S. P., Clarithromycin: a review of its antimicrobial activity, *Drugs*, 44, 117, 1992.

718. Levy, L., Enk, C. D., Zipris, D., and Cohen, I. R., Protection of mice against mycobacterial infection by lymphoid cell vaccination, *Isr. J. Med. Sci.*, 30, 22, 1994.

719. Mor, N., Lutsky, I., Weiss, L., Morecki, S., and Slavin, S., Resistance to mycobacteria in mice treated with reconstituted allogenic bone marrow cells following radiotherapy, *Int. J. Radiat. Oncol. Biol. Phys.*, 11, 79, 1985.

720. Gangadaharam, P. R. J., Lockhart, J. A., Awe, R. J., and Jenkins, D. E., Mycobacterial contamination through tap water, *Am. Rev. Respir. Dis.*, 113, 894, 1976.

721. Dizon, D., Mihailescu, C., and Bae, H. C., Simple procedure for detection of *Mycobacterium gordonae* in water causing false-positive acid-fast smears, *J. Clin. Microbiol.*, 3, 211, 1976.

722. Steere, A. C., Corrales, J., and von Graevenitz, A., A cluster of *Mycobacterium gordonae* isolates from bronchoscopy specimens, *Am. Rev. Respir. Dis.*, 120, 214, 1979.

723. Panwalker, A. P. and Fuhse, E., Nosocomial *Mycobacterium gordonae* pseudoinfection from contaminated ice machines, *Infect. Control*, 7, 67, 1986.

724. Stine, T. M., Harris, A. A., Levin, S., Rivera, N., and Kaplan, R. L., A pseudoepidemic due to atypical mycobacteria in a hospital water supply, *JAMA*, 258, 809, 1987.

725. Tokars, J. I., McNeil, M. M., Tablan, O. C., Chapin-Robertson, K., Patterson, J. E., Edberg, S. C., and Jarvis, W. R., *Mycobacterium gordonae* pseudoinfection associated with a contaminated antimicrobial solution, *J. Clin. Microbiol.*, 28, 2765, 1990.

726. Gonzalez, E. P., Crosby, R. M. N., and Walker, S. H., *Mycobacterium aquae* infection in a hydrocephalic child (*Mycobacterium aquae* meningitis), *Pediatrics*, 48, 947, 1971.

727. Sossi, N., Feldman, R. M., Feldman, S. T., Frueh, B. E., McGuire, G., and Davis, C., *Mycobacterium gordonae* keratitis after penetrating keratoplasty, *Arch. Ophthalmol.*, 109, 1064, 1991.

728. Moore, M. B., Newton, C., and Kaufman, H. E., Chronic keratitis caused by *Mycobacterium gordonae*, *Am. J. Ophthalmol.*, 102, 516, 1986.

729. Kurnik, P. B., Padmanabh, U., Bonatsos, C., and Cynamon, M. H., *Mycobacterium gordonae* as a human hepato-peritoneal pathogen, with a review of the literature, *Am. J. Med. Sci.*, 285, 45, 1983.

730. London, R. D., Damsker, B., Neibart, E. P., Knorr, B., and Bottone, E. J., *Mycobacterium gordonae*: an unusual peritoneal pathogen in a patient undergoing continuous ambulatory peritoneal dialysis, *Am. J. Med.*, 85, 703, 1988.

731. Carcaba, V., Carton, J. A., Fernandez Leon, A., and de Diego, I., Peritonitis por *Mycobacterium gordonae* en un paciente infectado por el virus de laimmunodeciencia humana, *Med. Clin. (Barcelona)*, 93, 598, 1989.

732. Lohr, D. C., Goeken, J. A., Doty, D. B., and Donta, S. T., *Mycobacterium gordonae* infection of a prosthetic aortic valve, *JAMA*, 329, 1528, 1978.

733. Jarikre, L. N., *Mycobacterium gordonae* genitourinary disease, *Genitourin. Med.*, 68, 45, 1992.

734. Shelley, W. B. and Folkens, A. T., *Mycobacterium gordonae* infection of the hand, *Arch. Dermatol.*, 120, 1064, 1984.

735. McIntyre, P., Blacklock, Z., and McCormack, J. G., Cutaneous infection with *Mycobacterium gordonae*, *J. Infect.*, 14, 71, 1987.

736. Gengoux, P., Portaels, F., Lachapelle, J. M., Minnikin, D. E., Tennstedt, D., and Tamigneau, P., Skin granulomas due to *Mycobacterium gordonae*, *Int. J. Dermatol.*, 26, 181, 1987.

737. Gribetz, A. R., Damsker, B., Bottone, E. J., Kirschner, P. A., and Teirstein, A. S., Solitary pulmonary nodules due to nontuberculous mycobacterial infection, *Am. J. Med.*, 70, 39, 1981.

738. Nathan, V., Mehta, J. B., and Dralle, W., Rifabutin in the treatment of cavitary lung disease due to *Mycobacterium gordonae*, *South. Med. J.*, 86, 839, 1993.

739. Hasegawa, T., Tada, K., and Ishii, M., Pulmonary infection caused by *Mycobacterium gordonae* (*M. gordonae*) in a healthy middle-aged male, *Nippon Kyobu Shikkan Gakkai Zasshi*, 30, 343, 1992.

740. Guarderas, J., Alvarez, S., and Berk, S. L., Progressive pulmonary disease caused by *Mycobacterium gordonae*, *South. Med. J.*, 79, 505, 1986.

741. Kumar, U. N. and Varkey, B., Pulmonary infection caused by *Mycobacterium gordonae*, *Br. J. Dis. Chest*, 74, 189, 1980.

742. Craig, C. P. and Kreitzer, S. M., Non-tuberculous mycobacterial infections: human infections due to *Mycobacterium gordonae, Infect. Dis. Rev.*, 6, 79, 1980.

743. Clague, H., Hopkins, C. A., Roberts, C., and Jenkins, P. A., Pulmonary infection with *Mycobacterium gordonae* in the presence of bronchial carcinoma, *Tubercle*, 66, 61, 1985.

744. Douglas, J. G., Calder, M. A., Choo-Kang, Y. F. J., and Leitch, A. G., *Mycobacterium gordonae*: a new pathogen? *Thorax*, 41, 152, 1986.

745. de Gracia, J., Vidal, R., Martin, N., Bravo, C., Gonzalez, T., and Riba, A., Pulmonary disease caused by *Mycobacterium gordonae, Tubercle*, 70, 135, 1989.

746. Aguado, J. M., Gomez-Garcés, J. L., Manrique, A., and Soriano, F., Pulmonary infection by *Mycobacterium gordonae* in an immunocompromised patient, *Diagn. Microbiol. Infect. Dis.*, 7, 261, 1987.

747. Lessnau, K. D., Milanese, S., and Talavera, W., *Mycobacterium gordonae*: a treatable disease in HIV-positive patients, *Chest*, 104, 1779, 1993.

748. Barber, T. W., Craven, D. E., and Farber, H. W., *Mycobacterium gordonae*: a possible opportunistic respiratory tract pathogen in patients with advanced human immunodeficiency virus, type 1 infection, *Chest*, 100, 716, 1991.

749. Chan, J., McKitrick, J. C., and Klein, R. S., *Mycobacterium gordonae* in the acquired immuno-deficiency syndrome, *Ann. Intern. Med.*, 101, 400, 1984.

750. Nakagawa, S., The flexor digitorum profundus tendon rupture caused by *Mycobacterium gordonae* tenosynovitis in a renal transplant recipient, *Rin Sei Ge*, 25, 665, 1990

751. Jarikre, L. N., Case report: disseminated *Mycobacterium gordonae* infection in a nonimmuno-compromised host, *Am. J. Med. Sci.*, 302, 382, 1991.

752. Turner, D. M., Ramsey, P. G., Ojemann, G. A., and Ralph, D. D., Disseminated *Mycobacterium gordonae* infection associated with glomerulonephritis, *West. J. Med.*, 142, 391, 1985.

753. Weinberger, M., Berg, S. L., Feuerstein, I. M., Pizzo, P. A., and Witebsky, F. G., Disseminated infection with *Mycobacterium gordonae*: report of a case and critical review of the literature, *Clin. Infect. Dis.*, 14, 1229, 1992.

754. Jackson, J., Leggett, J. E., Wilson, D. A., and Gilbert, D. N., *Mycobacterium gordonae* in fiberoptic bronchoscopes, *Am. J. Infect. Control*, 24, 19, 1996.

755. Wallace, C. G., Agee, P. M., and Demicco, D. D., Liquid chemical sterilization using peracetic acid: an alternative approach to endoscope processing, *ASAIO J.*, 41, 151, 1995.

756. MacCallum, P., Tolhurst, J. C., Buckle, G., and Sissons, H. A., A new mycobacterial infection in man, *J. Pathol. Bacteriol.*, 60, 93, 1948.

757. Muelder, K. and Nourou, A., Buruli ulcer in Benin, *Lancet*, 336, 1109, 1990.

758. van der Werf, T. S. and van der Graaf, W. T. A., Buruli ulcer in West Africa, *Lancet*, 336, 1440, 1990.

759. Lunn, H. F., Connor, D. H., Wilks, N. E., Barnley, G. R., Kamamunvi, F., Clancey, J. K., and Bee, J. D. A., Buruli (mycobacterial) ulceration in Uganda: a new focus of Buruli ulcer in Madi District, Uganda, *E. Afr. Med. J.*, 42, 275, 1965.

760. Hayman, J., Clinical features of *Mycobacterium ulcerans* infection, *Australas. J. Dermatol.*, 26, 67, 1985.

761. Hayman, J., *Mycobacterium ulcerans* infection, *Lancet*, 337, 124, 1991.

762. Uganda Buruli Group, Clinical features and treatment of preulcerative Buruli lesions (*Mycobacterium ulcerans* infection): report II, *Br. Med. J.*, 2, 390, 1970.

763. Hayman, J. and McQuenn, A., The pathology of *Mycobacterium ulcerans* infection, *Pathology*, 17, 594, 1985.

764. Darie, H., Djakeaux, S., and Cautoclaud, A., Therapeutic approach in *Mycobacterium ulcerans* infections, *Bull. Soc. Pathol. Exot.*, 87, 19, 1994.

765. Cornet, L., Richard-Kadio, M., N'Guessan, H. A., Yapo, P., Hossoko, H., Dick, R., and Casanelli, J. M., Treatment of Buruli's ulcers by excision-graft, *Bull. Soc. Pathol. Exot.*, 85, 355, 1992.

766. Brodt, H. R., Current therapy of atypical mycobacterial infections, *Immun. Infekt.*, 20, 39, 1992.

767. Christie, M., Suspected *Mycobacterium ulcerans* disease in Kiribati, *Med. J. Aust.*, 146, 600, 1987.

768. Exner, K. and Lemperle, G., Buruli ulcer — necrotizing infection of the hand of a plastic surgeon, *Handchir. Mikrochir. Plast. Chir.*, 19, 230, 1987.

769. Fehr, H., Egger, M., and Senn, I., Cotrimoxazole in the treatment of *Mycobacterium ulcerans* infection (Buruli ulcer) in West Africa, *Trop. Doct.*, 24, 61, 1994.

770. Song, M., Vincke, G., Vanachter, H., Benekens, J., and Achten, G., Treatment of cutaneous infection due to *Mycobacterium ulcerans*, *Dermatologica*, 171, 197, 1988.

771. Richmond, L. and Cummings, M. M., An evaluation of methods of testing the virulence of acid-fast bacilli, *Am. Rev. Tuberc.*, 62, 632, 1950.

772. Paramasivan, C. N., Govindan, D., Prabhakar, R., Somasundaram, P. R., Subbammal, S., and Tripathy, S. P., Species level identification of non-tuberculous mycobacteria from South Indian BCG trial area during 1981, *Tubercle*, 66, 9, 1985.

773. Kestle, D. G., Abbott, V. D., and Kubica, G. P., Differential identification of mycobacteria. II. Subgroup of groups II and III (Runyon) with different clinical significance, *Am. Rev. Respir. Dis.*, 95, 1041, 1967.

774. DeChairo, D. C., Kittredge, D., Meyers, A., and Corrales, J., Septic arthritis due to *Mycobacterium triviale*, *Am. Rev. Respir. Dis.*, 108, 1224, 1973.

775. Edwards, M. S., Huber, T. W., and Baker, C. J., *Mycobacterium terrae* synovitis and osteomyelitis, *Am. Rev. Respir. Dis.*, 117, 161, 1978.

776. Cianciulli, F. D., The radish bacillus (*Mycobacterium terrae*): saprophyte or pathogen? *Am. Rev. Respir. Dis.*, 109, 138, 1974.

777. Katz, D., *Mycobacterium terrae* tenosynovitis of the hand, *Ann. Chir. Main Memb. Super.*, 12, 136, 1993.

778. Weiszfeiler, G., Karassova, V., and Karczag, E., A new mycobacterium species: *Mycobacterium asiaticum* n. sp., *Acta Microbiol. Acad. Sci. Hung.*, 18, 247, 1971.

779. Blacklock, Z. M., Dawson, D. J., Kane, D. W., and McEvoy, D., *Mycobacterium asiaticum* as a potential pulmonary pathogen for humans: a clinical and bacteriologic review of five cases, *Am. Rev. Respir. Dis.*, 127, 241, 1983.

780. Taylor, L. Q., Williams, A. J., and Santiago, S., Pulmonary disease caused by *Mycobacterium asiaticum*, *Tubercle*, 71, 303, 1990.

781. Dawson, D. J., Blacklock, Z. M., Ashdown, L. R., and Bottger, E. C., *Mycobacterium asiaticum* as the probable causative agent in a case of olecranon bursitis, *J. Clin. Microbiol.*, 33, 1042, 1995.

782. Weitzman, I., Osadczyi, D., Corrado, M. L., and Karp, D., *Mycobacterium thermoresistibile*: a new pathogen for humans, *J. Clin. Microbiol.*, 14, 593, 1981.

783. Wolfe, J. M. and Moore, D. F., Isolation of *Mycobacterium thermoresistibile* following augmentation mammoplasty, *J. Clin. Microbiol.*, 30, 1036, 1992.

784. Neeley, S. P. and Denning, D. W., Cutaneous *Mycobacterium thermoresistibile* infection in a heart transplant recipient, *Rev. Infect. Dis.*, 11, 608, 1989.

785. Tsukamura, M., A new species of rapidly growing, scotochromogenic mycobacteria, *Mycobacterium neoaurum*, *Med. Biol. (Tokyo)*, 85, 229, 1972.

786. Holland, D. J., Chen, S. C. A., Chew, W. W. K., and Gilbert, G. L., *Mycobacterium neoaurum* infection of a Hickman catheter in an immunosuppressed patient, *Clin. Infect. Dis.*, 18, 1002, 1994.

787. Davison, M. B., McCormack, J. G., Blacklock, Z. M., Dawson, D. J., Tilse, M. H., and Crimmins, F. B., Bacteraemia caused by *Mycobacterium neoaurum*, *J. Clin. Microbiol.*, 26, 762, 1988.

788. Tsukamura, M., Kita, N., Otsuka, W., and Shimoide, H., A study of the taxonomy of the *Mycobacterium nonchromogenicum* complex and report of six cases of lung infection due to *Mycobacterium nonchromogenicum*, *Microbiol. Immunol.*, 27, 219, 1983.

789. Christensson, B., Olsson, B., Arner, M., and Miorner, H., Subcutaneous infection of the hand due to *Mycobacterium nonchromogenicum*, *J. Hand Surg. (Am.)*, 18, 130, 1993.

790. Casimir, M. T., Fainstein, V., and Papadopolous, N., Cavitary lung infection caused by *Mycobacterium flavescens*, *South. Med. J.*, 75, 253, 1982.

791. Chiodini, R. J., Van Kruiningen, H. J., and Merkal, R. S., Ruminant paratuberculosis (Johne's disease): the current status and future prospects, *Cornell Vet.*, 74, 218, 1984.

792. Fawcett, A. R., Goddard, P. J., McKelvey, W. A., Buxton, D., Reid, H. W., Greig, A., and Macdonald, A. J., Johne's disease in a herd of farmed red deer, *Vet. Rec.*, 136, 165, 1995.

793. Cocito, C., Gilot, P., Coene, M., de Kesel, M., Poupart, P., and Vannuffel, P., Paratuberculosis, *Clin. Microbiol. Rev.*, 7, 328, 1994.

794. Chiodini, R. J., Van Kruiningen, H. J., Merkal, R. S., Thayer, W. R., Jr., and Coutu, J. A., Characteristics of an unclassified *Mycobacterium* species isolated from patients with Crohn's disease, *J. Clin. Microbiol.*, 20, 966, 1984.

795. Chiodini, R. J., Van Kruiningen, H. J., Thayer, W. R., Jr., Merkal, R. S., and Coutu, J. A., Possible role of mycobacteria in inflammatory bowel disease. I. An unclassified *Mycobacterium* species isolated from patients with Crohn's disease, *Dig. Dis. Sci.*, 29, 1073, 1984.

796. Thayer, W. R., Jr., Coutu, J. A., Chiodini, R. J., Van Kruiningen, H. J., and Merkal, R. S., Possible role of mycobacteria in inflammatory bowel disease. II. Mycobacterial antibodies in Crohn's disease, *Dig. Dis. Sci.*, 29, 1080, 1984.

797. Przemioslo, R. T. and Ciclitira, P. J., Pathogenesis of Crohn's disease, *Q. J. Med.*, 88, 525, 1995.

798. Thompson, D. E., The role of mycobacteria in Crohn's disease, *J. Med. Microbiol.*, 41, 74, 1994.

799. Lisby, G., Andersen, J., Engbaek, K., and Binder, V., *Mycobacterium paratuberculosis* in intestinal tissue from patients with Crohn's disease demonstrated by a nested primer polymerase chain reaction, *Scand. J. Gastroenterol.*, 29, 923, 1994.

800. Thayer, W. R., The use of antimycobacterial agents in Crohn's disease, *J. Clin. Gastroenterol.*, 15, 5, 1992.

801. Molina, J. M., Anguiano, A., and Ferrer, O., Study on immune response of goats vaccinated with a live strain of *Mycobacterium paratuberculosis*, *Comp. Immunol. Microbiol. Infect. Dis.*, 19, 9, 1996.

802. Kreuzpaintner, G., Das, P. K., Stronkhorst, A., Slob, A. W., and Strohmeyer, G., Effect of intestinal resection on serum antibodies to the mycobacterial 45/48 kilodalton doublet antigen in Crohn's disease, *Gut*, 37, 361, 1995.

803. Kenefick, K. B., Adams, J. L., Steinberg, H., and Czuprynski, C. J., *In vivo* administration of a monoclonal antibody against the type I IL-1 receptor inhibits the ability of mice to eliminate *Mycobacterium paratuberculosis*, *J. Leukoc. Biol.*, 55, 719, 1994.

804. Mondal, D., Sinha, R. P., and Gupta, M. K., Effect of combination therapy in *Mycobacterium paratuberculosis* infected rabbits, *Indian J. Exp. Biol.*, 32, 318, 1994.

805. Adams, J., Follett, D., Hamilton, H., and Czuprynski, C., Effects of administration of anti-CD4 and anti-CD8 monoclonal antibodies on *Mycobacterium paratuberculosis* infection in intragastrically challenged mice, *Immunol. Lett.*, 35, 183, 1993.

806. Brumbaugh, G. W., Frelier, P. F., Roussel, A. J., Jr., and Thompson, T. D., Prophylactic effect of monensin sodium against experimentally induced paratuberculosis in mice, *Am. J. Vet. Res.*, 53, 544, 1992.

807. Chiodini, R. J., Kreeger, J. M., and Thayer, W. R., Use of rifabutin in treatment of systemic *Mycobacterium paratuberculosis* infection in mice, *Antimicrob. Agents Chemother.*, 37, 1645, 1993.

808. Rutgeerts, P., Geboes, K., Vantrappen, G., Van Isveldt, J., Peeters, M., Pennicks, F., and Vantrappen, G., Rifabutin and ethambutol do not help recurrent Crohn's disease in the neoterminal ileum, *J. Clin. Gastroenterol.*, 15, 24, 1992.

809. Prantera, C., Bothamley, G., Levenstein, S., Mangiarotti, R., and Argentieri, R., Crohn's disease and mycobacteria: two cases of Crohn's disease with high anti-mycobacterial antibody levels cured by dapsone therapy, *Biomed. Pharmacother.*, 43, 295, 1989.

810. Heller, R., Jaulhac, B., Charles, P., De Briel, D. et al., Identification of *Mycobacterium shimoidei* in a tuberculosis-like cavity by 16S ribosomal DNA direct sequencing, *Eur. J. Clin. Microbiol. Infect. Dis.*, 15, 172, 1996.

811. Emler, S., Praplan, P., Rohner, P., Auckenthaler, R., and Hirschel, B., Disseminated infection with *Mycobacterium celatum*, *Schweiz. Med. Wochenschr.*, 126, 1062, 1996.

812. Pitulle, C., Dorsch, M., Kazda, J., Wolters, J., and Stackebrandt, E., Phylogeny of rapidly growing members of the genus *Mycobacterium*, *Int. J. Syst. Bacteriol.*, 42, 337, 1992.

813. Kleepies, M., Kroppenstedt, R. M., Rainey, F. A., Webb, L. E., and Stackebrandt, E., *Mycobacterium hodleri* sp. nov., a new member of the fast-growing mycobacteria capable of degrading polycyclic aromatic hydrocarbons, *Int. J. Syst. Bacteriol.*, 46, 683, 1996.

9 Enterobacteriaceae

Enterobacteriaceae is a family of Gram-negative, facultatively anaerobic bacteria which are widely distributed worldwide in soil, water, plants, and animals, from insects to humans. They can be saprophytes or plant and animal parasites. Morphologically, the Enterobacteriaceae represent rod-shaped, usually (but not always) motile bacteria with peritrichous flagellae.

Many Enterobactcriaceae are the etiologic agents of a variety of diseases in plants, fish, cattle, and poultry. In humans, disease can originate by both invasive action and through production of toxins. Species which normally are not associated with human disease may often act as opportunistic pathogens. In fact, Enterobacteriaceae have been responsible for as many as half of the nosocomial infections reported annually in the United States, most frequently by species of the genera *Escherichia*, *Klebsiela*, *Enterobacter*, *Proteus*, *Providencia*, and *Serratia*.

9.1 *SHIGELLA* SPP.

9.1.1 INTRODUCTION

Shigella is a genus of Gram-negative facultatively anaerobic bacteria of the family *Enterobacteriaceae*. The bacterium is rod-shaped, nonmotile, and not encapsulated. It cannot utilize citrate as the only source of carbon and ferment carbohydrates with production of acid but not gas. On the basis of biochemical and antigenic studies, *Shigella* is differentiated into four distinct species: *S. dysenteriae* (subgroup A), *S. flexneri* (subgroup B), *S. boydii* (subgroup C), and *S. sonnei* (subgroup D). The normal habitat of these organisms is the gastrointestinal tract of humans and higher monkeys (chimpanzees). All species cause dysentery. In humans, the pathogen produces inflammation of the mucous membrane of the lower ileum and may extend to involve the lower ileum.

S. dysenteriae, which has been divided into 10 serologic types, does not ferment lactose or mannitol. It is a highly pathogenic organism causing severe dysentery which can be fatal in children. *S. dysenteriae* type 1 (Shiga bacillus) is the only *Shigella* spp. that can produce a soluble heat-labile neurotoxic exotoxin. *S. dysenteriae* type 2 (Schmitz bacillus) is serologically related to *Escherichia coli* (*S. alkalescens*) type 0112; it may cause occasionally epidemic diarrhea in humans. Other serological types of *S. dysenteriae* include types 3 to 7 (the Large-Sachs group of parashiga bacilli).

S. flexneri has six serotypes and two variants (X and Y) that are capable of fermenting mannitol but not lactose. They represent paradysentery bacilli of which type 2 produces an enterotoxin.

S. boydii is divided into 15 serotypes, all fermenting mannitol but not lactose. This species is common in tropical regions, where they produce severe diarrhea in humans.

S. sonnei, although serologically a homogeneous group, has two antigens (designated I and II) that may develop in varying proportions. It is capable of fermenting both mannitol and lactose (a relatively slow process lasting between 5 to 14 d). *S. sonnei* can cause mild (but frequently occurring) watery diarrhia of shorter duration.[1,2]

9.1.2 STUDIES ON THERAPEUTICS

9.1.2.1 *Trimethoprim-Sulfamethoxazole (Co-trimoxazole, TMP-SMX)*

DuPont et al.[3,4] have compared the anti-*Shigella* efficacy of trimethoprim given alone with a standard 5-d course treatment of trimethoprim-sulfamethoxazole (co-trimoxazole, TMP-SMX), and found both regimens to be equally effective. Bogaerts et al.[5] also compared the effects of TMP-SMX (160 mg TMP and 800 mg SMX, twice daily) with trimethoprim (300 mg, twice daily) in a 5-d therapy of adult patients with severe *Shigella* dysentery. Even though the patient population was small and did not allow for the conclusions to be statistically significant, excellent bacteriologic and clinical responses were obtained with both regimens, with the exception of patients infected with a trimethoprim-resistant strain of *S. dysenteriae* type 1.

When a trimethoprim-only therapy is applied, the case of a single-dose regimen vs. a standard 5-d therapy would be of interest to ascertain whether a single dose of the drug is less expensive than a standard 5-d therapy and also whether (as demonstrated for some urinary tract infections) a single-drug treatment is less conducive to development of drug resistance,[6-8] as well as less toxic.[9,10] In a randomized double-blind, placebo-controlled trial involving 53 patients with *Shigella* dysentery, Oldfield et al.[11] compared the therapeutic effect of a single dose of trimethoprim (600 mg) with a 5-d regimen of trimethoprim (200 mg, twice daily). While both dosage schedules were effective, there has been no significant statistical difference observed in the duration of diarrhea. Although only 3 of 57 (5%) of *Shigella* isolates were found to be resistant to trimethoprim in this particular trial, as proven in other studies,[12] resistance to trimethoprim has been much more widespread (see below).

9.1.2.2 Trimethoprim Resistance in Gram-Negative Bacteria

Because of its broad spectrum of activity and significant synergistic effect with sulfonamides, trimethoprim alone or in combinations with sulfamethoxazole and other sulfonamides, has been used in the clinic for over 25 years. However, over the intervening years trimethoprim resistance in Gram-negative bacteria has reached clinically significant proportions and has become a factor of immediate concern.[12-21] The problem of steadily increasing trimethoprim resistance has been especially alarming when considering pathogens, such as *Shigella* spp. which are responsible for a high rate of morbidity and mortality worldwide (Table 9.1).[21-23]

Gander and LaRocco[24] described a case of an AIDS patient with persistent shigellosis caused by *S. flexneri* who developed multiple resistance against trimethoprim-sulfamethoxazole, ampicillin, and tetracycline.

In general, there have been three important factors responsible for the development of trimethoprim resistance: (1) the emergence of stable resistance genes; (2) the presence of resistance vectors, such as epidemic strains, plasmids, or transposons; and (3) continuous or periodic selection pressure.[13,21]

9.1.2.2.1 *Emergence of stable trimethoprim resistance genes*

The mechanisms responsible for the emergence of stable trimethoprim resistance genes include: (1) qualitative (decreased affinity) or quantitative modifications of the chromosomal dihydrofolate reductase (DHFR); (2) the presence of new, trimethoprim-resistant DHFR; (3) impaired permeability; and (4) auxotrophy in thymine/thymidine.

The low-level trimethoprim resistance is usually associated with mutational events, such as decreased permeability, and quantitative or qualitative modifications of DHFR, the bacterial target of trimethoprim.[25] Plasmid-mediated low-level resistance, although rare, has also been observed.[26]

High-level resistance to trimethoprim is usually linked to plasmids (R factors) which encode an additional trimethoprim-resistant DHFR.[27,28] The major attributes of these plasmids include the ability to transfer from one bacterium to another, and to encode resistance to several unrelated

TABLE 9.1
Resistance to Trimethoprim-Sulfamethoxazole (TMP-SMX) Among *Shigella* spp. Worldwide[a]

Country	Year	Resistance (in %)	Total Strains Tested
Australia	1976–1979	26[b]	300
	1980–1983	31	86
Bangladesh	1980	0	1,018
	1984	55	890
India	1983	37	162
Sri Lanka	1980s	5	21
Thailand	1979–1984	35	1,033
	1986–1988	61.1	211
Philippines	1979–1984	8	96
U.S.	1978	1	355
	1990[c]	85	113
Mexico	1980	0	55
	1984	6	23
Chile	1983	25	85
	1987	37	100
Brazil	1983	23	57
Sudan	1984	18	133
Egypt	1980s	6	48
Finland	1980s[d]	6	1,211

[a] Data taken from Goldstein and Acar,[13,21] Hassan,[287] Murray,[12] and Hyams et al.[288]

[b] Data for TMP only.

[c] Data represent shigellosis (*S. dysenteriae, S. flexneri, S. boydii,* and *S. sonnei*) among military forces during operation Desert Shield, 1990.

[d] Most isolates were from travelers to the Black Sea and Mediterranean areas; there was an increase in resistance to TMP from 3% in 1975–1982 to 19% in 1984.

antibiotics. However, the plasmid-mediated transferable resistance to trimethoprim among highly resistant strains may frequently fluctuate.[29,30]

When first reported,[27] the plasmid-encoded trimethoprim resistance in Gram-negative bacteria was initially associated with extremely high minimum inhibitory concentration (MIC) values for trimethoprim (over 1000 mg/l). Later, the resistance mechanism was defined to be the result of plasmid-mediated production of an additional trimethoprim-resistant DHFR.[31,32] So far, in Gram-negative bacteria at least a dozen different plasmid-encoded DHFRs belonging to seven major groups (I to VII)[33] have been identified.

Transfer of *Shigella* R-plasmids *in vivo* has been rarely observed. In a recent report by Bratoeva and John,[34] strains of *S. dysenteriae* type 1 and *S. flexneri* type 5b have been isolated from a patient who developed dysentery and was treated with TMP-SMX for a short time. Both *Shigella* strains were multiresistant to the same antimicrobial agents, and each strain contained a 48-kb plasmid that conferred the entire resistance phenotype to a susceptible *E. coli*. Furthermore, the restriction endonuclease patterns of plasmid DNA from the respective strains were identical. The reported data corroborated the hypothesis that R-plasmid transfer may take place between nonpathogenic, fecal strains and pathogenic *Shigellae*, a process which might have been facilitated by inadequate treatment with TMP-SMX at the onset of the illness.[34]

9.1.2.2.2   Presence of resistant vectors

One partial explanation of the observed fluctuations in the transferability of high-level trimethoprim resistance is the presence of transposable elements (transposons) encoding resistance, which can jump from one plasmid to another plasmid, or on to the bacterial chromosome.[35] Tn7, the most common of the trimethoprim transposons, encodes resistance not only to trimethoprim (DHFR type Ia), but also to streptomycin and spectinomycin.[36,37] Tn4132 represents a second group of transposons which encodes resistance to trimethoprim alone and is clearly different from Tn7.[38] A third group of transposons is represented by Tn402, which encodes resistance to DHFR type II.[39]

In an attempt to define the fluctuations in transferability of high-level trimethoprim resistance in enterobacteria, Huovinen et al.[37] and Kraft et al.[40] studied the distribution and genetic location of Tn7 in the bacterial chromosome. One explanation of the general increase in the percentage of enterobacteria harboring Tn7[37,40] has been the premise that after the initial "infection" of the bacterial cell by a plasmid carrying Tn7, the transposon will jump and remain on the chromosome even when the initial plasmid has been cured spontaneously.[13]

9.1.2.2.3   Selection pressures

The last factor thought to be responsible for fluctuations in trimethoprim resistance is selection pressures. As was demonstrated that with the increased consumption of newer antimicrobial agents (cephalosporins and fluoroquinolones), the use of trimethoprim-sulfonamide combinations declined after 1982, and so did the percentage of trimethoprim-resistant strains.[13] In an interesting development, Amyes et al.[41,42] showed that ampicillin may select bacteria harboring plasmids encoding joint resistance to ampicillin and trimethoprim.

9.1.2.3   Fluoroquinolones

The fluoroquinolones represent the newest class of antimicrobial agents used in the treatment of shigellosis. In addition to being well absorbed after oral administration, the fluoroquinolones have large volumes of distribution with long elimination half-lives, making frequent dosing unnecessary. Thus, a 400-mg oral dose of norfloxacin produced peak fecal concentrations in the 207 to 2716 µg/g range;[43] the mean fecal concentrations of ciprofloxacin exceeded 500 µg/g at d 4 and 5 and up to 2 d after therapy.[44]

Another advantage of the fluoroquinolones has been the lack of plasmid-mediated resistance, and the inability of bacteria to transfer resistance to the drugs to other pathogenic Gram-negative organisms.[45]

An outbreak of acute bacillary dysentery due to multiple antibiotic-resistant *S. flexneri* IV in long-tailed macaques was treated successfully with enrofloxacin.[46] Once daily oral administration of 5 mg/kg enrofloxacin by gastric intubation produced 24-h serum concentrations above the MICs for the *Shigella* isolates from the outbreak.

9.1.2.4   Cephalosporins

A number of second- and third-generation orally active cephalosporins, showing good absorption by the gastrointestinal tract,[47,48] have been evaluated *in vitro* against multidrug-resistant shigellosis.[48-52]

While there has been significant progress in the development of parenteral cephalosporins in terms of higher stability against β-lactamases and broader antimicrobial activity, this goal has not been completely accomplished for orally active cephalosporins.[53,54] Structurally, the parenteral cephalosporins have a variety of side chains at the 3 and 7 positions of the cephalosporin molecule. In contrast, the requirement for good gastrointestinal absorption have limited the choice of side chains for oral cephalosporins; therefore, the number of distinct substituents at the 3 position has been very limited, and all substituents at the 7 position have been related to a native or modified phenylglycyl moiety. Attempts to deviate from this pattern have resulted in the synthesis of new orally active cephem derivatives with broader antimicrobial activity, especially against Gram-negative bacteria, but the new compounds still displayed decreased gastrointestinal absorption.[49,50,52,55]

Cephalexin, cephradine, and cefadroxil have only been partially stable against β-lactamases. Another compound, cefaclor, while not completely stable against plasmid β-lactamases, has been associated with a serum-sickness type illness in some children.[49]

Although most ampicillin-resistant *Shigellae* isolates were found susceptible to cephalexin, the latter failed to eradicate the pathogen in a randomized trial involving 154 infants and children with acute diarrhea.[56] Thus, after 5 d of treatment, cephalexin (80 mg/kg daily) failed to eradicate *Shigella* in 76% of the patients as compared with 28% in the ampicillin (100 mg/kg daily)-treated group with susceptible organisms; however, *Shigella* persisted in 78% of ampicillin-treated patients with resistant organisms. Furthermore, the diarrhea lasted more than 5 d in 43% of cephalexin-treated patients, in 56% of the ampicillin-receiving group with resistant organisms, but in only 9% of ampicillin-treated patients with susceptible organisms. The failure of cephalexin to eradicate *Shigella* and shorten the duration of shigellosis in most patients appeared to be the result of inadequate serum concentrations. Since the recommended daily dose of cephalexin is 25 to 50 mg/kg, in order to achieve adequate serum concentrations, it is doubtful that the patients could have tolerated dosages much larger than the 80 mg/kg (as used in this study).[56]

FK 027, an orally active cephem antibiotic, was found to be more active *in vitro* than cephalexin and cefaclor, showing MIC values against *S. disenteriae* A-1 Shiga, *S. flexneri* 1a EW-8, and *S. sonnei* I EW-33 of 0.78, 0.10, and 0.39 µg/ml, respectively; the corresponding values of cephalexin and cefaclor were 6.25, 6.25, and 3.13 µg/ml, and 3.13, 0.78, and 0.78 µg/ml, respectively.[56]

Cefixime (FR 17027) is a third-generation orally active aminothiazolyl cephalosporin derivative with an ethyl moiety at position 3 of the dihydrothiazine ring and a carboxyl group attached to the iminomethoxy portion of the acyl side chain.[49] The presence of an iminomethoxy group in the molecule confers greater stability against most plasmid-mediated and many chromosomal β-lactamases.[49,54] Cefixime was not hydrolyzed by the β-lactamases that hydrolyzed cefaclor, and achieved serum levels of 4 µg/ml after a 400-mg oral dose. When tested against 29 clinical isolates of *Shigella* spp., cefixime showed MIC_{50} and MIC_{90} values of 0.20 and 0.40 µg/ml; the corresponding values for cephalexin, cefaclor, and ceftizoxime were 6.3 and 12.5 µg/ml, 3.1 and 12.5 µg/ml, and 0.02 and 0.05 µg/ml, respectively.[49] Ashkenazi et al.[57] compared the clinical and bacteriologic efficacy of 5-d treatment with cefixime (8.0 mg/kg daily) with the response to TMP-SMX (10 to 50 mg/kg daily) in children with acute shigellosis (38 received cefixime and 39 received TMP-SMX). In the TMP-SMX group, 32 isolates were resistant and 7 were susceptible to TMP-SMX. Clinical response at day 5 showed cure, improvement, and failure in 89%, 8%, and 3%, respectively, in the cefixime group; and 25%, 44%, and 31%, respectively, in the

TMP-SMX-resistant group ($p <.001$). The response to treatment in the cefixime and the TMP-SMX-susceptible groups was similar. Overall, cefixime was superior to TMP-SMX in cases of high resistance rate to TMP-SMX.

Neu et al.[51] investigated the *in vitro* activity of ceftetrame (Ro 19-5247) and cefetamet (Ro 15-8074), two other orally active aminothiazolyl iminomethoxy cephalosporins having a side chain similar to that of cefotaxime β-acyl side chain. When tested against 15 *Shigella* spp. isolates, the MIC_{50} and MIC_{90} values of ceftetrame and cefetamet were 0.125 and 0.5 µg/ml, and 0.5 and 1.0 µg/ml, respectively. The corresponding MIC_{50} and MIC_{90} values of cephalexin, cefaclor, and cefotaxime were 8.0 and 16.0 µg/ml, 4.0 and 16.0 µg/ml, and 0.12 and 0.25 µg/ml, respectively. In general, cefotaxime was a more active antimicrobial agent than both ceftetrame and cefetamet. In turn, ceftetrame and cefetamet were more stable than cefaclor and cephalexin against β-lactamases and compared favorably with cefotaxime.[51]

Cefuroxime axetil, which is the acetoxyethyl ester of cefuroxime, has acted as a prodrug of cefuroxime. Thus, following its oral administration, cefuroxime axetil is deesterified in the intestinal mucosa and absorbed into the bloodstream as cefuroxime.[48] In adults, after oral digestion the peak serum concentrations of cefuroxime occurred in approximately 2 h.[58,59] When the drug was given with food, these concentrations were significantly higher.[60] In a separate study, Ginsburg et al.[48] have shown that the mean peak plasma concentrations of cefuroxime were reached between 90 and 120 min in all study patients (infants, children, and adults) independently of the fasting and feeding status. During the same study, the bioavailability of cefuroxime axetil was significantly enhanced in children (33 to 51% higher) after concomitant ingestion of cefuroxime axetil and infant formula or whole milk. Cefuroxime axetil differed from cephalexin and cephradine, the bioavailability of which was significantly reduced when coadministered with milk or infant formula.[61,62]

BMY 28100 is an orally active cephem derivative having a (Z)-propenyl side chain at position 3, and a *p*-hydroxyphenylglycyl substituent at position 7.[52] *In vitro* testing against 21 *Shigella* isolates have shown MIC_{50} and MIC_{90} values of 2.0 and 8.0 µg/ml. By comparison, the corresponding values of cefaclor and cephalexin were 2.0 and 16.0 µg/ml, and 8.0 and 16.0 µg/ml. In mice, after an oral dose of 50 mg/kg, the overall pharmacokinetic profile of BMY 28100 was comparable to that of cephalexin and more favorable than that of cefaclor.[52]

Ceftriaxone, a third-generation cephalosporin, has been shown to be highly active against *Shigella* strains with MIC values of 0.016 and 0.2 µg/ml.[63,64] Moreover, studies in excess of 500 *Shigella* isolates from various regions[63-73] revealed that all but two strains (both from Turkey)[70,71] were susceptible to ceftriaxone. An important advantage of ceftriaxone has been its long serum half-life (4.5 to 9 h).[74]

Controlled clinical trials[56,75,76] using cephalosporins for treatment of shigellosis have proven less hopeful in spite of promising *in vitro* activity. Thus, when compared with placebo for treatment of shigellosis in adult patients, intravenous administration of a single 1.0-g dose of ceftriaxone, while eliciting a moderate reduction in the frequency of stools and duration of fever, did not shorten the duration of diarrhea.[75]

In two reports, however, ceftriaxone has been found effective in the treatment of severe shigellosis in children. In a prospective randomized open study comprising 20 patients in each treated group, Varsano et al.[77] compared the efficacy of ceftriaxone (given in a single daily dose of 50 mg/kg for 5 d) and ampicillin (100 mg/kg divided in four equal doses for 5 d) in 40 children. Initially, both drugs were injected intravenously for 1 or 2 d, then continued either intramuscularly (ceftriaxone) or orally (ampicillin). All *Shigella* isolates were susceptible to ceftriaxone, while 28% were resistant to ampicillin. Ceftriaxone was found superior to ampicillin both in terms of clinical cure and eradication of *Shigella*: the duration of diarrhea was on average 2.5 d for the ceftriaxone-treated group vs. 6.8 d for the ampicillin-treated patients; at the end of the 5-d therapy, stool cultures for *Shigella* organisms were negative in 100% and 60% of the ceftriaxone- and ampicillin-treated patients, respectively.

In a trial involving 40 children with severe shigellosis, a 2-d course of ceftriaxone was found to be as beneficial as a 5-d course of the drug.[78] In another study, Park and Rogers[79] found *S. sonnei* completely susceptible to ceftriaxone, and recommended ceftriaxone therapy for treatment of severe shigellosis, especially in view of the high incidence of drug-resistant strains.

Parenteral administration of cefamandole (a second-generation cephalosporin) to nine patients with acute shigellosis was found to be ineffective, even though when tested *in vitro* cefamandole was more potent than cephalexin.[76] The latter (a first-generation cephalosporin) was also found ineffective against acute diarrhea in infants and children, as its serum concentration approximated the MIC value against the infecting strain of *Shigella*.[56]

The antishigellosis activity of DQ-2556, a new cephalosporin, was compared to that of other cephalosporins. Against 30 isolates of *Shigella* spp., DQ-2556 showed MIC_{50} and MIC_{90} values of <0.006 and 0.012 µg/ml; by comparison, the corresponding values of cefepim, cefpirome, cefuzonam, and ceftazidime were 0.012 and 0.10 µg/ml, 0.012 and 0.025 µg/ml, 0.025 and 0.10 µg/ml, and 0.10 and 0.20 µg/ml.[80]

In a prospective clinical trial lasting 5 d, ceftibutene was compared with TMP-SMX in the treatment of bacillary dysentery in children.[81] Both drugs were given orally, twice daily at doses of 4.5 mg/kg (ceftibutene), and 5.0 mg/kg and 25 mg/kg (for TMP and SMX, respectively). Six of 20 *Shigella* strains were resistant to TMP-SMX. The response of patients to ceftibutene and TMP-SMX appeared similar unless the pathogen was found to be TMP-SMX-resistant.

9.1.2.5   Amdinocillin Pivoxil (Mecillinam)

Amdinocillin pivoxil (mecillinam) is a β-lactam antibiotic which, contrary to other β-lactam derivatives, selectively bound to penicillin-binding proteins.[82,83] In addition to being more stable than ampicillin to most β-lactamases,[84] amdinocillin pivoxil was more efficient in penetrating the outer layer of bacterial cell envelopes.[85,86] Consequently, when compared with ampicillin, the resistance to amdinocillin pivoxil of most *Enterobacteriaceae* and *Shigella*, in particular, was less commonly seen;[87,88] cross-resistance, however, has been observed.[89]

One should note, however, that even though mecillinam has been highly active against *Shigella* strains,[88,90] its usefulness in the therapy of shigellosis has been hampered by the need for parenteral delivery. To this end, pivmecillinam (a prodrug, and the pivaloyloxymethyl ester of mecillinam) was not only well absorbed from the gastrointestinal tract but during or after absorption was rapidly hydrolyzed to mecillinam. This hydrolysis has been catalyzed by enzymes present in the blood and in many tissues, including the intestinal mucosa.[82,91,92]

Kabir et al.[93] evaluated, in a randomized, double-blind trial, the efficacy of mecillinam against acute shigellosis in 44 adult patients using ampicillin as an alternative therapy. Twenty-two patients received 400 mg of pivmecillinam, and 22 patients were given 500 mg of ampicillin for 5 d. The patients infected with strains susceptible to both antibiotics had mean durations of fecal excretion of *Shigella* strains of 1.2 and 1.4 d for pivmecillinam and ampicillin, respectively. The data obtained suggested that mecillinam was equipotent to ampicillin in the treatment of shigellosis.[93]

In a prospective randomized double-blind study, pivmecillinam was compared with co-trimoxazole (TMP-SMX), both given orally for 5 d to treat children with acute shigellosis (29 patients received pivmecillinam and 30 were treated with TMP-SMX).[94] Drug-resistant *Shigella* strains were isolated in 14% of the pivmecillinam group and in 21% of the TMP-SMX group. Persistence of diarrhea lasted on average 74 h and 73.8 h in the pivmecillinam and TMP-SMX groups, respectively. Overall, pivmecillinam has been found to be equipotent to co-trimoxazole in the therapy of acute shigellosis in children.

In another double-blind trial, 80 children (1 to 8 years of age) with acute shigellosis (bloody diarrhea of less than 3 d duration) were randomly assigned to receive either oral pivmecillinam (50 mg/kg daily) or nalidixic acid (60 mg/kg daily) for 5 d.[95] The stool frequency steadily decreased in both groups. There was no clinical failure in the pivmecillinam-treated patients and only three bacteriologic failures. By comparison, nalidixic acid failed to eradicate *Shigella* species in 10 patients, and clinical failures were observed in 11 of 37 patients receiving nalidixic acid, and in 2 of 26 patients infected with nalidixic acid-susceptible strains. The results of this study indicated that oral pivmecillinam was superior to nalidixic acid in the treatment of acute shigellosis in children, especially when the resistant strains are taken into account.

Ekwall and Svenungsson[96] evaluated the efficacy of a combination of pivmecillinam and pivampicillin (0.25 and 0.20 g, respectively, three times daily for 2 weeks) for the treatment of shigellosis. Twenty-three of 24 patients (96%) were found to be culture-negative after the treatment.

9.1.2.6 Azithromycin

The *in vitro* activity of azithromycin against enteric bacterial pathogens has been determined by agar dilution.[97] The antibiotic has been found highly effective against *Shigella* spp. with MIC_{90} value of 1.0 µg/ml; the corresponding values against *Salmonella* spp., *Campylobacter* spp., and *Escherichia coli* were 4.0, 0.125, and 2.0 µg/ml. The high intracellular concentrations achieved by azithromycin may be particularly relevant for enteric pathogens, such as *Shigella*, which typically invade cells as part of their infectious process.[97]

9.1.3 EVOLUTION OF THERAPIES AND TREATMENT OF SHIGELLOSIS

Bacillary dysentery is considered to be one of the major factors of childhood mortality, especially in developing countries,[98] in some cases causing more deaths than the watery diarrhea.[99,100] In a study conducted in Bangladesh, Bennish et al.[98] reported that of 9780 hospitalized shigellosis patients, 889 (9.1%) had died; of those, 32.3% occurred in children who were less than 1 year of age. In a multivariate analysis, younger age, decreased serum protein, altered consciousness, and thrombocytopenia were predictive of death.[98]

Bacteremia and metastatic foci during shigellosis have been rare and usually self-limiting.[101] In the majority of cases, *Shigella* bacteremia has been observed in tropical and subtropical regions[102-105] where malnutrition and immune deficiencies, especially in children, have been associated with high mortality rate.[105-108] However, the actual incidence of bacteremia could be higher than anticipated because often blood cultures have not been performed in most cases of acute or chronic diarrhea.[109,110] One limiting factor of *Shigella* bacteremia is the high sensitivity of the organism to complement-mediated serum bactericidal activity.[111]

Shigella bacteremia may lead to complications such as hematological disorders (hemoglobinopathy[112]), disseminated intravascular coagulation,[113] paroxysmal atrial tachycardia,[114] leukopenia, and hypogammaglobulinemia.[111]

Armor[115] reported a case in which *S. sonnei* induced both maternal disease (chorioamnionitis) and neonatal disease (pneumonia) in the immediate periparturitional period.

In terms of therapy, in addition to oral rehydration,[116,117] antimicrobial agents still remain an important part in the treatment of shigellosis. However, for several decades the steady and continuing increase in drug resistance towards commonly prescribed antimicrobial agents has remained a problem for the effective management of shigellosis.[118-120] After their introduction in the 1940s, the sulfonamides quickly became the drugs of choice against shigellosis[121-128] until an increased drug resistance led to their replacement by antibiotics such as the tetracyclines.

After the antibiotic therapy was introduced, the clinical course of shigellosis was shortened and the majority of patients were free of symptoms at the end of therapy;[129] for example, when given at a single dose of 2.5 g, tetracycline was effective against shigellosis.[130,131] During the 1960s, for the same reason — drug resistance — tetracycline was superseded by ampicillin, which in turn, because of the high incidence of bacteriologic failures both in children and adults[132,133] was displaced (in the 1970s) by trimethoprim-sulfamethoxazole.[134-136] Currently, due to widespread *Shigella* resistance, tetracycline and sulfonamides are no longer recommended for treatment of shigellosis.[106,137-140]

During the ensuing years, the increased resistance of *Shigella* to sulfamethoxazole[134,141,142] and the lack of synergy when *Shigella* strains have been found resistant to sulfamethoxazole,[141,143-145] reaffirmed the belief that on many occasions the therapeutic effect of trimethoprim-sulfamethoxazole was, in fact, most likely due to trimethoprim.[11] Nevertheless, both intravenous ampicillin and trimethoprim/sulfamethoxazole (TMP-SMX) have been shown to be effective against shigellosis and for the last 20 years or so these agents have been the drugs of choice.[64,76,129,146-151]

The recommended optimal dose and duration of therapy with ampicillin in most controlled trials have been 100 mg/kg, four times daily for 5 d.[149,152] However, shorter treatment regimens have proven to be effective as well. In one trial conducted by Gilman et al.,[153] the rate of clinical cure for 49 patients treated with a single daily dose of 100 mg/kg of ampicillin (maximum 4.0 g) was equivalent to the rate observed with a standard 5-d course (98% and 100%, respectively). The bacteriologic cure rates were, however, lower (80% and 95%, respectively), and correlated with the peak serum concentrations of the drug.

In some parts of the world, a progressive increase in resistance of *Shigella* strains to either ampicillin or trimethoprim when given alone, as well as in combination, have been reported.[154-161] Currently the resistance of *Shigellae* against ampicillin is so widespread that its therapeutic value is becoming very limited.

In common with other Gram-negative microorganisms, *Shigella* spp. contain a relatively heat-stable endotoxin which, when injected parenterally into small mammals causes diarrhea, weight loss, and inflammation of the intestinal wall. Early changes are manifested with generalized hyperemia and edema of the mucosa. As the surface tissue becomes necrotic and sloughs off, focal ulcerations may occur. The inflammatory process of the large bowel results in a frequent passage of copious liquid stools leading to significant loss of water and electrolytes (sodium and potassium), and the development of acidosis.[162] The *Shigella*-associated infection is essentially local and limited to the gut wall.

Although invasion of the bloodstream is an uncommon finding, extraintestinal shigellosis, mainly due to *S. dysenteriae* and *S. flexneri*, has been reported.[102,163-170] However, the events which may determine the pathogen's invasion of the bloodstream are not well understood. Under rare circumstances, *Shigella* bacteremia was diagnosed even in the absence of *Shigella* diarrhea.[171] Factors predisposing for *Shigella* bacteremia may include sickle cell anemia,[172] unusual susceptibility because of age (newborn infants), and impairment of the immune system.[173-175] Physical disruption of the epithelium resulting from infection with other organisms[176] or from biopsies may also become important.[177,178]

Salam and Bennish[106] have discussed the findings of eight clinical trials[75,109,143,146,179-182] where the effects of various antimicrobial agents against shigellosis (mainly *S. flexnery* and *S. dysenteriae* type 1) have been evaluated and compared with controls receiving either placebo or ineffective therapy (defined as treatment with antimicrobial drugs to which the *Shigella* isolate was resistant, or with orally administered nonabsorbable antimicrobial agents) (Table 9.2). In all but one of the trials,[179] antimicrobial therapy eliminated *Shigella* from stools faster than placebo or ineffective therapy.[106]

DuPont et al.[3] conducted three clinical trials to examine the efficacy of various combinations of antimicrobial drugs in the treatment of travelers' diarrhea among students in Mexico and the U.S. The results, shown in Table 9.3, demonstrated that most patients recovered by 48 h after initiation of treatment, and the drugs were well tolerated. What is most striking is the number of failures in the placebo-treated groups (71% in trials 1 and 2).

Therapy against acute *S. sonnei* is likely to be mostly beneficial if started early in the course of infection.[182] Neter et al.[177] described a unique case of *S. sonnei* bacteremia in a renal transplant recipient on concurrent immunosuppressive therapy. What was reported is a rare observation of

TABLE 9.2
Treatment of Shigellosis: Recommended Dose Regimens From
Controlled Clinical Trials[a]

Drug (Dose Regimen[b])	Shigella spp. Isolated	Clinical Outcome (in %)	Bacteriologic Outcome (in %)
Streptomycin (2.0 g daily, 4 times daily, orally)	S. flexneri S. boydii S. sonnei	—	67
Streptomycin (1.0 g daily, 4 times daily, orally) plus sulfaguanidine (8.0 g daily, 4 times daily, orally)	S. flexneri S. boydii S. sonnei	—	86
Streptomycin (1.0 g daily, 4 times daily, orally) plus sulfadimidine (4.0 g daily, 4 times daily, orally)	S. flexneri S. boydii S. sonnei	—	92
Ampicillin (100 mg/kg daily, 4 times daily, orally)	S. flexneri S. sonnei S. dysenteriae types 1 and 3	77–100 21[c]	92–100 77[c]
Ampicillin (500 mg/kg, 4 times daily, orally)	S. flexneri S. sonnei S. dysenteriae type 1 S. boydii	3.2 d[d]	83
Ampicillin (4.0 g as single dose, IV)	S. flexneri S. dysenteriae type 1	4.1 d[e]	1.1 d
Kanamycin (500 mg, b.i.d., intramuscularly)	S. flexneri S. sonnei S. boydii S. dysenteriae type 1	4.7 d	33
Amdinocillin pivoxil (children: 80 mg/kg daily, 4 times daily; adults: 400 mg/kg, 4 times daily)	Shigella spp.	—	—
TMP/SMX (20-80 mg TMP + 400 mg SMZ) (b.i.d., orally)	S. flexneri S. sonnei S. boydii	97[f]	94
Neomycin (100 mg/kg daily, 4 times daily, orally)	S. flexneri S. sonnei	40	13
Furazolidone (15–20 mg/kg, daily, 4 times daily, orally)	S. flexneri S. sonnei S. boydii	'60	53

TABLE 9.2 (continued)

Drug (Dose Regimen[b])	*Shigella* spp. Isolated	Clinical Outcome (in %)	Bacteriologic Outcome (in %)
Nalidixic acid (children: 55 mg/kg daily, 4 times daily, orally; adults: 1.0 g daily, 4 times daily, orally)	*S. flexneri* *S. dysenteriae* type 1	81	100
Sulfadiazine (120 mg/kg daily, 4 times daily, orally)	*S. flexneri* *S. sonnei* *S. dysenteriae* type 3	100 42[c]	100 42[c]

[a] Data taken from Haltalin et al.,[129,180,182] Stoker,[179] Tong et al.,[181] Lexomboon et al.,[143] Kabir et al.,[93] and Salam and Bennish.[146]

[b] Duration of treatment is 5 d, except for furazolidone (7 d).

[c] For patients with drug-resistant *Shigellae*.

[d] Mean number of days with diarrhea after therapy initiated (diarrhea not defined).

[e] Mean number of days with diarrhea after therapy initiated (diarrhea defined as > 2 unformed stools per day).

[f] Absence of fever and formed stools without blood or mucus after 48 h of therapy.

TABLE 9.3
Therapeutic Regimens for Shigellosis and Recovery Periods

Drugs	Regimen	Duration of Illness	No. of Patients Recovered/ No. of Patients Treated(%) at Indicated Time	
			48 h	72 h
Trial 1				
TMP-SMX	160 mg TMP + 800 mg SMX, b.i.d. for 5 d	16 h	9/9(100)	9/9(100)
TMP	200 mg, b.i.d. for 5 d	33 h	7/9(78)	8/9(89)
Placebo	b.i.d. for 5 d	110 h	0/5(0)	0/5(0)
Trial 2				
Furazolidone	100 mg, 4 times daily for 5 d	58 h	7/13(54)	9/13(69)
Ampicillin	500 mg, 4 times daily for 3 d	83 h	2/10(20)	4/10(40)
Trial 3				
Bicozamycin[a]	500 mg, 4 times daily for 3 d	37 h	10/13(77)	12/13(92)
Placebo	4 times daily for 3 d	90 h	2/12(25)	4/12(33)

[a]Bicozamycin is not currently available, nor is there evidence that it will be marketed in the foreseeble future.

Data taken from DuPont, H. L. et al., *Rev. Infect. Dis.*, 8(Suppl. 2), S217, 1986.

bloodstream invasion by *S. sonnei* which usually remains localized within the intestinal tract. Because of immunosuppression, there was only a modest antibody response against antigen O of the infecting microorganism; however, unexpectedly, the patient produced in high titer against a recently recognized antigen commonly shared by Gram-negative enteric bacteria.[183] The infection was resolved following treatment with chloramphenicol and lincomycin.[177]

In a double-blind clinical study conducted in Egypt, Bassily et al.[184] randomly assigned 109 adult patients with shigellosis to a short course with either norfloxacin (a single 800-mg dose), norfloxacin (400 mg twice daily for 3 d), or trimethoprim-sulfamethoxazole (160 mg and 800 mg, respectively, twice daily for 3 d). Five days after the start of all three regimens, diarrheal symptoms resolved in 86% to 97% of the patients, and bacteriologic failure (repeated positive stool cultures) occurred in only two patients. These recently published data indicated that short-course therapy with either norfloxacin or TMP-SMX can be used effectively to treat acute shigellosis in adult patients.

In another trial conducted in Africa, norfloxacin was used successfully in the therapy of trimethoprim-resistant *S. dysenteriae* type 1.[185] Several studies have suggested that a single dose of norfloxacin may be effective in the management of acute diarrhea, including a high drug concentration in stools 24 h after a 400-mg dose (200 to 2700 µg/g of stool) that remained elevated for 3 d after the dose,[43] the presence of enterohepatic recirculation of norfloxacin,[186] and the low MIC values for 90% of isolates of norfloxacin against enteropathogens (<0.1 µg/ml for *Shigella* spp.).[187,188]

Since the quinolones may reach high concentrations in stools after a single dose, the effectiveness of a single 800 mg dose of norfloxacin was compared with a 5-d treatment with TMP-SMX. In one randomized trial, adult patients with clinical dysentery received one of these regimens.[189] The clinical results and follow-up culture data were analyzed for those patients whose stool culture on presentation grew *Shigellae*. Fifty-five patients (26 treated with TMP-SMZ, and 29 treated with norfloxacin) whose bacterial isolates were susceptible to the antimicrobial agent given, have been compared by treatment group; there have been no significant differences observed in the duration of diarrhea (2.5 and 2.0 d for TMP-SMX and norfloxacin, respectively; $p = .200$), or the number of unformed stools after starting treatment (9.7 and 7.6 stools for TMP-SMX and norfloxacin, respectively; $p = .312$). The evidence of this trial demonstrated that one single dose of norfloxacin was as effective as a 5-d course of TMP-SMX.[189] Several other double-blind, placebo-controlled randomized clinical trials have confirmed the efficacy of norfloxacin in the treatment of diarrhea.[190-192]

Ciprofloxacin was found to be as effective as TMP-SMX in the treatment of shigellosis.[193] At doses of 500 mg given twice daily for 5 d, it consistently decreased the duration of diarrhea from 3–4 d to 1–2 d.[161,193-195] In this regard, it has been reported that a number of enteropathogens that showed resistance to TMP-SMX decreased the therapeutic efficacy of ciprofloxacin.[194,195] The benefits of a single-dose regimen vs. a 5-d therapy of ciprofloxacin have been discussed in several reports.[196-199]

In the therapy of shigellosis, when compared to ciprofloxacin alone, no tangible benefits were observed after loperamide (an antimotility drug) was administered concurrently with ciprofloxacin.[200] In contrast, in a double-blind, placebo-controlled, randomized clinical trial, Murphy et al.[201] reported that loperamide (4.0-mg initial dose followed by 2.0 mg after every loose stool, and as much as 16 mg daily) decreased the number of unformed stools and shortened the duration of diarrhea in shigella dysentery in adults treated with ciprofloxacin (500 mg twice daily) for 3 d.

While, in general, the fluoroquinolones have been effective in the treatment of shigellosis in adults, their use has been disapproved in children because of the adverse effects on cartilage.[202] Instead, for multidrug-resistant strains, nalidixic acid (three doses daily for 5 d) often remains as the only therapeutic alternative for children with shigellosis.[117] During an outbreak of shigellosis in Madagascar due to multidrug-resistant strains (*S. dysenteriae* type 1 and *S. flexneri*), a group of

25 children (aged 8 months to 12 years; mean age, 5.7 years) received three times pefloxacin at 12 mg/kg once daily for 3 d.[203] By the end of the second day, 19 of 25 children had no diarrhea, and stool cultures performed between 24 and 48 h after only one or two doses of pefloxacin had been administered, were negative for *Shigellae* in 21 of 25 patients. A second group of 13 children (mean age, 3.4 years) with bloody diarrhea caused by *S. sonnei, S. flexneri,* and *S. dysenteriae* (type 1) was treated with only one dose of pefloxacin (20 mg/kg); stools became normal in all cases by the end of the third day, and stool cultures performed between 5 and 8 d were negative of the pathogen in all cases.[203] Since the fluoroquinolones are capable of reaching high concentrations in the intestinal lumen for several days after oral administration,[204] it is likely that the eradication of *Shigellae* from stools may be achieved after only one dose.

Nalidixic acid, one of the original quinolone drugs, has been used to treat shigellosis when ampicillin- and/or TMP-SMX-resistant shigellosis (*S. dysenteriae* type 1) has been diagnosed.[118,205-209] In a controlled trial, Salam and Bennish[146] have found the clinical cure rate of nalidixic acid to be as effective as that of ampicillin, although the presence of *Shigella* in stools took longer to eradicate. While two other reports[209,210] corroborated the antishigellosis activity of nalidixic acid, results from a controlled trial in children by Haltalin et al.[211] have been contradictory.

Amdinocillin pivoxil (mecillinam) has also provided an alternative to ampicillin- and TMP-SMX-resistant *Shigella.*

Islam et al.[212] have compared the efficacy of gentamicin with nalidixic acid in the treatment of acute shigellosis in a double-blind trial of 79 children with bloody diarrhea of less than 72 h duration. Patients were randomly assigned to receive either gentamicin (30 mg/kg daily) or nalidixic acid (60 mg/kg daily) given orally in four equal doses for 5 d. Treatment failure was observed in 42% of the gentamicin-treated group as compared to none of those with nalidixic acid-sensitive *Shigella* spp. strains ($p = .0002$). The results of the study conclusively demonstrated the therapeutic ineffectiveness of oral gentamicin in the treatment of acute shigellosis.[212]

Furazolidone is probably effective in cases of mild to moderate shigellosis,[143,173] but should not be used for treatment of severe conditions.[213]

In a comparative study by Lionel et al.,[214] a single 2.5-g dose of tetracycline was found to be as effective as a 5-d course with the same drug; also, as effective as a combination of oral streptomycin and a sulfonamide (sulfadimidine).[179] Similarly, in a study of adult outpatients with a mild form of acute shigellosis, a single 800-mg dose of norfloxacin was equipotent to a 5-d course of trimethoprim-sulfamethoxazole.[189]

9.1.3.1 Absorbable Vs. Nonabsorbable Drugs in the Treatment of Shigellosis

Even though active *in vitro* and maintaining high concentrations in stool, nonabsorbable antimicrobial agents, such as streptomycin,[179] neomycin,[180] furazolidone,[143,213] and kanamycin,[215] were less effective against *Shigella* than absorbable drugs. Nunnery and Riley[216] have studied the antishigellosis effect of oral gentamicin in infants and children, but the reported results were not well defined and somewhat inconclusive. Even though *Shigella* was found to be susceptible *in vitro* to gentamicin,[140] as with other nonabsorbable drugs,[179,180,215] orally given gentamicin is unlikely to be effective. It may be possible to use gentamicin parenterally; however, such treatment would be appropriate only in seriously ill patients with access to hospital care.[106] It is of interest to mention that bicozamycin, which is a poorly absorbed drug, was found to be effective when given for only 3 d against shigellosis (Table 9.2).[3]

9.1.3.2 Shigellosis in HIV-Positive and AIDS Patients

In normal and otherwise healthy persons, shigellosis is usually self-limiting and if untreated will last between 1 and 30 d. However, because of their weakened immune status, in HIV-positive and

AIDS patients appropriate treatment is especially important since the infection may take a particularly virulent course characterized with prolonged diarrhea or extraintestinal manifestations such as bacteremia.[103,217]

S. flexneri has been diagnosed most frequently as the etiologic agent of diarrheal disease in immunocompetent homosexual men.[218] Surprisingly, there have been a relatively small number of cases of shigellosis in HIV-positive and AIDS patients. In a retrospective study by Nelson et al.,[219] during the period 1985–1990, of 526 HIV-positive patients investigated for diarrhea, only 7 patients (2 of them diagnosed with AIDS) have shown *Shigella* infection; species isolated included *S. flexneri, S. sonnei,* and *S. dysenteriae.* Ciprofloxacin was the drug of choice in all but two cases where ampicillin and neomycin were used.

Glypczynski et al.[103] described a case of *S. flexneri*-induced bacteremia in an AIDS patient. The strain, identified as serotype 3c, was susceptible to ampicillin, cefazoline, co-trimoxazole, chloramphenicol, and gentamicin, but resistant to tetracycline. Treatment with intravenous ampicillin at daily doses of 6.0 g for 10 d led to a rapid improvement but watery diarrhea with moderate intensity persisted. In another case, Gander and LaRocco[24] isolated a multiple drug-resistant *S. flexneri* in an HIV-positive patient with persistent diarrhea. The strain was resistant to ampicillin, tetracycline, ticarcillin, chloramphenicol, cephalothin, and trimethoprim-sulfamethoxazole, but susceptible to amikacin, gentamicin, tobramycin, cefamandole, cefazolin, cefoperazone, cefotaxime, cefoxitin, and cefuroxime, as well as a number of fluoroquinolones (ciprofloxacin, enoxacin, and norfloxacin). The patient's diarrhea was resolved by a 5-d course of antibiotic therapy; outpatient medication included 80 mg trimethoprim, 400 mg sulfamethoxazole, and 400 mg norfloxacin twice daily for 5 d.[24]

Antimicrobial susceptibility patterns, plasmid DNA content, and restriction enzyme digests of plasmid DNA were used to study 175 *Salmonella* and *Shigella* species isolated from predominantly HIV-positive adult patients from Kenya.[220] While all isolates were sensitive to ciprofloxacin, a significantly higher proportion of *Shigella* isolates were resistant to chloramphenicol, co-trimoxazole, tetracycline, and streptomycin as compared to *Salmonella* species. In addition to a 2- to 10-MDa range of plasmids, multiresistant *Shigella* spp. had a heavy 100- to 105-MDa plasmid. The data underscored the important role plasmid-encoded multidrug resistance plays in the spread of resistance among enteric bacteria.[220]

9.1.3.3 *Shigella* Endotoxins and Hematologic Abnormalities

Thrombotic thrombocytopenic purpura (TTP; thrombotic microangiopathy) has recently been diagnosed as one of several hematologic disorders occurring in HIV-positive patients.[221-223] It is a syndrome characterized by microangiopathic hemolytic anemia, thrombocytopenia, neurologic disorders, fever, and renal dysfunction. The pathophysiology of TTP seemed to correlate with the presence of circulating immune complexes that promote microthrombi formation. For the latter to occur, endothelial cell damage, leading to platelet adhesion and aggregation, and decrease in prostaglandin I_2 production play an important part.[224-227]

There have been several cases associating TTP with HIV-infected patients.[228-230] The etiology of such potentially fatal hematologic abnormality may well involve HIV-associated immune deficiency and/or opportunistic pathogen-related endotoxins. Thus, endothelial damage or direct platelet aggregation by endotoxins during infection, and immune complex-related endothelial damage have been postulated to play a role in the pathogenesis of secondary thrombotic microangiopathy.[221] Beris et al.[228] reported evidence from an HIV-infected patient which seemed to implicate *Shigella* endotoxins as part of the causative mechanism for this hematologic syndrome. The patient, who developed TTP during the course of rectosigmoiditis secondary to shigellosis, had elevated levels of immune complexes and the presence of *S. flexneri* known to produce endotoxins; both phenomena were associated with increased hemolysis and platelet consumption. In addition, during the acute microangiopathy, a mild form of acquired type II von Willebrand disease (a hemorrhagic diathesis characterized by prolonged bleeding time, deficiency of coagulation factor VIII, and often impairment of platelet adhesion on glass beads) was also diagnosed. Complete remission of TTP was achieved by aggressive treatment involving a combination of plasma exchange, fresh frozen plasma infusion, continuous prostacyclin perfusion, orally administered aspirin-dipyridamol, and intravenous injections of vincristine; the shigellosis responded to 500 mg of ciprofloxacin given twice daily for 10 d. Two months after diagnosis, the patient remained in remission on aspirin (100 mg daily) and dipyridamole (25 mg, t.i.d.).[228]

The hemolytic-uremic syndrome (HUS), as described by Gasser et al.,[231] is a disorder associated with hemolytic anemia, thrombocytopenia, and acute renal failure. There have been observations that the hemolytic anemia, which was often preceded by diarrhea, was associated with thrombotic renal microangiopathy[231] and mild disseminated intravascular coagulopathy.[232] These findings suggested the possibility of endotoxin derived from the gastrointestinal tract that produced a Schwartzman-like reaction in the renal microvasculature.[232,233] Although clinical studies failed to identify a circulating endotoxin after the onset of renal failure,[234,235] there have been occasional associations,[232,236,237] but not with one consistent infectious agent. A HUS secondary to shigellosis has been described by Ullis and Rosenblatt[113] as well as by others.[106,238,239] Rahaman et al.[239] have found that HUS was associated often with *S. dysenteriae* type 1 and leukemoid reactions, and that the complications occurred in children late in the course of the disease. Butler et al.[238] showed that prior treatment with antimicrobial drugs, the use of inappropriate antimicrobial drugs in hospital, and elevated leukocyte counts have been factors associated with the development of HUS during shigellosis.

Drugs that have been implicated in causing HUS include mitomycin[240] and penicillins;[241] the possible role of antimicrobial drugs as a risk factor for HUS might be either direct (to trigger HUS) or indirect (to allow time for the HUS to develop by preventing early deaths during severe illness).[238] In addition, antibiotic treatment may result in the release of *Shigella* endotoxin from dying bacteria, or the absorption of endotoxin or other bacterial products from lumenal bacteria other than *Shigella* through the ulcerated mucosa.[130,242,243]

Results by Koster et al.[169] showed circulating complexes in 10 of 20 patients with uncomplicated shigellosis, and in 4 of 6 patients with severe HUS. The occurrence of endotoxinemia before or during the onset of hemolysis may indicate that an endotoxin could be the mediator of renal cortical thrombosis. Histopathological similarities between the endotoxin-mediated experimental Shwartzman reaction and the hemolytic-uremic syndrome[233,244] supported this concept. The data of Koster et al.[169] lend credence to the hypothesis that severe colitis in shigellosis is very likely associated with circulating endotoxin(s) from the colon producing coagulopathy, renal microangiopathy, and hemolytic anemia.

Data from several recent reports[245-249] have raised important issues about the causes and treatment of HUS. For example, in addition to *Shigella* spp., it is now clear that Shiga-like toxin-producing *E. coli*[245,246] (types 0157:H7 and 011:HNM) can also be a cause of HUS. A second key issue is the potential for some antibiotics (ampicillin and nalidixic acid) used to treat *S. dysenteriae* type 1-induced dysentery to mediate HUS.[247,248] The elevated risk for HUS in patients with bloody diarrhea receiving antibiotic therapy should require careful monitoring of such patients.[249]

In conclusion, as opportunistic infections, such as shigellosis, become more frequent in patients with immunodeficiencies, pathogenic endotoxins released during such infections may well serve as triggering factors for the development of hematologic disorders and, therefore, should be monitored and treated aggressively.

9.1.3.4 Cutaneous Shigellosis

Stoll[250] has described a unique case of a purely cutaneous shigellosis in a homosexual man. The patient presented with a tender 1-cm furuncle on the dorsal penile shaft; there was also nontender left inguinal adenopathy. There was no gastrointestinal or urinary tract symptoms, but cultures of the penile lesions yielded *S. flexneri*. The shigellosis resolved completely after a 5-d therapy of double-strength TMP-SMX given twice daily.

Previously, cutaneous colonization with *Shigella* has been reported in infants with diaper dermatitis secondary to frequent watery stools.[251] Three cases of shigellosis in children associated with petechial or morbilliform rashes were also described with no mention of pustules, or cultures or biopsies of skin lesions performed.[252]

9.1.3.5 *Shigella* Osteomyelitis

Twum-Danso et al.[253] presented a case of *S. flexneri* osteomyelitis in an apparently healthy young man. The patient was successfully treated with ampicillin (500 mg every 6 h) for a period of 8 weeks. Previously, there had been only one case of *S. sonnei*-induced osteomyelitis reported, which occurred in a child with sickle cell anemia.[254]

9.1.3.6 Reactive Arthritis/Reiter's Syndrome and Enteric Bacterial Infections

Reactive arthritis, the dominant feature of Reiter's syndrome, has been associated with prior infection initiated by many different microorganisms, as evidenced by the presence of intra-articular bacterial antigens (bacteria, bacterial fragments, DNA, RNA, and bacterial lipopolysaccharides) in the joints of patients.[255] *S. flexneri*,[256] together with *Chlamidia trachomatis*,[257] *Campylobacter jejuni*,[258,259] and *Salmonella enteritidis*,[260,261] have all been detected in the joints. It is still unclear how these organisms have reached the joints and whether or not they persisted. However, the perseverance of synovitis might be explained by the establishment of reservoirs of bacteria at or near the site of primary infection.

Early reports[262-264] of short-term antibiotic therapy have indicated little success in the treatment of patients with reactive arthritis. In addition, the extensive use of sulfonamides in the therapy of dysentery failed to prevent the onset of enteric reactive arthritis and had no impact on the severity or course of arthritis.[265] The absence of clinical improvement following short-term antibiotic treatment of reactive arthritis, and the increasing evidence for the persistence of bacterial antigens, both in the joints and the site of primary infection provided impetus to studies utilizing prolonged antibiotic therapy.

Several uncontrolled trials,[266-268] have demonstrated the benefits of long-term treatment with sulfonamides or tetracyclines (doxycycline and minocycline). However, the interpretation of any beneficial effects from tetracycline therapy should be viewed with caution since these antibiotics are also known to inhibit collagenase activity,[269-271] to be effective scavengers of superoxide radicals, and for their ability to alter the cellular immune responses.[270]

In a double-blind, prospective, placebo-controlled trial, patients with reactive arthritis were given a 3-month course of lymecycline, a water-soluble tetracycline derivative.[272] The antibiotic eradicated *Chlamidia* as well as most strains of enteric Gram-negative bacteria. In another prospective study,[273] long-term antibiotic treatment resulted in a significant reduction in the frequency of associated attacks of synovitis. The beneficial response observed in patients with reactive arthritis receiving long-term antibiotic therapy may signify the importance of bacterial reservoirs present at or near the site of infection.

The presence of intra-articular bacterial antigens has provided little or no insight on the role cellular immunity might play in reactive arthritis.[255] However, the predominance of CD4+ lymphocytes in the inflammatory infiltrate in reactive arthritis has led to studies of CD4+ lymphocyte proliferation, both in mixed leukocyte cultures and when confronted with bacterial antigens *in vitro*. The results of lymphocyte proliferation, however, have been inconsistent[274] mainly because such experiments are difficult to interpret since they depend on many variables (antigen dose, reaction time, relative concentration of lymphocytes and antigen-presenting cells).[274-279] Furthermore, with the rising number of AIDS patients who are severely depleted of CD4+ lymphocytes and have developed severe reactive arthritis,[280] the potential role of CD4$^+$ lymphocytes in the immunopathogenic mechanism of this condition has been questioned. The finding that arthritis can be introduced in severe combined immunodeficiency (SCID) mice[281] has been another evidence casting doubt about the significance of CD4$^+$ cells in reactive arthritis.

9.1.3.7 Adjunct Therapies to Antimicrobial Agents in Shigellosis

The replacement of fluid deficit by oral rehydration, and nutritional support could be two major adjunctive therapies to antimicrobial regimens in the treatment of shigellosis.[106,116,117] However, such therapies cannot substantially reduce case-fatality rates as they do in cases of watery diarrhea.[282-284] The dehydration of patients with shigellosis has been attributed mainly to insensible fluid loss because of fever and decreased fluid intake due to anorexia, as well as the relatively modest loss of fluids through stools.[106] In addition, watery diarrhea may often precede symptoms of dysentery in children with shigellosis.[1] However, in the majority of cases, dehydration in shigellosis is not severe enough to warrant intravenous administration of fluids. According to Bennish et al.,[285] the relatively high sodium content of standard oral rehydration solutions (90 mmol/l) to a large degree would alleviate the severe hyponatremia that often is observed in *S. dysenteriae* type 1 infections.

Shigellosis is known to affect the nutritional status of patients in at least three ways: (1) metabolic effects of the infection; (2) loss of protein through the inflamed colonic mucosa; and (3) by a decrease in the caloric intake.[106] It has been postulated that the combination of these factors may be responsible for the retardation of growth observed in children following shigellosis.[286]

9.1.4 REFERENCES

1. Stoll, B. J., Glass, R. I., Huq, M. I., Khan, M. U., Banu, H., and Holt, J., Epidemiologic and clinical features of patients infected with *Shigella* who attended a diarrheal disease hospital in Bangladesh, *J. Infect. Dis.*, 146, 177, 1982.
2. Keusch, G. T., Formal, S. R., and Bennish, M. L., Shigellosis, in *Tropical and Geographical Medicine*, 2nd ed., Warren, K. S. and Mahmoud, A. A. F., Eds., McGraw-Hill, New York, 1990, 762.
3. DuPont, H. L., Ericsson, C. D., Reves, R. R., and Galindo, E., Antimicrobial therapy for traveler's diarrhea, *Rev. Infect. Dis.*, 8(Suppl. 2), S217, 1986.
4. DuPont, H. L., Reves, R. R., Galindo, E., Sullivan, P. S., Wood, L. V., and Mendiola, J. G., Treatment of travelers' diarrhea with trimethoprim/sulfamethoxazole and with trimethoprim alone, *N. Engl. J. Med.*, 307, 841, 1982.
5. Bogaerts, J., Habyalimana, J. B., Chevolet, T., and Vandepitte, J., Treatment of severe bacillary dysentery with trimethoprim alone, *Trans. R. Soc. Trop. Med. Hyg.*, 79, 203, 1985.
6. Tolkoff-Rubin, N. E., Weber, D., Fang, L. S. T., Kelly, M., Wilkinson, R., and Rubin, R. H., Trimethoprim-sulfamethoxazole for urinary tract infection in women, *Rev. Infect. Dis.*, 4, 444, 1982.
7. Counts, G. W., Stamm, W. E., McKevitt, M., Running, K., Holmes, K. K., and Turck, M., Treatment of cystitis in women with a single dose of trimethoprim-sulfamethoxazole, *Rev. Infect. Dis.*, 4, 484, 1982.
8. Anderson, J. D., Aird, M. Y., Johnson, A. M., Ree, R., Goresky, D., Brumwell, C. A., and Percicall-Smith, R. K. L., The use of a single 1 g dose of amoxycillin for the treatment of acute urinary tract infections, *J. Antimicrob. Chemother.*, 5, 481, 1979.
9. Neu, H. C., Trimethoprim alone for treatment of urinary tract infection, *Rev. Infect. Dis.*, 4, 366, 1982.
10. Kasanen, A. and Sundquist, H., Trimethoprim alone in the treatment of urinary tract infections: eight years of experience in Finland, *Rev. Infect. Dis.*, 4, 358, 1982.
11. Oldfield, E. C. III, Bourgeois, A. L., Omar, A.-K. M., and Pazzaglia, G. L., Empirical treatment of *Shigella* dysentery with trimethoprim: five-day course vs. single dose, *Am. J. Trop. Med. Hyg.*, 37, 616, 1987.
12. Murray, B. E., Resistance of *Shigella, Salmonella*, and other selected enteric pathogens, *Rev. Infect. Dis.*, 8(Suppl. 2), S172, 1986.

13. Goldstein, F. W. and Acar, J. F., Evolution and spread of trimethoprim resistance in gram-negative bacteria, *J. Med. Microbiol.*, 31, 1, 1990.

14. Huovinen, P., Renkonen, O.-V., Pulkkinen, L., Sunila, R., Grönroos, P., Klossner, M.-L., Virtanen, S., and Toivanen, P., Trimethoprim resistance of *Escherichia coli* in outpatients in Finland after ten years' use of plain trimethoprim, *J. Antimicrob. Chemother.*, 16, 435, 1985.

15. Towner, K. J. and Slack, R. C. B., Effect of changing selection pressures of trimethoprim resistance in Enterobacteriaceae, *Eur. J. Clin. Microbiol.*, 5, 502, 1986.

16. Reves, R. R., Murray, B. F., Pickering, L. K., Prado, D., Maddock, M., and Bartlett, A. V., Children with trimethoprim- and ampicillin-resistant fecal *Escherichia coli* in day care centers, *J. Infect. Dis.*, 156, 758, 1987.

17. Murray, B. E., Alvarado, T., Kim, K.-H., Vorachit, M., Jayanetra, P., Levine, M. M., Prenzel, I., Fling, M., Elwell, L., McCracken, G. H., Madrigal, G., Odio, C., and Trabulsi, L. R., Increasing resistance to trimethoprim-sulfamethoxazole among isolates of *Escherichia coli* in developing countries, *J. Infect. Dis.*, 152, 1107, 1985.

18. Young, H.-K., Jesudason, M. V., Koshi, G., and Amyes, S. G. B., Trimethoprim resistance amongst urinary pathogens in South India, *J. Antimicrob. Chemother.*, 17, 615, 1986.

19. Wylie, B., Amyes, S. G. B., Young, H.-K., and Koornhof, H. J., Identification of a novel plasmid-encoded dihydrofolate reductase mediating high-level resistance to trimethoprim, *J. Antimicrob. Chemother.*, 22, 429, 1988.

20. Urbina, R., Prado, V., and Canelo, E., Trimethoprim resistance in enterobacteria isolated in Chile, *J. Antimicrob. Chemother.*, 23, 143, 1989.

21. Goldstein, F. W. and Acar, J. F., Epidemiology of resistance to diaminopyridines, *J. Chemother.*, 5, 453, 1993.

22. Harnett, N., High level of resistance to trimethoprim, cotrimoxazole and other antimicrobial agents among clinical isolates of *Shigella* species in Ontario, Canada — an update, *Epidemiol. Infect.*, 109, 463, 1992.

23. Heikkilä, E., Slitonen, A., Jahkola, M., Fling, M., Sundsrtöm, L., and Huovinen, P., Increase of trimethoprim resistance among Shigella species, 1975–1988: analysis of resistance mechanisms, *J. Infect. Dis.*, 161, 1242, 1990.

24. Gander, R. M. and LaRocco, M. T., Multiple drug-resistance in *Shigella flexneri* isolated from a patient with human immunodeficiency virus, *Diagn. Microbiol. Infect. Dis.*, 8, 193, 1987.

25. Goldstein, F. W., Mécanismes de résistance aux sulfamides et au triméthoprime, *Bull. Inst. Pasteur*, 75, 109, 1977.

26. Young, H.-K. and Thompson, C. J., Plasmid-encoded trimethoprim-resistant dihydrofolate reductases in gram-negative bacteria, *J. Med. Microbiol.*, 31, 7, 1990.

27. Fleming, M. P., Datta, N., and Gruneberg, R. N., Trimethoprim resistance determined by R factors, *Br. J. Med.*, 1, 726, 1972.

28. Amyes, S. G. B., The success of plasmid-encoded drug resistance genes in clinical bacteria: an examination of plasmid-mediated ampicillin and trimethoprim resistance genes and their resistance mechanisms, *J. Med. Microbiol.*, 28, 73, 1989.

29. Amyes, S. G. B., Epidemiology of trimethoprim resistance, *J. Antimcrob. Chemother.*, 18(Suppl. C), 215, 1986.

30. Amyes, S. G. B., Doherty, C. J., and Young, H.-K., High-level trimethoprim resistance in urinary bacteria, *Eur. J. Clin. Microbiol.*, 5, 287, 1986.

31. Amyes, S. G. B. and Smith, J. T., R-factor trimethoprim resistance mechanism: an insusceptible target site, *Biochem. Biophys. Res. Commun.*, 58, 412, 1974.

32. Sköld, O. and Width, A., A new dihydrofolate reductase with low trimethoprim sensitivity induced by an R factor mediating high resistance to trimethoprim, *J. Biol. Chem.*, 249, 4324, 1974.

33. Towner, K. J., DNA probes for trimethoprim-resistant dihydrofolate reductases, *J. Med. Microbiol.*, 31, 9, 1990.

34. Bratoeva, M. P. and John, J. F., Jr., *In vivo* R-plasmid transfer in a patient with a mixed infection of shigella dysentery, *Epidemiol. Infect.*, 112, 247, 1994.

35. Towner, K. J., Venning, B. M., and Pinn, P. A., Occurrence of transposable trimethoprim resistance in clinical isolates of *Escherichia coli* devoid of self-transmissible resistance plasmids, *Antimicrob. Agents Chemother.*, 21, 336, 1982.

36. Barth, P. T., Datta, N., Hedges, R. W., and Grinter, N. J., Transposition of a deoxyribonucleic acid sequence encoding trimethoprim and streptomycin resistance from R483 to other replicons, *J. Bacteriol.*, 125, 800, 1976.

37. Huovinen, P., Pulkkine, L., Helin, H.-L., Mäkilä, M., and Toivanen, P., Emergence of trimethoprim resistance in relation to drug consumption in a Finnish hospital from 1971 through 1984, *Antimicrob. Agents Chemother.*, 29, 73, 1986.

38. Young, H.-K. and Amyes, S. G. B., Characterization of a new transposon-mediated trimethoprim-resistant dihydrofolate reductase, *Biochem. Pharmacol.*, 34, 4334, 1985.

39. Shapiro, J. A. and Sporn, P., Tn402: a new transposable element determining trimethoprim resistance that inserts in bacteriophage lambda, *J. Bacteriol.*, 129, 1632, 1977.

40. Kraft, C. A., Timbury, M. C., and Platt, D. J., Distribution and genetic location of Tn7 in trimethoprim-resistant *Escherichia coli*, *J. Med. Microbiol.*, 22, 125, 1986.

41. Amyes, S. G. B., McMillan, C. J., and Drysdale, J. L., Transferable trimethoprim resistance amongst hospital isolates, in *New Trends in Antibiotics: Research and Therapy*, Grassi, G. G. and Sabath, L. D., Eds., Elsevier/North Holland, Amsterdam, 1981, 325.

42. Amyes, S. G. B., The detection and incidence of transferable trimethoprim resistance, *Health Bull.*, 41, 100, 1983.

43. Cofsky, R. D., DuBouchet, L., and Landesman, S. H., Recovery of norfloxacin in feces after administration of a single oral dose to human volunteers, *Antimicrob. Agents Chemother.*, 26, 110, 1984.

44. Robinson, A., Wu, A. H. B., Ericsson, C. D., Johnson, P. C., and DuPont, H. L., *In vitro* activity of ciprofloxacin (CIP) against bacterial enteropathogens, in *Proc. 25th Intersci. Conf. Antimicrob. Agents Chemother.*, Minneapolis, American Society for Microbiology, Washington D.C., 1985.

45. Burman, L. G., Apparent absence of transferable resistance to nalidixic acid in pathogenic gram-negative bacteria, *J. Antimicrob. Chemother.*, 3, 509, 1977.

46. Line, A. S., Paul-Murphy, J., Aucoin, D. P., and Hirsh, D. C., Enrofloxacin treatment of long-tailed macaques with acute bacillary dysentery due to multiresistant *Shigella flexneri* IV, *Lab. Anim. Sci.*, 1992, 240, 1992.

47. Jones, R. N., Antimicrobial activity, spectrum and pharmacokinetics of old and new orally administered cephems, *Antimicrob. Newsl.*, 5, 1, 1988.

48. Ginsburg, C. M., McCracken, G. H., Jr., Petruska, M., and Olson, K., Pharmacokinetics and bactericidal activity of cefuroxime axetil, *Antimicrob. Agents Chemother.*, 28, 504, 1985.

49. Neu, H. C., Chin, N.-X., and Labthavikul, P., Comparative *in vitro* activity and β-lactamase stability of FR 17027, a new orally active cephalosporin, *Antimicrob. Agents Chemother.*, 26, 174, 1984.

50. Kamimura, T., Kojo, H., Matsumoto, Y., Mine, Y., Goto, S., and Kuwahara, S., *In vitro* and *in vivo* antibacterial properties of FK 027, a new orally active cephem antibiotic, *Antimicrob. Agents Chemother.*, 25, 98, 1984.

51. Neu, H. C., Chin, N.-X., and Labthavikul, P., *In vitro* activity and β-lactamase stability of two oral cephalosporins, ceftetrame (Ro 19-5247) and cefetamet (Ro 15-8047), *Antimicrob. Agents Chemother.*, 30, 423, 1986.

52. Leitner, F., Pursiano, T. A., Buck, R. E., Tsai, Y. H., Chisholm, D. R., Misiek, M., Desiderio, J. V., and Kessler, R. E., BMY 28100, a new oral cephalosporin, *Antimicrob. Agents Chemother.*, 31, 238, 1987.

53. Neu, H. C., The new beta-lactamase-stable cephalosporins, *Ann. Intern. Med.*, 97, 408, 1982.

54. Neu, H. C., Structure-activity relations of new beta-lactam compounds and *in vitro* activity against common bacteria, *Rev. Infect. Dis.*, 5(Suppl. 2), 319, 1983.

55. Brittain, D. C., Scully, B. E., Hirose, T., and Neu, H. C., The pharmacokinetic and bactericidal characteristics of oral cefixime, *Clin. Pharmacol. Ther.*, 38, 590, 1985.

56. Nelson, J. D. and Haltalin, K. C., Comparative efficacy of cephalexin and ampicillin for shigellosis and other types of acute diarrhea in infants and children, *Antimicrob. Agents Chemother.*, 7, 415, 1975.

57. Ashkenazi, S., Amir, J., Waisman, Y., Rachmel, A., Garty, B. Z., Samra, Z., Varsano, I., and Nitzan, M., A randomized, double-blind study comparing cefixime and trimethoprim-sulfamethoxazole in the treatment of childhood shigellosis, *J. Pediatr.*, 123, 817, 1993.

58. Harding, S. M., Williams, P. E. O., and Ayrton, J., Pharmacology of cefuroxime as the 1-acetoxyethyl ester in volunteers, *Antimicrob. Agents Chemother.*, 25, 78, 1984.

59. Sommers, D. K., Van Wyk, M., Williams, P. E. O., and Harding, S. M., Pharmacokinetics and tolerance of cefuroxime axetil in volunteers during repeated dosing, *Antimicrob. Agents Chemother.*, 25, 344, 1984.

60. Williams, P. E. O. and Harding, S. M., The absolute bioavailability of oral cefuroxime axetil in male and female volunteers after fasting and after food, *J. Antimicrob. Chemother.*, 13, 191, 1984.

61. Ginsburg, C. M. and McCracken, G. H., Jr., Pharmacokinetics of cephradine suspension in infants and children, *Antimicrob. Agents Chemother.*, 16, 74, 1979.

62. McCracken, G. H., Ginsburg, C. M., Clahsen, J. C., and Thomas, M. K., Pharmacologic evaluation of orally administered antibiotics in infants and children: effect of feeding on bioavailability, *Pediatrics*, 62, 738, 1978.

63. Lolekha, S., Poonyarit, P., Hongvistigul, W., Manatsathit, S., and Eambokalap, B., Treatment of shigellosis with a single dose of ceftriaxone, in *Progress in Therapy of Bacterial Infection*, Excerpta Medica, Amsterdam, 1983, 86.

64. Neu, H. C., Meropol, J., and Fu, K. P., Antibacterial activity of ceftriaxone (Ro 13-9904), a beta-lactamase-stable cefalosporin, *Antimicrob. Agents Chemother.*, 19, 414, 1981.

65. Angehrn, P., Probst, P. J., Reiner, R., and Then, R. L., Ro 13-9904, a long-acting broad-spectrum cephalosporin: *in vitro* and *in vivo* studies, *Antimicrob. Agents Chemother.*, 18, 913, 1980.

66. Kabir, I., Bulter, T., and Khanam, A., Comparative efficacy of single intravenous dose of ceftriaxone and ampicillin for shigellosis in a placebo-controlled trial, *Antimicrob. Agents Chemother.*, 29, 645, 1986.

67. Ling, J., Kam, K. M., Lam, A. W., and French, G. L., Susceptibilities of Hong Kong isolates of multiple resistant *Shigella* spp. to 25 antimicrobial agents, including ampicillin plus sulbactam and new 4-quinolones, *Antimicrob. Agents Chemother.*, 32, 20, 1988.

68. Hui-Lin, Z., Yi, L., Nai-Chang, Z., and An-Hua, H., A comparison of the *in vitro* properties of ceftriaxone with those of cephalosporins, *Chinese J. Antibiot.*, 13, 341, 1988.

69. Hohl, P., Von Graevenitz, Z., and Zollinzer-Iten, J., *In vitro* activity of Ro 19-5247 (T-2525) against intestinal pathogens glucose non-fermentive gram-negative rods: Legionella and Serratia, *Chemioterapia (Firenze)*, 6(Suppl. 2), 98, 1988.

70. Ceyhan, M., Dilmeu, U., Korten, V., and Mert, A., Shigella diarrhea and treatment, *Lancet*, 2, 45, 1988.

71. Korten, V., Mert, A., Ovunc, K., Ceyhan, M., Acar, S., and Ulas, T., Serotypes and drug resistance of *Shigella* strains isolated in Emtimesgut, Turkey in 1987, *Microbiyoloji Bulteni*, 22, 89, 1988.

72. Shawar, R., La Rocco, M., and Cleary, T. G., Comparative *in vitro* activity of ceftibuten (Sch 39720) against bacterial enteropathogens, *Antimicrob. Agents Chemother.*, 33, 781, 1989.

73. Mitra, A. K., Kabir, I., and Hossain, M. A., Piramecillinam-resistant *Shigella disenteriae* type 1 infection in Bangladesh, *Lancet*, 335, 1461, 1990.

74. Richards, D. M., Hell, R. C., Brogden, R. N., Speight, T. M., and Avery, G. S., Ceftriaxone: a review of its antibacterial activity, pharmacological properties and therapeutic use, *Drugs*, 27, 469, 1984.

75. Kabir, I., Butler, T., and Khanam, A., Comparative efficacies of single intravenous doses of ceftriaxone and ampicillin for shigellosis in a placebo-controlled trial, *Antimicrob. Agents Chemother.*, 29, 645, 1986.

76. Orenstein, W. A., Ross, L., Overturf, G. D., Wilkins, J., Redfield, D. R., and Underman, A., Antibiotic treatment of acute shigellosis: failure of cefamandole compared with trimethoprim/sulfamethoxazole and ampicillin, *Am. J. Med. Sci.*, 282, 27, 1981.

77. Varsano, I., Eidlitz-Marcus, T., Nussinovitch, M., and Elian, I., Comparative efficacy of ceftriaxone and ampicillin for treatment of severe shigellosis in children, *J. Pediatr.*, 118, 627, 1991.

78. Eidlitz-Marcus, T., Cohen, Y. H., Nussinovitch, M., Elian, I., and Varsano, I., Comparative efficacy of two- and five-day courses of ceftriaxone for treatment of severe shigellosis in children, *J. Pediatr.*, 123, 822, 1993.

79. Park, J. W. and Rogers, P. L., Treatment of shigellosis, *J. Pediatr.*, 119, 841, 1991.

80. Ishida, Y., Miyazaki, S., Yamaguchi, K., and Goto, S., *In vitro* and *in vivo* activity of DQ-2556, a new cephalosporin, *Chemotherapy*, 41, 5, 1995.

81. Prado, D., Lopez, E., Liu, H., Devoto, S., Woloj, M., Contrini, M., Murray, B. E., Gomez, H., and Cleary, T. G., Ceftibutene and trimethoprim-sulfamethoxazole for treatment of *Shigella* and enteroinvasive *Escherichia coli* disease, *Pediatr. Infect. Dis. J.*, 11, 644, 1992.

82. Spratt, B. G., Comparison of the binding properties of two 6-β-amidinopenicillanic acid derivatives that differ in their physiological effects on *Escherichia coli*, *Antimicrob. Agents Chemother.*, 11, 161, 1977.

83. Spratt, B. G., The mechanism of action of mecillinam, *J. Antimicrob. Chemother.*, 3(Suppl. B), 13, 1977.

84. Kucers, A. and Bennett, N. M., *The Use of Antibiotics. A Comprehensive Review With Clinical Emphasis*, 4th ed., J. B. Lippincott, Philadelphia, 1987, 256.

85. Tybring, L. and Melchior, N. H., Mecillinam (FL 1060), a 6-β-amidinopenicillanic acid derivative: bactericidal action and synergy *in vitro*, *Antimicrob. Agents Chemother.*, 8, 271, 1975.

86. Richmond, M. H., *In vitro* studies with mecillinam on *Escherichia coli* and *Pseudomonas aeruginosa*, *J. Antimicrob. Chemother.*, 3(Suppl. B), 29, 1977.

87. Uwaydah, M. and Osseiran, M., Susceptibility of recent *Shigella* isolates to mecillinam, ampicillin, tetracycline, chloramphenicol, and cotrimoxazole, *J. Antimicrob. Chemother.*, 7, 619, 1981.

88. Hansson, H. B., Walder, M., and Juhlin, I., Susceptibility of shigellae to mecillinam, nalidixic acid, trimethoprim, and five other antimicrobial agents, *Antimicrob. Agents Chemother.*, 19, 271, 1981.

89. Neu, H. C., Mecillinam, a novel penicillanic acid derivative with unusual activity against gram-negative bacteria, *Antimicrob. Agents Chemother.*, 9, 793, 1976.

90. Lund, F., Roholt, K., Tybring, L., and Godtfredsen, W. O., Mecillinam and pivmecillinam — β-lactam antibiotics with high activity against gram negative bacilli, in *Chemotherapy*, Vol. 5, William, J. D. and Geddes, A. M., Eds., Plenum Press, New York, 1976, 159.

91. Lerman, S. J., Waller, J. M., and Simms, D. H., Resistance of *Shigellae* to ampicillin and other antibiotics: South Bronx, New York (1971 and 1972), *J. Pediatr.*, 83, 500, 1973.

92. Roholt, K., Pharmacokinetic studies with mecillinam and pivmecillinam, *J. Antimicrob. Chemother.*, 3(Suppl. B), 71, 1977.

93. Kabir, I., Rahaman, M. M., Ahmed, S. M., Akhter, S. Q., and Butler, T., Comparative efficacies of pivmecillinam and ampicillin in acute shigellosis, *Antimicrob. Agents Chemother.*, 25, 643, 1984.

94. Prado, D., Liu, H., Velasquez, T., and Cleary, T. G., Comparative efficacy of pivmecillinam and co-trimoxazole in acute shigellosis in children, *Scand. J. Infect. Dis.*, 25, 713, 1993.

95. Alam, A. N., Islam, M. R., Hossain, M. S., Mahalanabis, D., and Hye, H. K., Comparison of pivmecillinam and nalidixic acid in the treatment of acute shigellosis in children, *Scand. J. Gastroenterol.*, 29, 313, 1994.

96. Ekwall, E. and Svenungsson, B., Pivampicillin/pivmecillinam in the treatment of shigella carriers, *Scand. J. Infect. Dis.*, 22, 623, 1990.

97. Gordillo, M. E., Singh, K. V., and Murray, B. E., *In vitro* activity of azithromycin against bacterial enteric pathogens, *Antimicrob. Agents Chemother.*, 37, 1203, 1993.

98. Bennish, M. L., Harris, J. R., Wojtyniak, B. J., and Struelens, M., Death in shigellosis: incidence and risk factors in hospital patients, *J. Infect. Dis.*, 161, 500, 1990.

99. Ronsmans, C., Bennish, M. L., and Wierzba, T., Diagnosis and management of dysentery by community health workers, *Lancet*, 2, 552, 1988.

100. Chen, L. C., Control of diarrheal disease morbidity and mortality: some strategic issues, *Am. J. Clin. Nutr.*, 31, 2284, 1978.

101. Squires, R. H., Keating, J. P., Rosenblum, J. L., Askin, F., and Ternberg, J. L., Splenic abscess and hepatic dysfunction caused by *Shigella flexneri*, *J. Pediatr.*, 98, 429, 1981.

102. Faucon, R. and Dulcoux, M., Septicémies a Shigella: a propos de deux nouvelle observation, *Méd. Trop.*, 24, 537, 1964.

103. Glypczynski, Y., Hansen, W., Jonas, C., and Deltenre, M., *Shigella flexneri* bacteraemia in a patient with acquired immune deficiency syndrome, *Acta Clin. Belg.*, 40, 388, 1985.

104. De Mol, P., Brasseur, D., Schatterman, E., and Kassam, S., Shigella and shigellaemia, *Scand. J. Infect. Dis.*, 13, 75, 1981.

105. Scragg, J. N., Rubidge, C. J., and Appelbaum, P. C., Shigella infection in African and Indian children with special reference to shigella septicemia, *J. Pediatr.*, 93, 796, 1978.

106. Salam, M. A. and Bennish, M. L., Antimicrobial therapy for shigellosis. *Rev. Infect. Dis.*, 13(Suppl. 4), S322, 1991.

107. The burden of disease resulting from children, in *New Vaccine Development: Establishing Priority*, Vol. 2, *Diseases of Importance in Developing Countries.*, Katz, S. L., Ed., National Academy Press, Washington, D.C., 1986, 165.

108. Bennish, M. L., Harris, J. R., Wojtyniak, B. J., and Struelens, M., Death in shigellosis: incidence and risk factors in hospitalized patients, *J. Infect. Dis.*, 161, 500, 1990.

109. Reed, W. P. and Albright, E. L., Serum factors responsible for killing of shigella, *Immunology*, 26, 205, 1974.

110. D'Auria, A., Shigella bacteremia, *Clin. Microbiol. Newsl.*, 4, 131, 1981.

111. Gray, J. A. and Gilmour, H. M., Fatal *Shigella flexneri* bacteraemia with disseminated intravascular coagulation, leucopenia and hypogammaglobulinemia, *J. Infect.*, 1, 277, 1979.

112. Evans, H. E., Sampath, A., Douglass, F., and Baki, A., Shigella bactaeremia in a patient with sickle cell anemia, *Am. J. Dis. Child.*, 123, 238, 1972.

113. Ullis, K. C. and Rosenblatt, R. M., Shiga Bacillus dysentery complicated by bacteremia and disseminated intravascular coagulation, *J. Pediatr.*, 83, 90, 1973.

114. Fernhoff, F. M. and Plotkin, S. A., Extraintestinal shigellosis: bacteremia and paroxysmal atrial tachycardia: *Shigella sonnei* in a three-year-old boy, *Clin. Pediatr.*, 12, 302, 1973.

115. Armor, S. A., Periparturitional shigellosis, *Nebr. Med. J.*, 75, 239, 1990.

116. World Health Organization, The Management of Diarrhoea and Use of Oral Rehydration Therapy: a Joint WHO/UNICEF Statement, 2nd ed., World Health Organization, Geneva, 1985.

117. World Health Organization, A Manual for the Treatment of Acute Diarrhoea for Use by Physicians and Other Senior Health Workers, publication no. WHO/CDD/SER/80.2 Rev. 1, World Health Organization, Geneva, 1984.

118. Lima, A. A., Lima, N. L., Pinho, M. C., Barros, E. A., Jr., Teixeira, M. J., Martins, M. C. V., and Guerrant, R. L., High frequency of strains multiply resistant to ampicillin, trimethoprim-sulfamethoxazole, streptomycin, chloramphenicol, and tetracycline isolated from patients with shigellosis in northeastern Brazil during the period 1988 to 1993, *Antimicrob. Agents Chemother.*, 39, 256, 1995.

119. Patwari, A. K., Multidrug resistant *Shigella* infections in children, *J. Diarrhoeal Dis. Res.*, 12, 182, 1994.

120. Rawashdeh, M. O., Ababneh, A. M., and Shurman, A. A., Shigellosis in Jordanian children: a clinico-epidemiologic prospective study and susceptibility to antibiotics, *J. Trop. Pediatr.*, 40, 355, 1994.

121. Anderson, D. E. W., Cruickshank, R., and Walker, J., The treatment of bacillary (Flexner) dysentery with sulphanilylguanidine, *Br. Med. J.*, 2, 497, 1941.

122. Cooper, M. L., Zucker, R. L., and Wagoner, S., Sulfathiazole for acute diarrhea and dysentery of infants and children, *JAMA*, 117, 1520, 1941.

123. Marshall, E. K., Bratton, A. C., Edwards, L. B., and Walker, E., Sulfanilylguanidine in the treatment of acute bacillary dysentery in children, *Bull. Johns Hopkins Hosp.*, 68, 94, 1941.

124. Reitler, R. and Marberg, K., Note on the treatment of acute bacillary dysentery with sulphapyridine, *Br. Med. J.*, 1, 277, 1941.

125. Fairley, N. H. and Boyd, J. S. K., Treatment of bacillary dysentery with sulphaguanidine, *Lancet*, 1,20, 1942.

126. Hardy, A. V., Watt, J., Peterson, J., and Schlosser, E., Studies of the acute diarrheal disease. VIII. Sulfaguanidine in the control of *Shigella dysenteriae* infections, *Public Health Rep.*, 57, 529, 1942.

127. Hardy, A. V., Burns, W., and Decapito, T., Studies of the acute diarrheal disease. X A. Cultural observations on the relative efficacy of sulfonamides in *Shigella dysenteriae* infections, *Public Health Rep.*, 58, 689, 1943.

128. Hardy, A. V. and Cummins, S. D., Studies of the acute diarrheal diseases. X B. A preliminary note on the clinical response to sulfadiazine therapy, *Public Health Rep.*, 58, 693, 1943.

129. Haltalin, K. C., Nelson, J. D., Ring, R. III, Sladoje, M., and Hinton, L. V., Double-blind treatment study of shigellosis comparing ampicillin, sulfadiazine, and placebo, *J. Pediatr.*, 70, 970, 1967.

130. Pickering, L. K., DuPont, H. L., and Olarte, J., Single-dose tetracycline therapy for shigellosis in adults, *JAMA*, 239, 853, 1978.

131. Lionel, N. D. W., Abeyasekera, F. J. B., Samarasinghe, H. G., Goonewardena, C. V., and Tawil, G. S., A comparison of a single dose and five-day course of tetracycline therapy in bacillary dysentery, *J. Trop. Med. Hyg.*, 72, 170, 1969.

132. Gilman, R. H., Spira, W., Rabbani, H., Ahmed, W., Islam, A., and Rahaman, M. M., Single-dose ampicillin therapy for severe shigellosis in Bangladesh, *J. Infect. Dis.*, 143, 164, 1981.

133. Meyer, P. W. and Lerman, S., Rise and fall of shigella antibiotic resistance, *Antimicrob. Agents Chemother.*, 17, 101, 1980.

134. Nelson, J. D., Kusmiesz, H., Jackson, L. H., and Woodman, E., Trimethoprim-sulfamethoxazole therapy for shigellosis, *JAMA*, 235, 1239, 1976.

135. Nelson, J. D., Kusmiesz, H., and Jackson, L. H., Comparison of trimethoprim-sulfamethoxazole and ampicillin therapy for shigellosis in ambulatory patients, *J. Pediatr.*, 89, 491, 1976.

136. Barada, F. A., Jr. and Guerrant, R. L., Sulfamethoxazole-trimethoprim versus ampicillin in treatment of acute invasive diarrhea in adults, *Antimicrob. Agents Chemother.*, 17, 961, 1980.

137. Marberg, K., Altmann, G., and Ashkol-Bruck, A., Observations on resistance to sulfadiazine and antibiotics in shigellosis, *Am. J. Trop. Med. Hyg.*, 7, 51, 1958.

138. Ross, S., Controni, G., and Khan, W., Resistance of shigellae to ampicillin and other antibiotics: its clinical and epidimiological implications, *JAMA*, 221, 45, 1972.

139. Weissman, J. B., Gangarosa, E. J., and DuPont, H. L., Changing needs in the antimicrobial therapy of shigellosis, *J. Infect. Dis.*, 127, 611, 1973.

140. Shahid, N. S., Rahaman, M. M., Haider, K., Banu, H., and Rahman, N., Changing pattern of resistant Shiga bacillus (*Shigella dysenteriae* type 1) and *Shigella flexneri* in Bangladesh, *J. Infect. Dis.*, 152, 1114, 1985.

141. Hanson, H. B., Walder, M., and Juhlin, I., Susceptibility of shigellae to mecillinam, nalidixic acid, trimethoprim, and five other antimicrobial agents, *Antimicrob. Agents Chemother.*, 19, 271, 1981.

142. Franzen, C., Experience of co-trimoxazole in the treatment of *Salmonella* and *Shigella* infections, *Scand. J. Infect. Dis.*, 8(Suppl.), 79, 1976.

143. Lexomboon, U., Mansuwan, P., Duangmani, C., Benjadol, P., and McMinn, M. T., Clinical evaluation of co-trimoxazole and furazolidone in treatment of shigellosis in children, *Br. Med. J.*, 1, 23, 1972.

144. Lewis, E. L., Anderson, J. D., and Lacey, R. W., A reappraisal of the antibacterial action of co-trimoxazole *in vitro*, *J. Clin. Pathol.*, 27, 87, 1974.

145. Jarvis, K. J. and Scrimgeour, G., *In vitro* sensitivity of *Shigella sonnei* to trimethoprim and sulfamethoxazole, *J. Med. Microbiol.*, 3, 554, 1970.

146. Salam, M. A. and Bennish, M. L., Therapy of shigellosis. I. Randomized, double-blind trial of nalidixic acid in childhood shigellosis, *J. Pediatr.*, 3, 901, 1988.

147. Haltalin, K. C., Nelson, J. D., Kusmiesz, H. T., and Hinton, L. V., Comparison of intramuscular and oral ampicillin therapy for shigellosis, *J. Pediatr.*, 73, 617, 1968.

148. Nelson, J. D., Kusmiesz, H., and Shelton, S., Oral or intravenous trimethoprim-sulfamethoxazole therapy for shigellosis, *Rev. Infect. Dis.*, 4, 546, 1982.

149. Haltalin, K. C., Nelson, J. D., Kusmiesz, H. T., and Hinton, L. V., Optimal dosage of ampicillin for shigellosis, *J. Pediatr.*, 74, 627, 1969.

150. Chang, M. J., Dunkle, L. M., Van Reken, D., Anderson, D., Wong, M. L., and Feigin, R. D., Trimethoprim-sulfamethoxazole compared to ampicillin in the treatment of shigellosis, *Pediatrics*, 59, 726, 1977.

151. Yunus, M., Rahman, A. S. M. M., Farooque, A. S. G., and Glass, R. I., Clinical trial of ampicillin vs. trimethoprim sulphamethoxazole in the treatment of *Shigella* dysentery, *J. Trop. Med. Hyg.*, 85, 195, 1982.

152. Gilman, R. H., Koster, F., Islam, S., McLaughlin, J., and Rahaman, M. M., Randomized trial of high- and low-dose ampicillin therapy for treatment of severe dysentery due to *Shigella dysenteriae* type 1, *Antimicrob. Agents Chemother.*, 17, 402, 1980.

153. Gilman, R. H., Spira, W., Rabbani, H., Ahmed, W., Islam, A., and Rahaman, M. M., Single-dose ampicillin therapy for severe shigellosis in Bangladesh, *J. Infect. Dis.*, 143, 164, 1981.

154. Pal, S. C., Epidemic bacillary dysentery in West Bengal, India, *Lancet*, 1, 1462, 1984.

155. Bennish, M., Eusof, A., Kay, B., and Wierzba, T., Multiresistant *Shigella* infections in Bangladash, *Lancet*, 2, 441, 1985.

156. Frost, J. A., Willshaw, G. A., Barclay, E. A., and Rowe, B., Plasmid characterization of drug-resistant *Shigella dysenteriae* 1 from an epidemic in Central Africa, *J. Hyg. (Cambridge)*, 94, 163, 1985.

157. Centers for Disease Control, Multiply resistant shigellosis in a day-care-center — Texas, *Morbid. Mortal. Wkly. Rep.*, 35, 753, 1986.

158. Centers for Disease Control, Nationwide dissemination of multiply resistant *Shigella sonnei* following common-source outbreak, *Morbid. Mortal. Wkly. Rep.*, 36, 633, 1987.

159. Gross, R. J., Threlfall, E. J., Ward, L. R., and Rowe, B., Drug resistance in *Shigella dysenteriae*, *Shigella flexneri* and *Shigella boydii* in England and Wales: increasing incidence of resistance to trimethoprim, *Br. J. Med.*, 288, 784, 1984.

160. Macaden, R. B., Gokul, N., Pereira, P., and Bhat, P., Bacillary dysentery due to multi-drug resistant *Shigella dysenteriae*, *Indian J. Med. Res.*, 71, 178, 1980.
161. Pichler, H., Diridl, G., Stickler, K., and Wolf, D., Clinical efficacy of ciprofloxacin compared with placebo in bacterial diarrhea, *Am. J. Med.*, 82(Suppl. 4A), 329, 1987.
162. Cheever, F. S., Shigellosis, in *Cecil-Loeb Textbook of Medicine*, 11th ed., Beeson, P. B. and McDermott, W., Eds., W. B. Saunders, Philadelphia, 250, 1963.
163. Barrett-Connor, E. and Connor, J. D., Extraintestinal manifestations of shigellosis, *Am. J. Gastroenterol.*, 53, 234, 1970.
164. Barrett-Connor, E. and Connor, J. D., Skin lesions and shigellosis, *Am. J. Trop. Med.*, 18, 555, 1969.
165. Horney, J. T., Schwarzmann, S. W., and Galambos, J. T., Shigella hepatitis, *Am. J. Gastroenterol.*, 66, 146, 1976.
166. Jao, R. L. and Jackson, G. G., Asymptomatic urinary tract infection with *Shigella sonnei* in chronic faecal carrier, *N. Engl. J. Med.*, 268, 1165, 1963.
167. Kim, M. H. and Hugues, W. T., Shigellosis and associated disease in infants and children, *J. Ky. Med. Assoc.*, 66, 542, 1968.
168. Ryan, J. M. and Riley, H. D., Shigella keratitis, a case report, *J. Pediatr.*, 74, 294, 1969.
169. Koster, F., Levin, J., Walker, L., Tung, K. S. K., Gilman, R. H., Rahaman, M. M., Majid, M. A., Islam, S., and Williams, R. C., Haemolytic uremic syndrome after shigellosis: relation to endotoxaemia and circulating immune complexes, *N. Engl. J. Med.*, 289, 927, 1978.
170. Morduchowicz, G., Huminer, D., Siegman-Igra, Y., Drucker, M., Block, D. S., and Pittik, D. S., Shigella bacteraemia in adults — a report of five cases and review of the literature, *Arch. Intern. Med.*, 147, 2034, 1987.
171. Graber, C. D., Browning, D., and Davis, J. S., Shigellemia without *Shigella* diarrhea, report of a case, *Am. J. Clin. Pathol.*, 46, 221, 1966.
172. Evans, H. E., Sampath, A. C., Douglass, F., and Baki, A., Shigella bacteremia in a patient with sickle cell anemia, *Am. J. Dis. Child.*, 123, 238, 1972.
173. Fish, C. H. and Jones, G., Furazolidone in the treatment of institutional shigellosis, *Am. J. Ment. Defic.*, 73, 214, 1968.
174. Kraybill, E. N. and Controni, G., Septicemia and enterocolitis due to *Shigella sonnei* in a newborn infant, *Pediatrics*, 42, 529, 1968.
175. Whitfield, C. and Humphries, J. M., Meningitis and septicemia due to shigellae in a newborn infant, *J. Pediatr.*, 70, 805, 1967.
176. Grater, C. D., Browning, D., and Davis, J. S., Shigellaemia without *Shigella* diarrhoea: report of a case, *Am. J. Clin. Pathol.*, 46, 221, 1966.
177. Neter, E., Merrin, C., Surgalla, M. J., and Wajsman, Z., *Shigella sonnei* bacteraemia: unusual antibody response from immunosuppressive therapy following renal transplantation, *Urology*, 4, 198, 1974.
178. Kazal, H. L., Sohn, N., Carrasco, J. I., Robilotti, J. G., and Delaney, W. E., The gay bowel syndrome: clinico-pathologic correlation in 260 cases, *Ann. Clin. Lab. Sci.*, 6, 184, 1976.
179. Stoker, D. J., Treatment of bacillary dysentery: with special reference to stosstherapy with tetracycline, *Br. Med. J.*, 1, 1179, 1962.
180. Haltalin, K. C., Nelson, J. D., Hinton, L. V., Kusmiesz, H. T., and Sladoje, M., Comparison of orally absorbable and nonabsorbable antibiotics in shigellosis. A double-blind study with ampicillin and neomycin, *J. Pediatr.*, 72, 708, 1968.
181. Tong, M. J., Martin, D. G., Cunningham, J. J., and Gunning, J. J., Clinical and bacteriological evaluation of antibiotic treatment in shigellosis, *JAMA*, 214, 1841, 1970.
182. Haltalin, K. C., Kusmiesz, H. T., Hinton, L. V., and Nelson, J. D., Treatment of acute diarrhea in outpatients: double-blind study comparing ampicillin and placebo, *Am. J. Dis. Child.*, 124, 554, 1972.
183. Neter, E. and Whang, H. Y., The common antigen of gram-negative enteric bacteria, in *Cellular Antigens*, Novotny, A., Ed., Springer-Verlag, New York, 1972, 14.
184. Bassily, S., Hyams, K. C., el-Masry, N. A., Farid, Z., Cross, E., Bourgeois, A. L., Ayal, E., and Hibbs, R. G., Short-course norfloxacin and trimethoprim-sulfamethoxazole treatment of shigellosis and salmonellosis in Egypt, *Am. J. Trop. Med. Hyg.*, 51, 219, 1994.
185. Rogerie, F., Ott, D., Vandenpitte, J., Verbist, L., Lemmens, P., and Habiyaremye, I., Comparison of norfloxacin and nalidixic acid for treatment of dysentery caused by *Shigella* dysenteriae type 1 in adults, *Antimicrob. Agents Chemother.*, 29, 883, 1986.

186. Corcione, F. and Giordano, B., Biliary pharmacokinetics of norfloxacine, *Chemioterapia*, 4(Suppl. 2), 494, 1985.
187. O'Hare, M. D., Flemingham, D., Ridgeway, G. L., and Gruneberg, R. N., The comparative *in vitro* activity of twelve 4-quinolone antimicrobial agents against enteric pathogens, *Drug Exp. Clin. Res.*, 11, 253, 1985.
188. Shungu, D. L., Weinberg, E., and Gadebusch, H. H., *In vitro* antibacterial activity of norfloxacin and other agents against gastrointestinal tract pathogens, *Antimicrob. Agents Chemother.*, 23, 86, 1983.
189. Gotuzzo, E., Oberhelman, R. A., Maguifia, C., Berry, S. J., Yi, A., Guzman, M., Ruiz, R., Leon-Barua, R., and Sack, R. B., Comparison of a single-dose treatment with norfloxacin and standard 5-day treatment with trimethoprim-sulfamethoxazole for acute shigellosis in adults, *Antimicrob. Agents Chemother.*, 33, 1101, 1989.
190. Bhattacharya, M. K., Nair, G. B., Sen, D., Paul, M., Debnath, A., Nag, A., Dutta, D., Dutta, P., Pal, S. C., and Bhattacharya, S. K., Efficacy of norfloxacin for shigellosis: a double blind randomized clinical trial, *J. Diarrhoeal Dis. Res.*, 10, 146, 1992.
191. Wiström, J., Jetborn, M., Ekwall, E., Norlin, K., Söderquist, B., Strömberg, A., Lundholm, R., Hogevik, H., Lagergren, L., Englund, G., Norrby, R., and the Swedish Study Group, Empiric treatment of acute diarrheal disease with norfloxacin: a randomized, placebo-controlled study, *Ann. Intern. Med.*, 117, 202, 1992.
192. Bhattacharya, S. K., Bhattacharya, M. K., Dutta, P., Sen, D., Rasaily, R., Moitra, A., and Pal, S. C., Randomized clinical trial of norfloxacin for shigellosis, *Am. J. Trop. Med. Hyg.*, 45, 683, 1991.
193. Ericsson, C. D., Johnson, P. C., DuPont, H. L., Morgan, D. R., Bitsura, J. M., and De la Cabada, F. J., Ciprofloxacin of trimethoprim-sulfamethoxazole as initial therapy for travelers' diarrhea, *Ann. Intern. Med.*, 106, 216, 1987.
194. Ericsson, C. D., DuPont, H. L., Mathewson, J. J., West, M. S., Johnson, P. C., and Bitsura, J. M., Treatment of travelers' diarrhea with sulfamethoxazole and trimethoprim and loperamide, *JAMA*, 263, 257, 1990.
195. Goodman, L. J., Trenholme, G. M., Kaplan, R. L., Segreti, J., Hines, D., Petrak, R., Nelson, J. A., Mayer, K. W., Landau, W., Parkhurst, G. W., and Levin, S., Empiric antimicrobial therapy of domestically acquired acute diarrhea in urban adults, *Arch. Intern. Med.*, 150, 541, 1990.
196. Bennish, M. L., Salam, M. A., Khan, W. A., and Khan, A. M., Treatment of shigellosis. III. Comparison of one- or two-dose ciprofloxacin with standard 5-day therapy: a randomized, blinded trial, *Ann. Intern. Med.*, 117, 727, 1992.
197. Bhattacharya, S. K., Bhattacharya, M. K., Dutta, D., Dutta, P., Paul, M., Sen, D., Sarkar, S., Saha, A., and Pal, S. C., Single-dose ciprofloxacin for shigellosis in adults, *J. Infect.*, 25, 117, 1992.
198. Williams, H. M. and Richards, J., Single-dose ciprofloxacin for shigellosis, *Lancet*, 335, 1343, 1990.
199. Kaya, I. S., Dilmen, U., and Senses, D. A., Danger of antibiotic resistance in shigellosis, *Lancet*, 336, 186, 1990.
200. Taylor, D. N., Sanchez, J. L., Candler, W., Thornton, S., McQueen, C., and Echeverria, P., Treatment of travelers' diarrhea: ciprofloxacin plus loperamide compared with ciprofloxacin alone, *Ann. Intern. Med.*, 114, 731, 1991.
201. Murphy, G. S., Bodhidatta, L., Echeverria, P., Tansuphaswadikul, S., Hoge, C. W., Imlarp, S., and Tamura, K., Ciprofloxacin and loperamide in the treatment of bacillary dysentery, *Ann. Intern. Med.*, 118, 582, 1993.
202. Fontaine, O., Antibiotics in the management of shigellosis in children: what role for quinolones? *Rev. Infect. Dis.*, 11(Suppl. 5), S1145, 1989.
203. Guyon, P., Cassel-Beraud, A.-M., Rakotonirina, G., and Gendrel, D., Short-term pefloxacin therapy in Madagascan children with shigellosis due to multiresistant organisms, *Clin. Infect. Dis.*, 19, 1172, 1994.
204. Pecquet, S., Ravoire, S., and Andremont, A., Faecal excretion of ciprofloxacin after a single oral dose and its effect on faecal bacteria in healthy volunteers, *J. Antimicrob. Chemother.*, 26, 125, 1990.
205. Frost, J. A., Rowe, B., and Vandepitte, J., Acquisition of trimethoprim resistance in epidemic strain of *Shigella dysenteriae* type 1 from Zaire, *Lancet*, 1, 963, 1982.
206. Parry, H. E., Nalidixic acid for shigellosis, *Lancet*, 2, 1206, 1983.
207. Malengreau, M., Nalidixic acid in *Shigella dysenteriae* outbreaks, *Lancet*, 2, 172, 1984.

208. Bose, R., Nashipuri, J. N., Sen, P. K., Datta, P., Bhattacharya, S. K., Datta, D., Sen, D., and Bhattacharya, M. K., Epidemic of dysentery in West Bengal: clinician's enigma, *Lancet*, 2, 1160, 1984.

209. Moorhead, P. J. and Parry, H. E., Treatment of Sonne dysentery, *Br. Med. J.*, 2, 913, 1965.

210. Hansson, H. B., Barkenius, G., Cronberg, S., and Juhlin, I., Controlled comparison of nalidixic acid or lactulose with placebo in shigellosis, *Scand. J. Infect. Dis.*, 13, 191, 1981.

211. Haltalin, K. C., Nelson, J. D., and Kusmiesz, H. T., Comparative efficacy of nalidixic acid and ampicillin for severe shigellosis, *Arch. Dis. Child.*, 48, 305, 1973.

212. Islam, M. R., Alam, A. N., Hossain, M. S., Mahalanabis, D., and Hye, H. K., Double-blind comparison of oral gentamicin and nalidixic acid in the treatment of acute shigellosis in children, *J. Trop. Pediatr.*, 40, 320, 1994.

213. Haltalin, K. C. and Nelson, J. D., Failure of furazolidone therapy in shigellosis, *Am. J. Dis. Child.*, 123, 40, 1972.

214. Lionel, N. D. W., Abeyasekera, F. I. B., Samarasinghe, H. G., Goonewardena, C. V., and Tawil, G. S., A comparison of a single dose and a five-day course of tetracycline therapy in bacillary dysentery, *J. Trop. Med. Hyg.*, 72, 170, 1969.

215. Nelson, J. D. and Haltalin, K. C., *In-vitro* susceptibility of *E. coli, Shigellae* and *Salmonellae* to kanamycin and therapeutic implications, *Ann. NY Acad. Sci.*, 132, 1006, 1966.

216. Nunnery, A. W. and Riley, H. D., Jr., Gentamicin: clinical and laboratory studies in infants and children, *J. Infect. Dis.*, 119, 460, 1969.

217. Mandell, W. and Neu, H. C., *Shigella* bacteremia in adults, *JAMA*, 255, 3116, 1986.

218. Quinn, T. C., Stam, W. E., Goodell, S. E., Mkrtichian, E., Benedetti, J., Corey, L., Schuffler, M. D., and Holmes, K. K., The polymicrobial origin of intestinal infection in homosexual men, *N. Engl. J. Med.*, 309, 576, 1983.

219. Nelson, M. R., Shanson, D. C., Hawkins, D., and Gazzard, B. G., *Shigella* in HIV infection, *AIDS*, 5, 1031, 1991.

220. Kariuki, S., Gilks, C., Brindle, R., Batchelor, B., Kimari, J., and Waiyaki, P., Antimicrobial susceptibility and presence of extrachromosomal deoxyribonucleic acid in *Salmonella* and *Shigella* isolates from patients with AIDS, *East Afr. Med. J.*, 71, 292, 1994.

221. Leaf, A. N., Laubenstein, L. J., Raphael, B., Hochster, H., Baez, L., and Karpatkin, S., Thrombotic thrombocytopenic purpura associated with human immunodeficiency virus type 1 (HIV-1) infection, *Ann. Intern. Med.*, 109, 194, 1988.

222. Meisenberg, B. R., Robinson, W. L., Mosley, C. A., Duke, M. S., Rabetoy, G. M., and Kosty, M. P., Thrombotic thrombocytopenic purpura in human immunodeficiency (HIV)-seropositive males, *Am. J. Hematol.*, 27, 212, 1988.

223. Shepard, K. V. and Bukowski, R. M., The treatment of thrombotic thrombocytopenic purpura with exchange transfusion, plasma infusion, and plasma exchange, *Semin. Hematol.*, 24, 178, 1987.

224. Kwann, H. C., The pathogenesis of thrombotic thrombocytopenic purpura, *Semin. Thromb. Hemost.*, 3, 184, 1979.

225. Meister, R. J., Sacher, R. A., and Phillips, T., Immune complexes in thrombotic thrombocytopenic purpura, *Ann. Intern. Med.*, 90, 717, 1979.

226. Hensby, C. N., Lewis, P. J., Hilgrad, P., Mufti, G. J., Hows, J., and Webster, J., Prostacycline deficiency in thrombotic thrombocytopenic purpura, *Lancet*, 2, 748, 1979.

227. Remuzzi, G., Rossi, E., Misiani, R., Marchesi, D., Mecca, G., de Gaetano, G., and Donati, M. B., Prostacycline and thrombotic microangiopathy, *Semin. Thromb. Hemost.*, 6, 391, 1980.

228. Beris, P., Dunand, V., Isoz, C., and Reynard, C., Association of thrombotic thrombocytopenic purpura and human immunodeficiency virus infection, *Nouv. Rev. Fr. Hematol.*, 32, 277, 1990.

229. Jokela, J., Flynn, T., and Henry, K., Thrombotic thrombocytopenic purpura in a human immunodeficiency virus (HIV)-seropositive homosexual man, *Am. J. Hematol.*, 25, 341, 1987.

230. Nair, J. M. G., Bellevue, R., and Dosik, H., Thrombotic thrombocytopenic purpura in patients with the acquired immunodeficiency syndrome (AIDS)-related complex, *Ann. Intern. Med.*, 109, 209, 1988.

231. Gasser, C., Gautier, E., Steck, A., Siebenmann, R. E., and Oechslin, R., Hämolytrisch-urämische syndrome: bilaterale nierenrindennekrosen bei akuten erworben hämolytischen anämien, *Schweiz. Med. Wochenschr.*, 85, 905, 1955.

232. Gianantonio, C., Vitacco, M., Mendilaharzu, F., Rutty, A., and Mendilaharzu, J., The hemolytic-uremic syndrome, *J. Pediatr.*, 64, 478, 1964.

233. Hammond, D. and Lieberman, E., The hemolytic uremic syndrome: renal cortical thrombotic micro-angiopathy, *Arch. Intern. Med.*, 126, 816, 1970.

234. van Wieringen, P. M. V., Monnens, L. A. H., and Bakkeren, J. A. J. M., Hemolytic-uremic syndrome: absence of circulating endotoxin, *Pediatrics*, 58, 561, 1976.

235. Kaplan, B. S. and Koornhof, H. J., Hemolytic-uraemic syndrome: failure to demonstrate circulating endotoxin, *Lancet*, 2, 1424, 1969.

236. Glasgow, L. A. and Balduzzi, P., Isolation of Coxsackie virus group A, type 4, from a patient with hemolytic-uremic syndrome, *N. Engl. J. Med.*, 273, 754, 1965.

237. Mettler, N. E., Isolation of a microtatobiote from patients with the hemolytic-uremic syndrome and thrombotic thrombocytopenic purpura and from mites in the United States, *N. Engl. J. Med.*, 281, 1023, 1969.

238. Butler, T., Islam, M. R., Azad, M. A. K., and Jones, P. K., Risk factors for development of hemolytic uremic syndrome during shigellosis, *J. Pediatr.*, 110, 894, 1987.

239. Rahaman, M. M., Jamiul Alam, A. K. M., Islam, M. R., Greenough, W. B. III, and Lindenbaum, J., Shiga bacillus dysentery associated with marked leukocytosis and erythrocyte fragmentation, *Johns Hopkins Med. J.*, 136, 65, 1975.

240. Lyman, N. W., Michaelson, R., Viscuso, R. L., Winn, R., Mulgaonkar, S., and Jacobs, M. G., Mitomycin-induced hemolytic-uremic syndrome, *Arch. Intern. Med.*, 143, 1617, 1983.

241. Brandslund, I., Peterson, P. H., Strunge, P., Hole, P., and Worth, P., Haemolytic-uraemic syndrome and accumulation of haemoglobin-haptoglobin complexes in plasma in serum sickness caused by penicillin drugs, *Haemostasis*, 9, 193, 1980.

242. Shenep, J. L. and Mogan, K. A., Kinetics of endotoxin release during antibiotic therapy for experimental gram-negative bacterial sepsis, *J. Infect. Dis.*, 150, 380, 1984.

243. Butler, T., Rahman, H., Al-Mahmud, K. A., Islam, M., Bardhan, P., Kabir, I., and Rahman, M. M., Animal model of hemolytic uremic syndrome of shigellosis: lipopolysaccharides of *Shigella disenteriae* 1 and *Shigella flexneri* produce leukocyte-mediated renal cortical necrosis in rabbits, *Br. J. Exp. Pathol.*, 66, 7, 1985.

244. Lanzkowsky, P. and McCrory, W., Disseminated intravascular coagulation as a possible factor in the pathogenesis of thrombotic microangiopathy (hemolytic-uremic syndrome), *J. Pediatr.*, 70, 460, 1967.

245. Cameron, A. S., Beers, M. Y., Walker, C. C., Rose, N., Anear, E., Manatakis, Z., Kirke, K., Calder, I., Jenkins, F., Goldwater, P. N., Paton, A., Paton, J., Jureidini, K., Hoffman, A., Henning, P., Hansman, D., Lawrence, A., Miller, R., Ratcliff, R., Doyle, R., Murray, C., Davos, D., Cameron, P., Seymour-Murray, J., Lanser, J., Selvey, L., and Beaton, S., Community outbreak of hemolytic uremic syndrome attributable to *Escherichia coli* 0111:NM — South Australia, *Morbid. Mortal. Wkly. Rep.*, 44, 550, 1995.

246. Goldwater, P. N. and Bettelheim, K. A., Hemolytic uremic syndrome due to Shiga-like toxin producing *Escherichia coli* 048:H21 in South Australia, *Emerging Infect. Dis.*, 1, 132, 1995.

247. Bin Saeed, A. A. A., El Bushra, H. E., and Al-Hamdan, N. A., Does treatment of bloody diarrhea due to *Shigella dysenteriae* type 1 with ampicillin precipitate hemolytic uremic syndrome? *Emerging Infect. Dis.*, 1, 134, 1955.

248. Al-Qarawi, S., Fontaine, R. E., and Al-Qahtani, M.-S., An outbreak of hemolytic uremic syndrome associated with antibiotic treatment of hospital inpatients for dysentery, *Emerging Infect. Dis.*, 1, 138, 1995.

249. Beers, M. and Cameron, S., Hemolytic uremic syndrome, *Emerging Infect. Dis.*, 1, 154, 1995.

250. Stoll, D. M., Cutaneous shigellosis, *Arch. Dermatol.*, 122, 22, 1986.

251. Montes, L. F., Pittillo, R. F., Hunt, D., Narkates, A. J., and Dillon, H. C., Microbial flora of infant's skin: comparison of types of microorganisms between normal skin and diaper dermatitis, *Arch. Dermatol.*, 103, 400, 1971.

252. Barrett-Connor, E. and Connor, J. D., Skin lesions and shigellosis, *Am. J. Trop. Med. Hyg.*, 18, 555, 1969.

253. Twum-Danso, K., Marwah, S., and Ahlberg, A., *Shigella* osteomyclitis in a fit young man, *Trop. Geogr. Med.*, 45, 88, 1993.

254. Rubin, H. M., Eardley, W., and Nichols, B. L., *Shigella sonnei* osteomyelitis and sickle cell anaemia, *Am. J. Dis. Child.*, 114, 83, 1968.

255. Hughes, R. A. and Keat, A. C., Reiter's syndrome and reactive arthritis: a current view, *Semin. Arthritis Rheum.*, 24, 190, 1994.

256. Paronen, I., Reiter's disease: a study of 344 cases observed in Finland, *Acta Med. Scand.*, 212(Suppl.), 1, 1948.

257. Keat, A., Thomas, B. J., and Taylor-Robinson, D., Chlamydial infection in the aetiology of arthritis, *Br. Med. Bull.*, 39, 168, 1983.

258. Urman, J. D., Zurier, R. B., and Rothfield, N. F., Reiter's syndrome associated with *Campylobacter* fetus infection, *Ann. Intern. Med.*, 86, 444, 1977.

259. Weir, W., Keat, A. C., and Welsby, P. D., Reactive arthritis associated with *Campylobacter* infection of the bowel, *J. Infect. Dis.*, 1, 281, 1979.

260. Warren, C. P. W., Arthritis associated with *Salmonella* infections, *Ann. Rheum. Dis.*, 29, 483, 1970.

261. Hannu, T. J. and Leirisalo-Repo, M., Clinical picture of reactive *Salmonella* arthritis, *J. Rheumatol.*, 15, 1668, 1988.

262. Short, C. L., Arthritis in the Mediterranean theatre of operation, *N. Engl. J. Med.*, 236, 468, 1947.

263. Noer, C. H. R., An "experimental" epidemic of Reiter's syndrome, *JAMA*, 197, 693, 1966.

264. Fowler, W. and Knight, G. H., Value of treatment in Reiter's disease, *Br. J. Vener. Dis.*, 32, 2, 1956.

265. Levy, B., Arthritis in venereal disease with particular reference to aetiology, *Med. J. Malaya*, 5, 42, 1950.

266. Rosenthal, L., Lagergren, C., and Olhagen, B., A clinical and roentgenological follow-up study of patients with uro-arthritis and pelvospondylitis, *Acta Rheum. Scand.*, 17, 3, 1971.

267. Pott, H.-G., Wittenborg, A., and Junge-Hulsing, G., Long-term antibiotic treatment in reactive arthritis, *Lancet*, 1, 245, 1988.

268. Panayi, G. S. and Clark, B., Minocycline in the treatment of patients with Reiter's syndrome, *Clin. Exp. Rheumatol.*, 7, 100, 1989.

269. Greenwald, R. A., Golub, L. M., Lavietes, B., Ramamurthy, N. S., Gruber, B., Laskin, R. S., and McNamara, T. F., Tetracyclines inhibit human synovial collagenase *in vivo* and *in vitro*, *J. Rheumatol.*, 14, 28, 1987.

270. Pruzanski, W. and Vader, P., Should tetracyclines be used in arthritis? *J. Rheumatol.*, 19, 1495, 1992.

271. Lauhio, A., Sorsa, T., Lindy, O., Suomalainen, K., Saari, H., Golub, L. M., and Konttinen, Y. T., The anticollagenolytic potential of lymecycline in the long-term treatment of reactive arthritis, *Arthritis Rheum.*, 35, 195, 1992.

272. Lauhio, A., Leirisalo-Repo, M., Lähdevirta, J., Saikku, P., and Repo, H., Double-blind placebo-controlled study of three-month treatment with lymecycline in reactive arthritis, with special reference to Chlamydia arthritis, *Arthritis Rheum.*, 34, 6, 1991.

273. Bardin, T., Enel, C., Cornelis, F., Salski, C., Jorgensen, C., Ward, R., and Lathrop, G. M., Antibiotic treatment of venereal disease and Reiter's syndrome in a Greenland population, *Arthritis Rheum.*, 35, 190, 1992.

274. Keat, A. C. and Knight, S. C., Do synovial fluid cells indicate the cause of reactive arthritis? *J. Rheumatol.*, 17, 1257, 1990.

275. Hermann, E., Mayet, W.-J., Lohse, A. W., Grevenstein, J., Mayer zum Büschenfelde, K.-H., and Fleischer, B., Proliferative response of synovial fluid and peripheral blood mononuclear cells to arthritogenic and non-arthritogenic microbial antigens and to the 65-kDa mycobacterial heat-shock protein, *Med. Microbiol. Immunol.*, 179, 215, 1990.

276. Harding, B. and Knight, S. C., The distribution of dendritic cells in the synovial fluid of patients with arthritis, *Clin. Exp. Immunol.*, 63, 594, 1986.

277. Stagg, A. J., Harding, B., Hughes, R. A., Keat, A., and Knight, S. C., The distribution and functional properties of dendritic cells in patients with seronegative arthritis, *Clin. Exp. Immunol.*, 84, 66, 1991.

278. Knight, S. C. and Stagg, A. J., Antigen-presenting cell types, *Curr. Opin. Immunol.*, 5, 374, 1993.

279. Stagg, A. J., Harding, B., Hughes, R. A., Keat, A., and Knight, S. C., Peripheral blood and synovial fluid T-cells differ in their responses to alloantigens and recall antigens presented by dendritic cells, *Clin. Exp. Immunol.*, 84, 72, 1991.

280. Rowe, I. F. and Keat, A. C. S., Human immunodeficiency virus infection and the rheumatologist, *Ann. Rheum. Dis.*, 48, 89, 1989.

281. Schaible, U. E., Kramer, M. D., Musteanu, C., and Simon, M. M., The severe combined immuno-deficiency (SCD) mouse: a laboratory model for the analysis of Lyme arthritis and carditis, *J. Exp. Med.*, 170, 1427, 1989.

282. Mahalanabis, D., Choudhuri, A. B., Bagchi, N. G., Bhattacharya, A. K., and Simpson, T. W., Oral fluid therapy of cholera among Bangladesh refugees, *Johns Hopkins Med. J.*, 132, 197, 1973.

283. Rahaman, M. M., Aziz, K. M. S., Patwari, Y., and Munshi, M. H., Diarrhoeal mortality in two Bangladesh villages with and without community-based oral rehydration therapy, *Lancet*, 2, 809, 1979.

284. National Control of Diarrheal Diseases Project, Impact of the National Control of Diarrhoeal Diseases project on infant and child mortality in Dakahlia, Egypt, *Lancet*, 2, 145, 1988.

285. Bennish, M. L., Kabir, I., Khan, A., Azad, A., and Robertson, G., Hyponatremia in shigellosis: incidence and mechanism, in *Proc. 28th Int. Conf. Antimicrob. Agents Chemother.*, American Society for Microbiology, Washington, D.C., Abstr. 38, 1988.

286. Black, R. E., Brown, K. H., and Becker, S., Effects of diarrhea associated with specific enteropathogens on the growth of children in rural Bangladesh, *Pediatrics*, 73, 799, 1984.

287. Hassan, H. S., Sensitivity of *Salmonella* and *Shigella* to antibiotics and chemotherapeutic agents in Sudan, *J. Trop. Med. Hyg.*, 88, 243, 1985.

288. Hyams, K. C., Bourgeois, A. L., Merrell, B. R., Rozmajzl, P., Escamilla, J., Thornton, S. A., Wasserman, G. M., Burke, A., Echeverria, P., Green, K. Y., Kapikian, A. Z., and Woody, J. N., Diarrheal disease during operation Desert Shield, *N. Engl. J. Med.*, 325, 1423, 1991.

9.2 SALMONELLA SPP.

9.2.1 INTRODUCTION

Salmonella is a genus of Gram-negative, facultatively anaerobic bacteria of the family Enterobacteriaceae. Morphologically, they are nonspore-forming rods, usually motile with peritrichous flagella. These bacteria utilize citrate as the sole source of carbon, and generally ferment glucose but not sucrose or lactose.

Salmonella is divided into species or serotypes on the basis of O (somatic), Vi (capsular), and H (flagellar) antigens. The somatic antigen is the basis for further separation into serogroups not contained in another group. Usually agglutination tests with pooled (polyvalent) antisera for groups A through E and Vi antigen can detect 95% of the serotypes recovered from humans and animals.

There are several species of *Salmonella* pathogenic to humans causing enteric fevers (typhoid and paratyphoid), septicemias, and gastroenteritis. The most frequent clinical manifestation has been food poisoning. According to recent data,[1] more than 60% of animal-protein processing plants and 37% of vegetable-processing plants tested positive for *Salmonella*.

In the most straightforward classification, *Salmonella* has been divided into typhoidal and nontyphoidal species. Some of the most common *Salmonella* species include:

1. *S. arizonae,* which has been found originally in reptiles[21] and turtles but also in fowls and other domestic animals, dried egg powder, dairy products, and meat; it causes gastroenteritis, enteric fever, bacteremia, and local infections
2. *S. choleraesius,* a group C species pathogenic to both humans and animals, that has been associated with paratyphoid fever, gastroenteritis, and septicemia in humans
3. *S. enteritidis* (also known as *Gärtner bacillus*), a species containing groups A-D serotypes and consisting of more than 1500 different serotypes, each of which is known by an individual name; in humans, it may produce parathyphoid fever, septicemia, and gastro-enteritis
4. *S. heidelberg* (also *S. enteritidis* serotype *heidelberg*)

5. *S. typhi* (also known as *typhoid bacillus*), a group D serotype that has been associated with typhoid fever in humans, and is transmitted by water or food contaminated by human excreta; *S. typhi* is further subdivided into V strains containing the Vi (virulence) antigen, V-W strains that have partially lost their Vi antigen, and W strains which do not contain the Vi antigen
6. *S. typhimurium* (also *S. enteritidis* serotype *typhimurium*)

Immunity to salmonella infections is usually short-lived, and susceptibility to identical serotypes has been documented.[2] Several vaccines against *S. typhi* have already been developed.[55-57]

Enhanced severity of salmonella disease has been observed in patients with different hemolytic anemias (especially those with sickle cell anemia in the U.S.), collagen vascular disease, immuno-suppression, malaria, and HIV infection.[9,17-21] The rapid increase in the number of immuno-compromised patients mainly due to the rise of the older population, HIV infection, and immuno-suppressed cancer patients, has contributed to the worldwide increase in the incidence of salmonellosis.[9]

Bacteremia and dissemination occurs only rarely in adolescent children and adults, but has been diagnosed in 5 to 40% of infants with gastroenteritis. Localized infections, which occur in up to 10% of patients with bacteremia, affect most often the meninges, skeletal system, heart, and the kidneys. Enteric fever is caused mainly by *S. typhi*, but has also been associated with several other salmonella species.[2]

9.2.2 EVOLUTION OF THERAPIES AND TREATMENT OF *SALMONELLA* INFECTIONS

Severe salmonella infections are diagnosed most frequently in patients with defective cell-mediated immunity or HIV infection.[9,18,24,30] Currently, a recurrent salmonella bacteremia in HIV-infected individuals[30,32] is considered to be diagnostic for AIDS.[31] Extraintestinal infections caused by non-typhoid salmonella usually have afflicted debilitated and immunocompromised patients.[68]

While *Salmonella* infections in immunocompromised hosts have been very frequent, the choice of therapy has been relatively very limited because of the intrinsic antibiotic resistance of these bacteria.[7,8,14] In addition, immunocompromised patients are often afflicted by renal and hematologic disorders which will further limit the choice of appropriate therapy.

Ciprofloxacin, a 4-quinolone carboxylic antibiotic, known for its broad antibacterial activity,[3,4] has been used successfully in the treatment of salmonellosis. Oral administration of ciprofloxacin resulted in blood and tissue concentrations markedly higher than MICs and as late as 8 h after a single oral dose.[5] This favorable pharmacokinetic profile, coupled with the capability to penetrate into phagocytic cells (granulocytes and macrophages),[10,11] has made ciprofloxacin potentially useful in the treatment of infections by intracellular pathogens, such as *Salmonella* in immunocompromised patients.[12,13]

Following is a description of various therapeutic modalities applied to infections caused by different *Salmonella* species.

9.2.2.1 *Salmonella typhimurium*

Esposito et al.[6] have used ciprofloxacin to treat *S. typhimurium* infection in an immunocompromised patient. Oral administration of 500 mg of the drug every 8 h eliminated the pathogen from feces cultures 2 d after initiation of therapy.

Patton et al.[15] have described a dramatic recovery after ciprofloxacin treatment of a multiple β-lactam antibiotic (ceftazidime, imipenem, mecillinam)-resistant *S. typhimurium* septicemia in an immunocompromised patient with acute lymphoblastic leukemia. The therapy consisted of an initial 17-d course of intravenous ciprofloxacin (a 400-mg loading dose followed by 200 mg given every 12 h), followed by oral administration at 250 mg every 8 h for 46 d.

Bogers et al.[16] have applied combined antibiotic and surgical therapy to treat a mediastinal rupture of a thoraco-abdominal mycotic aneurysm caused by *S. typhimurium* in a patient receiving immunosuppressive therapy following kidney transplantation. After the initial antibiotic treatment consisting of co-trimoxazole (1920 mg daily, then changed to amoxycillin at 6.0 g daily because of temporary deterioration in the kidney function) and surgical intervention (local debridement and implantation of an aortic prosthesis), a lifelong antibiotic treatment was required because of continuing immunosuppressive therapy and history of recurrent *S. typhimurium* bacteremia and periprosthetic problems.[16]

9.2.2.2 *Salmonella arizonae*

S. arizonae (previously referred to as *Arizona hinshawii*) is an uncommon human pathogen which was first identified in reptiles,[21] and then reported to be the causative agent in a case of human gastroenteritis in 1944.[20] There are more than 400 serotypes of *S. arizonae*. Very often, the disease is contracted through the ingestion of rattlesnake meat (which is known to be a common Hispanic folk remedy[35]) by individuals suffering from chronic medical conditions, including HIV infection.[25-29,36-42]

S. arizonae is considered to be an opportunistic pathogen in immunocompromised patients.[38] Clinical manifestations have been similar to those of other salmonella infections, namely septicemia, enteric fever, gastroenteritis, anorexia, and localized infections, such as cholecystitis, meningitis, arthritis, urinary tract infections, osteomyelitis, or combinations of these.[22,45,46] The pathogen tends to cause systemic infections in patients with underlying diseases,[3,23,24,28,29] such as neoplasms, systemic lupus erythematosus, cardiac disease, AIDS, diabetes, connective tissue diseases, and sickle cell anemia in patients treated with immunosuppressive therapy.[9,18,20,23,24,28,44]

In early reports,[20,23,30] treatment of *S. arizonae*-induced disease has been guided by the susceptibility of the organism, and most commonly involved the use of ampicillin or trimethoprim-sulfamethoxazole (TMP-SMX). However, HIV-infected patients may often develop adverse side effects to TMP-SMX.[33] Other antibiotics, such as chloramphenicol, cefamandole, kanamycin, and rifampin, have also been used on different occasions and with variable success.[30]

Ciprofloxacin, ampicillin, cephalotin, and amikacin were reported to be effective.[44] Thus, Noskin and Clarke[22] successfully treated *S. arizonae* bacteremia in an HIV-positive patient with ampicillin (2.0 g every 4 h). Upon discharge, to prevent recurrence, the patient received suppressive therapy with oral ampicillin (500 mg, b.i.d.) and later ciprofloxacin (500 mg, b.i.d.).

A case of systemic invasion of *S. arizonae* causing endogenous endophthalmitis in an immunocompromised patient without clinically apparent gastrointestinal symptoms was described by Caravalho et al.[34] The initial treatment with intravenous gentamicin was later switched to a 3-week regimen of topical tobramycin and a double-dose of oral TMP-SMX following the parenteral therapy.

Cortes et al.[43] reported a case of a patient with metastatic carcinoma (and a remote history of rattlesnake meat ingestion) who developed recurrent *S. arizonae* bacteremia and reactivation of tuberculosis after receiving corticosteroid and radiation therapies. The patient received a combination of TMP-SMX and ciprofloxacin.

9.2.2.3 *Salmonella dublin*

S. enteritidis serotype *dublin* is a group D salmonella species with distinct biochemical features that do not include fermentation of arabinose or utilization of citrate or acetate.[50] This pattern is unique among group D *Salmonella* and can be used to identify *S. dublin*. The pathogen is host-specific for cattle but it can also infect humans,[47,48] mostly after consumption of contaminated raw milk.[49,51,52]

S. dublin could present a high risk for immunocompromised hosts and usually causes severe illness with fever, diarrhea, and bacteremia; abdominal pain, nausea, and genitourinary symptoms have also been reported.[51-53] During 1971–1975, there was a fivefold increase in the annual incidence of *S. dublin* infections in humans just in California alone.[51] These organisms affected more often older people (50 years and older) and females than males.[51,52] About 50% of the affected patients had chronic underlying diseases, such as malignancies (metastatic abscesses), diabetes, peptic ulcers, and collagen vascular disease.[51-53] Approximately 65% to 80% of the patients with *S. dublin* infection will require hospitalization, and the mortality rate of the disease has reached about 20%.[47]

To further complicate treatment, drug resistance by *S. dublin* has been well documented. Thus, in one study conducted between 1978 and 1982, 15 out of 34 *S. dublin* isolates have been resistant to ampicillin, carbenicillin, and tetracycline, but 5 isolates were resistant only to ampicillin and carbenicillin, and one isolate was resistant to ampicillin, carbenicillin, chloramphenicol, sulfamethoxazole, and tetracycline.[50] Reports from Europe have also demonstrated increasing incidence of resistance to antibiotics, in particular, chloramphenicol.[54] Unlike other nontyphoid salmonella whose antibiotic resistance in animals seemed to be unrelated to resistance in humans, the antibiotic resistance of *S. dublin* isolates in humans paralleled the resistance pattern of isolates recovered from animals.[50]

The high frequency of *S. dublin* resistance and the potential for serious head and neck infection in immunocompromised patients make early diagnosis and treatment of this pathogen highly important. Bello and Pien[47] described a *S. dublin*-associated neck abscess in a diabetic patient who was treated with intravenous ampicillin (2.0 g every 4 h). Surgical debridement and further therapy with oral amoxicillin (1.0 g, t.i.d.) completely resolved the neck mass over a 2-week period.

9.2.2.4   *Salmonella choleraesius*

S. choleraesius is a highly invasive serotype that usually causes a septicemia syndrome and is most often recovered from blood but not stools.[58] It is considered to be one of the most virulent *Salmonella* spp. responsible for the highest incidence of fatal infections in humans.[59-61] Rhame et al.[65] reported a fatal outcome from *S. choleraesuis*-associated septicemia in immunocompromised patients that occurred in a single medical facility outbreak over a 6-month period.

Rarely a cause of meningitis in adults,[60] *Salmonella*-associated meningitis is predominantly a disease in infants. Even though the overall incidence of *Salmonella* meningitis is low, the mortality rate has been exceedingly high, mostly because of difficulties in sterilizing the cerebrospinal fluid, disease-related complications (cerebral abscesses, subdural empyema, and ventriculitis), hydrocephalus, and frequent relapses.[46,62]

Treatment of *Salmonella* meningitis has not been well defined, but ampicillin and chloramphenicol seem to be the most effective drugs. Recently, Kanchanapongkul[58] has reported a case of *S. choleraesius* meningitis in a patient with systemic lupus erythematosus — the treatment was successful and included a 2-week course of intravenous ceftriaxone (2.0 g daily), followed after hospital discharge by oral ciprofloxacin (400 mg, b.i.d.).

9.2.2.5   *Salmonella heidelberg*

By some accounts, *S. heidelberg* is the third most common serotype implicated in salmonellosis. It is the causative agent of 7% of all salmonella infections,[63] and nearly 9% of bacteremic salmonellosis.[64] Heal et al.[66] described a case of a thrombocytopenic and leukopenic patient with multiple myeloma who died from complications of *S. heidelberg* septicemia as the result of transfusion of contaminated platelets; treatment with ampicillin was unsuccessful.

9.2.2.6 *Salmonella enteritidis*

Navarro et al.[67] reported a fatal case of septic thrombophlebitis due to *S. enteritidis* in a patient with gastric adenocarcinoma with metastasis who developed a septic focus in a saphanous vein. Metastatic septic foci may appear anywhere in the organism, including the vascular system.

In an unusual case, a patient with leukemia who initially developed staphylococcal parotitis during his hospitalization, subsequently developed parotitis due to *S. enteritidis*.[69]

9.2.3 REFERENCES

1. Editorial. Food notes on immunosuppression; Salmonella, *J. Am. Vet. Med. Assoc.*, 206, 935, 1995.
2. Stutman, H. R., Salmonella, shigella, and campylobacter: common bacterial causes of infectious diarrhea, *Pediatr. Ann.*, 23, 538, 1994.
3. Wise, R., Haas, R., and Edwards, L. J., *In vitro* activity of Bay O 9867, a new quinolone derivative, compared with those of other antimicrobial agents, *Antimicrob. Agents Chemother.*, 23, 559, 1983.
4. Shrine, L., Saunders, J., Trynor, R., and Koornhof, H. J., A laboratory assessment of ciprofloxacin and comparable antimicrobial agents, *Eur. J. Clin. Microbiol.*, 3, 328, 1984.
5. Crump, B., Wise, R., and Dent, J., Pharmacokinetics and tissue penetration of ciprofloxacin, *Antimicrob. Agents Chemother.*, 3, 355, 1983.
6. Esposito, S., Gaeta, G. B., Galante, D., and Barba, D., Successful treatment with ciprofloxacin of *Salmonella typhimurium* infection in an immunocompromised host, *Infection*, 13, 288, 1985.
7. Bryan, J. P., Rocka, H., and Scheld, W. M., Problems in salmonellosis: rationale for clinical trials with newer β-lactam agents and quinolones, *Rev. Infect. Dis.*, 8, 189, 1986.
8. Buchwald, D. S. and Blaser, M. S., A review of human salmonellosis. II. Duration of excretion following infection with nontyphi salmonella, *Rev. Infect. Dis.*, 6, 345, 1984.
9. Wolfe, M. S., Armstrong, D., Louria, D. B., and Blevins, A., Salmonellosis in patients with neoplastic disease: a review of 100 episodes at Memorial Cancer Center over a 13-year period, *Arch. Intern. Med.*, 128, 546, 1971.
10. Easmon, C. S. F. and Crane, J. P., Uptake of ciprofloxacin by human neutrophils, *J. Antimicrob. Chemother.*, 16, 67, 1985.
11. Easmon, C. S. F. and Crane, J. P., Uptake of ciprofloxacin by macrophages, *J. Clin. Pathol.*, 38, 442, 1985.
12. Easmon, C. S. F. and Blowers, A., Ciprofloxacin treatment of systemic salmonella infection in sensitive and resistant mice, *J. Antimicrob. Chemother.*, 16, 615, 1985.
13. Brunner, H. and Zeiler, H.-J., Oral ciprofloxacin treatment for *Salmonella typhimurium* infection of normal and immunocompromised mice, *Antimicrob. Agents Chemother.*, 32, 57, 1988.
14. Smith, S. M., Palumbo, P. E., and Edelson, P. T., Salmonella strains resistant to multiple antibiotics, *Pediatr. Infect. Dis. J.*, 3, 455, 1984.
15. Patton, W. N., Smith, G. M., Leyland, M. J., and Geddes, A. M., Multiply resistant *Salmonella typhimurium* septicaemia in an immunocompromised patient successfully treated with ciprofloxacin, *J. Antimicrob. Chemother.*, 16, 667, 1985.
16. Bogers, A. J. J., van't Wout, J. W., Manger Cats, V., Quaegebeur, J. M., and Huysmans, H. A., Mediastinal rupture of a thoracoabdominal mycotic aneurysm caused by *Salmonella typhimurium* on an immunocompromised patient, *Eur. J. Cardio-thorac. Surg.*, 1, 116, 1987.
17. Nadelman, R. B., Mathier-Wagh, U., Yancovitz, S. R., and Mildvan, D., Salmonella bacteremia associated with the acquired immunodeficiency syndrome (AIDS), *Arch. Intern. Med.*, 145, 1968, 1985.
18. Black, P. H., Kunz, L. J., and Swartz, M. N., Salmonellosis: a review of some unusual aspects, *N. Engl. J. Med.*, 262, 811, 1960.
19. Fischl, M. A., Dickinson, G. M., Sinave, C., Pitchenik, A. E., and Clearly, T. J., Salmonella bacteremia as manifestation of acquired immunodeficiency syndrome, *Arch. Intern. Med.*, 146, 113, 1986.
20. Guckian, J. C., Byers, E. H., and Perry, J. E., *Arizona* infection in man, *Arch. Intern. Med.*, 119, 170, 1967.

21. Caldwell, M. E. and Ryerson, D. L., Salmonellosis in certain reptiles, *J. Infect. Dis.*, 65, 242, 1939.

22. Noskin, G. A. and Clarke, J. T., *Salmonella arizonae* bacteremia as the presenting manifestation of human immunodeficiency virus infection following rattlesnake meat ingestion, *Rev. Infect. Dis.*, 12, 514, 1990.

23. Petru, M. A. and Richman, D. D., *Arizona hinshawii* infection of an atherosclerotic abdominal aorta, *Arch. Intern. Med.*, 141, 537, 1981.

24. Jacobson, M. A., Hahn, S. M., Gerberding, J. L., Lee, B., and Sande, M. A., Ciprofloxacin for salmonella bacteremia in the acquired immunodeficiency syndrome (AIDS), *Ann. Intern. Med.*, 110, 1027, 1989.

25. Marzouk, J. B., Joseph, P., Lee, T. Y., Livermore, T., and Benjamin, R., *Arizona hinshawii* septicemia associated with rattlesnake powder — California, *Morbid. Mortal. Wkly. Rep.*, 32, 464, 1983.

26. Fainstein, V., Yancey, R., Trier, R., and Bodey, G. P., Overwhelming infection in a cancer patient caused by *Arizona hinshawii*: its relation to snake pill ingestion, *Am. J. Infect. Control*, 4, 147, 1982.

27. McIntyre, K. E., Malone, J. M., Richards, E., and Axline, S. G., Mycotic aortic pseudoaneurysm with aortoenteric fistula caused by *Arizona hinshawii*, *Surgery*, 91, 173, 1982.

28. Riley, K. B., Antoniskis, D., Maris, R., and Leedom, J. M., Rattlesnake capsule-associated *Salmonella arizonae* infections, *Arch. Intern. Med.*, 148, 1207, 1988.

29. Johnson, R. H., Lutwick, L. I., Huntley, G. A., and Vosti, K. L., *Arizona hinshawii* infections, *Ann. Intern. Med.*, 85, 587, 1976.

30. Sperber, S. J. and Schleupner, C. J., Salmonellosis during infection with human immunodeficiency virus, *J. Infect. Dis.*, 9, 925, 1987.

31. Centers for Disease Control, Revision of the CDC surveillance case definition for acquired immunodeficiency syndrome, *Morbid. Mortal. Wkly. Rep.*, 36(Suppl.), 3S, 1987.

32. Glaser, J. B., Morton-Kute, L., Berger, S. R., Weber, J., Siegal, F. P., Lopez, C., Robbins, W., and Landesman, S. H., Recurrent *Salmonella typhimurium* bacteremia associated with the acquired immunodeficiency syndrome, *Ann. Intern. Med.*, 102, 189, 1985.

33. Gordin, F. M., Simon, G. L., Wofsy, C. B., and Mills, J., Adverse reactions to trimethoprim-sulfamethoxazole in patients with the acquired immunodeficiency syndrome, *Ann. Intern. Med.*, 100, 495, 1984.

34. Caravalho, J., Jr., McMillan, V. M., Ellis, R. B., and Betancourt, A., Endogenous endophthalmitis due to *Salmonella arizonae* and *Hafnia alvei*, *South. Med. J.*, 83, 325, 1990.

35. Bhatt, B. D., Zuckerman, M. J., Foland, J. A., Guerra, L. G., and Polly, S. M., Rattlesnake meat ingestion — a common Hispanic folk remedy, *West. J. Med.*, 149, 605, 1988.

36. Fleishman, S., Haake, D. A., and Lovett, M. A., *Salmonella arizona* infections associated with ingestion of rattlesnake capsules, *Arch. Intern. Med.*, 149, 701, 1989.

37. Bhatt, B. D., Zuckerman, M. J., Foland, J. A., Polly, S. M., and Marwah, R. K., Disseminated *Salmonella arizona* infection associated with rattlesnake meat production, *Am. J. Gastroenterol.*, 84, 433, 1989.

38. Babu, K., Sonnenberg, M., Kathpalia, S., Ortega, P., Swiatlo, A. L., and Kocka, F. E., Isolation of salmonellae from dried rattlesnake preparations, *J. Clin. Microbiol.*, 28, 361, 1990.

39. Casner, P. R. and Zuckerman, M. J., *Salmonella arizonae* in patients with AIDS along the U.S.-Mexican border, *N. Engl. J. Med.*, 323, 198, 1990.

40. Cone, L. A., Boughton, W. H., Cone, L. A., and Lehv, L. H., Rattlesnake capsule-induced *Salmonella arizonae* bacteremia, *West. Med. J.*, 153, 315, 1990.

41. Waterman, S. H., Juarez, G., Carr, S. J., and Kilman, L., *Salmonella arizona* infections in Latinos associated with rattlesnake folk medicine, *Am. J. Public Health*, 80, 286, 1990.

42. Woolf, G. M. and Runyon, B. A., Spontaneous *Salmonella* infection of high-protein noncirrhotic ascites, *J. Clin. Gastroenterol.*, 12, 430, 1990.

43. Cortes, E., Zuckerman, M. J., and Ho, H., Recurrent *Salmonella arizona* infection after treatment for metastatic carcinoma, *J. Clin. Gastroenterol.*, 14, 157, 1992.

44. Kraus, A., Guerra-Bautista, G., and Alarcon-Segovia, D., *Salmonella arizona* arthritis and septicemia associated with rattlesnake ingestion by patients with connective tissue diseases: a dangerous complication of folk medicine, *J. Rheumatol.*, 18, 1328, 1991.

45. Medina, F., Fraga, A., and Lavalle, C., *Salmonella* septic arthritis in systemic lupus erythematosus: the importance of chronic carrier state, *J. Rheumatol.*, 16, 203, 1989.

46. Cohen, J. I., Bartlett, J. A., and Corey, R. G., Extra-intestinal manifestations of *Salmonella* infections, *Medicine (Baltimore)*, 66, 349, 1987.

47. Bello, E. F. and Pien, F. D., *Salmonella dublin* neck abscess, *Arch. Otolaryngol.*, 111, 476, 1985.

48. Guilloteau, L. A., Lax, A. J., MacIntyre, S., and Wallis, T. S., The *Salmonella dublin* virulence plasmid does not modulate early T-cell responses in mice, *Infect. Immun.*, 64, 222, 1996.

49. Richwald, G. A., Greenland, S., Johnson, B. J., Goldstein, E. J. C., and Plichta, D. T., Assessment of the excess risk of *Salmonella dublin* infection associated with the use of certified raw milk, *Public Health Rep.*, 103, 489, 1988.

50. Fierer, J. and Fleming, W., Distinctive biochemical features of *Salmonella dublin* isolated in California, *J. Clin. Microbiol.*, 17, 552, 1983.

51. Taylor, D. N., Bied, J. M., Munro, J. S., and Feldman, R. A., *Salmonella dublin* infections in the United States, 1979–1980, *J. Infect. Dis.*, 146, 322, 1982.

52. Werner, S. B., Humphrey, G. L., and Kamei, I., Association between raw milk and human *Salmonella dublin* infection, *Br. Med. J.*, 2, 238, 1979.

53. Fierer, J., Invasive *Salmonella dublin* infections associated with drinking raw milk, *West. J. Med.*, 138, 665, 1983.

54. Cherubin, C. E., Antibiotic resistance of *Salmonella* in Europe and the United States, *Rev. Infect. Dis.*, 3, 1105, 1981.

55. Levine, M. M., Taylor, D. N., and Ferreccio, C., Typhoid vaccines come of age, *Pediatr. Infect. Dis. J.*, 8, 374, 1989.

56. Typhoid immunization. Recommendations of the Advisory Committee of Immunization Practices, Centers for Disease Control, *Morbid. Mortal. Wkly. Rep.*, 43, 1, 1994.

57. Editorial, A single shot at *Salmonella typhi*: a new typhoid vaccine with pediatric advantages, *Pediatrics*, 96, 348, 1995.

58. Kanchanapongkul, J., *Salmonella*: a rare cause of meningitis in an adult, *Southeast Asian J. Trop. Med. Public Health*, 26, 195, 1995.

59. Saphra, I. and Wassermann, M., *Salmonella choleraesuis*: a clinical and epidemiological evaluation of 329 infections identified between 1940 and 1954 in the New York Salmonella Center, *Am. J. Med. Sci.*, 228, 525, 1954.

60. Allison, M. J., Dalton, H. P., Escobar, M. R., and Martin, C. J., *Salmonella choleraesuis* infections in man: a report of 19 cases and a critical literature review, *South. Med. J.*, 62, 593, 1969.

61. Hook, E. W., *Salmonella* species (including typhoid fever), in *Principles and Practice of Infectious Diseases*, 3rd ed., Mandell, G. L., Douglas, R. G., Jr., and Bennett, J. E., Eds., Churchill Livingstone, New York, 1990, 1700.

62. Bryan, J. P., Rocha, H., and Scheld, W. M., Problems in salmonellosis: rationale for clinical trials with newer beta-lactam agents and quinolones, *Rev. Infect. Dis.*, 8, 189, 1986.

63. Centers for Disease Control, Human *Salmonella* isolates: United States, 1982, *Morbid. Mortal. Wkly. Rep.*, 32, 598, 1983.

64. Blaser, M. J. and Feldman, R. A., *Salmonella* bacteremia: reports to the Centers for Disease Control, 1968–1979, *J. Infect. Dis.*, 143, 743, 1981.

65. Rhame, F. S., Root, R. K., MacLowry, J. D., Davidsman, T. A., and Bennett, J. V., *Salmonella* septicemia from platelet transfusion: study of an outbreak to a hematogenous carrier of *Salmonella choleraesuis*, *Ann. Intern. Med.*, 78, 633, 1973.

66. Heal, J. M., Jones, M. E., Forey, J., Chaudhry, A., and Stricof, R. L., Fatal *Salmonella* septicemia after platelet transfusion, *Transfusion*, 27, 2, 1987.

67. Navarro, M., Almirante, B., Bellmunt, J., and Jolis, L., Fatal septic thrombophlebitis due to *Salmonella enteritidis*, *Eur. J. Microbiol. Infect. Dis.*, 8, 82, 1989.

68. Ramos, J. M., Garcia-Corbeira, P., Aguado, J. M., Arjona, R., Alés, J. M., and Soriano, F., Clinical significance of primary vs. secondary bacteremia due to nontyphoid *Salmonella* in patients without AIDS, *Clin. Infect. Dis.*, 19, 777, 1994.

69. Georgilis, K., Hadjiloukas, L., Petrocheilou, V., and Mavrikakis, M., Parotitis due to *Salmonella enteritidis*, *Clin. Infect. Dis.*, 19, 798, 1994.

9.3   *YERSINIA ENTEROCOLITICA*

9.3.1 Introduction

Yersinia enterocolitica is a facultatively anaerobic, Gram-negative coccoid bacteria which is motile at 25°C and nonmotile at 37°C, and like other Enterobacteriaceae species, it ferments glucose and is oxidase-negative.[1]

Y. enterocolitica is one of the rapidly emerging human enteric pathogens associated with a wide spectrum of clinical and immunological manifestations.[2] It has been isolated worldwide from both clinical and nonclinical specimens,[3-6] but seems to be more commonly distributed in cooler climatic regions.[4,7]

Different *Yersinia* serotypes vary in their virulence.[3,4,8-11] Serotypes O:3, O:8, and O:9 are considered to be the most virulent ones, causing outbreaks of disease worldwide. For reasons still not well understood, it seems that serotypes O:3 and O:9 have predominated in Europe, whereas serotype O:8 has been the causative agent of most infections in the U.S.[4,12-16]

Laird and Cavanaugh[17] have observed an important correlation between autoagglutination and the virulence of *Yersinia* — that is, virulent strains, when fed to adult mice, autoagglutinated when grown at 36°C in tissue culture media, whereas strains that did not autoagglutinate were found to be avirulent.

Although enterotoxin is produced by most clinical isolates of *Yersinia*,[18] its involvement in the pathogenesis of disease is unlikely. However, the expression of plasmid-encoded proteins of the outer membranes of *Yersinia* has served as an important determinant of pathogenicity.[19-21]

For the majority of bacteria, iron is an essential growth factor which is obtained by most microorganisms through the release of high-affinity, low-molecular-weight iron chelators, known as siderophors. After binding ferric iron (Fe^{3+}), the siderophores re-enter the bacteria.[22] However, *Y. enterocolitica* is one bacteria that cannot synthesize siderophores,[23,24] but instead is endowed with siderophore receptors and can use as growth factors either siderophores delivered by other bacteria[23] (such as deferoxamine B, which is released by *Streptomyces pilosus*[23,25]), exogenous siderophores, or hemin.[23] This enables *Y. enterocolitica* to grow in the intestine where siderophores of bacterial origin are abundant. However, in tissues and organic fluids, the bacterium must compete with iron-binding proteins (transferin, lactoferrin), and multiplication would only be possible when there is an iron overload and supply is adequate, or when there are exogenous siderophores present.[25-27] Since both iron overloading and increased levels of deferoxamine were found to substantially increase the virulence of *Yersinia* (likely by attenuating the bactericidal activity of the serum[24,25,28]), the two conditions are considered to be independent predisposing factors for systemic infection with *Y. enterocolitica*.[2] Furthermore, excess iron has also been found to inhibit the chemotactic[29] and bactericidal[30] properties of the leukocytes. Some investigators,[25,27] however, have suggested that the apparent susceptibility to *Yersinia* infections of patients with severe iron overload should be attributed to excessive deferoxamine therapy, rather than the iron overload itself.

Transmission of *Y. enterocolitica* to human occurs primarily by ingestion of contaminated food (especially pork meat[31]), water, and milk.[32] Transmission from dogs, cats, and swine has also been reported.[33-38] In several cases, nosocomially acquired infection has also been documented,[39-41] as well as infection by transfusion of contaminated blood products.[42-45]

Together with several well-recognized syndromes (enterocolitis and pseudoappendicular syndrome), a wide array of uncommon clinical manifestations have been associated with *Yersinia* infections depending on the age, and the physical and immune status of the hosts.[2] Postinfection manifestations include arthritis, erythema nodosum, focal extraintestinal infections, and bacteremia. Overall, *Yersinia* infections most commonly occur in younger age groups.[32,46]

Yersinia enterocolitica-induced enterocolitis, which has an incubation period between 1 and 11 d,[9,24,31,33,39,47] is usually manifested by diarrhea, a low-grade fever, and abdominal pain.[5,6,33,46,48,49]

In most cases, the infection has been self-limited, but complications have also occurred including appendicitis,[5,50,51] diffuse ulceration and inflammation of the small intestine and colon,[33] intestinal perforation,[52] peritonitis,[53-57] ileocolic intussusception,[58] toxic megacolon,[59] cholangitis,[60] and mesenteric-vein thrombosis with gangrene of the small bowel.[61]

The pseudoappendicular syndrome caused by *Y. enterocolitica* is commonly characterized with fever, abdominal pain, tenderness of the right lower quadrant, and leukocytosis,[62,63] as well as nausea, vomiting, and diarrhea in some patients.[31,51,62,64]

Bacteremia caused by the pathogen is frequently observed in patients with predisposing underlying disease, such as immunosuppressive therapy, cirrhosis, hemochromatosis, acute iron poisoning, transfusion-dependent blood dyscrasias, deferoxamine therapy, diabetes mellitus, and malnutrition,[13,14,26,65-69] or the patients have been in an iron-overloaded state.[2] While the frequency of cirrhosis[70] strongly indicated that the liver played a critical role in the host defense against *Yersinia*, most of the predisposing underlying diseases (idiopathic hematochromatosis,[13,14] "Bantu siderosis",[13] thalassemia major,[13,25,27] chronic hemodialysis,[25] and iron poisoning[13,26]) have been associated with iron overload.

A wide array of complications may occur following bacteremic invasion of *Y. enterocolitica* into extraintestinal sites: hepatic and splenic abscesses,[13,14,71,72] rupture of vascular prosthesis,[72] endocarditis,[65,73,74] mycotic aneurysm,[75] infection of intravenous catheters,[76] meningitis,[32,77,78] peritonitis,[77] osteomyelitis,[79] septic arthritis,[80] pulmonary infiltrates,[80-82] lung abscess,[75] empyema,[83] renal abscess,[84] panophthalmitis,[78] cutaneous pustules,[78] bullous skin lesions,[85] reactive arthropathy and erythema nodosum,[86-92] Reiter's syndrome,[86,87] myocarditis,[87,89,93] and glomerulonephritis,[89,94,95] have all been observed as a result of bacteremia.[2]

9.3.2   HOST IMMUNE DEFENSE AGAINST *YERSINIA ENTEROCOLITICA*

In recent studies, Autenrieth et al.[96-98] have provided direct evidence that during cellular immune response against parenteral *Y. enterocolitica* infection in C57BL/6 mice, the T lymphocytes have been involved in the host reaction against the pathogen, and that a specific T cell-dependent immune response is required for an efficient defense mechanism against the extracellular *Y. enterocilitica*. This finding has been somewhat surprising for a microorganism which is presumed to multiply extracellularly in infected tissues,[99-102] and thereby should be eliminated primarily by nonspecific cellular (phagocytes), and/or nonspecific or specific humoral (complement, antibodies) immune responses.[103]

In further studies, Autenrieth et al.[98] have also found that *in vivo* neutralization of interferon-γ or tumor necrosis factor-α by specific antibodies prior to, or during, the infection of mice, had abrogated resistance to *Y. enterocolitica*, suggesting that macrophages, possibly activated by T lymphocytes, were still an important component of the host immune response in primary *Yersinia* infection.[104]

9.3.3   EVOLUTION OF THERAPIES AND TREATMENT OF *Y. ENTEROCOLITICA* INFECTIONS

In several reports,[105-109] *Y. enterocolitica* was found susceptible *in vitro* to trimethoprim-sulfamethoxazole (TMP-SMX), quinolones, tetracyclines, aminoglycosides, chloramphenicol, colistin, polymyxin, kanamycin, and the third generation of cephalosporins (cefamandole, cefoxitin). The bacterium was usually resistant to first-generation cephalosporins, erythromycin, and penicillins.[105-107] In general, patients with *Y. enterocolitica*-induced uncomplicated enterocolitis, as well as pseudoappendicular syndrome did not respond effectively to antimicrobial therapy.[35,49,105,110,111]

In an experimental mouse model of systemic *Y. enterocolitica* infection, doxycycline and gentamicin were effective in inhibiting the proliferation of serotype O:8, while cefotaxime and imipenem have been ineffective.[112]

TMP-SMX has failed to shorten the clinical or bacteriologic course of the infection, in a placebo-controlled, double-blind clinical trial of children with *Y. enterocolitica*-induced enterocolitis.[113]

Capron et al.[54] have described a case of spontaneous *Y. enterocolitica*-induced peritonitis leading to idiopathic hemochromatosis. The patient was successfully treated with oral doxycycline at 400 mg daily for 2 months. While abdominal symptoms and ascites progressively disappeared, 6 months later agglutinins against the pathogen (serotype 9) were positive at 1:640 dilution; treatment of idiopathic hemochromatosis with intermittent phlebotomy was started.

In another case of spontaneous peritonitis due to *Y. enterocolitica* that has developed in a patient with secondary alcoholic hemochromatosis, the therapy consisted of intravenous administration of cefoxitin (2.0 g/8 h) and gentamicin (80 mg/8 h), transfusion of packed red cells, oral lactulose, paromomycin, and cimetidine; after 1 week of treatment, the cell count of ascitic fluid was 80 cells/mm^3 (88% mononuclears), the pH was 7.41, and cultures showed no growth of the pathogen.[114]

Boemi et al.[38] have described three cases of *Y. enterocolitica* (biotype 4, serogroup O:3, phage type VIII) peritonitis in children affected by thalassemia major. In all cases, the infection was resolved by treatment with either cefoxitin and gentamicin (20-d regimen), netilmicin (15-d regimen), or tobramycin (9-d regimen).

As a general recommendation, patients with systemic and focal extraintestinal infections, as well as enterocolitis in immunocompromised hosts should be treated with antimicrobial agents.[2] In this regard, Cover and Aber[2] have suggested withholding deferoxamine and treatment with doxycycline or TMP-SMX for complicated *Yersinia* gastrointestinal and focal extraintestinal infections. A combination of doxycycline and an aminoglycoside was considered more appropriate for the treatment of *Y. enterocolitica*-induced bacteremia until antimicrobial susceptibility tests have been performed.[2]

9.3.3.1   *Y. enterocolitica* Infections in AIDS Patients

Nearly all of the patients with *Y. enterocolitica*-induced bacteremia have had underlying diseases, particulary cirrhosis, hemochromatosis, anemia, and immunodeficiencies (malignancy, diabetes mellitus, renal transplants, and recently, AIDS[115]). However, even with appropriate therapy, the mortality rate in patients with *Yersinia*-induced bacteremia has exceeded 30%.

Y. enterocolitica is known to invade the epithelial cells in the intestinal mucosa and peritoneal macrophages. Consequently, the bacteria will proliferate within the macrophages and then eventually will infiltrate the regional lymph nodes by transport into these cells.[116,117] Virulent *Yersinia* strains are often resistant to the bactericidal activity of normal human serum.[118]

Infection with HIV, which interferes with the CD4$^+$ lymphocyte functions and replicates in the macrophages, would precipitate impaired antigen presentation and/or impaired monokine production,[119] and thereby predispose the patient to the development of disseminated infection with *Yersinia*.[115] Cohen and Rodday[115] have described a case of an AIDS patient with *Y. enterocolitica* bacteremia who was treated initially with intravenous TMP-SMX. After the patient became defervescent and the diarrhea resolved, TMP-SMX was given orally but the patient developed fever and a macular rash. Oral ciprofloxacin was applied thereafter, and although blood and stool cultures were negative, the fever persisted both during and after completion of the ciprofloxacin therapy.[115]

In a recent report, Flament-Saillour et al.[120] described an AIDS patient with *Y. enterocolitica*-induced peritonitis with a history of cirrhosis due to chronic B/delta hepatitis. The patient was successfully treated with oral ofloxacin (400 mg daily) for 3 weeks, and no recurrence of fever or ascites was noted after 6 months of follow-up examination.

9.3.4 REFERENCES

1. Bottone, E. J., *Yersinia enterocolitica*: a panoramic view of a charismatic microorganism, *Crit. Rev. Microbiol.*, 5, 211, 1977.
2. Cover, T. L. and Aber, R. C., *Yersinia enterocolitica*, *N. Engl. J. Med.*, 321, 16, 1989.
3. Hoogkamp-Korstanje, J. A., de Koning, J., and Samson, J. P., Incidence of human infection with *Yersinia enterocolitica* serotypes O:3, O:8, and O:9 and the use of indirect immunofluorescence in diagnosis, *J. Infect. Dis.*, 153, 138, 1986.
4. Van Noyen, R., Vandepitte, J., Wauters, G., and Selderslaugh, R., *Yersinia enterocolitica*: its isolation by cold enrichment from patients and healthy subjects, *J. Clin. Pathol.*, 34, 1052, 1981.
5. Marks, M. I., Pai, C. H., Lafleur, L., Lackman, L., and Hammerberg, O., *Yersinia enterocolitica* gastroenteritis: a prospective study of clinical, bacteriologic, and epidemiologic features, *J. Pediatr.*, 96, 26, 1980.
6. Marriott, D. J., Taylor, S., and Dorman, D. C., *Yersinia enterocolitica* infection in children, *Med. J. Austr.*, 143, 489, 1985.
7. Mollaret, H. H., Bercovier, H., and Alonso, J. M., Summary of the data received at the WHO Reference Center for *Yersinia enterocolitis*, *Contrib. Microbiol. Immunol.*, 5, 174, 1979.
8. Keet, E. E., *Yersinia enterocolitica* septicemia: source of infection and incubation period identified, *NY State J. Med.*, 74, 2226, 1974.
9. Lassen, J., *Yersinia enterocolitica* in drinking-water, *Scand. J. Infect. Dis.*, 4, 125, 1972.
10. Thompson, J. S. and Gravel, M. J., Family outbreak of gastroenteritis due to *Yersinia enterocolitica* serotype O:3 from well water, *Can. J. Microbiol.*, 32, 700, 1986.
11. Aber, R. C., McCarthy, M. A., Berman, R., DeMelfi, T., and Witte, E., An outbreak of *Yersinia enterocolitica* gastrointestinal illness among members of a Brownie troop in Centre County, Pennsylvania, *Proc. 22nd Intersci. Conf. Antimicrob. Agents Chemother.*, American Society for Microbiology, Washington, D.C., 1982.
12. Kay, B. A., Wachsmuth, K., Gemski, P., Feeley, J. C., Quan, T. J., and Brenner, D. J., Virulence and phenotype characterization of *Yersinia enterocolitica* isolated from humans in the United States, *J. Clin. Microbiol.*, 17, 128, 1983.
13. Bouza, E., Dominguez, A., Meseguer, M., Buzon, L., Boixeda, D., Revillo, M. J., de Rafael, L., and Martinez-Beltran, J., *Yersinia enterocolitica* septicemia, *Am. J. Clin. Pathol.*, 74, 404, 1980.
14. Rabson, K. and Wauters, G., Pyraminidase activity in *Yersinia enterocolitica* and related organisms, *J. Clin. Microbiol.*, 21, 980, 1985.
15. Butler, T., *Plague and other Yersinia Infections*, Plenum Press, New York, 1983.
16. Braude, A. I., Davis, C. E., and Fierer, J., *Infectious Diseases and Medical Microbiology*, W. B. Saunders, Philadelphia, 1986, 339.
17. Laird, W. J. and Cavanaugh, D. C., Correlation of autoagglutination and virulens of Yersiniae, *J. Clin. Microbiol.*, 11, 430, 1980.
18. Pai, C. H., Mors, V., and Toma, S., Prevalence of enterotoxigenicity in human and nonhuman isolates of *Yersinia enterocolitis*, *Infect. Immun.*, 22, 334, 1978.
19. Cornelis, G., Laroche, Y., Balligand, G., Sory, M. P., and Wauters, G., *Yersinia enterocolitica*, a primary model for bacterial invasiveness, *Rev. Infect. Dis.*, 9, 64, 1987.
20. Skurnik, M. and Poikonen, K., Experimental intestinal infection of rats by *Yersinia enterocolitis* O:3: a follow-up study with specific antibodies to the virulence plasmid specified antigens, *Scand. J. Infect. Dis.*, 18, 355, 1986.
21. Martinez, R. J., Plasmid-mediated and temperature-regulated surface properties of *Yersinia enterocolitica*, *Infect. Immun.*, 41, 921, 1983.
22. Finkelstein, R. A., Sciortino, C. V., and McIntosh, M. A., Role of iron in microbe-host interactions, *Rev. Infect. Dis.*, 5(Suppl. 4), S759, 1983.
23. Perry, R. D. and Brubaker, R. R., Accumulation of iron by Yersiniae, *J. Bacteriol.*, 137, 1290, 1979.
24. Robins-Browne, R. M., Rabson, A. R., and Koornhof, H. J., Generalized infection with *Yersinia enterocolitica* and the role of iron, *Contrib. Microbiol. Immunol.*, 5, 277, 1970.
25. Robins-Browne, R. M. and Prpic, J. K., Effects of iron and desferrioxamine on infections with *Yersinia enterocolitica*, *Infect. Immun.*, 47, 774, 1985.

26. Melby, K., Slordahl, S., Gutteberg, T. J., and Nordbo, S. A., Septicaemia due to *Yersinia enterocolitica* after oral overdoses of iron, *Br. Med. J.*, 285, 467, 1982.

27. Scharnetzky, M., König, R., Lakomek, M., Tillmann, W., and Schröter, W., Prophylaxis of systemic yersinosis in thalassaemia major, *Lancet*, 1, 791, 1984.

28. Smith, R. E., Carey, A. M., Damare, J. M., Hetrick, F. M., Johnstone, R. W., and Lee, W. H., Evaluation of iron dextran and mucin for enhancement of the virulence of *Yersinia enterocolitica* serotype O:3 in mice, *Infect. Immun.*, 34, 550, 1981.

29. Becroft, D. M. O., Dix, M. R., and Farmer, K., Intramuscular iron-dextran and susceptibility of neonates to bacterial infections, *Arch. Dis. Child.*, 52, 778, 1977.

30. Gladstone, G. P. and Walton, E., The effect of iron and haematin on the killing of staphylococci by rabbit polymorphs, *Br. J. Exp. Pathol.*, 52, 452, 1971.

31. Tauxe, R. V., Vandepitte, J., Wauters, G., Martin, S. M., Goossens, V., De Mol, P., Van Noyen, R., and Thiers, G., *Yersinia enterocolitica* infections and pork: the missing link, *Lancet*, 1, 1129, 1987.

32. Tacket, C. O., Narain, J. P., Sattin, R., Lofgren, J. P., Konigsberg, C., Rendtorff, R. C., Rausa, A., Davis, B. R., and Cohen, M. L., A multistate outbreak of infections caused by *Yersinia enterocolitis* transmitted by pasteurized milk, *JAMA*, 251, 483, 1984.

33. Gutman, L. T., Ottesen, E. A., Quan, T. J., Noce, P. S., and Katz, S. L., An inter-familial outbreak of *Yersinia enterocolitis* enteritis, *N. Engl. J. Med.*, 288, 1372, 1973.

34. Ahvonen, P. and Rossi, T., Familial occurrence of *Yersinia enterocolitis* infection and acute arthritis, *Acta Paediatr. Scand.*, 206(Suppl.), 121, 1970.

35. Ahvonen, P., Human yersiniosis in Finland. II. Clinical features, *Ann. Clin. Rev.*, 4, 39, 1972.

36. Rabson, A. R., Koornhof, H. J., Notman, J., and Maxwell, W. G., Hepatosplenic abscesses due to *Yersinia enterocolitis*, *Br. Med. J.*, 4, 341, 1972.

37. Wilson, H. D., McCormick, J. B., and Feeley, J. C., *Yersinia enterocolitica* infection in a 4-month-old infant associated with infection in household dogs, *J. Pediatr.*, 89, 767, 1976.

38. Boemi, G., Chiesa, C., DiLorenzo, M., Patti, G., Marrocco, G., and Midulla, M., *Yersinia enterocolitica* peritonitis, *Gastroenterology*, 89, 927, 1985.

39. Toivanen, P., Toivanen, A., Olkkonen, L., and Aantaa, S., Hospital outbreak of *Yersinia enterocolitica* infection, *Lancet*, 1, 801, 1973.

40. Ratnam, S., Mercer, E., Picco, B., and Butler, R., A nosocomial outbreak of diarrheal disease due to *Yersinia enterocolitica* serotype O:5, biotype 1, *J. Infect. Dis.*, 145, 242, 1982.

41. McIntyre, M. and Nnochiri, E., A case of hospital-acquired *Yersinia enterocolitica* gastroenteritis, *J. Hosp. Infect.*, 7, 299, 1986.

42. Stenhouse, M. A. and Lilner, L. V., *Yersinia enterocolitica*: a hazard in blood transfusion, *Transfusion*, 22, 396, 1982.

43. Bjune, G., Ruud, T. E., and Eng, J., Bacterial shock due to transfusion with *Yersinia enterocolitica* infected blood, *Scand. J. Infect. Dis.*, 16, 411, 1984.

44. Wright, D. C., Sells, I. F., Vinton, K. J., and Pierce, R. N., Fatal *Yersinia enterocolitica* sepsis after blood transfusion, *Arch. Pathol. Lab. Med.*, 109, 1040, 1985.

45. Galloway, S. J. and Jones, P. D., Transfusion acquired *Yersinia enterocolitica*, *Aust. NZ J. Med.*, 16, 248, 1986.

46. Tacker, C. O., Ballard, J., Harris, N., Allard, J., Nolan, C., Quan, T., and Cohen, M. L., An outbreak of *Yersinia enterocolitis* infections caused by contaminated tofu (soybean curd), *Am. J. Epidemiol.*, 121, 705, 1985.

47. Esseveld, H., Human infections with *Yersinia enterocolitica*, *Antonie van Leeuwenhoek*, 35, 240, 1969.

48. Simmonds, S. D., Noble, M. A., and Freeman, H. J., Gastrointestinal features of culture-positive *Yersinia enterocolitica* infection, *Gastroenterology*, 92, 112, 1987.

49. Snyder, J. D., Christenson, E., and Feldman, R. A., Human *Yersinia enterocolitica* infections in Wisconsin: clinical, laboratory and epidemiologic features, *Am. J. Med.*, 72, 768, 1982.

50. Fukushima, H., Ito, Y., Saito, K., Kuroda, K., Inoue, J., Tsubokura, M., and Otsuki, K., Intrafamilial cases of *Yersinia enterocolitica* appendicitis, *Microbiol. Immun.*, 25, 71, 1981.

51. Nilehn, B. and Sjostrom, B., Studies on *Yersinia enterocolitica*: occurrence in various groups of acute abdominal disease, *Acta Pathol. Microbiol. Scand.*, 71, 612, 1967.

52. Moeller, D. D. and Burger, W. E., Perforation of the ileum in *Yersinia enterocolitica* infection, *Am. J. Gastroenterol.*, 80, 19, 1985.

53. Chiesa, C., Pacifico, L., and Aronoff, S. C., Implication of *Yersinia* species in primary peritonitis, *Am. J. Dis. Child.*, 139, 751, 1985.

54. Capron, J.-P., Capron-Chivrac, D., Tossou, H., Delamarre, J., and Eb, F., Spontaneous yersinia enterocolitica peritonitis in idiopathic hemochromatosis, *Gastroenterology*, 87, 1372, 1984.

55. Rabson, A. R. and Koornhof, H. J., *Yersinia enterocolitica* infections in South Africa, *S. Afr. Med. J.*, 46, 798, 1972.

56. Hansan, W., Demarteau-Laurent, C., and Yourassowsky, E., Mise en évidence de *Y. enterocolitica* dans le liquide d'ascite, *Med. Mal. Infect.*, 5, 231, 1975.

57. Fischer, D., Karsenti, P., and Paraf, A., Péritonite spontanée du cirrhotique a *Yersinia enterocolitica*, *Nouv. Presse Med.*, 10, 2292, 1981.

58. Burchfield, D. J., Rawlings, D., and Hamrick, H. J., Intussusception associated with *Yersinia enterocolitica* gastroenteritis, *Am. J. Dis. Child.*, 137, 803, 1983.

59. Stuart, R. C., Leahy, A. L., Cafferkey, M. T., and Stephens, R. B., *Yersinia enterocolitica* infection and toxic megacolon, *Br. J. Surg.*, 73, 590, 1986.

60. Rush, O., Sayed, H. I., Whitby, J. L., and Wall, W. J., Cholangitis caused by *Yersinia enterocolitica*, *Can. Med. Assoc. J.*, 123, 1017, 1980.

61. Leino, R. E., Renvall, S. Y., Lipasti, J. A., and Toivanen, A. M., Small-bowel gangrene caused by *Yersinia enterocolitica* III, *Br. Med. J.*, 280, 1419, 1980.

62. Olinde, A. J., Lucas, J. F., Jr., and Miller, R. C., Acute yersiniosis and its surgical significance, *South Med. J.*, 77, 1539, 1984.

63. Jepsen, O. B., Korner, B., Lauritsen, K. B., Hancke, A.-B., Andersen, L., Henrichsen, S., Brenoe, E., Christiansen, P. M., and Jahansen, A., *Yersinia enterocolitica* infection in patients with acute surgical abdominal disease: a prospective study, *Scand. J. Infect. Dis.*, 8, 189, 1976.

64. Zenyoji, H., Maruyama, T., Sakai, S., Kimura, S., Mizuno, T., and Momose, T., An outbreak of enteritis due to *Yersinia enterocolitica* occurring at a junior high school, *Jpn. J. Microbiol.*, 17, 220, 1973.

65. Foberg, U., Fryden, A., Kihlstrom, E., Persson, K., and Weiland, O., *Yersinia enterocolitica* septicemia: clinical and microbiological aspects, *Scand. J. Infect. Dis.*, 18, 269, 1986.

66. Mofenson, H. C., Caraccio, T. R., and Sharieff, N., Iron sepsis: *Yersinia enterocolitica* septicemia possibly caused by an overdose of iron, *N. Engl. J. Med.*, 316, 1092, 1987.

67. Gallant, T., Freedman, M. H., Vellend, H., and Francombe, W. H., Yersinia sepsis in patients with iron overload treated with deferoxamine, *N. Engl. J. Med.*, 314, 1643, 1986.

68. Chiu, H. Y., Flynn, D. M., Hoffbrand, A. V., and Politis, D., Infection with *Yersinia enterocolitica* in patients with iron overload, *Br. Med. J.*, 292, 97, 1986.

69. Boelaert, J. R., van Landuyt, H. W., Valcke, Y. J., Cantinieaux, B., Lornoy, W. F., Vanherweghem, J.-L., Moreillon, P., and Vendepitte, J. M., The role of iron overload in *Yersinia enterocolitica* and *Yersinia pseudotuberculosis* bacteremia in hemodialysis patients, *J. Infect. Dis.*, 156, 384, 1987.

70. Beucler, A., Rocher, G., and Seyer, J. L., Septicémies a *Yersinia enterocolitica* et *Yersinia pseudotuberculosis*: a propos de 236 cas, *Med. Mal. Infect.*, 13, 18, 1983.

71. Viteri, A. L., Howard, P. H., May, J. L., Ramesh, G. S., and Roberts, J. W., Hepatic abscess due to *Yersinia enterocolitica* without bacteremia, *Gastroenterology*, 81, 592, 1981.

72. Verhaegen, J., Dedeyne, G., Vansteenbergen, W., and Vandepitte, J., Rupture of vascular prosthesis in a patient with *Yersinia enterocolitica* bacteremia, *Diagn. Microbiol. Infect. Dis.*, 3, 451, 1985.

73. Appelbaum, J. S., Wilding, G., and Morse, L. J., *Yersinia enterocolitica* endocarditis, *Arch. Intern. Med.*, 143, 2150, 1983.

74. Urbano-Marquez, A., Estruch, R., Agusti, A., Jimenez de Anta, M. T., Ribalta, T., Grau, J. M., and Rozman, C., Infectious endocarditis due to *Yersinia enterocolitica*, *J. Infect. Dis.*, 148, 940, 1983.

75. Plotkin, G. R. and O'Rourke, J. N., Jr., Mycotic aneurysm due to *Yersinia enterocolitica*, *Am. J. Med. Sci.*, 281, 35, 1981.

76. Linares, J., Sitges-Serra, A., Garau, J., Perez, J. L., and Martin, R., Pathogenesis of catheter sepsis: a prospective study with quantitative and semiquantitative cultures of catheter hub and segments, *J. Clin. Microbiol.*, 21, 357, 1985.

77. Marx, R. S. and Johnson, J. E. III, *Yersinia enterocolitica* meningitis with septicemia and spontaneous peritonitis, *NC Med. J.*, 40, 691, 1979.

78. Sonnenwirth, A. C., Bacteremia with and without meningitis due to *Yersinia enterocolitica*, *Edwardsiella tarda, Comamonas terrigena*, and *Pseudomonas maltophilia*, *Ann. NY Acad. Sci.*, 174, 488, 1970.

79. Sebes, J. I., Mabry, E. H. III, and Rabinowitz, J. G., Lung abscess and osteomyelitis of rib due to *Yersinia enterocolitica, Chest*, 69, 546, 1976.

80. Taylor, B. G., Zafarzai, M. Z., Humphreys, D. W., and Manfredi, F., Nodular pulmonary infiltrates and septic arthritis associated with *Yersinia enterocolitica* bacteremia, *Am. Rev. Respir. Dis.*, 116, 525, 1977.

81. Ettensohn, D. B. and Roberts, N. J., Jr., *Yersinia enterocolitica* pneumonia, *NY State J. Med.*, 81, 791, 1981.

82. Sodervik, H., Syrjala, H., and Raisanen, S., Interstitial pneumonia and sepsis caused by *Yersinia enterocolitica* serotype 3, *Scand. J. Infect. Dis.*, 18, 241, 1986.

83. Clarridge, J., Roberts, C., Peters, J., and Musher, D., Sepsis and empyema caused by *Yersinia enterocolitica, J. Clin. Microbiol.*, 17, 936, 1983.

84. Saliou-Diallo, G. I., Kim, A., Pike, J., and Rao, G. M., Fatal *Yersinia enterocolitica* septicemia in a compromised host, *J. Kans. Med. Soc.*, 80, 558, 1979.

85. Olbrych, T. G., Zarconi, J., File, T. M., Jr., Traeger, S. M., and Tan, J. S., Bullous skin lesions associated with *Yersinia enterocolitica* septicemia, *Am. J. Med. Sci.*, 287, 38, 1984.

86. Ahvonen, P., Sievers, K., and Aho, K., Arthritis associated with *Yersinia enterocolitica* infection, *Acta Rheumatol. Scand.*, 15, 232, 1969.

87. Laitinen, O., Tuuhea, J., and Ahvonen, P., Polyarthritis associated with *Yersinia enterocolitica* infection: clinical features and laboratory findings in nine cases with severe joint symptoms, *Ann. Rheum. Dis.*, 31, 34, 1972.

88. Dequeker, J., Jamar, R., and Walravens, M., HLA-B27, arthritis and *Yersinia enterocolitica* infection, *J. Rheumatol.*, 7, 706, 1980.

89. Leino, R. and Kalliomaki, J. L., Yersiniosis as an internal disease, *Ann. Intern. Dis.*, 81, 458, 1974.

90. Aho, K., Ahvonen, P., Lassus, A., Sievers, K., and Tiilikanen, A., HLA-27 in reactive arthritis: a study of yersinia arthritis and Reiter's disease, *Arthritis Rheum.*, 17, 521, 1974.

91. Laitinen, O., Leirisalo, M., and Skylv, G., Relation between HLA-B27 and clinical features in patients with yersinia arthritis, *Arthritis Rheum.*, 20, 1121, 1977.

92. Olson, D. N. and Finch, W. R., Reactive arthritis associated with *Yersinia enterocolitica* gastroenteritis, *Am. J. Gastroenterol.*, 76, 524, 1981.

93. Agner, E., Larsen, J. H., and Leth, A., *Yersinia enterocolitica* carditis as a differential diagnosis — and the prognosis of this disease, *Scand. J. Rheumatol.*, 7, 26, 1978.

94. Friedberg, M., Dennenberg, T., Brun, C., Larsen, J. H., and Larsen, S., Glomerulonephritis in infections with *Yersinia enterocolitica* O-serotype 3. II. The incidence and immunological features of *Yersinia* infection in a consecutive glomerulonephritis population, *Acta Med. Scand.*, 209, 103, 1981.

95. Dennenberg, T., Friedberg, M., Samuelsson, T., and Winblad, S., Glomerulonephritis in infections in *Yersinia enterocolitica* O-serotype 3. I. Evidence for glomerular involvement in acute cases of yersiniosis, *Acta Med. Scand.*, 209, 97, 1981.

96. Autenrieth, I. B., Hantschmann, P., Heymer, B., and Heesemann, J., Immunohistological characterization of the cellular immune response against *Yersinia enterocolitica* in mice: evidence for the involvement of T lymphocytes, *Immunobiology*, 187, 1, 1993.

97. Autenrieth, I. B., Tingle, A., Reske-Kunz, A., and Heesemann, J., T lymphocytes mediate protection against *Yersinia enterocolitica* in mice: characterization of murine T-cell clones specific for *Y. enterocolitica, Infect. Immun.*, 60, 1140, 1992.

98. Autenrieth, I. B., Vogel, U., Preger, S., Heymer, B., and Heesemann, J., Experimental *Yersinia enterocolitica* infection in euthymic and T-cell-deficient athymic nude C57BL/6 mice: comparison of time course, histomorphology, and immune response, *Infect. Immun.*, 61, 2585, 1993.

99. Hanski, C., Kutschka, U., Schmoranzer, H. P., Naumann, M., Stallmach, A., Hahn, H., Menge, H., and Riecken, E. O., Immunohistochemical and electron microscopic study of interaction of *Yersinia enterocolitica* serotype O8 with intestinal mucosa during experimental enteritis, *Infect. Immun.*, 57, 673, 1989.

100. Lian, C. J., Hwang, W. S., and Pai, C. H., Plasmid-mediated resistance to phagocytosis in *Yersinia enterocolitica, Infect. Immun.*, 55, 1176, 1987.

101. Rosqvist, R., Bolin, I., and Wolf Watz, H., Inhibition of phagocytosis in *Yersinia pseudotuberculosis*: a virulence plasmid-encoded ability involving the Yop2b protein, *Infect. Immun.*, 56, 2139, 1988.

102. Simonet, M., Richard, S., and Berche, P., Electron microscopic evidence for *in vivo* extracellular localization of *Yersinia pseudotuberculosis* harboring the pYV plasmid, *Infect. Immun.*, 58, 841, 1990.

103. Hahn, H. and Kaufmann, S. H. E., The role of cell-mediated immunity in bacterial infections, *Rev. Infect. Dis.*, 3, 1221, 1981.

104. Autenrieth, I. B. and Heesemann, J., *In vivo* neutralization of tumor necrosis factor alpha and interferon-gamma abrogates resistance to *Yersinia enterocolitica* in mice, *Med. Microbiol. Immunol.*, 181, 333, 1992.

105. Hoogkamp-Korstanje, J. A., Antibiotics in *Yersinia enterocolitica* infections, *J. Antimicrob. Chemother.*, 20, 123, 1987.

106. Raevuori, M., Harvey, S. M., Pickett, M. J., and Martin, W. J., *Yersinia enterocolitica*: in vitro antimicrobial susceptibility, *Antimicrob. Agents Chemother.*, 13, 888, 1978.

107. Ahmedy, A., Vidon, D. J., Delmas, C. L., and Lett, M. C., Antimicrobial susceptibilities of food-isolated strains of *Yersinia enterocolitica*, *Y. intermedia*, *Y. frederiksenii*, and *Y. kristensenii*, *Antimicrob. Agents Chemother.*, 28, 351, 1985.

108. Hornstein, M. J., Jupeau, A. M., Scavizzi, M. R., Philippon, A. M., and Grimont, P. A., *In vitro* susceptibilities of 126 clinical isolates of *Yersinia enterocolitica* to 21 beta-lactam antibiotics, *Antimicrob. Agents Chemother.*, 27, 806, 1985.

109. Gaspar, M. C. and Soriano, F., Susceptibility of *Yersinia enterocolitica* to eight beta-lactam antibiotics and clavulanic acid, *J. Antimicrob. Chemother.*, 8, 161, 1981.

110. Cornelis, G., Wauters, G., and Vanderhaeghe, H., Presence de β-lactamase chez *Yersinia enterocolitica*, *Ann. Microbiol. (Paris)*, 124B, 139, 1973.

111. Black, R. E., Jackson, R. J., Tsai, T., Medvedsky, M., Shayegani, M., Feeley, J. C., MacLeod, K. I. E., and Wakelee, A. M., Epidemic *Yersinia enterocolitica* infection due to contaminated chocolate milk, *N. Engl. J. Med.*, 298, 76, 1978.

112. Scavizzi, M. R., Alonso, J. M., Philippon, A. M., Jupeau-Vessieres, A. M., and Guiyoule, A., Failure of newer beta-lactam antibiotics for murine *Yersinia enterocolitica* infection, *Antimicrob. Agents Chemother.*, 31, 523, 1987.

113. Pai, C. H., Gillis, F., Tuomanen, E., and Marks, M. I., Placebo-controlled double-blind evaluation of trimethoprim-sulfamethoxazole treatment of *Yersinia enterocolitica* gastroenteritis, *J. Pediatr.*, 104, 308, 1984.

114. de Cuenca-Moron, B., Solis-Herruzo, J. A., Moreno, D., Guijarro, C., Gentil, A. A., and Castellano, G., Spontaneous bacterial peritonitis due to *Yersinia enterocolitica* in secondary alcoholic hemochromatosis, *J. Clin. Gastroenterol.*, 11, 675, 1989.

115. Cohen, J. I. and Rodday, P., *Yersinia enterocolitica* bacteremia in a patient with the acquired immunodeficiency syndrome, *Am. J. Med.*, 86, 254, 1989.

116. Une, T., Studies on the pathogenesis of *Yersinia enterocolitica*. I. Experimental infection in rabbits, *Microbiol. Immunol.*, 21, 349, 1977.

117. Une, T., Studies on the pathogenesis of *Yersinia enterocolitica*. II. Interaction with cultured cells *in vitro*, *Microbiol. Immunol.*, 21, 365, 1977.

118. Pai, C. H. and deStephano, I., Serum resistance associated with virulence in *Yersinia enterocolitica*, *Infect. Immun.*, 35, 605, 1982.

119. Levy, J., Mysteries of HIV: challenges for therapy and prevention, *Nature*, 333, 519, 1988.

120. Flament-Saillour, M., de Truchis, P., Risbourg, M., and Nordmann, P., *Yersinia enterocolitica* peritonitis in a patient infected with the human immunodeficiency virus, *Clin. Infect. Dis.*, 18, 655, 1994.

10. *Campylobacter* spp.

10.1 INTRODUCTION

Campylobacter is a genus of motile Gram-negative microaerophilic to anaerobic bacteria with a curved or spiral-rod shape and a single polar flagellum at one or both ends. Originally classified as a member of the genus *Vibrio* as *Vibrio fetus*, *Campylobacter* comprises several species and subspecies.

In humans and animals, the bacterium is found in the oral cavity, gastrointestinal tract, and the reproductive organs. Some of the species are pathogenic in humans, causing enteritis and systemic diseases. Such factors as advanced age, a dysfunctional gastrointestinal tract, or underlying immune deficiency would enhance the risk of infection with *Campylobacter* spp. Thus, *C. coli* is the cause of diarrhea in humans. *C. cinaedi* and *C. fennelliae* (previously described as *Campylobacter*-like organisms[1,2]) are known to effect proctitis and diarrhea in immunocompetent homosexual men.

C. fetus (*Vibrio fetus*), a microaerophilic species and most commonly a bloodstream isolate, consists of several subspecies. *C. fetus* is associated with febrile illness[3] as well as thrombophlebitis, endocarditis, infected aortic aneurysm, septic arthritis, and osteomyelitis. *C. fetus* ssp. *fetus/intestinalis* are occasional human pathogens capable of causing systemic infection, especially in immunocompromised hosts and young children. *C. fetus* ssp. *jejuni* (*C. jejuni*, *Vibrio coli*, *V. jejuni*) is a common pathogen associated with acute bacterial gastroenteritis in humans. Currently, the thermophilic campylobacters *C. coli* and *C. jejuni* are recognized to be among the most important causes for diarrhea in both immunocompetent and immunocompromised hosts.[4-6]

C. laridis is also a thermophilic organism[7] causing usually self-limiting illness characterized by diarrhea, crampy abdominal pain, and mild fevers.[8,9] It is distinguished from *C. jejuni* by its nalidixic acid resistance, hyppurate hydrolysis, and anaerobic growth in the presence of trimethylamine-*N*-oxide (however, some rare nalidixic acid-resistant *C. jejuni* isolates have also been reported).[10,11]

C. pylori (*Helicobacter pylori*) is a species associated with gastritis and pyloric ulcers in humans. *C. sputorum* ssp. *sputorum* is nonpathogenic and found in the human oral cavity.

10.2 STUDIES ON THERAPEUTICS

10.2.1 MACROLIDE ANTIBIOTICS

Erythromycin and the newer macrolide antibiotics have been the subject of a renewed clinical interest because of their therapeutic effect against opportunistic pathogens which are becoming more prevalent in immunocompromised patients, and because of their excellent tissue penetration and potential immunomodulating properties. Some of the newer macrolides may also offer the possibility of once-daily dosing, resistance to acid degradation in the stomach without enteric coating, and reduced gastrointestinal side effects.[12]

Macrolide antibiotics have been used widely in the therapy of a number of clinically significant infections caused by Gram-positive and Gram-negative pathogens, including *Campylobacter*-associated enteritis.[13] In addition to erythromycin, which for several decades has been the drug of choice for many infections, newer macrolide antibiotics have brought new aspects into the treatment of infections. In general, erythromycin exhibits excellent tissue penetration with high tissue-to-plasma concentration ratios, thereby allowing for greater drug concentration at the site of action.[12]

Erythromycin has been used extensively in treatment of campylobacter enteritis. However, in a recent prospective study of children in Nigeria over a 10-year period,[14] the sensitivity of clinical strains of *C. jejuni/coli* to erythromycin has decreased from 70.8% to 20.7%. In addition, *C. jejuni* biotype 1, which in earlier studies accounted for 52.5% of all isolates in children under 2 years of age, increased to 87.5% in this study.

Williams et al.[15] have assessed the bacteriologic and clinical benefits of early treatment of *C. jejuni*-related enteritis. In contrast to its bacteriologic effectiveness by rapidly eliminating the organism from stools, erythromycin did not reduce the duration or severity of diarrhea, abdominal pain, or other symptoms.

Clarithromycin, a 14-membered macrolide, when compared to erythromycin, has displayed enhanced serum and tissue concentrations, longer serum elimination half-life, and improved patient tolerability allowing for twice-daily dosing.[13,16] In adults, the usual doses are 250 to 500 mg (b.i.d.) given orally. In pediatric patients, clarithromycin is administered in suspension at 7.5 mg/kg daily (maximum: 250 mg), b.i.d.[13] For example, in a pediatric trial, the clinical efficacy of clarithromycin against campylobacter enteritis was reported to be 98.9% (87 of 88 patients).[13] The safety profile of clarithromycin has been evaluated in children (aged 6 months to 15 years; mean 5.8 years) at doses ranging from 2.38 to 15 mg/kg, b.i.d. (mean 7.44 mg/kg, twice daily). Adverse side effects were mainly gastrointestinal and included mild to moderate nausea, vomiting, and diarrhea.[12,17,18]

Rokitamycin, another new 16-membered macrolide antibiotic, when tested in animal models, produced higher and more persistent serum concentrations than other macrolides because of its better oral absorption and increased antimicrobial potency of its primary metabolites.[19,20] Rokitamycin was found effective in pediatric patients (n = 100) with campylobacter enteritis; the results were compared with those in similar patients not treated with rokitamycin (n = 63), or treated with erythromycin (n = 11) or fosfomycin (n = 26).[21] The average recovery period from bloody stool for the rokitamycin-treated group was 1.2 d as compared to 5.5, 2.8, and 1.7 d for the untreated, erythromycin- and fosfomycin-treated groups, respectively. Eradication of *Campylobacter* spp. from the stool in almost all cases occurred within 2 d after treatment initiation.[21] The recommended daily dose regimens of rokitamycin are 20 to 40 mg/kg with adverse side effects of 1.9%.[12]

The *in vitro* activity of azithromycin against enteric bacterial pathogens has been determined in agar dilution. The antibiotic was very active against *Campylobacter* spp. showing an MIC_{90} value of 0.125 µg/ml.[22] The high intracellular concentration achieved by azithromycin might be particularly useful against this pathogen.

10.2.1.1 *Campylobacter* spp. Resistance to Macrolide Antibiotics

C. jejuni resistance to erythromycin is plasmid-mediated.[23] Taylor et al.[24] who had studied erythromycin-resistant campylobacter infections in Thailand found that of 23 *C. jejuni* strains isolated from patients before treatment, 15 (65%) were erythromycin-resistant (MIC ≥8 µg/ml). Moreover, drug resistance was far worse in strains acquired in an institutional setting (e.g., orphanages) than the community-acquired strains (53% vs. 11%). It was also found that erythromycin resistance can occur independently of tetracycline resistance.

It has been reported[25] that resistance to high-level tetracycline (32 to 128 µg/ml) was mediated by a plasmid of 45 to 50 kb; the HincII and AccI fragments of this plasmid, where the tetracycline resistance determinant has been located, were shown to be conserved.

Two studies conducted in the U.S. and Europe suggested that animal *C. jejuni* and *C. coli* isolates have been more resistant to antibiotics than the corresponding isolates from human *Campylobacter*.[26,27]

10.2.1.2   Effects of Macrolide Antibiotics on the Immune System

The beneficial interaction of macrolide antibiotics with various cellular and humoral components of the immune system may form the basis of important new therapeutic strategies against opportunistic infections in patients with impaired immune functions such as those with AIDS.[12] Thus, a number of studies[28-33] have demonstrated that macrolides can effectively penetrate into polymorphonuclear leukocytes, macrophages, and lymphocytes. Such ability may be particularly important for therapies against opportunistic intracellular pathogens, such as *Toxoplasma*, *Mycobacterium*, *Chlamydia*, *Legionella*, *Listeria*, and *Brucella*. For example, Anderson et al.[34] have reported intraphagocytic antimicrobial activity for erythromycin and roxithromycin. Other findings[29,35-37] also corroborated the presence of significant intracellular concentrations and activity of erythromycin. In addition, the latter appeared not to affect adversely the bactericidal oxidative metabolism of the polymorphonuclear leukocytes.[36,37] However, contrary to a previous report,[12] van Rensburg et al.[37] and Naess and Solberg[38] did not find erythromycin to potentiate phagocytosis.

Several conflicting reports have appeared with regard to the effects of macrolides on the chemotaxis of polymorphonuclear leukocytes. Data supporting enhancement of chemotaxis[35,37,39] have been contradicted by either macrolides diminishing chemotaxis[36] or having no effect.[38,40]

Further studies on the impact of erythromycin on the immune functions have demonstrated that it increased the amount of membrane receptors on polymorphonuclear leukocytes and lymphocytes, but did not increase the proportion of lymphocytes rosetting with erythrocyte-antibody cells and erythrocyte-antibody-complement cells, nor did it affect the lymphocyte response to mitogens.[38] In addition, erythromycin did not alter the levels of IgG, IgA, IgM, and complement (total hemolytic complement, C3, C4).[37]

10.2.2   FLUOROQUINOL-4-ONES

The introduction of fluoroquinolones into the armory of antibacterial chemotherapy opened a new and important avenue for the treatment of bacterial enteritis.[41-44] When compared to the structurally similar nalidixic acid, the fluoroquinol-4-ones differ by having a quinolone ring in place of the 1,8-naphthyridine system. In addition, they have a 1-piperazinyl group at position 7 to instill antipseudomonal activity, and a fluorine substituent at C-6.

The therapeutic efficacy of the fluoroquinolones coupled with their favorable pharmacokinetic properties have proved beneficial against enteropathic bacteria. Thus, norfloxacin and ciprofloxacin have been found effective in suppressing and eliminating potentially pathogenic aerobic Gram-negative bacteria colonizing the alimentary canal of neutropenic patients with acute leukemia, thereby reducing infection-associated morbidity and mortality due to sepsis.[45]

The oral bioavailability of the fluoroquinolones was found to be between 78% and 84%,[46-60] and their elimination half-life was in the range of 2 to 4 h for norfloxacin, and 8 to 11.5 h for pefloxacin. The protein binding of the fluoroquinolones was less than that of the nonfluorinated congeners. Excretion has been primarily by the kidneys in the active unchanged form.[47-60]

In cases of empiric treatment of gastroenteritis, however, the use of fluoroquinolones has been controversial.[61] Persistent and recurrent disease, especially in immunocompromised patients, as well as drug resistance have been widely reported to contradict earlier reports of high microbiological eradication rates.[62-65]

A significant drug interaction of the fluoroquinolones that deserves attention may occur after concurrent administration of theophylline — the result has been an increased toxicity and serum levels of the latter.[46] In addition, oral anticoagulants when used in combination with pefloxacin produced prolongation of the prothrombine time. Other unwarranted drug interactions include rifampin and chloramphenicol which can antagonize the therapeutic efficacy of the fluoroquinolones.[46]

Norfloxacin is a fluoroquinolone carboxylic acid with broad antibacterial activity.[66-68] Its pharmacokinetic profile[47-49] showed peak serum levels of 1.5 mg/l following absorption of 400 mg from the gastrointestinal tract;[69] peak levels in urine and stool reached up to 400 mg/l and 773 mg/kg, respectively.[69,70] An oral recommended dose of 400 mg (b.i.d. or t.i.d.) has been found effective against urinary tract infections and acute gastroenteritis. The drug was well tolerated with low incidence (<3%) of adverse side effects (nausea, headache, dizziness, rash, elevation of liver enzymes, and eosinophilia).[67] However, the clinical benefits of norfloxacin against campylobacter enteritis have been modest. Thus, Wiström et al.[71] found that in the case of campylobacteriosis, the difference in the cure rate between norfloxacin and placebo on the last treatment day was only 14%. The therapy was further limited by the development of resistance (persisting in six of nine campylobacter strains tested). In addition, a relatively high frequency (6%) of resistant *Campylobacter* strains has been reported.[71] The prophylactic use of norfloxacin in travelers' diarrhea has been studied by Wiström et al.[72]

Ciprofloxacin, a better absorbed fluoroquinolone agent, has shown pharmacokinetic properties similar to that of norfloxacin.[48-55,58-60] During 7 d of therapy at usual dose regimens, it produced fecal levels comparable to those of norfloxacin.[73] In a double-blind, randomized, placebo-controlled trial in adult subjects with campylobacter enteritis, ciprofloxacin was used at 500 mg (b.i.d.) for 5 d.[74] It reduced the duration of illness from 2.2–2.6 d in the placebo-treated group to 1.1–1.4 d ($p > .01$) in those randomized patients receiving the drug.[74,75]

In vitro and *in vivo* evaluation of AT-4140, a 6,8-difluoro-4-oxoquinoline-3-carboxylic acid derivative, has demonstrated broad and potent antibacterial activities.[76] When tested against 13 clinical isolates of *C. jejuni*, the MIC_{50} values of AT-4140, ciprofloxacin, and ofloxacin were 0.025, 0.1, and 0.2 µg/ml, respectively; the corresponding MIC_{90} values were 0.1, 0.39, and 0.78 µg/ml, respectively.

The pharmacokinetic profile of AT-4140 showed good oral absorption, relatively long plasma half-life, and good tissue distribution. Thus, in human studies, single oral doses of 400 to 800 mg produced peak plasma levels of 0.44 to 1.39 µg/ml with half-lives of approximately 16 h; by comparison, the corresponding half-lives of ciprofloxacin, ofloxacin, enoxacin, and norfloxacin were 3.3–4.9, 7.0, 6.2, and 3–4 h, respectively.[76] In contrast to existing fluoroquinolones, which have been clinically administered twice or three times daily, the long plasma half-life of AT-4140 seems to support once-a-day treatment.

DU-6859a, a new fluoroquinolone agent, was compared with ciprofloxacin in agar dilution susceptibility tests against enteric pathogens. The drug showed increased activity compared with ciprofloxacin against *Campylobacter* spp. isolates.[77]

AM-1155 is a 6-fluoro-8-methoxyquinolone with a wide spectrum of antibacterial activity.[78] As compared with ciprofloxacin, AM-1155 was two- to fourfold more active against *C. jejuni*.

10.2.2.1 *Campylobacter* Resistance to Fluoroquinolones

Although susceptible to fluoroquinolones,[79-81] both *C. jejuni* and *C. coli* have developed resistance to these agents.[63,82-90] In a retrospective study, Reina et al.[90,91] have determined the emergence of a steadily increasing resistance to nalidixic acid (unfluorinated 1,8-naphthyridine) and fluoroquinolones (ciprofloxacin) in thermophilic *C. jejuni* and *C. coli* strains collected from feces. Overall, 11.8% and 10.7% of *C. jejuni* clinical strains isolated during 1987–1991 were found resistant to nalidixic acid and ciprofloxacin, respectively.[91]

Other studies have also indicated a rapid emergence of resistance by *Campylobacter* species to ciprofloxacin,[63,85,92-94] ofloxacin,[82] and norfloxacin.[89,93,95] Gopal Rao[96] described the development of spontaneous resistance to ciprofloxacin in a strain of *C. jejuni* in a patient with persistent enteritis. The reason for such spontaneous resistance to fluoroquinolones may be explained either as a spontaneous mutation in the bacterial chromosome, or as a secondary cross-resistance to therapy with unrelated antibiotics.[97]

10.2.3 Mechanism of Fluoroquinolone Resistance

Detailed understanding of the mechanisms of the *Campylobacter* resistance to fluoroquinolines is important for the development of preventive strategies. Currently, two major mechanisms have been defined: (1) alterations in the bacterial DNA gyrase, the molecular target of the quinolone action; and (2) reduction of drug accumulation in the cells.[98]

10.2.3.1 Alterations in Bacterial DNA Gyrase

Bacterial DNA gyrase is a type II topoisomerase, an enzyme common for eubacteria, archaebacteria, viruses, and eukaryotes. In general, the role of topoisomerase enzymes is essential for DNA replication and recombination. In this regard, the DNA gyrase has been unique in its ability to insert superhelical turns (negative supercoils) into covalently closed double-stranded bacterial DNA molecules.[99] The process of supercoiling involves the concerted action of two gyrase subunits A which mediate transient double-strand breakage and rejoining, and two subunits B which provide energy by ATP hydrolysis for regeneration of the enzyme conformation to initiate the next cycle of DNA cleavage, strand passage, and rejoining of the broken strands.[98] What the fluoroquinolones do is to suppress the rejoining of the broken strands by forming stable ternary complexes with the bacterial gyrase and DNA; the subunits A will attach covalently to the cleaved DNA ends through tyrosine ester bonds.[100-102]

This unique feature of bacterial type II topoisomerases, such as DNA gyrase, to insert negative supercoils into DNA may well account for the *selective* action of the fluoroquinolones on bacteria since isolated mammalian topoisomerase enzymes studied up to date have been highly resistant to inhibition by quinol-4-ones.[66]

Two genes, *gyr*A and *gyr*B are coding for subunits A and B, respectively.[103-108] So far, several mutations, namely, *nal*A, *nfx*A, *nor*A, and *cfx*A, resulting in resistance to nalidixic acid[109-111] (a nonfluorinated 1,8-naphthyridine derivative) and fluoroquinolones,[112-114] have been mapped at the *gyr*A locus. All mutations were found to be confined within a highly conserved region, the "quinolone resistance-determining region" (QRDR).[115-117] However, despite increasing the resistance towards quinolones, these mutations did not change the bacterial susceptibilities to several structurally unrelated drugs.[116]

The isolation of DNA gyrase that was less sensitive to inhibition by ciprofloxacin from a ciprofloxacin-resistant *C. jejuni* isolate did signify that ciprofloxacin resistance in this organism has also been associated with alteration in the DNA gyrase.[83] Further data by Gootz and Martin[118] on quinolone-resistant *C. jejuni* mutants also strongly implied that alteration of the subunit A of DNA gyrase has been responsible for the observed resistance.

Cambau et al.[119] have identified in *Mycobacterium tuberculosis* the chromosomal DNA of an ofloxacin-resistant mutant (MTB2; MIC = 32 μg/ml). Comparison of the nucleotide sequences of the 150-bp fragments (within the QRDR of *gyr*A) obtained by polymerase chain reaction (PCR) revealed a point mutation in MTB2 leading to the substitution of histidine (basic) for aspartic acid (acidic) at a position corresponding to residues involved also in the quinolone resistance of *C. jejuni* (Asp90).[119] Another point to emphasize is that while in *Escherichia coli* mutations led to clinical resistance towards unfluorinated quinolones but not fluoroquinolones, in *C. jejuni* the observed resistance was associated with fluoroquinolones.[106]

In general, clinical resistance against fluoroquinolones is seldom found in intrinsically highly susceptible pathogens (Enterobacteriaceae) and entails a combination of at least two mutations. By comparison, pathogens which have moderate intrinsic susceptibility (*C. jejuni*, *Pseudomonas aeruginosa*, and *Staphylococcus aureus*) would require only one mutation to become clinically resistant.[105,120] As a result, the development of drug resistance during therapy may be the consequence of either acquisition of already resistant strains (such as the case of susceptible species), or the selection of mutants as was the case of less susceptible species.[98]

In contrast to mutations in *gyr*A, the *gyr*B gene mutations have been shown to be of lesser importance for the formation of drug resistance.[98]

10.2.3.2   Reduction of Quinolone Accumulation

In order to reach the intracellular DNA gyrase as their target, the quinolones must penetrate the bacterial cell wall. Clinical resistance because of reduced drug accumulation has been associated with at least one of two different mechanisms: (1) an energy-independent, passive mechanism which is based either on structural alterations, or a reduced expression of outer membrane protein (OPM) porins (water-filled protein pores) that facilitate the passage of hydrophilic quinolone compounds (such as ciprofloxacin and ofloxacin) through the outer bacterial membrane (e.g., Gram-negative organisms); and/or (2) an energy-requiring, active efflux mechanism of quinolones.[98]

10.2.3.2.1   *Reduced accumulation of quinolones due to impaired*
permeability of the outer cell membrane

Most studies to determine the mechanism of reduced quinolone accumulation have been done on *E. coli*. The latter has two major porins, OMP F and OMP C, forming pores of 1.2 and 1.0 nm, respectively.[121] Although loss of either porin by inactivation of the respective structural genes (*omp*F and *omp*C) would diminish the accumulation of hydrophilic quinolones, in *E. coli* the major portal of entry is OMP F (as evidenced by the 50% reduction of drug accumulation following *omp*F mutations).[122] Moreover, since the OMP F porin lacks specificity, other unrelated drugs (tetracycline, chloramphenicol, β-lactams) besides quinolones, may also use it to enter the bacterial cell; consequently, the loss of OMP F resulted in parallel resistance to all of these compounds.[122,123] In addition to mutations in the structural *omp*F gene, mutations at several unrelated loci[112,121,124-129] have also been proven to reduce the amount of the OMP F porin, thereby decreasing drug accumulation.

Data by Segreti et al.[83] have shown that the mechanism of fluoroquinolone resistance of *C. jejuni* appeared not related to the acquisition of plasmids or to alteration in OPMs, including the 45-kDa OPM that is considered the major porin of this organism.[130] The fact that naturally occurring *C. jejuni* mutants did not differ from the ciprofloxacin-susceptible isolates in MICs of nonquinolone antimicrobials lent additional support to no alterations of OPMs.[83]

10.2.3.2.2   *Reduced accumulation of quinolones resulting from increased*
efflux out of the cell

Cohen et al.[123] provided the first evidence for reduced accumulation of quinolones due to increased efflux out of the cells. Using energized inverted membrane vesicles of *E. coli*, these investigators have demonstrated that accumulation of hydrophilic (but not hydrophobic) quinolones did occur. The observed process was saturable, thereby indicating carrier-mediated drug transport. However, even at very low quinolone concentrations (0.04 mg/l) their intracellular presence was still detectable.[124] It was then postulated that additional factors (unspecific binding to intracellular compounds such as double-stranded DNA,[131] or difference between the intracellular and extracellular pH[98]) may have counteracted to keep the quinolones inside the cell. These and other findings lend support to the hypothesis that the efflux of quinolones, but not the influx, is an energy-requiring transport process.[132]

10.3   EVOLUTION OF THERAPIES AND TREATMENT OF
CAMPYLOBACTERIOSIS

In vitro susceptibility testing has revealed that most *Campylobacter* species were sensitive to tetracycline, doxycycline, gentamicin, chloramphenicol, and rifampin, whereas a significant number were shown to be resistant to erythromycin.[133] The fluoroquinolones (ciprofloxacin, ofloxacin, norfloxacin) have also been very effective because of their broad antimicrobial activity, minimal toxicity, and easy oral administration.[134] However, similarly to the macrolide antibiotics, fluoro-quinoline-resistant campylobacter organisms are likely to emerge.

10.3.1 *Campylobacter jejuni/coli*-Associated Enteritis

Campylobacter enteritis has been commonly diagnosed among children in developing countries[135] where *C. jejuni* may be excreted by up to 40% of children under 5 years of age.[135-138] This pool of largely asymptomatic excreters of an opportunistic enteric pathogen is of special concern since diarrhea affects most HIV-positive and AIDS patients. According to Thea et al.,[139] HIV-infected Zairian infants have an 11-fold increased risk of dying from diarrhea as compared to uninfected infants, thereby making it the major cause for mortality among HIV-infected children in Africa.

C. *jejuni* and *C. coli* are among the most frequently isolated causative agents in bacterial enteritis.[6] Their transmission in humans has most often been caused by drinking of contaminated water or ingestion of unpasteurized milk, and contact with domestic animals suffering from diarrhea.[6,140,141] In the general population, the diarrhea is usually self-limiting and lasts 2 to 5 d, but occasionally it can persist for 2 weeks or longer. Although in the majority of cases, fluid replacement without antibiotics would be sufficient treatment, in more serious cases specific therapy may be indicated. Macrolide antibiotics and fluoroquinolone antibacterials (ciproxloxacin, norfloxacin, ofloxacin) have been shown to be effective either prophylactically[72] or as therapy, where they may shorten the duration of diarrhea by 1 to 2 d.[142,143] The combination of trimethoprim-sulfamethoxazole, which has been used extensively in other enteric infections (shigellosis, severe travelers' diarrhea), has not been effective against *C. jejuni* because of drug resistance.[144]

In an earlier study, Nolan et al.[145] analyzed retrospectively the conditions of 82 patients with *C. jejuni*-associated enteritis to ascertain the efficacy of antimicrobial agents (erythromycin, tetracycline, metronidazole, sulfasalazine, ampicillin, trimethoprim-sulfamethoxazole, and doxycycline) and drugs that inhibited the gastrointestinal motility. The latter included lomotil (a combination of atropine and diphenoxylate), dicyclomine, and donnatal (a combination of phenobarbital, atropine, and hyoscyamine). The data obtained showed that while treatment with either erythromycin or tetracycline shortened the illness, the antimotility drugs impeded the resolution of infection.

According to a study by Robins-Browne et al.,[16] when antibiotic treatment of infants and young children with acute nonspecific gastroenteritis was required because of febrile, bloody, or prolonged diarrhea, erythromycin has been recommended since most *Campylobacter* strains were susceptible to it. It was further suggested that the antibiotic had displayed relatively little tendency to select for plasmid-mediated antibiotic resistance.

However, in a number of clinical trials, both in adults and children, erythromycin did not significantly alter the clinical course of *Campylobacter* infections,[146-151] although in some studies[152,153] it was indicated that children with *C. jejuni*-associated bloody diarrhea after receiving erythromycin early in the course of illness improved sooner than children given placebo. On the negative side, in a prospective trial of acute diarrhea in infants, daily regimens of erythromycin ethylsuccinate (40 mg/kg, divided in four doses) for 5 d had no effect on *C. jejuni/coli*.[24] The observed lack of efficacy might have been the result of drug resistance, since out of 23 strains isolated from the infants before treatment, 15 (65%) were found to be erythromycin-resistant (MIC >8 μg/ml).

In several cases, *C. jejuni* has been isolated from the bile of patients who have undergone surgical therapy for cholecystitis.[6] In a related study, Verbruggen et al.[154] identified *C. fetus* as the cause of acute cholecystitis in a middle-aged male patient.

C. *jejuni*-associated peritonitis was also described as a spontaneous bacterial infection in a patient with cirrhosis and massive ascites due to alcoholism,[155] and in patients undergoing continuous ambulatory peritoneal dialysis. In some cases, the patients frequently had associated diarrhea preceding the peritonitis.[156]

It is not unusual that *C. jejuni* enteritis (as much as 3% of patients) may be followed by Reiter's syndrome or reactive arthritis.[157] The latter most often presented as asymmetric oligoarticular disease affecting the knees, ankles, or wrists.[157] Rarely, *C. jejuni* has also been associated with septic arthritis, osteomyelitis, and prosthetic joint infections in immunocompromised patients.[6] Nonspecific myalgias occur in 19% to 69% of patients with *C. jejuni* enteritis.[6]

The occurrence of *Campylobacter*-associated sepsis has been linked to nutritional therapy.[158] Soonattrakul et al.[159] also described a case of an elderly woman with *Campylobacter* septicemia after ingestion of blended raw beef liver. The reported mortality of septicemia has been as high as 21%.[160]

Dermatologic manifestations, such as erysipelas-like cellulitis resulting from *C. jejuni* infection, have been diagnosed in patients with hypogammaglobulinemia,[161] and cellulitis was diagnosed in a patient with Bruton's (X-linked) agammaglobulinemia and in a patient with vascular disease.[162]

Pines et al.[163] reported a case of recurrent abortion in a patient with *C. jejuni* infection.

10.3.2 *CAMPYLOBACTER FETUS*-ASSOCIATED INFECTIONS

C. fetus ssp. *fetus*-associated endocarditis has been seldomly reported.[164] Nevertheless, the pathogen can cause severe endocarditis and thrombophlebitis because of its tendency to affect the vascular endothelium.

Righter and Woods[165] reported the case of a patient with *C. fetus* ssp. *fetus*-induced aortic aneurysm who recovered successfully after one-stage surgical repair and antibiotic therapy with erythromycin.

Carbone et al.[166] reported four cases of thrombophlebitis and cellulitis due to *C. fetus* ssp. *fetus*. Usually, such vascular infection with thrombophlebitis has been observed predominantly in adult male patients with underlying debilitating or immunocompromising illnesses.[167] Because the mortality from this condition may reach as high as 32%, empiric therapy with erythromycin, combined with an aminoglycoside or chloramphenicol has been recommended in suspect patients pending results of blood cultures.[166]

Kato et al.[168] reported a case of *C. fetus*-related infection of an abdominal aortic aneurysm which was treated surgically followed by antibiotic therapy consisting of intravenous infusion of fosfomycin and gentamicin and oral administration of minocycline. *C. fetus*, which in this particular case was cultured from the aneurysmal wall and intraluminal thrombi, should be considered in all situations involving infectious aneurysm in elderly or debilitated patients.

C. fetus ssp. *fetus*-related fetal loss or neonatal sepsis during pregnancy has also been reported. In one such instance, the infection was treated successfully with ampicillin and gentamicin.[169] Although rare, similar infections involving other *Campylobacter* spp. (*C. jejuni/coli*) have also been described. Even though all of the mothers survived, the fetal/neonatal mortality reached 80%. The pathogenesis of this campylobacter infection probably involved maternal bacteremia originating from the bowel with subsequent fetoplacental involvement.[169]

Morooka et al.[170] reported a nosocomial outbreak of *C. fetus* ssp. *fetus*-associated meningitis in a neonatal intensive care unit where asymptomatic carriers may have played a role in the transmission of infection.

The recommended treatment of *C. fetus* infections was with antibiotics.[171,172] *In vitro* testing of 22 antibiotics against 22 clinical isolates of *C. fetus* showed that combinations of ampicillin with cefazolin or gentamicin exhibited the highest synergistic effect.[172] Kato et al.[173] have described a case of *C. fetus* ssp. *fetus*-related meningitis in which the patient (with underlying chronic alcoholism and diabetes mellitus) did not respond to treatment with piperacillin and cefotaxime, but did respond to ampicillin and moxalactam and remained free of recurrent illness for 1 month after discontinuation of therapy.

In a review of *C. fetus*-related septic arthritis, Joly et al.[174] reported that most of the patients tended to be elderly with preexisting diseased joints and underlying illnesses such as alcoholism, cirrhosis, cancer, or diabetes. There was little radiographic evidence of bone destruction, and most patients have been cured with no recurrence of infection.

C. fetus ssp. *intestinalis*, which usually resides in the gastrointestinal tracts of cattle and sheep, has occasionally caused human disease affecting most often the elderly and debilitated patients. Diarrhea, however, was not a common presentation in *C. intestinalis* infections. Instead, sporadic cases of bacteremia, thrombophlebitis, and endocarditis have been reported in debilitated patients diagnosed with *C. intestinalis* infections.

Rao and Ralston[175] have described a case of *C. intestinalis*-induced meningitis in a kidney transplant recipient which was possibly associated with nutritional therapy. The sepsis was successfully treated with chloramphenicol (initial dose of 1.0 g every 4 h for 2 d, IV; then 1.0 g every 6 h for 2 weeks, IV); to prevent relapse, 1.0 g of erythromycin was administered daily (in divided doses) for 4 weeks. Wens et al.[176] identified the same subspecies as the cause of peritonitis followed by septicemia in a patient treated by continuous ambulatory peritoneal dialysis; parenteral tobramycin followed by oral erythromycin achieved a complete cure of this unusual complication.

In a randomized, placebo-controlled trial, Petruccelli et al.[177] have studied the efficacy of loperamide given with long- and short-course ciprofloxacin therapy of travelers' diarrhea; 41% of pretreatment stool specimen cultures were attributed to *Campylobacter*. Patients received 750 mg of ciprofloxacin with placebo, 750 mg of ciprofloxacin with loperamide, or a 3-d course of 500 mg of ciprofloxacin (b.i.d.) with loperamide. While not delivering a remarkable therapeutic advantage, loperamide appears to be safe for treatment of *Campylobacter* enteritis; there was a clinical relapse in 2 of 54 patients due to ciprofloxacin resistance.

10.3.3 *CAMPYLOBACTER* INFECTIONS IN HIV-POSITIVE AND AIDS PATIENTS

In several reports, the role and treatment of *Campylobacter* infections in HIV-positive and AIDS patients have been extensively discussed.[11,82,178-181]

In general, immunocompromised patients, such as those with malignant neoplasms, hypogammaglobulinemia, recipients of corticosteroid therapy, and AIDS patients appeared predisposed to chronic or recurrent *C. jejuni*-associated enterocolitis.[181-183] One should note that in some cases, chronic *Campylobacter* infections in immunocompromised hosts can be mistaken for colitis or Crohn's disease.[11,82,179,181] AIDS patients, who have a decreased population of T helper lymphocytes in their intestinal mucosa,[184] often suffer from chronic diarrheal disease and in many cases the infection-causing enteropathogen is not identified.[185] It has also been postulated that direct HIV-1 infection of the gut mucosa may be responsible for malabsorption and cause of disease.[186] Therefore, careful microbiological examination of stool samples for *Campylobacter* spp. should be very beneficial in diagnosing nonspecific colitis and chronic, seemingly pathogen-negative, diarrhea in HIV-positive patients.[187]

Although *C. jejuni* infection is known to occur frequently in young adults[3] and immunocompetent homosexual men,[188] it has also been diagnosed in HIV-positive patients.[179,189] In fact, bacteremia has been significantly more common in AIDS patients infected with *C. jejuni* than in otherwise healthy controls with *C. jejuni* infection.[178]

Funke et al.[190] have reported a case of an AIDS patient where identical isolates of *C. jejuni* susceptible, and later resistant, to macrolide antibiotics were isolated from feces before and after treatment with clarithromycin. Results from rRNA gene restriction analysis and serotyping have indicated that development of resistance rather than simultaneous infection with a susceptible and resistant strain has been responsible for this phenomenon. This finding was the first reported case of *in vivo* development of resistance by *C. jejuni* in a patient treated with a macrolide antibiotic.

Perlman et al.[181] described *C. jejuni* infection in four HIV-positive patients, of whom three had persistent and severe infection. Two treatment regimens were applied: (1) erythromycin (500 mg orally, every 6 h for 2 weeks); since fever and liquid stools persisted, oral tetracycline

(500 mg, every 8 h) was initiated, leading to partial healing of ileal ulcers, and (2) tetracycline (500 mg orally, every 6 h for 4 weeks). Although initially the bacteria were susceptible, during the course of treatment erythromycin-resistant isolates developed. All four patients had significantly elevated serum total IgA levels; as for the IgG and IgM levels, the ratios of *Campylobacter*-specific to total immunoglobulins were not markedly different from those in immunocompetent controls.[181]

Peterson et al.[191] described a unique case of prosthetic hip infection and bacteremia due to *C. jejuni* in a hemophiliac AIDS patient. The patient received extensive antibiotic treatment lasting for 8 weeks and consisting of intravenous gentamicin (80 mg or 1.5 mg/kg every 12 h) and ciprofloxacin (400 mg every 12 h) for a 17-d course; however, due to renal failure, gentamicin was substituted with intravenous erythromycin (500 mg every 6 h) and the ciprofloxacin dosage was reduced to 200 mg every 24 h. In this case, the observed severity of manifestations of osteomyelitis (lucency in the mural cavity of the femur and erosion of the cortex around the femoral component of the hip prosthesis) was in contrast to a previous report[174] of *C. fetus*-induced septic arthritis in which the immunocompetent patients showed little evidence of bone destruction.

Evans and Riley[11] reported a case of an HIV-positive patient for whom quinolone treatment of an initial *C. jejuni* infection was associated with development of colitis due to ciprofloxacin-resistant *C. laridis*. An initial 10-d course of ciprofloxacin led to complete abatement of symptoms; however, because of disease recurrence, the therapy was changed to intravenous doxycycline. *C. laridis* has been usually sensitive to aminoglycosides, ampicillin, erythromycin, norfloxacin, and tetracycline, but may develop resistance to cephalosporins, penicillin G, trimethoprim, trimethoprim-sulfamethoxazole, and vancomycin.[8,9]

Two other campylobacter species, *C. cinaedi* and *C. fennelliae*, have also been associated with enteritis in immunocompetent homosexual men.[181] The infection by these organisms, which is very often asymptomatic and rarely the cause of bacteremia,[192-196] could be manifested with diarrhea, abdominal cramps, and proctitis. Both species have been identified in HIV-positive individuals too.[188,192,196-198] Phenotypic characterization of clinical isolates has been based on morphology, motility, growth characteristics, and biochemical reactions.[133,199,200]

Sacks et al.[180] have used ciprofloxacin for the successful eradication of *C. cinaedi*-induced bacteremia in an HIV-positive homosexual man. The initial therapy, consisting of a 2-week course of oral erythromycin (500 mg every 6 h), followed by a 2-week course of oral tetracycline (500 mg every 6 h), and then intravenous erythromycin (1.0 g every 6 h), did not resolve the fever and persistent malaise, and blood cultures remained *Campylobacter*-positive. However, a 2-week course of oral ciprofloxacin (500 mg every 12 h) led to resolution of fever and diarrhea in 4 d, with pathogen-negative blood cultures.[180] In a separate case reported by Cimolai et al.,[192] an AIDS patient presented with fever, diarrhea, and *C. cinaedi*-positive blood cultures; the patient responded to treatment with tobramycin, cefazolin, and erythromycin. Decker et al.[201] have also described a case of an HIV-positive patient with *C. cinaedi*-related bacteremia which was resistant to erythromycin (500 mg orally, every 6 h for 12 d) but was successfully treated with oral ciprofloxacin (500 mg every 12 h for 1 week); it is of interest to mention that contrary to other reports of *C. cinaedi*-associated illness, the patient did not present with diarrhea or gastrointestinal disorders.

In HIV-positive patients, *C. fennelliae*-associated infection has been first documented by Ng et al.[196] Later, Kemper et al.[197] described *C. fennelliae*-like organisms as an important but concealed cause of bacteremia in a patient with AIDS.

In another report,[193] two homosexual men with bacteremia associated with *Campylobacter*-like organisms, who presented with fever, immunodeficiency, and concurrent tuberculosis, had received a predominantly antituberculosis multidrug regimen, which made it difficult to assess the effectiveness of any other single drug.

10.3.3.1   *Helicobacter pylori*-Induced Infections in HIV-Positive Patients

Battan et al.[202] have conducted a controlled study on HIV-infected patients undergoing upper endoscopy to evaluate the prevalence of *Helicobacter pylori* (*C. pylori*) infection, to correlate its presence with histologic and endoscopic findings, and to determine the behavior of this organism in the HIV-infected population. In general, the data collected indicated that HIV-infected patients were not more likely than other patients with upper gastrointestinal symptoms to be infected with *H. pylori*, or to develop type B chronic gastritis, and that in HIV-seropositive patients *H. pylori* remained noninvasive. Dorrell et al.[203] described an AIDS patient who in addition to *Candida albicans* infection, had presented with active chronic gastritis and nonspecific duodenitis. The patient received treatment consisting of oral amoxycillin (500 mg every 8 h) and metronidazole (400 mg every 8 h) for 2 weeks, as well as a course of bismuth (20 ml/240 mg, b.i.d.) for 1 month. The patient responded with a dramatic resolution of symptoms. These and other findings[204] strongly suggested that cell-mediated immune deficiency caused by HIV infection does not appear to increase the risk of infection with *H. pylori*.

10.4   HOST IMMUNE RESPONSE TO CAMPYLOBACTERIOSIS

Infection with *C. jejuni* is known to trigger a significant host immune response.[205] Furthermore, it was also demonstrated that repeated natural infections markedly elevated the antibody titer.[205,206] Immunocompetent hosts would normally produce *C. jejuni*-specific immunoglobulins in both serum[207] and intestinal fluids,[208] and elevated levels of preexisting antibodies may protect against symptomatic expression of infection.[209] Epidemiological data have indicated that humans become resistant only to clinical disease but not to intestinal colonization by the pathogen.[206]

AIDS patients with *Campylobacter* infection often present with elevated levels of serum immunoglobulins[210] which is likely due to polyclonal activation of B cells.[211] Findings by Perlman et al.,[181] coupled with the observation that patients with hypogammaglobulinemia suffered with severe and persistent *C. jejuni* infection,[5] implied that humoral immunity should be a major factor in controlling intestinal *Campylobacter* infections in immunocompromised hosts.[212]

The use of exogenous cytokines is considered to be one of the nonspecific ways to augment the ongoing specific immune response and to enhance the immune competency of the host. In a recent study, Baqar et al.[213] investigated the effects of several oral recombinant interleukins (rIL-2, rIL-5, and rIL-6) on the course of *C. jejuni* infection and the development of mucosal immunity in mice. Within 48 h of infection, the rIL-6-treated mice showed greater than 3-log-unit reduction in the number of *Campylobacter* shed in the feces. Although at somewhat slower clearance rate, colonization levels have been similarly reduced in rIL-5-treated animals, whereas treatment with rIL-2 had no significant effect on colonization levels as compared to controls. Furthermore, rIL-6 also elicited the most potent intestinal and systemic *C. jejuni*-specific IgA responses. Upon rechallenge, while the initial colonization in all cytokine-treated groups was approximately 2-log-units lower than that of controls, over time only rIL-2 was capable of controlling the local infection.[213] While these experiments provided no clear evidence for the mechanism(s) by which the infection was controlled in rIL-6-treated animals, it has been previously demonstrated that rIL-6 increased the antibody-dependent cellular cytotoxicity of polymorphonuclear leukocytes.[214] Based on the collected data, it appears that rIL-6 had the most potent effect on the elimination of *C. jejuni* from the intestines. In summary, although by different mechanisms, all three interleukins seem to play important roles in modulating the induction and/or expression of anti-*C. jejuni* immunity, thereby affecting the clinical course of the infection.

In several studies, ankylosing spondylitis, a seronegative polyarthritis, has been strongly associated with HLA-B27. While the etiology and pathogenesis of this condition are still not well understood, the search for a microbial cause (especially an enteric infection) has been stimulated by the presence of increased levels of total serum IgA in patients with ankylosing spondylitis.[215] In addition, increased levels of total serum IgG and IgM, although less frequently, have also been observed.[216] Evidence has been presented[217] that certain pathogenic Gram-negative bacteria shared a common antigen which cross-reacted with HLA B27-positive cells thereby hinting at the possibility that this cross-reactivity may somehow be related to the pathogenesis of ankylosing spondylitis. To shed more light on the matter, Andreasen et al.[218] investigated 22 patients with active ankylosing spondylitis to assess the levels of specific serum IgG, IgA, and IgM titers against *C. jejuni/coli* before and during treatment with sulfasalazine. The results, which showed no increase in pathogen-related antibodies, seemed not to support the hypothesis that *C. jejuni/coli* plays any significant role in the pathogenesis of active ankylosing spondylitis.

10.5   *CAMPYLOBACTER JEJUNI* BACTEREMIA AND THE GUILLAIN-BARRÉ SYNDROME

There have been an increasing number of reports[219-226] of patients developing Guillain-Barré syndrome[227] following *C. jejuni* gastrointestinal infection. In the observed cases, usually symptoms of *C. jejuni*-associated diarrhea had preceded the onset of the Guillain-Barré syndrome by 5 to 10 d, and the severity of the syndrome varied greatly. In one of the reports, Mishu et al.[222] found more frequent serologic evidence associating the Guillain-Barré syndrome with previous *C. jejuni* infection than in patients with other neurological disorders or healthy controls. Further serologic evidence,[223] established the majority of *C. jejuni* organisms as being from the Penner serogroup 19.

Hagensee et al.[228] have reported a rare case of Guillain-Barré syndrome associated with *C. jejuni* bacteremia in a patient with chronic graft-versus-host disease (GVHD) who 1 year earlier underwent allogeneic bone marrow transplantation. It is not unusual to observe the Guillain-Barré syndrome, as well as other neuromuscular disorders (polymyositis, myasthenia gravis) in allogeneic bone marrow transplant recipients;[229-231] in addition, the Guillain-Barré syndrome has also been associated with high-dose preparative therapy of cytosine arabinoside, or immune dysfunction secondary to GVHD.[230,231] What made the report by Hagensee et al.[228] unusual was the fact that it was the first *C. jejuni*-related Guillain-Barré syndrome to occur in a bone marrow transplant recipient. The patient was treated intravenously with immunoglobulin and ciprofloxacin and had a partial recovery.

The exact pathologic mechanism of *C. jejuni*-associated Guillain-Barré syndrome is still unclear. Yuki et al.[225] have found that all such patients shared the HLA-B35 antigen as compared to only 14% of the general population. In another study by the same investigators,[226] 9 of 13 patients with *C. jejuni*-associated Guillain-Barré syndrome had the structurally related HLA types B35, B51, and Bw52. Yet another type, HLA-B7, was also found in these patients.[226,228] Further serologic evidence has identified infection with particular serotypes (O19 and O1) of *C. jejuni* to be more frequently associated with the Guillain-Barré syndrome.[222,226,228]

According to Hagensee et al.,[228] the pathophysiology of *C. jejuni*-associated Guillain-Barré syndrome may involve an HLA-related predisposition to develop immune response against antigens shared by *C. jejuni* and elements of the nervous system. Results from several other studies seem to corroborate this hypothesis. Thus, Yuki et al.[232] have found that patients with *C. jejuni*-associated Guillain-Barré syndrome had high titers of IgG antibodies against the axon-related ganglioside GM$_1$, and Fujimoto and Amako[224] were able to produce antisera against a particular *C. jejuni* isolate which in addition to eliciting the Guillain-Barré syndrome also cross-reacted with human PO myelin-specific proteins. This data, together with the clinical response observed in some patients treated intravenously with immunoglobulin and plasmapheresis,[227] supported a key role for the humoral response in the *C. jejuni*-associated Guillain-Barré syndrome.

10.6 REFERENCES

1. Totten, P. A., Fennell, C. L., Tenover, F. C., Wezenberg, J. M., Perine, P. L., Stamm, W. E., and Holmes, K. K., "*Campylobacter cinaedi*" (sp. nov.) and "*Campylobacter fennelliae*" (sp. nov.): two new *Campylobacter* species associated with enteric disease in homosexual men, *J. Infect. Dis.*, 151, 131, 1985.

2. Vandamme, P., Falsen, E., Rossau, R., Segers, P., Tytgat, R., and De Ley, J., Revision of *Campylobacter*, *Helicobacter* and *Wolinella* taxonomy: emendation of generic descriptions and proposal of *Arcobacter* gen.*nov*, *Int. J. Syst. Bacteriol.*, 41, 88, 1991.

3. Riley, L. W. and Finch, M. J., Results of the first year of national surveillance of *Campylobacter* infections in the United States, *J. Infect. Dis.*, 151, 956, 1985.

4. Blaser, M. J. and Reller, L. B., *Campylobacter* enteritis, *N. Engl. J. Med.*, 305, 1443, 1981.

5. LeBar, W. D., Menard, R. R., and Check, F. E., Hypogammaglobulinemia and recurrent *Campylobacter jejuni* infection, *J. Infect. Dis.*, 152, 1099, 1985.

6. Peterson, M. C., Clinical aspects of *Campylobacter jejuni* infections in adults, *West. J. Med.*, 161, 148, 1994.

7. Benjamin, J., Leaper, S., Owen, R. J., and Skirrow, M. B., Description of *Campylobacter laridis*, a new species comprising the nalidixic acid resistant thermophilic *Campylobacter* (NARTC) group, *Curr. Microbiol.*, 8, 231, 1980.

8. Tauxe, R. V., Patton, C. M., Edmonds, P., Barrett, T. J., Brenner, D. J., and Blake, P. A., Illness associated with *Campylobacter laridis*, a newly recognized *Campylobacter* species, *J. Clin. Microbiol.*, 21, 222, 1985.

9. Simor, A. E. and Wilcox, L., Enteritis associated with *Campylobacter laridis*, *J. Clin. Microbiol.*, 25, 10, 1987.

10. Goosens, H. and Butzler, J. P., Isolation and identification of *Campylobacter* spp., in *Campylobacter jejuni: Current Status and Future Trends*, Nachamkin, I., Blaser, M. J., and Tompkins, L. S., Eds., American Society for Microbiology, Washington, D.C., 1992, 93.

11. Evans, T. G. and Riley, D., *Campylobacter laridis* colitis in a human immunodeficiency virus-positive patient treated with a quinolone, *Clin. Infect. Dis.*, 15, 172, 1992.

12. Kirst, H. A. and Sides, G. D., New directions for macrolide antibiotics: pharmacokinetics and clinical efficacy, *Antimicrob. Agents Chemother.*, 23, 1419, 1989.

13. Adam, D., Clinical use of the new macrolides, azalides, and streptogramins in pediatrics, *J. Chemother.*, 4, 371, 1992.

14. Baker, A. O. and Adefeso, A. O., The changing patterns of *Campylobacter jejuni/coli* in Lagos, Nigeria after ten years, *East Afr. Med. J.*, 71, 437, 1994.

15. Williams, M. D., Schorling, J. B., Barrett, L. J., Orgel, I., Koch, R., Shields, D. S., and Guerrant, R. L., Early treatment of *Campylobacter jejuni* enteritis, *Antimicrob. Agents Chemother.*, 33, 248, 1989 (correction in *Antimicrob. Agents Chemother.*, 33, 248, 1989).

16. Robins-Browne, R. M., Coovadia, H. M., Bodasing, M. N., and Mackenjee, M. K. R., Treatment of acute nonspecific gastroenteritis of infants and young children with erythromycin, *Am. J. Trop. Med. Hyg.*, 32, 886, 1983.

17. O'Sullivan, N. and Wise, R., Macrolide, lincosamide, and streptogramin antibiotics, *Curr. Opinion Infect. Dis.*, 3, 743, 1990.

18. Stahlmann, R. and Lode, H., Clarithromycin — ein neues macrolidantibiotikum, *Arzneimittelther.*, 9, 225, 1991.

19. Hara, K., Rokitamycin, *J. Antibiot.*, 40, 1851, 1987.

20. Sakakibara, H., Okekawa, O., Fujisawa, T., Aizawa, M., and Omura, S., Acyl derivatives of 16-membered macrolides. II. Antibacterial activities and serum levels of 3'-*O*-acyl derivatives of leucomycin, *J. Antibiot.*, 34, 1011, 1981.

21. Motohiro, T., Fujii, R., Sasaki, H., Koga, T., Sakata, Y., and Yamashita, A., A comparative study of the efficacy of rokitamycin vs. those of erythromycin and fosfomycin against pediatric *Campylobacter* enteritis, *Proc. 17th Int. Congr. Chemother.*, Berlin, Abstr., 1991.

22. Gordillo, M. E., Singh, K. V., and Murray, B. E., *In vitro* activity of azithromycin against bacterial enteric pathogens, *Antimicrob. Agents Chemother.*, 37, 1203, 1993.

23. Taylor, D. E., De Grandis, S. A., Karmali, M. A., and Fleming, P. C., Transmissible plasmids from *Campylobacter jejuni*, *Antimicrob. Agents Chemother.*, 19, 831, 1981.

24. Taylor, D. N., Blaser, M. J., Echeverria, P., Pitarangsi, C., Bodhidatta, L., and Wang, W.-L. L., Erythromycin-resistant *Campylobacter* infections in Thailand, *Antimicrob. Agents Chemother.*, 31, 438, 1987.

25. Taylor, D. E., Chang, N., Garner, R. S., Sherburne, R., and Mueller, L., Incidence of antibiotic resistance and characterization of plasmids in *Campylobacter jejuni* strains isolated from clinical sources in Alberta, Canada, *Can. J. Microbiol.*, 32, 28, 1986.

26. Elharrif, Z. F., Megraud, F., and Marchand, A.-M., Susceptibility of *Campylobacter jejuni* and *Campylobacter coli* to macrolides and related compounds, *Antimicrob. Agents Chemother.*, 28, 695, 1985.

27. Wang, W.-L. L., Reller, L. R., and Blaser, M. J., Comparison of antimicrobial susceptibility patterns of *Campylobacter jejuni* and *Campylobacter coli*, *Antimicrob. Agents Chemother.*, 26, 351, 1984.

28. Panteix, G., Harf, R., de Montclos, H., Verdier, M. F., Gaspar, A., and Leclercq, M., Josamycin pulmonary penetration determined by broncho-alveolar lavage in man, *J. Antimicrob. Chemother.*, 22, 917, 1988.

29. Anderson, R., van Rensburg, C. E. J., Joone, G., and Lukey, P. T., An in-vitro comparison of the intraphagocytic bioactivity of erythromycin and roxithromycin, *J. Antimicrob. Chemother.*, 20(Suppl. B), 57, 1987.

30. Dette, G. A. and Knothe, H., Kinetics of erythromycin uptake and release by human lymphocytes and polymorphonuclear leucocytes, *J. Antimicrob. Chemother.*, 18, 73, 1986.

31. Johnson, J. D., Hand, W. L., Francis, J. B., King-Thompson, N., and Corvin, R. W., Antibiotic uptake by alveolar macrophages, *J. Lab. Clin. Med.*, 95, 429, 1980.

32. Prokesh, R. C. and Hand, W. L., Antibiotic entry into human polymorphonuclear leukocytes, *Antimicrob. Agents Chemother.*, 21, 373, 1982.

33. Raghoebar, M., Lindeyer, E., van den Berg, W. B., and van Ginneken, C. A. M., On the mechanisms of association of the macrolide antibiotic erythromycin with isolated human polymorphonuclear leucocytes, *Biochem. Pharmacol.*, 37, 3221, 1988.

34. Anderson, R., Joone, G., and van Rensburg, C. E. J., An in-vitro evaluation of the cellular uptake and intraphagocytic bioactivity of clarithromycin (A-56268, TE-031), a new macrolide antimicrobial agent, *J. Antimicrob. Chemother.*, 22, 923, 1988.

35. Anderson, R., van Rensburg, C. E. J., Eftychis, H., Joone, G., and van Rensburg, A. J., Further studies on erythromycin effects on cellular immune functions *in vitro* and *in vivo*, *J. Antimicrob. Chemother.*, 10, 409, 1982.

36. Nelson, S., Summer, W. R., Terry, P. B., Warr, G. A., and Jakab, G. J., Erythromycin-induced suppression of pulmonary antibacterial defenses: a potential mechanism of superinfection in the lung, *Am. Rev. Respir. Dis.*, 136, 1207, 1987.

37. van Rensburg, C. E. J., Anderson, R., Joone, G., van der Merwe, M., and van Rensburg, A. J., Effects of erythromycin on cellular and humoral immune functions *in vitro* and *in vivo*, *J. Antimicrob. Chemother.*, 8, 467, 1981.

38. Naess, A. and Solberg, C. O., Effects of two macrolide antibiotics on human leukocyte membrane receptors and functions, *Acta Pathol. Microbiol. Immunol. Scand.*, 96, 503, 1988.

39. Aho, P. and Mannisto, P. T., Effects of two erythromycins, doxycycline and phenoxymethylpenicillin on human leucocyte chemotaxis *in vitro*, *J. Antimicrob. Chemother.*, 21(Suppl. D), 29, 1988.

40. Forsgren, A. and Schmeling, D., Effects of antibiotics on chemotaxis of human leukocytes, *Antimicrob. Agents Chemother.*, 11, 580, 1977.

41. Neu, H. C., Clinical use of quinolones, *Lancet*, 2, 1319, 1987.

42. Waldvogel, F. A., Clinical role of the quinolones today and in the future, *Eur. J. Clin. Microbiol. Infect. Dis.*, 8, 1075, 1989.

43. DuPont, H. L., Use of quinolones in the treatment of gastrointestinal infections, *Eur. J. Clin. Microbiol. Infect. Dis.*, 10, 325, 1991.

44. Eggleston, M. and Park, S.-Y., Review of the 4-quinolones, *Infect. Control*, 8, 119, 1987.

45. Bow, E. J. and Louie, T. J., Emerging role of quinolone in the prevention of Gram-negative bacteremia in neutropenic cancer patients and in the treatment of enteric infections, *Clin. Invest. Med.*, 12, 61, 1989.

46. Rubinstein, E., Segv, S., and Lev, B., The 4-quinolones: a promising new class of antibiotics, *Hosp. Ther.*, 8, 39, 1986.

47. Hughes, P. J., Webb, D. B., and Ascher, A. W., Pharmacokinetics of norfloxacin (MK 366) in patients with impaired kidney function — some preliminary results, *J. Antimicrob. Chemother.*, 13(Suppl. B), 55, 1984.

48. Wise, R., Norfloxacin — a review of pharmacology and tissue preparation, *J. Antimicrob. Chemother.*, 13(Suppl. B), 59, 1984.

49. Adhami, Z. N., Wise, R., Weston, D., and Crump, B., The pharmacokinetics and tissue penetration of norfloxacin, *J. Antimicrob. Chemother.*, 13, 87, 1984.

50. Höffken, G., Lode, H., Prinzing, C., Borner, K., and Koeppe, P., Pharmacokinetics of ciprofloxacin after oral and parenteral administration, *Antimicrob. Agents Chemother.*, 27, 375, 1985.

51. Hoogkamp-Korstanje, J. A. A., Van Oort, H. J, Schipper, J. K., and van der Wal, T., Intraprostatic concentration of ciprofloxacin and its activity against urinary pathogens, *J. Antimicrob. Chemother.*, 14, 641, 1984.

52. Crump, B., Wise, R., and Dent, J., Pharmacokinetics and tissue penetration of ciprofloxacin, *Antimicrob. Agents Chemother.*, 24, 784, 1983.

53. Wise, R., Lockley, R. M., Webberly, M., and Dent, J., Pharmacokinetics of intravenously administered ciprofloxacin, *Antimicrob. Agents Chemother.*, 26, 208, 1984.

54. Gonzalez, M. A., Uribe, F., Moisen, S. D., Fuster, A. P., Selen, A., Welling, P. G., and Painter, B., Multiple-dose pharmacokinetics and safety of ciprofloxacin in normal volunteers, *Antimicrob. Agents Chemother.*, 26, 741, 1984.

55. Boelaert, J., Vlacke, Y., Schurgers, M., Daneels, R., Rosseneu, M., Rosseel, M. T., and Bogaert, M. G., The pharmacokinetics of ciprofloxacin in patients with impaired renal function, *J. Antimicrob. Chemother.*, 16, 87, 1985.

56. Tsuei, S. D., Darragh, A. S., and Brick, I., Pharmacokinetics and tolerance of enoxacin in healthy volunteers administered at a dosage of 400 mg daily for 14 days, *J. Antimicrob. Chemother.*, 14(Suppl. C), 71, 1984.

57. Wise, R., Lockley, R., Dent, J., and Webberly, M., Pharmacokinetics and tissue penetration of enoxacin, *Antimicrob. Agents Chemother.*, 26, 17, 1984.

58. Tartaglione, T. A., Raffalovich, A. C., Poynor, W. J., Espinel-Ingroff, A., and Kerkering, T. M., Pharmacokinetics and tolerance of ciprofloxacin after sequential increasing oral doses, *Antimicrob. Agents Chemother.*, 29, 62, 1986.

59. Brittain, D. C., Scully, B. E., McElrath, M. J., Steinman, R., Labthavikul, P., and Neu, H. C., The pharmacology of orally administered ciprofloxacin, *Drugs Experim. Clin. Res.*, 11, 339, 1985.

60. Bergan, T., Torsteinsson, S. B., Kolstad, I. M., and Johnsen, S., Pharmacokinetics of ciprofloxacin after intravenous and increasing oral doses, *Eur. J. Clin. Microbiol.*, 5, 187, 1986.

61. Editorial, Quinolones in acute non-travelers' diarrhoea, *Lancet*, 336, 282, 1990.

62. Piddock, L. V., Whale, K., and Wise, R., Quinolone resistance in salmonella: clinical experience, *Lancet*, 335, 1459, 1990.

63. Goodman, L. J., Trenholme, G. M., Kaplan, R. L., Segreti, J., Hines, D., Petrak, R., Nelson, J. A., Mayer, K. W., Landau, W., Parkhurst, G. W., and Levin, S., Empiric antimicrobial therapy of domestically acquired acute diarrhea in urban adults, *Arch. Intern. Med.*, 150, 541, 1990.

64. Carlstedt, G., Dahl, P., Niklasson, P. M., Gullberg, K., Banck, G., and Kahlmeter, G., Norfloxacin treatment of salmonellosis does not shorten the carrier stage, *Scand. J. Infect. Dis.*, 22, 553, 1990.

65. Neill, M. A., Opal, S. M., Heelan, J., Giusti, R., Cassidy, J. E., White, R., and Mayer K. H., Failure of ciprofloxacin to eradicate convalescent fecal excretion after acute salmonellosis: experience during an outbreak in health care workers, *Ann. Intern. Med.*, 114, 195, 1991.

66. Percival, A., Ed., *Quinolones — Their Future in Clinical Practice*, Royal Society of Medicine Services, London, 1986.

67. Wang, C., Sabbaj, J., Corrado, M., and Hoagland, V., World-wide clinical experience with norfloxacin: efficacy and safety, *Scand. J. Infect. Dis.*, 48(Suppl.), 81, 1986.

68. Ruiz-Palacios, G. M., Norfloxacin in the treatment of bacterial enteric infections, *Scand. J. Infect. Dis.*, 81(Suppl.), 55, 1986.

69. Cofsky, R. D., DuBouchet, L., and Landesman, S. H., Recovery of norfloxacin in feces after administration of a single oral dose to human volunteers, *Antimicrob. Agents Chemother.*, 26, 110, 1984.

70. Swanson, B. N., Boppana, V. K., Ulosses, P. H., Rotmensch, H. H., and Ferguson, R. K., Norfloxacin dispository after sequentially increasing oral doses, *Antimicrob. Agents Chemother.*, 23, 284, 1983.

71. Wiström, J., Jertborn, M., Ekwall, E., Norlin, K., Söderquist, B., Strömberg, A., Lundholm, R., Hogevik, H., Lagergren, L., Englund, G., Norrby, S. R., and the Swedish Study Group, Empiric treatment of acute diarrheal disease with norfloxacin: a randomized, placebo-controlled trial, *Ann. Intern. Med.*, 117, 202, 1992.

72. Wiström, J., Norrby, S. R., Burman, L. G., Lundholm, R., Jellheden, B., and Englund, G., Norfloxacin versus placebo for prophylaxis against travellers' diarrhoea, *J. Antimicrob. Chemother.*, 20, 563, 1987.

73. Bramfitt, W., Franklin, I., Grady, D., Hamilton-Miller, J. M. T., and Illife, A., Changes in the pharmacokinetics of ciprofloxacin and fecal flora during administration of a 7-day course to human volunteers, *Antimicrob. Agents Chemother.*, 26, 757, 1984.

74. Pichler, H., Diridl, G., and Wolf, D., Ciprofloxacin in the treatment of acute bacterial diarrhea, *Eur. J. Clin. Microbiol.*, 5, 241, 1986.

75. Pichler, H. E. T., Diridl, G., Stickler, K., and Wolf, D., Clinical efficacy of ciprofloxacin compared with placebo in bacterial diarrhea, *Am. J. Med.*, 82(Suppl. 4A), 329, 1987.

76. Nakamura, S., Minami, A., Nakata, K., Kurobe, N., Kuono, K., Sakaguchi, Y., Kashimoto, S., Yoshida, H., Kojima, T., Ohue, T., Fujimoto, K., Nakamura, M., Hashimoto, M., and Shimizu, M., *In vitro* and *in vivo* antibacterial activities of AT-4140, a new broad-spectrum quinolone, *Antimicrob. Agents Chemother.*, 33, 1167, 1989.

77. Tomayko, J. F., Korten, V., and Murray, B. E., DU-6859a, a new fluoroquinolone agent: comparative *in vitro* activity against enteric pathogens and multiresistant outpatient *Escherichia coli*, *Diagn. Microbiol. Infect. Dis.*, 20, 45, 1994.

78. Hosaka, M., Yasue, T., Fukuda, H., Tomizawa, H., Aoyama, H., and Hirai, K., *In vitro* and *in vivo* antibacterial activities of AM-1155, a new 6-fluoro-8-methoxyquinolone, *Antimicrob. Agents Chemother.*, 36, 2108, 1992.

79. Goossens, H., De Mol, P., Cougnau, H., Levy, J., Grados, O., Ghysels, G., Aremye Innocent, H., and Butzler, J. P., Comparative *in vitro* activities of aztreonam, ciprofloxacin, norfloxacin, HR 810 (a new cephalosporin), RU 28965 (a new macrolide) and other agents against enteropathogens, *Antimicrob. Agents Chemother.*, 27, 388, 1985.

80. Lariviere, L. A., Gandreau, C. L., and Turgeon, F. F., Susceptibilities of clinical isolates of *Campylobacter jejuni* to twenty-five antimicrobial agents, *J. Antimicrob. Chemother.*, 18, 681, 1986.

81. Hirschl, A. M., Wolf, D., Berger, J., and Rotter, M. L., *In vitro* susceptibilities of *Campylobacter jejuni* and *Campylobacter coli* isolated in Austria to erythromycin and ciprofloxacin, *Zentralbl. Bakteriol. Hyg. (A)*, 272, 443, 1990.

82. Bernard, E., Roger, P. M., Carles, D., Bonaldi, V., Fournier, J. P., and Dellamonica, P., Diarrhea and *Campylobacter* infections in patients infected with the human immunodeficiency virus, *J. Infect. Dis.*, 159, 143, 1989.

83. Segreti, J., Gootz, T. D., Goodman, L. J., Parkhurst, G. W., Quinn, J. P., Martin, B. A., and Trenholme, G. M., High-level quinolone resistance in clinical isolates of *Campylobacter jejuni*, *J. Infect. Dis.*, 165, 667, 1992.

84. Wang, W.-L. L., Reller, L. B., and Blaser, M. J., Comparison of antimicrobial susceptibility patterns between *Campylobacter jejuni* and *Campylobacter coli*, *Antimicrob. Agents Chemother.*, 26, 351, 1984.

85. Endtz, H. P., Mouton, R. P., van der Reyden, T., Ruijs, G. J., Biever, M., and van Klingeren, B., Fluoroquinolone resistance in *Campylobacter* spp. isolated from human stools and poultry products, *Lancet*, 335, 787, 1990.

86. Taylor, D. E., Ng, L. K., and Lior, H., Susceptibility of *Campylobacter* species to nalidixic acid, enoxacin and other DNA-gyrase-inhibitors, *Antimicrob. Agents Chemother.*, 28, 708, 1985.

87. Walder, M., Sandstedt, K., and Ursing, J., Phenotypic characteristics of thermotolerant *Campylobacter* from human and animal sources, *Curr. Microbiol.*, 9, 291, 1983.

88. Vanhoof, R., Vanderlinden, M. P., Dierickx, R., Lauwers, S., Yourassowsky, E., and Butzler, J. P., Susceptibility of *Campylobacter fetus* subsp. *jejuni* to twenty nine antimicrobial agents, *Antimicrob. Agents Chemother.*, 14, 553, 1978.

89. Altwegg, M., Burnens, A., Zollinger-Iten, J., and Penner, J. L., Problems in identification of *Campylobacter jejuni* associated with acquisition of resistance to nalidixic acid, *J. Clin. Microbiol.*, 25, 1807, 1987.

90. Reina, J. and Alomar, P., Fluoroquinolone-resistance in thermophilic *Campylobacter* spp. isolated from stools of Spanish patients, *Lancet*, 336, 186, 1990.

91. Reina, J., Borrell, N., and Serra, A., Emergence of resistance to erythromycin and fluoroquinolones in thermotolerant *Campylobacter* strains isolated from feces 1987–1991, *Eur. J. Clin. Microbiol. Infect. Dis.*, 11, 1163, 1992.

92. Mirelis, B., Miro, E., Navarro, F., Ogalla, C. A., Bonal, J., and Prats, G., Increased resistance to quinolone in Catalonia, Spain, *Diagn. Microbiol. Infect. Dis.*, 16, 137, 1993.

93. Adler-Mosca, H., Lüthy-Hottenstein, J., Martinetti Lucchini, G., Burnens, A., and Altwegg, M., Development of resistance to quinolones in five patients with norfloxacin or ciprofloxacin, *Eur. J. Clin. Microbiol. Infect. Dis.*, 10, 953, 1991.

94. Anderson, J. J., *In vitro* susceptibility of *Campylobacter jejuni* and *Campylobacter coli* isolated in Denmark to fourteen antimicrobial agents, *Acta Pathol. Microbiol. Immunol. Scand.*, 95, 189, 1987.

95. Wretlind, B., Strömberg, A., Ostlund, L., Sjögren, E., and Kauser, B., Rapid emergence of quinolone resistance in Campylobacter jejuni in patients treated with norfloxacin, *Scand. J. Infect. Dis.*, 24, 685, 1992.

96. Gopal Rao, G., Development of spontaneous resistance to ciprofloxacin in a strain of *Campylobacter jejuni*, *J. Antimicrob. Chemother.*, 28, 317, 1991.

97. Cohen, S. P., McMurry, L. M., Hooper, D. C., Wolfson, J. S., and Levy, J. S., Cross-resistance to fluoroquinolones in multiple-antibiotic resistant (Mar) *Escherichia coli* selected by tetracycline or chloramphenicol decreased drug accumulation associated with membrane changes in addition to OmpF reduction, *Antimicrob. Agents Chemother.*, 33, 1318, 1989.

98. Wiedemann, B. and Heisig, P., Mechanisms of quinolone resistance, *Infection*, 22(Suppl. 2), S73, 1994.

99. Cozzarelli, N. R., DNA gyrase and supercoiling of DNA, *Science*, 207, 953, 1980.

100. Gellert, M., DNA topoisomerases, *Annu. Rev. Biochem.*, 50, 879, 1981.

101. Wang, J. C., DNA topoisomerases, *Annu. Rev. Biochem.*, 54, 665, 1985.

102. Reece, R. J. and Maxwell, A., DNA gyrase: structure and function, *Crit. Rev. Biochem. Mol. Biol.*, 26, 335, 1991.

103. Bachmann, B. J. and Low, K. B., Linkage map of *Escherichia coli* K-12, edition 6, *Microbiol. Rev.*, 44, 1, 1980.

104. Moyira, S., Ogasawara, N., and Yoshikawa, H., Structure and function of the replication origin of the *Bacillus subtilis* chromosome. III, *Nucleic Acids Res.*, 13, 2251, 1985.

105. Swanberg, S. L. and Wang, J. C., Cloning and sequencing of the *Escherichia coli gyr*A gene coding for the A subunit of DNA gyrase, *J. Mol. Biol.*, 197, 729, 1987.

106. Wyckoff, E., Natalie, D., Nolan, J. M., Lee, M., and Hsieh, T.-S., Structure of the *Drosophila* DNA topoisomerase II gene: nucleotide sequence and homology among DNA topoisomerases II, *J. Mol. Biol.*, 205, 1, 1989.

107. Dimri, G. P. and Das, H. K., Cloning and sequence analysis of *gyr*A gene of *Klebsiella pneumoniae*, *Nucleic Acids Res.*, 18, 151, 1990.

108. Wang, Y., Huang, W. M., and Taylor, D. E., Cloning and nucleotide sequence of the *Campylobacter jejuni gyr*A gene and characterization of quinolone resistance mutations, *Antimicrob. Agents Chemother.*, 37, 457, 1993.

109. Hane, M. W. and Wood, T. H., *Escherichia coli* K-12 mutants resistant to nalidixic acid: genetic mapping and dominance studies, *J. Bacteriol.*, 99, 238, 1969.

110. Sugino, A., Peebles, C. L., Kreuzer, K. N., and Cozzarelli, N. R., Mechanism of action of nalidixic acid: purification of *Escherichia coli nal*A gene product and its relationship to DNA gyrase and a novel nicking-closing enzyme, *Proc. Natl. Acad. Sci. U.S.A.*, 74, 4767, 1977.

111. Gellert, M., Mizuuchi, K., O'Dea, M. H., Itoh, T., and Tomizawa, J.-L., Nalidixic acid resistance: a second genetic character involved in DNA gyrase activity, *Proc. Natl. Acad. Sci. U.S.A.*, 74, 4772, 1977.

112. Hooper, D. C., Wolfson, J. S., Souza, K. S., Tung, C., McHugh, G. L., and Swartz, M. N., Genetic and biochemical characterization of norfloxacin resistance in *Escherichia coli*, *Antimicrob. Agents Chemother.*, 29, 639, 1986.

113. Hirai, K., Aoyama, H., Suzue, S., Irikura, T., Iyobe, S., and Mitsubishi, S., Isolation and characterization of norfloxacin-resistant mutants of *Escherichia coli* K-12, *Antimicrob. Agents Chemother.*, 30, 248, 1986.

114. Hooper, D. C., Wolfson, J. S., Ng, E. Y., and Swartz, M. N., Mechanism of action of and resistance to ciprofloxacin, *Am. J. Med.*, 82(Suppl. 4A), 12, 1987.

115. Horowitz, D. S. and Wang, J. C., Mapping the active site tyrosine of *Escherichia coli* DNA gyrase, *J. Biol. Chem.*, 262, 5339, 1987.

116. Yoshida, H., Bogaki, M., Nakamura, M., and Nakamura, S., Quinolone resistance-determining region in the DNA gyrase *gyr*A gene of *Escherichia coli*, *Antimicrob. Agents Chemother.*, 34, 1271, 1990.

117. Wang, Y., Huang, W. M., and Taylor, D. E., Cloning and nucleotide sequence of the *Campylobacter jejuni gyr*A gene and characterization of quinolone resistance mutations, *Antimicrob. Agents Chemother.*, 37, 457, 1993.

118. Gootz, T. D. and Martin, B. A., Characterization of high-level quinolone resistance in *Campylobacter jejuni*, *Antimicrob. Agents Chemother.*, 35, 840, 1991.

119. Cambau, E., Sougakoff, W., Besson, M., Truffot-Pernot, C., Grosset, J., and Jarlier, V., Selection of *gyr*A mutant of *Mycobacterium tuberculosis* resistant to fluoroquinolones during treatment with ofloxacin, *J. Infect. Dis.*, 170, 479, 1994.

120. Yoshida, H., Nakamura, M., Bogaki, M., and Nakamura, S., Proportion of DNA gyrase mutants among quinolone-resistant strains of *Pseudomonas aeruginosa*, *Antimicrob. Agents Chemother.*, 34, 1273, 1990.

121. Nikaido, H. and Rosenberg, E. Y., Porin channels in *Escherichia coli*: studies with liposomes reconstituted from purified proteins, *J. Bacteriol.*, 153, 241, 1983.

122. Chapman, J. S., Bertasso, A., and Georgopapadakou, N. H., Fleroxacin resistance in *Escherichia coli*, *Antimicrob. Agents Chemother.*, 33, 239, 1989.

123. Cohen, S. P., Hooper, D. C., Wolfson, J. S., Souza, K. S., McMurry, L. M., and Levy, S. B., Endogenous active efflux of norfloxacin in susceptible *Escherichia coli*, *Antimicrob. Agents Chemother.*, 32, 1187, 1988.

124. Kumar, S., Properties of adenyl cyclase and cyclic adenosine 3',5'-monophosphate receptor protein-deficient mutants of *Escherichia coli*, *J. Bacteriol.*, 125, 545, 1976.

125. Scott, N. W. and Harwood, C. R., Studies on the influence of the cyclic AMP system on major outer membrane proteins of *Escherichia coli*, *FEMS Microbiol. Lett.*, 9, 95, 1980.

126. Hooper, D. C., Wolfson, J. S., Souza, K. S., Ng, E. Y., McHugh, G. L., and Swartz, M. N., Mechanisms of quinolone resistance in *Escherichia coli*: characterization of *nfx*B and *nfx*C, two mutant resistance loci decreasing norfloxacin accumulation, *Antimicrob. Agents Chemother.*, 33, 283, 1989.

127. Cohen, S. P., McMurry, L. M., Hooper, D. C., Wolfson, J. S., and Levy, S. B., Cross-resistance to fluoroquinolones in multiple-antibiotic-resistant (Mar) *Escherichia coli* selected by tetracycline or chloramphenicol: decreased drug accumulation associated with membrane changes in addition to OmpF reduction, *Antimicrob. Agents Chemother.*, 33, 1318, 1989.

128. Greenberg, J. T., Chou, J. H., Monach, P. A., and Demple, B., Activation of oxidative stress genes by mutations at the *sox*Q/*cfx*B/*mar*A locus of *Escherichia coli*, *J. Bacteriol.*, 173, 4433, 1991.

129. Hooper, D. C., Wolfson, J. S., Bozza, M. A., and Ng, E. Y., Genetics and regulation of outer membrane protein expression by quinolone resistance loci *nfx*B, *nfx*C, and *cfx*B, *Antimicrob. Agents Chemother.*, 36, 1151, 1992.

130. Logan, S. M. and Trust, T. J., Outer membrane characteristics of *Campylobacter jejuni*, *Infect. Immun.*, 38, 898, 1982.

131. Shen, L. L. and Pernet, A. G., Mechanism of inhibition of DNA gyrase by analogues of nalidixic acid: the target of the drugs is DNA, *Proc. Natl. Acad. Sci. U.S.A.*, 82, 307, 1985.

132. Piddock, L. J. V., Mechanism of quinolone uptake into bacterial cells, *J. Antimicrob. Chemother.*, 27, 399, 1991.

133. Flores, B. M., Fennell, C. L., Holmes, K. K., and Stamm, W. E., *In vitro* susceptibilities of *Campylobacter*-like organisms to twenty antimicrobial agents, *Antimicrob. Agents Chemother.*, 28, 188, 1985.

134. Shah, P. M., Enzensberger, R., Glogau, O., and Knothe, H., Influence of oral ciprofloxacin or ofloxacin on the fecal flora of healthy volunteers, *Am. J. Med.*, 82(Suppl. 4A), 333, 1987.

135. Richardson, N. J., Koornhof, H. J., and Bokkenheuser, V. D., Long-term infections with *Campylobacter fetus* subsp. *jejuni*, *J. Clin. Microbiol.*, 13, 846, 1981.

136. Blaser, M. J., Glass, R. I., Huq, M. I., Stoll, B., Kibriya, G. M., and Alim, A. R. M. A., Isolation of *Campylobacter fetus* spp. *jejuni* from Bangladeshi children, *J. Clin. Microbiol.*, 12, 744, 1980.

137. Bokkenheuser, V. D., Richardson, N. J., Bryner, J. H., Roux, D. J., Schutte, A. B., Koornhof, H. J., Freiman, I., and Hartman, E., Detection of enteric campylobacteriosis in children, *J. Clin. Microbiol.*, 9, 227, 1979.

138. Rajan, D. P. and Mathan, V. I., Prevalence of *Campylobacter fetus* spp. *jejuni* in healthy populations in Southern India, *J. Clin. Microbiol.*, 15, 749, 1982.

139. Thea, D. M., St. Louis, M. E., Atido, U., Kanjinga, K., Kembo, B., Matondo, M., Tshiamala, T., Kamenga, C., Davachi, F., Brown, C., Rand, W. M., and Keusch, G. T., A prospective study of diarrhea and HIV-1 infection among 429 Zairian infants, *N. Engl. J. Med.*, 329, 1696, 1993.

140. Guerrant, R. L., Lahita, R. G., Winn, W. C., and Roberts, R. B., Campylobacteriosis in man: pathogenic mechanisms and review of 91 blood stream infections, *Am. J. Med.*, 65, 584, 1978.

141. Rettig, P. J., Campylobacter infections in human beings, *J. Pediatr.*, 94, 855, 1979.

142. Wiström, J., Jertborn, M., Hedström, S. A., Alestig, K., Englund, G., Jellheden, B., and Norrby, S. R., Short-term self-treatment of travelers' diarrhoea with norfloxacin: a placebo-controlled study, *J. Antimicrob. Chemother.*, 23, 905, 1989.

143. Rademaker, C. M. A., Hoepelman, I. M., Wolfhagen, M. J. H. M., Beumer, H., Rozenberg-Arska, M., and Verhoef, J., Results of a double-blind placebo-controlled study using ciprofloxacin for prevention of travelers' diarrhea, *Eur. J. Clin. Microbiol. Infect. Dis.*, 8, 690, 1989.

144. DuPont, H. L., Ericsson, C. D., Robinson, A., and Johnson, P. C., Current problems in antimicrobial therapy for bacterial enteric infection, *Am. J. Med.*, 82(Suppl. 4A), 324, 1987.

145. Nolan, C. M., Johnson, K. E., Coyle, M. B., and Faler, K., *Campylobacter jejuni* enteritis: efficacy of antimicrobial and antimotility drugs, *Am. J. Gastroenterol.*, 78, 621, 1983.

146. Anders, B. J., Lauer, B. A., Paisley, J. W., and Reller, L. B., Double-blind placebo controlled trial of erythromycin for treatment of *Campylobacter enteritis*, *Lancet*, 1, 131, 1982.

147. Karmali, M. A. and Fleming, P. C., *Campylobacter enteritis* in children, *J. Pediatr.*, 94, 527, 1979.

148. Mandal, B. K., Ellis, M. E., Dunbar, E. M., and Whale, K., Double-blind placebo-controlled trial of erythromycin in the treatment of clinical campylobacter infection, *J. Antimicrob. Chemother.*, 13, 619, 1984.

149. Pai, C. H., Gillis, F., Tuomanen, E., and Marks, M. I., Erythromycin in treatment of *Campylobacter enteritis* in children, *Am. J. Dis. Child.*, 137, 286, 1983.

150. Pitkanen, T., Pettersson, T., and Ponka, A., Effect of erythromycin on the excretion of *Campylobacter fetus* subspecies *jejuni*, *J. Infect. Dis.*, 145, 128, 1982.

151. Robins-Browne, R. M., Mackenjee, M. K. R., Bodasing, M. N., and Coovadia, H. M., Treatment of *Campylobacter*-associated enteritis with erythromycin, *Am. J. Dis. Child.*, 137, 282, 1983.

152. Salazar-Lindo, E., Sack, R. B., Chea-Woo, E., Kay, B. A., Piscoya, Z. A., Leon-Barua, R., and Yi, A., Early treatment with erythromycin of *Campylobacter jejuni*-associated dysentery in children, *J. Pediatr.*, 109, 357, 1986.

153. Schwartz, R. H., Early treatment with erythromycin for *Campylobacter jejuni*-associated diarrhea, *J. Pediatr.*, 110, 165, 1987.

154. Verbruggen, P., Creve, U., Hubens, A., and Verhaegen, J., *Campylobacter fetus* as a cause of acute cholecystitis, *Br. J. Surg.*, 73, 46, 1986.

155. NcNeil, N. I., Buttoo, S., and Ridgeway, G. L., Spontaneous bacterial peritonitis due to *Campylobacter jejuni*, *Postgrad. Med. J.*, 60, 487, 1984.

156. Wood, C. J., Fleming, V., Turnbridge, J., Thomson, N., and Atkins, R. C., Campylobacter peritonitis in continuous ambulatory peritoneal dialysis: report of eight cases and a review of the literature, *Am. J. Kidney Dis.*, 19, 257, 1992.

157. Keat, A., Reiter's syndrome and reactive arthritis in perspective, *N. Engl. J. Med.*, 309, 1606, 1983.

158. Centers for Disease Control, Campylobacter sepsis associated with nutritional therapy — California, *Morbid. Mortal. Wkly. Rep.*, 30, 294, 1981.

159. Soonattrakul, W., Anderson, B. R., and Bryner, J. H., Raw liver as a possible source of vibrio fetus septicemia in man, *Am. J. Med. Sci.*, 261, 245, 1971.

160. Schmidt, U., Chmel, H., Kaminski, G., and Sen, P., The clinical spectrum of campylobacter fetus infections: report of five cases and review of the literature, *Q. J. Med.*, 196, 431, 1980.

161. Kerstens, P. J. S. M., Endtz, H. P., Meis, J. F. G. M., Oyen, W. J. G., Koopman, R. J. I., van den Broek, P. J., and van der Meer, J. W. M., Erysipelas-like skin lesions associated with *Campylobacter jejuni* septicemia in patients with hypogammaglobulinemia, *Eur. J. Clin. Microbiol. Infect. Dis.*, 11, 842, 1992.

162. Spelman, D. W., Davidson, N., Buckmaster, N. D., Spicer, W. J., and Ryan, P., Campylobacter bacteremia: a report of 10 cases, *Med. J. Aust.*, 145, 503, 1986.

163. Pines, A., Goldhammer, E., Bregman, J., Kaplinsky, N., and Frankl, O., Campylobacter enteritis associated with recurrent abortion in gammaglobulinemia, *Acta Obstet. Gynecol. Scand.*, 62, 279, 1983.

164. Farrugia, D. C., Eykyn, S. J., and Smyth, E. G., *Campylobacter fetus* endocarditis: two case reports and review, *Clin. Infect. Dis.*, 18, 443, 1994.

165. Righter, J. and Woods, J. M., *Campylobacter* and endovascular lesion, *Can.. Surg.*, 28, 451, 1985.

166. Carbone, K. M., Heinrich, M. C., and Quinn, T. C., Thrombophlebitis and cellulitis due to *Campylobacter fetus* spp. *fetus*: report of four cases and a review of the literature, *Medicine (Baltimore)*, 64, 244, 1985.

167. Francioli, P., Herzstein, J., Grob, J. P., Valloton, J.-J., Mombelli, G., and Glauser, M. P., *Campylobacter fetus* subspecies *fetus* bacteremia, *Arch. Intern. Med.*, 145, 289, 1985.

168. Kato, R., Ohta, T., Kazui, H., Kondo, M., Naiki, M., and Tsuchioka, H., *Campylobacter fetus* infection of abdominal aortic aneurysm, *J. Cardiovasc. Surg. (Torino)*, 31, 756, 1990.

169. Simor, A. E., Karmali, M. A., Jadavji, T., and Roscoe, M., Abortion and perinatal sepsis associated with campylobacter infection, *Rev. Infect. Dis.*, 8, 397, 1986.

170. Morooka, T., Takeo, H., Yasumoto, S., Mimatsu, T., Yukitake, K., and Oda, T., Nosocomial meningitis due to *Campylobacter fetus* subspecies *fetus* in a neonatal intensive care unit, *Acta Pediatr. Jpn.*, 34, 530, 1992.

171. Morooka, T., Oda, T., and Shigeoka, H., *In vitro* evaluation of antibiotics for treatment of meningitis caused by *Campylobacter fetus* subspecies *fetus*, *Pediatr. Infect. Dis. J.*, 8, 653, 1989.

172. Goosens, H., Coignau, H., Vlaes, L., and Butzler, J. P., In-vitro evaluation of antibiotic combinations against *Campylobacter fetus*, *J. Antimicrob. Chemother.*, 24, 195, 1989.

173. Kato, H., Wakasugi, H., Mukuta, T., Furukawa, M., Yokota, M., Yamada, Y., Funakoshi, A., and Abe, M., *Campylobacter fetus* subspecies *fetus* meningitis with chronic alcoholism and diabetes mellitus, *Jpn. J. Med.*, 29, 542, 1990.

174. Joly, P., Boissonnas, A., Fournier, R., Khalifa, P., Vedel, G., Cremer, G. A., Languepin, A., Kerboull, M., and Laroche, C., Septic arthritis caused by *Campylobacter fetus*, *Rev. Rhum. Mal. Osteoartic.*, 53, 223, 1986.

175. Rao, K. V. and Ralston, R. A., Meningitis due to *Campylobacter fetus intestinalis* in a kidney transplant recipient, *Am. J. Nephrol.*, 7, 402, 1987.

176. Wens, R., Dratwa, M., Potvliege, C., Hansen, W., Tielemans, C., and Collart, F., *Campylobacter fetus* followed by septicemia in a patient on continuous ambulatory peritoneal dialysis, *J. Infect.*, 10, 249, 1985.

177. Petruccelli, B. P., Murphy, G. S., Sanchez, J. L., Walz, S., DeFraites, R., Gelnett, J., Haberberger, R. L., Echeverria, P., and Taylor, D. N., Treatment of traveler's diarrhea with ciprofloxacin and loperamide, *J. Infect. Dis.*, 165, 557, 1992.

178. Sorvilo, F. J., Lieb, L. E., and Waterman, S. H., Incidence of campylobacteriosis among patients with AIDS in Los Angeles County, *J. Acquir. Immune Defic. Syndr.*, 4, 598, 1991.

179. Dworkin, B., Wormser, G. P., Abdoo, R. A., Cabello, F., Aguero, M. E., and Sivak, S. L., Persistence of multiply antibiotic-resistant *Campylobacter jejuni* in a patient with the acquired immune deficiency syndrome, *Am. J. Med.*, 80, 965, 1986.

180. Sacks, L. V., Labriola, A. M., Gill, V. J., and Gordin, F. M., Use of ciprofloxacin for successful eradication of bacteremia due to *Campylobacter cinaedi* in a human immunodeficiency virus-infected person, *Rev. Infect. Dis.*, 13, 1066, 1991.

181. Perlman, D. M., Ampel, N. M., Schifman, R. B., Cohn, D. L., Patton, C. M., Aguirre, M. L., Wang, W.-L. L., and Blaser, M. J., Persistent *Campylobacter jejuni* infections in patients with human immunodeficiency virus (HIV), *Ann. Intern. Med.*, 108, 540, 1988.

182. Lambert, J. R., Karmali, M. A., and Newman, A., Campylobacter enteritis, *Ann. Intern. Med.*, 91, 929, 1979.
183. Kaldor, J., Pritchard, H., Serpell, A., and Metcalf, W., Serum antibodies in campylobacter enteritis, *J. Clin. Microbiol.*, 18, 1, 1983.
184. Rodgers, V. D., Fassett, R., and Kagnoff, M. F., Abnormalities in the intestinal mucosal T cells in homosexual populations including those with the lymphadenopathy syndrome and acquired immunodeficiency syndrome, *Gastroenterology*, 90, 552, 1986.
185. Rodgers, V. D. and Kagnoff, M. F., Gastrointestinal manifestations of the acquired immunodeficiency syndrome, *West. J. Med.*, 146, 57, 1987.
186. Nelson, J. A., Wiley, C. A., Reynolds-Kohler, C., Reese, C. E., Margaretten, W., and Levy, J. A., Human immunodeficiency virus detected in bowel epithelium from patients with gastrointestinal symptoms, *Lancet*, 1, 259, 1988.
187. Connolly, G. M., Forbes, A., and Gazzard, B. G., Investigation of seemingly pathogen-negative diarrhoea in patients infected with HIV 1, *Gut*, 31, 886, 1990.
188. Quinn, T. C., Goodell, S. E., Fennell, C. L., Wang, S.-P., Schuffler, M. D., Holmes, K. K., and Stamm, W. E., Infections with *Campylobacter jejuni* and *Campylobacter*-like organisms in homosexual men, *Ann. Intern. Med.*, 101, 187, 1984.
189. Guerin, J. M., Hoang, C., Galian, A., Lavergne, A., Lebiez, E., and Bitoun, A., Severe diarrhea in a patient with AIDS, *JAMA*, 256, 591, 1986.
190. Funke, G., Baumann, R., Penner, J. L., and Altwegg, M., Development of resistance to macrolide antibiotics in an AIDS patient treated with clarithromycin for *Campylobacter jejuni* diarrhea, *Eur. J. Clin. Microbiol. Infect. Dis.*, 13, 612, 1994.
191. Peterson, M. C., Farr, R. W., and Castiglia, M., Prosthetic hip infection and bacteremia due to *Campylobacter jejuni* in a patient with AIDS, *Clin. Infect. Dis.*, 16, 439, 1993.
192. Cimolai, N., Gill, M. J., Jones, A., Flores, B., Stamm, W. E., Laurie, W., Madden, B., and Shahrabadi, M. S., "*Campylobacter cinaedi*" bacteremia: case report and laboratory findings, *J. Clin. Microbiol.*, 25, 942, 1987.
193. Pasternak, J., Bolivar, R., Hopfer, R. L., Fainstain, V., Mills, K., Rios, A., Bodey, G. P., Fennell, C. L., Totten, P. A., and Stamm, W. E., Bacteremia caused by *Campylobacter*-like organisms in two male homosexuals, *Ann. Intern. Med.*, 101, 339, 1984.
194. Wilcox, C. M., Byford, B. A., Forsmark, C. E., Hadley, W. K., Cello, J. P., and Jacobson, M. A., *Campylobacter*-like organisms are uncommon pathogens in patients infected with the human immunodeficiency virus, *J. Clin. Microbiol.*, 28, 2370, 1990.
195. Aboulafia, D., Mathisen, G., and Mitsujasu, R., Case report: aggressive Kaposi's sarcoma and *Campylobacter* bacteremia in a female with transfusion associated AIDS, *Am. J. Med. Sci.*, 301, 256, 1991.
196. Ng, V. L., Hadley, W. K., Fennell, C. L., Flores, B. M., and Stamm, W. E., Successive bacteremias with "*Campylobacter cinaedi*" and "*Campylobacter fennelliae*" in a bisexual male, *J. Clin. Microbiol.*, 25, 2008, 1987.
197. Kemper, C. A., Mickelsen, P., Morton, A., Walton, B., and Deresinski, S. C., Helicobacter (*Campylobacter*) *fennelliae*-like organisms as an important but occult cause of bacteraemia in a patient with AIDS, *J. Infect.*, 26, 97, 1993.
198. Quinn, T. C., Stamm, W. E., Goodell, S. E., Mkrtichian, E., Benedetti, J., Corey, L., Schuffler, M. D., and Holmes, K. K., The polymicrobiological origin of intestinal infections in homosexual men, *N. Engl. J. Med.*, 309, 576, 1983.
199. Barrett, T. J., Patton, C. M., and Morris, G. K., Differentiation of *Campylobacter* species using phenotypic characterization, *Lab. Med.*, 19, 96, 1988.
200. Fennell, C. L., Totten, P. A., Quinn, T. C., Patton, D. L., Holmes, K. K., and Stamm, W. E., Characterization of *Campylobacter*-like organisms isolated from homosexual men, *J. Infect. Dis.*, 149, 58, 1984.
201. Decker, C. F., Martin, G. J., Barham, W. B., and Paparello, S. F., Bacteremia due to *Campylobacter cinaedi* in a patient infected with the human immunodeficiency virus, *Clin. Infect. Dis.*, 15, 178, 1992.
202. Battan, R., Ravigione, M. C., Palagiano, A., Boyle, J. F., Sabatini, M. T., Sayad, K., and Ottaviano, L. J., *Helicobacter pylori* infection in patients with acquired immune deficiency syndrome, *Am. J. Gastroenterol.*, 85, 1576, 1990.

203. Dorrell, L., Wardropper, A. G., and Ong, E. L. C., *Helicobacter pylori* infection in an HIV-seropositive patient with diarrhoea, *AIDS*, 7, 900, 1993.
204. Francis, N. D., Logan, R. P. H., Walker, M. M., Polson, R. J., Boylston, A. W., Pinching, A. J., Harris, J. R. W., and Baron, J. H., *Campylobacter pylori* in the upper gastrointestinal tract of patients with HIV infection, *J. Clin. Pathol.*, 43, 60, 1990.
205. Black, R. E., Levine, M. M., Clements, M. L., Hughes, T. P., and Blaser, M. J., Experimental *Campylobacter jejuni* infection in humans, *J. Infect. Dis.*, 157, 472, 1988.
206. Blaser, M. J., Black, R. E., Duncan, D. J., and Amer, J., *Campylobacter jejuni*-specific serum antibodies are elevated in healthy Bangladeshi children, *J. Clin. Microbiol.*, 21, 164, 1985.
207. Kosunen, T. U., Pitkanen, T., Pettersson, T., and Ponka, A., Clinical and serological studies in patients with *Campylobacter fetus* ssp. *jejuni* infection. II. Serological findings, *Infection*, 9, 279, 1981.
208. Winsor, D. K., Jr., Mathewson, J. J., and DuPont, H. L., Western blot analysis of intestinal secretory immunoglobulin A response to *Campylobacter jejuni* antigens in patients with naturally acquired *Campylobacter* enteritis, *Gastroenterology*, 90(Part 1), 1217, 1986.
209. Blaser, M. J., Sazie, E., and Williams, L. P., Jr., The influence of immunity on raw milk-associated *Campylobacter* infection, *JAMA*, 257, 43, 1987.
210. Chess, Q., Daniels, J., North, E., and Macris, N. T., Serum immunoglobulin elevation in the acquired immunodeficiency syndrome (AIDS): IgG, AgA, IgM, and IgD, *Diagn. Immunol.*, 2, 148, 1984.
211. Lane, H. C., Masur, H., Edgar, L. C., Whalen, G., Rook, A. H., and Fauci, A. S., Abnormalities in B-cell activation and immunoregulation in patients with the acquired immunodeficiency syndrome, *N. Engl. J. Med.*, 309, 453, 1983.
212. Johnson, R. J., Nolan, C., Wang, S.-P., Shelton, W. R., and Blaser, M. J., Persistent *Campylobacter jejuni* infection in an immunocompromised patient, *Ann. Intern. Med.*, 100, 832, 1984.
213. Baqar, S., Pacheco, N. D., and Rollwagen, F. M., Modulation of mucosal immunity against *Campylobacter jejuni* by orally administered cytokines, *Antimicrob. Agents Chemother.*, 37, 2688, 1993.
214. Borish, L., Rosenbaum, R., Albury, L., and Clark, S., Activation of neutrophils by recombinant interleukin-6, *Cell. Immunol.*, 121, 280, 1989.
215. Cowling, P., Ebringer, R., and Abringer, A., Association of inflammation with raised serum IgA in ankylosing spondylitis, *Ann. Rheum. Dis.*, 39, 545, 1973.
216. McGuigan, L. E., Geczy, A. F., and Edmonds, J. P., The immunopathology of ankylosing spondylitis — a review, *Semin. Arthr. Rheum.*, 15, 81, 1985.
217. Prendergast, J. K., Sullivan, J. S., Geczy, A., Upfold, L. I., Edmonds, J. P., Bashir, H. V., and Reiss-Levy, E., Possible role of enteric organisms in the pathogenesis of alkylosing spondylitis and other sero-negative arthropathies, *Infect. Immun.*, 41, 935, 1983.
218. Andreasen, J. J., Ringsdal, V. S., and Helin, P., No signs of *Campylobacter jejuni/coli*-related antibodies in patients with active ankylosing spondylitis, *APMIS*, 99, 735, 1991.
219. Rhodes, K. M. and Tattersfield, A. E., Guillain-Barré syndrome associated with Campylobacter infection, *Br. Med. J.*, 285, 173, 1982.
220. Ropper, A. H., Campylobacter diarrhea and Guillain-Barré syndrome, *Arch. Neurol.*, 45, 655, 1988.
221. Kaldor, J. and Speed, B. R., Guillain-Barré syndrome and *Campylobacter jejuni*: a serological study, *Br. Med. J.*, 288, 1867, 1984.
222. Mishu, B., Llyas, A. A., Koski, C. L., Vriesendorp, F., Cook, S. D., Mithen, F. A., and Blaser, M. J., Serologic evidence of previous *Campylobacter jejuni* infection in patients with the Guillain-Barré syndrome, *Ann. Intern. Med.*, 118, 947, 1993.
223. Kuroki, S., Saida, T., Nukina, M., Haruta, T., Yoshioka, M., Kobayashi, Y., and Nakanishi, H., *Campylobacter jejuni* strains from patients with Guillain-Barré syndrome belong mostly to Penner serogroup 19 and contain β-N-acetylglucosamine residues, *Ann. Neurol.*, 33, 243, 1993.
224. Fujimoto, S. and Amako, K., Guillain-Barré syndrome and *Campylobacter jejuni* infection, *Lancet*, 335, 1350, 1990.
225. Yuki, N., Sato, S., Itoh, T., and Miyatake, T., HLA-B35 and acute axonal polyneuropathy following *Campylobacter* infection, *Neurology*, 41, 1561, 1991.
226. Yuki, N., Sato, S., Fujimoto, S., Yamada, S., Tsujino, Y., Kinoshita, A., and Itoh, T., Serotype of *Campylobacter jejuni*, HLA and the Guillain-Barré syndrome, *Muscle Nerve*, 15, 968, 1992.
227. England, J., Guillain-Barré syndrome, *Annu. Rev. Med.*, 41, 1, 1990.

228. Hagensee, M. E., Benyunes, M., Miller, J. A., and Spach, D. H., *Campylobacter jejuni* bacteremia and Guillain-Barré syndrome in a patient with GVHD after allogeneic BMT, *Bone Marrow Transplant.*, 13, 349, 1994.

229. Johnson, N. T., Crawford, S. W., and Sargur, M., Acute demyelinating polyneuropathy with respiratory failure following high-dose systemic cytosine arabinoside and marrow transplantation, *Bone Marrow Transplant.*, 2, 203, 1987.

230. Eliashiv, S., Bremmer, T., Abramsky, O., Shahin, R., Agai, E., Naparstek, E., and Steiner, I., Acute inflammatory demyelinating polyneuropathy following bone marrow transplantation, *Bone Marrow Transplant.*, 8, 315, 1991.

231. Bolger, G. B., Sullivan, K. M., Spence, A. M., Appelbaum, F. R., Johnston, R., Sanders, J. E., Deeg, H. J., Witherspoon, R. P., Doney, K. C., Nims, J., Thomas, E. D., and Storb, R., Myasthenia gravis after allogeneic bone marrow transplantation: relationship to chronic graft-versus-host disease, *Neurology*, 36, 1087, 1986.

232. Yuki, N., Yoshino, H., Sato, S., and Miyatake, T., Acute axonal polyneuropathy associated with anti-GM_1 antibodies following *Campylobacter* enteritis, *Neurology*, 40, 1900, 1990.

11 Non-Cholera *Vibrio* spp.

11.1 INTRODUCTION

The genus *Vibrio* represents a group of Gram-negative, facultatively anaerobic, actively motile bacteria with one or two polar flagella. They include the cholera vibrios which are highly pathogenic to humans, and the non-cholera marine vibrios. The latter are free-living microorganisms found in the normal warm marine flora of the coastal U.S.[1-3] Molluscan shellfish (oysters, clams, mussels, and scallops) are filter feeders and concentrate *Vibrio* spp. in their tissues. According to Klontz et al.,[4] 5% to 10% of molluscan seafood at retail outlets contains *Vibrio* spp.

In humans, the main portal of entry for *Vibrio* spp. is the intestinal tract and infection can be contracted from eating raw shellfish or drinking contaminated water. The majority of patients with primary vibrio septicemia have had a recent history of eating undercooked seafood, especially raw oysters. Thorough cooking in many cases can prevent vibrio infections.[5] Those which are pathogenic to humans include the cholera vibrios (*V. cholerae* O1, *V. cholerae* O139, and other *V. cholerae* non-O1), as well as *V. parachaemoliticus*, and *V. vulnificus*.[6-8]

In general, infections caused by *V. vulnificus*, *V. parahaemolyticus*, and possibly *V. cholerae* non-O1 are more likely to induce primary septicemia either in patients with a preexisting liver disease, such as chronic hepatic hepatitis, cirrhosis, and iron-storage disease, or in patients with immune deficiencies.[9-11] In such patients, the extraintestinal vibrio infections can often result in serious disability or death.[9,10] However, there have been no reports of an increased risk of infection with *V. cholerae* O1 in HIV-positive patients.[8]

Vibrio vulnificus (previously referred to as *Beneckea vulnifica*[12]), a recently identified lactose-positive, halophilic marine organism, is a highly virulent, invasive species isolated from many tissues.[1,13-15] Its presence in seawater, which is not related to pollution levels, was determined in 95% of marine sites surveyed,[1] and in approximately 50% of oysters sampled during selected summer and fall months.[16] The highly pathogenic, virulent strains produce a potent enterotoxin and agglutinate a specific polyvalent (O1) antiserum. Serotypes which do not agglutinate to O1 antiserum have been generally associated with a milder diarrheal disease. In addition, *V. vulnificus* also produces an extracellular toxin which was found to be hemolytic and lethal for mice when injected intravenously or intraperitoneally, as well as toxic to tissue-cultured cells.[17,18]

Human infection with *V. vulnificus* is identified with two distinct clinical syndromes: primary septicemia and wound infection (accompanied by secondary sepsis).[9] The association of both these syndromes with raw oyster consumption (septicemia) and salt water exposure (wound infection) has been well documented.[9]

In the majority of cases, the incubation period for a raw oyster-associated primary septicemia, or gastrointestinal illness has been less than 24 h.[10] Primary septicemia is characterized by chills, fever, and prostration. In addition, hypotension and secondary cutaneous lesions may develop within 36 h of the onset of disease.[9] Pollack et al.[19] demonstrated the presence of antibodies to the homologous isolate in patients with *V. vulnificus*-induced septicemia.

Between 60% and 70% of patients with primary septicemia had been diagnosed with preexisting liver disease; the remaining cases involved immunocompromised patients (diabetes mellitus, hematologic malignancies) or patients with iron overload disorders.[7,10,11,20] Desenclos et al.[21] presented evidence suggesting that persons with reduced gastric acidity are at increased risk for primary septicemia. The latter is associated with 45% to 60% mortality rate, with most deaths occurring within 48 h of hospitalization even with appropriate treatment. The mortality rate may even approach 100% when patients presented with hypotension.[7,10,11,22]

There has been evidence suggesting that *V. vulnificus* possesses antiphagocytic surface antigen that confers resistance to neutrophil phagocytosis, thus contributing to its virulence.[23] Some of the *Vibrio* strains were found to be not susceptible to bactericidal action of normal serum by neither of the pathways of complement activation.[24] Moreover, there is also evidence that *V. vulnificus* produces extracellular products having proteolytic, collagenolytic, and elastase activities which would allow for its rapid invasion of body tissues.[17,18,25-27]

The second clinical syndrome associated with *V. vulnificus* is the wound infection. This is a relatively uncommon but potentially severe condition which may occur in equal frequency both in healthy individuals and in patients with underlying illness. Manifestations often observed include fever, pain and swelling at the wound site, and cellulitis.[10] About 50% of patients would require surgical debridement or amputation.[9,28] The overall mortality rate from *V. vulnificus*-induced wound infections may reach as high as 25%, with patients with liver disease, iron overload, or immune deficiencies accounting for the vast majority of deaths (65% to 75%).[10,20]

Even though the reported number of HIV-infected individuals who had acquired vibrio infections is relatively small,[29,30] such patients appeared to be at increased risk of acquiring the invasive disease.[9]

11.2   TREATMENT OF *VIBRIO VULNIFICUS* INFECTIONS

Treatment with antibiotics seemed to be effective against *Vibrio*-induced septicemia. Thus, case-fatality rates increased with greater delays between the onset of illness and initiation of antibiotic treatment.[10] Most *V. vulnificus* strains have been found to be susceptible *in vitro* to a number of antimicrobial agents, including amikacin, ampicillin, carbenicillin, cefoxitin, cephalothin, chloramphenicol, gentamicin, kanamycin, tetracycline, trimethoprim-sulfamethoxazole, and tobramycin.[30,31] Resistance to colistin and clindamycin has been reported.[13]

Based on data from mouse models, Morris and Tenney,[32] as well as others,[10,31] have recommended the use of tetracycline (or chloramphenicol) alone or in combination with an aminoglycoside (gentamicin) against *V. vulnificus* infection.[6,32] The use of gentamicin may not be warranted since *in vivo* studies in mice have shown that it had little activity against *V. vulnificus* except in very large doses (8 mg/kg);[31] *in vitro*, gentamicin proved also not to be very effective ($MIC_{90} = 8$ μg/ml).[33]

Chin et al.[30] reported successful treatment with intravenous ampicillin and gentamicin of a patient with AIDS-related complex, liver disease, and *V. vulnificus*-induced septicemia complicated with peritonitis, sepsis, and gastroenteritis associated with the pathogen.

In addition to antibiotic therapy, *V. vulnificus*-induced septicemia will require extensive supportive care consisting of administration of appropriate fluids for shock, adequate monitoring, and aggressive management of other symptoms, such as gastrointestinal bleeding.[6]

11.3   REFERENCES

1. Kelly, M. T. and Avery, D. M., Lactose-positive *Vibrio* in seawater: a cause of pneumonia and septicemia in a drowning victim, *J. Clin. Microbiol.*, 11, 278, 1980.
2. Tilton, R. C. and Ryan, R. W., Clinical and ecological characteristics of *Vibrio vulnificus* in the northeastern United States, *Diagn. Microbiol. Infect. Dis.*, 6, 109, 1987.
3. Kelly, M. T. and Stroh, E. M., Occurrence of *Vibrionaceae* in natural and cultivated oyster populations in the Pacific Northwest, *Diagn. Microbiol. Infect. Dis.*, 9, 1, 1988.

4. Klontz, K. C., Williams, L., Baldy, L. M., and Campos, M., Raw oyster- associated *Vibrio* infections: linking epidemiologic data with laboratory testing of oysters obtained from a retail outlet, *J. Food Protection*, 56, 997, 1993.

5. Blake, P. A., Vibrios on the half shell: what the walrus and the carpenter didn't know, *Ann. Intern. Med.*, 99, 558, 1983.

6. Morris, J. M. and Black, R. E., Cholera and other vibrios in the United States, *N. Engl. J. Med.*, 312, 343, 1985.

7. Blake, P. A., Merson, M. H., Weaver, R. E., Hollis, D. G., and Heublein, P. C., Disease caused by a marine vibrio: clinical characteristics and epidemiology, *N. Engl. J. Med.*, 300, 1, 1979.

8. Angulo, F. J. and Swerdlow, D. L., Bacterial enteric infections in persons infected with human immunodeficiency virus, *Clin. Infect. Dis.*, 21(Suppl. 1), S84, 1995.

9. Whitman, C. M. and Griffin, P. M., Commentary: preventing *Vibrio vulnificus* infection in the high-risk patient, *Infect. Dis. Clin. Practice*, 2, 275, 1993.

10. Klontz, K. C., Lieb, S., Schreiber, M., Janowski, H. T., Baldy, L. M., and Gunn, R. A., Syndromes of *Vibrio vulnificus* infections: clinical and epidemiologic features in Florida cases, 1981–1987, *Ann. Intern. Med.*, 109, 318, 1988.

11. Tacket, C. O., Brenner, F., and Blake, P. A., Clinical features and an epidemiological study of *Vibrio vulnificus* infections, *J. Infect. Dis.*, 149, 558, 1984.

12. Reichelt, J. L., Baumann, P., and Baumann, L., Study of genetic relationships among marine species of the genus *Beneckea* and *Photobacterium* by means of *in vitro* DNA/DNA hybridization, *Arch. Microbiol.*, 110, 101, 1976.

13. Blake, P. A., Merson, M. H., Weaver, R. E., Hollis, D. G., and Heublein, P. C., Disease caused by a marine vibrio: clinical characteristics and epidemiology, *N. Engl. J. Med.*, 300, 1, 1979.

14. Ghosh, H. K. and Bowen, T. E., Halophilic *Vibrio* from human tissue infections on the Pacific coast of Australia, *Pathology*, 12, 397, 1980.

15. Kelly, M. T. and McCormick, W. F., Acute bacterial myositis caused by *Vibrio vulnificus*, *JAMA*, 246, 72, 1981.

16. Tamplin, M., Roderick, G. E., Blake, N. J., and Cuba, T., Isolation and characterization of *Vibrio vulnificus* from two Florida estuaries, *Appl. Environ. Microbiol.*, 44, 1466, 1982.

17. Kreger, A. and Lockwood, D., Detection of extracellular toxin(s) produced by *Vibrio vulnificus*, *Infect. Immun.*, 33, 583, 1981.

18. Maneval, D. R., Wright, A. C., Marley, G. M., Patniak, R., and Morris, J. G., Characterization of an extracellular cytotoxin and other possible virulence factors of *Vibrio vulnificus*, *Proc. 24th Intersci. Conf. Antimicrob. Agents Chemother.*, American Society for Microbiology, Washington, D.C., 1984.

19. Pollack, S. J., Parrish, E. F. III, Barrett, T. J., Dretler, T. J., and Morris, J. G., Jr., *Vibrio vulnificus* septicemia: isolation of organism from stool and demonstration of antibodies by indirect immuno-fluorescence, *Arch. Intern. Med.*, 143, 837, 1983.

20. Bonner, J. R., Coker, A. S., Berryman, C. R., and Pollock, H. M., Spectrum of vibrio infections in a Gulf Coast community, *Ann. Intern. Med.*, 99, 464, 1983.

21. Desenclos, J. A., Klontz, K. C., Wolfe, L. E., and Hoercherl, S. A., The risk of vibrio illness in the Florida raw oyster eating population, 1981–1988, *Am. J. Epidemiol.*, 134, 290, 1991.

22. Johnstone, J. M., Becker, S. F., and McFarland, L. M., Man and the sea, *JAMA*, 253, 2850, 1985.

23. Kreger, A., DeChatelet, L., and Shirley, P., Interaction of *Vibrio vulnificus* with human polymorpho-nuclear phagocytosis, *J. Infect. Dis.*, 144, 244, 1981.

24. Carruthers, M. M. and Kabat, W. J., *Vibrio vulnificus* (lactose-positive *Vibrio*) and *Vibrio parahaemolyticus* differ in their susceptibilities to human serum, *Infect. Immun.*, 32, 964, 1981.

25. Smith, C. G. and Merkel, J. R., Collagenolytic activity of *Vibrio vulnificus*: potential contribution to its invasiveness, *Infect. Immun.*, 35, 1155, 1982.

26. Poole, M. D., Bowdre, J. H., and Klapper, D., Elastase produced by *Vibrio vulnificus*: *in vitro* and *in vivo* effects, *Proc. 82nd Annu. Meet. Am. Soc. Microbiol.*, Atlanta, American Society for Microbiology, Washington, D.C., 1982.

27. Carruthers, M. M. and Kabat, W. J., Isolation, purification, and characterization of a protease from *Beneckea vulnifica* (lactose-positive vibrio, *Vibrio vulnificus*), *Proc. 81st Annu. Meet. Am. Soc. Microbiol.*, Dallas, American Society for Microbiology, Washington, D.C., 1981.

28. Castillo, L. E., Winslow, D. L., and Pankey, G. A., Wound infection and septic shock due to *Vibrio vulnificus*, *Am. J. Trop. Med. Hyg.*, 30, 844, 1981.
29. Altekruse, S., Hyman, F., Klontz, K., Timbo, B., and Tollefson, L., Foodborne bacterial infections in individuals with the human immunodeficiency virus, *South. Med. J.*, 87, 169, 1994.
30. Chin, K. P., Lowe, M. A., Tong, M. J., and Koehler, A. L., *Vibrio vulnificus* after raw oyster ingestion in a patient with liver disease and acquired immune deficiency syndrome-related complex, *Gastroenterology*, 92, 796, 1987.
31. Bowdre, J. H., Hull, J. H., and Cocchetto, D. M., Antibiotic efficacy against *Vibrio vulnificus* in the mouse: superiority of tetracycline, *J. Pharmacol. Exp. Ther.*, 225, 595, 1983.
32. Morris, J. G., Jr. and Tenney, J., Antibiotic for *Vibrio vulnificus* infection, *JAMA*, 253, 1121, 1985.
33. Morris, J. G., Tenney, J. H., and Drusano, G. L., *In vitro* susceptibility of pathogenic *Vibrio* species to nofloxacin and six other antimicrobial agents, *J. Antimicrob. Chemother.*, 28, 442, 1985.

12 *Listeria monocytogenes*

12.1 INTRODUCTION

Listeria monocytogenes (also referred to as *Corinebacterium infantisepticum* and *Corinebacterium parvulum*) is a motile Gram-positive bacillus with pathogenic activity in mammals, birds, and fish. It belongs to a genus (*Listeria*) which has uncertain affiliation but closely resembles the organisms of the family Corinebacteriaceae.

In humans, the *L. monocytogenes* exhibits marked tropism for the central nervous system and the placenta. It is the etiologic agent of listeriosis, a rare but serious infectious disease in immuno-compromised hosts.[1,2] As many as 5% of the general population harbor *Listeria* in their intestinal tract.[3,4]

L. monocytogenes infection has an incubation period of 3 to 90 d, with an average of 3 to 4 weeks. An estimated 1840 cases of serious illness have been associated with this pathogen in the U.S. alone each year.[5,6] The overall mortality rate from listeriosis is between 30% and 62%.[7-9] In patients with listerial brain abscesses mortality can reach 57% of the population,[10] whereas in AIDS patients it was reported to be 29%.[11] In renal transplant recipients, the mortality was reported to approach 38%.[12]

A preceding gastrointestinal infection or disruption causing inflamed bowel mucosa may facilitate blood stream invasion by the pathogen.[13] Primarily, listeriosis affects individuals with deficient cell-mediated immunity,[13] often the very young, the elderly, patients on immunosuppressive therapy, cancer patients, and pregnant women. For example, *L. monocytogenes* has been the most common cause of bacterial meningitis in cancer patients.[14] AIDS patients because of their severe immuno-deficiency may be highly susceptible to invasive *Listeria* infections,[13,15-21] especially those patients with CD4+ cell counts below 50/μl.[11] By comparison with the general population, HIV-infected patients are 60 times more likely to acquire listeriosis.[11] Because of serious immunodeficiencies, in patients with full-blown AIDS the risk has been even higher (150 to 280 times).[1,3,11,15] Surprisingly though, the overall incidence of listeriosis in HIV-positive patients has been relatively low. The risk in such patients can be best determined from large population-based studies.

Listeriosis during pregnancy is not uncommon and may occur even in the absence of overt immune deficiency.[22] It is usually mild and rarely fatal unless other risk factors are present. The first maternal death by listerial bacteremia of a pregnant woman with AIDS was reported by Wetli et al.[23,24] *In utero* infections by *L. monocytogenes* have occurred transplacentally resulting in abortions, stillbirths, or premature births. When acquired during birth, listeriosis can cause cardio-respiratory distress, diarrhea, vomiting, and meningitis.

In adults, listeria infection, either as the result of an outbreak or sporadic, has been primarily foodborne.[3,25-27] It is typically associated with meningitis, endocarditis, and disseminated granulomatous lesions.

12.2 HOST IMMUNE DEFENSE AGAINST LISTERIOSIS

L. monocytogenes infections have been strongly associated with the presence of cellular deficiency as evidenced by the increased incidence in immunosuppressed patients receiving corticosteroid therapy.[14] The pathogen, which is a facultative intracellular parasite, is capable of surviving in the macrophages.[28] The listericidal activity of the macrophages would depend on the cell activation either by direct prior immunization or a nonspecific antigen stimulation. Although in the early stage of the infection, nonimmune macrophages lack listericidal activity, they still are capable of limiting multiplication in the lymphoreticular system. Following this initial phase of the infection, lymphokine-mediated activation of the macrophages will result in eradication of the pathogen.[22] The corticosteroids are known to exert deleterious effects on the macrophages and neutrophils by impairing chemotaxis, chemokinesis, and bactericidal activity,[29] and to interfere directly with their antilisterial activity.[30]

Another factor in the host defenses against *Listeria* is the viability of T lymphocyte functions.[22] Thus, *in vivo* studies have shown that antilisterial resistance could be parleyed by injection of immune spleen cells. Alternatively, treatment of spleen cells with antilymphocyte serum would block the development of resistance. Studies by Mackaness[31] and Mackaness and Hill[32] on the effects of specific antisera to thymus-derived lymphocytes in T cell-depleted mice confirmed the need for intact T lymphocyte functions in the host response to *Listeria*. The studies of Mackaness and Hill[31,32] as well as other investigators,[33] have demonstrated that sensitized T lymphocytes directed the eradication of *L. monocytogenes* by producing soluble cytokines which, in turn, will activate the microbicidal activity of the macrophages.

The endogenously produced tumor necrosis factor-α (TNF-α) was also found essential in the defense against *L. monocytogenes*.[22] Pretreatment of mice with antibody to TNF-α inhibited the generation of activated macrophages and converted a nonlethal listeriosis into a lethal infection.[34] In view of the infrequent occurrence of listeriosis in AIDS patients, the ability of TNF-α to restrict the infection is intriguing since these patients are known to have elevated TNF-α levels as a result of nonspecific macrophage activation, and therefore this cytokine may have a protective effect on the development of overt illness.[22] On the other hand, elevated TNF-α levels may also be viewed as a marker of chronic macrophage activation,[35,36] and there has been no evidence to suggest that elevated TNF-α levels would be more protective than normal levels.[22]

A T cell-independent mechanism of macrophage activation by interferon-γ has also been reported. Thus, in a study of *Listeria*-infected immunodeficient mice, IFN-γ was shown to be produced by cells other than T lymphocytes.[37,38]

12.3   LISTERIOSIS IN AIDS PATIENTS

In AIDS patients, *Listeria*-induced infections are seldom diagnosed and are most often observed in the late stages of the disease when CD4+ cell counts are usually well below normal.[11,13,15-17,20,39-48] In 1984, the first case of *L. monocytogenes* infection in an HIV-infected patient was reported by Real et al.[40] At least 16 different serotypes have been isolated from HIV-infected patients, with serotypes 1/2a, 1/2b, and 4b being the most prevalent (in over 90% of the population).[7] Listeriosis usually presents as meningitis,[13,17,20,44] meningoencephalitis,[13,41] primary bacteremia,[13,16,39,40,42,45,46] and/or infection of the contents of the pregnant uterus; other manifestations have been rare.[2,15,43,48]

In general, the clinical symptoms of listeriosis in HIV-infected patients did not differ significantly from those in other patients, except for the high incidence of brain abscesses and cerebritis seen in renal transplant recipients.[12,14,49] In one report, meningitis accounted for 71% of listerial infections among HIV-positive patients.[11]

Several hypotheses have been proposed to explain the rare occurrence of listeriosis in AIDS patients. It is possible that multiple courses of prophylactic antibiotic medications taken by AIDS patients to prevent the progression of HIV and prevent other opportunistic infections might alter the gastrointestinal flora and even eradicate the microorganism. Thus, trimethoprim-sulfamethoxazole, commonly given to prevent *Pneumocystis carinii* infections, has also been a very effective treatment against *L. monocytogenes*.[50] In another hypothesis, it has been postulated that contrary to predisposed immunocompromised patients who receive corticosteroid therapy that impair random movement, chemotaxis, and bactericidal activity of macrophages and polymorphonuclear cells, in AIDS patients the activity of nonimmune macrophages and granulocytes relatively has been retained intact.[6,44] Another factor could be the possibility that a T cell subset other than CD4+ cells may be responsible for the antilisterial immune response.[6]

It was also thought possible that genetic factors may play a role in the human defense against listeriosis.[6] Thus, it was postulated that one reason for the inability of AIDS patients to resist opportunistic infections has been their impaired (decreased) expression of class II histocompatibility gene proteins (such as HLA-DR), which are needed for successful antigen presentation and antigen-induced T lymphocyte activation.[51] It is relevant to mention that studies in experimental animals have demonstrated that protection against *Listeria* appeared restricted not by class II, but class I antigens.[52]

Furthermore, most opportunistic infections in HIV-positive patients are caused by either endogenous reactivation of latent pathogens (*Pneumocystis carinii, Toxoplasma gondii,* cytomegalovirus, mycobacteria, and herpes simplex virus), or from the inability of the host immune defenses to resist pathogens to which exposure is common.[15] However, *Listeria* is not known to remain latent in human macrophages for prolonged periods of time after the initial asymptomatic infection, and widespread exposure to *L. monocytogenes* in nonepidemic situations has been infrequent and of transitory nature.[2]

12.4 TREATMENT OF LISTERIOSIS

Listeriosis usually responds to antimicrobial therapy with no reports of recurrent infection.[15,22,53] In general, treatment with antibiotics (penicillin, ampicillin, amoxicillin), alone or in combination with aminoglycoside (gentamicin), is usually recommended (Table 12.1).[15] On several occasions, trimethoprim-sulfamethoxazole (TMP-SMX) was also reported to be effective when administered at concentrations attainable in serum and cerebrospinal fluid.[54-56] Berenguer et al.[15] have treated successfully an HIV-positive patient with a 21-d course of intravenous trimethoprim-sulfamethoxazole (5.0 mg of TMP/25 mg of SMX, four times daily).

One patient with a brain abscess caused by *L. monocytogenes* was treated with penicillin, chloramphenicol, and surgical drainage of the abscess.[48] *Listeria*-induced endocarditis responded to penicillin and netilmicin, combined with surgery.[43]

TABLE 12.1
Recommended Therapies of Listeriosis in AIDS Patients

Listeria Infection	Treatment	Ref.
Meningitis	Ampicillin (2.0 g every 4 h, IV)	17
	Ampicillin (2.0 g every 4 h, IV)	42
	TMP-SMX (160 mg of TMP) every 6 h	
Meningoencephalitis	Amoxycillin (12 g daily, IV; then 6 g daily, IV)	41
	Ampicillin (15 g daily, IV)	39
Brain abscess	Penicillin, chloramphenicol	48
Bacteremia	Ampicillin (3.0 g every 4 h, IV) Gentamicin (80 mg every 8 h, IV)	20
	Ampicillin (12 g daily, IV)	40
	Amoxycillin, gentamicin, sulfadiazine, pyrimethamine	45
	Penicillin	40
	Vancomycin	47
Endocarditis	Penicillin, netilmicin	43

12.5 REFERENCES

1. Angulo, F. J. and Swerdlow, D. L., Bacterial enteric infections in patients infected with human immunodeficiency virus, *Clin. Infect. Dis.*, 21(Suppl. 1), S84, 1995.
2. Armstrong, D., Listeria monocytogenes, in *Principles and Practice of Infectious Diseases*, 3rd ed., Mandell, G. L., Douglas, R. G., and Bennett, J.E., Eds., Chirchill Livingstone, New York, 1990, 1587.
3. Schuchat, A., Deaver, K. A., Wenger, J. D., Plikaytis, B. D., Mascola, L., Pinner, R. W., Reingold, A. L., Broome, C. V., and the Listeria Study Group, Role of foods in sporadic listeriosis. I. Case-control study of dietary risk factors, *JAMA*, 267, 2041, 1992.
4. Schlech, W. F. III, New perspectives on the gastrointesinal mode of transmission in invasive *Listeria monocytogenes* infection, *Clin. Invest. Med.*, 7, 321, 1984.
5. Altekruse, S., Hyman, F., Klontz, K., Timbo, B., and Tollefson, L., Foodborne bacterial infections in individuals with the human immunodeficiency virus, *South. Med. J.*, 87, 169, 1994.
6. Jacobs, J. L. and Murray, H. W., Why is *Listeria monocytogenes* not a pathogen in the acquired immunodeficiency syndrome? *Arch. Intern. Med.*, 146, 1299, 1986.
7. Gellin, B. G. and Broome, C. V., Listeriosis, *JAMA*, 261, 1313, 1989.
8. Cherubin, C. E., Marr, J. S., Sierra, M. F., and Becker, S., Listeria and gram-negative bacillary meningitis in New York City, 1972–1979: frequent causes of meningitis in adults, *Am. J. Med.*, 71, 199, 1981.
9. Pollock, S. S., Pollock, T. M., and Harrison, M. J. G., Infection of the central nervous system by *Listeria monocytogenes*: a review of 54 adult and juvenile cases, *Q. J. Med.*, 211, 331, 1984.
10. Dee, R. R. and Lorber, B., Brain abscess due to *Listeria monocytogenes*: case report and literature review, *Rev. Infect. Dis.*, 8, 968, 1986.
11. Jurado, R. L., Farley, M. M., Pereira, E., Harvey, R. C., Schuchat, A., Wenger, J. D., and Stevens, D. S., Increased risk of meningitis and bacteremia due to *Listeria monocytogenes* in patients with human immunodeficiency virus infection, *Clin. Infect. Dis.*, 17, 224, 1993.
12. Stamm, A. M., Desmukes, W. E., Simmons, B. P., Cobbs, C. G., Elliot, A., Budrich, P., and Harmon, J., Listeriosis in renal transplant recipients: report of an outbreak and review of 1-2 cases, *Rev. Infect. Dis.*, 4, 665, 1982.
13. Mascola, L., Lieb, L., Chiu, J., Fannin, S. L., and Linnan, M. J., Listeriosis: an uncommon opportunistic infection in patients with acquired immunodeficiency syndrome: report of five cases and a review of the literature, *Am. J. Med.*, 84, 162, 1988.
14. Niemen, R. E. and Lorber, B., Listeriosis in adults: a changing pattern: report of eight cases and review of the literature 1968–1978, *Rev. Infect. Dis.*, 2, 2, 1980.
15. Berenguer, J., Solera, J., Diaz, M. D., Moreno, S., Lopez-Herce, J. A., and Bouza, E., Listeriosis in patients infected with human immunodeficiency virus, *Rev. Infect. Dis.*, 13, 115, 1991.
16. Read, E. J., Orenstein, J. M., Chorba, T. L., Schwartz, A. M., Simon, G. L., Lewis, J. H., and Schulof, R. S., *Listeria monocytogenes* sepsis and small cell carcinoma of the rectum: an unusual presentation of the acquired immunodeficiency syndrome, *Am. J. Clin. Pathol.*, 83, 385, 1985.
17. Gould, I. A., Belok, L. C., and Handwerger, S., *Listeria monocytogenes*: a rare cause of opportunistic infection in the acquired immunodeficiency syndrome (AIDS) and a new cause of meningitis in AIDS: a case report, *AIDS Res.*, 2, 231, 1986.
18. Whimbley, E., Gold, J. W. M., Polsky, B., Dryjanski, J., Hawkins, C., Blevins, A., Brannon, P., Kiehn, T. E., Brown, A. E., and Armstrong, D., Bacteremia and fungemia in patients with the acquired immunodeficiency syndrome, *Ann. Intern. Med.*, 104, 511, 1986.
19. Schattenkerk, J. K. M., Klopping, C., Speelman, J. D., van Ketel, R. J., and Danner, S. A., Complications of the acquired immunodeficiency syndrome, 104, 726, 1986.
20. Koziol, K., Rielly, K. S., Bonin, R. A., and Salcedo, J. R., *Listeria monocytogenes* meningitis in AIDS, *Can. Med. Assoc. J.*, 135, 43, 1986.
21. Centers for Disease Control and Prevention, 1993 revised classification system for HIV infection and expanded surveillance case definition for AIDS among adolescents and adults, *Morbid. Mortal. Wkly. Rep.*, 41(RR-17), 1, 1992.
22. Decker, C. F., Simon, G. L., DiGioia, R. A., and Tuazon, C. U., Listeria monocytogenes infections in patients with AIDS: report of five cases and review, *Rev. Infect. Dis.*, 13, 413, 1991.

23. Wetli, C. V., Roldan, E. O., and Fojaco, R. M., Listeriosis as a cause of maternal death: an obstetric complication of the acquired immunodeficiency syndrome (AIDS), *Am. J. Obstet. Gynecol.*, 147, 7, 1983.

24. Wetli, C. V., Roldan, E. O., and Fojaco, R. M., Listeriosis in AIDS: an unfounded assumption, *Am. J. Obstet. Gynecol.*, 149, 805, 1984.

25. Schlech, W. F., Lavigne, P. M., Bortolussi, R. A., Allen, A. C., Haldane, E. V., Wort, A. J., Hightower, A. W., Johnsone, S. E., King, S. H., Nicholls, E. S., and Broome, C. V., Epidemic listeriosis: evidence for transmission by food, *N. Engl. J. Med.*, 308, 203, 1983.

26. Pinner, R. W., Schuchat, A., Swaminathan, B., Heyes, P. S., Deaver, K. A., Weaver, R. E., Plikaytis, B. D., Reeves, M., Broome, C. V., Wenger, J. D., and the Listeria Study Group, Role of foods in sporadic listeriosis. II. Microbiologic and epidemiologic investigation, *JAMA*, 267, 2046, 1992.

27. Linnan, M. J., Mascola, L., Lou, X. D., Goulet, V., May, S., Salminen, C., Hird, D. W., Yonekura, M. L., Hayes, P., Weaver, R., Audurier, M. L., Plikaytis, B. D., Fannin, S. L., Kleks, A., and Broome, C. V., Epidemic listeriosis associated with Mexican-style cheese, *N. Engl. J. Med.*, 319, 823, 1988.

28. Mackaness, G. B., Cellular resistance to infection, *J. Exp. Med.*, 116, 381, 1962.

29. Rinehart, J. J., Balcerzak, S. P., Sagone, A. L., and Lobuglio, A. F., Effects of corticosteroids on human monocyte function, *J. Clin. Invest.*, 54, 1337, 1974.

30. North, R. J., The action of cortisone acetate on cell-mediated immunity to infection: suppression of host cell proliferation and alteration of cellular composition of infected foci, *J. Exp. Med.*, 134, 1485, 1971.

31. Mackaness, G. B., The influence of immunologically committed lymphoid cells on macrophage activity *in vivo*, *J. Exp. Med.*, 129, 973, 1969.

32. Mackaness, G. B. and Hill, W. C., The effect of anti-lymphocyte globulin on cell-mediated resistance to infection, *J. Exp. Med.*, 129, 993, 1969.

33. Simon, H. B. and Sheagren, J. N., Cellular immunity *in vitro*. I. Immunologically mediated enhancement of macrophage bactericidal capacity, *J. Exp. Med.*, 133, 1377, 1971.

34. Nakane, A., Minagawa, T., and Kato, K., Endogenous tumor necrosis factor (cachectin) is essential to host resistance against *Listeria monocytogenes* infection, *Infect. Immun.*, 56, 2563, 1988.

35. Wright, S. C., Jewett, A., Mitsuyasu, R., and Bonavida, B., Spontaneous cytotoxicity and tumor necrosis factor production by peripheral blood monocytes from AIDS patients, *J. Immunol.*, 141, 99, 1988.

36. Moellering, R. C., Jr., Medoff, G., Leech, I., Wennersten, C., and Kunz, L. J., Antibiotic synergism against *Listeria monocytogenes*, *Antimicrob. Agents Chemother.*, 1, 30, 1972.

37. Bancroft, G. J., Schreiber, R. D., Bosma, G. C., Bosma, M. J., and Unanue, E. R., T cell-independent mechanism of macrophage activation by interferon-gamma, *J. Immunol.*, 139, 1104, 1987.

38. Newborg, M. F. and North, R. J., On the mechanism of T cell independent anti-*Listeria* resistance in nude mice, *J. Immunol.*, 124, 571, 1980.

39. Thiel, M., Kindt, R., Schmidt, H., Schassan, H., and Horst-Schmidt-Kliniken Potel, J., Listeriensepsis bei AIDS, *Dtsch. Med. Wochenschr.*, 111, 316, 1986.

40. Real, F. X., Gold, J. W. M., Krown, S. E., and Armstrong, D., *Listeria monocytogenes* bacteremia in the acquired immunodeficiency syndrome, *Ann. Intern. Med.*, 101, 883, 1984.

41. Schattenkerk, J. K. M. E., Klöpping, C., Speelman, J. D., Van Ketel, R. J., and Danner, S. A., Complications of the acquired immunodeficiency syndrome, *Ann. Intern. Med.*, 104, 726, 1986.

42. Harvey, R. L. and Chandrasekar, P. H., Chronic meningitis caused by *Listeria* in a patient infected with human immunodeficiency virus, *J. Infect. Dis.*, 157, 1091, 1988.

43. Riancho, J. A., Echevarria, S., Napal, J., Duran, R. M., and Macias, J. G., Endocarditis due to *Listeria monocytogenes* and human immunodeficiency virus infection, *Am. J. Med.*, 85, 737, 1988.

44. Beninger, P. R., Savoia, M. C., and Davis, C. E., Listeria monocytogenes meningitis in a patient with AIDS-related complex, *J. Infect. Dis.*, 158, 1396, 1988.

45. Bizet, C., Mechali, D., Rocourt, J., and Fraisse, F., Listeria monocytogenes bacteraemia in AIDS, *Lancet*, 1, 501, 1989.

46. Patey, O., Nedelec, C., Emond, J. P., Mayorga, R., N'Go, N., and Lafaix, C., *Listeria monocytogenes* septicemia in an AIDS patient with a brain abscess, *Eur. J. Clin. Microbiol. Infect. Dis.*, 8, 746, 1989.

47. Katner, H. P. and Joiner, T. A., *Listeria monocytogenes* sepsis from an infected indwelling I.V. catheter in a patient with AIDS, *South. Med. J.*, 82, 94, 1989.

48. Harris, J. O., Marquez, J., Swerdlow, M. A., and Magana, I. A., *Listeria* brain abscess in the acquired immunodeficiency syndrome, *Arch. Neurol.*, 46, 250, 1989.

49. Louria, D. B., Hensle, T., Armstrong, D., Collins, H. S., Blevins, A., Krugman, D., and Buse, M., Listeriosis complicating malignant disease: a new complication, *Ann. Intern. Med.*, 67, 261, 1967.

50. Spitzer, P. G., Hammer, S. M., and Karchmer, A. W., Treatment of *Listeria monocytogenes* infection with trimethoprim-sulfamethoxazole: case report and review of the literature, *Rev. Infect. Dis.*, 8, 427, 1986.

51. Fahey, J. L., Immunologic alterations, in Gotlieb, M. S. (moderator), The acquired immunodeficiency syndrome, *Ann. Intern. Med.*, 99, 208, 1983.

52. Jungi, T. W., Gill, T. J., Kunz, H. W., and Jungi, R., Genetic control of cell-mediated immunity in the rat, *J. Immunogenet.*, 9, 445, 1982.

53. Kales, C. P. and Holzman, R. S., Listeriosis in patients with HIV infection: clinical manifestations and response to therapy, *J. Acquir. Immun.*, 3, 139, 1990.

54. Tuazon, C. U., Shamsuddin, D., and Miller, H., Antibiotic susceptibility and synergy of clinical isolates of *Listeria monocytogenes*, *Antimicrob. Agents Chemother.*, 21, 525, 1982.

55. Winslow, D. L. and Pankey, G. A., *In vitro* activities of trimethoprim and sulfamethoxazole against *Listeria monocytogenes*, *Antimicrob. Agents Chemother.*, 22, 51, 1982.

56. Larsson, S., Walder, M. H., Cronberg, S. N., Forsgren, A. B., and Moestrup, T., Antimicrobial susceptibilities of *Listeria monocytogenes* strains isolated from 1958 to 1982 in Sweden, *Antimicrob. Agents Chemother.*, 28, 12, 1985.

13 Gastrointestinal Infections in the Immunocompromised Host

13.1 INTRODUCTION

The gastrointestinal (GI) tract is the largest lymphoid organ in the human body and, therefore, any defects in the cellular and/or humoral immune responses may be a strong predisposing factor to a multitude of enteric viral, fungal, bacterial, and protozoan pathogens, as seen in some of the preceding chapters.[1-5]

The identification of enteric pathogens in the GI tract has been especially important in patients with AIDS where the HIV-induced immunodeficiency greatly facilitates the possibility of opportunistic infections. For example, GI disorders have occurred in 30% to 50% of North American and European AIDS patients, and in nearly 90% of patients in developing countries. In AIDS patients, the initial symptoms of diarrhea include nausea, anorexia, malaise, and other mononucleosis-like manifestations at the time of seroconversion.[6] In full-blown AIDS, depending on the particular pathogen, diarrhea is manifested with large stool volumes, presence of blood, and abdominal pain.[7] In cases of chronic diarrhea, often the illness is accompanied by inanition and cachexia. In African patients with AIDS, this condition, referred to as "slim disease," could be superimposed on underlying GI infections caused by some tropical pathogens.[8]

Several viruses have been identified as enteric pathogens in patients with T cell deficiencies from causes other than AIDS, such as chemotherapy before bone marrow transplantation or severe combined immunodeficiency syndrome (SCID).[42-44] Novel viruses such as rotavirus, adenovirus, calicivirus, and astrovirus have been diagnosed in chronic diarrheal disease in children with SCID,[74,75] and in bone marrow transplant recipients. In the latter case, rotaviral and adenoviral infections were associated with markedly increased mortality.[76]

In the majority of AIDS patients, the causative agent(s) of GI infections can be identified (Table 13.1), and appropriate treatment may reduce the severity and frequency of gastrointestinal infections.[9,10] Although less often and with minimal inflammation, the human immunodeficiency virus (HIV) itself has also been found to infect mononuclear cells in lamina propria of the intestine in 30% to 39% of patients,[11-13] and in lamina propria of the esophagus in 36% of patients.[1] This, coupled with the fact that several studies of AIDS patients with GI manifestations have demonstrated the presence of villous atrophy, crypt hyperplasia, the occurrence of lactase deficiency and malabsorption, all in the absence of identifiable pathogens,[3,9,12,14-16,41] has raised the possibility that patients with AIDS may still develop an HIV-associated enteropathy caused by functional changes in the small bowel mucosa[12] as well as malabsorption.[3,14,15]

Furthermore, with the progression of AIDS disease, the CD4+ T cell population will continue to decline (including the number of CD4+ T cells in the mucosal population of the lamina propria[17-19]) leading to impaired cytotoxic T cell responses. The infection of mononuclear phagocytes by HIV also results in the activation and functional impairment of the monocyte-macrophages,[19-21] entailing monocytes passing through the mucosa and possibly residential macrophages. As a consequence of the altered functions of both cytotoxic T cells and macrophages,

TABLE 13.1

Gastrointestinal Pathogens in Immunocompromised Hosts

Pathogen	Clinical Manifestations
Fungi	
Candida albicans	Esophagus
Histoplasma capsulatum	Colon
Viruses	
Cytomegalovirus	Esophagus, stomach, colon
Herpes simplex virus	Esophagus, rectum
Adenovirus	Colon
Rotavirus	Small intestine
Astravirus	Small intestine
Calicivirus	Small intestine
Bacteria	
Mycobacterium avium-intracellulare (MAC)	Stomach, small intestine, colon
Campylobacter sp.	Diarrhea, possible bacteremia
Salmonella sp.	Diarrhea, septicemia
Shigella sp.	Diarrhea
Clostridium difficile	Colon
Listeria monocytogenes	Meningitis, bacteremia
Vibrio sp. (non-cholerae)	Possible bacteremia
Protozoa	
Cryptosporidium	Diarrhea
Isospora belli	Diarrhea
Microsporidia (*Enterocytozoon bieneusi*)	Diarrhea
Giardia lamblia	Diarrhea
Entameba histolytica	Diarrhea

Data collected from Ref. 1, 45, 46, and 79.

the GI tract becomes more susceptible to infection by such opportunistic pathogens as cytomegalovirus, various bacteria, and protozoa.[1]

Together with cellular immune responses, the systemic and mucosal immunity has a substantial role in the defense against enteropathogens. The ability to control GI infections greatly depends on the strength of the immune response which can profoundly influence the course of enteric infections, especially in immunocompromised hosts. In this context, while several studies have demonstrated the ability of AIDS patients to maintain some elements of immunologic memory by expressing humoral immunity to specific organisms[22-25] acquired earlier in life, which persist after HIV infection, specific systemic antibody responses to new infections and vaccines remain depressed in all stages of AIDS,[2,22,26-30] thereby limiting the capability of these patients to mount a viable response to acute infections as well as to vaccines devised to prevent them. For example, reduced levels of antibodies have been observed in AIDS patients against newly acquired infections caused by *Campylobacter jejuni*,[31] *Giardia lamblia*,[32] *Mycobacterium avium-intracellulare* (MAC),[33] and *Salmonella* spp.[34] Moreover, even when present, specific antibodies to chronic or reactivated enteric pathogens may be ineffective in controlling diseases caused by *Cryptosporidium*,[35,36] cytomegalovirus,[22] and *Shigella flexneri*.[37] In the latter case, both humoral and cell-mediated immunity are required to control the infection.[38-40]

The identification of some unusual serotypes of enteric adenoviruses in AIDS patients[45,46] has suggested that other novel viruses may well be present in these patients.[47] In this regard, a number of new assays have been instrumental in extending the diagnostic means available, including the polyacrylamide-gel electrophoresis (PAGE) to detect atypical rotaviruses[48] and picobirnaviruses,[49] enzyme immunoassay to detect astroviruses,[50] and a concentration technique to increase the sensitivity of detecting viral agents in fecal specimens by direct electron microscopy.[44,51] The results have shown that viruses may have been more common in HIV-associated diarrhea than was previously thought. Viruses have been found significantly more often in stools of AIDS patients with diarrhea than in specimens from patients without diarrhea. In addition, two novel viruses, astroviruses and picobirnavirus, have been detected in fecal specimens of HIV-infected patients.[45] While the results of Grohmann et al.[45] and others have shown that astrovirus,[52-54] calicivirus,[45] rotavirus,[43,55,56,77] and adenovirus[42,43,45,48,55,77] should be recognized as potential agents of diarrhea in AIDS patients, the association of picobirnavirus with diarrhea in these patients is still not conclusive.

13.2 THERAPEUTIC STRATEGIES FOR ENTERIC INFECTIONS

The evolution of therapies and current recommendations for treatment of various enteric infections in immunocompromised patients are described in details throughout this treatise in the corresponding chapters discussing individual enteric infections.

It should be strongly emphasized that enteric diseases in severely ill patients, such as those with AIDS, could be caused by a wide array of pathogens which will make empirical antimicrobial therapy difficult to implement. It is important, therefore, that patients while being evaluated, be given supportive therapy with rehydration, electrolyte supplementation, and drug regimens to inhibit intestinal secretion or motility. Although treatment with anti-motility drugs may be considered controversial for certain bacterial diarrheas (bloody diarrhea, fecal leukocytes, abdominal pain), in the majority of cases, significant symptomatic benefit may result from therapy with loperamide, diphenoxylate, paregoric, or Kaopectate®.[1]

In patients with AIDS, major problems that need to be addressed are the recurrence of diarrheal infection after termination of therapy, and the emergence of drug-resistant pathogens (cytomegalovirus,[57] herpes simplex virus,[58,59] *Campylobacter* spp.,[60] and *Shigella* spp.[61]). Other enteric pathogens, such as *Cryptosporidium, Microsporidia*, and to a great extent *Mycobacterium avium-intracellulare* (MAC) cannot be cured with the currently available antimicrobial agents.

Even though in 80% to 87% of AIDS-associated diarrhea, the causative pathogen(s) of the diarrhea is identified, enteropathies characterized with malabsorption, small-bowel mucosal abnormalities, and no identifiable pathogens have been observed in patients with profuse diarrhea.[12] Two drugs, octreotide and 5-acetylsalicylic acid (5-ASA), have been reported to be of some benefit in treating profuse diarrheal disease.

Octreotide, a synthetic cyclic octapeptide congener of somatostatin, was found to be effective in the treatment of patients with severe refractory diarrhea caused by pancreatic cholera (the Vipoma syndrome), carcinoid syndrome, and diabetic diarrhea,[62-64] as well as AIDS-associated diarrhea.[65-69] In these situations, the drug was reported to decrease the jejunal secretion of water and electrolytes, and to increase the absorption of water and electrolytes by the jejunal mucosa.

In a prospective, multicenter clinical trial, Cello et al.[70] studied the efficacy and safety of octreotide in the treatment of 51 AIDS patients with profuse refractory diarrhea (over 500 ml liquid stool daily). The patients received subcutaneously 50 µg of octeotride every 8 h for 48 h; when the stool volume was not reduced to less than 250 ml/daily, the dose was increased stepwise to 100, 250, and 500 µg. The results of this short-term therapy were somewhat disappointing, with a response rate reaching only 41%. However, since 61% of the patients with no identifiable enteric pathogens responded partially or completely to octreotide, the drug may still be of some benefit to such patients.

According to Londong et al.,[71] long-term octreotide treatment may be even less efficient because of diminished efficacy caused by downregulation of receptors. In contrast, during a 2-year period, Miranda-Ruiz et al.[72] have observed a 70% response rate to octreotide in 70 AIDS patients with severe, chronic hypersecretory diarrea (more than 10 daily evacuations and 2 to 7 l of daily stool volume). The patients received conventional antibiotic therapy in addition to 200 µg of octreotide given subcutaneously every 6 h for a minimum of 1 month; 10 patients received octreotide intermitently for up to 15 months.

Tierney et al.[73] investigated the efficacy of 5-ASA in the treatment of HIV-associated inflammatory bowel disease (mucosal inflammation) in the absence of identifiable enteric pathogens. The patients received orally 6 g of 5-ASA for 2 months. Diarrheal symptoms stabilized or improved in seven of nine patients, and the mucosal production of p24 antigen decreased significantly over a 2-month period.

13.2.1 PREVENTION OF ENTERIC INFECTIONS

In immunocompetent patients, antimicrobial therapy can lengthen the shedding period of *Salmonella* spp. in the stool and, therefore, is not usually recommended.[78] There have been no controlled studies on the antimicrobial treatment of HIV-positive patients with salmonella gastroenteritis. However, it has been recommended that HIV-infected patients receive antimicrobial therapy with ciprofloxacin (500 to 750 mg twice daily) to prevent extraintestinal infection.[78] In the case of *Campylobacter* infections, again ciprofloxacin (500 mg twice daily) has been recommended instead of erythromycin.[78] HIV-infected patients with salmonella septicemia would require long-term therapy with ciprofloxacin (500 to 750 mg twice daily) to prevent recurrence. Possible preventive therapy in children includes trimethoprim-sulfamethoxazole, ampicillin, cefotaxime, ceftriaxone, or chloramphenicol.

13.3   REFERENCES

1. Smith, P. D., Quinn, T. C., Strober, W., Janoff, E. N., and Masur, H., Gastrointestinal infections in AIDS, *Ann. Intern. Med.*, 116, 63, 1992.
2. Malebranche, R., Arnoux, E., Guérin, J. M., Pierre, G. D., Laroche, A. C., Péan-Guichard, C., Elie, R., Morisset, P. H., Spira, J. G., Mandeville, R., Drotman, P., Seemayer, T., and Dupuy, J.-M., Acquired immunodeficiency syndrome with severe gastrointestinal manifestations in Haiti, *Lancet*, 2, 873, 1983.
3. Dworkin, B., Wormser, G. P., Rosenthal, W. S., Heier, S. K., Braunstein, M., Weiss, L., Jankowski, R., Levy, D., and Weiselberg, S., Gastrointestinal manifestations of the acquired immunodeficiency syndrome: a review of 22 cases, *Am. J. Gastroenterol.*, 80, 774, 1985.
4. Colebunders, R., Francis, H., Mann, J. M., Bila, K. M., Izaley, L., Kimputu, L., Behets, F., Van der Groen, G., Quinn, T., Curran, J. W., and Piot, P., Persistent diarrhea, strongly associated with HIV infection in Kinshasa, *Am. J. Gastroenterol.*, 82, 859, 1987.
5. Janoff, E. N. and Smith, P. D., Perspectives on gastrointestinal infections in AIDS, *Gastroenterol. Clin. North Am.*, 17, 451, 1988.
6. Cooper, A. D., Gold, J., Maclean, P., Donovan, B., Finlayson, R., Barnes, T. G., Michelmore, H. M., Brooke, P., Penny, R., and the Sydney AIDS Study Group, Acute AIDS retrovirus infection: definition of a clinical illness associated with seroconversion, *Lancet*, 1, 537, 1985.
7. Smith, P. D. and Janoff, E. N., Infectious diarrhea in human immunodeficiency virus infection, *Gastroenterol. Clin. North Am.*, 17, 587, 1988.
8. Serwadda, D., Mugerwa, R. D., Sewankambo, N. K., Lwegaba, A., Carswell, J. W., Kirya, G. L., Bayley, A. C., Downing, R. G., Tedder, R. S., Clayden, S. A., Weiss, R. A., and Dalgleish, A. G., Slim disease: a new disease in Uganda and its association with HTLV-III infection, *Lancet*, 2, 849, 1985.
9. Smith, P. D., Lane, H. C., Gill, V. J., Quinnan, G. V., Fauci, A. S., and Masur, H., Intestinal infections in patients with the acquired immunodeficiency syndrome (AIDS): etiology and response to therapy, *Ann. Intern. Med.*, 108, 328, 1988.

10. Laughon, B. E., Druckman, D. A., Vernon, A., Quinn, T. C., Polk, B. F., Modlin, J. F., Yolken, R. H., and Bartlett, J. G., Prevalence of enteric pathogens in homosexual men with and without acquired immunodeficiency syndrome, *Gastroenterology*, 94, 984, 1988.

11. Fox, C. H., Kotler, D. P., Tierney, A. R., Wilson, C. S., and Fauci, A. S., Detection of HIV-1 RNA in the lamina propria of patients with AIDS and gastrointestinal disease, *J. Infect. Dis.*, 159, 467, 1989.

12. Ullrich, R., Zeitz, M., Heise, W., L'age, M., Höffken, G., and Riecken, E. O., Small intestinal structure and function in patients infected with human immunodeficiency virus (HIV): evidence for HIV-induced enteropathy, *Ann. Intern. Med.*, 111, 15, 1989.

13. Jarry, A., Cortez, A., Rene, E., Muzeau, F., and Brousse, N., Infected and immune cells in the gastrointestinal tract of AIDS patients: an immunohistochemical study of 127 cases, *Histopathology*, 16, 133, 1990.

14. Gillin, J. S., Shike, M., Alcock, N., Urmacher, C., Krown, S., Kurtz, R. C., Lightdale, C. J., and Winawer, S. J., Malabsorption and mucosal abnormalities of the small intestine in the acquired immunodeficiency syndrome, *Ann. Intern. Med.*, 102, 619, 1985.

15. Kotler, D. P., Gaetz, H. P., Lange, M., Klein, E. B., and Holt, P. R., Enteropathy associated with the acquired immunodeficiency syndrome, *Ann. Intern. Med.*, 101, 421, 1984.

16. Harriman, G. R., Smith, P. D., Horne, M. K., Fox, C. H., Koenig, S., Lack, E. E., Lane, H. C., and Fauci, A. S., Vitamin B_{12} malabsorption in patients with acquired immunodeficiency syndrome, *Arch. Intern. Med.*, 149, 2039, 1989.

17. Rodgers, V. D., Fassett, R., and Kagnoff, M. F., Abnormalities in intestinal mucosal T cells in homosexual populations including those with the lymphadenopathy syndrome and acquired immuno-deficiency syndrome, *Gastroenterology*, 90, 552, 1986.

18. Ellakany, S., Whiteside, T. L., Schade, R. R., and van Thiel, D. H., Analysis of intestinal lymphocyte subpopulations in patients with acquired immunodeficiency syndrome, *J. Clin. Pathol.*, 87, 356, 1987.

19. Smith, P. D., Ohura, K., Masur, H., Lane, H. C., Fauci, A. S., and Wahl, S. M., Monocyte function in the acquired immunodeficiency syndrome: defective chemotaxis, *J. Clin. Invest.*, 74, 2121, 1984.

20. Allen, J. B., McCartney-Francis, N., Smith, P. D., Simon, G., Gartner, S., Wahl, L. M., Popovic, M., and Wahl, S. M., Expression of interleukin 2 receptors by monocytes from patients with acquired immunodeficiency syndrome and induction of monocyte interleukin 2 receptors by human immuno-deficiency virus-1 *in vitro*, *J. Clin. Invest.*, 85, 192, 1990.

21. Baldwin, G. C., Fleischmann, J., Chung, Y., Koyanagi, Y., Chen, I. S., and Golde, D. W., Human immunodeficiency virus causes mononuclear phagocyte dysfunction, *Proc. Natl. Acad. Sci. U.S.A.*, 87, 3933, 1990.

22. Quinn, T. C., Piot, P., McCormick, J. B., Feinsod, F. M., Taelman, H., Kapita, B., Stevens, W., and Fauci, A. S., Serologic and immunologic studies in patients with AIDS in North America and Africa, *JAMA*, 257, 2617, 1987.

23. Quinn, G. V., Jr., Masur, H., Rook, A. H., Armstrong, G., Frederick, W. R., Epstein, J., Manischewitz, J. F., Macher, A. M., Jackson, L., Ames, J., Smith, H. A., Parker, M., Pearson, G. R., Parrillo, J., Mitchell, C., and Straus, S. E., Herpesvirus infections in the acquired immune deficiency syndrome, *JAMA*, 252, 72, 1984.

24. Luft, B. J., Brooks, R. G., Conley, F. K., Maccabe, R. E., and Remington, J. S., Toxoplasmic encephalitis in patients with acquired immune deficiency syndrome, *JAMA*, 252, 913, 1984.

25. Janoff, E. N., Hardy, W. D., Smith, P. D., and Wahl, S. M., Levels, specificity and affinity of IgG specific for recall antigens in patients with HIV, *J. Immunol.*, 147, 2130, 1991.

26. Janoff, E. N., Douglas, J. M., Jr., Gabriel, M., Blaser, M. J., Davidson, A. J., Cohn, D. L., and Judson, F. N., Class-specific antibody response to pneumococcal capsular polysaccharides in men infected with human immune deficiency virus type 1, *J. Infect. Dis.*, 158, 983, 1988.

27. Ammann, A. J., Schiffman, G., Abrams, D., Volberding, P., Ziegler, J., and Conant, M., B-cell immunodeficiency in acquired immune deficiency syndrome, *JAMA*, 251, 1447, 1984.

28. Lane, H. C., Depper, J. M., Greene, W. C., Whalen, G., Waldmann, T. A., and Fauci, A. S., Qualitative analysis of immune function in patients with the acquired immunodeficiency syndrome, *N. Engl. J. Med.*, 313, 79, 1985.

29. Lane, H. C., Masur, H., Edgar, L. C., Whalen, G., Rook, A. H., and Fauci, A. S., Abnormalities of B-cell activation and immunoregulation in patients with the acquired immunodeficiency syndrome, *N. Engl. J. Med.*, 309, 453, 1983.

30. Ragni, M. V., Ruben, F. L., Winklestein, A., Spero, J. A., Bontempo, F. A., and Lewis, J. H., Antibody responses to immunization of patients with hemophilia with and without evidence of human immunodeficiency virus (human T-lymphotropic virus type III) infection, *J. Lab. Clin. Med.*, 109, 545, 1987.

31. Perlman, D. M., Ampel, N. M., Schiffman, R. B., Cohn, D. L., Patton, C. M., Aguirre, M. L., Wang, W. L., and Blaser, M. J., Persistent *Campylobacter jejuni* infections in patients infected with the human immunodeficiency virus, *Ann. Intern. Med.*, 108, 540, 1988.

32. Janoff, E. N., Smith, P. D., and Blaser, M. J., Acute antibody responses to *Giardia lamblia* are depressed in patients with the acquired immunodeficiency syndrome, *J. Infect. Dis.*, 157, 798, 1988.

33. Winter, S. M., Bernard, E. M., Gold, J. W., and Armstrong, D., Humoral response to disseminated infection by *Mycobacterium avium-intracellulare* in acquired immunodeficiency syndrome, *J. Infect. Dis.*, 151, 523, 1985.

34. Tagliabue, A., Nencioni, L., Mantovani, A., Lazzarin, A., Villa, L., Romano, M., Rossini, S., Foppa, C. U., Fanetti, G., Masello, L. C., and Poli, G., Impairment of *in vitro* natural antibacterial activity in HIV- infected patients, *J. Immunol.*, 141, 2607, 1988.

35. Campbell, P. N. and Current, W. L., Demonstration of serum antibodies to *Cryptosporidium* spp. in normal and immunodeficient humans with confirmed infections, *J. Clin. Microbiol.*, 18, 165, 1983.

36. Ungar, B. L., Soave, R., Fayer, R., and Nash, T. E., Enzyme immunoassay detection of immunoglobulin M and G antibodies to *Cryptosporidium* in immunocompetent and immunocompromised persons, *J. Infect. Dis.*, 153, 570, 1986.

37. Blaser, M. J., Hale, T. L., and Formal, S. B., Recurrent shigellosis complicating human immunodeficiency virus infection: failure of pre-existing antibodies to confer protection, *Am. J. Med.*, 86, 105, 1989.

38. Klimpel, G. R., Niesel, D. W., and Klimpel, K. D., Natural cytotoxic effector cell activity against *Shigella flexneri*-infected HeLa cells, *J. Immunol.*, 136, 1081, 1986.

39. Morgan, D. R., DuPont, H. L., Gonik, B., and Kohl, S., Cytotoxicity of human peripheral blood and colostral leukocytes against *Shigella* species, *Infect. Immun.*, 46, 25, 1984.

40. Dinari, G., Hale, T. L., Austin, S. W., and Formal, S. B., Local and systemic antibody responses to *Shigella* infections in rhesus monkeys, *J. Infect. Dis.*, 155, 1065, 1987.

41. Heise, W., Mostertz, P., Arasteh, K., Skörde, J., and L'age, M., Gastrointestinale befunde bei der HIV-infektion, *Dtsch. Med. Wochenschr.*, 113, 1588, 1988.

42. Saulsbury, F. T., Winkelstein, J. A., and Yolken, R. H., Chronic rotavirus infection in immunodeficiency, *J. Pediatr.*, 97, 61, 1980.

43. Yolken, R. H., Bishop, C. A., Townsend, T. R., Bolyard, E. A., Bartlett, J., Santos, G. W., and Saral, R., Infectious gastroenteritis in bone-marrow-transplant recipients, *N. Engl. J. Med.*, 306, 1010, 1982.

44. LeBaron, C. W., Furutan, N. P., Lew, J. F., Allen, J. R., Gouvea, V., Moe, C., and Monroe, S. S., Viral agents of gastroenteritis. Public health importance and outbreak management, *Morbid. Mortal. Wkly. Rep.*, 39(RR-5), 1, 1990.

45. Grohmann, G. S., Glass, R. I., Pereira, H. G., Monroe, S. S., Hightower, A. W., Weber, R., Bryan, R. T., and the Enteric Opportunistic Infections Working group, Enteric viruses and diarrhea in HIV-infected patients, *N. Engl. J. Med.*, 329, 14, 1993.

46. Hierholzer, J. C., Adrian, T., Anderson, L. J., Wigand, R., and Gold, J. W. M., Analysis of antigenically intermediate strains of subgenus B and D adenoviruses from AIDS patients, *Arch. Virol.*, 103, 99, 1988.

47. Hierholzer, J. C., Wigand, R., Anderson, L. J., Adrian, T., and Gold, J. W. M., Adenoviruses from patients with AIDS: a plethora of serotypes and a description of five new serotypes of subgenus D (types 43-47), *J. Infect. Dis.*, 158, 804, 1988.

48. Bridger, J. C., Novel rotaviruses in animal and man, *Ciba Found. Symp.*, 128, 5, 1987.

49. Pereira, H. G., Fialho, A. M., Flewett, T. H., Teixeira, J. M., and Andrade, Z. P., Novel viruses in human faeces, *Lancet*, 2, 103, 1988.

50. Moe, C. L., Allen, J. R., Monroe, S. S., Gary, H. E., Jr., Humphrey, C. D., Herrmann, J. E., Blacklow, N. R., Carcamo, C., Koch, M., Kim, K.-H., and Glass, R. I., Detection of astrovirus in pediatric stool samples by immunoassay and RNA probe, *J. Clin. Microbiol.*, 29, 2390, 1991.

51. Grohmann, G., Glass, R. I., Gold, J., James, M., Edwards, P., Borg, T., Stine, S. E., Goldsmith, C., and Monroe, S. S., Outbreak of human calicivirus gastroenteritis in a day-care center in Sidney, Australia, *J. Clin. Microbiol.*, 29, 544, 1991.

52. Lew, J. F., Moe, C. L., Monroe, S. S., Allen, J. R., Harrison, B. M., Forrester, B. D., Stine, S. E., Woods, P. A., Hierholzer, J. C., Herrmann, J. E., Blacklow, N. R., Bartlett, A. V., and Glass, R. I., Astrovirus and adenovirus associated with diarrhea in children in day care center, *J. Infect. Dis.*, 164, 673, 1991.

53. Herrmann, J. E., Taylor, D. N., Echeverria, P., and Blacklow, N. R., Astroviruses as a cause of gastroenteritis in children, *N. Engl. J. Med.*, 324, 1757, 1991.

54. Cruz, J. R., Bartlett, A. V., Herrmann, J. E., Caceres, P., Blacklow, N. R., and Cano, F., Astrovirus-associated diarrhea among Guatemalan ambulatory rural children, *J. Clin. Microbiol.*, 30, 1140, 1992.

55. Gray, J. R. and Rabeneck, L., Atypical mycobacterial infection in the gastrointestinal tract in AIDS patients, *Am. J. Gastroenterol.*, 84, 1521, 1989.

56. Thea, D. M., Glass, R. I., Grohmann, G. S., Perriens, J., Ngoy, B., Kapita, B., Atido, U., Mabaluko, M., and Keusch, G. T., Prevalence of enteric viruses among hospitalized AIDS patients in Kinshasa, Zaire, *Trans. R. Soc. Trop. Med. Hyg.*, 87, 263, 1993.

57. Erice, A., Chou, S., Biron, K. K., Stanat, S. C., Balfour, H. A., Jr., and Jordan, M. C., Progressive disease due to ganciclovir-resistant cytomegalovirus in immunocompromised patients, *N. Engl. J. Med.*, 320, 289, 1989.

58. Oliver, N. M., Collins, P., Van der Meer, J., and Van't Wout, J. W., Biological and biochemical characterization of clinical isolates of herpes simplex virus type 2 resistant to acyclovir, *Antimicrob. Agents Chemother.*, 33, 635, 1989.

59. Sacks, S. L., Wanklin, R. J., Reece, D. E., Hicks, K. A., Tyler, K. L., and Coen, D. M., Progressive esophagitis from acyclovir-resistant herpes simplex, *Ann. Intern. Med.*, 111, 893, 1989.

60. Dworkin, B., Wormser, G. P., Abdoo, R. A., Cabello, F., Aguero, M. E., and Sivak, S. L., Persistence of multiply antibiotic-resistant *Campylobacter jejuni* in a patient with the acquired immunodeficiency syndrome, *Am. J. Med.*, 80, 965, 1986.

61. Gander, R. M. and LaRocco, M. T., Multiple drug-resistance in *Shigella flexneri* isolated from a patient with human immunodeficiency virus, *Diagn. Microbiol. Infect. Dis.*, 8, 193, 1987.

62. Vinik, A. I., Tsai, S. T., Moattari, A. R., Cheung, P., Ackhauser, F. E., and Cho, K., Somatostatin analogue (SMS 201-995) in the management of gastroenteropancreatic tumors and diarrhea syndromes, *Am. J. Med.*, 81(Suppl. 6B), 23, 1986.

63. Kvols, L. K., Metastatic carcinoid tumors and the carcinoid syndrome: a selective review of chemotherapy and hormonal therapy, *Am. J. Med.*, 81(Suppl. 6B), 49, 1986.

64. Williams, S. T., Woltering, E. A., O'Dorisio, T. M., and Fletcher, W. S., Effect of octeotride acetate on pancreatic exocrine function, *Am. J. Surg.*, 157, 459, 1989.

65. Katz, M. D., Erstad, B. L., and Rose, C., Treatment of severe cryptosporidium-related diarrhea with octeotride in a patient with AIDS, *Drug Intell. Clin. Pharm.*, 22, 134, 1988.

66. Clotet, B., Sirera, G., Cofan, F., Monterola, J. M., Tortosa, F., and Fox, M., Efficacy of the somatostatin analogue (SMS-201-995), sandostatin for cryptosporidial diarrhoea in patients with AIDS, *AIDS*, 3, 857, 1989.

67. Füessl, H. S., Zoller, W. G., Kochen, M. M., Bogner, J. R., Heinrich, B., Matuschke, A., and Goebel, F. D., Treatment of secretory diarrhea in AIDS with the somatostatin analogue SMS 201-995, *Klin. Wochenschr.*, 67, 452, 1989.

68. Robinson, E. N., Jr. and Fogel, R., SMS 201-995, a somatostatin analogue, and diarrhea in the acquired immunodeficiency syndrome (AIDS), *Ann. Intern. Med.*, 109, 680, 1988.

69. Cook, D. J., Kelton, J. G., Stanisz, A. M., and Collins, S. M., Somatostatin treatment for cryptosporidial diarrhea in a patient with the acquired immunodeficiency syndrome, *Ann. Intern. Med.*, 108, 708, 1988.

70. Cello, J. P., Grendell, J. H., Basuk, P., Simon, D., Weiss, L., Wittner, M., Rood, R. P., Wilcox, C. M., Forsmark, C. E., Read, A. E., Satow, J. A., Weikel, C. S., and Beaumont, C., Effect of octeotride on refractory AIDS-associated diarrhea: a prospective, multicenter clinical trial, *Ann. Intern. Med.*, 115, 705, 1991.

71. Londong, W., Angerer, M., Kutz, K., Landgraf, R., and Londong, V., Diminishing efficacy of octreotide (SMS 201-995) on gastric functions of healthy subjects during one-week administration, *Gastroenterology*, 96, 713, 1989.

72. Miranda-Ruiz, R., Feregrino-Gouos, M., Alvarado Diez, R., Castanon, G. J., Gallegos-Perez, H., and Aid Lidt, G., Experience of two years in therapy of AIDS hypersecretory diarrhea with octreotide, *Proc. Xth Int. Conf. AIDS*, Yokohama, 1994, Abstr. PB0177.

73. Tierney, A. R., Reka, S., Hecker, L., Cohen, S., Clayton, F., and Kotler, D. P., Treatment of HIV-associated inflammatory bowel disease with oral 5-ASA, *Proc. VIIIth Int. Conf. AIDS*, Amsterdam, 1992, Abstr. PoB 3725.

74. Chrystie, I. L., Booth, I. W., Kidd, A. H., Marxhall, W. C., and Banatvala, J. E., Multiple faecal virus excretion in immunodeficiency, *Lancet*, 1, 282, 1982.

75. Madeley, C. R., Epidemiology of gut viruses, in *Viruses and the Gut*, Farthing, M. J. G., Ed., Smith Kline and French Laboratories, Welwyn Garden City, U.K., 1988, 5.

76. Yolken, R. H., Bishop, C. A., Townsend, T. R., Bolyard, E. A., Bartlett, J., Santos, G. W., and Saral, R., Infectious gastroenteritis in bone-marrow-transplant recipients, *N. Engl. J. Med.*, 306, 1010, 1982.

77. Cinningham, A. L., Grohmann, G. S., Harkness, J., Law, C., Marriott, D., Tindall, E., and Cooper, D. A., Gastrointestinal viral infections in homosexual men who were symptomatic and seropositive for human immunodeficiency virus, *J. Infect. Dis.*, 158, 386, 1988.

78. Angulo, F. J. and Swerdlow, D. L., Bacterial enteric infections in persons infected with human immunodeficiency virus, *Clin. Infect. Dis.*, 31(Suppl. 1), S84, 1995.

14 Neisseriaceae

The Neisseriaceae is a family of Gram-negative, aerobic cocci and rod-shaped bacteria occurring singly or as pairs, short chains, or masses. These organisms, which may exist either as saprophytes or parasites, have been divided into four genera, *Acinetobacter*, *Kingella*, *Moraxella*, and *Neisseria*.

14.1 *ACINETOBACTER* SPP.

14.1.1 INTRODUCTION

Acinetobacter is a genus of bacteria belonging to the family Neisseriaceae. They represent aerobic, nonfermentative, nonmotile, Gram-negative, usually paired (diploid formation) coccobacilli. The organisms are oxidase-negative and catalase-positive. Over the last 30 years or so, there have been many extensive changes in the taxonomy of these organisms resulting in their classification into various genera (*Moraxella*, *Achromobacter*, *Acinetobacter*, etc.).[1-4] Since 1984 genetic evidence (based on phenotypic characters and identification of genotypic species using genetic transformations, DNA hybridization, and RNA sequence comparison[5,6]) has been provided for the relatedness of all Gram-negative, oxidase-negative, nonmotile, aerobic coccobacilli to be included in the genus *Acinetobacter*.[1,5] Of the currently recognized 17 genomic species and 19 biotypes of *Acinetobacter*, there are two clinically important species: *A. calcoaceticus* (previously known as *A. anitratus*, *Herellea vaginicola*, *Mima-Herellea*, etc.) and *A. baumannii*. The designation "*Acinetobacter calcoaceticus*" is widely used in the medical literature and remains as the reference name according to *Bergey's Manual of Systematic Bacteriology*.[7-14]

Acinetobacter spp. are extensively distributed in nature (soil and water)[1,15,16] as free-living saprophytes. These organisms have been isolated as commensals from the skin, throat, axillae, groin, toe webs, and various secretions of healthy subjects.[8,17-20] Less frequently, *Acinetobacter* can also colonize the normal intestine.[21] However, *Acinetobacter* spp. are not part of the normal human intestinal flora.[22]

In hospitals, the pathogen may be found frequently in moist environments such as room humidifiers,[23] tap water, sinks, in ventilatory equipment which form aerosols, vascular catheters,[19,20,24-31] as well as in nonsterile pharmaceuticals. The seasonal increase in the incidence of infections (late summer and early winter) may be related to temperature and humidity.[16,19,32,33] Another place of *Acinetobacter* colonization has been equipment that is used in respiratory illness therapies.[24] Transmission of acinetobacter organisms to patients via the hands of hospital personnel has been observed[26,27,34-41] and experimentally demonstrated.[16,34,42-46]

Pulsed-field gel electrophoresis has been used to investigate the epidemiology of hospital outbreaks of *Acinetobacter* infections.[47-50] A combination of biotype, antibiotype, and genome fingerprinting by macrorestriction analysis and polymerase chain reaction (PCR) amplification of inter-repeat sequences to delineate transmission of multiresistant *A. baumannii* has been used to detect nosocomial outbreaks of multiresistant *A. baumannii*.[51]

Dijkshoorn et al.[52] have studied the cell envelope protein profiles of *A. calcoaceticus* strains isolated in hospitals by sodium dodecyl sulfate-polyacrylamide gel electrophoresis.

As nosocomial pathogens, *Acinetobacter* spp. have been an important cause of morbidity and mortality among debilitated patients in intensive care units[37,42-45,53] and immunocompromised patients.[11,16,19,20,24-26,35,51,54-59]

Acinetobacter spp. have also been recognized as opportunistic pathogens with increasing pathogenic importance known to provoke outbreaks of pneumonia,[26,28,60-65] and severe primary infections including tracheobronchitis, meningitis,[19,66-86] endocarditis,[87] peritonitis,[88] skin and soft tissue infections, urinary tract infections,[89] bacteremia,[90,91] and burn[30] and wound infections, especially in immunocompromised hosts.[11,19,23,24,34,55,87-89,92-100] By some accounts,[101] *A. baumannii* has been ranked fourth among the recognized causes of pneumonia in hospitalized patients. Clinical manifestations of bloodstream acinetobacter infections may range from benign transient bacteremia to fulminant disease with septic shock associated with an overall mortality ranging from 17% to 46%.[8,36,59,96,102-109] *A. baumannii* bloodstream infections have been most common among patients with severely impaired host immune defense and breakdown of natural defense barriers (skin and mucous membranes),[16] and in general, were hospital-acquired.[8,36,96,102]

Predisposing factors for severe infections include serious underlying disease, malignancies, burns, immunosuppression, major surgery, and age (elderly and neonates).[8,93] Prolonged and wide use of antimicrobial agents may also contribute to *Acinetobacter* infections due to resistance.[19,33,34,83,106]

The respiratory tract is the most common site of infection.[16,19,20,25,26,35,56,94,105,110] Although results from several studies have indicated that most clinical isolates of *A. baumannii* reflected colonization rather than infection,[34,111] recent reports have suggested that this species causes more serious and often fatal nosocomial infections.[16,19,20,26,35,56,111-115] The acquisition of *A. baumannii* has been associated also with the length of stay in the intensive care unit in excess of that due to the underlying disease alone.[49,50]

There have also been reports of community-acquired *A. baumannii* infections.[16,19,109,116-118] The community-acquired acinetobacter pneumonias, although rare, were fulminant and also with high mortality rate.[119]

14.1.2 EVOLUTION OF THERAPIES AND TREATMENT OF *ACINETOBACTER* INFECTIONS

Because of their frequent multiple resistance to broad-spectrum antibiotics (β-lactams and aminoglycosides), acinetobacters are sometimes difficult to treat, and combination drug therapy is commonly recommended.

Very few β-lactam antibiotics are still clinically effective. Imipenem is by far the most active drug against *Acinetobacter* infections.[120,121] Other therapeutic choices often include combination of ticarcillin with sulbactam (the latter, a β-lactamase inhibitor, has also shown anti-acinetobacter activity by itself),[35] as well as ceftazidime.

Amikacin remains the most active of the aminoglycoside antibiotics, as resistance to it has developed with a relatively low frequency compared to other aminoglycosides.[122] Nevertheless, a significant correlation has been established between the extent of amikacin consumption and the occurrence of amikacin-resistant *Acinetobacter* spp.[122] The aminoglycoside antibiotics can also be used against acinetobacter when given in combination with β-lactams (ticarcillin, ceftazidime, or imipenem).[24,123]

Urban et al.[56] reported that 20 isolates, all resistant to imipenem, aminoglycosides, and β-lactams, responded favorably to a combination of ampicillin and sulbactam. Most likely the beneficial effect was due to sulbactam.

The reported resistance of acinetobacter to imipenem[56] seemed to run contrary to several studies[19,35,57] that suggested that imipenem had more potent activity against *Acinetobacter* spp. than any other antimicrobial agent, and often was the only effective drug.[35]

In vitro susceptibility experiments by Chow et al.[124] have demonstrated synergistic effects between ciprofloxacin and broad-spectrum β-lactam antibiotics or aminoglycosides. In a further study by Leonov et al.,[13] patients with multidrug-resistant *A. calcoaceticus* bacteremia responded favorably to treatment with eiher ciprofloxacin alone or in combination with amikacin (the only two drugs that showed *in vitro* activity against the clinical strains isolated). Ciprofloxacin was administered intravenously at 200 mg every 12 h. Upon improvement of the patient's condition, oral ciprofloxacin (750 mg, b.i.d.) was started. In combination therapy with amikacin, the latter was administered at doses of 7.5 mg/kg with intervals adjusted to creatinine clearance. The treatment, which lasted 2 to 4 weeks, was successful in all patients who received it.[13]

Go et al.[37] have described a nosocomial outbreak of infections due to imipenem-resistant *A. baumannii*. The pathogen was susceptible to polymyxin B and sulbactam.

The clinical course of *A. johnsonii*-associated infections, because of the low virulence of this species, has been usually benign and in most instances fever had partially resolved by the time the organism was identified.[31] Seifert et al.[31] effectively used various antimicrobial agents alone (mezlocillin, cefuroxime, or ciprofloxacin) or in combinations (gentamicin–flucloxacillin, ampicillin–gentamicin, piperacillin–gentamicin, mezlocillin–gentamicin, pyrimethamine–spiramycin, tobramycin–clindamycin, cefotaxime–tobramycin, and amoxicillin–clavulanic acid–gentamicin) to treat 13 cases of *A. johnsonii* bacteremia.

Smego[105] utilized aminoglycosides alone (tobramycin, gentamicin, and amoxicillin) or in combination with a second agent (gentamicin sulfate–oxacillin sodium, tobramycin–erythromycin, tobramycin–carbenicillin disodium, gentamicin–ampicillin sodium, and tobramycin–carbenicillin) to treat successfully *A. calcoaceticus* bacteremia in 16 patients.

14.1.2.1 *Acinetobacter* Resistance to Antibiotics

There are several hypotheses on how *Acinetobacter* spp. develop resistance to antimicrobial agents. The mechanisms suggested include the presence of aminoglycoside-modifying enzymes (such as 6′-*N*-acetyltransferase and aminoglycoside-3′-*O*-phosphotransferase type V),[35,57] cephalosporinase, β-lactamase enzymes of types TEM-1 and TEM-2,[57] and plasmid coding.[16,25] It should be noted that resistance may change rapidly during the same outbreak because of the loss or acquisition of plasmid coding for antimicrobial resistance or the appearance of chromosomal mutants.[25] It is relevant to mention that findings by Johnson et al.[20] did not corroborate the loss or acquisition of plasmid coding as a mechanism of resistance.

In early reports,[34,94,125] the majority of *Acinetobacter* strains that have been studied showed susceptibility to ampicillin, cephalosporins, minocycline, and gentamicin, and only 3.4% were resistant to carbenicillin. However, in subsequent years a higher proportion of acinetobacter became resistant to most of the commonly used antibacterial drugs,[16,20,25,27,35,37,56,60,99,112] including aminopenicillins, ureidopenicillins, ampicillin,[8] first- and second-generation cephalosporins,[8] cephamycins (cefoxitin),[12] gentamicin,[8] aminoglycosides-aminocyclitols,[8,38,125,126] chloramphenicol, ciprofloxacin,[8] and tetracyclines.[24] The differences in susceptibility values that have been reported in various countries (Japan, Germany,[35] Spain,[95] and France[12,125]) have been largely due to different environment and usage factors. *Acinetobacter* isolates usually susceptible to aminoglycosides in the past, have become resistant to pefloxacin.

Resistance to imipenem, which so far has been the most active drug against acinetobacter (*in vitro* susceptibility in some studies[8] of up to 100% of strains tested), was limited (0.5% to 5.0%).[24] In one study,[37] imipenem resistance developed after increased use of imipenem in patients with cephalosporin-resistant *Klebsiella* infections.[127] The imipenem resistance appeared to have derived from a prior multiresistant clone, in contrast to another clone which retained susceptibility to several antibiotics.[37]

Several mechanisms have been suggested to explain the acinetobacter resistance to imipenem, including reduced outer-membrane permeability,[128] altered penicillin-binding proteins,[129] and carbapenemase production.[130]

Polymyxin B and sulbactam were found effective against imipenem-resistant *A. baumannii*.[37] However, the recently reported resistance of *A. baumannii* strains to sulbactam leaves the polymyxins (colistimethate and polymyxin B) as the only alternative treatment available.[131]

Different *Acinetobacter* spp. also showed differences in the degree of their susceptibilities. Thus, *A. lwoffii* (formerly *Mima polymorpha*) strains were more susceptible to β-lactams than *A. baumannii*, and *A. haemolyticus* was highly resistant to aminoglycosides.[2,24] Other species, such as *A. junii* and *A. johnsonii*,[6,31,132,133] also isolated from a hospital environment but with low virulence,[31] and therefore, less frequently involved in nosocomial outbreaks, have also been found to be less resistant to antibiotics.[31]

In a study by Okpara and Maswoswe,[112] all of the 107 *A. baumannii* isolates studied were susceptible to a combination of imipenem and cilastatin, but showed resistance to cephalosporins, broad-spectrum penicillins, quinolones, and aztreonam; only 9 isolates were susceptible to one or more aminoglycosides.

In general, *Acinetobacter* spp. are naturally resistant to cephalosporins and kanamycin, and can frequently acquire plasmid-mediated resistance to penicillins, chloramphenicol, and aminoglycosides.[134-136] Several aminoglycoside-modifying enzymes have been reported in *Acinetobacter* spp. capable of conferring resistance to gentamicin, sisomicin, and tobramycin.[137] In addition, enzymatic resistance to amikacin was found to depend on the synthesis of 6'-*N*-acetyltransferase type 4, or 3'-*O*-phosphotransferase (APH(3')-VI).[138]

Krcméry et al.[139] have found *Acinetobacter* strains able to transfer resistance to amikacin, gentamicin, and cefamandole to *P. aeruginosa* or Enterobacteria.

14.1.3 REFERENCES

1. Juni, E., Genus III. *Acinetobacter* Brisou and Prévot 1954, 727[AL], in *Bergey's Manual of Systematic Bacteriology*, Vol. 1, Krieg, N. R. and Hold, J. G., Eds., Williams and Wilkins, Baltimore, 1984, 303.
2. Leduc, A., Fonaine, J., Brazeau, M., Panisset, L. C., and Montplaisir, S., Le bactériologiste clinique face a un probleme de classification: *Moraxella, Achromobacter, Acinetobacter, Can. J. Microbiol.*, 15, 655, 1969.
3. Bovre, K. and Henriksen, S. D., Minimal standards for description of new taxa within the genera *Moraxella* and *Acinetobacter*: proposal by the subcommittee on *Moraxella* and allied bacteria, *Int. J. Syst. Bacteriol.*, 26, 92, 1976.
4. Juni, E., Interspecies transformation of *Acinetobacter*: genetic evidence for a ubiquitous genus, *J. Bacteriol.*, 112, 917, 1972.
5. Bouvet, P. J. M. and Grimont, P. A. D., Taxonomy of the genus Acinetobacter with the recognition of *Acinetobacter baumannii* sp. nov., *Acinetobacter haemolyticus* sp. nov., *Acinetobacter johnsonii* sp. nov., and *Acinetobacter junii* sp. nov., and emmended descriptions of *Acinetobacter calcoaceticus* and *Acinetobacter lwoffi*, *Int. J. Syst. Bacteriol.*, 36, 228, 1986.
6. Bouvet, P. J. M. and Grimont, P. A. D., Identification and biotyping of clinical isolates of *Acinetobacter*, *Ann. Inst. Pasteur Microbiol.*, 138, 569, 1987.
7. Alexander, M., Rahman, M., Taylor, M., and Noble, W., A study of the value of electrophoresic and other techniques for typing *Acinetobacter calcoaceticus*, *J. Hosp. Infect.*, 12, 273, 1988.
8. Seifert, H., Strate, A., and Pulverer, G., Nosocomial bacteremia due to *Acinetobacter baumannii*: clinical features, epidemiology, and predictors of mortality, *Medicine (Baltimore)*, 74, 340, 1995.
9. Bleschemidt, B., Borneleit, P., and Kleber, H. P., Purification and characterization of an extracellular β-lactamase produced by *Acinetobacter calcoaceticus*, *J. Gen. Microbiol.*, 138, 1197, 1992.
10. Gerner-Smidt, P., Frequency of plasmids in strains of *Acinetobacter calcoaceticus*, *J. Hosp. Infect.*, 14, 23, 1989.

11. Gerner-Smidt, P., Ribotyping of *Acinetobacter calcoaceticus-Acinetobacter baumannii* complex, *J. Clin. Pathol.*, 30, 2680, 1992.

12. Joly-Guillou, M. L., Vallée, E., Bergogne-Bérézin, E., and Philippon, A., Distribution of beta-lactamases and phenotype analysis in clinical isolates of *Acinetobacter calcoaceticus*, *J. Antimicrob. Chemother.*, 22, 597, 1988.

13. Leonov, Y., Schlaeffer, F., Karpuch, J., Bourvin, A., Shemesh, Y., and Lewinson, G., Ciprofloxacin in the treatment of nosocomial multiply resistant *Acinetobacter calcoaceticus* bacteremia, *Infection*, 18, 234, 1990.

14. Sato, K. and Nakae, T., Outer membrane permeability of *Acinetobacter calcoaceticus* and its implication in antibiotic resistance, *J. Antimicrob. Chemother.*, 28, 35, 1991.

15. Baumann, A., Isolation of *Acinetobacter* from soil and water, *J. Bacteriol.*, 96, 39, 1968.

16. Bergogne-Bérézin, E., Joly-Guillou, K. L., and Vieu, J. F., Epidemiology of nosocomial infections due to *Acinetobacter calcoaceticus*, *J. Hosp. Infect.*, 10, 105, 1987.

17. Noble, W. C., Hope, Y. M., Midgley, G., Moore, M. K., Patel, S., Virani, Z., and Lison, E., Toewebs as a source of Gram-negative bacilli, *J. Hosp. Infect.*, 8, 248, 1986.

18. Taplin, D., Rebell, G., and Zaias, N., The human skin as a source of *Mima-Herellea* infections, *JAMA*, 186, 952, 1963.

19. Siegman-Igra, Y., Bar-Yosef, S., Gorea, A., and Avram, J., Nosocomial acinetobacter meningitis secondary to invasive procedures: report of 25 cases and review, *Clin. Infect. Dis.*, 17, 843, 1993.

20. Johnson, D. R., Love-Dixon, M. A., Brown, W. J., Levine, D. P., Downes, F. P., and Hall, W. N., Delayed detection of an increase in resistant acinetobacter at a Detroit hospital, *Infect. Control Hosp. Epidemiol.*, 13, 394, 1992.

21. Timsit, J. F., Garrait, V., Misset, B., Goldstein, F. W., Renaud, B., and Carlet, J., The digestive tract is a major site for *Acinetobacter baumannii* colonization in intensive care unit patients, *J. Infect. Dis.*, 168, 1336, 1993.

22. Grehn, M. and Graevenitz, A., Search for *Acinetobacter* subsp. *anitratus* enrichment in fecal samples, *J. Clin. Microbiol.*, 8, 342, 1978.

23. Smith, P. W. and Massanari, R. M., Room humidifiers as the source of *Acinetobacter* infections, *JAMA*, 237, 795, 1977.

24. Bergogne-Bérézin, E., Outbreaks caused by bacteria with novel multiple resistance: towards zero therapeutic options? The increasing significance of outbreaks of *Acinetobacter* spp.: the need for control and new agents, *J. Hosp. Infect.*, 30(Suppl.), 441, 1995.

25. Bergogne-Bérézin, E. and Joly-Guillou, M. L., Hospital infection with *Acinetobacter* spp.: an increasing problem, *J. Hosp. Infect.*, 18(Suppl. A), 250, 1991.

26. Hartstein, A. L., Rashad, A. L., Liebler, J. M., Actis, L. A., Freeman, J., Rourke, J. W., Jr., Stibolt, T. B., Tolmasky, M. E., Ellis, G. R., and Crosa, J. H., Multiple intensive care unit outbreak of *Acinetobacter calcoaceticus* subspecies *anitratus* respiratory infection and colonization associated with contaminated, reusable ventilator circuits and resuscitation bags, *Am. J. Med.*, 85, 624, 1988.

27. Holton, J., A report of a further hospital outbreak caused by multiresistant *Acinetobacter anitratus*, *J. Hosp. Infect.*, 3, 305, 1982.

28. Cunha, B. A., Klimek, J. J., Gracewski, J., McLaughlin, J. C., and Quintiliani, R., A common source of outbreak of acinetobacter pulmonary infections traced to Wright respirometers, *Postgrad. Med. J.*, 56, 169, 1980.

29. Smith, P. W. and Massanari, R. M., Room humidifier as a source of acinetobacter infections, *JAMA*, 56, 169, 1977.

30. Sherertz, R. J. and Sullivan, M. L., An outbreak of infections with *Acinetobacter calcoaceticus* in burn patients: contamination of patients' mattresses, *J. Infect. Dis.*, 151, 252, 1985.

31. Seifert, H., Strate, A., Schulze, A., and Pulverer, G., Vascular catheter-related bloodstream infection due to *Acinetobacter johnsonii* (formerly *Acinetobacter calcoaceticus* var. *lwoffii*): report of 13 cases, *Clin. Infect. Dis.*, 17, 632, 1993.

32. Ramphal, R. and Kluge, R. M., *Acinetobacter calcoaceticus* variety *anitratus*: an increasing nosocomial problem, *Am. J. Med. Sci.*, 277, 57, 1979.

33. Ratailliau, H. F., Hightower, W. A., Dixon, R. E., and Allen, J. R., *Acinetobacter calcoaceticus*: a nosocomial pathogen with an unusual seasonal pattern, *J. Infect. Dis.*, 139, 371, 1979.

34. French, G. L., Casewell, M. W., Roncoroni, A. J., Knight, S., and Phillips, I., A hospital outbreak of antibiotic-resistant *Acinetobacter anitratus*: epidemiology and control, *J. Hosp. Infect.*, 1, 125, 1980.

35. Seifert, H., Baginski, R., Schulze, A., and Pulverer, A., Antimicrobial susceptibility of *Acinetobacter* species, *Antimicrob. Agents Chemother.*, 37, 750, 1993.

36. Chen, Y. C., Chang, S. C., Hsieh, W. C., and Luh, K. T., *Acinetobacter calcoaceticus* bacteremia: analysis of 48 cases, *J. Formos. Med. Assoc.*, 90, 958, 1991.

37. Go, E. S., Urban, C., Burns, J., Kreiswirth, B., Elsner, W., Mariano, N., Mosinka-Snipas, K., and Rahal, J. J., Clinical and molecular epidemiology of acinetobacter infections sensitive only to polymixin B and sulbactam, *Lancet*, 344, 1329, 1994.

38. Peacock, J. E., Sorrell, L., Sottile, F. D., Price, L. C., and Rutala, W. A., Nosocomial respiratory tract colonization and infection with aminoglycoside-resistant *Acinetobacter calcoaceticus* var. *anitratus*: epidemiologic characteristics and clinical significance, *Infect. Control Hosp. Epidemiol.*, 9, 302, 1988.

39. Wise, K. A. and Tosolini, F. A., Epidemiological surveillance of *Acinetobacter* species, *J. Hosp. Infect.*, 16, 319, 1990.

40. Gerner-Smidt, P., Endemic occurrence of *Acinetobacter calcoaceticus* biovar. *anitratus* in an intensive care unit, *J. Hosp. Infect.*, 10, 265, 1987.

41. Allen, K. D. and Green, H. T., Hospital outbreak of multi-resistant *Acenitobacter anitratus*: an airborne mode of spread? *J. Hosp. Infect.*, 9, 110, 1987.

42. Humphreys, H., Towner, K. J., Crowe, M., Webster, C., and Winter, R., Acinetobacter infections, intensive care units, and handwashing, *Lancet*, 345, 121, 1995.

43. Schröcksnadel, H., Flörl, C., Dapunt, O., and Dierich, M. P., Acinetobacter infections, intensive care units, and handwashing, *Lancet*, 345, 121, 1995.

44. Inglis, T., Acinetobacter infections, intensive care units, and handwashing, *Lancet*, 345, 122, 1995.

45. Trilla, A., Vila, J., Zaragoza, M., and Salles, M., Acinetobacter infections, intensive care units, and handwashing, *Lancet*, 345, 123, 1995.

46. Ashley, D. and Watson, R., Acinetobacter infections, intensive care units, and handwashing, *Lancet*, 345, 123, 1995.

47. Gouby, A., Carles-Nurit, M.-J., Bouziges, N., Bourg, G., Mesnard, R., and Bouvet, P. J. M., Use of pulsed-field gel electrophoresis for investigation of hospital outbreak of *Acinetobacter baumannii*, *J. Clin. Microbiol.*, 30, 1588, 1992.

48. Mulin, B., Talon, D., Viel, J. F., Vincent, C., Leprat, R., Thouverez, M., and Michel-Briand, Y., Risk factors for nosocomial colonization with multiresistant *Acinetobacter baumannii*, *Eur. J. Clin. Microbiol. Infect. Dis.*, 14, 569, 1995.

49. Scerpella, E. G., Wanger, A. R., Armitige, L., Anderlini, P., and Ericsson, C. D., Nosocomial outbreak caused by a multiresistant clone of *Acinetobacter baumannii*: results of the case-control and molecular epidemiologic investigations, *Infect. Control Hosp. Epidemiol.*, 16, 92, 1995.

50. Lortholary, O., Fagon, J.-Y., Buu Hoi, A., Slama, M. A., Pierre, J., Giral, P., Rosenzweig, R., Gutmann, L., Safar, M., and Acar, J., Nosocomial acquisition of multiresistant *Acinetobacter baumannii*: risk factors and prognosis, *Clin. Infect. Dis.*, 20, 790, 1995.

51. Struelens, M. J., Carlier, E., Maes, N., Serruys, E., Quint, W. G. V., and van Belkum, A., Nosocomial colonization and infection with multiresistant *Acinetobacter baumannii*: outbreak delineation using DNA macrorestriction analysis and PCR-fingerprinting, *J. Hosp. Infect.*, 25, 15, 1993.

52. Dijkshoorn, L., Michel, M. F., and Degener, J. E., Cell envelope protein profiles of *Acinetobacter calcoaceticus* strains isolated in hospitals, *J. Med. Microbiol.*, 23, 313, 1987.

53. Regev, R., Dolfin, T., Zelig, I., Givoni, S., and Wolach, B., Acinetobacter septicemia: a threat to neonates? Special aspects in a neonatal intensive care unit, *Infection*, 21, 394, 1993.

54. Cefai, C., Richards, J., Gould, F. K., and McPeake, P., An outbreak of *Acinetobacter* respiratory tract infection, resulting from incomplete disinfection of ventilatory equipment, *J. Hosp. Infect.*, 5, 117, 1990.

55. Joly-Guillou, M. L., Decré, D., Wolff, M., and Bergogne-Bérézin, E., *Acinetobacter* spp.: clinical epidemiology in 89 intensive care units: a retrospective study in France during 1991, *2nd Int. Conf. Prevention of Infection (CIPI)*, Nice, France, May 1992, Abstr. CJ1.

56. Urban, C., Go, E., Mariano, N., Berger, B. J., Avraham, I., Rubin, D., and Rahal, J. J., Effect of sulbactam on infections caused by imipenem-resistant *Acinetobacter calcoaceticus* biotype *anitratus*, *J. Infect. Dis.*, 167, 448, 1993.

57. Vila, J., Marcos, A., Marco, F., Abdalla, S., Vergara, Y., Reig, R., Gomez-Lus, R., and Jimenez de Anta, T., *In vitro* antimicrobial production of beta-lactamases, aminoglycoside-modifying enzymes, and chloramphenicol acetyltransferase by and susceptibility of clinical isolates of *Acinetobacter baumannii*, *Antimicrob. Agents Chemother.*, 37, 138, 1993.

58. Jones, R. N., The current and future impact of antimicrobial resistance among nosocomial bacterial pathogens, *Diagn. Microbiol. Infect. Dis.*, 15, 3S, 1992.

59. Rolston, K., Guan, Z., Bodey, G. P., and Elting, L., *Acinetobacter calcoaceticus* septicemia in patients with cancer, *South. Med. J.*, 78, 647, 1985.

60. Castle, M., Tenney, J. H., Weinstein, M. P., and Eickhoff, T. C., Outbreak of a multiply resistant acinetobacter in a surgical intensive care unit: epidemiology and control, *Heart Lung*, 7, 641, 1978.

61. Buxton, A. E., Anderson, R. L., Werdegar, D., and Atlas, E., Nosocomial respiratory tract infection and colonization with *Acinetobacter calcoaceticus*: epidemiologic characteristics, *Am. J. Med.*, 65, 507, 1978.

62. Stone, J. W. and Das, B. C., Investigation of an outbreak of infection with *Acinetobacter calcoaceticus* in a special care baby unit, *J. Hosp. Infect.*, 7, 42, 1986.

63. Vandenbroucke-Grauls, C. M. J. E., Kerver, A. J. H., Rommes, J. H., Jansen, R., den Dekker, C., and Verhoef, J., Endemic *Acinetobacter anitratus* in a surgical intensive care unit: mechanical ventilators as reservoirs, *Eur. J. Clin. Microbiol. Infect. Dis.*, 7, 485, 1988.

64. Vila, J., Almela, M., and Jimenez de Anta, M. T., Laboratory investigation of hospital outbreak caused by two different multiresistant *Acinetobacter calcoaceticus* subsp. *anitratus* strains, *J. Clin. Microbiol.*, 27, 1086, 1989.

65. Carlquist, J. F., Conti, M., and Burke, J. P., Progressive resistance in a single strain of *Acinetobacter calcoaceticus* recovered during a nosocomial outbreak, *Am. J. Infect. Control*, 10, 43, 1982.

66. De Borg, G. G., Mima polymorpha in meningitis, *J. Bacteriol.*, 55, 764, 1948.

67. Robinson, R. G., Garrison, R. G., and Brown, R. W., Evaluation of the clinical significance of the genus *Herellea*, *Ann. Intern. Med.*, 60, 19, 1964.

68. Donald, W. D. and Doak, W. M., Mimeae meningitis and sepsis, *JAMA*, 200, 111, 1967.

69. de Fonseca, I., Acinetobacter anitratus as the causal agent of nosocomial infections in a maternity hospital: a report of five cases, *Ceylon Med. J.*, 26, 121, 1981.

70. Morgan, M. E. I. and Hart, C. A., Acinetobacter meningitis: acquired infection in a neonatal intensive care unit, *Arch. Dis. Child.*, 57, 557, 1982.

71. Lim, V. K. and Talib, A., A case of neonatal meningitis caused by *Acinetobacter calcoaceticus* var. *anitratus*, *Med. J. Malaysia*, 37, 11, 1982.

72. Mukhopadhyay, M. and Mukherjee, A. K., *Mima polymorpha* meningitis in a neonate, *J. Indian Med. Assoc.*, 87, 217, 1989.

73. Yogev, R., Ventriculitis from *Acinetobacter calcoaceticus* variant *anitratus*, *J. Neurol. Neurosurg. Psychiatr.*, 42, 475, 1979.

74. Wirt, T. C., McGee, Z. A., Oldfield, E. H., and Meacham, W. F., Intraventricular administration of amikacin for complicated gram-negative meningitis and ventriculitis, *J. Neurosurg.*, 50, 95, 1979.

75. Ghoneim, A. T. M. and Halaka, A., Meningitis due to *Acinetobacter calcoaceticus* variant *anitratus*, *J. Hosp. Infect.*, 1, 359, 1980.

76. Berk, S. L. and McCabe, W. R., Meningitis caused by *Acinetobacter calcoaceticus* var. *anitratus*: a specific hazard in neurosurgical patients, *Arch. Neurol.*, 38, 95, 1981.

77. Cherubin, C. E., Marr, J. S., Sierra, M. F., and Becker, S., Listeria and gram-negative bacillary meningitis in New York City, 1972–1979: frequent causes of meningitis in adults, *Am. J. Med.*, 71, 199, 1981.

78. Berkowitz, F. E., *Acinetobacter* meningitis — a diagnostic pitfall: a report of 3 cases, *S. Afr. Med. J.*, 61, 448, 1982.

79. Kobayashi, T. K., Yamaki, T., Yoshino, E., Terawaki, S., Tara, K., Nishida, K., and Sawaragi, I., Meningitis with *Acinetobacter calcoaceticus* in cerebrospinal fluid: a case report, *Acta Cytol.*, 27, 281, 1983.

80. Mombelli, G., Klastersky, J., Coppens, L., Daneau, D., and Nubourgh, Y., Gram-negative bacillary meningitis in neurosurgical patients, *J. Neurosurg.*, 59, 634, 1983.

81. Mayhall, C. G., Archer, N. H., Lamb, V. A., Spadora, A. C., Baggett, J. W., Ward, J. D., and Narayan, R. K., Ventriculostomy-related infections: a prospective epidemiologic study, *N. Engl. J. Med.*, 310, 553, 1984.

82. Gerner-Smidt, P., Hansen, L., Knudsen, A., Siboni, K., and Sogaard, I., Epidemic spread of *Acinetobacter calcoaceticus* in a neurosurgical department analyzed by electronic data processing, *J. Hosp. Infect.*, 6, 166, 1985.

83. Mancebo, J., Domingo, P., Blanch, L., Coll, P., Net, A., and Nolla, J., Post-neurosurgical and spontaneous gram-negative bacillary meningitis in adults, *J. Infect. Dis.*, 18, 533, 1986.

84. Alien, K. D. and Green, H. T., Hospital outbreak of multi-resistant *Acinetobacter anitratus*: an airborne mode of spread? *J. Hosp. Infect.*, 9, 110, 1987.

85. Kelkar, R., Gordon, S. M., Giri, N., Rao, K., Ramakrishnan, G., Saikia, T., Nair, C. N., Kurkure, P. A., Pai, S. K., Jarvis, W. R., and Advani, S. H., Epidemic iatrogenic *Acinetobacter* spp. meningitis following administration of intrathecal methotrexate, *J. Hosp. Infect.*, 14, 233, 1989.

86. Segev, S., Rosen, N., Joseph, G., Elran, H. A., and Rubinstein, E., Pefloxacin efficacy in gram-negative bacillary meningitis, *J. Antimicrob. Chemother.*, 26(Suppl. B), 187, 1990.

87. Gradon, J. D., Chapnick, E. K., and Lutwick, L. I., Infective endocarditis of a native valve due to *Acinetobacter*: case report and review, *Clin. Infect. Dis.*, 14, 1145, 1992.

88. Abrutyn, E., Goodhart, G. L., Roos, K., Anderson, R., and Buxton, A., *Acinetobacter calcoaceticus* outbreak associated with peritoneal dialysis, *Am. J. Epidemiol.*, 107, 328, 1978.

89. Lowes, J. A., Smith, J., Tabaqchali, S., and Shaw, E. J., Outbreak of infection in a urological ward, *Br. Med. J.*, 280, 722, 1980.

90. Kiehn, T. E. and Armstrong, D., Changes in the spectrum of organisms causing bacteremia and fungemia in immunocompromised patients due to venous access devices, *Eur. J. Clin. Microbiol. Infect. Dis.*, 9, 869, 1990.

91. Seifert, H. and Baginski, R., The clinical significance of *Acinetobacter baumannii* in blood cultures, *Int. J. Med. Microbiol.*, 277, 210, 1992.

92. Bergogne-Bérézin, E., *Acinetobacter* spp., saprophytic organisms of increasing pathogenic importance, *Zbl. Bakteriol.*, 281, 389, 1994.

93. Schloesser, R. L., Laufkoetter, E. A., Lehners, T., and Mietens, C., An outbreak of *Acinetobacter calcoaceticus* infection in neonatal care unit, *Infection*, 18, 230, 1990.

94. Glew, R. H., Moellering, R. C., and Kunz, L. J., Infections with *Acinetobacter calcoaceticus* (*Herellea vaginicola*): clinical and laboratory studies, *Medicine (Baltimore)*, 56, 79, 1977.

95. Vila, J., Almela, M., and Jimenez de Anta, M. T., Laboratory investigation of a hospital outbreak caused by two different multiresistant *Acinetobacter calcoaceticus* subsp. *anitratus* strains, *J. Clin. Microbiol.*, 27, 1086, 1989.

96. Beck-Sagué, C. M., Jarvis, W. R., Brook, J. H., Culver, D. H., Potts, A., Gay, E., Shotts, B. W., Hill, B., Anderson, R. L., and Weinstein, M. P., Epidemic bacteremia due to *Acinetobacter baumannii* in five intensive care units, *Am. J. Epidemiol.*, 132, 723, 1990.

97. Fagon, J. V., Chastre, J., Domart, Y., Troullet, J. L., Pierre, J., Darne, C., and Gibert, C., Nosocomial pneumonia in patients receiving continuous mechanical ventilation: prospective analysis of 52 episodes with use of a protected specimen brush and quantitative culture techniques, *Am. Rev. Respir. Dis.*, 139, 877, 1989.

98. Galvao, C., Swartz, R., Rocher, L., Reynolds, J., Starmann, B., and Wilson, D., Acinetobacter peritonitis during chronic peritoneal dialysis, *Am. J. Kidney Dis.*, 14, 101, 1989.

99. Joly-Guillou, M. L., Bergogne-Bérézin, E., and Vieu, J. F., Epidemiologie et résistance aux antibiotiques des *Acinetobacter* en millieu hospitalier, *Presse Med.*, 19, 357, 1990.

100. Gervich, D. H. and Grout, C. S., An outbreak of nosocomial *Acinetobacter* infections from humidifiers, *Am. J. Infect. Control*, 13, 210, 1985.

101. Jarvis, W. R. and Martone, W. J., Predominant pathogens in hospital infections, *J. Antimicrob. Chemother.*, 29(Suppl. A), 19, 1992.

102. Gomez Garcés, J. L. and Fernandez, M. L., Significado clinico de las bacteremias por *Acinetobacter calcoaceticus*, *Enferm. Infecc. Microbiol. Clin.*, 10, 622, 1990.

103. Moreno, S., Vicente, T., Armas, M., Bernaldo de Quiros, J. C. L., Rodriguez-Creixems, M., and Bouza, E., Bacteremia nosocomial por *Acinetobacter*, *Enferm. Infecc. Microbiol. Clin.*, 8, 606, 1990.

104. Raz, R., Alroy, G., and Sobel, J. D., Nosocomial bacteremia due to *Acinetobacter calcoaceticus*, *Infection*, 10, 168, 1982.

105. Smego, R. A., Endemic nosocomial *Acinetobacter calcoaceticus* bacteremia: clinical significance, treatment, and prognosis, *Arch. Intern. Med.*, 145, 2174, 1985.

106. Tilley, P. A. G. and Roberts, F. J., Bacteremia with *Acinetobacter* species: risk factors and prognosis in different settings, *Clin. Infect. Dis.*, 18, 896, 1994.

107. Fagon, J. Y., Chastre, J., Hance, A. J., Montravers, P., Novara, A., and Gibert, C., Nosocomial pneumonia in ventilated patients: a cohort study evaluating attributable mortality and hospital stay, *Am. J. Med.*, 94, 281, 1993.

108. Weinstein, M. P., Murphy, J. R., Reller, L. B., and Lichtenstein, K. A., The clinical significance of positive blood cultures: a comprehensive analysis of 500 episodes of bacteremia and fungemia in adults. II. Clinical observations, with special reference to factors influencing prognosis, *Rev. Infect. Dis.*, 5, 54, 1983.

109. Rudin, M. L., Michael, J. R., and Huxley, E. J., Community-acquired acinetobacter pneumonia, *Am. J. Med.*, 67, 39, 1979.

110. Bergogne-Bérézin, E., Joly, M. L., Berthelot, G., Fichelle, A., and Vieu, J. F., Epidemiologie d'*Acinetobacter calcoaceticus*, *Nouv. Presse Med.*, 9, 3351, 1980.

111. Rosenthal, S. L., Sources of *Pseudomonas* and *Acinetobacter* species found in human culture materials, *Am. J. Clin. Pathol.*, 62, 807, 1974.

112. Okpara, A. U. and Maswoswe, J. J., Emergence of multidrug-resistant isolates of *Acinetobacter baumannii*, *Am. J. Hosp. Pharm.*, 51, 2671, 1994.

113. Dijkshoorn, L., van Dalen, R., van Ooyen, A., Biji, D., Tjernberg, I., Michel, M. F., and Horrevorts, A. M., Endemic acinetobacter in intensive care units: epidemiology and clinical impact, *J. Clin. Pathol.*, 46, 533, 1993.

114. Myer, K. H. and Zinner, S. H., Bacterial pathogen of increasing significance in hospital-acquired infections, *Rev. Infect. Dis.*, 7(Suppl. 3), S371, 1985.

115. Finland, M., Emergence of antibiotic resistance in hospitals 1935–1975, *Rev. Infect. Dis.*, 1, 4, 1979.

116. Barnes, D. J., Naraqi, S., and Igo, J. D., Community-acquired acinetobacter pneumonia in adults in Papua New Guinea, *Rev. Infect. Dis.*, 10, 636, 1988.

117. Guerrero, M. L. F., Fernandez, J. L. D., Prieto, J. M., Garces, J. L., and Diaz, F. J., Community-acquired acinetobacter pneumonia, *Chest*, 78, 670, 1980.

118. Cordes, L. G., Brink, E. W., Checko, P. J., Lentnek, A., Lyons, R. W., Hayes, P. S., Wu, T. C., Tharr, D. G., and Fraser, D. W., A cluster of acinetobacter pneumonia in foundry workers, *Ann. Intern. Med.*, 95, 688, 1981.

119. Bernasconi, E., Wiist, J., Speich, R., Flury, G., and Krause, M., "Community-acquired" acinetobacter-pneumonie, *Schweiz. Med. Wochenshr.*, 123, 1566, 1993.

120. Vallée, E., Joly-Guillou, M. L., and Bergogne-Bérézin, E., Activité comparative de l'imipeneme, du céfotaxime et de la ceftazidime vis-a-vis d'Acinetobacter calcoaceticus, *Presse Med.*, 19, 588, 1990.

121. Suh, B., Shapiro, T., Jones, R., Satishchandran, V., and Truant, A. L., In vitro activity of β-lactamase inhibitors against clinical isolates of *Acinetobacter* species, *Diagn. Microbiol. Infect. Dis.*, 21, 111, 1995.

122. Buisson, Y., Tran Van Nhieu, G., Ginot, L., Bouvet, P., Schill, H., Driot, L., and Meyran, M., Nosocomial outbreaks due to amikacin-resistant tobramycin-sensitive *Acinetobacter* species: correlation with amikacin usage, *J. Hosp. Infect.*, 15, 83, 1990.

123. Jedlickova, Z., Tesarikova, E., and Vymola, F., Concerning the sensitivity of *Acinetobacter calcoaceticus*, *J. Hyg. Epidemiol. Microbiol. Immunol.*, 34, 73, 1990.

124. Chow, A. W., Wong, J., and Bartlett, K. H., Synergistic interactions of ciprofloxacin and extended spectrum beta-lactams or aminoglycosides against *Acinetobacter calcoaceticus* ss. *anitratus*, *Diagn. Microbiol. Infect. Dis.*, 9, 213, 1988.

125. Bergogne-Bérézin, E. and Joly-Guillou, M. L., An underestimated nosocomial pathogen, *Acinetobacter calcoaceticus*, *J. Antimicrob. Chemother.*, 16, 535, 1985.

126. Lambert, T., Gerbaud, G., Bouvet, P., Vieu, J. F., and Courvalin, P., Dissemination of amikacin resistance gene aphA6 in *Acinetobacter* spp., *Antimicrob. Agents Chemother.*, 34, 1244, 1990.

490 Infectious Diseases in Immunocompromised Hosts

127. Gould, I. M., MacKenzie, F., and Thomson, C., Acinetobacter infections, intensive care units, and handwashing, *Lancet*, 345, 122, 1995.
128. Sato, K. and Nakae, T., Outer membrane permeability of *Acinetobacter calcoaceticus* and its implementation in antibiotic resistance, *J. Antimicrob. Chemother.*, 28, 35, 1991.
129. Gehrlein, M., Leying, H., Cullmann, W., Wendt, S., and Opferkuch, N., Imipenem resistance in *Acinetobacter baumannii* is due to altered penicillin-binding proteins, *Chemotherapy*, 37, 405, 1991.
130. Paton, R., Miles, R. S., Hood, J., and Ainyes, S. H. G. B., ARI 1: beta- lactamase-mediated imipenem resistance in *Acinetobacter baumannii*, *Int. J. Antimicrob. Agents*, 2, 81, 1993.
131. Wood, C. A. and Reboli, A. C., Infections caused by imipenem-resistant *Acinetobacter calcoaceticus* biotype *anitratus*, *J. Infect. Dis.*, 168, 1602, 1993.
132. Traub, W. H., Serotyping of clinical isolates of Acinetobacter: serovars of genospecies 3, *Int. J. Med. Microbiol.*, 273, 12, 1990.
133. Bouvet, P. J. M., Jeanjean, S., Vieu, J. F., and Dijkshoorn, L., Species, biotype, and bacteriophage type determinations compared with cell envelope protein profiles for typing *Acinetobacter* strains, *J. Clin. Microbiol.*, 28, 170, 1990.
134. Murray, B. and Moellering, R., Aminoglycoside-modifying enzymes among clinical isolates of *Acinetobacter calcoaceticus* subsp. *anitratus* (*Herellea vaginicola*): explanation for high-level aminoglycoside resistance, *Antimicrob. Agents Chemother.*, 15, 190, 1979.
135. Devaud, M., Kayser, F., and Bachi, B., Transposon-mediated multiple antibiotic resistance in *Acinetobacter* strains, *Antimicrob. Agents Chemother.*, 22, 323, 1982.
136. Dowding, J. E., Novel aminoglycoside-modifying enzyme from a clinical isolate of *Acinetobacter*, *J. Gen. Microbiol.*, 110, 239, 1979.
137. Bergogne-Bérézin, E., Joly, M. L., Moreau, N., and Legoffic, F., Aminoglycoside-modifying enzymes in clinical isolates of *Acinetobacter calcoaceticus*, *Curr. Microbiol.*, 4, 361, 1980.
138. Lambert, T., Gerbaud, G., and Courvalin, P., Transferable amikacin resistance in *Acinetobacter* spp. due to a new 3′-aminoglycoside phosphonotransferase, *Antimicrob. Agents Chemother.*, 32, 15, 1988.
139. Krcméry, V., Langsadl, L., Antal, M., and Seckarova, A., Transferable amikacin and cefandamole resistance: *Pseudomonas maltophilia* and *Acinetobacter* strains as possible reservoirs of R plasmids, *J. Hyg. Epidemiol. Microbiol. Immunol.*, 28, 141, 1985.

14.2 *MORAXELLA* SPP.

14.2.1 INTRODUCTION

Bacteria of the genus *Moraxella* represent plump Gram-negative bacilli or coccobacilli which have a marked tendency to form pairs (diplo-arrangement).[1] Together with *Neisseria gonorrhea* and *N. meningitides*, *Moraxella* spp. belong to the family Neisseriaceae. They are short, aerobic, oxidase-positive, nonpigmented organisms found as parasites and pathogens on the mucous membranes of mammals. The genus *Moraxella* includes two subgenera: *Moraxella* occurring as rods, and *Moraxella* (*Branhamella*) occurring as cocci.

Among the human pathogens, *M.* (*Branhamella*) *catarrhalis* is a normal inhabitant of the nasal cavity and nasopharynx, occasionally causing respiratory disease and otitis media (called also *Neisseria catarrhalis*).

M. liquefaciens (*M. lacunata*) is the etiologic agent of conjunctivitis and corneal infections in humans (known also as the *diplococcus of Morax-Axenfeld* or *Haemophilus duplex*). *M. nonliquefaciens* has also been associated as a possible cause of human conjunctivitis and keratitis.[2]

As has been the case with *M. nonliquefaciens* and *M. osloensis*, based on standard microbiologic methods, differentiating the phenotypic characteristics of one *Moraxella* species from those of another may be difficult. Using genetic transformation methodology, Bövre[3] demonstrated that certain strains formerly assumed to be related to *M. nonliquefaciens* were genetically distinct and classified as *M. osloensis*.

Together with *M. lacunata* and *M. osloensis*, *M. nonliquefaciens* has been implicated, although not very frequently, in more serious infections, such as endophthalmitis,[1,4] endocarditis,[5] sepsis,[6] and meningitis.[7]

14.2.2 β-LACTAMASE PRODUCTION BY *M. NONLIQUEFACIENS*

van Bijsterveld[8] found aerobic organisms like *Moraxella* to be susceptible to penicillin. Nevertheless, penicillin resistance has already started to emerge.[9]

β-Lactamase production by *M. nonliquefaciens* has been observed,[10,11] with the enzyme being plasmid-mediated and similar to the β-lactamase (BRO-1) produced by *M. catarrhalis*.[9,12-14] The ability to produce BRO-1 can be transfered by conjugation from *M. nonliquefaciens* to *B. catarrhalis*, as well as within *B. catarrhalis*.[15,16] Further observations have established that bacterial strains capable of producing β-lactamase can also colonize the upper respiratory tract without the ecological support of antibiotics.[17,18] It is true, however, that penicillin antibiotics can cause a selection of β-lactamase producing pathogens as well as commensals in the upper respiratory tract.[17-20]

14.2.3 EVOLUTION OF THERAPIES AND TREATMENT OF *MORAXELA NONLIQUEFACIENS* INFECTION

Given the fact that *Moraxella* strains producing β-lactamase may reach as high as 85%,[21] therapy of *Moraxella* infections may necessitate the re-evaluation of antibiotic therapy.[22] Currently, amoxicillin–clavulanic acid, macrolides, quinolones, and third-generation cephalosporins have been recommended as treatment for *Moraxella* infections.[23]

Acute or suppurative bacterial thyroiditis are rather uncommon conditions.[24] It was highly unusual when Sudar et al.[25] described what is believed to be the first case of acute thyroiditis caused by *M. nonliquefaciens*. The patient was treated successfully with a 3-week course of intravenous cephradine, followed by another 3 weeks with oral ciprofloxacin. An infection of the thyroid gland can be the result of either direct extension from an infection in the surrounding tissue, spread of contaminated material through a persistent thyroglossal duct, or by direct trauma.[25] Other routes of infection include lymphatics or hematogenous spread.[24] The clinical symptoms of acute bacterial thyroiditis are manifested by fever, tenderness of the thyroid, local heat and dermal erythema, and fluctuation in the case of abscess.[25]

In another first case, *M. nonliquefaciens* was implicated as the causative agent of a septic arthritis in a patient undergoing hemodialysis.[23] While the pathogen showed resistance to ampicillin, the systemic infection was resolved successfully with a 6-week course of intravenous ceftriaxone (2.0 g after each dialysis).

14.2.3.1 *M. nonliquefaciens* Endophthalmitis

Treatment strategies for *M. nonliquefaciens*-associated endophthalmitis should include antibiotics and a dose and route of administration that will assure sufficient therapeutic intravitreous levels for an adequate period of time.[26] In this regard, antibiotics given subconjunctivally did not provide adequate intravitreous concentrations.[27,28] Then, intravitreous administration (first evaluated in 1978)[29] was recommended, and standard doses of many antibiotics were formulated over the past 10 years or so.[30] In addition, vitrectomy[31] may have to be performed within 36 h of the onset of symptoms[32] to remove from the vitreous those substances known to induce inflammation and endotoxin due to Gram-negative bacilli in order to prevent inflammatory membrane formation and secondary retinal detachment.[26,33]

Systemic antibiotics have shown variable intravitreous penetration. Barza[28] has found that when inflammation was not present, penicillins and cephalosporins were capable of achieving 1% of systemic levels in the vitreous after intravenous injection. However, when inflammation was present, antibiotic vitreous levels may vary, even to exceed 10% of serum levels. For example, the vitreous levels of gentamicin were 20% to 30% of systemic levels when given by continuous infusion in the presence of ocular inflammation.[28] Gentamicin, which binds to the pigmented choroid and the retina, may decrease availability to the vitreous.[26]

There is still little knowledge about the vitreous levels in inflamed human eyes with single parenteral dosing.[26] It seemed that because the infection and inflammation originated in the retinal vessels, systemic antibiotics tended to enter the vitreous more readily in patients with endogenous endophthalmitis.[27,28] Among the various antibiotics, ceftriaxone, imipenem, and ceftazidime were found to achieve adequate intravitreous levels when given systemically.[34-36]

Sufficient intravitreous levels of antibiotics should be of particular importance in cases of resistant Gram-negative bacilli. Studies have shown that ceftriaxone had vitreous levels of 11% and 24% of serum levels at 1 to 4 h and 12 to 13 h, respectively.[34] The corresponding values for imipenem were 16% at 3.9 h (after a 1.0-g systemic dose),[35] and 4% and 16% for ceftazidime at 1 h and 5 h (after an intravenous dose of 50 mg/kg), respectively.[36] The optimum duration of systemic therapy for endophthalmitis caused by Gram-negative bacilli has been established to be between 10 and 14 d.[27,37]

Evidence from several studies has demonstrated that patients treated with both vitrectomy and intravitreously injected antibiotics have a better visual outcome as compared to patients who have not been treated with both.[29,38,39] Thus, by one report,[29] 46% of patients receiving both procedures had a visual outcome of 20/100 or better.

Ebright et al.[1] have reported the first case of endophthalmitis caused by *M. nonliquefaciens* in an immunocompromised patient. Most likely the infection did occur through contact lens following minor trauma. The patient, a renal transplant recipient, was receiving immunosuppressive therapy (prednisone, azathioprine) at the time of infection. The latter was successfully treated, initially with 100 μg gentamicin and 2.5 mg cephaloridine into the eye, and then with aqueous penicillin G (2 million units every 4 h) for 2 weeks. The organism was identified as a strain of *M. nonliquefaciens* because of the ability of its DNA to readily transform a hypoxanthine auxotroph of *M. nonlique-faciens* to prototrophy (hypoxanthine independence) using a transformation assay system previously applied to identify *M. osloensis* (DNA from this organism failed to transform a tryptophan auxotroph of *M. osloensis* to prototrophy).[40]

Lobue et al.[41] also reported a case of *M. nonliquefaciens*-induced endophthalmitis following trabeculectomy.[42,43] The latter procedure is a surgical alternative for control of glaucoma refractory to medication and laser treatment.[44,45] Since the reported incidence of endophthalmitis after trabeculectomy has been very low,[46-49] the two reported cases of fulminant *Moraxella* endophthalitis are highly unusual. The applied treatment in one case included intravitreal administration of gentamicin (400 μg), clindamycin (450 μg), and dexamethazone (360 μg). The patient also received intravenously gentamicin (80 mg) and clindamycin (300 mg every 6 h), and oral prednisone (60 mg daily). In the second case, the patient was treated with intravitreal injections of gentamicin (0.3 mg), cephaloridine (0.5 mg), and dexamethazone (36 mg), as well as systemic gentamicin (80 mg t.i.d.) and cefazolin (1.0 mg every 6 h); tobramycin eyedrops were administered every 2 h, as were prednisolone acetate (1.0%) eyedrops. In both cases, the patients recovered completely.[41]

Kanski[50] also recommended that treatment of postoperative bacterial endophthalmitis should include high doses of antibiotics and corticosteroids administered concomitantly by systemic, intravitreal, and subconjunctival routes.

Sherman et al.[51] treated a bleb-associated endophthalmitis caused by a β-lactamase-positive strain of *M. nonliquefaciens* with a vitreous tap and intravitreal injections of tobramycin (100 μg) and cefazolin (2.25 mg), followed by a pars plana vitrectomy. The patient was subsequently treated with intravenous cefuroxime and topical fortified tobramycin and prednisolone acetate. In addition, since the postoperative course was complicated by a dense fibrin reaction, the patient received topical and systemic antibiotics and corticosteroids, and intracameral tissue-plasminogen activator. Four months after the initial manifestation, there was still residual ischemic damage to the retina, but the visual acuity had improved to 20/200.[51]

In another case of *M. nonliquefaciens* endophthalmitis,[26] a pars plana vitrectomy was followed by intravitreous amikacin (400 µg) and vancomycin (1.0 mg). Parenteral cefazolin (3.0 g daily) and gentamicin (240 mg daily) were also administered; the same antibiotics were injected subconjunctivally and given topically. A repeated vitrectomy was done, followed by intravitreous injections of ceftriaxone (2.0 mg) and gentamicin (100 µg); the parenteral antibiotic was changed to intravenous ceftriaxone (4.0 g daily) for 10 d. The patient responded poorly and lost vision in one eye.[26]

14.2.4 REFERENCES

1. Ebright, J. R., Lentino, J. R., and Juni, E., Endophthalmitis caused by *Moraxella nonliquefaciens*, *Am. J. Clin. Pathol.*, 77, 362, 1982.
2. Henriksen, S. D., Moraxella acinetobacter and mimeae, *Bact. Rev.*, 37, 522, 1973.
3. Bövre, K., Studies on transformation in *Moraxella* and organisms assumed to be related to *Moraxella*, *Acta Pathol. Microbiol. Scand.*, 62, 239, 1964.
4. Cooperman, E. W. and Friedman, A. H., Exogenous *Moraxella liquefaciens* endophthalmitis, *Ophthalmologica (Basel)*, 171, 177, 1975.
5. Silberfarb, P. M. and Lawe, J. E., Endocarditis due to *Moraxella liquefaciens*, *Arch. Intern. Med.*, 122, 512, 1968.
6. Butzler, J. B., Hansen, W., Cadranel, S., and Henriksen, S. D., Stomatitis with septicemia due to *Moraxella osloensis*, *J. Pediatr.*, 84, 721, 1974.
7. Berger, U. and Kreissel, M., Meningitis durch *Moraxella osloensis*, *Infection*, 166, 1974.
8. van Bijsterveld, O. P., Host-parasite relationship and taxonomic position of *Moraxella* and morphologically related organisms, *Am. J. Ophthalmol.*, 76, 543, 1973.
9. Wallace, R. J., Jr., Steingrube, V. A., Nash, D. R., Hollis, D. G., Flanagan, C., Brawn, B. A., Labidi, A., and Weaver, R. E., BRO beta-lactamases of *Branhamella catarrhalis* and *Moraxella* subgenus *Moraxella*, including evidence for chromosomal beta-lactamase transfer by conjugation in *B. catarrhalis*, *M. nonliquefaciens*, and *M. lacunata*, *Antimicrob. Agents Chemother.*, 33, 1845, 1989.
10. Rosenthal, S. L., Freundlich, L. F., Gilardi, G. L., and Clodomar, F. Y., *In vitro* antibiotic sensitivity of *Moraxella* species, *Chemotherapy*, 24, 360, 1978.
11. Mölstad, S., Arvidsson, E., Eliasson, I., Hovelius, B., Kamme, C., and Schalén, C., Production of beta-lactamase by respiratory tract bacteria in children: relationship to antibiotic use, *Scand. J. Prim. Health Care*, 10, 16, 1992.
12. Kamme, C., Vang, M., and Stahl, S., Intrageneric and intergeneric transfer of *Branhamella catarrhalis* beta-lactamase production, *Scand. J. Infect. Dis.*, 16, 153, 1984.
13. Malmvall, B.-E., Brorsson, J.-E., and Johnsson, J., *In vitro* sensitivity to penicillin V and beta-lactamase production of *Branhamella catarrhalis*, *J. Antimicrob. Chemother.*, 3, 374, 1977.
14. Percival, A., Corkill, J. E., Rowlands, J., and Sykes, R. B., Pathogenicity of and beta-lactamase production by *Branhamella (Neisseria) catarrhalis*, *Lancet*, 2, 1175, 1977.
15. Eliasson, I. and Kamme, C., Upper respiratory tract infections: ecological and therapeutic aspects of β-lactamase production with special reference to *Branhamella catarrhalis*, *Drugs*, 31(Suppl. 3), 116, 1986.
16. Kamme, C., Eliasson, I., Kahl-Knutsson, B., and Vang, M., Plasmid-mediated beta-lactamase in *Branhamella catarrhalis*, *Drugs*, 31(Suppl. 3), 55, 1986.
17. Brook, I. and Gober, A. E., Emergence of beta-lactamase producing aerobic and anaerobic bacteria in the oropharynx of children following penicillin chemotherapy, *Clin. Pediatr.*, 23, 338, 1984.
18. Scheifele, D. W. and Fussell, S. J., Ampicillin-resistant *Haemophilus influenzae* colonizing ambulatory children, *Am. J. Dis. Child.*, 135, 406, 1981.
19. Freijd, A. A. and Rynnel-Dagöö, B., Isolation of nasopharyngeal beta-lactamase producing *Haemophilus influenzae* in relation to antibiotic treatment of acute otitis media in infants, *Acta Otolaryngol. (Stockholm)*, 95, 351, 1983.

20. Karma, P., Luotonen, J., Pukander, J., Sipilä, M., Herva, E., and Grönroos, P., *Haemophilus influenzae* in acute otitis media, *Acta Otolaryngol. (Stockholm)*, 95, 105, 1983.

21. Catlin, B. W., *Branhamella catarrhalis*: an organism gaining respect as a pathogen, *Clin. Microbiol. Rev.*, 3, 293, 1990.

22. Mölstad, S., Eliasson, I., Hovelius, B., Kamme, C., and Schalén, C., Beta-lactamase production in the upper respiratory tract flora in relation to antibiotic consumption: a study in children attending day nurseries, *Scand. J. Infect. Dis.*, 20, 329, 1988.

23. Johnson, D. W., Lum, G., Nimmo, G., and Hawley, C. M., *Moraxella nonliquefaciens* septic arthritis in a patient undergoing hemodialysis, *Clin. Infect. Dis.*, 21, 1039, 1995.

24. Berger, S. A., Zonszein, J., Villamena, P., and Mittman, N., Infectious diseases of the thyroid gland, *Rev. Infect. Dis.*, 5, 108, 1983.

25. Sudar, J. M., Alleman, M. J. A., Jonkers, G. J. P. M., de Groot, R., and Jongejan, C., Acute thyroiditis caused by *Moraxella nonliquefaciens*, *Neth. J. Med.*, 45, 170, 1994.

26. Schmidt, M. E., Smith, M. A., and Levy, C. S., Endophthalmitis caused by unusual gram-negative bacilli: three case reports and review, *Clin. Infect. Dis.*, 17, 686, 1993.

27. Hibberd, P. L., Schein, O. D., and Baker, A. S., Intraocular infections: current therapeutic approach, *Curr. Clin. Top. Infect. Dis.*, 11, 118, 1991.

28. Barza, M., Treatment of bacterial infections of the eye, *Curr. Clin. Top. Infect. Dis.*, 1, 158, 1980.

29. Peyman, G. A., Vastine, D. W., and Raichand, M., Symposium: postoperative endophthalmitis: experimental aspects and their clinical application, *Ophthalmology*, 85, 374, 1978.

30. Carney, M. and Peyman, G. A., Vitrectomy in endophthalmitis, *Ophthalmol. Clin.*, 27, 127, 1987.

31. Haymet, T., Results in the treatment of bacterial endophthalmitis, *Aust. NZ J. Ophthalmol.*, 13, 401, 1985.

32. Peyman, G. A., Raichand, M., and Bennett, T. O., Management of endophthalmitis pars plana vitrectomy, *Br. J. Ophthalmol.*, 64, 472, 1980.

33. Hadden, O. B., Vitrectomy in the management of endophthalmitis, *Aust. J. Ophthalmol.*, 9, 27, 1981.

34. Sharir, M., Giora, T., Kneer, J., and Rubinstein, E., The intravitreal penetration of ceftriaxone in man following systemic administration, *Invest. Ophthalmol. Vis. Sci.*, 30, 2179, 1989.

35. Axelrod, J. L., Newton, J. C., Klein, R. M., Bergen, R. L., and Sheikh, M. Z., Penetration of imipenem into human aqueous and vitreous humor, *Am. J. Ophthalmol.*, 104, 649, 1987.

36. Walstad, R. A., Blika, S., Thurmann-Nielsen, E., and Halrorsen, T. B., The penetration of ceftazidime into the rabbit eye, *Scand. J. Infect. Dis.*, 19, 131, 1987.

37. Shrader, S. K., Band, J. D., Lauter, C. B., and Murphy, P., The clinical spectrum of endophthalmitis incidence, predisposing factors, and features influencing outcome, *J. Infect. Dis.*, 162, 115, 1990.

38. Ramsey, J. J., Newsom, D. L., Sexton, D. J., and Harms, W. K., Endophthalmitis: current approaches, *Ophthalmology*, 89, 1055, 1982.

39. Baum, J., Peyman, G. A., and Barza, M., Intravitreal administration of antibiotic in the treatment of bacterial endophthalmitis. III, *Consensu. Surv. Ophthalmol.*, 26, 204, 1982.

40. Juni, E., Simple genetic transformation assay for rapid diagnosis of *Moraxella osloensis*, *Appl. Microbiol.*, 27, 16, 1974.

41. Lobue, T. D., Deutsch, T. A., and Stein, R. M., *Moraxella nonliquefaciens* endophthalmitis after trabeculectomy, *Am. J. Ophthalmol.*, 99, 343, 1985.

42. Cairns, J. E., Trabeculectomy: preliminary report of a new method, *Am. J. Ophthalmol.*, 66, 673, 1968.

43. Watson, P., Trabeculectomy: a modified ab externo technique, *Ann. Ophthalmol.*, 2, 199, 1970.

44. Watson, P. G. and Barnett, F., Effectiveness of trabeculectomy in glaucoma, *Am. J. Ophthalmol.*, 79, 831, 1975.

45. D'Ermo, F., Bonomi, L., and Doro, D., A critical analysis of long-term results of trabeculectomy, *Am. J. Ophthalmol.*, 88, 829, 1979.

46. Hattenhauer, J. M. and Lipsich, M. P., Late endophthalmitis after filtering surgery, *Am. J. Ophthalmol.*, 72, 1097, 1971.

47. Tabbara, K. F., Late infections following filtering producers, *Ann. Ophthalmol.*, 8, 1228, 1976.

48. Freedman, J., Gupta, M., and Bunke, A., Endophthalmitis after trabeculectomy, *Arch. Ophthalmol.*, 96, 1017, 1978.

49. Lewis, R. and Phelps, C., Trabeculectomy versus thermosclerectomy: a five-year follow-up, *Arch. Ophthalmol.*, 91, 339, 1974.

50. Kanski, J., Treatment of late endophthalmitis associated with filtering blebs, *Arch. Ophthalmol.*, 91, 339, 1974.
51. Sherman, M. D., York, M., Irvine, A. R., Langer, P., Cevallos, V., and Whitcher, J. P., Endophthalmitis caused by β-lactamase-positive *Moraxella nonliquefaciens*, *Am. J. Ophthalmol.*, 115, 674, 1993.

14.3 *NEISSERIA* SPP.

14.3.1 INTRODUCTION

Neisseria is a genus of Gram-negative, oxidase and catalase-producing diplococci that are classified in the family Neisseriaceae, along with *Kingella, Moraxella,* and *Acinetobacter* species. These aerobic or facultatively anaerobic organisms are frequent respiratory (oropharynx, nasopharynx) and genitourinary tract commensals in humans. Although many of them are not ordinarily regarded as pathogens, some may cause infections especially in immunocompromised hosts. The organisms are usually coffee-bean-shaped and paired.

N. meningitidis, which is the specific etiologic agent of epidemic cerebrospinal meningitis, is differentiated serologically into four main groups (A-D) and several provisional groups; group C is the most important pathogen, also known as *meningococcus. N. sicca* is a species characterized by dry grayish or slimy white or yellow colonies.

Over the years, *N. sicca* has been reported to cause serious infections, especially in immuno-compromised patients, such as meningitis,[1,2] pneumonia,[3-5] inflammatory spondylitis,[6] osteomyelitis,[7] urethritis,[8] Waterhouse-Fridrichsen syndrome,[9] a case of fatal frontal sinusitis,[10] bacteremia,[11] and endocarditis.[1,12-21]

Although the clinical manifestations of endocarditis associated with *N. sicca* are not significantly different from those of other *Neisseria*-induced endocarditis, they include a fairly acute onset of symptoms and high fever, a delayed diagnosis, and a high rate of multiple embolic phenomena.[12,20,22]

All reported cases of *N. sicca*-induced pneumonitis occurred in patients with decreased immune responses either due to corticosteroid therapy[4] or old age.[3,5] In the latter case, the emergence of *N. sicca* as the etiologic agent of community-acquired pneumonia is very likely due to the relative immunodeficiency induced by aging.[5,23]

Although primary necrotizing fasciitis is usually due to *Streptococcus* group A, several cases in which *N. meningitidis* was the causative agent have been reported, including one in an immunocompetent patient.[24] In the latter case (caused by a group A pathogen), a nonsteroidal anti-inflammatory therapy might have been the predisposing factor. The involvement of two distant sites strongly suggested hematogenous dissemination of the microorganism.[24]

Studies by Orren et al.[25] indicated that complement deficiency may be associated with the increased susceptibility to *N. meningitidis*-associated meningococcal disease.

14.3.2 TREATMENT OF *NEISSERIA* INFECTIONS

In antimicrobial susceptibility testing conducted by Heiddal et al.,[20] *N. sicca* was found resistant to clindamycin, vancomycin, and trimethoprim-sulfamethoxazole, but sensitive to penicillin, ampicillin, cefuroxime, aztreonam, sulfonamides, erythromycin, chloramphenicol, tetracycline, and gentamicin. However, Gris et al.[5] found *N. sicca* resistant to penicillin and erythromycin. In the several studies conducted, the MIC values (in micrograms per milliliter) for *N. sicca* have been determined as follows: penicillin, 0.5[20] and 0.78;[22] ampicillin, 0.2,[12,21] 0.4,[12] and 0.5;[20] gentamicin, 0.02,[12] 0.8,[12] 1.0,[21] and 2.0;[20] cephalotin, 3.12;[22] cefuroxime, 2.0;[20] ceftriaxone, 0.06;[20] aztreonam, 0.03;[21] and ciprofloxacin, 1.0.[20]

Oral cefaclor at 1.5 g daily produced dramatic improvement of *N. sicca* pneumonia and bronchiectasis in a 76-year-old immunocompromised patient.[5] Another cephalosporin derivative, cefalotin, was also found to be effective.

Heiddal et al.[20] successfully treated native-valve endocarditis due to *N. sicca* with a 6-week course of intravenous ceftriaxone and aztreonam. In another case of native-valve endocarditis, the therapeutic regimen consisted of a 4-week course with ampicillin and gentamicin, followed by a 2-week course of aztreonam.

Various other drugs used in the therapy of *N. sicca*-induced endocarditis include sulfonamide,[17] penicillin,[18] combinations of penicillin with either sulfonamide,[19] or streptomycin,[22] and combinations of ampicillin–gentamicin,[26] cefazolin–vancomycin–gentamicin,[12] ampicillin–penicillin–gentamicin,[12] and penicillin–gentamicin–aztreonam.[20]

14.3.3 REFERENCES

1. Bansmer, C. and Brem, J., Acute meningitis caused by *Neisseria sicca*, *N. Engl. J. Med.*, 238, 596, 1948.
2. Kienitz, M. and Ritzerfeld, W., Meningitis purulenta und sepsis mit nachweis von *Neisseria sicca*, *Z. Med. Mikrobiol. Immunol.*, 152, 55, 1966.
3. Alcid, D. V., *Neisseria sicca* pneumonia, *Chest*, 77, 123, 1980.
4. Gilrane, T., Tracy, J. D., Greenlee, R. M., Schelpert, J. W. III, and Brandstetter, R. D., *Neisseria sicca* pneumonia: report of two cases and review of the literature, *Am. J. Med.*, 78, 1038, 1985.
5. Gris, P., Vincke, G., Delmez, J. P., and Dierckx, J. P., *Neisseria sicca* pneumonia and bronchiectasis, *Eur. Respir. J.*, 2, 685, 1989.
6. Mella, B., Inflammatory spondylitis, *J. Neurosurg.*, 22, 393, 1965.
7. Doern, G. V., Blacklow, N. R., Gantz, N. M., Aucoin, P., Fischer, R. A., and Parker, D. S., *Neisseria sicca* osteomyelitis, *J. Clin. Microbiol.*, 16, 595, 1982.
8. Wilkinson, A. E., Occurrence of neisseria other than gonococcus in the genital tract, *Br. J. Vener. Dis.*, 28, 24, 1952.
9. Leon, A. P., *Cepas de Neisseria meningitidis* de grupo derologico, nuevo o no clasificado y *Neisseria faringis sicca* aisladas de casos del sindrome Waterhouse-Friderichsen de un brote epidemico en Mexico, *Rev. Invest. Salud Publica*, 31, 68, 1971.
10. Moon, T., Lin, R. Y., and Jahn, A. F., Fatal frontal sinusitis due to *Neisseria sicca* and *Eubacterium lentum*, *J. Otolaryngol.*, 15, 193, 1986.
11. Herbert, D. A. and Ruskin, J., Are the "nonpathogenic" Neisseriae pathogenic? *Am. J. Clin. Pathol.*, 75, 739, 1981.
12. Thornhill-Jones, M., Li, M. W., Canawati, H. N., Ibrahim, M. Z., and Sapico, F. I., *Neisseria sicca* endocarditis in intravenous drug abusers, *West. J. Med.*, 142, 255, 1985.
13. Schultz, O. T., Acute vegetative endocarditis with multiple secondary foci of involvement due to *Micrococcus pharyngitidis-siccae*, *JAMA*, 71, 1739, 1918.
14. Graef, I., De La Chapelle, C. E., and Vance, M. C., *Micrococcus pharyngis siccus* endocarditis, *Am. J. Pathol.*, 8, 347, 1932.
15. Goldstein, J. D., Endocarditis due to a *Neisseria pharyngis* organism, *Am. J. Med. Sci.*, 187, 672, 1934.
16. Shiling, M. S., Bacteriology of endocarditis with report of two unusual cases, *Ann. Intern. Med.*, 13, 476, 1939.
17. Weed, M. R., Clapper, M., and Myers, G. B., Endocarditis caused by *Micrococcus pharyngis siccus*: recovery after treatment with heparin and sulfapyridine, *Am. Heart J.*, 25, 547, 1943.
18. Hudson, R., *Neisseria pharyngis* bacteremia in a patient with subacute bacterial endocarditis, *J. Clin. Pathol.*, 10, 195, 1957.
19. Linde, Z. M. and Heinz, H. S., Bacterial endocarditis following surgery for congenital heart disease, *N. Engl. J. Med.*, 263, 65, 1960.
20. Heiddal, S., Sverrisson, J. T., Yngvason, F. E., Cariglia, N., and Kristinsson, K. G., Native-valve endocarditis due to *Neisseria sicca*: case report and review, *Clin. Infect. Dis.*, 16, 667, 1993.
21. Lopez-Vélez, R., Fortun, J., de Pablo, C., and Martinez Beltran, J., Native-valve endocarditis due to *N. sicca*, *Clin. Infect. Dis.*, 18, 660, 1994.
22. Gay, R. M. and Sevier, R. E., *Neisseria sicca* endocarditis: report of a case and review of the literature, *J. Clin. Microbiol.*, 8, 729, 1978.
23. Roberts-Thomson, I. C., Whittingham, S., and Youngchaiyud, U., Aging immune response and mortality, *Lancet*, 2, 24, 1968.

24. Mentec, H., Chosidow, O., Lafaurie, P., Darmon, J. Y., Simon, M., Roujeau, J. C., and Brun-Buisson, C. H., Necrotizing fasciitis, caused by *Neisseria meningitidis*, simultaneously involving an arm and a leg, *Ann. Dermatol. Venereol.*, 120, 889, 1993.

25. Orren, A., Caugant, D. A., Fijen, C. A. P., Dankert, J., van Schalkwyk, E. J., Poolman, J. T., and Coetzee, G. J., Characterization of strains of *Neisseria meningitidis* recovered from complement-sufficient and complement-deficient patients in the Western Cape province, South Africa, *J. Clin. Microbiol.*, 32, 2185, 1994.

26. Ghoneim, A. T. and Tandon, A. P., Prosthetic valve endocarditis due to *Neisseria sicca*: a case report, *Indian Heart J.*, 31, 246, 1979.

15 Pseudomonadaceae

The Pseudomonadaceae family of bacteria comprises Gram-negative, aerobic, straight or curved motile rods with polar flagella. They are widely distributed in soil, and fresh and salt water. It is divided into four genera: *Pseudomonas*, *Xanthomonas*, *Frateuria*, and *Zoogloea*.

Two pseumonads, *Burkholderia cepacia* and *Stenotrophomonas maltifolia,* have recently emerged as opportunistic pathogens in immunocompromised hosts. One of the most striking properties of these two species has been their ability to develop resistance to a wide variety of antimicrobial agents, thus leaving very limited options for effective therapies.

15.1 BURKHOLDERIA (PSEUDOMONAS) CEPACIA

15.1.1 Introduction

Pseudomonas cepacia (also known as *P. multivorans* and *P. kingii*) is a phytopathogen of the genus *Pseudomonas*, which was originally described as the cause of the soft rot in onions.[1] Although classified as pseudomonad, this bacterium is only distantly related to *P. aeruginosa*. Other related species include the plant pathogen *P. gladioli*, and the human pathogens *P. mallei*, *P. pseudomallei*, and *P. picketii*.[2] In 1992, Yabuuchi et al.[3] proposed that *P. cepacia,* together with six other pseudomonads of the same RNA homology group, be classified as a new genus, *Burkholderia*.

B. cepacia are ubiquitous Gram-negative bacteria of the family Pseudomonadaceae, found in soil, water, and plants. They are aerobic, motile by polar flagella, glucose-nonfermenting organisms which cannot only proliferate under conditions of minimal nutrition, but can also survive in the presence of certain disinfectants.[4,5] *B. cepacia* isolated even from distilled water appeared to differ both morphologically and physiologically from their laboratory subcultured counterparts.[4]

By some accounts,[6] *Pseudomonas* spp. have surpassed staphylococci as the cause of hospital-associated nosocomial infections in both frequency and severity. Thus, over the past decade or so, *B. cepacia* has been increasingly associated as the etiologic agent of nosocomial infections in chronically ill or severely debilitated immunocompromised hosts,[7-9] in patients in intensive care units,[10] and in patients receiving antibiotic or immunosuppressive therapies.[11-16] The presence of *B. cepacia* in the hospital environment has been shown to lead to colonization and infection.[11-13] For example, equipment used in wound, urinary tract,[17] cardiac, and respiratory instrumentation therapies have been identified as primary sources of infection,[18-22] as were hospital water supplies, and physiologically saline and disinfectant solutions.[18,19,23 26] Of the *B. cepacia*-contaminated disinfectant solutions, special attention must be given to various diluted aqueous quaternary ammonium disinfectants,[5,21,23,27-32] which because of the danger of nosocomial *B. cepacia* infections, have even been recommended for elimination by the Centers for Disease Control.[33]

Nosocomial outbreaks of *B. cepacia* infections have also been attributed to contamination of reusable electronic ventilator temperature probes in intensive care units,[34] thermometers used in cascade ventilation,[10] ventilator temperature sensors,[35] contaminated heparin flushes of central venous catheters inserted into oncology patients,[9] contamination of automatic peritoneal dialysis machines,[36] inappropriate use of chlorhexidine,[37] and bacteremia after open heart surgery due to contaminated pressure transducers.[38]

Snell et al.[39] have reported excessive morbidity and mortality associated with *B. cepacia* after lung transplantation, especially when the bacterium was isolated for the first time after transplantation; the predisposing factors in that particular setting are still unknown.[2]

Although considered to have a low virulence, *B. cepacia* may become potentially a lethal pathogen in the immunocompromised host,[13] causing a variety of respiratory tract infections,[40,41] such as necrotizing and other forms of pneumonia[14,42,43] and lung abscess.[15]

Since the early 1980s, *B. cepacia* infections have emerged as very serious and a steadily emerging problem in patients with cystic fibrosis.[33,44-49] Furthermore, these organisms have been shown capable of colonizing and infecting human soft tissue[18,50] and the urinary tract,[21,23] causing meningitis, endocarditis, pneumonia, and most significantly bacteremia.[7-9,27,28,51] The latter complication may frequently result in endocarditis,[26,52] as reported in both hospitalized patients and heroin addicts.[26,52]

In a study by Yamaguchi et al.,[42] among the predisposing factors leading to *B. cepacia*-induced pneumonia epidemics among patients with hematologic malignancies and solid tumors have been acute leukemia, malignant lymphomas, lung cancer, and myelodysplastic syndrome.

15.1.2 TREATMENT OF *B. CEPACIA* INFECTIONS

The clinical course of *B. cepacia* pneumonia is characterized by high fever and elevation of the C-reactive protein.[42] Treatment of the infection may be difficult because of the nearly universal resistance of this organism to commonly used antipseudomonal agents.[44,53,54]

Historically, the most effective agents against *B. cepacia* infections have been chloramphenicol and trimethoprim-sulfamethoxazole (TMP-SMX, co-trimoxazole), even though their clinical efficacy has been somewhat limited.[55,56]

Furthermore, often the treatment of *B. cepacia* pulmonary infections may be complicated by discrepancies between the observed *in vitro* susceptibility and the clinical response to antibiotic therapy. For example, although ceftazidime, temocillin, imipenem, and ciprofloxacin exerted *in vitro* activity against *B. cepacia*, their clinical efficacy has been rather limited.[57-61] On a more promising side, using killing curves, Kerr[60] has found the combination of ceftazidime and temocillin to exert synergistic activity against 70% of *B. cepacia* isolates.

One of the factors that have complicated the issue of antibiotic susceptibility was the fact that patients were often colonized or infected with multiple clones of the pathogen, very few of which have actually been selected for antimicrobial susceptibility testing.[54] For example, in spite of high *in vitro* activity of ceftazidime against *B. cepacia*,[62] Gold et al.[57] have found that only 7 of 14 patients treated showed a favorable clinical response; moreover, none of the patients showed any appreciable bacteriologic response. Even in patients who responded to therapy, the pathogen was rarely, if ever, eradicated.[57,63]

Yamaguchi et al.[42] used two drug regimens to treat *B. cepacia*-associated pneumonia in 14 immunocompromised patients: (1) intravenous ceftazidime at 4.0 g daily (pneumonia resolved in 9 of 12 patients), and (2) intravenous minocycline at 200 mg daily (pneumonia resolved in 7 of 10 patients). Despite therapy, 4 of the patients still died of respiratory failure caused by the pathogen, while 10 patients survived.

15.1.2.1 *B. cepacia* Colonization and Infection of Patients with Cystic Fibrosis

Patients with cystic fibrosis have a distinctive bacterial flora in the respiratory tract, with *P. aeruginosa* being the most common microorganism isolated.[64-66] However, there has been a progressive escalation in the incidence of *B. cepacia* being isolated from such patients either alone or in combination with *P. aeruginosa*.[33,44-47,67,68]

The spread of *B. cepacia* through the previously stable cystic fibrosis population has become increasingly alarming.[33,47,69-74] Moreover, in many patients infected with *B. cepacia*, the clinical course of the disease has been different from that seen with *P. aeruginosa*.[33] Thus, patients infected with *B. cepacia* may experience greater impairment of their pulmonary functions. While in some cases such events may produce only asymptomatic carriage or a slow decline in the respiratory function, in some 20% of patients, an accelerated fatal decline in pulmonary function has been observed, accompanied by necrotizing pneumonia and bacteremia.[2,44,75] In addition, a syndrome characterized by high fever, severe progressive respiratory failure, leukocytosis, and elevated erythrocyte sedimentation rate has also occurred.[44]

The factors responsible for *B. cepacia* colonization and subsequent tissue damage are not well understood, and a direct pathogenic role for *B. cepacia* is yet to be proven.[2] Sajjan et al.[76] have described a 22-kDa pilin-associated protein which acted as mucin-binding adhesin for *B. cepacia*. Gessner and Mortensen[77] have suggested a possible pathogenic role for such factors as hemolysin, lipase, lecinthinase, and proteases.

Isles et al.[44] have proposed three distinct clinical patterns for patients with cystic fibrosis infected with *B. cepacia*: (1) chronic asymptomatic carriage of the bacteria either alone or in combination with *P. aeruginosa*; (2) progressive deterioration over a period of several months with recurrent fever, progressive weight loss, and repeated hospital admissions; and (3) rapid, usually fatal deterioration in previously mildly affected patients.

Females otherwise in good clinical conditions who acquired *B. cepacia* appeared to be at special risk of developing severe and unexpected pulmonary complications that often may result in death;[48,49] the prevalence may approach 40%.[76] Males, on the other hand, regardless of their clinical condition, appeared less likely to experience an immediate decline in their clinical condition.[33]

The overwhelming evidence for the existence of person-to-person transmission of *B. cepacia* may warrant limiting contact between patient and outpatient populations.[2,69,78-84]

Treatment of *B. cepacia* in patients with cystic fibrosis has been difficult because of its resistance to antibiotics, and eradication is seldom achieved despite aggressive antibiotic therapy.[62] Nevertheless, combinations of temocillin with aminoglycosides[61] and ceftazidime[60] have shown some encouraging results.

In addition, some carbapenem antibiotics have displayed promising *in vitro* activity.[56] Simpson et al.[85] have found that imipenem in combination with BRL 42715 (a β-lactamase inhibitor) decreased by eightfold the values of the MICs for 23 of 24 *B. cepacia* isolates. The combinations of imipenem with clavulanic acid, sulbactam, or tazobactam were ineffective, suggesting the possibility that many strains of *B. cepacia* may have produced carbapenemases.

15.1.3 DRUG RESISTANCE OF *PSEUDOMONAS* SPP.

Because of their genetic and physiologic properties, *Pseudomonas* spp. are one of the most antibiotic-resistant bacteria. This property allows them to survive environmental conditions which are lethal to many other bacteria, by selecting highly resistant clones. Resistance of *Pseudomonas* spp. to a wide array of β-lactam antibiotics, aminoglycosides, and quinolones has been steadily increasing and may be the result of different mechanisms.[54,86-88]

15.1.3.1 Resistance to β-Lactam Antibiotics

With their inherent low toxicity and potent antibacterial activity, the β-lactam antibiotics (penicillins and cephalosporins) have been widely used against *Pseudomonas* infections since their introduction into the clinic in the 1960s. However, in recent years, the resistance to such drugs as carbenicillin and piperacillin has risen substantially (from 7% and 0% in 1974 to 70% and 30% in 1984, respectively).[54]

The mechanism for this resistance has been the acquisition of plasmids that encode β-lactamase.[89] β-Lactamase enzymes, which are very common in Gram-negative microorganisms, are produced constitutively. However, their level of expression may vary with the copy number of the plasmid or with the relative rate of transcription and translation into an active protein. Predominantly, the β-lactamases are penicillinases that easily hydrolyze penicillin and ampicillin; carbenicillin is hydrolyzed at a slower rate. Two of these β-lactamases, TEM 1 and TEM 2, are the most common enzymes in *Pseudomonas*.[90] Another group of β-lactamases, the CARB enzymes (initially thought to be *Pseudomonas*-specific) can efficiently hydrolyze ticarcillin, mezlocillin, azlocillin, and piperacillin.[91]

The *Pseudomonas* genes encoding these enzymes have been found on transposons, facilitating their dissemination among a population of bacteria. Furthermore, genes encoding aminoglycoside and other antibiotic resistance may be linked in a single transposable unit along with the β-lactamase, thus making one single genetic event, even at a low frequency, responsible for the introduction and maintenance of a wide variety of antibiotic-resistant phenotypes in a population.[54] In addition, transposons may jump to another plasmid or to a chromosomal location in another organism. Since the common, very large IncP-2 plasmids of *Pseudomonas* are persistently maintained, even in the absence of antibiotic selection,[92] location of a transposon on either site may result in the establishment of multidrug-resistant microorganisms with minimal tendency to revert to a more antibiotic-susceptible phenotype.[54]

All *Pseudomonas* species are capable of producing a chromosomal β-lactamase which is a cephalosporinase by activity.[93] Contrary to plasmid-mediated enzymes, however, the chromosomal enzymes are inducible; that is, under normal conditions these enzymes are repressed and, generally, because of insufficient amounts, not able to produce clinically significant antibiotic resistance. However, after exposure to β-lactam antibiotics (including newer third-generation cephalosporins), *Pseudomonas* organisms can be induced to express very large amounts of this chromosomal β-lactamase.[94] Screening of clinical isolates of *B. cepacia* from patients with cystic fibrosis revealed that many strains were capable of either producing the chromosomal enzyme constitutively or being very readily induced to produce high levels of β-lactamase.[54]

Another mechanism to convey antibiotic resistance was described by Godfrey et al.[95] These investigators found that certain *Pseudomonas* strains highly resistant to ticarcillin and piperacillin did not produce significant amounts of β-lactamase. Instead, these strains were shown to alter the penicillin-binding proteins. The latter are critical for bacterial cell wall synthesis and are usual targets for β-lactam drugs. In these strains, the target enzymes (assayed collectively as penicillin-binding proteins) have decreased affinity for penicillins, thereby protecting the cell from the lethal action of the β-lactam antibiotics.

A third type of resistance mechanism may involve altering the permeability to β-lactam drugs.[54] Thus, Nicas and Hancock[96] have identified in some laboratory mutants of *P. aeruginosa* absent or modified porin channels through which β-lactam antibiotics enter the bacterial cell. The ability to permeate through these channels is a major determinant of antimicrobial drug susceptibility, and a significant factor for bacterial cell survival.[54]

15.1.3.2   Resistance to Aminoglycosides

In general, the resistance mechanisms of *Pseudomonas* spp. to aminoglycosides display patterns similar to those for β-lactam antibiotics, namely, (1) *Pseudomonas* spp. being able to produce aminoglycoside-modifying enzymes capable of inactivating the drug; (2) the aminoglycoside target, the ribosome, may be mutated to prevent binding of the drug; (3) the accumulation of aminoglycosides may be altered by the microorganism; and (4) decreasing the amount of aminoglycoside entering the microbial cell.[54]

The production of aminoglycoside-modifying enzymes is likely the most common mechanism of drug resistance found in clinical isolates.[97] Thus, a variety of enzymes (acetyltransferases, phosphoryltransferases, and adenylyltransferases) may be produced by plasmid-encoded genes located very often on transposable elements. Some of these enzymes may be very specific in their activity, such as modifying the cyclitol moiety or the deoxystreptamine ring of the aminoglycoside molecule. In many instances one single strain may produce (or one single plasmid may encode) more than one class of aminoglycoside-modifying enzymes, thus making the organism, for example, resistant to one aminoglycoside drug but susceptible to another by virtue of different drug-specific classes of enzyme being produced.[98]

Another potential mechanism of aminoglycoside resistance involves mutations affecting the ribosomal structure. For example, mutagenized strains with altered ribosomes that did not bind aminoglycosides have been selected in laboratory experiments.[54] The so-called "small colony" variant is another common mutation leading to decresased uptake of the aminoglycoside and drug resistance.[99] Since the aminoglycosides bind and enter the bacterial cell wall due to differences in the electric potential across the outer membrane, *Pseudomonas* mutants have been found to affect the cellular energy systems, such as deficient cytochromes and nitrite reductase causing clinically significant resistance.[100,101]

In addition to entering the bacterial cell through porins, *Pseudomonas* spp. are also being accumulated directly through the outer membrane by displacing Mg^{2+}, which stabilizes the phosphate-rich lipopolysaccharide of *Pseudomonas*.[102]

15.1.3.3 Resistance to Quinolones

Quinolone derivatives, such as ciprofloxacin, have been used in the treatment of *Pseudomonas* infections with some success.[103] Their mechanism of action involves interference with bacterial topoisomerases, the enzymes that nick and uncoil supercoiled DNA helixes to allow DNA replication. It has been shown that resistance to quinolones did not develop in one-step mutation, thus allowing longer periods of therapy. However, *Pseudomonas* strains resistant to quinolones have been selected gradually during therapy. While the mechanism of resistance is still not well understood, the resistant isolates seem to become again susceptible to the drug after therapy has been suspended for a time.[54]

15.1.3.4 Resistance to Other Antibiotics

The susceptibility of clinical isolates of *Pseudomonas* spp. to such antibiotics as tetracyclines, chloramphenicol, and trimethoprim-sulfamethoxazole (TMP-SMX), although variable, may develop swiftly. For example, *B. cepacia*, which may be susceptible to TMP-SMX initially, has rarely responded to treatment.[54]

15.1.4 REFERENCES

1. Burkholder, W. H., Sour skin, a bacterial rot of onion bulbs, *Phytopathology*, 50, 115, 1950.
2. Spencer, R. C., The emergence of epidemic, multiple-antibiotic-resistant *Stenotrophomonas* (*Xanthomonas*) *maltophilia* and *Burkholderia* (*Pseudomonas*) *cepacia*, *J. Hosp. Infect.*, 30(Suppl.), 453, 1995.
3. Yabuuchi, E., Kosako, Y., Oyaizu, H., Yano, I., Hotta, H., Hashimoto, Y., Ezaki, T., and Arakawa, M., Proposal of *Burkholderia* gen. nov. and transfer of seven species of the genus *Pseudomonas* group II to the new genus, with the type species *Burkholderia cepacia* (Pelleroni and Holmes 1981) comb. nov., *Microbiol. Immunol.*, 36, 1251, 1992.
4. Carson, L. A., Favero, M. S., Bond, W. W., and Petersen, N. J., Morphological, biochemical, and growth characteristics of *Pseudomonas cepacia* from distilled water, *Appl. Microbiol.*, 25, 476, 1973.

5. Dixon, R. E., Kaslow, R. A., Mackel, D. C., Fulkerson, C. C., and Mallison, G. F., Aqueous quaternary ammonium antiseptics and disinfectants: use and misuse, *JAMA*, 236, 2415, 1976.

6. Rogers, D. E., The changing pattern of life-threatening microbial disease, *N. Engl. J. Med.*, 261, 677, 1959.

7. Goldman, D. A. and Klinger, J. D., *Pseudomonas cepacia*: biology, mechanisms of virulence, epidemiology, *J. Pediatr.*, 108, 806, 1986.

8. Holmes, B., The identification of *Pseudomonas cepacia* and its occurrence in clinical material, *J. Appl. Bacteriol.*, 61, 299, 1986.

9. Pegues, D. A., Carson, L. A., Anderson, R. L., Norgard, M. J., Argent, T. A., Jarvis, W. R., and Woernle, C. H., Outbreak of *Pseudomonas cepacia* bacteremia in oncology patients, *Clin. Infect. Dis.*, 16, 407, 1993.

10. Conly, J. M., Klass, L., and Larson, L., *Pseudomonas cepacia* colonization and infection in intensive care units, *Can. Med. Assoc. J.*, 134, 363, 1986.

11. Sobel, J. D., Hashman, N., Reinharz, G., and Merzbach, D., Nosocomial *Pseudomonas cepacia* infection associated with chlorhexidine contamination, *Am. J. Med.*, 73, 183, 1982.

12. Pallent, L. J., Hugo, D. J., Grant, D. J. W., and Davies, A., *Pseudomonas cepacia* as contaminant and infective agent, *J. Hosp. Infect.*, 4, 9, 1983.

13. Randall, C., The problem of *Pseudomonas cepacia* in a hospital, *Can. J. Public Health*, 71, 119, 1980.

14. Rosenstein, B. J. and Hall, D. E., Pneumonia and septicemia due to *Pseudomonas cepacia* in a patient with cystic fibrosis, *Johns Hopkins Med. J.*, 147, 188, 1980.

15. Poe, R. H., Marcus, H. R., and Emerson, G. L., Long abscess due to *Pseudomonas cepacia*, *Annu. Rev. Respir. Dis.*, 115, 861, 1977.

16. Holmes, A., Jiang, R.-J., Sun, L. et al., Emergence of epidemic strains of *Burkholderia cepacia* involving both CF and non-CF populations, Proc. 36th Intersci. Conf. Antimicrob. Agents Chemother., American Society for Microbiology, Washington, D.C., Abstract J32, 1996, 224.

17. Keizur, J. J., Lavin, B., and Heidich, R. B., Iatrogenic urinary tract infection with *Pseudomonas cepacia* transrectal ultrasound guided needle biopsy of the prostate, *J. Urol.*, 149, 523, 1993.

18. Basset, D. C. J., Stokes, K. J., and Thomas, W. R. G., Wound infection with *Pseudomonas multivorans*: a water-borne contaminant of disinfectant solutions, *Lancet*, 1, 1188, 1970.

19. Burdon, D. W. and Whitby, J. L., Contamination of hospital disinfectants with *Pseudomonas* species, *Br. Med. J.*, 2, 153, 1967.

20. Gilardi, G. L., Characterization of EO-1 strains (*Pseudomonas kingii*) isolated from clinical specimens and the hospital environment, *Appl. Microbiol.*, 20, 521, 1970.

21. Hardy, P. C., Ederer, G. M., and Matsen, J. M., Contamination of commercially packaged urinary catheter kits with the pseudomonad EO-1, *N. Engl. J. Med.*, 282, 33, 1970.

22. Reinharz, J. A., Pierce, A. K., Mays, B. B., and Sanford, J. P., The potential role of inhalation therapy equipment in nosocomial pulmonary infection, *J. Clin. Invest.*, 44, 831, 1965.

23. Mitchell, R. G. and Hayward, A. C., Postoperative urinary-tract infections caused by contaminated irrigating fluid, *Lancet*, 1, 793, 1966.

24. Phillips, I., Eykyn, S., Curtis, M. A., and Snell, J. J. S., *Pseudomonas cepacia* (*multivorans*) septicaemia in an intensive-care unit, *Lancet*, 1, 375, 1971.

25. Speller, D. C. E., Stephens, M. E., and Viant, A. C., Hospital infection by *Pseudomonas cepacia*, *Lancet*, 1, 798, 1971.

26. Norrega, E. R., Rubinstein, E., Simberkoff, M. S., and Rahal, J. J., Sub-acute and acute endocarditis due to *Pseudomonas cepacia* in heroin addicts, *Am. J. Med.*, 59, 29, 1975.

27. Weinstein, R. A., Emori, T. G., Anderson, R. L., and Stamm, W. E., Pressure transducers as a source of bacteremia after open heart surgery: report of an outbreak and guidelines for prevention, *Chest*, 69, 338, 1976.

28. Plotkin, S. A. and Austrian, R., Bacteremia caused by *Pseudomonas* sp. following the use of materials stored in solutions of a cationic surface active agent, *Am. J. Med. Sci.*, 235, 621, 1958.

29. Frank, M. J. and Schaffner, W., Contaminated aqueous benzalkonium chloride: an unnecessary hospital infection hazard, *JAMA*, 236, 2418, 1976.

30. Kaslow, R. A., Mackal, D. C., and Mallison, G. F., Nosocomial pseudobacteremia: positive blood cultures due to contaminated benzalkonium antiseptics, *JAMA*, 236, 2407, 1976.

31. Jumaa, P. A. and Chattopadhyay, B., Pseudobacteraemia, *J. Hosp. Infect.*, 27, 167, 1994.

32. Dixon, R. E., Kaslow, R. A., Mackel, D. C., Fulkerson, C. C., and Mallison, G. F., Aqueous quarternary ammonium antiseptics and disenfectants: use and misuse, *JAMA,* 236, 2415, 1976.

33. Thomassen, M. J., Demko, C. A., Klinger, J. D., and Stern, R. C., *Pseudomonas cepacia* colonization among patients with cystic fibrosis: a new opportunist, *Am. Rev. Respir. Dis.*, 131, 791, 1985.

34. Weems, J. J., Nosocomial outbreak of *Pseudomonas cepacia* associated with contamination of reusable electronic ventilator temperature probes, *Infect. Control Hosp. Epidemiol.*, 14, 583, 1993.

35. Berthelot, P., Grattard, F., Mahul, P., Jospe, R., Pozzetto, B., Ros, A., Gaudin, O. G., and Auboyer, C., Ventilator temperarature sensors: an unusual source of *Pseudomonas cepacia* in nosocomial infection, *J. Hosp. Infect.*, 25, 33, 1993.

36. Berkelman, R. L., Godley, J., Weber, J. A., Anderson, R. L., Lerner, M., Petersen, N. J., and Allen, J. R., *Pseudomonas cepacia* peritonitis associated with contamination of automatic peritoneal dialysis machines, *Ann. Intern. Med.*, 96, 456, 1982.

37. Sobel, J. D., Hashman, N., Reinherz, G., and Merzbach, D., Nosocomial *Pseudomonas cepacia* infection associated with chlorhexidine contamination, *Am. J. Med.*, 73, 183, 1982.

38. Weinstein, R. A., Emori, T. G., Anderson, R. L., and Stamm, W. E., Pressure transducers as a source of bacteremia after open heart surgery: report of an outbreak and guidelines for prevention, *Chest*, 69, 338, 1976.

39. Snell, G. I., de Hoyos, A., Krajden, M., Winton, T., and Maurer, J. R., *Pseudomonas cepacia* in lung transplant recipients with cystic fibrosis, *Chest*, 103, 466, 1993.

40. Pederman, M. M., Marso, E., and Pickett, M. J., Pathogenicity and antibiotic susceptibility, *Am. J. Clin. Pathol.*, 54, 178, 1970.

41. Dailey, R. H. and Banner, E. J., Necrotizing pneumonitis due to *Pseudomonas* "eugonic oxidizer - group I", *N. Engl. J. Med.*, 279, 361, 1968.

42. Yamaguchi, Y., Fujita, J., Takigawa, K., Negayama, K., Nakazawa, T., and Takahara, J., Clinical features of *Pseudomonas cepacia* pneumonia in an epidemic among immunocompromised patients, *Chest*, 103, 1706, 1993.

43. Pierce, A. K., Edmonson, E. B., McGee, G., Ketchersid, J., Loudon, R. C., and Sanford, J. P., An analysis of factors predisposing to Gram-negative bacillary necrotizing pneumonia, *Am. Rev. Respir. Dis.*, 94, 309, 1966.

44. Isles, A., Maclusky, I., Corey, M., Gold, M., Prober, C., Fleming, P., and Levison, H., *Pseudomonas cepacia* infection in cystic fibrosis, *J. Pediatr.*, 104, 206, 1984.

45. Thomassen, M. J., Demko, C. A., Doershuk, C. F., Stern, R. C., and Klinger, J. D., *Pseudomonas cepacia*: decrease in colonization in patients with cystic fibrosis, *Am. Rev. Respir. Dis.*, 134, 669, 1986.

46. Tablan, O. C., Chorba, T. L., Schidlow, D. V., White, J. W., Hardy, K. A., Gilligan, P. H., Morgan, W. M., Carson, L. A., Martone, W. J., Jason, J. M., and Jarvis, W. R., *Pseudomonas cepacia* colonization in patients with cystic fibrosis: risk factors and clinical outcome, *J. Pediatr.*, 107, 382, 1985.

47. Tablan, O. C., Martone, W. J., Doershuk, C. F., Stern, R. C., Thomassen, M. J., Klinger, J. D., White, J. W., Carson, L. A., and Jarvis, W. R., Colonization of the respiratory tract with *Pseudomonas cepacia* in cystic fibrosis: risk factors, *Chest*, 91, 527, 1987.

48. Editorial, *Pseudomonas cepacia* — more than a harmless commensal? *Lancet*, 339, 1385, 1992.

49. Goven, J. R. W. and Nelson, J. W., Microbiology of cystic fibrosis lung infections: themes and issues, *J. R. Soc. Med.*, 86(Suppl. 20), 11, 1993.

50. Taplan, D., Basset, D. C. J., and Mertz, P. M., Foot lesions associated with *Pseudomonas cepacia*, *Lancet*, 2, 1568, 1971.

51. Yabuuichi, E., Miyajima, N., Hotta, H., Abiyana, A., and Tanaka, N., *Pseudomonas cepacia* from blood of a burn patient, *Med. J. Osaka Univ.*, 21, 1, 1970.

52. Neu, H. C., Garvey, G. J., and Beach, M. P., Successful treatment of *Pseudomonas cepacia* endocarditis in a heroin addict with trimethoprim-sulfamethoxazole, *J. Infect. Dis.*, 128(Suppl.), 768, 1973.

53. Gold, R., Jin, E., Levison, H., Isles, A., and Fleming, P. C., Ceftazidime alone and in combination in patients with cystic fibrosis: lack of efficacy in treatment of severe respiratory infections caused by *Pseudomonas cepacia*, *J. Antimicrob. Chemother.*, 12A, 331, 1983.

54. Prince A., Antibiotic resistance of *Pseudomonas* species, *J. Pediatr.*, 108, 830, 1986.

55. Nord, C. E., Wadstrom, T., and Wretlind, B., Synergistic effect of colonization of sulfamethoxazole, trimethoprim and colistin against *Pseudomonas maltophilia* and *Pseudomonas cepacia*, *Antimicrob. Agents Chemother.*, 6, 521, 1974.

56. Lewin, C., Doherty, C., and Govan, J. R. W., *In vitro* activities of meropenem, PD 127391, PD 131628, ceftazidime, chloramphenicol, co-trimoxazole and ciprofloxacin against *Pseudomonas cepacia*, *Antimicrob. Agents Chemother.*, 37, 123, 1993.

57. Gold, R., Jin, E., Levison, H., Isles, A., and Fleming, P., Ceftazidime in patients with cystic fibrosis: lack of efficacy in treatment of severe respiratory infections caused by *P. cepacia*, *J. Antimicrob. Chemother.*, 12(Suppl. B), 331, 1983.

58. Aronoff, S. C. and Klinger, J. D., *In vitro* activities of aztreonam, piperacillin, and ticarcillin combined with amikacin against amikacin-resistant *Pseudomonas aeruginosa* and *P. cepacia* isolates from children with cystic fibrosis, *Antimicrob. Agents Chemother.*, 25, 279, 1984.

59. Bhakta, D. R., Leader, I., Jacobson, R., Robinson, D. B., Honicky, R. E., and Kumar, A., Antibacterial properties of investigational, new and commonly used antibiotics against isolates of *Pseudomonas cepacia* in Michigan, *Chemotherapy*, 38, 319, 1991.

60. Kerr, J. R., *In vitro* activity of drug combinations of ceftazidime, cefotaxime, cefuroxime, ciprofloxacin, chloramphenicol, imipenem and temocillin against clinical isolates of *Pseudomonas cepacia* from patients with cystic fibrosis, *Int. J. Antimicrob. Agents*, 3, 205, 1993.

61. Taylor, R. F. H., Gaya, H., and Hodson, M. E., Temocillin and cystic fibrosis: outcome of intravenous administration in patients infected with *Pseudomonas cepacia*, *J. Antimicrob. Chemother.*, 29, 341, 1992.

62. Fleming, P. C. and Knie, B., Activity of ceftazidime against *Pseudomonas aeruginosa* from bacteraemic and fibrocystic patients, *J. Antimicrob. Chemother.*, 8(Suppl. B), 169, 1981.

63. Hyatt, A. C., Chipps, B. E., Humor, K. M., Mellitis, D. F., Lietman, P. S., and Rosenstein, B. J., A double-blind trial of anti-*Pseudomonas* chemotherapy of acute respiratory exacerbations in patients with cystic fibrosis, *J. Pediatr.*, 99, 307, 1981.

64. Taussig, L. M. and Landau, L. I., Cystic fibrosis, *Semin. Respir. Med.*, 1, 167, 1979.

65. Hoiby, N., *Pseudomonas aeruginosa* infection in cystic fibrosis, *Acta Pathol. Microbiol. Scand.*, 262(Suppl.), 1, 1977.

66. Corey, M. L., Longitudinal studies in cystic fibrosis, in *Perspectives in Cystic Fibrosis*, Sturgess, J. M., Ed., Canadian Cystic Fibrosis Foundation, 1980, 246.

67. Blessing, J., Walker, J., Maybury, B., Yeager, A. S., and Lewiston, J., *Pseudomonas cepacia* and *maltophilia* in the cystic fibrosis patient, *Am. Rev. Respir. Dis.*, 119, 262, 1979.

68. Nolan, G., McIvor, P., Levison, H., Fleming, P., Corey, M., and Gold, M., Antibiotic prophylaxis in cystic fibrosis: inhaled cephaloridine as adjunct to oral therapy, *J. Pediatr.*, 101, 626, 1982.

69. Burdge, D. R., Nakielna, E. M., and Noble, M. A., Case control and vector studies of nosocomial acquisition of *Pseudomonas cepacia* in adult patients with cystic fibrosis, *Infect. Control Hosp. Epidemiol.*, 14, 127, 1993.

70. Gilligan, P. H., Microbiology of airway disease in patients with cystic fibrosis, *Clin. Microbiol. Rev.*, 4, 35, 1991.

71. Govan, J. R. W. and Nelson, J. W., Microbiology of lung infection in cystic fibrosis, *Br. Med. Bull.*, 48, 912, 1992.

72. Govan, J. R. W. and Glass, S., The microbiology and therapy of cystic fibrosis lung infections, *Rev. Med. Microbiol.*, 1, 19, 1990.

73. Nelson, J. W., Doherty, C. J., Brown, P. H., Greening, A. P., Kaufmann, M. E., and Govan, J. R. W., *Pseudomonas cepacia* in inpatients with cystic fibrosis, *Lancet*, 33B, 1525, 1991.

74. Smith, D. L., Smith, G. G., Gunnery, L. B., and Stableforth, D. E., *Pseudomonas cepacia* infection in cystic fibrosis, *Lancet*, 339, 252, 1992.

75. Rosenstein, B. J. and Hall, D. E., Pneumonia and septicaemia due to *Pseudomonas cepacia* in a patient with cystic fibrosis, *Johns Hopkins Med. J.*, 147, 188, 1980.

76. Sajjan, S. U., Corey, M., Karmali, M. A., and Forstner, J. F., Binding of *Pseudomonas cepacia* to human intestinal mucin and respiratory mucin from patients with cystic fibrosis, *J. Clin. Invest.*, 89, 648, 1992.

77. Gessner, A. R. and Mortensen, J. E., Pathogenic factors of *Pseudomonas cepacia*, *J. Clin. Microbiol.*, 33, 115, 1990.

78. Govan, J. R. W., Brown, P. H., Maddison, J., Doherty, C. J., Nelson, J. W., Dodd, M., Greening, A. P., and Webb, A. K., Evidence for the transmission of *Pseudomonas cepacia* by social contact in cystic fibrosis, *Lancet*, 342, 15, 1993.

79. LiPuma, J. J., Dasen, S. E., Nielsen, D. W., Stern, R. C., and Stull, T. L., Person-to-person transmission of *Pseudomonas cepacia* from patients with cystic fibrosis, *Lancet*, 336, 1094, 1990.

80. Millar-Jones, L., Paule, A., Saunders, A., and Goodchild, M. C., Transmission of *Pseudomonas cepacia* among cystic fibrosis patients, *Lancet*, 340, 491, 1992.

81. Simmonds, E. J., Conway, S. P., Ghonheim, A. T. M., Ross, H., and Littlewood, J. M., *Pseudomonas cepacia*: a new pathogen in patients with cystic fibrosis referred to a large centre in the United Kingdom, *Arch. Dis. Child.*, 65, 647, 1990.

82. Smith, D. L., Gunnery, L. B., Smith, E. G., Stableforth, D. E., Kaufmann, M. E., and Pitt, T. L., Epidemic of *Pseudomonas cepacia* in an adult cystic fibrosis unit: evidence of person to person transmission, *J. Clin. Microbiol.*, 31, 3017, 1993.

83. Taylor, R. F. H., Dalla Costa, L., Kaufmann, M. E., Pitt, T. L., and Hodson, M. E., *Pseudomonas cepacia* pulmonary infection in adults with cystic fibrosis: is nosocomial acquisition occurring? *J. Hosp. Infect.*, 21, 199, 1992.

84. Walters, S. and Smith, E. G., *Pseudomonas cepacia* in cystic fibrosis: transmissibility and its application, *Lancet*, 342, 3, 1993.

85. Simpson, I. N., Hunter, R., Govan, J. R., and Nelson, J. W., Do all *Pseudomonas cepacia* produce carbapenemases? *J. Antimicrob. Chemother.*, 32, 339, 1993.

86. Gilligan, P. H., Gage, P. A., Bradshaw, L. M., Schidlow, D. V., and DeCicco, B. J., Isolation medium for the recovery of *Pseudomonas cepacia* from respiratory secretions of patients with cystic fibrosis, *J. Clin. Microbiol.*, 22, 5, 1985.

87. Tablan, O. C., Carson, L. A., Cusick, L. B., Bland, L. A., Marton, W. J., and Jarvis, W. R., Laboratory proficiency test results on use of selective media for isolating *Pseudomonas cepacia* from simulated sputum specimens of patients with cystic fibrosis, *J. Clin. Microbiol.*, 25, 485, 1987.

88. Beckman, W. and Lessie, T. C., Response of *Pseudomonas cepacia* to β-lactam antibiotics: utilization of penicillin G as the carbon source, *J. Bacteriol.*, 140, 1126, 1979.

89. Sykes, R. B. and Matthew, M. H., The beta-lactamases of gram-negative bacteria and their role in resistance to beta-lactam antibiotics, *J. Antimicrob. Chemother.*, 2, 115, 1976.

90. Jacoby, G. A. and Matthew, M., The distribution of beta-lactamase genes on plasmids found in *Pseudomonas*, *Plasmid*, 2, 41, 1979.

91. Jacoby, G. A. and Sutton, L., Activity of beta-lactam antibiotics against *Pseudomonas aeruginosa* carrying R plasmids determining different beta-lactamases, *Antimicrob. Agents Chemother.*, 16, 243, 1979.

92. Prince, A. S. and Barlam, T., Isolation of a DNA fragment containing replication functions from the IncP2 megaplasmid pMG2, *J. Bacteriol.*, 161, 792, 1985.

93. Sabath, L. D., Jago, M., and Abraham, E. P., Cephalosporinase and penicillinase activities of a beta-lactamase from *Pseudomonas pyocyanea*, *Biochem. J.*, 96, 739, 1965.

94. Vu, H. and Nikaido, H., Role of beta-lactam hydrolysis in the mechanism of resistance of a beta-lactamase-constitutive *Enterobacter cloacae* strain to expanded-spectrum beta-lactams, *Antimicrob. Agents Chemother.*, 27, 393, 1985.

95. Godfrey, A. J., Bryan, L. E., and Rabin, H. R., Beta-lactam-resistant *Pseudomonas aeruginosa* with modified penicillin-binding protein emerging during cystic fibrosis treatment, *Antimicrob. Agents Chemother.*, 19, 705, 1981.

96. Nicas, T. I. and Hancock, R. E., *Pseudomonas aeruginosa* outer membrane permeability: isolation of a porin protein F-deficient mutant, *J. Bacteriol.*, 153, 281, 1983.

97. Davies, J., Resistance to aminoglycosides: mechanisms and frequency, *Rev. Infect. Dis.*, 5(Suppl. 2), S261, 1983.

98. Prince, A. S. and Jacoby, G. A., Cloning the gentamicin resistance gene from a *Pseudomonas aeruginosa* plasmid in *Escherichia coli* enhances detection of aminoglycoside modification, *Antimicrob. Agents Chemother.*, 22, 525, 1982.

99. Bryan, L. E., Haraphongse, R., and van den Elzen, H. M., Gentamicin resistance in clinical isolates of *Pseudomonas aeruginosa* associated with decreased gentamicin accumulation and no detectable enzymatic modification, *J. Antibiot.*, 29, 743, 1976.

100. Bryan, L. E. and Kwan, S., Aminoglycoside-resistant mutants of *Pseudomonas aeruginosa* deficient in cytochrome d nitrite reductase, and aerobic transport, *Antimicrob. Agents Chemother.*, 19, 958, 1981.
101. Bryan, L. E., Aminoglycoside resistance, in *Antimicrobial Drug Resistance*, Bryant, L. E., Ed., Academic Press, New York, 1984, 254.
102. Hancock, R. W., Raffle, V. J., and Nicas, T. I., Involvement of the outer membrane in gentamicin and streptomycin uptake and killing in *Pseudomonas aeruginosa*, *Antimicrob. Agents Chemother.*, 19, 777, 1981.
103. Chin, N. X. and Neu, H. C., Ciprofloxacin, a quinolone carboxylic acid compound active against aerobic and anaerobic bacteria, *Antimicrob. Agents Chemother.*, 25, 319, 1984.

15.2 *STENOTROPHOMONAS (XANTHOMONAS) MALTOPHILIA*

15.2.1 INTRODUCTION

Stenotrophomonas (Xanthomonas) maltophilia is one of several new microorganisms that have recently emerged as potentially important opportunistic/nosocomial pathogens, especially in debilitated and immunocompromised patients.[1-5] The incidence of clinical isolation of this organism is on the rise (especially in hospital settings), possibly in part because of its unusual resistance to various commonly used broad-spectrum antimicrobial agents.[5-9] Several reports[10-12] have suggested that *S. maltophilia* is the most frequently isolated pseudomonad from clinical material after *P. aeruginosa*. For example, during the period 1981–1984, the annual isolation rate in just one institution, the University of Virginia Hospital, rose from 7.1 to 14.1 per 10,000 patients discharged.[13] In a report by Gardner et al.,[14] 97% of all clinical isolates were hospital-acquired, and 92% of the infected patients had received antecedent antibiotic therapy.

S. maltophilia was first described in 1960 by Hugh and Ryschenkow[15] as *Pseudomonas maltophilia*. In 1983, Swings et al.[16] determined that sufficient genetic and biochemical differences with pseudomonads existed to reclassify the organism as a distinct genus, *Xanthomonas*. However, in 1993, the name *Stenotrophomonas* was suggested for a new genus to include *X. maltophilia* as its single species under the name *Stenotrophomonas maltophilia*.[17]

S. maltophilia is a motile, free-living, Gram-negative, aerobic bacillus with multitrichous polar flagellae.[18,19] Like *P. aeruginosa*, *S. maltophilia* does not ferment lactose. It oxidizes maltose and, usually, dextrose and xylose.[1] Enzymes such as elastase, esterase, hyaluronidase, hemolysin, lipase, mucinase, and RNase may be potentially important factors in the virulence of *S. maltophilia*.[4]

The pathogen has been isolated from various human, animal, and environmental sources, such as water, soil, sewage, raw milk, frozen fish, rabbit and human feces, and hospital disinfectant solutions.[15,20,21] In a report by Agger et al.[22] of 23 patients with wound infections resulting from injuries by corn-harvesting machines, one third were caused by *S. maltophilia*.

As compared with *P. aeruginosa*, the pathogenic and virulence factors in *S. maltophilia* infections are still not fully understood, although both are considered to be opportunistic pathogens.[1] One distinct difference between the two organisms has been the ability of *P. aeruginosa* to produce specific virulent hemolysins that promote tissue invasion and necrosis — *S. maltophilia* does not produce these enzymes. However, a strain of *S. maltophilia* associated with a case of bacteremia and ecthyma gangrenosum was shown to produce protease and elastase,[23] similar to the exoenzyme profile of *P. aeruginosa*.

Clinical isolates of *S. maltophilia* have been recovered from multiple sites,[24] including blood,[13] urine,[13,21] respiratory secretions,[24] cerebrospinal fluid, pericardial fluid, pus, and wound swabs.[25,26]

The frequency of *S. maltophilia* infections in patients with cystic fibrosis has been on the rise.[24,27,28] Thus, in a cystic fibrosis pediatric population, the *S. maltophilia* prevalence rate was 10%; in addition, all children were co-infected with *P. aeruginosa*.[29]

Other clinical manifestations associated with *S. maltophilia* include endocarditis (overall mortality rate of 40%),[6,30-35] meningitis,[6,36-39] primary bacteremia,[40-42] pneumonia,[14,43,44] urinary tract infections,[25,26] ecthyma gangrenosum,[6,23] mastoiditis,[45] epididymitis,[46] cellulitis,[47] abscesses,[25] intravenous line-associated bacteremia,[48] infections of traumatic and postoperative wounds,[12,22,25,26,49] bloodstream infections,[40-42,50] and eye infections.[39,46,51]

The single most important predisposing factor for acquiring *S. maltophilia* infection has been the presence of a compromised immune system.[5,52] Other predisposing factors include patients undergoing mechanical ventilation in shock-trauma intensive care units receiving antimicrobial therapy,[53] and patients on imipenem chemotherapy.[7]

In a match-control study using multivariate techniques, Elting et al.[7] have examined the factors predisposing to clinically significant nosocomial infection with *S. maltophilia*. During a 6-month period, 16 cases of unusually severe infections were diagnosed in cancer patients; 8 patients had disseminated infection, and 6 died as a result of the infection. In the latter cases, all patients had taken imipenem. Among the predisposing factors examined, therapy with broad-spectrum antibiotics and indwelling central venous catheterization were found to significantly increase susceptibility to infection. However, exposure to imipenem was the single most important risk factor.[7,54-57]

In immunocompromised hosts, the infection occasionally may become disseminated.[7] It has been observed among patients with obstructive pulmonary disorders, diabetes, and malignant neoplasms, as well as in patients undergoing open heart surgery and prosthetic valve replacement.[6,13,26,41,48,58] Fatal infections with *S. maltophilia* have been reported on several occasions.[6,13,59]

Evidence supporting the association of *S. maltophilia* with host immune defects was presented by Nagai.[58] It was found that patients with malignant lesions had predilection for being infected or colonized by *S. maltophilia* — the pathogen has been isolated from the site of the lesion in 39 (48%) of 82 patients.[31] Even though the pathogenicity of *S. maltophilia* has not always occurred in the presence of malignancies,[21,30,32,60] it was suggested that an altered microenvironment owing to anaerobic glycolysis from tumor destruction may select for the emergence of certain pathogens, such as *S. maltophilia*, *in situ*.[58]

15.2.2 Drug Development and Treatment of *S. Maltophilia* Infections

In vitro susceptibility studies[31,41,43,61] have shown *S. maltophilia* to be susceptible to doxycycline, chloramphenicol, moxalactam, and especially trimethoprim-sulfamethoxazole (TMP-SMX, co-trimoxazole).[5,7,8,13,62] Khardori et al.[3] have examined the susceptibilities of 45 clinical and 3 environmental isolates of *S. maltophilia* to newer antibiotics by broth microdilution. The quinolones PD117596, PD117558, PD127391, A-56620, amifloxacine, and fleroxacin were the most active agents tested, with 70% to 99% of the isolates being susceptible; all isolates were resistant to trospectomycin. The new aminoglycosides SCH 24120 and SCH 22591 were active against 12% and 1% of the isolates, respectively.[3]

The synergistic effects of various drug combinations against *S. maltophilia* have been explored in several *in vitro* studies.[61,63-67] According to Jacobs et al.,[63] and Traub and Spohr,[64] the combination of ticarcillin and clavulanic acid was synergistic against six strains of *S. maltophilia*, with a MIC value fourfold lower than that of ticarcillin alone. Zuravleff and Yu[41] found synergistic *in vitro* activity with the combination of TMP-SMX, carbenicillin, and rifampin, as well as when gentamicin replaced TMP-SMX in this combination.

In another *in vitro* study,[68] the addition of ciprofloxacin to either a third-generation cephalosporin or a broad-spectrum penicillin was synergistic or additive against 28 strains of *S. maltophilia*. However, the *in vivo* efficacy of these combinations and the potential for emergence of resistance is not known.

At present, the TMP-SMX is considered the best therapeutic option against infections by *S. maltophilia*.[7,66] In a study by Morrison et al.,[13] the pathogen demonstrated 100% susceptibility to TMP-SMX. However, a significant number of patients cannot tolerate this combination because of hypersensitivity reactions.[3]

15.2.2.1 Resistance to Antimicrobial Agents

One of the most striking observations with *S. maltophilia* is the unusual resistance to a broad array of antimicrobial agents.[1,66] It has often shown resistance to antimicrobial agents used as first-line drugs during the initial therapy of Gram-negative bacterial infections, including those active against *P. aeruginosa*.[5,7,8,13,41,42,61,62,67-69]

In an earler report, Gilardi[25] found that 22 clinical isolates of *S. maltophilia* displayed a high degree of native resistance to various aminoglycosides, β-lactams, and tetracyclines. Neu et al.[66] also found resistance to antibiotics in 50 clinical isolates of *S. maltophilia*. While all isolates were resistant to imipenem, CGP 31608, aztreonam, and carumonam, the majority showed resistance to azlocillin, piperacillin, mezlocillin, ticarcillin, cefotaxime, ceftizoxime, ceftriaxone, cefoperazone, and ceftazidime.

Mett et al.[70] proposed two mechanisms that might explain the resistance to β-lactams: changes in the low outer membrane permeability, and constitutive overproduction of β-lactamases. The change of permeability, making the membrane impervious to antimicrobial drugs, may be the result of a decrease in production of an outer membrane protein necessary for the porins to function.[71] With regard to the second hypothesis, Saino et al.[72] have isolated two distinct β-lactamases, designated as L1 and L2. L1, which is a Zn-containing penicillinase that is not inhibited by clavulanic acid, was found to hydrolyze imipenem. The second β-lactamase, L2 is a cephalosporinase which was reported active even against ceftizoxime and aztreonam.[73] However, the production of both L1 and L2 was rapidly suppressed when *S. maltophilia* was grown in the presence of β-lactams.

In spite of reduced permeability and the presence of β-lactamases, some strains of *S. maltophilia* have shown susceptibility *in vitro* to a number of third-generation cephalosporins, such as ceftazidime, cefoperazone, and the β-lactam moxalactam.[1]

The mechanisms of *S. maltophilia* resistance to aminoglycosides is less clear. Plasmid-mediated resistance has been described in two studies.[31,74] Differences in the susceptibility towards aminoglycosides at 30°C (mostly resistant) and at 37°C (mostly sensitive) have also been reported.[75,76] The observed dissimilarity has been attributed to changes in the outer membrane profiles (OMPs), which correlated with temperature-dependent resistance to gentamicin.[77] In separate studies, it was found that the OMPs of *S. maltophilia* may vary according to the medium composition, which in turn, may account for the medium-dependent susceptibility to β-lactam antibiotics, other than imipenem.[70,78] Results reported by Cullman[79] demonstrated that the OMP profile of *S. maltophilia* contributed to its resistance to most antibiotics.

All strains of *S. maltophilia* were resistant to imipenem because of the presence of a Zn-containing penicillinase.[80] The latter, a L1 β-lactamase, which degrades carbapenem antibiotics, requires Zn^{2+} for its activity and stability.[81] This reliance on Zn^{2+} should be taken into account and the content of zinc ions in the susceptibility test media should be monitored.[82]

S. maltophilia was found resistant against nearly all of the 4-quinolones, including norfloxacin and ciprofloxacin.[83] Again, the mechanism of resistance has not been clearly delineated.

15.2.3 REFERENCES

1. Marshall, W. F., Keating, M. R., Anhalt, J. P., and Steckelberg, J. M., *Xanthomonas maltophilia*: an emerging nosocomial pathogen, *Mayo Clin. Proc.*, 64, 1097, 1989.
2. Neu, H. C., Unusual nosocomial infections, *Disease-A-Month*, 30, 1, 1984.

3. Khardori, N., Reuben, A., Rosenbaum, B., Rolston, K., and Bodey, G. P., *In vitro* susceptibility of *Xanthomonas* (*Pseudomonas*) *maltophilia* to newer antimicrobial agents, *Antimicrob. Agents Chemother.*, 34, 1609, 1990.

4. Spenser, R. C., The emergence of epidemic, multiple-antibiotic-resistant *Stenotrophomonas* (*Xanthomonas*) *maltophilia* and *Burkholderia* (*Pseudomonas*) *cepacia*, *J. Hosp. Infect.*, 30(Suppl.), 453, 1995.

5. Khardori, N., Elting, L., Wong, E., Schable, B., and Bodey, G., Nosocomial infections due to *Xanthomonas maltophilia* (*Pseudomonas maltophilia*) in patients with cancer, *Rev. Infect. Dis.*, 12, 997, 1990.

6. Muder, R. R., Yu, V. L., Dummer, J. S., Vinson, C., and Lumish, R. M., Infections caused by *Pseudomonas maltophilia*, *Arch. Intern. Med.*, 147, 1672, 1987.

7. Elting, L. S., Khardori, N., Bodey, G. P., and Fainstein, V., Nosocomial infection caused by *Xanthomonas maltophilia*: a case-control study of predisposing factors, *Infect. Control Hosp. Epidemiol.*, 11, 134, 1990.

8. Aoun, M., Van der Auwera, P., Devleeshouwer, C., Daneau, D., Seraj, N., Meunier, F., and Gerain, J., Bacteremia caused by non *aeruginosa Pseudomonas* species in a cancer centre, *J. Hosp. Infect.*, 22, 307, 1992.

9. Elting, L. S. and Bodey, G. P., Septicaemia due to *Xanthomonas* species and non-*aeruginosa Pseudomonas* species: increasing incidence of catheter-related infections, *Medicine (Baltimore)*, 69, 296, 1990.

10. Holmes, B., Lapage, S. P., and Easterling, B. G., Distribution in clinical material and identification of *Pseudomonas maltophilia*, *J. Clin. Pathol.*, 32, 66, 1979.

11. Rosenthal, S. L., Sources of *Pseudomonas* and *Acinetobacter* species found in human culture materials, *Am. J. Clin. Pathol.*, 62, 807, 1974

12. Pederson, M. M., Marso, E., and Pickett, M. J., Non-fermentative bacilli associated with man. III. Pathogenicity and antibiotic susceptibility, *Am. J. Clin. Pathol.*, 54, 178, 1970.

13. Morrison, A. J., Jr., Hoffmann, K. K., and Wenzel, R. P., Associated mortality and clinical characteristics of nosocomial *Pseudomonas maltophilia* in a university hospital, *J. Clin. Microbiol.*, 24, 52, 1986.

14. Gardner, P., Griffin, W. B., Swartz, M. N., and Kunz, L. J., Non-fermentative gram-negative bacilli of nosocomial interest, *Am. J. Med.*, 48, 735, 1970.

15. Hugh, R. and Ryschenkow, E., An *Alcaligenes*-like *Pseudomonas* species, *Bacteriol. Proc.*, 60, 78, 1960.

16. Swings, J., De Vos, P., Van den Mooter, M., and De Ley, J., Transfer of *Pseudomonas maltophilia* Hugh 1981 to the genus *Xanthomonas* as *Xanthomonas maltophilia* (Hugh 1981) comb. nov., *Int. J. Syst. Bacteriol.*, 33, 409, 1983.

17. Palleroni, N. J. and Bradbury, J. F., *Stenotrophomonas* a new bacterial genus for *Xanthomonas maltophilia* (Hugh 1980) Swings et al., *Int. J. Syst. Bacteriol.*, 43, 606, 1993.

18. Stanier, R. Y., Palleroni, N. J., and Doudoroff, M., The aerobic pseudomonads: a taxonomic study, *J. Gen. Microbiol.*, 43, 159, 1966.

19. Clark, W. A., Hollis, D. G., Weaver, R. E., and Riley, P., *Identification of Unusual Pathogenic Gram-negative Aerobic and Facultative Anaerobic Bacteria*, Centers for Disease Control, Atlanta, GA, 1985.

20. High, R. and Ryschenkow, E., *Pseudomonas maltophilia*, an *Alcaligenes*-like species, *J. Gen. Microbiol.*, 26, 123, 1961.

21. Wishart, M. W. and Riley, T. V., Infection with *Pseudomonas maltophilia* hospital outbreak due to contaminated disinfectant, *Med. J. Aust.*, 2, 710, 1976.

22. Agger, W. A., Coybill, T. H., Busch, H., Landercasper, J., and Callister, S. M., Wounds caused by corn-harvesting machines: an unusual source of infection due to Gram-negative bacilli, *Rev. Infect. Dis.*, 8, 927, 1986.

23. Bottone, E. J., Reitano, M., Janda, J. M., Troy, K., and Cuttner, J., *Pseudomonas maltophilia* exoenzyme activity as correlate in pathogenesis of ecthyma gangrenosum, *J. Clin. Microbiol.*, 24, 995, 1986.

24. Klinger, J. D. and Thomassen, M. J., Occurrence and antimicrobial susceptibility of gram-negative nonfermentative bacilli in cystic fibrosis patients, *Diagn. Microbiol. Infect. Dis.*, 3, 149, 1985.

25. Gilardi, G. L., *Pseudomonas maltophilia* infections in man, *Am. J. Clin. Pathol.*, 51, 58, 1969.

26. Gilardi, G. L., Infrequently encountered *Pseudomonas* species causing infection in humans, *Ann. Intern. Med.*, 77, 211, 1972.

27. Bauernfeind, A., Bertele, R. M., Harms, K., Hörl, G., Jungwirth, R., Petermüller, C., Przyklenk, B., and Weisslein-Pfister, C., Qualitative and quantitative microbiological analysis of sputa of 102 patients with cystic fibrosis, *Infection*, 15, 270, 1987.

28. Karpati, F., Malmborg, A.-S., Alfredson, H., Hjelte, L., and Starndvik, B., Bacterial colonization with *Xanthomonas maltophilia* — a retrospective study in a cystic fibrosis patient population, *Infection*, 22, 258, 1994.

29. Gladman, G., Connor, P. J., Williams, R. F., and David, T. J., Controlled study of *Pseudomonas cepacia* and *Pseudomonas maltophilia* in cystic fibrosis, *Arch. Dis. Child.*, 67, 192, 1992.

30. Semel, J. D., Trenholme, G. M., Harris, A. A., Jupa, J. E., and Levin, S., *Pseudomonas maltophilia* pseudosepticemia, *Am. J. Med.*, 64, 403, 1978.

31. Yu, V. L., Rumans, L. W., Wing, E. J., McLeod, R., Sattler, F. N., Harvey, R. M., and Deresinski, S. C., *Pseudomonas maltophilia* causing heroin-associated infective endocarditis, *Arch. Intern. Med.*, 138, 1667, 1978.

32. Yeh, T. J., Anabtawi, I. N., Cornett, V. E., White, A., Stern, W. H., and Ellison, R. G., Bacterial endocarditis following open-heart surgery, *Ann. Thorac. Surg.*, 3, 29, 1967.

33. Dismukes, W. E., Karchmer, A. W., Buckley, M. J., Austen, W. G., and Swattz, M. N., Prosthetic valve endocarditis: analysis of 38 cases, *Circulation*, 48, 365, 1973.

34. Fischer, J. J., *Pseudomonas maltophilia* endocarditis after replacement of the mitral valve: a case study, *J. Infect. Dis.*, 128(Suppl.), S771, 1973.

35. Subbannayya, K., Ramnarayan, K., Shivananda, P. G., Shatapathy, P., and Mathai, A., *Pseudomonas maltophilia* endocarditis, *Indian J. Pathol. Microbiol.*, 27, 311, 1984.

36. Trump, D. L., Grossman, S. A., Thompson, G., and Murray, K., CSF infections complicating the management of neoplastic meningitis: clinical features and results of therapy, *Arch. Intern. Med.*, 142, 583, 1982.

37. Patrick, S., Hindmarch, J. M., Hague, R. V., and Harris, D. M., Meningitis caused by *Pseudomonas maltophilia*, *J. Clin. Pathol.*, 28, 741, 1975.

38. Denis, F., Sow, A., David, M., Chiron, J.-P., Samb, A., and Diop Mar, I., Etude de deux cas de méningites a *Pseudomonas maltophilia* observés au Sénégal, *Bull. Soc. Med. Afr. Noire Lang Fr.*, 22, 135, 1977.

39. Devy, J. N. S., Venkatesh, A., and Shivananda, P. G., Neonatal infections due to *Pseudomonas maltophilia*, *Indian Pediatr.*, 21, 72, 1984.

40. Narasimhan, S. L., Gopaul, D. L., and Hatch, L. A., *Pseudomonas maltophilia* bacteremia associated with a prolapsed mitral valve, *Am. J. Clin. Pathol.*, 68, 304, 1977.

41. Zuravleff, J. J. and Yu, V. L., Infections caused by *Pseudomonas maltophilia* with emphasis on bacteremia: case reports and a review of the literature, *Rev. Infect. Dis.*, 4, 1236, 1982.

42. Sonnewirth, A. C., Bacteremia with and without meningitis due to *Yersinia enterocolitica*, *Edwardsiella tarda*, *Comamonas terrigena*, and *Pseudomonas maltophilia*, *Ann. NY Acad. Sci.*, 174, 488, 1970.

43. Sarkar, T. K., Gilardi, G., Aguam, A. S., Josephson, J., and Leventhal, G., Primary *Pseudomonas maltophilia* infection of the lung, *Postgrad. Med. J.*, 65, 253, 1979.

44. Feeley, T. W., du Moulin, G. C., Hedley-Whyte, J., Bushnell, L. S., Gilbert, J. P., and Feingold, D. S., Aerosol polymyxin and pneumonia in seriously ill patients, *N. Engl. J. Med.*, 293, 471, 1975.

45. Harlowe, H. D., Acute mastoiditis following *Pseudomonas maltophilia* infection: case report, *Laryngoscope*, 82, 882, 1972.

46. Sutter, V. L., Identification of *Pseudomonas* species isolated from hospital environment and human sources, *Appl. Microbiol.*, 16, 1532, 1968.

47. Von Graevenitz, A., Uber die isolierung von *Pseudomonas maltophilia* aus klinischem untersuchungsmaterial, *Med. Welt*, 1, 177, 1965.

48. Schoch, P. E. and Cunha, B. A., *Pseudomonas maltophilia*, *Infect. Control Hosp. Epidemiol.*, 8, 169, 1987.

49. Dyte, P. H. and Gillians, J. A., *Pseudomonas maltophilia* infection in an abattoir worker, *Med. J. Aust.*, 1, 444, 1977.

50. Fritsche, D., Lütticken, R., and Böhmer, H., *Pseudomonas maltophilia* as an agent of infection in man, *Zentralbl. Bakteriol. Hyg. Mikrobiol. Abt. 1 Orig. Reihe A*, 229, 89, 1974.

51. Ben-Tovim, T., Eylan, E., Romano, A., and Stein, R., Gram-negative bacteria isolated from external eye infections, *Infection*, 2, 162, 1974.

52. Victor, M. A., Arpi, M., Braun, B., Jonsson, V., and Hansen, M. M., *Xanthomonas maltophilia* bacteremia in immunocompromised hematological patients, *Scand. J. Infect. Dis.*, 26, 163, 1994.

53. Villarino, M. E., Stevens, L. E., Schable, B., Mayers, G., Miller, J. M., Burke, J. P., and Jarvis, W. R., Risk factors for epidemic *Xanthomonas maltophilia* infection/colonization in intensive care patients, *Infect. Control Hosp. Epidemiol.*, 13, 201, 1992.

54. Trumbore, D., Pontzer, R., Levinson, M. E., Kaye, D., Cynamon, M., Liu, C., Hinthorn, D. R., Tan, J. S., and File, T. M., Multicenter study of the clinical efficacy of imipenem/cilastatin for treatment of serious infections, *Rev. Infect. Dis.*, 7(Suppl. 3), S476, 1985.

55. Diaz-Mitoma, F., Harding, G. K. M., Louie, T. J., Thomson, M., James, M., and Ronald, A. R., Prospective randomized comparison of imipenem/cilastatin and cefotaxime for treatment of lung, soft tissue and renal infections, *Rev. Infect. Dis.*, 7(Suppl. 3), S452, 1985.

56. Garau, J., Martin, R., Bouza, E., Romero, J., Garaia Rodriguez, J. A., Perea, E., Martinez Luengas, F., Gobernado, M., and Montero, R., Imipenem in the treatment of severe bacterial infections in seriously ill patients, *J. Antimicrob. Chemother.*, 18(Suppl. E), 131, 1986.

57. Bodey, G. P., Elting, L. S., Jones, P., Alvarez, M. E., Rolston, K., and Fainstein, V., Imipenem/cilastatin therapy of infections in cancer patients, *Cancer*, 60, 255, 1987.

58. Nagai, T., Association of *Pseudomonas maltophilia* with malignant lesions, *J. Clin. Microbiol.*, 20, 1003, 1984.

59. Durbec, O., Albanese, J., Brunel, M., Soula, F., and Granthil, C., Septicémie foudroyante a *Pseudomonas maltophilia* au course d'un traitement par imipéneme et amikacin, *Presse Med.*, 18, 227, 1989.

60. Fisher, M. C., Long, S. S., Roberts, E. M., Dunn, J. M., and Balsara, R. K., *Pseudomonas maltophilia* bacteremia in children undergoing open heart surgery, *JAMA*, 246, 1571, 1981.

61. Felegie, T. P., Yu, V. L., Rumans, L. W., and Yee, R. B., Susceptibility of *Pseudomonas maltophilia* to antimicrobial agents, singly and in combination, *Antimicrob. Agents Chemother.*, 16, 833, 1979.

62. Vartivarian, S., Anaisse, E., Bodey, G., Sprigg, H., and Rolston, K., A changing pattern of susceptibility of *Xanthomonas maltophilia* to antimicrobial agents: implication for therapy, *Antimicrob. Agents Chemother.*, 38, 624, 1994.

63. Jacobs, M. R., Aronoff, S. C., Johenning, S., and Yamabe, S., Comparative activities of the β-lactamase inhibitors YTR 830, clavulanate and sulbactam combined with extended-spectrum penicillins against ticarcillin-resistant Enterobacteriaceae and pseudomonads, *J. Antimicrob. Chemother.*, 18, 177, 1986.

64. Traub, W. H. and Spohr, M., Comparative disk and broth dilution susceptibility test results with ticarcillin and timentin against *Pseudomonas aeruginosa* and *Pseudomonas maltophilia*, *Chemotherapy*, 33, 340, 1987.

65. Yu, V. L., Felegie, T. P., Yee, R. B., Pasculle, A. W., and Taylor, F. H., Synergistic interaction *in vitro* with use of three antibiotics simultaneously against *Pseudomonas maltophilia*, *J. Infect. Dis.*, 142, 602, 1980.

66. Neu, H. C., Saha, G., and Chin, N.-X., Resistance of *Xanthomonas maltophilia* to antibiotics and the effect of beta-lactamase inhibitors, *Diagn. Microbiol. Infect. Dis.*, 12, 283, 1989.

67. Nord, C.-E., Wadstrom, T., and Wretlind, B., Synergistic effect of combinations of sulfamethoxazole, trimethoprim, and colistin against *Pseudomonas maltophilia* and *Pseudomonas cepacia*, *Antimicrob. Agents Chemother.*, 6, 521, 1974.

68. Chow, A. W., Wong, J., and Bartlett, K. H., Synergistic interactions of ciprofloxacin and extended-spectrum β-lactams or aminoglycosides against multiply drug-resistant *Pseudomonas maltophilia*, *Antimicrob. Agents Chemother.*, 32, 782, 1988.

69. Moody, M. R., Young, V. M., and Kenton, D. M., *In vitro* antibiotic susceptibility of pseudomonads other than *Pseudomonas aeruginosa* recovered from cancer patients, *Antimicrob. Agents Chemother.*, 2, 344, 1972.

70. Mett, H., Rosta, S., Schacher, B., and Frei, R., Outer membrane permeability and β-lactamase content in *Pseudomonas maltophilia* clinical isolates and laboratory mutants, *Rev. Infect. Dis.*, 10, 765, 1988.

71. Büscher, K. H., Cullmann, W., Dick, W., Wendt, S., and Opferkuch, W., Imipenem resistance in *Pseudomonas aeruginosa* is due to diminished expression of outer membrane proteins, *J. Infect. Dis.*, 156, 681, 1987.

72. Saino, Y., Kobayashi, F., Inoue, M., and Mitsuhashi, S., Purification and properties of inducible penicillin β-lactamase isolated from *Pseudomonas maltophilia*, *Antimicrob. Agents Chemother.*, 22, 564, 1982.

73. Saino, Y., Inoue, M., and Mitsuhashi, S., Purification and properties of an inducible cephalosporinase from *Pseudomonas maltophilia* GN12873, *Antimicrob. Agents Chemother.*, 25, 362, 1984.
74. Krcméry, V., Antal, M., Langsadl, L., and Knothe, H., Transferable amikacin resistance in *Pseudomonas maltophilia* and *Acinetobacter calcoaceticus*, *Infection*, 13, 89, 1985.
75. Wheat, P. F., Winstanley, T. G., and Spencer, R. C., Effect of temperature on antimicrobial susceptibility of *Pseudomonas aeruginosa*, *J. Clin. Pathol.*, 38, 1055, 1985.
76. Townsend, R., Winstanley, T. G., and Spencer, R. C., In-vitro susceptibility of *Xanthomonas maltophilia* to aztreonam and clavulanic acid as a test for the presumptive identification of the species, *J. Hosp. Infect.*, 18, 324, 1991.
77. Wilcox, M. H., Winstanley, T. G., and Spencer, R. C., Outer-membrane protein profiles of *Xanthomonas maltophilia* isolates displaying temperature-dependent susceptibility to gentamicin, *J. Antimicrob. Chemother.*, 33, 663, 1994.
78. Bonfiglis, G. and Livermore, D. M., Zinc ions and medium dependent-susceptibility to β-lactams in *Xanthomonas maltophilia*, *J. Antimicrob. Chemother.*, 33, 181, 1994.
79. Cullman, W., Antibiotic susceptibility and outer membrane proteins of clinical *Xanthomonas maltophilia*, *Chemotherapy*, 37, 246, 1991.
80. Dufresne, J., Vezina, G., and Levesque, R. C., Cloning and expression of the imipenem-hydrolyzing β-lactamase operon for *Pseudomonas maltophilia* in *Escherichia coli*, *Antimicrob. Agents Chemother.*, 32, 819, 1988.
81. Bicknell, R., Emanuel, E. L., Gagnon, J., and Waley, S. G., The production and molecular properties of the zinc β-lactamase of *Pseudomonas maltophilia* IID 1275, *Biochem. J.*, 229, 791, 1985.
82. Hawkey, P. M., Birkenhead, D., Kerr, K. G., Newton, K. E., and Hyde, W. A., Effect of divalent cations in bacteriological media on the susceptibility of *Xanthomonas maltophilia* to imipenem with special reference to zinc ions, *J. Antimicrob. Chemother.*, 31, 47, 1993.
83. Phillips, I. and King, A., Comparative activity of the 4-quinolones, *Rev. Infect. Dis.*, 10(Suppl. 1), S70, 1988.

16 Rickettsiaceae

The tribe Rickettsieae, family Rickettsiaceae, order Rickettsiales, is made up of pleomorphic, mostly intracellular bacteria divided into three genera, *Coxiella*, *Rickettsia*, and *Rochalimeae (Bartonella)*.

These microorganisms can be rod-shaped to coccoid, and often pleomorphic cells with typical cell wall and no flagella. Rickettsieae are Gram-negative and can only multiply inside host cells. Widespread in nature, they have been found intracytoplasmatically or free in the lumen of the gut in arthropods (lice, fleas, ticks, and mites), by which these bacteria are transmitted to vertebrate hosts (humans and other mammals). Among the human diseases caused by Rickettsia, typhus fever, spotted fever, scrub typhus (tsutsugamushi disease), and the Rocky Mountain fever, have been most frequently observed.

Ehrlichieae is another tribe classified in the family Rickettsiaceae and made up of rickettsia-like microorganisms adapted to existence in invertebrates, mainly arthropods, and pathogenic to certain mammals, including humans. It comprises three genera, *Cowdria*, *Ehrlichia*, and *Neorickettsia*.

16.1 *BARTONELLA* SPP.

16.1.1 INTRODUCTION

Severely immunocompromised patients, such as those with AIDS, are at unusually high risk of developing *Bartonella* infections after coming in tramautic contact (scratches or bites) with domesticated cats, considered to be a major reservoir of these microorganisms.[1] Formerly known as *Rochalimeae*, the four species of this genus (*R. quintana*, *R. henselae*, *R. elizabethae*, and *R. vinsonii*) are currently recognized as more closely associated to *B. bacilliformis*, which is the sole member of the genus *Bartonella*.[2] Since the genus *Bartonella* was described before *Rochalimeae*, the former designation took precedence over the latter.[1] Two major *Bartonella* spp., *B. quintana* and *B. henselae*, have been isolated from HIV-infected patients, as causing bacillary angiomatosis,[3,4] relapsing bacteremia with fever, endocarditis, as well as angiomatous lesions involving the skin, liver, lung, spleen, bone, and the brain.[1,5-7]

B. quintana was first identified as an HIV-associated opportunistic pathogen in 1990, when Relman et al.[8] found that it was the causative agent of lesions in AIDS patients with bacillary angiomatosis (a vascular proliferative response in the skin and extracutaneous organs).[9] In addition, the bacteria were isolated from HIV-infected patients with relapsing febrile illness,[10] and with peliosis hepatis (a disorder characterized by blood-filled peliotic changes in the hepatic or splenic parenchyma).[11]

From a clinical standpoint, it is important to differentiate between the *Bartonella*-associated syndromes of bacteremia (occurring in the absence of focal vascular proliferative response in tissue) and tissue infection (bacillary angiomatosis, poliosis hepatis), which are associated with angiogenic response.[4]

Only recently characterized as a distinct species,[12,13] *B. henselae* has also been isolated from tissue of HIV-positive patients with bacillary angiomatosis and peliosis hepatis.[3,12,14] *B. henselae* can also produce relapsing bacteremia with fever, and endocarditis.[1] Serological studies have confirmed that *B. hanselae* was the cause of the "cat-scratch disease".[15-17]

Bartonella infections in HIV-positive patients, if not diagnosed promptly, may become fatal.[18] The severity of *Bartonella* infections appeared to increase with the fall of CD4+ cell counts. Koehler and Tappero[7] found the mean CD4+ cell count of 15 HIV-positive patients infected with *Bartonella* to be 57/mm^3. In another study,[19] when compared to controls, 42 HIV-infected patients with *Bartonella*-associated bacillary angiomatosis had a statistically significant CD4+ cell count of less than 200/mm^3.

In immunocompromised hosts, *Bartonella* infections may also result from reactivation, rather than primary infection, as demonstrated by Tappero et al.,[20] who have identified low-titer antibodies to *Bartonella* spp. in banked sera obtained from HIV-infected patients before the diagnosis of bacillary angiomatosis was made, and increased titers at the time of diagnosis.

16.1.2 EVOLUTION OF THERAPIES AND TREATMENT OF *BARTONELLA* INFECTIONS

When treated with antibiotics, immunocompromised patients with bacillary angiomatosis and peliosis hepatis responded well to medication.[1,4] Following on an earlier report[3] of complete resolution of lesions in an HIV-positive patient treated empirically with erythromycin for bacillary angiomatosis, erythromycin has been successfully used in the therapy of both bacillary angiomatosis and bacillary peliosis.[3,5-7,12,13,21-32] Usually erythromycin is given orally at 500 mg four times daily; however, it could be administered intravenously in cases of severe disease.[8]

Oral doxycycline at doses of 100 mg b.i.d. was also reported to be consistently successful in the treatment of bacillary angiomatosis and bacillary peliosis in AIDS patients.[3,8,10,11,13,14,33-38]

The use of another antibiotic, tetracycline also resulted in the resolution of *B. henselae*-induced lesions in an HIV-infected patient with bacillary angiomatosis,[14] as well as in the resolution of *B. henselae* bacteremia in two immunocompetent patients.[10]

Tappero et al.[21] successfully treated cutaneous bacillary angiomatosis in an immunocompetent patient with minocycline.

One potential drawback observed after the first several doses of antibiotic therapy was the occurrence of exacerbated systemic symptoms and fever (the Jarisch-Herxheimer reaction) — pretreatment with antipyretics may attenuate this response.[14]

The therapeutic efficacy of other antimicrobial drugs in the treatment of bacillary angiomatosis has also been studied. However, with the possible exception of rifampin,[22,34,39-41] the results have been inconclusive.[4]

In spite of their *in vitro* activity against *Bartonella* spp., penicillin, penicillinase-resistant penicillins, aminopenicillins, and first-generation cephalosporins had no activity against bacillary angiomatosis lesions caused by *B. henselae* and *B. quintana*.[14,22,25,30,31,34,42]

Some of the third-generation cephalosporins, however, appeared to be effective against *Bartonella* infections in HIV-infected patients. Thus, a pregnant woman with cutaneous bacillary angiomatosis responded with complete resolution of lesions after a 2-week therapy with ceftizoxime,[43] and another patient with *B. quintana*-induced endocarditis responded to a 5-week treatment with ceftriaxone.[5] The latter, however, failed to cure bacillary angiomatosis of the lymph node.[44]

Blood *Bartonella* infections tended to produce relapses regardless of the immune status of the patient, and on many occasions such relapses occurred in spite of antibiotic therapy.[10,12,45]

Skin and bone lesions resulting from bacillary angiomatosis have also been reported.[14,25,30,31,42,46] In addition, relapses were most likely to occur in cases where short-term antibiotic therapies have been applied. Even though there has been no indication that long-term antibiotic therapy would have been more beneficial, treating bacillary angiomatosis with prolonged antibiotic regimens has been recommended.[8]

16.1.3 REFERENCES

1. Regnery, R. L., Childs, J. E., and Koehler, J. E., Infections associated with *Bartonella* species in persons infected with human immunodeficiency virus, *Clin. Infect. Dis.*, 21(Suppl. 1), S94, 1995.
2. Brenner, D. J., O'Connor, S. P., Winkler, H. H., and Steigerwalt, A. G., Proposals to unify the genera *Bartonella* and *Rochalimaea*, with descriptions of *Bartonella quintana* comb. nov., *Bartonella vinsonii* comb. nov., *Bartonella henselae* comb. nov., and *Bartonella elizabethae* comb. nov., and to remove the family *Bartonellaceae* from the order Rickettsiales, *Int. J. Syst. Bacteriol.*, 43, 777, 1993.
3. Stoler, M. H., Bonfiglio, T. A., Steigbigel, R. T., and Pereira, M., An atypical subcutaneous infection associated with acquired immunodeficiency syndrome, *Am. J. Clin. Pathol.*, 80, 714, 1983.
4. Koehler, J. E. and Tappero, J. W., Bacillary angiomatosis and bacillary peliosis in patients infected with human immunodeficiency virus, *Clin. Infect. Dis.*, 17, 612, 1993.
5. Spach, D. H., Callis, K. P., Paauw, D. C., Hauze, Y. B., Schoenknecht, F. D., Welch, D. F., Rosen, H., and Brenner, D. J., Endocarditis caused by *Rochalimaea quintana* in a patient infected with human immunodeficiency virus, *J. Clin. Microbiol.*, 31, 692, 1993.
6. Hadfield, T. L., Warren, R., Kass, M., Brun, E., and Levy, C., Endocarditis caused by *Rochalimaea henselae*, *Hum. Pathol.*, 24, 1140, 1993.
7. Koehler, J. E. and Tappero, J. W., Bacillary angiomatosis and bacillary peliosis in patients infected with human immunodeficiency virus, *Clin. Infect. Dis.*, 17, 612, 1993.
8. Relman, D. A., Loutit, J. S., Schmidt, T. M., Falkow, S., and Tompkins, L. S., The agent of bacillary angiomatosis: an approach to the identification of uncultured pathogens, *N. Engl. J. Med.*, 323, 1573, 1990.
9. LeBoit, P. E., Berger, T. G., Egbert, B. M., Beckstead, J. H., Yen, T. S. B., and Stober, M. H., Bacillary angiomatosis: the histopathology and differential diagnosis of a pseudoneoplastic infection in patients with human immunodeficiency virus disease, *Am. J. Surg. Pathol.*, 13, 909, 1989.
10. Slater, L. N., Welch, D. F., Hensel, D., and Goody, D. W., A newly recognized fastidious gram-negative pathogen as a cause of fever and bacteremia, *N. Engl. J. Med.*, 323, 1587, 1990.
11. Perkocha, L. A., Geaghan, S. M., Yen, T. S. B., Nishimura, S. L., Chan, S. P., Garcia-Kennedy, R., Honda, G., Stoloff, A. C., Klein, H. Z., Goldman, R. L., Van Meter, S., Ferrell, L. D., and LeBoit, P. E., Clinical and pathological features of bacillary peliosis hepatis in association with human immunodeficiency virus infection, *N. Engl. J. Med.*, 323, 1581, 1990.
12. Regnery, R. L., Anderson, B. E., Clarridge, J. E. III, Rodriguez-Barradas, M. C., Jones, D. C., and Carr, J. H., Characterization of a novel *Rachalimaea* species, *R. henselae* sp. nov., isolated from blood of a febrile, HIV-positive patient, *J. Clin. Microbiol.*, 30, 265, 1992.
13. Welch, D. F., Pickett, D. A., Slater, L. N., Steigerwalt, A. G., and Brenner, D. J., *Rochalimaea henselae* sp. nov., a cause of septicemia, bacillary angiomatosis, and parenchymal bacillary peliosis, *J. Clin. Microbiol.*, 30, 275, 1992.
14. Koehler, J. E., Quinn, F. D., Berger, T. G., LeBoit, P. E., and Tappero, J. W., Isolation of *Rochalimaea* species from cutaneous and osseous lesions of bacillary angiomatosis, *N. Engl. J. Med.*, 327, 1625, 1992.
15. Regnery, R. L., Olson, J. G., Perkins, B. A., and Bibb, W., Serological response to "*Rochalimaea henselae*" antigen in suspected cat-scratch disease, *Lancet*, 339, 1443, 1992.
16. Dolan, M. J., Wong, M. T., Regnery, R. L., Jorgensen, J. H., Garcia, M., Peters, J., and Drehner, D., Syndrome of *Rachalimaea henselae* adenitis suggesting cat scratch disease, *Ann. Intern. Dis.*, 118, 331, 1993.
17. Schmidt, M. J., Robinson, L. E., Regnery, R. L., Olson, J. G., and Childs, J. E., Encephalopathy and liver lesions in patients with cat-scratch disease, *Proc. 33rd Intersci. Conf. Antimicrob. Agents Chemother.*, session 127, New Orleans, American Society for Microbiology, Washington, D.C., 1993.
18. Cockerell, C. J., Whitlow, M. A., Webster, G. F., and Friedman-Klen, A. E., Epithelioid angiomatosis: a distinct vascular disorder in patients with the acquired immunodeficiency syndrome or AIDS-related complex, *Lancet*, 2, 654, 1987.
19. Mohle-Boetani, J., Reingold, A., LeBoit, P., Berger, T., Wenger, J., and Tappero, J., Bacillary angiomatosis: spectrum of disease and clinical characteristics in HIV+ patients, *Proc. 32nd Intersci. Conf. Antimicrob. Agents Chemother.*, Anaheim, American Society for Microbiology, Washington D.C., Abstr. 372, 1992.

20. Tappero, J., Regnery, R., Koehler, J., and Olson, J., Detection of serologic response to *Rochalimaea henslae* in patients with bacillary angiomatosis (BA) by immunofluorescent antibody (IFA) testing, *Proc. 32nd Intersci. Conf. Antimicrob. Agents Chemother.*, Anaheim, American Society for Microbiology, Washington, D.C., Abstr. 674, 1992.

21. Tappero, J. W., Koehler, J. E., Berger, T. G., Cockerell, C. J., Lee, T.-H., Busch, M. P., Stites, D. P., Mohle-Boetani, J., Reingold, A. L., and LeBoit, P. E., Bacillary angiomatosis and bacillary splenitis in immunocompromised adults, *Ann. Intern. Med.*, 118, 363, 1993.

22. LeBoit, P. E., Berger, T. G., Egbert, B. M., Yen, T. S. B., Stoler, M. H., Bonfiglio, T. A., Strauchen, J. A., English, C. K., and Wear, D. J., Epithelioid haemangioma-like vascular proliferation in AIDS: manifestation of cat-scratch disease bacillus infection? *Lancet*, 1, 960, 1988.

23. Slater, L. N., Welch, D. F., and Min, K.-W., *Rochalimeae henselae* bacillary angiomatosis and peliosis hepatis, *Arch. Intern. Med.*, 152, 602, 1992.

24. Spach, D. H., Panther, L. A., Thorning, D. R., Dunn, J. E., Plorde, J. J., and Miller, R. A., Intracerebral bacillary angiomatosis in a patient infected with human immunodeficiency virus, *Ann. Intern. Med.*, 116, 740, 1992.

25. Berger, T. G., Tappero, J. W., Kaymen, A., and LeBoit, P. E., Bacillary (epithelioid) angiomatosis and concurrent Kaposi's sarcoma in acquired immunodeficiency syndrome, *Arch. Dermatol.*, 125, 1543, 1989.

26. Rudikoff, D., Phelps, R. G., Gordon, R. E., and Bottone, E. J., Acquired immunodeficiency syndrome-related bacillary vascular proliferation (epithelioid angiomatosis): rapid response to erythromycin therapy, *Arch. Dermatol.*, 125, 706, 1989.

27. Milam, M., Balerdi, M. J., and Toney, J. F., Epithelioid angiomatosis secondary to disseminated cat scratch disease involving the bone marrow and skin in a patient with acquired immune deficiency syndrome: a case report, *Am. J. Med.*, 88, 180, 1990.

28. Cairo, I., Hulsebosch, H.-J., and van der Wouw, P. A., Bacillary angiomatosis, *Br. J. Dermatol.*, 125, 292, 1991.

29. Tappero, J. W., Mohle-Boetani, J., Koehler, J. E., Swaminathan, B., Berger, T. G., LeBoit, P. E., Smith, L. L., Wenger, J. D., Pinner, R. W., Kemper, C. A., and Reingold, A. L., The epidemiology of bacillary angiomatosis and bacillary peliosis, *JAMA*, 269, 770, 1993.

30. van der Wouw, P. A., Hadderingh, R. J., Reiss, P., Hulsebosch, H.-J., Walford, N., and Lange, J. M. A., Disseminated cat-scratch disease in a patient with AIDS, *AIDS*, 3, 751, 1989.

31. Szaniawski, W. K., Don, P. C., Bitterman, S. R., and Schachner, J. R., Epithelioid angiomatosis in patients with AIDS, *J. Am. Acad. Dermatol.*, 23, 41, 1990.

32. Goodman, P. and Balachandran, S., Bacillary angiomatosis in a patient with HIV infection, *Am. J. Roentgenol.*, 160, 207, 1993.

33. Tappero, J. W. and Koehler, J. E., Cat scratch disease and bacillary angiomatosis, *JAMA*, 266, 1938, 1991.

34. Koehler, J. E., LeBoit, P. E., Egbert, B. M., and Berger, T. G., Cutaneous vascular lesions and disseminated cat-scratch disease in patients with the acquired immunodeficiency syndrome (AIDS) and AIDS-related complex, *Ann. Intern. Med.*, 109, 449, 1988.

35. Kemper, C. A., Lombard, C. M., Deresinski, S. C., and Tompkins, L. S., Visceral bacillary epithelioid angiomatosis. Possible manifestations of disseminated cat scratch disease in the immunocompromised host: a report of two cases, *Am. J. Med.*, 89, 216, 1990.

36. Mui, B. S. K., Mulligan, M. E., and George, W. L., Response of HIV-associated disseminated cat scratch disease to treatment with doxycycline, *Am. J. Med.*, 89, 229, 1990.

37. Herts, B. R., Rafii, M., and Spiegel, G., Soft-tissue and osseous lesions caused by bacillary angiomatosis: unusual manifestations of cat-scratch fever in patients with AIDS, *Am. J. Roentgenol.*, 157, 1249, 1991.

38. Pilon, V. A. and Echols, R. M., Cat-scratch disease in a patient with AIDS, *Am. J. Clin. Pathol.*, 92, 236, 1989.

39. Knobler, E. H., Silvers, D. N., Fine, K. C., Lefkowitch, J. H., and Grossman, M. E., Unique vascular skin lesions associated with human immunodeficiency virus, *JAMA*, 260, 524, 1988.

40. Hall, A. V., Roberts, C. M., Maurice, P. D., McLean, K. A., and Shousha, S., Cat-scratch disease in a patient with AIDS: atypical skin manifestation, *Lancet*, 2, 453, 1988.

41. Lopez-Elzaurdia, C., Fraga, J., Sols, M., Burgos, E., Sanchez-Garcia, M., and Garcia-Diez, A., Bacillary angiomatosis associated with cytomegalovirus infection in a patient with AIDS, *Br. J. Dermatol.*, 125, 175, 1991.

42. Marasco, W. A., Lester, S., and Parsonnet, J., Unusual presentation of cat scratch disease in a patient positive for antibody to the human immunodeficiency virus, *Rev. Infect. Dis.*, 11, 793, 1989.

43. Riley, L. E. and Tuomala, R. E., Bacillary angiomatosis in a pregnant patient with acquired immunodeficiency syndrome, *Obstet. Gynecol.*, 79, 818, 1992.

44. Slater, L. N. and Min, K.-W., Polypoid endobronchial lesions: a manifestation of bacillary angiomatosis, *Chest*, 102, 972, 1992.

45. Lucey, D., Dolan, M. J., Moss, C. W., Garcia, M., Hollis, D. G., Wegner, S., Morgan, G., Almeida, R., Leong, D., Greisen, K. G., Welch, D. F., and Slater, L. N., Relapsing illness due to *Rochalimae henselae* in immunocompetent hosts: implication for therapy and new epidemiologic association, *Clin. Infect. Dis.*, 14, 683, 1992.

46. Krekorian, T. D., Radner, A. B., Alcorn, J. M., Haghighi, P., and Fang, F., Biliary obstruction caused by epithelioid angiomatosis in a patient with AIDS, *Am. J. Med.*, 89, 820, 1990.

16.2 EHRLICHIA SPP.

16.2.1 INTRODUCTION

The tribe *Ehrlichieae* contains obligate intracellular bacterial parasites with a tropism for leukocytes.[1] It comprises three genera, *Ehrlichia*, *Cowdria*, and *Neorickettsia*. As of 1984,[2] the genus *Cytoecetes*, which consists of parasites developing in granulocytes, has been incorporated into the genus *Ehrlichia*.[3] Like Rickettsieae, at least four members of the tribe *Ehrlichieae* are known to be vector-borne.[2]

Recent genetic studies have shown significant similarities (85.7%) in the sequences of the 16S rRNA in *Ehrlichia risticii* and *Rickettsia prowazekii*, the etiologic agent of the epidemic typhus. Both microorganisms belong to the α subdivision of the purple bacteria.[4]

E. canis, *E. sennetsu*, *E. phagocytophila*, *E. equi*, *E. chaffeensis*, and *E. risticii* are the five best characterized species of the genus *Ehrlichia*.[1] Depending on the particular species, the *Ehrlichia* organisms can infect circulating monocytes, granulocytes, lymphocytes, or platelets and thus can be transmitted by or isolated from blood.[1]

Morphologically, members of the tribe *Ehrlichieae* represent small Gram-negative cocci, generally round but sometimes pleomorphic, especially in tissue cultures. They do not appear to contain significant amounts of peptidoglycan,[5,6] and most commonly have been found in membrane-lined vacuoles within the cytoplasm of infected eukaryotic host cells, primarily leukocytes.

In nature, *Ehrlichieae* organisms are known to infect specific species of animal hosts (domestic and wild Canidae, horse, sheep, cattle, bison). However, the natural hosts of *E. sennetsu* are humans.[1]

Pathogen-induced host immunosuppression has been associated with infection by two *Ehrlichia* species, *E. risticii* and *E. phagocytophila*. Thus, in addition to generalized immunosuppression in mice[7] and horses,[8] class II histocompatibility antigen (Ia antigen) induction on the surface of *E. risticii*-infected macrophages was suppressed in response to interferon-γ (used *in vitro*),[9] suggesting inhibition of antigen-specific T cell activation. In the case of *E. phagocytophila* infection, both suppression of the humoral immune response[10] and reduced neutrophil function[11] have been well documented.

The incubation period for ehrlichial infections (ehrlichiosis) is between 1 and 3 weeks. Major symptoms include fever, depression, and anorexia.[1] Disease progression apparently is dependent on the size of the inoculum; that is, only higher dosages of *Ehrlichia* spp. can cause disease, whereas the innate defense mechanisms appear to eliminate lower dosages of *Ehrlichia* organisms from the host.[7] In contrast to infection with the tribe *Rickettsieae*, in human ehrlichiosis hematologic abnormalities are pronounced,[12-14] as well as increased serum hepatic aminotransferase activities.[12,13] Additionally, augmentation of the α2-globulin levels has been reported in *E. sennetsu* infection.[15]

Although persistent infections in animals by *Ehrlichia* spp. have been well documented,[16] persistent infections in humans have been rare. Dumler et al.[17] have reported a serologically proven acute infection with *E. chaffeensis* in which the patient's condition, despite therapy with tetracycline and chloramphenicol, progressively worsened, resulting in multiple secondary infections and gastrointestinal hemorrhage, and finally death. This case represented the first definitive evidence that *E. chaffeensis* is capable of establishing persistent human infection and suggested a role for this pathogen in the induction of immune compromise associated with a fatal outcome.[17]

The report of Pearce et al.,[18] which described bone marrow hypoplasia in a patient with ehrlichiosis, has raised the question whether unrecognized human ehrlichial infection may be a cause of aplastic anemia, as has been the case with chronic canine ehrlichiosis.

Contrary to rickettsia, host cells infected with *E. risticii, E. sennetsu, E. canis,* or *C. ruminantium* have shown little cytolysis until the cytoplasm has been completely filled with infecting organisms and the cell burst.[1] However, ehrlichiosis appeared to occur not only by cell lysis but also through exocytosis, by fusion of the vacuole membrane with the plasma membrane. Furthermore, the entrance of *Ehrlichia* spp. into new host cells was found not always to be preceded by lysis of infected host cells. To this end, *in vitro* experiments have demonstrated that in intestinal epithelial cells, which create a monolayer tightly connected by circumferential zones of intercellular junctions, the ehrlichial organisms have been transmitted between adjacent cells by a coupled exocytosis in one cell and endocytosis in an adjacent cell.[19]

Among the members of the tribe *Ehrlichieae, E. sennetsu*, isolated from mice, from a patient's blood, bone marrow, and lymph node,[20-22] is the first species known to cause human infection in nature. Sennetsu ehrlichiosis, which has been documented in Japan since the late 19th century[23] and recently in Malaysia,[24,25] is manifested by an acute febrile illness with lethargy, pronounced hematologic abnormalities, lymphocytosis, and postauricular and posterior cervical lymphodenopathy.[1] Laboratory findings included leukopenia, with an increase in neutrophils at the initial disease stage, and both a relative and an absolute increase in lymphocytes (accompanied by the appearance of atypical cells) in the late febrile to convalescent stages.[1] While the mode of transmission of *E. sennetsu* is not known, a fish parasite has been suspected as a vector since the disease was associated with the consumption of a particular raw fish.[26]

Since the late 1980s, more than 200 cases of ehrlichiosis have been confirmed in the U.S.,[13,27-34] and at least three fatalities have been associated with the infection.[13,32]

In 1987, Maeda et al.[14] described a human infection caused by *E. canis*, the etiologic agent of canine ehrlichiosis (tropical canine pancytopenia), with clinical symptoms similar to those of patients with the Rocky Mountain spotted fever, except that there was no rash. In dogs, the brown dog tick (*Rhipicephalus sanguineus*) is the vector.[35] Since *R. sanguineus* feeds infrequently on humans,[36] the possibility was raised that an antigenically similar, but distinct, agent may be the cause of illness in case-patients, or an unrecognized mechanism of transmission.[37]

In humans, after an incubation period of 12 to 14 d, *E. canis* infection caused acute febrile illness with encephalopathy, mild hepatitis, acute tubular necrosis, anemia, and thrombocytopenia, followed by inclusions in the patient's circulating leukocytes. The inclusions disappeared 4 d after the beginning of antimicrobial therapy.[14] In general, the laboratory and pathologic findings in humans have been remarkably similar to those of canine ehrlichiosis.[38-41]

16.2.2 EVOLUTION OF THERAPIES AND TREATMENT OF EHRLICHIOSIS

The large number of hospitalizations and the serious, even fatal, complications associated with human ehrlichiosis have underscored the severity of this infection in some patients.[13] The cytopenia associated with *Ehrlichia* infections is produced by bone marrow hypoplasia which may be severe. Therefore, prompt antimicrobial therapy is required prior to serologic studies, especially in immunocompromised or splenectomized patients, as well as in HIV-positive patients who may develop a more overwhelming rickettsial infection.[18,42,43]

Several *in vitro* studies have been conducted to determine the susceptibilities of *Ehrlichia* spp. to various antimicrobial agents. Thus, *E. risticii* was found susceptible to tetracyclines but not erythromycin and nalidixic acid.[44] On the other hand, *E. sennetsu* has been susceptible to doxycycline and ciprofloxacin but resistant to erythromycin, penicillin, and chloramphenicol.[45] Similarly to other rickettsiae, *Ehrlichia* spp. were resistant to aminoglycosides.

In animal studies, tetracyclines have been reported to be effective in the treatment of *E. equi*,[46] *E. phagocytophila*,[47] *E. ondiri*,[48] *E. canis*,[16,49] and *C. ruminantium* infections.[50]

In human ehrlichiosis,[13,14,25] as well as in the canine disease,[16] oxytetracycline and doxycycline were found to effectively correct pyrexia within 24 to 48 h.

A combination of trimethoprim and sulfadimidine-sulfamethylphenazole,[47] or chloramphenicol[51] were also reported to be effective against *E. phagocytophila* infection.

Chloramphenicol seems to be as effective as tetracyclines and should be considered as an alternative drug in patients for whom treatment with tetracyclines has been contraindicated.[13]

Maeda et al.[14] initially treated a patient with *E. canis* infection with chloramphenicol. However, when the chloramphenicol levels were over the 100-µg/ml level and the patient's anemia and thrombocytopenia persisted, the therapy was changed to intravenous doxycycline (100 mg every 34 h); the patient subsequently recovered.

16.2.3 REFERENCES

1. Rikihisa, Y., The tribe *Ehrlichiae* and ehrlichial diseases, *Clin. Microbiol. Rev.*, 4, 286, 1991.
2. Ristic, M. and Huxsoll, D., Tribe II. *Ehrlichiae*, in *Bergey's Manual of Systematic Bacteriology*, Vol. 1, Krieg, N. R. and Holt, J. G., Eds., Williams and Wilkins, Baltimore, 1984, 704.
3. Tyzzer, E. E., *Cytoecetes microti*, N.G.N. sp., a parasite developing in granulocytes and infective to small rodents, *Parasitology*, 30, 242, 1938.
4. Weisburg, W. G., Dobson, M. E., Samuel, J. E., Dasch, G. A., Mallavia, L. P., Baca, O., Mandelco, L., Sechrest, J. E., Weiss, E., and Woese, C. R., Phylogenetic diversity of the rickettsiae, *J. Bacteriol.*, 171, 4202, 1989.
5. Rikihisa, Y., Ultrastructure of rickettsiae with special emphasis on ehrlichia, in *Ehrlichiosis: a Vector-Borne Disease of Animals and Humans*, Williams, J. C. and Kakoma, I., Eds., Kluwer Academic, Boston, 1991, 22.
6. Rikihisa, Y., Perry, B. D., and Cordes, D. O., Rickettsial link with acute equine diarrhea, *Vet. Rec.*, 115, 390, 1984.
7. Rikihisa, Y., Johnson, G. J., and Burger, C. J., Reduced immune responsiveness and lymphoid depletion in mice infected with *Ehrlichia risticii*, *Infect. Immun.*, 55, 2215, 1987.
8. Rikihisa, Y., Johnson, G. C., and Reed, S. M., Immune responses and intestinal pathology of ponies experimentally infected with Potomac horse fever, in *Proceedings of a Symposium on Potomac Horse Fever*, Veterinary Learning Systems, Lawrenceville, NJ, 1988, 27.
9. Messick, J. B. and Rikihisa, Y., Suppression of 1-A^d on P388D$_1$ cells by *Ehrlichia risticii* infection in response to gamma interferon, *75th Annu. Meet. Fed. Am. Soc. Exp. Biol.*, Atlanta, Abstr. 5684, 1991, p. A1351.
10. Batungbacal, M. R. and Scott, G. R., Suppression of the immune response to clostridial vaccine by tick-borne fever, *J. Comp. Pathol.*, 92, 409, 1982.
11. Woldehiwet, Z., The effect of tick-borne fever on some functions of polymorphonuclear cells of sheep, *J. Comp. Pathol.*, 97, 481, 1987.
12. Centers for Disease Control, Human ehrlichiosis — United States, *Morbid. Mortal. Wkly. Rep.*, 37, 270, 1988.
13. Eng, T. R., Harkess, J. R., Fishbein, D. B., Dawson, J. E., Greene, C. N., and Satalowich, E. T., Epidemiologic, clinical and laboratory findings of human ehrlichiosis in the United States, *JAMA*, 264, 2251, 1988.
14. Maeda, K., Markowitz, N., Hawley, R. C., Ristic, M., Cox, D., and McDade, J. E., Human infection with *Ehrlichia canis*, a leukocytic rickettsia, *N. Engl. J. Med.*, 316, 853, 1987.
15. Tachibana, N., Sennetsu fever: the disease, diagnosis, and treatment, in *Microbiology — 1986*, Winkler, H. and Ristic, M., Eds., American Society for Microbiology, Washington, D.C., 1986, 205.

16. Buhles, W. C., Huxsoll, D. L., and Ristic, M., Tropical canine pancytopenia: clinical, hematologic, and serologic response of dogs to *Ehrlichia canis* infections, tetracycline therapy, and challenge inoculation, *J. Infect. Dis.*, 130, 357, 1974.

17. Dumler, J. S., Sutker, W. L., and Walker, D. H., Persistent infection with *Ehrlichia chaffeensis*, *Clin. Infect. Dis.*, 17, 903, 1993.

18. Pearce, C. J., Conrad, M. E., Nolan, P. E., Fishbein, D. B., and Dawson, J. E., Ehrlichiosis: a cause of bone marrow hypoplasia in humans, *Am. J. Hematol.*, 28, 53, 1988.

19. Rikihisa, Y., Growth of *Ehrlichia risticii* in human colonic epithelial cells, in *Rickettsiology: Current Issues and Perspectives*, Hechemy, K., Paretsky, D., Walker, D. H., and Mallavia, L. P., Eds., The New York Academy of Sciences, New York, 1990, 104.

20. Misao, T. and Kobayashi, Y., Studies on infectious mononucleosis (glandular fever). I. Isolation of etiologic agent from blood, bone marrow, and lymph node of a patient with infectious mononucleosis by using mice, *Kyushu Med. Sci.*, 6, 145, 1955.

21. Kakoma, I., Carson, C. A., and Ristic, M., Direct and indirect lymphocyte participation in the immunity and immunopathology of tropical canine pancytopenia — a review, *Comp. Immun. Microbiol. Infect. Dis.*, 3, 291, 1980.

22. Kakoma, I., Carson, C. A., Ristic, M., Stephenson, E. M., Hildebrandt, P. K., and Huxsoll, D. L., Platelet migration inhibition as an indicator of immunologically mediated target cell injury in canine ehrlichiosis, *Infect. Immun.*, 20, 242, 1978.

23. Misao, T. and Katsuta, K., Epidemiology of infectious mononucleosis, *Jpn. J. Clin. Exp. Med.*, 33, 73, 1956.

24. Ristic, M., Current strategies in research on ehrlichiosis, in *Ehrlichiosis: a Vector-Borne Disease of Animals and Humans*, Williams, J. C. and Kakoma, I., Eds., Kluwer Academic, Boston, 1990, 136.

25. Weiss, E., Dasch, G. A., Williams, J. C., and Kang, Y.-H., Biological properties of the genus *Ehrlichia*: substrate utilization and energy metabolism, in *Ehrlichiosis: a Vector-Borne Disease of Animals and Humans*, Williams, J. C. and Kakoma, I., Eds., Kluwer Academic, Boston, 1990, 59.

26. Fukuda, T., Sasahara, T., and Kitao, T., Studies on the causative agent of Hyuganetsu disease. XI. Characteristics of rickettsia-like organism isolated from metacercaria of *Stellantchasmus falcatus* parasitic in grey mullet, *J. Jpn. Assoc. Infect. Dis.*, 47, 474, 1973.

27. Fishbein, D. B., Kemp, A., Dawson, J. E., Green, N. E., Redus, M. A., and Fields, D. H., Human ehrlichiosis: prospective active surveillance in febrile hospitalized patients, *J. Infect. Dis.*, 160, 803, 1989.

28. Fishbein, D. B., Dawyer, L. A., Holland, C. J., Hayes, E. B., Okoroanyanwu, W., Williams, D., Sikes, R. K., Ristic, M., and McDade, J. E., Unexplained febrile illness after exposure to ticks, *JAMA*, 257, 3100, 1987.

29. Harkess, J. R., Ewing, S. A., Crutcher, J. M., Kudlac, J., McKee, G., and Istre, G. R., Human ehrlichiosis in Oklahoma, *J. Infect. Dis.*, 159, 576, 1989.

30. Petersen, L. R., Sawyer, L. A., Fishbein, D. B., Kelley, R. W., Thomas, R. J., Magnarelli, L. A., Redus, M., and Dawson, J. E., An outbreak of ehrlichiosis in members of an army reserve unit exposed to ticks, *J. Infect. Dis.*, 159, 562, 1989.

31. Taylor, J. P., Betz, T. G., Fishbein, D. B., Roberts, M. A., Dawson, J., and Ristic, M., Serological evidence of possible human infection with *Ehrlichia* in Texas, *J. Infect. Dis.*, 158, 217, 1988.

32. Walker, D. H., Taylor, J. P., Buie, J. S., and Dearden, C., Fatal human ehrlichiosis, *Proc. 89th Annu. Meet. Am. Soc. Microbiol.*, American Society for Microbiology, Washington, D.C., Abstr. D76, 1989, 95.

33. McDade, J. E., Ehrlichiosis — a disease of animals and humans, *J. Infect. Dis.*, 161, 609, 1990.

34. Dawson, J. E., Anderson, B. E., Fishbein, D. B., Sanchez, J. L., Goldsmith, C. S., Wilson, K. H., and Duntley, C. W., Isolation and characterization of an *Ehrlichia* spp. from a patient diagnosed with human ehrlichiosis, *J. Clin. Microbiol.*, 29, 2741, 1991.

35. Ristic, M., Pertinent characteristics of leukocytic rickettsiae of humans and animals, in *Microbiology 1986*, Leive, L., Bonzentree, P. S., Morello, J. A., Silver, S. D., and Wu, H., Eds., American Society for Microbiology, Washington, D.C., 1986, 182.

36. Harwood, R. F. and James, M. T., *Entomology in Human and Animal Health*, Macmillan, New York, 1979, 385.

37. Rohrbach, B. W., Harkess, J. R., Ewing, S. A., Kudlac, J., McKee, G. L., and Istree, G. R., Epidemiologic and clinical characteristics of persons with serologic evidence of *E. canis* infection, *Am. J. Public Health*, 80, 442, 1990.

38. Greene, C. E. and Harvey, J. W., Canine ehrlichiosis, in *Clinical Microbiology and Infectious Disease of the Dog and Cat*, Greene, C. E., Ed., W. B. Saunders, Philadelphia, 1984, 545.

39. Kuehn, N. F. and Gaunt, S. D., Clinical and hematologic findings in canine ehrlichiosis, *J. Am. Vet. Med. Assoc.*, 186, 355, 1985.

40. Hildebrandt, P. K., Conroy, J. D., McKee, A. E., Nyindo, M. B. A., and Huxsoll, D. L., Ultrastructure of *Ehrlichia canis*, *Infect. Immun.*, 7, 265, 1973.

41. Dumler, J. S., Brouqui, P., Aronson, J., Taylor, J. P., and Walker, D. H., Identification of ehrlichia in human tissue, *N. Engl. J. Med.*, 325, 1109, 1991.

42. Kallick, C. A., Levin, S., and Reddi, K. T., Association of a rickettsia-like agent identified in human bone marrow failure with *Ehrlichia canis* and tropical canine pancytopenia, *Proc. 13th Intersci. Conf. Antimicrob. Agents Chemother.*, American Sociaty for Microbiology, Washington, D.C., 1973, 1.

43. Kallick, C., Thadhani, K., Ristic, M., Keesler, R. H., and Levin, S., Association of acquired immune deficiency syndrome (AIDS) with *Ehrlichia*-like organisms, *Proc. 23rd Intersci. Conf. Antimicrob. Agents Chemother.*, American Society for Microbiology, Washington, D.C., 1983, 121.

44. Rikihisa, Y. and Jiang, B. M., *In vitro* susceptibility of *Ehrlichia risticii* to eight antibiotics, *Antimicrob. Agents Chemother.*, 32, 986, 1988.

45. Brouqui, P. and Raoult, D., *In vitro* susceptibility of *Ehrlichia sennetsu* to antibiotics, *Antimicrob. Agents Chemother.*, 34, 1593, 1990.

46. Madigan, J. E. and Gribble, D., Equine ehrlichiosis in northern California: 49 cases (1968–1981), *J. Am. Vet. Med. Assoc.*, 190, 445, 1987.

47. Anika, S. M., Nouws, J. F. M., VanGogh, H., Nieuwenhuijis, J., and Vree, T. B., Chemotherapy and pharmacokinetics of some antimicrobial agents in healthy dwarf goats and those infected with *Ehrlichia phagocytopenia* (tick-borne fever), *Res. Vet. Sci.*, 41, 386, 1986.

48. Haig, D. A. and Danskin, D., The aetiology of bovine petechial fever (Ondiri disease), *Res. Vet. Sci.*, 3, 129, 1962.

49. Amyx, H. L., Huxsoll, D. L., Zeiler, D. C., and Hildebrandt, P. K., Therapeutic and prophylactic value of tetracycline in dogs infected with the agent of tropical canine pancytopenia, *J. Am. Vet. Med. Assoc.*, 159, 1428, 1971.

50. Bezuidenhout, J. D., Recent research findings on cowdriosis, in *Ehrlichiosis: a Vector-Borne Disease of Animals and Humans*, Williams, J. C. and Kakoma, I., Eds., Kluwer Academic, Boston, 1990, 125.

51. Anika, S. M., Nouws, J. F. M., Vree, T. B., and van Miert, A. S. J. P. A. M., The efficacy and plasma disposition of chloramphenicol and spiramycin in tick-borne fever-infected dwarf goats, *J. Vet. Pharmacol. Ther.*, 9, 433, 1986.

17 Alcaligenaceae

17.1 ALCALIGENES XYLOSOXIDANS

17.1.1 Introduction

The family Alcaligenaceae consists of the genera *Alcaligenes* and *Bordetella*. *Alcaligenes* is a widespread genus of Gram-negative, aerobic, rod-shaped, alkaline-producing bacteria found often in the intestine of vertebrates and as part of the normal skin flora. The genus *Alcaligenes* has three clinically relevant species: *A. faecalis* (synonymous with *A. odorans*), *A. piechaudii*, and *A. xylosoxidans*. Furthermore, *A. xylosoxidans* has been divided into two subspecies, *A. xylosoxidans* subsp. *xylosoxidans* and *A. xylosoxidans* subsp. *denitrificans*.[1-4]

A. *xylosoxidans* subsp. *xylosoxidans* is a nonfermentative, motile, oxidase- and catalase-positive, peritrichous flagellated rod, which can produce acid from xylose.[5,6] In addition to xylose oxidation, the peritrichous flagella have been helpful to distinguish *Alcaligenes* from *Pseudomonas* species.[7] The taxonomic classification of *Alcaligenes xylosoxidans* subsp. *xylosoxidans* has been controversial. Over the years, *Alcaligenes xylosoxidans* subsp. *xylosoxidans* has been synonymous with *Alcaligenes denitrificans* subsp. *xylosoxidans*, *Alcaligenes ruhlandii*, and CDC group Vd.[8,9] The bacterium is no longer subdivided into types IIIa and IIIb on the basis of nitrate reduction.[6,10] In 1971, Yabuuchi et al.[11] proposed the name *Achromobacter xylosoxidans* as a new species. However, this name has not been universally accepted, and a number of investigators expressed disagreement,[7,12-14] including the *Bergey's Manual of Determinative Bacteriology*. Gilardi[15] and Tatum et al.[6] considered *A. xylosoxidans* to be distinct from other nonfermentative Gram-negative rods. For the sake of clearing the taxonomic confusion, it should be mentioned that the designation "*Achromobacter*" has been used historically to define Gram-negative, asporogenous, peritrichously flagellated bacteria that are oxidase-positive, can aerobically acidify carbohydrates, and do not produce 3-ketolactose from lactose.[16,17]

The reservoir of *Alcaligenes* spp. is still unknown.[18,19] *A. xylosoxidans* subsp. *xylosoxidans* is most commonly found in water, which may explain its presence in otitis media.[20,21] It was also isolated from purulent human ear discharge,[21,22] and may be part of the normal large-intestine flora.

17.1.2 Evolution of Therapies and Treatment of *Alcaligenes xylosoxidans* Infections

Although infrequently, *A. xylosoxidans* subsp. *xylosoxidans* has been the etiologic agent of sometimes life-threatening opportunistic infections, such as pneumonia, bacteremia, and meningitis in patients with underlying immune deficiencies,[5,7,18,23-29] premature infants,[30-33] as well as the cause of nosocomial septicemia in immunocompromised patients, generally arising from contaminated hemodialysis or intravenous fluids (diagnostic tracer materials).[34] Olsen and Hoeprich[35] and Lofgren et al.[36] have described postoperative prosthetic aortic valve endocarditis due to *S. xylosoxidans* subsp. *xylosoxidans*.

In addition to ear fluid, *A. xylosoxidans*. subsp. *xylosoxidans* has also been isolated from a wide array of clinical specimens (swabs of eye, ear, and pharynx, blood, cerebrospinal fluid, bile, peritoneal fluid, bronchial washings, urine, feces, pus, and wound cultures),[10,21,23,25,29,37-40] some of which have been linked to nosocomial infections.[21,23,24]

Even though *A. xylosoxidans* subsp. *xylosoxidans* has been often isolated from the aqueous environment of infected patients,[18,23] direct evidence linking this bacterium to the source of infection has been difficult to obtain, especially in newborns. Boukadida et al.[41] described a lethal neonatal meningitis that was directly induced by the cutaneous use of aqueous eosin solutions heavily contaminated by *A. xylosoxidans*. Since the pathogen was also resistant to various antiseptics, such as chlorhexidine,[18,26] cetrimide, and quaternary ammonium derivatives,[23] antiseptic solutions can eventually become a source of serious infections in immunocompromised hosts.

It is clear from the increased incidence that *A. xylosoxidans* should no longer be considered nonpathogenic, and generalized infections caused by this organism, if not treated appropriately, may be severe and very often fatal.[7,15,31,32,40,42-48]

A. xylosoxidans subsp. *xylosoxidans* was found to be susceptible to a number of antimicrobial agents, including ticarcillin, ticarcillin–clavulanic acid, cefrazidime, imipenem, colistin, trimethoprim-sulfamethoxazole (TMP-SMX), but was resistant to cefotaxime, fosfomycin, amikacin, gentamicin, and tobramycin.[41] In general, most strains exhibited high-level resistance to first- and second-generation cephalosporins and aminoglycosides.[49]

Several studies[42,50-52] have shown susceptibilities against a broad spectrum of penicillins and the newer third generation of cephalosporins. Thus, the MIC_{50} values of penicillins, azlocillin and piperacillin were 0.5 µg/ml or less;[50] moxalactam, ceftazidime, and imipenem were also found active.[51] According to Legrand and Anaissie,[42] the range of MIC values varied from 0.06 to 128 µg/ml for cefoperazone, piperacillin, and ticarcillin; from 0.015 to 32 µg/ml for amikacin, ceftazidime, cefotaxime, cefoxitin, ceftizoxime, aztreonam, and imipenem; from 0.03 to 64 µg/ml for ceftriaxone and ciprofloxacin; and from 0.0187/0.0378 to 4.0/76 µg/ml for TMP-SMX.

In an earlier report, Dworzack et al.[5] have described a community-acquired bacteremic *A. xylosoxidans* subsp. *xylosoxidans* infection in a patient with idiopathic IgM deficiency, who was successfully cured with a synergistic combination of carbenicillin (50 m/kg, intravenously, every 4 h) and kanamycin (7.5 mg/kg, intramuscularly, b.i.d.).

IgM deficiency, which may be a predisposing factor to *Alcaligenes*-induced bacteremia, has been reported to occur in association with atopy,[53] the Wiscott-Aldrich syndrome,[54] protein-losing enteropathy,[55,56] and some malignancies (plasma cell myeloma, hepatoma, and chronic lymphocytic leukemia).[56] In addition, isolated idiopathic IgM deficiency has been observed in patients with meningococcemia,[57-60] recurrent *Pseudomonas* infections,[61] and autoimmune hemolytic anemia.[62]

Shigeta et al.[26] presented six cases of bacterial ventriculitis due to *A. xylosoxidans* subsp. *xylosoxidans* after craniotomy or cranial trepanation had been performed. With one exception, where the patient relapsed repeatedly with ventriculitis, in all remaining patients the duration of infection was relatively short and they recovered with appropriate chloramphenicol intraperitoneal therapy (500 mg or 1.0 g daily).

Lofgren et al.[36] have described a fatal case of prosthetic valve endocarditis due to *A. xylosoxidans* subsp. *xylosoxidans* despite treatment with TMP-SMX and moxalactam. In another case, the patient with community-acquired *A. xylosoxidans* bacteremic pneumonia, after initially responding to treatment with ceftazidime (2.0 g, b.i.d.) and TMP-SMX (15 mg/kg of trimethoprim daily), became increasingly hypoxemic and died 12 d after admission; *A. xylosoxidans* subsp. *xylosoxidans* was persistently cultured from the sputum.[63]

Patients with severe renal deficiencies requiring dialysis have increased risk to become infected from contaminated dialysis solutions, and have developed wound infections, peritonitis, and bacteremia due to *Alcaligenes*.[17]

In several studies,[42,47,64] the link between cancer and infections with *A. xylosoxidans* subsp. *xylosoxidans* have been discussed. Based on a review of 30 cases of nosocomial *A. xylosoxidans* infections in cancer patients which were traced to a contaminated antibiotic-containing mouthwash,

Gröschel et al.[47] concluded that such patients have a particular predilection for infection with this organism. Legrand and Anaissie[42] also evaluated 10 cases of *Alcaligenes xylosoxidans* subsp. *xylosoxidans* bacteremia in cancer patients and found that in the limited number of patients studied, antineoplastic chemotherapy and neutropenia seemed not be predisposing factors. Rather, the infections might have been related to contamination of central venous catheters or the result of gastrointestinal (GI) pathology where mucositis and breakdown of the intestinal barrier following chemotherapy had allowed invasion via the bloodstream by the pathogen, which is known to be part of the normal flora of the GI tract in humans.[6] All patients who received antibacterial therapy consisting of one or two β-lactam antibiotics, or TMP-SMX, ceftazidime, or ticarcillin alone have recovered.[42] The potential role of contaminated indwelling central venous catheters in such infections was further corroborated by Cieslak and Raszka,[64] who described a central venous catheter-associated *A. xylosoxidans* subsp. *xylosoxidans* bacteremia in a child with an advanced AIDS disease who was not neutropenic. The infection was successfully resolved with a 2-week course of amikacin and ceftazidime infused through the Broviac catheter, which was not removed.[64] The amikacin–ceftazidime combination seemed to be synergistic despite the resistance of the isolate to amikacin alone.

Neonatal infections with *A. xylosoxidans* subsp. *xylosoxidans* have been associated with bacteremia/septicemia, as well as infections of the central nervous system, including ventriculitis and meningitis.[24,26,30,33,65-67] The severity of such neonatal infections may reach an overall mortality rate as high as 60%.[65] Treatment regimens included combinations of antibiotics, such as chloramphenicol, cephaloridine, ampicillin, erythromycin, kanamycin, and streptomycin.

Sepkowitz et al.[24] have treated successfully an infant with *A. xylosoxidans* subsp. *xylosoxidans* meningitis with intravenously given carbenicillin (300 mg/kg daily) and moxalactam (100 mg/kg loading dose, followed by 50 mg/kg, four times daily). Pan et al.[68] have presented the first instance of neonatal meningitis with transient diabetes insipidus caused by *A. xylosoxidans*. After a 4-week course with imipenem and TMP-SMX, the patient stabilized but with sequelae of hydrocephalus and hearing impairment.

The first case of *A. xylosoxidans* subsp. *xylosoxidans* chronic otitis media with cholesteatoma in an immunocompetent child was described by Bénaoudia et al.[69] The patient recovered after 1 week of treatment with intravenous piperacillin (300 mg/kg daily). In two previously reported cases of chronic ear discharge with cholesteatoma,[70,71] this organism was not associated as pathogen.

A corneal ulcer that developed in a patient wearing therapeutic soft contact lens has been linked to *A. xylosoxidans* subsp. *xylosoxidans* infection. The patient did not have a preexisting microbial keratitis and was not receiving corticosteroid therapy.[67]

Haqque et al.[72] have described a case of continuous ambulatory peritoneal dialysis (CAPD)-associated peritonitis due to *Alcaligens xylosoxidans* subsp. *denitrificans*. The therapy, which consisted of once-daily intraperitoneal administration of gentamicin (8.0 mg/l in each exchange) together with oral ciprofloxacin (500 mg, b.i.d.), failed to eradicate the organism. The CAPD catheter was removed and the patient after receiving intravenous piperacillin was switched to hemodialysis and eventually recovered. In a previously described case of CAPD peritonitis caused by *A. xylosoxidans* subsp. *denitrificans*,[73] the patient was initially treated with intraperitoneal tobramycin (20 mg/l of dialysate once daily) and cephalotin (250 mg/l of dialysate) for 3 d. Although the peritoneal effluent became clear and the patient was without symptoms, the peritonitis recurred in about 2 to 3 weeks. The treatment was changed to TMP-SMX (a loading dose of 80 mg TMP and 400 mg SMX in 1.0 l dialysate, followed by 5.0 mg and 25 mg, respectively, per liter of dialysate for 10 d), with subsequent clinical and bacteriologic cure.

A case of septicemia in a patient with aortic valve insufficiency caused by *A. xylosoxidans* subsp. *denitrificans* was also described by Unoki et al.[74]

A clinical evaluation for efficacy and safety of sultamicillin in patients with meibomianitis (inflammation of the meibomian glands) due to *A. xylosoxidans* subsp. *xylosoxidans* and

A. xylosoxidans subsp. *denitrificans* has been carried out by Ooishi and Miyao.[75] The antibiotic showed lower MIC values than ampicillin and was especially useful against bacteria resistant to both ampicillin and cefaclor.

17.2 *OCHROBACTRIM ANTHROPI*

17.2.1 INTRODUCTION AND TAXONOMY

Ochrobactrim anthropi is a recently named[76] bacterial species with confusing history and taxonomy.[77] Previously known as CDC group Vd, *O. anthropi* is an oxidase-producing, Gram-negative, non-lactose-fermenting bacillus that oxidizes glucose and grows readily on McConkey agar.[9,78,79] Taxonomically, for the last 20 years or so, *O. anthropi* has been closely associated with the genus *"Achromobacter"*, which as defined by Tatum et al.[6] is comprised of Gram-negative, rod-shaped species with strictly aerobic metabolism and ability to oxidize carbohydrates and produce oxidase but not 3-ketolactose. Originally, it included four taxa: *"Achromobacter xylosoxidans"* groups IIIa and IIIb, and *"Achromobacter"* species biotypes 1 and 2.[6] However, after several taxonomic revisions,[2,12,80] these organisms were reclassified to the genus *Alcaligenes* as *A. xylosoxidans*, which left *"Achromobacter"* with official standing as a taxonomic entity but without member organisms. It has, therefore, been suggested,[3] that the name *"Achromobacter"* be placed in quotation marks.[77]

Despite the ambivalent status of the genus *"Achromobacter"*, a number of *"Achromobacter"*-like organisms continue to be isolated from clinical specimens, and their sometimes unsubstantiated taxonomic classification keep adding more confusion to the nomenclature. For example, according to a classification by the Centers for Disease Control (CDC), the *"Achromobacter"* species biotypes 1 and 2 (conferred by Tatum et al.[6]) have been referred to as groups Vd-1 and Vd-2, respectively, and a third organism, Vd-3 (now known as *Agrobacterium radiobacter*[81]) has been added to this group. However, even this classification was already in doubt after the suggestion[82] that *Agrobacterium radiobacter* may be identical with *Agrobacterium tumefaciens*.

Holmes and Dawson,[83] after reevaluating *"Achromobacter"*-like organisms, were able to organize them into six groups (termed *"Achromobacter"* groups A–F) based on phenotypic characteristics. According to this arrangement, since there has been no difference between *"Achromobacter"* species biotypes 1 and 2 (corresponding to the CDC goups Vd-1 and Vd-2), these two species were both assigned to group A. Subsequently, the CDC combined the two biotypes as Vd,[84] and ensuing analysis[85] supported this classification. Further studies[3] have established that *"Achromobacter"* groups C and D were essentially biotypes of group A, and that group E organisms were a biotype of group B. Finally, group F organisms were found to be distinctly different from all other groups to the extent that their proper inclusion in any of the other groups seemed unwarranted.

Morphologically, *Ochrobactrim anthropi* (formerly CDC group Vd) has been closely associated with *Alcaligenes xylosoxidans* subsp. *xylosoxidans*, as well as with *Agrobacterium radiobacter* and *"Achromobacter"* group B. Further, it superficially resembles pseudomonads in that it is motile and obligately aerobic. However, there have been several distinct features that might be used to differentate these species.[77] Thus, while all were capable of producing acid from glucose and xylose, *O. anthropi* did so in a weak and delayed fashion.[3] *Alcaligenes* may be distinguish from the other taxa by its ability to grow on cetrimide and by its inability to hydrolyze urea. *Agrobacterium radiobacter* may be set apart by its ability to oxidize lactose and to form 3-ketolactose.[86,87] Other distinct features of *A. radiobacter* include the rapid hydrolysis of urea, *O*-nitrophenyl-β-D-galactopyranoside and esculin, and the presence of an inducible cephalosporinase and an aminoglycoside acetyltransferase.[88]

Finally, *"Achromobacter"* group B may be separated from *O. anthropi* and *A. xylosoxidans* subsp. *xylosoxidans* by virtue of a positive *O*-nitrophenyl-β-D-galactopyranoside test,[89] as well as by its ability to hydrolyze esculin, and it may be differentiated from *A. radiobacter* by its lack of H$_2$S production when tested on lead acetate paper.[76,77,81,82,84,85,87]

17.2.2 TREATMENT OF *OCHROBACTRIM ANTHROPY* INFECTION

Although *O. anthropi* has been isolated from human clinical specimens and environmental and hospital water sources and inhalation therapy equipment,[90] it was rarely found to be patho-genic.[27,77,91-94] However, the organism appears to be increasingly recognized as a human opportu-nistic pathogen associated with intravascular catheters and unpredictable multiple antibiotic resis-tance. With very few exceptions,[95] all reported cases of *O. anthropi* involved immunocompromised patients.[27,77,91,93,96,97]

Antibacterial sensitivity testing has shown the organism to be susceptible to imipenem, mox-alactam, gentamicin, TMP-SMX, tetracycline, and rifampin with MIC values of 3.1, 12.5, 1.6 to 2.0, 0.5 to 2.0, 0.2 to 8.0, and 2.0 to 12.5 µg/ml, respectively.[27,91,92] The organism was generally resistant to β-lactam antibiotics, with MIC values of over 64 µg/ml for ampicillin, ticarcillin, mezlocin, azlocillin, and piperacillin, and over 32 µg/ml for cefazolin, cefamandole, cefuroxime, cefotixin, ceftriaxone, cefotaxime, cefoperazone, and ceftazidime.[91] However, despite *in vitro* sus-ceptibility to imipenem in initial isolates, on several occasions treatment with this agent failed to eradicate the organism and had to be changed eventually to amikacin.[96]

The first human infection with *O. anthropi* was reported by Appelbaum and Campbell[27] in the form of a pancreatic abscess in an elderly immunocompromised patient with a preexistent multiple debilitating condition. While the infection responded to treatment with gentamicin, the patient died from unrelated respiratory failure. In another case, a patient with astrocytoma and postoperative chemotherapy with *bis*-chloroethylnitrosourea (resulting in steroid-responsive cerebral edema and chronic pancytopenia) developed an *O. anthropi* infection.[92] The bacteremia was resolved after antibiotic therapy with gentamicin (270 mg daily) and TMP-SMX (80 mg of TMP and 400 mg of SMX, each given intravenously eight times a day) for 2 weeks.

A case of *O. anthropy*-associated osteochondritis complicating a nail-puncture wound of the foot in an immunocompetent patient was successfully treated with TMP-SMX (10 mg/kg of TMP daily divided equally every 6 h, intravenously) and gentamicin (6.6 mg/kg daily divided equally every 6 h) and surgical debridement and irrigation of the infected site; postoperative oral therapy with TMP-SMX (160 mg of TMP and 800 mg of SMX) every 6 h was implemented for 1 week.[91]

Van Horn et al.[93] have described a patient with urinary tract infection and bacteremia caused by *O. anthropi* complicating Hodgkin's disease. The patients responded completely to a combination of norfloxacin (400 mg orally, b.i.d.), amikacin (500 mg intravenously, b.i.d.), and TMP-SMX (320/1600 mg orally, four times daily).

Cieslak et al.[77] have reported the first case of central venous catheter-related sepsis caused by *O. anthropi* in a child undergoing chemotherapy for retinoblastoma. In a separate study,[94] seven cases of *O. anthropi* bacteremia were also associated with central venous catheter-related sepsis. The infection responded to treatment with either gentamicin or ciprofloxacin–imipenem.

Kern et al.[96] have found that despite *in vitro* susceptibility of *O. anthropi* to imipenem, the latter failed to eradicate the pathogen in a leukemic patient.

Three cases of *O. anthropi* meningitis were diagnosed among pediatric patients who underwent neurosurgical procedures in which pericardial grafts were contaminated with the organism.[95]

17.3 *AGROBACTERIUM RADIOBACTER*

Agrobacterium is a genus of bacteria belonging to the family Rhizobiaceae and comprising four species: *A. tumefaciens, A. radiobacter, A. rhizogenes,* and *A. rubi*.[87] Morphologically, they are small, Gram-negative, aerobic, flagellated rods, found in soil, or in the roots or stems of plants. Except for *A. radiobacter,* which is not a phytopathogen,[81,98] the remaining *Agrobacterium* spp. initiate host cell proliferation on various plants causing hypertrophy (galls) on the plant stems.[99,100]

While most clinical isolates (pleural exudates, blood, sputum, urine, nose swabs, artificial kidney, and contaminated serum and vaccine) of *A. radiobacter* are believed to be nonpathogenic,[101] its clinical significance is still not fully documented.[102-114] However, even with its low pathogenicity, *A. radiobacter* can still become opportunistic in immunocompromised hosts (including HIV-positive patients), especially in those with indwelling intravenous catheters.[103,105,112,114]

An initial report[102] has described an *A. radiobacter*-associated prosthetic valve endocarditis in a patient with multiple positive blood cultures. In the majority of the remaining cases,[103-105,107,108] the infections occurred in patients with central venous catheters, which on several occasions had to be removed.[104,105,109,114] In general, patients with *A. radiobacter* infection were predominantly immunocompromised because of disease (lymphoma, leukemia, ovarian carcinoma[103]) or cytotoxic chemotherapy. In two other reports, *A. radiobacter* bacteremia has been associated with peritonitis in patients undergoing continuous ambulatory peritoneal dialysis,[110,113] and urinary tract infection.[111]

Roilides et al.[103] have described the first case of an HIV-1-infected person, a child with a central venous catheter, who developed bacteremia due to *A. radiobacter.* The isolate was susceptible to ampicillin, cephalothin, imipenem, gentamicin, TMP-TMX, and ceftriaxone, with MIC values of less than 8.0 μg/ml, but was moderately resistant to ceftazidime (MIC = 32 μg/ml), tobramycin, and amikacin.

In the various cases described, the treatment of *A. radiobacter* bacteremia for the most part was effective and involved conventional dose regimens of either ceftriaxone (50 mg/kg daily, intravenously),[103] cefotaxime,[106,108] gentamicin,[111] and combinations of gentamicin–TMP-SMX,[110] imipenem–TMP-SMX,[103] imipenem–cilastin,[105] or amikacin–piperacillin (500 mg, b.i.d. and 3.0 g every 4 h, respectively).[114]

17.4 "*ACHROMOBACTER*" GROUP B

The status of "*Achromobacter*" group B as a human pathogen is even less settled.[3,77] Several clinical isolates, some of them recovered from patients with endocarditis, have been reported by Holmes et al.[3] One well-documented case of "*Achromobacter*" group B infection has been described by McKinley et al.[115] in a late replacement valve endocarditis. The isolates were sensitive to aminoglycosides, cephalosporins, amoxycillin–clavulanic acid, ciprofloxacin, erythromycin, and tetracycline, but resistant to penicillins, sulfonamides, trimethoprim, and rifampicin. Intravenous therapy with cefuroxime (1.5 g, t.i.d.) and gentamicin (the dosage was controlled by the need to achieve peak serum concentrations of 5 to 10 mg/l and troughs of less than 2.0 mg/l) for 6 weeks has been successful.[115]

17.5 REFERENCES

1. Holt, J. G., Krieg, N. R., Sneart, P. H. A., and Staley, J. T., Eds., *Bergey's Manual of Determinative Bacteriology,* 9th ed., Williams and Wilkins, Baltimore, 1994, pp. 75, 121.
2. Kiredjian, M., Holmes, B., Kersters, K., Guilvout, I. and De Ley, J., *Alcaligenes piechaudii,* a new species from human clinical specimens and the environment, *Int. J. Syst. Bacteriol.,* 36, 282, 1986.
3. Holmes, B., Costas, M., Wood, A. C., and Kersters, K., Numerical analysis of electrophoretic protein patterns of "*Achromobacter*" group B, E, and F strains from human blood, *J. Appl. Bacteriol.,* 68, 495, 1990.
4. Kersters, K. and De Ley, J., Genus *Alcaligenes* Castellani and Chalmers 1919, in *Bergey's Manual of Systematic Bacteriology,* Vol. 1, Krieg, N. R., Ed., Williams and Wilkins, Baltimore, 1984, 361.
5. Dworzack, D. L., Murray, C. M., Hodges, G. R., and Barnes, W. G., Community-acquired bacteremic *Achromobacter xylosoxidans* type IIIa pneumonia in a patient with idiopathic IgM deficiency, *Am. J. Clin. Pathol.,* 70, 712, 1978.

6. Tatum, H. W., Ewing, W. H., and Weaver, R. E., Miscellaneous gram-negative bacteria, in *Manual of Clinical Microbiology*, 2nd ed., Lennette, E., Spaulding, E. H., and Truant, J. P., Eds., American Society for Microbiology, Washington, D.C., 1974, 270.

7. Igra-Siegman, Y., Chmel, H., and Cobbs, C., Clinical and laboratory characteristics of *Achromobacter xylosoxidans* infection, *J. Clin. Microbiol.*, 11, 141, 1980.

8. Gilardi, G. L., Microbiological Terminology Update. II. Clinically Significant Gram-Negative Rods and Cocci (Excluding Rickettsiales, Enterobacteriaceae and Anaerobes), North General Hospital, New York, 1988.

9. Chester, B. and Cooper, L. H., *Achromobacter* species (CDC group Vd): morphological and biochemical characterization, *J. Clin. Microbiol.*, 9, 425, 1979.

10. King, E. O., The Identification of Unusual Pathogenic Gram-Negative Bacteria, National Communicable Disease Center, Atlanta, 1964.

11. Yabuuchi, E., Yano, I., Goto, S., Tanimura, E., Ito, T., and Ohyama, A., Description of *Achromobacter xylosoxidans* Yabuuchi and Ohyama, *Int. J. Syst. Bacteriol.*, 24, 470, 1971.

12. Hendrie, M. S., Holding, A. J., and Shewan, J. M., Emended description of the genus *Alcaligenes* and of *Alcaligenes faecalis* and proposal that the generic name *Achromobacter* be rejected: status of the named species of *Alcaligenes* and *Achromobacter*, *Int. J. Syst. Bacteriol.*, 24, 534, 1974.

13. Holding, A. J. and Shewan, J. M., Genus *Alcaligenes* Castellani and Chalmers 1919, in *Bergey's Manual of Determinative Bacteriology*, 8th ed., Buchanan, R. E. and Gibbons, N. E., Eds., Williams and Wilkins, Baltimore, 1974, 273.

14. Yamasato, K., Akagawa, M., Oishi, N., and Kuraishi, H., Carbon substrate assimilation profiles and other taxonomic features of *Alcaligenes faecalis*, *Alcaligenes ruhlandii* and *Achromobacter xylosoxidans*, *J. Gen. Appl. Microbiol.*, 28, 193, 1981.

15. Gilardi, G. L., Identification of miscellaneous glucose nonfermenting gram negative bacteria, in *Glucose Nonfermenting Gram-Negative Bacteria in Clinical Microbiology*, Gilardi, G. L., Ed., CRC Press, West Palm Beach, FL, 1978, 45.

16. Dees, S. B. and Moss, C. W., Identification of *Achromobacter* species by cellular fatty acid and by production of keto acids, *J. Clin. Microbiol.*, 8, 61, 1978.

17. Schloch, P. A. and Cunha, B. A., Nosocomial *Achromobacter xylosoxidans* infections, *Infect. Control Hosp. Epidemiol.*, 9, 84, 1988.

18. Holmes, B., Snell, J. S., and Lapage, S. P., Strains of *Achromobacter xylosoxidans* from clinical material, *J. Clin. Pathol.*, 30, 595, 1977.

19. von Graevenitz, A., Clinical role of infrequently encountered nonfermenters, in *Glucose Nonfermenting Gram-Negative Bacteria in Clinical Microbiology*, Gilardi, G. L., Ed., CRC Press, West Palm Beach, FL, 1978, 119.

20. Spear, J. B., Fuhrer, J., and Kirby, B. D., *Achromobacter xylosoxidans* (*Alcaligenes xylosoxidans* subsp. *xylosoxidans*) bacteremia associated with a well-water source: case report and review of the literature, *J. Clin. Microbiol.*, 26, 598, 1988.

21. Yabuuchi, E. and Ohyama, A., *Achromobacter xylosoxidans* n. sp. from human ear discharge, *Jpn. J. Microbiol.*, 15, 477, 1971.

22. Wintermeyer, S. M. and Nahata, M. C., *Alcaligenes xylosoxidans* subsp. *xylosoxidans* in children with chronic otorrhea, *Otolaryngol. Head Neck Surg.*, 114, 332, 1996.

23. Reverdy, M. E., Freney, J., Fleurette, J., Coulet, M., Surgot, M., Marmet, D., and Ploton, C., Nosocomial colonization and infection by *Achromobacter xylosoxidans*, *J. Clin. Microbiol.*, 19, 140, 1984.

24. Sepkowitz, D. V., Bostic, D. E., and Maslow, M. J., *Achromobacter xylosoxidans* meningitis: case report and review of the literature, *Clin. Pediatr.*, 26, 483, 1987.

25. Decré, D., Arlet, G., Danglot, C., Lucet, J. C., Fournier, G., Bergogne- Bérézin, E., and Phillipon, A., A beta-lactamase-overproducing strain of *Alcaligenes denitrificans* subsp. *xylosoxidans* isolated from a case of meningitis, *J. Antimicrob. Chemother.*, 30, 769, 1992.

26. Shigeta, S., Yasunaga, Y., Honsumi, K., Okamura, H., Kumata, R., and Endo, S., Cerebral ventriculitis associated with *Achromobacter xylosoxidans*, *J. Clin. Pathol.*, 31, 156, 1978.

27. Appelbaum, P. C. and Campbell, D. B., Pancreatic abscess associated with *Achromobacter* group Vd biovar 1, *J. Clin. Microbiol.*, 12, 282, 1980.

28. Shigeta, S., Higa, K., Ikeda, M., and Endo, S., A purulent meningitis caused by *Achromobacter xylosoxidans*, *Igaku No Ayumi*, 88, 336, 1974.

29. Pien, F. D. and Higa, H. Y., *Achromobacter xylosoxidans* isolates in Hawaii, *J. Clin. Microbiol.*, 7, 239, 1978.
30. Foley, J. F., Gravelle, C. R., Englehard, W. E., and Chin, T. D. Y., *Achromobacter* septicemia fatalities in prematures, *Am. J. Dis. Child.*, 101, 279, 1961.
31. Sindhu, S. S., *Achromobacter* meningitis in the newborn, *J. Singapore Pediatr. Soc.*, 13, 31, 1971.
32. Lee, S. L. and Tan, K. L., *Achromobacter* meningitis in the newborn, *Singapore Med. J.*, 13, 261, 1972.
33. Namnyak, S. S., Holmes, B., and Fathalla, S. E., Neonatal meningitis caused by *Achromobacter xylosoxidans*, *J. Clin. Microbiol.*, 22, 470, 1985.
34. McGuckin, M. B., Thorpe, R. J., Koch, K. M., Alavi, A., Staum, M., and Abrutyn, E., An outbreak of *Achromobacter xylosoxidans* related to diagnostic tracer producers, *Am. J. Epidemiol.*, 115, 785, 1982.
35. Olsen, D. A. and Hoeprich, P. D., Postoperative infection of an aortic prosthesis with *Achromobacter xylosoxidans*, *West. J. Med.*, 136, 153, 1982.
36. Lofgren, R. P., Nelson, A. E., and Crossley, K. B., Prosthetic valve endocarditis due to *Achromobacter xylosoxidans*, *Am. Heart J.*, 101, 502, 1981.
37. Yabuuchi, E., Ito, T., Tanimura, E., Yamamoto, N., and Ohyama, A., *In vitro* antimicrobial activity of ceftizoxime against glucose-nonfermentative gram-negative rods, *Antimicrob. Agents Chemother.*, 20, 136, 1981.
38. Appelbaum, P. C., Stavitz, J., Bentz, M. S., and von Kuster, L. C., Four methods of identification of gram-negative nonfermenting rods: organisms more commonly encountered in clinical specimens, *J. Clin. Microbiol.*, 12, 271, 1980.
39. Toki, N. and Kitaura, H., A case of suppurative skin disease which is thought to be due to *Achromobacter xylosoxidans*, *Nippon Hifuka Gakkai Zasshi*, 90, 843, 1980.
40. Manzella, J. P., *Achromobacter xylosoxidans* bacteremia, *Digest. Dis. Sci.*, 32, 781, 1987.
41. Boukadida, J., Monastiri, K., Snoussi, N., Jeddi, M., and Berche, P., Nosocomial neonatal meningitis by *Alcaligenes xylosoxidans* transmitted by aqueous eosin, *Pediatr. Infect. Dis. J.*, 12, 696, 1993.
42. Legrand, C. and Anaissie, E., Bacteremia due to *Achromobacter xylosoxidans* in patients with cancer, *Clin. Infect. Dis.*, 14, 479, 1992.
43. Dubey, L., Krasinski, K., and Hernanz-Schulman, M., Osteomyelitis secondary to trauma or infected contiguous soft tissue, *Pediatr. Infect. Dis. J.*, 7, 26, 1988.
44. Welk, S. W., Achromobacter pneumonia, *West. Med. J.*, 136, 349, 1982.
45. Puthucheary, S. D. and Ngeow, Y. F., Infections with *Achromobacter xylosoxidans* from clinical material, *Singapore Med. J.*, 27, 58, 1986.
46. Chandrasekar, P. H., Arathoon, E., and Levine, D. P., Infections due to *Achromobacter xylosoxidans*: case report and review of the literature, *Infection*, 14, 279, 1986.
47. Gröschel, D., Codey, L. D., and Tiemann, C., Nosocomial infections with *Achromobacter xylosoxidans* in cancer patients, *Proc. 19th Intersci. Conf. Antimicrob. Agents Chemother.*, American Society for Microbiology, Washington, D.C., Abstr. 378, 1979.
48. D'Amato, R. F., Salemi, M., Mathews, A., Cleri, D. J., and Reddy, G., *Achromobacter xylosoxidans* (*Alcaligenes xylosoxidans* subsp. *xylosoxidans*) meningitis associated with a gunshot wound, *J. Clin. Microbiol.*, 26, 2425, 1988.
49. Fass, R. J. and Barnishan, J., In-vitro susceptibilities of nonfermentative gram-negative bacilli other than *Pseudomonas aeruginosa* to 32 antimicrobial agents, *Rev. Infect. Dis.*, 2, 841, 1980.
50. Fass, R. J., Statistical comparison of the antibacterial activities of broad-spectrum penicillins against gram-negative bacilli, *Antimicrob. Agents Chemother.*, 24, 156, 1983.
51. Strandberg, D. A., Jorgensen, J. H., and Drutz, D. J., Activities of aztreonam and new cephalosporins against infrequently isolated gram-negative bacilli, *Antimicrob. Agents Chemother.*, 24, 282, 1983.
52. Moody, J. A., Peterson, L. R., and Gerding, D. N., In-vitro activities of ureidopenicillins alone and in combination with amikacin and three cephalosporin antibiotics, *Antimicrob. Agents Chemother.*, 26, 256, 1984.
53. Kaufman, H. S. and Hobbs, J. R., Immunoglobulin deficiencies in an atopic population, *Lancet*, 2, 1061, 1970.
54. Wintrobe, M. M., Lee, G. R., Boggs, D. R., Bithell, T. C., Foerster, J., Athens, J. W., and Lukens, J. N., *Clinical Hematology*, 7th ed., Lea and Febiger, Philadelphia, 1974, 1387.

55. Asquith, P., Thompson, R. A., and Cooke, W. T., Serum immunoglobulins in adult celiac disease, *Lancet*, 2, 129, 1969.
56. McKelvey, E. M. and Fahey, J. L., Immunoglobulin changes in disease: quantitation on the basis of heavy polypeptide chains, IgG, IgA and IgM, and of light polypeptide chains, type K and type L, *J. Clin. Invest.*, 44, 1778, 1965.
57. Fass, R. J. and Saslaw, S., Chronic meningococcemia: possible pathogenic role of IgM deficiency, *Arch. Intern. Med.*, 130, 943, 1972.
58. Hobbs, J. R., Milner, R. D. G., and Watt, P. J., Gamma-m deficiency predisposing to meningococcal septicemia, *Br. Med. J.*, 4, 583, 1967.
59. Jones, D. M., Tobin, B. M., and Butterworth, A., Three cases of meningococcal infection in a family, associated with a deficient immune response, *Arch. Dis. Child.*, 48, 742, 1973.
60. Kelly, S., Storm, E., and Juckett, D., Immunoglobulin M in meningococcemia, *NY State J. Med.*, 70, 1298, 1970.
61. Faulk, W. P., Kiyasu, W. S., Cooper, M. D., and Fudenberg, H. H., Deficiency of IgM, *Pediatrics*, 47, 399, 1971.
62. Stoelings, G. B. A., van Munster, P. J. J., and Slooff, J. P., Antibody deficiency syndrome and autoimmune hemolytic anemia in a boy with isolated IgM deficiency: dysimmunoglobulinemia type 5, *Acta Paediatr. Scand.*, 58, 352, 1969.
63. Mandell, W. F., Garvey, G. J., and Neu, H. C., *Achromobacter xylosoxidans* bacteremia, *Rev. Infect. Dis.*, 9, 1001, 1987.
64. Cieslak, T. J. and Raszka, W. V., Catheter-associated sepsis due to *Alcaligenes xylosoxidans* in a child with AIDS, *Clin. Infect. Dis.*, 16, 592, 1993.
65. Doxiadis, S. A., Pavlatou, M., and Chryssostomidou, O., *Bacillus faecalis alcaligenes* septicemia in the newborn, *J. Pediatr.*, 56, 648, 1960.
66. Shigeta, S., Higa, K., Ikeda, M., and Endo, S., A purulent meningitis caused by *Achromobacter xylosoxidans*, *Igaku No Ayumi*, 88, 336, 1974.
67. Fiscella, R. and Noth, J., *Achromobacter xylosoxidans* corneal ulcer in a therapeutic soft contact lens wearer, *Cornea*, 8, 267, 1989.
68. Pan, C. H., Wang, H. Z., Hsieh, K. S., and Liu, Y. C., *Alcaligenes xylosoxidans* neonatal meningitis: a case report, *Chung Hua I Hsueh Tsa Chih (Taipei)*, 57, 301, 1996.
69. Bénaoudia, F., Francois, M., Brahimi, N., Narcy, P., and Bingen, E., *Alcaligenes xylosoxidans*-associated infection in an infant with cholesteatoma, *Pediatr. Infect. Dis. J.*, 14, 637, 1995.
70. Bluestone, C. D., Current management of chronic suppurative otitis media in infants and children, *Pediatr. Infect. Dis. J.*, 7, 137, 1988.
71. Fliss, D. M., Meidan, N., Dagan, R., and Leiberman, A., Aerobic bacteriology of chronic suppurative otitis media without cholesteatoma in children, *Ann. Otol. Rhinol. Laryngol.*, 101, 866, 1992.
72. Haqque, S. S., Roth, M., and Bailie, R., Unsuccessful treatment of CAPD peritonitis caused by *Alcaligenes xylosoxidans* subsp. *denitrificans*, *Renal Failure*, 17, 611, 1995.
73. Morrison, A. J. and Boyce, K., Peritonitis caused by *Alcaligenes denitrificans* subsp. *xylosoxidans*: case report and review of the literature, *J. Clin. Microbiol.*, 24, 879, 1986.
74. Unoki, T., Nakamura, I., and Kunihiro, M., A case of septicemia caused by *Alcaligenes denitrificans* subsp. *xylosoxidans* and a review of the literature, *Kansenshogaku Zasshi*, 60, 627, 1986.
75. Ooishi, M. and Miyao, M., A clinical evaluation of sultamicillin fine granules in the treatment of meibomianitis, *Jpn. J. Antibiot.*, 41, 2059, 1988.
76. Holmes, B., Popoff, M., Kiredjian, M., and Kersters, K., *Ochrobactrim anthropi* gen. nov., sp. nov. from human clinical specimens and previously known as group Vd, *Int. J. Syst. Bacteriol.*, 38, 406, 1988.
77. Cieslak, T. J., Robb, M. L., Drabick, C. J., and Fischer, G. W., Catheter-associated sepsis caused by *Ochrobactrim anthropi*: report of a case and review of related nonfermentative bacteria, *Clin. Infect. Dis.*, 14, 902, 1992.
78. Oberhofer, T. R. and Howard, B. J., Nonfermentative gram-negative bacteria, in *Clinical and Pathogenic Microbiology*, Howard, B. J., Klaas, J. III, and Rubin, S. J., Eds., C. V. Mosby, St. Louis, 1987, 329.
79. Rubin, S. J., Granato, P. A., and Wasilauskas, B. L., Glucose-nonfermenting gram-negative bacteria, in *Manual of Clinical Microbiology*, 4th ed., Lennette, E. H., Balows, A., Hausler, W. J., Jr., and Shadomy, H. J., Eds., American Society for Microbiology, Washington, D.C., 1985, 330.

80. Yabuuchi, E. and Yano, I., *Achromobacter* gen. nov. and *Achromobacter xylosoxidans* (ex Yabuuchi and Ohyama 1971) nom. rev., *Int. J. Syst. Bacteriol.*, 31, 477, 1981.

81. Riley, P. S. and Weaver, R. E., Comparison of thirty-seven strains of Vd-3 bacteria with *Agrobacterium radiobacter*: morphological and physiological observations, *J. Clin. Microbiol.*, 5, 172, 1977.

82. Holmes, B. and Roberts, P., The classification, identification, and nomenclature of agrobacteria, *J. Appl. Bacteriol.*, 50, 443, 1981.

83. Holmes, B. and Dawson, C. A., Numerical taxonomic studies on *Achromobacter* isolates from clinical material, in *Gram Negative Bacteria of Medical and Public Health Importance: Taxonomy, Identification, Application, Lille, May 25–27, 1983*, Leclerc, H., Ed., Les Editions INSERM, 114, 331, 1983.

84. Clark, W. A., Hollis, D. G., Weaver, R. E., and Riley, P., Identification of Unusual Pathogenic Gram-Negative Aerobic and Facultatively Anaerobic Bacteria, U.S. Department of Health and Human Services, Centers for Disease Control, Atlanta, 1985, 334.

85. Holmes, B., Pinning, C. A., and Dawson, C. A., A probability matrix for the identification of gram-negative, aerobic, nonfermentative bacteria that grow on nutrient agar, *J. Gen. Microbiol.*, 132, 1827, 1986.

86. Bernarts, M. J. and De Ley, J., A biochemical test for crown-gall bacteria, *Nature*, 197, 406, 1963.

87. Kersters, K., De Ley, J., Sneath, P. H. A., and Sackin, M., Numerical taxonomic analysis of *Agrobacterium*, *J. Gen. Microbiol.*, 78, 227, 1973.

88. Martinez, J. L., Martinez-Suarez, J., Culebras, E., Perez-Diaz, J. C., and Bacquero, F., Antibiotic inactivating enzymes from a clinical isolate of *Agrobacterium radiobacter*, *J. Antimicrob. Chemother.*, 23, 283, 1989.

89. Oberhofer, T. R., Rowen, J. W., and Cunningham, G. F., Characterization and identification of gram-negative, nonfermentative bacteria, *J. Clin. Microbiol.*, 5, 208, 1977.

90. Moffet, H. L. and Williams, T., Bacteria recovered from distilled water and inhalation therapy equipment, *Am. J. Dis. Child.*, 114, 7, 1967.

91. Barson, W. J., Cromer, B. A., and Marcon, M. J., Puncture wound osteochondritis of the foot caused by CDC group Vd, *J. Clin. Microbiol.*, 25, 2014, 1987.

92. Kish, M. A., Buggy, B. P., and Forbes, B. A., Bacteremia caused by *Achromobacter* species in an immunocompromised host, *J. Clin. Microbiol.*, 19, 947, 1984.

93. Van Horn, K. G., Gedris, C. A., Ahmed, T., and Wormser, G. P., Bacteremia and urinary tract infection associated with CDC group Vd biovar 2, *J. Clin. Microbiol.*, 27, 201, 1989.

94. Grandsen W. R. and Eykyn, S. J., Seven cases of bacteremia due to *Ochrobactrim anthropi*, *Clin. Infect. Dis.*, 15, 1068, 1992.

95. *Ochrobactrim anthropi* meningitis associated with cadaveric pericardial tissue processed with a contaminated solution — Utah, 1994, *Morbid. Mortal. Wkly. Rep.*, 45, 671, 1996.

96. Kern, W. V., Oethinger, M., Kaufhold, A., Rozdzinski, E., and Marre, R., *Ochrobactrim anthropi* bacteremia: report of four cases and short review, *Infection*, 21, 306, 1993.

97. Haditsch, M., Binder, L., Tschurtschenthaler, G., Watschinger, R., Zauner, G., and Mittermayer, H., Bacteremia caused by *Ochrobactrim anthropi* in an immunocompromised child, *Infection*, 22, 291, 1994.

98. Hofer, A. W., A characterization of *Bacterium radiobacter* (Beijerinck and van Delden) Löhnis, *J. Bacteriol.*, 41, 193, 1941.

99. Allen, O. N., Holding, A. J., and Genus, I. I., Agrobacterium Conn. 1942, 359.Nom. gen. cons. Opiin. 33, Jud. Comm. 1970, 10, in *Bergey's Manual of Determinative Bacteriology*, 8th ed., Williams and Wilkins, Baltimore, 1974, 264.

100. Lippincott, J. A. and Lippincott, B. B., The genus *Agrobacterium* and plant tumorigenesis, *Annu. Rev. Microbiol.*, 29, 377, 1975.

101. Lautrop, H., *Agrobacterium* spp. isolated from clinical specimens, *Acta Pathol. Microbiol. Scand. Suppl.*, 187, 63, 1967.

102. Plotkin, G. R., *Agrobacterium radiobacter* prosthetic valve endocarditis, *Ann. Intern. Med.*, 93, 839, 1980.

103. Roilides, E., Mueller, B. U., Letterio, J. J., Butler, K., and Pizzo, P. A., *Agrobacterium radiobacter* bacteremia in a child with human immunodeficiency virus infection, *Pediatr. Infect. Dis. J.*, 10, 337, 1991.

104. Blumberg, D. A. and Cherry, J. D., *Agrobacterium radiobacter* and CDC group Ve-2 bacteremia, *Diagn. Microbiol. Infect. Dis.*, 12, 351, 1989.

105. Potvliege, C., Vanhuynegem, L., and Hansen, W., Catheter infection caused by an unusual pathogen, *Agrobacterium radiobacter*, *J. Clin. Microbiol.*, 27, 2120, 1989.

106. Freney, J., Gruer, L. D., Bornstein, N., Kiredjian, M., Guilvout, I., Letouzey, M. N., Combe, C., and Fleurette, J., Septicemia caused by *Agrobacterium* sp., *J. Clin. Microbiol.*, 22, 683, 1985.

107. Wilson, A. P. R., Ridgway, G. L., Ryan, K. E., and Patterson, K. P., Unusual pathogens in neutropenic patients, *J. Hosp. Infect.*, 11, 398, 1988.

108. Cain, J. R., A case of septicemia caused by *Agrobacterium radiobacter*, *J. Infect.*, 16, 205, 1988.

109. Ekelund, B., Johnsen, C. R., and Nielesen, P. B., Septicemia with *Agrobacterium* species from a permanent vena cephalica catheter, *Acta Pathol. Immunol. Scand.*, 95, 323, 1987.

110. Swann, R. A., Foulkes, S. J., Holmes, B., Young, J. B., Mitchell, R. G., and Reeders, S. T., "*Agrobacterium* yellow group" and *Pseudomonas paucimobilis* causing peritonitis in patients receiving continuous ambulatory peritoneal dialysis, *J. Clin. Pathol.*, 38, 1293, 1985.

111. Alós, J. I., de Rafael, L., Gonzalez-Palacios, R., Aguilar, J. M., Allona, A., and Baquero, F., Urinary tract infection probably caused by *Agrobacterium radiobacter*, *Eur. J. Clin. Microbiol.*, 4, 596, 1985.

112. Fernandez-Guerrero, M. L., Fernandez-Clua, M. A., Fernandez-Ortega, F., Gomez-Garces, J. L., and Navarro, A., *Agrobacterium radiobacter* bacteremia: study of 2 cases and review of the literature, *Enferm. Infecc. Microbiol. Clin.*, 13, 157, 1995.

113. Rodby, R. A. and Glick, E. J., *Agrobacterium radiobacter* peritonitis in two patients maintained on chronic peritoneal dialysis, *Am. J. Kidney Dis.*, 18, 402, 1991.

114. Hammerberg, O., Bialkowska-Hobrzanska, H., and Gopaul, D., Isolation of *Agrobacterium radiobacter* from a central venous catheter, *Eur. J. Clin. Microbiol. Infect. Dis.*, 10, 450, 1991.

115. McKinley, K. P., Laundy, T. J., and Masterson, R. G., *Achronobacter* group B replacement valve endocarditis, *J. Infect.*, 20, 262, 1990.

18 *Leuconostoc* spp.

Leuconostoc spp. are Gram-positive, saprophytic, facultative anaerobic microorganisms belonging to genus II of the family *Streptococcaceae*. Morphologically, they represent spherical but often lenticular, nonmotile cells, some species of which form dextran.[1,2] *Leuconostoc* spp. are found on herbage, vegetables, dairy products, wine, and sugar solutions.

Not until 1985 were *Leuconostoc* spp., which have been used in the diary, wine, and pickling industries, considered pathogenic for humans, when Buu-Hoi et al.[3] reported the isolation of two highly vancomycin-resistant *Leuconostoc* strains (MIC values of 512 and 1024 µg/ml, respectively) from clinical specimens of two immunocompromised patients. In the past, although not very often, resistance to vancomycin among cocci has been reported,[10] especially by *Streptococcus mutans*, *S. bovis*, *S. sanguis* II, and enterococci.[6,9,11-14]

Later, Rubin et al.[4] described a case of an infant receiving vancomycin who developed bacteremia caused by a vancomycin-resistant *Leuconostoc mesenteroides*; the vancomycin therapy had been initiated to treat a prior catheter-associated *Staphylococcus epidermidis* bacteremia. The subsequent 2-week course with intravenous penicillin was successful. In addition to penicillin (MIC = 1.0 µg/ml), all isolates were inhibited by clindamycin, cefazolin, and erythromycin, and although none elaborated β-lactamase, the minimal bactericidal concentration (MBC) values indicated that *Leuconostoc* bacteria were tolerant to penicillin (MBC >64 µg/ml).[4]

Subsequently, vancomycin-resistant *Leuconostoc* spp. isolates have been recovered from the cerebrospinal fluid of a previously healthy patient with pyogenic meningitis,[16] from blood cultures of four infants,[17] and the peritoneal isolate of a patient with systemic sclerosis.[18]

Powdered formula, an economic form of infant feeding commonly used in institutional settings, may become contaminated with microorganisms and serve as a source of nosocomial infections. In one such case, Noriega et al.[19] have reported *L. mesenteroides*-associated bacteremia from an instant formula contaminated by the blender that was used to rehydrate it.

Giacometti et al.[20] have isolated *L. citreum* from the lung of an AIDS patient who later died from acute respiratory failure. The isolate showed no zone of culture inhibition with a 30 µg vancomycin disk. Previously, Giraud et al.[21] reported a case of fatal *Leuconostoc* infection in an adult bone marrow transplant recipient.

In two separate studies,[3,22] the antimicrobial susceptibilities of *Leuconostoc* spp. have been determined. When tested in the agar dilution assay, eight strains of *L. sanguis* II, *L. mesenteroides*, and *L. lactis* were found highly resistant to vancomycin, teichomycin, sulfonamide, and fosfomycin (MIC = 512 to 1024, 256 to 1024, 256 to 2048, and >2048 µg/ml, respectively).[3] Penicillin G and ampicillin were more active than cephalothin, trimethoprim, cefotaxime, streptomycin, and kanamycin (MIC = 0.12 to 1.0, 0.5 to 2.0, 1.0 to 8.0, 2.0 to 8.0, 2.0 to 16, 1.0 to 16, and 2.0 to 16 µg/ml, respectively), whereas cefoxitin and pefloxacin were inactive (MIC = 32 to 128 and 16 to 128 µg/ml, respectively). All strains were susceptible to tetracycline, minocycline, chloramphenicol, rifampin, gentamicin, tobramycin, netilmicin, and amikacin (MIC = 1.0 to 8.0, 0.5 to 2.0, 4.0 to 8.0, 0.25 to 2.0, 0.12 to 2.0, 0.5 to 2.0, 0.12 to 1.0, and 0.25 to 2.0 µg/ml, respectively). Erythromycin and clindamycin were highly active against all strains (MIC = 0.03 to 0.06 µg/ml for both drugs).

Overall, resistance to vancomycin, sulfonamide, and fosfomycin appears to be a common trait in the genus *Leuconostoc*.[3,22] Combinations of penicillin G (5.0 µg/ml) with either streptomycin (8.0 µg/ml) or gentamicin (2.0 µg/ml) had synergistic activity in six of eight strains tested.[3]

In view of the rising population of immunocompromised patients and the spread of opportunistic/nosocomial infections, it is of great importance that testing for vancomycin susceptibility, especially of streptococci, staphylococci,[7] and *Lactobacillus* spp.[5] isolated from patients receiving vancomycin be performed promptly. *Leuconostoc* spp. as opportunistic pathogens, at least in immunocompromised patients, can be responsible for severe infections.[21]

18.1 TREATMENT OF *LEUCONOSTOC* SPP. INFECTIONS AND THE PROBLEM OF RESISTANCE TO VANCOMYCIN

Vancomycin is a glycopeptide antibiotic with highly potent antibacterial activity, used widely in the treatment of Gram-positive infections in penicillin-sensitive patients, *Clostridium difficile*-associated enterocolitis, methicillin-intolerant *Staphylococcus aureus*, etc.[8,9] With the increased use of vancomycin, the likelihood of encountering infections caused by vancomycin-resistant *Leuconostoc* spp. has become a distinct possibility.[4] In this regard, the recovery of vancomycin-resistant "streptococci" should convey a high degree of suspicion that the causative agent may, in fact, be *Leuconostic* spp.[5,6] As Horowitz et al.[15] have found, the latter can be easily confused on morphological appearance and fermentation reactions with more common isolates, such as α-hemolytic streptococci.

18.2 REFERENCES

1. Garvie, E. I., Separation of species of the genus *Leuconostoc* and diffferentiation of the Leuconostocs from other lactic acid bacteria, *Methods Microbiol.*, 16, 147, 1984.
2. Garvie, E. I., Genus *Leuconostoc*, in *Bergey's Manual of Systematic Bacteriology*, Vol. 2, Sneath, P. H. A., Mair, N. S., Sharpe, M. E., and Holt, J. G., Eds., Williams and Willkins, Baltimore, 1986, 1071.
3. Buu-Hoi, A., Branger, C., and Acar, J. F., Vancomycin-resistant streptococci or *Leuconostoc* sp., *Antimicrob. Agents Chemother.*, 28, 458, 1985.
4. Rubin, L. G., Veliozzi, E., Shapiro, J., and Isenberg, H. D., Infection with vancomycin-resistant "streptococci" due to *Leuconostoc* species, *J. Infect. Dis.*, 157, 216, 1988.
5. Thornsberry, C. and Facklam, R. R., Vancomycin resistant streptococci? Probably not, *Antibiotic Newslett.*, 1, 63, 1984.
6. Shlaes, D. M., Marino, J., and Jacobs, M. R., Infection caused by vancomycin-resistant *Streptococcus sanguis* II, *Antimicrob. Agents Chemother.*, 25, 527, 1984.
7. Schwalbe, R. S., Stapleton, J. T., and Gilligan, P. H., Emergence of vancomycin resistance in coagulase-negative staphylococci, *N. Engl. J. Med.*, 316, 927, 1987.
8. Watanakunakorn, C., The antimicrobial action of vancomycin, *Rev. Infect. Dis.*, 3, S210, 1981.
9. Geraci, J. E. and Hermans, P. E., Vancomycin, *Mayo Clin. Proc.*, 58, 88, 1983.
10. Edwards, D., *Antimicrobial Drug Action*, University Park Press, Baltimore, 1980, 131.
11. Baker, C. N. and Thornsberry, C., Antimicrobial susceptibility of *Streptococcus mutans* isolated from patients with endocarditis, *Antimicrob. Agents Chemother.*, 5, 268, 1974.
12. Bourgault, A. M., Wilson, W. R., and Washington, J. A., Antimicrobial susceptibilities of species of viridans streptococci, *J. Infect. Dis.*, 140, 316, 1979.
13. Harder, E. J., Wilkowske, C. J., Washington, J. A., and Geraci, J. E., *Streptococcus mutans* endocarditis, *Ann. Intern. Med.*, 80, 364, 1974.
14. Thornsberry, C., Baker, C. N., and Facklam, L. L., Antibiotic susceptibility of *Streptococcus bovis* and other group D streptococci causing endocarditis, *Antimicrob. Agents Chemother.*, 5, 228, 1974.
15. Horowitz, H. W., Handwerger, S., van Horn, K. G., and Wormser, G. P., *Leuconostoc*, an emerging pathogen, *Lancet*, 2, 1329, 1987.
16. Coovadia, Y. M., Solwa, Z., and van den Ende, J., Meningitis caused by vancomycin-resistant *Leuconostoc* sp., *J. Clin. Microbiol.*, 25, 1784, 1987.

17. Coovadia, Y. M., Solwa, Z., and van den Ende, J., Potential pathogenicity of *Leuconostoc*, *Lancet*, 1, 306, 1988.

18. Dyas, A. and Chauhan, N., Vancomycin-resistant *Leuconostoc*, *Lancet*, 1, 306, 1988.

19. Noriega, F. R., Kotloff, K. L., Martin, M. A., and Schwalbe, R. S., Nosocomial bacteremia caused by *Enterobacter sakazakii* and *Leuconostoc mesenteroides* resulting from extrinsic contamination of infant formula, *Pediatr. Infect. Dis. J.*, 9, 447, 1990.

20. Giacometti, A., Ranaldi, R., Siquini, F. M., and Scalise, G., *Leuconostoc citreum* isolated from lung in AIDS patient, *Lancet*, 342, 622, 1993.

21. Giraud, P., Altal, M., Lemouzy, J., Huguet, F., Schlaifer, D., and Pris, J., Leuconostoc, a potential pathogen in bone marrow transplantation, *Lancet*, 341, 1481, 1993.

22. Orberg, P. K. and Sandine, W. E., Common occurrence of plasmid DNA and vancomycin resistance in *Leuconostoc* spp., *Appl. Environ. Microbiol.*, 48, 1129, 1984.

19 *Treponema pallidum*

19.1 INTRODUCTION

As stated by Scheck and Hook,[1] "acknowledging the important role of host response (cellular and humoral immunity) in the pathogenesis and resolution of clinical neurosyphilis syndrome, it is likely that CNS involvement in syphilis patients with concomitant HIV infection may present progress, and respond to therapy differently than in individuals without HIV infection". Because of the frequency of CNS invasion by *T. pallidum* in the early stage of syphilis,[2,3] the possibility exists for the CNS to serve as a sheltered depot in which the spirocheta may be protected from host defense or antimicrobial therapy. However, the HIV-associated immunodeficiency would make neurosyphilis more common and more difficult to treat in HIV-infected patients than in those without HIV coinfection.[1]

The inability of HIV infected patients to mount an adequate immunologic response in preventing the recrudescence of neurosyphilis after treatment should not been underestimated.[4] The impact of the immunosuppressive effect of HIV infection on the natural history of syphilis was evident from the report of Horowitz et al.,[5] describing a patient who was treated for primary syphilis and yet only 4 years later relapsed into delusional behavior. In the pre-HIV era, with no therapy at all, the mean length of time to progression to this kind of neurosyphilis exceeded 15 years, and the aforementioned 4-year course of illness was essentially unknown.[4]

Based on careful review of the available data on neurosyphilis before and after the spread of the HIV epidemic, Musher et al.[6] concluded that "HIV infection affects concurrent syphilis, causing a failure to respond to treatment within the expected time; relapse of infection after treatment; and the frequent appearance of early neurosyphilis after therapy with conventional dosage of penicillin. Hence, it is deemed important to discuss the *Treponema pallidum* involvement in CNS in a separate chapter."

Treponema pallidum is a species of the genus *Treponema* of the family Spirochaetaceae. These are Gram-negative, microanaerophilic, elongated spiral microorganisms that exhibit motility with a flexing, bending, and snapping motion, and divide by transverse fission. The outer surfaces have a polar flagella that winds around the organism.[7] They propel themselves by spinning around their longitudinal axis.

In humans, *Treponema* are found in the oral, intestinal, and genital mucosa. *T. pallidum* subsp. *pallidum* was first described in 1905 by Schaudin and Hoffman[8] as the causative agent of venereal, nonvenereal, and congenital syphilis. Only limited replication of *T. pallidum* has been achieved in cell culture systems.[9] The spirocheta is usually cultivated in rabbits or guinea pigs for research purposes.

Most likely, *T. pallidum* enters the body through minute abrasions of the skin or mucous membranes. Its attachment to host cells involves the participation of mucopolysaccharides.[10,11]

T. pallidum almost certainly can reach the CNS before the development of skin lesions diagnostic of the secondary stage of the disease.[1,12] It has been found within axons of cutaneous nerves in chancres.[13] Spirochetas are present in the cerebrospinal fluid of 15% to 40% of all patients with early syphilis,[2,14] and yet, by some accounts,[12,15] of all patients with syphilis only 10% or less will develop neurosyphilis.

19.1.1 Host Immune Response to *Treponema pallidum*

The immune response to *T. pallidum* in early syphilis is triggered by a combination of stimulatory and suppressive signals.[11] Treponemal antigens are processed and presented to T helper lymphocytes by macrophages and other antigen-presenting cells. T cells, in turn, secrete lymphokines to upregulate the T lymphocyte response.[9] Treponemas are opsonized by specific neutralizing antibodies which facilitate their ingestion and destruction by activated macrophages.[16] However, because of the relatively inert nature of its cell surface, *T. pallidum* may evade the host's initial immunologic response resulting in dissemination to peripheral sites.[16]

Immunity to reinfection with *T. pallidum* does develop,[17] and serum antibodies to the pathogen may be used for diagnostic purposes.[11,18,19]

Several hypotheses have been advanced to explain the persistence of *T. pallidum* against the host immunologic response.[9] Thus, the existence of an immunosuppressive stage in secondary syphilis involving interference with the host's cell-mediated immunity in spite of high spirocheta titers, has been postulated.[10] In a second hypothesis, host-associated protein binding to the surface of treponemas has been suggested to play a role.[20,21] Furthermore, antigens may be concealed within the immunologically inert components on the treponemal surface, such as mucopolysaccharides or membrane lipids.[22,23] Yet other investigators have suggested an immunoprotective niche,[24] or a failure to trigger the oxidative metabolic burst in macrophages.[25]

The manifestations of tertiary syphilis have been explained in part as the result of a hypersensitivity response,[26] although treponemas themselves have been recovered in gummata.[27]

19.1.2 Central Nervous System Involvement in Syphilis

Most of the current knowledge of neurosyphilis has been derived from earlier studies. The earliest symptomatic evidence of neurosyphilis, syphilitic meningitis, usually appears 1 to 2 years after the infection. It seems that the spirocheta lays dormant in the cerebrospinal fluid (CSF) causing minimal reaction after the primary infection before proceding to cause the neurological manifestations of tertiary syphilis.[12]

All CNS involvement of treponema is the result of vascular or meningeal inflammation.[28-30] In general, the CNS involvement of treponema may be divided into two major categories: early involvement of the CNS, which is limited to the meninges (presenting as latent syphilis, acute syphilitic meningitis, and meningovascular syphilis), and later parenchymal involvement (presenting as tabes dorsalis and general paresis).[1,12] Since all syndromes of neurosyphilis start as meningitis, meningeal inflammation remains a component in all of its forms.[28,31,32] Clinical manifestations of some of the most commonly observed syndromes of neurosyphilis are presented below.

19.1.2.1 *Asymptomatic Neurosyphilis*

Asymptomatic neurosyphilis is defined by the lack of symptoms or signs in spite of CSF pleocytosis or positive serology. The number of asymptomatic patients who will develop symptomatic syphilis increases with the passage of time.[33]

19.1.2.2 *Meningeal Neurosyphilis*

This syndrome, which usually occurs most often during the 2 years of infection, is characterized by signs of meningeal irritation with stiff neck, headache, nausea, and vomiting; the patients stay afibrile. Cranial neuropathies affecting mostly facial and auditory nerves are common — sensorineural deafness occurred in up to 20% of patients with acute syphilitic meningitis.[32] CSF examination shows increased pressure, pleocytosis, moderate elevation of protein, and positive serologies in the CSF and serum.[12] Only a small percentage of patients with meningeal neurosyphilis will actually develop severe illness. The acute form results from perivascular lymphocytic and plasma cell infiltration of the meninges.[28]

19.1.2.3 *Meningovascular Neurosyphilis*

Both meningeal and vascular components are present in patients with meningovascular neurosyphilis.[3] Although abrupt onset of neurologic deficits in patients with meningovascular syphilis is common, cerebrovascular neurosyphilis is associated with slowly progressive vascular insufficiency, usually of the middle cerebral artery.[28] While meningovascular neurosyphilis may appear at any time, it takes on average 7 years after the infection to emerge. In general, meningovascular neurosyphilis rarely involves arterial vessels supplying the spinal cord,[28,34] but when it does the resulting damage is irreversible.[35-38]

19.1.2.4 *Parenchymal Neurosyphilis*

The success of modern antimicrobial therapy made late parenchymal syphilis a relatively seldom-occurring syndrome.[1] Nevertheless, patients with symptomatic neurosyphilis may develop tabes dorsalis or general paresis indicating a parenchymal involvement by the organism.[1,12]

19.1.2.5 *Tabes Dorsalis*

Tabes dorsalis, also referred to as locomotor ataxia or tabetic neurosyphilis, common in the pre-penicillin therapy era, has been rarely diagnosed in most developed countries.[39] Of all the neurosyphilis syndromes, tabes dorsalis has the longest latency, occurring 15 to 25 years after the primary infection.[28] It is characterized by lancinating "lightning" pains, paresthesias, diminished deep tendon reflexes, progressive ataxia, and bowel and bladder dysfunctions. Among other symptoms, pupillary abnormalities are uniform, and optic atrophy, areflexia, and hypotonia are common.[1] Pathologically, tabes dorsalis is characterized by leptomeningeal infiltration by spirochetes involving the pre-ganglionic portion of dorsal nerve roots. If not adequately treated, the inflammatory changes will progress to atrophic changes of the posterior columns of the spinal cord and the posterior nerve roots.[1]

19.1.2.6 *General Paresis*

Treponema-induced paretic neurosyphilis (dementia paralytica) represents a chronic meningoencephalitis resulting in severe disruption of the function of the cerebral cortex, leading to general degeneration of the patient's mental and physical state.[28] Prior to modern antimicrobial therapy, paretic neurosyphilis was reported to affect 5% to 10% of all first admissions to psychiatric hospitals,[40,41] reaching a peak incidence in untreated patients approximately 10 to 20 years after the primary infection.[28,42,43] Dementia becomes the most prominent feature of the late stages of the disease, together with seizures[39] and paralytic manifestations (hemiparesis, monoplegia, aphasia) followed by complete immobilization.

19.1.2.7 *Gummatous Neurosyphilis*

Gummatous neurosyphilis, the most uncommon syndrome of neurosyphilis, is the result of intense inflammation culminating in gumma formation.[28,44] Gummatous lesions are symptoms of late tissue reaction to syphilis[45] manifested as areas of necrosis surrounded by a densely cellular connective tissue mixed with epithelioid and giant cells. CNS gummas are reported to arise commonly from pia matter and subsequently invade the brain substance or spinal cord; brain involvement, although described, is relatively uncommon.[1]

19.2   EVOLUTION OF THERAPIES AND TREATMENT OF SYPHILIS

Clinical cure of early syphilis implies the resolution of lesions. Biological cure, on the other hand, means total eradication of treponema. The latter, however, might be impossible to achieve even when clinical cure is evident since viable organisms may persist in sites such as the anterior eye chambers, the endolymph, and the CSF. It is likely that these organisms may replicate slowly, thereby making eradication conditional to a prolonged course of therapy.[9]

The therapy objectives for neurosyphilis are closely associated with the clinical stage of the disease. However, after the introduction of penicillin and the subsequent widespread use of antibiotics, the clinical manifestations of the disease may have changed.[43,45-51] Thus, the occurrence of general paresis and tabes dorsalis (parenchymatous neurosyphilis) has become less common,[43,47,52-54] while the number of patients with asymptomatic neurosyphilis has increased, as did such clinical manifestations as seizures and ocular or auditory involvements.[39,45,47] According to data by Hotson,[47] and corroborated by other researchers as well,[43,45] the widespread use of oral antibiotics had unintentionally changed neurosyphilis into a progressive, partially treated meningitis resulting in "partial rather than fully developed manifestations as the rule."

In general, treatment of neurosyphilis was less successful when parenchymal tissue destruction had occurred (as in general paresis or tabes dorsalis) as compared with meningovascular and meningitic disease.[55]

One important task during treatment of patients with asymptomatic neurosyphilis is to bring back to normal, or at least improve, the CSF abnormalities, thereby reducing the risk for disease progression to symptomatic neurosyphilis.[1]

The introduction of penicillin into the clinic had a profound effect on the outcome of neurosyphilis resulting in a dramatic decrease of the number of patients entering mental hospitals.[56] No other antibiotic has led to lower failure rates than penicillin.[9] For example, patients with seropositive primary syphilis after treatment with 2.4 to 2.5 million units of intramuscular benzathine penicillin had a cumulative retreatment rate (because of either reinfection or treatment failure) of 4% over an observation period of 12 to 21 months.[57,58]

Early studies have included such formulations as amorphous penicillin, penicillin G, penicillin in beeswax or peanut oil (sustained-release preparations), procaine penicillin, procaine penicillin G in 2% aluminum monostearate, and benzathine penicillin G.

However, even though penicillin has been widely used, the optimal dose and duration of therapy with various penicillin formulations still remain somewhat controversial.[12,59] Thus, while a dose regimen of 2.4×10^6 units of benzathine penicillin G given intramuscularly once a week for 3 weeks has been extensively used in the clinic,[60] Mohr et al.[61] were unable to determine any detectable drug levels in the CSF in 12 of 13 patients. Currently, this dose regimen is no longer recommended by the World Health Organization (WHO).[62] Similarly, treatment with procaine penicillin G alone did not result in measurable levels in CSF.[12] Current recommendation is that benzathine penicillin should not be used in the treatment of any type of neurosyphilis.[9]

At present, the recommended therapy for neurosyphilis is intravenous penicillin G, given at 2 to 4 million units every 4 h (total of 12 to 14 million units).[63] This regimen consistently attained CSF levels higher than treponemacidal levels (0.03 IU/ml). The current recommendation for treatment with aqueous penicillin G is for 4 million units to be administered intravenously every 4 h for 2 weeks.[12]

In an alternative treatment, procaine penicillin G may be applied daily intramuscularly at 2.4 million units with oral probenicid at 500 mg.

Several reports have indicated that the response of syphilitic meningitis to penicillin therapy is prompt, with resolution of symptoms within several days to weeks.[64-66] Becker[67] reported return to normal from hearing deficits following treatment with high dose of intravenous penicillin G.

However, treatment failure may occur as recurrent hearing loss returns within several months after initial therapy.

Neafie and Marty[68] have diagnosed a case of syphilitic gastritis in a patient with overt symptoms of neurosyphilis. After a 2-week course of intravenous penicillin G (3×10^6 U given every 4 h), the patient was discharged. Gastric involvement in syphilis may occur during the primary, secondary, and tertiary stages of the disease due to spirochetemia.[69-73]

The activity of amoxicillin, another β-lactam antibiotic, has been evaluated in the treponemal immobilization assay. At a concentration of 0.42 µg/ml, it showed potency equivalent to that of penicillin (0.018 µg/ml);[74] in a rabbit orchitis model, the corresponding value was 0.11 µg/ml.[75] When amoxicillin (2.0 g) was given concomitantly with probenicid (500 mg), it produced a mean serum concentration of 4.0 µg/ml after 8 h;[76] for a dose regimen consisting of 3.0 g of amoxicillin and 1.0 g of probenicid, the mean serum concentration was 10.31 µg/ml after 8 h.[77]

In a clinical trial of patients with latent syphilis, the mean trough CSF concentration of amoxicillin on the second day of therapy (2.0 g amoxicillin given every 8 h, and 500 mg of probenicid given every 6 h) was 0.32 µg/ml.[75] In a similar treatment with seven patients, consisting of 1.0 g amoxicillin (six times daily) and 500 mg probenicid (four times daily), the lowest trough CSF levels were 0.5 µg/ml.[74] Onada[78] reported successful treatment of 30 patients with primary and secondary syphilis using a 4-week course of oral amoxicillin at 250 mg every 6 h.

A number of tetracycline antibiotics have also been studied for activity against *T. pallidum*. Thus, in a tissue culture system, the minimum inhibitory concentration (MIC) and minimum bactericidal concentration (MBC) values of tetracycline · HCl were 0.2 and 0.5 µg/ml, respectively.[79] Furthermore, clinical strains of treponema were as sensitive to tetracyclines as the laboratory Nichols' strain.[80] Schroeter et al.[81] used a total dose of 30 g of tetracycline · HCl to treat patients with primary or secondary syphilis; the cumulative retreatment rate was 9.2% at 1 year, and 12.7% at 2 years post-treatment.

Two other tetracycline analogs, aurcomycin and terramycin, have been shown to penetrate the blood-brain barrier and brain when taken every 6 h.[82] A third analog, doxycycline, produced significantly higher CSF and brain levels than oxytetracycline and tetracycline.[83,84] In a small study, treatment with doxycycline given at 200 mg daily for 28 d (with repeat courses three or four times over 1 year) resulted in a 90% and 100% clinical success rate in the therapy of primary and secondary syphilis, respectively.[85]

Doxycycline, which has been shown to reach treponemacidal CSF levels at 400 mg daily, may be an alternative for tetracycline.[86] For nonpregnant patients allergic to penicillin, a 30-d course of oral tetracycline (500 mg, four times daily) has been recommended,[12] or doxycycline at 200 to 400 mg daily for 28 d.[9]

While penicillin is still the drug of choice,[63] the antitreponemal efficacy of a third-generation cephalosporin antibiotic, ceftriaxone, has also been examined. After intramuscular administration, the serum half-life of ceftriaxone was approximately 8 h.[87] Its MIC value and 50% treponema immobilization concentration were determined to be 0.0006 and 0.01 µg/ml, respectively,[88,89] and the mean trough CSF level in rabbits treated with 7.5 mg/kg (every 12 h for 7 to 10 d) was 0.018 µg/ml.[89] In a rabbit model of cutaneous syphilis, ceftriaxone was slightly less active than intravenous penicillin G with respective 50% curative doses of 0.96 and 0.29 mg/kg per day, given for 5 d.[90]

An intramuscular bolus of 125 mg of ceftriaxone was used to treat incubating syphilis; 25 of 27 patients receiving the therapy did not develop early syphilis after 3 months.[91] In the same clinical trial, treatment of primary and secondary syphilis resulted in clinical cure in all 10 patients treated with 250 mg daily of ceftriaxone for 10 d, as well as all 6 patients who received 500 mg on five alternate days. In two other studies, 14 patients with primary and secondary syphilis were successfully treated with 1.0 g ceftriaxone administered on four alternate days.[87] Daily dose of 2.0 g of the antibiotic given for 2 or 5 d was successful in the treatment of primary syphilis.[92]

Cefmetazole, a cephamycin-type cephalosporin, has been reported as effective as benzathine penicillin in the treatment of active syphilis in a rabbit model.[93]

Several macrolide antibiotics have also been investigated for activity against *T. pallidum*. In a cell culture system, erythromycin showed MIC and MBC values each of 0.005 µg/ml.[94] However, erythomycin did not penetrate efficiently into the CSF.[82,95] In a rabbit model using the Nichols' strain of *T. pallidum*, the median time for lesions to become dark-field negative was significantly greater when the rabbits were treated with erythromycin than with benzathine penicillin.[96] Cumulative retreatment rates of up to 37% were described after the use of 1.0 to 2.0 g of erythromycin daily in patients with primary syphilis.[97] By comparison, dose regimens consisting of 2.0 and 3.0 g daily of erythromycin base for 10 d produced cumulative retreatment rates of 26.8% and 10.9% after 1 year, and 29.9% and 21.3% after 2 years, respectively.[81]

However, a number of investigators have reported clinical failures following erythromycin therapy of early syphilis.[98-102] After failure to respond to erythromycin, Stamm et al.[98] have recovered from a patient with secondary syphilis a treponema strain resistant to both erythromycin and roxithromycin.

Azithromycin, one of the newer macrolide antibiotics tested for activity against *T. pallidum* showed longer half-life and much greater tissue penetration than erythromycin. However, a treponema strain resistant to both azithromycin and erythromycin has also been isolated.[101] Lukehart et al.[103] have compared the activities of azithromycin (at daily doses of 7.5 to 30 mg/kg) and benzathine penicillin (200,000 units given weekly for 2 weeks) in a rabbit model of syphilis. The lesions became dark-field negative in the penicillin-treated rabbits earlier than in the azithromycin-treated rabbits.[103]

Spiramycin, another macrolide antibiotic, strongly inhibited both clinical and the Nichols' strains of *T. pallidum*; by comparison, clindamycin did not show activity.[98]

Alder et al.[104] have studied the effects of clarithromycin against experimental *T. pallidum* infection in hamsters. The therapy was effective when the antibiotic was administered subcutaneously once or twice daily for 1 week at 1 or 8 d after the infection. Combination of clarithromycin and benzathine penicillin G did not appear to be synergistic. The 14-hydroxy metabolite of clarithromycin was also found to be equally effective.

Chloramphenicol was shown to produce adequate CSF levels as well as favorable response in penicillin-allergic patients.[105] Romanowsky et al.[106] have treated successfully paretic neurosyphilis using intravenous chloramphenicol at 4.0 g daily for 2 weeks.

When tested in a syphilis rabbit model, several quinolones took substantially longer to cure chancres than penicillin. However, the decrease in the reagin titers following high-dose treatment with norfloxacin was equivalent to that of penicillin.[107] Ofloxacin seemed to have no effect against treponema in a rabbit model of incubating syphilis.[80]

19.2.1 Syphilis in HIV-Infected Patients

The HIV infection and syphilis, both being complex sexually transmitted diseases, can interact on several levels,[108] such as modification of the risk for acquisition and transmission of HIV,[109-111] changes in the clinical manifestationss of HIV infection,[108,112,113] increased frequency of recommended therapy failures among HIV-infected patients,[114] and conversely, the potential modifications in occurrence of manifestations and therapeutic response of neurosyphilis in HIV-infected patients.[2,6,114-117] The incidence of neurosyphilis-associated manifestations may be higher and the time to presentation of clinical symptoms swifter in HIV-positive patients as compared with patients without HIV.[116]

Furthermore, HIV-infected patients have been reported to fail treatment for early syphilis and then seen to progress rapidly to tertiary neurosyphilis, usually vascular or meningeal disease.[114,115,118,119] Severe syphilitic encephalitis and artheritis have been diagnosed in an HIV-infected patient in whom the CSF reagin test remained negative.[120] Ocular disorders associated with syphilis, such as uveitis, papillitis, vitreitis, optic neuritis, and retinitis, have also been described in HIV-positive patients.[113,121-123]

Overall, the currently available information, which is based on several case reports[63,114,124] and small case series,[116,125] has been generally insufficient, thus emphasizing the need for large-scale and prospective studies comparing the CNS involvement of syphilis in patients with and without HIV infection.[1]

19.2.2 ANTIBIOTIC TREATMENT OF NEUROSYPHILIS IN IMMUNOCOMPROMISED HOSTS

The optimal antibiotic regimens for immunocompromised patients with neurosyphilis is not well defined, and is currently under active examination. Results from a number of studies have suggested that, in general, the presently recommended therapy for early syphilis may not be effective in patients with HIV infection.[6,114,115,118,119,126-132]

Initial treatment with 4.8–7.2 million units of benzathine penicillin G, rather than the currently accepted 2.4 million units, has been recommended for early syphilis. However, in a study by Gordon et al.,[133] patients with HIV infection have relapsed after therapy, even with 7.2 million units. Furthermore, the same group[133] has examined the effects of high-dose regimens of penicillin G in HIV-infected individuals with symptomatic neurosyphilis — in the trial, 11 patients (5 of them already treated previously for early syphilis with benzathine penicillin G) received intravenously 18 to 24 million units daily of penicillin G for 10 d.

The results of Gordon et al.,[133,134] questioning the clinical efficacy of high-dose penicillin G regimens in HIV-infected patients, have been challenged by several groups of investigators[135-138] who attribute the apparent lack of clinical efficacy to the use of inadequately sensitive and specific markers measuring the response to treatment.

The reported problems with the efficacy of antibiotic treatment of neurosyphilis in HIV-infected patients, with or without immunosuppression still need to be substantiated by further studies.[138] In this regard, the current status of serologic testing after therapy for syphilis has been addressed in several studies.[139-141]

Cusini et al.[142] have described a case of atypical early syphilis in an HIV-infected homosexual male presenting with a slowly developing nodule on the wrist, followed after 2 months by a few scattered, large papular lesions. The lesions healed after treatment consisting of intravenous aqueous crystalline penicillin G (6 million units, b.i.d. for 5 d), followed by intramuscular benzathine penicillin G (2.4 million units per week for 21 d).

Ceftriaxone has also been evaluated for treatment of neurosyphilis in HIV-infected patients.[108] Korting et al.[88] have found that ceftriaxone effectively penetrated the blood-brain barrier and produced high serum levels following daily (or every other day) administration of 50 to 100 mg for 5 to 10 d. Additional studies have demonstrated that ceftriaxone was clinically effective in small numbers of patients with incubating syphilis, primary and secondary syphilis, and in neurosyphilis.[143]

In a recent study, Dowell et al.[144] have evaluated the response to ceftriaxone of HIV-infected patients with late latent or asymptomatic neurosyphilis. The antibiotic was given to 43 patients (47% of them had received prior treatment of 2.4 to 7.2 million units of benzathine penicillin within the last 3 years) at daily doses of 1.0 to 2.0 g for 10 to 14 d. Positive response to ceftriaxone was observed in only 65% of the patients, while 12% remained serum-fast and 21% had serologic evidence of relapse. Overall, a substantial 27% failure rate has been observed.[144] Marra et al.[89] have also reported a significant degree of failure of ceftriaxone in the treatment of experimental neurosyphilis.

19.2.3 BIOPHARMACOLOGY OF PENICILLIN CHEMOTHERAPY OF SYPHILIS

One characteristic feature of the treponemal cell wall biosynthesis is the cross-linking between N-acetyl muramic acid groups catalyzed by transpeptidases. Acting as a competitive inhibitor, penicillin interferes with this process by becoming tightly bound to the enzyme.[145] Cunningham et al.[146] have identified treponemal proteins capable of binding penicillin. While it has been hypothesized that penicillin can be effective only during active replication of *T. pallidum* when the construction of new cell walls is taking place,[147] it has been suggested that nonreplicating organisms may also be affected because of the need to continually repair and replace cell wall components between divisions.[148] Collart et al.[147] have found that *T. pallidum* remained virulent even after incubation with high concentrations of penicillin for up to 72 h.

19.2.3.1 Pharmacokinetics of Penicillin

Norris and Edmonson[94] have determined in cell culture the MIC of penicillin as 0.0005 μg/ml; the corresponding MBC value was 0.0025 μg/ml. Nell[79] has estimated that after 18 h of incubation, concentrations of 0.001 to 0.003 μg/ml of penicillin would be required to reduce the mobility of a *T. pallidum* suspension to 50%. Furthermore, the rate at which the pathogen was immobilized *in vitro* had increased proportionally to penicillin concentrations of up to 0.1 μg/ml, when a plateau was reached.[79] In a rabbit model of syphilitic orchitis, the plateau occurred at penicillin serum concentrations of 0.36 μg/ml.

In vitro clearance levels in rabbit serum were estimated to be between 0.005 μg/ml and 0.01 μg/ml of penicillin.[149] According to a recommendation by WHO for penicillin therapy,[150] a minimum drug serum level of 0.018 μg/ml (0.03 U/ml) would be necessary to provide a four- to sixfold safety margin for individual variations in the pharmacokinetics.

It appears that in early syphilis when rapid division of treponema occurs, 8 d is the optimum length of time for treatment with penicillin.[151] While the recommended dose regimen of benzathine penicillin G for treatment of early syphilis is 2.4 million units,[152,153] subtreponemacidal serum concentrations of less than 0.018 μg/ml have been found between days 3 and 6 after dosing.[154-156] It has also been reported[155] that such subtreponemacidal levels were more likely to occur in younger patients. In several studies,[33,157-159] 600,000 units of daily doses of procain penicillin seemed to provide consistently adequate peak serum penicillin concentrations.

The levels that penicillin can achieve in CSF are not synonymous with its brain tissue levels.[9] There is scarce information about penicillin human brain tissue levels after parenteral administration. Thus, Wellman et al.[82] have obtained brain tissue at prefrontal leucotomy in patients with uninflamed meninges; the investigators did not detect any penicillin at 4 or 24 h after an intramuscular injection of 600,000 U of procain penicillin.

Although the penetration of penicillin into CSF can be increased by fever,[160] fever therapy is no longer an option.[9] However, when the blood-brain barrier is defective, such as in meningitic, meningovascular, or paretic states, leakage of penicillin into the CSF can occur.[161] As reported by Weikhardt,[162] as little as 200,000 U of penicillin daily for 30 d, can successfully treat general paresis in some patients.

Of the various penicillin formulations, benzathine penicillin consistently failed to produce treponemacidal concentrations in the CSF.[61,154,156] By comparison, procaine penicillin daily at 600,000 U only infrequently produced treponemacidal levels in CSF.[157-159]

It has been shown[163] that 1.8 and 2.4 million units daily of procaine penicillin given concomitantly with probenicid (500 mg, every 6 h) can produce treponemacidal concentrations in the CSF. On the other hand, Van der Valk et al.[164] have found subtreponemacidal concentrations of penicillin in the CSF of 17 of 40 patients within 24 h after receiving 2.4 million units of procaine penicillin with probenicid 500 mg four times daily. It might have been possible to obtain higher levels of penicillin after several days of treatment to allow penicillin to accumulate within the CNS when a steady state is reached. According to Dunlop,[165] 500,000 units of procaine penicillin and probenicid 500 mg every 6 h produced treponemacidal concentrations. The beneficial effect of probenicid is perceived to result from its ability to increase the half-life of penicillin in the brain and serum.[166]

Intravenous penicillin G, at daily doses of 5 to 24 millions, consistently produced treponemacidal CSF levels.[61,157,159]

19.2.3.2 Allergic Reactions to Penicillin and Desensitization

Adverse reactions to penicillin are more likely to occur during parenteral administration rather than oral treatment, and with longer rather than short courses of treatment.[167] In addition, allergic response to benzathine penicillin have been observed more often than with other penicillin formulations.[55]

However, desensitization can be implemented even in patients with past history of severe reactions to penicillins. This may be an important issue with pregnant women for whom tetracyclines have been contraindicated and erythromycin may not be efficacious.[9] Usually, desensitization begins with small doses of oral penicillin, doubling the dose every 15 min for 3 to 4 h. Such initial treatment would enable subsequent full implementation of intravenous penicillin therapy without the danger of anaphylaxis, and with lower incidence of other allergic reactions.[168-170]

19.2.4 THE JARISCH-HERXHEIMER REACTION

Soon after initiation of treatment, a large number of patients with early syphilis may present with the Jarisch-Herxheimer reaction (JHR), a syndrome characterized with fever, malaise, and exacerbation of skin manifestations.[171] By some accounts, JHR occurred in 26% of patients with secondary syphilis treated with benzathine penicillin,[172] and in 65% of those treated with the faster released aqueous procaine penicillin.[173]

The mechanism of JHR is still not clearly understood. The roles of endotoxin,[172,174] and extravascular complement[171,175] have been proposed and then largely discounted. The release of tumor necrosis factor and other lymphokines have been correlated with JHR and may account for most of its features.[176] In addition, it has also been suggested that a deficiency of endogenous opioids may be a contributory factor.[177] Furthermore, the severity of JHR may be linked to the rate of release of the therapeutic agent into tissues and bacteria and the speed of its action.[178]

In active neurosyphilis, JHR has a delayed onset but is more prolonged. It is characterized mainly with lower maximum temperature than that observed in early syphilis; however, dementia, psychosis, meningismus, and cranial nerve lesions may become worse in 2% of patients.[179] In pregnant patients with latent syphilis, primary or secondary syphilis, the symptoms may include increased uterine contractions and decreased fetal movements, fetal heart abnormalities, and intrauterine death.[180]

Treatment of JHR with systemic steroids may alleviate only the fever mainly in cases of cardiovascular or neurosyphilis.[179] Meptazinol, an analgesic drug with opioid antagonistic properties, when administered intravenously at doses of 300 to 500 mg to patients treated for louse-borne relapsing fever, reduced the clinical severity of JHR; naloxone and steroids had no measurable effect.[181]

19.3   REFERENCES

1. Scheck, D. N. and Hook E. W. III, Neurosyphilis, *Infect. Dis. Clin. North Am.*, 8(4), 769, 1994.
2. Lukehart, S. A., Hook, E. W. III, Baker-Zander, S. A., Collier, A. C., Critchlow, C. W., and Handsfield, H. H., Invasion of the central nervous system by *Treponema pallidum*: implications for diagnosis and therapy, *Ann. Intern. Med.*, 109, 855, 1988.
3. Wile, U. J. and Stokes, J. H., Involvement of the central nervous system during the primary stage of syphilis, *JAMA*, 64, 979, 1913.

4. Musher, D. M. and Baughn, R. E., Neurosyphilis in HIV-infected persons, *N. Engl. J. Med.*, 331, 1516, 1994.

5. Horowitz, H. W., Valsamis, M. P., Wicher, V., Abbruscato, F., Larsen, S. A., Wormser, G. P., and Wicher, K., Cerebral syphilitic gumma confirmed by the polymerase chain reaction in a man with human immunodeficiency virus infection, *N. Engl. J. Med.*, 331, 1488, 1994.

6. Musher, D. M., Hamill, R. J., and Baughn, R. E., Effect of human immunodeficiency virus (HIV) infection on the course of syphilis and on the response to treatment, *Ann. Intern. Med.*, 113, 872, 1990.

7. Strugnell, R., Cockayne, A., and Penn, C. W., Molecular and antigenic analysis of Treponemas, *Crit. Rev. Microbiol.*, 17, 231, 1990.

8. Schaudin, F. N. and Hoffman, E., Vorlaufiger bericht uber das vorkommen von spirochaeten in syphilitischen krankheitsproduckten und bei papillomen, *Arbeiten Aus Dem K Gesundheitsamte*, 22, 527, 1905.

9. Goldmeier, D. and Hay, P., A review and update on adult syphilis, with particular reference to its treatment, *Int. J. STD AIDS*, 4, 70, 1993.

10. Sell, S. and Norris, S. J., The biology, pathology and immunology of syphilis, *Int. Rev. Exp. Pathol.*, 24, 203, 1983.

11. Fitzgerald, T. J., Pathogenesis and immunology of *Treponema pallidum*, *Annu. Rev. Microbiol.*, 35, 29, 1981.

12. Pachner, A. R., Spirochetal diseases of the CNS, *Neurol. Clin.*, 4, 207, 1986.

13. Sell, S. and Salman, J., Demonstration of *Treponema pallidum* in axons of cutaneous nerves in experimental chancres of rabbits, *Sex. Transm. Dis.*, 19, 1, 1992.

14. Chesney, A. M. and Kemp, J. E., Incidence of *Spirochaeta pallida* in cerebro-spinal fluid during early stage of syphilis, *JAMA,* 83, 1725, 1924.

15. Clark, E. G. and Danbolt, N., The Oslo study of the natural course of untreated syphilis, *Med. Clin. North Am.*, 48, 613, 1964.

16. Baker-Zander, S. A. and Lukehart, S. A., Macrophage mediated killing of opsonized *Treponema pallidum*, *J. Infect. Dis.*, 165, 69, 1992.

17. Magnuson, H. G., Thomas, E. W., Olansky, S., Kaplan, S. J., de Mello, L., and Cutler, J. C., Inoculation of syphilis in human volunteers, *Medicine (Baltimore)*, 35, 33, 1956.

18. Bishop, N. B. and Miller, J. N., Humoral immunity in experimental syphilis. II. The relationship of neutralizing factors in immune serum to acquired resistance, *J. Immunol.*, 117, 197, 1976.

19. Fitzgerald, T. J. and Johnson, R. C., Mucopolysaccharidases of *Treponema pallidum*, *Infect. Immun.*, 24, 261, 1979.

20. Alderete, J. F. and Baseman, J. B., Surface associated host proteins on virulent *Treponema pallidum*, *Infect. Immun.*, 26, 1048, 1979.

21. Marchitto, K. S., Kindt, T. J., and Norgard, M. V., Monoclonal antibodies directed against major histocompatibility complex antigens bind to the surface of *Treponema pallidum* isolated from infected rabbits or humans, *Cell Immunol.*, 101, 633, 1986.

22. Fitzgerald, T. J., Miller, J. N., Repesh, L. A., Rice, M., and Urquart, A., Binding of glycosaminoglycans to the surface of *Treponema pallidum* and subsequent effects on complement interacting between antigen and antibody, *Genitourin. Med.*, 61, 13, 1985.

23. Penn, C. W., Pathogenicity and immunology of *Treponema pallidum*, *J. Med. Microbiol.*, 24, 1, 1987.

24. Medici, M. A., The immunoprotective niche: a new pathogenic mechanism for syphilis, the systemic mycoses and other infectious diseases, *J. Theoret. Biol.*, 36, 617, 1972.

25. Wilson, C. B., Tsai, V., and Remington, J. S., Failure to trigger the oxidative metabolic burst by normal macrophages, *J. Exp. Med.*, 151, 328, 1980.

26. Marshak, L. C. and Rothman, S., Skin testing with purified suspension of *Treponema pallidum*, *Am. J. Syphilis*, 35, 35, 1951.

27. Turner, T. B., Hardy, P. H., and Newman, B., Infectivity tests in syphilis, *Br. J. Vener. Dis.*, 45, 183, 1969.

28. Merritt, H. H., Adams, R. D., and Solomon, H. C., *Neurosyphilis*, Oxford University Press, New York, 1946.

29. Izzat, N. N., Bartruff, J. K., Glicksman, J. M., Holder, W. R., and Knox, J. M., Validity of the VDRL test on cerebrospinal fluid contaminated by blood, *Br. J. Vener. Dis.*, 47, 162, 1971.

30. Simon, R. P., Neurosyphilis, *Arch. Neurol.*, 42, 606, 1985.

31. Holmes, M. D., Brant-Zawadzki, M. M., and Simon, R. P., Clinical features of meningovascular syphilis, *Neurology*, 34, 553, 1984.
32. Merritt, H. H. and Moore, M., Acute syphilitic meningites, *Medicine (Baltimore)*, 14, 119, 1935.
33. Lukehart, S. A. and Holmes, K. K., Syphilis, in *Harrison's Principles of Internal Medicine*, 12th ed., Wilson, J.D., Braunwald, E., Isselbacher, K. J., Petersdorf, R. G., Martin, J. B., Fauci, A. S., and Root, R. K., Eds., McGraw-Hill, New York, 1991, 651.
34. Adams, R. D. and Merritt, H. H., Meningeal and vascular syphilis of the spinal cord, *Medicine (Baltimore)*, 23, 181, 1944.
35. Harrigan, E. P., McLaughlin, T. J., and Feldman, R. G., Transverse myelitis due to meningovascular syphilis, *Arch. Neurol.*, 41, 337, 1984.
36. Lowenstein, D. H., Mills, C., and Simon, R. P., Acute syphilis transverse myelitis: unusual presentation of meningovascular syphilis, *Genitourin. Med.*, 63, 333, 1987.
37. Silber, M. H., Syphilitic myelopathy, *Genitourin. Med.*, 65, 338, 1989.
38. Terry, P. M., Glancy, G. R., and Graham, A., Meningovascular syphilis of the spinal cord presenting with incomplete Brown-Sequard syndrome: case report, *Genitourin. Med.*, 65, 189, 1989.
39. Swartz, M., Neurosyphilis, in *Sexually Transmitted Diseases*, 2nd ed., Holmes, K. K., Mardh, P. A., and Sparling, P. F., Eds., McGraw-Hill, New York, 1990, 231.
40. Catterall, R. D., Neurosyphilis, *Br. J. Hosp. Med.*, 17, 585, 1977.
41. Moore, M. and Merritt, H. H., Role of syphilis of the nervous system in the production of mental disease, *JAMA*, 107, 1292, 1936.
42. Hahn, R. D., Webster, B., Weickhardt, G. et al., Penicillin treatment of general paresis (dementia paralytica), *Arch. Neurol. Psychiatr.*, 81, 557, 1959.
43. Hooshmand, H., Escobar, M. R., and Kopf, S. W., Neurosyphilis: a study of 121 patients, *JAMA*, 219, 726, 1972.
44. Kulla, L., Russell, S., Smith, T. W., Zito, J. L., and Davidson, R., Neurosyphilis presenting as a focal mass lesion: a case report, *Neurosurgery*, 14, 234, 1984.
45. Burke, J. M. and Schaberg, D. R., Neurosyphilis in the antibiotic era, *Neurology*, 35, 1368, 1985.
46. Healthfield, K. W. G., The decline of neurolues, *Practitioner*, 217, 753, 1976.
47. Hotson, J. R., Modern neurosyphilis: a partially treated chronic meningitis, *West. J. Med.*, 135, 191, 1981.
48. Joffe, R., Black, M. M., and Floyd, M., Changing clinical picture of neurosyphilis: report of seven unusual cases, *Br. Med. J.*, 1, 211, 1968.
49. Joyce-Clark, N. and Molteno, A. C. B., Modified neurosyphilis in the Cape Peninsula, *S. Afr. Med. J.*, 53, 10, 1978.
50. Kofman, O., The changing pattern of neurosyphilis, *Can. Med. Assoc. J.*, 74, 807, 1956.
51. Anonymous, Modified neurosyphilis, *Br. Med. J.*, 2, 647, 1978.
52. Jordan, K., Marino, J., and Damast, M., Bilateral oculomotor paralysis due to neurosyphilis, *Ann. Neurol.*, 3, 90, 1978.
53. Lanigan-O'Keefe, L. M., Return to normal of Argyll Robertson pupils after treatment, *Br. Med. J.*, 2, 1191, 1977.
54. Luxon, L., Lees, A. J., and Greenwood, R. J., Neurosyphilis today, *Lancet*, 1, 90, 1979.
55. Wilner, E. and Brody, J. A., Prognosis of general paresis after treatment, *Lancet*, 2, 1370, 1968.
56. Schmidt, R. P. and Conyea, E. F., Neurosyphilis, in *Clinical Neurology*, Baker, A. B. and Baker, L. H., Eds., Harper and Row, New York, 1980, 1.
57. Smith, C. A., Kamp, M., Olansky, S., and Price, E. V., Benzathine penicillin G in the treatment of syphilis, *Bull. WHO*, 15, 1087, 1956.
58. Shafer, J. K. and Smith, C. A., Treatment of early infectious syphilis with *N,N*-bibenzylethylene-diamine dipenicillin G, *Bull. WHO*, 10, 619, 1954.
59. Whiteside, C. M., Persistence of neurosyphilis despite multiple treatment regimens, *Am. J. Med.*, 87, 225, 1989.
60. Mandell, G. L., Alexander, E. R., Arndt, K. A. et al., Sexually transmitted diseases treatment guidelines, *Morbid. Mortal. Wkly. Rep.*, 31, 50S, 1982.
61. Mohr, J. A., Griffiths, W., Jackson, R., Saadah, H., Bird, P., and Riddle, J., Neurosyphilis and penicillin levels in cerebrospinal fluid, *JAMA*, 236, 2208, 1976.
62. Wilcox, R. R., Treatment of syphilis, *Bull. WHO*, 59, 655, 1981.

63. Centers for Disease Control and Prevention, 1993 Sexually transmitted diseases treatment guidelines, *Morbid. Mortal. Wkly. Rep.*, 42(No. RR-14), 27, 1993.

64. Bayne, L. L., Schmidley, J. W., and Goodin, D. S., Acute syphilis meningitis: its occurrence after clinical and serologic cure of secondary syphilis with penicillin G, *Arch. Neurol.*, 43, 137, 1986.

65. Fiumara, N. J. and Newburg, M., Untreated relapsing secondary syphilis with meningitis, *J. Am. Acad. Dermatol.*, 20, 682, 1989.

66. Byrne, T. N., Bose, A., Sze, G., and Waxman, S. G., Syphilitic meningitis causing paraparesis in an HIV-negative woman, *J. Neurol. Sci.*, 103, 48, 1991.

67. Becker, G. D., Late syphilis: otologic symptoms and results of the FTA- ABS test, *Arch. Otolaryngol.*, 102, 729, 1976.

68. Neafie, R. C. and Marty, A. M., Unusual infections in humans, *Clin. Microbiol. Rev.*, 6, 34, 1993.

69. Eusterman, G. B., Gastric syphilis: observation based on 93 cases, *JAMA*, 96, 173, 1931.

70. Sachar, D. B., Klein, R. S., Swerdlow, F., Bottone, E., Khilnani, M. T., Waye, J. D., and Wisniewski, M., Erosive syphilitic gastritis: dark-field and immunofluorescent diagnosis from biopsy specimen, *Ann. Intern. Med.*, 80, 512, 1974.

71. Chung, K. Y., Lee, G. M., Chon, C. Y., and Lee, J. B., Syphilitic gastritis: demonstration of *Treponema pallidum* with the use of fluorescent treponemal antibody absorption complement and immunoperoxidase stains, *J. Am. Acad. Dermatol.*, 21, 183, 1989.

72. Shy, S. W., Lai, Y. S., Lee, W. H., and Tseng, H. H., Ulceronodular gastritis in secondary syphilis, *J. Infect.*, 22, 277, 1991.

73. Rank, E. L., Goldenberg, S. A., Hasson, J., Cartun, R. W., and Grey, N., *Treponema pallidum* and *Helicobacter pylori* recovered in a case of chronic active gastritis, *Am. J. Clin. Pathol.*, 97, 116, 1992.

74. Faber, W. R., Bos, J.D., Rietra, P. J. G. M., Fass, H., and Van Eijk, R. V. W., Treponemacidal levels of amoxycillin in cerebrospinal fluid, *Sex. Transm. Dis.*, 10, 148, 1983.

75. Morrison, R. E., Harrison, S. M., and Tramont, E. C., Oral amoxycillin, an alternative treatment for neurosyphilis, *Genitourin. Med.*, 61, 359, 1985.

76. Vitti, T. G. H., Gurwitt, M. J., and Ronald, A. R., Pharmacological studies of amoxycillin in non fasting adults, *J. Infect. Dis.*, 129(Suppl.), S149, 1974.

77. Barbhaiya, R., Thin, R. N., Turner, P., and Wadsworth, J., Clinical pharmacological studies of amoxycillin: effect of probenicid, *Br. J. Vener. Dis.*, 55, 211, 1979.

78. Onada, Y., Clinical evaluation of amoxycillin in treatment of syphilis, *J. Int. Med. Res.*, 7, 539, 1979.

79. Nell, E. E., Comparative sensitivities of treponemas of syphilis, yaws, and bejel to penicillin *in vitro*, with observations on factors affecting its treponemal actions, *Am. J. Syph.*, 38, 92, 1954.

80. Veller-Fornasa, C., Tarantello, M., Cipriani, R., Guerra, L., and Peserico, A., Effect of ofloxacin on *Treponema pallidum* in incubating experimental syphilis, *Genitourin. Med.*, 63, 214, 1987.

81. Schroeter, A. L., Lucas, J. B., Price, E. V., and Falcone, V. H., Treatment for early syphilis and reactivity of serologic tests, *JAMA*, 221, 471, 1972.

82. Wellman, W. E., Dodge, H. W., Jr., Heilman, F. R., and Petersen, F. C., Concentration of antibiotics in the brain, *J. Clin. Lab. Med.*, 43, 275, 1954.

83. Anderson, H. and Alestig, K., The penetration of doxycilline into CSF, *Scand. J. Infect. Dis.*, 9(Suppl.), 17, 1976.

84. Barza, M., Brown, R. B., Shanks, C., Gamble, C., and Weinstein, L., Relation between lipophilicity and pharmacological behavior on minocycline, doxycycline, tetracycline and oxytetracycline in dogs, *Antimicrob. Agents Chemother.*, 8, 713, 1975.

85. Onada, Y., Therapeutic effect of oral doxycycline on syphilis, *Br. J. Vener. Dis.*, 55, 110, 1979.

86. Yim, C. W., Flynn, N. M., and Fitzgerald, F. T., Penetration of oral doxycycline into the cerebrospinal fluid of patients with latent or neurosyphilis, *Antimicrob. Agents Chemother.*, 28, 347, 1985.

87. Schöfer, H., Vogt, H. J., and Milbradt, R., Ceftriaxone for the treatment of primary and secondary syphilis, *Chemotherapy*, 35, 140, 1989.

88. Korting, H. C., Walther, D., Riethmuller, V., and Meurer, M., Comparative *in vitro* susceptibility of *Treponema pallidum* to ceftriaxone, *Chemotherapy*, 32, 352, 1986.

89. Marra, C. M., Slatter, V., Tartaglione, T. A., Baker-Zander, S. A., and Lukehart, S. A., Evaluation of aqueous penicillin G and ceftriaxone for experimental neurosyphilis, *J. Infect. Dis.*, 165, 396, 1992.

90. Johnson, R. C., Bey, R. F., and Wolgamot, S. J., Comparison of the activities of ceftriaxone and penicillin G against experimentally induced syphilis in rabbits, *Antimicrob. Agents Chemother.*, 21, 984, 1982.

91. Hook, E. W. III, Roddy, R. C., and Handsfield, H. H., Ceftriaxone therapy for incubating and early syphilis, *J. Infect. Dis.*, 158, 881, 1988.

92. Moorthy, T. T., Lee, C. T., Lim, K. B., and Tan, T., Ceftriaxone for the treatment of primary syphilis in man: a preliminary study, *Sex. Transm. Dis.*, 14, 116, 1987.

93. Baker-Zander, S. A. and Lukehart, S. A., Efficacy of cemetazole in the treatment of active syphilis in the rabbit model, *Antimicrob. Agents Chemother.*, 33, 1465, 1989.

94. Norris, S. J. and Edmonson, D. G., *In vitro* system to determine MICs and MBCs of antimicrobial agents against *Treponema pallidum* subspecies *pallidum* (Nichols strain), *Antimicrob. Agents Chemother.*, 32, 68, 1988.

95. Everett, E. D. and Strausbaugh, L. J., Antimicrobial agents and the central nervous system, *Neurosurgery*, 6, 691, 1980.

96. Whiteside Yim, C., Flynn, N. M., and Fitzgerald, F. T., Detection of oral doxycycline into the cerebrospinal fluid of patients with latent or neurosyphilis, *Antimicrob. Agents Chemother.*, 28, 347, 1985.

97. Elliot, W. C., Treatment of primary syphilis, *J. Am. Vener. Dis. Assoc.*, 3, 128, 1976.

98. Stamm, L. V., Stapleton, J. T., and Bassford, P. J., *In vitro* assay to demonstrate high level erythromycin resistance of a clinical isolate of *Treponema pallidum*, *Antimicrob. Agents Chemother.*, 32, 164, 1988.

99. Hashisaki, P., Wertzberger, G. G., Conrad, G. L., and Nichols, C. R., Erythromycin failure in the treatment of syphilis in a pregnant woman, *Sex. Transm. Dis.*, 10, 36, 1983.

100. Duncan, W. C., Failure of erythromycin to cure secondary syphilis in a patient infected with the human immunodeficiency virus, *Acta Dermatol.*, 125, 82, 1989.

101. Stamm, L. V. and Parrish, E. A., *In vitro* activity of azithromycin and CP-63,956 against *Treponema pallidum*, *J. Antimicrob. Chemother.*, 25(Suppl. A), 11, 1990.

102. Fenton, L. J. and Light, I. J., Congenital syphilis after maternal treatment with erythromycin, *Obstet. Gynecol.*, 47, 492, 1976.

103. Lukehart, S. A., Fohn, M. J., and Baker-Zander, S. A., Efficacy of azithromycin for therapy of active syphilis in the rabbit model, *J. Antimicrob. Chemother.*, 25(Suppl. A), 91, 1990.

104. Alder, J., Jarvis, K., Mitten, M., Shipkowitz, N. L., Gupta, P., and Clement, J., Clarithromycin therapy of experimental *Treponema pallidum* infections in hamsters, *Antimicrob. Agents Chemother.*, 37, 864, 1993.

105. Romansky, M. J., Olansky, S., Taggart, S. R. et al., Chloromycetin in the treatment of various types of syphilis, *Am. J. Syph. Gonorrhea Vener. Dis.*, 35, 234, 1951.

106. Romanowsky, B., Starreveld, E., and Jarema, A. J., Treatment of neurosyphilis with chloramphenicol: a case report, *Br. J. Vener. Dis.*, 59, 225, 1983.

107. Andriole, V. T., An update on the efficacy of ciprofloxacin in animal models of infection, *Am. J. Med.*, 87(Suppl. 5A), 325, 1989.

108. Hook, E. W. III, Syphilis and HIV infection, *J. Infect. Dis.*, 160, 530, 1989.

109. Darrow, W. W., Echenberg, D. F., Jaffe, H. W., O'Malley, P. M., Byers, R. H., Getchell, J. P., and Curran, J. W., Risk factors for human immunodeficiency virus (HIV) infection in homosexual man, *Am. J. Public Health*, 77, 479, 1987.

110. Quinn, T. C., Glasser, D., Cannon, R. O., Matuszak, D. L., Dunning, R. W., Kline, R. L., Campbell, C. H., Israel, E., Fauci, A. S., and Hook, E. W. III, Human immunodeficiency virus infection among patients attending clinics for sexually transmitted disease, *N. Engl. J. Med.*, 318, 197, 1988.

111. Stamm, W. E., Handsfield, H. H., Rompalo, A. M., Ashley, R. L., Roberts, P. L., and Corey, L., The association between genital ulcer disease and acquisition of HIV infection in homosexual man, *JAMA*, 260, 1429, 1988.

112. Hicks, C. B., Benson, P. M., Lupton, G. P., and Tramont, E. C., Seronegative secondary syphilis in a patient infected with the human immunodeficiency virus (HIV) with Kaposi's sarcoma: a diagnostic dilemma, *Ann. Intern. Med.*, 107, 492, 1987.

113. Radolf, J. D. and Kaplan, R. P., Unusual manifestations of secondary syphilis and abnormal humoral immune response to *Treponema pallidum* antigens in a homosexual man with asymptomatic human immunodeficiency virus infection, *J. Am. Acad. Dermatol.*, 18, 423, 1988.

114. Berry, C. D., Hooton, T. M., Collier, A. C., and Lukehart, S. A., Neurologic relapse after benzathine penicillin therapy for secondary syphilis in a patient with HIV infection, *N. Engl. J. Med.*, 316, 1587, 1987.

115. Johns, D. R., Tierney, M., and Felsenstein, D., Alteration in the natural history of neurosyphilis by concurrent infection with the human immunodeficiency virus, *N. Engl. J. Med.*, 316, 1569, 1987.

116. Katz, D. A., Berger, J. R., and Duncan, R. C., Neurosyphilis: a comparative study of the effects of infection with human immunodeficiency virus, *Arch. Neurol.*, 50, 243, 1993.

117. Tramont, E. C., Syphilis in the AIDS era, *N. Engl. J. Med.*, 316, 1600, 1987.

118. Musher, D. M., Syphilis, neurosyphilis, penicillin, and AIDS, *J. Infect. Dis.*, 163, 1201, 1991.

119. Katz, D. A. and Berger, J. R., Neurosyphilis in acquired immunodeficiency syndrome, *Arch. Neurol.*, 46, 895, 1989.

120. Morgello, S. and Laufer, H., Quaternary neurosyphilis, *Lancet*, 2, 1549, 1988.

121. McLeish, W. M., Pulido, J. S., Holland, S., Culbertson, W. W., and Winward, K., The ocular manifestations of syphilis in the human immunodeficiency virus type I infected host, *Ophthalmology*, 97, 196, 1990.

122. Levy, J. H., Liss, R. A., and Maguire, A. M., Neurosyphilis and oculosyphilis in patients with concurrent human immunodeficiency virus infection, *Retina*, 9, 175, 1989.

123. Tramont, E. C., Controversies regarding the natural history and treatment of syphilis in HIV disease, *AIDS Clin. Rev.*, 6, 97, 1991.

124. Berger, J. R., Moskowitz, L., Fischl, M., and Kelley, R. E., The neurologic complications of AIDS: frequently the initial manifestation, *Neurology*, 34(Suppl. 1), 134, 1984.

125. Gourevitch, M. N., Selwyn, P. A., Davenny, K., Buono, D., Schenbaum, E. E., Klein, R. S., and Friedland, G. H., Effects of HIV infection on the serologic manifestations and response to treatment of syphilis in intravenous drug users, *Ann. Intern. Med.*, 118, 350, 1993.

126. Tien, R. D., Gean-Marton, A. D., and Mark, A. S., Neurosyphilis in HIV carriers: MR findings in six patients, *Am. J. Roentgenol.*, 158, 1325, 1992.

127. Salloum, E., Pella, P., Horn, D., and Hewlett, D., Stroke due to neurosyphilis: first manifestations of human immunodeficiency virus infections in two homosexual men, *Infect. Dis. Clin. Pract.*, 1, 43, 1992.

128. Harris, R. L., Rutecki, P. A., Donovan, D. T., Bradshaw, M. W., and Williams, T. W., Jr., Fever, headache, and hearing loss in a young homosexual man, *Hosp. Pract. (Off. Ed.)*, 20, 167, 1985.

129. Clark, R. and Carlisle, J. T., Neurosyphilis and HIV infection, *South. Med. J.*, 81, 1204, 1988.

130. Lanska, M. J., Lanska, D. J., and Schmidley, J. W., Syphilitic polyradiculopathy in an HIV-positive man, *Neurology*, 38, 1297, 1988.

131. Kase, C. S., Levitz, S. M., Wolinsky, J. S., and Sulis, C. A., Pontine pure motor hemiparesis due to meningovascular syphilis in human immunodeficiency syndrome virus-positive patients, *Arch. Neurol.*, 45, 832, 1988.

132. Smith, M. E. and Canalis, R. F., Otologic manifestations of AIDS: the otosyphilis connection, *Laryngoscope*, 99, 365, 1989.

133. Gordon, S. M., Eaton, M. E., George, R., Larsen, S., Lukehart, S. A., Kuypers, J., Marra, C. M., and Thompson, S., The response of symptomatic neurosyphilis to high-dose intravenous penicillin G in patients with human immunodeficiency virus infection, *N. Engl. J. Med.*, 331, 1469, 1994.

134. Gordon, S. M., Eaton, M. E., and Lukehart, S. A., Neurosyphilis in patients with human immunodeficiency virus infection, *N. Engl. J. Med.*, 332, 1170, 1995.

135. Tramont, E. C., Neurosyphilis in patients with human immunodeficiency virus infection, *N. Engl. J. Med.*, 332, 1169, 1995.

136. Rodriguez-Bano, J., Izquierdo, G., and Muniain, M. A., Neurosyphilis in patients with human immunodeficiency virus infection, *N. Engl. J. Med.*, 332, 1169, 1995.

137. Gourevitch, M. N., Klein, R. S., and Schoenbaum, E. E., Neurosyphilis in patients with human immunodeficiency virus infection, *N. Engl. J. Med.*, 332, 1170, 1995.

138. Horowitz, H., Wormser, G. P., and Wicher, K., Neurosyphilis in patients with human immunodeficiency virus infection, *N. Engl. J. Med.*, 332, 1171, 1995.

139. Romanowski, B., Sutherland, R., Fick, G. H., Mooney, D., and Love, E. J., Serologic response to treatment of infectious syphilis, *Ann. Intern. Med.*, 114, 1005, 1991.

140. Lukehart, S. A., Serologic testing after therapy for syphilis: is there a test for cure? *Ann. Intern. Med.*, 114, 1057, 1991.

141. Müller, F., Specific immunoglobulin M and G antibodies in the rapid diagnosis of human treponemal infections, *Diagn. Immunol.*, 4, 1, 1986.
142. Cusini, M., Zerboni, R., Muratori, S., Monti, M., and Alessi, E., Atypical early syphilis in an HIV-infected homosexual male, *Dermatologica*, 177, 300, 1988.
143. Hook, E. W. III, Baker-Zander, S. A., Moskovitz, B. L., Lukehart, S. A., and Handsfield, H. H., Ceftriaxone therapy for asymptomatic syphilis: case report and Western blot analysis of serum and cerebrospinal fluid IgG response to therapy, *Sex. Transm. Dis.*, 13, 185, 1986.
144. Dowell, M. E., Ross, P. G., Musher, D. M., Cate, T. R., and Baughn, R. E., Response of latent syphilis or neurosyphilis to ceftriaxone therapy in persons infected with human immunodeficiency virus, *Am. J. Med.*, 93, 481, 1992.
145. Wilcox, R. R., Changing patterns of treponemal disease, *Br. J. Vener. Dis.*, 50, 169, 1974.
146. Cunningham, T. M., Miller, J. N., and Lovett, M. A., Identification of *Treponema pallidum* penicillin proteins, *J. Bacteriol.*, 169, 5298, 1987.
147. Collart, P., Pechere, J. C., Francheschini, P., and Dunoyer, P., Persisting virulence of *Treponema pallidum* after incubation with penicillin in Nelson-Mayer medium, *Br. J. Vener. Dis.*, 48, 29, 1972.
148. Rein, M. F., Biopharmacology of syphilis therapy, *J. Am. Vener. Dis. Assoc.*, 3, 109, 1976.
149. Eagle, H. R., Fleischman, R., and Musselman, A. D., The effective concentration of penicillin *in vitro* and *in vivo* for streptococcus, pneumococcus and *Treponema pallidum*, *J. Bacteriol.*, 59, 625, 1950.
150. Isdoe, O., Guthe, T., and Wocox, R. R., Penicillin in the treatment of syphilis, *Bull. WHO*, 47(Suppl.), 5, 1972.
151. Eagle, H. and Musselman, A. D., The spirocheticidal action of penicillin *in vitro* and its temperature coefficient, *J. Exp. Med.*, 80, 493, 1944.
152. Hook, E. W. III and Marra, C. M., Acquired syphilis in adults, *N. Engl. J. Med.*, 326, 1060, 1992.
153. Anonymous, Sexually transmitted diseases treatment guidelines, *Morbid. Mortal. Wkly. Rep.*, 38(Suppl. 8), 1, 1989.
154. Frenz, G., Neilsen, P. B., Esperson, F., Czartovyski, A., and Aastrup, H., Penicillin concentrations in blood and spinal fluid after a single intramuscular injection of penicillin G benzathine, *Eur. J. Clin. Microbiol.*, 3, 147, 1984.
155. Collart, P., Poitevin, M., Milovanovic, A., Herlin, A., and Durel, J., Kinetic study of serum penicillin concentrations after single doses of benzathine and benethamine penicillin in young and old people, *Br. J. Vener. Dis.*, 56, 355, 1980.
156. Polnikorn, N., Witoonpanich, R., Vorachit, M., Vejjajiva, S., and Vijjajiva, A., Penicillin concentration in cerebrospinal fluid after different treatment regimens for syphilis, *Br. J. Vener. Dis.*, 56, 363, 1980.
157. Goh, B. T., Smith, G. W., Samarasinghe, L., Singh, V., and Lim, K. S., Penicillin concentrations in serum and cerebrospinal fluid after intramuscular injection of aqueous procaine penicillin 0.6 MU with and without probenicid, *Br. J. Vener. Dis.*, 60, 371, 1984.
158. Goldmeier, D. and Waterworth, P. M., Penetration of penicillin into the cerebrospinal fluid of patients with latent syphilis, *Pharmatherapeutica*, 1, 14, 1981.
159. Löwenhagen, G. B., Brorson, J. E., and Kaijer, B., Penicillin concentrations in cerebrospinal fluid and serum after intramuscular, intravenous and oral administration to syphilitic hospitals, *Arch. Dermatovener. (Stockholm)*, 63, 53, 1983.
160. Dewhurst, K. and Todd, J., The effect of fever on the penetration of penicillin into the cerebrospinal fluid, *Int. J. Neuropsychiatr.*, 1, 257, 1965.
161. Barling, R. W. A. and Selkon, J. B., The penetration of antibiotics into cerebrospinal fluid and brain tissue, *J. Antimicrob. Chemother.*, 4, 203, 1978.
162. Weikhardt, G. D., Penicillin therapy in general paresis, *Am. J. Psychiatr.*, 105, 63, 1948.
163. Dunlop, E. M. C., Al-Egaily, S. S., and Hovang, E. T., Production of treponemacidal concentration of penicillin in cerebrospinal fluid, *Br. Med. J.*, 283, 646, 1981.
164. Van der Valk, P. M. G., Kraai, E. J., van Voorst Vader, P. C., Haaxma-Reiche, H., and Snijder, J. A. M., Penicillin concentrations in cerebrospinal fluid (CSF) during repository treatment regimens for syphilis, *Genitourin. Med.*, 64, 223, 1988.
165. Dunlop, E. M. C., Survival of treponemas after treatment: comments, clinical conclusions and recommendations, *Genitourin. Med.*, 61, 293, 1985.
166. Fishman, R. A., Blood brain and CSF barriers to penicillin and related organic acids, *Arch. Neurol.*, 15, 113, 1966.

167. Adkinson, N. F., Risk factors for drug allergy, *J. Allergy Clin. Immunol.*, 74, 567, 1984.
168. Sullivan, T. J., Antigen specific desensitization of patients allergic to penicillin, *J. Allergy Clin. Immunol.*, 69, 500, 1982.
169. Stark, B. J., Gross, G. N., Lumry, W. R., and Sullivan, T. J., Oral desensitization of penicillin-allergic patients, *J. Allergy Clin. Immunol.*, 73, 112, 1984.
170. Wendel, G. D., Stark, B. J., Jamison, R. B., Molina, R. D., and Sullivan, T. J., Penicillin allergy and desensitization in serious infections in pregnancy, *N. Engl. J. Med.*, 312, 1229, 1985.
171. Warrall, D. A., Perine, P. L., Krause, D. W., Bing, D. H., and MacDougal, S. J., Pathophysiology and immunology of the Jarisch-Herxheimer like reaction in louse borne relapsing fever: comparison of tetracycline and slow release penicillin, *J. Infect. Dis.*, 147, 898, 1983.
172. Shenep, J. L., Feldman, S., and Thornton, D., Evaluation for endotoxemia in patients receiving penicillin therapy for secondary syphilis, *JAMA*, 256, 388, 1986.
173. Anderson, J., Mindel, A., Tovey, S. J., and Williams, P., Primary and secondary syphilis, 20 years' experience. III. Diagnosis, treatment and follow-up, *Genitourin. Med.*, 65, 239, 1989.
174. Bryceson, A. D. M., Clinical pathology of the Jarisch-Herxheimer reaction, *J. Infect. Dis.*, 133, 696, 1976.
175. Fulford, K. W. M., Johnson, N., Loveday, C., Storey, J., and Tedder, R. S., Changes in intravascular complement and antitreponemal antibody titres preceding the Jarisch-Herxheimer reaction in secondary syphilis, *Clin. Exp. Immunol.*, 24, 483, 1976.
176. Remicke, D. G., Negussie, Y., Deforge, L. E., Kunkel, S. L., Eyon, A., and Griffin, G. E., Cytokine production during the Jarisch-Herxheimer reaction (JH-R), *FASEB J.*, 5, 7552, 1991.
177. Wright, D. J. M., Endogenous opioid reaction in the Jarisch-Herxheimer reaction, *Lancet*, 1, 1135, 1983.
178. Rottenberg, R., Treatment of neurosyphilis, *J. Am. Vener. Dis. Assoc.*, 3, 153, 1976.
179. Brown, S. T., Adverse reactions in syphilis therapy, *J. Am. Vener. Dis. Assoc.*, 3, 172, 1976.
180. Klein, V. R., Cox, S. M., Mitchell, M. D., and Wendel, G. D., The Jarisch-Herxheimer reaction complicating syphilotherapy in pregnancy, *Obstet. Gynecol.*, 75, 375, 1990.
181. Teklu, B., Habte-Michael, A., Warrell, D. A., White, N. J., and Wright, D. J. M., Meptazinol diminishes the Jarisch-Herxheimer reaction of relapsing fever, *Lancet*, 1, 835, 1983.

20 *Mycoplasma* spp.

20.1 INTRODUCTION

Mycoplasma is a genus of bacteria classified in the family Mycoplasmataceae, order Mycoplasmatales, class Mollicutes. These microorganisms represent highly pleomorphic, Gram-negative, spherical to ovoid-shaped cells bound by a single triple-layered membrane but lacking a rigid cell wall. The mycoplasmas differ from viruses in that they do not require a host cell for replication but instead divide by binary fusion. The mycoplasmas need cholesterol or another sterol in order to maintain growth. They are parasites and pathogens, widely distributed on the mucous membranes of humans, animals, and birds, as well as common contaminants of animal cell cultures.

Among the various species of *Mycoplasma*, *M. buccale* is a common inhabitant of the oropharynx of nonhuman primates, and *M. faucium* is a species found occasionally in the oropharynx of humans and frequently in the oropharynx of nonhuman primates. *M. pneumoniae*, *M. hominis*, *M. fermentans*, and *M. orale* have all been associated with human infections involving the respiratory tract as well as extrapulmonary sites, such as the reproductive tracts of both male and females. Recent reports have indicated that in some immunocompromised patients, such as those with AIDS, some of these organisms[1] (*M. fermentans*,[1-5] *M. penetrans*,[6-8] and *M. pirum*[9]) can act as cofactors in the progression of HIV infection.[10]

The description of atypical pneumonia as a clinical entity was first applied in 1938 by Reimann to characterize an unusual form of "tracheobronchopneumonia" and severe symptoms.[11] Currently, the term "atypical pneumonia" implies a generally benign illness in which systemic complaints often are more prominent than respiratory ones.[12-18] A pathological definition of pneumonia is that of inflammation of the lung parenchyma, distal to the terminal bronchioles, and comprising the respiratory bronchioles, alveolar ducts, alveolar sacs, and alveoli.[19]

20.1.1 *MYCOPLASMA PNEUMONIAE*

Among the various microorganisms implicated in atypical pneumonia (*Chlamidia psittaci*, *Chlamidia pneumoniae*, *Coxiella burnetii*, *Francisella tularensis*, *Legionella pneumophilia*, influenza A and B viruses, adenovirus, and the respiratory syncytial virus),[20-23] *Mycoplasma pneumoniae* has been described as the etiologic agent of various respiratory (intractable cough, bullous myringitis, sinusitis, pharyngitis with cervical adenopathy) and extrapulmonary (hemolytic anemia, CNS complications, myopericarditis, erythema multiforme, and Stevens-Johnson syndrome) conditions.[12] By some estimates,[24] approximately 20% of all cases of pneumonia in the general population and 50% of those in persons living in close quarters or community-acquired (i.e., military barracks, dormitories, nursing homes), have been caused by *M. pneumoniae*.[25] Preexisting immunity to the infection is not long-lasting.[26]

M. pneumoniae was first discovered by Eaton et al.[27] in 1944 and became known as the Eaton's agent until Chanock et al.[28,29] gave it its current name and established it as the primary cause of atypical pneumonia.

M. pneumoniae is the smallest free-living organism[30] that can grow both aerobically and anaerobically.[31] It is a motile bacterium that can attach itself to the respiratory epithelium by using a specialized terminal organelle called the PI protein.[31,32] It is spread from person to person, mainly through contact with infected droplets or aerosol transmission.[16,17]

Immune-mediated mechanisms probably play a role in *M. pneumoniae* infections. Thus, Luby[32] has demonstrated in animal models that while inflammatory changes developed slowly prior to exposure, they evolved much more quickly after reinfection. Furthermore, *M. pneumoniae* has been shown to stimulate the B and T cell mitogenic activity and to inhibit cell-mediated immunity.[29] During the acute phase of atypical pneumonia, the levels of IgG immune complex (IgG-IC) were at their highest stage which correlated with the pulmonary involvement. No IgG-IC has been found in the serum of patients not having pneumonia.[33] *M. pneumoniae* has been occasionally responsible for formation of autoantibodies.[31,34]

Clinically, the respiratory manifestations of *M. pneumoniae* infections are primarily associated with mild pneumonia, tracheobronchitis, and pharyngitis.[12,35] The onset of disease is usually characterized with headache, malaise, and a low-level fever,[32] as well as with an intractible, nonproductive cough. Hilar adenopathy has been found in up to 22% of patients.[36]

In the absence of direct evidence of mycoplasmal invasion, it has been postulated that extrapulmonary manifestations of mycoplasmal infection may have to be the consequence of an autoimmune phenomenon involving either humoral or cellular immunity.[37-40] Several findings have lent credence to that hypothesis. For example, mycoplasmas have been known to stimulate various host responses, such as autoantibody production, antigen-antibody complex formation, T cell proliferation, and polyclonal B cell activation.[41-43] The presence of autoantibodies to brain and other host tissues has suggested a link between *M. pneumoniae* and extrapulmonary disease.[37] Such antibodies have been produced during mycoplasmal pneumonia and most evidence implies that they are stimulated by antigens cross-reactive with host tissues, such as the I antigen on erythrocytes and glycolipids in brain tissue.[37]

CNS involvement is a major extrapulmonary complication evolving from *M. pneumoniae* infections which occur in approximately 7% of patients with pneumonia.[44] The organisms have been isolated from the cerebrospinal fluid.[14] Meningoencephalitis, aseptic meningitis, transverse myelitis, neuropathies, cerebrovascular thrombosis, cerebellar ataxia, cranial nerve palsies, striatal lesions leading to acute neurologic dysfunction, and sensorineural hearing loss have been reported.[24,31,45-55] The mortality rates from CNS involvement by *Mycoplasma* may reach as high as 10% of patients, with residual neurologic effects being common.[24] *M. pneumoniae* has also been described as a cause of the Guillain-Barré syndrome.[56]

Dermatologic complications arising from extrapulmonary involvement of *M. pneumoniae* infections usually consist of erythematous maculopapular or vesicular rash.[12] In addition, *M. pneumoniae* has been known to be a cause of the Stevens-Johnson syndrome (a bullous form of erythema multiforme) which, if present in the absence of pneumonia, should signal a search for the bacteria.[57-63]

Among other extrapulmonary involvements of *M. pneumoniae*, nonspecific gastrointestinal symptoms have been common.[44] Cardiac disease, although infrequent,[46,64] included myocarditis, pericarditis,[38,65-69] congestive heart failure, hemipericardium, and complete heart block.[24] In addition, *M. pneumoniae* has been isolated from the synovial fluid of a patient with pneumonia and polyarthritis.[70] Leinikki et al.[71] have found that antibodies to *M. pneumoniae* may rise in noninfectious pancreatitis, possibly because of a cross reaction between the mycoplasmal lipid antigen and the pancreatic tissue. In several reports, *M. pneumoniae* has also been associated with ocular infections.[72-75]

20.1.2 *MYCOPLASMA GENITALIUM*

M. genitalium, which was first isolated from the urethra in nongonococcal urethritis (NGU) by Tully et al.,[76] is known to colonize the lower genital tract of both male and female primates. Later, the organism was also isolated together with *M. pneumoniae* from throat specimens with mycoplasmal pneumonia.[77,78] The discovery of both organisms from the human respiratory tract was facilitated by structural similarities (shared epitopes) of their adhesins,[79] the surface proteins that mediate the attachment of mycoplasma to the host epithelial cells. In addition, there has been evidence[80] of shared cross reaction in serological tests between *M. pneumoniae* and *M. genitalium*, including shared membrane proteins and cross-reacting epitopes between their adhesin proteins.[78,79] Definite diagnosis and characterization of the *Mycoplasma* organisms in pulmonary infection may necessitate identification by culture or DNA probe from respiratory secretions or normally sterile body fluids and tissues.[81] In this regard, the commercial cDNA probe procedures may have deficiencies (detecting levels only from 50,000 to 100,000 organisms),[82] thereby precluding clear distinction between *M. pneumoniae* and *M. genitalium*. Proper diagnostic techniques may require the use of genome amplification procedures, involving use of the full nucleotide sequence of dominant adhesin proteins of both organisms (which are known) and the selection as primers of gene fragments specific for each organism.[83-85] Another diagnostic approach may involve the use of unique epitopes on the adhesins[79] or other components of these two mycoplasmas[86] as antigens in serological testing.

20.2 STUDIES ON THERAPEUTICS

20.2.1 FLUOROQUINOLONES

The fluoroquinolones (4-oxoquinolines) are a class of antibiotics structurally related to nalidixic acid (a 1,8-naphthyridine analog), and known for their antibacterial activity primarily by inhibiting the subunit A of the bacterial DNA gyrase.[87-90] The latter enzyme is a type II topoisomerase which controls the shape and functioning of the bacterial DNA through its unique supercoiling and relaxing activities.[91,92] By introducing negative superhelical twists into double-stranded DNA, the DNA gyrase allows DNA replication and facilitates DNA synthesis, repair, recombination, and transposition.[93,94] The inhibition of DNA gyrase will lead to uncontrolled synthesis of mRNA and protein, extensive filamentation and vacuole formation, and degradation of chromosomal DNA by the exonucleases, ultimately resulting in bacterial destruction.[90,95,96]

While the early quinolones had a relatively limited scope of antibacterial activity, low potency, high frequency of spontaneous bacterial resistance, low serum drug concentrations, and short half-lives, the newer 6-fluoro-3-carboxyquinol-4-one derivatives displayed broad antibacterial activity against a wide variety of Gram-negative and Gram-positive aerobic and facultative anaerobic bacteria, and bacterial strains multiresistant to β-lactam antibiotics and aminoglycosides.[87,97] In addition to their high potency and low incidence of resistance, the fluoroquinolones have a much better pharmacokinetic profile as evidenced by their high oral bioavailability, extensive tissue penetration, low protein binding, and long elimination half-lives.[98] However, with the possible exception of ofloxacin and pefloxacin, the ability of the fluoroquinolones to penetrate into the cerebrospinal fluid has been limited. In the case of pefloxacin, its concentration in the synovial fluid was similar to that in the serum.[99]

In general, the fluoroquinolones tended to accumulate in the macrophages and polymorphonuclear leukocytes.[100]

20.2.1.1 *In Vitro* Potency and *In Vivo* Efficacy of Fluoroquinolones

The *in vitro* activity of the fluoroquinolones against *M. pneumoniae* has been extensively studied.[98,101-108] While *M. pneumoniae* was not susceptible to the progenitor nalidixic acid,[109] the antimicrobial potency clearly improved with the fluoroquinolones. Thus, the minimum inhibitory concentration (MIC_{90}) values of norfloxacin, pefloxacin, ciprofloxacin, ofloxacin, defloxacin, lomefloxacin, fleroxacin, sparfloxacin, PD 127391, and WIN 57272 were 12.5,[110] 2.0,[105] 1.0 to 2.0,[101,104-106] 1.0 to 2.0,[102,105] 8.0,[104] 4.0 to 8.0,[102,108] 8.0,[102] 0.125 to 0.25,[102,107] 0.031,[107] and 0.125[102] µg/ml, respectively; sparfloxacin, PD 127391, and WIN 57272 were considered highly active *in vitro*.[103] The MIC$_{90}$ value of temafloxacin against *M. pneumoniae* was 2.0 µg/ml (0.125 to 4.0 µg/ml).[104,111] Ciprofloxacin was reported bactericidal against *M. pneumoniae* at a concentration of 1.0 µg/ml.[112] The latter was also shown to be effective *in vitro* against *M. hominis*.[101,113,114]

Temafloxacin was also significantly active against *M. hominis* — in two comparative *in vitro* studies, its mean MIC$_{90}$ was 0.125 µg/ml.[89] Other fluoroquinolones active *in vitro* against *M. hominis* included norfloxacin, sparfloxacin, ciprofloxacin, ofloxacin, lomefloxacin, enoxacin, and fleroxacin with MIC$_{90}$ values of 8.0,[115,116] 0.06,[107,117] 0.5 to 2.0,[116,118,119] 1.0 to 2.0,[116,118] 2.0 to 8.0,[108,116,118,119] 8.0,[116] and 2.0 µg/ml,[116] respectively.

Arai et al.[120] investigated the *in vivo* efficacies of temafloxacin, ofloxacin, and ciprofloxacin against *M. pneumoniae* in an experimental hamster pneumonia model. The animals were infected intrathecally and sacrificed 18 h after the final medication. Drug efficacies were determined by the colony-forming units (CFU) of *M. pneumoniae* in the lungs. Temafloxacin and ofloxacin, but not ciprofloxacin, were active when oral administration of 200 mg/kg (once daily) for 5 d was initiated 24 h after infection. Furthermore, continuous administration for 15 d of temafloxacin, but not ofloxacin or ciprofloxacin, significantly reduced the number of viable *M. pneumoniae* in the lungs. The data obtained suggested that temafloxacin and ofloxacin have been effective in the acute phase of the infection and, in addition, that temafloxacin was also effective in the late stage of infection when progressive lung alterations and continuous increases in mycoplasmal growth did occur.[120]

20.2.1.2 Ofloxacin

Structurally, ofloxacin represents a pyridonecarboxylic acid analog of nalidixic acid. It possesses a tricyclic (1,2,3-*de*)-1,4-benzoxazine ring system which differentiates ofloxacin from the other fluoroquinolones. Furthermore, the presence of a C-3-methyl group on the oxazine ring has created an asymmetric center, the spatial orientation of which plays an important role in determining the antimicrobial activity of the molecule. Thus, against Gram-positive and Gram-negative bacteria, (–)-ofloxacin was found to be as much as 100-fold more active than the (+)-enantiomer, and about twice as active as the racemic mixture.[121] In addition, the combination of C-7-piperazinyl ring and the C-6-fluorine substitution improved the oral bioavailability and antibacterial activity of ofloxacin.[96]

The pharmacokinetics of ofloxacin have been characterized by nearly complete bioavailability (95% to 100%), with peak serum concentrations in the range of 2 to 3 mg/l after a 400-mg oral dose, and an average half-life of 5 to 8 h.[96] This extended half-life allows for twice-daily dosing.[122]

Compared with other fluoroquinolones, the ofloxacin elimination has been more dependent on renal clearance, which in turn, may necessitate more frequent dosage adjustments in patients with impaired renal function. One advantage of ofloxacin over other fluoroquinolones is that it is less likely to affect the pharmacokinetics of companion drugs (e.g., theophylline),[123,124] which commonly interact with fluoroquinolones such as ciprofloxacin and enoxacin.[96]

20.2.1.3 Temafloxacin

Among the unique structural features of temafloxacin, a 6-fluoro-7-piperazino-4-quinolone derivative,[125] its *N*-(2,4-difluoro)phenyl ring is thought to be responsible for confering activity against Gram-positive bacteria and water solubility,[126,127] whereas the C-3-methyl group on the piperazinyl ring interfered with the GABA receptor binding, thereby minimizing the potential for CNS effects.[128] The lower lipid solubility of temafloxacin has further limited its ability to cross the blood-brain barrier, thus reducing adverse CNS effects.[129]

Initially, the adverse side effects of temafloxicin were reported to be relatively mild in nature (nausea, dizziness, and headache) for doses of up to 600 mg, b.i.d. given over 7 to 28 d.[125] In 1992, however, the drug was withdrawn from clinical evaluation worldwide because of severe side effects.

20.2.1.4 Compound Q-35

Compound Q-35 is a new fluoroquinolone derivative with broad-spectrum activity against various respiratory pathogens,[130,131] including *M. pneumoniae*.[132] The addition of a 3-methylaminopiperidine ring and a methoxy substituent to the quinolone moiety has structurally differentiated compound Q-35 from other fluoroquinolone compounds.

The *in vitro* potency and *in vivo* efficacy of Q-35 against *M. pneumoniae* suggested myco-plasmacidal activity.[132] The MIC_{50} and minimum bactericidal concentration (MBC_{50}) values were 0.39 and 0.78 μg/ml, respectively. The efficacy of Q-35 was also investigated and compared with that of other fluoroquinolones (ofloxacin, ciprofloxacin) in a hamster model of experimental pneumonia which measured the CFU of *M. pneumoniae* in the lungs. Q-35 and ofloxacin showed efficacy following oral administration of 200 mg/kg daily for 5 d, initiated 24 h after infection, while ciprofloxacin was inactive. Continuous administration of Q-35 for 10 d significantly reduced the number of viable *M. pneumoniae* in the lungs.[132] In addition to being active in the early stage of the infection, like temofloxacin, Q-35 was also effective in the middle and late stages of mycoplasmosis.

20.2.1.5 Bacterial Resistance to Fluoroquinolones

Unfortunately, bacterial resistance to fluoroquinolones has developed quickly, mainly through a single-step mutation in the structure of DNA gyrase.[93] In addition, drug resistance may have also developed from decreased drug permeation, increased efflux, or a combination of both. Compared to older quinolones, however, resistance to the newer generation of fluoroquinolones has been seen less frequently.[93,133,134]

Even though plasmid-mediated resistance has been common in many antibiotics, it has not yet been observed with the quinolones.[94,135]

20.2.2 Macrolide Antibiotics

The newly developed macrolide antibiotics differ from erythromycin in the size of the lactone ring and/or its substitution pattern.[136] For example, roxithromycin, dirithromycin, clarithromycin, and flurithromycin all possess a 14-membered lactone ring, whereas azithromycin contains a 15-membered ring, and rokitamycin and miokamycin belong to the 16-membered ring class of macrolides.[137,138]

Some of the newer macrolides have been semisynthetic derivatives derived from the natural products after structural modifications. Thus, 6-*O*-methylerythromycin A (clarithromycin) and 6,11-di-*O*-methylerythromycin A (TE-032), which have been prepared by modifying the C-6-hydroxyl group of erythromycin,[139] showed much better acid stability[140] than the parent erythromycin, which is labile at gastric pH. Another example is RP 59500, a macrolide congener which has been recently developed by structural modifications of pristinamycin (a streptogramin analog).[141]

The major advantage of the newer macrolides over erythromycin has been their improved pharmacokinetic profiles, rather than their *in vitro* potency.[142,143] Erythromycin, although capable of reaching high tissue concentrations, still has poor gastric acid stability and a short half-life, necessitating administration four times daily. While to date, no *M. pneumoniae* strain has been found to be resistant to erythromycin, its effectiveness has been limited by erratic absorption patterns and occasional gastrointestinal intolerance, especially after prolonged use.[144]

Contrary to erythromycin, the newer macrolides possess greater oral bioavailability, longer serum half-lives, higher tissue-to-serum concentration ratios, and especially the ability to sustain high levels in pulmonary tissue or bronchial mucosa[145] that exceeded the MICs for many respiratory pathogens, including *M. pneumoniae*. In addition, some of the macrolides (e.g., clarithromycin[146]) can attain a higher peak concentrations in the serum.

Overall, because of their better pharmacokinetic profiles, the newer macrolide antibiotics can be administered at lower daily doses and at less frequent intervals (once or twice daily) than would be possible with erythromycin.[103]

Since some of the mycoplasmas (*M. fermentans*) can become intracellular,[147] the ability of certain macrolides (e.g., azithromycin, clarithromycin) to penetrate easily into phagocytic cells[148,149] should further increase their therapeutic potential.

The *in vitro* activity of the macrolide antibiotics has been extensively studied.[102,104,108,150-153] The results from the various studies have been very consistent, showing high antimycoplasmal potency, although no direct bactericidal effect against *M. pneumoniae*.[103] The MIC_{90} values of erythromycin, roxithromycin, clarithromycin, azithromycin, rokitamycin, miokamycin, pristinamycin, josamycin, and RP 59500 were in the range of <0.004 to 0.062,[102,108,110,150] <0.01 to 0.03,[151,152] 0.008 to 0.05,[104,108,110,150,152,154] 0.002 to 0.01,[108,152] 0.016 to 0.125,[153] <0.01,[151] 0.05,[151] 0.125,[154] and 0.1 μg/ml,[141] respectively.

20.2.2.1   Clarithromycin

Structurally, clarithromycin represents the 6-*O*-methyl analog of erythromycin.[139] It is well absorbed after oral administration (68% bioavailability). Clarithromycin is 65% to 70% bound to serum proteins, and produces more predictable plasma concentration levels than the parent erythromycin, with a peak concentration at about 2 h.

The major metabolite of clarithromycin is the 14-hydroxyclarithromycin.[155] The latter was not only found to exert equally potent antimicrobial activity, but against certain bacteria, such as *Haemophilus influenzae*, to be even more effective.[156,157] Furthermore, the two compounds are additive, or occasionally synergistic.[149]

Clarithromycin is given orally at doses of 250 to 500 mg, twice daily, depending on the nature and severity of the infection.[149] It has been well tolerated, with less than 3% of patients experiencing nausea, diarrhea, abdominal pain or discomfort, dyspepsia, and taste disorder.

O'Connor and Fris[158] have studied the interactions of clarithromycin and carbamazepine (an anticonvulsant drug prescribed for treatment of tonic-clonic and complex partial seizure disorder). When the two drugs were given together, clarithromycin markedly increased the serum concentrations of carbamazepine, thereby necessitating lowering of the carbamazepine dosage by 30% to 50% during such treatment. Similarly to erythromycin,[159] clarithromycin may interfere with the carbamazepine metabolism through the cytochrome P-450 oxidase enzyme system, resulting in increased carbamazepine serum levels.

20.2.2.2   Roxithromycin

Roxithromycin is an ether-oxime derivative of erythromycin.[160] While the *in vitro* activity of roxithromycin is broader in its scope than that of erythromycin, it is slightly less than that of the *O*-methyl derivative, clarithromycin. In general, its MIC_{90} values of 2.0 mg/l or less, and 2.0 to 4.0 mg/l are indicative, respectively, of full and moderate susceptibility to this antibiotic. Against *M. pneumoniae*, *M. hominis*, and *Ureaplasma urealyticum*, the MIC_{90} values of roxithromycin were 0.03,[152] >55.58,[152,161] and 3.14 mg/l, respectively.[152,161]

The antimicrobial mechanism of action of roxithromycin involved bacterial growth inhibition by binding to the 50S bacterial ribosomal subunit and disrupting the protein synthesis. In drug-resistant bacterial strains, alteration in the ribosomal subunit prevented binding.[162] This pattern of drug resistance has been observed in all of the 14-membered ring macrolides, and nearly complete cross-resistance between roxithromycin and erythromycin has been reported *in vitro*.[163]

There have been conflicting reports with regard to the effects of roxithromycin on *in vitro* and *ex vivo* human macrophage chemotaxis.[164-167] Studies have found either no effect[164] or stimulation of human neutrophil locomotion.[165-167] Furthermore, roxithromycin appeared not to impede the normal cytokine production by monocytes.[168]

While roxithromycin was weakly and nonspecifically bound to albumin (15.6% to 26.7%), it is strongly, specifically, and saturably bound to α1-acid glycoprotein. The maximum value of protein binding was 96.4% and was reached at concentrations of 2.5 mg/l.[169]

The peak plasma concentrations (C_{max}) of roxithromycin following oral administration of 150-mg dose were in the range 6.61 to 7.9 mg/l,[169-171] and between 9.1 and 11.02 mg/l after a 300-mg dose. On average, the C_{max} levels were reached 1.3 to 2.2 h after the ingestion of the 300-mg dose,[172,173] although in one study[174] it took 3.3 h. When compared to single doses of clarithromycin (500 mg) and azithromycin (500 mg), a 300-mg dose of roxithromycin produced higher C_{max} levels.[160]

The mean elimination half-lives of roxithromycin at 150-mg and 300-mg doses were 8.4 and 15.5 h, respectively,[170,171,175] and considerably longer than that of erythromycin (1.5 to 3 h).[176]

Since administration of roxithromycin 15 min after a standard meal may result in reduced bioavailability,[171,172] it has been recommended that the antibiotic is given at least 15 min before ingestion of food.[160,177] In most clinical protocols, roxithromycin has been used at 300 mg daily, divided into two doses; however, once daily administration has also been evaluated and found equally effective.[178]

20.2.2.3 Azithromycin

Azithromycin (CP-62,993, XZ-450) is a 15-membered macrolide (9-deoxo-9a-aza-9a-methyl-9a-homoerythromycin) analog of erythromycin,[179,180] which was shown to possess a broad antimicrobial activity.[181-187] Azithromycin differs from erythromycin in that it contains a methyl-substituted nitrogen at C-9 of the lactone ring.

The azalide structure of azithromycin has been found to be more stable than erythromycin in the low pH environment of the stomach,[188] thereby contributing to its improved bioavailability.[189] The amphiphilic nature of the azalide molecule may also contribute to the rapid accumulation of azithromycin within cells (macrophages and polymorphonuclear cells), which would serve as delivery vehicles of the antibiotic to the site of infection.[148,190-193]

In general, the pharmacokinetics of azithromycin, as compared with other macrolides (clarithromycin and roxithromycin), are characterized by low, but prolonged serum concentrations and high tissue concentrations.[188] Thus, the azithromycin concentrations in most tissue samples were in the 1.0 to 9.0 mg/kg range between 12 h and 3 d after administration of a single 500-mg oral dose.[189]

The serum protein binding of the antibiotic was concentration-dependent and varied between 50% and 12%.[182]

When tested *in vitro* against *M. pneumoniae*, azithromycin showed a MIC value of 0.001 mg/l, as compared to 0.008 mg/l for erythromycin and tetracycline, and 0.25 mg/l for doxycycline.[194]

20.2.2.4 Flurithromycin

Flurithromycin is a fluorinated macrolide antibiotic with antibacterial spectrum similar to that of erythromycin, as demonstrated in *in vitro* tests.[195] The drug also showed good bioavailability and tissue distribution.[196] Flurithromycin appeared to be tolerated differently than other conventional macrolides. It has been found that its influence on the hepatic enzymes was much less than that of erythromycin.[197] In addition, flurithromycin elicited a marked reduction or even abolition of intestinal flora without overgrowth of pathogenic species.[198]

The hepatic and intestinal effects of flurithromycin and erythromycin in female Sprague-Dawley rats have been investigated by Benoni et al.[199] The antibiotic was given orally at 30 to 100 mg/kg. Contrary to erythromycin, which is known to significantly decrease the levels of hepatic drug-metabolizing enzymes (cytochrome b5, cytochrome P-450, and aminopyrine N-demethylase) by forming a cytochrome P-450-Fe(II) metabolite complex,[200] flurithromycin did not interact with the hepatic drug-metabolizing enzymes, possibly by not forming the P-450-Fe(II) metabolite complex.[201] Furthermore, erythromycin is known to moderately influence the intestinal microbial flora. This effect by erythromycin may have some clinical implications by enabling resistant bacteria to overgrow and induce intestinal side effects.[202,203] By comparison, flurithromycin had marked inhibitory effect on some bacterial species (e.g., *Bacteroides*) which are known for their ability to facilitate the colonization of the intestines by pathogenic bacteria.[199]

20.2.2.5 Dirithromycin

Dirithromycin is a new macrolide with spectrum of antimicrobial activity similar to that of erythromycin but with enhanced pharmacokinetic properties, which include relatively high tissue concentrations but low plasma concentrations. *In vivo*, dirithromycin is converted into erythromycylamine, a metabolite which itself has shown potent antimicrobial activity and long half-life of 20 to 50 h.[204] As a result, dirithromycin can be administered at once-daily dose.

20.2.2.6 Terdecamycin

Terdecamycin is a new macrolide antibiotic that is a chemically modified analog of the sedecamycin. It showed highly potent activity against mycoplasmas in animal models. When tested against an experimentally induced *M. hyopneumoniae* infection in pigs, terdecamycin at 50 ppm and 200 ppm significantly alleviated the symptoms of pneumonia.[205]

20.2.3 ROLE OF HORMONES IN GENITAL MYCOPLASMAS

Studies by Furr and Taylor-Robinson[206,207] have demonstrated that the proportion of mice that can be infected intravaginally with *M. pulmonis* was larger when the animals were pretreated with progesterone, as were both the number of organisms recovered and the duration of infection. However, when the mice were treated with estrogen, such enhancement did not occur. Conversely, infection of the murine genital tract by either *M. hominis* or *Ureaplasma urealyticum* was enhanced by pretreating mice with estrogen[208-210] but not with progesterone. These findings have raised the possibility that genital mycoplasmal infections may be controlled by treating mice during infection with the hormone that did not induce susceptibility or enhance infection. Indeed, when progesterone-treated TO or BALB/c mice have been infected intravaginally with *M. pulmonis*, and then given estradiol (which changed their reproductive cycle to the estrous phase), the pathogen for the most part was eradicated.[211] The majority of mice not treated with estradiol continued to shed organisms from the vagina for at least 91 d. In a separate experiment by the same investigators, estradiol-treated BALB/c mice were infected intravaginally with *M. hominis*, and treated 1 month later with progesterone (which changed their reproductive cycle to the diestrous phase). The treatment resulted in pathogen eradication in all mice within 1 month; the majority of mice not given progesterone continued to shed organisms for at least 167 d.[211]

The results of these studies have suggested the possibility of hormones to influence vaginal mycoplasmal infections by changing the vaginal colonization pattern following hormonal changes.[212] As demonstrated in mice, in animals already colonized by mycoplasmas, reversion of the cycle by hormone treatment to the phase that was known not to be conducive to vaginal colonization was soon followed by loss of the organisms.[211]

20.3 EVOLUTION OF THERAPIES AND TREATMNET OF MYCOPLASMA INFECTIONS

20.3.1 MYCOPLASMA PNEUMONIAE INFECTIONS

After attachment to the respiratory epithelium, *M. pneumoniae* produces hydrogen peroxide and superoxide, causing injury to the epithelial cells and their associated cilia. The resulting ciliostasis may explain, at least in part, the observed prolonged cough associated with *M. pneumoniae* infections.[24,31]

In human pulmonary infections, *M. pneumoniae* may be suppressed by proper antibiotic treatment but still may remain viable even in convalescence.[213] The antibodies did not eliminate the carrier state.[32]

There have been no reports in the literature to suggest that *M. pneumoniae* infections are opportunistic. However, such infections may be more severe in immunocompromised hosts as compared to healthy individuals.[214,215]

Tetracycline and erythromycin have been found to be equally effective in the treatment of *M. pneumoniae* infections.[12] Although prolonged therapy may be needed (2 to 3 weeks),[31] both antibiotics were capable of reducing the duration of respiratory symptoms.

Recommended dose regimens for *M. pneumoniae* pneumonia in adults consisted of erythromycin (0.5 g, t.i.d.), or tetracycline (250 to 500 mg, four times daily), or doxycycline (100 mg, b.i.d.) given for 10 to 14 d.[18,216] In severe illness, the doses may be increased and the duration of treatment extended to 3 weeks. Intravenous administration of erythromycin has also been suggested in more serious conditions. For children less than 8 years old, oral erythromycin has been the drug of choice at doses of 30 to 50 mg/kg daily for 10 to 14 d.[18]

Since ciprofloxacin has shown variable activity against *M. pneumoniae*,[217] it is not recommended for therapy against this organism.[218,219]

An enhanced therapeutic efficacy has been envisioned for the newer generation of macrolide antibiotics (clarithromycin, azithromycin, roxithromycin, and dirithromycin) and fluoroquinolones (norfloxacin, pefloxacin, ciprofloxacin, ofloxacin, enoxacin, lomefloxacin, temafloxacin, and sparfloxacin) because of their improved microbiologic and pharmacokinetic properties, such as better absorption by the gastrointestinal tract than erythromycin, resulting in higher concentrations in tissue and cells.[103,220,221]

In a double-blind, multicenter and randomized trial, Cassell et al.[150] have evaluated the clinical efficacy of clarithromycin against community-acquired *M. pneumoniae* pneumonia and compared it with that of erythromycin. Patients received clarithromycin at either 250 or 500 mg, b.i.d., or erythromycin at either 250 or 500 mg, four times daily, for a maximum of 14 d; approximately one third of the patients received the higher dosages. Both drugs were effective in the treatment of pneumonia with no statistically significant or clinically important differences.[150] The findings of Cassell et al.[150] were corroborated by results from another multicenter, double-blind trial conducted in Canada and Sweden, where patients with community-acquired pneumonia were randomized to receive either oral clarithromycin at 250 mg, b.i.d., or oral erythromycin (500 mg, four times daily) for 7 to 14 d,[222] and by an earlier study by Anderson et al.[223] who demonstrated that clarithromycin and erythromycin had comparable clinical success rates (over 90%) among patients with community-acquired pneumonia.

Results from a 10-d randomized, comparative study of the efficacy and tolerance of roxithromycin (300 mg daily) and doxycycline (100 mg daily) in the treatment of women with positive endocervical cultures for *Chlamydia trachomatis* and *Mycoplasma* spp., have shown that *M. hominis* was eradicated in 100% of the cases by doxycycline and in 85% of cases by roxithromycin.[224] Against *U. urealyticum* the corresponding values were 73% and 87% for roxithromycin and doxycycline, respectively. However, the incidence of side effects for doxycycline were significantly more than that recorded for roxithromycin.

One of the first studies using azithromycin in the treatment of atypical pneumonia was conducted by Schönwald et al.[225] In an open, randomized, multicenter trial, its clinical efficacy was compared to that of erythromycin. Azithromycin was administered for 5 d at a dosage of 250 mg twice daily on day 1, and 250 mg once daily on days 2 to 5; erythromycin was given for 10 d at 500 mg, four times daily. Of the 50 patients treated with azithromycin, *M. pneumoniae* and *Chlamydia psittaci* were recovered from 31 and 8 patients, respectively; the corresponding numbers in the 44 patients treated with erythromycin were 24 and 8, respectively. With no therapeutic failures in each group, and very few side effects, azithromycin appeared to be as effective as erythromycin in the treatment of atypical pneumonia. In a follow-up study by the same investigators,[226] all 84 patients with atypical pneumonia were treated with a total dose of 1.5 g. The 41 patients of group A were treated with azithromycin for 3 d at 500 mg once daily, whereas 43 patients of group B received a 5-d course starting with 250 mg, b.i.d. on day 1, followed by 250 mg once daily on days 2 to 5. All patients were clinically cured by day 4, with most of them becoming afibrile within 48 h of starting treatment. Overall, the 1.5-g total dose of azithromycin was equally effective when administered either as a 3- or 5-d regimen.[226]

The efficacy and safety of azithromycin vs. erythromycin in the treatment of acute non-nosocomial infections of the upper and lower respiratory tract in children have been investigated in an open, randomized and multicenter trial.[227] Azithromycin was administered to 77 patients at a dose of 10 mg/kg daily (once daily for 3 d), or 10 mg/kg daily on day 1 followed by 5.0 mg/kg daily on days 2 to 5; erythromycin was given to 74 patients as an oral suspension at 50 mg/kg daily, t.i.d. for at least 7 d. Both drugs were administered at least 1 h before, or 2 h after, meals. While clinical cure was achieved in 94.8% of the azithromycin group, and in 83.3% of the erythromycin group, there was no statistically significant difference in clinical efficacy. Patients with *M. pneumoniae* had a very favorable clinical response to either antibiotic treatment.[227]

The clinical efficacy and safety of dirithromycin and erythromycin were compared in patients with bacterial pneumonia mainly due to *M. pneumoniae* and *Legionella pneumophilia*.[228,229] Patients were randomized to receive either dirithromycin as a single daily dose of 500 mg or erythromycin at 250 mg, four times daily for 10 to 14 d. The response rates in both trials were recorded post-therapy and late post-therapy (2 to 3 weeks after completion of treatment). The results were similar, averaging between 92.0/94.5% and 98.7% for the dirithromycin-treated patients, and between 90.3% and 100% for the erythromycin-receiving group.

In several studies, ofloxacin has been evaluated for treatment of lower respiratory tract infections (pneumonia, acute bronchitis, and exacerbations of chronic obstructive pulmonary disease[230]).[231-234] Thus, in one open, noncomparative trial, the drug was given orally at 400 mg, twice daily for 10 d to patients with community-acquired pneumonia or pathogen-confirmed bronchitis, including three cases of atypical pneumonia due to *M. pneumoniae* which were successfully treated.[232] Peugeot et al.[231] used the same dose regimen (400 mg, b.i.d.) to treat lower respiratory tract infections (pneumonia, bronchitis) caused by *M. pneumonia*, *Legionella pneumophilia*, and in most cases *Chlamydia pneumoniae*, and compared the results with erythromycin (400 mg every 6 h). Clinical cure was achieved with ofloxacin in 63% of patients with pneumonia and in 83% of patients with bronchitis, while clinical cure with erythromycin was achieved in 46% of patients with pneumonia and 54% of patients with bronchitis. Mild gastrointestinal and CNS side effects were observed in several patients receiving either of the two drugs.[231]

In an open, multicenter trial, Mouton et al.[235] have assessed the efficacy of intravenous ofloxacin therapy (200 mg, b.i.d.) followed, when appropriate, by oral administration at the same dose. Dosage adjustments were made in cases of renal failure. Clinical cure against the various pathogens involved (including *M. pneumoniae*) was achieved in 93.5% of patients, suggesting that intravenously administered ofloxacin was an effective treatment for a range of infections due to susceptible organisms.

The clinical efficacy of temafloxacin against lower respiratory tract infections has been compared with those of other quinolone drugs (ciprofloxacin and amoxicillin).[236,237] When administered at 600 mg, b.i.d., temafloxacin compared favorably to ciprofloxacin (500 mg or 750 mg, b.i.d.)[237] and amoxicillin (500 mg, t.i.d.)[236] in achieving clinical cure. However, due to its severe adverse side effects, temafloxacin was withdrawn from worldwide markets in 1992.[238]

Salmi et al.[240,241] studied the clinical efficacy of brodimoprim,[239] an antimicrobial diamino-pyrimidine analog, in the treatment of acute respiratory tract infections. The drug, when given at 400 mg as a loading dose, followed by 200 mg daily, for 10 d, was equally effective to a regimen of doxycycline consisting of 200 mg as a loading dose, followed by 100 mg daily for 10 d.

The spectrum of *M. pneumoniae* CNS infections is variable and may range from mild men-ingismus to severe irreversible neurological impairment.[46,49-51,55,242-245] Cases of acute choreoathetoid movement (an encephalitic disorder) have been relatively rare.[49,52] While CNS involvement in association with *M. pneumoniae* has been observed both with and without respiratory symptoms,[46,243,246] there have been two reports of 45% and 52% incidence of mycoplasmal respiratory infection preceding neurologic involvement.[46,50]

The pathologic mechanism(s) of *M. pneumoniae* encephalitis is still unclear and may involve either a direct invasion of the CNS,[247,248] an autoimmune reaction,[41,249] or a neurotoxin effector released by the mycoplasma itself.[37] With regard to the latter possibility, *M. neurolyticum* and *M. gallisepticum* were found to produce neurotoxin-related neurologic disease in animals; so far, however, no neurotoxin has been associated with *M. pneumoniae*.[244]

Among the various extrapulmonary manifestations of *M. pneumoniae*, development of hemolytic anemia may result from cold hemagglutinin production (an autoimmune disorder).[12,250-254] Cold hemagglutinins are IgM antibodies directed against the Ia antigen on the red blood cell membrane.[252,255,256] The mechanism by which *M. pneumoniae* stimulates the synthesis of autoantibody with anti-Ia antibody specificity is thought to involve either alteration of the erythrocyte Ia antigen by *M. pneumoniae* or antigenic identity between *M. pneumoniae* and erythrocytes.[252,257] Significant hemolysis has been reported to occur, usually in the late stage of infection and only with high titers.[31,250,251,253,254,258] Hemolytic anemia due to cold hemagglutinins is usually classified as either primary (idiopathic) or secondary. While no underlying disorder has been clearly linked to the primary disease, the secondary form has been associated with lympho-proliferative diseases and certain infections (mononucleosis, listeriosis, mumps, subacute bacterial endocarditis, syphilis, trypanosomiasis, malaria, influenza, and infections with *Legionella*, *M. pneumoniae*, cytomegalovirus, and adenoviruses).[255,256,259] Infection with *M. pneumoniae* is by far the most common.[254]

Fink et al.[260] have reported a case of cold hemagglutinin disease complicating *M. pneumoniae* infection in a pediatric cancer patient undergoing cytotoxic chemotherapy. The course of disease was mild (as had been observed in other cases[26,250]) and treatment with josamycin for 10 d and oral prednisolone was successful. Chu et al.[254] have shown association between corticosteroid therapy and decreased severity of the cold hemagglutinin hemolytic anemia. Atkinson et al.[261] have demonstrated in an animal model that high-dose corticosteroids increased the survival of erythrocytes coated with IgM and the C3 complement by decreasing sequestration in the endothelial system. Clinically, high-dose corticosteroids have alleviated hemolysis due to low-titer cold hemagglutinins, most likely by altering the macrophage-complement receptor function.[253]

Idiopathic thrombocytopenic purpura is characterized by thrombocytopenia due to immune-mediated destruction of platelets.[262] Bacterial[263] and protozoal (malaria)[264] infections may occasion-ally be responsible for thrombocytopenia in patients with intermittent or chronic idiopathic thrombo-cytopenic purpura. Veenhoven et al.[265] have described such a case where the thrombocytopenia was associated with *M. pneumoniae*. After treatment with erythromycin for 2 weeks and with prednisone (60 mg daily) for 9 d, the infection was gradually resolved.

Rapid clinical improvement of pericarditis secondary to *M. pneumoniae* infection has been achieved with erythromycin at daily doses of 50 mg/kg.[67-69]

20.3.2 *MYCOPLASMA HOMINIS* INFECTIONS

In women, *M. hominis* is a well-recognized pathogen affecting the genitourinary tract,[25] and the etiologic agent of postpartum fever,[266-268] cesarian section wound infection,[239,269] pyelonephritis,[270,271] and the likely cause of pelvic inflammatory disease.[272] During delivery, the organism may be acquired, causing meningitis,[273] brain abscess,[274] and eye infections.[275] Furthermore, *M. hominis* bacteremia has been reported after abortion and childbirth.[266,267,276] While the majority of reports describing *M. hominis* septicemia following abortion or childbirth have emphasized the benign nature of the infection (even in a severely immunocompromised patient with malignant lymphoma who recovered without antibiotic treatment[277]), Young and Cox[276] have reported a nearly fatal case of puerperal fever due to *M. hominis* following childbirth.

When given at 200 mg, b.i.d. for 10 d, ofloxacin achieved a cure rate of 86% (n = 50) in patients with urogenital infection due to *M. hominis*, and 55% (n = 43) for *Ureaplasma urealyticum*.[88]

The clinical efficacy of ofloxacin was tested and compared with that of erythromycin in a prospective double-blind trial in patients with nongonococcal urethritis with special emphasis on the occurrence of *M. hominis* and *U. urealyticum* infections.[278] The male patients were randomized to receive either ofloxacin (200 mg, b.i.d.) or erythromycin (500 mg, b.i.d.) for 1 week. The clinical efficacy on day 15 was 77.4% in the erythromycin group and 84.3% in the ofloxacin group. While the difference in efficacy was not significant, side effects (mostly gastrointestinal complaints) in patients of the erythromycin group occurred more often (38.5% vs. 21.3% in the ofloxacin group).

The efficacy and safety of ofloxacin (200 mg, b.i.d. for 7 d) were compared with those of metronidazole (400 mg, b.i.d. for 7 d) in the treatment of bacterial vaginosis mainly due to *M. hominis*, *Gardnerella vaginalis*, *Mobiluncus* spp., and *Bacteroides* spp.[279] Diagnostic cure was significantly better in the metronidazole group (56% of patients), as compared with 23% in the ofloxacin-receiving group (*p* = .001). The difference in efficacy was associated with the higher eradication rates for *G. vaginalis* (100% for metronidazole vs. 56% for ofloxacin) and *Bacteroides* spp. (97% and 49%, respectively). Against *M. hominis* the corresponding values for metronidazole and ofloxacin were 56% and 45%, respectively.[279]

In another comparative study, a 7-d course of oral erythromycin (500 mg, b.i.d.) was assessed against oral metronidazole (400 mg, b.i.d.) also administered for 7 d.[280] Again, the results confirmed the clinical superiority of metronidazole in the therapy of bacterial vaginitis: treatment failure occurred in 81% of patients given erythromycin, as compared with only 17% in the metronidazole-receiving group (*p* <.001).

The overall results of the aforementioned studies[279,280] have reaffirmed that metronidazole, at 400 to 500 mg twice daily for 7 d, is the drug of choice for treatment of bacterial vaginitis,[281-284] even though relapse with metronidazole has been fairly common, with at least 20% of patients requiring further treatment within 3 to 4 weeks.[285] Shorter metronidazole therapy has also been encouraged in order to increase compliance and decrease the side effects associated with systemic metronidazole use.[286] A single 2.0-g dose has shown a 69% to 72% cure rate assessed at 4 or more weeks after therapy.[283,284,286] The use of metronidazole as 0.75% gel,[287] tablet,[288] or sponge[289] for treatment of bacterial vaginosis has also been recommended.

The therapeutic efficacy of clindamycin has also been investigated.[290-294] In one study, of the three doses of the antibiotic (0.1%, 1%, or 2% cream) applied intravaginally, the 2% clindamycin application had the greatest effect on the bacterial vaginosis-associated flora resulting in a 94% clinical cure rate.[290] In a double-blinded, randomized trial,[291] similar intravaginal administration of clindamycin (0.1%, 1%, and 2% cream) twice daily for 5 d eradicated and/or decreased the counts of *Gardnerella vaginalis*, *Mobiluncus* spp., and *M. hominis* in 92% of patients, as compared with only 11% in the placebo group (*p* <.0001). There were no significant differences in the clinical cure rates for the 0.1%, 1%, and 2% dose regimens (89%, 88%, 100%, respectively).[291]

The clinical efficacy of ampicillin–sulbactam vs. clindamycin in the treatment of postpartum endomyometritis has been investigated by Martens et al.[295] in an open, randomized, and comparative study. In addition to *Mycoplasma* spp. and *Bacteroides bivius*-associated bacteremia (22%), the most frequent endometrial isolates were *Streptococcus faecalis*, *Escherichia coli*, and *Ureaplasma urealyticum*. Both ampicillin (2.0 g) and sulbactam (1.0 g) were administered intravenously every 6 h, while the clindamycin regimen (900 mg) was given intravenously every 8 h. The resulting clinical cure rates were similar in both groups (83% in the ampicillin–sulbactam group and 88% in the clindamycin group); however, there were more treatment failures against *Mycoplasma* in the ampicillin–sulbactam group.

Rare cases of sternal wound *M. hominis* infections and bacteremia in immunocompetent patients following cardiothoracic surgery[296,297] and prosthetic valve endocarditis[298] have also been described. Since *M. hominis* is known to colonize the upper respiratory tract in only 1% to 3% of healthy individuals,[299] intubation of the respiratory tract or contamination of the wound by respiratory secretions were less likely to have caused these infections.[297]

There have been relatively few *M. hominis* infections in male patients, such as following multiple trauma[300] and surgical interventions of the urinary tract.[301,302]

A combination treatment of intravenous tetracycline (500 mg, four times daily) and erythromycin (1.0 g, four times daily) for 7 d, followed by oral doxycycline (100 mg) for an additional 6 weeks was used by Smyth and Weinbren[296] to eradicate a *M. hominis* sternal wound infection.

Luttrell et al.[303] have described two cases of septic arthritis due to *M. hominis*. The treatment consisted of either oral doxycycline (100 mg, b.i.d.) in one case where the patient did not survive, or combination of vancomycin, gentamicin, and doxycycline in the other. Septic arthritis due to *M. hominis*, which has been diagnosed mainly during the postpartum period in immunosuppressed hosts, or in patients who had recently undergone urinary tract surgery,[300,304-316] has been very difficult to distinguish from septic arthritis caused by other bacteria.[303] In nearly half of the reported cases of septic arthritis, the patients have been immunocompromised[307,309] as the result of immuno-suppressive medication,[308-310,313] hematologic malignancies,[312,313] hypogammaglobulinemia,[313,315,317] and common variable immunodeficiency.[318] In three cases, the patients who were receiving chronic immunosuppressive medication relapsed despite antimycoplasma therapy.[309,310,314]

Webster et al.[319] have demonstrated that the presence of antibody has been critical for inhibition of mycoplasmal growth *in vitro* and that mycoplasmas, including *M. hominis*, when phagocytosed by neutrophils in the absence of antibody, were not eradicated.

Clough et al.[309] have reported a *M. hominis*-associated septic arthritis and bacteremia in a patient with systemic lupus erythematosus. The pathogen was resistant to treatment with various antimicrobial agents, including doxycycline, clindamycin, and ciprofloxacin. However, resolution was achieved by a combination of chemotherapy with temafloxacin (600 mg, b.i.d. orally) and doxycycline (100 mg, b.i.d. orally), arthroscopic drainage of the persistently infected joint, several intravenous infusions of immunoglobulins (which led to increase in the levels of antibodies specific to *M. hominis*), and finally discontinuation of steroid medication.

Several cases of postoperative *M. hominis* infections in liver[320-323] and renal[324] transplant recipients have also been reported. In such cases, treatment with doxycycline[321,322] or ciprofloxacin[320,323] has been recommended. It was recognized that *M. hominis* infections might have been related to the immunosuppression of the organ transplant recipients[277,297] and pericarditis.[38]

Roberts et al.[325] have described a case of *M. hominis*-related respiratory disease in a severely immunocompromised patient with X-linked hypogammaglobulinemia.

Unlike *M. pneumoniae*-induced pneumonia, the one due to *M. hominis* has been extremely rare in immunocompetent individuals.

20.3.3 MYCOPLASMA FERMENTANS (INCOGNITUS STRAIN) INFECTIONS

The newly recognized human pathogenic mycoplasma, *M. fermentans* (incognitus strain) was found to cause a fatal systemic infection in experimental primates.[326] It has also caused systemic infections in patients with AIDS, as well as in HIV-negative individuals.[2,3,147,326-328] *M. fermentans* infections in AIDS patients appeared to be related to dysfunctional deficits of various organ systems (thymus, liver, spleen, lymph node, kidney, and brain), causing dementia, hepatitis, and nephropathy.[3,329]

M. fermentans has also been reported to produce fatal infection in previously healthy non-AIDS patients.[147,330] Postmortem histopathological examination revealed fulminant necrosis involving the lymph nodes, spleen, lungs, adrenal gland, heart, and/or brain.[330] For example, studies by Bauer et al.[329] of tissues recovered from HIV-positive patients with AIDS-associated nephropathy have demonstrated that parenchymal cells such as the epithelial cells of glomeruli and tubules in the kidney were infected with *M. fermentans*. Furthermore, the largest concentrations of mycoplasma were in the basement membranes and in the proteinaceous casts of the infected kidneys. By comparison, kidneys of AIDS patients without disease-associated nephropathy did not reveal similar infection of the parenchymal cells or casts in the renal tubules.[329] Using a highly sensitive and specific polymerase chain reaction (PCR) assay,[5,9] Dawson et al.[4] have identified a high prevalence of *M. fermentans* in the urine of HIV-positive patients.

The pathogenesis of *M. fermentans* infection has been unusual in that despite fulminant tissue necrosis, there has been lymphocyte depletion and an apparent lack of cellular immune response or inflammatory reaction in the infected tissues. To explain this uncommon phenomenon, Lo et al.[147] have postulated that infection with *M. fermentans* may have resulted in either damage to key component of the host's immune system, or that the pathogen may possess special biological properties to elude immunosurveillance by the infected hosts.

In a case of systemic *M. fermentans* in a previously healthy non-AIDS patient, treatment with doxycycline at daily doses of 300 mg for 6 weeks led to full recovery.[330]

20.3.4 MYCOPLASMA PENETRANS INFECTIONS

Unlike most other mycoplasmas, *M. penetrans* has two unusual morphologic features: it is an elongated flask-shaped organism, with two unique but sharply divided internal compartments. While the tip-like compartment is densely packed with fine granules, the body compartment is loosely filled with coarse granules consistent with ribosomal structures.[7] This characteristic feature has also been seen in *M. iowae*,[331] one of two species that were phylogenetically most closely related to *M. penetrans*. Other properties of *M. penetrans* include adherence, hemadsorption, and cytadsorption, and the ability to invade many different types of mammalian cells. This mycoplasma requires cholesterol for its growth, and is capable of fermenting glucose. It also hydrolyzes arginine, but does not hydrolyze urea.[7] The latter biochemical property of *M. penetrans* is shared by *M. iowae* and only a few other mycoplasma species (*M. alvi*, *M. sualvi*, *M. moatsii*, *M. pirum*, and *M. fermentans*).

Lo et al.[1,7] have isolated *M. penetrans* from the urine and urogenital tract of patients with AIDS. The organism has pathogenic properties associated with its *in vivo* virulence. Because *M. penetrans* was identified and isolated from the urogenital tracts of HIV-infected patients, the most likely route of its transmission might have been through sexual contact.

Antibody to this novel mycoplasma was not common among sexually active patients without HIV infection. Thus, using an enzyme-linked immunosorbent assay and Western blotting, Wang et al.[8] have detected more than 100 times higher frequence of antibodies to *M. penetrans* in serum from AIDS patients (40%) as compared with only 0.3% from HIV-negative controls. *M. penetrans*-specific antibodies has also been identified in the serum of 20% of HIV-infected, but symptom-free individuals. The antibodies' major immunoreactivity was directed against P35 and P38, the two major lipid-associated membrane protein antigens of the organism.[8]

20.4 MYCOPLASMAS AS COFACTORS PROMOTING AIDS

There has been evidence supporting the hypothesis that *M. fermentans* may exert a direct impact in promoting AIDS by enhancing the HIV cytocidal effects on CD4$^+$ lymphocytes.[332]

It has been previously shown by Lemaitre et al.[333,334] that HIV-1-infected cultures when treated with antimycoplasmal antibiotics had a significantly reduced cytocidal effect by HIV on T cells, even though they continued to produce high titers of HIV-1. The investigators postulated that a procaryotic agent, most likely a mycoplasma, may have been responsible for the observed increase in the cytocidal effect of the HIV-infected cultures. These results have been further corroborated by the finding that antigens of a killed mycoplasma (*Acholeplasma laidlawii*) could stimulate HIV-1 production (p24 antigen and infectious particles) in HIV-1-infected cells.[335]

The aforementioned research, as well as studies with *M. fermentans* and *M. pirum* have strongly indicated that mycoplasmas may indeed be involved as cofactors increasing the development of AIDS in HIV-positive patients.[10,336-339]

20.5 *IN VITRO* SUSCEPTIBILITY OF *MYCOPLASMA* SPP. TO ANTIMICROBIAL AGENTS AND CLINICAL SIGNIFICANCE

Antimicrobial agents, in general, confer their activities by inhibiting bacterial cell wall synthesis, as well as the cell membrane, folic acid, or protein synthesis, or by interfering with the transfer of genetic information.[340,341]

Because *Mycoplasma* spp. lack rigid cell walls, they are not expected to be sensitive to antibiotics that can impair the cell wall biosynthesis (penicillins and cephalosporins), as well as to agents that interfere with either folic acid synthesis (sulfonamides), bacterial protein biosynthesis (tetracyclines, macrolides, aminoglycosides, and chloramphenicol) or inhibit DNA gyrase (topoisomerase), such as the fluoroquinolones. However, even though antibiotics were not mycoplasmacidal and did not eradicated mycoplasmas from the host, clinical improvement has been observed in some instances despite the persistence of mycoplasmas. In other cases, however, clinical improvement was dependent upon the interaction of the antimicrobial agent and an intact host immune system.[340]

Jao and Finland[342] have found *M. pneumoniae* susceptible to a number of antimicrobial agents, with erythromycin and the tetracyclines shown to exert clinical benefits by reducing the symptoms of respiratory illness in patients with *M. pneumoniae* infections. However, the clinical response was not associated with the elimination of the pathogen from the respiratory secretions.[213] Furthermore, while administration of antimicrobial agents with *in vitro* activity against *M. pneumoniae* to family contacts of persons with mycoplasmal pneumonia prevented the development of clinical disease, it did not prevent infection among such contacts.[343]

M. genitalium, which shares many features with *M. pneumoniae*, was found by Renaudin et al.[109] to have similar susceptibility *in vitro* as *M. pneumoniae* to various macrolides, tetracyclines, and fluoroquinolones.

M. hominis strains have been generally resistant to erythromycin, aminoglycosides, β-lactams, vancomycin, sulfonamides, and trimethoprim.[344,345] *In vitro* susceptibility testing has shown sensitivities to tetracyclines,[297,344,346,347] lincomycin, and clindamycin,[348] and moderate susceptibility to chloramphenicol and rifampin. However, in several studies, an increasing *M. hominis* resistance to tetracyclines (including doxycycline) has been well documented.[344,345,349,350] In some instances, the tetracycline resistance of *M. hominis* has been related to its acquisition of DNA sequences homologous to the streptococcal ^{TET}M plasmid.[309,351] To this end, tetracycline-resistant isolates of *Ureaplasma* (family Mycoplasmataceae), a closely associated genus of pleomorphic, Gram-negative bacteria that also lack bacterial cell walls, have also been recovered.[352] Roberts and Kenny[353,354] and others[355-357] have shown that these tetracycline-resistant ureaplasmas also contained the ^{TET}M plasmid.

Several groups of investigators[102,104,358,359] have studied the activity of a number of newer macrolide antibiotics, such as spectinomycin and trospectomycin (a spectinomycin analog) against *M. hominis*. Using the agar dilution method, Echaniz Avilés et al.[358] have found that 120 strains of *M. hominis* were 100% resistant to erythromycin, azithromycin, clarithromycin, and roxithromycin, with MIC values in the range of 32 to 256, 32 to 256, 32 to 128, and 32 to 256 mg/l, respectively; by comparison, the corresponding values of the two most active compounds, spectinomycin and trospectomycin, were 8 to 62 and 2 to 128 mg/l, which translated to 30% and 10% resistance, respectively.

In vitro, *M. fermentans* has been shown to be resistant to penicillin, ampicillin, and erythromycin, but susceptible to tetracycline, doxycycline, chloramphenicol, and ciprofloxacin, with MIC values of 0.5 µg/ml or less.[360] Contrary to *M. pneumoniae*, which was very susceptible to erythromycin (MIC = 0.0073 µg/ml), two strains of *M. fermentans* (PG18 and the incognitus strain) were resistant, with MIC values of 31.2 and 43 µg/ml, respectively.

Since the peak serum concentration of erythromycin has been determined to be about 1.1 µg/ml,[361] the reported *in vitro* data were very much in agreement with the observed clinical results, where *M. pneumoniae* infection (but not *M. fermentans*) has responded to treatment with erythromycin.

Poulin et al.[10] have also investigated *in vitro* the antibiotic susceptibility of *M. fermentans*, and compared it with that of other AIDS-associated mycoplasmas (*M. penetrans* and *M. pirum*). Strains of all three mycoplasmas were susceptible to doxycycline, tetracycline, clindamycin, and clarithromycin at the attainable serum levels of 1.6, 1.6, 2.0, and 3.4 µg/ml, respectively.

20.6 REFERENCES

1. Lo, S.-C., Hayes, M. M., Wang, R. Y.-H., Pierce, P. F., Kotani, H., and Shih, J. W.-K., Newly discovered mycoplasma isolated from patients infected with AIDS, *Lancet*, 338, 1415, 1991.
2. Lo, S.-C., Shih, J. W.-K., Yang, N.-Y., Ou, C.-Y., and Wang, R. Y., A novel virus-like infectious agent in patients with AIDS, *Am. J. Trop. Med. Hyg.*, 40, 213, 1989.
3. Lo, S.-C., Dawson, M. S., Wong, D. M., Newton, P. B. III, Sonoda, M. A., Engler, W. F., Wang, R. Y.-H., Shih, J. W.-K., Alter, H. J., and Wear, D. J., Identification of *Mycoplasma incognitus* infection in patients with AIDS: an immunohistochemical, *in situ* hybridization and ultrastructural study, *Am. J. Trop. Med. Hyg.*, 41, 601, 1989.
4. Dawson, M. S., Hayes, M. M., Wang, R. Y.-H., Armstrong, D., Kundsin, R. B., and Lo, S.-C., Detection and isolation of *Mycoplasma fermentans* from urine of HIV-1 infected patients, *Arch. Pathol. Lab. Med.*, 117, 511, 1993.
5. Wang, R. Y.-H., Hu, W. S., Dawson, M. S., Shih, J. W.-K., and Lo, S.-C., Selective detection of *Mycoplasma fermentans* by polymerase chain reaction and by using a nucleotide sequence within the insertion sequence-like element, *J. Clin. Microbiol.*, 30, 245, 1992.
6. Behbahani, N., Blanchard, A., Cassell, G. H., and Montagnier, L., Phylogenetic analysis of *Mycoplasma penetrans*, isolated from HIV infected patients, *FEMS Microbiol. Lett.*, 109, 63, 1993.
7. Lo, S.-C., Hayes, M. M., Tully, J. G., Wang, R. Y.-H., Kotani, H., Pierce, P. F., Rose, D. L., and Shih, J. W., *Mycoplasma penetrans* sp. nov., from the urogenital tract of patients with AIDS, *Int. J. Syst. Bacteriol.*, 42, 357, 1992.
8. Wang, R. Y.-H., Shih, J. W., Grandinetti, T., Pierce, P. F., Hayes, M. M., Wear, D. J., Alter, H. J., and Lo, S.-C., High frequency of antibodies to *Mycoplasma penetrans* in HIV-infected patients, *Lancet*, 340, 1312, 1992.
9. Grau, O., Kovacic, R., Griffais, R., and Montagnier, L., Development of a selective and sensitive polymerase chain reaction assay for the detection of *Mycoplasma pirum*, *FEMS Microbiol. Lett.*, 106, 327, 1993.
10. Poulin, S. A., Perkins, R. E., and Kundsin, R. B., Antibiotic susceptibilities of AIDS-associated mycoplasmas, *J. Clin. Microbiol.*, 32, 1101, 1994.

11. Reimann, H. A., An acute infection of the respiratory tract with atypical pneumonia, *JAMA,* 111, 2377, 1938.
12. Martin, R. E. and Bates, J. H., Atypical pneumonia, *Infect. Dis. Clin. North Am.*, 5, 585, 1991.
13. Cunha, B. A. and Quintiliani, R., The atypical pneumonia: a diagnostic and therapeutic approach, *Postgrad. Med. J.*, 66, 96, 1979.
14. Donowitz, G. R. and Mandell, G. L., Acute pneumonia, in *Principles and Practice of Infectious Disease*, 3rd ed., Mandell, G. L., Douglas, R. G., and Bennett, J. M., Eds., Churchill Livingston, New York, 1990, 540.
15. George, R., Aiskind, M., Rasch, J., and Rasch, J. R., *Mycoplasma* and adenovirus pneumonias: comparison with other atypical pneumonias in a military population, *Ann. Intern. Med.*, 65, 931, 1966.
16. Johnson, D. H. and Cunha, B. A., Atypical pneumonias: clinical and extrapulmonary features of *Chlamydia*, *Mycoplasma*, and *Legionella* infections, *Postgrad. Med. J.*, 93, 69, 1993.
17. Sue, D. Y., Community-acquired pneumonia in adults, *West. J. Med.*, 161, 383, 1994.
18. Schlick, W., The problems of treating atypical pneumonia, *J. Antimicrob. Chemother.*, 31(Suppl. C), 111, 1993.
19. Hirschmann, J. V. and Murray, J. F., Pneumonia and lung abscess, in *Harrison's Principles of Internal Medicine*, 11th ed., Wilson, J. D., Braunwald, E., Isselbacher, K. J., Petersdorf, R. G., Martin, J. B., Fauci, A. S., and Root, R. K., Eds., McGraw-Hill, New York, 1987, 1075.
20. Ruuskanen, O., Nohynek, H., Ziegler, T., Capeding, R., Rikalainen, H., Huovinen, P., and Leinonen, M., Pneumonia in childhood: etiology and response to antimicrobial therapy, *Eur. J. Clin. Microbiol. Infect. Dis.*, 11, 217, 1992.
21. Stark, J. M., Lung infections in children, *Curr. Opin. Pediatr.*, 5, 273, 1993.
22. Fass, R. J., Aetiology and treatment of community-acquired pneumonia in adults: a historical perspective, *J. Antimicrob. Chemother.*, 32(Suppl. A), 17, 1993.
23. Woodhead, M., Pneumonia in the elderly, *J. Antimicrob. Chemother.*, 34(Suppl. A), 85, 1994.
24. Cassell, G. and Cole, B., Mycoplasmas as agents of human disease, *N. Engl. J. Med.*, 304, 80, 1981.
25. Wendel, P. J. and Wendel, G. D., Jr., Sexually transmitted diseases in pregnancy, *Semin. Perinatol.*, 17, 443, 1993.
26. Foy, H. M., Kenny, G., Cooney, M., and Allen, I. D., Long-term epidemiology of infections with *Mycoplasma pneumoniae*, *J. Infect. Dis.*, 139, 681, 1979.
27. Eaton, M. D., Meiklejohn, G., and van Herick, W., Studies on the etiology of primary atypical pneumonia: a filterable agent transmissible to cotton rats, hamsters, and chick embryos, *J. Exp. Med.*, 79, 649, 1944.
28. Chanock, R. M., Hauflick, L., and Barile, M. F., Growth on artificial medium of an agent associated with atypical pneumonia and its identification as a PPLO, *Proc. Natl. Acad. Sci. U.S.A.*, 48, 41, 1962.
29. Chanock, R. M., Mufson, M. A., Bloom, H. H., James, W. D., Fox, H. H., and Kingston, J. R., Eaton agent pneumonia, *JAMA,* 175, 213, 1961.
30. Collier, A. M. and Clyde, W. A., Relationships between *Mycoplasma pneumoniae* and human respiratory epithelium, *Infect. Immun.*, 3, 694, 1971.
31. Couch, R. B., *Mycoplasma pneumoniae* (primary atypical pneumonia), in *Principles and Practice of Infectious Disease*, 3rd ed., Mandell, G. L., Douglas, R. G., and Bennett, J. M., Eds., Churchill Livingstone, New York, 1990, 1446.
32. Luby, J. P., Southwestern Internal Medical Conference: pneumonias in adults due to Mycoplasma, Chlamidiae, and viruses, *Am. J. Med. Sci.*, 294, 45, 1987.
33. Mizutani, H. and Mizutani, H., Immunoglobulin M rheumatoid factor in patients with mycoplasmal pneumonia, *Am. Rev. Respir. Dis.*, 134, 1237, 1986.
34. Cotton, E. M., Strampfer, M. J., and Cunha, B. A., *Legionella* and *Mycoplasma* pneumonia: a community hospital experience with atypical pneumonias, *Clin. Chest Med.*, 12, 237, 1987.
35. Mufson, M. A., Manko, M. A., Kingston, J. R., and Channock, R. M., Eaton agent pneumonia — clinical features, *JAMA,* 178, 369, 1961.
36. MacFarlane, J. T., Miller, A. C., Smith, W. H., Morris, A. H., and Rose, D. H., Comparative radiographic features of community acquired legionnaires' disease, pneumococcal pneumonia, mycoplasma pneumonia, and psittacosis, *Thorax*, 39, 28, 1984.

37. Fernald, G. W., Immunological mechanisms suggested in the association of *Mycoplasma pneumoniae* and extrapulmonary disease: a review, *Yale J. Biol. Med.*, 56, 475, 1983.
38. Kenney, R. T., Li, J. S., Clyde, W. A., Wall, T. C., O'Connor, C. M., Campbell, P. T., Van Trigt, P., and Corey, G. R., Mycoplasmal pericarditis: evidence of invasive disease, *Clin. Infect. Dis.*, 17(Suppl. 1), S58, 1993.
39. Lind, K., Manifestations and complications of *Mycoplasma pneumoniae* disease: a review, *Yale J. Biol. Med.*, 56, 461, 1983.
40. Chen, S., Tsai, C. C., and Nouri, S., Carditis associated with *Mycoplasma pneumoniae* infection, *Am. J. Dis. Child.*, 140, 471, 1986.
41. Biberfield, G. and Norberg, R., Circulating immune complexes in *Mycoplasma pneumoniae* infection, *J. Immunol.*, 112, 413, 1974.
42. Loomes, L. M., Uemura, K.-I., and Feizi, T., Interaction of *Mycoplasma pneumoniae* with erythrocyte glycolipids of I and i antigen types, *Infect. Immun.*, 47, 15, 1985.
43. Fernald, G. W., Immunologic interactions between host cells and mycoplasmas: an introduction, *Rev. Infect. Dis.*, 49(Suppl.), S201, 1982.
44. Mansel, J., Rosenow, E. C. III, and Martin, J. W., Jr., *Mycoplasma pneumoniae* pneumonia, *Chest*, 95, 639, 1989.
45. Nishioka, K., Masuda, Y., Okada, S., Takata, N., Tasaka, S., and Ogura, Y., Bilateral sensorineural hearing loss associated with *Mycoplasma pneumoniae* pneumonia, *Laryngoscope*, 97, 1203, 1987.
46. Pönkä, A., Carditis associated with *Mycoplasma pneumoniae* infection, *Acta Med. Scand.*, 206, 77, 1979.
47. Thomas, N. H., Collins, J. E., Robb, S. A., and Robinson, R. O., *Mycoplasma pneumoniae* infection and neurological disease, *Arch. Dis. Child.*, 69, 573, 1993.
48. Cimolai, N., Mycoplasma pneumoniae, *Arch. Dis. Child.*, 71, 281, 1994.
49. Beskind, D. L. and Keim, S. M., Choreoathetotic movement disorder in a boy with *Mycoplasma pneumoniae* encephalitis, *Ann. Emerg. Med.*, 23, 1375, 1994.
50. Lehtokoski-Lehtiniemi, E. and Koskiniemi, M., *Mycoplasma pneumoniae* encephalitis: a severe entity in children, *Pediatr. Infect. Dis. J.*, 8, 651, 1989.
51. Lind, K., Zoffman, H., and Larssen, S. O., *Mycoplasma pneumoniae* infections associated with affection of the central nervous system, *Acta Med. Scand.*, 205, 325, 1979.
52. Al-Mateen, M., Gibbs, M., Dietrich, R., Mitchell, W. G., and Menkes, J. H., Encephalitis lethargica-like illness in a girl with mycoplasma infection, *Neurology*, 38, 1155, 1988.
53. Saitoh, S., Wada, T., Narita, M., Kohsaka, S., Mizukami, S., Togashi, T., and Kajii, N., *Mycoplasma pneumoniae* infection may cause striatal lesions leading to acute neurologic dysfunction, *Neurology*, 43, 2150, 1993.
54. Thomas, N. H., Collins, J. E., Robb, S. A., and Robinson, R. O., *Mycoplasma pneumoniae* infection and neurologic disease, *Arch. Dis. Child.*, 69, 573, 1993.
55. Evans, M. R. W. and Marshall, A. J., Recovery from mycoplasma meningoencephalitis, credited to penicillin allergy, *Lancet*, 335, 1100, 1990.
56. Hodges, G. R. and Perkins, R. L., Landry-Guillain-Barré syndrome associated with *Mycoplasma pneumoniae* infection, *JAMA*, 210, 2088, 1969.
57. Adunsky, A., Steiner, Z. P., Eframian, A., and Klajman, A., Stevens-Johnson syndrome associated with *Mycoplasma pneumoniae* infection, *Cutis*, 40, 123, 1987.
58. Ludlam, G. B., Bridges, J. B., and Benn, E. C., Association of Stevens-Johnson syndrome with antibody for *Mycoplasma pneumoniae*, *Lancet*, 2, 958, 1964.
59. Foy, H. M., Kenny, G. E., and Koler, J., *Mycoplasma pneumoniae* in Stevens-Johnson syndrome, *Lancet*, 2, 550, 1966.
60. Sanders, D. Y. and Johnson, H. W., Stevens-Johnson syndrome associated with *Mycoplasma pneumoniae* infection, *Am. J. Dis. Child.*, 121, 243, 1971.
61. Sontheimer, R. D., Garibaldi, R. A., and Krueger, G. G., Stevens-Johnson syndrome associated with *Mycoplasma pneumoniae* infections, *Arch. Dermatol.*, 114, 241, 1978.
62. Levy, M. and Shear, N. H., *Mycoplasma pneumoniae* infections and Stevens-Johnson syndrome, *Clin. Pediatr.*, 30, 42, 1991.
63. Salmon, P. and Rademaker, M., Erythema multiforme associated with an outbreak of *Mycoplasma pneumoniae* function, *NZ Med. J.*, 106, 449, 1993.

64. Sands, M. J., Saty, J. E., Turner, J. E., Jr., and Soloff, L. A., Pericarditis and perimyocarditis associated with active *Mycoplasma pneumoniae* infection, *Ann. Intern. Med.*, 86, 544, 1977.

65. Greyston, J. T., Alexander, E. R., Kenny, G. E., Clarke, E. R., Fremont, J. C., and MacColl, W. A., *Mycoplasma pneumoniae* infections: clinical and epidemiologic studies, *JAMA*, 191, 369, 1965.

66. Naftalin, J. M., Wellisch, G., Kahana, Z., and Diengott, D., *Mycoplasma pneumoniae* septicemia, *JAMA*, 228, 565, 1974.

67. Belaguer, A., Boronat, M., and Carrascosa, A., Successful treatment of pericarditis associated with *Mycoplasma pneumoniae* infection, *Pediatr. Infect. Dis. J.*, 9, 141, 1990.

68. Cahen, R., Orgiazzi, J., Loiffet, O., Gardere, J., and Despierres, G., Pericardite aiguë isolée due probablement a *Mycoplasma pneumoniae*, *Nouv. Presse Med.*, 8, 525, 1979.

69. Lopez Vivancos, J., Vilaseca, J., Arnau, J. M., and Guardia, J., Pleuropericarditis por *Mycoplasma pneumoniae*, *Med. Clin. (Barcelona)*, 83, 694, 1984.

70. Davis, C. P., Cochran, S., Lisse, J., Buck, G., DiNuzzo, A. R., Weber, T., and Reinharz, J. A., Isolation of *Mycoplasma pneumoniae* from synovial fluid samples in a patient with pneumonia and polyarthritis, *Arch. Int. Med.*, 148, 969, 1988.

71. Leinikki, P. O., Panzar, R., and Tykka, H., Immunoglobulin M antibody response against *Mycoplasma pneumoniae* lipid antigen in patients with acute pancreatitis, *J. Clin. Microbiol.*, 8, 113, 1978.

72. Murray, H. W., Masur, H., Senterfit, L. B., and Roberts, R. B., The protean manifestations of *Mycoplasma pneumoniae* infection in adults, *Am. J. Med.*, 58, 229, 1975.

73. Tuazon, C. U. and Murray, H. W., Atypical pneumoniae, in *Respiratory Infections: Diagnosis and Management*, 2nd ed., Pennington, J. E., Ed., Raven Press, New York, 1988, 346.

74. Salzman, M. B., Sood, S. K., Slavin, M. L., and Rubin, L. G., Ocular manifestations of *Mycoplasma pneumoniae* infection, *Clin. Infect. Dis.*, 14, 1137, 1992.

75. Cordonnier, M., Caspers-Velu, L. E., Jacquemin, C., Van Nechel, C., and Tombroff, M., Bilateral optic neuropathy and white dot syndrome following a mycoplasmal infection, *Br. J. Ophthalmol.*, 77, 673, 1993.

76. Tully, J. G., Taylor-Robinson, D., Cole, R. M., and Rose, D. L., A newly discovered mycoplasma in the human urogenital tract, *Lancet*, 1, 1288, 1981.

77. Tully, J. G. and Baseman, J. B., Mycoplasma, *Lancet*, 337, 1296, 1991.

78. Baseman, J. B., Dallo, S. F., Tully, J. G., and Rose, D. L., Isolation and characterization of *Mycoplasma genitalium* strains from the human respiratory tract, *J. Clin. Microbiol.*, 26, 2266, 1988.

79. Morrison-Plummer, J., Lazzell, A., and Baseman, J. B., Shared epitopes between *Mycoplasma pneumoniae* major adhesin protein P1 and a 140 kilodalton protein of *Mycoplasma genitalium*, *Infect. Immun.*, 55, 49, 1987.

80. Taylor-Robinson, D., Furr, P. M., and Tully, J. G., Serological cross-reaction between *Mycoplasma genitalium* and *M. pneumoniae*, *Lancet*, 1, 527, 1983.

81. Hauger, S. B., Approach to the pediatric patient with HIV infection and pulmonary symptoms, *J. Pediatr.*, 119, S26, 1991.

82. Shaw, S. B., DNA probes for the detection of *Legionella* species, *Mycoplasma pneumoniae*, and members of the *Mycobacterium tuberculosis* complex, in *DNA Probes in Infectious Diseases*, CRC Press, Boca Raton, FL, 1989, 101.

83. Bernet, C., Garret, M., de Barbeyrac, B., Bébéar, C., and Bonnet, J., Detection of *Mycoplasma pneumoniae* by using the polymerase chain reaction, *J. Clin. Microbiol.*, 27, 2492, 1989.

84. Jensen, J. S., Uldum, S. A., Sondergard-Andersen, J., Vuust, J., and Lind, K., Polymerase chain reaction for detection of *Mycoplasma genitalium* in clinical samples, *J. Clin. Microbiol.*, 29, 46, 1991.

85. Palmer, H. M., Gilroy, C. B., Furr, P. M., and Taylor-Robinson, D., Development and evaluation of the polymerase chain reaction to detect *Mycoplasma genitalium*, *FEMS Microbiol. Lett.*, 77, 199, 1991.

86. Morrison-Plummer, J., Jones, D. H., Daly, K., Tully, J. G., Taylor-Robinson, D., and Baseman, J. B., Molecular characterization of *Mycoplasma genitalium* species-specific and cross-reactive determination: identification of an immunodominant protein of *M. genitalium*, *Isr. J. Med. Sci.*, 23, 453, 1987.

87. von Rosenstiel, N. and Adam, D., Quinolone antibacterials: an update of their pharmacology and therapeutic use, *Drugs*, 47, 872, 1994.

88. Ziegler, C., Stary, A., Mailer, H., Kopp, W., Gebhart, W., and Söltz-Szöts, J., Quinolones as an alternative treatment of chlamydial, mycoplasma, and gonococcal urogenital infections, *Dermatology*, 185, 128, 1992.

89. Tartaglione, T. A. and Hooton, T. M., The role of fluoroquinolones in sexually transmitted disease, *Pharmacotherapy*, 13, 189, 1993.

90. Crumplin, G. C., The mechanism of action of quinolones, in *Quinolones — Their Future in Clinical Practice*, Percival, A., Ed., International Congress and Symposium Series, Royal Society of Medicine Services, London, 1986, 1.

91. Drlica, K., Coughlin, S., and Gennaro, M. L., Mode of action of quinolones: biochemical aspects, in *The New Generation of Quinolones*, Siporin, C., Heifetz, C. L., and Domagala, J. M., Eds., Marcel Dekker, New York, 1990, 45.

92. Sonstein, S. A., Mode of action of quinolones: antibacterial aspects, in *The New Generation of Quinolones*, Siporin, C., Heifetz, C. L., and Domagala, J. M., Eds., Marcel Dekker, New York, 1990, 63.

93. Crumplin, G. C. and Odell, M., Development of resistance to ofloxacin, *Drugs*, 34(Suppl. 1), 1, 1987.

94. Wolfson, J. S. and Hooper, D. C., The fluoroquinolones: structures, mechanisms of action and resistance, and spectra of activity *in vitro*, *Antimicrob. Agents Chemother.*, 28, 581, 1985.

95. Rohatgi, K. and Courtright, J. B., Major change in the structure and morphology of the bacterial nucleotide after treatment of cells with quinolones, in *The New Generation of Quinolones*, Siporin, C., Heifetz, C. L., and Domagala, J. M., Eds., Marcel Dekker, New York, 1990, 317.

96. Lamp, K. C., Bailey, E. M., and Rybak, M. J., Ofloxacin clinical pharmacokinetics, *Clin. Pharmacokinet.*, 22, 32, 1992.

97. Shah, P. M. and Frech, K., Overview of clinical experience with quinolones, in *Quinolones — Their Future in Clinical Practice*, Percival, A., Ed., International Congress and Symposium Series, Royal Society of Medicine Services, London, 1986, 29.

98. Finch, R. G. and Gabbay, F. J., The 6-fluoroquinolones *in vitro* activity, pharmacokinetic behaviour and *in vivo* considerations, in *Quinolones — Their Future in Clinical Practice*, Percival, A., Ed., International Congress and Symposium Series, Royal Society of Medicine Services, London, 1986, 17.

99. Prieur, B., Di Menza, C., and Charlot, J., Passage de la péflocine dans le liquide articulaire, *Presse Med.*, 14, 2019, 1985.

100. Hooper, D. C. and Wolfson, J. S., Fluoroquinolone antimicrobial agents, *N. Engl. J. Med.*, 324, 384, 1991.

101. Renaudin, H., Quentin, C., de Barbeyrac, B., and Bébéar, C., Activité *in vitro* de nouvelle quinolones sur les mycoplasmes pathogènes pour l'homme, *Pathol. Biol.*, 36, 496, 1988.

102. Kenny, G. E. and Cartwright, F. D., Susceptibility of *Mycoplasma pneumoniae* to several new quinolones, tetracycline and erythromycin, *Antimicrob. Agents Chemother.*, 35, 587, 1991.

103. Bébéar, C., Dupon, M., Renaudin, H., and de Barbeyrac, B., Potential improvements in therapeutic options for mycoplasmal respiratory infections, *Clin. Infect. Dis.*, 17(Suppl. 1), S202, 1993.

104. Waltes, K. B., Cassell, G. H., Canupp, K. C., and Fernandes, P. B., *In vitro* susceptibilities of mycoplasma and ureaplasmas to new macrolides and aryl-fluoroquinolones, *Antimicrob. Agents Chemother.*, 32, 1500, 1988.

105. Stopler, T., Gerichter, C. B., and Branski, D., Antibiotic-resistant mutants of *Mycoplasma pneumoniae*, *Isr. J. Med. Sci.*, 16, 169, 1980.

106. Cassell, G. H., Waites, K. B., Pate, M. S., Canupp, K. C., and Duffy, L. B., Comparative susceptibility of *Mycoplasma pneumoniae* to erythromycin, ciprofloxacin, and lomefloxacin, *Diagn. Microbiol. Infect. Dis.*, 12, 433, 1989.

107. Waites, K. B., Duffy, L. B., Schmid, T., Crabb, D., Pate, M. S., and Cassell, G. H., *In vitro* susceptibilities of *Mycoplasma pneumoniae*, *Mycoplasma hominis*, and *Ureaplasma urealyticum* to sparfloxacin and PD 127391, *Antimicrob. Agents Chemother.*, 35, 1181, 1991.

108. Renaudin, H. and Bébéar, C., Comparative *in vitro* activity of azithromycin, clarithromycin, erythromycin and lomefloxacin against *Mycoplasma pneumoniae* and *Ureaplasma urealyticum*, *Eur. J. Clin. Microbiol. Infect. Dis.*, 9, 838, 1990.

109. Renaudin, H., Tully, J. G., and Bébéar, C., *In vitro* susceptibilities of *Mycoplasma genitalium* to antibiotics, *Antimicrob. Agents Chemother.*, 36, 870, 1992.

110. Osada, Y. and Ogawa, H., Antimycoplasmal activity of ofloxacin (DL-8280), *Antimicrob. Agents Chemother.*, 23, 509, 1983.

111. Hardy, D. G., Activity of temafloxacin and other fluoroquinolones against typical and atypical community-acquired respiratory tract pathogens, *Am. J. Med.*, 91(Suppl. 6A), 12, 1991.

112. Brunner, H. and Zeiler, H.-Z., Chemotherapy of experimental *Mycoplasma pneumoniae* infection in hamsters and host response, in *Recent Advances in Mycoplasmology* (Zentralblätt für Bakteriologie, Suppl. 20), Stanek, G., Cassell, G. H., and Whitcomb, R. F., Eds., Gustav Fischer Verlag, Stuttgart, 1990, 83.

113. Furneri, P. M., Tempera, G., Caccamo, F., and Speciale, A. M., *In vitro* activity of ciprofloxacin against clinical isolates and standard strains of mycoplasmas and chlamidiae, *Rev. Infect. Dis.*, 10(Suppl.), S55, 1988.

114. Ridgway, G. L., Mumtaz, G., Gabriel, F. G., and Oriel, J. D., The activity of ciprofloxacin and other 4-quinolones against *Chlamydia trachomatis* and mycoplasmas *in vitro*, *Eur. J. Clin. Microbiol.*, 3, 344, 1984.

115. Simon, C. and Lindner, U., *In vitro* activity of norfloxacin against *Mycoplasma hominis* and *Ureaplasma urealyticum*, *Eur. J. Clin. Microbiol.*, 2, 479, 1983.

116. Kenny, G. E., Hooton, T. M., Roberts, M. C., Cartwright, F. D., and Hoyt, J., Susceptibilities of genital mycoplasmas to newer quinolones as determined by the agar dilution method, *Antimicrob. Agents Chemother.*, 33, 103, 1989.

117. Richard, P. and Gutmann, L., Sparfloxacin and other new fluoroquinolones, *J. Antimicrob. Chemother.*, 30, 739, 1992.

118. Robbins, M. J., Baskerville, A. J., and Sanghrajka, M., Comparative *in vitro* activity of lomefloxacin, a difluoro-quinolone, *Diagn. Microbiol. Infect. Dis.*, 12, 65S, 1989.

119. Hoban, D., DeGagne, P., and Witwicki, E., *In vitro* activity of lofloxacin against *Chlamydia trachomatis*, *Neisseria gonorrhoeae*, *Haemophillus ducreyi*, *Mycoplasma hominis*, and *Ureaplasma urealyticum*, *Diagn. Microbiol. Infect. Dis.*, 12, 83S, 1989.

120. Arai, S., Gohara, Y., Akashi, A., Kuwano, K., Nishimoto, M., Yano, T., Oizumi, K., Takeda, K., and Yamaguchi, T., Effects of new quinolones on *Mycoplasma pneumoniae*-infected hamsters, *Antimicrob. Agents Chemother.*, 37, 287, 1993.

121. Hayakawa, I., Atarashi, S., Yokohama, S., Imamura, M., Sakano, K., and Furukawa, M., Synthesis and antibacterial activities of optically active ofloxacin, *Antimicrob. Agents Chemother.*, 29, 163, 1986.

122. Lode, H., Höffken, G., Olschewski, P., Sievers, B., Kirch, A., Borner, K., and Koeppe, P., Pharmacokinetics of ofloxacin after parenteral and oral administration, *Antimicrob. Agents Chemother.*, 31, 1338, 1987.

123. Gregoire, S. L., Grasela, T. H., Freer, J. P., Tack, K. J., and Schentaz, J. J., Inhibition of theophilline clearance by coadministered ofloxacin without alteration of theophilline effects, *Antimicrob. Agents Chemother.*, 31, 375, 1987.

124. Wijnands, W. J. A., Vree, T. B., and Van Herwaarden, C. L. A., The influence of quinolone derivatives on theophilline clearance, *Br. J. Clin. Pharmacol.*, 22, 677, 1986.

125. Pankey, G. A., Temafloxacin: an overwiew, *Am. J. Med.*, 91(Suppl. 6A), 166S, 1991.

126. Nye, K., Shi, Y. G., Andrews, J. M., Ashby, J. P., and Wise, R., The *in vitro* activity, pharmacokinetics and tissue penetration of temafloxacin, *J. Antimicrob. Chem.*, 24, 415, 1989.

127. Granneman, G. R., Carpenter, P., Morrison, P. J., and Pernet, A., Pharmacokinetics of temafloxacin in humans after single oral doses, *Antimicrob. Agents Chemother.*, 35, 436, 1991.

128. Persival, A., Impact of chemical structure on quinolone potency, spectrum, and side effects, *J. Antimicrob. Chemother.*, 28(Suppl. C), 1, 1991.

129. Inatsuchi, H., Kawamura, N., Nishizawa, K., Masuda, A., and Tanaka, M., The penetration of new quinolones into cerebrospinal fluid, *Proc. 3rd Int. Conf. on New Quinolones*, July 1990, Vancouver, Canada, Abstr. 362.

130. Ito, T., Otsuki, M., and Nishino, T., *In vitro* antibacterial activity of Q-35, a new fluoroquinolone, *Antimicrob. Agents Chemother.*, 36, 1708, 1992.

131. Matsumoto, M., Kojima, K., Nagano, H., Matsubara, S., and Yokota, T., Photostability and biological activity of fluoroquinolones substituted at the 8 position after UV irradiation, *Antimicrob. Agents Chemother.*, 36, 1715, 1992.

132. Gohara, Y., Arai, S., Akashi, A., Kuwano, K., Tseng, C.-C., Matsubara, S., Matumoto, M., and Furudera, T., *In vitro* and *in vivo* activities of Q-35, a new fluoroquinolone, against *Mycoplasma pneumoniae*, *Antimicrob. Agents Chemother.*, 37, 1826, 1993.

133. Torres, A., Fernandez-Roblas, R., Méndez, R., and Soriano, F., Comparative activity of ofloxacin and seven other antimicrobials against urea-splitting microorganisms, *Infection*, 14(Suppl. 4), S233, 1986.

134. Kaatz, G. W., Seo, S. M., Barriere, S. L., Albrecht, L. M., and Rybak, M. J., Efficacy of ofloxacin in experimental *Staphylococcus aureus* endocarditis, *Antimicrob. Agents Chemother.*, 34, 257, 1990.

135. Courvalin, P., Plasmid-mediated 4-quinolone resistance: a real or apparent absence? *Antimicrob. Agents Chemother.*, 34, 681, 1990.

136. Kirst, H. A. and Sides, G. D., New directions for macrolide antibiotics: structural modifications and *in vitro* activity, *Antimicrob. Agents Chemother.*, 33, 1413, 1989.

137. Kirst, H. A., New macrolides: expanded horizons for an old class of antibiotics, *J. Antimicrob. Chemother.*, 28, 787, 1991.

138. Ball, P., The future role and importance of macrolides, *J. Hosp. Infect.*, 19(Suppl. A), 47, 1991.

139. Morimoto, S., Takahashi, Y., Watanabe, Y., and Omura, S., Chemical modification of erythromycin. I. Synthesis and antibacterial activity of 6-*O*-methylerythromycin A, *J. Antibiot.*, 37, 187, 1984.

140. Morimoto, S., Misawa, Y., Adachi, T., Nagate, T., Watanabe, Y., and Omura, S., Chemical modification of erythromycins. II. Synthesis and antibacterial activity of *O*-alkyl derivatives of erythromycin A, *J. Antibiot.*, 43, 286, 1990.

141. Renaudin, H., Boussens, B., and Bébéar, C., *In vitro* activity of RP 59500 against Mycoplasma, *Proc. 31st Intersci. Conf. Antimicrob. Agents Chemother.*, American Society for Microbiology, Washington, D.C., Abstr. 897, 1991.

142. Kirst, H. A. and Sides, G. D., New directions for microlide antibiotics: pharmacokinetics and clinical efficacy, *Antimicrob. Agents Chemother.*, 33, 1419, 1989.

143. Wise, R., The development of macrolides and related compounds, *J. Antimicrob. Chemother.*, 23, 299, 1989.

144. Washington, J. A. and Wilson, W. R., Erythromycin: a microbial and clinical perspective after 30 years of clinical use (second of two parts), *Mayo Clin. Proc.*, 60, 271, 1985.

145. Fernandes, P. B., The macrolide revival: thirty-five years after erythromycin, *Antimicrob. Newsl.*, 4, 25, 1987.

146. Fernandes, P. B., Bailer, R., Swanson, R., Hanson, C. W., McDonald, E., Ramer, N., Hardy, D., Shipkowitz, N., Bower, R. R., and Gade, E., *In vitro* and *in vivo* evaluation of A-56268 (TE-031), a new macrolide, *Antimicrob. Agents Chemother.*, 30, 865, 1986.

147. Lo, S.-C., Dawson, M. S., Newton, P. B. III, Sonoda, M. A., Shih, J. W.- K., Engler, W. F., Wang, R. Y.-H., and Wear, D. J., Association of the virus-like infectious agent originally reported in patients with AIDS with acute fatal disease in previously healthy non-AIDS patients, *Am. J. Trop. Med. Hyg.*, 41, 364, 1989.

148. McDonald, P. J. and Pruul, H., Phagocyte uptake and transport of azithromycin, *Eur. J. Clin. Microbiol. Infect. Dis.*, 10, 828, 1991.

149. Phillips, I., Acar, J., Baquero, F., Bergan, T., Forsgren, A., and Wiedemann, B., ESGAB breakpoint determination: clarithromycin, *Eur. J. Clin. Microbiol. Infect. Dis.*, 10, 993, 1991.

150. Cassell, G. H., Drnec, J., Waites, K. B., Pate, M. S., Duffy, L. B., Watson, H. L., and McIntosh, J. C., Efficacy of clarithromycin against *Mycoplasma pneumoniae*, *J. Antimicrob. Chemother.*, 27(Suppl. A), 47, 1991.

151. Bébéar, C., Renaudin, H., Maugein, J., de Barbeyrac, B., and Clerc, M.-T., Pristinamycin and human mycoplasmas: *in vitro* activity compared with macrolides and lincosamides, *in vivo* efficacy in *Mycoplasma pneumoniae* experimental infection, in *Recent Advances in Mycoplasmology* (Zentralblätt für Bakteriologie, Suppl. 20), Stanek, G., Cassell, G. H., Tully, J. G., and Whitcomb, R. F., Eds., Gustav Fischer Verlag, Stuttgart, 1990, 77.

152. Felmingham, D., Robbins, M. J., Sanghrajka, M., Leakey, A., and Ridgway, G. L., The *in vitro* activity of some 14-, 15- and 16-membered macrolides against *Staphylococcus* spp., *Legionella* spp., *Mycoplasma* spp. and *Ureaplasma urealyticum*, *Drugs Exp. Clin. Res.*, 17, 91, 1991.

153. Hara, K., Suyama, N., Yamaguchi, K., Kohno, S., and Saito, A., Activity of macrolides against organisms responsible for respiratory infection with emphasis on *Mycoplasma* and *Legionella*, *J. Antimicrob. Chemother.*, 20(Suppl. B), 75, 1987.

154. Morimoto, S., Nagate, T., Sugita, K., Ono, T., Numata, K., Miyachi, J., Misawa, Y., Yamada, K., and Omura, S., Chemical modification of erythromycins. III. *In vitro* and *in vivo* antibacterial activities of new semisynthetic 6-*O*-methylerythromycin A, TE-031 (clarithromycin) and TE-032, *J. Antibiot.*, 43, 295, 1990.

155. Hardy, D. J., Extent and spectrum of the antimicrobial activity of clarithromycin, *Pediatr. Infect. Dis. J.*, 12, S99, 1993.

156. Klein, J. O., Clarithromycin: where do we go from here? *Pediatr. Infect. Dis. J.*, 12, S148, 1993.

157. Guay, D. R. P. and Craft, H. C., Overview of the pharmacology of clarithromycin suspension in children, *Pediatr. Infect. Dis. J.*, 12, S106, 1993.

158. O'Connor, N. K. and Fris, J., Clarithromycin-carbamazepine interaction in a clinical setting, *J. Am. Board Fam. Pract.*, 7, 489, 1994.

159. Ketter, T. A., Post, R. M., and Worthington, K., Principles of clinically important drug interactions with carbamazepine. I, *J. Clin. Psychopharmacol.*, 11, 198, 1991.

160. Markham, A. and Faulds, D., Roxithromycin: an update of its antimicrobial activity, pharmacokinetic properties and therapeutic use, *Drugs*, 48, 297, 1994 (correction in *Drugs*, 48, 793, 1994).

161. Ferreruela, R. M., Alcaraz, M. J., Farga, M. A. et al., Activity of new macrolides against genitourinary and respiratory mycoplasmas, *Rev. Esp. Quimioter.*, 4, 209, 1991.

162. Paulsen, O., Roxithromycin — a macrolide with improved pharmacokinetic properties, *Drugs Today*, 27, 193, 1991.

163. Barlam, T. and Neu, H. C., *In vitro* comparison of the activity of RU 28965, a new macrolide, with that of erythromycin against aerobic and anaerobic bacteria, *Antimicrob. Agents Chemother.*, 25, 529, 1984.

164. Carlone, N. A., Cuffini, A. M., Tullio, V., and Sassella, D., Comparative effects of roxithromycin and erythromycin on cellular immune functions *in vitro*. II. Chemotaxis and phagocytosis of ³H-*Staphylococcus aureus* by human macrophages, *Microbios*, 58, 17, 1989.

165. Anderson, R., Erythromycin and roxithromycin potentiate human neutrophil locomotion *in vitro* by inhibition of leukoattractant: activated superoxide generation and autooxidation, *J. Infect. Dis.*, 159, 966, 1989.

166. Satake, N., Nagai, S., Nishimura, K., and Izumi, T., The effect of roxithromycin (RXM, erythromycin derivative) on blood neutrophil mobility toward FMLP in patients with diffuse bronchiectasis and idiopathic pulmonary fibrosis, *Eur. Respir. J.*, 5(Suppl. 15), 142, 1992.

167. Akamatsu, H., Sasaki, H., Matoba, Y. et al., Effects of roxithromycin on neutrophil chemotaxis and phagocytosis *in vitro*, *Ensho*, 14, 59, 1994.

168. Bailly, S., Pocidalo, J.-J., Fay, M., and Gougerot-Pocidalo, M. A., Differential modulation of cytokine production by macrolides: interleukin-6 production is increased by spiramycin and erythromycin, *Antimicrob. Agents Chemother.*, 35, 2016, 1991.

169. Zini, R., Fournet, M. P., Barre, J. et al., *In vitro* study of roxithromycin binding to serum proteins and erythrocytes in humans, *Br. J. Clin. Pract.*, 42(Suppl. 55), 54, 1988.

170. Kees, F., Grobecker, H., Fourtillian, J. B. et al., Comparative pharmacokinetics of single dose roxithromycin (150 mg) versus erythromycin stearate (500 mg) in healthy volunteers, *Br. J. Clin. Pract.*, 42(Suppl. 55), 51, 1988.

171. Puri, S. K. and Lassman, H. B., Roxithromycin: a pharmacokinetic review of a macrolide, *J. Antimicrob. Chemother.*, 20(Suppl. B), 89, 1987.

172. Lassman, H. B., Puri, S. K., Ho, I., Sabo, R., and Mezzino, M. J., Pharmacokinetics of roxithromycin (RU 965), *J. Clin. Pharmacol.*, 28, 141, 1988.

173. Nilsen, O. G., Aamo, T., Zahlsen, K., and Svarva, P., Macrolide pharmacokinetics and dose scheduling of roxithromycin, *Diagn. Microbiol. Infect. Dis.*, 15(Suppl. 4), 71S, 1992.

174. Boeckh, M., Lode, H., and Höffken, G., Pharmacokinetics of roxithromycin and influence of H2-blockers and antacids on gastrointestinal absorption, *Eur. J. Clin. Microbiol. Infect. Dis.*, 11, 465, 1992.

175. Tremblay, D., Jaeger, H., Fourtillan, J. B. et al., Pharmacokinetics of three single doses (150, 300, 450 mg) of roxithromycin in young volunteers, *Br. J. Clin. Pract.*, 42(Suppl. 55), 49, 1988.

176. Nilsen, O. G., Comparative pharmacokinetics of macrolides, *J. Antimicrob. Chemother.*, 20(Suppl. 20), 81, 1987.

177. Tremblay, D., Meyer, B., Saint-Salvi, B., and Robinet, D., Influence of food on bioavailability of roxithromycin (RU 965), *Acta Pharmacol. Toxicol.*, 59(Suppl. 5), 191, 1986.

178. Pechère, J.-C., Clinical evaluation of roxithromycin 300 mg once daily as an alternative to 150 mg twice daily, *Diagn. Microbiol. Infect. Dis.*, 15(Suppl. 4), 111S, 1992.

179. Girard, A. E., Girard, D., English, A. R., Gootz, T. D., Cimochowsky, C. R., Faiella, J. A., Haskell, S. L., and Retsema, J. A., Pharmacokinetic and *in vivo* studies with azithromycin (CP-62,993). A new macrolide with an extended half-life and excellent tissue distribution, *Antimicrob. Agents Chemother.*, 31, 1948, 1987.

180. Retsema, J. A., Girard, A., Schelkly, W., Manousos, M., Anderson, M., Bright, G., Borovoy, R., Brennan, L., and Mason, R., Spectrum and mode of action of azithromycin (CP-62,993), a new 15-membered-ring macrolide with improved potency against Gram-negative organisms, *Antimicrob. Agents Chemother.*, 31, 1939, 1987.

181. Lode, H. and Schaberg, T., Azithromycin in lower respiratory tract infections, *Scand. J. Infect. Dis. Suppl.*, 83, 26, 1992.

182. Barry, A. L., Jones, R. N., and Thornberry, C., *In vitro* activity of azithromycin (CP-92,993), clarithromycin (A-56,268, TE 031), erythromycin, roxithromycin and clindamycin, *Antimicrob. Agents Chemother.*, 32, 752, 1988.

183. Fernandes, P. B. and Hardy, D. J., Comparative *in vitro* potencies of nine macrolides, *Drugs Exp. Clin. Res.*, 14, 445, 1988.

184. Goldstein, F. W., Emirian, M. F., Controt, A., and Acar, J. F., Bacteriostatic and bactericidal activity of azithromycin against *Haemophilus influenzae*, *J. Antimicrob. Chemother.*, 25(Suppl. A), 25, 1990.

185. Maskell, J. P., Sefton, A. M., and Williams, J. D., Comparative *in vitro* activity of azithromycin and erythromycin against Gram-positive cocci, *Haemophilus influenzae* and anaerobes, *J. Antimicrob. Chemother.*, 25(Suppl. A), 19, 1990.

186. Edelstein, P. H. and Edelstein, M. A. C., *In vitro* activity of azithromycin against clinical isolates of *Legionella* species, *Antimicrob. Agents Chemother.*, 35, 180, 1991.

187. Ridgway, G. L., Mumtaz, G., and Fenelon, L., The *in vitro* activity of clarithromycin and other macrolides against the type strain of *Chlamydia pneumoniae* (TWAR), *J. Antimicrob. Chemother.*, 27(Suppl. A), 43, 1991.

188. Foulds, G., Shephard, R. M., and Johnson, R. D., The pharmacokinetics of azithromycin in human serum and tissue, *J. Antimicrob. Chemother.*, 25(Suppl. A), 73, 1990.

189. Fiese, E. F. and Steffen, S. H., Comparison of the acid stability of azithromycin and erythromycin A, *J. Antimicrob. Chemother.*, 25(Suppl. A), 39, 1990.

190. Pascual, A., Lopez Lopez, G., Aragon, J., and Perea, E. J., Effect of azithromycin and erythromycin on human polymorphonuclear leukocyte function against *Staphylococcus aureus*, *Chemotherapy*, 36, 422, 1990.

191. Shentag, J. J. and Ballow, Ch., Tissue-directed pharmacokinetics, *Am. J. Med.*, 91(Suppl. 3A), 5S, 1991.

192. Gladue, R. P., Bright, G. M., Isaacson, R. E., and Newborg, M. F., *In vitro* and *in vivo* uptake of azithromycin (CP-62,993) by phagocytic cells: possible mechanism of delivery and release at sites of infection, *Antimicrob. Agents Chemother.*, 33, 277, 1989.

193. Morris, D. L., De Souza, A., Jones, J. A., and Morgan, W. E., High and prolonged pulmonary tissue concentrations of azithromycin following a single oral dose, *Eur. J. Clin. Microbiol. Infect. Dis.*, 10, 859, 1991.

194. Rylander, M. and Hallander, H. O., *In vitro* comparison of the activity of doxycycline, tetracycline, erythromycin and a new macrolide, CP-62,993, against *Mycoplasma pneumoniae*, *Mycoplasma hominis* and *Ureaplasma urealyticum*, *Scand. J. Infect. Dis. Suppl.*, 53, 12, 1988.

195. Gialdroni Grassi, G. et al., *In vitro* activity of flurithromycin, a novel macrolide antibiotic, *Chemioterapia*, 5, 177, 1986.

196. Bonardi, G., Del Soldato, P., and Lepore, A. M., Bioavailability of flurithromycin after p.o. and i.v. dosing in healthy volunteers, *Acta Pharmacol. Toxicol.*, 59, 291, 1986.

197. Villa, P., Corti, F., Guaitani, A., Bartosek, I., Casacci, F., De Marchi, F., and Pacei, E., Effects of a new fluorinated macrolide (P-0501A) and other erythromycins on drug metabolizing enzymes in rat liver, *J. Antibiot.*, 39, 463, 1986.

198. Benoni, G., Cuzzolin, L., Del Soldato, P., Lepore, A. M., and Velo, G. P., The influence of erythromycin and flurithromycin on the normal gastrointestinal flora of humans, *Chemioterapia*, 6(Suppl. 2), 341, 1987.

199. Benoni, G., Cuzzolin, L., Leone, R., and Fracasso, M. E., Hepatic and intestinal effects of flurithromycin and erythromycin in the rat, *J. Chemother.*, 4, 271, 1992.

200. Larrey, D., Tinel, M., and Pessayre, D., Formation of inactive cytochrome P-450-Fe(II)-metabolite complexes with several erythromycin derivatives but not with josamin and midecamycin in rats, *Biochem. Pharmacol.*, 32, 1487, 1983.

201. Villa, P., Corti, F., Guaitani, A., Bartosek, I., Casacci, F., De Marchi, F. and Pacei, E., Effects of *in vivo* treatment with a new fluorinate macrolide (P-0501A) and other erythromycins on drug clearance and hepatic functions in perfused rat liver, *J. Antibiot.*, 39, 463, 1986.

202. Sakata, H., Fujita, K., and Yoshioka, H., The effect of antimicrobial agents on faecal flora of children, *Antimicrob. Agents Chemother.*, 29, 225, 1986.

203. Wiegertsma, N., Jansen, G., and Van der Waaij, D., Effect of twelve antimicrobial drugs on the colonization resistance of the digestive tract of mice and on endogenous potentially pathogenic bacteria, *J. Hyg.*, 88, 221, 1982.

204. Sides, G. D., Cerimele, B. J., Black, H. R., Busch, U., and DeSante, K. A., Pharmacokinetics of dirithromycin, *J. Antimicrob. Chemother.*, 31(Suppl. C), 31, 65, 1992.

205. Ueda, Y., Ohtsuki, S., Narukawa, N., and Takeda, K., Effect of terdecamycin on experimentally induced *Mycoplasma hyopneumoniae* in pigs, *J. Vet. Med. B*, 41, 283, 1994.

206. Furr, P. M. and Taylor-Robinson, D., Enhancement of experimental *Mycoplasma pulmonis* infection of the mouse genital tract by progesteron treatment, *J. Hyg.*, 92, 139, 1984.

207. Taylor-Robinson, D. and Furr, P. M., The interplay of host and organism factors in infection of the mouse genital tract by *Mycoplasma pulmonis*, *J. Hyg.*, 95, 7, 1985.

208. Furr, P. M. and Taylor-Robinson, D., The establishment and persistence of *Ureaplasma urealyticum* on oestradiol-treated female mice, *J. Med. Microbiol.*, 29, 111, 1989.

209. Furr, P. M. and Taylor-Robinson, D., Oestradiol-induced *Mycoplasma hominis* infection of the genital tract of female mice, *J. Gen. Microbiol.*, 135, 2743, 1989.

210. Furr, P. M., Hetherington, C. M., and Taylor-Robinson, D., The susceptibility of germ-free, oestradiol-treated mice to *Mycoplasma hominis*, *J. Med. Microbiol.*, 30, 233, 1989.

211. Taylor-Robinson, D. and Furr, P. M., Elimination of mycoplasma from the murine genital tract by hormone treatment, *Epidemiol. Infect.*, 105, 163, 1990.

212. Taylor-Robinson, D. and Munday, P. E., Mycoplasmal infection of the female genital tract and its complications, in *Genital Tract Infections in Women*, Hare, M. J., Ed., Churchill Livingston, Edinburgh, 1988, 228.

213. Smith, C. B., Friedewald, W. T., and Chanock, R. M., Shedding of *Mycoplasma pneumoniae* after tetracycline and erythromycin therapy, *N. Engl. J. Med.*, 276, 1172, 1967.

214. Dearth, J. C. and Rhodes, K. H., Infectious mononucleosis complicated by severe *Mycoplasma pneumonia* infection, *Am. J. Dis. Child.*, 134, 744, 1980.

215. Foy, H. M., Ochs, H., Davis, S. D., Kenny, G. E., and Luce, R. R., *Mycoplasma pneumoniae* infections in patients with immunodeficiency syndromes: report of four cases, *J. Infect. Dis.*, 127, 388, 1973.

216. Janknegt, R., Wijnands, W. J. A., and Stobberingh, E. E., Antimicrobial practice: antibiotic policies in Dutch hospitals for the treatment of pneumonia, *J. Antimicrob. Chemother.*, 34, 431, 1994.

217. Thys, J. P., Quinolones in the treatment of bronchopulmonary infections, *Rev. Infect. Dis.*, 10(Suppl. 1), 212, 1988.

218. Frieden, T. R. and Mangi, R. J., Inappropriate use of oral ciprofloxacin, *JAMA*, 264, 1438, 1990.

219. Neu, H. C., Ciprofloxacin: an overview and prospective appraisal, *Am. J. Med.*, 82(Suppl. 4A), 395, 1987.

220. Neu, H. C., The development of macrolides: clarithromycin in perspective, *J. Antimicrob. Chemother.*, 27(Suppl. A), 1, 1991.

221. Schentag, J. J. and Ballow, C. H., Tissue-directed pharmacokinetics, *Am. J. Med.*, 91(Suppl. 3A), 5, 1991.

222. Chien, S.-M., Pichotta, P., Siepman, N., Chan, C. K., and the Canada-Sweden Clarithromycin-Pneumonia Study Group, Treatment of community-acquired pneumonia: a multicenter, double-blind, randomized study comparing clarithromycin with erythromycin, *Chest*, 103, 697, 1993.

223. Anderson, G., Esmonde, T. S., Coles, S., Macklin, J., and Carnegie, A., A comparative safety and efficacy study of clarithromycin and erythromycin stearate in community acquired pneumonia, *J. Antimicrob. Chemother.*, 27S(A), 117, 1991.

224. van Schouwenburg, J., de Bruyn, O., Fourie, E., van Rensburg, J., Rodruques, A., and Pickard, I., A randomized, comparative study of the efficacy and tolerance of roxithromycin and doxycycline in the treatment of women with positive endocervical cultures for *Chlamydia trachomatis* and *Mycoplasma* spp. in an *in vitro* fertilization program, *Diagn. Microbiol. Infect. Dis.*, 15, 1295, 1992.

225. Schönwald, S., Gunjaca, M., Kolacny-Babic, L., Car, V., and Gosev, M., Comparison of azithromycin and erythromycin in the treatment of atypical pneumonia, *J. Antimicrob. Chemother.*, 25(Suppl. A), 123, 1990.

226. Schönwald, S., Skerk, V., Petricevic, I., Car, V., Majerus-Music, Lj., and Gunjaca, M., Comparison of three-day and five-day courses of azithromycin in the treatment of atypical pneumonia, *Eur. J. Clin. Microbiol. Infect. Dis.*, 10, 877, 1991.

227. Manfredi, R., Jannuzzi, C., Mantero, E., Longo, L., Schiavone, R., Tempesta, A., Pavesio, D., Pecco, P., and Chido, F., Clinical comparative study of azithromycin versus erythromycin in the treatment of acute respiratory tract infections in children, *J. Chemother.*, 4, 364, 1992.

228. Jacobson, K., Clinical efficacy of dirithromycin in pneumonia, *J. Antimicrob. Chemother.*, 31(Suppl. C), 121, 1993.

229. Liippo, K., Tala, E., Piolijoki, H., Brückner, O.-J., Rodrig, J., and Smits, J. P. H., A comparative study of dirithromycin and erythromycin in bacterial pneumonia, *J. Infect.*, 28, 131, 1994.

230. Isada, C. M., Pro: antibiotics for chronic bronchitis with exacerbations, *Semin. Respir. Infect.*, 8, 243, 1993.

231. Peugeot, R. L., Lipsky, B. A., Hooton, T. M., and Pecoraro, R. E., Treatment of lower respiratory infections in outpatients with ofloxacin compared with erythromycin, *Drugs Exp. Clin. Res.*, 17, 253, 1991.

232. Gentry, L. O., Lipsky, B., Farber, M. O., Tucker, B., and Rodriguez-Gomez, G., Oral ofloxacin therapy for lower respiratory tract infection, *South. Med. J.*, 85, 14, 1992.

233. Maesen, F. P. V., Davies, B. L., Baur, C., and Sumajow, C. A., Clinical, microbiological and pharmacokinetic studies on ofloxacin in acute purulent exacerbations of chronic respiratory disease, *J. Antimicrob. Chemother.*, 18, 629, 1986.

234. Le Chevalier, B., Beaycaire, G., Mouton, Y., and Study Group, Efficacy and safety of oral ofloxacin for treatment of pneumonia, *Rev. Infect. Dis.*, 11(Suppl. 5), S1223, 1989.

235. Mouton, Y., Leroy, O., Beuscart, C., Sivery, B., Senneville, E., Chidiac, C., Beaucaire, G., and Vincent du Laurier, M., Efficacy of intravenous ofloxacin: a French multicentre trial in 185 patients, *J. Antimicrob. Chemother.*, 26(Suppl. D), 115, 1990.

236. Carbon, C., Léophonte, P., Petitpretz, P., Chauvin, J. P., and Hazebroucq, J., Efficacy and safety of temafloxacin versus those of amoxicillin in hospitalized adults with community-acquired pneumonia, *Antimicrob. Agents Chemother.*, 36, 833, 1992.

237. Chodosh, S., Temafloxacin compared with ciprofloxacin in mild to moderate lower respiratory tract infections in ambulatory patients: a multicenter, double-blind, randomized study, *Chest*, 100, 1497, 1991.

238. Norrby, S. R. and Pernet, A. G., Assessment of adverse events during drug development: experience with temafloxacin, *J. Antimicrob. Chemother.*, 28(Suppl. C), 111, 1991.

239. Marchese, A., Debbia, E. A., and Schito, G. C., Brodiprim: effects of sub-MICs on virulence traits of respiratory pathogens, *Proc. 34th Intersci. Conf. Antimicrob. Agents Ohemother.*, American Society for Microbiology, Washington, D. C., Abstract E45, 1994, 158.

240. Salmi, H. A., Lehtomäki, K., and Kylmämaa, T., Comparison of brodimoprim and doxycycline in acute respiratory tract infections: a double-blind clinical trial, *Drugs Exp. Clin. Res.*, 12, 349, 1986.

241. Salmi, H. A., Brodimoprim in acute respiratory tract infections, *J. Chemother.*, 5, 532, 1993.

242. Carstenen, H. and Nilsson, K.-O., Neurological complications associated with *Mycoplasma pneumoniae* infection in children, *Neuropediatrics*, 18, 57, 1987.

243. Lerer, R. J. and Kalavsky, S. M., Central nervous system disease associated with *Mycoplasma pneumoniae* infection: report of five cases and review of the literature, *Pediatrics*, 58, 658, 1973.

244. Agustin, E. T., Gill, V., and Cunha, B. A., *Mycoplasma pneumoniae* meningoencephalitis complicated by diplopia, *Heart Lung*, 23, 436, 1994.

245. Hodges, G. R., Fass, R. J., and Saslaw, S., Central nervous system disease associated with *Mycoplasma pneumoniae* infection, *Arch. Intern. Med.*, 130, 277, 1972.

246. Urquhart, G. E. D., *Mycoplasma pneumoniae* infection and neurological complications, *Br. Med. J.*, 2, 1512, 1979.

247. Kasahara, I., Otsubo, Y., Yanase, T., Oshima, H., Ichimaru, H., and Nakamura, M., Isolation and characterization of *Mycoplasma pneumoniae* from cerebrospinal fluid of a patient with pneumonia and meningoencephalitis, *J. Infect. Dis.*, 152, 823, 1985.

248. Abramovitz, P., Schvartzman, P., Harel, D., Lis, I., and Naot, Y., Direct invasion of the central nervous system by *Mycoplasma pneumoniae*: a report of two cases, *J. Infect. Dis.*, 155, 482, 1987.

249. Fisher, R. S., Clark, A. W., Wolinsky, J. S., Parhad, I. M., Moses, H., and Mardiney, M. R., Postinfection leukoencephalitis complicating *Mycoplasma pneumoniae* infection, *Arch. Neurol.*, 40, 109, 1983.

250. Murray, H. W., Masur, H., Senterfit, L. B., and Roberts, R. B., The protean manifestations of *Mycoplasma pneumoniae* infection in adults, *Am. J. Med.*, 58, 229, 1975.

251. Turtzo, D. F. and Ghatak, P. K., Acute hemolytic anemia with *Mycoplasma pneumoniae* pneumonia, *JAMA*, 236, 1140, 1976.

252. Feizi, T., Monotypic cold agglutinins in infection by Mycoplasma pneumoniae, *Nature*, 215, 540, 1967.

253. Schreiber, A. D., Herskovitz, B. S., and Goldwein, M., Low-titer cold-hemagglutinin disease, *N. Engl. J. Med.*, 296, 1490, 1977.

254. Chu, C.-S., Braun, S. R., Yarbro, J. W., and Hayden, M. R., Corticosteroid treatment of hemolytic anemia associated with *Mycoplasma pneumoniae* pneumonia, *South. Med. J.*, 83, 1106, 1990.

255. Packman, C. H. and Leddy, J. P., Cryopathic hemolytic syndromes, in *Hematology*, Williams, W. J., Beutler, E., Erslev, A. J., and Lichtman, M. A., Eds., McGraw-Hill, New York, 1983, 642.

256. Case records of the Massachusetts General Hospital, weekly clinicopathological exercises: case 39-1983, *N. Engl. J. Med.*, 309, 782, 1983.

257. Deas, J. E., Jenney, F. A., Lee, L. T., and Howe, C., Immune electron microscopy of cross-reactions between *Mycoplasma pneumoniae* and human erythrocytes, *Infect. Immun.*, 24, 211, 1979.

258. Jacobson, L. B., Longstreth, G. F., and Edgington, T. S., Clinical and immunologic features of transient cold agglutinin hemolytic anemia, *Am. J. Med.*, 54, 514, 1973.

259. Wintrobe, M. M., Lee, G. R., Boggs, D. R., Bithell, T. C., Foester, J., Athens, J. W., and Lukens, J. N., Eds., *Clinical Hematology*, 8th ed., Lea and Febiger, Philadelphia, 1981.

260. Fink, F. M., Dengg, K., Kilga-Nogler, S., Schönitzer, D., and Berger, H., Cold haemagglutinin disease complicating *Mycoplasma pneumoniae* infection in a child under cytotoxic cancer treatment, *Eur. J. Pediatr.*, 151, 435, 1992.

261. Atkinson, J. P., Schreiber, A. D., and Frank, M. M., Effects of corticosteroids and splenectomy on the immune clearance and destruction of erythrocytes, *J. Clin. Invest.*, 52, 1509, 1973.

262. McMillan, R., Immune thrombocytopenia, *Clin. Haematol.*, 12, 69, 1983.

263. Veenhofen, W. A., Halie, M. R., Stijnen, P. J., and Nieweg, H. O., Bacterial infections and thrombocytopenia in chronic idiopathic thrombocytopenic purpura, *Acta Haematol.*, 62, 159, 1979.

264. Kelton, J. G., Keystone, J., Neame, P. B., Moore, J., Gauldie, J., and Jensen, J. B., The mechanism of malaria-induced thrombocytopenia, *Clin. Res.*, 30, 320A, 1982.

265. Veenhoven, W. A., Smithuis, R. H. M., and Kerst, A. J. F. A., Thrombocytopenia associated with mycoplasma pneumoniae infection, *Neth. J. Med.*, 37, 75, 1990.

266. Wallace, R. J., Jr., Alpert, S., Brown, K., Lin, J. S. L., and McCormack, W. M., Isolation of *Mycoplasma hominis* from patients with post partum fever, *Obstet. Gynecol.*, 51, 181, 1978.

267. McCormack, W. M., Lee, Y. H., and Lin, J. S., Genital mycoplasmas in post partum fever, *J. Infect. Dis.*, 127, 193, 1973.

268. Tully, J. G. and Smith, L. G., Post partum septicaemia with *Mycoplasma hominis*, *JAMA*, 204, 827, 1968.

269. Russell, F. E. and Fallon, P. J., Mycoplasma and the urogenital tract, *Lancet*, 1, 1295, 1978.

270. Thomsen, A. C., Occurrence and pathogenicity of *Mycoplasma hominis* in the upper urinary tract: a review, *Sex. Transm. Dis.*, 10, 323, 1983.

271. Thomsen A. C. and Lindskov, H. O., Diagnosis of *Mycoplasma hominis* pyelonephritis by demonstration of antibodies in urine, *J. Clin. Microbiol.*, 9, 681, 1979.

272. Mardh, P.-A. and Weström, L., Antibodies to *Mycoplasma hominis* in patients with genital infections and in healthy controls, *Br. J. Vener. Dis.*, 46, 390, 1970.

273. Hyjelm, E., Jonsell, G., Linglof, T., Mardh, P.-A., Moller, B., and Sedin, G., Meningitis in a newborn infant caused by *Mycoplasma hominis*, *Acta Paediatr. Scand.*, 69, 415, 1980.

274. Siber, G. R., Alpert, S., Smith, A. L., Lin, J. S. L., and McCormack, W. M., Neonatal central nervous system infection due to *Mycoplasma hominis*, *J. Paediatr.*, 90, 625, 1977.

275. Jones, D. M. and Tobin, B., Neonatal eye infections due to *Mycoplasma hominis*, *Br. J. Med.*, 3, 467, 1968.

276. Young, M. J. and Cox, R. A., Near fatal puerperal fever due to *Mycoplasma hominis*, *Postgrad. Med. J.*, 66, 147, 1990.

277. Friis, H., Plesner, A., Scheibel, J., Justesen, T., and Lind, K., *Mycoplasma hominis* septicaemia, *Br. Med. J.*, 286, 2013, 1983.

278. Moller, B. R., Herrmann, B., Ibsen, H. H. B., Halkier-Sorensen, L., From, E., and Mardh, P.-A., Occurrence of *Ureaplasma urealyticus* and *Mycoplasma hominis* in non-gonoccocal urethritis before and after treatment in a double-blind trial of ofloxacin versus erythromycin, *Scand. J. Infect. Dis.*, 68, 31, 1990.

279. Nayagam, A. T., Smith, M. D., Ridgway, G. L., Allason-Jones, E., Robinson, A. J., and Stock, J., Comparison of ofloxacin and metronidazole for the treatment of bacterial vaginosis, *Int. J. Sex. Transm. Dis. AIDS*, 3, 204, 1992.

280. Wathne, B., Holst, E., Hovelius, B., and Mardh, P.-A., Erythromycin versus metronidazole in the treatment of bacterial vaginosis, *Acta Obstet. Gynecol. Scand.*, 72, 470, 1993.

281. Sexually transmitted diseases treatment guidelines, United States Department of Health and Human Services, Centers for Disease Control, Atlanta, 38(Suppl. 8), 32, 1989.

282. Schmitt, C., Sobel, J. D., and Meriwether, C., Bacterial vaginosis: treatment with clindamycin cream versus oral metronidazole, *Obstet. Gynecol.*, 79, 1020, 1992.

283. Eschenbach, D. A., Critchlow, C. W., Watkins, H., Smith, K., Spiegel, C. A., Chen, K. C. S., and Holmes, K. K., A dose-duration study of metronidazole for the treatment of nonspecific vaginosis, *Scand. J. Infect. Dis. Suppl.*, 40, 73, 1983.

284. Swedberg, J., Steiner, J. F., Deiss, F., Steiner, S., and Driggers, D. A., Comparison of single dose versus one week course of metronidazole for symptomatic bacterial vaginosis, *JAMA*, 254, 1046, 1985.

285. Lossick, J. G., Treatment of sexually transmitted vaginosis/vaginitis, *Rev. Infect. Dis.*, 12(Suppl. 6), S665, 1990.

286. Lugo-Miro, V. I., Green, M., and Mazur, L., Comparison of different metronidazole therapeutic regimens for bacterial vaginosis, *JAMA*, 268, 92, 1992.

287. Hillier, S. L., Lipinski, C., Briselden, A. M., and Eschenbach, D. A., Efficacy of intravaginal 0.75% metronidazole gel for the treatment of bacterial vaginosis, *Obstet. Gynecol.*, 81, 963, 1993.

288. Bistoletti, P., Fredricsson, B., Hagstrom, B., and Nord, C.-E., Comparison of oral and vaginal metronidazole therapy for nonspecific bacterial vaginosis, *Gynecol. Obstet. Invest.*, 21, 144, 1986.

289. Edelman, D. A. and North, B. B., Treatment of bacterial vaginosis with intravaginal sponges containing metronidazole, *J. Reprod. Med.*, 34, 341, 1989.

290. Hillier, S., Krohn, M. A., Watts, D. H., Wolner-Hanssen, P., and Eschenbach, D., Microbiologic efficacy of intravaginal clindamycin cream for the treatment of bacterial vaginosis, *Obstet. Gynecol.*, 76, 407, 1990.

291. Hill, G. B. and Livengood, C. H., Bacterial vaginosis — associated microflora and effects of topical intravaginal clindamycin, *Am. J. Obstet. Gynecol.*, 171, 1198, 1994.

292. Hillier, S. L., Krohn, M. N., Rabe, L. K., Klebanoff, S. J., and Eschenbach, D. A., The normal vaginal flora, H_2O_2-producing lactobacilli, and bacterial vaginosis in pregnant women, *Clin. Infect. Dis.*, 16(Suppl. 4), S273, 1992.

293. Martius, J., Krohn, M. A., Hillier, S. L., Stamm, W. E., Holmes, K. K., and Eschenbach, D. A., Relationships of vaginal *Lactobacillus* sp., cervical *Chlamydia trachomatis*, and bacterial vaginosis to preterm birth, *Obstet. Gynecol.*, 71, 89, 1988.

294. Krohn, M. A., Hillier, S. L., and Eschenbach, D. A., Comparison of methods for diagnosing bacterial vaginosis among pregnant women, *J. Clin. Microbiol.*, 27, 1266, 1989.

295. Martens, M. G., Faro, S., Hammill, H. A., Smith, D., Riddle, G., and Maccato, M., Ampicillin/ sulbactam versus clindamycin in the treatment of postpartum endomyometritis, *South. Med. J.*, 83, 408, 1990.

296. Smyth, E. G. and Weinbren, M. J., *Mycoplasma hominis* sternal wound infection and bacteraemia, *J. Infect.*, 26, 315, 1993.

297. Steffenson, D. O., Dummer, J. S., Granick, M. S., Pasculle, A. W., Griffith, B. P., and Cassell, G. H., Sternotomy infections with *Mycoplasma hominis*, *Ann. Intern. Med.*, 106, 204, 1987.

298. Cohen, J. I., Sloss, L. J., Kundsin, R., and Golightly, L., Prosthetic valve endocarditis by *Mycoplasma hominis*, *Am. J. Med.*, 86, 819, 1989.

299. Mufson, M., *Mycoplasma hominis*: a review of its role as a respiratory tract pathogen of humans, *Sex. Transm. Dis.*, 10, 335, 1983.

300. Ti, T. Y., Dan, M., Stemke, G. W., Robertson, J., and Goldsand, G., Isolation of *Mycoplasma hominis* from the blood of men with multiple trauma and fever, *JAMA*, 247, 60, 1982.

301. Di Girolami, P. C. and Madoff, S., *Mycoplasma hominis* septicaemia, *J. Clin. Microbiol.*, 16, 566, 1982.

302. Simberkoff, M. S. and Toharsky, B., Mycoplasmaemia in adult male patients, *JAMA*, 236, 2522, 1976.

303. Luttrell, L. M., Kanj, S. S., Corey, G. R., Lins, R. E., Spinner, R. J., Mallon, W. J., and Sexton, D. J., *Mycoplasma hominis* septic arthritis: two case reports and review, *Clin. Infect. Dis.*, 19, 1067, 1994.

304. Verinder, D. G. R., Septic arthritis due to *Mycoplasma hominis*: a case report and review of the literature, *J. Bone Joint Surg.*, 60-B, 224, 1978.

305. Kayser, S. and Bhend, H. J., Lumbar pain caused by mycoplasma infection, *Infection*, 20, 97, 1992.

306. Madoff, S. and Hooper, D. C., Nongenitourinary infections caused by *Mycoplasma hominis* in adults, *Rev. Infect. Dis.*, 10, 602, 1988.

307. Meyer, R. D. and Clough, W., Extragenital *Mycoplasma hominis* infections in adults: emphasis on immunosuppression, *Clin. Infect. Dis.*, 17(Suppl. 1), S243, 1993.

308. Nylander, N., Tan, M., and Newcombe, D. S., Successful management of *Mycoplasma hominis* septic arthritis involving a cementless prosthesis, *Am. J. Med.*, 87, 348, 1989.

309. Clough, W., Cassell, G. H., Duffy, L. B., Rinaldi, R. Z., Bluestone, R., Morgan, M. A., and Meyer, R. D., Septic arthritis and bacteremia due to *Mycoplasma* resistant to antimicrobial therapy in a patient with systemic lupus erythematosus, *Clin. Infect. Dis.*, 15, 402, 1992.

310. Sneller, M., Wellborne, F., Barile, M. F., and Plotz, P., Prosthetic joint infection with *Mycoplasma hominis*, *J. Infect. Dis.*, 153, 174, 1986.

311. Olson, L. D., Shane, S. W., Karpas, A. A., Cunningham, T. M., Probst, P. S., and Barile, M. F., Monoclonal antibodies to surface antigens of a pathogenic *Mycoplasma hominis* strain, *Infect. Immun.*, 59, 1683, 1991.

312. McDonald, M. I., Moore, J. O., Harrelson, J. M., Browning, C. P., and Gallis, H. A., Septic arthritis due to *Mycoplasma hominis*, *Arthritis Rheum.*, 26, 1044, 1983.

313. McMahon, D. K., Dummer, J. S., Pasculle, A. W., and Cassell, G. H., Extragenital *Mycoplasma hominis* infections in adults, *Am. J. Med.*, 89, 275, 1990.

314. Burdge, D. R., Reid, G. D., Reeve, C. E., Robertson, J. A., Stemke, G. W., and Bowie, W. R., Septic arthritis due to dual infection with *Mycoplasma hominis* and *Ureaplasma urealyticum*, *J. Rheum.*, 15, 366, 1988.

315. Taylor-Robinson, D., Thomas, B. J., Furr, P. M., and Keat, A. C., The association of *Mycoplasma hominis* with arthritis, *Sex. Transm. Dis.*, 10(Suppl.), 341, 1983.

316. Kim, S. K., *Mycoplasma hominis* septic arthritis, *Ann. Plast. Surg.*, 20, 163, 1988.

317. Roifman, C. M., Pandu Rao, C., Lederman, H. M., Lavi, S., Quinn, P., and Gelfand, E. W., Increased susceptibility to Mycoplasma infection in patients with hypogammaglobulinemia, *Am. J. Med.*, 80, 590, 1986.

318. Jorup-Ronstrom, C., Ahl, T., Hammarstrom, L., Smith, C. I. E., Rylander, M., and Hallander, H., Septic osteomyelitis and polyarthritis with *Ureaplasma* in hypogammaglobulinemia, *Infection*, 17, 301, 1989.

319. Webster, A. D. B., Furr, P. M., Hughes-Jones, N. C., Gorick, B. D., and Taylor-Robinson, D., Critical dependence on antibody for defense against mycoplasmas, *Clin. Exp. Immunol.*, 71, 383, 1988.

320. Haller, M., Forst, H., Ruckdeschel, G., and Pratschke, E., *Mycoplasma hominis* in liver transplantation, *Surgery*, 113, 359, 1993.

321. Jacobs, F., Van de Stadt, J., Gelin, M., Nonhoff, C., Gay, F., Adler, M., and Thys, J.-P., *Mycoplasma hominis* infection of perihepatic hematomas in a liver transplant recipient, *Surgery*, 111, 98, 1992.

322. Jacobs, F. and Thys, J.-P., *Mycoplasma hominis* in liver transplantation: reply, *Surgery*, 113, 359, 1993.

323. Haller, M., Forst, H., Ruckdeschel, G., Denecke, H., and Peter, K., Peritonitis due to *Mycoplasma hominis* and *Ureaplasma urealyticum* in a liver transplant recipient, *Eur. J. Clin. Microbiol. Infect. Dis.*, 10, 172, 1991.

324. Mokhbat, J. E., Peterson, P. K., Sabath, L. D., and Robertson, J. A., Peritonitis due to *Mycoplasma hominis* in a renal transplant recipient, *J. Infect. Dis.*, 146, 713, 1982.

325. Roberts, D., Murray, A. E., Pratt, B. C., and Meigh, R. E., *Mycoplasma hominis* as a respiratory pathogen in X-linked hypogammaglobulinaemia, *J. Infect. Dis.*, 18, 175, 1989.

326. Lo, S.-C., Wang, R. Y., Newton, P. B. III, Yang, N.-Y., Sonoda, M. A., and Shih, J. W.-K., Fatal infection of silvered leaf monkeys with a virus-like infectious agent (VLIA) derived from a patient with AIDS, *Am. J. Trop. Med. Hyg.*, 40, 399, 1989.

327. Saillard, C., Carle, P., Bové, M., Bébéar, C., Lo, S.-C., Shih, J. W.-K., Wang, R. Y.-H., Rose, D. L., and Tully, J. G., Genetic and serologic relatedness between *Mycoplasma fermentans* strains and a mycoplasma recently identified in tissues of AIDS and non-AIDS patients, *Res. Virol.*, 141, 385, 1990.

328. Lo, S.-C., Shih, J. W.-K., Newton, P. B. III, Wong, D. M., Hayes, M. M., Benish, J. R., Wear, D. J., and Wang, R. Y.-H., Virus-like infectious agent (VLIA) is a novel pathogenic mycoplasma: *Mycoplasma incognitus*, *Am. J. Trop. Med. Hyg.*, 41, 586, 1989.

329. Bauer, F. A., Wear, D. J., Angritt, P., and Lo, S.-C., *Mycoplasma fermentans* (incognitus strain) infection in the kidneys of patients with acquired immunodeficiency syndrome and associated nephropathy: a light microscopic, immunohistochemical, and ultrastructural study, *Hum. Pathol.*, 22, 63, 1991.

330. Lo, S.-C., Buchholz, C. L., Wear, D. J., Hohm, R. C., and Marty, A. M., Histopathology and doxycycline treatment in a previously healthy non-AIDS patient systematically infected by *Mycoplasma fermentans* (incognitus strain), *Modern Pathol.* 4, 750, 1991.

331. Mirsalimi, S. M., Rosendal, S., and Julian, R. T., Colonization of the intestine of turkey embryos exposed to *Mycoplasma iowae*, *Avian Dis.*, 33, 310, 1989.

332. Lo, S.-C., Tsai, S., Benish, J. R., Shih, J. W.-K., Wear, D. J., and Wong, D. M., Enhancement of HIV-1 cytocidal effects of CD4+ lymphocytes by the AIDS-associated mycoplasma, *Science*, 251, 1074, 1991.

333. Lemaitre, M., Guétard, D., Hénin, Y., Montagnier, L., and Zerial, A., Protective activity of tetracycline analogs against the cytopathic effect of the human immunodeficiency viruses in CEM cells, *Res. Virol.*, 141, 5, 1990.

334. Lemaitre, M., Hénin, Y., Destouesse, F., Ferrieux, C., Montagnier, L., and Blanchard, A., Role of mycoplasma infection in the cytopathic effect induced by human immunodeficiency virus type 1 in infected cell lines, *Infect. Immun.*, 60, 742, 1992.

335. Chowdhurg, M. I. H., Koyanagi, Y., Kobayashi, S., Yamamoto, N., Munakata, T., and Akai, S., Mycoplasma and AIDS, *Lancet*, 336, 247, 1990.

336. Wright, K., Research news: mycoplasma in the AIDS spotlight, *Science*, 248, 682, 1990.

337. Anonymous, Mycoplasma and AIDS: what connections? *Lancet*, 337, 20, 1991.

338. Montagnier, L., Blanchard, A., Guétard, D., Berneman, D., Lemaitre, M., Di Rienzo, A.-M., Chamaret, S., Hénin, Y., Bahraoui, E., Dauguet, C., Axler, C., Firstetter, M., Roue, R., Pialoux, G., and Dupont, D., A possible role of mycoplasmas as co-factors in AIDS, in *Retroviruses of Human AIDS and Related Animal Diseases: Proceedings of the Colloque des Cent Gardes*, Girard, M. and Valette, L., Eds., Fondation M. Mérieux, Lyon, France, 1990, 9.

339. Katseni, V. L., Gilroy, C. B., Ryait, B. K., Ariyoshi, K., Bieniasz, P. D., Weber, J. N., and Taylor-Robinson, D., *Mycoplasma fermentans* in individuals seropositive and seronegative for HIV-1, *Lancet*, 341, 271, 1993.

340. McCormack, W. M., Susceptibility of mycoplasmas to antimicrobial agents: clinical implications, *Clin. Infect. Dis.*, 17(Suppl. 1), S200, 1993.

341. Georgiev, V. St., Treatment and developmental therapeutics of *Mycobacterium avium* complex (MAC) infections, *Int. J. Antimicrob. Agents*, 4, 247, 1994.

342. Jao, R. L. and Finland, M., Susceptibility of *Mycoplasma pneumoniae* to 21 antibiotics *in vitro*, *Am. J. Med. Sci.*, 253, 639, 1967.

343. Jensen, K. J., Senterfit, L. B., Scully, W. E., Conway, T. J., West, R. F., and Drummy, W. W., *Mycoplasma pneumoniae* infections in children: an epidemiologic appraisal in families treated with oxytetracycline, *Am. J. Epidemiol.*, 86, 419, 1967.

344. Braun, P., Klein, J. O., and Kass, E. H., Susceptibility of genital mycoplasmas to antimicrobial agents, *Appl. Microbiol.*, 19, 62, 1970.

345. Bygdeman, S. M. and Mardh, P.-A., Antimicrobial susceptibility and susceptibility testing of *Mycoplasma hominis*: a review, *Sex. Transm. Dis.*, 10(Suppl.), 366, 1983.

346. Harwick, H. J. and Fekety, F. R., The antibiotic susceptibility of *Mycoplasma hominis*, *J. Clin. Pathol.*, 22, 434, 1969.

347. Shaw, D. R. and Lin, J., Extragenital *Mycoplasma hominis*: a report of 2 cases, *Med. J. Aust.*, 148, 144, 1988.

348. Myhre, E. B. and Mordh, P. A., Treatment of extragenital infections caused by *Mycoplasma hominis*, *Sex. Transm. Dis.*, 11, 382, 1983.

349. Koutsky, L. A., Stamm, W. E., Brunham, R. C., Stevens, C. E., Cole, B., Hale, J., Davick, P., and Holmes, K. K., Persistence of *Mycoplasma hominis* after therapy: importance of tetracycline resistance and coexisting vaginal flora, *Sex. Transm. Dis.*, 10(Suppl.), 374, 1983.

350. Cummings, M. C. and McCormack, W. M., Increase in resistance of *Mycoplasma hominis* to tetracyclines, *Antimicrob. Agents Chemother.*, 34, 2297, 1990.

351. Roberts, M. C., Koutsky, L. A., Holmes, K. K., LeBlanc, D. J., and Kenny, G. E., Tetracycline-resistant *Mycoplasma hominis* strains contain streptococcal ^{TET}M sequences, *Antimicrob. Agents Chemother.*, 28, 141, 1985.

352. Stimson, J. B., Hale, J., Bowie, W. R., and Holmes, K. K., Tetracycline-resistant *Ureaplasma urealyticum*: a cause of persistent nongonococcal urethritis, *Ann. Intern. Med.*, 94, 192, 1981.

353. Roberts, M. C. and Kenny, G. E., Dissemination of the *tetM* tetracycline resistant determinant to *Ureaplasma urealyticum*, *Antimicrob. Agents Chemother.*, 29, 350, 1986.

354. Roberts, M. C. and Kenny, G. E., *TetM* tetracycline-resistant determinants in *Ureaplasma urealyticum*, *Pediatr. Infect. Dis. J.*, 5, S338, 1986.

355. Evans, R. T. and Taylor-Robinson, D., The incidence of tetracycline-resistance strains of *Ureaplasma urealyticum*, *J. Antimicrob. Chemother.*, 4, 57, 1978.

356. Robertson, J. A., Stemke, G. W., Maclelland, S. G., and Taylor, D. E., Characterization of tetracycline-resistant strains of *Ureaplasma urealyticum*, *J. Antimicrob. Chemother.*, 21, 319, 1988.

357. Robertson, J. A., Coppola, J. E., and Heisler, O. R., Standardized method for determining antimicrobial susceptibility of strains of *Ureaplasma urealyticum* and their response to tetracycline, erythromycin and rosaramicin, *Antimicrob. Agents Chemother.*, 20, 53, 1981.

358. Echaniz Avilés, G., Conde Gonzalez, C., Juarez Figueroa, L., Barahas, N. C., Tamayo Legoreta, E., and Calderon Jaimes, E., *In vitro* activity of several antimicrobial agents against genital mycoplasmas, *Clin. Ther.*, 14, 688, 1992.

359. Yancey, R. J. and Klein, L. K., In-vitro activity of trospectomycin sulphate against mycoplasma and ureaplasma species isolated from humans, *J. Antimicrob. Chemother.*, 21, 731, 1988.

360. Hayes, M. M., Wear, D. J., and Lo, S.-C., *In vitro* antimicrobial susceptibility testing for the newly identified AIDS-associated *Mycoplasma*: *Mycoplasma fermentans* (incognitus strain), *Arch. Pathol. Lab. Med.*, 115, 464, 1991.

361. Sande, M. A. and Mandell, G. L., Antimicrobial agents, in *Goodman and Gilman: The Pharmacological Basis of Therapeutics*, 7th ed., Gilman, A. G., Goodman, L. S., Rall, T. W., and Murad, F., Eds., Macmillan, New York, 1170, 1985.

Section III

Parasitic Infections

21 Introduction

Traditionally, medical parasitology has included the study of three major groups of organisms: parasitic protozoa, parasitic helminths (worms), and those arthropods that directly cause disease or act as vectors of various pathogens.[1] Typically, a parasite is an organism that simultaneously injures and derives sustenance from another living organism.

Parasitic protozoa are single-cell eukaryotic organisms comprising the simplest forms of the animal kingdom. Their unicellular free-living structure ranges in size from submicroscopic to macroscopic — most parasitic protozoa in humans are less than 50 μm in size, with the smallest (mainly intracellular forms) measuring between 1.0 to 10 μm. Currently, the protozoa are divided into seven phyla: Sarcomastigophora, Labyrinthomorphpha, Apicomplexa, Microspora, Acetospora, Myxozoa, and Ciliophora.[2]

The life cycle stages of protozoa differ both in structure and activity. Trophozoite is a general term used to described the active, feeding, and multiplying stage of most protozoa, which in the majority of parasitic species is also associated with their pathogenesis. A variety of terms are utilized to depict different stages of Apicomplexa, such as tachyzoite and bradyzoite for *Toxoplasma gondii*, merozoite (the form resulting from fission of a multinucleate schizont), as well as sexual stages, such as gametocytes and gametes. Furthermore, some protozoa produce cysts, which represent stages containing one or more infective forms, and have protective membranes or a thickened wall. The cysts, which must survive outside the host, usually have more resistant walls than those that form in tissues.[2-4]

Binary fission, the most common pattern of reproduction, is asexual — the organelles are duplicated and the protozoan then divides into two complete organisms. Protozoa of the phylum Apicomplexa are characterized with both sexual and asexual reproduction patterns. In some protozoa, the life cycle is rather complex requiring two different host species to complete; others require only a single host. In the latter case, a single infective protozoan entering a susceptible host has the potential to produce an enormous population.[2]

Parasitic infections commonly result in tissue damage leading to disease.[5] In chronic parasitic infections the tissue damage is frequently the result of an immune response to the parasite and/or to host antigens. However, tissue damage may also occur from toxic protozoal products and/or to mechanical damage. Very often, the parasites may avoid the killing effect of the immune system in immunocompetent hosts by using an array of escape mechanisms, such as: (1) *antigenic masking*, in which a parasite covers itself with host antigens to escape immune detection; (2) *blocking of serum factors*, where some parasites acquire a coating of antigen-antibody complexes or non-cytotoxic antibodies that will sterically block the binding of specific antibody or lymphocytes to the parasite surface antigens; (3) *intracellular location* which by concealing the parasite antigens will protect the parasites from the direct effects of the host's immune response and/or delay detection by the immune system; (4) *antigenic variation*, in which some protozoa will change their surface antigens during the course of infection, thereby escaping the immune response to the original antigens; and (5) *immunosuppression*, where a protozoan infection will generally produce some degree of host immunosuppression, in which reduced immune responses may delay detection of antigenic variants, and a reduced ability of the immune system may be slow to inhibit the growth of and/or to kill parasites.[5-7]

Different hypotheses have been suggested to explain the immunosuppression observed during the course of parasitic infections, including (1) the presence in the infected hosts of parasite or host substances that nonspecifically will stimulate the growth of antibody-protecting B lymphocytes, rather than stimulating the proliferation of specific anti-parasite B cells; (2) proliferation of suppressor T lymphocytes and/or macrophages that inhibit the immune system; and (3) production by the parasite of specific immune suppressor substances.[5,8,9]

21.1   REFERENCES

1. Olson, L. J., Parasitology, in *Medical Microbiology*, 3rd ed., Baron, S., Ed., Churchill Livingston, New York, 965, 1991.
2. Yaeger, R. G., Protozoa: structure, classification, growth, and development, in *Medical Microbiology*, 3rd ed., Baron, S., Ed., Churchill Livingston, New York, 967, 1991.
3. Englund, P. T. and Sher, A., Eds., *The Biology of Parasitism. A Molecular and Immunological Approach*, Alan R. Liss, New York, 1988.
4. Beaver, P. C. and Jung, R. C., Eds., *Animal Agents and Vectors of Human Disease*, 5th ed., Lea and Fabiger, Philadelphia, 1985.
5. Seed, J. R., Protozoa: pathogenesis and defenses, in *Medical Microbiology*, 3rd. ed., Baron, S., Ed., Churchill Livingston, New York, 1991, 973.
6. Aggarwal, A. and Nash, T. E., Antigen variation of *Giardia lamblia in vivo*, *Infect. Immun.*, 56, 1420, 1988.
7. Capron, A. and Dessaint, J. P., Molecular basis of host-parasite relationship: towards the definition of protective antigens, *Immunol. Rev.*, 112, 27, 1989.
8. Denis, M. and Chadee, K., Immunopathology of *Entamoeba histolytica* infections, *Parasitol. Today*, 4, 247, 1988.
9. Dyer, M. and Tait, A., Control of lymphoproliferation by *Theilera anulata*, *Parasitol. Today*, 3, 309, 1987.

22 Eucococcidiida

Over the last 10 years or so, the reported incidence of cryptosporidiosis and isosporiasis, two invasive opportunistic/nosocomial infections in man, has risen dramatically. A large population of immunocompromised patients because of underlying diseases such as hematologic malignancies and acquired immunodeficiency syndrome (AIDS), or patients undergoing cancer chemotherapy or immunosuppressive therapy, are particularly susceptible to the effects of these infections. With the spread of the AIDS epidemic, the subject of actual and potential therapy of cryptosporidiosis became increasingly important and of considerable interest to clinicians. The causative agents of cryptosporidiosis and isosporiasis are two parasites, *Cryptosporidium* spp. and *Isospora belli*, respectively. The pathogens represent two genera of coccidian protozoans classified in the suborder Eimeriina, order Eucococcidiida. Taxonomically both coccidian protozoa are related to *Toxoplasma gondii* and *Plasmodium* spp.

22.1 *CRYPTOSPORIDIUM* SPP.

22.1.1 INTRODUCTION

Cryptosporidium (family Cryptosporiidae, suborder Eimeriina, order Eucococcidiida) was initially described by Tyzzer in 1907.[1] The first cases of human cryptosporidiosis were reported in 1976.[2,3]

Morphologically, these protozoan parasites, which are relatively small (2 to 6 μm, depending on the stage of development), complete their life cycle in a single host.[4] The pathogenic mechanism by which *Cryptosporidium* causes diarrhea is presently unknown. After ingestion of the oocyst, intestinal bile acids and proteases act to liberate the motile sporozoites into the intestinal lumen.[5] The sporozoites will attach to the microvillous surface and interact with enterocytes before penetrating the plasma membrane of mucosal cells by invagination.[6] In the intestinal epithelium, parasites replicate within parasitophorous vacuoles by both asexual multiplication and sexual differentiation.[7] The asexual multiplication will produce meronts which contain merozoites. The merozoites infiltrate the intestinal lumen and reinvade the epithelial cells. Gamogony will occur when some of the merozoites rather than undergoing merogony, will develop into microgametocytes (male form) and macrogametocytes (female form). Fertilization of macrogametocytes will result in new oocyst production.[8] Oocysts represent the infective stage of the parasite and are spread mainly by fecal/oral routes. Some oocysts, however, may rupture into the intestinal lumen, resulting in a cycle of autoinfection.[9] It takes between 3 and 5 d for the life cycle of *Cryptosporidium* to complete.[10,11] The endogenous stages of the parasite in the brush border of the epithelial cells are detected usually by histologic means using H&E-stained intestinal specimens fixed within 1 to 2 h after death.[12,13]

Oocysts can be seen microscopically in direct fecal smears or intestinal contents stained with Kinyoun's carbolfuchsin, modified acid-fast stain, Giemsa stain, as well as a number of other stains.[14-17] Chichino et al.[18] described two new rapid extemporaneous negative-staining methods to detect *Cryptosporidium* oocysts in stools by using light-green and merbromine in 1% and 2% aqueous solution, respectively. Oocysts were found in fecal specimens or intestinal contents even 24 h after death of the host, and can be preserved for weeks when kept moist and stored at 4°C.[12,19]

In cases of intestinal cryptosporidiosis, the feces may contain 10^5 to 10^7/ml *Cryptosporidium* oocysts. On occasion, shedding is detected several hours before the onset of cryptosporidial diarrhea and as late as 2 weeks after symptoms have resolved.[12]

The molecular mechanism(s) and specific proteins involved in the initial interaction between *Cryptosporidium* sporozoites and the intestinal epithelial cells are not known. Lectins, carbohydrate-binding proteins, have been thought to mediate a number of cell–cell interactions including those between parasite and hosts. In an earlier study, Thea et al.,[20] using a hemagglutination assay, demonstrated that *C. parvum* sporozoites exhibited surface-associated lectin activity. In subsequent experiments, Joe et al.[21] defined the carbohydrate specificity of this lectin and determined its role in *in vitro* attachment and invasion of host cells by the sporozoites. Of 12 monosaccharides tested, galactose (Gal) and *N*-acetylgalactosamine (GalNAc) were identified as the strongest inhibitors of hemagglutination. Furthermore, to determine whether the lectin exhibited a preference for specific glycosidic linkages, several Gal-containing disaccharides were evaluated for their inhibitory effect. Two disaccharides, Gal(β1-3)GalNAc and Gal(α1-4)Gal were found to be the most inhibitory. To this end, it should be noted that the blood group antigen-related P_1 glycoprotein contains Gal(α1-4)Gal as the terminal sugar moiety, and Gal and GalNAc are constituents of bovine submaxillary mucin (BSM) and two other glycoproteins, fetuin and oromucoid.[21] Further experiments have shown that the surface-associated lectins have the potential to adhere to host cell receptors as an early event in the pathogenesis of *C. parvum*. Thus, BSM and fetuin (both inhibitors of the *C. parvum* Gal/GalNAc lectin) reduced the attachment and invasion of sporozoites to MDCK cells, thereby suggesting that the *C. parvum* sporozoite lectin may play a role in the initial parasite-host cell interaction.

Prior to 1982, cryptosporidiosis was considered to be an infrequent parasitic disease occurring mainly in animals and with only eight reported cases in humans.[4,22-25] In the last several years, however, because of improved diagnostic techniques and the raising tide of the AIDS epidemic, and the immunosuppressed population in general, *Cryptosporidium*-induced infections are considered to be one of the world's most commonly found causes of diarrheal illness in humans, especially infants and children,[26-28] the elderly,[29,30] and AIDS patients in particular.[31-42]

Cryptosporidial infections are not limited to gastrointestinal illness only. Respiratory, conjunctival, gastric, and gall blader infections caused by *Cryptosporidium* have also been reported,[12,13,42-48] whereas Ito and Kawata[49] have presented a case of liver cryptosporidiosis. Acute pancreatitis in HIV-infected patients due to *Cryptosporidium* infection has also been reported.[50]

Respiratory cryptosporidiosis is caused by the invasion of *C. parvum* into the epithelial lining of the airways. Various symptoms of respiratory infection include cough, wheezing, croup, shortness of breath, and hoarseness, and the presence of oocysts in the sputum, tracheal aspirates, bronchoalveolar lavage fluid, brush biopsy specimens, and the alveolar exudate from lung biopsy.[51-53] Similarly to cryptosporidial diarrhea, the most severe and life-threatening cases of respiratory cryptosporidiosis occur in immunocompromised patients,[43,54] such as those infected with HIV.[31] Thus, Meynard et al.[55] have reported a fatal case of pulmonary cryptosporidiosis in an AIDS patient who died 2 months after the onset of respiratory symptoms.

Gross et al.[56] described a case of an AIDS patient having multiple cryptosporidial infection of the biliary tree, pancreas, respiratory tract, and the bowel.

Cron and Sherry[57] have described a pediatric patient with Reiter's syndrome secondary to cryptosporidial gastroenteritis. In another complication associated with cryptosporidiosis, several cases of benign pneumatosis cystoides intestinalis among AIDS patients have been reported.[58] This association suggests that cryptosporidial infection may be pathogenically involved in the pneumatosis and not being merely incidental.

Results from histologic examination of mice by Tatar et al.[59] have indicated that stress and/or *Helicobacter felis* activated *Cryptosporidium muris* and caused gastric inflammation, the extent of which depended on the duration of the stress.

Rose[60] described three outbreaks of waterborne disease attributed to *Cryptosporidium*, with two of them linked to drinking water, and the third to surface water. Other investigators[61-68] have also reported outbreaks of cryptosporidiosis associated with water. Experiments by Fayer and Nerad[69] demonstrated that oocysts of *C. parvum* in water can retain viability and infectivity after freezing and that oocysts may survive longer at freezing temperatures as low as $-20°C$.[70]

In this regard, the effects of disinfection of drinking water with ozone or chlorine dioxide on the survival of *C. parvum* oocysts have been examined.[71,72] Disinfection of *C. parvum* oocysts by pulsed light treatment has also been proposed.[73] Low-molecular-weight gases (ammonia, ethylene oxide, and methyl bromide) may also serve as potential disinfectants for *C. parvum* oocysts where soil, rooms, buildings, tools, or instruments might be contaminated with the parasites.[74] High-temperature short-time conditions (71.1°C for 5 to 15 s) used in commercial pasteurization have been sufficient to destroy the infectivity of *C. parvum* oocysts.[75]

Based on environmental occurrence, the risk of *Cryptosporidium* transmission by the water route may be equal to, or greater than, that of *Giardia*. Shepherd and Wyn-Jones[76] have evaluated and optimized methods for the simultaneous detection of *C. parvum* and *Giardia* cysts from water, including cartridge or membrane filtrations, and calcium carbonate flocculation. The knowledge of the hydrophobic and cell surface charge properties of *C. parvum* is important for the appropriate choice of various flocculation treatments, membrane filters, and cleaning agents in connection with the oocyst recovery.[77] Rochelle et al.[78] have developed a rapid procedure for detection of *Cryptosporidium* using *in vitro* cell culture combined with polymerase chain reaction (PCR).

Cryptosporidiosis outbreaks among school children after coming into contact with calves during educational farm outings have also been reported,[79,80] as well as a foodborne outbreak of diarrheal illness associated with *C. parvum*.[81,82]

In the immunocompetent host, cryptosporidial infections result in a self-limited, flu-like gastrointestinal disorder[83-86] which resolves spontaneously in 1 to 4 weeks;[11,86,87] patients will develop immunity and recover completely from the infection. The highest incidence of cryptosporidiosis has been reported in infant populations of the tropical and subtropical zones during the warmer months of the year.[88,89]

In immunocompromised hosts, however, *Cryptosporidium* usually produces a severe and prolonged illness with high morbidity, which in AIDS patients has been clearly associated with the CD4+ counts.[33,90-92] The mortality rate of cryptosporidiosis in immunocompromised patients is also high:[93] in adults, it is associated mainly with AIDS patients[4,94,95] and children having hypogammaglobulinemia,[96,97] severe combined immunodeficiency (SCID),[98,99] or patients receiving immunosuppressive therapy for malignancies[100-103] or renal transplant recipients.[104]

With regard to epidemiology, cryptosporidial infections in immunocompetent hosts are more prevalent in underdeveloped countries (4% to 32%) as compared with developed nations (0.6% to 20%).[105] Among AIDS patients, cryptosporidiosis was found much more prevalent in Africa and Haiti (50%) than it is in the U.S. (3% to 4%). With the spread of the AIDS epidemic, especially in Asia, these numbers are expected to increase. Furthermore, within the AIDS population, children and homosexual men have had higher incidence of cryptosporidiosis than heterosexual persons (predominantly intravenous drug abusers).[105]

Clinical manifestations of gastrointestinal cryptosporidiosis include watery diarrhea (as much as 17 l of watery stools a day[106]), cramping, epigastric abdominal pain, weight loss, anorexia, flatulence, and malaise; while nausea, vomiting, and myalgias may also be present, fever is generally uncommon. The symptoms usually develop insidiously and increase in severity as immune competence deteriorates.[105] In AIDS patients, the observed elevation of serum levels of alkaline phosphatase and γ-glutamyl transpeptidase (while the levels of serum transaminase and bilirubin remain normal) is likely to be associated with cryptosporidial infection, although other factors causing such abnormalities may not be ruled out. Davis et al.[107] presented clinical, pathologic, and radiographic evidence from an immunodeficient child with chronic cryptosporidiosis of the biliary tract, that were consistent with primary sclerosing cholangitis (PSC), a rare and incurable disorder of unknown ethiology. It may well be that chronic cryptosporidial infection of the biliary tract is one etiological mechanism producing PSC in immunocompromised children who were unable to resolve infections of the biliary tract.

Cases of asymptomatic *Cryptosporidium* infections have also been described,[86,108,109] including in HIV-infected patients.[108,110]

22.1.2 HOST IMMUNE RESPONSE TO CRYPTOSPORIDIAL INFECTIONS

In a study aimed at determining the role of gut intraepithelial lymphocytes (IEL) to cryptosporidial disease, McDonald et al.[111] used SCID mice infected with *C. muris*. SCID mice receiving no lymphoid cells developed chronic infections and excreted large numbers of oocysts until the end of the experiment. By comparison, SCID mice injected with IEL from immune animals were able to overcome the infection, produced fewer oocysts, and recover sooner than mice which received IEL or mesenteric lymph node cells from naive BALB/c donors. However, depletion of CD4$^+$ cells from immune IEL abrogated the ability to transfer immunity to SCID mice, while depletion of CD8$^+$ cells only marginally reduced the protective capacity of immune IEL. Furthermore, control SCID mice which received no lymphocytes had ≤1% CD4$^+$ cells in the IEL from the small intestine, whereas the IEL from SCID mice recovered from infection as a result of injection with immune IEL, contained 15% CD4$^+$ cells. The results of these experiments strongly suggested that the ability to control cryptosporidial infection correlated with the presence of protective CD4$^+$ cells in the gut epithelium.[111] In a separate study,[112] mice deficient in either $\alpha\beta$ or $\gamma\delta$ T cells were found to be more susceptible to *C. parvum* infection than were the control mice. Of the two subpopulations, however, the $\alpha\beta$ T cells were more important for resistance than their $\gamma\delta$ counterparts. Results from a separate study by the same investigators,[113] indicated that in BALB/c mice there was correlation between the development of immunity to *C. muris* infection and both a parasite antigen-specific proliferative response and Th1 and Th2 cytokine production by spleen cells.

The cases of two diabetic patients with normal CD4$^+$ cell counts who developed chronic cryptosporidial diarrhea, which is usually seen in patients with low CD4$^+$ cell counts, suggested that some immune defect(s) other than cellular might be involved in the pathogenesis of cryptosporidiosis.[114]

Tatalick and Perryman[115,116] have tested the hypothesis that adoptive transfer of immune spleen cell subsets from immunocompetent BALB/c mice immunized with *C. parvum* antigen would prevent initial infection or terminate persistent infection in SCID mice. In particular, these investigators evaluated the protective effect of surface antigen-1 (SA-1) immune lymphocyte subsets and naive cell subsets. Cell donor mice were immunized with either solubilized *C. parvum* oocysts and sporozoites (positive control) or a surface antigen-1 (SA-1) enriched *C. parvum* antigen fraction. In summary, the results have shown that intravenous injection of either naive or immune CD4$^+$ T and B lymphocytes combined, or CD4$^+$ T lymphocytes alone, terminated persistent *C. parvum* infection in SCID mice. Intestinal infectivity scores were markedly reduced by 9 d postengraftment in all animals and continued to decline throughout the remainder of the experiments. Furthermore, flow cytometric analysis demonstrated significantly increased CD4$^+$ T lymphocytes in the spleen of recipient SCID mice when compared with infected SCID mice receiving no cells. *C. parvum*-specific antibody was detected on day 12 postengraftment in mice receiving SA-1 immune CD4$^+$ T and B lymphocytes but was not detectable in mice receiving naive cell subsets.[115] The SA-1 antigen have been defined as those antigens recognized by the neutralizing monoclonal antibody 17.41, and a SA-1 enriched fraction may be obtained by immunoaffinity chromatography.[116]

22.1.3 EVOLUTION OF THERAPIES AND TREATMENT OF CRYPTOSPORIDIOSIS

Sporadic cryptosporidial diarrhea in children is a relatively mild disease that is easily managed with oral rehydration alone.[117-119] In immunocompromised patients, however, the diarrhea may develop into a chronic, debilitating, and often fatal illness.[120] It leads to fluid and electrolyte abnormalities, malnutrition, and significant weight loss.[105,121-126] For example, in one study of AIDS patients, 96% of patients experienced weight loss, while 55% had diarrhea.[127] In another report,[128] the diarrhea was present in 60% of the AIDS population.

Currently, there is no effective chemotherapy of cryptosporidial diarrhea in immunocompromised patients.[129-134] Moreover, the lack of clinical improvement in such patients following chemotherapy alone may be the result, at least partially, of the presence of multiple concurrent infections and therapies aggravating the already existing immune deficiencies.[135]

There is also no known treatment for pulmonary cryptosporidiosis, a rare complication of intestinal cryptosporidiosis in AIDS patients.

Over the years, a number of therapeutic approaches to cure cryptosporidiosis have been attempted using different agents, including macrolide antibiotics, peptides, as well as immunotherapy. So far, the results have been rather disappointing.

22.1.3.1 Macrolide Antibiotics

Among the macrolide antibiotics, most notably spiramycin has been tested extensively both *in vitro* and *in vivo* for its clinical efficacy against cryptosporidiosis.[136] In several anecdotal reports,[56,137-146] spiramycin was described as useful against cryptosporidial diarrhea and with relatively low incidence of toxic side effects, most often gastrointestinal irritation and hypersensitivity reaction.[105,145,147]

Gross et al.[56] used spiramycin to treat one AIDS patient with multiple-system-involvement cryptosporidial infection; 1.0 g of the antibiotic was administered every 8 h for a period of 8 weeks. While a slight decrease in the alkaline phosphatase level was observed (from 771 to 575 IU/l), stool specimens continued to be positive for cryptosporidial oocysts. After completion of therapy, the patient became afibrile, felt well, and formed stools; however, the alkaline phosphatase level remained five times normal and the patient continued to pass oocysts in the stools.[56]

According to Moskovitz et al.,[141] 28 of 37 patients with cryptosporidial diarrhea (the majority with AIDS) when given 3.0 g of spiramycin daily, responded favorably, as defined by the reduction in the daily number of bowel movements to less than 50% of baseline and fewer than five. In 12 cases, the cryptosporidial oocysts were eradicated from the stools, and the drug, overall, was well tolerated.[141]

In an uncontrolled study conducted by Connolly et al.,[148] 15 AIDS patients with cryptosporidial diarrhea were given either erythromycin or spiramycin (500 mg, four times daily, orally). Although the treatment was limited because of unwarranted side effects, most of the patients were reported to respond favorably by having greater than 50% reduction of stool volume; however, contrary to a previous report,[149] spiramycin did not eradicate the pathogen. In a randomized, double-blind, placebo-controlled study involving 44 otherwise healthy children, spiramycin was described as effective against acute diarrhea caused by *C. parvum*.[150,151] The antibiotic was given at 100 mg/kg daily (in two divided doses) for 10 d; compared to placebo-receiving patients, the results showed reduced symptoms of diarrhea ($p = .002$) and excretion of *Cryptosporidium* oocysts ($p = .032$).

With regard to data reporting therapeutic efficacy of spiramycin against cryptosporidiosis, especially in immunocompromised hosts, it is important to emphasize that, so far, all results about its clinical merits have originated mainly from uncontrolled trials involving very limited numbers of patients, and therefore, should be viewed still as premature and with justified skepticism — the accuracy of such reports must be evaluated in and corroborated by multicenter placebo-controlled trials. To lend credence to such skepticism, in a number of reports,[152-155] spiramycin was described as completely ineffective against gastrointestinal cryptosporidiosis. Thus, in a double-blind, placebo-controlled trial involving infants and young children (some of them immunocompromised) with cryptosporidial diarrhea, Wittenberg et al.[154,155] found spiramycin lacking activity.

Some contributing factors to the perceived clinical efficacy of spiramycin may be traced to the observed tendency of the infection to disappear spontaneously,[156] or to clinical improvement[157] due to concomitant discontinuation of immunosuppressive medication,[142,143] as well as to better control of cryptosporidial diarrhea in the early stage of AIDS as opposed to cryptosporidiosis in advanced stages of AIDS where the state of immune deficiency is much worse.[158]

In a recent report, Weikel et al.[159] described that two of three AIDS patients with cryptosporidiosis receiving high doses of spiramycin developed acute intestinal injury as the likely result of direct damage to the epithelium by the drug.

A multicenter, placebo-controlled clinical trial of chronic cryptosporidiosis in AIDS patients treated with spiramycin is currently under way and will undoubtedly shed more light on its clinical efficacy; preliminary data from the trial indicated that when administered orally at 1.0 g, three times daily, the antibiotic is nontoxic and may reduce the severity of cryptosporidial diarrhea.[105]

The chemotherapeutic effect of azithromycin, another macrolide antibiotic, against *Cryptosporidium* infection was studied in prednisolone-immunosuppressed 7-week-old female ICR mice.[160] The drug was administered once daily at 400 mg/kg, 13 h postinoculation for 3 d. Compared to controls, the oocyst production of the azithromycin-treated mice was markedly reduced.[160] In dexamethasone-immunosuppressed rats infected with *C. parvum*, azithromycin consistently prevented ileal infection, while spiramycin was ineffective.[161] In addition, the observed activity was dose-related and a daily dose of 200 mg/kg was the minimum one that prevented infection; the latter, however, reappeared after therapy was ceased.[161]

Dupont et al.[162] have reported a favorable outcome in an AIDS patient with pulmonary cryptosporidiosis after treatment with azithromycin — what made this particular case unusual was the presence of extracellular invasive forms of the parasite in the bronchoalveolar lavage of the patient. Hicks et al.[163] have described a successful outcome in three of four pediatric AIDS patients (a marked decrease in stool volume and frequency within 36 h of initiating therapy, and resolution of diarrhea within 5 d) after treatment with azithromycin for severe diarrheal illness solely due to *C. parvum*; the fourth required prolonged therapy with azithromycin to achieve clearance. In another report, Vargas et al.[164] described two pediatric patients with cancer who received azithromycin for *Cryptosporidium*-associated diarrhea that was unresponsive to supportive care. One child had choleriform diarrhea requiring daily fluid replacement of up to 65% of his total body weight; the other had protracted diarrhea and wasting. In both cases, administration of azithromycin resulted in prompt clinical improvement.

In a retrospective study, Jordan[165] compared the incidence of cryptosporidial enteritis in AIDS patients (n = 63) receiving prophylactic clarithromycin (500 mg, b.i.d.) for *Mycobacterium avium* complex (MAC) with patients (n = 73) not treated with clarithromycin who served as the control group. None of the patients who received clarithromycin developed cryptosporidial enteritis compared with four patients (all with CD4$^+$ of less than 25 cells/mm^3) from the control group. In a subsequent 2-year follow-up study of an additional 217 AIDS patients with CD4$^+$ of <50 cells/mm^3 receiving clarithromycin (500 mg, b.i.d.) as MAC prophylaxis, no patient developed cryptosporidial enteritis. These results provided strong evidence supporting the use of clarithromycin in AIDS patients as prophylaxis against both MAC and cryptosporidiosis.[165] Cama et al.[166] have examined the therapeutic efficacy of clarithromycin and its 14-hydroxy metabolite in acute and chronic *C. parvum* infections in mice. While significant parasite reductions were detected at ileal and hepatic levels by both compounds, no parasite eradication was observed in any of the studies, and the *C. parvum* presence at the colonic and ceccal levels was not markedly reduced either.

Roxithromycin, a macrolide antibiotic previously found active against *Isospora* and *Toxoplasma* infections, was devoid of activity against intestinal cryptosporidiosis in AIDS patients.[167]

The anticryptosporidial activity of five macrolide antibiotics (azithromycin, clarithromycin, erythromycin, oleandomycin, and spiramycin) was evaluated in a dexamethasone-immunosuppressed rat model.[168] All macrolides reduced the severity of the ileal infection; however, their effect on the cecal infection was variable, depending on the antibiotic and the applied dose.

Giacometti et al.[169] have also examined the efficacy of four macrolides (azithromycin, clarithromycin, roxithromycin, and spiramycin) alone and with combination with pyrimethamine, dapsone, atovaquone, artemisin, and minocycline against *C. parvum* oocysts. The macrolide concentrations studied were 0.25, 0.5, 1.0, 2.0, 4.0, 8.0, 16.0, and 32 µg/ml, and those for the other agents were: artemisin, 0.02, 0.2, and 2.0 µg/ml; atovaquone, 0.2, 2.0, and 20 µg/ml; minocycline, 0.2, 2.0, and 20 µg/ml; dapsone, 0.1, 1.0, and 10 µg/ml; and pyrimethamine, 0.005, 0.05, and 0.5 µg/ml. The results have shown that azithromycin and clarithromycin at ≥16 µg/ml, and roxithromycin at 32 µg/ml were inhibitory. Neither artemisin, atovaquone, nor dapsone had any significant inhibitory effect on *C. parvum*, but minocycline at concentrations of 20 µg/ml was significantly active, whereas pyrimethamine at a concentration of 0.5 µg/ml was inhibitory. Of all macrolide combinations with the other drugs, only the activities of azithromycin, clarithromycin, and roxithromycin each was improved when combined with either minocycline at ≥2.0 µg/ml, or pyrimethamine at concentration of 0.5 µg/ml.[169]

22.1.3.2 Paromomycin

Recently, paromomycin, a poorly absorbed per os aminoglycoside antibiotic known for its activity against *Giardia* and amebic intestinal infections, has been tested for activity against cryptosporidiasis both in experimental animal models and in humans.[170-187]

Gatlie et al.[188] have found paromomycin able to control the symptoms of gastrointestinal cryptosporidiosis and to eradicate the parasite in some patients without evidence of serious toxicity. Clezy et al.[189] used paromomycin in five HIV-infected patients with gastrointestinal cryptosporidiosis. The drug was administered at 1.5 g daily (divided in six equal doses) or 2.0 g daily (divided in five equal doses) depending on the patient's weight (over 60 kg, or less than 60 kg, respectively). The patients were evaluated on a 2-weekly basis mainly to monitor symptoms of diarrhea and changes in the weight. Within 24 h of commencing the therapy, four patients had reduction in diarrhea (to 1–3 semiformed bowel actions daily), and in one patient the bowel movements returned to normal after 1 week of medication. The control of diarrhea was maintained in all patients during the first 4 weeks of therapy, but four of five patients continued to have detectable oocysts in stools during the treatment. Paromomycin was tolerated well, with serum levels reaching over 6.2 mg/l (lower limit of detection).[189]

Hoepelman[90,190] and others[186] have recommended for therapy with paromomycin an initial regimen of 500 mg of the drug given four times daily for 2 to 3 weeks followed by a maintenance therapy with 500 mg b.i.d. to prevent relapse.

In a prospective, randomized, double-blind trial, the therapeutic efficacy of paromomycin was tested against cryptosporidiosis in 10 AIDS patients.[182] Patients were randomized to receive either paromomycin or placebo; after 14 d, they were switched to the other treatment for 14 additional days. During the paromomycin treatment phase, oocyst excretion decreased from 314×10^6 to 109×10^6 per 24 h ($p < .02$). The oocyst excretion increased for the four patients initially on placebo as compared with a median decrease of $128 \times 10^6/24$ h for the six patients initially treated with paromomycin ($p < .02$). Furthermore, stool frequency also decreased more in those treated with the antibiotic (3.6 fewer vs. 1.25 fewer/24 h; $p < .05$). The overall trend was in favor of drug over placebo for stool weight, stool character, and the Karnofsky score, leading to improvement in both clinical and parasitologic parameters of cryptosporidiosis in AIDS patients. The results presented by White et al.[182] elicited extensive comments from other investigators.[171-173]

Mohri et al.[177] described an AIDS patient with hemophilia A and intractable diarrhea and fever, who, approximately 2 months after admission, developed respiratory infection and hypoxia due to *Cryptosporidium* but was successfully treated with paromomycin inhalation.

Samson and Brown[58] successfully treated cryptosporidiosis in an AIDS patient with a combination of paromomycin and clofazimine.

However, results from the evaluation of high-dose regimens of paromomycin against cryptosporidiosis in a dexamethazone-treated rat model were not so encouraging.[191] While the drug was effective at ≥50 mg/kg daily for ileal infection, and at ≥200 mg/kg daily for cecal infection, at 1 and 3 weeks after cessation of treatment, a persistent cryptosporidial infection was demonstrated in all rats. These results confirmed the therapeutic limitations of this compound because of its potential toxicity at high doses and its inability to eradicate the infection.

Tan et al.[192] have reported a paromomycin-associated pancreatitis in HIV-related cryptosporidiosis — the observed hyperamylasemia (abnormally high elevation of amylase in the blood serum) resolved with discontinuation of treatment and recurred when paromomycin medication was reinstituted. Another potential drawback of long-term, high-dose paromomycin therapy in AIDS patients has been its poor systemic absorption following oral administration.[193]

22.1.3.3 Somatostatin and Analogs

Somatostatin (a tetradecapeptide factor inhibiting the release of somatotropin) has been found useful in the treatment of secretory diarrhea related to various diseases, such as Zollinger-Ellison syndrome,[194] Verner-Morrison syndrome,[195,196] the carcinoid syndrome,[197] glucagonomas,[195] and ileostomy.[198] Somatostatin is known to prolong the intestinal transit time and to induce the net intestinal water and electrolyte reabsorption in patients with diarrhea. Since the native form of somatostatin has a short half-life (3 to 4 min) necessitating its intravenous administration,[199] analogs with longer half-life were subsequently developed.[200]

For the past several years attention has focused on one somatostatin analog, octreotide (sandostatin, SMS 201-995) for its activity against cryptosporidial diarrhea in AIDS patients.[201-205] Structurally, octreotide is a small peptide comprising eight amino acid residues that share homology with a four-amino acid sequence present in somatostatin.[206] The biological activity of octreotide mimicked to a great extent that of endogenous somatostatin, especially its potent ability to inhibit the release of vasoactive intestinal peptide, and/or its action on the intestinal mucosal target tissue.[207,208] Octreotide has a longer half-life (90 to 120 min) and duration of activity of up to 8 h.[209,210]

Katz et al.[210] have used octreotide to treat one 26-year-old hemophiliac patient with AIDS and cryptosporidiosis. The patient showed clinical improvement following continuous intravenous administration of the drug. The therapy lasted for 40 d (75 µg/ml of octreotide and 3000 ml/d of parenteral nutrition). Noticeable improvement in the nutritional and immune status of AIDS patients with cryptosporidial diarrhea following therapy with octeotride was reported in several other studies as well.[167,211]

Clotet et al.[212] treated four AIDS patients subcutaneously with progressively escalating doses of octreotide starting with 50 µg (until a maximum dose of 500 µg) every 8 h. The minimum dose controlling symptoms was maintained for 15 d, and if partial response was observed (reduction greater than 50% in symptoms and number of stools passed daily), a maintenance therapy was initiated; only one of the patients responded completely. Füessl et al.[213,214] used octreotide to treat secretory diarrhea in AIDS patients by injecting the drug subcutaneously twice daily at doses of either 50 or 100 µg.

In an open-label, multicenter, controlled clinical trial involving 49 AIDS patients with profuse diarrhea, octreotide was administered subcutaneously for 14 d (50 µg every 8 h for 3 d, then 100 µg, 250 µg, and 500 µg every 8 h for 3 d each, if no response to prior dose was observed).[215] Four patients responded completely and 13 partially, for an overall rate of 34.7%. After ceasing the therapy, diarrhea recurred in all patients who had initially responded.[215]

Fanning et al.[216] reported results from a pilot-escalating study of 17 nonconsecutive HIV-positive patients given subcutaneous octreotide for refractory diarrhea. The outcome of the trial was quite modest: of the 11 patients who completed the therapy, only 5 responded and were ultimately maintained on long-term octreotide medication (dose range of 50 to 250 μg); while 3 of the patients remained stable on the same dose regimen, the remaining 2 have had their diarrhea worsened and required further increase in drug dosage.

Moroni et al.[217] have examined the effect of octeotride on the bowel frequency of 13 patients with AIDS-associated refractory diarrhea. All patients received 100 μg t.i.d. of subcutaneous octeotride for 1 week; those patients who did not improve were given 250 μg, t.i.d. for an additional 1 week. The bowel frequency returned to normal in one patient, and decreased by more than 50% in seven others; one patient improve at the higher dose.

In general, octreotide was well tolerated and its toxicity was limited to mild adverse reactions, such as pain at the injection site, nausea, abdominal pain, and discomfort or bloating.[209,218]

In a study conducted by Nousbaum et al.,[201] the resolution of cryptosporidial infection in one immunosuppressed patient receiving AZT and the somatostatin analog octreotide was not attributed to the prior improvement of immune functions by the effects of AZT, but rather to the efficacy of octreotide — the progressive disappearance of diarrhea, malabsorption, and cryptosporidia in stools coincided with the octreotide medication.

In the broader context of *Cryptosporidium*-induced diarrhea, especially the inability to treat this condition in AIDS patients, the probable mode of action of octreotide deserves special consideration. Severe manifestations of watery diarrhea observed in AIDS patients have been frequently associated with infection by cryptosporidia. This, however, has not always been the case since the immunodeficiency virus itself may directly cause mucosal hypersecretory response[210] which would result in enteropathy[219-221] and diarrhea. Furthermore, an HIV invasion into the enterochromaffin cells of the intestinal mucosa (which is known to occur[219-221]), may create a local deficiency of somatostatin. Such deficiency, if developed, may explain the beneficial effect of octreotide in ameliorating the cryptosporidial diarrhea in some AIDS patients.[167]

Alternatively, the protein coat of HIV was found to contain amino acid sequences that are homologous with the vasoactive intestinal peptide (VIP).[222] Based on the fact that VIP is an effective stimulant of intestinal fluid secretion,[223] Gaginella and O'Dorisio[207] advanced the hypothesis that HIV may activate the VIP receptors, thereby triggering, at least partially, a diarrheal response.

The mechanism of action of octreotide on the cryptosporidial diarrhea, while still not fully elucidated, may involve a nonspecific effect on the gastrointestinal mucosal fluid and electrolyte secretion.[210] The fact that both somatostatin and octreotide inhibited the effect of VIP on the intestinal secretion may provide one aspect of the mechanism of action of octreotide, namely, its ability to act on the membrane receptor which recognizes VIP. In one report,[224] somatostatin itself was also found effective against refractory cryptosporidial diarrhea in a patient with AIDS.

Although it is still possible that octeotride may prove to be useful against some cases of AIDS-associated intestinal cryptosporidiosis, this will require not only stringently conducted placebo-controlled trials, but also the participation of homogeneous patient populations with regard to their probable cause of diarrhea and better compliance with stool collections.[225]

22.1.3.4 Lytic Peptides

A number of naturally occurring lytic peptides (cecropins[226] and megainins[227]) have shown promising antimicrobial activity.[228] Structurally, the lytic peptides represent generally small (less than 36 amino acid residues; molecular weight <4000) amphipathic proteins that fold into helices with hydrophilic and hydrophobic faces; the latter will facilitate their interactions with cell membranes.[226] Cecropin, megainin, and some of their synthetic analogs were found to form ion channels in both cell membranes and synthetic planar lipid membranes.[229-231] Recently, Arrowood et al.[232] have found two synthetic lytic peptides, Shiva-10 (molecular weight of 2537) and Hecate-1 (molecular weight of 2537) that exerted anticryptosporidial activity *in vitro*. One concern regarding the antiparasitic activity of lytic peptides *in vivo* is their potential enteric and/or systemic toxicities.[228]

22.1.3.5   Other Experimental Therapeutics

In addition to macrolide antibiotics, a number of other drugs were studied for activity against cryptosporidiosis,[233-237] including azidothymidine, α-difluoromethylornithine, paromomycin, halofuginone, corticosteroids, diclazuril, and sulfonamides. In all cases, however, the number of patients treated was usually limited, and in most instances the reported results could not be reproduced; in addition, some of the drugs displayed unacceptable toxicities.

According to Chandrasekar,[238] a remarkable recovery of an AIDS patient with intractable chronic cryptosporidial diarrhea occurred following treatment with azidothymidine (AZT). The medication was initiated at a dose of 200 mg every 4 h; after 1 week, the dose of AZT was decreased to 100 mg every 4 h. Results from stool smears, after 22 d of therapy were negative for cryptosporidia.[238] In another study,[148] three AIDS patients with cryptosporidial diarrhea when given AZT for more than 3 months, responded with cessation of diarrhea and no cryptosporidia isolated from stools. The observed clinical, parasitologic, and histological resolution of intestinal cryptosporidiosis after treatment with AZT is thought to be a secondary effect to an overall improvement of cell-mediated immune functions caused by suppression of the HIV by AZT.[238,239]

Greenberg et al.[239] tried a therapy in which one patient (AIDS complicated with severe cryptosporidial diarrhea and malabsorption) received, in addition to AZT (500 mg, every 8 h; parenteral administration), a low-dose (500 mg, every 8 h) of parenteral acyclovir. Previously, the combination of AZT and acyclovir has been found synergistic *in vitro* and results from one clinical trial suggested its feasibility for treatment of AIDS.[240]

α-Difluoromethylornithine (eflornithine, DFMO) is a drug known as an irreversible inhibitor of ornithine decarboxylase and capable of suppressing the biosynthesis of putrescine and other polyamines.[241] It has been used successfully in the treatment of parasitic protozoal infections.[242-244] Soave et al.[245] reported that three of five patients with AIDS, when medicated with DFMO, showed some palliation of their diarrheal symptoms, with one of the patients having both clinical and parasitological response. Rolston et al.[246] have treated 22 patients with AIDS and severe cryptosporidial diarrhea with DFMO. Of the 17 evaluable patients, only 5 had complete resolution of diarrhea and negative follow-up stool examination for *Cryptosporidium*; 7 of the patients did not respond, and the remaining 5 had either partial resolution, or responded but then relapsed after cessation of therapy.[246] The observed toxicity (bone marrow suppression, hearing impairment, and gastrointestinal intolerance) of DFMO has been serious enough to compromise its intended clinical use.

Sinefungin, a 6-amino-9*H*-purine antibiotic derived from *Streptomyces griseolus*, was found effective at oral daily doses of 2.0 to 10 mg/kg against experimental *C. parvum* infection in immunosuppressed rats, as evidenced by the suppression of oocyst shedding.[247] The activity was dose-related and correlated with oocyst disappearance from the ileal sections.[248] However, relapses occurred after discontinuation of therapy, suggesting that the drug did not clear the parasites from the biliary tract.

Assan et al.[249] have reported a case of hypoglycemia after mefloquine therapy (1.5 g over a 2-d period) for severe gastrointestinal cryptosporidiosis in a cachectic AIDS patient with protracted diarrhea. Other structurally related antimalarial drugs (quinine and its isomer, quinidine) have been well known for causing iatrogenic hypoglycemia due to excessive insulin secretion.

The therapeutic efficacy of halofuginone against *C. parvum* in calves[250,251] and immunosuppressed rats was also tested.[252] In calves, the drug was given orally at doses of 30 to 500 μg/kg over a period of 3 to 14 d. Results showed that at doses of 60 μg/kg and up, oocysts were no longer detected in 98% of the animals 5 to 6 d after the start of treatment, and calves remained negative for at least 7 d after withdrawal; however, from days 7 to 10, some of the animals excreted oocysts again. Overall, a dose of 60 to 125 μg/kg given over 7 d was the most appropriate.[250] Halofuginone was also found to be inhibitory *in vitro* by reducing the multiplication of *C. parvum* by more than 90% when applied at high concentrations.[253]

Treatment of dexamethasone-immunosuppressed rats with dehydroepiandrosterone (DHEA) resulted in a significant reduction of cryptosporidial activity as evidenced by the reduced oocyst shedding and colonization of host tissues by parasites.[254,255] Treatment with dexamethasone alone caused a decrease in both the T and B lymphocytes and natural killer (NK) cell responses, and antibody production. With the exception of NK cell activity, all changes reversed following administration of DHEA.[254] Since HIV-infected patients exhibited increased levels of circulating glucocorticosteroids and diminished levels of DHEA,[256] the potentiation of immune functions by DHEA is being clinically investigated.[257]

Loria et al.[258] have compared the activity of DHEA with two of its metabolites, androstenediol and androstenetriol (produced by C_7 β-hydroxylation of androstenediol) and found that although the three analogs acted in a similar manner *in vivo*, *in vitro* their effects were dramatically different, with only androstenetriol potentiating the cellular response by increasing lymphocyte activation and counteracting the immunosuppressive activity of hydrocortisone.

When administered at daily doses of 200 mg/kg (for body weight of less than 50 kg) or 400 mg (body weight over 50 kg), diclazuril had no obvious beneficial effect on the severe cryptosporidial infection in nine seriously ill AIDS patients.[259] However, Menichetti et al.[260] reported successful treatment of cryptosporidial diarrhea in one AIDS patient with 100 mg of oral diclazuril given every 12 h for 10 d; after 5 d of medication, the watery bowel movements decreased to only two daily and the oocyst count revealed no more than one element every 10 high-power fields.

In an open-label phase I prospective trial conducted in Canada, severely immunocompromised AIDS patients (mean CD4+ cell count of 44×10^6 cells/l) with refractory cryptosporidiosis showed only a modest, short-lived response to letrazuril given at an initial oral dose of 50 mg. Treatment was continued for ≥10 d and for as long as there was a response; all patients had previously failed to respond to paromomycin treatment.[261] In another Canadian open-label, prospective study,[262] AIDS patients (mean CD4+ cell count of 30×10^6 cells/l) with symptomatic intestinal cryptosporidiosis were treated with letrazuril daily in escalating oral doses of 50 to 100 mg for 6 weeks — 50% of the patients experienced an improvement with no serious dose-related toxicities. The pharmacokinetics of letrazuril were examined by Victor et al.[263]

Arprinocid [6-amino-9-(2-chloro-6-fluorobenzyl)purine], an anticoccidial agent, when used prophylactically in mice, markedly reduced the oocyst excretion with no histologic evidence of infection.[264] Against experimental cryptosporidiosis in hamsters, arprinocid exerted activity on the parasite by inhibiting dihydrofolate reductase and glucose-6-phosphate dehydrogenase, in what appeared to be a parasitistatic rather than parasiticidal effect. At the dosages used, however, arprinocid was unable to completely abolish the propagation of parasites if applied after the establishment of infection in 12-d old hamster neonates.[264]

Lasalocid (a coccidiostatic ionophorous, transport-inducing antibiotic), when used at a dose of 8.0 mg/kg, was found effective, but toxic, against experimental cryptosporidial infections in calves.[265-267] In another study,[160] lasalocid was given daily at doses of 64 or 128 mg/kg to prednisolone-immunosuppressed ICR mice; compared to controls, the drug effectively reduced the oocyst production. Rehg[268] has compared the activity of lasalocid and two other ionophorous antibiotics, monensin and salinomycin, in dexamethazone-immunosuppressed rats infected with *C. parvum*. When applied prophylactically, lasalocid prevented infection in a dose-dependent manner, whereas monensin and salinomycin were ineffective. Therapeutically, lasalocid eliminated established overt infections of the intestine, although it persisted in the common bile duct, and intestinal infection recurred after treatment was ceased.[268]

Maduramicin and alborixin, two polyether ionophores at 3.0 mg/kg daily have also shown antisporidial activity (96% and 71% reduction of oocyst shedding, respectively, after 3 weeks of treatment) but also some toxicity as demonstrated by weight loss.[269]

Recently, Forney et al.[270-272] studied the anticryptosporidial potential of a number of serine proteinase inhibitors (α-1-antitrypsin, antipain, aprotinin, leupeptin, methoxysuccinyl-ala-ala-provaline chloromethylketone, soybean trypsin inhibitor, and phenylmethylsulfonyl fluoride). In a bovine fallopian tube epithelial cell culture,[273] leupeptine and the soybean trypsin inhibitor were the most active compounds reducing the parasite numbers to 40% to 50% of the control mean at 500 mg/ml.[271]

According to Rehg,[274] diethyldithiocarbamate was the only immunomodulator of seven evaluated to show activity against *C. parvum* in immunosuppressed rats. When administered prophylactically, diethyldithiocarbamate at daily oral doses of ≥ 75 mg/kg markedly ($p \leq .05$) reduced the severity of ileal infection, and at doses of ≥ 300 mg daily, it significantly ($p \leq .05$) inhibited the infection of the biliary tract. Overall, the activity of diethyldithiocarbamate may prove beneficial for cryptosporidiosis of the small intestine but not for the large intestine or biliary tract.

The intact microtubule function within *C. parvum* is essential for parasite infectivity. In an attempt to elucidate the cellular mechanisms by which anti-microtubular drugs, such as colchicin and vinblastin, are able to inhibit host cell infections,[275] Wiest et al.[276] have investigated the effect of colchicin on the microtubule organization of *C. parvum*. Their results have demonstrated that while colchicin did not block excystation by the microtubules, it disrupted the microtubule network within the *C. parvum* sporozoites. Therefore, anti-microtubular agents may become beneficial by blocking *C. parvum* infection of host cells at latter stages during infection, such as through inhibition of parasite invasion or survival within the parasitophorous vacuole.[276]

In an open-label safety study, Davis et al.[277] have examined the efficacy and pharmacokinetics of nitazoxanide, a nitrothiazole benzamide with broad-spectrum antimicrobial activity, against AIDS-related cryptosporidial diarrhea. Thirty AIDS patients were assigned to receive, in order of enrollment, daily oral doses of either 0.5, 1.0, 1.5, or 2.0 g of the drug for 4 weeks. Patients with persistent cryptosporidial diarrhea were given up to 2.0 g daily of nitazoxanide for an additional 4 weeks. Preliminary data from 22 patients who completed at least 4 weeks of therapy have revealed that 15 (68%) had a reduction of bowel movement frequency: 2 of 6 patients (33%), 7 of 7 (100%), 4 of 6 (67%), and 2 of 3 (67%) at 0.5, 1.0, 1.5, and 2.0 g daily, respectively. Of the nine patients (41%) who showed parasitologic improvement, oocyst shedding decreased by at least two grades or became undetectable in four patients (18%). Furthermore, higher doses of nitazoxanide appeared to be associated with higher peak and trough plasma nitazoxanide metabolite levels, and with greater reduction in the bowel movement frequency. There has been no significant toxicity observed at daily doses as high as 2.0 g of the drug. Overall, nitazoxanide displayed favorable clinical profile, but was less effective parasitologically, thereby necessitating longer duration of treatment and/or higher dose regimens.[277]

Some sulfonamide drugs (sulfadimethoxine, sulfamethazine) when evaluated in immuno-suppressed rats, showed prophylactic activity against *C. parvum*.[278,279] Greenfield et al.[280] have evaluated the prophylactic efficacy of bismuth subsalicylate against *C. parvum* in immunodeficient mice.

Arrowood et al.[281] have found five dinitroaniline herbicides (trifluralin, profluralin, nitralin, pen-dimethalin, and fluchloralin) exhibiting significant anticryptosporidial activity *in vitro*, with IC_{50} values ranging from 0.19 μM for the most active, pendimethalin, to 4.5 μM for the least effective, nitralin.

So far, more than 100 antimicrobial agents, antibiotics, and anthelminthics have been tested for activity against cryptosporidiosis.[136,138,264,281,282] The overwhelming majority of these drugs were found ineffective (e.g., included clopidol, sulfamethoxazole, diloxanide, furazolidone, metronida-zole, pentamidine, piperazine, pyrimethamine, thiobendazole, robenidine, quinine, amphotericin B, β-lactams, clindamicin, colistin, erythromycin, gentamicin, ketoconazole, monensin, oxytetracy-cline, sulfonamides, trimethoprim, bleomycin, cholestyramine, levamisole, quinacrine, chloroquine, and primaquine).[283]

22.1.3.6 Immunotherapy of Cryptosporidiosis

The lack of effective anticryptosporidial chemotherapy in immunocompromised patients on one hand, and the importance of the immune system in determining the host's response towards invading pathogens on the other, have prompted the evaluation of some immunotherapeutic approaches for prevention and treatment of cryptosporidiosis.

A number of polyclonal and monoclonal antibodies capable of neutralizing the infectivity of cryptosporidial sporozoites and merozoites have already been produced.[284-286] In one study, daily oral treatment of BALB/c athymic (nude) mice infected with *C. parvum* with monoclonal antibody (MAb) 17.41 for 10 d, significantly reduced (p <.005) the number of parasites in the intestinal tract, but did not affect the number of organisms in the biliary system.[286,287] Apparently, antibodies targeted directly at the biliary system will be needed in order to minimize or prevent cryptosporidial replication in the gall bladder and bile ducts.[286]

Langer and Riggs[288] have found that neutralizing monoclonal antibodies protected against *C. parvum* infection by inhibiting sporozoite attachment and invasion. The protective antibodies have defined a distinct, conserved epitope on an epical complex exoantigen of *C. parvum*.[289]

Adoptive transfer of BALB/c thymocytes, spleen, and bone marrow cells to severe combined immunodeficient (SCID) mice experimentally infected with *C. parvum*, resulted in functional immunologic reconstitution followed by complete eradication of the cryptosporidial infection; oocyst shedding was undetectable 2 weeks after reconstitution.[290] However, mice reconstituted with human peripheral blood lymphocytes did not show a comparable decrease in oocyst shedding, although the noticeable decline in the intensity of shedding which took place 4 weeks after reconstitution persisted through week 7; the observed finding suggested that human cells may have had a transient effect upon the infection.[290] Kuhls et al.[291] have observed an improved survival rate in SCID mice with cryptosporidiosis after adoptively transferring CD4$^+$ and CD4$^-$, CD8$^-$, and B220$^-$ BALB/c splenocytes.

Some of the novel immunotherapeutic approaches towards treatment of cryptosporidiosis include the use of cow's milk globulin[292] and hyperimmune bovine colostrum.[98,293]

Initial reports have indicated that bovine colostrum obtained from cows that were naturally infected with *Cryptosporidium*, when administered orally to three patients with cryptosporidiosis, failed to exert any beneficial effect.[294] However, Tzipori et al.[98,295] demonstrated that a specially produced hyperimmune bovine colostrum (HBC) was effective in three patients (one of them with AIDS) with intestinal cryptosporidiosis. *In vitro* evaluation,[296] as well as controlled experiments in animal models and neonatal calves, confirmed the immunotherapeutic activity of HBC as evidenced by the reduction of parasite load.[297,298]

This potentially new anticryptosporidial therapy was tested successfully by Ungar et al.[299] in one AIDS patient with fulminant cryptosporidial diarrhea by passively transferring large amounts of immune elements present in HBC to the affected host; the patient showed remission of diarrhea and elimination of *Cryptosporidium* oocysts from stool specimens. Nord et al.[300] conducted a randomized, double-blind, controlled pilot study in five AIDS patients with cryptosporidial diarrhea. HBC was administered by continuous nasogastric infusion at 20 ml/h (approximately 30 mg total immunoglobulin/ml) for 10 d. Although the study was hampered by such factors as the small number of patients, significant difference among patients (oocyst load and severity of diarrhea at the onset of the trial), and the inability to obtain adequate baseline information about daily stool volumes before treatment was started, the overall results have demonstrated that HBC may prove to be effective in treating patients with cryptosporidiosis.[300]

In a prospective study, Greenberg and Cello[301] have evaluated the safety and efficacy of colostrum-derived bovine immunoglobulin concentrate in the treatment of *C. parvum*-induced severe chronic diarrhea in AIDS patients. The treatment lasted for 21 d, with the medication given either in powder or capsule form. Patients receiving the powder form experienced a significant decrease in mean stool weight, from 1158 ± 114 g/d at baseline, to 595 ± 63 g/d ($p = .04$) at the end of treatment, and 749 ± 123 g/d ($p = .03$) 1 month after completion of therapy. The stool frequency also decreased from 6.6 ± 0.6 bowel movements per day at study entry, to 5.4 ± 0.7 during treatment ($p = .04$), and 5.4 ± 0.9 during observation ($p = .12$). Patients who received the medication in capsule form showed no improvement. While showing certain benefits, the optimal dosage, duration of therapy, and overall efficacy of bovine immunoglobulin concentrate need to be determined in placebo-controlled trials.[301]

The active ingredient(s) of HBC are presently unknown. However, it may be possible that the bovine IgG_1 immunoglobulin, which is very closely related to human IgA, may elicit a protective effect similar to the one already postulated for bovine IgG_1 in enteropathogenic and enterotoxigenic *E. coli*-related diarrheas, and enteric infection caused by rotavirus.[302-305] It is also plausible that the active ingredient of HBC is a cytokine.

Doyle et al.[306] have determined the major *C. parvum* sporozoite antigens that were recognized on Western blots (immunoblots) by the hyperimmune bovine colostrum. Nineteen of the surface *C. parvum* membrane proteins, which were radioiodinated and immunoprecipitated, were identified as the target of the protective colostral immunoglubulin preparation.

Some potential mechanisms of action that may explain the early clinical response to HBC and decrease in the number of detectable oocysts, include blocking of intestinal receptor sites with interruption of the extracellular autoinfectious life cycle stages, and/or providing a critical substance absent because of diminished population of CD4+ cells which activates some intact function(s) of the immune response.[299]

So far, attempts to produce large quantities of HBC for immunotherapy have been modestly successful.[297,298,307,308] Cama and Sterling[309] described an alternative method which may overcome some of the limitations associated with large-scale production of HBC, by using egg yolks from hyperimmunized hens (HEY).[309-313] The main immunoglobulin present in HEY, IgY,[314] has been known for its considerable temperature and acid resistance.[315] Although the concentration of IgY in HEY is lower than the reported concentration of IgG_1 in HBC, the new procedure will offer the advantages of continuous production, easy collection and storage, and the feasibility of large-scale manufacturing.[309] When administered orally to neonatal mice, HEY led to a significant reduction ($p \leq .001$) in the number of parasites.[309]

Hoskins et al.[316] have studied the effect of HBC raised against *C. parvum*, on the *C. wrairi*-induced infection in guinea pigs. The results have shown oocyst shedding to be markedly reduced in animals inoculated intraintestinally with *C. wrairi* sporozoites previously incubated with HBC raised to *C. parvum*; however, oocyst shedding did not occur when the guinea pigs were treated orally with HBC, and the treatment was begun simultaneously with inoculation of *C. wrairi* oocysts. While the lack of activity of orally administered HBC indicated that HBC may have a limited beneficial effect on established cryptosporidial infections, its continuous infusion may prove to be more effective therapy than a fractional dose regimen.[316]

Fourteen AIDS patients with symptomatic cryptosporidiosis were treated with either a specific bovine dialyzable leukocyte extract (immune DLE) prepared from lymph node lymphocytes of calves immunized with cryptosporidia, or with a nonspecific (nonimmune) DLE prepared from nonimmunized calves.[317,318] Of the seven patients who received immune DLE, six gained weight and had a decrease in bowel movement frequency; eradication of oocysts from stools was observed in five patients. By comparison, six of seven recipients of nonimmune DLE showed no decrease in bowel movements and in four of them no clearing of oocysts from stools was observed; five of the patients continued to lose weight. When five of the nonimmune DLE recipients were treated with immune DLE, four experienced a decrease in bowel movement frequency and considerable weight gain, with eradication of oocysts from stools in two patients.[317] Even though sustained symptomatic improvement of patients given immune DLE was evident, the lack of an appropriate cryptosporidial antigen would only allow a postulation that the observed microbiologic and clinical improvements were indeed caused by the immune-DLE-induced augmentation of cellular immunity towards *C. parvum*. In this regard, DLE has been found to contain an antigen-binding product of T helper lymphocytes that enhanced the cell-mediated immune responses in man.[319,320] In several studies, DLE was found beneficial in the treatment of various bacterial, fungal, and viral infections,[321-323] as well as against parasites such as *Eimeria bovis* in cattle[324] and *Eimeria ferrisi* in mice.[325]

Chung et al.[326] reported a failure to treat one patient with congenital dysgammaglobulinemia type I[327] (deficient IgG, IgA, and elevated IgM levels) and persistent cryptosporidiosis, over a 13-week period with oral bovine transfer factor from calves immunized with cryptosporidia; the addition of spiramycin toward the end of therapy was not beneficial either.

In an attempt to broaden the scope of immunotherapeutic approaches for treatment of cryptosporidiosis, Borowitz and Saulsbury[328] administered human serum immune globulin to one child who experienced a prolonged cryptosporidial infection while receiving maintenance therapy for acute leukemia. The therapy appeared to be effective, with symptoms ceasing after the child received 2.5 g of human serum immune globulin through a nasogastric tube on two consecutive days. Several previous studies have demonstrated that orally given human serum immune globulin was effective in prevention and treatment of infectious gastroenteritis in children with primary immunodeficiency diseases[329] and recipients of bone marrow transplants.[330]

Acute cryptosporidiosis has been usually associated with production of IgM and IgG serum antibodies against the parasite.[331] The important role of such antibodies during normal immune responses was described in several reports of chronic cryptosporidiosis in children with congenital immunoglobulin deficiency but intact cellular immunity.[96-98] Since seroepidemiologic studies have indicated that between 30% and 80% of healthy adults will produce serum antibody to *Cryptosporidium*,[332-334] it is very likely then that the commercially available human serum immune globulin may contain substantial amounts of IgG antibody to the parasite, thereby making it a valuable source of passive immunity in patients with chronic cryptosporidial infection.[328]

Kern et al.[333] studied the effects of recombinant interleukin-2 (rIL-2) against cryptosporidiosis in patients having AIDS or persistent lymphadenopathy syndrome (LAS). Increasing doses of rIL-2 (from 10^3 U/m^2 to 10^6 U/m^2) were administered as an intravenous bolus injection. Two of the patients with severe intestinal cryptosporidiosis had their diarrhea ceased under the treatment with rIL-2, and not occurring during the following 2 months. At the high-dose level, the rIL-2 caused some minor adverse reactions, such as fever, chills, and malaise or vomiting.[333] The observed anticryptosporidial effect of rIL-2 was likely due to its ability to enhance immune responses to foreign antigens[335,336] by acting as a second messenger of T lymphocyte activation.[336,337] After its release from IL-2-producer lymphocytes (mainly within the T4$^+$ subsets), IL-2 facilitates an adequate reaction by the T responder lymphocytes against infectious pathogens or allogeneic malignant cells.[335,336,338]

The activity of recombinant murine interferon-γ (IFN-γ) against *C. parvum* infection was evaluated in immunosuppressed rats.[339] Daily intraperitoneal injections of at least 125,000 U/kg significantly ($p < .05$) reduced the intensity of subsequent ileal infection, and at 500,000 U/kg, IFN-γ inhibited the colonization of the biliary tract. Furthermore, when administered for 11 d to rats with established *C. parvum* infection, IFN-γ substantially ($p < .05$) reduced the number of parasites in the small intestine, but was ineffective against infection of the biliary tract and large intestine.[339]

Since studies in murine models have confirmed the anticryptosporidial activity of IFN-γ, and IL-12 has been known for its ability to induce IFN-γ production, Urban et al.[340] have examined the effect of IL-12 to prevent or cure cryptosporidial infection in neonatal BALB/c and SCID mice. Treatment of both immunocompetent and immunodeficient mice with IL-12 before experimental inoculation with cryptosporidial oocysts prevented or greatly reduced the severity of infection — the intestinal epithelial cell invasion and/or early intracellular development of cryptosporidiosis was inhibited by exogenous IL-12. Furthermore, the protective effect of IL-12 was completely blocked by anti-IFN-γ monoclonal antibodies. Also, established infections were associated with elevated IFN-γ gene expression and were not ameliorated by IL-12 treatment, even though such treatment further enhanced IFN-γ gene expression. Overall, the study results provided tangible evidence that treatment with exogenous IL-12 can prevent cryptosporidial infection through an IFN-γ-dependent, specific immune system-independent mechanism, and that endogenous IL-12 production has a role in limiting the infection.[340]

Kuhls et al.[341] have cast doubt about the ability of IFN-γ (10,000 IU) to alter the course of *C. parvum* infection in newborn SCID mice. IFN-γ did not reverse the initial susceptibility of the neonatal SCID mice to cryptosporidiosis, and continued treatment at 10,000 IU weekly did not alter survival.

Capetti et al.[342] studied the therapeutic efficacy of recombinant human granulocyte-macrophage colony-stimulating factor (rHuGM-CSF) in HIV-positive patients (CD4+ counts of <50 cells/mm³) with paromomycin-resistant cryptosporidiosis. rHuGM-CSF was given subcutaneously at 300 mg daily for 14 d, then every other day for an additional 14 d, together with zidovudine (500 mg) and paromomycin. The patients showed prompt clinical response to rHuGM-CSF (cessation of diarrhea in 2 d), but relapsed when therapy was discontinued.

22.1.3.7   Alternative Therapies For Cryptosporidiosis

In addition to chemotherapy, one important aspect in the management of cryptosporidial infections in immunodeficient patients has been the need to provide supportive care by decreasing the intestinal motility and maintaining a proper fluid and electrolyte balance by giving patients oral rehydration reduced-osmolarity solutions[343] containing glucose, sodium bicarbonate, and potassium,[105,344] and parenteral feeding.[121,345] Furthermore, in immunocompromised hosts, the reversal of underlying immune deficiencies by discontinuation of immunosuppressive therapy has led to successful recovery from cryptosporidiosis.[3,100,104,135,142] In one case described by Holley and Thiers,[346] the patient, with bullous pemphigoid, did not have cryptosporidia in the stools until after the initiation of immunosuppressive therapy with steroids and azathioprine. It was postulated that the patient had reactivation of a latent infection, possibly representing a previously asymptomatic carrier state. The medication, which involved daily doses of 80 mg prednisone, was sufficient to cause immuno-suppression by eliciting T cell depletion and dysfunction[347,348] that had not only indirectly affected the humoral responses,[349] but also interfered with the antibody binding and monocyte IgG and complement receptor functions.[350]

22.1.3.8   Development of *In Vitro* and *In Vivo* Assays of Cryptosporidiosis

One obstacle that has been hampering efforts at developing novel chemotherapeutic agents against cryptosporidial infections was the lack of adequate *in vitro* and *in vivo* assays for evaluation of potential drug candidates.

Recently, Flanigan et al.[296] described an *in vitro* model of *C. parvum* infection involving the human intestinal epithelial cell line HT29.74.[351,352] In another study, Gut et al.[8] have developed an *in vitro* culture system using Madin-Darby canine kidney (MDCK) cells as host cells;[353] the assay provided access to both the asexual and sexual intracellular stages of *C. parvum*.

McDonald et al.[253] have found that sporozoites of *C. parvum* which were excysted *in vitro* from oocysts isolated from calves or patients with AIDS, underwent development in monolayers of the mouse fibroblast cell line L929; asexual multiplication was predominant (especially between 24 and 48 h after the infection), although a relatively small number of gametocytes was also present.

A new viability assay for *Cryptosporidium* and *Eimeria* sporozoites, which involved the use of both acridine orange and bisbenzamide, was shown to be more rapid, easier to perform, and less subjective than procedures used before; the assay has been applied to investigate the efficacy of respiratory inhibitors and the pH on the sporozoites.[354]

A chemiluminescence immunoassay was developed to detect *C. parvum* growth in MDCK cell cultures, which were plated at an optimal density of 1×10^4 cells/well and maintained as a monolayer for 4 d prior to infection with 2×10^4 parasites/well.[355] The Merifluor immunofluorescent assay was also used for the blinded detection of *Cryptosporidium* and *Giardia* in sodium acetate formalin-fixed stools.[356]

Recently, Edlind et al.[357] have proposed expression of *C. parvum* β-tubulin sequences in yeast as a potential model for drug development.

Among the recently developed animal models, Rehg et al.[358] characterized a dexamethasone-immunosuppressed rat model of chronic cryptosporidial infection, while Brasseur et al.[359] described a rodent model of persistent *Cryptosporidium* infection suitable for screening of drug candidates.

Mead et al.[360] have developed murine models of chronic cryptosporidial infections in congenitally SCID and nude mice with features similar to that of persistent infections observed in immunodeficient patients.

Several immunodeficient rodent models are currently in use in which persistent, largely asymptomatic *C. parvum* infections can be established. Piglets, to the contrary, develop a self-limiting diarrheal infection. Taking advantage of the currently available animal models, Tzipori et al.[170] have developed a testing sequence in which SCID mice were used initially to test drugs for inhibitory activity against *C. parvum*, after which the drug's therapeutic potential was further evaluated in piglets. Paromomycin and hyperimmune bovine colostrum-immunoglobulin were selected to evaluate this system in which the suckling SCID mice were infected with *C. paravum*. In suckling SCID mice *C. paravum* tended to cause infections associated with the villus surface, whereas in weaned and in older SCID mice, the infections were more frequently localized in abscessed crypts. Since the rates of oocyst shedding in suckling SCID mice were 50 to 200 times higher than in weaned mice, the former would make a considerably more sensitive model for drug testing. Treatment with paromomycin, which even in high doses was not toxic in both SCID mice (3.0 g/kg daily) and piglets (500 mg/kg daily), was very effective against villus surface infections in suckling mice; however, the drug showed markedly lower activity against infections localized in inaccessible sites, such as abscessed crypts and stomach pits present in weaned and adult SCID mice. In piglets, the therapeutic efficacy of paromomycin depended on the severity of the diarrheal illness. Thus, while mild and moderate diarrhea and infection caused by one *C. parvum* isolate were cleared, paromomycin was ineffective in severely sick piglets infected with a second isolate, presumably because of a rapid transit time through the gut. In contrast to paromomycin, hyperimmune bovine colostrum-immunoglobulin treatment reduced the rate of *C. parvum* infection moderately in SCID mice and only slightly in piglets, again probably because of a rapid transit time through the gut and inactivation in the stomach.[170]

A two-phase SCID mouse model preconditioned with anti-IFN-γ monoclonal antibody has been developed by Tzipori at al.[361] IFN-γ (1.0 mg injected into newly weaned SCID mice 2 h before challenge with *C. parvum* oocysts) markedly exacerbated the course of the infection for ≥47 d compared with challenged mice that received an equivalent dose of irrelevant antibody. The extent and distribution of mucosal infection were profound, involving the stomach and several segments of the small and large intestines. The acute phase which lasted for the first 25 d after the challenge involved infection of the gut, followed by a chronic phase which consistently involved, in addition, infection of the hepatobiliary tract.

Meulbroek et al.[54] described an immunosuppressed rat model of respiratory cryptosporidiosis. Lewis rats, which were first immunosuppressed by subcutaneous injection of methylprednisolone acetate and then inoculated intratracheally with 10^6 *C. parvum* oocysts, were able to develop a reproducible infection consisting of all known developmental stages of the parasite confined in the epithelium lining airways from the trachea to the terminal bronchioles; the developmental stages were morphologically indistinguishable from those seen in gut epithelium.[54]

Perryman and Bjorneby[286] suggested the use of SCID foals as one reliable large animal model of clinical cryptosporidiosis.

In order to identify better animal models for infection, Enriquez and Sterling[362] examined *C. parvum* infection in 19 different strains of mice representing twelve H-2 haplotypes, and one gerbil, *Meriones unguiculatus*. Fecal samples and histologic specimens from the intestines taken on day 7 after the infection indicated that only the beige mouse (C57BL/6J-bg[J]) harbored a significant number of parasites, although it was still considerably lower than the one observed in neonatal mice.[362]

Novak and Sterling[363] have investigated the susceptibility dynamics of *C. parvum* in neonatal BALB/c mice. The susceptibility decreased until 14 d of age (19 d of age at sacrifice) when the mice could no longer be infected; the parasite load in the infected mice was also diminished from 235.6 parasites per high-power field (9 d of age at sacrifice) to 0.25 (18 d of age at sacrifice).[363]

It may be said that the animal models presently available, combined with the success of Current and coworkers[10,364] in culturing *Cryptosporidium* through its complete life cycle in cell culture[10] and hen eggs,[364] should provide some useful options for preclinical evaluation of drugs active against experimental cryptosporidiosis.

One drawback of some murine models of cryptosporidiosis developed earlier, was that only neonatal mice (1 to 4 d old) were susceptible to cryptosporidia, and that the infected mice, in general, failed to develop clinical signs of the disease.[365,366] The experimental infections in livestock, although mimicking human disease more closely, still exhibited distinct differences, such as extensive colonic involvement in lambs and the lack of diarrhea in most infected piglets.[367-369]

Miller et al.[370] made the observation that clinical, histologic, and parasitologic manifestations of cryptosporidiosis in infant nonhuman primates corresponded closely to those found in young children. Consequently, a reproducible experimental model of cryptosporidiosis was developed in pigtailed macaques (*Macaca nemestrina*) by inoculation with either 2×10^5 or 10 oocysts through a nasogastric tube; the result was the development of clinical enteritis concomitant with fecal passage of large numbers of cryptosporidial oocysts.[371]

22.1.4 REFERENCES

1. Tyzzer, E. E., A sporozoan found in the peptic glands of the common mouse, *Proc. Soc. Exp. Biol.*, 5, 12, 1907.
2. Nime, F. A., Burek, J. D., Page, D. L., Holscher, M. A., and Yardley, J. H., Acute enterocolitis in a human being infected with the protozoan *Cryptosporidium*, *Gastroenterology*, 70, 592, 1976.
3. Meisel, J. L., Perera, D. R., Meligro, C., and Rubin, C. E., Overwhelming water diarrhea associated with *Cryptosporidium* in an immunosuppressed patient, *Gastroenterology*, 70, 1156, 1976.
4. Berkowitz, C. D., AIDS and parasitic infections, including *Pneumocystis carinii* and cryptosporidiosis, *Pediatr. Clin. North Am.*, 32, 933, 1985.
5. Current, W. L. and Reese, N. C., A comparison of endogenous development of three isolates of *Cryptosporidium* in suckling mice, *J. Protozool.*, 33, 98, 1986.
6. Kuhls, T. L,, Mosier, D. A., and Crawford, D. L., Effects of carbohydrates and lectins on cryptosporidial sporozoite penetration of cultured cell monolayers, *J. Protozool.*, 38, 74S, 1991.
7. Wilson, M. E. and Pearson, R. D., Parasitic diseases of normal hosts in North America, *Hosp. Pract. (Off)*, 21, 164A-164D, 164I-164L, 164P-164Q, 1986.
8. Gut, J., Petersen, C., Nelson, R., and Leech, J., *Cryptosporidium parvum*: *in vitro* cultivation in Madin-Darby canine kidney cells, *J. Protozool.*, 38, 72S, 1991.
9. Current, W. L., The biology of *Cryptosporidium*, in *Parasitic Infections*, Leech, J. H., Sande, M. A., and Root, R. K., Eds., Churchill Livingston, New York, 1988, 109.
10. Current, W. L. and Haynes, T. B., Complete development of *Cryptosporidium* in cell culture, *Science*, 224, 603, 1984.
11. Navin, T. R. and Juranek, D. D., Cryptosporidiosis — clinical, epidemiologic and parasitologic review, *Rev. Infect. Dis.*, 6, 313, 1984.
12. Moon, H. W. and Woodmansee, D. B., Cryptosporidiosis, *J. Am. Vet. Med. Assoc.*, 189, 643, 1986.
13. Angus, K. W., Cryptosporidiosis in man, domestic animals and birds: a review, *J. R. Soc. Med.*, 76, 62, 1983.
14. Kirkpatrick, C. E., *Cryptosporidium* infections as a cause of calf diarrhea, *Vet. Clin. North Am. Food. Anim. Pract.*, 1, 515, 1985.

15. Anderson, B. C., Quick and easy diagnosis of cryptosporidiosis and John's disease, *Vet. Med.*, 80, 87, 1985.
16. Current, W. L., Human enteric coccidia. I. *Cryptosporidium*, *Clin. Microbiol.*, 7, 167, 1985.
17. Garcia, L. S., Bruckner, D. A., Brewer, T. C., and Shimizu, R. Y., Techniques for the recovery and identification of *Cryptosporidium* oocysts from stool specimens, *J. Clin. Microbiol.*, 18, 185, 1983.
18. Chichino, G., Bruno, A., Cevini, C., Atzori, C., Gatti, S., and Scaglia, M., New rapid methods of *Cryptosporidium* oocysts in stools, *J. Protozool.*, 38, 212S, 1991.
19. Yang, S., Healey, M. C., and Du, C., Infectivity of preserved *Cryptosporidium parvum* oocysts for immunosuppressed adult mice, *FEMS Immunol. Med. Microbiol.*, 13, 141, 1996.
20. Thea, D. M., Pereira, M. E. A., Kotler, D., Sterling, C. R., and Keusch, G. T., Identification and partial purification of a lectin on the surface of the sporozoite of *Cryptosporidium parvum*, *J. Parasitol.*, 78, 886, 1992.
21. Joe, A., Hamer, D. H., Kelley, M. A., Pereira, M. E. A., Keusch, G. T., Tsipori, S., and Ward, H. D., Role of a Gal/GalNAc-specific sporozoite surface lectin in *Cryptosporidium parvum*-host cell interaction, *J. Eukaryot. Microbiol.*, 41, 44S, 1994.
22. Current, W. L. and Blagburn, B. L., *Cryptosporidium* and *Microsporidia*: some closing comments, *J. Protozool.*, 38, 244S, 1991.
23. Current, W. L. and Garcia, L. S., Cryptosporidiosis, *Clin. Microb. Rev.*, 4, 325, 1991.
24. Garcia, L. S. and Current, W. L., Cryptosporidiosis: clinical features and diagnosis, *Crit. Rev. Clin. Lab. Sci.*, 27, 439, 1989.
25. Current, W. L. and Garcia, L. S., Cryptosporidiosis, *Clin. Lab. Med.*, 11, 873, 1991.
26. Bhan, M. K., Bhandari, N., Bhatnagar, S., and Bahl, R., Epidemiology and management of persistent diarrhoea in children of developing countries, *Indian J. Med. Res.*, 104, 103, 1996.
27. Assefa, T., Mohammed, H., Abebe, A., Abebe, S., and Tafesse, B., Cryptosporidiosis in children seen at the children's clinic of Yakatit 12 Hospital, Addis Ababa, *Ethiop. Med. J.*, 34, 43, 1996.
28. Fraser, D., Naggan, L., El-On, J., Deckelbaum, R. J., and Dagan, R., Risk factors for symptomatic and asymptomatic *Cryptosporidium* (CR) and *Giardia lamblia* (GL) infection in a cohort of Israeli bedouin children, *Proc. 36th Intersci. Conf. Antimicrob. Agents Chemother.*, American Society for Microbiology, Washington, D.C., Abstr. K153, 1996.
29. Neill, M. A., Rice, S. K., Ahmad, N. V., and Flanigan, T. P., Cryptosporidiosis: an unrecognized cause of diarrhea in elderly hospitalized patients, *Clin. Infect. Dis.*, 22, 168, 1996.
30. Gerba, C. P., Rose, J. B., and Haas, C. N., Sensitive populations: who is at the greatest risk? *Int. J. Food Microbiol.*, 30, 113, 1996.
31. Poirot, J. L., Deluol, A. M., Antoine, M., Heyer, F., Cadranel, J., Meynard, J.-L., Meyochas, M.-C., Girard, P.-M., and Roux, P., Broncho-pulmonary cryptosporidiosis in four HIV-infected patients, *J. Eukaryot. Microbiol.*, 43, 78S, 1996.
32. Farthing, M. J., Kelly, M. P., and Veitch, A. M., Recently recognized microbial enteropathies and HIV infection, *J. Antimicrob. Chemother.*, 37(Suppl. B), 61, 1996.
33. Greenberg, P. D., Koch, J., and Cello, J. P., Diagnosis of *Cryptosporidium parvum* in patients with severe diarrhea and AIDS, *Dig. Dis. Sci.*, 41, 2286, 1996.
34. Manatsathit, S., Tansupasawasdikul, S., Wanachiwanawin, D., Setawarin, S., Suwanagool, P., Prakasvejakit, S., Leelakusolwong, S., Eampokalap, B., and Kachintorn, U., Causes of chronic diarrhea in patients with AIDS in Thailand: a prospective clinical and microbiological study, *J. Gastroenterol.*, 31, 533, 1996.
35. Tarimo, D. S., Killewo, J. Z., Minjas, J. N., and Msamanga, G. I., Prevalence of intestinal parasites in adult patients with enteropathic AIDS in north-eastern Tanzania, *East Afr. Med. J.*, 73, 397, 1996.
36. Ghorpade, M. V., Kulkarni, S. A., and Kulkarni, A. G., Cryptosporidium, Isospora and Strongyloides in AIDS, *Natl. Med. J. India*, 9, 201, 1996.
37. Lanjewar, D. N., Rodrigues, C., Saple, D. G., Hira, S. K., and DuPont, H. L., Cryptosporidium, Isospora and Strongyloides in AIDS, *Natl. Med. J. India*, 9, 17, 1996.
38. Dieng, T., Ndir, O., Diallo, S., Coll-Seck, A. M., and Dieng, Y., Prevalence of *Cryptosporidium* sp. and *Isospora belli* in patients with acquired immunodeficiency syndrome (AIDS) in Dakar (Senegal), *Dakar Med.*, 39, 121, 1994.
39. Gunthard, M., Meister, T., Luthy, R., and Weber, R., Intestinal cryptosporidiosis in HIV infection: clinical features, course and therapy, *Dtsch. Med. Wochenschr.*, 121, 686, 1996.

40. Moolasart, P., Eampokalap, B., Ratanasrithong, M., Kanthasing, P., Tansupaswaskul, S., and Tanchanpong, C., Cryptosporidiosis in HIV infected patients in Thailand, *Southeast Asian J. Trop. Med. Public Health*, 26, 335, 1995.

41. Esfandiari, A., Jordan, W. C., and Brown, C. P., Prevalence of enteric parasitic infection among HIV-infected attendees of an inner city AIDS clinic, *Cell. Mol. Biol. (Noisy-le-grand)*, 41(Suppl. 1), S19, 1995.

42. Lopez-Velez, R., Tarazona, R., Garcia Camacho, A., Gomez-Mampaso, E., Guerrero, A., Moreira, V., and Villanueva, R., Intestinal and extraintestinal cryptosporidiosis in AIDS patients, *Eur. J. Clin. Microbiol. Infect. Dis.*, 14, 677, 1995.

43. Forgacs, P., Tarshis, A., Ma, P., Federman, M., Mele, L., Silverman, M. L., and Shea, J.A., Intestinal and bronchial cryptosporidiosis in an immunodeficient homosexual man, *Ann. Intern. Med.*, 99, 793, 1983.

44. Guarda, L. A., Stein, S. A., Cleary, K. A., and Ordonez, N. G., Human cryptosporidiosis in the acquired immune deficiency syndrome, *Arch. Pathol. Lab. Med.*, 107, 562, 1983.

45. Pitlik, S. D., Fainstein, V., Rios, A., Guarda, L., Mansell, P. W. A, and Hersh, E. M., Cryptosporidial cholecystitis, *N. Engl. J. Med.*, 308, 967, 1983.

46. Blumberg, R. S., Kelsey, P., Perrone, T., Dickersin, R., Laguaglia, M., and Ferruci, J., Cytomegalovirus- and *Cryptosporidium*-associated acalculous gangrenous cholecystitis, *Am. J. Med.*, 76, 1118, 1984.

47. French, A. L., Beaudet, L. M., Benator, D. A., Levy, C. S., Kassa, M., and Orenstein, J. M., Cholecystectomy in patients with AIDS: clinicopathologic correlations in 107 cases, *Clin. Infect. Dis.*, 21, 852, 1995.

48. Mifsud, A. J., Bell, D., and Shafi, M. S., Respiratory cryptosporidiosis as a presenting feature of AIDS, *J. Infect.*, 28, 227, 1994.

49. Ito, A. and Kawata, K., Liver cryptosporidiosis, *Ryoikibetsu Shokogun Shirizu*, 7, 75, 1995.

50. Talens, A., Montoya, E., Cubells, M. L., Garcia Novales, J. et al., Acute pancreatitis and acquired immunodeficiency syndrome, *Rev. Esp. Enferm. Dig.*, 88, 155, 1996.

51. Goodstein, R. F., Colombo, C. S., Illfelder, M. A., and Skaggs, R. E., Bronchial and gastrointestinal cryptosporidiosis in AIDS, *J. Am. Osteopath. Assoc.*, 89, 195, 1989.

52. Hjyling, N. and Jensen, B. N., Respiratory cryptosporidiosis in HIV-positive patients, *Lancet*, 2, 590, 1988.

53. Kibbler, C. C., Smith, A., Hamilton-Dutoit, S. J., Milbum, H., Pattinson, J. K., and Prentice, H. G., Pulmonary cryptosporidiosis occurring in a bone marrow transplant patient, *Scand. J. Infect. Dis.*, 19, 581, 1987.

54. Meulbroek, J. A., Novilla, M. N., and Current, W. L., An immunosuppressed rat model of cryptosporidiosis, *J. Protozool.*, 38, 113S, 1991.

55. Meynard, J. L., Meyohas, M. C., Binet, D., Chouaid, C., and Frottier, J., Pulmonary cryptosporidiosis in the acquired immunodeficiency syndrome, *Infection*, 24, 328, 1996.

56. Gross, T. L., Wheat, J., Bartlett, M., and O'Connor, K. W., AIDS and multiple system involvement with *Cryptosporidium*, *Am. J. Gastroenterol.*, 8, 456, 1986.

57. Cron, R. Q. and Sherry, D. D., Reiter's syndrome associated with cryptosporidial gastroenteritis, *J. Rheumatol.*, 22, 1962, 1995.

58. Samson, V. E. and Brown, W. R., Pneumatosis cystoides intestinalis in AIDS-associated cryptosporidiosis: more than incidental finding? *J. Clin. Gastroenterol.*, 22, 311, 1996.

59. Tatar, G., Haziroglu, R., and Hascelik, G., *Helicobacter felis* as a cofactor alone or together with stress in cryptosporidial activation in mice, *J. Int. Med. Res.*, 23, 473, 1995.

60. Rose, J. B., Occurrence and significance of *Cryptosporidium* in water, *J. Am. Water Works Assoc.*, 80, 53, 1988.

61. Dworkin, M. S., Goldman, D. P., Wells, T. G., Kobayashi, J. M., and Herwaldt, B. L., Cryptosporidiosis in Washington State: an outbreak associated with well water, *J. Infect. Dis.*, 174, 1372, 1996.

62. Kuroki, T., Watanabe, Y., Asai, Y., Yamai, S. et al., An outbreak of waterborne cryptosporidiosis in Kanagawa, Japan, *Kansenshogaku Zasshi*, 70, 132, 1996.

63. Osewe, P., Addiss, D. G., Blair, K. A., Hightower, A., Kamb, M. L., and Davis, J. P., Cryptosporidiosis in Wisconsin: a case-control study of post-outbreak transmission, *Epidemiol. Infect.*, 117, 297, 1996.

64. Addiss, D. G., Pond, R. S., Remshak, M., Juranek, D. D., Stokes, S., and Davis, J. P., Reduction of risk of watery diarrhea with point-of-use water filters during a massive outbreak of waterborne *Cryptosporidium* infection in Milwaukee, Wisconsin, 1993, *Am. J. Trop. Med. Hyg.*, 54, 549, 1996.

65. Goldstein, S. T., Juranek, D. D., Ravenholt, O., Hightower, A. W., Martin, D. G., Mesnik, J. L., Griffiths, S. D., Bryant, A. J., Reich, R. R., and Herwaldt, B. L., Cryptosporidiosis: an outbreak associated with drinking water despite state-of-the-art water treatment, *Ann. Intern. Med.*, 124, 459, 1996.

66. Kramer, M. H., Herwaldt, B. L., Craun, G. F., Calderon, R. L., and Juranek, D. D., Surveillance for waterborne-disease outbreaks — United States, 1993–1994, *Morbid. Mortal. Wkly. Rep. (CDC Surveill. Summ.)*, 45, 1, 1996.

67. Bridgman, S. A., Robertson, R. M., Syed, O., Speed, N., Andrews, N., and Hunter, P. R., Outbreak of cryptosporidiosis associated with a disinfected groundwater supply, *Epidemiol. Infect.*, 115, 555, 1995.

68. Mackenzie, W. R., Kazmierczak, J. J., and Davis, J. P., An outbreak of cryptosporidiosis associated with a resort swimming pool, *Epidemiol. Infect.*, 115, 545, 1995.

69. Fayer, R. and Nerad, T., Effects of low temperatures on viability of *Cryptosporidium parvum* oocysts, *Appl. Environ. Microbiol.*, 62, 1431, 1996.

70. Fayer, R., Trout, J., and Nerad, T., Effects of a wide range of temperatures on infectivity of *Cryptosporidium parvum* oocysts, *J. Eukaryot. Microbiol.*, 43, 64S, 1996.

71. Peeters, J. E., Mazas, E. A., Masschelein, W. J., Villacorta Martinez de Maturana, I., and Debacker, E., Effect of disinfection of drinking water with ozone or chlorine dioxide on survival of *Cryptosporidium parvum* oocysts, *Appl. Environ. Microbiol.*, 55, 1519, 1989.

72. Owens, J. H., Miltner, R. J., Schaefer, F. W. III, and Rice, E. W., Pilot-scale ozone inactivation of *Cryptosporidium*, *J. Eukaryot. Microbiol.*, 41, 56S, 1994.

73. Arrowood, M. J., Xie, L. T., Riegner, K., and Dunn, J., Disinfection of *Cryptosporidium parvum* oocysts by pulsed light treatment evaluated in an *in vitro* cultivation model, *J. Eukaryot. Microbiol.*, 43, 88S, 1996.

74. Fayer, R., Graczyk, T. K., Cranfield, M. R., and Trout, J. M., Gaseous disinfection of *Cryptosporidium parvum* oocysts, *Appl. Environ. Microbiol.*, 62, 3908, 1996.

75. Harp, J. A., Fayer, R., Pesch, B. A., and Jackson, G. J., Effect of pasteurization on infectivity of *Cryptosporidium parvum* oocysts in water and milk, *Appl. Environ. Microbiol.*, 62, 2866, 1996.

76. Shepherd, K. M. and Wyn-Jones, A. P., An evaluation of methods for the simultaneous detection of *Cryptosporidium* oocysts and *Giardia* cysts from water, *Appl. Environ. Microbiol.*, 62, 1317, 1996.

77. Drozd, C. and Schartzbrod, J., Hydrophobic and electrostatic cell surface properties of *Cryptosporidium parvum*, *Appl. Environ. Microbiol.*, 62, 12227, 1996.

78. Rochelle, P. A., Ferguson, D. M., Handojo, T. J., De Leon, R., Stewart, M. H., and Wolfe, R. L., Development of a rapid detection procedure for *Cryptosporidium*, using *in vitro* cell culture combined with PCR, *J. Eukaryot. Microbiol.*, 43, 72S, 1996.

79. Evans, M. R. and Gardner, D., Cryptosporidiosis outbreak associated with an educational farm holiday, *Commun. Dis. Rep. CDR Rev.*, 6, R50, 1996.

80. Sayers, G. M., Dillon, M. C., Connolly, E., Thornton, L. et al., Cryptosporidiosis in children who visited an open farm, *Commun. Dis. Rep. CDR Rev.*, 6, R140, 1996.

81. Centers for Disease Control and Infections, Foodborne outbreak of diarrheal illness associated with *Cryptosporidium parvum*-Minnesota, 1995, *JAMA*, 276, 1214, 1996.

82. Foodborne outbreak of diarrheal illness associated with *Cryptosporidium parvum*-Minnesota, 1995, *Morbid. Mortal. Wkly. Rep.*, 45, 783, 1996.

83. Anderson, B. C., Donndelinger, T., Wilkins, R. M., and Smith, J., Cryptosporidiosis in a veterinary student, *J. Am. Vet. Med. Assoc.*, 180, 408, 1982.

84. Baxby, D., Hart, C. A., and Blundell, N., Shedding of oocysts by immunocompetent individuals with cryptosporidiosis, *J. Hyg.*, 95, 708, 1985.

85. Brasseur, P., Lemeteil, D., and Mallet, E., La cryptosporidiose chez l'enfant immunocompetent, *Presse Med.*, 16, 177, 1987.

86. Current, W. L., Reese, N. C., Ernest, J. V., Bailey, W. S., Heyman, M. B., and Weinstein, W. M., Human cryptosporidiosis in immunocompetent and immunodeficient persons, *N. Engl. J. Med.*, 308, 1252, 1983.

87. Reese, N. C., Current, W. L., Ernest, J. V., and Bailey, W. S., Cryptosporidiosis of man and calf: a case report and results of experimental infections in mice and rats, *Am. J. Trop. Med. Hyg.*, 31, 226, 1982.

88. Casemore, D. P., The epidemiology of human cryptosporidiosis, in *Cryptosporidiosis. Proc. 1st Int. Workshop*, Edinburgh, Angus, K. W. and Blewett, D. A., Eds.,1988, 65.

89. Malla, N., Sehgal, R., Ganguly, N. K., and Mahajan, R. C., Cryptosporidiosis — the Indian scene, *Indian J. Pediatr.*, 56, 6, 1989.

90. Hoepelman, A. I., Current therapeutic approaches to cryptosporidiosis in immunocompromised patients, *J. Antimicrob. Chemother.*, 37, 871, 1996.

91. Colford, J. M., Jr., Tager, I. B., Hirozawa, A. M., Lemp, G. F., Aragon, T., and Petersen, C., Cryptosporidiosis among patients infected with human immunodeficiency virus: factors related to symptomatic infection and survival, *Am. J. Epidemiol.*, 144, 807, 1996.

92. Heyworth, M. F., Parasitic diseases in immunocompromised hosts: cryptosporidiosis, isosporiasis, and strongyloidiasis, *Gastroenterol. Clin. North Am.*, 25, 691, 1996.

93. Issacs, D., *Cryptosporidium* and diarrhea, *Arch. Dis. Child.*, 60, 608, 1985.

94. Malenbranche, R., Arnous, E., Guerin, J. M., Pierre, G. D., Laroche, A. C., Pean-Guichard, C., Elie, R., Morisset, P. H., Spira, T., Mandeville, R., and Seemayer, T., Acquired immunodeficiency syndrome with severe gastrointestinal manifestations, *Lancet*, 2, 873, 1983.

95. Vakil, N. B., Schwartz, S. M., Buggy, B. P., Brummitt, C. F., Kherellah, M., Letzer, D. M., Gilson, I. H., and Jones, P. G., Biliary cryptosporidiosis in HIV-infected people after the waterborne outbreak of cryptosporidiosis in Milwaukee, *N. Engl. J. Med.*, 334, 19, 1996.

96. Lasser, K. H., Lewin, K. J., and Ryning, F. W., Cryptosporidial enteritis in a patient with congenital hypogammaglobulinaemia, *Hum. Pathol.*, 10, 234, 1979.

97. Sloper, K. S., Dourmashkin, R. R., Bird, R. B., Slavin, G., and Webster, A. D. B., Chronic malabsorption due to cryptosporidiosis in a child with immunoglobulin deficiency, *Gut*, 23, 80, 1982.

98. Tzipori, S., Robertson, D., and Chapman, C., Remission of diarrhea due to cryptosporidiosis in an immunodeficient child treated with hyperimmune bovine colostrum, *Br. Med. J.*, 293, 1276, 1986.

99. Kocoshis, S. A., Cibull, M. L., Davis, T. E., Hinton, J. T., Seip, M., and Banwell, J. G., Intestinal and pulmonary cryptosporidiosis in an infant with severe combined immunoglobulin deficiency, *J. Pediatr. Gastroenterol. Nutr.*, 3, 149, 1984.

100. Miller, R. A., Holmberg, R. E., and Clausen, C. R., Life-threatening diarrhoea caused by *Cryptosporidium* in a child undergoing therapy for acute lymphocytic leukaemia, *J. Pediatr.*, 103, 256, 1983.

101. Lewis, I. J., Hart, C. A., and Baxby, D., Diarrhoea due to *Cryptosporidium* in acute lymphoblastic leukaemia, *Arch. Dis. Child.*, 60, 60, 1985.

102. Foot, A. B., Oakhill, A., and Mott, M. G., Cryptosporidiosis and acute leukaemia, *Arch. Dis. Child.*, 65, 236, 1990.

103. Gentile, G., Venditti, M., Micozzi, A., Caprioli, A., Donelli, G., Tirindelli, C., Meloni, G., Arcese, W., and Martino, P., Cryptosporidiosis in patients with hematologic malignancies, *Rev. Infect. Dis.*, 13, 842, 1991.

104. Weisburger, W. R., Hutcheson, D. F., Yardley, J. H., Roche, J.C., Hillis, W. D., and Charache, P., Cryptosporidiosis in an immunosuppressed renal-transplant recipient with IgA deficiency, *Am. J. Clin. Pathol.*, 72, 473, 1979.

105. Soave, R., Cryptosporidiosis and isosporiasis in patients with AIDS, *Infect. Dis. Clin. North Am.*, 2, 485, 1988.

106. Gelb, A. and Miller, S., AIDS and gastroenterology, *Am. J. Gastroenterol.*, 81, 619, 1986.

107. Davis, J. J., Heyman, M. B., Ferrell, L., Kerner, J., Kerlan, R., Jr., and Thaler, M. M., Sclerosing cholangitis associated with chronic cryptosporidiosis in a child with a congenital immunodeficiency disorder, *Am. J. Gastroenterol.*, 82, 1196, 1987.

108. Pettoello-Mantovani, M., Di Martino, L., Dettori, G., Vajro, P., Scotti, Ditullio, M. T., and Guandalini, S., Asymptomatic carriage of intestinal *Cryptosporidium* in immunocompetent and immunodeficient children: a prospective study, *Pediatr. Infect. Dis. J.*, 14, 1042, 1995.

109. Mercado, R. and Garcia, M., Asymptomatic cryptosporidiosis in an infant, *Bol. Chil. Parasitol.*, 49, 71, 1994.

110. Zar, F., Geiseler, P. J., and Brown, V. A.. Asymptomatic carriage of *Cryptosporidium* in the stool of a patient with acquired immunodeficiency syndrome, *J. Infect. Dis.*, 151, 195, 1985.

111. McDonald, V., Robinson, H. A., Kelly, J. P., and Bancroft, G. J., Immunity to *Cryptosporidium muris* infection in mice is expressed through gut CD4+ intraepithelial lymphocytes, *Infect. Immun.*, 64, 2556, 1996.

112. Waters, W. R. and Harp, J. A., *Cryptosporidium parvum* infection in T-cell receptor (TCR)-alpha- and TCR-delta-deficient mice, *Infect. Immun.*, 64, 1854, 1996.

113. Tilley, M., McDonald, V., and Bancroft, G. J., Resolution of cryptosporidial infection in mice correlates with parasite-specific lymphocyte proliferation associated with both Th1 and Th2 cytokine secretion, *Parasite Immunol.*, 17, 459, 1995.

114. Trevino-Perez, S., Luna-Castanos, G., Matilla-Mattilla, A., and Nieto-Cisneros, L., Chronic diarrhea and *Cryptosporidium* in diabetic patients with normal lymphocyte subpopulation: 2 case reports, *Gac. Med. Mex.*, 131, 219, 1995.

115. Tatalick, L. M. and Perryman, L. E., Effect of surface antigen-1 (SA-1) immune lymphocyte subsets and naive cell subsets in protecting SCID mice from initial and persistent infection with *Cryptosporidium parvum*, *Vet. Immunol. Immunopathol.*, 47, 43, 1995.

116. Tatalick, L. M. and Perryman, L. E., Attempts to protect severe combined immunodeficient (SCID) mice with antibody enriched for reactivity to *Cryptosporidium parvum* surface antigen-1, *Vet. Parasitol.*, 58, 281, 1995.

117. Shield, J., Baumer, J.H., Dawson, J. A., and Wilkinson, P. J., Cryptosporidiosis — an educational experience, *J. Infect.*, 21, 297, 1990.

118. Daoud, A. S., Zaki, M., Pugh, R. N., al-Mutairi, G., al-Ali, F., and el-Saleh, Q., Cryptosporidium gastroenteritis in immunocompetent children from Kuwait, *Trop. Geogr. Med.*, 421, 113, 1990.

119. Miron, D. and Kenes, Y., Cryptosporidiosis in children, *Harefuah*, 118, 315, 1990.

120. Levine, M. M., Antimicrobial therapy for infectious diarrhea, *Rev. Infect. Dis.*, 8(Suppl. 2), S207, 1986.

121. Gerberding, J. L., Diagnosis and management of HIV-infected patients with diarrhoea, *J. Antimicrob. Chemother.*, 23(Suppl. A), 83, 1989.

122. Cone, L. A., Woodward, D. R., Potts, B. E., Byrd, R. G., Alexander, R. M., and Last, M. D., An update on the acquired immunodeficiency syndrome (AIDS): associated disorders of the alimentary tract, *Dis. Colon Rectum*, 29, 60, 1986.

123. Santangelo, W. C. and Krejs, G.L., Gastrointestinal manifestations of the acquired immunodeficiency syndrome, *Am. J. Med. Sci.*, 292, 328, 1986.

124. Cello, J. P., Gastrointestinal manifestations of HIV infection, *Infect. Dis. Clin. North Am.*, 2, 387, 1988.

125. Laughon, B. E., Druckman, D. A., Vernon, A., Quinn, T. C., Polk, B. F., Moldin, J. F., Yolken, R. H., and Bartlett, J. G., Prevalence of enteric pathogens in homosexual men with and without acquired immunodeficiency syndrome, *Gastroenterology*, 94, 984, 1988.

126. Smith, P. D., Lane, H. C., Gill, V. J., Manischewitz, J. F., Quinnan, G. V., Fauci, A. S., and Masur, H., Intestinal infections in patients with the acquired immunodeficiency syndrome (AIDS): etiology and response to therapy, *Ann. Intern. Med.*, 108, 328, 1988.

127. Dworkin, B., Wormser, G. P., Rosenthal, W. S., Heier, S. K., Braunstein, M., Weiss, L., Jankowski, R., Levy, D., and Weiselberg, S., Gastrointestinal manifestations of the acquired immunodeficiency syndrome: a review of 22 cases, *Am. J. Gastroenterol.*, 80, 774, 1985.

128. Gold, J. W., Clinical spectrum of infections in patients with HTLV-III-associated diseases, *Cancer Res.*, 49(Suppl. 9), 4652s, 1985.

129. Soave, R., Cryptosporidiosis and isosporiasis in patients with AIDS, *Infect. Dis. Clin. North Am.*, 2, 485, 1988.

130. Connolly, G. M., Dryden, M.S., Shanson, D. C., and Gazzard, B. G., Cryptosporidial diarrhoea in AIDS and its treatment, *Gut*, 29, 593, 1988.

131. Soave, R. and Johnson, W. D., Jr., *Cryptosporidium* and *Isospora belli* infections, *J. Infect. Dis.*, 157, 225, 1988.

132. Hudson, R., No treatment for cryptosporidiosis in AIDS patients, *J. Am. Osteopath. Assoc.*, 89, 716, 1989.

133. Soave, R., Treatment strategies for cryptosporidiosis, *Ann. NY Acad. Sci.*, 616, 442, 1990.

134. Georgiev, V. St., Opportunistic infections: treatment and developmental therapeutics of cryptosporidiosis and isosporiasis, *Drug Dev. Res.*, 28, 445, 1993.

135. Centers for Disease Control, Cryptosporidiosis: assessment of chemotherapy of males with acquired immunodeficiency syndrome (AIDS), *Morbid. Mortal. Wkly. Rep.*, 31, 589, 1982.

136. Brasseur, P., Lemeteil, D., and Ballet, J. J., Anti-cryptosporidial activity screened with an immuno-suppressed rat model, *J. Protozool.*, 38, 230S, 1991.

137. Pilla, A. M., Rybak, M. J., and Chandrasekar, P. H., Spiramycin in the treatment of cryptosporidiosis, *Pharmacotherapy*, 7, 188, 1987.

138. Centers for Disease Control, Update: treatment of cryptosporidiosis in patients with acquired immuno-deficiency syndrome (AIDS), *Morbid. Mortal. Wkly. Rep.*, 33, 117, 1984.

139. Portnoy, D., Whiteside, M. E., Buckley, E., and MacLeod, C. L., Treatment of intestinal crypto-sporidiosis with spiramycin, *Ann. Intern. Med.*, 101, 202, 1984.

140. Decaux, G. M. and Devroeda, C., Acute colitis related to spiramycin, *Lancet*, 2, 993, 1978.

141. Moskovitz, B. L., Stanton, T. L., and Kusmierek, J. J., Spiramycin therapy for cryptosporidial diarrhoea in immunocompromised patients, *J. Antimicrob. Chemother.*, 22(Suppl. B), 189, 1988.

142. Collier, A. C., Miller, P. A., and Meyers, J. D., Cryptosporidiosis after marrow transplantation: person-to-person transmission and treatment with spiramycin, *Ann. Intern. Med.*, 101, 205, 1984.

143. Mead, G. M., Sweetenham, J. W., Ewins, D. L., Furlong, M., and Lowes, J. A., Intestinal crypto-sporidiosis: a complication of cancer treatment, *Cancer Treat. Rep.*, 70, 769, 1986.

144. Fafard, J. and Lalonde, R., Long-standing symptomatic cryptosporidiosis in a normal man: clinical response to spiramycin, *J. Clin. Gastroenterol.*, 12, 190, 1990.

145. Galvano, G., Cattaneo, G., and Reverso-Giovantin, E., Chronic diarrhea due to *Cryptosporidium*: the efficacy of spiramycin treatment, *Pediatr. Med. Chir.*, 15, 297, 1993.

146. Wilmsmeyer, B., Dopfer, R., Hoppe, J. E., and Niethammer, D., Cryptosporidium enteritis, *Monatsschr. Kinderheilkd.*, 141, 130, 1993.

147. Descotes, J., Vial, T., Delattre, D., and Evreux, J.-C., Spiramycin: safety in man, *J. Antimicrob. Chem.*, 22, 207, 1988.

148. Connolly, G. M., Dryden, M. S., Shanson, D. C., and Gazzard, B. G., Cryptosporidial diarrhoea in AIDS and its treatment, *Gut*, 29, 593, 1988.

149. Kotler, D. P., Gaetz, H. P., Lange, M., Klein, E. B., and Holt, P. R., Enteropathy associated with the acquired immunodeficiency syndrome, *Ann. Intern. Med.*, 101, 421, 1984.

150. Saez-Llorens, X., Odio, C. M., Umana, M. A., and Morales, M. V., Spiramycin vs. placebo for treatment of acute diarrhea caused by *Cryptosporidium*, *Pediatr. Infect. Dis. J.*, 8, 136, 1989.

151. Saez-Llorens, X., Spiramycin for treatment of *Cryptosporidium* enteritis, *J. Infect. Dis.*, 160, 342, 1989.

152. Casemore, D.P., Sands, R. L., and Curry, A., *Cryptosporidium* species: a "new" human pathogen, *J. Clin. Pathol.*, 38, 1321, 1985.

153. Woolf, G. M., Townsend, M., and Guyatt, G., Treatment of cryptosoridiosis with spiramycin in AIDS: an "N of 1", *J. Clin. Gastroenterol.*, 9, 632, 1987.

154. Wittenberg, D. F., Miller, N. M., and van den Ende, J., Spiramycin is not effective in treating *Cryptosporidium* diarrhea in infants: results of a double-blind randomized trial, *J. Infect. Dis.*, 159, 131, 1989.

155. Wittenberg, D. F., Spiramycin for treatment of *Cryptosporidium* enteritis, *J. Infect. Dis.*, 160, 342, 1989.

156. Berkowitz, C. D. and Seidel, J. S., Spontaneous resolution of cryptosporidiosis in a child with acquired immunodeficiency syndrome, *Am. J. Dis. Child.*, 139, 967, 1985.

157. Markus, M. B., Spiramycin and coccidiosis, *Med. J. Aust.*, 147, 472, 1987.

158. Current, W. L., *Cryptosporidium*: its biology and potential for environmental transmission, *Crit. Rev. Environ. Control*, 17, 21, 1986.

159. Weikel, C., Lazenby, A., Belitsos, P., McDewitt, M., Fleming, H. E., Jr., and Barbacci, M., Intestinal injury associated with spiramycin therapy of *Cryptosporidium* infection in AIDS, *J. Protozool.*, 38, 147S, 1991.

160. Kimata, I., Uni, S., and Iseki, M., Chemotherapeutic effect of azithromycin and lasalocid on *Crypto-sporidium* infection in mice, *J. Protozool.*, 38, 232S, 1991.

161. Rehg, J. E., Activity of azithromycin against cryptosporidia in immunosuppressed rats, *J. Infect. Dis.*, 163, 1293, 1991.

162. Dupont, C., Bougnoux, M. E., Turner, L., Rouveix, E., and Dorra, M., Microbiological findings about pulmonary cryptosporidiosis in two AIDS patients, *J. Clin. Microbiol.*, 34, 227, 1996.

163. Hicks, P., Zwiener, R. J., Squires, J., and Savell, V., Azithromycin therapy for *Cryptosporidium parvum* infection in four children infected with human immunodeficiency virus, *J. Pediatr.*, 129, 297, 1996.

164. Vargas, S. L., Shenep, J. L., Flynn, P. M., Pui, C. H., Santana, V. M., and Hughes, W. T., Azithromycin for treatment of severe *Cryptosporidium* diarrhea in two children with cancer, *J. Pediatr.*, 123, 154, 1993.

165. Jordan, W. C., Clarithromycin prophylaxis against *Cryptosporidium* enteritis in patients with AIDS, *J. Natl. Med. Assoc.*, 88, 425, 1996.

166. Cama, V. A., Marshall, M. M., Shubitz, L. F., Ortega, Y. R., and Sterling, C. R., Treatment of acute and chronic *Cryptosporidium parvum* infection in mice using clarithromycin and 14-OH clarithromycin, *J. Eukaryot. Microbiol.*, 41, 25S, 1994.

167. Kreinik, G., Burstein, O., Landor, M., Bernstein, L., Weiss, L. M., and Wittner, M., Successful management of intractable cryptosporidial diarrhea with intravenous octreotide, a somatostatin analog, *AIDS*, 5, 765, 1991.

168. Rehg, J. E., Anti-cryptosporidial activity of macrolides in immunosuppressed rats, *J. Protozool.*, 38, 228S, 1991.

169. Giacometti, A., Cirioni, O., Del Prete, S. M., Barchiesi, F., and Scalise, G., *In vitro* anti-cryptosporidial activity of macrolides alone and in combination with other drugs, *Proc. 36th Intersci. Conf. Antimicrob. Agents Chemother.*, American Society for Microbiology, Washington, D.C., Abstr. E70, 1996.

170. Tzipori, S., Rand, W., Griffiths, J., Widmer, G., and Crabb, J., Evaluation of an animal model system for cryptosporidiosis: therapeutic efficacy of paromomycin and hyperimmune bovine colostrum-immunoglobulin, *Clin. Diagn. Lab. Immunol.*, 1, 450, 1994.

171. Cirioni, O., Giacometti A., Balducci, M., Drenaggi, D., Del Prete, M. S., and Scallise, G., Anti-cryptosporidial activity of paromomycin, *J. Infect. Dis.*, 172, 1169, 1995.

172. Verdon, R., Polianski, J., Gaudebout, C., and Pocidalo, J. J., Paromomycin for cryptosporidiosis in AIDS, *J. Infect. Dis.*, 171, 1070, 1995.

173. Tzipori, S., Griffiths, J., and Theodus, C., Paromomycin treatment against cryptosporidiosis in patients with AIDS, *J. Infect. Dis.*, 171, 1069, 1995.

174. Mancassola, R., Reperant, J. M., Naciri, M., and Chartier, C., Chemoprophylaxis of *Cryptosporidium parvum* infection with paromomycin in kids and immunological study, *Antimicrob. Agents Chemother.*, 39, 75, 1995.

175. Jimenez-Beatty Navarro, M. D., de la Fuente Aguado, J., Sopena Arguelles, B., and Martinez Vazquez, C., Paromomycin in the treatment of cryptosporidiosis, *Rev. Clin. Esp.*, 195, 62, 1995.

176. Healey, M. C., Yang, S., Rasmussen, K. R., Jackson, M. K., and Du, C., Therapeutic efficacy of paromomycin in immunosuppressed adult mice infected with *Cryptosporidium parvum*, *J. Parasitol.*, 81, 114, 1995.

177. Mohri, H., Fujita, H., Asakura, Y., Katoh, K., Okamoto, R., Tanabe, J., Harano, H., Noguchi, T., Inayama, Y., and Amano, T., Case report: inhalation therapy of paromomycin is effective for respiratory infection and hypoxia by cryptosporidium with AIDS, *Am. J. Med. Sci.*, 309, 60, 1995.

178. Verdon, R., Polianski, J., Gaudebout, C., Marche, C., Garry, L., and Pocidalo, J.-J., Evaluation of curative anticryptosporidial activity of paromomycin in a dexamethazone-treated rat model, *Antimicrob. Agents Chemother.*, 38, 1681, 1994.

179. Scaglia, M., Atzori, C., Marchetti, G., Orso, M., Maserati, R., Orani, A., Novati, S., and Olliaro, P., Effectiveness of aminosidine (paromomycin) sulfate in chronic *Cryptosporidium* diarrhea in AIDS patients: an open, uncontrolled, prospective clinical trial, *J. Infect. Dis.*, 170, 1349, 1994.

180. Rehg, J. E., A comparison of anticryptosporidial activity of paromomycin with that of other aminoglycosides and azithromycin in immunosuppressed rats, *J. Infect. Dis.*, 170, 934, 1994.

181. Youssef, M. M., Hammam, S. M., abou Samra, L. M., and Khalifa, A. M., Aminosidine sulphate in experimental cryptosporidiosis, *J. Egypt. Soc. Parasitol.*, 24, 239, 1994.

182. White, A. C., Jr., Chappell, C. L., Hayat, C. S., Kimball, K. T., Flanigan, T. P., and Goodgame, R. W., Paromomycin for cryptosporidiosis in AIDS: a prospective, double-blind trial, *J. Infect. Dis.*, 170, 419, 1994.

183. Forester, G., Sidhom, O., Nahass, R., and Andavolu, R., AIDS-associated cryptosporidiosis with gastric structure and a therapeutic response to paromomycin, *Am. J. Gastroenterol.*, 89, 1096, 1994.

184. Wallace, M. R., Nguyen, M. T., and Newton, J. A., Jr., Use of paromomycin for the treatment of cryptosporidiosis in patients with AIDS, *Clin. Infect. Dis.*, 17, 1070, 1993.

185. Anand, A., Cryptosporidiosis in patients with AIDS, *Clin. Infect. Dis.*, 17, 297, 1993.

186. Fichtenbaum, C. J., Ritchie, D. J., and Powderly, W. G., Use of paromomycin for treatment of cryptosporidiosis in patients with AIDS, *Clin. Infect. Dis.*, 16, 298, 1993.

187. Goodgame, R. W., Genta, R. M., White, A. C., and Chappell, C. L., Intensity of infection in AIDS-associated cryptosporidiosis, *J. Infect. Dis.*, 167, 704, 1993.

188. Gatlie, J., Jr., Piot, D., Hawkins, K., Bernal, A., Clemmons, J., and Stool, E., Treatment of gastro-intestinal cryptosporidium, *Proc. VIth Int. Conf. AIDS*, San Francisco, 1990, Abstr. 2121.

189. Clezy, K., Gold, J., Blaze, J., and Jones, P., Paromomycin for the treatment of cryptosporidial diarrhoea in AIDS patients, *AIDS*, 5, 1146, 1991.

190. Hoepelman, I. M., Human cryptosporidiosis, *Int. J. STD AIDS*, 7(Suppl. 1), 28, 1996.

191. Verdon, R., Polianski, J., Gaudebout, C., Marche, C., Garry, L., Carbon, C., and Jones, P. G., Evaluation of high-dose regimen of paromomycin against cryptosporidiosis in the dexamethasone-treated rat model, *Antimicrob. Agents Chemother.*, 39, 2155, 1995.

192. Tan, W. W., Chapnick, E. K., Abter, E. I., Haddad, S., Zimbalist, E. H., and Lutwick, L. I., Paromomycin-associated pancreatitis in HIV-related cryptosporidiosis, *Ann. Pharmacother.*, 29, 22, 1995.

193. Bissuel, F., Cotte, L., de Montclos, M., Rabodonirina, M., and Trepo, C., Absence of systemic absorption of oral paromomycin during long-term, high-dose treatment for cryptosporidiosis in AIDS, *J. Infect. Dis.*, 170, 749, 1994.

194. Bonfils, S., Ruszniewski, P., Costil, V., Laucournet, H., Vatier, J., Rene, E., and Mignon, M., Prolonged treatment of Zollinger-Ellison syndrome by long-acting somatostatin, *Lancet*, 1, 554, 1986.

195. Ch'ng, J. L., Anderson, J. V., Williams, S. J., Carr, D.H., and Bloom, S. R., Remission of symptoms during long term treatment of metastatic pancreatic endocrine tumours with long-acting somatostatin analogue, *Br. Med. J.*, 292, 981, 1986.

196. Maton, P. N., O'Dorisio, T. M., Howe, B. A., McArthur, K. E., Howard, H. M., Cherner, J. A., Malarkey, T. B., Collen, M. J., Gardner, J. D., and Jensen, R. T., Effect of a long-acting somatostatin analogue (SMS 201- 995) in a patient with pancreatic cholera, *N. Engl. J. Med.*, 312, 17, 1985.

197. Dharmsathaphorn, K., Sherwin, R. S., Cataland, S., Jaffe, B., and Dobbins, J., Somatostatin inhibits diarrhea in the carcinoid syndrome, *Ann. Intern. Med.*, 92, 68, 1980.

198. Williams, N. S., Cooper, J. C., Axon, A. T. R., King, R. F. G. J., and Barker, M., Use of a long-acting somatostatin analogue in controlling life threatening ileostomy diarrhoea, *Br. Med. J.*, 289, 1027, 1984.

199. Sheppard, M., Shapiro, B., Pimstone, B., Kronheim, M. B., and Gregory, M., The metabolic clearance and plasma half disappearance time of exogenous somatostatin in man, *J. Clin. Endocrinol. Metab.*, 49, 50, 1979.

200. Bauer, W., Briner, U., Doepfner, W., Haller, R., Huguenin, R., Marbach, P., Petcher, T. J., and Pless, J., SMS 201-995: a very potent and selective octapeptide analogue of somatostatin with prolonged action, *Life Sci.*, 31, 1133, 1982.

201. Nousbaum, J. B., Robaszkiewicz, M., Cauvin, J. M., Garre, M., and Gouerou, H., Treatment of intestinal cryptosporidiosis with zidovudine and SMS 201-995, a somatostatin analog, *Gastro-enterology*, 101, 874, 1989.

202. Casals, A., Lorente, L., Jou, B., and Clotet, A., Usefulness of a somatostatin analog in the treatment of chronic severe diarrhea caused by *Cryptosporidium*, *Med. Clin. (Barcelona)*, 92, 358, 1989.

203. Santos, G. I., Mur Gimeno, P., Herreros Fernandez, M., and del Arco Galan, C., The usefulness of somatostatin analog SMS 201-995 in treating *Cryptosporidium*-induced diarrhea associated with the acquired immunodeficiency syndrome, *Med. Clin. (Barcelona)*, 95, 796, 1990.

204. Robinson, E. N., Jr. and Fogel, R., SMS 201-995, a somatostatin analogue, and diarrhea in the acquired immunodeficiency syndrome (AIDS), *Ann. Intern. Med.*, 109, 680, 1988.

205. Oehler, R. and Loos, U., Therapy of severe AIDS-associated diarrhea with the somatostatin analog octreotide, *Med. Klin.*, 88, 45, 1993.

206. Longnecker, S. M., Somatostatin and octreotide: literature review and description of therapeutic activity in pancreatic neoplasia, *Drug Intell. Clin. Pharm.*, 22, 1, 1988.

207. Gaginella, T. S. and O'Dorisio, T. M., Octreotide: entering the new era of peptidomimetic therapy, *Drug Intell. Clin. Pharm.*, 22, 154, 1988.

208. Santangelo, W. C., O'Dorisio, T. M., Kim, J. G., Severino, G., and Krejs, G., VIPoma syndrome: effect of a synthetic somatostatin analogue, *Scand. J. Gastroenterol.*, 21, 187, 1986.

209. Gorden, P., Somatostatin and somatostatin analogue (SMS 201-995) in the treatment of hormone-secreting tumors of the pituitary and gastrointestinal tract and non-neoplastic diseases of the gut, *Ann. Intern. Med.*, 110, 35, 1989.

210. Katz, M. D., Erstad, B. L., and Rose, C., Treatment of severe *Cryptosporidium*-related diarrhea with octreotide in a patient with AIDS, *Drug Intell. Clin. Pharm.*, 22, 134, 1988.

211. Simon, D., Weiss, L., Tanowitz, H. B., and Wittner, M., Resolution of *Cryptosporidium* infection in an AIDS patient after improvement of nutritional and immune status with octreotide, *Am. J. Gastroenterol.*, 86, 615, 1991.

212. Clotet, B., Sierra, G., Cofan, F., Monterola, J. M., Tortosa, F., and Foz, M., Efficacy of the somatostatin analogue (SMS 201-995), sandostatin, for cryptosporidial diarrhea in patients with AIDS, *AIDS*, 3, 857, 1989.

213. Füessl, H. S., Heinlein, H., and Goebel, F. D., Symptomatische behandlung unstillbarer diarrhoen bei AIDS mit dem somatostatin-analog SMS 201-995, *Klin. Wochenschr.*, 66(Suppl. 13), 240, 1988.

214. Füessl, H. S., Zoller, W. G., Kochen, M. M., Bogner, J.R., Heinrich, B., Matuschke, A., and Goebel, F. D., Treatment of secretory diarrhea in AIDS with the somatostatin analogue SMS 201-995, *Klin. Wochenschr.*, 67, 452, 1989.

215. Cello, J. P., Grendell, J. H., Basuk, P., Simon, D., Weiss, L., Rood, R., Wilcox, C., Forsmark, C., Read, A., Satow, J., Weikel, C., and Beaumont, C., Controlled clinical trial of octreotide (sandostatin) for refractory AIDS-associated diarrhea, *Gastroenterology*, 98, A163, 1990.

216. Fanning, M., Monte, M., Sutherland, L. R., Broadhead, M., Murphy, G. F., and Harris, A. G., Pilot study of sandostatin (octreotide) therapy of refractory HIV-associated diarrhea, *Dig. Dis. Sci.*, 36, 476, 1991.

217. Moroni, M., Esposito, R., Cernuschi, M., Franzetti, F., Carosi, G. P., and Fiori, G. P., Treatment of AIDS-related refractory diarrhoea with octreotide, *Digestion*, 54(Suppl. 1), 30, 1993.

218. Crawford, F. G. and Vermund, S. H., Human cryptosporidiosis, *Crit. Rev. Microbiol.*, 16, 113, 1988.

219. Nelson, J. A., Wiley, C. A., Reynolds-Kohler, C., Reese, C. E., Margaretten, W., and Levy, J. A., Human immunodeficiency virus detected in bowel epithelium from patients with gastrointestinal symptoms, *Lancet*, 1, 259, 1988.

220. Levy, J. A., Margaretten, W., and Nelson, J., Detection of HIV in enterochromaffin cells in the rectal mucosa of an AIDS patient, *Am. J. Gastroenterol.*, 84, 787, 1989.

221. Bigornia, E., Simon, D., Weiss, L., Tanowitz, H., Jones, J., Wittner, M., and Lyman, W., Detection of HIV-1 viral protein and genomic sequences in enterochromaffin cells of HIV-1-seropositive patients, *Am. J. Gastroenterol.*, 85, 1264, 1990.

222. Ruff, M. R., Martin, B. M., Guins, E. I., Farrar, W. L., and Pert, C.B., CD4 receptor-binding peptides that block HIV infectivity cause human monocyte chemotaxis: relationship to vasoactive intestinal polypeptide, *FEBS Lett.*, 211, 17, 1987.

223. Gaginella, T. S., Hubel, K. A., and O'Dorisio, T. M., Vasoactive intestinal polypeptide and intestinal chloride secretion, in *Vasoactive Intestinal Peptide*, Said, I., Ed., Raven Press, New York, 1982, 211.

224. Cook, D. J., Kelton, J. G., Stanisz, A. M., and Collins, S. M., Somatostatin treatment for cryptosporidial diarrhea in a patient with the acquired immunodeficiency syndrome (AIDS), *Ann. Intern. Med.*, 108, 708, 1988.

225. Friedman, L. S., Somatostatin therapy for AIDS diarrhea: muddy waters, *Gastroenterology*, 101, 1446, 1991.

226. Boman, H. G. and Hultmark, D., Cell-free immunity in insects, *Annu. Rev. Microbiol.*, 41, 103, 1987.

227. Zasloff, M., Magainins, a class of antimicrobial peptides from *Xenopus* skin: isolation, characterization of two active forms, and partial cDNA sequence of a precursor, *Proc. Natl. Acad. Sci. U.S.A.*, 84, 5449, 1987.

228. Arrowood, M. J., Jaynes, J. M., and Healey, M. C., Hemolytic properties of lytic peptides active against the sporozoites of *Cryptosporidium parvum*, *J. Protozool.*, 38, 161S, 1991.

229. Christensen, B., Fink, J., Merrifield, R. B., and Mauzerall, D., Channel-forming properties of cecropins and related model compounds incorporated into planar lipid membranes, *Proc. Natl. Acad. Sci. U.S.A.*, 85, 5072, 1988.

230. Duclohier, H., Molle, G., and Spach, G., Antimicrobial peptide magainin-I from *Xenopus* skin forms anion-permeable channels in planar lipid bilayers, *Biophys. J.*, 56, 1017, 1989.

231. Westerhoff, H. V., Juretic, D., Hendler, R. W., and Zasloff, M., Magainins and the disruption of membrane-linked free-energy transduction, *Proc. Natl. Acad. Sci. U.S.A.*, 86, 6597, 1989.

232. Arrowood, M.J., Jaynes, J. M., and Healey, M. C., *In vitro* activities of lytic peptides against the sporozoites of *Cryptosporidium parvum*, *Antimicrob. Agents Chemother.*, 35, 224, 1991.

233. Fayer, R. and Ungar, B. L. P., Cryptosporidium ssp. and cryptosporidiosis, *Microbiol. Rev.*, 50, 458, 1986.

234. Janoff, E. N. and Reller, L.B., Cryptosporidium species, a protean protozoan, *J. Clin. Microbiol.*, 25, 967, 1987.

235. Kern, P., Toy, J., and Dietrich, M., Preliminary clinical observation with recombinant interleukin-2 in patients with AIDS or LAS, *Blut*, 50, 1, 1985.

236. Soave, R. and Armstrong, D., *Cryptosporidium* and cryptosporidiosis, *Rev. Infect. Dis.*, 8, 1012, 1986.

237. Sogni, P., Coutarel, P., Chaussade, S., Michopoulos, S., Dupouy-Camet, P., Merrouche, Y., Gaudric, M., Couturier, D., and Guerre, J., Effect of azidothymidine on cryptosporidial diarrhea in a patient with acquired immunodeficiency syndrome, *Gastroenterol. Clin. Biol.*, 13, 1087, 1989.

238. Chandrasekar, P. H., "Cure" of chronic cryptosporidiosis during treatment with azidothymidine in a patient with acquired immunodeficiency syndrome, *Am. J. Med.*, 83, 187, 1987.

239. Greenberg, R.E., Mir, R., Bank, S., and Siegal, F. P., Resolution of intestinal cryptosporidiosis after treatment of AIDS with AZT, *Gastroenterology*, 97, 1327, 1989.

240. Surbone, A., Yarchoan, R., McAtee, N., Blum, M. R., Maha, M., Allain, J. P., Thomas, R. V., Mitsuya, H., Nusinoff Lehrman, S., Leuther, M., Pluda, J. M., Jacobsen, F. K., Kessler, H. A., Myers, C. E., and Broder, S., Treatment of the acquired immune deficiency syndrome (AIDS) and AIDS-related complex with a regimen of 3'-azido-2',3'-dideoxythymidine (azidothymidine or zidovudine) and acyclovir, *Ann. Intern. Med.*, 108, 534, 1988.

241. Sjordsma, A. and Schechter, P. J., Chemotherapeutic implications of polyamine biosynthesis inhibition, *Clin. Pharmacol. Ther.*, 35, 287, 1984.

242. McCann, P. P., Bacchi, C. J., Hanson, W. L., Cain, G. D., Nathan, H. C., Hutner, S. H., and Sjoerdsma, A., Effect on parasitic protozoa of α-difluoromethylornithine, an inhibitor of ornithine decarboxylase, in *Advances in Polyamine Research*, Vol. 3, Caldarera, C. M., Zappia, V., and Bachrach, U., Eds., Raven Press, New York, 1981, 97.

243. Sjoerdsma, A., Golden, J. A., Schachter, P. J., Barlow, J. L. R., and Santi, D. V., Successful treatment of lethal protozoal infections with the ornithine decarboxylase inhibitor, α-difluoroornithine, *Trans. Assoc. Am. Physicians*, 97, 70, 1984.

244. Campbell, W. C., The chemotherapy of parasitic infections, *J. Parasitol.*, 72, 45, 1986.

245. Soave, R., Sjoerdsma, A., and Cawein, M. J., Treatment of cryptosporidiosis in AIDS patients with DFMO, *Proc. 1st Int. Conf. AIDS*, Atlanta, 1985, Abstr. 30.

246. Rolston, K. V. I., Fainstein, V., and Bodey, G. P., Intestinal cryptosporidiosis treated with eflornithine: a prospective study among patients with AIDS, *J. Acquir. Immune Defic. Syndr.*, 2, 426, 1989.

247. Brasseur, F., Favennec, L., Lemeteil, D., Roussel, F., and Ballet, J. J., An immunosuppressed rat model for evaluation of anti-*Cryptosporidium* activity of sinefungin, *Folia Parasitol. (Praha)*, 41, 13, 1994.

248. Brasseur, P., Lemeteil, D., and Ballet, J. J., Curative and preventive anticryptosporidium activities of sinefungin in an immunosuppressive adult rat model, *Antimicrob. Agents Chemother.*, 37, 889, 1993.

249. Assan, R., Perronne, C., Chotard, L., Larger, E., and Vildé, J.-L., Mefloquine-associated hypoglycaemia in a cachectic AIDS patient, *Diabetes Metabol.*, 21, 54, 1995.

250. Villacorta, I., Peeters, J.E., Vanopdenbosch, E., Ares-Mazas, E., and Theys, H., Efficacy of halofuginone lactate against *Cryptosporidium parvum* in calves, *Antimicrob. Agents Chemother.*, 35, 283, 1991.

251. Naciri, M., Mancassola, R., Yvore, P., and Peeters, J. E., The effect of halofuginone lactate on experimental *Cryptosporidium parvum* infections in calves, *Vet. Parasitol.*, 45, 199, 1993.

252. Rehg, J. E., The activity of halofuginone in immunosuppressed rats infected with *Cryptosporidium parvum*, *J. Antimicrob. Chemother.*, 35, 391, 1995.

253. McDonald, V., Stables, R., Warhurst, D. C., Barer, M. R., Blewett, D. A., Chapman, H. D., Connolly, G. M., Chiodini, P. L., and McAdam, K. P., *In vitro* cultivation of *Cryptosporidium parvum* and screening for anticryptosporidial drugs, *Antimicrob. Agents Chemother.*, 34, 1498, 1990.

254. Rasmussen, K. R., Martin, E. G., Arrowood, M. J., and Healey, M. C., Effects of dexamethasone and dehydroepiandrosterone in immunosuppressed rats infected with *Cryptosporidium parvum*, *J. Protozool.*, 38, 157S, 1991.

255. Rasmussen, K. R., Martin, E. G., and Healey, M. C., Effects of dehydroepiandrosterone in immuno-suppressed rats infected with *Cryptosporidium parvum*, *J. Parasitol.*, 79, 364, 1993.

256. Merril, C. R., Harrington, M.G., and Sunderland, T., Plasma dehydroepiandrosterone on endocrine-metabolic parameters in postmenopausal women, *J. Clin. Endocrinol. Metab.*, 71, 696, 1990.

257. Esparza, J., Report of a WHO informal consultation on preclinical and clinical aspects of the use of immunomodulators in HIV infection, *AIDS*, 4, 1, 1990.
258. Loria, R. M., Padgett, D. A., and Huynh, P. N., Regulation of the immune response by dehydro-epiandrosterone and its metabolites, *J. Endocrinol.*, 150(Suppl.), S209, 1996.
259. Connolly, G. M., Youle, M., and Gazzard, B. G., Diclazuril in the treatment of severe cryptosporidial diarrhoea in AIDS patients, *AIDS*, 4, 700, 1990.
260. Menichetti, F., Moretti, M. V., Marroni, M., Papili, R., and Di Candilo, F., Diclazuril for crypto-sporidiosis in AIDS, *Am. J. Med.*, 90, 271, 1991.
261. Loeb, M., Walach, C., Phillips, J., Fong, I., Salit, I., Rachlis, A., and Walmsley, S., Treatment with letrazuril of refractory cryptosporidial diarrhea complicating AIDS, *J. Acquir. Immune Defic. Syndr. Hum. Retrovirol.*, 10, 48, 1995.
262. Harris, M., Deutsch, G., MacLean, J. D., and Tsoukas, C. M., A phase I study of letrazuril in AIDS-related cryptosporidiosis, *AIDS*, 8, 1109, 1994.
263. Victor, G. H., Conway, B., Hawley-Foss, N. C., Manion, D., and Sahai, J., Letrazuril therapy for cryptosporidiosis: clinical response and pharmacokinetics, *AIDS*, 7, 438, 1993.
264. Kim, C. W., Chemotherapeutic effect of arprinocid in experimental cryptosporidiosis, *J. Parasitol.*, 73, 663, 1987.
265. Whitlock, R. H., Therapeutic strategies involving antimicrobial treatment of the gastrointestinal tract of large animals, *J. Am. Vet. Med. Assoc.*, 185, 1210, 1984.
266. Moone, H. C., Woode, G. N., and Ahrens, F. A., Attempted chemoprophylaxis of cryptosporidiosis in calves, *Vet. Rec.*, 110, 181, 1982.
267. Fisher, O., Attempted therapy and prophylaxis of cryptosporidiosis in calves by administration of sulfamidine, *Acta Vet. (Brno)*, 52, 183, 1983.
268. Rehg, J. E., Anticryptosporidial activity of lasalocid and other ionophorous antibiotics in immuno-suppressed rats, *J. Infect. Dis.*, 168, 1566, 1993.
269. Mead, J. R., You, X., Pharr, J. E., Belenkaya, Y., Arrowood, M. J., Fallon, M. T., and Schinazi, R. F., Evaluation of maduramicin and alborixin in a SCID mouse model of chronic cryptosporidiosis, *Antimicrob. Agents Chemother.*, 39, 854, 1995.
270. Forney, J. R., Yang, S., and Healey, M. C., Anticryptosporidial potential of alpha-1-antitrypsin, *J. Eukaryot. Microbiol.*, 43, 63S, 1996.
271. Forney, J. R., Yang, S., Du, C., and Healey, M. C., Efficacy of serine protease inhibitors against *Cryptosporidium parvum* infection in a bovine fallopian tube epithelial cell culture system, *J. Parasitol.*, 82, 638, 1996.
272. Forney, J. R., Yang, S., and Healey, M. C., Interaction of the human serine protease inhibitor alpha-1-antitrypsin with *Cryptosporidium parvum*, *J. Parasitol.*, 82, 496, 1996.
273. Yang, S., Healey, M. C., Du, C., and Zhang, J., Complete development of *Cryptosporidium parvum* in bovine fallopian tube epithelial cells, *Infect. Immun.*, 64, 349, 1996.
274. Rehg, J. E., Effect of diethyldithiocarbamate on *Cryptosporidium parvum* infection in immuno-suppressed rats, *J. Parasitol.*, 82, 158, 1996.
275. Wiest, P. M., Johnson, J. H., and Flanigan, T. P., Microtubule inhibitors block *Cryptosporidium parvum* infection of a human enterocyte cell line, *Infect. Immun.*, 61, 4888, 1993.
276. Wiest, P. M., Dong, K. L., Johnson, J. H., Tzipori, S., Boeklheide, K., and Flanigan, T. P., Effect of colchicine on microtubules in *Cryptosporidium parvum*, *J. Eukaryot. Microbiol.*, 41, 66S, 1994.
277. Davis, L. J., Soave, R., Dudley, R. E., Fessel, J. W., Faulkner, S., and Mamakos, J. P., Nitazoxanide (NTZ) for AIDS-related cryptosporidial diarrhea (CD): an open-label safety, efficacy and pharmaco-kinetic study, *Proc. 36th Intersci. Conf. Antimicrob. Agents Chemother.*, American Society for Micro-biology, Washington, D.C., Abstr. LM50, 1996.
278. Rehg, J. E., Hancock, M. L., and Woodmansee, D. B., Anticryptosporidial activity of sulfadimethoxine, *Antimicrob. Agents Chemother.*, 32, 1907, 1988.
279. Rehg, J. E., Anticryptosporidial activity is associated with specific sulfonamides in immunosuppressed rats, *J. Parasitol.*, 77, 238, 1991.
280. Greenfield, R. A., Mosier, D. A., Crawford, D. L., Abrams, V. L., and Kuhls, T. L., Bismuth subsalicylate prophylaxis of *Cryptosporidium parvum* infection in immunodeficient mice, *J. Eukaryot. Microbiol.*, 43, 69S, 1996.

281. Arrowood, M. J., Mead, J. R., Xie, L., and You, X., *In vitro* anticryptosporidial activity of dinitroaniline herbicides, *FEMS Microbiol. Lett.*, 136, 245, 1996.

282. Tzipori, S., Cryptosporidiosis in perspective, *Adv. Parasitol.*, 27, 63, 1988.

283. Hart, A. and Baxby, D., Management of cryptosporidiosis, *J. Antimicrob. Chemother.*, 15, 3, 1985.

284. Bjorneby, J. M., Riggs, M. W., and Perryman, L. E., *Cryptosporidium parvum* merozoites share neutralization-sensitive epitopes with sporozoites, *J. Immunol.*, 145, 298, 1990.

285. Riggs, M. W., McGuire, T. C., Mason, P. H., and Perryman, L. E., Neutralization-sensitive epitopes are exposed on the surface of *Cryptosporidium parvum* sporozoites, *J. Immunol.*, 143, 1340, 1989.

286. Perryman, L. E. and Bjorneby, J. M., Immunotherapy of cryptosporidiosis in immunodeficient animal models, *J. Protozool.*, 38, 98S, 1991.

287. Bjorneby, J. M., Hunsaker, B. D., Riggs, M. W., and Perryman, L. E., Monoclonal antibody immunotherapy in nude mice persistently infected with *Cryptosporidium parvum*, *Infect. Immun.*, 59, 1172, 1991.

288. Langer, R. C. and Riggs, M. W., Neutralizing monoclonal antibody protects against *Cryptosporidium parvum* infection by inhibiting sporozoite attachment and invasion, *J. Eukaryot. Microbiol.*, 43, 76S, 1996.

289. Riggs, M. W., Yount, P. A., Stone, A. L., and Langer, R. C., Protective monoclonal antibodies define a distinct, conserved epitope on an apical complex exoantigen of *Cryptosporidium parvum* sporozoites, *J. Eukaryot. Microbiol.*, 43, 74S, 1996.

290. Mead, J. R., Arrowood, M. J., Healey, M. C., and Sidwell, R. W., Cryptosporidial infections in SCID mice reconstituted with human or murine lymphocytes, *J. Protozool.*, 38, 59S, 1991.

291. Kuhls, T. L., Mosier, D. A., Crawford, D. L., Abrams, V. L., and Greenfield, R. A., Improved survival of severe combined immunodeficiency (SCID) mice with cryptosporidiosis by adoptively transferring CD4$^+$ and CD4$^-$ CD8$^-$ B220$^-$ BALB/c splenocytes (Spls), *J. Eukaryot. Microbiol.*, 43, 71S, 1996.

292. Kotler, D. P., Preliminary observations of the effect of cow's milk globulin upon intestinal cryptosporidiosis in AIDS, *Proc. IIIrd Int. Conf. AIDS*, Washington, D.C., Abstr., 1987.

293. Perryman, L. E., Riggs, M. W., Mason, P. H., and Fayer, R., Kinetics of *Cryptosporidium parvum* sporozoite neutralization by monoclonal antibodies, immune bovine serum, and immune bovine colostral antibodies, *Infect. Immun.*, 58, 257, 1990.

294. Saxon, A. and Weinstein, W., Oral administration of bovine colostrum anti-cryptosporidia antibody fails to alter the course of human cryptosporidiosis, *J. Parasitol.*, 73, 413, 1987.

295. Tzipori, S., Robertson, D., Chapman, C., and White, L., Chronic cryptosporidial diarrhoea and hyperimmune cow colostrum, *Lancet*, 2, 344, 1987.

296. Flanigan, T., Marshall, R., Redman, D., Kaetzel, C., and Ungar, B., *In vitro* screening of therapeutic agents against *Cryptosporidium*: hyperimmune cow colostrum is highly inhibitory, *J. Protozool.*, 38, 225S, 1991.

297. Fayer, R., Perryman, L. E., and Riggs, M. W., Hyperimmune bovine colostrum neutralizes *Cryptosporidium* sporozoites and protects mice against challenge, *J. Parasitol.*, 75, 151, 1989.

298. Fayer, R., Andrews, B., Ungar, B. L. P., and Blagburn, B., Efficacy of hyperimmune bovine colostrum for prophylaxis of cryptosporidiosis in neonatal calves, *J. Parasitol.*, 75, 393, 1989.

299. Ungar, B. L. P., Ward, D. J., Fayer, R., and Quinn, C. A., Cessation of *Cryptosporidium*-associated diarrhea in an acquired immunodeficiency syndrome patient after treatment with hyperimmune bovine colostrum, *Gastroenterology*, 98, 486, 1990.

300. Nord, J., Ma, P., DiJohn, D., Tzipori, S., and Tacket, C.O., Treatment with bovine hyperimmune colostrum of cryptosporidial diarrhea in AIDS patients, *AIDS*, 4, 581, 1990.

301. Greenberg, P. D. and Cello, J. P., Treatment of severe diarrhea caused by *Cryptosporidium parvum* with oral bovine immunoglobulin concentrate in patients with AIDS, *J. Acquir. Immune Defic. Syndr. Hum. Retrovirol.*, 13, 348, 1996.

302. Mietens, C., Keinhorst, H., Hilpert, H., Gerber, H., Amster, H., and Pahud, J. J., Treatment of infantile *E. coli* gastroenteritis with specific bovine anti-*E. coli* milk immunoglobulins, *Eur. J. Pediatr.*, 132, 239, 1979.

303. Brussow, H., Hilpert, H., Walther, I., Sidoti, J., Mietens, C., and Bachmann, P., Bovine milk immunoglobulin for passive immunity to infantile rotavirus gastroenteritis, *J. Clin. Microbiol.*, 25, 982, 1987.

304. Hilpert, H., Brussow, H., Mietens, C., Sidoti, J., Lerner, L., and Werchau, H., Use of bovine milk concentrate containing antibody to rotavirus to treat rotavirus gastroenteritis in infants, *J. Infect. Dis.*, 156, 158, 1987.

305. Tacket, C. O., Losonsky, G., Link, H., Hoany, Y., Guesry, P., Hilpert, H., and Levine, M. M., Protection by milk immunoglobulin concentrate against oral challenge with enterotoxigenic *Escherichia coli*, *N. Engl. J. Med.*, 318, 1240, 1988.

306. Doyle, P. S., Crabb, J., and Petersen, C., Anti-*Cryptosporidium parvum* antibodies inhibit infectivity *in vitro* and *in vivo*, *Infect. Immun.*, 61, 4079, 1993.

307. Fayer, R., Guidry, A., and Blagburn, B. L., Immunotherapeutic efficacy of bovine colostral immuno-globulins from a hyperimmunized cow against cryptosporidiosis in neonatal mice, *Infect. Immun.*, 58, 2962, 1990.

308. Fayer, R., Tilley, M., Upton, S. J., Guidry, A. J., Thayer, D. W., Hildreth, M., and Thomson, J., Production and preparation of hyperimmune bovine colostrum for passive immunotherapy of cryptosporidiosis, *J. Protozool.*, 38, 38S, 1991.

309. Cama, V. A. and Sterling, C. R., Hyperimmune hens as a novel source of anti-*Cryptosporidium* antibodies suitable for passive immune transfer, *J. Protozool.*, 38, 42S, 1991.

310. Gottstein, B. and Hemmeler, E., Egg yolk immunoglobulin Y as an alternative antibody in the serology of echinococcosis, *Z. Parasitenkd.*, 71, 273, 1985.

311. Vieira, J., Oliveira, M., Russo, E., Maciel, R., and Pereira, A., Egg yolk as a source of antibodies for human parathyroid hormone (hPTH) radioimmunoassay, *J. Immunoassay*, 5, 121, 1984.

312. Bartz, C. R., Conklin, R. H., Tunstall, C. B., and Steele, J. H., Prevention of murine rotavirus with chicken egg yolk immunoglobulins, *J. Infect. Dis.*, 142, 439, 1980.

313. Otake, S., Nishihara, Y., Makimura, M., Hatta, H., Kim, M., Yamamoto, T., and Hirasawa, M., Protection of rats against dental caries by passive immunization with hen-egg-yolk antibody (IgY), *J. Dent. Res.*, 70, 162, 1991.

314. Leslie, G. A. and Clem, L. W., Phylogeny and immunoglobulin structure and function, *J. Exp. Med.*, 130, 1337, 1969.

315. Losch, U., Schranner, I., Wanke, R., and Jurgens, L., The chicken egg, an antibody source, *J. Vet. Med.*, 33, 609, 1986.

316. Hoskins, D., Chrisp, C. E., Suckow, M. A., and Fayer, R., Effect of hyperimmune bovine colostrum raised against *Cryptosporidium parvum* on infection of guinea pigs by *Cryptosporidium wrairi*, *J. Protozool.*, 38, 185S, 1991.

317. McMeeking, A., Borkowsky, W., Klesius, P. H., Bonk, S., Holzman, R. S., and Lawrence, H. S., A controlled trial of bovine dialyzable leukocyte extract for cryptosporidiosis in patients with AIDS, *J. Infect. Dis.*, 161, 108, 1990.

318. Louie, E., Borkowsky, W., Klesius, P. H., Haynes, T. B., Gordon, S., Bonk, S., and Lawrence, H. S., Treatment of cryptosporidiosis with oral bovine transfer factor, *Clin. Immunol. Immunopathol.*, 44, 329, 1987.

319. Borkowsky, W. and Lawrence, H. S., Antigen-specific inducer factor in human leukocyte dialysates: a product of T_H cells which binds to anti-V region and anti-Ia region antibodies, in *Immunology of Transfer Factor*, Kirkpatrick, C. H., Burger, D. R., and Lawrence, H. S., Eds., Academic Press, New York, 1983, 75.

320. Jeter, W. S., Kibler, R., Soli, T. C., and Stephens, C. A., Oral administration of bovine and human dialyzable transfer factor to human volunteers, in *Immune Regulators in Transfer Factor*, Kahn, A., Kirkpatrick, C. H., and Hill, N. O., Eds., Academic Press, New York, 1979, 451.

321. Lawrence, H. S., Transfer factor in cellular immunity, *Harvey Lecture Series 68*, Academic Press, New York, 1974, 239.

322. Schulkind, M. L. and Ayoub, E. M., Transfer factor and its clinical applications, in *Advances in Pediatrics*, Barness, L. A., Ed., Year Book Medical, Chicago, 1980, 89.

323. Jones, J. F., Jeter, W. S., Fulginiti, V. A., Munnich, L. L., Pritchett, R. F., and Wedgwood, R. J., Treatment of childhood combined Epstein-Barr virus/cytomegalovirus infection with oral bovine transfer factor, *Lancet*, 2, 122, 1991.

324. Klesius, P. H. and Kristensen, F., Bovine transfer factor: effect on bovine and rabbit coccidiosis, *Clin. Immunol. Immunopathol.*, 7, 240, 1977.

325. Klesius, P. H., Quals, D. F., Elston, A. L., and Fudenberg, H. H., Effects of bovine transfer factor (TFd) in mouse coccidiosis (*Eimeria ferrisi*), *Clin. Immunol. Immunopathol.*, 10, 214, 1987.

326. Chung, H. H., Shaw, D., Klesius, P., and Saxon, A., Inability of oral bovine transfer factor to eradicate cryptosporidial infection in a patient with congenital dysgammaglobulinemia, *Clin. Immunol. Immunopathol.*, 50, 402, 1989.

327. Schlegel, R. J. and Kirkpatrick, C. H., Immune deficiency diseases: the dysgammaglobulinemias, in *Immunology II*, Bellanti, J. A., Ed., W. B. Saunders, Philadelphia, 1978, 653.

328. Borowitz, S. M. and Saulsbury, F. T., Treatment of chronic cryptosporidial infection with orally administered human serum immune globulin, *J. Pediatr.*, 119, 593, 1991.

329. Losonsky, G. A., Johnson, J. P., Winkelstein, J. A., and Yolken, R. H., Oral administration of human serum immunoglobulin in immunodeficient patients with viral gastroenteritis, *J. Clin. Invest.*, 76, 2362, 1985.

330. Tutschka, P. J., The use of immunoglobulin in bone marrow transplantation, *J. Clin. Immunol.*, 10(Suppl.), 88, 1990.

331. Ungar, B. L. P., Soave, R., Fayer, R., and Nash, T. E., Enzyme immunoassay detection of immunoglobulin M and G antibodies to *Cryptosporidium* in immunocompetent and immunocompromised persons, *J. Infect. Dis.*, 153, 570, 1986.

332. Tzipori, S. and Campbell, I., Prevalence of cryptosporidium antibodies in 10 animal species, *J. Clin. Microbiol.*, 14, 455, 1981.

333. Kern, P., Toy, J., and Dietrich, M., Preliminary clinical observations with recombinant interleukin-2 in patients with AIDS or LAS, *Blut*, 50, 1, 1985.

334. Ungar, B. P. L., Milligan, M., and Nutman, T. B., Serologic evidence of cryptosporidium infection in US volunteers before and during Peace Corps service in Africa, *Arch. Intern. Med.*, 149, 894, 1989.

335. Donahue, J. H., Resenstein, M., Chang, A. E., Lotze, M. T., Robb, R. J., and Rosenberg, S. A., The systemic administration of purified interleukin 2 enhances the ability of sensitized murine lymphocytes to cure a disseminated syngeneic lymphoma, *J. Immunol.*, 132, 2123, 1984.

336. Ruscetti, F. W. and Gallo, R. C., Human T-lymphocyte growth factor: regulation of growth and function of T lymphocytes, *Blood*, 57, 379, 1981.

337. Wagner, H., Kronke, M., Solbach, W., Scheurich, P., Rollinghoff, M., and Pfizenmaier, K., Murine T cell subsets and interleukins: relationships between cytotoxic T cells, helper T cells and accessory cells, *Clin. Haematol.*, 11, 607, 1982.

338. Pearlstein, K. T., Palladino, M. A., Welte, K., and Vilcek, J., Purified human interleukin-2 enhances induction of immune interferon, *Cell Immunol.*, 80, 1, 1983.

339. Rehg, J. E., Effect of interferon-gamma in experimental *Cryptosporidium parvum* infection, *J. Infect. Dis.*, 174, 229, 1996.

340. Urban, J. F., Jr., Fayer, R., Chen, S. J., Gause, W. C., Gately, M. K., and Finkelman, F. D., IL-12 protects immunocompetent and immunodeficient neonatal mice against infection with *Cryptosporidium parvum*, *J. Immunol.*, 156, 263, 1996.

341. Kuhls, T. L., Mosier, D. A., Abrams, V. L., Crawford, D. L., and Greenfield, R. A., Inability of interferon-gamma and aminoguanidine to alter *Cryptosporidium parvum* infection in mice with severe combined immunodeficiency, *J. Parasitol.*, 80, 480, 1994.

342. Capetti, A., Bonfanti, P., Rizzardini, G., and Milazzo, F., Can rHuGM-CSF help treating drug-resistant cryptosporidiosis in AIDS, *Proc. 36th Intersci. Conf. Antimicrob. Agents Chemother.*, American Society for Microbiology, Washington, D.C., Abstr. G33, 1996.

343. Lentidoro, I., Anastasio, E., Pensabene, L., Apollini, M., and Guandalini, S., Oral rehydration in infants with acute diarrhea: using a new preparation of reduced osmolarity, *Pediatr. Med. Chir.*, 18, 67, 1996.

344. Posada, G., Pizarro, D., and Mohs, E., Oral rehydration in children with *Cryptosporidium muris* infection, *Bol. Med. Hosp. Infant Mex.*, 44, 740, 1987.

345. Wu, K. Z., Chew, S. K., Oh, H. M., Lin, R. V., Allen, D. M., and Monteiro, E. H., Acquired immunodeficiency syndrome and *Cryptosporidium* infection, *Singapore Med. J.*, 35, 418, 1994.

346. Holley, H. P., Jr. and Thiers, B. H., Cryptosporidiosis in a patient receiving immunosuppressive therapy: possible activation of latent infection, *Dig. Dis. Sci.*, 31, 1004, 1986.

347. Katz, P., Immunosuppressive therapy, in *Advances in Internal Medicine*, Stollerman, G. H., Ed., Year Book Medical, Chicago, 1984, 167.

348. Fauci, A. S., Mechanisms of the immunosuppressive and anti-inflammatory effects of gluco-corticosteroids, *J. Immunopharmacol.*, 1, 1, 1978.

349. Fauci, A. S., Haynes, B. F., and Katz, P., Drug-induced T- and B-lymphocyte and monocyte dysfunction, in *Infections In the Abnormal Host*, Grieco, M. H., Ed., Yorke Medical Books, Brooklyn, NY, 1980, 163.

350. Schreiber, A. D., Parsons, J., McDermott, P., and Cooper, R. A., Effect of corticosteroids on the human monocyte IgG and complement receptors, *Clin. J. Invest.*, 56, 1189, 1975.

351. Aji, T., Flanigan, T. P., Marshall, R., Kaetzel, C., and Aikawa, M., Ultrastructural study of asexual development of *Cryptosporidium parvum* in a human intestinal cell line, *J. Protozool.*, 38, 82S, 1991.

352. Flanigan, T. P., Aji, T., Marshall, R., Soave, R., Aikawa, M., and Kaetzel, C., Asexual development of *Cryptosporidium parvum* within a differential human enterocyte cell line, *Infect. Immun.*, 59, 234, 1991.

353. Villacorta, I., de Graaf, D., Charlier, G., and Peeters, J. E., Complete development of *Cryptosporidium parvum* in MDBK cells, *FEMS Microbiol. Lett.*, 142, 129, 1996.

354. Brown, S. M., McDonald, V., Denton, H., and Coombs, G. H., The use of a new viability assay to determine the susceptibility of *Cryptosporidium* and *Eimeria* sporozoites to respiratory inhibitors and extremes of pH, *FEMS Microbiol. Lett.*, 142, 203, 1996.

355. You, X., Arrowood, M. J., Lejkowski, M., Xie, L., Schinazi, R. F., and Mead, J. R., A chemi-luminescence immunoassay for evaluation of *Cryptosporidium parvum* growth *in vitro*, *FEMS Microbiol. Lett.*, 136, 251, 1996.

356. Grigoriew, G. A., Walmsley, S., Law, L., Chee, S. L., Yang, J., Keystone, J., and Krajden, M., Evaluation of the Merifluor immunofluorescent assay for the detection of *Cryptosporidium* and *Giardia* in sodium acetate formalin-fixed stools, *Diagn. Microbiol. Infect. Dis.*, 19, 89, 1994.

357. Edlind, T., Li, J., and Katiyar, S., Expression of *Cryptosporidium parvum* beta-tubulin sequences in yeast: potential model for drug development, *J. Eukaryot. Microbiol.*, 43, 86S, 1996.

358. Rehg, J. E., Hancock, M. L., and Woodmansee, D. B., Characterization of a dexamethasone-treated rat model of cryptosporidial infection, *J. Infect. Dis.*, 158, 1406, 1988.

359. Brasseur, P., Lemeteil, D., and Ballet, J. J., Rat model for human cryptosporidiosis, *J. Clin. Microbiol.*, 26, 1037, 1988.

360. Mead, J. R., Arrowood, M. J., Sidwell, R. W., and Healey, M. C., Chronic *Cryptosporidium parvum* infections in congenitally immunodeficient SCID and nude mice, *J. Infect. Dis.*, 163, 1297, 1991.

361. Tzipori, S., Rand, W., and Theodos, C., Evaluation of a two-phase SCID mouse model preconditioned with anti-interferon-gamma monoclonal antibody for drug testing against *Cryptosporidium parvum*, *J. Infect. Dis.*, 172, 1160, 1995.

362. Enriquez, F. J. and Sterling, C. R., *Cryptosporidium* infections in inbred strains of mice, *J. Protozool.*, 38, 100S, 1991.

363. Novak, S. M. and Sterling, C. R., Susceptibility dynamics in neonatal BALB/c mice infected with *Cryptosporidium parvum*, *J. Protozool.*, 38, 102S, 1991.

364. Current, W. L. and Long, P. L., Development of human and calf *Cryptosporidium* in chicken embryos, *J. Infect. Dis.*, 148, 1108, 1983.

365. Sherwood, K., Angus, K. W., Snodgrass, D. R., and Tzipori, S., Experimental cryptosporidiosis in laboratory mice, *Infect. Immun.*, 38, 471, 1982.

366. Pohjola, S. and Lindberg, L. A., Experimental cryptosporidiosis in mice, calves and chicken, *Acta Vet. Scand.*, 27, 80, 1986.

367. Tzipori, S., Angus, K. W., Campbell, I., and Gray, E. W., Experimental infection of lambs with *Cryptosporidium* isolated from a human patient with diarrhoea, *Gut*, 23, 71, 1982.

368. Sanford, S. E., Enteric cryptosporidial infection in pigs: 184 cases (1981–1985), *J. Am. Vet. Med. Assoc.*, 190, 695, 1987.

369. Tzipori, S., Angus, K. W., Campbell, I., and Clerihew, L. W., Diarrhea due to *Cryptosporidium* infection in artificially reared lambs, *J. Clin. Microbiol.*, 14, 100, 1981.

370. Miller, R. A., Bronsdon, M. A., Kuller, L., and Morton, W. R., Clinical and parasitologic aspects of cryptosporidiosis in nonhuman primates, *Lab. Anim. Sci.*, 40, 42, 1990.

371. Miller, R. A., Bronsdon, M. A., and Morton, W. R., Experimental cryptosporidiosis in a primate model, *J. Infect. Dis.*, 161, 312, 1990.

22.2   *ISOSPORA* SPP.

22.2.1   INTRODUCTION

Isospora spp. are apicomplexan protozoan parasites that are taxonomically related to *Cryptosporidium, Toxoplasma,* and *Sarcocystis* spp., all members of the family Eimeriidae (suborder Eimeriina). Two species of *Isospora, I. belli* and *I. hominis,* have been found in humans.[1]

The life cycle of *Isospora* is similar to that of other enteric coccidia. It involves a multistep asexual stage (merogony), followed by sexual reproduction (gamogony) and the subsequent development of oocysts. The latter, when released into the environment, are usually unsporulated and noninfective, requiring maturation to become infective.[1-3]

The mechanism of *I. belli*-induced infections is still not well understood.[3] The disease is transmitted usually by oocysts through fecal contamination of the environment, food, or water. Unsporulated oocysts, initially noninfective in the large intestine or the perianal area, may become infective within 20 to 24 h at 25 to 29°C.[3,4] Immunocompromised hosts, especially AIDS patients, are particularly at risk to the effects of these parasites.[5]

Morphologically, the intestinal lesions are characterized by villous atrophy incorporating flattened, blunted, or fused villi, focal necrosis of epithelial cells, crypt hyperplasia, as well as infiltration of the lamina propria by eosinophils, mononuclear and inflammatory cells.[6-8] It is not clear whether the mucosal damage is related to the mechanical entry and exit of the parasites from the host cell, or is mediated by parasite metabolites such as toxins, or it is related to a hypersensitivity reaction caused by the presence of parasitic antigens.[3]

The *Isospora* oocysts are identified in acid-fast- or auramine-stained fecal smears and are easily distinguishable from *Cryptosporidium* because of their ellipsoidal shape and larger size.[9] Serological identification is not available for *Isospora.*

Because of their impaired immune responses, patients with AIDS seem to be at higher risk of being infected with *Isospora.*[10-14] According to one report,[15] *Isospora* infections have been observed in 15% of Haiti's AIDS population. By another account,[9] in the U.S., only 0.2% of AIDS patients had the infection. Isosporiasis is also often associated with traveller's diarrhea in many regions of Africa, South America, and Southeast Asia.[16-19]

Using data from a surveillance registry conducted over an 8-year period, Sorvillo et al.[20] have found that AIDS patients receiving continuous prophylactic medication of trimethoprim-sulfamethoxazole against *Pneumocystic carinii* pneumonia have been less likely to develop primary infection to express latent isosporiasis because of its anti-isosporidial effect.

Clinical manifestations of isosporiasis may range from acute, but self-limited gastroenteritis in the immunocompetent host to chronic, usually intermittent illness in immunodeficient patients.[2,7–9,12,21-26] The clinical signs and symptoms of isosporiasis are frequently indistinguishable from those of cryptosporidiosis. Charcot-Leyden crystals and high fat content in stool specimens, as well as peripheral eosinophilia are among the common signs of the infections.[9] In one AIDS patient, *Isospora* parasites were identified in the lymph nodes, in what appeared to be perhaps the only reported case of extraintestinal involvement of this protozoan.[25]

22.2.2   EVOLUTION OF THERAPIES AND TREATMENT OF ISOSPORIASIS

Contrary to cryptosporidiosis, isosporiasis is treated rather successfully. For example, clinical and parasitologic cure has been achieved within 1 week after initiation of oral therapy with trimethoprim-sulfamethoxazole (co-trimoxazole).[9,13,15,24-29]

Lumb and Hardiman[3] described a rapid response of two AIDS patients with isosporidial diarrhea (one of them also with concurrent cryptosporidiosis) to treatment with co-trimoxazole (960 mg, four times daily) for 10 d. However, the diarrhea recurred after cessation of treatment, thereby necessitating a maintenance therapy.[3]

DeHovitz et al.[15] have recommended chronic medication with trimethoprim-sulfadoxine to prevent recurrence of isosporiasis.[13]

High risk of adverse reactions in AIDS patients treated with co-trimoxazole has been reported.[30]

Deluol et al.[31] described somewhat disappointing results from treatment of 11 AIDS patients with isosporiasis. Thus, sulfamethoxazole appeared to be the only drug found effective; however, a prolonged parasitologic surveillance was required in order to detect frequent relapses and to assess the long-term efficacy of the drug.

Therapies for isosporiasis consisting of metronidazole and quinacrine have also been reported.[21-23]

Amprolium, a coccidiostatic agent,[32] was also used to treat isosporiasis. In one AIDS patient, increasing doses (10 to 90 mg/kg, daily) of amprolium were applied to control the infection, but the drug caused polyneuropathy.[33]

Other agents that have been used to treat isosporiasis included diclazuril and furazolidone.[34-36] Diclazuril, a benzeneacetonitrile derivative active against *Eimeria* infections in animals, was found effective against *I. belli* infection in AIDS patients.[35]

22.2.3 REFERENCES

1. Levine, N. D., Taxonomy and life cycles, in *The Biology of the Coccidia*, Long, P. L., Ed., University Park Press, Baltimore, 1982, 1.
2. Faust, E. C., Russell, P. F., and Jung, R. C., *Craig and Faust's Clinical Parasitology*, 8th ed., Lea and Febiger, Philadelphia, 1974, 177.
3. Lumb, R. and Hardiman, R., *Isospora belli* infection: a report of two cases in patients with AIDS, *Med. J. Aust.*, 155, 194, 1991.
4. Morakote, N., Muangimpong, Y., Somboon, P., and Khamboonruang, C., Acute human isosporiasis in Thailand: a case report, *S.E. Asian J. Trop. Med. Public Health*, 18, 107, 1987.
5. Shein, R. and Gelb, A., *Isospora belli* in a patient with acquired immunodeficiency syndrome, *J. Clin. Gastroenterol.*, 6, 525, 1984.
6. Marcial-Seoane, M. A. and Serrano-Olmo, J., Intestinal infection with *Isospora belli*, *P. R. Health Sci.*, 14, 137, 1995.
7. Brandborg, L., Goldberg, S. B., and Briedenbach, W. C., Human coccidiosis — a possible cause of malabsorption: the life cycle in small-bowel mucosal biopsies as a diagnostic feature, *N. Engl. J. Med.*, 283, 1306, 1970.
8. Trier, J. S., Moxey, P. C., Schimmel, E. M., and Robles, E., Chronic intestinal coccidiosis in man; intestinal morphology and response to treatment, *Gastroenterology*, 66, 923, 1974.
9. Soave, R., Cryptosporidiosis and isosporiasis in patients with AIDS, *Infect. Dis. Clin. North Am.*, 2, 485, 1988.
10. Rogowska-Szadkowska, D., Parasitic infectons in AIDS, *Wiad. Parazytol.*, 42, 145, 1996.
11. Risse, J. H., Adam, G., Langen, H. J., Biesterfeld, S., and Hoffmann, R., Intestinal strongyloidiasis and isosporiasis in AIDS, *Rofo. Fortschr. Geb. Rontgenstr. Neuen Bildgeb. Verfahr.*, 161, 564, 1994.
12. Chaika, N. A., Isosporiasis and AIDS, *Med. Parazitol. (Mosk.)*, 3, 45, 1993.
13. Shekhar, K. C., Ng, K. P., and Rokiah, I., Human isosporiasis in an AIDS patient — report of first case in Malaysia, *Med. J. Malaysia*, 48, 355, 1993.
14. Wittner, M., Tanowitz, H. B., and Weiss, L. M., Parasitic infections in AIDS patients: cryptosporidiosis, isosporiasis, microsporidiosis, cyclosporiasis, *Infect. Dis. Clin. North Am.*, 7, 569, 1993.
15. DeHovitz, J. A., Pape, J. W., Boncy, M., and Johnson, W. D., Jr., Clinical manifestation in patients with acquired immunodeficiency syndrome, *N. Engl. J. Med.*, 315, 87, 1986.
16. Skinner, J. I., Human infection with *Isospora belli* in England: a case report, *J. Med. Microbiol.*, 5, 271, 1972.
17. Sorvillo, F., Lieb, L., Iwakoshi, K., and Waterman, S. H., *Isospora belli* and the acquired immunodeficiency syndrome, *N. Engl. J. Med.*, 322, 131, 1990.
18. Butler, T. and De Boer, W. G. R. M., *Isospora belli* infection in Australia, *Pathology*, 13, 593, 1981.
19. Shaffer, N. and Moore, L., Chronic traveller's diarrhea in a normal host due to *Isospora belli*, *J. Infect. Dis.*, 159, 596, 1989.

20. Sorvillo, F. J., Lieb, L. E., Seidel, J., Kerndt, P., Turner, J., and Ash, L. R., Epidemiology of isosporiasis among persons with acquired immunodeficiency syndrome in Los Angeles County, *Am. J. Trop. Med. Hyg.*, 53, 656, 1995.

21. Faust, E. C., Giraldo, L. E., Caicedo, G., and Bonfante, R., Human isosporiasis in the Western Hemisphere, *Am. J. Trop. Med. Hyg.*, 10, 343, 1961.

22. Forthal, D. N. and Guest, S. S., *Isospora belli* enteritis in three homosexual men, *Am. J. Trop. Med. Hyg.*, 33, 1060, 1984.

23. Liebman, W. M., Thaler, M. M., DeLorimier, A., Brandborg, L. L., and Goodman, J., Intractable diarrhea of infancy due to intestinal coccidiosis, *Gastroenterology*, 78, 579, 1980.

24. Ma, P., Kaufman, D., and Montana, J., *Isospora belli* diarrheal infection in homosexual men, *AIDS Res.*, 1, 327, 1984.

25. Restrepo, C., Macher, A. M., and Radany, E. H., Disseminated extraintestinal isosporiasis in a patient with acquired immune deficiency syndrome, *Am. J. Clin. Pathol.*, 87, 536, 1987.

26. Westerman, E. L. and Christensen, R. P., Chronic *Isospora belli* infection treated with co-trimoxazole, *Ann. Intern. Med.*, 91, 413, 1979.

27. Gorricho Mendevil, J., Torres Sopena, L., Paradineiro Somoza, J. C., and Moles Calandre, B., Treatment of recurrent *Isospora belli* diarrhea, *Rev. Esp. Enferm. Dig.*, 87, 612, 1995.

28. Gerberding, J. L., Diagnosis and management of HIV-infected patients with diarrhoea, *J. Antimicrob. Chemother.*, 23(Suppl. A), 83, 1989.

29. Gelb, A. and Miller, S., AIDS and gastroenterology, *Am. J. Gastroenterol.*, 81, 619, 1986.

30. Pape, J. W., Verdier, R. I., and Johnson, W. D., Jr., Treatment and prophylaxis of *Isospora belli* infection in patients with the acquired immunodeficiency syndrome, *N. Engl. J. Med.*, 320, 1044, 1989.

31. Deluol, A. M., Cenac, J., Michon, C., Matheron, S., Coulaud, J. P., and Savel, J., 11 cases of isosporiasis (*Isospora belli*) in patients with AIDS, *Bull. Soc. Pathol. Exot. Filiales*, 81, 64, 1988.

32. Rogers, E. F., Clark, R. L., Pessolano, A. A., Becker, H. J., Leanza, W. J., Sarett, L. H., Cuckler, A. C., McManus, E., Garzillo, M., Malanga, C., Ott, W. H., Dickinson, A. M., and Van Iderstine, A., *J. Am. Chem. Soc.*, 82, 2974, 1960.

33. Veldhuyzen van Zanten, S. J. O., Lange, J. M. A., Laarman, H. P., Reitra, P. J. G. M., and Danner, S. A., Amprolium for coccidiosis in AIDS, *Lancet*, 2, 345, 1984.

34. Limson-Pobre, R. N., Merrick, S., Gruen, D., and Soave, R., Use of diclazuril for the treatment of isosporiasis in patients with AIDS, *Clin. Infect. Dis.*, 20, 201, 1995.

35. Kayembe, K., Desmet, P., Henry, M. C., and Stoffels, P., Diclazuril for *Isospora belli* infection in AIDS, *Lancet*, 1, 1397, 1989.

36. Weiss, L. M., Perlman, D. C., Sherman, J., Tanowitz, H., and Wittner, M., *Isospora belli* infection: treatment with pyrimethamine, *Ann. Intern. Med.*, 101, 474, 1988.

22.3   *TOXOPLASMA GONDII*

22.3.1   INTRODUCTION

Toxoplasma is a genus of coccidian protozoa classified into the suborder Eimeriina, order Eucoccidiida, comprising intracellular parasites of many organs and tissues of birds and mammals, including humans. The only known complete hosts of these parasites are cats and other Felidae, in which both asexual and sexual developmental cycles occur in the intestinal epithelium, culminating in the passage of oocysts in the feces. The intestinal stages do not occur in other hosts.

Toxoplasma gondii is considered to be the causative agent of toxoplasmosis. It is a widespread intracellular parasite infecting a wide range of birds and mammals, including humans. The sexual cycle of the organism takes place in the intestinal epithelium of the cat, which is the definitive host. *T. gondii* exists in three forms: tachyzoite, tissue cysts (pseudocysts), and oocysts.

T. gondii was first discovered in 1908 by Nicolle and Manceaux[1] in a North African rodent, and by Splendore[2] in Brazilian rabbits. Inside the host cells (reticuloendothelial system and CNS), the protozoan multiplies by a peculiar type of longitudinal binary fission called endodyogeny, which involves the formation of two daughter cells within a mother cell. Next, the daughter cells surround themselves with their own membranes and leave the mother cell after disruption of its envelope. Under certain conditions, large cysts (about 150 µm in diameter) are produced, comprising thousands of single cells.[3] The asexual cycle of the parasite also includes the formation of trophozoites and bradyzoites. The mean generation time of trophozoites does not exceed 6 h,[4] whereas for bradyzoites it may reach 3 weeks.[5] Bradyzoites are generally enclosed within the cyst walls,[6] which may also protect them from the action of some drugs.

Although highly similar in structure, tachyzoites and bradyzoites differ by the relative amount of certain organelles and by specific surface or cytoplasmic molecules.[7] Differences in structure and contents also exist between parasitophorous vacuoles and cysts.[7]

T. gondii tachyzoites execute a complex and little understood combination of rapid movements (a clockwise torque that causes torsion, spinning, and pivoting; and a longitudinal pull that contracts, bends, and tilts the parasite) to reach and penetrate human or other animal cells. It has been postulated that these forces might have resulted from the action of an actin-myosin system enveloping the twisted framework of microtubules characteristic of these parasites.[8] Similarly to most intracellular parasites, T. gondii avoids lysing the host cells during invasion by wrapping itself in a vacuolar membrane. This parasitophorous vacuole membrane (PMV), which is often retained to serve as a critical transport interface between the parasite and the host cell cytoplasm, is derived from either the host cell membrane or from lipids secreted by the parasite. Suss-Toby et al.[9] have determined that in the case of T. gondii, the PMV consisted primarily of invaginated host cell membrane. Furthermore, the formation and closure of a fission pore connecting the extracellular medium and the vacuolar space was detected as the PMV pinched off. This final stage of parasite entry was accomplished without any breach in cell membrane integrity.[9] The potential role of five surface proteins of T. gondii tachyzoites in host cell invasion was investigated; at least two proteins, SAG1 and SAG2, were shown to be involved in the invasion process.[10]

The initial attachment of Toxoplasma tachyzoites to target host cells was found to be dependent on the host cell development cycle by binding specifically to a host cell receptor which has been upregulated in the mid-S phase of the cell cycle — the parasite attachment increased as the host cells proceeded from the G_1 phase to the mid-S phase, and then decreased as the cells entered the G_2-M boundary.[11]

While persistence of Toxoplasma cysts within host tissues may contribute to maintenance of immunity against reinfection, their presence may also represent, under certain conditions, a potential danger for reactivation of infection, especially in immunocompromised patients and infants with congenital toxoplasmosis.[12]

Transmission of infection is caused by ingestion of either parenteral cysts (trophozoites) from raw, infected meat, or oocysts from feces of domestic pets (cats), by transplantation of infected organs,[13,14] tainted blood transfusion,[15] or even accidental inoculation in a laboratory setting.[16] In immunocompetent hosts, toxoplasmosis is asymptomatic and benign.[17,18] The incidence of the disease is most frequent between 16 and 25 years of age.[19]

Human toxoplasmosis is expressed either as congenital or acquired. Congenital toxoplasmosis is present in newborn infants and is characterized by encephalitis, rash, jaundice, and hepatomegally, usually associated with chorioretinitis, hydrocephalus, and microcephaly, and with high mortality rate.[20-22] T. gondii can be transmitted from mother to fetus during primary maternal infection acquired after, or possibly, slightly before conception.[23] The incidence of congenital toxoplasmosis is highest in the third trimester, whereas severity is most pronounced when maternal infection is acquired during the first trimester.[23] Studies of congenital toxoplasmosis in twins confirmed the definite role of the placenta in the modalities and mechanism of fetal contamination by Toxoplasma.[24] When infection occurs during late pregnancy, it is generally associated with delayed development of ocular lesions in infants who are seropositive at birth.[25] Many children with congenital toxoplasmosis have significant retinal damage at birth and consequent loss of vision. Nonetheless, vision may be remarkably good even in the presence of large macular scars, and active lesions may become quiescent with treatment.[26] A general serological screening of pregnant women for toxoplasmosis should be done early,[27] and its treatment during pregnancy[28-32] should require special consideration of drug toxicity to the fetus, in particular when therapy is initiated during the first two trimesters where damage to the fetus (embryopathies) is most likely to happen.[33]

D'Ercole et al.[34] have described the case of a patient with systemic lupus erythematosus, treated with corticosteroids, who presented during two consecutive pregnancies with serological reactivation of toxoplasmosis associated with fetal lesions. This case is indicative of the increasing number of immunocompromised pregnant women with immunity to *T. gondii* that may pose a higher risk of reactivation of maternal toxoplasmosis and congenital infection.

After comparing lymphocyte surface phenotypes and functions in pediatric patients with congenital toxoplasmosis (ages 1 month to 5 years) as well as uninfected babies, recently infected and chronically infected adults, McLeod et al.[35] have concluded that specific deficiencies in the cell-mediated immune responses towards *Toxoplasma* lysate antigens (TLA) may account for the significant organ damage observed in infants and children with congenital toxoplasmosis. Pyrimethamine and sulfonamide treatment did not alter the lymphocyte response to TLA, neither there was a correlation between concomitant serum pyrimethamine levels and lymphocyte blastogenic responses to TLA.[35]

By and large, acquired (i.e., noncongenital) toxoplasmosis is manifested by lymphadenopathy, fatigue or malaise, fever, sore throat, headache, myocardial disease, chorioretinitis, and seizures.[17] The lymphadenopathy is most likely to be cervical (97%) with lymph nodes being usually enlarged, rubbery, and nontender. Lymphadenopathy may be also febrile, nonfebrile, or subclinical.[19] One definition advanced by Theologides and Kennedy[36] postulates three clinical syndromes for acquired toxoplasmosis, namely, (1) glandular toxoplasmosis, manifested as infectious mononucleosis (but with the absence of a heterophile antibody); (2) miliary toxoplasmosis, seen as a "typhus"-like syndrome associated with maculopapular exanthema, atypical pneumonia, myocarditis, and nonfocal neurological symptoms (lymphadenopathy may not be always present), followed by slow convalescence or death; and (3) localized toxoplasmosis, presented as granulomatous uveitis, cardiomyopathy, and/or granulomatous meningoencephalitis.[6,37]

Chorioretinitis associated with toxoplasmosis is believed to be the most often encountered infection of the posterior segment of the eye which may also lead to blindness.[38-40] Encysted *T. gondii* bradyzoites when persisting in ocular tissues may cause recurrence of the disease. Chemotherapeutic eradication of encysted bradyzoites from chronically infected tissues is usually hampered by the structure of the cyst walls as well as the organism's low metabolism. Wei et al.[41] described an AIDS patient who presented with precipitous visual loss secondary to optic nerve toxoplasmosis as the primary complaint, which subsequently led to the diagnosis of toxoplasmic papilitis and life-threatening cerebral involvement as an initial manifestation of AIDS. Herrera Rubio et al.[42] have discussed a case of aspecific chorioretinitis as initial manifestation of HIV infection and diffuse *Toxoplasma* encephalitis.

Cerebral toxoplasmosis is manifested by fever, encephalitis, convulsions, delirium, lymphadenopathy, and mononuclear pleocytosis, followed by death. In the brain, *T. gondii* multiplies in the neurons and other cells, causing cellular and interstitial necrosis. Occasionally, the infarction necrosis may lead to formation of extensive lesions.[19,43] Bamford[18] described one case of toxoplasmosis with symptoms suggesting the presence of space-occupying cerebral lesions and meningitis. As previously reported,[1] the majority of such space-occupying toxoplasmic lesions were associated with immune disorders (Hodgkin's disease, multiple myeloma, and leukemia) and ensuing therapy with immunosuppressive drugs.

Until recently, toxoplasmic encephalitis (TE) was diagnosed predominantly in immunocompromised patients with malignancies of the reticuloendothelial system or organ transplant recipients.[14,44,45] However, after the advent of the AIDS epidemic TE has become one of the most common causes of encephalitis in this population.[46-52] While toxoplasmosis comprised about 75%

of all cases of nonviral infections in AIDS patients,[47] the incidence of CNS toxoplasmosis alone was estimated to range between 3% and 44%.[25,46,49] It is believed that the occurrence of TE in AIDS patients has most likely been the result of reactivation of a latent infection rather than diagnosed as acute acquired infection.[21] A study encompassing 31 medical centers and 61 patients with AIDS concluded that presently the overall prognosis of TE is poor — the median survival time following initiation of therapy was 4 months.[53] Clinically, TE is characterized mainly with neurological disorders such as seizures, mental status change, coma, confusion, psychosis, anemia, as well as focal neurological abnormalities (hemiparesis, hemiplegia, hemisensory loss, cranial nerve palsies, aphasia, ataxia, and alexia), and meningeal symptoms.[48,54,55] Computerized axial tomography (CAT) has been of considerable help in diagnosing TE — mild to severe edema is observed on CAT scan in almost every patient.[48] Lesions were rounded, single or multiple, and isodense or hypodense.[49] Furthermore, contrast studies have revealed the presence of ring or nodular enhancement in over 90% of patients.[56] Recently, magnetic resonance imaging (MRI) is being used to detect lesions not demonstrated by CAT.[44] It is recommended, therefore, that MRI be performed in seropositive AIDS patients with neurological signs or symptoms even though the CAT scan has not produced evidence for TE.[44] Tuazon,[57] Altes et al.,[58] and Carrazana et al.[59] have reviewed the diagnosis and treatment strategies of CNS toxoplasmosis in AIDS patients.

Artigas et al.[60] have described two cases of AIDS patients who after being successfully treated for cerebral toxoplasmosis presented a few weeks later with fatal neurologic abnormalities characterized with enlargement of the cerebral ventricles, severe ventriculoencephalitis with large ependymal and subependymal necrosis, and numerous pseudomembranes within the ventricle lumen. This form of diffuse meningo-encephalo-ventriculo-myelitis, which appeared unique to AIDS, upon immunohistochemical examination revealed the presence of miriads of tachyzoites within and around the necrotic areas.

Pulmonary toxoplasmosis in AIDS patients is the second most frequent localization after the brain.[61-63] Its frequency is estimated to be between 0.2% and 3.7%, and it is seldom identified prior to autopsy. Clinical manifestations include severe interstitial pneumonitis occurring in profoundly immunodeficient patients.[64] Disseminated *T. gondii* infection may also present with fulminant pneumonia.[65] In a retrospective and descriptive study of *T. gondii*-induced pneumonia in AIDS patients, Oksenhendler et al.[66] discussed the clinical presentation, diagnostic procedures, results of therapy, and hypotheses on the pathophysiology of the infection.

Cardiac[67,68] and liver[69-71] toxoplasmosis have been described in only a limited number of patients.

Besnier et al.[72] have described a case of toxoplasmosis disseminated in the bladder of an AIDS patient.

Another rare case of reversible anterior bilateral opercular syndrome (Foix-Chavany-Marie syndrome) secondary to cerebral *Toxoplasma* abscesses has been described in an AIDS patient by Grassi et al.[73]

22.3.1.1 Tachyzoite-Bradyzoite Interconversion

There is a limited knowledge about the metabolic activities of *Toxoplasma* trophozoites vs. bradyzoites. Both bradyzoites and tachyzoites contained high activities of phosphofructokinase (specific for pyrophosphate rather than ATP), pyruvate kinase, and lactate dehydrogenase, suggesting that energy metabolism in both developmental stages may be centered around a high glycolytic flux linked to lactate production.[74] However, the markedly higher activity of pyruvate kinase and lactate dehydrogenase in bradyzoites also indicated that lactate production has been particularly important for this form. These results were consistent with the bradyzoites lacking a functional tricarboxylic acid (TCA) cycle and respiratory chain and also suggestive of their lack of susceptibility to atovaquone.[74]

In their pursuit to elucidate a possible mechanism(s) for triggering the differentiation of tachyzoite to bradyzoite form, Tomavo and Boothroyd[75] studied *Toxoplasma* mutants resistant to atovaquone. These investigators found that at least one atovaquone-resistant mutant of *Toxoplasma* has been predisposed to a bradyzoite pattern of gene expression suggesting that the mitochondrion may be involved in the differentiation process. Further experiments have demonstrated that atovaquone-resistant *T. gondii* mutants were also hypersensitive to clindamycin, which is thought to act on the putative plastid organelle of this protozoan. Similarly to *Plasmodium*, *Toxoplasma* apparently possesses an organellar-like genome (approximately 35 kb), which is highly homologous to chloroplast DNA in plants, especially algae.[76] At present, the actual subcellular of this DNA in any of these parasites is not known. Nevertheless, the presence of such a genome clearly indicates a novel plastid-like organelle.

The studies of Tomavo and Boothroyd[75] on atovaquone-resistant *T. gondii* mutants suggested that the mitochondrial and plastid functions are interconnected and that the reliance of the parasite on the mitochondrial function differed in the bradyzoite vs. tachyzoite form, as seen by the ability of *T. gondii* to respond to certain drug pressures by differentiating to a form that is less affected by that drug's action. In particular, the results of Bohne et al.[77] and Tomavo and Boothroyd[75] confirmed that inhibition of the mitochondrial function of *T. gondii* specifically induced the differentiation of tachyzoites to bradyzoites *in vitro*.

The kinetics of stage-specific protein expression during tachyzoite-bradyzoite conversion have been studied both *in vitro*[78] and *in vivo*.[79] In the mouse brain during infection with *T. gondii*, the kinetics and patterns of expression of bradyzoite-specific proteins have shown that 6 d after the ingestion of cysts, parasites found in the brain were expressing only tachyzoite-specific proteins (anti-SAG1 antibodies were used as a marker).[79] The expression of the bradyzoite-specific protein Pb36 was first noted after 9 d in vacuoles containing mixed parasites simultaneously expressing SAG1 and Pb36 or cysts containing parasites expressing only the bradyzoite marker. One important observation was the multiplication of cysts in foci, suggesting that the immune suppression triggered the release of parasites from preexisting cysts but that factors inducing bradyzoite development remained fully effective in driving parasites into this pathway.[79] Under stress conditions, such as incubation at alkaline pH, the expression of the tachyzoite-specific antigen SAG1 gradually decreased and finally disappeared during the conversion from tachyzoites into bradyzoites. In contrast, the expression of the bradyzoite-specific antigen BAG1 increased during this differentiation process.[80]

22.3.2 HOST IMMUNE RESPONSE TO *TOXOPLASMA GONDII*

Humoral toxicity has been known to be involved in development of resistance towards acute toxoplasmosis.[81,82] However, it is not known whether antibodies play a protective role in resistance against the development of toxoplasmic encephalitis.

At least two types of humoral antibodies, complement-fixing and cytoplasm-modifying, are produced against *T. gondii*. IgM antibodies, although not common, were detected in as many as 20% of all AIDS patients with CNS toxoplasmosis.[44] According to Proempeler et al.,[83] reviewing 2206 cases of pregnant women, *Toxoplasma*-specific IgM antibodies were detected in only 69 patients (3.1%). So far, serological diagnosis of toxoplasmosis has not been very helpful.

The role of cell-mediated immunity in the resistance towards infections caused by intracellular parasites such as *T. gondii* has been extensively studied, both against acute toxoplasmosis[84,85] and the development of toxoplasmic encephalitis.[86-88] Thus, mononuclear phagocytes were found to be an important part of the efferent limb of the cellular control of such infections.[89-94] The mechanism of action of phagocytes involves the participation of potent oxygen intermediates (hydrogen peroxide, hydroxyl radical, oxygen anion), which are generated during the phagocytic respiratory burst[95-98] under various stimulatory conditions.[99-103] Murray and Cohn[104] presented evidence for the susceptibility of *T. gondii* to such oxygen intermediates released by the macrophages. *In vitro* data indicated that hydroxyl radicals and singlet oxygen, when formed in a cell-free system, were the primary toxoplasmacidal agents, whereas the oxygen anion and hydrogen peroxide acted as precursors. Additional results by Murray et al.[105] demonstrated the presence of an oxygen-dependent antimicrobial mechanism of action for mononuclear phagocytes beyond the production of oxygen anion and hydrogen peroxide, further underscoring the oxygen intermediates as an important part of the macrophage resistance towards *T. gondii*.

Locksley and Klebanoff[106] also discussed the role of oxygen-dependent microbicidal systems in leukocytes in host defenses against major nonerythrocytic intracellular protozoa, such as *T. gondii*. While the hydrogen peroxide-halide-peroxidase microbicidal system was uniformly cidal to *T. gondii in vitro*, the toxicity of peroxidase-independent oxygen product(s) was more variable. Studies to date showed that phagocytes (e.g., neutrophils and monocytes) which possess substantial activity against *T. gondii* contain granule peroxidase and are able to generate a vigorous respiratory burst. To the contrary, the absence of granule peroxidase caused a markedly diminished respiratory burst, which left resident macrophages vulnerable to invasion by the protozoan.[106] Consequently, in the absence of antibody, the parasite will not only be capable of entering such macrophages, but also will survive and replicate within the intracellular environment. Enhancement of antitoxoplasma activity of resident macrophages can be accomplished by either activation of these cells through exposure to sensitized T cell products, or by the introduction of exogenous peroxidase into the vacuole.[106]

Both CD4+ and CD8+ cytotoxic T lymphocytes have been part of the human immune response to *T. gondii* infection. Studying factors which may influence the stimulation of these cells, Purner et al.[107] found that both antigen-pulsed and *Toxoplasma*-infected antigen-presenting cells (APC) induced T cell proliferation. The *Toxoplasma*-infected APC elicited strong proliferation of CD4+ T cells, but little or no proliferation of CD8+ T cells, unless high antigen loads were used. Furthermore, the *Toxoplasma*-infected APC stimulated specific cytotoxicity poorly or not at all due to the death of stimulated cultures, whereas antigen-pulsed APC elicited a substantial specific cytotoxicity. Nonetheless, specific CD8+ memory T cells were demonstrated, and rare CD8+ *Toxoplasma*-specific cytotoxic T lymphocytes have been subcloned.[107]

Cytokines, in particular interferon-γ (IFN-γ) and interleukin-12 (IL-12),[108-110] play an important role in host protection against infections with obligate intracellular parasites, such as *T. gondii*.[111-113] The relationship between IFN-γ and IL-12 in generating innate immune responses and resistance to acute *T. gondii* infection was evaluated in *T. gondii*-exposed IFN-γ knockout mice.[114] The data obtained revealed distinct functions for IL-12 and IFN-γ in host resistance to the protozoan: IL-12 preceded and initiated the synthesis of IFN-γ, while the latter directly controlled the parasite growth and diminished the contributions of IL-4- and IL-5-producing T cell subsets. In the absence of endogenous IFN-γ, the mice developed unimpaired IL-12 responses to *T. gondii* while failing to control acute infection.[114]

To analyze the role of IFN-γ in the early phase of toxoplasmosis, IFN-γ receptor-deficient (IFN-γ R0/0) mice were orally infected with low-virulence *Toxoplasma*. The mice died from the disease up to day 10 postinfection, whereas immunocompetent wild-type mice developed chronic toxoplasmosis. These and related experiments have demonstrated that IFN-γ was absolutely required for the efficient activation of macrophages, which have been of critical importance in the defense against toxoplasmosis.[115]

The CD4+ T cells are known to be heterogeneous (Th1 and Th2) with regard to cytokine secretion.[116] The Th1 cells preferentially secrete IL-1 and IFN-γ, whereas Th2 cells predominantly produce IL-4, IL-5, IL-6, and IL-10.[117-120] IL-4 has been reported to exert a dominant effect in determining the pattern of cytokine (Th2-type) produced by CD4+ T lymphocytes upon subsequent antigen stimulation *in vitro*.[121-124] In addition, IL-4 is one of the cytokines which downregulates the production of IFN-γ by the Th1 subset of CD4+ T cells. Since IFN-γ is a critical factor in mediating resistance towards *T. gondii*,[82] Suzuki et al.[125] have examined the role of IL-4 in the pathogenesis of toxoplasmic encephalitis using IL-4-targeted mutant (IL-4$^{-/-}$) mice. Whereas control mice survived, IL-4$^{-/-}$ mice all died from 6 to 20 weeks after peroral infection with cysts of the ME49 strain of *T. gondii*. These and other results from this study indicated that IL-4 has been protective against the development of toxoplasmic encephalitis by preventing formation of *T. gondii* cysts and proliferation of tachyzoites in the brain. The impaired ability of IL-4$^{-/-}$ mice in the late stage of *T. gondii* infection to produce IFN-γ most likely contributed to their susceptibility to development of severe toxoplasmic encephalitis.[125]

Bala et al.[126] have investigated the ability of *T. gondii* to trigger cytokine synthesis in humans. For this purpose, human peripheral blood mononuclear cells (PBMC) obtained from both HIV-seronegative and HIV-seropositive subjects were exposed *in vitro* to the soluble *T. gondii* tachyzoite antigen STAg, and the levels of IL-1, IL-6, IL-12, GM-CSF, and TNF-α were measured by the enzyme-linked immunosorbent assay. High levels of different cytokines were detected in the PBMC cultures from both HIV-positive and HIV-negative patients with *T. gondii*. The observed ability of STAg to trigger various cytokine response (including TNF-α) *in vitro* and the fact that this tachyzoite antigen also dramatically enhanced HIV replication *in vitro* (as measured by the effect on reverse transcriptase activity), have raised the possibility that the growth of the parasite in immunodeficient individuals may potentiate retroviral replication though the action of these cytokines (such as TNF-α) and thereby serve as a cofactor for AIDS development.[126]

Infection of mice with *T. gondii* elicited both a protective Th1 and immune downregulatory Th2 cytokine response.[108] Among Th1-type cytokines so far studied, IFN-γ, IL-2, and IL-12[127] appeared to be the major mediators against acute parasitic infections. Thus, exogenous IL-12 when given at the time of acute toxoplasmic infection, elicited an increase in the natural killer (NK) cell population and enhanced the production of IFN-γ.[128,129] Sharma et al.[130] have found that exogenously administered IL-2 also protected mice against a sublethal challenge by *T. gondii*. Shirahata et al.[131] have also reported enhancement by recombinant human IL-2 of host resistance to *T. gondii* infection in pregnant mice. The explicit mechanism by which IL-2 regulates host protection against the protozoan has not been determined, but it is assumed that it may be needed for priming and maintaining the cell-mediated host response — there has been evidence showing that a marked decrease in the production of IL-2 will take place in mice 7 d after infection.[132-134]

The major function of another interleukin, IL-7, (a monomeric protein produced by bone marrow stromal cells[135,136] and fetal thymus) is to induce the proliferation of pre-B lymphocytes and CD4$^+$ and CD8$^+$ T cells, and to enhance the cytotoxicity of cytotoxic lymphocytes[137] and NK cells.[138,139] Inbred mice when infected with a lethal dose of *T. gondii* and then treated with IL-7 twice daily beginning at the time of infection survived, whereas mice either treated after infection or not treated died.[140] Phenotypic analysis of splenocytes identified an expansion of NK (asialo GM1$^+$) cells and CD8$^+$ T cell populations. Furthermore, *in vivo* depletion of these cell populations has shown that cells expressing these phenotypes were important for maintaining protection against the parasite. Also, IFN-γ depletion resulted in complete reversal of the protective effect of IL-7 administration, whereas *in vivo* depletion of endogenous IL-7 enhanced susceptibility to infection. Further analysis by semiquantitative reverse-transcriptase polymerase chain reaction has demonstrated that IL-7 enhanced the IFN-γ response and reversed the parasite-mediated downregulatory response on IL-2.

The function of IL-10 synthesis was examined during early infection with the avirulent *T. gondii* ME-49 strain in IL-10-deficient (knockout) mice.[141] In contrast to controls which displayed 100% survival, the IL-10-deficient mice succumbed within the first 2 weeks of the infection, with no evidence of enhanced parasite proliferation. Furthermore, the mortality in the IL-10 knockout mice was associated with enhanced liver pathology characterized by increased cellular infiltration and intense necrosis. The levels of IL-12 and IFN-γ in the sera of infected IL-10-deficient animals were four- to sixfold higher than those in sera from controls, as were mRNA levels for IFN-γ, IL-1β,

TNF-α, and IL-12 in lung tissue. Taken together, the results of the study suggested that endogenous IL-10 synthesis played an important role *in vivo* in downregulating monokine and IFN-γ responses to acute intracellular infection, thereby preventing host immunopathology.[141]

Interleukin-15 (IL-15) is a new cytokine[142] which resembles IL-2 in its biological activities. It was shown to stimulate a wide range of immune cells, including lymphocyte-activated killer (LAK) cells,[143] $\gamma\delta$ T cells,[144] NK cells,[145] and B cells.[146] In addition, IL-15 was demonstrated to increase the proliferation of PBMC from HIV-infected patients in response to HIV-specific antigens.[147] Unlike IL-2, however, IL-15 is not produced by lymphocytes, but instead (at least among cells of the immune system) it appeared to be secreted predominantly by monocytes/macrophages.[148] Although the sequence of IL-15 is not homologous with that of IL-2, it uses components of IL-2R for binding and signal transduction.[149] Khan and Kasper[150] have studied the effect of IL-15 on prevention of murine infection with *T. gondii*. IL-15 was able to stimulate the production and proliferation of CD8$^+$ T cells that have been exposed to parasite antigen. CD8$^+$ T lymphocytes, which have been known to proliferate in response to active parasite infection,[85,87,151,152] did not increase in numbers when soluble *T. gondii* lysate antigen alone was used for immunization. However, in the presence of both exogenous recombinant IL-15 and parasite lysate antigen, there has been near doubling in the number of toxoplasmacidal antigen-specific CD8$^+$ T cells.[150]

Cells synthesize heat shock proteins (hsps) in response to various noxious stimuli, including elevation of body temperature.[153,154] In addition, hsps also serve as major immunogens that can elicit both cellular[155,156] and humoral immunity[157,158] in association with several infectious states. While protective immunity against *T. gondii* is mediated mainly by T cell-dependent immune responses[159,160] in patients with acute toxoplasmosis, $\gamma\delta$ T cells seemed to participate in the first line of defense against infection[161,162] and to increase their numbers in the peripheral blood.[163,164] Nagasawa et al.[165] have shown that the induction of hsp65 (a heat shock protein and a known ligand for $\gamma\delta$ cells[166,167]) within and on host macrophages, has correlated closely with protection against *Toxoplasma* infection in mice. In subsequent studies in mice, Hisaeda et al.[168] have also demonstrated that $\gamma\delta$ T lymphocytes (having both the Thy-1$^+$ and Thy-1$^-$ phenotypes) played an important role in the expression of hsp65 within and on host peritoneal macrophages in an IFN-γ-independent manner; concurrently, there has been an increase in the number of T cells bearing the $\gamma\delta$ receptor with Thy-1$^+$ and Thy-1$^-$ phenotypes in the peritoneal cavity and spleen. Further studies by Hisaeda et al.[169] in mice infected with *T. gondii* have demonstrated that extrathymic rather than intrathymic $\gamma\delta$ T cells played the important role of protecting the mice from *T. gondii* and the expression of hsp65 protein.

In a separate study, Kasper et al.[170] have shown that adoptive transfer of $\gamma\delta$ T cells into microglobulin-β_2-deficient mice that have been depleted of both CD4$^+$ and NK cells, prolonged the survival against acute parasite challenge when compared with nontransferred controls. These and other related experiments,[170] in turn, have confirmed that $\gamma\delta$ T cells have been an important factor in the development of protective immunity during the early stages of infection with *T. gondii*.

Several studies have indicated the importance of IFN-γ not only for inhibition of *T. gondii* multiplication, but also for the stage differentiation (tachyzoite-bradyzoite interconversion) process of this parasite.[77,171] In an effort to further determine the extent to which parasitic and host cell-dependent factors are important for triggering the conversion between tachyzoites and bradyzoites, Gross and Bohne[172] have established that activation with IFN-γ significantly reduced the replication rate of the protozoan, confirming previous findings.[173] Whereas activation with IFN-γ host cell-dependently suppressed the growth of *T. gondii* by either tryptophan starvation in human fibroblasts or by nitric oxide release in murine macrophages, the inhibition of the parasite's mitochondrial function has been the common trigger for stage differentiation[7] (see Section 22.3.1.1).

Chemokines are members of the cytokine family that signal through seven transmembrane domain receptors and whose principal activity is as chemotactic factors.[174] With the exception of lymphotactin, the chemokines contain four invariable cysteine residues in one of two patterns:

(1) the CC pattern, in which the two cysteines are adjacent, and (2) the CXC pattern, in which the two cysteines are separated with a single residue. Within the human CXC chemokines, there is a subgroup of neutrophil chemotactic factors (IL-8, the GRO proteins, NAP-2, ENA-78, and GCP-2) which contain, in close proximity to their NH_2 terminals, a protein sequence known as ELR. The presence of ELR has been shown to be crucial for binding of these neutrophil chemotactic factors to IL-8 receptors.[175] Those of the human CXC chemokines that lack the ELR sequence include such proteins as the platelet factor-4, SDF-1, HuMig, and IP-10, none of which have activity on neutrophils. Among the latter group of CXC chemokines, the relationship between HuMig and IP-10 has been particularly close. Thus, a pairwise comparison of their protein sequences has revealed 37% identity over the 76 amino acids of the mature proteins that were comparable. In addition, the genes of HuMig and IP-10 (*Humig* and *IP-10*, respectively) have been shown to be adjacent on chromosome 4q21.21, with their respective codons separated by less than 16 kb, suggesting close evolutionary relationship.[176] Furthermore, mouse and human *mig* and *crg-2* (the mouse homolog of *IP-10*), and *IP-10* have all been inducible by rIFN-γ.[177] Both HuMig[178] and IP-10,[179] and the mouse homologs MuMig and Crg-2 (both also IFN-γ-inducible), have all been shown to be T cell chemotactic factors *in vitro*.

Amichay et al.[176] have analyzed the expression of the genes *Mumig*, *crg-2*, and *IFN-γ* during experimental infections with *T. gondii*. While all three genes were induced in multiple organs, during the acute phase of the infection as well as after intraperitoneal injection of rIFN-γ, the levels of *Mumig* mRNA in the liver were as high or higher than its levels in any other organ. In contrast, the organs showing the highest expression of *crg-2* and *IFN-γ* varied among the experimental models, with induction of these latter genes colocalizing. Furthermore, IFN-γ was necessary for the induction of *Mumig* during the infection with *T. gondii*; by comparison, the induction of *crg-2* was not completely dependent on IFN-γ. Moreover, the pattern of induction of *crg-2* was consistent with Crg-2 acting primarily locally, whereas the pattern for *Mumig* induction suggested that MuMig may have a systemic role during the infection. The data of Amichay et al.[176] have demonstrated that the close relationships between IFN-γ and Mig and Crg-2/IP-10, described previously *in vitro*, also hold during complex immune responses *in vivo*. Although the physiologic roles of Mig and Crg-2/IP-10 still remain not clearly defined, the dramatic induction of *Mumig* and *crg-2* mRNAs in response to rIFN-γ to more than 400-fold of baseline levels in a mouse macrophage cell line *in vitro*, suggested that Mig and Crg-2/IP-10 mediated a subset of the effects of IFN-γ, a cytokine that is particularly critical for effective cell-mediated immunity against *T. gondii* infection.[176]

Khalil and Rashwan[180] have found the levels of TNF-α in the sera of patients with toxoplasmosis significantly higher as compared to healthy controls — acute infection was associated with the highest levels of TNF-α, indicating that it may play a role in its pathogenesis. In chronic infection, the level of TNF-α correlated with the IHA antibody titer, suggesting that antibodies against *T. gondii* may participate in the TNF-α production.

22.3.3   STUDIES ON THERAPEUTICS

22.3.3.1   Pyrimethamine–Sulfonamide Combinations

Sheffield and Melton[181] have studied the activity of pyrimethamine and sulfadiazine on the fine structure and multiplication of *T. gondii* RH strain in rhesus monkey kidney cell structures. The drugs were added 4 h after infection either alone or in combination. Pyrimethamine (1.0 µg/ml) blocked multiplication and caused significant morphologic changes — the parasites were rounded, often with fragmented nucleus, and their division was inhibited as seen by the abnormal daughter membrane formation during endodyogeny. No effect was present in sulfadiazine-treated *T. gondii* when concentrations of up to 50 µg/ml were used. When a combination of both drugs was applied (0.1 µg/ml of pyrimethamine and 0.5 µg/ml of sulfadiazine), the effect was synergistic.[181,182] The latter finding was corroborated by Harris et al.,[183] who by measuring the incorporation of [^{3}H]uracil into *Toxoplasma*-infected, differentiated L_6E_9 rat myocytes, found that low-dose pyrimethamine (0.1 µg/ml) and sulfadiazine (25 µg/ml) acted in a synergistic manner to suppress the *Toxoplasma* growth.

Werner and Egger[184] have evaluated the efficacy of fansidar (a combined preparation of sulfadoxine and pyrimethamine in a 20:1 ratio) in experimental mouse models of acute and chronic toxoplasmosis. The drug, which was administered to mice daily for 5 d beginning 6 h after the infestation with *T. gondii*, was found to be effective on all forms of the proliferative and cyst-forming stages. Compte et al.[185,186] have compared the therapeutic efficacy of fansidar with that of pyrimethamine-sulfadiazine in the treatment of ocular congenital toxoplasmosis with recurrences; fansidar was found to be the less effective medication.

Other combinations, comprising pyrimethamine–sulfamonomethoxine and pyrimethamine–sulfamethoxypyrazine (20 mg/kg pyrimethamine and 200 mg/kg sulfonamide), were also tested and found effective in preventing death.[184] However, when administration was not initiated until 3 d postinfection, only fansidar (given for 5 d) was able to completely eradicate parasites from some animals.[184] Pregnant women infected with *T. gondii* gave birth to normal children after being treated with fansidar; post-treatment serological examination revealed a reduction of the IgG titers.[187]

Metakelfin (combination of sulfamethoxypyrazine, 20 mg/kg and pyrimethamine, 1.0 mg/kg) was more effective in treating mice infected with *T. gondii* than either drug applied alone.[188] Sulfamethoxypyrazine-longum, a long-acting form of the drug, when administered at doses of 125 to 200 mg/kg led mice to full recovery from experimental toxoplasmosis.[188] Metakelfin at 25 mg/kg given daily to mice with experimental toxoplasmosis for a period of 2 weeks, was 100% effective in controlling the infection; 1-week treatment was inadequate.[189] When metakelfin was administered as early as 4 h postinfection, no cysts were detected in brain tissues.[189]

Following therapy of *Mastomys natalensis* chronically infected with *T. gondii* strain ALT with sulfamethoxypyrazine–pyrimethamine, the brains were studied for structural alterations in cysts by light and electron microscopy.[190] Changes were found in the cyst walls, bradyzoites, and more significantly, in the endodyogeny stages — the degree of damage was proportional to the intensity of the bradyzoite metabolism.[190]

A combination of sulfamethoxydiazine and pyrimethamine eliminated all *Toxoplasma* forms (zoites and cysts, including young cysts) in NMRI mice, when treatment was commenced no later than day 5 postinfection; if, however, administration begun on day 7, there was no curative effect.[191] Usually older cysts in the brain will not respond to therapy, likely because of their low metabolism that does not allow the drugs to interfere with essential metabolic processes.[191]

The pyrimethamine pharmacokinetics in HIV-infected patients seropositive to *T. gondii* have been investigated by Jacobson et al.[192] In general, there have been no differences in the pharmacokinetic parameters of pyrimethamine in HIV-infected patients compared with those of non-HIV-positive patients, as well as no change in the pharmacokinetics of zidovudine in these patients.

22.3.3.2 Trimethoprim–Sulfonamide Combinations

Over the years, combinations of trimethoprim and sulfamethoxazole (co-trimoxazole, bactrim, septrim, sumetrolim) were studied extensively both *in vitro* and *in vivo*, as well as in humans as therapy for toxoplasmosis.

Trimethoprim, which possesses a mechanism of action similar to that of pyrimethamine, is however, less toxic to the bone marrow.[193,194] The enzymatic locus of action of trimethoprim is the enzyme dihydrofolate reductase.[195] Dihydrofolate (FAH_2) and triphosphopyridine nucleotide (TPNH) bind to DHFR in a sequential but nonobligatory order. FAH_2 is then reduced to tetrahydrofolate (FAH_4), and both molecules will leave DHFR in a random manner. Results from a study of the inhibition kinetics of trimethoprim have shown that the drug bound to DHFR at the same site as did FAH_2 and was completely displaced by it. While trimethoprim may bind to DHFR in the absence of TPNH, there was evidence suggesting that the complex trimethoprim-TPNH-DHFR dissociated to a lesser degree than did the trimethoprim-DHFR complex.[195]

The ultimate and critical target of chemotherapy with trimethoprim and sulfamethoxazole is the pool of tetrahydrofolate cofactors (structurally, representing FAH_4/one-carbon fragment complexes) present in microbial cells.[196] These cofactors participate in one or more biosynthetic reactions by donating their one-carbon units to generate various products and regenerating FAH_4 or dihydrofolate (FAH_2) in the process. In order to keep the system functional, FAH_2 must be reconverted, with the help of dihydrofolate reductase (DHFR), back to FAH_4.

Based on their affinity to trimethoprim and other antifolate drugs, the various DHFRs have been divided into bacterial (high affinity for trimethoprim), mammalian (low affinity for trimethoprim), and a transition group. It is this difference of affinity that will determine the selectivity, and ultimately, the usefulness of antifolate drugs as anti-infective agents.

Co-trimoxazole, at concentrations as low as 60 µg/ml, inhibited the replication of *T. gondii* within HeLa cells and mouse peritoneal macrophages; the inhibition reached 100% following 18 h of treatment at 37°C.[197] More prolonged exposure of the parasite resulted in its eradication from the cellular monolayers.[197] Further experiments by Nguyen and Stadtsbaeder[198] have demonstrated that the replication of *T. gondii* in cultured human monocytes was totally suppressed after 24 h of exposure to trimethoprim–sulfamethoxazole (1.6 or 2.0 µg/ml, and 56.0 or 70.0 µg/ml, respectively); no cytotoxic effect on the monocytes was noted. Given alone, neither of the two drugs was found effective.[198]

The effect of co-trimoxazole on the interaction between mitochondria and parasitophorous vacuoles in macrophages *in vitro* was also investigated.[199]

Grossman and Remington[200] showed that *in vitro*, trimethoprim alone at concentrations of 10 to 20 µg/ml caused death of intracellular *T. gondii*. Sulfamethoxazole by comparison, at concentrations as high as 100 µg/ml had no meaningful effect against the intracellular parasites. When the two drugs were used as combination (2.0 µg/ml of trimethoprim and 50.0 µg/ml of sulfamethoxazole), a significant synergistic effect took place. Another trimethoprim–sulfamethoxazole combination (200 mg/kg of each drug) given by gavage protected 87% of mice with 50,000 LD_{100} of *T. gondii*.[200]

In a number of studies,[201,202] trimethoprim when applied alone was found virtually inactive against *T. gondii in vivo*, whereas its combinations with sulfamethoxazole were, again, effective against murine[202] and human[203-205] toxoplasmosis. Thus, a nearly 100% survival rate was noted in mice fed with sulfamethoxazole (800 mg/100 ml of drinking water) and trimethoprim (160 mg/100 ml of drinking water) starting 3 to 4 d before infection with *T. gondii* and continuing for 20 d afterwards.[206] In addition, the combination of the two drugs provided immunity (having both humoral and cellular characteristics) against reinfection.[206]

In a mouse model of experimental toxoplasmosis, Terragna et al.[207-211] found that daily doses of 1.0 to 2.0 mg of trimethoprim and 5.0 to 10 mg of sulfamethoxazole led to survival rates of 76% to 100%;[207] the observed protective effect was dose-dependent and the highest survival rate (91.3%) was demonstrated with the intermediate dosage.[202,207]

As compared to oral sulfamethoxazole alone (50 to 200 mg/kg), oral septrim (trimethoprim–sulfamethoxazole in a 1:5 ratio) resulted in higher survival of mice with experimental toxoplasmosis; in the same study, oral trimethoprim (10 to 40 mg/kg) alone, did not have antitoxoplasmic effect.[212] In a separate report,[213] daily medication with septrim at 600 mg/kg led to a 35% survival rate in mice infected with *T. gondii*; a 50% survival was observed following a similar treatment with 500 mg/kg daily of sulfamethoxazole.

Nguyen and Stadtsbaeder[214] compared the therapeutic efficacy of co-trimoxazole, pyrimethamine–sulfadiazine, and spiramycin during the proliferative and chronic phases of infection in mice inoculated with *T. gondii* (Beverley avirulent strain). The results of their study indicated that co-trimoxazole and pyrimethamine–sulfadiazine were superior to spiramycin during the proliferative phase, but neither drug was effective against tissue cysts in chronically infected mice. The treatment (all drugs administered in drinking water) was started either immediately after the avirulent infection (evolution phase) or 15 d later (chronic phase), and continued for 42 d at daily doses (approximate mean concentrations) of 923 mg/kg (co-trimoxazole), 4.8 + 240 mg/kg (pyrimethamine–sulfadiazine), and 962 mg/kg (spiramycin). Oral pyrimethamine alone (25 mg/kg daily for 7 d, starting 24 h after inoculation) eliminated cysts in the brain of mice.[215]

With regard to various *T. gondii* strains, it should be mentioned that the pathology of infection caused in mice by the avirulent Beverley strain of *T. gondii* is considered to be very similar to that in humans; that is, the infection is latent or subclinical by nature, with encystment in tissues during the chronic phase.

In further experiments, Nguyen and Stadtsbaeder[216] have compared the effectiveness of co-trimoxazole and spiramycin in female mice infected in midpregnancy with the Beverley strain of *T. gondii*. Therapeutically, co-trimoxazole was more beneficial than spiramycin as seen by the statistically significant increase in the rate of both successful delivery and offspring survival.[216] Moreover, results based on antitoxoplasma antibody determination in offsprings indicated a better *in utero* control of congenital infection by co-trimoxazole than by spiramycin. Both drugs were administered in drinking water at concentrations of 9.6 mg/kg (co-trimoxazole) and 10 mg/ml (spiramycin) beginning 5 d after *Toxoplasma* inoculation.[216] Since in pregnant women spiramycin did not readily cross the placental barrier,[217] its effectiveness in treatment of fetuses infected *in utero* has been questioned.[218]

A combination of trimethoprim and sulfamoxole was applied by Maier and Piekarski[219] to treat albino mice infected with the virulent BK strain of *T. gondii* for 20 d. Results showed a marked reduction of mortality with no antibodies formed and no detectable cysts in the brain of treated animals. When compared to trimethoprim–sulfamethoxazole, the combination of trimethoprim and sulfamoxole had a slightly better therapeutic effect.[219]

Attempts by Feldman[201] to cure infection of *T. gondii* (RH strain) in mice with trimethoprim–sulfisoxazole (alone or in 1:4 combination) were unsuccessful; the drugs were administered either in drinking water or by injection.

22.3.3.3 Miscellaneous Sulfonamides

Rabbits inoculated with *T. gondii* (RH strain) were treated with 2-sulfamoyl-4,4′-diaminodiphenyl sulfone (SDDS) by intraperitoneal administration of 150 mg/kg daily for 2 weeks, beginning 48 h after the infection. The drug produced complete cure and immunity against the infection.[220] In a similar study, Kumar et al.[221] asserted that at daily oral doses of >100 mg/kg administered for 1 to 2 weeks, SDDS protected rabbits infected with *T. gondii*; the presence of 2-mercaptoethanol-sensitive (hemagglutinin antigen/HA) antibodies which persisted for 4 to 6 weeks has been observed.

In a mouse model of acute toxoplasmosis, SDDS (130 mg/kg) when given for 7 d in combination with either sulfadiazine (100 mg/kg) or pyrimethamine (1.0 mg/kg), markedly augmented the mean survival time; the dosing started 24 h after intraperitoneal injection of 2×10^4 parasites.[222,223] Treatment of chronic infection (*T. gondii* Beverley strain) for 40 d with SDDS–pyrimethamine and SDDS–sulfamonomethoxine eradicated cysts from 50% and 46.2% of mice, respectively; when given 2 d before infection, and for 7 d afterwards, both combinations completely prevented infection.[222] Experiments by Werner and Catar[223] showed that while SDDS–pyrimethamine and SDDS–sulfamonomethoxine effectively eliminated the parasite in the proliferative and cyst-forming stages of toxoplasmosis, the combinations had no effect on older cysts with resting metabolism (even after 3 weeks of therapy with once-daily oral doses). Overall, the combination of SDDS and pyrimethamine was more potent than that with sulfamonomethoxine.[223]

Another sulfonamide derivative, sulfamethoxypyrazine was used to treat mice infected with *T. gondii* at daily doses of 83.3 and 166.5 mg/kg.[224] After receiving the lower dose, 72% of the animals survived as compared to only 64% for the higher dose. In both groups, the survival rate was higher than that of controls.[225]

Histochemical examination of rats revealed that after 15 d of treatment with daily doses of 166.5 mg/kg (divided and injected subcutaneously twice daily), sulfamethoxypyrazine enhanced mitochondrial swelling and fatty degeneration of T. gondii.[225] The therapeutic effect of sulfamethoxy-pyrazine against toxoplasmosis in mice was synergistically potentiated by prevaccination with killed T. gondii (RH strain).[226] For example, after oral administration of 8.0 mg daily for 4 weeks, the drug prolonged the survival by 47%; following prevaccination, however, the survival rate was augmented by 83%.[226]

Werner et al.[227] investigated the efficacy of sulfamethoxypyrazine (alone, or in combination with pyrimethamine and spiramycin) in experimental toxoplasmosis in NMRI mice. A minimal single dose of 50 mg/kg of sulfamethoxypyrazine was needed to maintain an adequate drug serum levels for 2 weeks; nonetheless, alone, the drug was unable to eliminate the parasite from host tissues.[227] Increased potency was achieved by combined medication with pyrimethamine (50 mg/kg daily of each drug) commencing 48 h postinfection — mice were parasite-free 4 weeks after the infection. The combination of sulfamethoxypyrazine and spiramycin, although limiting the spread of the protozoan (most pronounced during early infection) did not prevent cyst formation.[227] Brus et al.[228] reported that a complete cure of experimental toxoplasmosis in mice was achieved by a 10-d oral treatment with 125 to 150 mg/kg of sulfamethoxypyrazine starting on the day of infection.

Mice treated with sulfamonomethoxine and killed Toxoplasma organisms were protected against the infection to a greater extent than from either one of them when applied alone.[229] Orally ingested sulfamonomethoxine (500 mg/kg daily for 2 to 3 weeks) was more potent in prolonging the life of mice infested by T. gondii, than either spiramycin, acetylspiramycin, or pyrimethamine.[230] Combinations of sulfamonomethoxine with any of the latter three drugs were also effective but not nearly as much as sulfamonomethoxine given alone.[230] According to Brus et al.,[228] oral doses of 50 to 150 mg/kg of sulfamonomethoxine administered for 10 d were sufficient to provide complete cure of murine experimental toxoplasmosis. Similar results were produced with 150 mg/kg of sulfamonoethoxine, the ethyl analog of sulfamonomethoxine.[228]

An emulsion consisting of 3-sulfamido-3-methoxypyrazine and 2,4-diamino-5-(p-chlorophenyl)-6-ethylpyrimidine was injected subcutaneously into mice infected with T. gondii — the combination was effective in eradicating the parasite.[231] Side effects included a gradually increasing leukopenia as well as gradual rise of alpha- and gamma-globulin levels at the expense of beta-globulin.

In NMRI mice inoculated intraperitoneally with brain suspension from mice chronically infected with T. gondii (20 to 30 cysts = 200,000 trophozoites), only sulfatolomide and pyrimethamine, when given alone on the day of infection, provided curative effect.[191]

If used in conventional dosage, sulfisoxazole was found therapeutically ineffective in treating toxoplasmosis.[232] Its median effective dose was usually 20 times greater than that of sulfadiazine and nearly 100 times greater than that of sulfamethazine. In immunodeficient patients, a prolonged treatment with sulfisoxazole was required in order to acquire immunity.[18]

In an earlier study, Shitova and Novitskaya[233] found combinations of sulfadimesine with either aminoquinol or pyrimethamine to be very effective in mouse experimental toxoplasmosis.

When administered concomitantly at a dose of 100 mg/kg, dimethylsulfoxide (DMSO) slightly enhanced the curative effect of 2-methoxy-3-sulfamylamidopyrazine to mice infected with T. gondii.[234] Under similar conditions, sulfadiazine (100 mg/kg) provided a complete cure.[234]

22.3.3.4 Macrolide Antibiotics

22.3.3.4.1 Spiramycin

According to some studies,[235] the mechanism of action of spiramycin was similar to the mechanism by which erythromycin and other related macrolides exert their antibacterial activity. Spiramycin is thought to inhibit the parasite protein synthesis by binding to some ribosomal components of *T. gondii,* thereby preventing the elongation of the peptide chain.[236,237] While erythromycin bound to the 50*S* ribosomal unit of bacteria, it did not bind to mammalian 80*S* ribosomes, and that may explain its selective toxicity for bacteria.[238] Furthermore, erythromycin effectively suppressed the binding to the ribosome of both donor and acceptor substrates.[239] Spiramycin acted primarily by stimulating the dissociation of peptidyl-tRNA from ribosomes during toxoplasmosis.[239] Another hypothesis was based on the premise that spiramycin confers its antitoxoplasmic activity by a nonribosomal mode of action involving the possibility of an immunomodulating effect.[236]

The pharmacokinetics of spiramycin were investigated after single and repeated administrations.[240] After entering the blood circulation, spiramycin disappeared rapidly and was retained in the liver, lung, spleen, and kidney for a considerable period of time — its concentrations increased steadily with prolonged administration.[241] Twenty-four hours after a single oral dose of 500 mg/kg, the concentration of the antibiotic in the spleen reached 164 µg/ml.[197] Following intravenous administration of a single 500-mg dose during 1-h infusion, the peak serum concentrations of spiramycin were 1.54 to 3.10 mg/l. The antibiotic was rapidly and widely distributed in the body with higher ratios of tissue/serum concentrations in the bucco-dental, pulmonary, and prostatic tissues and skin. The terminal elimination half-life of spiramycin was about 5 h.[240]

The antitoxoplasmic activity of acetylspiramycin, an analog of spiramycin, has also been investigated.[241] In acutely infected mice, combinations of acetylspiramycin with either obioactin or sulfamethoxypyrazine prevented *Toxoplasma* organisms from encysting in brain and heart tissues.[242] If administered alone, acetylspiramycin was effective only in heart but not brain tissues. All of the drugs tested failed to act in chronically infected mice. Overall, the combination acetylspiramycin–obioactin was the most potent, leading to a 52.4% reduction in the cyst counts in brain.[242]

22.3.3.4.2 Roxithromycin

Roxithromycin (RU 28965), an ether oxime derivative of erythromycin, was reported effective in mice against lethal dosing of virulent *T. gondii* (RH strain).[243] The therapy (daily oral dose of 10 mg) when initiated at either 24 h before, or 2 h and 24 h after the infection with 2×10^3 tachyzoites, protected mice by 90%, 8%, and 50%, respectively, as compared with 0% in untreated controls.[243] The protozoan was isolated from less than 20% of the roxithromycin-treated mice.[230]

In earlier studies, Jones et al.[244] and Barlam and Neu[245] tested *in vitro* the activity of roxithromycin. The antibiotic, when used against *T. gondii* in murine peritoneal macrophage cultures, showed an IC_{50} value of 54 µ*M*.[246] It decreased the number of infected cells, the number of tachyzoites per vacuole, and the number of cells containing rosettes (i.e., clusters of more than eight tachyzoites).[246] Chang and Pechère[247] found that roxithromycin was efficient against acute peritoneal murine toxoplasmosis. Thus, after five daily doses of 540 and 360 mg/kg (beginning 24 h after challenge), the antibiotic produced 100% and 50% survival rates, respectively.[247] After 14 doses starting 3 h after challenge, the 50%-survival dose was 360 mg/kg daily. *T. gondii* was recovered from the brain in 59% and 28% of surviving mice treated with 5 and 14 doses, respectively.[246]

Luft[248] reported that roxithromycin protected mice against lethal infections induced by an extremely virulent RH strain and by the C56 strain of *T. gondii*; given 2 h after infection, the drug protected over 80% of the mice. At doses of less than 250 µg/ml, roxithromycin had no effect on the proliferation of the parasite in murine peritoneal macrophage cultures.[246]

Concomitant administration of roxithromycin and IFN-γ proved to be synergistic in a murine model of TE.[249]

The efficacy of roxithromycin alone and in combination with pyrimethamine or sulfadiazine has been investigated *in vitro* and in a murine model of acute toxoplasmosis.[250] In MRC5 fibroblast tissue cultures, roxithromycin inhibited the *Toxoplasma* growth at concentrations of ≥0.02 mg/l;

the IC_{50} value was estimated to be 1.34 mg/l. There was no synergistic effect observed *in vitro* for its combinations with pyrimethamine or sulfadiazine. In mice infected with 10^4 tachyzoites of the virulent RH strain, roxithromycin was used orally for 10 d from day 1 after infection. When administered alone at daily doses of 50 or 200 mg/kg, roxithromycin slightly prolonged the survival compared with untreated controls, but was strikingly synergistic with both pyrimethamine and sulfadiazine at subtherapeutic daily doses of 12.5 and 100 mg/kg, respectively. The combination regimens led to marked reduction in parasite numbers in blood and tissue compared with any of the agents used alone.[250]

22.3.3.4.3   Azithromycin

Structurally, azithromycin (CP-62,993, XZ-450) represents a 15-membered macrolide (9-deoxo-9a-aza-9a-methyl-9a-homoerythromycin).[251,252] It is a new macrolide antibiotic with a broad spectrum of antimicrobial activity, which has been actively investigated against various opportunistic pathogens, including *T. gondii*.[253,254]

In vitro, in murine peritoneal macrophage cultures, azithromycin had an IC_{50} value of 140 μM against *T. gondii*.[246]

Azithromycin was shown to inhibit the growth of *T. gondii* tachyzoites *in vitro*, but the effect was only observed with prolonged incubation with the antibiotic, revealing its delayed mode of action on the protozoan.[255] The mechanism of action of azithromycin very likely involves inhibition of the parasitic protein synthesis although the site of action and fixation in the parasite has not been clearly demonstrated. Azithromycin has also been shown effective against intracystic bradyzoites *in vitro*, but its long-term administration to chronically infected mice failed to reduce the mean number of brain cysts.[255]

There has been an additive effect *in vitro* when azithromycin was applied in combination with either pyrimethamine or sulfadiazine. Furthermore, a remarkable synergistic effect was observed *in vivo* when these combinations were tested against acute murine toxoplasmosis.[255]

In models of acute toxoplasmosis, while the effect of azithromycin on brain infection was limited, it cleared parasites from blood and lungs of infected mice, resulting in a significant protection of treated animals compared with controls.[255]

At daily oral doses of 200 mg/kg administered for 10 d, the antibiotic successfully protected mice against death caused by intraperitoneal inoculation of *T. gondii*.[256,257] The same dosage regimen led to 80% survival of mice infected intracerebrally with the protozoan, demonstrating that active concentrations of the drug may be attained in the inflamed central nervous system.[256]

In a murine model of lethal chronic toxoplasmosis, prolonged administration of azithromycin at 100 mg/kg daily for 100 d protected all mice compared with 19 of 25 control animals which died ($p < .001$).[258] The concentrations of azithromycin in the brains of five animals ranged from 0.7 to 2.3 $\mu g/g$, with no evidence of accumulation even after 100 doses.

Araujo and Remington[259] have found synergistic activity between azithromycin and IFN-γ in murine toxoplasmosis. Combined treatment for 10 d with azithromycin (75 mg/kg daily) and IFN-γ (2.0 μg daily) resulted in 40% protection of mice given lethal inoculum of *T. gondii*. When administered alone, azithromycin protected mice by less than 10%.[259]

A parallel study on the *in vivo* activity of azithromycin, roxithromycin, and spiramycin against *T. gondii* showed azithromycin to be significantly more active against acute toxoplasmosis even when roxithromycin and spiramycin were given at twice its dose.[260] Thus, a daily dose of 200 mg/kg of azithromycin administered for 10 d was sufficient to achieve 100% survival of mice inoculated with as high as 1×10^5 tachyzoites. Also, 90% of mice inoculated with strain MO (isolated from an AIDS patient) survived when treated the same, but only 40% of mice injected with the same inoculum of the SOU strain (isolated from an AIDS patient) survived. Drug concentrations in the brain were nearly 10-fold higher than those in the serum after daily treatment with 200 mg/kg of azithromycin for 10 d. Overall, azithromycin attained high concentrations in the liver, spleen, and heart which exceeded concurrent serum levels by 25- to 200-fold.[260]

22.3.3.4.4   Rifamycins

Rifabutin is a semisynthetic derivative of rifamycin S, which has shown activity alone and in combinations with other drugs in murine models of systemic toxoplasmosis and toxoplasmic encephalitis.[261] Mice infected with a lethal inoculum of *T. gondii* tachyzoites or cysts were protected 100% by rifabutin at doses of 300 or 400 mg/kg administered for 10 d; doses of 100 and 200 mg/kg of the drug protected 10% to 40% and 80% of mice, respectively. Combinations of nonprotective (50 mg/kg) or slightly protective (100 mg/kg) doses of rifabutin with doses of sulfadiazine, pyrimethamine, clindamycin, or atovaquone, which did not confer any protection against death from toxoplasmosis when administered alone, resulted in remarkable enhancement of the *in vivo* activities of all of these drugs.[261]

The *in vitro* and *in vivo* activity of rifabutin against *T. gondii* have also been investigated by Olliaro et al.[262] and Brun-Pascaud et al.[263] Using either a low-virulence or a high-virulence strain of *T. gondii* (subcultured in drug-free conditions after exposure to various drug concentrations), no parasite growth was observed after subculture at 1 month after exposure to 6.0 mg/l of rifabutin for the low virulence and 12 mg/kg for the high virulence strain.[262] The IC_{50} of rifabutin was 26.5 mg/l in a different series of experiments using an enzyme-linked immunoassay. In an acute murine model of toxoplasmosis, survival was significantly improved when mice received a 12-d treatment with 50, 100, or 200 mg/kg daily of rifabutin starting 5 d before infection with a high-virulence strain of parasites. Combination therapy with rifabutin–clarithromycin (at 25, 50, and 100 mg/kg daily of each drug) also led to markedly improved survival. The calculated ED_{50} values for rifabutin and rifabutin–clarithromycin were 160.5 and 114.8, respectively.[262]

The efficacy of rifabutin in combination with atovaquone, clindamycin, pyrimethamine, or sulfadiazine for treatment of toxoplasmic encephalitis in mice was also examined.[264] In order to determine whether any synergistic effect existed, doses of each drug that were not effective in reducing inflammation in the brain of mice with TE when used alone were used in combination with a dose of rifabutin which was minimally effective. Only the combinations of rifabutin–atovaquone and rifabutin–clindamycin showed statistically significant reduction in brain inflammation.

Rifapentine, another semisynthetic analog of rifamycin, was also investigated for activity against *T. gondii in vitro* and *in vivo*.[265] The antibiotic, which inhibited the intracellular replication of the parasite, was not toxic to the host cells. Mice infected either intraperitoneally with tachyzoites of the RH strain or orally with tissue cysts of the C56 strain were protected by rifapentine with degree of activity similar to that of atovaquone but apparently higher than that induced by rifabutin.[265]

22.3.3.4.5   Other macrolide antibiotics

Compound A-56268 is a new 6-*O*-methyl derivative of erythromycin with a longer serum half-life than the parent compound.[266] Chang and Pechère[246] demonstrated that in murine peritoneal macrophage cultures, A-56268 blocked the incorporation of [^{3}H]uracil by the virulent R strain of *T. gondii* with an IC_{50} value of 147 μM. When given by gavage to mice with acute toxoplasmosis at 300 mg/kg for 9 d, A-56268 led to 100% survival.[267] Moreover, 41.6% of the surviving mice were free from cerebral infection with the parasite. The drug was inhibitory rather than cidal against the protozoan.[267]

Another macrolide antibiotic, josamycin, at daily doses of 600 to 2400 mg/kg, administered orally for 45 d, did not show any activity against the *Toxoplasma* virulent RH and avirulent PV strains in mice.[268]

At concentrations of 50 µg/ml, rifampin exerted a marked inhibitory effect against *Toxoplasma* replication *in vitro* in mammalian cell cultures.[269] However, in experimental toxoplasmosis in mice, oral or intraperitoneal administration did not render any protection against the *T. gondii*.[269]

Treatment of experimental toxoplasmosis with clarithromycin-based combination regimens with minocycline or pyrimethamine led to 100% cure of active and latent infection caused by RH or TS4 *T. gondii* tachyzoites.[270] The proposed therapeutic modality could be especially useful since clarithromycin-based combinations can also provide safe and effective treatment against *Mycobacterium avium* complex infections associated with AIDS patients.

22.3.3.5 Clindamycin

There have been some peculiar kinetics in the clindamycin action against *T. gondii*, mainly with regard to its delayed effect on the replication of the tachyzoites.[271] Fichera et al.[272] have investigated the replication of *T. gondii* tachyzoites as a function of time after the addition of clindamycin. Thus, when intracellular tachyzoites were treated with up to 20 μM of clindamycin (over 1000 times the 50% inhibitory concentration) they exhibited doubling (replication) times indistinguishable from those of controls (approximately 7 h). Next, the drug-treated parasites emerged from the infected cells and established parasitophorous vacuoles inside new host cells as efficiently as the untreated controls; however, the replication time within the second vacuole was dramatically slowed. Furthermore, the growth inhibition within the second vacuole did not require the continuing presence of the drug, but it was dependent solely on the concentration and duration of drug treatment in the first (previous) vacuole. The susceptibility of intracellular parasites to nanomolar concentrations of clindamycin contrasted sharply with that of extracellular tachyzoites, which were completely resistant to treatment, even through several cycles of subsequent intracellular replication. This peculiar phenotype, in which drug effects have been observed only in the second infectious cycle, has also been associated with the actions of azithromycin and chloramphenicol, but not with the activity of cycloheximide, tetracycline, and anisomycin. While these findings provided new and unusual insights into the mode of action of clindamycin and other macrolide antibiotics against *T. gondii*, the relevant target for their action still remains unknown.[272]

The effects of clindamycin alone or in combination with pyrimethamine on the proliferation of *T. gondii* in cultured mammalian cells, and its effect on the parasite's RNA and protein synthesis, have been investigated by Blais et al.[273] After treating infected macrophages with clindamycin and clindamycin–pyrimethamine for 48 h, the IC_{50} for parasite growth were 32.50 ± 1.30 and 10.78 ± 0.56 µg/ml, respectively. When free tachyzoites were pre-exposed to clindamycin for 4 h, the reduction of parasite infectivity was proportional to the amount of drug — 100 ng/ml of clindamycin reduced the infectivity of *T. gondii* to $46.5\% \pm 8.5\%$ of that of untreated controls. Furthermore, at 40 µg/ml, clindamycin reduced the protein synthesis by $56.2\% \pm 6.0\%$, but did not affect the RNA synthesis after a 4-h exposure of free parasite tachyzoites to the drug.[273]

Administration of clindamycin hydrochloride (alone or in combination with corticosteroids) to cats with toxoplasmic retinochoroiditis resulted in total resolution of clinical manifestations.[274] In another study,[275] treatment with clindamycin resolved recurrent toxoplasmosis and decreased the pathogen's titers in cats with inflammatory intestinal disease and prior medication with immunosuppressive drugs. The antibiotic reduced mortality by 44% when used prophylactically ($p < .001$) in chronic toxoplasmic infection in mice, but appeared to be less effective when used to treat clinically apparent reactivation.[276]

McMaster et al.[277] investigated the effects of clindamycin and *N*-demethyl-4'-pentylclindamycin (U-24) in mice infected with *T. gondii* (RH strain). The two antibiotics were administered by gavage or mixed in diet for 1 to 14 consecutive days after injection of trophozoites. All mice were cured when fed by gavage with 50 mg/kg of U-24 for 8 d, or 400 mg/kg of clindamycin for 11 d.[277]

Clindamycin was found to be efficient in treating acute and chronic toxoplasmosis in a mouse model, and in preventing congenital transmission during acute stage of infection in the mother.[278] In addition, clindamycin was effective in eradicating the parasites from host tissues (spleen, liver, and blood) during chronic (latent) infection. When calculated on a mg/kg basis, the most effective dosage of clindamycin in mice appeared to be higher than that applied conventionally in humans; that is, approximately 250 mg/kg per 24 h in mice, as compared with approximately 15 to 30 mg/kg per 24 h in man. However, when doses were equated on a comparable surface area basis (a more reliable measurement), the dose for mice (750 mg/m^3) was much closer to the human dose (550 to 1100 mg/m^3).[278]

Thiermann et al.[279] observed that even though clindamycin, at daily doses of 8 mg for 12 d, increased the survival rate in mouse model of experimental toxoplasmosis, residual *Toxoplasma* organisms remained in 8 of 10 mice; by comparison, pyrimethamine–sulfamethoxypyridazine combination cured all infected animals with no residual parasites left 40 d later. When injected intraperitoneally to mice with *Toxoplasma* trophozoites, clindamycin provided 80% protection from death.[280] In murine toxoplasmic encephalitis, it reduced the mortality in cortisone-treated mice by 100%.[281] Other reports have indicated that clindamycin was also effective in treating ocular toxoplasmosis,[282,283] toxoplasmic myocarditis,[284] and cerebral toxoplasmosis.[285-288]

Terragna et al.[289] described antitoxoplasmic activity for a combination of clindamycin and sulfadiazine — *in vivo*, the combination elicited cure rates ranging between 80% and 100%.

22.3.3.6 Tetracyclines

The activity of various tetracycline antibiotics in acute experimental toxoplasmosis in mice have been studied at length.[290-295] One of them, minocycline, is a semisynthetic, broad-spectrum antibiotic which in addition to being antibacterial,[296] has also displayed antimalarial activity.[297,298] In one study,[299] Swiss-Webster mice were treated with minocycline once daily for 12 d beginning 2 h after infection — as compared to controls, the observed survival and cure rates were 100% and 40%, respectively, when minocycline was administered at 100 mg/kg daily; the corresponding rates were 0% and 0% when pyrimethamine was given at a daily dose of 8.5 mg/kg. Combination of minocycline and pyrimethamine at the same doses resulted in 100% and 50% survival and cure rates, respectively.

Absolute survival and cure rates were attained when minocycline was administered to mice twice daily at 100 mg/kg for 12 d. The serum levels of the antibiotic in normal mice after a single oral dose of 50 or 100 mg/kg peaked after 1 h at 1.8 mg/l and 10 mg/l, respectively, and showed an extended half-life.[299]

A combination of minocycline (daily dose of 50 mg/kg) and sulfadiazine (daily dose of 100 mg/kg) after being fed by gavage for a period of 2 weeks, protected mice 100% after inoculation of 50,000 LD$_{100}$ of *T. gondii* (RH strain).[300] In similar experiments, minocycline alone at 50 mg/kg daily gave only 50% protection. One reason for the observed lower percentage survival rate might have been the poor penetration of minocycline through the blood-brain barrier, resulting in inability to eradicate the parasite from the brain tissues of chronically infected mice.[300] The potency of the minocycline–sulfadiazine combination was equal to that of pyrimethamine (12.5 mg/kg daily)–sulfadiazine (100 mg/kg daily).[300]

Intraperitoneal (but not oral) administration of minocycline or doxycycline (both antibiotics given at daily doses of 13.3 mg/kg for 2 weeks) was effective against toxoplasmosis in mice.[301] In the same model, oxytetracycline was inactive. Indorf and Pegram[302] have used doxycycline in the management of toxoplasmic encephalitis in a patient with AIDS.

Fertig et al.[303,304] have reported the treatment of one patient with toxoplasmosis[305] with 500 mg of tetracycline (four times daily) given for 3 weeks, followed by conventional therapy with pyrimethamine–sulfadiazine.

Garin et al.[295] used demethylchlortetracycline to treat toxoplasmosis in mice — dosing with 200 mg/kg daily resulted in 60% survival rate. Eyles and Coleman[292] have found that in acute murine toxoplasmosis, the mean curative dosage of chlortetracycline and tetracycline was approximately 1240 mg/kg daily.

22.3.3.7 Miscellaneous Antibiotics

Mitomycin C, at a dose of 0.1 mg/kg, was more potent against experimental toxoplasmosis in mice compared to the conventional dose of 0.05 mg/kg.[306]

Lonomycin A, a polyether antibiotic,[307,308] when tested *in vitro* in host cell cultures at a concentration of 0.01 μg/ml in TC-199 medium, elicited complete inhibition of *Toxoplasma* multiplication.[309]

Lasalocid, another polyether antibiotic isolated from *Streptomyces lasaliensis*, has been shown to be effective *in vitro* against *T. gondii*.[310] When added to cell cultures at 0.05 μg/ml, either prior to or after inoculation, the drug suppressed the proliferation of the parasite, but only partially blocked its penetration into the cell.[310]

Gentamicin (1.0 mg/kg) was found ineffective *in vivo* against experimental murine toxoplasmosis; in the same model, primaquine (0.25 mg/kg) also failed to act.[179]

22.3.3.8 Atovaquone

Atovaquone (*trans*-2-[4-(4-chlorophenyl)cyclohexyl]-3-hydroxy-1,4-naphthalenedione), an antiprotozoal drug,[311,312] acts primarily by inhibiting the mitochondrial cytochrome bc_1 complex. Atovaquone has been investigated as an alternative agent for oral use in the treatment of toxoplasmosis.[313]

Although the *in vitro* activity of the drug varied among different strains of *T. gondii* tachyzoites, Araujo et al.[314] have found that atovaquone inhibited six of seven strains (including those isolated from AIDS patients) at concentrations of 4.8×10^{-9} to 4.8×10^{-6} mol/l. Higher concentrations of atovaquone were needed to kill bradyzoites within cysts — while at a concentration of 2.8×10^{-6} mol/l the drug was ineffective, the incubation of *T. gondii* cysts obtained from infected mice with 2.8×10^{-4} mol/l of atovaquone for 1 to 8 d resulted in loss of viability of cysts.[314-316]

Romand et al.[317] have studied the *in vitro* potency and *in vivo* efficacy of atovaquone alone and in combinations with pyrimethamine, sulfadiazine, clarithromycin, and minocycline against *T. gondii*. *In vitro*, in MRC5 fibroblast tissue cultures, atovaquone inhibited the parasites at concentrations of ≥0.02 mg/l; the IC_{50} was 6.4×10^{-8} mol/l (0.023 mg/l). *In vivo*, mice were acutely infected intraperitoneally with 10^4 tachyzoites of the virulent RH strain of *T. gondii* and then treated perorally for 10 d from day 1 postinfection. The following drug regimens were investigated: atovaquone alone at 100 and 50 mg/kg daily; and the combinations of 50 mg/kg atovaquone with either 200 mg/kg sulfadiazine, 12.5 mg/kg pyrimethamine, 200 mg/kg clarithromycin, or 50 mg/kg minocycline. Compared with untreated mice, both dosages of atovaquone alone resulted in prolonged survival, concurrent with reduced parasite burdens in blood and tissues during the course of treatment. While in terms of survival, the combinations of atovaquone with the other drugs were more efficient than each drug administered alone, the parasite burdens in blood and organs were not reduced compared with those in mice treated with any of the agents alone.[317] In mice infected with the RH strain of *T. gondii*, treatment of atovaquone at 100 mg/kg daily for 10 d initiated 1 d postinfection, resulted in 100% survival.[314]

In a rat model, the activity of atovaquone against *T. gondii* seemed to be less promising.[318]

In chronically infected mice (1 to 3 months before initiation of treatment), atovaquone at daily doses of 100 or 200 mg/kg produced a steady decline in the number of *T. gondii* cysts found in the brain.[314,315,319] In addition to reducing the number of cysts, atovaquone decreased the size of the cysts[319] as well as perivascular inflammatory infiltrates and infiltrates in the meninges and parenchyma,[315,319] evidence that atovaquone had eradicated the cysts without causing cyst rupture or release of *Toxoplasma* antigens.[319] Ultrastructural examination after 4 weeks of treatment demonstrated a substantial increase in both the numbers of cysts with lysed and/or degenerated bradyzoites. It is probable that atovaquone acted predominantly against the metabolically active immature bradyzoites, rather than the mature organisms.[319]

The mechanism of action of atovaquone has been determined mainly in studies on *Plasmodium* spp.,[320,321] and to a lesser extent in *T. gondii*[322] and *Pneumocystis carinii*.[323] The drug was demonstrated to be a powerful and selective inhibitor of the *Plasmodium* mitochondrial respiratory chain, but had little activity on rat liver mitochondria *in vitro*.[321] Atovaquone acted by binding to the cytochrome bc_1 complex (complex III) of the respiratory chain causing inhibition of the pyrimidine biosynthesis. Such an action may be, in fact, the basis for its selectivity since mammalian cells (but not protozoa) are capable of bypassing the *de novo* pyrimidine synthesis. At higher concentrations, atovaquone was able to suppress the substrate-ubiquinone reductases of the respiratory chain as do other ubiquinone antagonists.[321] The activity of dihydroorotate dehydrogenase, a key enzyme in *de novo* pyrimidine synthesis in *Plasmodium falciparum*[324] and *P. carinii*[325] was also inhibited by atovaquone through the inhibition of electron transport. At least in *P. carinii*, the mechanism of action of atovaquone appeared to involve a linkage between the respiratory chain and the oxidative phosphorylation, and the ability of the drug to reduce the adenosine triphosphate (ATP) synthesis.[323]

22.3.3.9   Trimetrexate and Related Compounds

Trimetrexate, a lipid-soluble analog of methotrexate, was found to be a potent inhibitor of *T. gondii* dihydrofolate reductase, the presumed target of other folate inhibitors (pyrimethamine, trimethoprim).[326,327] Trimetrexate is an agent that does not require uptake by the folate carrier transport system, a major mechanism of cellular resistance both *in vitro* and *in vivo*.[328]

The IC_{50} value of trimetrexate for the DHFR of *T. gondii* was 500- and 10,000-fold less than those of pyrimethamine and trimethoprim, respectively.[329] Contrary to methotrexate, trimetrexate is rapidly taken up by *T. gondii* tachyzoites.[329] *In vitro* experiments have shown that *Toxoplasma* proliferation in murine peritoneal macrophages was completely abolished by exposure to 10^{-7} M of trimetrexate for 18 h;[326,330] the corresponding values for pyrimethamine and trimethoprim were 10^{-6} and 10^{-4} M, respectively.[326]

In order to exert its activity, methotrexate, a potent inhibitor of mammalian and bacterial DHFR itself (inhibition constant: [k_i] value of 10^{-11}), requires transport by a folate-specific membrane carrier that is found in mammalian cells.[330] Since *Toxoplasma* parasites lack a transmembrane transport system for physiologic folates (such as pteroyl glutamate), host toxicity could be prevented by co-administration of leucovorin (the reduced folate) without reversing the antiprotozoal activity of the antifolate drug.[330,331] Mammalian cells can utilize leucovorin (which bypasses the inhibition of DHFR by antifolates) while certain protozoa (*T. gondii*, for example) cannot.

In acutely infected BALB/c mice, trimetrexate alone (oral or intraperitoneal routes of administration) prolonged the survival rate, and in combination with sulfadiazine allowed 93% to 100% of the mice to survive.[326] Although in humans the half-life of trimetrexate (9.5 h) is considerably lower than that of pyrimethamine, apparently it still allows the drug to penetrate the central nervous system faster than pyrimethamine and may, therefore, be of more value for long-term therapy.[48]

Clinical experience with trimetrexate in the management of toxoplasmosis is rather limited. Thus, five of nine patients treated with the drug responded well for periods ranging between 2 weeks and 3 months; three of the patients failed to respond.[48]

Piritrexim (BW 301) is a lipid-soluble analog of trimetrexate. It showed shorter half-life (and therefore, potentially less toxicity) than trimetrexate.[332] Piritrexim inhibited the catalytic activity of DHFR with an IC_{50} value of 17 nM,[332] concentration that was 40- to over 1000-fold less than the corresponding values of trimethoprim and pyrimethamine, respectively. Furthermore, piritrexim was able to suppress the replication of *T. gondii* in mouse peritoneal macrophage culture at concentrations of 0.1 to 1.0 µM; leucovorin did not affect the ability of piritrexim to inhibit *Toxoplasma* proliferation. The addition of sulfadiazine to piritrexim appeared to enhance its potency in murine toxoplasmosis.[332,333]

The synthesis of a number of lipophilic antifolates (2,4-diaminopteridines, 2,4-diamino-5-methyl-5-deazapteridines, 2,4-diamino-5-unsubstituted-5-deazapteridines, and 2,4-diamino-quinazolines) that showed superior activity to trimetrexate and piritrexim against *T. gondii in vitro*, has been reported.[334] Structurally, each of these compounds possessed an aryl group attached to the 6-position of the heterocyclic moiety through a two-atom bridge (either CH_2NH, CH_2NMe, CH_2S, or CH_2CH_2). High levels of combined potency and selectivity as growth inhibitors of *T. gondii*, and as inhibitors of the microbial enzymes relative to the mammalian enzyme, were found only among the 5-methyl-5-deazapteridines.

Jackson et al.[335] have identified another four 6,7-disubstituted-2,4-diaminopteridines as inhibitors of a folate precursor, the *p*-aminobenzoic acid. In addition, these compounds also caused significant inhibition of *T. gondii* tachyzoite replication in Madin-Darby bovine kidney cells in the 0.1 to 10 μM concentration range, with three of these compounds (GR 92754, AH 10639, and AN 2504) being at least one order of magnitude more potent than pyrimethamine. Furthermore, GR 92754, AH 10639, and AH 2504 were substantially more potent and selective than pyrimethamine as inhibitors of *T. gondii* DHFR, with IC_{50} values ranging from 0.018 to 0.033 μM. Overall, GR 92754 was the most potent and selective anti-DHFR agent with superior activity against both *T. gondii* and *Pneumocystis carinii*.

22.3.3.10 Epiroprim

Epiroprim [2,4-diamino-5-(3,5-diethoxy-4-pyrrol-1-ylbenzyl)pyrimidine; Ro 11-8958, EPM] is a new selective inhibitor of microbial dihydrofolate reductase, with excellent activity against staphylococci, enterococci, pneumococci, and streptococci which was considerably better than trimethoprim.

The efficacy of epiroprim *in vitro* and in the treatment of acute *Toxoplasma* infection in mice, has been evaluatied.[336] While the IC_{50} of epiroprim for *T. gondii* DHFR (0.9 μM) was similar to that of pyrimethamine, it was 650-fold more selective than pyrimethamine for *T. gondii* DHFR compared with human DHFR. In mice acutely infected with the RH strain of *T. gondii*, intraperitoneally administered epiroprim (300 mg/kg daily, for 14 d) alone was ineffective. However, 100% survival was seen when it was combined with orally administered sulfadiazine (375 mg/kg daily), which alone was also ineffective. Increases in survival rates were observed in combinations with sulfadiazine at doses as low as 0.375 mg/kg daily.

The combination of epiroprim with dapsone was synergistic and showed *in vitro* activity superior to that of trimethoprim–sulfamethoxazole.[337] Orally administered epiroprim combined with dapsone also prolonged the survival of mice. Mehlhorn et al.[338] have also tested epiroprim alone and in combination with dapsone in mice, where epiroprim–dapsone led to complete cure of infection. However, even though synergistic (100% survival rate at daily doses of 50 mg/kg of each drug) the combination epiroprim–dapsone was only parasitostatic.[339] A 3-week therapy of chronically infected mice with either epiroprim (50 mg/kg daily), dapsone (50 mg/kg daily), or pyrimethamine (15 mg/kg daily) decreased the numbers of *T. gondii* cysts and the inflammation in their brains; the combination epiroprim–dapsone (both drugs each at 50 mg/kg daily) further reduced the number of brain cysts in comparison with the corresponding monotherapies.[339] Based on its overall efficacy and safety profile, epiroprim has been recommended as a potentially less toxic alternative to pyrimethamine for the treatment of toxoplasmosis.[336]

22.3.3.11 Purine Analogs

Arprinocid, an anticoccidial agent, was described to be highly efficient in the treatment of acute infection caused by *T. gondii* (RH strain).[340] The therapy was successful even when initiated as late as 72 h postinfection with as little as 100 μg daily of the drug.

Arprinocid is known to be a specific and competitive inhibitor of the transmembrane transport of hypoxanthine[341] and its incorporation into nucleic acids. This mode of action may be associated with the observed activity of arprinocid against *T. gondii*. Perroto et al.[342] demonstrated that neither formate nor glycine (both purine precursors) were incorporated into the nucleic acids of extracellular *T. gondii*, thereby asserting the notion that this parasite is not capable of *de novo* synthesis of purines. To compensate, the protozoan utilized hypoxanthine salvage as a source of purines.[343] The report of Wang et al.[344] related to the ability of arprinocid to inhibit DHFR of *Eimeria tenella* (a coccidian parasite closely associated with *Toxoplasma*) is adding another dimension to its mechanism of action.

Arprinocid and its *in vivo* metabolite, arprinocid-*N*-oxide, suppressed the growth of *T. gondii* in human fibroblast cultures.[345] The corresponding IC_{50} values were 20.0 and 2.0 μg/ml. For both agents, the host cells were less sensitive than the parasite. Addition of hypoxanthine to the culture did not reverse the inhibitory activity of either drug. *In vivo* experiments in mice with acute toxoplasmosis (*T. gondii* RH strain) showed that arprinocid at a daily oral dose of 136 μg protected against death. A mutant of *T. gondii* was isolated and found to be resistant to arprinocid, thus leaving the possibility open that the biologically active form of the drug may, in fact, be its *N*-oxide metabolite.[345]

22.3.3.12 Histone Deacetylase Inhibitors

A novel cyclic tetrapeptide fungal metabolite, apicidin [cyclo(*N*,*O*-methyl-L-tryptophanyl-L-isoleucinyl-D-pipecolinyl-L-2-amino-8-oxodecanoyl)], isolated from *Fusarium* spp., has shown a potent and broad-spectrum antiprotozoal activity *in vitro* against Apicomplexan parasites (*Plasmodium*, *Cryptosporidium*, *Toxoplasma*).[346] The activity of apicidin appeared to be due to a low nanomolar inhibition of the Apicomplexan histone deacetylase, resulting in the hyperacetylation of histones in treated parasites. Since the acetylation-deacetylation of the ε-amino group of specific histone residues is required, the inhibition of histone deacetylation would interfere with the transcriptional regulation of eukaryotic cells, thereby making it a central factor in the transcriptional control in eukaryotic cells. It is believed that the 2-amino-8-oxodecanoic acid residue of the cyclic tetrapeptide molecule mimics the ε-aminoacetylated lysine residues of histone substrates, leading to potent reversible inhibition of histone deacetylase. Other related cyclic tetrapeptide histone deacetylase inhibitors (HC-toxin[347] and trichostatin[348]) have also been evaluated and found to exert antiparasitic activity. Thus, apicidin, apicidin A, HC-toxin, and trichostatin, all competed with [³H]apicidin A (chosen to be the radiolabeled ligand because it was an equipotent congener/analog of apicidin) binding with IC_{50} values in the 4.0- to 50-n*M* range.[346] These results suggested that the inhibition of parasitic histone deacetylase may represent an attractive new target for the design and development of novel anti-Apicomplexan agents.[346]

22.3.3.13 Miscellaneous Derivatives With Anti-*Toxoplasma* Activity

5-Fluorouracil (5-FU), a known anticancer agent, when applied at 40 mg/kg displayed good activity against experimental murine toxoplasmosis.[306] By measuring the incorporation of [³H]uracil into *Toxoplasma*-infected, differentiated L6E9 rat myocytes, Harris et al.[183] have found that 5-FU was effective even at 0.01 μg/ml. A combination of 0.01 μg/ml of 5-FU and pyrimethamine (0.1 μg/ml) was synergistic and as potent as high-dose pyrimethamine (1.0 μg/ml).[183] When tested *in vitro*, 5-FU was found to be effective against *Toxoplasma* even at a concentration of 0.01 μg/ml.[173]

In an enzyme immunoassay developed by Derouin and Chastang,[349] difluoromethylornithine (a potent inhibitor of ornithine decarboxylase) was ineffective against *T. gondii* at concentrations of ≥25 m*M*. Other antitoxoplasma agents that were tested in the same enzyme immunoassay included pyrimethamtine, sulfadoxine, and (2*R*,5*R*)-6-heptyne-2,5-diamine (another ornithine decarboxylase inhibitor). Their inhibitory concentrations were ≥0.05 μg/ml, 30.0 μg/ml, and 2.0 m*M*, respectively.[349] Previously, Hofflin et al.[350] found difluoromethylornithine to be inactive against *Toxoplasma* at concentrations of 20.0 m*M*. Harris et al.[183] also reported difluoromethylornithine inactive *in vitro*, and with no additive effect with either pyrimethamine or sulfadiazine.

Diclazuril, a benzeneacetonitrile derivative, has been found effective *in vitro* and against acute toxoplasmosis in mice, alone[351] and in combination with pyrimethamine.[352] When administered at 10 mg/kg beginning 6 d after inoculation and given for 10 d, diclazuril protected 90% of the mice over a 56-d observation period; at doses of 1.0 and 0.5 mg/kg, the drug was effective in only 20% and 0% of mice, respectively. Treatment with diclazuril (1.0 or 0.5 mg/kg) combined with pyrimethamine (12.5 mg/kg) led to survival of all animals at the 56-d observation period; if the same dosages of diclazuril (1.0 and 0.5 mg/kg) were combined with 6.0 mg/kg pyrimethamine, the survival rates at day 56 were 30% and 0%, respectively.

A number of fluoroquinolones (ciprofloxacin, fleroxacin, ofloxacin, temafloxacin, and trovafloxacin) have been examined for activity against toxoplasmosis. Only trovafloxacin markedly inhibited intracellular replication without significant toxicity to the host cells. In a murine model of acute toxoplasmosis, daily doses of 100 or 200 mg/kg of trovafloxacin given for 10 d protected 100% of infected mice against death; at daily doses of 50 mg/kg, the protection was 90%.[353]

Robenidine is a guanidine derivative known for its coccidiostatic activity in poultry. Bakhtari and Jira[354] have tested robenidine in mice chronically infected with the avirulent cyst-forming HF strain of *T. gondii*. The drug was applied alone (at doses of 50 and 100 mg/kg), and in combination with two other antiprotozoal agents, pyrimethamine and sulfadoxine (at doses of 2.5 and 250 mg/kg, respectively). None of the drugs tested (alone or in combinations) was able to produce any meaningful effect on cyst-stage toxoplasmosis.

An intraperitoneal combination of robenidine and lactotrim (in 1:1 ratio) was more effective against murine toxoplasmosis (ED_{50} = 20 mg/kg) than robenidine administered alone by the same route (ED_{50} = 55 mg/kg).[355] In the same model, the intraperitoneal ED_{50} values of lactotrim alone and in combination with sulfamethoxazole were 11.0 and 8.0 mg/kg, respectively;[355] the combination was synergistic since sulfamethoxazole alone was inactive.

The penetration of *T. gondii*, *Sarcocystis* spp., and *Besnotia jellisoni* into cultured cells was markedly reduced by 0.1 mg of quinine sulfate/ml in the inoculum medium.[356] Against *T. gondii* in particular, the penetration was blocked by as little as 0.01 mg/ml of the drug. The incubation of *Toxoplasma* on cells in medium containing quinine prior to inoculation of the parasite in quinine-free medium, did not significantly inhibit its penetration — the organisms remained motile in the presence of quinine, and the few that entered the cells stayed intracellular.[356] It is likely that quinine interfered by inhibiting some enzyme functions or by producing surface phenomena in the cultured cells which obstructed the sporozoite penetration.[357]

Ethanolic extract of propolis showed lethal activity against *T. gondii* in BALB/c mice.[358] Propolis is a resinous substance found in beehives which is collected by bees from buds.

A single subcutaneous injection of muramyl dipeptide (80 mg/kg) to CBA mice one day before infection with *T. gondii* tachyzoites enhanced their resistance significantly.[359] The mechanism of action of muramyl dipeptide was unclear since it failed to augment the production of cytolytic antibodies, and to activate the peritoneal macrophages as well.

Araujo and Slifer[360] have examined the interaction between drugs and the nonionic block copolymers CRL 8131 and CRL 8142 in the treatment of toxoplasmosis in murine models of the disease. The block copolymers when used alone caused only slight prolongation of time to death, but not survival. However, a significant increase in the survival rates was observed when mice were treated with either of the copolymers with doses of sulfadiazine, pyrimethamine, clindamycin, or atovaquone, which did not prevent mortality when used alone. For example, the combinations of CRL 8131 with sulfadiazine or pyrimethamine resulted in 50% and 40% survival rates, respectively. Also, treatment of CRL 8131 with a dose of clindamycin that protected 40% of the mice when used alone resulted in 100% survival. Furthermore, treatment of toxoplasmic encephalitis with CRL 8131 plus an ineffective dose of atovaquone also reduced inflammation and numbers of *T. gondii* cysts in the brain. In related experiments, studies on the drug-enhancing activity of CRL 8131 revealed that mice immunized with *Toxoplasma* lysate plus copolymer had their lymphocyte proliferation responses to *T. gondii* antigens substantially higher than those in mice immunized with lysate alone, and challenge of immunized mice with a lethal inoculum of *T. gondii* resulted in significant survival. Furthermore, administration of CRL 8131 alone appeared to provoke downregulation in the production of IFN-γ and upregulation in the production of IL-2, but no difference was noted in the production of tumor necrosis factor-α between mice treated with CRL 8131 and controls.[360]

Krahenbuhl et al.[361] have used poloxamers (nonionic block copolymers composed of a central hydrophobic chain of polyoxypropylene flanked by two hydrophylic chains of polyoxyethylene) to test their ability to alter the course of acute infection caused by a highly virulent *T. gondii* in mice. The effect varied substantially with the length of the constituent chains of the poloxamers. The most effective preparations were highly effective when administered after infection providing dose-dependent protection against 10 to 1000 LD_{100} doses of the pathogen. The observed protection was more effective after multiple treatments compared with a single treatment.

Tachibana et al.[362] examined the activity of stearylamine-bearing liposomes against *T. gondii* (RH strain). When tachyzoites were treated *in vitro* with liposomes consisting of 20 mol% stearylamine and 80 mol% phosphatidylcholine (130 μg/ml of total lipids), over 95% of the parasites were killed within 90 min. In *in vivo* experiments, intraperitoneal injection of 10 mg of 30 mol% stearylamine/70 mol% phosphatidylcholine-containing liposomes to mice shortly before or after *T. gondii* challenge, afforded protection from death for more than 30 d to 70% to 80% of the liposome-treated mice; by comparison, untreated animals succumbed within 9 d.[362]

A study was conducted to determine the effect of flunixin meglumine on the endocrinologic response (as monitored by the plasma levels of 15-ketodihydro-$PGE_{2\alpha}$, progesterone, and estrone sulfate) of pregnant ewes receiving constant medication with the drug (1.0 mg/kg intramuscularly, twice daily) following infection with *T. gondii*.[363] The medication was started 1 d prior to infection and lasted until the end of the gestation period. No early abortions (less than 10 d after infection) were seen in the infected group. Overall, the endocrinologic changes reflected the pathological changes in the uterus and fetuses. Flunixin meglumine neither completely inhibited prostaglandin release during abortion nor inhibited the physiological change of the hormone before parturition, even though it depressed the prostaglandin release before abortion or parturition and eliminated fever.[363]

Using electron microscopy, the ultrastructural features of the cortisone effects on the early development and formation of *T. gondii* tissue cysts were studied in the brains of experimental mice on days 8 to 47 postinoculation.[364]

Pettersen[365] has shown that the destruction of *T. gondii* by pepsin-hydrochloric acid solution was due to the acid rather than the enzyme, as previously thought.

Hamadto et al.[366] found that neither praziquantel nor levamisole had any effect on acute toxoplasmosis in mice.

Clotrimazole, an antifungal agent, when tested in mice for activity against the asexual stages of replication of *T. gondii* (trophozoites and tachyzoites) was found ineffective.[367] The drug was also inactive in *in vitro* assays.

Chao et al.[368] examined the effects of morphine addiction on the pathogenesis of murine toxoplasmosis.

22.3.3.14   Development of Drug Testing Methodologies

Mack and McLeod[369] developed a new microassay for *in vitro* evaluation of activity against *T. gondii*, in which the amounts of reagents, cells, and trophozoites necessary to quantitate the biological effect were reduced significantly.

Although there have been inherent differences between humans and animals that can reduce the relevance of data obtained experimentally, the currently available animal models have greatly contributed to our understanding about various aspects of the mechanism of action, efficacy, and the safety of anti-*Toxoplasma* drugs.[370] With the possible exception of rats, which are partially resistant, *Toxoplasma* infection can be readily produced in most laboratory animals.

According to the parasitic strain used, the resulting infection can be acute, subacute, or chronic, and may be monitored by either the survival of animals, the histopathologic examination of lesions, or by titration of parasites in infected tissues using subinoculation to mice or tissue culture. The latter procedure has proven very beneficial to describe the kinetics of infection in host tissues and to assess the efficacy of drugs according to their pharmacokinetics and tissue distribution.[370]

The currently available animal models for evaluation of congenital toxoplasmosis and chorioretinitis have not been completely satisfactory, mainly due to the marked differences between the mode of infection in humans and in animals. In this regard, experiments performed in primates, while providing useful insights for the management of congenital toxoplasmosis, have been of limited value in assessing ocular toxoplasmosis.[370]

The pathogenesis of toxoplasmic encephalitis is still not clearly understood, and of the currently available animal models, no one has proven adequate in producing focal encephalitic lesions as observed in immunocompromised patients. Direct inoculation of tachyzoites into brain tissue can induce focal encephalitis, but this model has been difficult to use for large-scale studies. To this end, Arribas et al.[371] have developed a new murine model of toxoplasmic encephalitis based on the intracerebral inoculation of tachyzoites of the highly virulent RH strain of *T. gondii*. The intracerebral infection resulted in 100% mortality rate on day 5. The disease course has been characterized by the formation of large inflammatory abscessed infiltrates by day 2, which expanded throughout the remaining period of observation. In addition, numerous tachyzoites were detectable in the brain parenchyma by the second day of infection.

Even though cellular immunity has been credited with the control of toxoplasmosis at the chronic stage, the administration of immunosuppressive drugs did not usually result in focal brain reactivation. The latter can only be produced using antibodies against CD8+ and CD4+ T lymphocytes or IFN-γ. The use of genetically immunodeficient animals, while presenting another alternative, has been of limited interest for pharmacologic research since infection of nude or T cell-depleted mice usually results in a dissemination of infection.[370]

22.3.4 MODE OF ACTION AND PHARMACOKINETICS OF SULFONAMIDES AND ANTIFOLATE DRUGS

At present, the most effective therapy for toxoplasmosis, and TE in particular, consists of combined treatment of sulfonamides and pyrimethamine (or trimethoprim).

The mode of action of sulfonamides involves blocking the formation by the parasite of dihydrofolic acid from *p*-aminobenzoic acid (PABA). Since humans do not synthesize dihydrofolate from PABA (but instead directly reduce dietary folic acid to dihydrofolate), they suffer no metabolic insult from the use of sulfonamides.[372] However, both man and parasites enzymatically reduce dihydrofolate to tetrahydrofolate with the help of the enzyme dihydrofolate reductase (DHFR). The ultimate product of this conversion is folinic acid, a metabolically active form of folate.

Pyrimethamine and trimethoprim both inhibit the activity of DHFR and consequently abolish the production of tetrahydrofolate and folinic acid.[373] The beneficial effect of these drugs resides in their greater selectivity for the protozoan dihydrofolate reductase as opposed to that of the host. While trimethoprim is a powerful and specific inhibitor of bacterial DHFR, pyrimethamine is more specific for protozoa (*T. gondii*, *Plasmodium*).[374] Various combinations of pyrimethamine (or trimethoprim) and sulfonamides (or trisulfapyrimidines) were found to act synergistically in blocking the folic acid metabolism of replicating tachyzoites of *T. gondii*. Unfortunately, the cyst form of the protozoan remains very often unaffected and may rupture and reinitiate the process, thus contributing to the high incidence of relapses following discontinuation of chemotherapy.

Relapses are common in AIDS patients,[48,54,55,375] where the recurrence rate may reach as high as 80% of all patients.[44]

In general, sulfonamides are administered orally at a daily dosage of 75 mg divided in four equal doses.[372] Trisulfapyrimidines are the preferred form of sulfonamides. Determination of serum sulfonamide levels is necessary in order to assure the presence of adequate therapeutic levels of 12 to 15 mg/100 ml.[372] Excessive blood levels of sulfonamides may interfere with the fungicidal (and to a lesser extent, bactericidal) properties of the polymorphonuclear leukocytes by virtue of suppressing the myeloperoxidase-mediated pathways of the leukocytes. Such high drug levels are common, for example, in patients with renal dysfunctions.[376] The importance of any such leukocyte defect, of course, is much greater in immunodeficient hosts.

Pyrimethamine is given orally at 0.5 mg/kg daily in two divided doses; the dose, however, may be doubled in the first 2 to 3 d of treatment.[372] Used in this way, pyrimethamine would normally produce stable serum levels of about 0.5 µg/ml. Since less than 4% of the drug is excreted daily in the urine, serum levels may be present for several weeks after treatment has been terminated.[372] In the body, pyrimethamine is highly bound to proteins (87%), is lipophilic and has a half-life of 35 to 175 h; the drug appears to be cleared by hepatic metabolism.[377]

Weiss et al.[378] have examined the serum and cerebrospinal fluid (CSF) concentrations of pyrimethamine in AIDS patients with acute TE who have been receiving continuous daily treatment of the drug. Results have shown a partition coefficient for CSF/serum levels between 0.127 and 0.265 (12.7% to 26.5% of serum levels in CSF). In general, serum levels of >750 ng/ml in the presence of sulfonamides and >3000 ng/ml when pyrimethamine is used alone, may be necessary to successfully manage acute cerebral toxoplasmosis.[378] Luft and Remington[44] reported that after oral administration of 50 mg of pyrimethamine to patients with meningeal leukemia its plasma level reached 0.3 µg/ml with the CSF concentration being about 10 to 25% of that found in the serum.

In a number of reports,[379-382] the presence of panmyelopathy and pancytopenia has been attributed to pyrimethamine medication. In view of such findings, it is important that the peripheral blood count of patients be closely monitored — in the event of leukopenia (<1000 neutrophils/mm³) or a fall in platelets (<100,000/mm³), the chemotherapy should be stopped and intramuscular folinic acid initiated.[383,384] The toxicity may also be circumvented through a prophylactic use of intramuscular folinic acid (or calcium leucovorin) at a daily dose of 10 mg without interfering with the treatment of toxoplasmosis.[385] Since the therapy of TE in AIDS patients is a life-long treatment, the bone marrow toxicity of the pyrimethamine–sulfonamide regimen may preclude other therapies with antiviral drugs (such as azidothymidine) which are also known to exert bone marrow toxicity.

An isocratic high-performance liquid chromatography (HPLC) method to measure pyrimethamine extracted from plasma of infants has been reported; the measurement required lower volumes of plasma (100 µl) and showed increased sensitivity to pyrimethamine at 210 nm.[386] Roberts et al.[387] have developed two new assays for pyrimethamine analysis: an enzyme inhibition assay that can be run on an automated analyzer, and an improved HPLC method — the calibration range of both assays was 100 to 3000 µg/l.

22.3.5 Evolution of Therapies and Treatment of Toxoplasmosis

Current therapeutic strategies and future prospects for the treatment of congenital and acquired toxoplasmosis have been extensively reviewed.[388-393] One of the major problems confronting the development of successful anti-*Toxoplasma* agents has been the ability of the parasite to differentiate from the actively growing tachyzoite form, which is susceptible to drug action, into the chronic, almost latent bradyzoite state, which is not susceptible and, therefore, cannot be eradicated by any of the currently known antitoxoplasmic agents. Because the bradyzoites remain as a source of recrudescing infection, drug therapy must be maintained for the life of the patient.

The molecular signals and mechanism(s) involved in the tachyzoite-bradyzoite interconversion are not known.[75] Blocking this differentiation process would be a major breakthrough in the cure of toxoplasmosis by preventing reactivation of the latent forms, and thereby attenuating disease. Similarly, stimulating bradyzoites to differentiate back to the drug-sensitive tachyzoites would facilitate chemotherapy that may completely clear the body of the protozoan (see Sections 22.3.1.1 and 22.3.3.8).[75]

Therapy of congenital toxoplasmosis, in general, is based on spiramycin, which is capable of achieving high concentrations in the placenta; if the fetus is uninfected, pyrimethamine and sulfonamides are administered after the fourth month of pregnancy.[23] Lambotte[394] has found prenatal therapy of congenital toxoplasmosis to be beneficial in reducing the frequency of infant infection. Various options for prevention of ocular toxoplasmosis associated with congenital toxoplasmosis were discussed by Bloch-Michel.[395]

For primary therapy of toxoplasmosis in immunocompromised patients, in severe cases of the disease, and in congenital toxoplasmosis, treatment with a synergistic combination of pyrimethamine and sulfonamide (e.g., co-trimoxazole) has been widespread.[396]

Spiramycin, alone or in combination with pyrimethamine–sulfonamide, is used often in pregnant women with acute infection to prevent congenital toxoplasmosis.[389]

Clindamycin is utilized frequently for the management of acute flares of toxoplasmic chorioretinitis and as second-line therapy for toxoplasmic encephalitis in AIDS patients.[51,389] Holliman[397] discussed the effect of folate supplements in the therapy of cerebral toxoplasmosis, while Grange et al.[398] have surveyed the therapy of *T. gondii*-induced myocarditis in AIDS patients.

Immunomodulating drugs such as IFN-γ, alone or in combination with roxithromycin, were found effective in murine models of toxoplasmosis; interleukin-2 was also found to be effective in a murine model.[389]

When treating toxoplasmosis in immunocompromised patients, it is important to take into consideration the tendency of such patients to develop simultaneously other opportunistic diseases, such as cytomegalovirus infection and *Pneumocystis carinii* pneumonia.[372] If it occurs, the management of such conditions would, undoubtedly, be very difficult. In this regard, gross alterations of the host microbial flora, as a result of excessive antimicrobial medication and unduly prolonged treatment, must be avoided in order to prevent undesired superinfections.

In evaluating the antitoxoplasmic potency of drugs, Piketty et al.[399] recommended *in vivo* quantitation of parasites in the blood, lungs, and the brain of infected mice. At various intervals after infection, subcultures of serial dilutions of blood, lung, and brain homogenates were performed in fibroblast tissue cultures for determination of parasitic loads. Using this technique, the therapeutic potencies of pyrimethamine (18.5 mg/kg daily), sulfadiazine (375 mg/kg daily), and clindamycin (300 mg/kg daily), administered for 10 d (from day 1 or day 4 after infection), were assessed.

22.3.5.1   Pyrimethamine–Sulfonamide Combinations

Leport et al.[55] have treated 35 AIDS patients with TE with a combination of pyrimethamine–sulfadiazine over a 30-month period. The initial use of a higher daily dose of pyrimethamine (50 to 100 mg instead of the conventional 25-mg dose) was justified because of the poor prognosis of cerebral toxoplasmosis. In spite of the higher dose regimen, only 2 of the patients experienced hematologic toxicity that warranted discontinuation of pyrimethamine therapy, while 31 patients showed improvement. Furthermore, of the 24 patients who were evaluable for long-term therapy, 14 (58%) achieved complete resolution and 10 had late clinical and/or computed tomographic scan sequelae. Reintroduction of the combination therapy resulted in complete resolution of relapse in 8 of 10 cases.[55] Gonzalez-Clemente et al.[400] have also recommended the use of combination pyrimethamine–sulfadiazine for 3 to 6 weeks to treat acute episodes of toxoplasmic encephalitis.

Holliman[401] reported satisfactory response to sulfonamide–pyrimethamine medication of 20 AIDS patients with toxoplasmosis, although a high incidence of toxicity was present. Wanke et al.[54] found that 11 of 13 AIDS patients with CNS toxoplasmosis receiving pyrimethamine–sulfadiazine combination showed clinical and radiologic improvement; toxic side effects included neutropenia, fever, and rash. Autopsies performed in five patients revealed evidence of *T. gondii*.[54] In one report,[402] treatment of AIDS patients having toxoplasmosis with pyrimethamine–sulfadiazine was found to produce complications in 29%, and serious complications in 8% of treated cases.

There is lack of evidence to suggest that treatment with pyrimethamine prevented relapse of toxoplasmic encephalitis to occur. In this regard, cerebral toxoplasmosis resistant to pyrimethamine–sulfadiazine (1.0 g and 25 mg, respectively, four times daily) has been reported in AIDS patients.[403,404]

Contrary to previous reports,[405] which described successful therapy of cerebral toxoplasmosis using pyrimethamine and clindamycin in place of sulfadiazine (see Section 22.3.5.3.2), Bell et al.[406] observed progression of cerebral lesions in one patient receiving the pyrimethamine–clindamycin combination. It was this latter finding that necessitated sulfadiazine desensitization as a useful alternative. The sulfadiazine desensitization was carried out in three AIDS patients with cerebral toxoplasmosis and prior severe sulfonamide reactions (diffused maculopapular rash).[406] The achieved maximum tolerated daily doses were 2.0 g of the drug in one patient and 4.0 g for the remaining two patients. Side effects comprised transient fever, mild pruritis, and hyperglycemia (presumably exacerbated by the steroid given before desensitization).[406] Tenant-Flowers et al.[407] conducted a study to assess the efficacy of a sulfadiazine desensitization protocol to treat patients with AIDS and cerebral toxoplasmosis and known sulfonamide allergy, and to ensure that an adequate dose of sulfadiazine (2.0 to 4.0 g daily) was achieved rapidly (within 4 to 5 d). Moreover, the effect of concurrent corticosteroid therapy on the success rate of the sulfadiazine regimen was also evaluated. The proposed desensitization protocol employed the oral administration of gradually increasing increments of sulfadiazine every 3 h over a 5-d period. The overall success rate of desensitization was reported to be 62%; seven patients achieved a final dose of 4.0 g daily, and for three patients the dose was 2.0 g daily. The concurrent corticosteroid administration did not appear to affect the outcome in the number of patients studied (total of 16).[407] Gilquin et al.[408] have also described an efficient protocol to induce tolerance towards sulfadiazine in an AIDS patient using betamethasone and dexchlorpheniramine.

Leport et al.[409] have assessed results from potential interactions of multiple drug regimens (pyrimethamine–clindamycin, pyrimethamine–sulfadiazine, and pyrimethamine alone) administered to 35 AIDS patients receiving maintenance therapy for toxoplasmosis. Adverse side effects were associated with pyrimethamine in 10 cases, to clindamycin in 7, and to sulfadiazine in 8 patients.[409] Pedrol et al.[410] concluded that an intermittent (2 d per week) maintenance therapy for CNS toxoplasmosis with pyrimethamine–sulfadiazine combination was effective in preventing relapses in AIDS patients, although prospective randomized studies still remain to be done. The application of low-dose alternate-day pyrimethamine medication as a maintenance therapy for cerebral toxoplasmosis in AIDS was also discussed.[411]

A Swiss HIV cohort study[412] had the objective of determining whether a long-term maintenance therapy for cerebral toxoplasmosis may be protective also against *Pneumocystis carinii* pneumonia in patients with AIDS. The medication applied consisted of either pyrimethamine–sulfonamides (in 50% of patients), pyrimethamine–clindamycin (in 25%), or pyrimethamine alone (in 9% of patients). Overall, patients with cerebral toxoplasmosis showed a low risk of subsequently developing *P. carinii* pneumonia, most likely due to the chronic suppressive effects of pyrimethamine and sulfonamides.

Twelve patients with toxoplasmic chorioretinitis were treated with fansidar (pyrimethamine and sulfadoxine at 25 and 500 mg/kg, respectively), starting with a loading dose of two tablets of fansidar, followed by one tablet daily; prednisone (0.5 mg/kg daily) was added and gradually tapered off. The duration of treatment was 21 to 50 d (median, 28 d). In 83% of patients, the scar was considerably smaller than the original lesion (on average 25% of original lesion), with no side effects observed.[413]

A case of severe dermatomyositis in association with high serum *Toxoplasma* antibody titers responded to treatment with pyrimethamine and sulfadiazine.[414]

In utero treatment of congenital toxoplasmosis with pyrimethamine–sulfadiazine has also been reported.[415,416] Mothers in 52 cases of toxoplasmic fetopathy (group 1) were treated *in utero* with combination of pyrimethamine and sulfadiazine (or sulfisoxazole), and with spiramycin.[416] The results were compared with those obtained from 51 other infants with congenital toxoplasmosis whose mothers (group 2) had received spiramycin alone. Furthermore, patients of both groups received the same medication of pyrimethamine–sulfadiazine and spiramycin after birth. Parasitologic examination of the placenta was positive in 42% for group 1, and 76.6% for group 2, while specific IgM titers in newborns were detected in 17.4% and 69.2% of cases, respectively; these findings indicated that prenatal treatment with pyrimethamine–sulfonamides resulted in less progressive infection at birth.[416] The limitations of prenatal therapy of congenital toxoplasmosis with pyrimethamine–sulfadiazine combination[417] and its passage through the placenta[418] have also been explored.

Cottrell[419] has described the successful treatment of a 4-year-old child with acquired toxoplasmic encephalitis using a combination of pyrimethamine and sulfamidine for a period of 6 months. Acquired toxoplasmic encephalitis in children, although not common, was first reported in 1941.[420]

One case of toxoplasmosis complicated with myeloblastic leukemia was treated with pyrimethamine (50 mg daily) and sulfadimidine (1.0 g, three times daily); the therapy against myeloblastic anemia was started prior to that and consisted of cytosine arabinoside and daunorubicine.[421] After 2.5 weeks of treatment (and still with leukemia in no relapse), the patient suffered profound thrombocytopenia and neutropenia (due to bone marrow aplasia) from which the patient did not recover. The fatal outcome was attributed to the cumulative effect of antileukemia drugs and the combination pyrimethamine–sulfadimidine.[421] Commenting on this case, Price et al.[422] strongly suggested that pyrimethamine not only acted, as expected, as antagonist to dihydrofolate reductase, but also destroyed both normal and malignant stem cells during the DNA synthesis *S*-phase of the cell cycle. It is believed that prolonged administration of *S*-phase-active drugs will draw normal marrow stem cells out of their resting stage (G_0) and into the reproductive cycle. Such action will abolish the selective advantage of normal stem cells over malignant cells in response to chemotherapeutic drugs, thereby allowing the normally resting marrow cells to become vulnerable to antitumor agents (such as cytosine arabinoside and daunomycin) as they are being drawn into the cell cycle.[423-425]

Studying the mechanism of increased serum creatinine levels after administration of pyrimethamine and dapsone in healthy volunteers and HIV-infected patients, Opravil et al.[426] found that pyrimethamine inhibited the renal secretion of creatinine by what appeared to be a reversible inhibition of the renal tubular secretion of creatinine without affecting the glomerular filtration rate.

22.3.5.1.1 Acute renal failure to sulfadiazine therapy in AIDS patients

Acute renal failure due to crystal deposition of sulfadiazine in the urinary tract should be of growing concern if appropriate prophylactic measures have not been taken promptly.[427-439]

Carbone et al.[440] have observed the presence of sulfadiazine-associated obstructive nephropathy in one patient with AIDS. According to Becker et al.,[430] due to the high prevalence of potential risk factors, the incidence of sulfadiazine-associated renal impariment was 1.9% to 7.5% in patients with AIDS, compared with 1% to 4% in HIV-seronegative controls. Furthermore, its occurrence appeared to be delayed in HIV-infected individuals with a median of 3 weeks of medication compared with about 10 d in HIV-negative subjects; in conformance, the cumulative sulfadiazine dose at time of manifestation has doubled in AIDS patients (median of 84 g vs. 40 g in controls).

Molina et al.[441] reported four cases of AIDS patients with toxoplasmic encephalitis who developed sulfadiazine-induced crystalluria after receiving a combination of sulfadiazine and pyrimethamine. The crystalluria can be rapidly reversed by rehydration and urine alkalinization.[430,434,441,442] It was recommended that after high doses of sulfadiazine, patients be adequately hydrated and their urinary pH maintained above 7.5.[441] Diaz et al.[428] treated an AIDS patient with sulfadiazine-induced urolithiasis acute renal failure (acute lumbar pain, dysuria, urinary frequency, and hematuria) with intravenous fluids and alkalinization of the urine.

22.3.5.1.2 Adverse cutaneous reactions to pyrimethamine combinations in AIDS patients

The value of various clinical and laboratory parameters in predicting the occurrence of skin reactions in AIDS patients with toxoplasmic encephalitis induced by pyrimethamine combinations with either sulfadiazine or clindamycin, and the effects of continued therapy for patients with these reactions, have been studied retrospectively by Caumes et al.[443] Seventy-five percent of patients (18 of 25) treated with pyrimethamine–sulfadiazine developed cutaneous reactions after a mean of 11 d, whereas 58% (15 of 26) of patients who received pyrimethamine–clindamycin had cutaneous reactions after a mean of 13 d ($p = .56$). Nine (50%) of the 18 patients continued to receive pyrimethamine–sulfadiazine throughout the duration of hypersensitivity, compared with all 15 patients who were treated with pyrimethamine–clindamycin ($p = .002$). Thus, treatment throughout the duration of hypersensitivity is more likely to succeed for patients receiving the pyrimethamine–clindamycin combination, whereas therapy with pyrimetamine–sulfadiazine has been associated with more pronounced cutaneous side effects and a high risk of developing Lyell's syndrome and Stevens-Johnson syndrome.[443]

22.3.5.2 Trimethoprim–Sulfonamide Combinations

In patients with toxoplasmosis, therapy with trimethoprim (160 mg) and sulfamethoxazole (800 mg) daily for 10 d, resulted in a significant remission of symptoms.[444] Norrby et al.[205] treated five patients with lymphadenopathy due to toxoplasmosis with good therapeutic results by using co-trimoxazole for a period of 4 weeks. No adverse effects on the bone marrow were observed during a 3-month trial; however, a transient stomatitis was present, as well as allergic exanthema.[205] In another study, Norrby and Eilard[445] described one case of recurrent toxoplasmosis that required repeated (on three different occasions) treatment with co-trimoxazole. This and other reports[195,446] of recurrent toxoplasmosis (which seemed to be independent of the type of drug combination therapy), would necessitate the need for long-term monitoring of patients, especially in those cases where an immune deficiency is present (or might be developed) resulting in increased virulence of the *Toxoplasma* pathogen.

Williams and Savage[447] have described as dramatic the recovery of a child with generalized toxoplasmosis following therapy with co-trimoxazole (400 mg sulfamethoxazole and 80 mg trimethoprim, twice daily for 1 month). This result led to the recommendation that co-trimoxazole be used as the treatment of choice for acquired toxoplasmosis, especially in immunocompromised patients and cases of congenital toxoplasmosis. However, the recommendation of Williams and Savage[447] has been seriously questioned by Remington.[448]

Esposito et al.[449] described the use of co-trimoxazole in the management of cerebral encephalitis in AIDS patients showing severe hematologic damage caused by pyrimethamine and concurrent zidovudine therapy — the lesions completely resolved after 3 weeks of therapy. Solbreux et al.[450] conducted a retrospective study on the use of co-trimoxazole as diagnostic support and treatment of suspected cerebral toxoplasmosis in AIDS patients. The drug was reported to be effective, as evidenced by the improved clinical and radiological status. However, further prospective randomized therapeutic trials seem to be in order to confirm these observations.

Data by Jick[451] demonstrated that of 1121 hospitalized patients receiving trimethoprim–sulfamethoxazole, only 91 (8%) experienced side effects attributed to this combination; the most common adverse reactions were gastrointestinal upset (nausea, vomiting, anorexia, and diarrhea, 3.9%) and skin reactions (erythema, urticaria, and itch, 3.3%).

22.3.5.3   Antibiotic Therapy of Toxoplasmosis

22.3.5.3.1   Spiramycin

Over the years, spiramycin has been used extensively in the treatment of human congenital toxoplasmosis.[218,236,452-455] Fetuses infected with *T. gondii* often developed impaired vision or neurologic disorders, even after 5 years post-partum.[456] The risk of congenital infections due to acute toxoplasmosis acquired during the first trimester of pregnancy has been estimated at 15%.[236] Although such a risk is usually higher during the second (30%) and third (60%) trimesters, only acute toxoplasmosis acquired in the first trimester has been associated with severe congenital infections.[236] Alternating 3 weeks of therapy with oral spiramycin with 2 weeks of no treatment, resulted in a diminished incidence of congenital toxoplasmosis from 17% to 5%,[253] or from 61% to 23%.[218]

Hohfeld et al.[457] reported their experience in treating 98 cases of fetal *Toxoplasma* infection with spiramycin during pregnancy. Of the 52 pregnancies allowed to proceed, 43 were treated additionally with pyrimethamine and sulfonamides. After a mean follow-up period of 19 months, 41 infants showed evidence of subclinical toxoplasmosis. The therapeutic efficacy of the additional treatment with pyrimethamine and sulfonamides was evidenced by a marked reduction of severe congenital toxoplasmosis and the relative decrease in the ratio of benign to subclinical forms.[457]

In a clinical trial involving 67 patients, Chodos and Habegger-Chodos[458] described spiramycin as effective in treating posterior uveitis caused by *Toxoplasma*. However, Fajardo et al.[459] found that in 87 patients with posterior uveitis, therapy with combination pyrimethamine–sulfadiazine was superior to that of spiramycin (and/or steroids). In two other studies,[460,461] spiramycin was reported to be ineffective in treating toxoplasmic uveitis.

Timsit and Bloch-Michel[462] have studied 54 patients with active toxoplasmic chorioretinitis and found the therapy with pyrimethamine–sulfadiazine to be statistically more effective than a corresponding treatment with systemic steroids either given alone or in combination with spiramycin.

As reported by Descotes et al.,[463] there has been little serious toxicity associated with spiramycin. Contrary to other macrolide antibiotics, spiramycin was not damaging to the liver. It caused mild gastrointestinal disturbance, and allergic reactions were confined to transient skin eruptions.[463] Ostlere et al.[464] reported the development of allergy towards spiramycin during prophylactic treatment of fetal toxoplasmosis.

Kawakami et al.[465] have described a case of dermatomyositis in a patient with toxoplasmosis, which was successfully cured with prednisolone for the dermatomyositis and acetylspiramycin for toxoplasmosis. Facial erythema and cervical lymphadenopathy preceded myalgia and muscle weakness of the extremities.

22.3.5.3.2   Clindamycin and clindamycin–pyrimethamine combinations

Burke and Mills[284] described one case of acute toxoplasmic lymphadenitis treated with 600 mg daily of oral clindamycin. The therapy was continued for 28 d, after which the patient was apyrexial and clinically well.

Dannemann et al.[466] have used clindamycin with promising results to treat 15 AIDS patients with toxoplasmic encephalitis[467,468] as part of either primary or alternative therapy. Eleven of the patients responded by clinical or radiologic improvement after receiving the antibiotic either alone or in combination with pyrimethamine. Twelve patients continued to receive oral clindamycin as suppressive therapy on an outpatient basis. The adverse reactions of clindamycin were mainly diarrhea, reversible granulocytopenia, and skin reaction.[466] Westblom and Belshe[469] described as successful the treatment of cerebral toxoplasmosis in one AIDS patient using a combination of intravenous clindamycin (600 mg, every 6 h) and pyrimethamine (25 mg daily) for 37 d. There was clinical improvement and complete resolution of CAT scan abnormalities.

One side effect often associated with the use of clindamycin (as much as 80% of recorded cases) has been the development of colitis of the pseudomembranous type.[470] Marcos et al.[471] have provided a protocol for clindamycin desensitization in an AIDS patient.

Rolston[472,473] reported treatment of four AIDS patients with clindamycin (1200 to 1800 mg daily) and pyrimethamine (25 mg daily) — only oral clindamycin was used in the initial therapy (in an earlier study, Podzamczer and Gudiol[286] used the antibiotic intravenously). Three of four patients who responded to the initial 8-week regimen also remained symptom-free through a maintenance therapy with oral clindamycin (600 mg daily) and pyrimethamine (25 mg daily), three times weekly for a period of 6 to 8 months.[472] Previously, Kaplan et al.[287] recommended a dose regimen of 3600 mg clindamycin daily, whereas Rolston and Hoy[285] applied 1200 to 2400 mg of the drug daily to treat three AIDS patients with TE.

Ruf and Pohle[474] have found that in the treatment of AIDS patients with cerebral toxoplasmosis, combination regimens consisting of pyrimethamine, clindamycin, and spiramycin, and pyrimethamine–clindamycin proved to be equally effective, and that the addition of spiramycin did not provide additional benefit. Myelosuppressive side effects due to pyrimethamine prevented the addition of folinic acid at the start of the antitoxoplasmic therapy.

Dannemann et al.[475] reported interim results from an ongoing large-scale, prospective, randomized study to determine the potential role of clindamycin in the management of toxoplasmic encephalitis. Data were presented on 33 patients, 15 of whom received oral pyrimethamine and clindamycin (intravenously, then orally), and 18 of whom received pyrimethamine and sulfadiazine (both drugs given orally). The interim evaluation did not reveal any significant differences between the two regimens in the clinical and radiologic response. Both regimens caused similar adverse side effects; however, patients on pyrimethamine–clindamycin medication had more pronounced gastrointestinal side effects and more adverse hematologic reactions than those receiving pyrimethamine–sulfadiazine.[475] In a further report by Dannemann et al.,[476] a randomized unblinded phase II, multicenter clinical trial was conducted in California to compare the therapeutic efficacy of a combination of pyrimethamine and clindamycin to that of pyrimethamine and sulfadiazine. The study allowed for crossover in the event of failure or intolerance of the assigned regimen. The patients were treated for 6 weeks with pyrimethamine and folinic acid plus either sulfadiazine or clindamycin (the latter injected intravenously during the first 3 weeks). The results of several end points for efficacy, when taken together, indicated that the relative efficacies of clindamycin and sulfadiazine appeared to be approximately the same. Hence, the use of clindamycin should be considered as an acceptable alternative to sulfadiazine in patients unable to tolerate sulfadiazine.[476]

Through the European Network for the Treatment of AIDS, a multicenter trial was conducted to compare, again, the potency and safety of pyrimethamine (50 mg daily)-clindamycin (2.4 mg daily) and pyrimethamine (50 mg daily)–sulfadiazine (4.0 mg daily) for treatment and maintenance therapy of toxoplasmic encephalitis.[477] The preliminary results have demonstrated that 77% of the 148 patients evaluated responded completely or showed improvement with minor sequelae during therapy; 20% of the patients deteriorated. The adverse side effects consisted primarily of rash (52 patients), fever (31 patients), diarrhea (17 patients), and nausea (12 patients).

Fourteen AIDS patients with toxoplasmic encephalitis who were not treated with the standard regimen of pyrimethamine and sulfonamide because of previous history of bone marrow suppression and severe allergic reactions to sulfonamide, were given instead pyrimethamine–clindamycin combination (both drugs were administered orally).[478] The therapy comprised of pyrimethamine (first, a 100-mg loading dose, followed by 50 mg daily) and clindamycin (600 to 900 mg every

8 h); the duration of treatment was between 6 and 8 weeks. All patients received oral folinic acid (15 mg daily). Complete or partial response was evident in all 14 patients at the end of 2 months of primary therapy (10 of 14 patients showed complete resolution of clinical signs, and 8 of 14 patients showed complete resolution of neuroradiologic signs). All patients continued on a maintenance therapy of 25 mg daily of pyrimethamine, and 300 mg (every 6 h) or 450 mg (every 8 h) of clindamycin. Although no relapses were observed, symptoms that did not resolve at the end of the 2-month period of acute therapy tended to remain unchanged.[478]

Leport et al.[479] have also conducted an open study in AIDS patients with brain toxoplasmosis using pyrimethamine–clindamycin combination. Cohn et al.[480] reported no difference in the survival of AIDS patients with toxoplasmic encephalitis who were treated continuously with either pyrimethamine–sulfadiazine or pyrimethamine–clindamycin (median therapy of 311 and 422 d, respectively; $p = .25$).

A combination of 5-fluorouracil and clindamycin was also used to treat a case of cerebral toxoplasmosis in AIDS.[481]

22.3.5.3.3   Clarithromycin

Clarithromycin (1.5 to 2.0 g) combined with pyrimethamine (25 mg) was used successfully (regression of neurologic signs and encephalitic abnormalities) to treat cerebral toxoplasmosis in two AIDS patients.[482] The use of clarithromycin–pyrimethamine was suggested as an alternative treatment of toxoplasmosis in AIDS patients who cannot receive or tolerate sulfonamides.

The role of clarithromycin–minocycline combination treatment[483] and in maintenance[484] therapies of toxoplasmosis in AIDS patients was also examined.

Alba et al.[485] have also discussed the use of clarithromycin for the treatment of cerebral toxoplasmosis associated with HIV infection.

22.3.5.3.4   Azithromycin

A prospective study was conducted to evaluate azithromycin in combination with pyrimethamine for treatment of acute toxoplasmic encephalitis in AIDS patients.[486] Fourteen patients were given 75 mg of pyrimethamine and 500 mg azithromycin daily for 4 weeks. Of the eight patients who were evaluable for clinical response, five responded favorably, one had an intermediate response, and two patients did not respond. Based on the adverse effects observed (rash, abnormal liver function, vomiting, and hypoacousia), it seemed that the azithromycin dosage used in the combination was not optimal.

Godofsky[487] has also described the use of azithromycin in the treatment of cerebral toxoplasmosis.

22.3.5.3.5   Doxycycline

Two reports of treating cerebral toxoplasmosis with a combination of doxycycline and pyrimethamine have appeared.[488,489] Clinical improvement was described in a patient with AIDS and toxoplasmic encephalitis after daily treatment with doxycycline (400 mg) and pyrimethamine (25 mg) — CAT scanning of the brain showed complete resolution of two ring-enhanced lesions within 5 weeks of therapy.[489]

22.3.5.4   Atovaquone

So far, atovaquone has been studied in small numbers of patients (n = 5 to 24) with cerebral toxoplasmosis who were mostly unresponsive to conventional chemotherapy.[490-493] At doses of 750 mg, four times daily, atovaquone produced a complete or partial radiologic response in 37% to 87.5% of patients. In the largest trial involving 87 patients (results not published yet), after 6 weeks of treatment, 35% of the patients had a partial clinical response and 12% had the disease stabilized, although the mortality rate associated with the disease reached 40%, 18 weeks after initiation of therapy.[313]

Bouboulis et al.[494] used atovaquone to resolve successfully cerebral toxoplasmic lesions in a child and in an adult HIV-positive patient who failed to respond to conventional therapy with high-dose (3.0 mg/kg daily) pyrimethamine, as well as clindamycin and azithromycin. A rapid oral desensitization was initiated in the adult patient because of maculopapular rash developed during the attempted treatment with pyrimethamine.

Schimkat et al.[495] have described the successful treatment of bifocal ocular toxoplasmosis in an AIDS patient using 750 mg, t.i.d. of the drug — the infiltrates healed within 8 d, leaving retinochoroidal scars. During maintenance therapy (atovaquone at 750 mg, three times daily) two relapses occurred, but were successfully treated by increasing the dosage of atovaquone to 750 mg, four times daily, and the addition of trimethoprim–sulfamethoxazole and clindamycin–pyrimethamine, respectively.

Durand et al.[496] reported a treatment failure of atovaquone in one patient with cerebral toxoplamosis.

In an uncontrolled open-label study, Katlama et al.[497] have evaluated the efficacy and tolerance of atovaquone as a long-term maintenance therapy in patients with toxoplasmic encephalitis and intolerant to conventional anti-*Toxoplasma* drugs. The patients, who received 750 mg, four times daily, of the drug were followed up for a mean period of 1 year. While 17 patients (26%) experienced a toxoplasmic encephalitis relapse, the survival probability was 70% at 1 year after the episode of TE. The overall results suggested that atovaquone has been a well-tolerated and effective maintenance therapy in patients who were intolerant to conventional anti-*Toxoplasma* drugs.

22.3.5.5 Trimetrexate

The therapeutic efficacy of trimetrexate has been evaluated in nine sulfonamide-intolerant AIDS patients with biopsy-proven cerebral toxoplasmosis.[498] The patients received trimetrexate (30 to 280 mg/m² daily) plus leucovorin (20 to 90 mg/m², every 6 h) for 28 to 149 d. Radiographic responses were documented in eight patients, and clinical responses in five patients. Despite the improvement, however, all patients showed both clinical and radiographic deterioration within 12 to 109 d of their initial improvement. The activity of trimetrexate administered alone, although dramatic in sulfonamide-intolerant patients, has been transient in nature, thereby making this drug inappropriate as a single-agent therapy for AIDS-associated toxoplasmosis.[498]

22.3.5.6 Prophylaxis of Cerebral Toxoplasmosis

In a comparative study to evaluate the efficacy and safety of three regimens for primary prophylaxis of toxoplasmic encephalitis, Antinori et al.[499] have found co-trimoxazole (160 mg trimethoprim and 800 mg sulfamethoxazole every other day) significantly reducing the risk of TE. The combination dapsone–pyrimethamine (100 mg weekly dapsone and 25 mg biweekly pyrimethamine) was equally effective, whereas aerosolized pentamidine (300 mg monthly) was efficacious only against *Pneumocystis carinii* pneumonia. A similar finding was also reported by Nielsen et al.[500]

Klinker et al.[501] have used pyrimethamine alone (50 mg daily) as prophylaxis for toxoplasmic encephalitis in 56 patients with advanced HIV infection (38 patients with CD4+ counts of ≤200 cells/µl) and presence of serum IgG antibodies to *T. gondii*. All patients received folinic acid (7.5 mg daily) as supplement. During prophylaxis (697 months; mean, 12.5 ± 12.1) only one patient developed TE, and four patients had their treatment discontinued because of adverse side effects.

However, based on the results of a randomized trial in patients with advanced AIDS disease (absolute CD4+ counts of <200 cells/µl) who had been treated with trimethoprim–sulfamethoxazole for toxoplasmic encephalitis, additional prophylaxis for TE with pyrimethamine appeared unnecessary.[502] Still, Van Delden et al.[503] have attributed the continuing occurrence of toxoplasmic encephalitis among AIDS patients to the lack of prophylaxis — according to data obtained from a Swiss HIV cohort study, at least one half of the cases of TE could have been prevented with a combination of prophylaxis, better motivation of physician, and increased compliance of patients.

22.3.5.7 Management of Ocular Toxoplasmosis

The frequency of ocular toxoplasmosis in AIDS patients has been on the increase.[504] As reported by Chakroun et al.,[505] the incidence rose from 3.3% in 1983, to 6.1% in 1988, and 5.9% during the first trimester of 1989.

Blanc-Jouvan et al.[506] have described a case of *T. gondii*-associated chorioretinitis following liver transplantation. Peacock et al.[507] have identified bone marrow transplant recipients who are seropositive for antibody to *T. gondii* and have findings consistent with previous toxoplasma retinochoroiditis on pretransplant ophthalmologic examination, as yet another high-risk population for reactivation of ocular toxoplasmosis in the early post-transplant period.

In 1991, Engstrom et al.[508] conducted a survey on the current practices for management of ocular toxoplasmosis. The results have shown the use of systemic corticosteroids as part of the initial treatment regimen in 95% of cases. Systemic corticosteroids are usually administered to patients having their vision threatened.[16] Patients with unilateral focal chorioretinitis (without associated old scars in the posterior pole) presumably caused by acquired toxoplasmosis, when treated with systemic or periocular corticosteroids not accompanied by antiparasitic medication showed rapid increase of inflamation.[509]

The most often used therapy for ocular toxoplasmosis[510-513] consisted of combination of pyrimethamine, sulfadiazine, and corticosteroids (32% of cases),[514-516] or pyrimethamine, sulfa-diazine, clindamycin, and corticosteroids (27%);[517] adjunct therapies involving photocoagulation, cryotherapy, or vitrectomy have been used in 33% of the cases.[508] In a typical example, Psilas et al.[514] have reported positive response of patients with acute toxoplasmic chorioretinitis following treatment with sulfonamides, pyrimethamine, and corticosteroids for a period of 4 weeks.

Rothova et al.[518] conducted a perspective multicenter study to evaluate the efficacy of therapeutic strategies for treatment of ocular toxoplasmosis in 106 patients. Medication was given for at least 4 weeks and consisted of three combinations, namely, pyrimethamine, sulfadiazine, and cortico-steroids (group 1; 29 patients), clindamycin, sulfadiazine, and corticosteroids (group 2; 37 patients), and co-trimoxazole (trimethoprim–sulfamethoxazole) and corticosteroids (group 3; 8 patients); patients with peripheral retinal lesions remained without systemic therapy (group 4; 32 patients). Patients from group 1 received leucovorin (5.0 mg twice weekly). No difference in the duration of inflammatory activity was noticed between the separate groups of patients. The investigators concluded that independently of the therapy given, the size of the retinal focus was the most important factor in predicting the duration of inflammatory activity ($p < .05$). There was a 52% reduction in the size of the retinal inflammatory focus in the pyrimethamine-treated patients, as compared with only 25% of untreated cases. The most frequently observed side effects of pyrimethamine treatment included hematologic complications (thrombocytopenia and leukopenia, despite the leucovorin medication).[518]

Colin and Harie[519] have conducted a prospective, randomized study in 29 patients with presumed toxoplasmic retinochoroiditis to compare the efficacy of oral pyrimethamine–sulfadiazine with subconjunctival injections of clindamycin. Results from both treatments showed no difference in the mean visual acuity after completion of therapy, with mean healing times being similar (1.80 months for clindamycin, and 1.88 months for pyrimethamine–sulfadiazine). At the 14 months follow-up examination, recurrence of ocular toxoplasmosis developed in both groups — 21% (clindamycin) and 36% (pyrimethamine–sulfadiazine) of patients. In general, other than discomfort, the subconjunctival injection of clindamycin did not produce any significant adverse side effects, thus providing a useful alternative in the choice of anti-*Toxoplasma* ocular therapy.[519] A report by Hansen et al.[520] discussed the successful therapy of toxoplasmic retino-choroiditis following specific treatment with pyrimethamine, sulfamethoxydiazine, clindamycin, and spiramycin, in double or triple combinations.

After evaluating the data of 33 patients with active toxoplasmic retinochoroiditis that were followed up for 2 to 9 years, Theodossiadis et al.[521] found no real differences between treatment with argon laser and medication in terms of success rate, time of regression of lesion recurrences, and complications. The regression of the active lesion in the laser-treated group was accomplished in 25 to 50 d, whereas in the medication-treated group it took 50 to 150 d.

Atovaquone at oral doses of 750 mg, four times daily, resolved vitreal inflammation and improved visual acuity from 20/200 to 20/40 in a pediatric AIDS patient with toxoplasmic retinochoroiditis — there was no evidence of recurrence at 5-month follow-up examination.[522]

Tassignon et al.[523] have examined the intraocular penetration of anti-toxoplasmic drugs administered either by subconjunctival, retrobulbar, or intramuscular routes. Drug measurements were performed in the anterior chamber, the vitreous, and the retina-choroid of a healthy rabbit eye; the best results were obtained for spiramycin, trimethoprim–sulfamethoxazole, and clindamycin. The therapeutic efficacy on *Toxoplasma*-infected rabbit eye was investigated using an indirect method; pyrimethamine, and especially doxycycline, have shown the best results.[523]

Neuroretinitis is a distinct clinical entity consisting of moderate to severe visual loss, optic nerve head edema, macular exudate in a stellate pattern, and variable vitreous inflammation. Several cases of neuroretinitis associated with *T. gondii* infection have been described by Fish et al.[524] Treatment with systemic antibiotics and corticosteroids resulted in restoration of visual acuity to 20/25 or better, thereby suggesting that although rare, toxoplasmic neuroretinitis is a potentially treatable ocular disorder.

Falcone et al.[525] have described a case in which toxoplasmic papillitis was the initial manifestation of AIDS.

22.3.6 THE ROLE OF IMMUNOTHERAPY IN THE TREATMENT OF TOXOPLASMOSIS

Ultimately, the control of severe *Toxoplasma* infections will rest with the ability of the host to develop an adequate cell-mediated immune response. With the advance of recombinant lympho-kines, as well as drugs capable of enhancing the cell-mediated immunity, immunotherapy alone or in conjunction with specific chemotherapy will play an increasing role in the management of toxoplasmosis, especially in immunocompromised patients.[44,81]

IFN-γ with its pleiotropic adjuvant effects on host defenses plays an active role in the development of appropriate cell-mediated immune responses by the host.[526] Administration of IFN-γ can enhance the antibody production and survival time of mice infected with *Toxoplasma*.[527] Furthermore, IFN-γ also augments the activity of natural killer (NK) cells and activates the macrophages, making these cells important factors in the development of viable host resistance against *Toxoplasma*.[44]

Using a mouse model of acute toxoplasmosis, Shirahata et al.[528] have examined the effects of *in vivo* administration of monoclonal antibodies against T cell subsets and anti-asialo GM1 antibody on the course of infection and the early IFN-γ response. The data obtained suggested that the endogenous IFN-γ produced during the first several days of infection was critical for the generation of anti-*Toxoplasma* resistance. In addition, the results of the study suggested that CD8$^+$ T lymphocytes played a central role in the resolution of acute toxoplasmosis by participating in the endogenous production of IFN-γ and the development of protective immunity to *T. gondii*.

Gomez Marin et al.[529] have investigated the role of IFN-γ in protecting the monocytoid cell line THP1 against *T. gondii*. The addition of IFN-γ to cultured infected TNP1 cells reduced the number of parasitized cells without altering the intracellular multiplication during the first 24 h — the reduction was potentiated by bacterial lipopolysaccharide. In related experiments, the role of secretory phospholipase A_2 (sPLA$_2$), an enzyme important for the *T. gondii* cellular invasion, and its relation to IFN-γ-induced protection, was also examined. Treatment of cells or parasites with a specific inhibitor of sPLA$_2$ substantially reduced the number of infected cells at 6 h. Furthermore, the addition of exogenous sPLA$_2$ did not interfere with the protective effect of IFN-γ and conferred protection when used alone. The data obtained suggested that IFN-γ resisted cell invasion by *T. gondii* by suppressing the parasite production of phospholipase A_2.

In several reports, *T. gondii* was described to be both sensitive to, and inducer of, IFN-γ in chick and mouse models.[530-532] On the other hand, Ahronheim[533] presented data from a plaque assay which indicated the lack of interaction between the growth of parasite and the classical IFN system in human embryonic fibroblasts. Studies by Pfefferkorn and Guyre,[534] however, showed recombinant IFN-γ (but not IFN-α or -β) to have a potent antitoxoplasmic activity in human fibroblasts. It is thought that the antitoxoplasmic mode of action of IFN-γ is the result of its ability to induce the production of indoleamine dioxygenase, a powerful enzyme which degrades tryptophan within the host cells to *N*-formylkynurenine.[535] In the next step, a constitutive host cell formamidase will degrade the *N*-formylkynurenine to kynurenine, which in turn, will leak from the host cell into the medium. Consequently, a reduced concentration in the host cell of an essential amino acid, such as tryptophan, will impair the growth of *T. gondii*. The protozoan growth will be slowed down even more since intracellular parasites are separated from the host cell cytoplasm by the parasitophorous vacuolar membrane; because of that, relative to the cytoplasm, the intravacuolar concentration of tryptophan will be even lower. Nathan et al.[536] demonstrated that macrophages activated by IFN-γ will eliminate *T. gondii* by virtue of their enhanced oxidative metabolism.

The activity of recombinant IFN-γ in combination with either pyrimethamine or clindamycin has been examined in a murine model of acute toxoplasmosis.[537] A markedly higher survival rate was observed in mice treated with such combinations as compared to those receiving treatment with any of these drugs alone. As mentioned earlier, IFN-γ acted synergistically with the antibiotic roxithromycin[249] and azithromycin[259] when tested in a mouse model of toxoplasmic encephalitis.

Recently, considerable evidence has been accumulated to suggest that *in vivo* administration of interleukin-2 (IL-2) or culturing of certain cell types with IL-2 resulted in modulation of the immune response caused by IL-2. The latter was shown to facilitate the development of cytotoxic T cells[44,538,539] and tumor-specific cells,[540] and to enhance transplantation tolerance[541] and antigen-induced T cell proliferation.[44,542]

Toxoplasma infections are known to elicit both immune enhancement and immune suppression.[543-545] For example, splenocytes from mice acutely infected with *T. gondii* showed a decreased ability to produce IL-2 — administration of IL-2 resulted in reduction in the number of *Toxoplasma* cysts in the brain and marked increase in the survival rate.[44] In a related study,[546] a similar *in vivo* administration of IL-2 was shown to reverse the T cell unresponsiveness of *Mycobacterium bovis*-infected mice.

Sharma et al.[547] have reported that administration of recombinant IL-2 (rIL-2) induced a significant ($p < .01$) decrease in the mortality of mice infected with LD$_{100}$ dose of *T. gondii*. Furthermore, mice treated with rIL-2 had considerably lower (<0.005) concentrations of cysts in the brain.[547] No changes in the antibody response were noticed and IL-2 administration failed to reverse the suppression to concanavalin A- and lipopolysaccharide-induced transformation of lymphocytes in mice acutely infected with *T. gondii*. As suggested,[547] antibodies were unlikely to have participated in any major way in reversal by IL-2 of immunosuppression associated with *Toxoplasma* infection.

The well-known activity of NK cells to lyse parasites (e.g., *T. gondii*) directly[547,548] is enhanced by IL-2.[538] Hence, it would be reasonable to assume that the increased survival rate of *Toxoplasma*-infected mice by IL-2 was the result of enhanced NK cell activity against *Toxoplasma* tachyzoites.[547]

Huldt et al.[549] have provided experimental evidence that a toxoplasmic infection in mice can trigger changes in the anatomy and functions of the thymus; in addition, the protozoan may also interfere with the differentiation and migration of thymocytes.

Fegies and Guerrero[550] used levamisole to boost the immune response in five patients with toxoplasmosis. The drug, when given alone (at 150 mg daily for 3 d, every 14 d during a 2-month period), or in combination with trimethoprim–sulfamethoxazole (300 mg daily for 30 d) induced significant increase and normalization of the T lymphocyte counts, and consequently, an enhancement of the cellular immune response with suppression of antitoxoplasmic antibody titers. The lower T lymphocyte counts in *T. gondii*-infected patients correlated with the depressed thymus activity found in *T. gondii*-infected animals.[550] Later, however, the results of Fegies and Guerrero were contradicted by Zastera et al.,[551] who did not find any activity of levamisole against experimental toxoplasmosis in mice — the drug was administered in the stomach at the same doses and schedule (2.5 mg/kg for three consecutive days, every 2 weeks for a 2-month period), as described in Reference 550. The effect of levamisole on toxoplasmosis during pregnancy in guinea pigs was also investigated.[552]

It has been shown that macrophages that were specifically activated by *Toxoplasma*-sensitized lymphocytes possessed increased capacity to control the intracellular proliferation of the protozoan in cell cultures *in vitro*[269,290-292] as well as in immune animals.[553-556]

The SAG1 protein of *T. gondii* has been evaluated as a protective antigen in mucosal immunization with cholera toxin as an adjuvant.[557] Thus, as compared with controls, CBA/J mice after being intranasally immunized with a combination of SAG1 and cholera toxin exhibited significantly fewer cysts in the brain following oral infection with the 76K strain of *T. gondii*. This acquired protection, which lasted for 5 months, was characterized by high levels of serum anti-SAG1 IgG antibodies, as well as an enhanced systemic cellular response. Furthermore, a significant production of anti-SAG1 IgA was induced in the intestinal secretions of protected mice. The proposed intranasal immunization may prove useful in inducing the mucosal and systemic immune responses, thereby providing enhanced resistance against chronic toxoplasmosis.

Corynebacterium parvum and Bacillus Calmette-Guérin (BCG) both stimulated the lymphoreticular system and were used as nonspecific enhancers of host resistance.[558] Some polysaccharides were also found to be potent stimulants of reticuloendothelial cells[559] and were applied in experimental bacterial and protozoal infections.[558,560] Nguyen and Stadtsbaeder[558] have reported that polysaccharides, such as lentinan, the micro- and macromolecular forms of *Schizophyllan* and *Coriolus versicolor* extract, were effective *in vitro* against *T. gondii* (RH strain) by activating macrophages treated for 2 d with 500 µg/ml of polysaccharides prior to inoculation with the protozoan.

In cell culture experiments, Lyche et al.[561] have found that properdin was an important cofactor for activating antibodies against *Toxoplasma*, although by itself properdin did not show any antitoxoplasmic activity.[562] In addition to its antibody-activating effect, properdin appeared to have also the ability to disassociate antibodies attached to reactive sites on *Toxoplasma* parasites. Consequently, high concentrations of properdin may exert instead the opposite effect — that is, inhibiting the antibody effect on *Toxoplasma*.

22.3.7 Drug-Resistant Mutants of *Toxoplasma gondii*

As mentioned earlier,[345] drug-resistant mutants of *T. gondii* have been isolated and characterized. Experiments by Sander and Midtvedt[563] have established that mice infected with *T. gondii* (RH strain) have developed a sulfonamide-resistant mutant after being fed with a low sublethal dose (0.5 mg daily) of sulfamethoxazole for a prolonged period of time (290 d). In a related study, Lai et al.[564] have demonstrated the development of a sulfadiazine-resistant mutant of *T. gondii* by treating mice with approximately 8.0 mg of the drug for only 10 d. The mutant, however, was still susceptible to medication with pyrimethamine and spiramycin.

Pfefferkorn and Pfefferkorn[565] have found adenine arabinoside, which suppressed the DNA synthesis by *T. gondii*, to be more inhibitory to the protozoan than to human fibroblast host cell cultures. A single-step mutant of *T. gondii*, which was 50-fold more resistant to adenine arabinoside, was isolated after mutagenesis with *N*-methyl-*N'*-nitro-*N*-nitroguanidine. In another study by the same researchers,[566] a *T. gondii* mutant resistant to 5-fluorodeoxyuridine was also characterized.

Aphidicolin, a mycotoxin known to inhibit DNA polymerase-α, was able to block the growth of *T. gondii* in cofluent cultural human fibroblasts. Using mutagenesis by ethylnitrosourea, an aphidicolin-resistant mutant of the protozoan was isolated.[567] An increased deoxycytidine triphosphate pool present in the mutant was the probable explanation for its resistance towards aphidicolin. In mammalian cells, deoxycytidine triphosphate reversed competitively the inhibition of DNA synthesis by aphidicolin.[568] While many inhibitors of DNA synthesis either bind to the DNA template or block the production of the required deoxynucleotide triphosphates,[567] aphidicolin directly suppressed the DNA polymerization by DNA polymerase-α. The latter was responsible for nuclear DNA replication in eukaryotic cells.[567]

22.3.8 References

1. Nicolle, C. and Manceaux, L., Sur une infection a corps de Leishman (ou organismes voisins) su gondi, *C. R. Acad. Sci. (Paris)*, 147, 763, 1908.
2. Splendore, A., Un nuovo protozoa parasita dei conigli, *Rev. Soc. Sci. (Sao Paolo)*, 3, 109, 1908.
3. Grell, K. G., *Protozoology*, Springer, New York, 1973, 440.
4. Jones, T. C., Len, L., and Hirsch, J. G., Assessment of *in vitro* immunity against *Toxoplasma gondii*, *J. Exp. Med.*, 141, 466, 1975.
5. Beverley, J. K. A., A rational approach to the treatment of toxoplasmic uveitis, *Trans. Ophthal. Soc.*, 78, 109, 1958.
6. Frenkel, J. K., La toxoplasmose chez l'animal et chez l'homme, *Med. Hyg.*, 32, 323, 1974.
7. Fortier, B., Coignard-Chatain, C., Soete, M., and Dubremetz, J. F., Structure and biology of *Toxoplasma gondii* bradyzoites, *C. R. Seances Soc. Biol. Fil.*, 190, 385, 1996.
8. Frixione, E., Mondragon, R., and Meza, I., Kinematic analysis of *Toxoplasma gondii* motility, *Cell. Motil. Cytoskeleton*, 34, 152, 1996.
9. Suss-Toby, E., Zimmerberg, J., and Ward, G. E., *Toxoplasma* invasion: the parasitophorous vacuole is formed from host cell plasma membrane and pinches off via a fission pore, *Proc. Natl. Acad. Sci. U.S.A.*, 93, 8413, 1996.
10. Grimwood, J. and Smith, J. E., *Toxoplasma gondii*: the role of parasite surface and secreted proteins in host cell invasion, *Int. J. Parasitol.*, 26, 169, 1996.
11. Grimwood, J., Mineo, J. K., and Kasper, L. H., Attachment of *Toxoplasma gondii* to host cells is host cell cycle dependent, *Infect. Immun.*, 64, 4039, 1996.
12. Nguyen, B. T. and Stadtsbaeder, S., Comparative effects of cotrimoxazole (trimethoprim-sulfamethoxazole), pyrimethamine-sulfadiazine and spiramycin during avirulent infection with *Toxoplasma gondii* (Beverley strain) in mice, *Br. J. Pharmacol.*, 79, 923, 1983.
13. Renoult, E., Biava, M. F., Hulin, C., Frimat, L., Hestin, D., and Kessler, M., Transmission of toxoplasmosis by renal transplant: a report of four cases, *Transplant. Proc.*, 28, 181, 1996.
14. Gallino, A., Maggiorini, M., Kiowski, W., Martin, X., Wunderli, W., Schneider, J., Turina, M., and Follath, F., Toxoplasmosis in heart transplant recipients, *Eur. J. Clin. Microbiol. Infect. Dis.*, 15, 389, 1996.
15. Kimball, A. C., Kean, B. H., and Kellner, A., The risk of transmitting toxoplasmosis by blood transfusion, *Transfusion*, 5, 447, 1965.
16. Feldman, H. A., Toxoplasmosis, *N. Engl. J. Med.*, 279, 1370, 1968.
17. Jones, T. C., Kean, B. H., and Kimball, A. C., Acquired toxoplasmosis, *NY State J. Med.*, 69, 2237, 1969.
18. Bamford, C. R., Toxoplasmosis mimicking a brain abscess in an adult with treated scleroderma, *Neurology*, 25, 343, 1975.

19. Levine, N. D., *Protozoan Parasites of Domestic Animals and of Man,* Burgess Publishing, Minneapolis, 1973, 294.
20. Feldman, H. A., The clinical manifestations and laboratory diagnosis of toxoplasmosis, *J. Trop. Med. Hyg.,* 2, 420, 1953.
21. Feldman, H. A. and Miller, L. T., Congenital human toxoplasmosis, *Ann. NY Acad. Sci.,* 64, 180, 1956.
22. Conyn-van Spaendonck, M. A., van Knapen, F., and de Jong, P. T., Congenital toxoplasmosis, *Tijdschr. Kindergeneeskd.,* 58, 227, 1990.
23. Russo, M. and Calanti, B., Prevention of congenital toxoplasmosis, *Clin. Ter.,* 134, 383, 1990.
24. Couvreur, J., Thulliez, T., Daffos, F., Aufrant, C., Bompart, Y., Goumy, P., and Tournier, G., 6 cases of toxoplasmosis in twins, *Ann. Pediatr. (Paris),* 38, 63, 1991.
25. Wilson, C. B., Remington, J. S., Stagno, S., and Reynolds, D. W., Development of adverse sequelae in children born with subclinical congenital *Toxoplasma* infection, *Pediatrics,* 66, 767, 1980.
26. Mets, M. B., Holfels, E., Boyer, K. M., Swisher, C. N., Roizen, N., Stein, L., Stein, M., Hopkins, J., Withers, S., Mack, D., Luciano, R., Patel, D., Remington, J. S., Meier, P., and McLeod, R., Eye manifestations of congenital toxoplasmosis, *Am. J. Ophthalmol.,* 122, 309, 1996.
27. Krausse, T., Straube, W., Wiersbitzky, S., Hitz, V., and Kewitsch, A., Screening for toxoplasmosis in pregnancy — a pilot program in Northeast Germany, *Geburtshilfe Frauenheilkd.,* 53, 613, 1993 (see comment in *Geburtshilfe Frauenheilkd.,* 53, 648, 1993).
28. Dutto, G. N., Recent developments in the prevention and treatment of congenital toxoplasmosis, *Int. Ophthalmol.,* 13, 407, 1989.
29. Carin, J. P., Mojon, M., Piens, M. A., and Chevalier-Nuttall, I., Monitoring and treatment of toxoplasmosis in the pregnant woman, fetus and newborn, *Pediatrie,* 44, 705, 1989.
30. Jeannel, D., Costagliola, D., Niel, C., Hubert, B., and Danis, M., What is known about the prevention of congenital toxoplasmosis? *Lancet,* 336, 359, 1990.
31. Douche, C., Benabdesselam, A., Mokhtari, F., and Le Mer, Y., Value of prevention of congenital toxoplasmosis, *J. Fr. Ophthalmol.,* 19, 330, 1996.
32. Kuchar, A., Hayda, M., and Steinkogler, P. J., Congenital toxoplasmosis retinochoroiditis after primary infection of the mother in pregnancy, *Ophthalmologie,* 93, 190, 1996.
33. Griffith, E. L., The treatment of toxoplasmosis during pregnancy, *J. Am. Med. Wom. Assoc.,* 28, 140, 1973.
34. D'Ercole, C., Boubli, L., Franck, J., Casta, M., Harle, J.-R., Chagnon, C., Cravello, L., Leclaire, M., and Blanc, B., Recurrent congenital toxoplasmosis in a woman with lupus erythematosus, *Prenat. Diagn.,* 15, 1171, 1995.
35. McLeod, R., Mack, D. C., Boyer, K., Mets, M., Roizen, N., Swisher, C., Patel D., Beckman, E., Vitullo, D., Johnson, D., and Meier, P., Phenotypes and functions of lymphocytes in congenital toxoplasmosis, *J. Lab. Clin. Med.,* 116, 623, 1990.
36. Theologides, A. and Kennedy, B. J., Clinical manifestations of toxoplasmosis in the adult, *Arch. Intern. Med.,* 117, 536, 1966.
37. Frenkel, J. K., Advances in the biology of *Sporozoa, Z. Parasitenk.,* 45, 125, 1974.
38. Woods, A.C., Modern concepts of the etiology of uveitis, *Am. J. Ophthalmol.,* 50, 1170, 1960.
39. O'Connor, G. R., Ocular toxoplasmosis, *Jpn. J. Ophthalmol.,* 19, 1, 1975.
40. Pivetti-Pezzi, P., Accorinti, M., Tamburi, S., Ciapparoni, V., and Abdulaziz, M. A., Clinical features of toxoplasmic retinochoroiditis in patients with acquired immunodeficiency syndrome, *Ann. Ophthalmol.,* 26, 73, 1994.
41. Wei, M. E., Campbell, S. H., and Taylor, C., Precipitous visual loss secondary to optic nerve toxoplasmosis as an unusual presentation of AIDS, *Aust. NZ J. Ophthalmol.,* 24, 75, 1996.
42. Herrera Rubio, J., Farinas, M. C., Tejido, R., Garcia Palomo, J. D., and Tejido, R., Aspecific chorioretinitis as initial manifestation of HIV infection and diffuse *Toxoplasma* encephalitis, *Med. Clin. (Barcelona),* 106, 198, 1996.
43. Martin-Duverneuil, N., Cordoliani, Y. S., Sola-Martinez, M. T., Miaux, Y., Weill, A., and Chiras, J., Cerebral toxoplasmosis: neuroradiologic diagnosis and prognostic monitoring, *J. Neuroradiol.,* 22, 196, 1995.
44. Luft, B. J. and Remington, J. S., Toxoplasmic encephalitis, *J. Infect. Dis.,* 157, 1, 1988.
45. Rostaing, L., Baron, E., Fillola, O., Roques, C., Durand, D., Massip, P., Lloveras, J. J., and Suc, J. M., Toxoplasmosis in two renal transplant recipients: diagnosis by bone marrow aspiration, *Transplant. Proc.,* 27, 1733, 1995.

46. Luft, B. J. and Remington, J. S., Toxoplasmosis of the central nervous system, in *Current Clinical Topics in Infectious Diseases*, Vol. 6, Remington, J. S. and Swartz, M. N., Eds., McGraw-Hill, New York, 1985, 315.

47. Levy, R. M., Bredersen, D. E., and Rosenblum, M. L., Neurobiological manifestations of the acquired immunodeficiency syndrome (AIDS): experience of UCSF and review of the literature, *J. Neurosurg.*, 621, 475, 1985.

48. Tuazon, C. U., Toxoplasmosis in AIDS patients, *J. Antimicrob. Chemother.*, 23(Suppl. A), 77, 1989.

49. Ferrer, S., Fuentes, I., Domingo, P., Munoz, C. et al., Cerebral toxoplasmosis in patients with human immunodeficiency virus (HIV) infection: clinico-radiological and therapeutic aspects in 63 patients, *An. Med. Interna*, 13, 4, 1996.

50. Winstanley, P., Drug treatment of toxoplasmic encephalitis in acquired immunodeficiency syndrome, *Postgrad. Med. J.*, 71, 404, 1995.

51. Luft, B. J., Hafner, R., Korzun, A. H., Leport, C., Antoniskis, D., Bosler, E. M., Bourland, D. D. III, Uttamchandani, R., Fuhrer, J., Jacobson, J., Morlat, P., Vildé, J.-L., Remington, J. S., and the members of the ACTG 077p/ANRS 009 Study Team, Toxoplasmic encephalitis in patients with the acquired immunodeficiency syndrome. *N. Engl. J. Med.*, 329, 995, 1993.

52. Ferrer, S., Fuentes, I., Domingo, P., Munoz, C. et al., Cerebral toxoplasmosis in patients with human immunodeficiency virus (HIV) infection: clinico-radiological and therapeutic aspects in 63 patients, *An. Med. Interna*, 13, 4, 1996.

53. Haverkos, H. W. (coordinator), Assessment of therapy for *Toxoplasma* encephalitis. The TE Study Group, *Am. J. Med.*, 82, 907, 1987.

54. Wanke, C., Tuazon, C. U., Kovacs, A., Dina, T., Davis, D. O., Barton, N., Katz, D., Lunde, M., Levy, C., Conley, F. K., Lane, H. C., Fauci, A. S., and Mazur, H., *Toxoplasma* encephalitis in patients with acquired immune deficiency syndrome: diagnosis and response to therapy, *Am. J. Trop. Med. Hyg.*, 36, 509, 1987.

55. Leport, C., Raffi, F., Metherton, S., Katlama, C., Regnier, B., Saimot, A. G., Marche, C., Vedrenne, C., and Vildé J.-L., Treatment of central nervous system toxoplasmosis with pyrimethamine/sulfadiazine combination in 35 patients with acquired immunodeficiency syndrome: efficacy of long-term continuous therapy, *Am. J. Med.*, 84, 94, 1988.

56. Post, M. J. D., Kusunoglu, S. J., Hensley, C. T., Chan, J. C., Moskowitz, L. B., and Hoffman, T. A., Cranial CT in acquired immunodeficiency syndrome: spectrum of diseases and optimal contrast enhancement technique, *Am. J. Radiol.*, 145, 929, 1985.

57. Tuazon, C. U., Toxoplasmosis in AIDS patients, *J. Antimicrob. Chemother.*, 23(Suppl. A), 77, 1989.

58. Altes, J., Salas, A., Ricart, C., Villalonga, C., Riera, M., and Casquero, P., Cerebral toxoplasmosis in patients with AIDS, *Arch. Neurobiol. (Madrid)*, 52(Suppl. 1), 121, 1989.

59. Carrazana, E. J., Rossitch, E., Jr., and Samuels, M. A., Cerebral toxoplasmosis in the acquired immune deficiency syndrome, *Clin. Neurol. Neurosurg.*, 91, 291, 1989.

60. Artigas, J., Grosse, G., Niedobitek, F., Kassner, M., Risch, W., and Heise, W., Severe toxoplasmic ventriculomeningoencephalomyelitis in two AIDS patients following treatment of cerebral toxoplasmic granuloma, *Clin. Neuropathol.*, 13, 120, 1994.

61. Mortier, E., Poirot, J. L., Marteau, M., Febvre, M., Meynard, J. L., Duvivier, C., Maury, E., Picard, O., and Cabane, J., Pulmonary toxoplasmosis in patients with human immunodeficiency virus infection: 21 cases, *Presse Med.*, 25, 485, 1996.

62. Halme, M., Jokipil, L., Jokipil, A. M., Ristola, M., and Lahdevirta, J., *Toxoplasma* pneumonia in a patient with AIDS, *J. Infect.*, 31, 252, 1995.

63. Gadea, I., Cuenca, M., Benito, N., Pereda, J. M., and Soriano, F., Bronchoalveolar lavage for the diagnosis of disseminated toxoplasmosis in AIDS patients, *Diagn. Microbiol. Infect. Dis.*, 22, 339, 1995.

64. Knani, L., Bouslama, K., Varette, C., Gonzalez Canali, G., Cabane, J., Lebas, J., and Imbert, J. C., Pulmonary toxoplasmosis in AIDS: report of 3 cases, *Ann. Med. Interne (Paris)*, 141, 469, 1990.

65. Miller, R. F., Lucas, S. B., and Bateman, N. T., Disseminated *Toxoplasma gondii* infection presenting with a fulminant pneumonia, *Genitourin. Med.*, 72, 139, 1996.

66. Oksenhendler, E., Cadranel, J., Sarfati, C., Katlama, C., Datrym, A., Marche, C., Wolf, M., Roux, P., Derouin, F., and Clauvel, J. P., *Toxoplasma gondii* pneumonia in patients with the acquired immunodeficiency syndrome, *Am. J. Med.*, 88(5N), 18N, 1990.

67. Albrecht, H., Stellbrink, H. J., Fenske, S., Schafer, H., and Greten, H., Successful treatment of *Toxoplasma gondii* myocarditis in an AIDS patient, *Eur. J. Clin. Microbiol. Infect. Dis.*, 13, 500, 1994.
68. Duffield, J. S., Jacob, A. J., and Miller, II. C., Recurrent, life-threatening atrioventricular dissociation associated with toxoplasma myocarditis, *Heart*, 76, 453, 1996.
69. Mastroianni, A., Coronado, O., Scarani, P., Manfredi, R., and Chiodo, F., Liver toxoplasmosis and acquired immunodeficiency syndrome, *Recenti Prog. Med.*, 87, 353, 1996.
70. Bonacini, M., Kanel, G., and Alamy, M., Duodenal and hepatic toxoplasmosis in a patient with HIV infection: review of the literature, *Am. J. Gastroenterol.*, 91, 1838, 1996.
71. Kume, H. and Takai, T., Toxoplasmosis of the liver, *Ryoikibetsu Shokogun Shirizu*, 7, 93, 1995.
72. Besnier, J. M., Verdier, M., Cotty, F., Fétissof, F., Besancenez, A., and Choutet, P., Toxoplasmosis of the bladder in a patient with AIDS, *Clin. Infect. Dis.*, 21, 452, 1995.
73. Grassi, M. P., Borella, M., Clerici, F., Perin, C., Bini, M. T., and Mongoni, A., Reversible bilateral opercular syndrome secondary to AIDS-associated cerebral toxoplasmosis, *Ital. J. Neurol. Sci.*, 15, 115, 1994.
74. Denton, H., Roberts, C. W., Alexander, J., Thong, K. W., and Coombs, G. H., Enzymes of energy metabolism in the bradyzoites and tachyzoites of *Toxoplasma gondii*, *FEMS Microbiol. Lett.*, 137, 103, 1996.
75. Tomavo, S. and Boothroyd, J. C., Interconnection between organellar functions, development and drug resistance in the protozoan parasite, *Toxoplasma gondii*, *Int. J. Parasitol.*, 25, 1293, 1995.
76. Wilson, I., Gardner, M., Kaveri, R., and Williamson, D., Extrachromosomal DNA in the Apicomplexa, *NATO ASI Ser.*, H78, 51, 1993.
77. Bohne, W., Heesemann, J., and Gross, U., Reduced replication of *Toxoplasma gondii* is necessary for induction of bradyzoite-specific antigens: a possible role for nitric oxide in triggering stage conversion, *Infect. Immun.*, 62, 1761, 1994.
78. Soete, M. and Dubremetz, J. F., *Toxoplasma gondii*: kinetics of stage-specific protein expression during tachyzoite-bradyzoite conversion *in vitro*, *Curr. Top. Microbiol. Immunol.*, 219, 76, 1996.
79. Odaert, H., Soete, M., Fortier, B., Camus, D., and Dubremetz, J. F., Stage conversion of *Toxoplasma gondii* in mouse brain during infection and immunodepression, *Parasitol. Res.*, 82, 28, 1996.
80. Gross, U., Bohne, W., Lüder, C. G., Lugert, R., Seeber, F., Dittrich, C., Pohl, F., and Ferguson, D. J. P., Regulation of developmental differentiation in the protozoan parasite *Toxoplasma gondii*, *J. Eukaryot. Microbiol.*, 43, 114S, 1996.
81. Krahenbuhl, J. L. and Remington, J. S., The immunology of toxoplasma and toxoplasmosis, in *Immunology of Parasitic Infections*, Cohen, S. and Warren, K. S., Eds., Blackwell, Oxford, 1982, 356.
82. Wong, S.-Y. and Remington, J. S., Biology of *Toxoplasma gondii*, *AIDS*, 7, 299, 1993.
83. Proempeler, H. J., Vogt, A., and Petersen, E. E., Diagnosis of toxoplasmosis in pregnancy, *Geburtshilfe Franenheilkd.*, 49, 642, 1989.
84. Suzuki, Y. and Remington, J. S., Dual regulation of resistance against *Toxoplasma gondii* infection by Lyt-2+ and Lyt-1+, L3T4+ cells in mice, *J. Immunol.*, 140, 3943, 1988.
85. Gazzinelli, R. T., Hakim, F. T., Hieny, S., Shearer, G. M., and Sher, A., Synergistic role of CD4+ and CD8+ T lymphocytes in IFN-γ production and protective immunity induced by an attenuated *Toxoplasma gondii* vaccine, *J. Immunol.*, 146, 286, 1991.
86. Suzuki, Y., Joh, K., Kwon, O.-C., Yang, Q., Conley, F. K., and Remington, J. S., MHC class I gene(s) in the D/L region but not the TNF-α gene determines development of toxoplasmic encephalitis in mice, *J. Immunol.*, 153, 4651, 1994.
87. Brown, C. R. and MacLeod, R., Class I MHC genes and CD8+ T cells determine cyst number in *Toxoplasma gondii* infection, *J. Immunol.*, 145, 3438, 1990.
88. Gazzinelli, R., Xu, Y., Hieny, S., Cheever, A., and Sher, A., Simultaneous depletion of CD4+ and CD8+ T lymphocytes is required to reactivate chronic infection with *Toxoplasma gondii*, *J. Immunol.*, 149, 175, 1992.
89. Mackaness, G. B., Cellular resistance to infection, *J. Exp. Med.*, 116, 381, 1962.
90. North, R. J., Suppression of cell-mediated immunity to infection by an antimitotic drug: further evidence that migrant macrophages express immunity, *J. Exp. Med.*, 132, 535, 1970.
91. McLeod, R. and Remington, J. S., Studies on the specificity of killing of intracellular pathogens by macrophages, *Cell Immunol.*, 34, 156, 1977.
92. North, R. J., The concept of the activated macrophage, *J. Immunol.*, 121, 806, 1978.

93. Mauel, J., Buchmuller, Y., and Behin, R., Studies on the mechanism of macrophage activation. I. Destruction of intracellular *Leishmania enrietii* in macrophages activated by cocultivation with stimulated lymphocytes, *J. Exp. Med.*, 148, 393, 1978.

94. Nogueira, N. and Cohn, Z. A., *Trypanozoma cruzi*: *in vitro* induction of macrophage microbicidal activity, *J. Exp. Med.*, 148, 288, 1978.

95. Klebanoff, S. J., Antimicrobial mechanisms in neutrophilic polymorphonuclear leucocytes, *Semin. Hematol.*, 12, 117, 1975.

96. Johnson, R. B., Keele, B. B., Nisra, H. P., Lehmeier, J. E., Webb, L S., Baehner, R. L., and Rajagopalan, K. U., The role of superoxide anion generation in phagocytic bacterial activity: studies with normal and chronic granulomatous disease leukocytes, *J. Clin. Invest.*, 55, 1357, 1975.

97. Babior, B. M., Oxygen-dependent microbial killing by phagocytes, *N. Engl. J. Med.*, 298, 659, 1978.

98. Babior, B. M., Oxygen-dependent microbial killing by phagocytes, *N. Engl. J. Med.*, 298, 721, 1978.

99. Nathan, C. F. and Root, R. K., Hydrogen peroxide release from mouse peritoneal macrophages: dependence on sequential activation and triggering, *J. Exp. Med.*, 146, 1648, 1972.

100. Weiss, S. J., King, G. W., and LoBuglio, A. F., Evidence for hydroxyl radical generation by human monocytes, *J. Clin. Invest.*, 60, 370, 1977.

101. Drath, D. B. and Karnovsky, M. L., Superoxide production by phagocytic leukocytes, *J. Exp. Med.*, 141, 257, 1975.

102. Johnston, R. B., Jr., Godzik, C. A., and Cohn, Z. A., Increased superoxide anion production by immunologically activated and chemically elicited macrophages, *J. Exp. Med.*, 148, 115, 1978.

103. Reiss, M. and Roos, D., Difference in oxygen metabolism of phagocytosing monocytes and neutrophils, *J. Clin. Invest.*, 61, 480, 1978.

104. Murray, H. W. and Cohn, Z. A., Macrophage oxygen-dependent antimicrobial activity. I. Susceptibility of *Toxoplasma gondii* to oxygen intermediates, *J. Exp. Med.*, 150, 938, 1979.

105. Murray, H. W., Juangbhanich, C. W., Nathan, C. F., and Cohn Z. A., Macrophage oxygen dependent antimicrobial activity. II. The role of oxygen intermediates, *J. Exp. Med.*, 150, 950, 1979.

106. Locksley, R. M. and Klebanoff, S. J., Oxygen-dependent microbicidal systems of phagocytes and host defense against intracellular protozoa, *J. Cell. Biochem.*, 22, 173, 1983.

107. Purner, M. B., Berens, R. L., Nash, P. B., van Linden, A., Ross, E., Kruse, C., Krug, E. C., and Curiel, T. J., CD4-mediated and CD8-mediated cytotoxic and proliferative immune responses to *Toxoplasma gondii* in seropositive humans, *Infect. Immun.*, 64, 4330, 1996.

108. Kasper, L. H. and Boothroyd, J. C., *T. gondii* and toxoplasmosis, in *Immunology and Molecular Biology of Parasitic Infections*, 3rd ed., Warren, K. S. and Agabian, N., Eds., Blackwell Scientific, Cambridge, 1993, 269.

109. Scharton-Kersten, T., Denkers, E. Y., Gazzinelli, R., and Sher, A., Role of IL-12 in induction of cell-mediated immunity to *Toxoplasma gondii*, *Res. Immunol.*, 146, 539, 1995.

110. Scharton-Kersten, T., Caspar, P., Sher, A., and Denkers, E. Y., *Toxoplasma gondii*: evidence for interleukin-12-dependent and -independent pathways of interferon-gamma production induced by an attenuated parasite strain, *Exp. Parasitol.*, 84, 102, 1996.

111. Hunter, C. A., Subauste, C. S., and Remington, J. S., The role of cytokines in toxoplasmosis, *Biotherapy*, 7, 237, 1994.

112. Pelloux, H. and Ambroise-Thomas, P., Cytokine production by human cells after *Toxoplasma gondii* infection, *Curr. Top. Microbiol. Immunol.*, 219, 155, 1996.

113. Gazzinelli, R. T., Amichay, D., Scharton-Kersten, T., Grünwald, E. et al., Role of macrophage-derived cytokines in the induction and regulation of cell-mediated immunity to *Toxoplasma gondii*, *Curr. Top. Microbiol. Immunol.*, 219, 127, 1996.

114. Scharton-Kersten, T. M., Wynn, T. A., Denkers, E. Y., Bala, S., Grunvald, E., Hieny, S., Gazzinelli, R. T., and Sher, A., In the absence of endogenous IFN-gamma, mice develop unimpaired IL-12 responses to *Toxoplasma gondii* while failing to control acute infection, *J. Immunol.*, 157, 4045, 1996.

115. Deckert-Schlüter, M., Rang, A., Weiner, D., Huang, S., Wiestler, O. D., Hof, H., and Schlüter, D., Interferon-gamma receptor-deficiency renders mice highly susceptible to toxoplasmosis by decreased macrophage activation, *Lab. Invest.*, 75, 827, 1996.

116. Georgiev, V. St. and Albright, J. F., Cytokines and their role as growth factors and in regulation of immune responses, *Ann. NY Acad. Sci.*, 685, 584, 1993.

117. Mosmann, T. R., Cherwinski, H., Bond, M. W., Giedlin, M. A., and Coffman, R. L., Two types of murine helper T cell clone. I. Definition according to profiles of lymphokine activities and secreted proteins, *J. Immunol.*, 136, 2348, 1986.

118. Cherwinski, H. M., Schumacher, J. H., Brown, K. D., and Mosmann, T. R., Two types of mouse helper T cell clone. III. Further differences in lymphokine synthesis between Th1 and Th2 clones revealed by RNA hybridization, functionally monospecific bioassays, and monoclonal antibodies, *J. Exp. Med.*, 166, 1229, 1987.

119. Mosmann, T. R. and Coffman, R. L., Th1 and Th2 cells: different patterns of lymphokine secretion lead to different functional properties, *Annu. Rev. Immunol.*, 7, 145, 1989.

120. Fiorentino, D. F., Bond, M. W., and Mosmann, T. R., Two types of mouse T helper cells. IV. Th2 clones secrete a factor that inhibits cytokine production by Th1 clones, *J. Exp. Med.*, 170, 2081, 1989.

121. LeGros, G., Ben-Sasson, S. Z., Seder, R., Finkelman, F. D., and Paul, W. E., Generation of interleukin 4 (IL-4)-producing cells *in vivo* and *in vitro*: IL-2 and IL-4 are required for *in vitro* generation of IL-4-producing cells, *J. Exp. Med.*, 172, 921, 1990.

122. Swain, S. L., Weinberg, A. D., English, M., and Huston, G., IL-4 directs the development of Th2-like helper effectors, *J. Immunol.*, 145, 3796, 1990.

123. Betz, M. and Fox, B. S., Regulation and development of cytochrome *c*-specific IL-4-producing T cells, *J. Immunol.*, 145, 1046, 1990.

124. Seder, R. A., Paul, W. E., Davis, M. M., and de St. Groth, B. F., The presence of interleukin 4 during *in vitro* priming determines the lymphokine-producing potential of CD4[4] T cells from T cell receptor transgenic mice, *J. Exp. Med.*, 176, 1091, 1992.

125. Suzuki, Y., Yang, Q., Yang, S., Nguyen, N., Lim, S., Liesenfeld, O., Kojima, T., and Remington, J. S., IL-4 is protective against development of toxoplasmic encephalitis, *J. Immunol.*, 157, 2564, 1996.

126. Bala, S., Englund, G., Kovacs, J., Wahl, L., Martin, M., Sher, A., and Gazzinelli, R. T., *Toxoplasma gondii* soluble products induce cytokine secretion by macrophages and potentiate *in vitro* replication of a monotropic strain of HIV, *J. Eukaryot. Microbiol.*, 41, 7S, 1994.

127. Gazzinelli, R. T., Hayashi, S., Wysocka, M., Carrera, L., Kuhn, R., Muller, W., Roberge, F., Trinchieri, G., and Sher, A., Role of IL-12 in the initiation of cell mediated immunity by *Toxoplasma gondii* and its regulation by IL-10 and nitric oxide, *J. Eukaryot. Microbiol.*, 41, 9S, 1994.

128. Khan, I. A., Matsuura, T., and Kasper, L. H., Interleukin-12 enhances murine survival against acute toxoplasmosis, *Infect. Immun.*, 62, 1639, 1994.

129. Seder, R. A., Gazzinelli, R., Sher, A., and Paul, W. E., Interleukin 12 acts directly on CD4[+] T cells to enhance priming for interferon γ production and diminishes interleukin 4 inhibition of such priming, *Proc. Natl. Acad. Sci. U.S.A.*, 90, 10188, 1993.

130. Sharma, S. D., Hofflin, J. M., and Remington, J. S., *In vivo* recombinant IL-2 enhances survival against a lethal challenge with *T. gondii*, *J. Immunol.*, 135, 416, 1985.

131. Shirahata, T., Muroya, N., Ohta, C., Goto, H., and Nakane, A., Enhancement by recombinant human interleukin 2 of host resistance to *Toxoplasma gondii* infection in pregnant mice, *Microbiol. Immunol.*, 37, 583, 1993.

132. Haque, S., Khan, I., Haque, A., and Kasper, L. H., Impairment of the cellular immune response in acute murine toxoplasmosis: regulation of interleukin 2 production and macrophage-mediated inhibitory effects, *Infect. Immun.*, 62, 2908, 1994.

133. Khan, I. A., Matsuura, T., and Kasper, L. H., IL-10 mediates immunosuppression following acute infection with *T. gondii* in mice, *Parasite Immunol.*, 17, 185, 1995.

134. Candolfi, E., Hunter, C. A., and Remington, J. S., Mitogen- and antigen-specific proliferation of T cells in murine toxoplasmosis is inhibited by reactive nitrogen intermediates, *Infect. Immun.*, 62, 1995, 1994.

135. Namen, A. E., Schmeierer, A. E., March, C. J., Overell, R. W., Park, L. S., Urdal, D. L., and Mochizuki, D. Y., B cell precursor growth promoting activity: purification and characterization of a growth factor active on lymphocyte precursors, *J. Exp. Med.*, 167, 988, 1988.

136. Welch, P. A., Namen, A. E., Goodwin, R. G., Armitage, R., and Cooper, M. D., Human IL-7. a novel T cell growth factor, *J. Immunol.*, 143, 3562, 1989.

137. Hickman, C. J., Crim, J. A., Mostowski, H. S., and Siegel, J. P., Regulation of human cytotoxic T lymphocyte development by IL-7, *J. Immunol.*, 145, 2415, 1990.

138. Alderson, M. R., Sassenfeld, H. M., and Widmer, M. B., Interleukin 7 enhances cytolytic T lymphocyte generation and induces lymphokine-activated killer cells from human peripheral blood, *J. Exp. Med.*, 172, 577, 1990.

139. Lynch, D. H. and Miller, R. E., Induction of murine lymphokine-activated killer cells by recombinant IL-7, *J. Immunol.*, 145, 1983, 1990.

140. Kasper, L. H., Matsuura, T., and Khan, I. A., IL-7 stimulates protective immunity in mice against the intracellular pathogen, *Toxoplasma gondii*, *J. Immunol.*, 155, 4798, 1995.

141. Gazzinelli, R. T., Wysocka, M., Hieny, S., Scharton-Kersten, T., Cheever, A., Kühn, R., Müller, W., Trinchieri, G., and Sher, A., In the absence of endogenous IL-10, mice acutely infected with *Toxoplasma gondii* succumb to a lethal immune response dependent on CD4⁺ T cells and accompanied by overproduction of IL-12, IFN-gamma and TNF-alpha, *J. Immunol.*, 157, 798, 1996.

142. Grabstein, K. H., Eisenman, J., Shanebeck, K., Rauch, C., Srinivasan S., Fung, V., Beers, C., Richardson, J., Shoenborn, M. A., and Ahdieh, M., Cloning of a cell growth factor, that interacts with the beta chain of the interleukin-2 receptor, *Science*, 264, 965, 1994.

143. Gamero, A. M., Ussery, D., Reintgen, D. S., Puleo, C. A., and Djeu, J. Y., Interleukin 15 induction of lymphokine-activated killer cell function against autologous tumor cells in melanoma patient lymphocytes by a CD18- dependent, perforin-related mechanisms, *Cancer Res.*, 55, 4988, 1995.

144. Nishimura, H., Hiromatsu, K., Kobayashi, N., Grabstein, K. H., Paxton, R., Sugamura, K., Bluestone, J. A., and Yoshikai, Y., IL-15, a novel growth factor for murine gamma delta T cells induced by *Salmonella* infection, *J. Immunol.*, 156, 663, 1996.

145. Carson, W., Ross, M., Baiocchi, R., Marien, M. J., Boianni, B., Grabstein, K. H., and Caligiuri, M. A., Endogenous production of interleukin 15 by activated human monocytes is critical for optimal production of interferon-gamma by natural killer cells *in vitro*, *J. Clin. Invest.*, 96, 2278, 1995.

146. Armitage, R. J., Macduff, B. M., Eisenman, J., Paxton, R., and Grabstein, K. H., IL-15 has stimulatory activity for the induction of B cell proliferation and differentiation, *J. Immunol.*, 154, 483, 1995.

147. Seder, R. A., Grabstein, K. H., Berzofsky, J. A., and McDyer, J. F., Cytokine interactions in human immunodeficiency virus-infected individuals: roles of interleukin (IL)-2, IL-12, and IL-15, *J. Exp. Med.*, 182, 1067, 1995.

148. Doherty, T. M., Seder, R. A., and Sher, A., Induction and regulation of IL-15 expression in murine macrophages, *J. Immunol.*, 156, 735, 1996.

149. Carson, W. E., Giri, J. G., Lindemann, M. J., Linett, M. L., Ahdieh, M., Paxton, R., Anderson, D., Eisenmann, J., Grabstein, K., and Caligiuri, M. A., Interleukin (IL) 15 is a novel cytokine that activates human natural killer cells via components of the IL-2 receptor, *J. Exp. Med.*, 180, 1395, 1994.

150. Khan, I. A. and Kasper, L. H., IL-15 augments CD8⁺ T cell-mediated immunity against *Toxoplasma gondii* in mice, *J. Immunol.*, 157, 2103, 1996.

151. Subauste, C. S., Koniaris, A. H., and Remington, J. S., Murine CD8⁺ cytotoxic T lymphocytes lyse *Toxoplasma gondii*-infected cells, *J. Immunol.*, 147, 3955, 1991.

152. Khan, I. A., Ely, K. H., and Kasper, L. H., Antigen-specific CD8⁺ T cell clone protects against acute *Toxoplasma gondii* infection in mice, *J. Immunol.*, 152, 1856, 1994.

153. Lindquist, S., The heat-shock response, *Annu. Rev. Biochem.*, 55, 1151, 1986.

154. Schlesinger, M. S., Heat shock proteins, *J. Biol. Chem.*, 265, 12111, 1990.

155. Anzola, J., Luft, B. J., Gorgone, G., Dattwyler, R. J., Soderberg, C., Lahessmaa, R., and Peltz, G., *Borrelia burgdorferi* HSP70 homolog: characterization of an immunoreactive stress protein, *Infect. Immun.*, 60, 3704, 1992.

156. Estes, D. M., Turaga, P. S. D., Siever, K. M., and Teale, J. M., Characterization of an unusual cell type (CD4⁺CD3⁻) expanded by helminth infection and related to the parasite stress response, *J. Immunol.*, 144, 1846, 1993.

157. Engman, D. M., Dragon, E. A., and Donelson, J. D., Human humoral immunity to hsp70 during *Trypanosoma cruzi* infection, *J. Immunol.*, 144, 3987, 1990.

158. Hedstrom, R., Culpepper, J., Harrison, R. A., Agabian, N., and Newport, G., A major immunogen in *Schistosoma mansoni* infections is homologous to the heat-shock protein Hsp70, *J. Exp. Med.*, 165, 1430, 1987.

159. Nagasawa, H., Manabe, T., Maekawa, Y., Oka, M., and Himeno, K., Role of L3T4⁺ and Lyt-2⁺ T cell subsets in protective immune responses of mice against infection with a low or high virulent strain of *Toxoplasma gondii*, *Miicrobiol. Immunol.*, 35, 215, 1991.

160. Araujo, F. G., Depletion of CD4⁺ T cells but not inhibition of the protective activity of IFN-γ prevents cure of toxoplasmosis mediated by drug therapy in mice, *J. Immunol.*, 149, 3003, 1992.

161. Asarnow, D. M., Goodman, T., Lefrancois, L., and Allison, J. P., Distinct antigen receptor repertoires of two classes of murine epithelium-associated T cells, *Nature*, 341, 60, 1989.

162. Kaufmann, S. H. E. and Kabelitz, D., γδ lymphocytes and heat shock proteins, *Curr. Top. Microbiol. Immunol.*, 167, 191, 1991.

163. De Paoli, P., Basaglia, G., Gennari, D., Crovatto, M., Modolo, M. L., and Santini, G., Phenotypic profile and functional characteristics of human γ and δ cells during acute toxoplasmosis, *J. Clin. Microbiol.*, 30, 729, 1992.

164. Scalise, F., Gerli, R., Castellucci, G., Spinozzi, F., Fabietti, G. M., Crupi, S., Sensi, L., Britta, R., Vaccaro, R., and Bertotto, A., Lymphocytes bearing the γδ T-cell receptor in acute toxoplasmosis, *Immunology*, 76, 668, 1992.

165. Nagasawa, H., Oka, M., Maeda, K., Jian-Guo, C., Hisaeda, H., Ito, Y., Good, R. A., and Himeno, K., Induction of heat shock protein closely correlates with protection against *Toxoplasma gondii* infection, *Proc. Natl. Acad. Sci. U.S.A.*, 89, 3155, 1992.

166. Haregewoin, A., Soman, G., Hom, R. C., and Finberg, R. W., Human γδ⁺ cells respond to mycobacterial heat shock protein, *Nature*, 340, 309, 1989.

167. Kaur, I., Voss, S. D., Gupta, R. S., Schell, K., Fisch, P., and Sondel, P. M., Human peripheral γδ T cells recognize hsp60 molecules on Daudi Burkitt's lymphoma cells, *J. Immunol.*, 150, 2046, 1993.

168. Hisaeda, H., Nagasawa, H., Maeda, K., Maekawa, Y., Ishikawa, H., Ito, Y., Good, R. A., and Himeno, K., γδ T cells play an important role in hsp65 expression and acquiring protective immune responses against infection with *Toxoplasma gondii*, *J. Immunol.*, 154, 244, 1995.

169. Hisaeda, H., Sakai, T., Nagasawa, H., Ishikawa, H., Yosutomo, K., Maekawa, Y., and Himeno, K., Contribution of extrathymic gamma delta T cells to the expression of heat-shock protein and the protective immunity in mice infected with *Toxoplasma gondii*, *Immunology*, 88, 551, 1996.

170. Kasper, L. H., Matsuura, T., Fonseka, S., Arruda, J., Channon, J. Y., and Khan, I. A., Induction of gamma delta T cells during acute murine infection with *Toxoplasma gondii*, *J. Immunol.*, 157, 5521, 1996.

171. Adams, W. B., Hibbs, J. B., Jr., Taintor, R. R., and Krahenbuhl, J., Microbiostatic effect of murine-activated macrophages for *Toxoplasma gondii*: role for synthesis of inorganic nitrogen oxides from L-arginine, *J. Immunol.*, 144, 2725, 1990.

172. Gross, U. and Bohne, W., *Toxoplasma gondii*: strain- and host cell-dependent induction of stage differentiation, *J. Eukaryot. Microbiol.*, 41, 10S, 1994.

173. Pfefferkorn, E. R., Eckel, M., and Rebhun, S., Interferon-gamma suppresses the growth of *Toxoplasma gondii* in human fibroblasts through salvation for tryptophan, *Mol. Biochem. Parasitol.*, 20, 215, 1986.

174. Murphy, P., The molecular biology of leukocyte chemoattractant receptors, *Annu. Rev. Immunol.*, 12, 593, 1994.

175. Hebert, C. A., Vitangcol, R. V., and Baker, J. B., Scanning mutagenesis of interleukin-8 identifies a cluster of residues required for receptor binding, *J. Biol. Chem.*, 266, 18989, 1991.

176. Amichay, D., Gazzinelli, R., Karupiah, G., Moench, T. R., Sher, A., and Farber, J. M., Genes for chemokines MuMig and Crg-2 are induced in protozoan and viral infections in response to IFN-γ with patterns of tissue expression that suggest nonredundant roles *in vivo*, *J. Immunol.*, 157, 4511, 1996.

177. Farber, J. M., HuMig: a new human member of the chemokine family of cytokines, *Biochem. Biophys. Res. Commun.*, 192, 223, 1993.

178. Liao, F., Rabin, R. L., Yannelli, J. R., Koniaris, L. G., Vanguri, P., and Farber, J. M., Human Mig chemokine: biochemical and functional characterization, *J. Exp. Med.*, 182, 1301, 1995.

179. Taub, D. D., Lloyd, A. R., Conlon, K., Wang, J. M., Ortaldo, J. R., Harada, A., Matsushima, K., Kelvin, D. J., and Oppenheim, J. J., Recombinant human interferon-inducible protein 10 is a chemoattractant for human monocytes and T lymphocytes and promotes T cell adhesion to endothelial cells, *J. Exp. Med.*, 177, 1809, 1993.

180. Khalil, S. S. and Rashwan, E. A., Tumour necrosis factor-alpha (TNF- alpha) in human toxoplasmosis, *J. Egypt. Soc. Parasitol.*, 26, 53, 1996.

181. Sheffield, H. G. and Melton, M. L., Effect of pyrimethamine and sulfadiazine on the fine structure and multiplication of *Toxoplasma gondii* in cell cultures, *J. Parasitol.*, 61, 704, 1975.

182. Nguyen, B. T., Stadtsbaeder, S., and Horvat, F., Comparative effect of trimethoprim and pyrimethamine, alone and in combination with a sulfonamide on *Toxoplasma gondii*: *in vitro* and *in vivo* studies, in *Current Chemotherepy (Proc. 10th Int. Congr. Chemother.)*, Vol. 1, Siegenthaler, W. and Luethy, R., Eds., American Society for Microbiology, Washington, D.C., 1978, 137.

183. Harris, C., Salgo, M. P., Tanowitz, H. B., and Wittner, M., *In vitro* assessment of antimicrobial agents against *Toxoplasma gondii*, *J. Infect. Dis.*, 157, 14, 1988.

184. Werner, H. and Egger, I., Comparative chemotherapeutical studies on the effect of bactrim and other combined preparations on the proliferative and cyst-forming phase of *Toxoplasma gondii* in NMRI mice: experimental chemotherapy of toxoplasmosis, *Zentralbl. Bakteriol. Parasitenkd. Infektioskr. Hyg. Abt. 1: Orig. Reihe A*, 231, 349, 1975.

185. Compte, P., Verin, P., and Le Bras, M., Treatment of recurrent congenital ocular toxoplasmosis: our initial experience with fansidar, *Bull. Soc. Ophthalmol. Fr.*, 89, 567, 1989.

186. Compte, P., Verin, P., and Le Bras, M., Treatment of recurrent congenital ocular toxoplasmosis: our initial experience with fansidar, *Bull. Soc. Ophthalmol. Fr.*, 89, 571, 1989.

187. Barbosa, J. C. and Ferreira, I., Sulfadoxine-pyrimethamine (fansidar) in pregnant women with *Toxoplasma* antibody titers, in *Current Chemotherapy (Proc. 10th Int. Congr. Chemother.)*, Vol. 1, Siegenthaler, W. and Luethy, R., Eds., American Society for Microbiology, Washington, D.C., 1978, 134.

188. Herman, Z., Sokola, A., and Szaflarski, J., Tentative treatment of experimental toxoplasmosis in mice. VIII. Effect of sulfamethoxypyrazine-pyrimethamine combination and effect of sulfamethoxypyrazine-longum in the treatment of experimental toxoplasmosis in the mouse, *Acta Parasitol. Pol.*, 18, 483, 1970.

189. Gupta, S. L., Gautam, O. P., and Chhbra, M. B., Chemotherapeutic efficacy of some agents against experimental toxoplasmosis in mice, *Indian J. Med. Res.*, 74, 767, 1981.

190. Werner, H., Matuschka, F. R., and Branderburg, I., Structural changes of *Toxoplasma gondii* bradyzoites and cysts following therapy with sulfamethoxypyrazine-pyrimethamine: studies by light and electron microscopy: consequences for chemotherapy, *Zentralbl. Bakteriol. Parasitenkd. Infektionskr. Hyg. Abt. 1: Orig. Reihe A*, 245, 240, 1979.

191. Werner, H. and Dannemann, R., Experimentalle untersuchungen uber die wirksamkeit von therapeutika auf zoite zystenentwicklung von *Toxoplasma gondii* in NMRI-mausen, *Z. Tropenmed. Parasitol.*, 23, 63, 1972.

192. Jacobson, J. M., Davidian, M., Rainey, P. M., Hafner, R., Raasch, R. H., and Luft, B. J., Pyrimethamine pharmacokinetics in human immunodeficiency virus-positive patients seropositive for *Toxoplasma gondii*, *Antimicrob. Agents Chemother.*, 40, 1360, 1996.

193. Bushby, S. R. and Hitchings, G. H., Trimethoprim, a sulfonamide potentiator, *Postgrad. Med. J.*, 45(Suppl.), 72, 1969.

194. Udall, V., Toxicology of sulfonamide-trimethoprim combinations, *Postgrad. Med. J.*, 45(Suppl.), 42, 1969.

195. Burchall, J. J., Mechanism of action of trimethoprim-sulfamethoxazole. II, *J. Infect. Dis.*, 128(Suppl.), S437, 1973.

196. Hitchings, G. H., Mechanism of action of trimethoprim-sulfamethoxazole. I, *J. Infect. Dis.*, 128(Suppl.), S433, 1973.

197. Nguyen, B. T. and Stadtsbaeder, S., *In vitro* activity of cotrimoxazole on the intracellular multiplication of *Toxoplasma gondii*, *Pathol. Eur.*, 10, 307, 1975.

198. Nguyen, B. T. and Stadtsbaeder, S., *In vitro* effects of trimethoprim with and without sulfamethoxazole on *Toxoplasma gondii* RH in human monocytes (antitoxoplasma activity of trimethoprim-sulfamethoxazole), *Drugs Exp. Clin. Res.*, 4, 43, 1978.

199. Nguyen, B. T., Stadtsbaeder, S., and Horvat, F., Macrophages infectes par *Toxoplasma gondii* RH: influence *in vitro* du cotrimoxazole sur l'interaction mitochondries-vacuoles parasitophorique, *Nouv. Presse Med.*, 8, 2833, 1979.

200. Grossman, P. L. and Remington, J. S., The effect of trimethoprim and sulfamethoxazole on *Toxoplasma gondii in vitro* and *in vivo*, *Am. J. Trop. Med. Hyg.*, 28, 445, 1979.

201. Feldman, H. A., Effects of trimethoprim and sulfisoxazole alone and in combination on murine toxoplasmosis, *J. Infect. Dis.*, 128, S774, 1973.

202. Sander, J. and Midtvedt, T., The effect of trimethoprim on acute experimental toxoplasmosis in mice, *Acta Pathol. Microbiol. Scand. Sect. B*, 78, 664, 1970.

203. Domart, A., Robineau, M., and Carbon, C., La toxoplasmose acquise: une nouvelle chimiotherapie: l'association sulfamethoxazole-trimethoprim, *Nouv. Presse Med.*, 2, 321, 1973.

204. Mossner, G., Klinische ergebnisse mit dem kombinations — praparat sulfamethoxazol-trimethoprim, *Antimicrob. Anticancer Ther. (Proc. 6th Congr. Chemother.)*, 1, 966, 1970.

205. Norrby, R., Eilard, T., Svedhen, A., and Lycke, E., Treatment of toxoplasmosis with trimethoprim-sulphamethoxazole, *Scand. J. Infect. Dis.*, 7, 72, 1975.

206. Stadtsbaeder, S. and Calvin-Preval, M. C., Trimethoprim-sulfamethoxazole association during experimental toxoplasmosis in the mouse, *Acta Clin. Belg.*, 28, 34, 1973.

207. Terragna, A., Rossolini, A., Cellesi, C., Figura, N., and Barberi, A., Activity of the combination trimethoprim-sulfamethoxazole on experimental toxoplasmosis, *Arzneim.-Forsch.*, 23, 1328, 1973.

208. Cellesi, C., Barberi, A., and Terragna, A., Effect of the association trimethoprim-sulfamethoxazole in the experimental infection of mice by *Toxoplasma gondii*: histochemical study, *Boll. Ist. Sieroter. (Milan)*, 52, 70, 1973.

209. Terragna, A., Cellesi, C., and Barberi, A., Effect of the association trimethoprim-sulfamethoxazole in the experimental infection of mice by *Toxoplasma gondii*: histological and immunobiological studies, *Boll. Ist. Sieroter. (Milan)*, 52, 60, 1973.

210. Terragna, A., Cellesi, C., Rossolini, A., and Figura, N., Activity of trimethoprim-sulfamethoxazole (TMP-SMZ) combination in experimental rat toxoplasmosis, *G. Mal. Infett. Parassitol.*, 26, 861, 1974.

211. Terragna, A., Rossolini, A., Cellesi, C., and Figura, N., Use of a trimethoprim-sulfamethoxazole (TMP-SMZ) combination in experimental murine toxoplasmosis, *Gazz. Med. Ital.*, 133, 33, 1974.

212. Szaflarski, J., Sokola, A., and Herman, Z. S., Tentative treatment of experimental toxoplasmosis in mice. IX. Effect of trimethoprim, sulfamethoxazole and their combination septrin, *Acta Parasitol. Pol.*, 22, 22, 1974.

213. Csoka, R. and Szeri, I., Hungarian chemotherapeutic agents in the experimental toxoplasmosis of mice. II. Studies with sumetrolim, *Egeszsegtudomany*, 19, 302, 1975.

214. Nguyen, B. T. and Stadtsbaeder, S., Comparative effects of cotrimoxazole (trimethoprim-sulfamethoxazole), pyrimethamine-sulphadiazine and spiramycin during avirulent infection with *Toxoplasma gondii* (Beverley strain) in mice, *Br. J. Pharmacol.*, 79, 923, 1983.

215. Iseki, M., Nishibayashi, M., Asada, S., Aihara, Y., Morishita, Y., and Takada, S., Influences of drug administration on the cyst number in brain and the antibody titer of mice chronically infected with Beverley strain of *Toxoplasma gondii*, *Osaka Shiritsu Daigaka Igaku Zasshi*, 20, 395, 1971.

216. Nguyen, B. T. and Stadtsbaeder, S., Comparative effects of cotrimoxazole (trimethoprim-sulphamethoxazole) and spiramycin in pregnant mice infected with *Toxoplasma gondii* (Beverley strain), *Br. J. Pharmacol.*, 85, 713, 1985.

217. Garin, J. P., Pellerat, J., Maillard, M., and Woehrle-Hezez, R., Bases theoriques de la prevention par la spiramycine de la toxoplasmose congenitale chez la femme enceinte, *Presse Med.*, 76, 2266, 1968.

218. Desmonts, G. and Couvreur, J., Congenital toxoplasmosis: a prospective study of the offspring of 542 women who acquired toxoplasmosis during pregnancy. Pathophysiology of congenital disease, in *Proc. 6th European Congr. Perinat. Med., Vienna*, Thalhammer, O., Baumgarten, K., and Polak, A., Eds., Georg Thieme, Stuttgart, 1979, 51.

219. Maier, W. and Piekarski, G., Experimental studies on the activity of the combination sulfamoxole/trimethoprim (CN 3123) on the *Toxoplasma* infection in albino mice, *Arzneimit.-Forsch.*, 26, 620, 1976.

220. Gill, H. S. and Prakash, O., Effect of 2-sulfamoyl-4,4'-diaminodiphenyl sulfone, dimethyl chlortetracycline hydrochloride, spiramycin and berberine hydrochloride in rabbits experimentally infected with the RH strain of *Toxoplasma*, *Indian J. Med. Res.*, 58, 1197, 1970.

221. Kumar, P. S., Kumar, R., and Mohapatra, L. N., Effect of SDDS (2-sulfamoyl-4,4'-diaminodiphenyl sulfone) on experimental infection with *Toxoplasma gondii* in rabbits, *Indian J. Med. Res.*, 67, 908, 1978.

222. Gill, H. S. and Prakash, O., Chemotherapy and chemoprophylaxis of experimental toxoplasmosis, *Indian J. Med. Res.*, 60, 1022, 1972.

223. Werner, H. and Catar, G., On the effect of SDDS in combination with pyrimethamine or sulfa monomethoxine on cysts of *Toxoplasma gondii* in NMRI mice, *Tropenmed. Parasitol.*, 25, 313, 1974.

224. Terragna, A., Bassetti, D., Giovanelli, A., and Genta, V., Experimental determination of the protective effect of sulfamethoxypyrazine in mice treated with *Toxoplasma gondii*, *Minerva Med.*, 61, 1129, 1970.

225. Terragna A., Rossolini, A., and Genta, V., Sulfamethoxypyrazine in experimental infection of rats by *Toxoplasma gondii*: histochemical evaluation, *Ann. Sclavo*, 12, 281, 1970.

226. Aoki, T., Effect of sulfamethoxypyrazine and combined use of vaccine on acute toxoplasmosis in mice, *Kseichugaku Zasshi*, 20, 132, 1972.

227. Werner, H., Dannemann, R., and Egger, I., On the effect of ultra long-lasting sulfonamide, sulphamethoxypyrazine (Longum®, Kelfizina®) on the proliferative phase of replication of *Toxoplasma gondii* in NMRI mice: contribution to experimental chemotherapy of toxoplasmosis, *Zentralbl. Bakteriol. (Orig. A)*, 222, 126, 1972.

228. Brus, R., Chrusciel, T. L., Steffen, J., and Szaflarski, J., Antitoxoplasmic activity of sulfonamides with various radicals in experimental toxoplasmosis in mice, *Z. Tropenmed. Parasitol.*, 22, 98, 1971.

229. Morita, C., Izawa, H., and Soekawa, M., Effect of killed *Toxoplasma* and sulfamonomethoxine on experimental toxoplasmosis in mice, *Zentralbl. Veterinaermed. Reihe B*, 18, 15, 1971.

230. Tsai, C. S., Chiene, J. G., and Cross, J. H., Treatment of toxoplasmosis in mice: effects of spiramycin, acetylspiramycin, pyrimethamine and sulfamonomethoxine singly or in combinations, *Clin. J. Microbiol.*, 6, 31, 1973.

231. Zardi, O., Adorisio, E., Nobili, G., and Lattanzi, M. T., Effects of an association of 2-sulfamido-3-methoxypyrazine and 2,4-diamino-5(*p*-chlorophenyl)-6-ethylpyridine in experimental toxoplasmosis, *Clin. Ter.*, 57, 129, 1971.

232. Frenkel, J.K., Sulfisoxazole called suboptimal therapy in toxoplasmosis, *Neurology*, 25, 899, 1975.

233. Shitova, E. M. and Novitskaya, N. A., Results of treating experimental toxoplasmosis in mice with some chemotherapeutic drugs, *Farmakol. Toksikol.*, 29, 709, 1966.

234. Crusciel, T. L., Herman, Z. S., Sokola, A., Steffen, J., and Szaflarski, J., Tentative treatment of experimental toxoplasmosis. VII. Effect of some sulfonamides applied with DMSO (dimethyl sulfoxide) and doxycycline, methacycline, sanasil, amantadine and bithionol on the course of subacute toxoplasmosis, *Acta Parasitol. Pol.*, 18, 393, 1970.

235. Pestka, S., Inhibition of protein synthesis, in *Molecular Mechanisms of Protein Biosynthesis*, Weissbach, H. and Pestka, S., Eds., Academic Press, New York, 1977, 467.

236. Chang, H. R. and Pechère, J. C., Activity of spiramycin against *Toxoplasma gondii in vitro*, in experimental infections and in human infection, *J. Antimicrob. Chemother.*, 22(Suppl.), 87, 1988.

237. Menninger, J. R. and Otto, D. P., Erythromycin, carbomycin and spiramycin inhibit protein synthesis by stimulating the dissociation of peptidyl-tRNA from ribosomes, *Antimicrob. Agents Chemother.*, 21, 811, 1982.

238. Mao, J. C. H., Putterman, M., and Wiegand, R. G., Biochemical basis for selective toxicity of erythromycin, *Biochem. Pharmacol.*, 19, 391, 1970.

239. Brisson-Noel, A., Trien-Luot, P., and Courvalin, P., Mechanism of action of spiramycin and other macrolides, *J. Antimicrob. Chemother.*, 22(Suppl.), 13, 1988.

240. Frydman, A. M., Le Roux, Y., Desnottes, J. F., Kaplan, P., Djebber, F., Cournot, A., Duchier, J., and Gaillot, J., Pharmacokinetics of spiramycin in man, *J. Antimicrob. Chemother.*, 22(Suppl. B), 93, 1988.

241. Mas Bakal, P. and In'T Veld, N., Postponed spiramycin treatment of acute toxoplasmosis in white mice, *Trop. Geogr. Med.*, 17, 254, 1965.

242. Suzuki, N., Espinas, F. M., Sakurai, H., Saito, A., Sasaki, H., Kato, G., Manba, K., Taniguchi, K., Mochizuki, K., and Osaki, H., Studies on the activity of obioactin with acetylspiramycin on mice infected with *Toxoplasma gondii*, *Zentralbl. Bakteriol. Microbiol. Hyg. Ser. A*, 256, 367, 1984.

243. Chan, J. and Luft, B. J., Activity of roxithromycin (RU 28965), a macrolide, against *Toxoplasma gondii* infection in mice, *Antimicrob. Agents Chemother.*, 30, 323, 1986.

244. Jones, R. N., Barry, A. C., and Thornsberry, C., *In vitro* evaluation of three new macrolide antimicrobial agents, RU 28,965, RU 29,065 and RU 29,702, and comparisons with other orally administered drugs, *Antimicrob. Agents Chemother.*, 24, 209, 1983.

245. Barlam, T. and Neu, H. S., *In vitro* comparison of the activity of RU 28,965, a new macrolide, with that of erythromycin against aerobic and anaerobic bacteria, *Antimicrob. Agents Chemother.*, 25, 529, 1984.

246. Chang, H. R. and Pechère, J. C., *In vitro* effects of four macrolides (roxithromycin, spiramycin, azithromycin (CP-62,993, and A-56268) on *Toxoplasma gondii*, *Antimicrob. Agents Chemother.*, 32, 524, 1988.

247. Chang, H. R. and Pechère, J. C., Effect of roxithromycin on acute toxoplasmosis in mice, *Antimicrob. Agents Chemother.*, 31, 1147, 1987.

248. Luft, B. J., *In vivo* and *in vitro* activity of roxithromycin against *Toxoplasma gondii* in mice, *Eur. J. Clin. Microbiol.*, 6, 479, 1987.

249. Hofflin, J. M. and Remington, J. S., *In vivo* synergism of roxithromycin (RU 28,965), 31, 346, 1987.

250. Romand, S., Bryskier, A., Montot, M., and Derouin, F., In-vitro and in-vivo activities of roxithromycin in combination with pyrimethamine or sulphadiazine against *Toxoplasma gondii*, *J. Antimicrob. Chemother.*, 35, 821, 1995.

251. Girard, A. E., Girard, D., English, A. R., Gootz, T. D., Cimochowski, C.R., Faiella, J. A., Haskell, S. L., and Ratsema, J. A., Pharmacokinetic and *in vivo* studies with azithromycin (CP-62,993), a new macrolide with an extended half-life and excellent tissue distribution, *Antimicrob. Agents Chemother.*, 31, 1948, 1987.

252. Retsema, J., Girard, A., Schelkly, W., Manousos, M., Anderson, M., Bright, G., Borovoy, R., Brennan, L., and Mason, R., Spectrum and mode of action of azithromycin (CP-62,993), a new 15-membered ring macrolide with improved potency against gram-negative organisms, *Antimicrob. Agents Chemother.*, 31, 1939, 1987.

253. Coulaud, J. P., Azithromycin: new orientations, *Pathol. Biol. (Paris)*, 43, 547, 1995.

254. Lode, H., Borner, K., Koeppe, P., and Schaberg, T., Azithromycin — review of key chemical, pharmacokinetic and microbiological features, *J. Antimicrob. Chemother.*, 37(Suppl. C), 1, 1996.

255. Derouin, F., New pathogens and mode of action of azithromycin: *Toxoplasma gondii*, *Pathol. Biol. (Paris)*, 43, 561, 1995.

256. Araujo, F. G., Guptill, D. R., and Remington, J. S., Azithromycin, a new macrolide antibiotic with potent activity against *Toxoplasma gondii*, *Antimicrob. Agents Chemother.*, 32, 755, 1988.

257. Wise, R., The development of macrolides and related compounds, *J. Antimicrob. Chemother.*, 23, 299, 1989.

258. Dumas, J. L., Chang, R., Mermillod, B., Piguet, P. F., Compte, R., and Pechère, J. C., Evaluation of the efficacy of prolonged administration of azithromycin in a murine model of chronic toxoplasmosis, *J. Antimicrob. Chemother.*, 34, 111, 1994.

259. Araujo, F. G. and Remington, J. S., Synergistic activity of azithromycin and gamma interferon in murine toxoplasmosis, *Antimicrob. Agents Chemother.*, 35, 1672, 1991.

260. Araujo, F. G., Shepard, E. M., and Remington, J. S., *In vivo* activity of macrolide antibiotics azithromycin, roxithromycin and spiramycin against *Toxoplasma gondii*, *Eur. J. Clin. Microbiol. Infect. Dis.*, 10, 519, 1991.

261. Araujo, F. G., Slifer, T., and Remington, J. S., Rifabutin is active in murine models of toxoplasmosis, *Antimicrob. Agents Chemother.*, 38, 570, 1994.

262. Olliaro, P., Gorini, G., Jabes, D., Regazzetti, A., Rossi, R., Marchetti, A., Tinelli, C., and Della Bruna, C., In-vitro and in-vivo activity of rifabutin against *Toxoplasma gondii*, *J. Antimicrob. Chemother.*, 34, 649, 1994.

263. Brun-Pascaud, M., Chau, F., Rajagopalan-Levasseur, P., Derouin, F., and Girard, P. M., Evaluation of the activities of rifabutin combined with atovaquone or low-dose of cotrimoxazole for prevention of pneumocystosis and toxoplasmosis in a dual infection rat model, *J. Eukaryot. Microbiol.*, 43, 14S, 1996.

264. Araujo, F. G., Suzuki, Y., and Remington, J. S., Use of rifabutin in combination with atovaquone, clindamycin, pyrimethamine, or sulfadiazine for the treatment of toxoplasmic encephalitis in mice, *Eur. J. Clin. Microbiol. Infect. Dis.*, 15, 394, 1996.

265. Araujo, F. G., Khan, A. S., and Remington, A. A., Rifapentine is active *in vitro* and *in vivo* against *Toxoplasma gondii*, *Antimicrob. Agents Chemother.*, 40, 1335, 1996.

266. Fernandes, P. B., Bailer, R., Swanson, R., Hanson, C. H., McDonald, E., Ramer, N., Hardy, D., Shipkowitz, N., Bower, R. R., and Gade, E., *In vitro* and *in vivo* evaluation of A-56268 (TE-031), a new macrolide, *Antimicrob. Agents Chemother.*, 30, 865, 1986.

267. Chang, H. R., Rudareanu, F. C., and Pechère, J. C., Activity of A-56268 (TE-031), a new macrolide against *Toxoplasma gondii* in mice, *J. Antimicrob. Chemother.*, 22, 359, 1988.

268. Terragna, A., Canessa, A., and Terragna, F. M., Effect of josamycin on experimental toxoplasmosis in mice, *IRCS Med. Sci.*, 13, 310, 1985.

269. Remington, J. S., Yagura, T., and Robinson, W. S., The effect of rifampin on *Toxoplasma gondii*, *Proc. Soc. Exp. Biol. Med.*, 135, 167, 1970.

270. Alder, J., Hutch, T., Meulbroek, J. A., and Clement, J. C., Treatment of experimental *Toxoplasma gondii* infection by clarithromycin-based combination therapy with minocycline or pyrimethamine, *J. Acquir. Immune Defic. Syndr.*, 7, 1141, 1994.

271. Pfefferkorn, E. R. and Borotz, S. E., Comparison of mutants of *Toxoplasma gondii* selected for resistance to azithromycin, spiramycin, or clindamycin, *Antimicrob. Agents Chemother.*, 38, 31, 1994.

272. Fichera, M. E., Bhopale, M. K., and Roos, D. S., *In vitro* assays elucidate peculiar kinetics of clindamycin action against *Toxoplasma gondii*, *Antimicrob. Agents Chemother.*, 39, 1530, 1995.

273. Blais, J., Tardif, C., and Chamberland, S., Effect of clindamycin on intracellular replication, protein synthesis, and infectivity of *Toxoplasma gondii*, *Antimicrob. Agents Chemother.*, 37, 2571, 1993.

274. Lappin, M. R., Greene, C. E., Winston, S., Toll, S. L., and Epstein, M.E., Clinical feline toxoplasmosis: serologic diagnosis and therapeutic management of 15 cases, *J. Vet. Intern. Med.*, 3, 139, 1989.

275. Peterson, J. L., Willard, M. D., Lees, G. E., Lappin, M. R., Dieringer, T., and Floyd, E., Toxoplasmosis in two cats with intestinal disease, *J. Am. Vet. Med. Assoc.*, 199, 473, 1991.

276. Filice, G. A. and Pomeroy, C., Effect of clindamycin on pneumonia from reactivation of *Toxoplasma gondii* infection in mice, *Antimicrob. Agents Chemother.*, 35, 780, 1991.

277. McMaster, P. R. B., Powers, K. G., Finerty, J. F., and Lunde, M. N., The effect of two chlorinated lincomycin analogs against acute toxoplasmosis in mice, *Am. J. Trop. Med. Hyg.*, 22, 14, 1973.

278. Araujo, F. G. and Remington, J. S., Effect of clindamycin on acute and chronic toxoplasmosis in mice, *Antimicrob. Agents Chemother.*, 5, 647, 1974.

279. Thiermann, E., Atias, A., Olguin, J., Menard, E., and Lorca, M., Effect of clindamycin on experimental toxoplasmosis in mice, *Rev. Med. Chile*, 105, 433, 1977.

280. Terragna, A., Canessa, A., Terragna, F. M., and Corradino, L., Attivita della clindamicina e della josamicina nell'infezione sperimentale da *Toxoplasma gondii*, *Minerva Med.*, 75, 2305, 1984.

281. Hofflin, J. M. and Remington, J. S., Clindamycin in a murine model of toxoplasmic encephalitis, *Antimicrob. Agents Chemother.*, 31, 492, 1987.

282. Tabbara, K. F. and O'Connor, G. R., Treatment of ocular toxoplasmosis with clindamycin and sulfadizine, *Ophthalmology*, 87, 129, 1980.

283. Ferguson, J. G., Clindamycin therapy for toxoplasmosis, *Ann. Ophthalmol.*, 13, 95, 1981.

284. Burke, G. J. and Mills, A. F., Toxoplasmosis and clindamycin, *S. Afr. Med. J.*, 55, 156, 1979.

285. Rolston, K. V. I. and Hoy, J., Role of clindamycin in the treatment of central nervous system toxoplasmosis, *Am. J. Med.*, 83, 551, 1987.

286. Podzamczer, D. and Gudiol, F., Clindamycin in cerebral toxoplasmosis, *Am. J. Med.*, 84, 800, 1988.

287. Kaplan, L., Wofsy, C., and Volberding, P., Treatment of patients with acquired immune deficiency syndrome and associated manifestations, *JAMA*, 257, 1374, 1987.

288. Velimirovic, B., Toxoplasmosis in immunosuppression and AIDS, *Infection*, 12, 315, 1984.

289. Terragna, A., Canessa, A., and Melioli, G., Evaluation of antitoxoplasmic activity of drugs *in vitro* and *in vivo*, in *Recent Advancements in Chemotherapy (Proc. 14th Int. Congr. Chemother., Tokyo)*, Ishigami, J., Ed., Tokyo University Press, Tokyo, 1985, 2540.

290. Christen, W. and Thiermann, E., Quimioterapia experimental de la toxoplasmosis. II. Efecto de la acromicina sobre toxoplasmosis experimental del ration, *Bol. Inform. Parasitol. Chil.*, 8, 49, 1953.

291. Kass, E. and Steen, E., Aureomycin treatment of acute experimental toxoplasmosis in rabbits, *Acta Pathol. Microbiol. Scand.*, 28, 1965, 1951.

292. Eyles, D. E. and Coleman, N., Notes on the treatment of acute experimental toxoplasmosis of the mouse with chlorotetracycline and tetracycline, *Antibiot. Chemother.*, 4, 988, 1954.

293. Midtvedt, T., Acute experimental toxoplasmosis in mice treated with some new chemotherapeutics and antibiotics, *Acta Pathol. Microbiol. Scand.*, 61, 67, 1964.

294. Grassi, C. and Kass, E., Failure of tetramycin treatment in acute experimental toxoplasmosis, *Acta Pathol. Microbiol. Scand.*, 30, 304, 1952.

295. Garin, J. P., Perrin-Fayolle, M., and Paliard, P., Toxoplasmose experimentale de la souris: guerison clinique et anatomopathologique par la demethylchlortetracycline (DMCT), *Presse Med.*, 73, 531, 1965.

296. Brogden, R. N., Speight, T. M., and Avery, G. S., Minocycline: a review of its antibacterial and pharmacokinetic properties and therapeutic use, *Drugs*, 9, 251, 1975.

297. Colwell, E. J., Hockman, R. L., Intraprasert, R., and Tirabutana, C., Minocycline and tetracycline treatment of acute *Falciparum malaria* in Thailand, *Am. J. Trop. Med. Hyg.*, 21, 144, 1972.

298. Willerson, D., Rieckmann, K. H., Carson, P. E., and Frischer, H., Effects of minocycline against chloroquine-resistant *Falciparum malaria*, *Am. J. Trop. Med. Hyg.*, 21, 857, 1972.

299. Chang, H. R., Compte, R., Piguet, P. F., and Pechère, J. C., Activity of minocycline against *Toxoplasma gondii* infection in mice, *J. Antimicrob. Chemother.*, 27, 639, 1991.

300. Tabbara, K. F., Sakuragi, S., and O'Connor, G. R., Minocycline in the chemotherapy of murine toxoplasmosis, *Parasitology*, 84, 297, 1982.

301. Perea, E. J. and Daza, R. M., The effect of minocycline, doxycycline and oxytetracycline on experimental mouse toxoplasmosis, *Bull. Soc. Pathol. Exot. Ses. Fil.*, 69, 367, 1976.

302. Indorf, A. S. and Pegram, P. S., Use of doxycycline in the management of a patient with toxoplasmic encephalitis, *AIDS*, 8, 1633, 1994.

303. Fertig, A., Selwyn, S., and Tibble, M. J. K., Tetracycline and toxoplasmosis, *Br. Med. J.*, 2, 192, 1977.

304. Fertig, A., Selwyn, S., and Tibble, M. J. K., Tetracycline treatment in a food-borne outbreak of toxoplasmosis, *Br. Med. J.*, 1, 1064, 1977.

305. Grossman, P. L. and Remington, J. S., Tetracycline and toxoplasmosis, *Br. Med. J.*, 1, 1664, 1977.

306. Srivastava, A. K., Singh, B., Ali, M. S., and More, B. K., Chemotherapeutic efficacy of anticancer drugs against experimental toxoplasmosis in mice, *Indian Vet. J.*, 62, 401, 1985.

307. Otake, N., Koenuma, M., Miyamae, H., Sato, S., and Saito, Y., Studies on ionophorous antibiotics. III. The structure of Ionomycin A, a polyether antibiotic, *Tetrahedron Lett.*, 4147, 1975.

308. Otake, N., Koenuma, M., Miyamae, H., Sato, S., and Saito, Y., Studies on the ionophorous antibiotics. IV. Crystal and molecular structure of the thallium salt of Ionomycin A, *J. Chem. Soc. Perkin II*, 494, 1977.

309. Miyagami, T., Takei, Y., Matsumoto, Y., Otake, N., Mizone, K., Mizutani, T., Omura, S., Ozeki, M., and Suzuki, N., An *in vitro* study on the toxoplasmicidal activity of Ionomycin A in host cells, *J. Antibiot.*, 34, 218, 1981.

310. Melton, M. L. and Sheffield, H. G., Activity of the anticoccidial compound, lasalocid, against *Toxoplasma gondii* in cultured cells, *J. Parasitol.*, 61, 713, 1975.

311. Hudson, A. T., Randall, A. W., Fry, M., Ginger, C. D., Hill, B., Latter, V. S., McHardy, N., and Williams, R. B., Novel anti-malarial hydroxynaphthoquinones with potent broad spectrum antiprotozoal activity, *Parasitology*, 90, 45, 1985.

312. Haile, L. G. and Flaherty, J. F., Atovaquone: a review, *Ann. Pharmacokinet.*, 27, 1488, 1993.

313. Spencer, C. M. and Goa, K. L., Atovaquone: a review of its pharmacological properties and therapeutic efficacy in opportunistic infections, *Drugs*, 50, 176, 1995.

314. Araujo, F. G., Huskinson, J., and Remington, J. S., Remarkable *in vitro* and *in vivo* activities of the hydroxynaphthoquinone 566C80 against tachyzoites and tissue cysts of *Toxoplasma gondii*, *Antimicrob. Agents Chemother.*, 35, 293, 1991.

315. Araujo, F. G., Huskinson-Mark, J., Gutteridge, W. E., and Remington, J. S., *In vitro* and *in vivo* activities of the hydroxynaphthoquinone 566C80 against the cyst form of *Toxoplasma gondii*, *Antimicrob. Agents Chemother.*, 36, 326, 1992.

316. Huskinson-Mark, J., Araujo, J., and Remington, J. S., Evaluation of the effect of drugs on the cyst form of *Toxoplasma gondii*, *J. Infect. Dis.*, 164, 170, 1991.

317. Romand, S., Pudney, M., and Derouin, F., *In vitro* and *in vivo* activities of the hydroxynaphthoquinone atovaquone alone or combined with pyrimethamine, sulfadiazine, clarithromycin, or minocycline against *Toxoplasma gondii*, *Antimicrob. Agents Chemother.*, 37, 2371, 1993.

318. Brun-Pascaud, M., Chau, F., Simonpoli, A.-M., Girard, P.-M., Derouin, F., and Pocidalo, J. J., Experimental evaluation of combined prophylaxis against murine pneumocystosis and toxoplasmosis, *J. Infect. Dis.*, 170, 653, 1994.

319. Ferguson, D. J. P., Huskinson-Mark, J., Araujo, F. J., and Remington, J. S., An ultrastructural study of the effect of treatment with atovaquone in brains of mice chronically infected with the ME49 strain of *Toxoplasma gondii*, *Int. J. Exp. Pathol.*, 75, 111, 1994.

320. Seymour, K. K., Lyons, S. D., Phillips, L., Rieckemann, K. H., and Christopherson, R. I., Cytotoxic effects of inhibitors of *de novo* pyrimidine biosynthesis upon *Plasmodium falciparum*, *Biochemistry*, 33, 5268, 1994.

321. Fry, M. and Pudney, M., Site of action of the antimalarial hydroxynaphthoquinone, 2-[*trans*-4-(4'-chlorophenyl)cyclohexyl]-3-hydroxy-1,4-naphthoquinone (566C90), *Biochem. Pharmacol.*, 43, 1545, 1992.

322. Pfefferkorn, E. R., Borotz, S. E., and Nothnagel, R. F., Mutants of *Toxoplasma gondii* resistant to atovaquone (566C80) or decoquinate, *J. Parasitol.*, 79, 559, 1993.

323. Gutteridge, W. E., 566C80, an antimalarial hydroxynaphthoquinone with broad spectrum: experimental activity against opportunistic parasitic infections in AIDS patints, *J. Protozool.*, 38, S141, 1991.

324. Ittarat, I., Asawamahasakda, W., and Meshnick, S. P., The effects of antimalarials on the *Plasmodium falciparum* dihydroorotate dehydrogenase, *Exp. Parasitol.*, 79, 50, 1994.

325. Ittarat, I., Asawamahasakda, W., Bartlett, M. S., Smith, J. W., and Meshnick, S. R., Effects of atovaquone and other inhibitors on *Pneumocystis carinii* dihydroorotate dehydrogenase, *Antimicrob. Agents Chemother.*, 39, 325, 1995.

326. Kovacs, J. A., Allegra, C. J., Chabner, B. A., Swan, J. C., Drake, J., Lunde, M., Parrillo, J. E., and Mazur, H., Potent effect of trimetrexate, a lipid-soluble antifolate, on *Toxoplasma gondii*, *J. Infect. Dis.*, 155, 1027, 1987.

327. Allegra, C. J., Kovacs, J. A., Drake, J. C., Swan, J. C., Chabner, B. A., and Mazur, H., Potent *in vitro* and *in vivo* antitoxoplasma activity of the lipid-soluble antifolate trimetrexate, *J. Clin. Invest.*, 79, 478, 1987.

328. Marshall, J. L. and DeLap, R. J., Clinical pharmacokinetics and pharmacology of trimetrexate, *Clin. Pharmacokinet.*, 26, 190, 1994.

329. Kovacs, J. A., Allegra, J. C., Chabner, B. A., Drake, J. C., Swan, J. C., Parrillo, J. E., and Mazur, H., Potent *in vitro* and *in vivo* antitoxoplasma activity of the new lipid-soluble antifolate trimetrexate, *Clin. Res.*, 34, 522A, 1986.

330. Allegra, C. J., Kovacs, J. A., Drake, J. C., Swan, J. C., Chabner, B. A., and Mazur, H., Potent *in vitro* and *in vivo* antitoxoplasma activity of the lipid-soluble antifolate trimetrexate, *J. Clin. Invest.*, 79, 478, 1987.

331. U.S. Department of Health and Human Services, Treatment of *Toxoplasma gondii* and *Pneumocystis carinii* infections with trimetrexate, *U.S. Patent Appl.*, 865,055, 1986.

332. Kovacs, J. A., Allegra, C. J., Swan, J. C., Drake, J. C., Parrillo, J. E., Chabner, B. A., and Mazur, H., Potent antipneumocystic and antitoxoplasma activities of piritrexim, a lipid-soluble antifolate, *Antimicrob. Agents Chemother.*, 32, 430, 1988.

333. Araujo, F. G., Guptill, D. R., and Remington, J. S., *In vivo* activity of piritrexim against *Toxoplasma gondii*, *J. Infect. Dis.*, 156, 828, 1987.

334. Piper, J. P., Johnson, C. A., Krauth, C. A., Carter, R. L., Hosmer, C. A., Queener, S. F., Borotz, S. E., and Pfefferkorn, E. R., Lipophilic antifolates as agents against opportunistic infections. I. Agents superior to trimetrexate and piritrexim against *Toxoplasma gondii* and *Pneumocystis carinii* in *in vitro* evaluations, *J. Med. Chem.*, 39, 1271, 1996.

335. Jackson, H. C., Biggadike, K., McKilligin, E., Kinsman, O. S., Queener, S. F., Lane, A., and Smith, J. E., 6,8-Disubstituted 2,4-diaminopteridines: novel inhibitors of *Pneumocystis carinii* and *Toxoplasma gondii* dihydrofolate reductase, *Antimicrob. Agents Chemother.*, 40, 1371, 1996.

336. Martinez, A., Allegra, C. J., and Kovacs, J. A., Efficacy of epiprim (Ro 11-8958), a new dihydrofolate reductase inhibitor, in the treatment of acute *Toxoplasma* infection in mice, *Am. J. Trop. Med. Hyg.*, 54, 249, 1996.

337. Locher, H. H., Schlunegger, H., Hartman, P. G., Angehrn, P., and Then, R. L., Antibacterial activities of epiprim, a new dihydrofolate reductase inhibitor, alone and in combination with dapsone, *Antimicrob. Agents Chemother.*, 40, 1376, 1996.

338. Mehlhorn, H., Dankert, W., Hartman, P. G., and Then, R. L., A pilot study on the efficacy of epiprim against developmental stages of *Toxoplasma gondii* and *Pneumocystis carinii* in animal models, *Parasitol. Res.*, 81, 296, 1995.

339. Chang, H. R., Arsenijevic, D., Comte, R., Polak, A., Then, R. L., and Pechère, J. C., Activity of epiroprim (Ro 11-8958), a dihydrofolate reductase inhibitor, alone and in combination with dapsone against *Toxoplasma gondii*, *Antimicrob. Agents Chemother.*, 38, 1803, 1994.

340. Luft, B. J., Potent *in vivo* activity of arprinocid, a purine analogue, against murine toxoplasmosis, *J. Infect. Dis.*, 154, 692, 1986.

341. Wang, C. C., Tolman, R. L., Simashkevich, P. M., and Stotish, R. L., Arprinocid, an inhibitor of hypoxanthine-guanine transport, *Biochem. Pharmacol.*, 28, 2249, 1979.

342. Perroto, J., Keister, D. B., and Gelderman, A. H., Incorporation of precursors into toxoplasma DNA, *J. Protozool.*, 18, 470, 1971.

343. Pfefferkorn, E. R. and Pfefferkorn, L. C., *Toxoplasma gondii*: specific labeling of nucleic acids of intracellular parasites in Lesch-Nyhan cells, *Exp. Parasitol.*, 41, 95, 1977.

344. Wang, C. C., Simashkevich, P. M., and Stotish, R. L., Mode of anticoccidial action of arprinocid, *Biochem. Pharmacol.*, 28, 2241, 1979.

345. Pfefferkorn, E. R., Eckel, M. E., and McAdams, E., *Toxoplasma gondii*: *in vivo* and *in vitro* studies of a mutant resistant to arprinocid-*N*-oxide, *Exp. Parasitol.*, 65, 282, 1988.

346. Darkin-Rattray, S. J., Gurnett, A. M., Myers, R. W., Dulski, P. M., Crumley, T. M., Allocco, J. J., Cannova, C., Meinke, P. T., Colletti, S. L., Bednarek, M. A., Singh, S. B., Goetz, M. A., Dombrowski, A. W., Polishook, J. D., and Schmatz, D. M., Apicidin: a novel antiprotozoal agent that inhibits parasite histone deacetylase, *Proc. Natl. Acad. Sci. U.S.A.*, 93, 13143, 1996.

347. Liesch, J. M., Sweeley, C. C., Staffeld, G. D., Anderson, M. S., Weber, D. J., and Scheffer, R. P., Structure of HC-toxin, a cyclic tetrapeptide from *Helminthosporium carbonum*, *Tetrahedron*, 38, 45, 1982.

348. Yoshida, M., Kijima, M., Akita, M., and Beppu, T., Potent and specific inhibition of mammalian histone deacetylase both *in vivo* and *in vitro* by trichostatin A, *J. Biol. Chem.*, 265, 17174, 1990.

349. Derouin, F. and Chastang, C., Enzyme immunoassay to assess effect of antimicrobial agents on *Toxoplasma gondii* in tissue culture, *Antimicrob. Agents Chemother.*, 32, 303, 1988.

350. Hofflin, J. M., Guptill, D. R., Araujo, F. G., and Remington, J. S., Difluoromethylornithine and formycin B in toxoplasmosis, *J. Infect. Dis.*, 152, 1101, 1985.

351. Lindsay, D. S. and Blagburn, B. L., Activity of diclazuril against *Toxoplasma gondii* in cultured cells and mice, *Am. J. Vet. Res.*, 55, 530, 1994.

352. Lindsay, D. S., Rippey, N. S., and Blagburn, B. L., Treatment of acute *Toxoplasma gondii* infections in mice, *J. Parasitol.*, 81, 315, 1995.

353. Khan, A. A., Slifer, T., Araujo, F. G., and Remington, J. S., Travafloxacin is active against *Toxoplasma gondii*, *Antimicrob. Agents Chemother.*, 40, 1855, 1996.

354. Bakhtari, S. K. and Jira, J., Chemotherapy of experimental toxoplasmosis with special reference to robenidine, *Folia Parasitol. (Praha)*, 35, 193, 1988.

355. Adarve Garcia, E., Escario, J., and Martinez Fernandez, A. R., Antitoxoplasmic effect of lactotrim, sulfamethoxazole and robenidine, *An. R. Acad. Farm.*, 48, 519, 1982.

356. Fayer, R., Melton, M. L., and Sheffield, H. G., Quinine inhibition of host cell penetration by *Toxoplasma gondii*, *Besnotia iellisoni* and *Sarcocystis* sp. *in vitro*, *J. Parasitol.*, 58, 595, 1972.

357. Fayer, R. L., Quinine inhibition of host cell penetration by eimerian sporozoites *in vitro*, *J. Parasitol.*, 57, 901, 1971.

358. Starzyk, J., Scheller, S., Szaflarski, J., Moskwa, M., and Stojko, A., Biological properties and clinical application of propolis. II. Studies on the antiprotozoan activity of ethanol extract of propolis, *Arzneimit.-Forsch.*, 27, 1198, 1977.

359. Krahenbuhl, J. L., Sharma, S. D., Ferraresi, R. W., and Remington, J. S., Effect of muramyl dipeptide treatment on resistance to infection with *Toxoplasma gondii* in mice, *Infect. Immun.*, 31, 716, 1981.

360. Araujo, F. G. and Slifer, T., Nonionic block copolymers potentiate activities of drugs for treatment of infections with *Toxoplasma gondii*, *Antimicrob. Agents Chemother.*, 39, 2696, 1995.

361. Krahenbuhl, J. L., Fukutomi, Y., and Gu, L., Treatment of acute experimental toxoplasmosis with investigational poloxamers, *Antimicrob. Agents Chemother.*, 37, 2265, 1993.

362. Tachibana, H., Yoshihara, E., Kaneda, Y., and Nakae, T., Protection of *Toxoplasma gondii*-infected mice by stearylamine-bearing liposomes, *J. Parasitol.*, 76, 352, 1990.

363. Aiumlamai, S., Fredriksson, G., Uggla, A., Kindahl, H., and Edqvist, L. E., The effect of *Toxoplasma gondii* infection in flunixin meglumine treated pregnant ewes as monitored by plasma levels of 15-ketodihydroprostaglandin F_2 alpha, progesterone, oestrone sulphate and ultrasound scanning, *Zentralbl. Veterinarmed. (A)*, 37, 23, 1990.

364. Hulinska, D., Sykora, J., and Zastera, M., Effect of cortisone on *Toxoplasma gondii* infection studied by electron microscopy, *Folia Parasitol. (Praha)*, 37, 207, 1990.

365. Pettersen, E. K., Destruction of *Toxoplasma gondii* by HCl solution, *Acta Pathol. Microbiol. Scand. Sect. B*, 87, 217, 1979.

366. Hamadto, N. H., Rashed, S. M., Marii, N. E., Sobhy, M. M., el-Ridi, A. M., and el-Fakahany, A. F., The effect of some drugs on acute toxoplasmosis in mice, *J. Egypt. Soc. Parasitol.*, 19, 523, 1989.

367. Werner, H. and Piekarski, G., Die wirkung von clotrimazol auf den erreger der toxoplasmose, *Toxoplasma gondii, Arzneimit.-Forsch.*, 26, 53, 1976.

368. Chao, C. C., Sharp, B. M., Pomeroy, C., Filice, G. A., and Peterson, P.K., Effects of morphine addiction on the pathogenesis of murine toxoplasmosis, *Adv. Exp. Med. Biol.*, 288, 223, 1991.

369. Mack, D. C. and McLeod, R., New micromethod to study the effect of antimicrobial agents on *Toxoplasma gondii*: comparison of sulfadoxine and sulfadiazine individually and in combination with pyrimethamine and study of clindamycin, metronidazole and cyclosporine A, *Antimicrob. Agents Chemother.*, 26, 26, 1984.

370. Derouin, F., Lacroix, C., Sumyuen, M. H., Romand, S., and Garin, Y. J., Experimental models of toxoplasmosis: pharmacological applications, *Parasite*, 2, 243, 1995.

371. Arribas, J. R., de Diego, J. A., Gamallo, C., and Vazquez, J. J., A new murine model of severe acute toxoplasma encephalitis, *J. Antimicrob. Chemother.*, 36, 503, 1995.

372. McNamara, J. J., Antibiotic therapy in compromised hosts, *Calif. Med.*, 119, 49, 1973.

373. Bushby, S. R. M., Combined antibacterial action *in vitro* of trimethoprim and sulfonamides, *Postgrad. Med. J.*, 45(Suppl.), 10, 1969.

374. Hitchings, G. H., Folate antagonists as antibacterial and antiprotozoal agents, *Ann. NY Acad. Sci.*, 186, 444, 1971.

375. Wong, B., Gold, W., Brown, A., Lange, M., Fried, R., Grieco, M., Mildvan, D., Giron, J., Tapper, M. L., Lerner, C. W., and Armstrong, D., Central nervous system toxoplasmosis in homosexual men and parenteral drug users, *Ann. Intern. Med.*, 100, 36, 1984.

376. Lehrer, R. I., Inhibition by sulfonamides of the candidacidal activity of human neutrophils, *J. Clin. Invest.*, 50, 2498, 1971.

377. Cavallito, J. C., Nichol, C. A., Brenkman, W. D., Jr., DeAngelis, R. C., Stickney, D. R., Simmons, W. S., and Sigel, C. W., Lipid-soluble inhibitors of dihydrofolate reductase. I. Kinetics, tissue distribution and extent of metabolism of pyrimethamine, methoprim and etoprim in the rat, dog and man, *Drug Metab. Dispos.*, 6, 329, 1978.

378. Weiss, L. M., Harris, C., Berger, M., Tanowitz, H. B., and Wittner, M., Pyrimethamine concentrations in serum and cerebrospinal fluid during treatment of acute toxoplasma encephalitis in patients with AIDS, *J. Infect. Dis.*, 157, 580, 1988.

379. Sfetsos, M., Panmyelopathie nach daraprim-anwendung bei toxoplasmose, *Med. Klin.*, 65, 1039, 1970.

380. Karsentz, J., Gorin, N. C., Valensi, P., Mornet, M., Najman, A., and Duhamel, G., Pancytopenia following pyrimethamine treatment of toxoplasmosis, *Nouv. Presse Med.*, 9, 265, 1980.

381. Pajor, A., Pancytopenia in a patient given pyrimethamine and sulphamethoxydiazine during pregnancy, *Arch. Gynecol. Obstet.*, 247, 215, 1990.

382. Boudes, P., Zittoun, J., and Sobel, A., Acute pancytopenia induced by pyrimethamine during treatment of cerebral toxoplasmosis associated with AIDS: role of dihydrofolate reductase inhibitors, *Ann. Med. Interne (Paris)*, 141, 183, 1990.

383. Nye, F. J., Treating toxoplasmosis, *J. Antimicrob. Chemother.*, 5, 244, 1979.

384. Van Delden, C. and Hirschel, B., Folinic acid supplements to pyrimethamine-sulfadiazine for *Toxoplasma* encephalitis are associated with better outcome, *J. Infect. Dis.*, 173, 1294, 1996.

385. O'Connor, G. P., Management of ocular toxoplasmosis, *Bull. NY Acad. Med.*, 50, 192, 1974.

386. Zytkovicz, T. H., Salter, J., Hennigan, L., Timperi, R., Maguire, J., and Hoff, R., Isocratic reversed-phase HPLC method to measure pyrimethamine extracted from plasma of infants treated for toxoplasmosis, *Clin. Chem.*, 37, 1281, 1991.

387. Roberts, W. L., Reynolds, K. M., Heimer, R., Jatlow, P. I., and Raincy, P. M., Pyrimethamine analysis by enzyme inhibition and HPLC assays, *Am. J. Clin. Pathol.*, 104, 82, 1995.
388. Piens, M. A. and Garir, J. P., New perspectives in the chemoprophylaxis of toxoplasmosis, *J. Chemother.*, 1, 46, 1989.
389. McCabe, R. E. and Oster, S., Current recommendations and future prospects in the treatment of toxoplasma, *Drugs*, 38, 973, 1989.
390. Georgiev, V. St., Opportunistic/nosocomial infections: treatment and developmental therapeutics. Toxoplasmosis, *Med. Res. Rev.*, 13, 529, 1993.
391. Georgiev, V. St., Management of toxoplasmosis, *Drugs*, 48, 179, 1994.
392. Boyer, K. M., Diagnosis and treatment of congenital toxoplasmosis, *Adv. Pediatr. Infect. Dis.*, 11, 449, 1996.
393. Behbahani, R., Moshfeghi, M., and Baxter, J. D., Therapeutic approaches for AIDS-related toxoplasmosis, *Ann. Pharmacother.*, 29, 960, 1995 (see comment in *Ann. Pharmacother.*, 29, 1303, 1995).
394. Lambotte, R., Toxoplasmose congenitale: evaluation du benefice therapeutique prenatal, *J. Gynecol. Obstet. Biol. Reprod. (Paris)*, 5, 265, 1976.
395. Bloch-Michel, E., Ocular toxoplasmosis in 1989, *Bull. Soc. Belge Ophthalmol.*, 230, 53, 1989.
396. Finielz, P., Chuet, C., Ramdane, M., and Guiserix, J., Treatment of cerebral toxoplasmosis in AIDS with cotrimoxazole, *Presse Med.*, 24, 917, 1995.
397. Holliman, R. E., Folate supplements and the treatment of cerebral toxoplasmosis, *Scand. J. Infect. Dis.*, 21, 475, 1989.
398. Grange, F., Kinney, E. L., Monsuez, J. J., Rybojad, M., Derouin, F., Khuong, M. A., and Janier, M., Successful therapy for *Toxoplasma gondii* myocarditis in acquired immunodeficiency syndrome, *Am. Heart J.*, 120, 443, 1990.
399. Piketty, C., Derouin, F., Rouveix, B., and Pocidalo, J. J., *In vivo* assessment of antimicrobial agents against *Toxoplasma gondii* by quantitation of parasites in the blood, lungs, and brain of infected mice, *Antimicrob. Agents Chemother.*, 34, 1467, 1990.
400. Gonzalez-Clemente, J. M., Miró, J. M., Pedrol, E., Alvarez, R., Gateil, J. M., Mallolas, J., Graus, F., Mercader, J. M., Guelar, A., Jimenez de Anta, M. T. et al., Encephalic toxoplasmosis in patients with acquired immunodeficiency syndrome. A clinico-radiological study and the therapeutic results in 78 cases, *Med. Clin. (Barcelona)*, 95, 441, 1990.
401. Holliman, R. E., Clinical and diagnostic findings in 20 patients with toxoplasmosis and acquired immune deficiency syndrome, *J. Med. Microbiol.*, 35, 1, 1991.
402. Cimino, C., Lipton, R. B., Williams, A., Feraru, E., Harris, C., and Hirschfeld, A., The evaluation of patients with human immunodeficiency virus-related disorders and brain mass lesions, *Arch. Intern. Med.*, 151, 1381, 1991.
403. Langmann, P., Klinker, H., and Richter, E., Pyrimethamine-sulphadiazine resistant cerebral toxoplasmosis in AIDS, *Dtsch. Med. Wochenschr.*, 120, 780, 1995.
404. Huber, W., Bautz, W., Classen, M., and Schepp, W., Pyrimethamine-sulfadiazine resistant cerebral toxoplasmosis in AIDS, *Dtsch. Med. Wochenschr.*, 120, 60, 1995.
405. Luft, B. J., Brooks, R. G., Conley, P. K., McCabe, R. E., and Remington, J. S., Toxoplasmic encephalitis in patients with acquired immune deficiency syndrome, *JAMA*, 252, 913, 1984.
406. Bell, E. T., Tapper, M. L., and Pollock, A. A., Sulphadiazine desensitization in AIDS patients, *Lancet*, 1, 163, 1985.
407. Tenant-Flowers, M., Boyle, M. J., Carey, D., Marriott, D. J., Harkness, J. L., Penny, R., and Cooper, D. A., Sulphadiazine desensitization in patients with AIDS and cerebral toxoplasmosis, *AIDS*, 5, 311, 1991.
408. Gilquin, J., Magar, Y., Acar, J. F., and Blamontier, J., Induction de tolerance a la sulfadiazine chez un malade atteint de syndrome d'immunodeficit acquit, *Presse Med.*, 17, 2306, 1988.
409. Leport, C., Tournerie, C., Raguin, G., Fernandez-Martin, J., Niyongabo, T., and Vildé, J.-L., Long-term follow-up of patients with AIDS on maintenance therapy for toxoplasmosis, *Eur. J. Clin. Microbiol. Infect. Dis.*, 10, 191, 1991.
410. Pedrol, E., Gonzalez-Clemente, J. M., Gateil, J. M., Mallolas, J., Miró, J. M., Graus, F., Alvarez, R., Mercader, J. M., Berenguer, J., Jimenez de Anta, M. T., Valls, M. E., and Soriano, E., Central nervous system toxoplasmosis in AIDS patients: efficacy of an intermittent maintenance therapy, *AIDS*, 4, 511, 1990.

411. Bhatti, N. and Larson, E., Low-dose alternate-day pyrimethamine for maintenance therapy in cerebral toxoplasmosis complicating AIDS, *J. Infect.*, 21, 119, 1990.

412. Heald, A., Flepp, J. M., Chave, J. P., Malinverni, R., Ruttimann, S., Gabriel, V., Renold, C., Sugar, A., Hirschel, B., and the Swiss HIV Cohort Study, Treatment for cerebral toxoplasmosis protects against *Pneumocystis carinii* pneumonia in patients with AIDS, *Ann. Intern. Med.*, 115, 760, 1991.

413. Michalova, K., Rihova, E., and Havlikova, M., Fansidar in the treatment of toxoplasmosis, *Cesk. Slov. Oftalmol.*, 52, 173, 1996.

414. Harland, C. C., Marsden, J.R., Vernon, S. A., and Allen, B. R., Dermatomyositis responding to treatment of associated toxoplasmosis, *Br. J. Dermatol.*, 125, 76, 1991.

415. Couvreur, J., In utero treatment of congenital toxoplasmosis with a pyrimethamine-sulfadiazine combination, *Presse Med.*, 20, 1136, 1991.

416. Couvreur, J., Thulliez, P., Daffos, F., Aufrant, C., Bompard, Y., Gesquiere, A., and Desmonts, G., Fetal toxoplasmosis: in utero treatment with pyrimethamine sulfamides, *Arch. Fr. Pediatr.*, 48, 397, 1991.

417. Boulot, P., Pratlong, F., Sarda, P., Deschamps, F., Hedon, B., Laffargue, F., and Viaia, J. L., Limitations of prenatal treatment of congenital toxoplasmosis with a sulfadiazine-pyrimethamine combination, *Presse Med.*, 31, 570, 1990.

418. Dorangeon, P., Fay, R., Marx-Chemba, C., Leroux, B., Harika, G., Dupouy, D., Quereux, C., Choisy, H., Pinon, J. M., and Wahl, P., Transplacental passage of the pyrimethamine-sulfadoxine combination in the prenatal treatment of congenital toxoplasmosis, *Presse Med.*, 19, 2036, 1990.

419. Cottrell, A. J., Acquired toxoplasma encephalitis, *Arch. Dis. Child.*, 61, 84, 1986.

420. Sabin, A. B., Toxoplasmic encephalitis in children, *JAMA*, 116, 801, 1941.

421. Rose, M. S., Black, P. J., and Barkhan, P., Fatal outcome after combined therapy for myeloblastic leukaemia and toxoplasmosis, *Lancet*, 1, 600, 1973.

422. Price, I. A., Bondy, P. K., and Ferench, G. E., Fatal outcome after combined therapy for myeloblastic leukaemia and toxoplasmosis, *Lancet*, 1, 727, 1973.

423. Bruce, W. R., Meeker, B. E., and Valeriote, F. A., Comparison of the sensitivity of normal hematopoietic and transplanted lymphoma colony-forming cells to chemotherapeutic agents administered *in vivo*, *J. Natl. Cancer Inst.*, 37, 233, 1966.

424. Valeriote, F. A. and Bruce, W. R., Comparison of the sensitivity of hematopoietic colony-forming cells in different proliferative states to vinblastine, *J. Natl. Cancer Inst.*, 38, 393, 1967.

425. Bruce, W. R. and Meeker, B. E., Comparison of the sensitivity of hematopoietic colony-forming cells in different proliferative states to 5-fluorouracil, *J. Natl. Cancer Inst.*, 38, 401, 1967.

426. Opravil, M., Keusch, G., and Luthy, R., Pyrimethamine inhibits renal secretion of creatinine, *Antimicrob. Agents Chemother.*, 37, 1056, 1993.

427. Simon, D. I., Brosius, F. C. III, and Rothstein, D. M., Sulfadiazine crystalluria revisited: the treatment of *Toxoplasma* encephalitis in patients with acquired immunodeficiency syndrome, *Arch. Intern. Med.*, 150, 2379, 1990.

428. Diaz, F., Collazos, J., Mayo, J., and Martinez, E., Sulfadiazine-induced multiple urolithiasis and acute renal failure in a patient with AIDS and *Toxoplasma* encephalitis, *Ann. Pharmacother.*, 30, 41, 1996.

429. Rodriguez-Carballeira, M., Casagran, A., More, J., Argilaga, R., and Garcia, M., Acute renal insufficiency caused by sulfadiazine in a patient with cerebral toxoplasmosis and AIDS, *Enfer. Infecc. Microbiol. Clin.*, 14, 125, 1996.

430. Becker, K., Jablonowski, H., and Haussinger, D., Sulfadiazine-associated nephrotoxicity in patients with the acquired immunodeficiency syndrome, *Medicine (Baltimore)*, 75, 185, 1996.

431. Peh, C. A., Kimber, T. E., Shaw, D. R., and Clarkson, A.R., Acute renal failure due to sulphadiazine in a patient with acquired immunodeficiency syndrome (AIDS), *Aust. NZ J. Med.*, 25, 58, 1995.

432. Potter, J. L. and Kofron, W. G., Sulfadiazine/N^4-acetylsulfadiazine crystalluria in a patient with the acquired immune deficiency syndrome (AIDS), *Clin. Chim. Acta*, 230, 221, 1994.

433. Bressollette, L., Carlhant, D., Bellein, V., Morand, C., Mottier, D., and Riche, C., Crystalluria induced by sulfadiazine in an AIDS patient, *Therapy*, 49, 154, 1994.

434. Furrer, H., von Overbeck, J., Jaeger, P., and Hess, B., Sulfadiazine nephrolithiasis and nephropathy, *Schweiz. Med. Wochenschr.*, 124, 2100, 1994.

435. Marques, L. P., Madeira, E. P., and Santos, O. R., Renal alterations induced by sulfadiazine therapy in an AIDS patient, *Clin. Nephrol.*, 42, 68, 1994 (see comments in *Clin. Nephrol.*, 39, 254, 1993).

436. Kronawitter, U., Jacob, K., Zoller, W. G., Rauh, G., and Goebel, F. D., Acute kidney failure caused by sulfadiazine stones: a complication of the therapy of toxoplasmosis in AIDS, *Dtsch. Med. Wochenschr.*, 118, 1683, 1993.

437. Hein, R., Brunkhorst, R., Thon, W. F., Schedel, I., and Schmidt, R. E., Symptomatic sulfadiazine crystalluria in AIDS patients: a report of two cases, *Clin. Nephrol.*, 39, 254, 1993 (comment in *Clin. Nephrol.*, 42, 68, 1994).

438. Farinas, M. C., Echevarria, S., Sampedro, I., Gonzalez, A., Gonzalez, A., Pérez del Molino, A., and Gonzalez-Macias, J., Renal failure due to sulphadiazine in AIDS patients with cerebral toxoplasmosis, *J. Intern. Med.*, 233, 365, 1993.

439. Diaz, F., Collazos, J., Mayo, J., and Martinez, E., Sulfadiazine-induced multiple urolithiasis and acute renal failure in a patient with AIDS and *Toxoplasma* encephalitis, *Ann. Pharmacother.*, 30, 41, 1996.

440. Carbone, L. G., Bendixen, B., and Appel, G. B., Sulfadiazine-associated obstructive nephropathy occurring in a patient with the acquired immunodeficiency syndrome, *Am. J. Kidney Dis.*, 12, 72, 1988.

441. Molina, J. M., Belefant, X., Doco-Lacompte, T., Idatte, J. M., and Modai, J., Sulfadiazine induced crystalluria in AIDS patients with toxoplasma encephalitis, *AIDS*, 5, 587, 1991.

442. Oster, S., Hutchinson, F., and McCabe, R., Resolution of acute renal failure in toxoplasmic encephalitis despite continuance of sulfadiazine, *Rev. Infect. Dis.*, 12, 618, 1990.

443. Caumes, E., Bocquet, H., Guermonprez, G., Rogeaux, O., Bricaire, F., Katlama, C., and Gentililini, M., Adverse cutaneous reactions to pyrimethamine/sulfadiazine and pyrimethamine/clindamycin in patients with AIDS and toxoplasmic encephalitis, *Clin. Infect. Dis.*, 21, 656, 1995.

444. Lafrenz, M., Ziegler, K., Saender, R., Budde, E., and Naumann, G., Treatment of toxoplasmosis, *Muenchen. Med. Wochenschr.*, 115, 2057, 1973.

445. Norrby, R. and Eilard, T., Recurrent toxoplasmosis, *Scand. J. Infect. Dis.*, 8, 275, 1976.

446. Greenlee, J. E., Johnson, W. D., Jr., Campa, J. F., Adelman, L. S., and Sande, M. A., Adult and cerebellar ataxia, *Ann. Intern. Med.*, 82, 367, 1975.

447. Williams, M. and Savage, D. C. L., Acquired toxoplasmosis in children, *Arch. Dis. Child.*, 53, 829, 1978.

448. Remington, J. S., Acquired toxoplasmosis in children, *Arch. Dis. Child.*, 55, 80, 1980.

449. Esposito, R., Lazzarin, A., Orlando, G., Gallo, M., and Foppa, C. U., ABC of AIDS: treatment of infections and antiviral agents, *Br. Med. J. (Clin. Res.)*, 295, 668, 1987.

450. Solbreux, P., Sonnet, J., and Zech, F., A retrospective study about the use of cotrimoxazole as diagnostic support and treatment of suspected cerebral toxoplasmosis in AIDS, *Acta Clin. Belg.*, 45, 85, 1990.

451. Jick, H., Adverse reactions to trimethoprim-sulfamethoxazole in hospitalized patients, *Rev. Infect. Dis.*, 4, 426, 1982.

452. Martin, C. and Mahon, R., Traitment de la toxoplasmose, *Nouv. Presse Med.*, 2, 2202, 1974.

453. Desmonts, G. and Couvreur, J., Congenital toxoplasmosis: a prospective study of 378 pregnancies, *N. Engl. J. Med.*, 290, 1110, 1974.

454. Desmonts, G., Couvreur, J., and Thulliez, P., Prophylaxis of congenital toxoplasmosis: effects of spiramycin on placental injection, *J. Antimicrob. Chemother.*, 22(Suppl.), 193, 1988.

455. Fortier, B., Ajana, F., Pinto de Sousa, M. I., Aissi, E., and Camus, D., Prevention and treatment of materno-fetal toxoplasmosis, *Presse Med.*, 20, 1374, 1991.

456. Koppe, J. G., Loewer-Siegler, D. H., and De Roever-Bonnet, H., Results of 20-year follow-up of congenital toxoplasmosis, *Lancet*, 1, 254, 1986.

457. Hohfeld, P., Dattos, F., Thilliez, P., Aufrant, C., Couvreur, J., MacAleese, J., Descombey, D., and Forestier, F., Fetal toxoplasmosis: outcome of pregnancy and infant follow-up after in utero treatment, *J. Pediatr.*, 115, 765, 1989.

458. Chodos, J. B. and Habegger-Chodos, H. E., The treatment of ocular toxoplasmosis with spiramycin, *Arch. Ophthalmol.*, 65, 401, 1961.

459. Fajardo, R. V., Furguiele, F. P., and Leopold, J. M., Treatment of toxoplasmosis uveitis, *Arch. Ophthalmol.*, 67, 712, 1962.

460. Cassidy, J. V., Bahler, J. W., and Minken, M. V., Spiramycin for toxoplasmosis, *Am. J. Ophthalmol.*, 57, 227, 1964.

461. Canamucio, C. J., Hallet, J. W., and Leopold, J. M., Recurrence of treated toxoplasmic uveitis, *Am. J. Ophthalmol.*, 55, 1035, 1963.

462. Timsit, J. C. and Bloch-Michel, E., Efficacite de la chimiotherapie specifique dans la prevention des recidives des chorioretinitis toxoplasmiques dans les quatre annees qui suivent la traitment, *J. Fr. Ophthalmol.*, 10, 15, 1987.

463. Descotes, J., Vial, T., Delattre, D., and Evreux, J. C., Spiramycin: safety in man, *Antimicrob. Agents Chemother.*, 22(Suppl. B), 207, 1988.

464. Ostlere, L. S., Langtry, J. A., and Staughton, R. C., Allergy to spiramycin during prophylactic treatment of fetal toxoplasmosis, *Br. Med. J.*, 302, 970, 1991.

465. Kawakami, Y., Hayashi, J., Fujisaki, T., Tani, Y. et al., A case of toxoplasmosis with dermatomyositis, *Kansenshogaku Zasshi*, 69, 1312, 1995.

466. Dannemann, B. R., Israelski, D. M., and Remington, J. S., Treatment of toxoplasmic encephalitis with intravenous clindamycin, *Arch. Intern. Med.*, 148, 2477, 1988.

467. Remington, J. S. and Vildé, J.-L., Clindamycin for toxoplasma encephalitis in AIDS, *Lancet*, 338, 1142, 1991.

468. Santos Gil, I., Noguerado Asensio, A., del Arco Galan, C., and Garcia Polo, I., Clindamycin in the treatment of cerebral toxoplasmosis in a patient with AIDS, *Rev. Clin. Esp.*, 185, 47, 1989.

469. Westblom, T. U. and Belshe, R. B., Clindamycin therapy of cerebral toxoplasmosis in an AIDS patient, *Scand. J. Infect. Dis.*, 20, 561, 1988.

470. Goldsmith, J. M., Toxoplasmosis and clindamycin, *S. Afr. Med. J.*, 57, 37, 1980.

471. Marcos, C., Sopena, B., Luna, I., Gonzalez, R., de la Fuente, J., and Martinez-Vazquez, C., Clindamycin desensitization in an AIDS patient, *AIDS*, 9, 1201, 1995.

472. Rolston, K. V. I., Clindamycin in cerebral toxoplasmosis, *Am. J. Med.*, 85, 254, 1988.

473. Rolston, K. V., Treatment of acute toxoplasmosis with oral clindamycin, *Eur. J. Clin. Microbiol. Infect. Dis.*, 10, 181, 1991.

474. Ruf, B. and Pohle, H. D., Role of clindamycin in the treatment of acute toxoplasmosis of the central nervous system, *Eur. J. Clin. Microbiol. Infect. Dis.*, 10, 183, 1991.

475. Dannemann, B. R., McCutchan, J. A., Israelski, D. M., Antoniskis, D., Leport, C., Luft, B. J., Chiu, J., Vildé, J.-L., Nussbaum, J. N., Orellana, M., Heseltine, P. N. C., Leedom, J. M., Clumeck, N., Morlat, P., Remington, J. S., and the California Collaborative Treatment Group, Treatment of acute toxoplasmosis with intravenous clindamycin, *Eur. J. Clin. Microbiol. Infect. Dis.*, 10, 193, 1991.

476. Dannemann, B., MacCutchan, J. A., Israelski, D., Antoniskis, D., Leport, C., Luft, B., Nussbaum, J., Clumeck, N., Morlat, P., Chiu, J., Vildé, J.-L., Orellana, M. M., Feigal, D., Bartok, A., Heseltine, P., Leedom, J., Remington, J. S., and the California Collaborative Treatment Group, Treatment of toxoplasmic encephalitis in patients with AIDS: a randomized trial comparing pyrimethamine plus clindamycin to pyrimethamine plus sulfadiazine, *Ann. Intern. Med.*, 116, 33, 1992.

477. Katlama, C., Evaluation of the efficacy and safety of clindamycin plus pyrimethamine for induction and maintenance therapy of toxoplasmic encephalitis in AIDS, *Eur. J. Clin. Microbiol. Infect. Dis.*, 10, 189, 1991.

478. Foppa, C. U., Bini, T., Gregis, G., Lazzarin, A., Esposito, R., and Moroni, M., A retrospective study of primary and maintenance therapy of toxoplasmic encephalitis with oral clindamycin and pyrimethamine, *Eur. J. Clin. Microbiol. Infect. Dis.*, 10, 187, 1991.

479. Leport, C., Bastuji-Garin, S., Perronne, C., Salmon, D., Marche, C., Bricaire, F., and Vildé, J.-L., An open study of the pyrimethamine-clindamycin combination in AIDS patients with brain toxoplasmosis, *J. Infect. Dis.*, 160, 557, 1989.

480. Cohn, J. A., McMeeking, A., Cohen, W., Jacobs, J., and Holzman, R. S., Evaluation of the policy of empiric treatment of suspected *Toxoplasma* encephalitis in patients with acquired immunodeficiency syndrome, *Am. J. Med.*, 86, 521, 1989.

481. Dhiver, C., Milandre, C., Poizot-Martin, I., Drogoul, M. P., Gastaut, J. L., and Gastaut, J. A., 5-Fluoro-uracil-clindamycin for treatment of cerebral toxoplasmosis, *AIDS*, 7, 143, 1993.

482. Dalston, M. O., Tavares, W., Bazin, A. R., Hahn, M. D. et al., Clarithromycin combined with pyrimethamine in cerebral toxoplasmosis: a report of 2 cases, *Rev. Soc. Bras. Med. Trop.*, 28, 409, 1995.

483. Lacassin, F., Schaffo, D., Perronne, C., Longuet, P., Leport, C., and Vildé, J.-L., Clarithromycin-minocycline combination as salvage therapy for toxoplasmosis in patients infected with human immunodeficiency virus, *Antimicrob. Agents Chemother.*, 39, 276, 1995.

484. Sellal, A., Rabaud, C., Amiel, C., Hoen, B., May, T., and Canton, Ph., Maintenance treatment of cerebral toxoplasmosis in AIDS: role of clarithromycin-minocycline combination, *Presse Med.*, 25, 509, 1996.

485. Alba, D., Molina, F., Ripoli, M. M., and del Arco, A., Clarithromycin in the treatment of cerebral toxoplasmosis associated with HIV infection, *Rev. Clin. Esp.*, 192, 458, 1993.

486. Saba, J., Morlat, P., Raffi, F., Hazebroucq, V., Joly, V., Leport, C., and Vildé, J.-L., Pyrimethamine plus azithromycin for treatment of acute toxoplasmic encephalitis in patients with AIDS, *Eur. J. Clin. Microbiol. Infect. Dis.*, 12, 853, 1993.

487. Godofsky, E. W., Treatment of presumed cerebral toxoplasmosis with azithromycin, *N. Engl. J. Med.*, 330, 575, 1994.

488. Valencia, M. E., Laguna, F., Soriano, V., and Gonzalez Lahoz, J., Favorable course of cerebral toxoplasmosis treated with doxycycline and pyrimetamine, *Rev. Clin. Esp.*, 192, 197, 1993.

489. Hagberg, L., Palmertz, B., and Lindberg, J., Doxycycline and pyrimethamine for toxoplasmic encephalitis, *Scand. J. Infect. Dis.*, 25, 157, 1993.

490. Clumeck, N., Katlama, C., Ferrero, T. et al., Atovaquone (1,4-hydroxynaphthoquinone, 566C80) in the treatment of acute cerebral toxoplasmosis (CT) in AIDS patients, *Proc. 32nd Intersci. Conf. Antimicrob. Agents Chemother.*, American Society for Microbiology, Washington, D.C., Abstr. 1217, 1992.

491. Grundman, M., Torres, R. A., Thorn, M., Hriso, and Britton, D., Neuroradiologic response to 566C80 salvage therapy for CNS toxoplasmosis, *Proc. VIIth Int. Conf. AIDS*, Amsterdam, Abstr. PoB 3185, 1992.

492. Kovacs, J. A., NIAID-Clinical CIAIDSP: efficacy of atovaquone in treatment of toxoplasmosis in patients with AIDS, *Lancet*, 340, 637, 1992.

493. Lafeuillade, A., Pellegrino, P., Poggi, C., Profizi, N., Quilichini, R., Chonette, I., and Navarreté, M. S., Efficacité de l'atovaquone dans les toxoplasmoses résistantes du SIDA, *Presse Med.*, 22, 1708, 1993.

494. Bouboulis, D. A., Rubinstein, A., Shliozberg, J., Madden, J., and Frieri, M., Cerebral toxoplasmosis in childhood and adult HIV infection treated with 1,4-hydroxynaphthoquinone and rapid desensitization with pyrimethamine, *Ann. Allergy Asthma Immunol.*, 74, 491, 1995.

495. Schimkat, M., Althaus, C., Armbrecht, C., Jablonowski, H., and Sundmacher, R., Treatment of toxoplasmosis retinochoroiditis with atovaquone in an AIDS patient, *Klin. Monatsbl. Augenheilkd.*, 206, 173, 1995.

496. Durand, J. M., Cretel, E., Bagneres, D., Guillemot, E., Kaplanski, G., and Soubeyrand, J., Failure of atovaquone in the treatment of cerebral toxoplasmosis, *AIDS*, 9, 812, 1995.

497. Katlama, C., Mouthon, B., Gourdon, D., Lapierre, D., and Rousseau, F., Atovaquone as long-term suppressive therapy for toxoplasmic encephalitis in patients with AIDS and multiple drug intolerance, *AIDS*, 10, 1107, 1996.

498. Masur, H., Polis, M. A., Tuazon, C. U., Ogata-Arakaki, D., Kovacs, J. A., Katz, D., Hilt, D., Simmons, T., Feuerstein, I., Lundgren, B., Lane, H. C., Chabner, B. A., and Allegra, C. J., Salvage trial of trimetrexate-leucovorin for the treatment of cerebral toxoplasmosis in patients with AIDS, *J. Infect. Dis.*, 167, 1422, 1993.

499. Antinori, A., Murri, R., Ammassari, A., De Luca, A., Linzalone, A., Cingolani, A., Damiano, F., Maiuro, G., Vecchiet, J., Scoppettuolo, G., Tamburrini, E., and Ortona, L., Aerosolized pentamidine, cotrimoxazole and dapsone-pyrimethamine for primary prophylaxis of *Pneumocystis carinii* pneumonia and toxoplasmic encephalitis, *AIDS*, 9, 1343, 1995.

500. Nielsen, T. L., Jensen, B. N., Nelsing, S., Mathiesen, L. R., Skinhoj, P., and Nielsen, J. O., Randomized study of sulfamethoxazole-trimethoprim versus aerosolized pentamidine for secondary prophylaxis of *Pneumocystis carinii* pneumonia in patients with AIDS, *Scand. J. Infect. Dis.*, 27, 217, 1995.

501. Klinker, H., Langmann, P., and Richter, E., Pyrimethamine alone as prophylaxis for cerebral toxoplasmosis in patients with advanced HIV infection, *Infection*, 24, 324, 1996.

502. Jacobson, M. A., Besch, C. L., Child, C., Hafner, R., Matts, J. P., Muth, K., Wentworth, D. N., Neaton, J. D., Abrams, D., Rimland, D., Perez, G., Grant, I. H., Sarovalatz, L. D., Brown, L. S., Deyton, L., and the Terry Bairn Community Programs for Clinical Research on AIDS, Primary prophylaxis with pyrimethamine for toxoplasmic encephalitis in patients with advanced human immunodeficiency virus disease: results of a randomized trial, *J. Infect. Dis.*, 169, 384, 1994.

503. Van Delden, C., Gabriel, V., Sudre, P., Flepp, M., von Overbeck, J., Hirschel, B., and the Swiss HIV Cohort Study, Reasons for failure of prevention of *Toxoplasma* encephalitis, *AIDS*, 10, 509, 1996.

504. Tabbara, K. F., Ocular toxoplasmosis: toxoplasmic retinochoroiditis, *Int. Ophthalmol. Clin.*, 35, 15, 1995.

505. Chakroun, M., Meyohas, M. C., Pelosse, B., Zazoun, L., Vacherot, B., Derouin, F., and Leport, C., Ocular toxoplasmosis in AIDS, *Ann. Med. Interne (Paris)*, 141, 472, 1990.

506. Blanc-Jouvan, M., Boibieux, A., Fleury, J., Fourcade, N., Gandilhon, F., Dupouy-Camet, J., Peyron, F., and Ducerf, C., Chorioretinitis following liver transplantation: detection of *Toxoplasma gondii* in aqueous humor, *Clin. Infect. Dis.*, 22, 184, 1996.

507. Peacock, J. E., Jr., Greven, C. M., Cruz, J. M., and Hurd, D. D., Reactivation of toxoplasmic retinochoroiditis in patients undergoing bone marrow transplantation: is there a role for chemoprophylaxis? *Bone Marrow Transplant.*, 15, 983, 1995.

508. Engstrom, R. E., Jr., Holland, G. N., Nussenblatt, R. B., and Jabs, D. A., Current practices in the management of ocular toxoplasmosis, *Am. J. Ophthalmol.*, 111, 601, 1991.

509. Ronday, M. J., Luyendijk, L., Baarsma, G. S., Bollemeijer, J. G., Van der Lelij, A., and Rothova, A., Presumed acquired ocular toxoplasmosis, *Arch. Ophthalmol.*, 113, 1524, 1995.

510. Mittelviefhaus, H., Treatment of ocular toxoplasmosis. II. Therapeutic approaches, *Kinderarztl. Prax.*, 61, 154, 1993.

511. Mittelviefhaus, H., Treatment of ocular toxoplasmosis. I. Basic principles and diagnosis, *Kinderarztl. Prax.*, 61, 90, 1993.

512. Rothova, A., Ocular involvement in toxoplasmosis, *Br. J. Ophthalmol.*, 77, 371, 1993 (correction in *Br. J. Ophthalmol.*, 77, 683, 1993).

513. Rothova, A., Meenken, C., Buitenhuis, H. J., Brinkman, C. J., Baarsma, G. S., Boen-Tan, T. N., de Jong, P. T. V. M., Klaasen-Broekma, N., Schweitzer, C. M. C., Timerman, Z., de Vries, J., Zaal, M. J. W., and Kijlstra, A., Therapy of ocular toxoplasmosis, *Am. J. Ophthalmol.*, 115, 517, 1993.

514. Psilas, K., Petroutsos, G., and Aspiotis, M., Treatment of toxoplasmosis, *J. Fr. Ophthalmol.*, 13, 551, 1990.

515. Lebech, A. M., Lebech, M., Borme, K. K., and Mathiesen, L. R., Toxoplasmosis-chorioretinitis: clinical course and treatment of seven patients, *Ugeskr. Laeger*, 158, 3935, 1996.

516. Morlat, P., Vimard, E., Rabaud, C., Katlama, C. et al., Ocular toxoplasmosis in HIV infected patients: a French National Survey, *Proc. 35th Intersci. Conf. Antimicrob. Agents Chemother.*, American Society for Microbiology, Washington, D.C., Abstr. I35, 1995, 211.

517. Lam, S. and Tessler, H. H., Quadruple therapy for ocular toxoplasmosis, *Can. J. Ophthalmol.*, 28, 58, 1993.

518. Rothova, A., Buitenhuls, H. J., Meenken, C., Baarsma, G. S., Boen-Tan, T. N., de Jong, P. T., Schweitzer, C. M., Timmerman, Z., de Vries, J., Zaal, M. J., and Kijlstra, A., Therapy of ocular toxoplasmosis. *Int. Ophthalmol.*, 13, 415, 1989.

519. Colin, J. and Harie, J. C., Presumed toxoplasmic chorioretinitis: comparative study of treatment with pyrimethamine and sulfadiazine or clindamycin, *J. Fr. Ophthalmol.*, 12, 161, 1989.

520. Hansen, L. L., Nieuwenhuis, I., Hoeffken, G., and Heise, W., Retinitis in AIDS patients: diagnosis, follow-up and treatment, *Fortschr. Ophthalmol.*, 86, 232, 1988.

521. Theodossiadis, G. P., Koutsandrea, C., and Tzonou, A., A comparative study concerning the treatment of active toxoplasmic retinochoroiditis with argon laser and medication (follow-up 2–9 years), *Ophthalmologica*, 199, 77, 1989.

522. Lopez, J. S., de Smet, M. D., Masur, H., Mueller, B. U., Pizzo, P. A., and Nessenblatt, R. B., Orally administered 566C80 for treatment of ocular toxoplasmosis in a patient with the acquired immunodeficiency syndrome, *Am. J. Ophthalmol.*, 113, 331, 1992.

523. Tassignon, M. J., Brihaye, M., De Meuter, F., Vercruysse, A., Van Hoof, F., and De Wilde, F., Efficacy of treatments in experimental toxoplasmosis, *Bull. Soc. Belge Ophthalmol.*, 230, 59, 1989.

524. Fish, R. H., Hoskins, J. C., and Kline, L. B., Toxoplasmosis neuroretinitis, *Ophthalmology*, 100, 1177, 1993.

525. Falcone, P. M., Notis, C., and Merhige, K., Toxoplasmic papillitis as the initial manifestation of acquired immunodeficiency syndrome, *Ann. Ophthalmol.*, 25, 56, 1993.

526. Gallin, J. I., Farber, J. M., Holland, S. M., and Nitman, T. B., Interferon-gamma in the management of infectious diseases (clinical conference), *Ann. Intern. Med.*, 123, 216, 1995 (see comments in *Ann. Intern. Med.*, 124, 1095, 1996).

527. McCabe, R. E., Luft, B. J., and Remington, J. S., Effect of murine interferon gamma on murine toxoplasmosis, *J. Infect. Dis.*, 150, 961, 1984.

528. Shirahata, T., Yamashita, T., Ohta, C., Goto, H., and Nakane, A., CD8+ T lymphocytes are the major cell population involved in the early gamma interferon response and resistance to acute primary *Toxoplasma gondii* infection in mice, *Microbiol. Immunol.*, 38, 789, 1994.

529. Gomez Marin, J. E., Bonhomme, A., Guenounou, M., and Pinon, J. M., Role of interferon-gamma against invasion by *Toxoplasma gondii* in a human monocytic cell line (THP1): involvement of the parasite's secretory phospholipase A_2, *Cell Immunol.*, 169, 218, 1996.

530. Rytel, M. W. and Jones, T. C., Induction of interferon in mice infected with *Toxoplasma gondii*, *Proc. Soc. Exp. Biol. Med.*, 123, 859, 1966.

531. Freshman, M. M., Merigan, T. C., and Remington, J.S., *In vitro* and *in vivo* antiviral action of an interferon-like substance introduced by *Toxoplasma gondii*, *Proc. Soc. Exp. Biol. Med.*, 123, 862, 1966.

532. Remington, J. S. and Merigan, T. C., Interferon: protection of cells infected with an intracellular protozoan (*Toxoplasma gondii*), *Science*, 161, 804, 1968.

533. Ahronheim, G. A., *Toxoplasma gondii*: human interferon studies by plaque assay, *Proc. Soc. Exp. Biol. Med.*, 161, 522, 1979.

534. Pfefferkorn, E. P. and Guyre, P. M., Inhibition of growth of *Toxoplasma gondii* in cultured fibroblasts by human recombinant gamma interferon, *Infect. Immun.*, 44, 211, 1984.

535. Pfefferkorn, E. P., Interferon-gamma blocks the growth of *Toxoplasma gondii* in human fibroblasts by inducing the host cells to degrade tryptophan, *Proc. Natl. Acad. Sci. U.S.A.*, 81, 908, 1984.

536. Nathan, C. F., Murray, H. W., Wiebe, M. E., and Rubin, B. Y., Identification of interferon gamma as the lymphokine that activates human macrophages oxidative metabolism and antimicrobial activity, *J. Exp. Med.*, 158, 670, 1983.

537. Israelski, D. and Remington, J., Activity of gamma interferon in combination with pyrimethamine or clindamycin in treatment of murine toxoplasmosis, *Eur. J. Clin. Microbiol. Infect. Dis.*, 9, 358, 1990.

538. Hafeneider, S. H., Conlan, P. J., Henney, C. S., and Gillis, S., *In vivo* interleukin-2 administration augments the generation of alloreactive T lymphocytes and resident natural killer cells, *J. Immunol.*, 130, 222, 1983.

539. Wagner, H., Hardt, C., Heeg, K., Rolinghoff, M., and Pfizenmaier, K., T-cell-derived helper factor allows *in vivo* induction of cytotoxic T cells in nu/nu mice, *Nature*, 284, 278, 1980.

540. Cheever, M. A., Greenberg, P. D., Fefer, A., and Gillis, S., Augmentation of the antitumor therapeutic efficacy of long-term, cultured T-lymphocytes by *in vivo* administration of purified interleukin-2, *J. Exp. Med.*, 155, 968, 1983.

541. Malkovsky, M., Medawar, P. B., Hunt, F. R. S., Palmer, L., and Dore, C., A diet enriched in vitamin A acetate or *in vivo* administration of interleukin 2 can counteract a tolerogenic stimulus, *Proc. R. Soc. London*, 220, 439, 1984.

542. Hoffenbach, A., Lagrange, P. H., and Bach, M. A., Deficit of interleukin 2 production associated with impaired T-cell proliferation responses in *Mycobacterium lepraemurium* infection, *Infect. Immun.*, 39, 109, 1983.

543. Hibbs, J. B., Jr., Lambert, L. H., Jr., and Remington, J. S., Adjuvant induced resistance to tumor development in mice, *Proc. Soc. Biol. Med.*, 139, 1053, 1972.

544. Hauser, W. E., Jr., Sharma, S. D., and Remington, J. S., Natural killer cells induced by acute and chronic *Toxoplasma* infection, *Cell. Immunol.*, 69, 330, 1982.

545. Suzuki, Y., Watanabe, N., and Kobayashi, A., Non-specific suppression of primary antibody responses and presence of plastic-adherent suppressor cells in *Toxoplasma gondii*-infected mice, *Infect. Immun.*, 32, 30, 1981.

546. Coolizzi, V., *In vivo* and *in vitro* administration of interleukin-2- containing preparation reverses T-cell unresponsiveness in *Mycobacterium bovis* BCG-infected mice, *Infect. Immun.*, 45, 25, 1984.

547. Sharma, S. D., Hofflin, J. M., and Remington, J. S., *In vivo* recombinant interleukin 2 administration enhances survival against a lethal challenge with *Toxoplasma gondii*, *J. Immunol.*, 135, 4160, 1955.

548. Hatcher, F. M. and Kuhn, R. E., Natural killer (NK) cell activity against extracellular forms of *Trypanozoma cruzi*, in *NK Cells and Other Natural Effector Cells*, Herberman, R. B., Ed., Academic Press, New York, 1982, 1091.

549. Huldt, G., Gard, S., and Olovson, S. E., Effect of *Toxoplasma gondii* on thymus, *Nature*, 244, 301, 1973.

550. Fegies, M. and Guerrero, J., Treatment of toxoplasmosis with levamisole, *Trans. R. Soc. Trop. Med. Hyg.*, 71, 178, 1977.
551. Zastera, M., Fruehbauer, Z., and Pokorny, J., Levamisole therapy of experimental toxoplasmosis in white mice, *Cesk. Epidemiol. Mikrobiol. Immunol.*, 31, 94, 1982.
552. Youssef, M. Y., el-Ridi, A. M., Arafa, M. S., el-Sawy, M. T., and el- Sayed, W. M., Effect of levamisole on toxoplasmosis during pregnancy in guinea pigs, *J. Egypt. Soc. Parasitol.*, 15, 41, 1985.
553. Stadtsbaeder, S., Nguyen, B. T., and Calvin-Preval, M. C., Respective role of antibodies and immune macrophages during acquired immunity against toxoplasmosis in mice, *Ann. Immunol. (Inst. Pasteur)*, 126(C), 461, 1975.
554. Stadtsbaeder, S., Piter, L., and Clotuche De Bruyn, L., Immunisation contre la toxoplasmose chez la souris, *Lyon Medic.*, 225, 175, 1971.
555. Jones, T.C., Len, L., and Hirsch, J. G., Assessment *in vitro* of immunity against *Toxoplasma gondii*, *J. Exp. Med.*, 141, 466, 1975.
556. Remington, J. S., Krahenbuhl, J. L., and Mendenhall, J. W., A role for activated macrophages in resistance to infection with *Toxoplasma*, *Infect. Immun.*, 6, 829, 1972.
557. Debard, N., Buzoni-Gatel, D., and Bout, D., Intranasal immunization with SAG1 protein of *Toxoplasma gondii* in association with cholera toxin dramatically reduces development of cerebral cysts after oral infection, *Infect. Immun.*, 64, 2158, 1996.
558. Nguyen, B. T. and Stadtsbaeder, S., Comparative biological and antitoxoplasmic effects of particulate and water-soluble polysaccharides, *in vitro*, *Adv. Exp. Med. Biol.*, 121(A), 255, 1979.
559. Di Luzio, N. R., Pharmacology of the reticuloendothelial system — accent on glucan, *Adv. Exp. Med. Biol.*, 73(A), 412, 1976.
560. Delville, J. and Jacques, P. J., Therapeutic effect of yeast glucan in mice infected with *Mycobacterium leprae*, *Arch. Int. Physiol. Biochem.*, 85, 965, 1977.
561. Lyche, E., Lund, E., Strannegard, O., and Falsen, E., The effect of immune system and activator on the fertility of *Toxoplasma gondii* for cell culture, *Acta Pathol. Microbiol. Scand.*, 63, 206, 1965.
562. Strannegard, O. and Lyche, E., Properdin and the antibody-effect on *Toxoplasma gondii*, *Acta Pathol. Microbiol. Scand.*, 66, 227, 1966.
563. Sander, J. and Midtvedt, T., Development of sulphonamide resistance in *Toxoplasma gondii*, *Acta Pathol. Microbiol. Scand. (B) Microbiol. Immunol.*, 79, 531, 1971.
564. Lai, C. H., Tizard, I. R., and Ingram, D. C., Development of a sulphonamide resistant strain of *Toxoplasma gondii*, *Trans. R. Soc. Med. Hyg.*, 68, 257, 1974.
565. Pfefferkorn, E. R. and Pfefferkorn, L. C., Arabinosyl nucleosides inhibit *Toxoplasma gondii* and allow the selection of resistant mutants, *J. Parasitol.*, 62, 993, 1976.
566. Pfefferkorn, E. R. and Pfefferkorn, L. C., *Toxoplasma gondii*: characterization of a mutant resistant to 5-fluorodeoxyuridine, *Exp. Parasitol.*, 42, 44, 1977.
567. Pfefferkorn, E. R., Characterization of a mutant of *Toxoplasma gondii* resistant to aphidicolin, *J. Parasitol.*, 31, 306, 1984.
568. Oguro, M., Suzuki-Hori, C., Nagano, H., Mano, Y., and Ikegami, S., The mode of inhibitory action by aphidicolin on eukaryotic DNA polymerase, *Eur. J. Biochem.*, 97, 603, 1979.

23 Microsporidia

23.1 INTRODUCTION

Microsporidia is a nontaxonomic designation used commonly to describe a group of obligate intracellular parasites classified under the order Microsporida, phylum Microspora, class Microsporea. Their primary habitat is invertebrates, especially arthropods, although they were also found in lower and very rarely in higher vertebrates. Microsporida comprises two suborders: Pansporoblastina and Apansporoblastina.

First discovered by Nägeli in 1857 in silkworms,[1] microsporidia can be isolated in a wide array of invertebrates and all classes of vertebrates.[2-7] Currently, more than 100 microsporidial genera and nearly 1000 species have been identified. In addition to living organisms, microsporidia have been found also in ditch water.[8]

Morphologically, microsporidia are small unicellular parasites which are considered to be eukaryotic organisms because of the presence of a nucleus with a nuclear envelope, an intracytoplasmic membrane system, and chromosome separation on mitotic spindles.[3,9] However, they also share prokaryotic features: in addition to the small rRNA which is of prokaryotic size, they also lack mitochondria, peroxisomes, and Golgi membranes.[2] The microsporidia spores contain a characteristic extrusible polar tube which serves as a passage for inoculation of the infectious agent (sporoplasm) into host cells.

Some microsporidial species may develop in particular host cells of a single organ system, while others may cause systemic infections involving different organ systems.[2] *Enterocytozoon bieneusi* appears to exhibit a strong preference for small intestinal epithelium.[10] Its development occurs predominantly in the apical cytoplasm, especially in the Golgi region immediately above the nucleus.[11-13] It seems likely that this may be the preferred site of morphogenesis since as microsporidians lack mitochondria they must rely on those of the host cells which are particularly rich in this region of the cytoplasma.[14] It is of interest to note that *E. bieneusi* displays strong preference for infecting absorptive cells; only rarely it is seen in goblet or enterochromatin cells.[11]

In 1957, Matsubayashi et al.[15] diagnosed the first case of microsporidiosis in humans. Subsequently, several more cases were reported.[2,16-18] Initially, microsporidia species pathogenic to humans have been classified in five genera: *Enterocytozoon* spp. (*E. bieneusi*), *Encephalitozoon* spp. (*Encephalitozoon cuniculi, E. hellem*), *Septata* spp. (*Septata intestinalis*), *Nosema* spp. (*Nosema connori, N. corneum, N. ocularum*), and *Pleistophora* sp., as well as a number of unclassified microsporidial organisms collectively referred to as *Microsporidium* sp. (*Microsporidium ceylonensis*, and *M. africanum*). However, based on genetic and immunologic studies, recently, *Septata intestinalis* has been reclassified to *Encephalitozoon intestinalis*.[19] The potential sources and means of transmission of human microsporidial infections are still not very clear.[2] It is likely that parasites may be ingested via food contaminated with spores, which are resistant to environmental extremes and can survive for months, or via insect stings.[20,21] Inside the host, ingested spores travel to the intestine where the polar tubules of the parasite evert, penetrate the intestinal epithelial cells, and inject their cellular contents, or sporoplasm, into these host cells.[22] The latter eventually rupture and release spores that infect other nearby cells or travel hematogenously or via infected macrophages to other organs, such as liver, brain, and kidney.[3,17,23]

Microsporidia have been recognized as opportunistic pathogens[24,25] in immunocompromised patients[3,16,18,26,27] and those with AIDS,[16,18,23,26,28-31] and three new microsporidial species, *E. intestinalis,*[32-38] *E. hellem,*[20,39] and *E. bieneusi*[20,40] were first isolated from AIDS patients. In addition, *E. bieneusi* has also been isolated from immunocompetent patients[41,42] and from an immunocompromised patient secondary to organ transplantation.[2]

It should be noted that any imbalance of host-parasite interactions may result in proliferation and dissemination of the parasites, causing destruction of the host cells.[2] One unexpected occurrence during a case of dissemination of *E. hellem* has been the parasitic infestation of respiratory epithelial-lining cells extending from the proximal trachea distally into small-order conducting airways.[39]

Disease manifestations may vary depending on the infecting species, mode of infection, age of the host at the time of infection, and the competence of the host's immune response.[16,18] The number of sufficiently documented cases of microsporidiosis among non-HIV-infected patients is rather limited.[16-18,26] However, the number of cases of microsporidiosis in HIV-infected patients has been in the hundreds.[26] Thus, in HIV-positive patients, *E. bieneusi* has been associated with diarrhea and wasting syndrome,[40,43,44] cholecystitis and cholangitis,[45,46] bronchitis and pneumonia,[47] and sinusitis and rhinitis;[48,49] *E. cuniculi* with fulminant hepatitis,[50] peritonitis,[51] and disseminated infection;[52] *E. hellem* with keratoconjunctivitis and conjunctivitis,[20] disseminated infection (tubulointerstitial nephritis, ureteritis, cystitis, keratoconjuctivitis, and colonization of bronchial epithelium),[39,53] prostatic abscess,[54] and bronchiolitis and pneumonia;[55] *E. intestinalis* with diarrhea, and disseminated infection (tubulointerstitial nephritis, diarrhea, and cholecystitis);[32-35] *Pleistophora* sp. with myositis.[22] In addition, some undesignated *Encephalitozoon* species have been found to cause keratoconjunctivitis,[56] and sinusitis and nasal polyps.[57,58] Blanshard et al.[59] have recorded the first case in an AIDS patient of intestinal microsporidiosis involving simultaneous infection with two different types of microsporidia: *E. bieneusi* and a non-*E. bieneusi* microsporidian.

Enterocytozoon bieneusi is currently the most commonly recognized microsporidian species in humans.[60] With very few exceptions, it has been found predominantly in HIV-positive patients.[13,36,61,62] In 7% to 50% of severely immunodeficient patients (CD4+ cell counts below 100/mm³), *E. bieneusi* has been associated with chronic diarrhea which has been difficult to treat.[11,36,63-69] In HIV-infected patients with less severe cellular immunodeficiency (CD4+ cell counts above 100 to 200/mm³), *E. bieneusi* may cause a self-limiting diarrhea.[2] Overall, intestinal microsporidiosis likely accounts for approximately 15% to 30% of all cases of chronic diarrhea in AIDS patients.[21] The infection is localized to the small intestine with the jujenum (or ileum) seemingly more heavily infested than the duodenum.[70] Both electron and light microscopic studies suggested that the pathogenic mechanism involved in intestinal microsporidiosis involved the shedding of infected enterocytes containing large numbers of spores.[71] HIV-associated infections with other microsporidia are relatively less frequent.[29]

Encephalitozoon spp. have been isolated from corneal and conjunctival specimens of patients with keratoconjunctivitis.[20,26,56,58,72-78] In addition, *Encephalitozoon* infections[16,26] have been associated with bronchiolitis,[55] sinusitis,[48,58] nephritis,[79] cystitis or ureteritis,[39,79,80] hepatitis,[50] peritonitis,[51] and disseminated infection.[52,80] *Encephalitozoon intestinalis* was another microsporidial species diagnosed in intestinal and disseminated infections in HIV-positive patients.[34-36,48,64,81-83]

E. cuniculi was recently confirmed to infect humans, affecting AIDS[50-52,79,84,85] as well as HIV-seronegative patients.[15,86]

Myositis associated with *Pleistophora* sp. has been described in two immunocompromised patients.[22,87,88] In an early report, Margileth et al.[89] have described an infant with severe immunodeficiency to be heavily infected with *Nosema connori* with heavy involvement of the renal tubular epithelium. *Nosema* has since been identified as the causative agent of corneal infections in HIV-seronegative patients.[90,91]

In humans, the particular microsporidial species and the competence of the immune response may lead to different host-parasite interactions.[2] Usually, in otherwise healthy persons, microsporidial infections will develop into acute intestinal, self-limiting disease.[41] So far, systemic microsporidiosis has not been clearly documented in previously healthy patients. By comparison, patients with severe immunodeficiency are at highest risk for developing microsporidial disease. What is not well understood in such cases is whether the disease represents reactivation of latent infection acquired prior to the state of suppressed immunity, or whether microsporidiosis has been associated with recently acquired infection.[2]

The viability of the host cellular immune responses represents one critical aspect for preventing symptomatic microsporidiosis, which is predominantly associated with CD4+ cellular deficiency. It has been suggested,[18] that some species, such as E. bieneusi, may be natural parasites of humans, possibly causing a transient diarrhea but normally remaining below the threshold of detection. However, with progression of cellular immunodeficiency, reactivation of latent microsporidial infection may occur.

The role of humoral immune responses is yet to be fully understood, but similarly to other human opportunistic protozoal infections, microsporidian-specific antibodies alone may not be protective.[2]

The clinical manifestations of microsporidiosis include intestinal, ocular, muscular, and systemic disease. In HIV-infected individuals, chronic diarrhea coupled with wasting syndrome,[92-95] and disseminated infections[34,39,52,55,80,81] (particularly in patients with CD4+ cell counts below 50/mm^3) have been most frequently observed, whereas ocular microsporidiosis has been limited to the superficial epithelium of the cornea and conjuctiva.

23.2 OCULAR MICROSPORIDIOSIS

Encephalitozoon hellem[96] has been most often identified as the causative agent of ocular microsporidiosis.[20,73,75,78,97] It was isolated from conjunctival scrappings and corneal tissue of several male homosexual AIDS patients with keratconjunctivitis where it develops within parasitophorous vacuoles located in the most superficial layers of epithelial cells.

While keratitis may be severe, it rarely, if ever, leads to corneal ulceration.[78] A typical pattern of systemic E. hellem infection involves concomitant keratoconjunctival, urinary tract, and bronchial infection.[39,55,80] Associated clinical manifestations may include keratoconjunctival inflammation, cystitis, nephritis, renal failure, bronchitis, pneumonia, and possibly, progressive respiratory failure.[2]

In addition to E. hellem, Nosema spp. have been reported to infect human cornea.[98,99] Nosema corneum, the first human microsporidian isolated, has been recovered from the corneal stroma of an HIV-seronegative patient with keratitis and iritis,[90,91] and high Nosema algerae antibody titers were observed in humans with ocular microsporidiosis.[100]

23.3 HOST IMMUNE RESPONSE TO MICROSPORIDIA

Using an experimental model of E. cuniculi-infected BALB/c mice, Schmidt and Shadduck[101,102] demonstrated that host immune responses play a critical role in preventing lethal microsporidiosis. Thus, adoptive transfer of sensitized syngeneic T-enriched spleen cells protected athymic mice inoculated with E. cuniculi, where passive transfer of native T lymphocytes or hyperimmune antiserum failed to protect or prolong survival in the infected athymic mice. Further studies have shown that cytokines released by the sensitized T-enriched murine splenic lymphocytes activated thioglycollate-elicited macrophages to kill E. cuniculi in vitro. However, elicited macrophages treated with medium from nonsensitized lymphocytes failed to control E. cuniculi replication.

Furthermore, antibodies against *E. cuniculi* exerted an opsonization effect that may block parasite entry into nonphagocytic cells.[102]

Since microsporidia can evade intracellular killing and successfully reside within the macrophages, it has been of interest to determine whether the macrophage could be successfully converted from a susceptible host cell to an effector cell capable of eliminating the parasite and thereby serving as a mediator of resistance to microsporidia infection. Niederkorn and Shadduck[103] have investigated the roles of antibodies and complement in the capacity of rabbit mononuclear peritoneal macrophages to phagocytose *E. cuniculi in vitro*. While normal rabbit serum or cell culture medium had little effect on the rate of removal of parasites by rabbit peritoneal macrophages, treatment with immune rabbit serum or immune rabbit immunoglobulin G significantly ($p < .001$) increased phagocytosis of *E. cuniculi*. In addition, guinea pig complement was found to markedly ($p < .001$) enhance the phagocytosis of antibody-treated *E. cuniculi*. The results of the study suggested a role for antibody enhancement of phagocytosis and intracellular killing as a mechanism of resistance to microsporidiosis.[103]

Recent studies[104-107] have also indicated that reactive nitrogen intermediates, such as nitric oxide, were involved in the mechanisms by which microphages kill intracellular pathogens. To this end, Didier et al.[108] have found that thioglycollate-elicited BALB/c murine peritoneal macrophages could be activated by incubation with lipopolysaccharide (LPS) and murine recombinant interferon (rIFN)-γ to kill *E. cuniculi in vitro*. In further studies, Didier[104] examined the role of nitrogen intermediates in the killing of *E. cuniculi* by activated murine peritoneal macrophages. Nitric oxide is a short-lived product of L-arginine metabolism which is oxidized to generate relatively stable by-products, such as NO_2^- and NO_3^- in murine macrophages.[109,110] Thus, addition of the L-arginine analog, N^3-monomethyl-L-arginine (NMMA) at concentrations of 50, 100, and 250 μM significantly inhibited the nitrite synthesis and prevented microsporidia killing. Conversely, addition of exogenous L-arginine at concentrations of 5.0 mM or 10 mM reversed the NMMA-induced inhibition of parasite killing. These results strongly indicated that reactive nitrogen intermediates contributed to the killing of microsporidia by LPS + rIFN-γ-activated murine peritoneal macrophages *in vitro*.[104,111]

23.4   STUDIES ON THERAPEUTICS

23.4.1   FUMAGILLIN

Fumagillin is an oxiran-containing antibiotic isolated from *Aspergillus fumigatus*. In one early study,[112] fumagillin has been shown to control *Nosema*-induced infection in honeybees. In addition, fumagillin also inhibited the replication of *Encephalitozoon cuniculi* in infected cell cultures *in vitro*,[18,113,114] and in a rabbit model *in vivo*.[2] The 50% inhibitory concentration (IC_{50}) values of fumagillin against *E. cuniculi* in rabbit kidney cells was 0.00086 μg/ml.[114] By comparison, the corresponding values for thiabendazole, albendazole, and oxibendazole were 0.30, 0.0044, and 0.0015, respectively; itraconazole, toltrazuril, metronidazole, ronidazole, and ganciclovir were ineffective in this testing system.[114] *E. cuniculi* organisms grown in the presence of fumagillin were swollen and had electron-lucent cytoplasm. In addition, it appeared that the absolute number of cytoplasmic ribosomes decreased and bound ribosomes were released.[113] Ultrastructural studies have also suggested that following exposure to fumagillin, the fluid balance was affected, possibly by interference with plasma membrane functions.[113]

Jaronski[115] found that fumagillin inhibited microsporidial RNA synthesis at concentrations of 66 mg/l (in 5% sucrose solution). While the DNA was not affected, histological evidence showed an almost complete halt in the parasite's life cycle at the sporoblast stage (48 to 56 h postinfection).

While fumagillin has been shown to be fairly effective against various species of microsporidia,[112,116-119] lasting eradication of the microsporidian has not been achieved.[18,23] Relatively high dosage rates resulted in increased larval period and mortality and reduced larval weight, fecundity, and egg hatch.[116,118,119] It appeared that fumagillin acted by arresting protozoal multiplication inside host cells but was not directly toxic to the spores.[113]

So far, little therapeutic application of fumagillin has been found against human microsporidiosis. Diesenhouse et al.[120] have used topical fumagillin to treat microsporidial keratoconjunctivitis.

Studies by Lewis and Lynch[116] indicated that unwarranted toxicity may cast serious doubts on the therapeutic value of fumagillin.

23.4.2 ALBENDAZOLE

Albendazole (methyl-5-[propylthio]-2-benzimidazolecarbamate) possesses broad-spectrum anthelminthic activity against several intestinal nematode and cestode infections.[121] It has been successfully used in the treatment of giardiasis,[122] intestinal nematodes, and systemic helminth infections such as hydatid cyst disease.[123]

The minimal inhibitory concentrations of albendazole against *E. cuniculi* and *E. hellem* were 0.015 and 0.008 μg/ml, respectively; the corresponding IC_{50} values were 0.004 and 0.001 μg/ml.[124] Studies on its mechanism of action revealed selective binding to the colchicin-sensitive sites on microtubules, thereby preventing polymerization into microtubules (that is, new tubulin dimers from being added), and thus interfering with nutrient uptake and cell division.[123,125,126] The microtubules are important in the formation of spindles allowing nuclear division in the parasites. In microsporidia, the only known site for microtubule synthesis is in the intranuclear spindles. In the absence of spindles, chromosome segregation cannot take place, leading to clumping of chromatin.

Morphologically, albendazole altered the sporogony in concentrations inhibiting microsporidian growth.[124] Spores without developed inner content as well as numerous electron-dense formations were frequently observed. In addition, massive extrusion of polar tubes within the parasitophorous vacuoles also occurred. In view of the putative role of tubulins in polar tube eversion,[127] the microtubule-affecting albendazole may be associated with precocious polar tube extrusion, which may be the cause for the inhibition of propagation.[124]

Electron microscopic studies by Blanshard et al.[128] have shown higher incidence of abnormalities. In the meronts, cytoplasmic vacuoles were seen with some of them surrounded by incomplete membranes. The nuclei have been frequently irregular in outline with disruption of the nuclear membranes and electron-lucent vacuoles between the nucleoplasm and the membranes. In addition, there was proliferation of the rough endoplasmic reticulum, and membrane whorls were found in the cytoplasm. In the sporonts, some developing polar tubes have been swollen and pale. The enlarged parasites occasionally had incomplete or ballooned plasmalemmata, as well as abnormal lipid-like inclusion. The presence of abnormally enlarged spores with some of them containing multiple nuclei and sets of organelles suggested incomplete division of the sporonts.[128]

Haque et al.[129] have examined the antimicrosporidial activity of albendazole on an insect-infecting microsporidian, *Nosema bombycis in vitro* in *Spodoptera frugiperda* cells, and *in vivo* in a lepidopteran larva, *Helicoverpa (Heliotis) zea*. Albendazole caused a significant reduction in the percentage of infected *S. frugiperda* cells observed at concentrations of 5.3 μg/ml; however, recrudescence did take place after the drug was withdrawn from the cultures. Furthermore, the drug nearly eliminated established infections from 6th-instar larvae and pupae after consumption of 2.0 to 4.0 mg, and infections were not established at all when 4.0 mg of albendazole were consumed concurrently with the infective spores. However, even at the highest dose, albendazole had no deleterious effect on the growth and viability of *H. zea*. Ultrastructural changes in *N. bombycis* caused by albendazole included clumping of chromatin in the nuclei and highly aberrant sporogonic stages.[129]

The side effects of albendazole treatment have been rare but may include nausea, rash, reversible alopecia, neutropenia, and liver function abnormalities.[123] One impediment of albendazole use is its insolubility in water.[130]

23.4.3 BENOMYL

Hsiao and Hsiao[131] have found benomyl, another benzimidazole derivative, active against insect-infecting microsporidia. Benomyl was also reported to cause nuclear aberrations in meronts and sporonts of *Nosema heliothidis* in *H. zea* larvae.[132] In another development, Davidse[133] concluded that carbendazim, a breakdown product of benomyl, inhibited mitosis in fungi by interfering with the spindle formation. However, similarly to fumagillin, benomyl showed unwarranted toxicity that outweighed its beneficial effects.[134]

23.4.4 MICROSPORIDIAL TARGETS FOR CHEMOTHERAPEUTIC INTERVENTION

One of the characteristic features of eukaryotic cells is the presence of microtubules as major components of the mitotic spindle, and in some cases, the cytoskeleton and flagella or cilia.[135] The microtubules are formed by polymerization of tubulin, a dimeric protein comprised of α- and β-tubulin subunits, each approximately 440 amino acids long. Each tubulin subunit binds one molecule of GTP, and polymerization is followed by hydrolysis of the β-tubulin GTP. At present, the mechanisms that control the rapid polymerization and depolymerization of the spindle micro-tubules before and after mitosis are not very clear.[135]

Microsporidia develop exclusively intracellularly and have no metabolically active stages outside the host cell.[27] The unique life cycle involving a proliferative merogonic stage followed by a sporogonic stage completes with the production of distinctive and resistant infective spores. The latter, which are used to identify and distinguish microsporidia from other organisms, contain a tubular extrusion apparatus to inject the spores into the host cell.[27,60,136] This polar tubular apparatus consists of a highly coiled, hollow, polar tubule which upon appropriate environmental stimulation undergoes extrusion from the spore to attach to a suitable host cell and allow the infectious sporoplasm to pass through into the target cell where a new generation of microsporidial organisms is produced.

Recent studies by Leitch et al.[127] have suggested that the polar tubular apparatus may be a useful target for chemotherapeutic intervention. The capability of various agents to interfere with the polar tubular extrusion was investigated *in vitro* in an assay utilizing *E. hellem* cultured from an AIDS patient. Four agents, cytochalasin D, demecoline, nifedipine, and itraconazole were found to inhibit the polar tubular extrusion.[127]

In addition to GTP, several classes of drugs (colchicine, vinca alkaloids, and benzimidazoles) have been the most well-studied effectors of microtubule polymerization.[137] Within these active classes of compounds, the benzamidazoles (e.g., thiabendazole, benomyl, albendazole, albendazole sulfoxide, nocodazole, carbendazim, oxibendazole, etc.) have been unique in their ability to be selectively toxic to lower eukaryotes, such as microsporidia.[135] Based on biochemical and genetic analysis, the β-tubulin subunit in eukaryotes has been identified as their primary target. By isolating resistant mutants of susceptible fungi (e.g., *Aspergillus nidulans*) and sequencing their β-tubulin genes,[137-141] four different regions of the β-tubulin molecule were implicated in benzimidazole activity. These regions include amino acid residues 6, 165–167, 198–200, and 241. Katiyar et al.[135] have analyzed partial β-tubulin sequences from *E. hellem* and *E. cuniculi* for the presence of five amino acid residues previously implicated in benzimidazole susceptibility. The results have demonstrated that Glu-198 and, in particular, Phe-200 correlated with the benzimidazole suscep-tibility. *E. hellem* and *E. cuniculi* were very similar to each other over the region analyzed. Thus, in addition to Phe-167 and Arg-241, their β-tubulin subunits included Glu-198 and Phe-200, suggesting that both microsporidians would be susceptible to benzimidazole activity.[135]

23.5 EVOLUTION OF THERAPY AND TREATMENT OF MICROSPORIDIOSIS

At present, there is no established and effective therapy for microsporidiosis. Patients are often treated empirically, usually with several drugs. Accepted therapy, such as diet alterations and antidiarrheal medications, have often been ineffective in alleviating the diarrhea and malabsorption associated with intestinal microsporidiosis.[142]

Different agents, such as metronidazole, itraconazole, octreotide, primaquine, lomotil, sulfalazine, paromomycin, trimethoprim–sulfamethoxazole, sulfisoxazole, and loperamide, have been used to treat patients, with variable results.

In patients with *E. bieneusi*-elicited diarrhea, symptomatic management is carried out usually with standard nonspecific antidiarrheal drugs.[93] In cases of failure to respond, subcutaneous octeotride (a somatostatin analog) has been recommended at 100 to 500 µg, t.i.d.[143] For patients on parenteral nutrition, octreotide up to 500 µg (not to exceed 50 µg/h) may be added directly to the total parenteral nutrition.[144]

Matsubayashi et al.[15] have used sulfisoxazole to treat successfully *E. cuniculi* infection of the CNS. While trimethoprim–sulfamethoxazole and octreotide relieved diarrhea in a few cases,[93,143] neither drug was successful in eliminating the parasite from the gastrointestinal tract. On the other hand, therapy with trimethoprim–sulfamethoxazole followed by sulfadiazine was found effective against *Pleistophora*-associated myositis.[87,88]

Eeftinck Schattenkerk et al.[65] have observed pronounced improvement in 6 patients or disappearance of diarrhea in 4 patients in 10 of 13 patients treated empirically with metronidazole. With one exception (250 mg, b.i.d.), the drug was given at 500 mg, t.i.d. In four of the patients, the response was prolonged; however, repeat biopsies showed continued presence of microsporidia regardless of the response to metronidazole.[65] In another case, one patient with microsporidiosis treated similarly also showed transient improvement.[145] In an appatrent contradiction, a study by Blanshard and Gazzard[146] showed no improvement in four patients following metronidazole therapy.

A 4-week course with 400 mg of albendazole orally, twice daily, in six HIV-infected patients with intestinal *E. bieneusi* resulted in cessation of diarrhea and either weight gain or cessation of weight loss; three patients who relapsed after treatment received a 6-week course.[142] Molina et al.[69] have observed transient improvement in five AIDS patients treated with metronidazole (given at 1.5 mg daily), but a longer response in three patients treated with albendazole (at 800 mg daily). However, in all patients, the diarrhea recurred after the end of therapy, and spores of *E. bieneusi* were recovered from the stools of all patients.[69] At low concentrations albendazole may bind reversibly to its tubulin target in *E. bieneusi* which, in turn, may provide a partial explanation why diarrhea may return to pretreatment levels when the low-dose treatment is discontinued.[142]

Dieterich et al.[121] studied the effect of albendazole on 29 severely immunocompromised AIDS patients (peripheral blood CD4$^+$ lymphocyte counts ranging from 1 to 60 cells/mm^3) with intestinal microsporidiosis (persistent watery diarrhea, and a slow but progressive weight loss). At doses of 400 mg, b.i.d., albendazole was effective in substantially reducing diarrhea. In another study, Aarons et al.[147] described a case of *Encephalitozoon*-associated renal failure in an HIV-positive patient. Treatment with albendazole (400 mg, b.i.d.) led to disappearance of spores from the urine, clinical improvement, and return of renal function virtually to normal. One case of an AIDS patient with *Encephalitozoon*-associated disseminated microsporidiosis (intestinal, urinary, nasal, and ocular involvement) has been successfully treated with albendazole given at 400 mg, b.i.d.[148]

Weber et al.[149] described two patients with HIV-associated chronic diarrhea caused by *Encephalitozoon (Septata) intestinalis* who after receiving a 2-week course of 400 mg (b.i.d.) of albendazole became asymptomatic, with no parasites detected in stool specimens.

Itraconazole has been used to treat *Nosema* infections in invertebrates.[150] Yee et al.[75] found itraconazole (200 mg orally, twice daily) effective in the treatment of *E. cuniculi*-associated epithelial keratopathy in an AIDS patient. After 6 weeks of treatment, there was improvement of vision and reduction of foreign body sensation and punctuate staining; topical application of coltrin (intravenous trimethoprim–sulfisoxazole formulation) resulted in no significant improvement.[75]

However, Albrecht et al.[151] reported failure of itraconazole to prevent *E. bieneusi* infection in an AIDS patient who developed intestinal microsporidiosis while on a high-dose itraconazole therapy (200 mg, b.i.d.) for secondary prophylaxis against histoplasmosis; the serum level of itraconazole was determined at 7.9 μg/ml (levels above 2.0 μg/ml are considered to be therapeutic).

Metcalfe et al.[77] used propamidine isethionate (4,4'-diamidino-α,ω-diphenoxypropane isethionate) 0.1% eye drops (six times daily) to treat successfully *E. cuniculi*-associated kerato-conjunctivitis in an AIDS patient.

23.6 REFERENCES

1. Nägeli, K. W., Ueber die neue krankheit der seidenraupe und verwandte oraganismen, *Bot. Z.*, 15, 760, 1857.
2. Weber, R., Bryan, R. T., Schwartz, D. A., and Owen, R. L., Human microsporidial infections, *Clin. Microbiol. Rev.*, 7, 426, 1994.
3. Canning, E. U., Lom, J., and Dykova, I., *The Microsporidia of Vertebrates*, Academic Press, New York, 1986.
4. Sprague, V., Microspora, in *Synopsis and Classification of Living Organisms*, Vol. 1, Parker, S. B., Ed., McGraw-Hill, New York, 1982, 589.
5. Sprague, V., Becnel, J. J., and Hazard, E. I., Taxonomy of phylum Microspora, *Crit. Rev. Microbiol.*, 18, 285, 1992.
6. Sprague, V. and Vavra, J., Biology of microsporidia, in *Comparative Pathobiology*, Vol. 1, Bulla, L. A., Jr. and Cheng, T. C., Eds., Plenum Press, New York, 1976, 1.
7. Sprague, V. and Vavra, J., Systematics of the microsporidia, in *Comparative Pathobiology*, Vol. 2, Bulla, L. A., Jr. and Cheng, T. C., Eds., Plenum Press, New York, 1977, 1.
8. Avery, S. W. and Undeen, A. H., The isolation of microsporidia and other pathogens from concentrated ditch water, *J. Am. Mosq. Control Assoc.*, 3, 54, 1987.
9. Canning, E. U. and Hollister, W. S., *Enterocytozoon bieneusi* (Microspora): prevalence and pathogenicity in AIDS patients, *Trans. R. Soc. Trop. Med. Hyg.*, 84, 181, 1990.
10. Orenstein, J. M., Tenner, M., and Kotler, D. P., Localization of infection by the microsporidian *Enterocytozoon bieneusi* in the gastrointestinal tract of AIDS patients with diarrhea, *AIDS*, 6, 195, 1992.
11. Orenstein, J. M., Microsporidiosis in the acquired immunodeficiency syndrome, *J. Parasitol.*, 77, 843, 1991.
12. Cali, A. and Owen, R. I., Intracellular development of *Enterocytozoon*, a unique microsporidian found in the intestine of AIDS patients, *J. Protozool.*, 37, 145, 1990.
13. Orenstein, J. M., Chiang, J., Steinberg, W., Smith, P. D., Rotterdam, H., and Kotler, D. P., Intestinal microsporidiosis as a cause of diarrhea in human immunodeficiency virus-infected patients: a report of 20 cases, *Hum. Pathol.*, 21, 475, 1990.
14. Gourley, W. K. and Swedo, J. L., Intestinal infection by microsporidia *Enterocytozoon bieneusi* of patients with AIDS: an ultrastructural study of the use of human mitochondria by a protozoan, *Lab. Invest.*, 58, 35A, 1988.
15. Matsubayashi, H., Koike, T., Mikata, T., and Hagiwara, S., A case of *Encephalitozoon*-like body infection in man, *Arch. Pathol.*, 67, 181, 1959.
16. Bryan, R. T., Microsporidia, in *Principles and Practice of Infectious Diseases*, 3rd ed., Mandell, G. L., Douglas, R. G., and Bennett, J. E., Eds., Churchill Livingston, New York, 1990, 2130.
17. Bryan, R. T., Cali, A., Owen, R. L., and Spencer, H. C., Microsporidia: opportunistic pathogens in patients with AIDS, in *Progress in Clinical Parasitology*, Vol. 2, Sun, T., Ed., Field and Wood, Philadelphia, 1991, 1.
18. Canning, E. U. and Hollister, W. S., Human infections with microsporidia, *Rev. Med. Microbiol.*, 3, 35, 1992.
19. Hartskeerl, R. A., van Gool, T., Schuitema, A. R. J., Didier, E. S., and Terpstra, W. J., Genetic and immunological characterization of the microsporidian *Septata intestinalis* Cali, Kotler and Orenstein, 1993; reclassification to *Encephalitozoon intestinalis*, *Parasitology*, 110, 277, 1995.
20. Didier, E. S., Didier, P. J., Friedberg, D. N., Stenson, S. M., Orenstein, J. M., Yee, R. W., Tio, F. O., Davis, R. M., Vossbrinck, C., Millichamp, N., and Shadduck, J. A., Isolation and characterization of a new human microsporidian, *Encephalitozoon hellem* (n.sp.), from three AIDS patients with keratoconjunctivitis, *J. Infect. Dis.*, 163, 617, 1991.

21. Weber, R., Bryan, R. T., Owen, R. L., Wilcox, C. M., Gorelkin, L., and Visvesvara, G. S., Improved light-microscopical detection of microsporidia spores in stool and duodenal aspirates, *N. Engl. J. Med.*, 326, 161, 1992.

22. Chupp, G. L., Alroy, J., Adelman, L. S., Breen, J. C., and Skolnik, P. R., Myositis due to *Pleistophora* (Microsporidia) in a patient with AIDS, *Clin. Infect. Dis.*, 16, 15, 1993.

23. Shadduck, J. A., Human microsporidiosis and AIDS, *Rev. Infect. Dis.*, 11, 203, 1989.

24. Canning, E. U. and Hollister, W. S., Microsporidia of mammals — widespread pathogens or opportunistic curiosities? *Parasitol. Today*, 3, 267, 1987.

25. Canning, E. U. and Hollister, W. S., *In vitro* and *in vivo* investigations of human microsporidia, *J. Parasitol.*, 38, 631, 1991.

26. Bryan, R. T. and Weber, R., Microsporidia: emerging pathogens in immunodeficient persons, *Arch. Pathol. Lab. Med.*, 117, 1243, 1993.

27. Canning, E. U., Microsporidia, in *Parasitic Protozoa*, Vol. 6, 2nd ed., Kreier, J. P. and Baker, J. R., Eds., Academic Press, New York, 1993, 299.

28. Shadduck, J. A. and Greeley, E., Microsporidia and human infections, *Clin. Microbiol. Rev.*, 2, 158, 1989.

29. Orenstein, J. M., Tenner, M., Cali, A., and Kotler, D. P., A second species of microsporidia that causes intestinal disease in AIDS, *Immunol. Microbiol.*, 98, A467, 1990.

30. Kotler, D. P., Francisco, A., Clayton, F., Scholes, J. V., and Orenstein, J. M., Small intestinal injury and parasitic diseases in AIDS, *Ann. Intern. Med.*, 113, 444, 1990.

31. Wittner, M., Tanowitz, H. B., and Weiss, L. M., Parasitic infections in AIDS patients: cryptosporidiosis, isosporiasis, microsporidiosis, cyclosporiasis, *Infect. Dis. Clin. North Am.*, 7, 569, 1993.

32. Cali, A., Kotler, D. P., and Orenstein, J. M., *Septata intestinalis* n.g., n.sp., an intestinal microsporidian associated with chronic diarrhea and dissemination in AIDS patients, *J. Protozool.*, 40, 101, 1993.

33. Cali, A., Orenstein, J. M., Kotler, D. P., and Owen, R. L., A comparison of two microsporidian parasites in enterocytes of AIDS patients with chronic diarrhea, *J. Protozool.*, 38, S96, 1991.

34. Orenstein, J. M., Dieterich, D. T., and Kotler, D. P., Systemic dissemination by a newly recognized intestinal microsporidia species in AIDS, *AIDS*, 6, 1143, 1992.

35. Orenstein, J. M., Tenner, M., Cali, A., and Kotler, D. P., A microsporidian previously undescribed in humans, infecting enterocytes and macrophages, and associated with diarrhea in an acquired immunodeficiency syndrome patient, *Hum. Pathol.*, 23, 722, 1992.

36. Field, A., Hing, M., Milliken, S., and Marriott, D., Microsporidia in the small intestine of HIV infected patients: a new diagnostic technique and a new species, *Med. J. Aust.*, 158, 390, 1993.

37. Didier, E. S., Rogers, L. B., Orenstein, J. M., Baker, M. D., Vossbrinck, C. R., van Gool, T., Hartskeerl, R., Soave, R., and Beaudet, L. M., Characterization of *Encepahlitozoon* (*Septata*) *intestinalis* isolates cultured from nasal mucosa and bronchoalveolar lavage fluids of two AIDS patients, *J. Eukaryote Microbiol.*, 43, 34, 1996.

38. Kelly, P., McPhail, P., Ngwenya, B., Luo, N., Karew, A., Pankjurst, C., Drobniewski, F., and Farthing, M., *Septata intestinalis*: a new microsporidian in Africa, *Lancet*, 344, 271, 1995.

39. Schwartz, D. A., Bryan, R. T., Hewan-Lowe, K. O., Visvesvara, G. S., Weber, R., Cali, A., and Angritt, P., Disseminated microsporidiosis (*Encephalitozoon hellem*) and acquired immunodeficiency syndrome: autopsy evidence for respiratory acquisition, *Arch. Pathol. Lab. Med.*, 116, 660, 1992.

40. Desportes, I., Le Charpantier, Y., Galian, A., Bernard, F., Cochand- Priollet, B., Lavergne, A., Ravisse, P., and Modigliani, R., Occurrence of a new microsporidian, *Enterocytozoon bieneusi* n.g., n.sp. in the enterocytes of a human patient with AIDS, *J. Protozool.*, 32, 250, 1985.

41. Sandfort, J., Hannemann, A., Gelderblom, H., Stark, K., Owen, R. L., and Ruf, B., *Enterocytozoon bieneusi* infection in an immunocompetent patient who had acute diarrhea and who was not infected with the human immunodeficiency virus, *Clin. Infect. Dis.*, 19, 514, 1994.

42. Deluol, A.-M., Poirot, J.-L., Heyer, F., Roux, P., and Levy, D., Intestinal microsporidiosis: about clinical characteristics and laboratory diagnosis, *J. Eukaryote Microbiol.*, 41, 33S, 1994.

43. Dobbins, W. O. III and Weinstein, W. M., Electron microscopy of the intestine and rectum in acquired immunodeficiency syndrome, *Gastroenterology*, 88, 738, 1985.

44. Modigliani, R., Bories, C., Le Charpentier, Y., Salmeron, M., Messing, B., Galian, A., Rambaud, J. C., Lavergene, A., Cochand-Priollet, B., and Desportes, I., Diarrhoea and malabsorption in acquired immune deficiency syndrome: a study of four cases with special emphasis on opportunistic protozoan infections, *Gut*, 26, 179, 1985.

45. McWhinney, P. H. M., Nathwani, D., Green, S. T., Boyd, J. F., and Forrest, J. A. H., Microsporidiosis detected in association with AIDS-related sclerosing cholangitis, *AIDS*, 5, 1394, 1991.

46. Pol, S., Romana, C., Richard, S., Carnot, F., Dumont, J. L., Bouche, H., Pialoux, G., Stern, M., Pays, J. F., and Berthelot, P., *Enterocytozoon bieneusi* infection in acquired immunodeficiency syndrome-related sclerosing cholangitis, *Gastroenterology*, 102, 1778, 1992.

47. Weber, R., Kuster, H., Keller, R., Bächi, T., Spycher, M. A., Briner, J., Russi, E., and Lüthy, R., Pulmonary and intestinal microsporidiosis in a patient with the acquired immunodeficiency syndrome, *Am. Rev. Respir. Dis.*, 146, 1603, 1992.

48. Eeftinck Schattenkerk, J. K. M., van Gool, T., Schot, L. S., van den Bergh Weerman, M., and Dankert, J., Chronic rhinosinusitis, a new clinical syndrome in HIV-infected patients with microsporidiosis, *Workshop on Intestinal Microsporidia in HIV Infection*, Paris, Abstr., 1992.

49. Hartskeerl, R. A., Schuitema, A. R. J., van Gool, T., and Terpstra, J., Genetic evidence for the occurrence of extraintestinal *Enterocytozoon bieneusi* infections, *Nucleic Acids Res.*, 21, 4150, 1993.

50. Terada, S., Reddy, K. R., Jeffers, L. J., Cali, A., and Schiff, E. R., Microsporidian hepatitis in the acquired immunodeficiency syndrome, *Ann. Intern. Med.*, 107, 61, 1987.

51. Zender, H. O., Arrigoni, E., Eckert, J., and Kapanci, Y., A case of *Encephalitozoon cuniculi* peritonitis in a patient with AIDS, *Vet. Pathol.*, 92, 352, 1989.

52. De Groote, M. A., Visvesvara, G. S., Wilson, M. L., Pieniazek, N., Slemenda, S. B., Da Silva, A., Leitch, G. J., Bryan, R. T., and Reves, R., Polymerase chain reaction and culture confirmation of disseminated *Encephalitozoon cuniculi* infection in a patient with AIDS: successful therapy with albendazole, *J. Infect. Dis.*, 171, 1375, 1995.

53. Hollister, W. S., Canning, E. U., Colbourn, N. I., Curry, A., and Lacey, C. J. N., Characterization of *Encephalitozoon hellem* (Microspora) isolated from the nasal mucosa of a patient with AIDS, *Parasitology*, 107, 351, 1993.

54. Schwartz, D. A., Visvesvara, G., Weber, R., and Bryan, R. T., Male genital microsporidiosis and AIDS: prostatic abscess due to *Encephalitozoon hellem*, *J. Eukaryote Microbiol.*, 41, 61S, 1994.

55. Schwartz, D. A., Visvesvara, G. S., Leitch, G. J., Tasjian, L., Pollack, M., Holden, J., and Bryan, R. T., Pathology of symptomatic microsporidial (*Encephalitozoon hellem*) bronchiolitis in AIDS: a new respiratory pathogen diagnosed from lung biopsy, bronchoalveolar lavage, sputum, and tissue culture, *Hum. Pathol.*, 24, 937, 1993.

56. Centers for Disease Control, Microsporidial keratoconjunctivitis in patients with AIDS, *Morbid. Mortal. Wkly. Rep.*, 39, 188, 1990.

57. Canning, E. U., Curry, A., Lacey, C. J., and Fenwick, D., Ultrastructure of *Encephalitozoon* sp. infecting the conjunctival, corneal, and nasal epithelia of a patient with AIDS, *Eur. J. Parasitol.*, 28, 226, 1992.

58. Lacey, C. J. N., Clark, A., Frazer, P., Metcalfe, T., and Curry, A., Chronic microsporidian infection in the nasal mucosae, sinuses and conjunctivae in HIV disease, *Genitourin. Med.*, 68, 179, 1992.

59. Blanshard, C., Hollister, W. S., Peacock, C. S., Tovey, D. G., Ellis, D. S., Canning, E. U., and Gazzard, B. G., Simultaneous infection with two types of intestinal microsporidia in a patient with AIDS, *Gut*, 33, 418, 1992.

60. Cali, A., General microsporidian features and recent findings on AIDS isolates, *J. Protozool.*, 38, 625, 1991.

61. Orenstein, J. M., Zierdt, W., Zierdt, C., and Kotler, D. P., Identification of spores of *Enterocytozoon bieneusi* in stool and duodenal fluid from AIDS patients, *Lancet*, 336, 1127, 1990.

62. Ditrich, O., Lom, J., Dykova, I., and Vavra, J., First case of *Enterocytozoon bieneusi* in the Czech Republic: comments on the ultrastructure and teratoid sporogenesis of the parasite, *J. Eukaryote Microbiol.*, 41, 35S, 1994.

63. Cello, J. P., Grendell, J. H., Basuk, P., Simon, D., Weiss, L., Wittner, M., Rood, R. P., Wilcox, M., Forsmark, C. E., Read, A., Satow, J. A., Weikel, C. S., and Beaumont, R. N., Effect of octreotide on refractory AIDS-associated diarrhea, *Ann. Intern. Med.*, 115, 705, 1991.

64. van Gool, T., Snijders, F., Reiss, P., Eeftinck Schattenkerk, J. K. M., van den Bergh Weerman, M. A., Bartelsman, J. F. W. M., Bruins, J. J. M., Canning, E. U., and Dankert, J., Diagnosis of intestinal and disseminated microsporidial infections in patients with HIV by a new rapid fluorescence technique, *J. Clin. Pathol.*, 46, 694, 1993.

65. Eeftinck Schattenkerk, J. K. M., van Gool, T., van Ketel, R. J., Bartelsman, J. F. W. M., Kuiken, C. L., Terpstra, W. J., and Reiss, P., Clinical significance of small-intestinal microsporidiosis in HIV-1-infected individuals, *Lancet*, 337, 895, 1991.

66. Greenson, J. K., Belitsos, P. C., Yardley, J. H., and Bartlett, J. G., AIDS enteropathy: occult enteric infections and duodenal mucosal alterations in chronic diarrhea, *Ann. Intern. Med.*, 114, 366, 1991.

67. Lucas, S. B., Papadaki, L., Conlon, C., Sewankambo, N., Goodgame, R., and Serwadda, D., Diagnosis of intestinal microsporidiosis in patients with AIDS, *J. Clin. Pathol.*, 42, 885, 1989.

68. Michiels, J. F., Hofman, P., Saint Paul, M. C., and Loubière, R., Pathological features of intestinal microsporidiosis in HIV positive patients, *Pathol. Res. Pract.*, 189, 377, 1993.

69. Molina, J. M., Sarfati, C., Beauvais, B., Lémann, M., Lesourd, A., Ferchal, F., Casin, I., Lagrange, P., Modigliani, R., Derouin, F., and Modai, J., Intestinal microsporidiosis in human immunodeficiency virus-infected patients with chronic unexplained diarrhea: prevalence and clinical and biologic features, *J. Infect. Dis.*, 167, 217, 1993.

70. Orenstein, J. M., Tenner, M., and Kotler, D. P., Localization of infection by microsporidia *Enterocytozoon bieneusi* in the gastrointestinal tracts of AIDS patients, *Immunol. Microbiol.*, 98, A467, 1990.

71. Peacock, C. S., Blanshard, C., Tovey, D. G., Ellis, D. S., and Gazzard, B. G., Histological diagnosis of intestinal microsporidiosis in patients with AIDS, *J. Clin. Pathol.*, 44, 558, 1991.

72. Lowder, C. Y., Meisler, D. M., McMahon, J. T., Longworth, D. L., and Rutherford, I., Microsporidia infection of the cornea in a man seropositive for human immunodeficiency virus, *Am. J. Ophthalmol.*, 109, 242, 1990.

73. Friedberg, D. N., Stenson, S. M., Orenstein, J. M., Tierno, P. M., and Charles, N. C., Microsporidial keratoconjunctivitis in acquired immunodeficiency syndrome, *Arch. Ophthalmol.*, 108, 504, 1990.

74. Cali, A., Meisler, D. M., Rutherford, I., Lowder, C. Y., McMahon, J. T., Longworth, D. L., and Bryan, R. T., Corneal microsporidiosis in a patient with AIDS, *Am. J. Trop. Med. Hyg.*, 44, 463, 1991.

75. Yee, R. W., Tio, F. O., Martinez, J. A., Held, K. S., Shadduck, J. A., and Didier, E. S., Resolution of microsporidial epithelial keratopathy in a patient with AIDS, *Ophthalmology*, 98, 196, 1991.

76. Desser, S. S., Hong, H., and Yang, J., Ultrastructure of the development of a species of *Encephalitozoon* cultured from the eye of an AIDS patient, *Parasitol. Rev.*, 78, 677, 1992.

77. Metcalfe, T. W., Doran, R. M. L., Rowlands, P. L., Curry, A., and Lacey, C. J. M., Microsporidial keratoconjunctivitis in a patient with AIDS, *Br. J. Ophthalmol.*, 76, 177, 1992.

78. Schwartz, D. A., Visvesvara, G. S., Diesenhouse, M. D., Weber, R., Font, R. L., Wilson, L. A., Corrent, G., Serdarevic, O. N., Rosberger, D. F., Keenen, P. C., Grossniklaus, H. E., Hewan-Lowe, K., and Bryan, R. T., Pathologic features and immunofluorescent antibody demonstration of ocular microsporidiosis (*Encephalitozoon hellem*) in seven patients with acquired immunodeficiency syndrome, *Am. J. Ophthalmol.*, 115, 285, 1993.

79. Hollister, W. S., Canning, E. U., and Colbourn, N. I., A species of *Encephalitozoon* isolated from an AIDS patient: criteria for species differentiation, *Folia Parasitol.*, 40, 293, 1993.

80. Weber, R., Kuster, H., Visvesvara, G. S., Bryan, R. T., Schwartz, D. A., and Lüthy, R., Disseminated microsporidiosis due to *Encephalitozoon hellem*: pulmonary colonization, microhematuria and mild conjunctivitis in a patient with AIDS, *Clin. Infect. Dis.*, 17, 415, 1993.

81. Asmuth, D. M., DeGirolami, P. C., Federman, M., Ezratty, C. R., Pleskow, D. K., Desai, G., and Wanke, C. A., Clinical features of microsporidiosis in patients with AIDS, *Clin. Infect. Dis.*, 18, 819, 1993.

82. Wanke, C. A. and Mattia, A. R., A 36-year-old man with AIDS, increase in chronic diarrhea, and intermittent fever and chills, *N. Engl. J. Med.*, 329, 1946, 1993.

83. Franzen, C., Müller, A., Hartmann, P., Hegener, P., Salzberger, B., Diehl, V., and Fatkenheuer, G., Polymerase chain reaction for detection of microsporidian DNA in gastrointestinal biopsies of HIV-infected patients, *Proc. 36th Intersci. Conf. Antimicrob. Agents Chemother.*, American Society for Microbiology, Washington, D.C., Abstr. D61, 1996, 71.

84. Bergquist, R., Morfeldt-Mansson, L., Pehrson, P. O., Petrini, B., and Wasserman, J., Antibody against Encephalitozoon cuniculi in Swedish homosexual men, *Scand. J. Infect. Dis.*, 16, 389, 1984.

85. Didier, E. S., Vossbrinck, C. R., Baker, M. D., Rogers, L. B., Bertucci, D. C., and Shadduck, J. A., Identification and characterization of three *Encephalitozoon cuniculi* strains, *Parasitology*, 111, 4121, 1995.

86. Bergquist, N. R., Stinzing, G., Smedman, L., Waller, T., and Andersson, T., Diagnosis of encephalitozoonosis in man by serological studies, *Br. Med. J.*, 288, 902, 1984.

87. Ledford, D. K., Overman, M. D., Gonzalvo, A., Cali, A., Mester, S. W., and Lockey, R. F., Micro-sporidiosis myositis in a patient with the acquired immunodeficiency syndrome, *Ann. Intern. Med.*, 102, 628, 1985.

88. Macher, A. M., Neafie, R., Angritt, P., and Tuur, S. M., Microsporidial myositis and the acquired immunodeficiency syndrome (AIDS): a four-year follow-up, *Ann. Intern. Med.*, 109, 343, 1988.

89. Margileth, A. M., Strano, A. J., Chandra, R., Neafie, R., Blum, M., and McCully, R. M., Disseminated nosematosis in an immunologically compromised infant, *Arch. Pathol.*, 95, 145, 1973.

90. Shadduck, J. A., Meccoli, R. A., Davis, R., and Font, R. L., First isolation of a microsporidian from a human patient, *J. Infect. Dis.*, 162, 773, 1990.

91. Davis, R. M., Font, R. L., Keisler, M. S., and Shadduck, J. A., Corneal microsporidiosis: a case report including ultrastructural observations, *Ophthalmology*, 97, 953, 1990.

92. Bartlett, J. G., Belitsos, P. C., and Sears, C. L., AIDS enteropathy, *Clin. Infect. Dis.*, 15, 726, 1992.

93. Current, W. L. and Owen, R. L., Cryptosporidiosis and microsporidiosis, in *Enteric Infection: Mechanism, Manifestations, and Management*, Farthing, J. M. C. and Keusch, G. T., Eds., Chapman and Hall Medical, London, 1989, 223.

94. Guerrant, R. L. and Bobak, D. A., Medical progress: bacterial and protozoal gastroenteritis, *N. Engl. J. Med.*, 325, 327, 1991.

95. Smith, P. D., Quinn, T. C., Strober, W., Janoff, E. M., and Masur, H., Gastrointestinal infections in AIDS, *Ann. Intern. Med.*, 116, 63, 1992.

96. Didier, P. J., Didier, E. S., Orenstein, J. M., and Shadduck, J. A., Fine structure of a new human microsporidian, *Encephalitozoon hellem*, in culture, *J. Protozool.*, 38, 502, 1991.

97. Friedberg, D. N., Didier, E. S., and Yee, R. W., Microsporidial keratoconjunctivitis, *Am. J. Ophthalmol.*, 116, 380, 1993.

98. Ashton, N. and Wirasinha, P. A., Encephalitozoonosis (Nosematosis) of the cornea, *Br. J. Ophthalmol.*, 57, 669, 1973.

99. Pinnolis, M., Egbert, P. R., Font, R. L., and Winter, F. C., Nosematosis of the cornea, *Arch. Ophthalmol.*, 99, 1044, 1981.

100. Didier, E. S., Shadduck, J. A., Didier, P. J., Millichamp, N., and Vossbrinck, C. R., Studies on ocular microsporidia, *J. Protozool.*, 38, 635, 1991.

101. Schmidt, E. C. and Shadduck, J. A., Murine encephalitozoonosis model for studying the host-parasite relationship of a chronic infection, *Infect. Immun.*, 40, 936, 1983.

102. Schmidt, E. C. and Shadduck, J. A., Mechanisms of resistance to the intracellular protozoan *Encephalitozoon cuniculi* in mice, *J. Immunol.*, 133, 2712, 1984.

103. Niederkorn, J. Y. and Shadduck, J. A., Role of antibody and complement in the control of *Encephalito-zoon cuniculi* infections by rabbit macrophages, *Infect. Immun.*, 27, 995, 1980.

104. Didier, E. S., Reactive nitrogen intermediates implicated in the inhibition of *Encephalitozoon cuniculi* (phylum Microspora) replication in murine peritoneal macrophages, *Parasit. Immunol.*, 17, 405, 1995.

105. Granger, D. L., Macrophage production of nitrogen oxides in host defense against microorganisms, *39th Forum Immunol.*, 141, 570, 1991.

106. Nathan, C. F. and Hibbs, J. B., Jr., Role of nitric oxide synthesis in macrophage antimicrobial activity, *Curr. Opin. Immunol.*, 3, 65, 1991.

107. Liew, F. Y., The role of nitric oxide in parasitic diseases, *Ann. Trop. Med. Parasitol.*, 87, 637, 1993.

108. Didier, E. S., Varner, P. W., Didier, P. J., Aldras, A. M., Millichamp, N. J., Murphey-Corb, M., Bohm, R., and Shadduck, J. A., Experimental microsporidiosis in immunocompetent and immunodeficient mice and monkeys, *Folia Parasitol.*, 41, 1, 1994.

109. Green, L. C., Wagner, D. A., Glogowski, J., Skipper, P. L., Wishnok, J. S., and Tannenbaum, S. R., Analysis of nitrate, nitrite, and [^{15}N]nitrate in biological fluids, *Anal. Biochem.*, 126, 131, 1982.

110. Marletta, M. A., Yoon, P. S., Iyengar, R., Leaf, C. D., and Wishnok, J. S., Macrophage oxidation of L-arginine to nitrite and nitrate: nitric oxide is an intermediate, *Biochemistry*, 27, 8706, 1988.

111. Didier, E. S. and Shadduck, J. A., IFN-γ and LPS induce murine macrophages to kill *Encephalitozoon cuniculi in vitro*, *J. Eukaryote Microbiol.*, 41, 34S, 1994.

112. Katznelson, H. and Jamieson, C. A., Control of *Nosema* disease of honey bees with fumagillin, *Science*, 115, 70, 1952.

113. Shadduck, J. A., Effect of fumagillin on *in vitro* multiplication of *Encephalitozoon cuniculi*, *J. Protozool.*, 27, 202, 1980.

114. Franssen, F. F. J., Lumeij, J. T., and van Knapen, F., Susceptibility of *Encephalitozoon cuniculi* to several drugs *in vitro*, *Antimicrob. Agents Chemother.*, 39, 1265, 1995.

115. Jaronski, S. T., Cytochemical evidence for RNA synthesis inhibition by fumagillin, *J. Antibiot.*, 25, 327, 1972.

116. Lewis, L. C. and Lynch, R. E., Treatment of *Ostrinia nubilalis* larvae with fumagil B to control infections caused by *Perezia pyraustae*, *J. Invertebr. Pathol.*, 15, 43, 1970.

117. Fox, R. M. and Weiser, J., A microsporidian parasite of *Anopheles gambiae* in Liberia, *J. Parasitol.*, 45, 21, 1959.

118. Flint, H. M., Eaton, J., and Klassen, W., The use of fumidil-B to reduce microsporidian disease in colonies of the boll weevil, *Ann. Entomol. Soc. Am.*, 65, 942, 1972.

119. Wilson, G. G., The use of fumidil B to suppress the microsporidian *Nosema fumiferanae* in stock cultures of the spruce budworm, *Choristoneura fumiferana* (Lepidoptera: Tortricidae), *Can. Entomol.*, 106, 995, 1974.

120. Diesenhouse, M. D., Wilson, L. A., Corrent, G., Visvesvara, G. S., Grossniklaus, H. E., and Bryan, R. T., Treatment of microsporidial keratoconjunctivitis with topical fumagillin, *Am. Ophthalmol.*, 115, 293, 1993.

121. Dieterich, D. T., Lew, E. A., Kotler, D. P., Poles, M. A., and Orenstein, J. M., Treatment with albendazole for intestinal disease due to *Enterocytozoon bieneusi* in patients with AIDS, *J. Infect. Dis.*, 169, 178, 1994.

122. Dutta, A. K., Phadke, M. A., Bagada, A. C., Joshi, V., Gazder, A., Biswas, T. K., Gill, H. H., and Jagota, S. C., A randomised multicentre study to compare the safety and efficacy of albendazole and metronidazole in the treatment of giardiasis in children, *Indian J. Pediatr.*, 61, 689, 1994.

123. Horton, R. J., Chemotherapy of *Echinococcus* infection in man with albendazole, *Trans. R. Soc. Trop. Med. Hyg.*, 83, 97, 1989.

124. Ditrich, O., Kucerova, Z., and Koudela, B., *In vitro* sensitivity of *Encephalitozoon cuniculi* and *E. hellem* to albendazole, *J. Eukaryote Microbiol.*, 41, 37S, 1994.

125. Lacey, E., Mode of action of benzimidazoles, *Parasitol. Today*, 6, 112, 1990.

126. Russell, G. J., Gill, J. H., and Lacey, E., Binding of [³H]benzimidazole carbamates to mammalian brain tubulin and the mechanism of selective toxicity of the benzimidazole anthelmintics, *Biochem. Pharmacol.*, 43, 1095, 1992.

127. Leitch, G. J., Qing, H., Wallace, S., and Visvesvara, G. S., Inhibition of the spore polar filament extrusion of the microsporidium, *Encephalitozoon hellem*, isolated from an AIDS patient, *J. Eukaryote Microbiol.*, 40, 711, 1993.

128. Blanshard, C., Ellis, D. S., Dowell, S. P., Tovey, G., and Gazzard, B. G., Electron microscopic changes in *Enterocytozoon bieneusi* following treatment with albendazole, *J. Clin. Pathol.*, 46, 898, 1993.

129. Haque, Md. A., Hollister, W. S., Wilcox, A., and Canning, E. U., The antimicrosporidial activity of albendazole, *J. Invertebr. Pathol.*, 62, 171, 1993.

130. Townsend, L. B. and Wise, D. S., The synthesis and chemistry of certain anthelmintic benzimidazoles, *Parasitol. Today*, 6, 107, 1990.

131. Hsiao, T. H. and Hsiao, C., A novel drug for controlling a microsporidian disease of the alfalfa weevil, *J. Invertebr. Pathol.*, 22, 303, 1973.

132. Brooks, W. H., Cranford, J. D., and Pearce, L. W., Benomyl: effectiveness against the microsporidian *Nosema heliothidis* in the corn earworm, *J. Invertebr. Pathol.*, 31, 239, 1978.

133. Davidse, L. C., Antimitotic activity of methyl benzimidazole-2-yl carbamate (MCB) in *Aspergillus nidulans*, *Pestic. Biochem. Physiol.*, 3, 317, 1973.

134. Harvey, G. T. and Gaudet, P. M., The effects of benomyl on the incidence of microsporidia and the development performance of eastern spruce budworm (Lepidoptera, Tortricidae), *Can. Entomol.*, 109, 987, 1977.

135. Katiyar, S. K., Gordon, V. R., McLaughlin, G. L., and Edlind, T. D., Antiprotozoal activities of benzimidazoles and correlations with β-tubulin sequence, *Antimicrob. Agents Chemother.*, 38, 2086, 1994.

136. Cali, A. and Owen, R. L., Microsporidiosis, in *The Laboratory Diagnosis of Infectious Diseases: Principles and Practice*, Vol. 1, Balows, A., Hausler, W., and Lennette, E. H., Eds., Springer-Verlag, New York, 1988, 928.

137. Fujimura, M., Oeda, K., Inoue, H., and Kato, T., A single amino-acid substitution in the beta-tubulin gene of *Neurospora* confers both carbendazim resistance and diethofencarb sensitivity, *Curr. Genet.*, 21, 399, 1992.

138. Jung, M. K. and Oakley, B. R., Identification of an amino acid substitution in the *benA*, β-tubulin gene of *Aspergillus nidulans* that confers thiabendazole resistance and benomyl supersensitivity, *Cell Motil. Cytoskeleton*, 17, 87, 1990.

139. Jung, M. K., Wilder, I. B., and Oakley, B. R., Amino acid alterations in the *benA* (β-tubulin) gene of *Aspergillus nidulans* that confer benomyl resistance, *Cell Motil. Cytoskeleton*, 22, 170, 1992.

140. Ohrbach, M. J., Porro, E. B., and Yanofsky, C., Cloning and characterization of the gene for β-tubulin from a benomyl-resistant mutant of *Neurospora crassa* and its use as a dominant selectable marker, *Mol. Cell. Biol.*, 6, 2452, 1986.

141. Thomas, J. H., Neff, N. F., and Botstein, D., Isolation and characterization of mutations in the β-tubulin gene of *Saccharomyces cerevisiae*, *Genetics*, 112, 715, 1985.

142. Blanshard, C., Ellis, D. S., Tovey, D. G., Dowell, S., and Gazzard, B. G., Treatment of intestinal microsporidiosis with albendazole in patients with AIDS, *AIDS*, 6, 311, 1992.

143. Simon, D., Weiss, L. M., Tanowitz, H. B., Cali, A., Jones, J., and Wittner, M., Light microscopic diagnosis of human microsporidiosis and variable response to octreotide, *Gastroenterology*, 100, 271, 1991.

144. Kreinik, G., Burstein, O., Landor, E. W., Burnstein, L., Weiss, L. M., and Wittner, M., Successful treatment of intractable cryptosporidial diarrhea with intravenous octreotide (sandostatin), a somatostatin analog, *AIDS*, 5, 765, 1991.

145. Bernard, E., Michiels, J. F., Durant, J., Hoffman, P., Desalvador, F., Loubière, R., Le Fichoua, Y., and Dellamonica, P., Intestinal microsporidiosis due to *Enterocytozoon bieneusi*: a new case report in an AIDS patient, *Lancet*, 5, 606, 1991.

146. Blanshard, C. and Gazzard, B. G., Microsporidiosis in HIV-1-infected individuals, *Lancet*, 337, 1488, 1991.

147. Aarons, E. J., Woodrow, D., Hollister, W. S., Canning, E. U., Francis, N., and Gazzard, B. G., Reversible renal failure caused by a microsporidian infection, *AIDS*, 8, 1119, 1994.

148. Lecuit, M., Oksenhendler, E., and Sarfati, C., Use of albendazole for disseminated microsporidian infection in a patient with AIDS, *Clin. Infect. Dis.*, 19, 332, 1994.

149. Weber, R., Sauer, B., Spycher, M. A., Deplazes, P., Keller, R., Ammann, R., Briner, J., and Lüthy, R., Detection of *Septata intestinalis* in stool specimens and coprodiagnostic monitoring of successful treatment with albendazole, *Clin. Infect. Dis.*, 19, 342, 1994.

150. Liu, T. P. and Myrick, G. R., Deformities in the spore of *Nosema apis* as induced by itraconazole, *Parasitol. Res.*, 75, 498, 1989.

151. Albrecht, H., Stellbrink, H.-J., and Sobottka, I., Failure of itraconazole to prevent *Enterocytozoon bieneusi* infection, *Genitourin. Med.*, 71, 325, 1995.

24 *Leishmania* spp.

24.1 INTRODUCTION

Leishmania is a broad genus of flagellate protozoa (suborder Trypanosomatina, order Kinetoplastida) characterized by two morphologic stages in their life cycle: amastigote, found intracellularly in vertebrates (such as humans), and promastigote, found in the digestive tract of invertebrate hosts (such as phlebotomine sandfly) and in cultures. Some species of *Leishmania*, which has worldwide distribution, are known to be pathogenic in humans. Because all species are morphologically indistinguishable, they are classified either by their geographic origin, ecologic characteristics, or their tendency to cause visceral, cutaneous, or mucocutaneous leishmaniasis.

Parasites are usually recovered from the bone marrow, spleen, liver, and the lymph nodes. A case of atypical dissemination was reported by Yebra et al.,[1] who have isolated *Leishmania* amastigotes from clinically unaffected skin of an HIV-seropositive patient. The fact that the patient remained asymptomatic for several months despite heavy parasitization might have been the result of deeply impaired immunity.

A reported case of vaginal leishmaniasis in an immunocompetent patient,[2] and a case of a severe *Leishmania*-associated rectal lesion in a homosexual AIDS patient,[3] suggested that venereal transmission may also occasionally take place.[4]

In some classifications, *Leishmania* organisms have been divided in four major complexes comprising species and subspecies: *L. donovani*, *L. tropica*, *L. mexicana*, and *L. brasiliensis*. Some of the clinically more important species of these organisms include: *L. brasiliensis*, a taxonomic complex comprising the subspecies and species causing the cutaneous and mucocutaneous forms of leishmaniasis; *L. donovani*, a taxonomic complex comprising the subspecies causing the visceral forms of leishmaniasis; *L. donovani infantum* (*L. infantum*) a subspecies of the *L. donovani* complex responsible form the infantile form of leishmaniasis in the Mediterranean littoral, Near and Middle East, Sub-Saharan and East Africa, and China; *L. donovani chagasi*, a subspecies of the *L. donovani* complex; *L. tropica*, a taxonomic complex comprising species causing the Old World form of cutaneous leishmaniasis; *L. major*, a species of the *L. tropica* complex causing the rural form of the Old World cutaneous leishmaniasis; *L. tropica minor* (also *L. nilotica*), a species of the *L. tropica* complex causing the urban form of Old World leishmaniasis.

24.1.1 Visceral Leishmaniasis (Kala-azar)

Visceral leishmaniasis is a chronic and highly lethal (if untreated) disease caused by *L. donovani*, *L. infantum*, and *L. chagasi*. The parasites multiply in the endothelial cells and spread to the lymph nodes and then hematogenously throughout the body. These species can be distinguished only by differences in the epidemiology, clinical features, and response to treatment. The disease is endemic in parts of Southern Europe, the Middle East, Central Asia, Eastern China, the Indian subcontinent, and some areas of Africa (Kenya and Sudan) and Central and South America.

The incubation period of the disease is usually 2 to 4 months, but in some cases it may be as long as 10 years.[5] Recovery appears to be followed by a long-lasting immunity, and in immunocompetent persons, second infection is almost unknown.[6] However, animal studies by Aebischer et al.[7] conducted in immune hosts (i.e., resistant mice experimentally infected with *L. major*) have

705

shown that the parasites did not show any loss of virulence and were capable of inducing progressive disease in susceptible (immunocompromised) hosts.

Clinically, visceral leishmaniasis is characterized by fever, chronic consumption, splenomegaly, pancytopenia, and hypergammaglobulinemia.[8,9] Although it is relatively rarely diagnosed in immunosuppressed patients,[9,10] if left untreated visceral leishmaniasis is potentially fatal.[11-13] The most common underlying disorders in an immunocompromised host predisposing to visceral leishmaniasis include hematologic malignancies, systemic lupus erythematosus, renal transplantation, protein-calorie malnutrition, age, and immunosuppressive corticosteroid therapy.[10,11,14-22] Piarroux et al.[23] have suggested the use of a polymerase chain reaction (PCR) technique to amplify a repeated sequence from the *L. infantum* genome in an attempt to diagnose visceral leishmaniasis in immunocompromised hosts.

It is estimated that about 50% of all cases of visceral leishmaniasis are associated with an HIV co-infection, especially in areas where the endemic disease overlaps with the HIV epidemic (East Africa, South America, and Southern Europe, especially Spain).[1,4,24-43] Splenomegaly, which was seen in nearly all cases of visceral leishmaniasis in immunocompetent patients, has not always been observed in HIV-infected individuals. Another distinction between the two populations is that antibodies to *Leishmania*, which were present in about 95% of immunocompetent patients, were absent in significant part (66%, by some accounts) of HIV-infected patients tested.[44]

There is some evidence suggesting that after a primary infection, *Leishmania* amastigotes remain viable even in healthy people for long periods.[45] Latent infection can progress into overt and sometimes rapidly progressing disease under conditions of stress and immunosuppression.[11,46] Protracted chronic relapses of visceral leishmaniasis in HIV-infected patients (45.5% vs. 10% in immunocompetent patients) is very characteristic for this population.[4,47] Chenoweth et al.[48] reported a rare case of disseminated AIDS-related visceral leishmaniasis with initial presentation of pulmonary symptoms and pleural effusions. This unusual location has been previously reported in an immunocompromised patient,[49] leaving open the possibility of *Leishmania*-associated respiratory disease.[44]

24.1.2 Cutaneous Leishmaniasis

Cutaneous leishmaniasis is an endemic disease characterized by the development of cutaneous papules that evolve into nodules which then break down to form indolent ulcers. The latter heal by producing depressed scars. The disease has been classified into Old World and New World (American) forms.

Old World leishmaniasis is divided into three distinct types, according to clinical manifestation and epidemiology: (1) *rural*, an acute and rapidly evolving form characterized with mainly multiple lesions accompanied by inflammation and crusting; (2) *urban*, typified by a slowly developing single lesion persisting for a year or more; and (3) a type of cutaneous leishmaniasis caused by *L. aethiopica* and known by many names according to its locality or occurrence. It is endemic for the highlands of Kenya and Ethiopia, the Middle East, and the Indian subcontinent. Its lesions are less inflamed and more chronic (usually self-limited and lasting for several years) than those of the other forms.

The New World (American) leishmaniasis has been diagnosed throughout Central and South America, with the exception of Chile and Argentina. It is characterized by lesions that develop and heal similarly to those of the Old World leishmaniasis. However, the lesions tend to be less nodular and more ulcerative and destructive.

24.1.3 Mucocutaneous Leishmaniasis

Mucocutaneous leishmaniasis is one of the many varieties of the New World form which differ as to etiologic agent, vector, distribution, pathology, epidemiology, and clinical course and manifestations. The disease is caused by *L. brasiliensis* and is characterized by the chronic, progressive metastatic spread of lesions to the nasal, pharyngeal, and buccal mucosa that may occur months and even years after the initial appearance of the lesion (which has usually healed). The disease is often associated with mutilating destruction of the nasal septum, palate, lips, pharynx, and larynx.

24.1.4 DIFFUSE CUTANEOUS LEISHMANIASIS

This is a rare chronic form of cutaneous leishmaniasis observed in Africa (Kenya, Ethiopia), and Central and South America. It is characterized by the local and hematogeneous spread from a primary lesion to produce generalized nodular lesions similar to those observed in lepromatous leprosy in the skin, and sometimes involving the nasal mucosa and laryngopharinx.

24.2 EVOLUTION OF THERAPIES AND TREATMENT OF LEISHMANIASIS

In general, treatment of classical visceral leishmaniasis is not yet satisfactory (as much as 41% therapeutic failure[50]). Treatment of HIV-positive patients has yielded even worse results — therapeutic failures and relapses have occurred in over 50% of patients.[8] The impairment of host cell-mediated immunity (macrophage activation), and CD4+ lymphocyte depletion in the case of AIDS, is largely responsible for the lack of adequate production of interleukin (IL)-2 and interferon (IFN)-γ, thus allowing for the persistence of viable amastigotes and reduced efficacy of antimicrobial therapy.[51] Studies by Murray et al.[51] demonstrated that either of two T cell subsets, L3T4+ and Lyt-2+, were mainly responsible for mediating the *in vivo* execution of antileishmanial chemotherapy, although other cells, such as B lymphocytes or natural killer cells, may also play some role.

Since the 1940s, the most often prescribed therapy for visceral leishmaniasis involves pentavalent antimonials: sodium stibogluconate and *N*-methylglucamine (glucantime, meglumine antimoniate).[52,53] Medrano et al.[27] have recommended one of two therapeutic regimens: (1) glucantime at 20 mg/kg daily (alone or with allopurinol at 900 mg daily) for up to 20 d; and (2) pentamidine isothionate at 4.0 mg/kg daily for up to 15 d. Vigevani et al.[25] applied two 15-d courses of glucantime to treat successfully three cases of visceral leishmaniasis in HIV-infected patients.[9,25] In another study,[9] three 10-d courses with 50 mg/kg daily of glucantime were reported adequate to cure the infection. However, Verdejo et al.[54] raised the possibility of certain *Leishmania* strains becoming resistant to pentavalent antimonials. In addition, cardiac toxicity related to glucantime therapy has been reported.[8,55]

In immunocompetent patients, primary visceral leishmaniasis usually responds well to treatment with pentavalent antimonials (over 98%).[44,56] The recommended initial dose of sodium stibogluconate (pentostam) is 20 mg/kg daily, up to a maximum of 850 mg daily. However, because of their defective cell-mediated immunity,[57] HIV-infected patients did not respond to such treatment, showing a high mortality rate even after commencing therapy.[26,44] High doses of stibogluconate (up to 60 mg/kg daily) have been used successfully for the treatment of persistent relapsing leishmaniasis; however, toxicity was a problem.[58] The use of synergistic combinations of stibogluconate and allopurinol or paromomycin has also been recommended.[44,59] Berenguer et al.[12] treated successfully visceral leishmaniasis in HIV-infected patients with three 3-week courses of intramuscular pentavalent antimony at daily doses of 850 mg.

Alternatives to antimonial therapy include pentamidine, amphotericin B, and allopurinol.[44,60] Long-term prophylactic therapy with either allopurinol or *N*-methylglucamine has been recommended to prevent relapses in HIV-infected patients.[9]

24.2.1 LIPOSOMAL AMPHOTERICIN B

Highly lipophilic by nature, amphotericin B elicits a specific effect on *Leishmania* by its higher affinity for episterol precursors of ergosterol in the parasite cell membranes than for cholesterol in the mammalian cell membranes.[61] In a hamster model of visceral leishmaniasis, amphotericin B was found to be 200- to 400-fold more active than the pentavalent antimonials.[61] However, because of excessive toxicity its use has been limited only to cases of pentavalent antimony-resistant mucosal leishmaniasis[62,63] where a total dose of about 20 mg/kg has been recommended.[64] Mishra et al.[65] have shown that a low alternate daily dose of 0.5 mg/kg and a low total dose of 7.0 mg/kg cured visceral leishmaniasis in 59 of 60 pentavalent antimony-resistant patients.

When tested in animal models, a number of liposome-incorporated antimicrobial drugs, including amphotericin B, have been found more effective against visceral leishmaniasis because of their preferential uptake by the macrophages and delivery to the parasitophorous vacuole.[66-69] In mice infected with *L. donovani*, liposomal amphotericin B (AmBisome) was over fivefold more effective and more than 25-fold less toxic than conventional amphotericin B.[70] In a mouse model, three to seven doses of 3.0 mg/kg of amphotericin B produced 40- to 80-μg/g levels of the antibiotic in the liver and spleen, and 20 to 40% of the total dose has been recovered from these organs. The extensive half-life of AmBisome (about 2 weeks) suggested that liposomal amphotericin may be suitable for intermittent dosing.[71]

In two recent reports,[72,73] AmBisome has been shown effective in patients with visceral leishmaniasis. Thus, Baily et al.[72] treated an immunosuppressed but asymptomatic patient with leishmaniasis of the tongue with a relatively low-dose regimen of AmBisome (1.0 mg/kg daily for 15 d, followed by 4 d rest and another 6-d course of 0.75 mg/kg daily); although low-dose, the therapy was extremely effective.

In a multicenter clinical trial, Davidson et al.[73] applied AmBisome to treat visceral leishmaniasis in both immunocompetent and immunocompromised patients. Ten immunocompetent patients (6 children) received 1.0 to 1.38 mg/kg daily for 21 d, and 10 (9 children) were given 3.0 mg/kg daily for 10 d; all patients were cured without significant adverse side effects and without relapse during the 12 to 24 months of follow-up. Eleven adult immunocompromised patients (seven of them co-infected with HIV, including four already with AIDS) received 100 mg (1.38 to 1.85 mg/kg) daily for 21 d; all were initially considered cured, but eight relapsed clinically and parasitologically at 3 to 22 months of follow-up.[73]

Amphotericin B cholesterol dispersion (amphocil) is another lipid-associated formulation of amphotericin B consisting of disk-shaped particles.[67] Initial studies with amphocil showed efficacy in a mouse model[74] and in patients with visceral leishmaniasis in Brasil.[75]

24.2.2 Host Immune Response to Leishmaniasis

Leishmania is an intracellular protozoan that replicates exclusively in macrophages, thereby significantly influencing the host immune responses. Therefore, the complex interactions between the virulence factors inherent to the parasite and the genetically determined host-defense mechanisms play a significant role in the outcome of *Leishmania* infections.[9,76] Even though the role of serum factors in the pathogenesis of disease and in protecting against reinfection cannot be underestimated, the resolution of leishmaniasis is markedly dependent on the cell-mediated immune responses — T cells viability is critical in determining the outcome of the infection.[57] In both murine and human infections, strong T helper type 2 responses have been associated with leishmaniasis, and a decreased or absent T helper type 2 response has been associated with healing.[76]

A different immunological pattern is associated with cutaneous leishmaniasis — a strong delayed hypersensitivity and *in vitro* proliferative responses take place both during the disease and after healing.[76] In diffuse cutaneous leishmaniasis, the immunological response is characterized by significant *Leishmania*-specific antibody production in the absence of T cell proliferation or delayed hypersensitivity response to the parasite, and uncontrolled cutaneous lesions.[76]

In immunocompetent hosts, the T cells will respond to *Leishmania* antigens by proliferation and production of lymphokines, such as IFN-γ, IL-3, granulocyte-macrophage colony-stimulating factor (GM-CSF), and macrophage colony-stimulating factor (M-CSF), to activate the oxygen-dependent and -independent microbicidal systems in the macrophages to inhibit the intracellular replication of the parasite.[76-87] However, the production of IFN-γ has been reduced in patients with AIDS.[88] The viability of *Leishmania* amastigotes may likely depend on the failure of the T cells to produce IFN-γ in response to parasitic antigens. *In vitro* studies have demonstrated that IFN-γ was effective in killing *L. donovani*. In addition, enhanced T cell[89] and monocyte oxidative activities have been shown following the use of IFN-γ in AIDS patients.[90-92] So far the use of IFN-γ alone in the treatment of opportunistic infections have failed to meet expectations.[92,93] However, the effective use of IFN-γ as an adjunct to pentavalent antimonials in an experimental model of human macrophages,[94] and in a group of immunocompetent patients with refractory disease,[95] suggested that such combinations might be potentially useful as immunochemotherapy.

An ongoing clinical trial utilizing GM-CSF in combination with antimonial therapy has resulted in rapid reversal of both leukopenia and thrombocytopenia associated with active visceral leishmaniasis.[76]

During the active stage of leishmaniasis, the production of T lymphocyte decreases with broader suppression of lymphocyte functions.[57,77] While during active visceral leishmaniasis patients lack parasite-specific delayed hypersensitivity responses, after resolution of symptoms the lymphocyte titers increase to produce cytokines in response to leishmanial antigens.[77]

In the context of the overall role cytokines play in controlling macrophage activation, it should be noted that several cytokines, such as IL-4, IL-10, and transforming growth factor (TGF)-β exhibit regulatory or inhibitory activity of macrophage activation. In particular, TGF-β has been identified as an important component in establishing leishmanial infection, and IL-12 as a cytokine involved in protection.[76]

24.3 REFERENCES

1. Yebra, M., Segovia, J., Manzano, L., Vargas, J., and Bernaldo de Quiros, L., Disseminated-to-skin kala-azar and the acquired immunodeficiency syndrome, *Ann. Intern. Med.*, 108, 490, 1988.
2. Symmers, W. S. C., Leishmaniasis acquired by contagion: a case of marital infection in Britain, *Lancet*, 1, 127, 1960.
3. Rosenthal, P. J., Chaisson, R. E., Hadley, W. K., and Leech, J. H., Rectal leishmaniasis in a patient with the acquired immunodeficiency syndrome, *Am. J. Med.*, 84, 307, 1988.
4. Montalban, C., Calleja, J. L., Erice, A., Laguna, F., Clotet, B., Podzamczer, D., Cobo, J., Mallolas, J., Yebra, M., Gallego, A., and the Cooperative Group for the Study of Leishmaniasis in AIDS, Visceral leishmaniasis in patients infected with human immunodeficiency virus, *J. Infect.*, 21, 261, 1990.
5. Faust, E. C., Russell, P. T., and Jung, R. C., in *Craig and Faust's Clinical Pathology*, Lea and Febiger, Philadelphia, 1970, 89.
6. Manson-Bahr, P. E. C, in *Infectious Diseases*, Hoeprich, P. D., Ed., Harper and Row, Hagerstown, MD, 1972, 1127.
7. Aebischer, T., Moody, S. F., and Handman, E., Persistence of virulent *Leishmania major* in murine cutaneous leishmaniasis: a possible hazard for the host, *Infect. Immun.*, 61, 220, 1993.
8. Altés, J., Salas, A., Riera, M., Udina, M., Galmés, A., Balanzat, J., Ballesteros, A., Buades, J., Salva, F., and Villalonga, C., Visceral leishmaniasis: another HIV-associated opportunistic infection? Report of eight cases and review of the literature, *AIDS*, 5, 201, 1991.
9. Fernandez-Guerrero, M. L., Aguado, J. M., Buzon, L., Barros, C., Montalban, C., Martin, T., and Bouza, E., Visceral leishmaniasis in immunocompromised hosts, *Am. J. Med.*, 83, 1098, 1987.
10. Badaro, R., Carvalho, E. M., Rocha, H., Queiroz, A. C., and Jones, T. C., *Leishmania donovani*: an opportunistic microbe associated with progressive disease in three immunocompromised patients, *Lancet*, 1, 647, 1986.
11. Ma, D. D. F., Concannon, A. J., and Hayes, J., Fatal leishmaniasis in renal-transplant recipient, *Lancet*, 2, 311, 1979.

12. Berenguer, J., Moreno, S., Cerdenaro, E., Bernaldo de Quiros, J. C. L., Garcia de la Fuente, A., and Bouza, E., Visceral leishmaniasis in patients infected with human immunodeficiency virus (HIV), *Ann. Intern. Med.*, 11, 129, 1989.

13. Broeckaert, A., Michielsen, P., and Vandepitte, J., Fatal leishmaniasis in renal-transplant patient, *Lancet*, 2, 740, 1979.

14. Senaldi, G., Cadeo, G., Carnevale, G., diPerri, G., and Carosi, G., Visceral leishmaniasis as an opportunistic infection, *Lancet*, 1, 1094, 1984.

15. Harrison, L. H., Naidu, T. G., Drew, J. S., de Alencar, J. E., and Pearson, R. D., Reciprocal relationship between undernutrition and parasitic disease visceral leishmaniasis, *Rev. Infect. Dis.*, 8, 447, 1986.

16. Herne, N., Mediterranean kala-azar in two adults treated with immunosuppressive agents, *Rev. Med. Interne*, 1, 237, 1980.

17. Hauteville, D., Chagnon, A., Camille, R. I., Herne, N., and Verdier, M., Leishmaniose viscérale méditerraneénne chez un leucémique en remission, *Nouv. Presse Med.*, 9, 1713, 1980.

18. Gastaut, J. A., Blanc, A. P., Imbert, C. I., Sebahoun, G., and Carcassonne, Y., Leishmaniose viscérale méditerrenéenne de l'adulte au cours de la remission complete d'une leucémie aigue lymphoblastique, *Nouv. Presse Med.*, 10, 1332, 1981.

19. Troncy, I., Girard, D., Guyot, P. H., Bel, A., and Coeur, P. H., Leishmaniose viscérale méditerrenéenne mortelle sur terrain immunodéprime, *Nouv. Presse Med.*, 10, 3726, 1981.

20. Wallis, P. J. W. and Clark, C. J. M., Visceral leishmaniasis complicating systemic lupus erythematosus, *Ann. Rheum. Dis.*, 42, 201, 1983.

21. Frances, G., Merie Beral, H., Franceschini, P. H., Lessana-Leibowitch, M., and Escande, J. P., Kala-azar chez l'immunodéprime: a propos d'un cas revelé par des signes cutanés, *Presse Med.*, 13, 2433, 1984.

22. Martinez, J., Masa, C., and Maeztu, R., Visceral leishmaniasis as opportunistic infection, *Lancet*, 1, 1094, 1986.

23. Piarroux, R., Gambarelli, F., Dumon, H., Fontes, M., Dunan, S., Mary, C., Toga, B., and Quilici, M., Comparison of PCR with direct examination of bone marrow aspiration, myeloculture, and serology for diagnosis of visceral leishmaniasis in immunocompromised patients, *J. Clin. Microbiol.*, 32, 746, 1994.

24. Alvar, J., Gutierrez-Solar, B., Molina, R., Lopez-Velez, R., Garcia-Camacho, A., Martinez, P., Laguna, F., Cercenado, E., and Galmes, A., Prevalence of *Leishmania* infection among AIDS patients, *Lancet*, 339, 1427, 1992.

25. Vigevani, G. M., Galli, M., Rizzardini, G., Antinori, S., Almaviva, M., and Coen, M., Visceral leishmaniasis in HIV infection: a report of three cases, *AIDS*, 3, 674, 1989.

26. Alvar, J., Blazquez, J., and Najera, R., Association of visceral leishmaniasis and human immunodeficiency virus, *J. Infect. Dis.*, 160, 560, 1989.

27. Medrano, F. J., Hernandez-Quero, J., Jiménez, E., Pineda, J. A., Rivero, A., Sanchez-Quijano, A., Velez, I. D., Viciana, P., Castillo, R., Reyes, M. J., Carvajal, F., Leal, M., and Lissen, E., Visceral leishmaniasis in HIV-1-infected individuals: a common opportunistic infection in Spain? *AIDS*, 6, 1499, 1992.

28. World Health Organization, AIDS, leishmaniasis dangers of clash highlighted, *TDR News*, 36, 1, 1991.

29. De la Loma, A., Alvar, J., Martinez-Galliano, E., Blazquez, J., Alcala-Munoz, A., and Najera, R., Leishmaniasis or AIDS, *Trans. R. Soc. Trop. Med. Hyg.*, 79, 421, 1985.

30. Clauvel, J. P., Couder, L. J., Belmin, J., Daniel, M. T., Rabian, C., and Seligmann, M., Visceral leishmaniasis complicating acquired immunodeficiency syndrome (AIDS), *Trans. R. Soc. Trop. Med. Hyg.*, 80, 1010, 1986.

31. Martinez-Fernandez, R., Garcia-Diaz, J. D., Gutierrez-Sanchez, J., Riopérez-Carmena, E., Valdivieso-Varela, L., and Alonso-Navas, F., Leishmaniasis visceral en pacientes adictos a drogas por via parenteral, VIH positivos, *Med. Clin. (Barcelona)*, 88, 509, 1986.

32. Guix, J., Aguilar, E., Gabril, F., Labios, M., and Escrig, V., Leishmaniasis visceral, adiccion a drogas por via parenteral y seropositividad frente al HIV, *Enferm. Infecc. Microbiol. Clin.*, 5, 636, 1987.

33. Franco-Vicario, R., Beltran de Heredia, J. M., Rojo, P., and Hermosa, C., Leishmaniosis visceral acociada al sindrome de la inmunodeficiencia adquirida, *Med. Clin. (Barcelona)*, 88, 565, 1987.

34. Medrano Gonzalez, F., Aleman Lorenzo, A., and Beato Perez, J. L., Leishmaniosis visceral de curso fatal asociada a infection por HTLV-III, *Med. Clin. (Barcelona)*, 87, 780, 1986.

35. Olivan, A., Reparaz, J., Uriz, J., and Sola, J., Leishmaniasis e infeccion por HIV, *Enferm. Infecc. Microbiol. Clin.*, 7, 60, 1989.

36. Rivero, A., Santos, J., Marquez, M., Gavilan, J. C., and Carralero, C., Leishmaniasis visceral asociada a infeccion por el HIV, *Enferm. Infecc. Microbiol. Clin.*, 7, 59, 1989.

37. Laguna Cuesta, F., Garcia Aguado, C., Puente Puente, S., and Mateu Paris, B., Leishmaniasis visceral e infeccion por HIV: tres nuevos casos, *Rev. Clin. Esp.*, 184, 267, 1989.

38. Ribelles, M., Casals, A., Valls, J., and Clotet, B., Leishmaniasis visceral de evolution benigna en un paciente infectado por el virus de la inmunodeficiencia humana, *Med. Clin. (Barcelona)*, 92, 679, 1989.

39. Montalban, C., Martinez-Fernandez, R., Calleja, J. L., Garcia-Diaz, J. de D., Rubio, R., Dronda, F., Moreno, S., Yebra, M., Barros, C., Cobo, J., Martinez, M. C., Ruiz, F., and Costa, J. R., Visceral leishmaniasis (kala-azar) as an opportunistic infection in patients with the human immunodeficiency virus in Spain, *Rev. Infect. Dis.*, 11, 655, 1989.

40. Grau, J. M., Boch, X., Selgado, A. C., and Urbano-Marquez, A., Human immunodeficiency virus (HIV) and aplastic anemia, *Ann. Intern. Med.*, 110, 576, 1989.

41. Smith, D., Gazzard, B., Lindley, R. P., Darwish, A., Reed, C., Bryceson, D. M., and Evans, D. A., Visceral leishmaniasis (kala azar) in a patient with AIDS, *AIDS*, 3, 41, 1989.

42. Verdejo, J., Alvar, J., Polo, R. M., and Gonzalez-Lahoz, J. M., Leishmaniasis visceral asociada a anti-HTLV III positivo, *Rev. Clin. Esp.*, 180, 221, 1987.

43. Alvar, J., Verdejo, J., Osuna, A., and Najera, R., Visceral leishmaniasis in a patient seropositive for HIV, *Eur. J. Clin. Microbiol.*, 6, 604, 1987.

44. Peters, B. S., Fish, D., Golden, R., Evans, D. A., Bryceson, A. D. M., and Pinching, A., Visceral leishmaniasis in HIV infection and AIDS: clinical features and response to therapy, *Q. J. Med.*, 283, 1101, 1990.

45. Pampiglione, S., Manson-Bahr, P. E. C., Giungu, F., Giungu, G., Parenti, A., and Canestri, G., Studies on Mediterranean leishmaniasis. II. Asymptomatic cases of visceral leishmaniasis, *Trans. R. Soc. Trop. Med. Hyg.*, 68, 447, 1974.

46. Wong, B., Parasitic infections in immunocompromised hosts, *Am. J. Med.*, 76, 479, 1984.

47. Mariscal Sistiaga, F., Dominguez Moreno, B., Lenguas Portero, F., Martinez Forde, J. M., and Galvan Guijo, B., Kala-azar en el hospital de enfermedades infecciosa: revision de 104 casos, *Rev. Clin. Esp.*, 159, 47, 1980.

48. Chenoweth, C. E., Singal, S., Pearson, R. D., Betts, R. F., and Markovitz, D. M., Acquired immuno-deficiency syndrome-related visceral leishmaniasis presenting in a pleural effusion, *Chest*, 103, 648, 1993.

49. Geraci, J. E., Wilson, W. R., and Thompson, J. H., Jr., Visceral leishmaniasis (kala-azar) as a cause of fever of unknown origin, *Mayo Clin. Proc.*, 55, 455, 1980.

50. Marsden, P. D. and Jones, T. C., Clinical manifestations, diagnosis, and treatment of leishmaniasis, in *Human Parasitic Disease*, Vol. 1, *Leishmaniasis*, Ghang, K.-P., Bray, R. S., Ruitenberg, E. S., and McInnis, A. J., Eds., Elsevier, Amsterdam, 1985, 185.

51. Murray, H. W., Oca, M. J., Granger, A. M., and Schreiber, R. D., Requirement for T cells and effect of lymphokines in successful chemotherapy for an intracellular infection: experimental visceral leish-maniasis, *J. Clin. Invest.*, 83, 1253, 1989.

52. Bryceson, A. D. M., Therapy in man, in *The Leishmanias in Biology and Medicine*, Peters, W. and Killick-Kendrick, R., Eds., Academic Press, London, 1987, 848.

53. Herwaldt, B. L. and Berman, J. D., Recommendations for treating leishmaniasis with sodium stibo-gluconate (pentostam) and review of pertinent clinical studies, *Am. J. Trop. Med. Hyg.*, 46, 296, 1992.

54. Verdejo, J., Alvar, J., Polo, R. M., and Gonzalez-Lahoz, J. M., Glucantime-resistant visceral leish-maniasis in immunocompromised patients, *Am. J. Med.*, 85, 128, 1988.

55. Rizzi, M., Arici, C., Bonaccorso, C., and Gavazzeni, G., Visceral leishmaniasis in a patient with human immunodeficiency virus, *Trans. R. Soc. Trop. Med. Hyg.*, 82, 565, 1988.

56. Bryceson, A. D. M., Chulay, J. D., Ho, M., Mugambii, M., Were, J. B., Muigai, R., Chunge, C., Gachini, G., Meme, J., Anabwani, G., and Bhatt, S. M., Visceral leishmaniasis unresponsive to antimonial drugs. I. Clinical and immunological studies, *Trans. R. Soc. Trop. Med. Hyg.*, 79, 700, 1985.

57. Pearson, R. D., Wheeler, D. A., Harrison, L. H., and Kay, H. D., The immunobiology of leishmaniasis, *Rev. Infect. Dis.*, 5, 907, 1983.

58. Bryceson, A. D. M., Chulay, J. D., and Mugambi, M., Visceral leishmaniasis unresponsive to antimonial drugs. II. Response to high dose sodium stibogluconate or prolonged treatment with pentamidine, *Trans. R. Soc. Trop. Med. Hyg.*, 79, 705, 1985.

59. Chunge, C. N., Gachihi, G., Muigai, R., Wasunna, K., Rashid, J. R., Chulay, J. D., Anabwani, G., Oster, C. N., and Bryceson, A. D. M., Visceral leishmaniasis unresponsive to antimonial drugs. III. Successful treatment using combination of sodium stibogluconate plus allopurinol, *Trans. R. Soc. Trop. Med. Hyg.*, 79, 715, 1985.

60. Dellamonica, P., Bernard, E., Le Fichoux, Y., Politano, S., Carles, M., Durand, J., and Mondain, V., Allopurinol for treatment of visceral leishmaniasis in patients with AIDS, *J. Infect. Dis.*, 160, 904, 1989.

61. Berman, J. D., Hanson, W. L., Chapman, W. L., Alving, C. R., and Lopez Berestein, G., Antileishmanial liposome-encapsulated amphotericin B in hamsters and monkeys, *Antimicrob. Agents Chemother.*, 30, 847, 1986.

62. Sampaio, S. A. P., Godoy, J. T., Paiva, L., and Dillon, N. L., The treatment of American (Mucocutaneous) leishmaniasis with amphotericin B, *Arch. Dermatol.*, 82, 627, 1960.

63. Crofts, M. A., Use of amphotericin B in mucocutaneous leishmaniasis, *J. Trop. Med. Hyg.*, 79, 111, 1976.

64. World Health Organization, Control of Leishmaniasis, Techn. Report Ser. No. 793, World Health Organization, Geneva, 1990.

65. Mishra, M., Biswas, U. K., Jha, D. N., and Khan, A. B., Amphotericin versus pentamidine in antimony-unresponsive kala-azar, *Lancet*, 340, 1256, 1992.

66. Croft, S. L., Neal, R. A., and Rao, L. S., Liposomes and other drug delivery systems in the treatment of leishmaniasis, in *Leishmaniasis: The Current Status and New Strategies for Control*, Hart, D. T., Ed., Plenum Press, New York, 1989, 783.

67. Janknegt, R., de Marie, S., Bakker-Woudenberg, I. A. J. M., and Crommelin, D. J. A., Liposomal and lipid formulations of amphotericin B: clinical pharmacokinetics, *Clin. Pharmacokinet.*, 23, 279, 1992.

68. Bakker-Woudenberg, I. A. J. M., Lokerse, A. F., ten Kate, M. T., Melissen, P. M. B., van Vianen, W., and van Etten, E. W. M., Liposomes as carriers of antimicrobial agents of immunomodulatory agents in the treatment of infections, *Eur. J. Clin. Microbiol. Infect. Dis.*, 1, 61, 1993.

69. Heath, S., Chance, M. L., and New, R. R., Quantitative and ultrastructural studies on the uptake of drug loaded liposomes by mononuclear phagocytes infected with *Leishmania donovani*, *Mol. Biochem. Parasitol.*, 12, 49, 1984.

70. Croft, S. L., Davidson, R. N., and Thornton, E. A., Liposomal amphotericin B in the treatment of visceral leishmaniasis, *J. Antimicrob. Chemother.*, 28, 111, 1991.

71. Gradoni, L., Davidson, R. N., Orsini, S., Betto, P., and Giambenedetti, M., Activity of liposomal amphotericin B (AmBisome) against *Leishmania infantum* and tissue distribution in mice, *J. Drug Targeting*, 1, 311, 1993.

72. Baily, G. G., Pitt, M. A., Curry, A., Haboubi, N. Y., Tuffin, J. R., and Mandal, B. K., Leishmaniasis of the tongue treated with liposomal amphotericin B, *J. Infect.*, 28, 327, 1994.

73. Davidson, R. N., Di Martino, L., Gradoni, L., Giacchino, R., Russo, R., Gaeta, G. B., Pempinello, R., Scott, S., Raimondi, F., Cascio, A., Prestileo, T., Caldiera, L., Wilkinson, R. J., and Bryceson, A. D. M., Liposomal amphotericin B (ambisome) in Mediterranean visceral leishmaniasis: a multi-centre trial, *Q. J. Med.*, 87, 75, 1994.

74. Berman, J. D., Ksionski, G., Chapman, W. L., Waits, V. B., and Hanson, W. L., Activity of amphotericin B cholesterol dispersion (amphocil) in experimental visceral leishmaniasis, *Antimicrob. Agents Chemother.*, 36, 1987, 1992.

75. Dietze, R., Falquieto, A., Ksionski, G., Grogl, M., and Berman, J., Treatment of visceral leishmaniasis with amphocil (amphotericin B cholesterol dispersion), *Proc. 32nd Intersci. Conf. Antimicrob. Agents Chemother.*, Anaheim, American Society of Microbiology, Washington, D.C., 1992, 226.

76. Reed, S. G. and Scott, P., T-cell and cytokine responses in leishmaniasis, *Curr. Opin. Immunol.*, 5, 524, 1993.

77. Carvalho, E. M., Badaro, R., Reed, S. G., Johnson, W. D., Jr., and Jones, T. C., Absence of γ interferon and interleukin-2 production during active visceral leishmaniasis, *J. Clin. Invest.*, 76, 2066, 1985.

78. Murray, H. W., Spitalny, G. W., and Nathan, C. F., Activation of mouse peritoneal macrophages *in vitro* and *in vivo* by interferon-gamma, *J. Immunol.*, 134, 1619, 1985.

79. Murray, H. W., Rubin, B. Y., and Rothermel, C. D., Killing of intracellular *Leishmania donovani* by lymphokine-stimulated human mononuclear phagocytes: evidence that interferon-γ is the activating lymphokine, *J. Clin. Invest.*, 72, 1505, 1983.

80. Murray, H. W., Stern, J. J., Welte, K., Rubin, B. Y., Carriero, S. M., and Nathan, C. F., Experimental visceral leishmaniasis: production of interleukin 2 and interferon-γ, tissue immune reaction, and response to treatment with interleukin 2 and interferon-γ, *J. Immunol.*, 138, 2290, 1987.

81. Stern, J., Oca, M., Rubin, B. Y., Anderson, S., and Murray, H. W., Role of L3T4+ and Lyt-2+ cells in experimental visceral leishmaniasis, *J. Immunol.*, 140, 3971, 1988.

82. Murray, H. W., Interferon-gamma, the activated macrophage and host defense against microbial challenge, *Ann. Intern. Med.*, 108, 595, 1988.

83. Murray, H. W., Masur, H., and Keithly, J. S., Cell-mediated immune response in experimental visceral leishmaniasis. I. Correlation between resistance to *L. donovani* and lymphokine-generating capacity, *J. Immunol.*, 129, 344, 1982.

84. Murray, H. W. and Cartelli, D. M., Killing of intracellular *Leishmania donovani* by human mononuclear phagocytes: evidence for oxygen-dependent and -independent leishmanicidal activity, *J. Clin. Invest.*, 72, 32, 1983.

85. Sacks, D. L., Lal, S. L., Shrivastava, S. N., Blackwell, J., and Neva, F. A., An analysis of T cell responsiveness in Indian kala-azar, *J. Immunol.*, 138, 908, 1987.

86. Hoover, D. L., Nacy, C. A., and Meltzer, M. S., Human monocyte activation for cytotoxicity against intracellular *Leishmania donovani* amastigotes: induction of microbicidal activity by interferon-gamma, *Cell. Immunol.*, 94, 500, 1985.

87. Hoover, D. L., Finbloom, D. S., Crawford, R. M., Nacy, C. A., Gilbreath, M., and Meltzer, M. S., A lymphokine distinct from interferon-γ that activates human monocytes to kill *Leishmania donovani* in vitro, *J. Immunol.*, 136, 1329, 1986.

88. Murray, H. W., Rubin, B. Y., Masur, H., and Roberts, R. B., Impaired production of lymphokines and immune (gamma) interferon in the acquired immunodeficiency syndrome, *N. Engl. J. Med.*, 310, 883, 1984.

89. Parkin, J. M., Eales, L. J., Moshtael, O., Galazka, A. R., and Pinching, A. J., A preliminary report on the use of interferon-gamma in patients with the acquired immune syndrome, in *Clinical Aspects of AIDS and AIDS-Related Complex*, Staquet, M. J., Hemmer, R., and Baert, A. E., Eds., Oxford University Press, Oxford, 1986, 157.

90. Murray, H. W., Scavuzzo, D., Jacobs, J. L., Kaplan, M. H., Libby, D. M., Schindler, J., and Roberts, R. B., *In vitro* and *in vivo* activation of human mononuclear phagocytes by gamma interferon: studies with normal and AIDS monocytes, *J. Immunol.*, 138, 2457, 1987.

91. Pennington, J. E., Groopman, J. E., Small, G. J., Laubenstein, L., and Finberg, R., Effect of intravenous recombinant gamma-interferon on the respiratory burst of blood monocytes from patients with AIDS, *J. Infect. Dis.*, 153, 609, 1986.

92. Lane, H. C., Sherwin, S. A., Masur, H., Gelmann, E. P., Rook, A. H., Manischewitz, J. F., Quinnan, G. V., Smith, P., Wahl, S., Allyn, S. P., Higgins, S. E., Megill, M. E., and Fauci, A. S., A phase I trial of recombinant immune (gamma) interferon in patients with the acquired immunodeficiency syndrome, *Clin. Res.*, 33, 408A, 1985.

93. Miles, S. A., Martinez, O., Sherwin, S., Carden, J., and Mitsuyasu, R., Phase I trial of recombinant interferon gamma in AIDS-related Kaposi's sarcoma, *Proc. 2nd Int. Conf. AIDS*, Paris, 1989, 39.

94. Murray, H. W., Berman, J. D., and Wright, S. D., Immunochemotherapy for intracellular *Leishmania donovani* infection: γ-interferon plus pentavalent antimony, *J. Infect. Dis.*, 157, 973, 1988.

95. Badaro, R., Falcoff, E., Badaro, F. S., Carvalho, E. M., Pedral-Sampaio, D., Barral, A., Carvalho, J. S., Barral-Netto, M., Brandley, M., Silva, L., Bina, J. C., Teixeira, R., Falcoff, R., Rocha, H., Ho, J. L., and Johnson, W. D., Jr., Treatment of visceral leishmaniasis with pentavalent antimony and interferon gamma, *N. Engl. J. Med.*, 322, 16, 1990.

25 *Strongyloides stercoralis*

25.1 INTRODUCTION

Strongyloides stercoralis, the causative agent of strongyloidiasis, is an intestinal nematode classified in the genus Strongyloides. The latter are plasmids widely distributed as intestinal parasites in mammals. *S. stercoralis* (known also as *S. intestinalis, Anguillula intestinalis, A. stercoralis*) is a roundworm occurring mainly in tropical and subtropical countries.[1] In the U.S., strongyloidiasis is endemic in certain southern regions (eastern Kentucky, Tennessee, Louisiana, and southern Appalachia),[2-4] although cases have been reported in all major geographic areas of the country,[2,3,5-18] with fatal outcomes being reported in malnourished children from socioeconomically deprived circumstances.[13,19,20]

  S. stercoralis is uniquely capable of perpetuating itself both in the soil and within the human host.[21,22] The female worm and her larvae reside in the mucosa and submucosa of the small intestine where they effect diarrhea and ulceration (intestinal strongyloidiasis or Cochin-China disease). After the larvae are expelled from the infected individual through feces, they develop in the soil to become the threadlike filariform larvae which are capable of penetrating the human skin upon contact, causing distinct cutaneous lesions known as larva currens. The larvae may eventually be carried in the bloodstream to the lungs where they cause hemorrhage by rupturing the alveoli (pulmonary strongyloidiasis). From the lungs, *S. stercoralis* enters the trachea and esophagus and then invades the intestines, thus closing the endogenous cycle of development. The unusual auto-infection cycle of this parasite permits its persistence in the infected hosts to last indefinitely, often as a well-regulated, undetected parasitosis.[23,24]

  Because of the irregular larval output by the intestinal adult female parasites, the diagnostic sensitivity of stool examination may be low, thereby making the parasitologic diagnosis difficult.[25] Several serologic tests for the detection of antibodies directed against *S. stercoralis* antigens have been described.[26-31] Genta et al.[32] and others[33] have evaluated the diagnostic implications of parasite-specific immune responses in immunocompromised patients and found the presence of high levels of IgG antibodies against *S. stercoralis* filariform larval antigens that can be used for diagnostic purposes. In another study by Genta et al.,[34] most patients with strongyloidiasis were capable of mounting specific IgA responses against filariform larval antigens which were different from those recognized by IgG.

  Strongyloidiasis may be characterized with overwhelming proliferation of worms in the gastrointestinal tract and by maturation of noninfective rhabtidiform larvae into the infective filariform larvae before the latter are excreted into the stool. In addition, the worms can cause damage directly by invading tissues or by carrying with them intestinal microorganisms that cause secondary infections.[5,6,35-43]

  S. stercoralis, which inhabits the gastrointestinal tract of a substantial proportion of the human population, can cause a chronic and essentially asymptomatic infection showing little if any symptoms in the immunocompetent host.[18,44-49] However, in the presence of abnormalities in the immune responses[50,51] (mainly cellular[5,6,52,53] but also humoral immunity), hyperinfection may develop.[8,35,39,54-56]

Clinically, strongyloidiasis is often asymptomatic but may be manifested by abdominal pain, distention, or ileus, and by secondary infections due to enteric (bacterial or fungal) microorganisms.

25.2   STRONGYLOIDIASIS IN HIV-INFECTED PATIENTS

Opportunistic disseminated strongyloidiasis is an important cause for morbidity and mortality in immunocompromised patients.[1,6,57,58] Patients on corticosteroid therapy,[5,6,59,60] renal transplant recipients[61-65] or patients with renal deficiency,[35,39,66,67] patients with systemic lupus erythematosus,[50] asthma,[37,41] chronic dermatosis,[10,35,39,66] chronic infections (lepromatous leprosy,[35,50] tuberculoid leprosy,[50] and tuberculosis[35,39,68]), as well as those with neoplastic conditions (lymphoma, leukemia, and solid tumors),[6-9,35,36,40,50,66,69-71] protein-calorie malnutrition[10,19,35,44,72,73] (shown to compromise cell-mediated immunity[35,74]), chronic alcoholism,[11,75,76] and achlorhydria,[12,77,78] are at higher risk and may develop systemic strongyloidiasis. Kiyuna et al.[79] have reported a case of periarteritis nodosa associated with disseminated strongyloidiasis.

Patients infected with HIV[80,81] and the human T lymphotropic virus type 1 (HTLV-1) may be also at risk. A high prevalence of HTLV-1-directed antibodies has been found in carriers of *S. stercoralis*.[82] This phenomenon may be linked to selective immunosuppression by the retrovirus (as evidenced by the very low total serum levels of IgE) creating a favorable environment for nematode proliferation.[83] Furthermore, it has been also suggested that the *Strongyloides* infection may, in turn, contribute to the leukemogenesis by HTLV-1 in cases of adult T cell leukemia lymphoma.[84]

With the emergence of the AIDS epidemic, strongyloidiasis was expected to be one of the opportunistic infections affecting these patients.[1,85] Disseminated strongyloidiasis and the hyperinfection syndrome are among the opportunistic infections considered indicative of an underlying cell-mediated immunodeficiency in patients with AIDS. Surprisingly, however, at present only a very few cases of strongyloidiasis in AIDS patients have been described,[80,86,87] even though sexually active homosexual men are at increased risk for *S. stercoralis* infection, which can be acquired as a sexually transmitted disease. In the several cases reported in the literature,[81,85,88-90] the disease has been localized in the intestines with no dissemination, suggesting incidental rather than opportunistic infection.[1] As discussed by Petithory and Derouin[91] and Gachot et al.,[92] until more relevant data are accumulated, strongyloidiasis should no longer be considered an opportunistic infection in AIDS.

The underrepresentation of the hyperinfection among the opportunistic infections linked to AIDS may be explained, at least partially, with the specific immunodeficiency state of AIDS, which may be more conducive to reactivation of infection with unicellular protozoa (e.g., *Toxoplasma gondii*) rather than to proliferation of infections involving complex, multicellular worms.[86] Other factors, such as underdiagnosis and underreporting may also account for the small number of strongyloidiasis in AIDS patients.

According to Gompels et al.,[80] there was compelling evidence to suggest that the development of hyperinfection occurred only in a subset of doubly infected patients because of greater severity of HIV-induced immunodeficiency and the presence of an additional defect of the host defense, such as granulocytopenia. That is, that cell-mediated immunodeficiency due to HIV alone will not predispose to *Strongyloides* hyperinfection, but will also require reduced numbers or function of granulocytes.

The eosinophil count is typically elevated in immunocompetent patients,[32,93-97] but is usually absent in immunosuppressed patients with the hyperinfection syndrome.[32,93,94] As reported by Aziz,[44] as many as 94% of patients with strongyloidiasis showed peripheral blood eosinophilia as a symptom of the disease. Savage et al.[98] reported an unusual case of an immunosuppressed patient with strongyloidiasis who was minimally symptomatic but with a dramatic increase in his eosinophil count. While the mechanism of this phenomenon was unclear some synergistic association between the eosinophilopoietic effects of helminth infection[94,99] and chemotherapy[100] seemed plausible. In several other reports,[32,101-103] cases of immunosuppressed patients with mild strongyloidiasis and higher eosinophilic counts have also been described. Since there is no eosinophilia in AIDS patients, it may be the lack of eosinophils that is the most relevant factor to predisposition.[80]

While individuals with asymptomatic infection do not have raised IgE titers, it is often a feature in immunocompromised patients, such as AIDS.[80] It has been suggested that greater survival may be associated with higher IgE levels.[1]

25.3   CUTANEOUS MANIFESTATIONS OF STRONGYLOIDIASIS

During chronic uncomplicated infections and disseminated hyperinfections, *S. stercoralis* filariform larvae may migrate to the skin, causing a variety of lesions.[23,25,43,69,104-116] The most characteristic cutaneous manifestation of strongyloidiasis is larva currens.[22,23,117,118] This skin lesion, which was first described by Fulleborn,[119] is formed after the rapid intracutaneous migration of the parasite. It is often associated with a localized urticarial reaction.[5,104] The typical eruption represents an intensely pruritic linear or serpigenous urticarial lesion (usually one, but occasionally multiple), surrounded by a flare that moves intermittently at the rate of 5 to 15 cm/h. The attacks of larva currens are short and sporadic and last usually for several hours, with the patient remaining symptom-free for weeks or months between attacks.[104] They occur mostly on the buttocks, groin, and the trunk,[23,107,108,113,120] but the thighs, neck, and rarely, face and arms may also be affected.[23,107,121] The prevalence of larva currens remains low in America.[18,48,122]

Another cutaneous manifestation of strongyloidiasis is the massive migration of filiform larvae into the skin which may occur during dissemination in immunocompromised patients.[69,104,105,123] It is typically presented as rapidly progressing petechial and purpuric eruptions involving the trunk and proximal portions of the limbs.[104] Once the patient's superficial dermal vessels have been damaged, decrease in the platelet count and clotting factors contribute to the purpura.

Chronic urticaria is the third clearly described condition associated with strongyloidiasis.[24,106,110] This cutaneous manifestation, which has been diagnosed in as many as 66% of patients,[24] is characterized with fixed urticarial wheals lasting 1 to 2 d, usually affecting the buttocks and waistline.

25.4   CORTICOSTEROID THERAPY AS A PREDISPOSING FACTOR FOR STRONGYLOIDIASIS

One of the major stages of the development cycle of *S. stercoralis* within the human body is the transformation of rhabdiform larvae into invasive filariform larvae in the gut.[5] It takes between on average 24 to 48 h for this process to complete. There is evidence that the conversion of rhabdiform larve into the filariform can be altered by corticosteroid administration.[22] It has been established by several groups[124-126] that during corticosteroid administration in animals infected with *Nippostrongylus brasiliensis* or *S. ratti*, there has been an absolute rise in worm numbers and a fractional increase in invasive filariform larvae relative to rhabdiform larvae in the intestinal tracts. However, the mechanism of this augmentation of metamorphosis is poorly understood. Moreover, the corticosteroids may also reduce the local inflammation which, in turn, may further impair the containment of the parasites, allowing increased number of invasive filiform larvae to penetrate the gut wall and complete the endogenous autoinfection cycle. Finally, the immunosuppression activity of corticosteroids (or any other immunosuppressive drug, such as azathioprine and cyclophosphamide) will also help enhance the predisposition of the host to hyperinfection.[5]

25.5   TREATMENT OF STRONGYLOIDIASIS

Even though the morbidity and mortality rate is relatively high, especially in immunocompromised hosts with hyperinfection syndrome, those patients who receive prompt and adequate treatment have a reasonably favorable prognosis to survive.

Thiabendazole, a 2-(4-thiazolyl)benzimidazole antihelminthic agent, has been the drug of choice in the treatment of strongyloidiasis.[10] However, it is not available for parenteral administration. Thiabendazole has been especially effective in immunocompetent patients.[127,128] For uncomplicated gastrointestinal infections, the usual recommended dose has been 25 mg/kg b.i.d. for 2 or more days.[5,6,11,50,67,80,86] However, in immunocompromised patients, the therapy may take longer than that, as well necessitate higher doses.[5,6,114,129] Thus, Adam et al.[36] have found it necessary to use courses of 15 to 40 g of thiabendazole for over 10 to 15 d in order to achieve favorable response. Because of its adverse side effects (dizziness, hypotension, neurotoxicity, leukopenia,[130] and elevated hepatic enzymes[130,131]) in some patients, at least the prophylactic use of thiabendazole is controversial and did not receive wide acceptance.[132]

Scowden et al.[5] have treated a number of immunocompromised patients with strongyloidiasis using a combination of thiabendazole (15 to 25 mg/kg, b.i.d., orally or via a nasogastric tube) and metronidazole.

In two cases,[133,134] adult respiratory distress syndrome (ARDS) associated with *S. stercoralis* has been described with fatal outcome in spite of thiabendazole therapy. In one of the reported cases,[134] ARDS had developed after successful therapy of the parasitic disease and coincided with the rapid taper of the immunosuppressive corticosteroid therapy. In two previous reports by the same group,[135,136] treatment of pulmonary strongyloidiasis has been successful despite continued therapy with high-dose systemic corticosteroids. Persistent infections despite adequate antiparasitic therapy with thiabendazole have been associated with the development of lung abscesses[14] harboring the parasite. The lesions are refractory to oral medication and may result in death. To this end, surgical resection or drainage may be helpful.[5]

Savage et al.[98] treated strongyloidiasis in an immunosuppressed patient with albendazole (another benzimidazole antihelminthic agent) at daily doses of 400 mg given in four 3-d cycles. Two other reports[137,138] have corroborated the efficacy of this dose regimen. Hanck and Holzer[59] also reported the use of oral albendazole to treat an immunosuppressed patient on corticosteroid therapy, with severe diarrhea and dehydration because of strongyloidiasis. Dramatic improvement has been reported in a case of fulminating strongyloidiasis complicating kala-azar after treatment with albendazole.[139]

While the use of albendazole as primary worm therapy may reduce the need for thiabendazole, the latter in spite of its higher toxicity compared to albendazole, still remains the drug of choice in refractory strongyloidiasis.

Recent reports have indicated that ivermectin, a macrolide antibiotic primarily known for its activity against onchocerciasis, was also efficacious in the treatment of strongyloidiasis in immunocompetent patients with cure rates averaging 94%.[140] Torres et al.[81] have used ivermectin in HIV-infected patients with *S. stercoralis*-associated hyperinfection. Two regimens have been applied: a single 200-µg/kg daily oral dose, or the same dose given on a multiple schedule (on days 1, 2, 15, and 16). All seven patients who received multiple doses showed sustained clinical and parasitological cure, whereas one of two patients who were given the single dose relapsed promptly and fatally.

Other drugs that have been used in the treatment of strongyloidiasis were pyrvinium pamoate and mebendazole. Giannoulis et al.[141] treated a patient with disseminated strongyloidiasis with mebendazole (200 mg, b.i.d., over a 3-d period), with dramatic clinical improvement; the dose regimen was repeated in 2 and 5 weeks to completely eliminate the nematode from feces. However, some studies have suggested that while pyrvinium pamoate and mebendazole have been effective against hookworms (*Necator americana*, *Ancylostoma duodenale*, *A. caninum*, *A. brasiliensis*), their efficacy against strongyloidiasis is questionable.[96]

25.6   REFERENCES

1. Genta, R. M., Global prevalence of strongyloidiasis: critical review with epidemiologic insights into the prevention of disseminated disease, *Rev. Infect. Dis.*, 11, 755, 1989.

2. Fulmer, H. S. and Huempfner, H. R., Intestinal helminths in eastern Kentucky: a survey in rural counties, *Am. J. Trop. Med. Hyg.*, 14, 269, 1965.
3. Ophüs, W., A fatal case of strongyloidiasis in man, with autopsy, *Arch. Pathol.*, 8, 1, 1929.
4. Berk, S. L., Verghese, A., Alvarez, S., Hall, K., and Smith, B., Clinical and epidemiologic features of strongyloidiasis: a prospective study in rural Tennessee, *Arch. Intern. Med.*, 147, 1257, 1987.
5. Scowden, E. B., Schaffner, W., and Stone, W. J., Overwhelming strongyloidiasis: an unappreciated opportunistic infection, *Medicine (Baltimore)*, 57, 527, 1978.
6. Igra-Siegman, Y., Kapila, R., Sen, P., Kaminski, Z. C., and Louria, D. B., Syndrome of hyperinfection with *Strongyliodes stercoralis*, *Rev. Infect. Dis.*, 3, 397, 1981.
7. Pollock, T. W. and Perencevich, E. N., Hyperinfection with *Strongyloides stercoralis* in a patient with Hodgkin's disease, *J. Am. Ostheopath. Assoc.*, 76, 171, 1976.
8. Rogers, W. A., Jr. and Nelson, B., Strongyloidiasis and malignant lymphoma: "opportunistic infection" by a nematode, *JAMA*, 195, 685, 1966.
9. Buss, D. H., *Strongyloides stercoralis* infection complicating granulocytic leukemia, *NC Med. J.*, 32, 269, 1971.
10. Civantos, F. and Robinson, M. J., Fatal strongyloidiasis following corticosteroid therapy, *Am. J. Dig. Dis.*, 14, 643, 1969.
11. Cahill, K. M., Thiabendazole in massive strongyloidiasis, *Am. J. Trop. Med. Hyg.*, 16, 451, 1967.
12. Amir-Ahmadi, H., Braun, P., Neva, F. A., Gottlieb, L. S., and Zamcheck, N., Strongyloidiasis at the Boston City Hospital, *Am. J. Dig. Dis.*, 13, 959, 1968.
13. Smith, S. B., Schwartzman, M., Mencia, L. F., Blum, E. B., Krogstad, D., Nitzkin, J., and Healy, G. R., Fatal disseminated strongyloidiasis presenting as acute abdominal distress in an urban child, *J. Pediatr.*, 91, 607, 1977.
14. Seabury, J. H., Abadie, S., and Savoy, F., Jr., Pulmonary strongyloidiasis with lung abscess: ineffectiveness of thiabendazole therapy, *Am. J. Trop. Med. Hyg.*, 20, 209, 1971.
15. Cuni, L., Rosner, F., and Chawla, S. K., Fatal strongyloidiasis in immunosuppressed patients, *NY State J. Med.*, 77, 2109, 1977.
16. Cummins, R. O., Suratt, P. M., and Horwitz, D. A., Disseminated *Strongyloides stercoralis* infection, *Arch. Intern. Med.*, 138, 1005, 1978.
17. Berger, R., Kraman, S., and Paciotti, M., Pulmonary strongyloidiasis complicating therapy with corticosteroids, *Am. J. Trop. Med. Hyg.*, 29, 31, 1980.
18. Milder, J. E., Walzer, P. D., Kilgore, G., Rutherford, I., and Klein, M., Clinical features of *Strongyloides stercoralis* infection in an endemic area of the United States, *Gastroenterology*, 80, 1481, 1981.
19. Cookson, J. B., Montgomery, R. D., Morgan, H. V., and Tudor, R. W., Fatal paralytic ileus due to strongyloidiasis, *Br. Med. J.*, 4, 771, 1972.
20. Huchton, P. and Horn, R., Strongyloidiasis, *J. Pediatr.*, 55, 602, 1959.
21. Faust, E. C. and DeGroat, A., Internal autoinfection in human strongyloidiasis, *Am. J. Trop. Med.*, 20, 359, 1940.
22. Galliard, H., Pathogenesis of *Strongyloides*, *Helminthol. Abstr.*, 36, 247, 1967.
23. Gill, G. V. and Bell, D. R., *Strongyloides stercoralis* infection in former Far East prisoners of war, *Br. Med. J.*, 2, 572, 1979.
24. Grove, D. I., Strongyloidiasis in Allied prisoners of war in Southeast Asia, *Br. Med. J.*, 2, 598, 1980.
25. Pelletier, L. L., Chronic strongyloidiasis in World War II Far East ex-prisoners of war, *Am. J. Trop. Med. Hyg.*, 33, 55, 1984.
26. Carroll, S. M., Karthigasu, K. T., and Grove, D. I., Serodiagnosis of human strongyloidiasis by an enzyme-linked immunosorbent assay, *Trans. R. Soc. Trop. Med. Hyg.*, 75, 706, 1981.
27. Genta, R. M., Strongyloidiasis, in *Immunodiagnosis of Parasitic Diseases*, Walls, K. and Schantz, P., Eds., Academic Press, New York, 1986, 183.
28. Genta, R. M. and Weil, G. J., Antibodies to *Strongyloides stercoralis*: larval surface antigens in chronic strongyloidiasis, *Lab. Invest.*, 47, 87, 1982.
29. McRury, J., de Messias, I. T., Walzer, P. D., Huitger, T., and Genta, R. M., Specific IgE responses in human strongyloidiasis, *Clin. Exp. Immunol.*, 65, 631, 1986.
30. Neva, F. A., Gam, A. A., and Burke, J., Comparison of larval antigens in an enzyme-linked immunosorbent assay for strongyloidiasis in humans, *J. Infect. Dis.*, 144, 427, 1981.

31. Genta, R. M., Predictive value of an enzyme-linked immunosorbent assay (ELISA) for the sero-diagnosis of strongyloidiasis, *Am. J. Clin. Pathol.*, 89, 391, 1988.

32. Genta, R. M., Douce, R. W., and Walzer, P. D., Diagnostic implications of parasite-specific immune responses in immunocompromised patients with strongyloidiasis, *J. Clin. Microbiol.*, 23, 1099, 1986.

33. Abdul-Fattah, M. M., Nasr, M. E., Yousef, S. M., Ibraheem, M. I., Abdul-Wahhab, S. E., and Soliman, H. M., Efficacy of ELISA in diagnosis of strongyloidiasis among the immunocompromised patients, *J. Egypt. Soc. Parasitol.*, 25, 491, 1995.

34. Genta, R. M., Frei, D. F., and Linke, M. J., Demonstration and partial characterization of parasite-specific immunoglobulin A responses in human strongyloidiasis, *J. Clin. Microbiol.*, 25, 1505, 1987; published erratum: *J. Clin. Microbiol.*, 27, 1143, 1989.

35. Purtilo, D. T., Meyers, W. M., and Connor, D. H., Fatal strongyloidiasis in immunosuppressed patients, *Am. J. Med.*, 56, 488, 1974.

36. Adam, M., Morgan, O., Persaud, C., and Gibbs, W. N., Hyperinfection syndrome, with *Strongyloides stercoralis* in malignant lymphoma, *Br. Med. J.*, 1, 264, 1973.

37. Ali-Khan, Z. and Seemayer, T. A., Fatal bowel infection and sepsis: an unusual complication of systemic strongyloidiasis, *Trans. R. Soc. Trop. Med. Hyg.*, 69, 473, 1975.

38. Brown, H. W. and Perna, V. P., An overwhelming *Strongyloides* infection, *JAMA*, 168, 1648, 1958.

39. Cruz, T., Reboucas, G., and Rocha, H., Fatal strongyloidiasis in patients receiving corticosteroids, *N. Engl. J. Med.*, 275, 1093, 1966.

40. Kuberski, T. T., Gabor, E. P., and Boudreaux, D., Disseminated strongyloidiasis: a complication of the immunosuppressed host, *West. J. Med.*, 122, 504, 1975.

41. Higenbottam, T. W. and Heard, B. E., Opportunistic pulmonary strongyloidiasis complicating asthma treated with steroids, *Thorax*, 31, 226, 1976.

42. Liepman, M., Disseminated *Strongyloides stercoralis*, a complication of immunosuppression, *JAMA*, 231, 287, 1975.

43. Cadham, F. T., Infestation with *Strongyloides stercoralis* associated with severe symptoms, *Can. Med. Assoc. J.*, 29, 18, 1933.

44. Aziz, E. M., *Strongyloides stercoralis* infestation: review of the literature and report of 33 cases, *South. Med. J.*, 62, 806, 1969.

45. Rojas, R. A. M., *Pathology of Protozoal and Helminthic Diseases*, Williams and Wilkins, Baltimore, 1971, 713.

46. Scaglia, M., Brustia, R., Gatti, S., Bernuzzi, A. M., Strosselli, M., Malfitano, A., and Capelli, D., Autochthonous strongyloidiasis in Italy: an epidemiological and clinical review of 150 cases, *Bull. Soc. Pathol. Exot. Filiales*, 77, 328, 1984.

47. Genta, R. M., Gatti, S., Linke, M. J., Cevini, C., and Scaglia, M., Endemic strongyloidiasis in northern Italy: clinical and immunological aspects, *Q. J. Med.*, 258, 679, 1988.

48. Davidson, R. A., Strongyloidiasis: a presentation of 63 cases, *NC Med. J.*, 43, 23, 1982.

49. Davidson, R. A., Fletcher, R. H., and Chapman, L. E., Risk factors for strongyloidiasis: a case-control study, *Arch. Intern. Med.*, 144, 321, 1984.

50. Rivera, E., Maldonado, N., Velez-Garcia, E., Grillo, A. J., and Malaret, G., Hyperinfection syndrome with *Strongyloides stercoralis*, *Ann. Intern. Med.*, 72, 199, 1970.

51. Keller, R. and Keist, R., Protective immunity to *Nippostrongylus brasiliensis* in the rat: central role of the lymphocyte in worm expulsion, *Immunology*, 22, 767, 1972.

52. Neva, F. A., Biology and immunology of human strongyloidiasis, *J. Infect. Dis.*, 153, 397, 1986.

53. Genta, R. M., *Strongyloides stercoralis*: immunobiological considerations on an unusual worm, *Parasitol. Today*, 2, 241, 1986.

54. Wong, B., Parasitic diseases in immunocompromised hosts, *Am. J. Med.*, 76, 479, 1984.

55. Longworth, D. L. and Weller, P. F., Hyperinfection syndrome with strongyloidiasis, in *Current Clinical Topics in Infectious Diseases*, Remington, J. S. and Swartz, M. N., Eds., McGraw-Hill, New York, 1986, 1.

56. Willis, A. J. P. and Nwokolo, C., Steroid therapy and strongyloidiasis, *Lancet*, 1, 1396, 1966.

57. Smith, J. W., Strongyloidiasis, *Clin. Microbiol. Newslett.*, 13, 33, 1991.

58. Armstrong, D. and Paredes, J., Strongyloidiasis, in *Respiratory Disease in the Immunocompromised Host*, Shalamer, J., Pizzo, P. A., Parrillo, J. E., and Masur, H., Eds., J. B. Lippincott, Philadelphia, 1991, 428.

59. Hanck, Ch. and Holzer, B. R., Strongyloidiasis unter immunosuppressiver therapy, *Schweiz. Med. Wochenschr.*, 122, 899, 1992.
60. Stewart, J. B. and Heap, B. J., Fatal disseminated strongyloidiasis in an immunocompromised former war prisoner of the Japanese, *J. R. Army Med. Corps*, 131, 47, 1985,
61. Batoni, F. L., Ianhez, L. E., Saldanha, L. B., and Sabbaga, E., Acute respiratory insufficiency caused by disseminated strongyloidiasis in a renal transplant, *Rev. Inst. Med. Trop. Sao Paulo*, 18, 283, 1976.
62. Fagundes, L. A., Busato, O., and Brentano, L., Strongyloidiasis: fatal complication of renal transplantation, *Lancet*, 2, 439, 1971.
63. Meyers, A. M., Shapiro, D. J., Milne, F. J., Myburgh, J. A., and Rabkin, R., *Strongyloides stercoralis* hyperinfection in a renal allograft recipient, *S. Afr. Med. J.*, 50, 1301, 1976.
64. Scoggin, C. H. and Call, N. B., Acute respiratory failure due to disseminated strongyloidiasis in a renal transplant recipient, *Ann. Intern. Med.*, 87, 456, 1977.
65. DeVault, G. A., King, J. W., Rohr, M. S., Landreneau, M. D., Brown, S. T. III, and McDonald, J. C., Opportunistic infections with *Strongyloides stercoralis* in renal transplantation, *Rev. Infect. Dis.*, 12, 653, 1990.
66. Dwork, K. G., Jaffe, J. R., and Lieberman, H. D., Strongyloidiasis with massive hyperinfection, *NY State J. Med.*, 75, 1230, 1975.
67. Neefe, L. I., Pinilla, O., Garagusi, V. F., and Bauer, H., Disseminated strongyloidiasis with cerebral involvement, *Am. J. Med.*, 55, 832, 1973.
68. Nagalotimath, S. J., Ramaprasad, A. V., and Chandrashekhar, N. K., Fatal strongyloidiasis in a patient receiving corticosteroids, *Indian J. Pathol. Bacteriol.*, 17, 190, 1974.
69. Yim, Y., Kikkawa, Y., Tanowitz, H., and Wittner, M., Fatal strongyloidiasis in Hodgkin's disease after immunosuppressive therapy, *J. Trop. Med. Hyg.*, 73, 245, 1970.
70. Rassiga, A. L., Lowry, J. L., and Forman, W. B., Diffuse pulmonary infection due to *Strongyloides stercoralis*, *JAMA*, 230, 426, 1974.
71. Suzuki, T., Nara, N., Miyake, S., Eishi, Y., Sugiyama, E., and Aoki, N., Fatal strongyloidiasis latent over 42 years in the antineoplastic chemotherapy of a case with malignant lymphoma, *Jpn. J. Med.*, 28, 96, 1989.
72. Hartz, P. H., Human strongyloidiasis with internal autoinfection, *Arch. Pathol.*, 41, 601, 1946.
73. Yoeli, M., Most, H., Berman, H. H., and Scheinesson, G. P. II., The clinical picture and pathology of a massive *Strongyloides* infection in a child, *Trans. R. Soc. Trop. Med. Hyg.*, 57, 346, 1963.
74. Bistrian, B. R., Sherman, M., Blackburn, G. L., Marshall, R., and Shaw, C., Cellular immunity in adult marasmus, *Arch. Intern. Med.*, 137, 1408, 1977.
75. Gage, J. G., A case of *Strongyloides intestinalis* with larvae in the sputum, *Arch. Intern. Med.*, 7, 561, 1911.
76. Tullis, D. C. H., Bronchial asthma associated with intestinal parasites, *N. Engl. J. Med.*, 282, 370, 1970.
77. Giannella, R. A., Broitman, S. A., and Zamcheck, N., Influence of gastric acidity on bacterial and parasitic enteric infections, *Ann. Intern. Med.*, 78, 271, 1973.
78. Shikhobalova, N. P. and Semenova, N. E., On the problem of the clinical study and treatment of strongyloidiasis, *Trop. Dis. Bull.*, 41, 411, 1944.
79. Kiyuna, M., Toda, T., Tamamoto, T., Shimajiri, S., Shingaki, Y., Hokama, M., and Ohwan, I., An autopsy case of periarteritis nodosa associated with disseminated strongyloidiasis, *Rinsho Byori*, 42, 883, 1994.
80. Gompels, M., Todd, J., Peters, B., Main, J., and Pinching, A. J., Disseminated strongyloidiasis in AIDS: uncommon but important, *AIDS*, 5, 329, 1991.
81. Torres, J. R., Isturiz, R., Murillo, J., Guzman M., and Contreras, R., Efficacy of ivermectin in the treatment of strongyloidiasis complicating AIDS, *Clin. Infect. Dis.*, 17, 900, 1993.
82. Nakada, K., Kohakura, M., Komoda, H., and Hinuma, Y., High incidence of HTLV-I antibody in carriers of *Strongyloides stercoralis*, *Lancet*, 1, 633, 1984.
83. Newton, R. C., Limpuangthip, P., Greenberg, S., Gam, A., and Neva, F. A., *Strongyloides stercoralis* hyperinfection in a carrier of HTLV-1 virus with evidence of selective immunosuppression, *Am. J. Med.*, 92, 202, 1992.
84. Yamaguchi, K., Matutes, E., Catovsky, D., Galton, D. A. G., Nakada, K., and Takatsuki, K., Strongyloides stercoralis as candidate co-factor for HTLV-1-induced leukaemogenesis, *Lancet*, 2, 94, 1987.

85. Pialoux, G., Beriel, P., Caudron, J., Chousterman, M., and Meyrignac, C., Syndrome d'imminodépression acquise associé a une anduillulose sévere, *Presse Med.*, 13, 1960, 1984.
86. Maayan, S., Wormser, G. P., Widerhorn, J., Sy, E. R., Kim, Y. H., and Ernst, J. A., *Strongyloides stercoralis* hyperinfection in a patient with the acquired immune deficiency syndrome, *Am. J. Med.*, 83, 945, 1987.
87. Vieyra-Herrera, G., Becerril-Carmona, G., Padua-Gabriel, A., Jessurun, J., and Alonso-de Ruiz, P., *Strongyloides stercoralis* hyperinfection in a patient with the acquired immune deficiency syndrome, *Acta Cytol*, 32, 277, 1988.
88. René, E., Marche, C., Régnier, B., Saimot, A. G., Vittecoq, B., Matheron, S., Le Port, C., Bricaire, F., Bure, A., Brun-Vezinet, C., Coulaud, J. P., and Bonfils, S., Manifestations digestives du syndrome d'immunodéficience acquise (SIDA): étude chez 26 patients, *Gastroenterol. Clin. Biol.*, 9, 327, 1985.
89. Baird, J. K., De Vinatea, M. L., Macher, A. M., Sierra, J. A. R., and Lasala, G., AIDS: case for diagnosis series, *Milit. Med.*, 152, M17, 1987.
90. Hillyer, G. V. and Climent, C., Acquired immunodeficiency syndrome (AIDS) and parasitic disease in Puerto Rico, *Bol. Asoc. Med. PR*, 80, 312, 1988.
91. Petithory, J. C. and Derouin, F., AIDS and strongyloidiasis in Africa, *Lancet*, 1, 921, 1987.
92. Gachot, B., Bouvet, E., Bure, A., Decre, D. et al., HIV infection and malignant strongyloidiasis, *Rev. Prat.*, 40, 2129, 1990.
93. Pearson, R. D. and Guerrant, R. L., *Strongyloides* infections, in *Hunter's Tropical Medicine*, 7th ed., Strickland, G. T., Ed., W. B. Saunders, Philadelphia, 1991, 706.
94. Spry, C. J. F., *Eosinophils: A Comprehensive Review, and Guide to the Scientific and Medical Literature*, Oxford University Press, Oxford, 1988.
95. Moro-Furlani, A. M. and Krieger, H., Familial analysis of eosinophilia caused by helminthic parasites, *Genet. Epidemiol.*, 9, 185, 1992.
96. Fisher, D., McCary, F., and Currie, B., Strongyloidiasis in the Northern Territory, *Med. J. Aust.*, 159, 88, 1993.
97. Prociv, P., Strongyloidiasis in the Northern Territory, *Med. J. Aust.*, 159, 636, 1993.
98. Savage, D., Foadi, M., Haworth, C., and Grant, A., Marked eosinophilia in an immunosuppressed patient with strongyloidiasis, *J. Intern. Med.*, 236, 473, 1994.
99. Sher, A. and Coffman, R. L., Regulation of immunity to parasites by T cells and T cell-derived cytokines, *Annu. Rev. Immunol.*, 10, 385, 1992.
100. Thomson, A. W., Mathie, I. H., and Sewell, H. F., Cyclophosphamide-induced eosinophilia in the rat: concomitant changes in T-cell subsets, B cell and large granular lymphocytes within lymphoid tissues, *Immunology*, 60, 383, 1987.
101. Gherman, I., Oproiu, A., Aposteneau, G., Constantinescu, M., Cociasu, S., Pospai, D., and Enuica, V., Observations on 35 cases of strongyloidiasis hospitalized at a clinical digestive disease unit, *Rev. Med. Interna*, 41, 169, 1989.
102. Stey, C., Jost, J., and Lüthy, R., Extraintestinale strongyloidiasis bei erworbenem immunmangelsyndrom, *Dtsch. Med. Wochensch.*, 115, 1716, 1990.
103. Azab, M. E., Mohamed, N. H., Salem, S. A., Safar, E. H., Bebars, M. A., Sabry, N. M., and Mohamed, M. S., Parasitic infections associated with malignancy and leprosy, *J. Egypt. Soc. Parasitol.*, 22, 59, 1992.
104. von Kuster, L. C. and Genta, R. M., Cutaneous manifestations of strongyloidiasis, *Arch. Dermatol.*, 124, 1826, 1988.
105. Kalb, R. E. and Grossman, M. E., Periumbilical purpura in disseminated strongyloidiasis, *JAMA*, 256, 1170, 1986.
106. Napier, L. E., *Strongyloides stercoralis* infection. II. Strongyloidiasis among ex-prisoners of war, *J. Trop. Med. Hyg.*, 52, 46, 1949.
107. Arthur, R. P. and Sheley, W. B., Larva currens: a distinct variant of cutaneous larva migrans due to *Strongyloides stercoralis*, *Arch. Dermatol.*, 78, 186, 1958.
108. Cunlife, W. J. and Silva, L. G., Linear urticaria due to larva currens: strongyloidiasis, *Br. J. Dermatol.*, 80, 108, 1968.
109. Stone, O. J., Newell, G. B., and Mullins, J. F., Cutaneous strongyloidiasis: larva currens, *Arch. Dermatol.*, 106, 734, 1972.

110. Corsini, A. C., Strongyloidiasis and chronic urticaria, *Postgrad. Med. J.*, 58, 247, 1982.

111. Grove, D. I., Treatment of strongyloidiasis with thiabendazole: an analysis of toxicity and effectiveness, *Trans. R. Soc. Trop. Med. Hyg.*, 76, 114, 1982.

112. Pelletier, L. L. and Gabre-Kidan, T., Chronic strongyloidiasis in Vietnam veterans, *Am. J. Med.*, 78, 139, 1985.

113. Orecchia, G., Pazzaglia, A., Scaglia, M., and Rabbiosi, G., Larva currens following systemic steroid therapy in a case of strongyloidiasis, *Dermatologica*, 171, 366, 1985.

114. Gordon, S. M., Gal, A. A., Solomon, A. R., and Bryan, J. A., Disseminated strongyloidiasis with cutaneous manifestations in an immunocompromised host, *J. Am. Acad. Dermatol.*, 31, 255, 1994.

115. Bank, D. E., Grossman, M. E., Kohn, S. R., and Rabinowitz, A. D., The thumbprint sign: rapid diagnosis of disseminated strongyloidiasis, *J. Am. Acad. Dermatol.*, 23, 324, 1990.

116. Ronan, S. G., Reddy, R. L., Manaligod, J. R., Alexander, J., and Fu, T., Disseminated strongyloidiasis presenting as purpura, *J. Am. Acad. Dermatol.*, 21, 1123, 1989.

117. Smith, J. D., Goette, D. K., and Odom, R. B., Larva currens: cutaneous strongyloidiasis, *Arch. Dermatol.*, 112, 1161, 1976.

118. Proctor, E. M., Muth, H. A. V., Proudfoot, D. L., Allen, A. B., Fisk, R., Isaac-Renton, J., and Black, W. A., Endemic institutional strongyloidiasis in British Columbia, *Can. Med. Assoc. J.*, 136, 1173, 1987.

119. Fulleborn, F., Hautquaddeln und "autoinfektion" bei strongyloidestragen, *Arch. Schiffs Trop. Hyg.*, 30, 821, 1926.

120. Caplan, J. P., Creeping eruption and intestinal strongyloidiasis, *Br. J. Med.*, 1, 396, 1949.

121. Brumpt, L. C. and Sang, H. T., Larva currens seul signe pathognomonique de la strongyloidose, *Ann. Parasitol.*, 48, 319, 1973.

122. de Messias, I. T., Telles, F. Q., Boaretti, A. C., Sliva, S., Guimarres, L. M., and Genta, R. M., Clinical, immunological and epidemiological aspects of strongyloidiasis in an endemic area of Brasil, *Allergol. Immunopathol.*, 15, 37, 1987.

123. McLarnon, M. and Ma, P., Brain stem glioma complicated by *Strongyloides stercoralis*, *Ann. Clin. Lab. Sci.*, 2, 546, 1981.

124. Harley, J. P. and Gallicchio, V., Effect of cortisone on the establishment of *Nippostrongylus brasiliensis* in the rabbit, *J. Parasitol.*, 56, 271, 1970.

125. Moqbel, R., Effect of corticosteroids on experimental strongyloidiasis. Proc. Br. Soc. Parasitology, *Parasitology*, 69, xviii, 1974.

126. Ogilvie, B. M., Use of cortisone derivatives to inhibit resistance to *Nippostrongylus brasiliensis* and to study the fate of parasites in resistant hosts, *Parasitology*, 55, 723, 1965.

127. Franz, K. H., Clinical trials with thiabendazole against human strongyloidiasis, *Am. J. Trop. Med. Hyg.*, 12, 211, 1963.

128. Most, H., Treatment of common parasitic infections of man encountered in the United States. I, *N. Engl. J. Med.*, 287, 495, 1972.

129. Kramer, M. R., Gregg, P., Goldstein, M., Llamas, R., and Krieger, B. P., Disseminated strongyloidiasis in AIDS and non-AIDS immunocompromised hosts: diagnosis by sputum and bronchoalveolar lavage, *South. Med. J.*, 83, 1226, 1990.

130. Schumaker, J. D., Band, J. D., Lensmeyer, G. L., and Craig, W. A., Thiabendazole treatment of severe strongyloidiasis in a hemodialyzed patient, *Ann. Intern. Med.*, 89, 644, 1978.

131. Royle, G., Fraser-Moodie, A., and Jones, M. W., Hyperinfection with *Strongyloides stercoralis* in Great Britain, *Br. J. Surg.*, 61, 498, 1974.

132. Bush, A., Gabriel, R., Gatus, S. J., and Thornton, J. G., Recurrent hyperinfestation with Strongyloides stercoralis in a renal allograft patient, *Br. Med. J.*, 286, 52, 1983.

133. Cook, G. A., Rodriguez, A., Silva, H., Rodriguez-Iturbe, B., and Bohorquez de Rodriguez, H., Adult respiratory distress secondary to strongyloidiasis, *Chest*, 92, 1115, 1987.

134. Thomson, J. R. and Berger, R., Fatal adult respiratory distress syndrome following successful treatment of pulmonary strongyloidiasis, *Chest*, 99, 772, 1991.

135. Berger, R., Kramm, S., and Paciotti, M., Pulmonary strongyloidiasis complicating therapy with corticosteroids, *Am. J. Trop. Med. Hyg.*, 29, 31, 1980.

136. Thomson, J. R. and Berger, R., *Strongyloides stercoralis* infection: a review of 66 cases, *South. Med. J.*, 82(Suppl.), 7, 1989.

137. Bidulph, J., Mebendazole and albendazole for infants, *Pediatr. Infect. Dis. J.*, 5, 373, 1990.

138. Currie, B., Why does Australia have no national drug policy? *Med. J. Aust.*, 157, 210, 1992.

139. Nandy, A., Addy, M., Patra, P., and Bandyopashyay, A. K., Fulminating strongyloidiasis complicating Indian kala-azar, *Trop. Geogr. Med.*, 47, 139, 1995.

140. Naquira, C., Jimenez, G., Guerra, J. G., Bernal, R., Nalin, D. R., Neu, D., and Aziz, M., Ivermectin for human strongyloidiasis and other intestinal helminths, *Am. J. Trop. Med. Hyg.*, 40, 304, 1989.

141. Giannoulis, E., Arvanitakis, C., Zaphirolopoulos, A., Nakos, V., Karkavelas, G., and Haralambidis, S., Disseminated strongyloidiasis with uncommon manifestations in Greece, *J. Trop. Med. Hyg.*, 89, 171, 1986.

26 *Cyclospora* spp.

26.1 INTRODUCTION

Organisms of the genus *Cyclospora* were first observed by Eimer in 1870 in the intestine of the mole.[1] The genus was created in 1881 by Schneider,[2] who described *C. glomerica* from a myriapod. Schaudinn[3] has also been credited with the first life-cycle study of *C. caryolitica* from moles, in which the parasite was described to develop in the intestinal epithelium and produce severe enteritis. In the ensuing years, *Cyclospora* spp. have been isolated from snakes,[4] insectivores,[5-8] rodents,[9] and most recently humans.[10] However, the first probable reported observation of *Cyclospora* infection in humans was by Ashford,[11] who in 1979 isolated the still-unnamed organisms from three patients of Papua New Guinea — although morphologically similar to *Cyclospora*, the isolated parasites were thought to possibly represent a new species of *Isospora* since four sporozoites were tentatively identified within each sporocyst. In 1986, Soave et al.[12] reported four cases of patients who had travelled to Haiti and Mexico and presented with enteritis caused by parasites similar to *Cyclospora*. The consensus that has emerged from 1990 to early 1993 was that the organism was possibly related to the cyanobacteria,[13-19] and the name "cyanobacterium-like body" has become widely adopted. Subsequently, Ortega et al.[10] succeeded in inducing sporulation of cyanobacterium-like bodies obtained from Peruvian patients, and conducted ultrastructural studies, which revealed the presence of organelles characteristic of coccidian protozoa of the phylum Apicomplexa and the genus *Cyclospora*. Based on these characteristics the name *Cyclospora cayetanensis* has been proposed.[20] Molecular phylogenetic analysis of rDNA sequences also revealed that the human-associated *C. cayetanensis* is closely related to members of the Eimeria genus.[21]

Subsequently, numerous reports have documented new cases worldwide and confirmed the association of diarrheal illness with *C. cayetanensis*.[22-64]

Sporulation characteristics combined with light and electron microscopic[65-67] identification of the life cycle stages of *Cyclospora* sp. provided evidence that these organisms require only a single host to complete their entire life cycle. In humans, the habitat of *Cyclospora* is the enterocyte of the small intestine.[19,67] All four asexual stages of *Cyclospora* (sporozoite, trophozoite, schizont, and merozoite) were observed within the parasitophorous vacuoles located in the apical supranuclear region of the enterocytes.[67] By inducing sporulation and excystation of oocysts (sexual stage) experimentally, the oocysts of *Cyclospora* were found to contain two sporocysts, with each sporo-cyst containing two sporozoites.[10] By comparison, the *Isospora* oocysts contain two sporocysts, but each of them has four sporozoites. *Cryptosporidium* has no sporocyst stage — instead, each oocyst consists of four naked sporozoites. Electron microscopic studies have shown that the unsporulated oocysts of *Cyclospora* possess an outer fibrillar coat, a cell wall and cell membrane, and light and dark granules,[10,15] whereas sporozoites within the sporocysts have a membrane-bound nucleus and micronemes.[10]

Various modes of transmission of the parasite to humans have been suggested.[11,13,14] However, it appears that cyclosporiasis can be contracted through consumption of fecally contaminated water supplies or food.[16,23,28,35,68,69] Some patients have been infected from accidental ingestion of aquarium water and from swimming in Lake Michigan.[22] It seems likely that water supplies may be contaminated by bird droppings.[16,70] Person-to-person transmission is unlikely because excreted oocysts require days to weeks, under favorable environmental conditions, to sporulate and become infectious.[40]

Cyclosporiasis has been diagnosed in immunocompetent adults,[17,22,38] in children,[10,17,71] immunocompromised (especially those with HIV infection) patients,[13,14,22,53,56,58] and on rare occasions in asymptomatic carriers.[10,17,23,58,72,73] The most typical signs of *C. cayetenensis* disease include persistent, acute, or chronic watery, nonbloody diarrhea, which begins days or weeks after infection.[17,23,40] The onset may be abrupt or gradual,[17] with such symptoms as nausea, vomiting, anorexia, bloating, abdominal cramping, increased gas, watery diarrhea, fatigue, and malaise.[11,12,17,22-24,28,30] In immunocompetent hosts, the diarrhea appeared to be prolonged but self-limited, lasting on average between 3 and 6 weeks, according to the various reports.[10,12,16,17,22,23] Although *Cyclospora*-associated diarrhea may be acute or chronic, the latter appeared to occur more frequently.[19,22,23,72,74] The resolution of symptoms seemed to correlate with the disappearance of the organisms from the stool, although diarrhea may persist after parasites are no longer detected.[31]

In immunocompromised patients, such as those with AIDS or diabetes,[74] the diarrhea tends to be persistent, unremitting, and more prolonged (for up to 15 weeks),[22,23] with higher morbidity (profound loss of weight and fatigue),[74] and recurrence after therapy is completed.[30,39] According to data by Pape et al.,[39] *Cyclospora*-induced diarrhea may be considered an opportunistic infection in HIV-infected individuals because it preceded the development of AIDS in 37% of patients.

After studying the difference in the clinical course of cyclosporiasis in patients with and without AIDS, Sifuentes-Osornio et al.[74] have suggested a possible extraintestinal involvement (acalculous cholecystitis) of *Cyclospora* in AIDS patients. While these investigators did not provide direct evidence of biliary infection due to *C. cayetenensis*, other *Cyclospora* spp. have been found in the biliary tract of moles,[8] which is an indirect proof of tissue tropism by these parasites.

The mechanism by which *Cyclospora* causes diarrhea has not been fully defined. In an earlier hypothesis,[75] it was suggested that similarly to cyanobacterium intoxication, *Cyclospora* produces an okadaic acid-like toxin capable of inhibiting phosphatase and modifying an array of cellular functions, including smooth muscle contractility and enteric neurotransmitter secretion. Now that *Cyclospora* has been identified as a coccidian parasite, this assumption seems less likely. Currently, cyclosporiasis is known to be associated with an inflammatory process in the small bowel[76] resulting in villus fusion and atrophy, which may reduce the surface area available for absorption and thus cause diarrhea.[74] This hypothesis has been supported by findings of impaired xylose absorption in patients with *Cyclospora* infection.[76,77]

26.1.1 HOST IMMUNE RESPONSE TO *CYCLOSPORA*

Little is known about the host immune response to *C. cayetanensis*. Its oocysts did not react with monoclonal antibody specific for *Cryptosporidium parvum*.[10,17] Although Long et al.[15] have found that patients passing *Cyclospora* in the stool have produced antibodies against these organisms, recurrent disease has been reported, indicating that infection did not provide lasting immunity.[23]

26.2 TREATMENT OF CYCLOSPORIASIS

A number of antibiotics have been used in the treatment of cyclosporiasis, including metronidazole, norfloxacin, ciprofloxacin, quinacrine, nalidixic acid, tinidazole, diloxanide, spiramycin, and azithromycin, but without apparent benefit.[11,12,17,22,34,78] Orally administered trimethoprim–sulfamethoxazole (TMP-SMX, co-trimoxazole) has been clearly efficacious.[40] The recommended dosage regimens have been, for adults, 160 mg of TMP and 800 mg of SMX, twice daily; and for children, daily oral doses of 5.0 and 25 mg/kg of TMP and SMX, respectively, twice daily.[79] Currently, a 31-d course of co-trimoxazole has been recommended,[80] although uncontrolled data collected for treatment of *Isospora belli* infections have suggested that as little as 2 d of treatment may be sufficient for immunocompetent patients.[81,82] Treatment regimens for patients who cannot tolerate sulfa drugs have not yet been identified.[40]

In a randomized, double-blind, placebo-controlled trial recently completed in Nepal,[83] 960 mg of co-trimoxazole (160 mg of TMP, and 800 mg of SMX) when administered twice daily for 7 d, eradicated the parasites in approximately 90% of immunocompetent adults, with no signs of relapse among treated patients followed for an additional 7 d.

In the largest trial so far of HIV-infected patients with cyslosporiasis, co-trimoxazole (160 mg of TMP, and 800 mg of SMX) was given orally four times daily for 10 d — both clinical improvement (cessation of symptoms in mean of 2.5 d) and parasitologic efficacy have been reported.[39] Secondary prophylaxis was successful with only a single relapse in a group of 12 patients taking co-trimoxazole prophylaxis for a mean of 7 months.

26.3 REFERENCES

1. Eimer, T., Ueber die ei- oder kugelförmigen sogennanten psorospermien der wirbeltiere, *Stubber's Verlangshandlung*, Würzburg, Germany, 1870, 1.
2. Schneider, A., Sur les psorospermies oviformes ou coccidies, espèces nouvelles ou peuconnues, *Arch. Zool. Exp. Gen.*, 9, 387, 1881.
3. Schaudinn, F., Studien über krankheitserregende protozoen. I. *Cyclospora caryolitica* Schaud., der erreger der perniciosen enteritis des maulwurfs, *Arbeit. Kaisereisch. Gesundheits.*, 18, 378, 1902.
4. Pellérdy, L. P., *Coccidia and Coccidiosis*, 2nd ed., Verlag Paul Parey, Berlin, 1965, 959.
5. Pellérdy, L. P. and Tanyi, J., *Cyclospora talpae* N. sp. (Protozoa: Sporozoa) from the liver of *Talpa europaea*, *Folia Parasitol. (Praha)*, 15, 275, 1968.
6. Duszynski, D. W. and Wattam, A. R., Coccidian parasites (Apicomplexa: Eimeridae) from insectivores. IV. Four new species in *Taipa europaea* from England, *J. Protozool.*, 35, 58, 1988.
7. Ford, P. L. and Duszynski, D. W., Coccidian parasites (Apicomplexa: Eimeridea) from insectivores. VI. Six new species from the eastern mole, *Scalopus aquaticus*, *J. Protozool.*, 35, 223, 1988.
8. Mohamed, H. A. and Molyneux, D. H., Developmental stages of *Cyclospora talpae* in the liver and bile duct of the mole (*Talpa europeae*), *Parasitology*, 101, 345, 1990.
9. Ford, P. L., Duszynski, D. W., and McAllister, C. T., Coccidia (Apicomplexa) from heteromyid rodents in the Southwestern United States, Baja California, and Northern Mexico with three new species from *Chaetodipus hispidus*, *J. Parasitol.*, 76, 325, 1990.
10. Ortega, Y. R., Sterling, C. R., Gilman, R. H., Cama, V. A., and Diaz, F., *Cyclospora* species: a new protozoan pathogen in humans, *N. Engl. J. Med.*, 328, 1308, 1993.
11. Ashford, R. W., Occurrence of an undescribed coccidian in man in Papua New Guinea, *Ann. Trop. Med. Parasitol.*, 73, 497, 1979.
12. Soave, R., Dubey, J. P., Ramos, L. J., and Tummings, M., A new intestinal pathogen? *Clin. Res.*, 34, 533A, 1986.
13. Hart, A. S., Ridinger, M. T., Soundarajan, R., Peters, C. S., Swiatlo, A. L., and Kocka, F. E., Novel organism associated with chronic diarrhea in AIDS, *Lancet*, 335, 169, 1990.
14. Long, E. G., Ebrahimzadeh, A., White, E. H., Swisher, B., and Callaway, C. S., Alga associated with diarrhea in patients with acquired immunodeficiency syndrome and in travelers, *J. Clin. Microbiol.*, 28, 1101, 1990.
15. Long, E. G., White, E. H., Carmichael, W. W., Quinlisk, P. M., Raja, R., Swisher, B. L., Daugharty, H., and Cohen, M. T., Morphologic and staining characteristics of a cyanobacterium-like organism associated with diarrhea, *J. Infect. Dis.*, 164, 199, 1991.
16. Centers for Disease Control, Outbreaks of diarrheal illness associated with cyanobacteria (blue-green algae)-like bodies, Chicago and Nepal, 1989 and 1990, *Morbid. Mortal. Wkly. Rep.*, 40, 325, 1991.
17. Shlim, D. R., Cohen, M. T., Eaton, M., Rajah, R., Long, E. G., and Ungar, B. L. P., An alga-like organism associated with an outbreak of prolonged diarrhea among foreigners in Nepal, *Am. J. Trop. Med. Hyg.*, 45, 383, 1991.

18. Weekly Epidemiological Record, Diarrhoeal diseases — outbreaks associated with cyanobacteria (blue-green algae)-like bodies: United States and Nepal, *Epidemiol. Rec.*, 33, 241, 1991.

19. Bendall, R. P., Lucas, S., Moody, A., Tovey, G., and Chiodini, P. L., Diarrhoea associated with cyanobacterium-like bodies: a new coccidian enteritis in man, *Lancet*, 341, 590, 1993.

20. Ortega, Y. R., Gilman, R. H., and Sterling, C. R., A new coccidian parasite (Apicomplexa: Eimeridae) from humans, *J. Parasitol.*, 80, 625, 1994.

21. Relman, D. A., Schmidt, T. M., Gajadhar, A., Sogin, M., Cross, J., Yoder, K., Sethabutr, O., and Echeverria, P., Molecular phylogenetic analysis of *Cyclospora*, the human intestinal pathogen, suggests that it is closely related to Eimeria species, *J. Infect. Dis.*, 173, 440, 1996.

22. Wurtz, R. M., Kocka, F. E., Peters, C. S., Weldon-Linne, C. M., Kuritza, A., and Yungbluth, P., Clinical characteristics of seven cases of diarrhea associated with a novel acid-fast organism in the stool, *Clin. Infect. Dis.*, 16, 136, 1993.

23. Hoge, C. W., Shlim, D. R., Rajah, R., Triplett, J., Shear, M., Rabold, J. G., and Echeverria, P., Epidemiology of diarrheal illness associated with coccidian-like organism among travelers and foreign residents in Nepal, *Lancet*, 341, 1175, 1993.

24. McDougall, R. J. and Tandy, M., Coccidian/cyanobacterium-like bodies as a cause of diarrhea in Australia, *Pathology*, 25, 375, 1993.

25. Connor, B. A., Shlim, D. R., Scholes, J. V., Rayburn, J. L., Reidy, J., and Rajah, R., Pathologic changes in the small bowel in nine patients with diarrhea associated with a coccidia-like body, *Ann. Intern. Med.*, 119, 377, 1993.

26. Berlin, O. G. W., Novak, S. M., Porschen, R. K., Long, E. G., Stelma, G. N., and Schaeffer, F. W. III, Recovery of *Cyclospora* organisms from patients with prolonged diarrhea, *Clin. Infect. Dis.*, 18, 606, 1994.

27. Butcher, A. R., Lumb, R., Coulter, E., and Nielsen, D. J., Coccidian/cynobacterium-like body associated diarrhea in an Australian traveller returning from overseas, *Pathology*, 26, 59, 1994.

28. Brennan, M. K., MacPherson, D. W., Palmer, J., and Keystone, J. S., Cyclosporiasis: a new cause of diarrhea, *Can. Med. Assoc. J.*, 155, 1293, 1996.

29. Soave, R. and Johnson, W. D., Jr., Cyclospora: conquest of an emerging pathogen, *Lancet*, 345, 667, 1995.

30. Farthing, M. J. G., Kelly, M. P., and Veitch, A. M., Recently recognized microbial enteropathies and HIV infection, *J. Antimicrob. Chemother.*, 37(Suppl. B), 61, 1996.

31. Wurtz, R., *Cyclospora*: a newly identified intestinal pathogen in humans, *Clin. Infect. Dis.*, 18, 620, 1994.

32. Hoge, C. W., Shlim, D. R., and Echeverria, P., Cyanobacterium-like Cyclospora species, *N. Engl. J. Med.*, 329, 1504, 1993.

33. Flynn, P. M., Emerging diarrheal pathogens: *Cryptosporidium parvum, Isospora belli, Cyclospora* species, and Microsporidia, *Pediatr. Ann.*, 25, 480, 1996.

34. Gascon, J., Corachan, M., Bombi, J. A., Valls, M. E., and Bordes, J. M., Cyclospora in patients with traveller's diarrhea, *Scand. J. Infect. Dis.*, 27, 511, 1995.

35. Huang, P., Weber, J. T., Sosin, D. M., Griffin, P. M., Long, E. G., Murphy, J. J., Kocka, F., Peters, C., and Kallick, C., The first reported outbreak of diarrheal illness associated with *Cyclospora* in the United States, *Ann. Intern. Med.*, 123, 409, 1995.

36. Chiodini, P. L., A "new" parasite: human infection with *Cyclospora cayetanensis*, *Trans. R. Soc. Trop. Med. Hyg.*, 88, 369, 1994.

37. Sinniah, B., Rajeswari, B., Johari, S., Ramakrishnan, K., Wan Yusoff, S., and Rohela, M., *Cyclospora* sp. causing diarrhea in man, *Southeast Asian J. Trop. Med. Public Health*, 25, 221, 1994.

38. Ooi, W. W., Zimmerman, S. K., and Needham, C. A., *Cyclospora* species as a gastrointestinal pathogen in immunocompetent hosts, *J. Clin. Microbiol.*, 33, 1267, 1995.

39. Pape, J. W., Verdier, R.-I., Boncy, M., Boncy, J., and Johnson, W. D., Jr., *Cyclospora* infection in adults infected with HIV, *Ann. Intern. Med.*, 121, 654, 1994.

40. Chambers, J., Somerfeldt, S., Mackey, L., Nichols, S., Ball, R., Roberts, D., Dufford, N., Reddick, A., and Gibson, J., Outbreaks of *Cyclospora cayetanensis* infection — United States, 1996, *Morbid. Mortal. Wkly. Rep.*, 276, 183, 1996.

41. Booy, R. and Tudor-Williams, G., Co-trimoxazole for cyclospora infection, *Lancet*, 345, 1303, 1995.

42. Soave, R., *Cyclospora*: an overview, *Clin. Infect. Dis.*, 23, 429, 1996.

43. Anonymous, *Cyclospora* infections on the increase, *J. Ark. Med. Soc.*, 93, 143, 1996.

44. Clarke, S. C. and McIntyre, M., The incidence of *Cyclospora cayetanensis* in stool samples submitted to a district general hospital, *Epidemiol. Infect.*, 117, 189, 1996.

45. Crowley, B., Path, C., Moloney, C., and Keane, C. T., *Cyclospora* species — a cause of diarrhoea among Irish travellers to Asia, *Ir. Med. J.*, 89, 110, 1996.

46. Lammers, H. A., van Gool, T., and Eeftinck Schattenkerk, J. K., Two patients with diarrhea caused by *Cyclospora cayetanensis*, *Ned. Tijdschr. Geneeskd.*, 140, 890, 1996.

47. Centers for Disease Control, Update: outbreaks of *Cyclospora cayetanensis* infection — United States and Canada, 1996, *Morbid. Mortal. Wkly. Rep.*, 45, 611, 1996.

48. Wanachiwanawin, D., Lertlaituan, P., Manatsathit, S., Tunsupasawasdikul, S., Suwanagool, P., and Thakerngpol, K., *Cyclospora* infection in an HIV infected patient with ultrastructural study, *Southeast Asian J. Trop. Med. Public Health*, 26, 375, 1995.

49. Albert, M. J., Kabir, I., Azim, T., Hossain, A., Ansaruzzaman, M., and Unicomb, L., Diarrhea associated with *Cyclospora* sp. in Bangladesh, *Diagn. Microbiol. Infect. Dis.*, 19, 47, 1994.

50. van Gool, T. and Dankert, J., Three emerging protozoal infections in The Netherlands: *Cyclospora*, *Diantamoeba*, and *Microspora* infections, *Ned. Tijdschr. Geneeskd.*, 140, 155, 1996.

51. Lontie, M., Degroote, K., Michaels, J., Bellers, J., Mangelschots, E., and Vandepitte, J., *Cyclospora* sp.: a coccidian that causes diarrhoea in travellers, *Acta Clin. Belg.*, 50, 288, 1995.

52. Chacin-Bonilla, L., *Cyclospora*: a pathogenic parasite in humans, *Invest. Clin.*, 36, 43, 1995.

53. Robinson, R. D., Parasitic infections associated with HIV/AIDS in the Carribean, *Bull. Pan. Am. Health Organ.*, 29, 129, 1995.

54. Purych, D. B., Perry, I. L., Bulawka, D., Kowalewska-Grochowska, K. T., and Oldale, B. L., A case of *Cyclospora* infection in an Albertan traveller, *Can. Commun. Dis. Rep.*, 21, 88, 1995.

55. Weber, R. and Deplazes, P., New parasitic diseases in man: infections caused by Microsporida and *Cyclospora* species, *Schweiz. Med. Wochenschr.*, 125, 909, 1995.

56. Raguin, C., Heyer, F., Rousseau, C., Aerts, J., Desplaces, N., and Deluol, A., *Cyclospora* infection in an HIV infected patient, *Presse Med.*, 24, 1134, 1995.

57. Zerpa, R., Uchima, N., and Huicho, L., *Cyclospora cayetanensis* associated with watery diarrhoea in Peruvian patients, *J. Trop. Med. Hyg.*, 98, 325, 1995.

58. Maggi, P., Brandonisio, O., Larocca, A. M., Rollo, M. et al., *Cyclospora* in AIDS patients: not always an agent of diarrhoeic syndrome, *New Microbiol.*, 18, 73, 1995.

59. Deluol, A. M., Junod, C., Poirot, J. L., Heyer, F., N'Go, Y., and Cosnes, J., Travellers diarrhea associated with *Cyclospora* sp., *J. Eukaryote Microbiol.*, 41, 32S, 1994.

60. Junod, C., Deluol, A. M., Cosnes, J., and Bauer, P., *Cyclospora*, a new coccidium agent of travelers' diarrhea, *Presse Med.*, 23, 1312, 1994.

61. Clarke, S. C. and McIntyre, M., Human infection with *Cyclospora*, *J. Infect.*, 29, 112, 1994.

62. Casemore, D. P., *Cyclospora*: another "new" pathogen, *J. Med. Microbiol.*, 41, 217, 1994.

63. Markus, M. B. and Frean, J. A., Occurrence of human *Cyclospora* infection in sub-Saharan Africa, *S. Afr. Med. J.*, 83, 862, 1993.

64. Rijpstra, A. C. and Laarman, J. J., Repeated findings of unidentified small *Isospora*-like coccidia in faecal specimens from travelers returning to The Netherlands, *Trop. Geogr. Med.*, 45, 280, 1993.

65. Nhieu, J. T. V., Nin, F., Fleury-Feith, J., Chaumette, M.-T., Schaeffer, A., and Bretagne, S., Identification of intracellular stages of *Cyclospora* species by light microscopy of thick sections using hematoxylin, *Hum. Pathol.*, 27, 1107, 1996.

66. Deluol, A.-M., Teilhac, M. F., Poirot, J.-L., Heyer, F., Beaugerie, L., and Chatelet, F.-P., *Cyclospora* sp.: life cycle studies in patient by electron microscopy, *J. Eukaryote Microbiol.*, 43, 128S, 1996.

67. Sun, T., Ilardi, C., Asnis, D., Bresciani, A., Goldenberg, S., Roberts, B., and Teichberg, S., Light and electron microscopic identification of *Cyclospora* species in the small intestine, *Clin. Microbiol. Infect. Dis.*, 195, 216, 1996.

68. Rabold, J. G., Hoge, C. W., Shlim, D. R., Kefford, C., Rajah, R., and Echeverria, P., *Cyclospora* outbreak associated with chlorinated drinking water, *Lancet*, 344, 1360, 1994.

69. Connor, B. A. and Shlim, D. R., Foodborne transmission of *Cyclospora*, *Lancet*, 346, 1634, 1995.

70. Wurtz, R. M., Kocka, F. E., Kallick, C., Peters, C., and Dacumos, F., Blue green algae associated with a diarrheal outbreak, *Proc. 91st Meet. Am. Soc. Microbiol.*, American Society for Microbiology, Washington, D.C., Abstr. C-21, 1991.

71. Hoge, C. W., Echeverria, P., Rajah, R., Jacobs, J., Malthouse, S., Chapman, E., Jimenez, L. M., and Shlim, D., Prevalence of *Cyclospora* species and other enteric pathogens among children less than 5 years of age in Nepal, *J. Clin. Microbiol.*, 33, 3058, 1995.

72. Pollock, R. C., Bendall, R. P., Moody, A., Chiodini, P. L., and Churchill, D. R., Traveller's diarrhoea associated with a cyanobacterium-like bodies: a new coccidium enteritis in man, *Lancet*, 340, 556, 1992.

73. Goodgame, R. W., Understanding intestinal spore-forming protozoa: Cryptosporidia, Microsporidia, Isospora, and Cyclospora, *Ann. Intern. Med.*, 124, 429, 1996.

74. Sifuentes-Osornio, J., Porras-Cortés, G., Bendall, R. P., Morales-Villareal, F., Reyes-Teran, G., and Ruiz-Palacios, G. M., *Cyclospora cayetanensis* infection in patients with and without AIDS: biliary disease as another clinical manifestation, *Clin. Infect. Dis.*, 21, 1092, 1995.

75. Karaki, H., Traveller's diarrhoea associated with cyanobacterium-like bodies, *Lancet*, 340, 1159, 1992.

76. Connor, B. A., Shlim, D. R., Scholes, J. V., Rayburn, J. L., Reidy, J., and Rajah, R., Pathologic changes in the small bowel in nine patients with diarrhea associated with a coccidia-like body, *Ann. Intern. Med.*, 119, 377, 1993.

77. Bendall, R. P. and Chiodini, P. L., Intestinal malabsorption associated with human *Cyclospora* infection, *Proc. 1st Biannual Conf. Federation Infectious Societies (London)*, Federation of Infectious Societies, Manchester, U.K., Abstr. 817, 1994.

78. Shear, M., Connor, B. A., Shlim, D. R., Taylor, D. N., and Rabold, J. G., Azithromycin treatment of cyclospora infections, *Gastroenterology*, 106(Suppl. 4), 772A, 1994.

79. Madico, G., Gilman, R. H., Miranda, E., Cabrera, L., and Sterling, C. R., Treatment of *Cyclospora* infections with co-trimoxazole, *Lancet*, 342, 122, 1993.

80. Anonymous, Drugs for parasitic infections, *Med. Lett.*, 35, 111, 1993.

81. Westerman, E. L. and Christensen, R. P., Chronic *Isospora belli* infection treated with co-trimoxazole, *Ann. Intern. Med.*, 91, 413, 1979.

82. DeHovitz, J. A., Pape, J. W., Bongy, M., and Johnson, W. D., Jr., Clinical manifestations and therapy of *Isospora belli* infection in patients with the acquired immunodeficiency syndrome, *N. Engl. J. Med.*, 315, 87, 1986.

83. Hoge, C. W., Shlim, D. R., Ghimire, M., Rabold, J. G., Pandey, P., Walch, A., Rajah, R., Gaudio, P., and Echeverria, P., Placebo-controlled trial of co-trimoxazole for cyclospora infections among travellers and foreign residents in Nepal, *Lancet*, 345, 691, 1995.

27 Arthropod Infestations in HIV-Infected Patients

The human immunodeficiency virus (HIV) is a lymphotropic human retrovirus that has been currently classified into two types: HIV-1 (the causative agent of nearly all infections in the U.S. and Europe) and HIV-2 (associated with infections mainly in West Africa and isolated cases elsewhere).

Primary HIV infections are usually asymptomatic. In the 10% to 20% of primary infections which are symptomatic, the presentation is of an acute febrile illness with varying severity depending on the route of infection and the size of the viral inoculum. Following the primary infection, the HIV enters its latent stage. However, some patients develop persistent generalized lymphadenopathy which may be associated with constitutional symptoms. In both asymptomatic patients and those with generalized lymphadenopathy, HIV disease may progress to AIDS-related complex (ARC) characterized with such symptoms as fever, weight loss, persistent diarrhea, oropharyngeal candidiasis, herpes zoster, and oral hairy leukoplakia. Most of these patients, as well as asymptomatic patients and patients with generalized lymphadenopathy will develop AIDS, which is defined by profound immunodeficiency leading to the occurrence of opportunistic infections and neoplasia (Kaposi's sarcoma, lymphoma, squamous cell carcinoma). The CD4 T helper lymphocyte count is used as an indirect marker to monitor the HIV-induced immunodeficiency.

The prevalence of cutaneous manifestations during the course of HIV infections has been recognized as an important factor for the early diagnosis of HIV disease and prompt initiation of therapy to delay its progression and to prevent opportunistic infections.[1,2] Skin manifestations caused by infectious agents represent one of three major groups of dermatologic disorders associated with the HIV infection (Table 27.1). The other two groups are neoplastic disorders and a miscellaneous group which includes papulosquamous, papular, vascular, autoimmune, oral, and drug-related skin disorders (Table 27.2).[1,2]

The majority of cutaneous manifestations listed in Table 27.1, due to their increased frequency not only in HIV-infected individuals but in a large population of other immunocompromised patients, will be discussed in the various chapters referring to the particular opportunistic pathogen. Some arthropod infestations which complicate HIV disease and other immune deficiencies will be discussed in the context of this chapter.

27.1 SCABIES (SARCOPTIDOSIS)

The causative agent of scabies is *Sarcoptes scabiei*, the itch mite in humans, an acarid belonging to the genus *Sarcoptes*. In domestic (horses, cows, dogs, and pigs) and wild animals, *S. scabiei* causes mange. Scabies is a contagious dermatitis that is transmitted by close contact and is characterized by a papular eruption over tiny, raised sinuous burrows (cuniculi) excavated by the female mite in the superficial layers of the skin where she lays her eggs and deposits her irritating excreta.[3]

TABLE 27.1
Cutaneous Infections in HIV-Positive Patients

Viral infections
    Herpes simplex virus types 1 and 2
    Cytomegalovirus
    Varicella zoster virus
    Epstein-Barr virus
    Human papilloma virus
    Moluscum contagiosum

Bacterial infections
    Staphylococcus aureus infections
    Bacillary angiomatosis
    Mycobacterioses
      Leprosy
      Mycobacterium tuberculosis
      Mycobacterium haemophilium/M. fortuitum
      Mycobacterium avium-intracellulare
      Bacille Calmette-Guérin (BCG)
    Syphilis

Fungal infections
    Candidiasis
    Pityrosporum infections
    Dermatophytoses
    Dessiminated mycoses
      Cryptococcosis
      Coccidioidomycosis
      Histoplasmosis
      Sporotrichosis

Arthropod infestations
    Scabies
    Demodicidosis
Protozoan Infections
    Extrapulmonary pneumocystosis
    Leishmaniasis
    Cutaneous toxoplasmosis

Sarcoptidosis is manifested by intense pruritus (linear papulovesicles located in flexural and intertriginous areas), and occasionally eczema (from scratching) and secondary bacterial infection. A rare, but more severe, form is the crusted (Norwegian) scabies which is characterized by heavy infestation of *S. scabiei*, and is observed in mentally retarded and senile patients, as well as patients with severe systemic disease and in immunocompromised individuals.

The crusted (Norwegian) scabies was first described in 1868 by Danielsen and Boeck[4] in Norwegian patients with Hansen's disease, but was later diagnosed in mentally handicapped individuals as well as patients with Down's syndrome,[5] tabes dorsalis, and syringomyelia.[6] There has been increased incidence of crusted scabies in immunocompromised patients (impaired humoral and cell-mediated immunity,[7,8] diabetes[9]), patients suffering from hematologic malignancy (T cell leukemia,[10,11] lymphatic,[12] and monocytic leukemia[13]), and patients receiving immunosuppressive therapy (renal transplant recipients,[6,14-16] lupus erythematosus,[17] vasculitis,[18] and high-potency topical corticosteroids[19,20]).

TABLE 27.2
Noninfectious Skin Manifestations
in HIV Disease

Papulosquamous eruptions
  Seborrheic dermatitis
  Psoriasis vulgaris
  Reiter's syndrome
  Xeroderma/acquired ichthyosis
  Erythroderma

Papular eruptions
  Papular eruptions in AIDS
  HIV-associated eosinophilic folliculitis

Vascular disorders
  Thrombocytic purpura
  Vasculitis
  Lymphomatoid granulomatosis
  Hyperalgesic pseudothrombophlebitis
  Linear telangiecthema

Autoimmune disorders
  Vitiligo
  Sicca syndrome

Oral manifestations
  Oropharyngeal candidiasis

Hair alterations
Nail changes

Norwegian scabies is manifested by a marked crusting dermatitis of the hands and feet with subungual horny debris, erythematous scaling plaques on the neck, scalp, and trunk that may become generalized, and usually lymphadenopathy, eosinophilia, elevated levels of IgE,[21] and decreased levels of IgA.[22] Even though unsanitary living conditions certainly may be related to crusted scabies,[23] in some patients personal hygiene was found not to be a significant factor in altering the rate of mite proliferation.[24]

Topical treatment with gamma benzene hexachloride lotion or permethrin is usually effective for scabies. In crusted scabies, total-body application may be required.[2]

Both pruritic linear papulovesicles and the hyperkeratotic papules of Norwegian scabies have been described in association with AIDS.[24-26] With progressive deterioration of their immune responses, HIV-infected patients become more vulnerable to crusted scabies presenting with generalized hyperkeratosis resembling psoriasis vulgaris, keratoderma blenorrhagica of Reiter's syndrome, or Darier's disease.[2]

Glover et al.[24] have described a fatal case of Norwegian scabies in an AIDS patient who died with bacteremia, pericarditis, and pneumonia. The patient failed to respond to therapy consisting of intravenous nafcillin, normal saline solution, packed red blood cells, and topical 1% lindane lotion.

Fisher and Warner[26] found that postscabies dermatitis after successful treatment may be a problem in AIDS patients — its treatment may be difficult and frustrating because of the severe itching and dermatitis.

27.2 DEMODICIDOSIS

Demodex folliculorum is the causative agent of demodicidosis, a pruritic papulonodular eruption occurring on the scalp, face, and neck of HIV-infected patients.[2,27] The pathogen belongs to a genus of mites or acarids (family *Demodicidae*) found in the hair of humans and in sebaceous secretions, especially of the face and nose. Skin biopsies have shown a dense lymphoeosinophilic inflammatory infiltrate in the papillary and midreticular dermis and occasionally in a perifollicular arrangement.[2] It is important that demodicidosis is differentiated from other nonspecific papular eruptions observed during AIDS, such as eosinophilic folliculitis and *Pityrosporum* folliculitis. Treatment of this skin disorder is usually by topical application of gamma benzene hexachloride lotion or permethrin creame.[2]

In the first record of opportunistic demodicidosis associated with AIDS, Dominey et al.[27] have described a distinctive papulonodular variant of this infestation in two AIDS patients. It was characterized by pruritus, abrupt onset, numerous mites on skin scraping and biopsy samples, and rapid response to 1% gamma benzene hexachloride lotion or 1% permethrin cream. Impaired immune responses might have allowed these normally commensal organisms to proliferate in the skin to the point of causing disease. In an alternative hypothesis, Soeprono and Schinella[28] suggested that the development of eosinophilic pustular folliculitis is an unusual hypersensitivity response to mite.

27.3 REFERENCES

1. Dover, J. S. and Johnson, R. A., Cutaneous manifestations of human immunodeficiency virus infection. I, *Arch. Dermatol.*, 127, 1383, 1991.
2. Dover, J. S. and Johnson, R. A., Cutaneous manifestations of human immunodeficiency virus infection. II, *Arch. Dermatol.*, 127, 1549, 1991.
3. Brown, H. W., Arthropods and Human Disease, in *Cecil-Loeb Textbook of Medicine*, Beeson, P. B. and McDermott, W., Eds., W. B. Saunders, Philadelphia, 1963, 444.
4. Danielsen, D. C. and Boeck, W., Quoted by Hebra, F., in *Diseases of the Skin*, New Sydenham Society, London, 1868.
5. Alligood, T., Fix, L. W., and Samoredin, C., Norwegian scabies: a case report and review of the literature, *W. Va. Med. J.*, 77, 33, 1981.
6. Patterson, W. D., Allen, B. R., and Beveridge, G. W., Norwegian scabies during immunosuppressive therapy, *Br. Med. J.*, 4, 211, 1973.
7. Dick, G. F., Burgdorf, W. H. C., and Gentry, W. C., Jr., Norwegian scabies in Bloom's syndrome, *Arch. Dermatol.*, 115, 212, 1979.
8. Sadick, N., Kaplan, M. H., Pahwa, S. G., and Sarngadharan, M. G., Unusual features of scabies complicating human T-lymphotropic virus type III infection, *J. Am. Acad. Dermatol.*, 15, 482, 1986.
9. Pitz, R. J., Tur, E., Brenner, S., and Krakowski, A., Norwegian scabies following topical corticosteroid therapy, *Isr. J. Med. Sci.*, 17, 1165, 1981.
10. Suzumiya, J., Sumiyoshi, A., Kuroki, T., and Inoue, S., Crusted (Norwegian) scabies with adult T-cell leukemia, *Arch. Dermatol.*, 121, 903, 1985.
11. Arata, J., Ohara, A., Yamamoto, Y., Ikeda, M., and Kobayashi, M., Coexistence of unusual scabies and pneumocytosis in a patient without any underlying disease, *J. Dermatol.*, 11, 89, 1984.
12. Dostrovsky, A., Raubitschek, F., and Sagher, F., Scabies norvegica and lymphatic leukemia, *Dermatologica*, 113, 26, 1956.
13. Evans, D. I., Norwegian scabies and monocytic leukemia, *Br. Med. J.*, 4, 613, 1973.
14. Espy, P. D. and Jolly, H. W., Jr., Norwegian scabies: occurrence in a patient undergoing immuno-suppression, *Arch. Dermatol.*, 112, 193, 1976.
15. Wolf, R., Wolf, D., Viskoper, R. J., and Sandbank, M., Norwegian-type scabies mimicking contact dermatitis in an immunosuppressed patient, *Postgrad. Med. J.*, 78, 228, 1985.
16. Youshock, E. and Glaser, S. D., Norwegian scabies in a renal transplant patient, *JAMA*, 246, 2608, 1981.

17. Mikheev, G. N., Development of hyperkeratotic or Norwegian scabies in two patients with lupus erythematosus, *Vestn. Dermatol. Venerol.*, 4, 57, 1987.
18. Neste, D. A., Minne, G., Thomas, P., and Gosselin, X., Hyperkeratotic (Norwegian) scabies and onychomycosis in an immunosuppressed patient, *Dermatologica*, 170, 142, 1985.
19. Clayton, R. and Farrow, S., Norwegian scabies following topical steroid therapy, *Postgrad. Med. J.*, 51, 647, 1975.
20. Macmillan, A. L., Unusual feature of scabies associated with topical fluorinated steroids, *Br. J. Dermatol.*, 87, 496, 1972.
21. Burks, J. W., Jung, R., and George, W. M., Norwegian scabies, *Arch. Dermatol.*, 74, 131, 1956.
22. Hancock, B. W. and Ward, A. M., Serum immunoglobulin in scabies, *J. Invest. Dermatol.*, 63, 482, 1974.
23. Mellanby, K., *Scabies*, Oxford University Press, London, 1943.
24. Glover, R., Young, L., and Goltz, R. W., Norwegian scabies in acquired immunodeficiency syndrome: report of a case resulting in death from associated sepsis, *J. Am. Acad. Dermatol.*, 16, 396, 1987.
25. Kaplan, M. H., Sadick, N., McNutt, N. S., Meltzer, M., Sarngadharan, M. G., and Pahwa, S., Dermatologic findings and manifestations of acquired immunodeficiency syndrome (AIDS), *J. Am. Acad. Dermatol.*, 16, 485, 1987.
26. Fisher, B. K. and Warner, L. C., Cutaneous manifestations of the acquired immunodeficiency syndrome, *Int. J. Dermatol.*, 26, 615, 1987.
27. Dominey, A., Rosen, R., and Tschen, J., Papulonodular demodicidosis associated with acquired immunodeficiency syndrome, *J. Am. Acad. Dermatol.*, 20, 197, 1989.
28. Soeprono, F. F. and Schinella, R. A., Eosinophilic pustular folliculitis in patients with acquired immunodeficiency syndrome, *J. Am. Acad. Dermatol.*, 14, 1020, 1986.

Section IV

Fungal Infections

28 Introduction

During the last two decades or so, the incidence of fungal infections has increased dramatically. Deep-seated mycoses are creating serious problems for clinicians working with certain populations of patients, such as those with cancer, the immunocompromised, and physiologically compromised.[1,2]

With ever-expanding application of immunosuppressive therapy, the role host factors (the T lymphocyte system) play in the defense against systemic fungal infections is currently the subject of intensive studies, and new approaches for antifungal therapy are being investigated.

The need for effective antifungal drugs has been felt more and more acutely with the emergence of the AIDS pandemic and the AIDS-related complex (ARC), which are nearly always associated with opportunistic fungal infections.

Another factor facilitating the spread of opportunistic mycoses has been the significant improvement achieved in the management of bacterial infections.

At present, the majority of antifungal agents available to clinicians, in addition to having some unacceptable side effects, are, by mechanism of action, fungistatic. Such a mode of action, for the most part, requires prolonged periods of treatment, and relapses after treatment is ceased are frequent. Since both human and fungal cells are, by nature, eukaryotic, prolonged antifungal chemotherapy is damaging to host cells too. Overcoming an obstacle such as this presents a fundamental challenge to scientists in their quest for safer, more selective, and effective antifungal agents.[1,2]

28.1 GENERAL CHARACTERISTICS OF FUNGI

The fungi are a group of mostly aerobic, heterotrophic, nonmotile eukaryotic organisms with well-defined cell wall but devoid of chlorophyll, which reproduce by spores.[3] The spores, which can be generated either sexually or asexually, represent propagating units without embryo. After germination, the spores produce such diverse forms as molds and yeasts. These two forms are not always mutually exclusive, and a fungus can exist in either a mold or yeast form under proper growth conditions.

In molds, the spores germinate to generate branching filaments known as hyphae, which may be divided into cells by septa. In its most complex form, usually seen in fungi of Basidiomycota, the septa have a barrel-shaped central apparatus called dolipore. While not all of the fungal hyphae may have septa, regardless of its presence or absence, the filaments usually elongate by apical growth. It should be noted, however, that all fungal parts have the potential for growth. A mass of hyphae is called mycellium, which on macroscopic examination appears distinctly fuzzy.[3] Most fungal hyphae are capable of indefinite growth under favorable conditions, which for most pathogenic species *in vitro* is 25 to 35°C, and acidic pH (6.0 to 6.8). While light is not required for fungal growth, its presence may influence sexual and asexual sporulation in many fungi.

In the yeast form, the spores germinate to produce round, oval, or elongated single cells that reproduce mainly by budding (some by fission) to generate moist or mucoid colonies.[3] Occasionally, the bud will remain attached to the mother cell and undergo continuous budding (without separation) to generate chains of elongated cells known as pseudohyphae.

The sexual reproduction of fungi is initiated by conjugation of two cells (differentiated or undifferentiated) within the same thallus (that is, the actively growing vegetative organism as distinguished from reproductive or resting portions), or two cells from opposite mating types. Typically, the sexual reproduction consists of three stages: (1) plasmogamy (union of two protoplasts); (2) karyogamy (fusion of two nuclei); and (3) meiosis. In the majority of sexually reproducing fungi, the diploid stage is transient and is followed immediately by meiotic division to yield haploid spores. In fungal species devoid of sexual stage, the hyphae remain haploid and generate spores only by mitosis.[3]

A number of pathogenic fungi will exist in the yeast form (parasitic) in host tissues but in hyphal (mycelial) form (saprobic) *in vitro*. Such fungi are known as dimorphic. However, not all dimorphic pathogens will have yeast forms *in vivo*. For example, *Coccidioides immitis* grows as a spherule with endosporulation in host tissues, while agents of chromoblastomycosis will form round structures called sclerotic bodies that divide by internal septation of different planes.

28.2 FUNGAL TAXONOMY

The basic taxonomic fungal rank is the species. Species are organized into hierarchical systems of genera, families, orders, classes, and phyla (or divisions).[3] The kingdom of fungi is comprised of four phyla: Zygomycota, Ascomycota, Basidiomycota, and the form-phylum Deuteromycota (Fungi Imperfecti). Each of the phyla is divided into two or more classes as follows: (1) Zygomycota: Zygomycetes and Trichomycetes; (2) Ascomycota: Ascomycetes and Hemiascomycetes; (3) Basidiomycota: Holobasidiomycetes and Heterobasidiomycetes; and (4) Deuteromycota: Blastomycetes, Coelomycetes, and Hyphomycetes.

The Fungi Imperfecti is a group of fungi classified in the form-phylum Deuteromycota. They have septate hyphae and are currently known to reproduce only by means of conidia. No sexual state (teleomorph) is known, hence the name Fungi Imperfecti. Many Deuteromycota are the same as some anamorphs of Ascomycota and also have some basidiomycetous affinities. It is surmised, therefore, that the majority of Fungi Imperfecti may be defined as anamorphs of ascomycetous fungi whose teleomorphs are still undiscovered or have been lost during their evolution.[3]

28.3 REFERENCES

1. Georgiev, V. St., *Antifungal Drugs*, (Ann. NY Acad. Sci., Vol. 544), The New York Academy of Sciences, New York, 1988.
2. Georgiev, V. St., Fungal infections and the search for novel antifungal agents, *Ann. NY Acad. Sci.*, 544, 1, 1988.
3. Kwon-Chung, K. J. and Bennett, J. E., *Medical Mycology*, Lea and Febiger, Philadelphia, 1992, 3.

29 Fungal Cell Envelope and Mode of Action of Antimycotic Agents

Antifungal drugs currently used in clinical practice against systemic mycoses include polyene antibiotics (e.g., amphotericin B), azole derivatives (e.g., ketoconazole, fluconazole, itraconazole), and 5-fluorocytosine.[1,2] With the exception of the latter, all other agents act by mechanisms aimed at disrupting the integrity of the fungal cell membrane be either interfering with the biosynthesis of membrane sterols or inhibiting sterol functions.[4-6]

29.1 FUNGAL CELL WALL

The fungal cell envelope consists of cell wall and cell membrane. The cell wall, which is essential for the survival of the fungus, is not present in mammalian cells. It is a rigid stratified structure consisting generally of chitinous microfibrils embedded in a matrix of small polysaccharides, proteins, lipids, inorganic salts, and pigments that provide skeletal support and shape of the protoplast.[7] The cell wall determines the shape of the fungal cell and confers rigidity and strength to the cell. Furthermore, because of its limited porosity, the fungal cell wall serves as a permeability barrier for large molecules. Structurally, it is a multilayer formation comprised largely of carbohydrates, such as glucans, chitin, and mannoproteins. The latter create a surface layer which penetrates the wall to some depth and shields the glucans from attack by Z-glucanase.[8] Some mannan-containing exoenzymes may be concentrated in the periplasmic space next to the plasmalema.[9,10]

The cell wall glucans represent mixtures of branched β-1,3- and β-1,6-linked glucose polymers.[11] The glycosyl units within the glucans are arranged as long coiling chains of β-(1,3)-linked residues, with occasional side chains involving β-(1,6)-linkage.[6] Moreover, three β-(1,3) chains positioned in parallel can associate to generate a triple helix, and aggregation of such helices will further produce a network of water-insoluble fibrils capable of retaining the shape of the yeast cell. Even in chitin-rich filamentous aspergilli, the β-(1,3)-glucan is necessary to conserve the integrity of the cell wall.[12,13] However, it appeared that in *Cryptococcus neoformans*, the β-(1,3)-linked glucose units may not provide structural support of the cell wall since they apparently exist only as side chains on β-(1,6)-glucan polymers.[14]

Glucans are synthesized on the cytoplasmic surface of the plasma membrane, and then extruded and deposited on the outer surface of the cell wall as microfibrils, which subsequently congregate to form crystalline structures.[4,6,11] It has also been suggested that a predominantly β-(1,6)-glucan layer is deposited near the cell surface where it may serve as a barrier protecting the β-(1,3)-glucans. The reason that such deposition was postulated has been the need to remove the β-(1,6)-glucans from intact cells prior to solubilization of β-(1,3)-glucans.[11]

In most fungi, the β-(1,3)-glucan units are produced with the help of glucan synthase. Based on functional analysis (but not physical examination[15]), the glucan synthase is comprised of at least two subunits.[16,17] One of the subunits, which is confined within the plasma membrane, is believed to be the catalytic subunit because it is protected from heat denaturation by the substrate,

UDP-glucose (UDP-Glc). The second subunit binds GTP and associates with and activates the catalytic subunit.[15]

The stimulation of glucan biosynthesis by nucleotides that might be involved in the regulation of glucan synthase *in vivo* was investigated in detail by Shematek and Cabib,[18] and some structural requirements for an activator of this enzyme, and hypothetical sites of interaction with it, have emerged.[19] Guanosine triphosphate (GTP) was found to be the most potent activator of glucan synthase, with an $S_{0.5}$ (concentration needed for half-maximal stimulation) value of 0.2 μM; by comparison, the corresponding value for adenosine triphosphate (ATP) was approximately 100-fold higher.[18] In addition to nucleoside triphosphates, there have been other effective stimulants of glucan synthase — albeit at higher concentrations, guanosine diphosphate, some inorganic pyrophosphates, and higher polyphosphates have also stimulated the enzyme.[19]

Various structural requirements for stimulating the glucan synthase activity have been determined.[19] For example, conversion of the terminal phosphate group of the nucleoside triphosphates to methyl ester, or attaching it to another nucleoside molecule reduced the potency by competitively inhibiting the stimulatory effect. Other findings suggested that either glucan synthase itself or a regulatory subunit of the enzyme may possess, in addition to an activation site that interacts with the terminal phosphate group, also a binding site for the nucleoside residue of the stimulatory molecule.[11,19] Other structural analogs of ATP and GTP, which carried imino or methylene groups in place of the α,β- or β,γ-oxygen, have also demonstrated enzyme-activating properties with $S_{0.5}$ values similar to those of the parent nucleosides. Compounds having a sulfur atom attached to the terminal phosphate group were also found to be active.[19] When used in the same experiment, adenosine-β,γ-imino-triphosphate and guanosine-β,γ-imino-triphosphate did not show any additive effect, suggesting interaction with the same domain of the enzyme.[19]

The fungal cell wall mannoproteins are built of branched mannose polymers attached to the protein through an *N*-acetylglucosamine-*N*-acetylglucosamine group. All linkages are α, with the exception of those between the two *N*-acetylglucosamine residues and between the mannose and *N*-acetylglucosamine, which are β.[20] In the outermost region of the yeast cell wall, the mannoproteins appeared to be covalently bound to β-(1,3)-glucan since β-(1,3)-glucanase is required to solubilize them.

Chitin, the third major polysaccharide of the fungal cell wall consists predominantly of unbranched chains of β-(1→4)-2-acetamido-2-deoxy-D-glucose, also known as *N*-acetyl-D-glucosamine (GlcNAc).[11] Similarly to glucans, chitin is synthesized at the cytoplasmic surface of the plasma membrane and then extruded and deposited on the outer surface.[8] More than 90% of chitin in a normal yeast wall was found in the region of the bud scars in the form of an annulus with an external thinner rim and a thin central plate,[11] with the remainder dispersed over the whole cell wall.[21,22] The distribution of chitin in the cell wall deviates according to the fungal species and may be as low as <1% in the yeast form of *Candida albicans*[23-25] to 10% to 20% for *Blastomyces dermatitidis, Histoplasma capsulatum, Coccidioides immitis,*[26,27] and the mycelial form of *C. albicans.*[24] Duran et al.[28] have provided evidence that chitin synthase, the enzyme catalyzing the formation of this polysaccharide, has been confined exclusively within the plasma membrane. Fungal chitin synthases[29-31] have been present in cell homogenates largely as zymogens.[23,32]

Some fungal walls also contain chitosan, an extensively deacylated form of chitin.[24]

29.2. FUNGAL CELL MEMBRANE

The cell membrane is the second major structural component of the fungal cell envelope.[4] Functionally, it represents a barrier between the cytoplasm and the environment, regulating the transport of molecules in and out of the fungal cell.[5] One important feature of the cell membrane is to serve as a matrix for the membrane-bound enzymes, such as the glucan- and chitin synthases.

Structurally, the cell membrane is a lipid bilayer with phosphatidyl choline, phosphatidyl ethanolamine, and ergosterol (or in certain cases, zymosterol) being its major components. Kaneko et al.[33] have studied the lipid composition of 30 different species of yeasts and found that the greater part of them contained 7% to 15% total lipids and 3% to 6% total phospholipids per dry cell weight. Qualitatively, all of the yeast membranes studied had similar neutral lipid constituents (triglycerides, sterol esters, free fatty acids, and free sterols) and polar components (phosphatidyl choline, phosphatidyl ethanolamine, phosphatidyl serine, phosphatidyl inositol, cardiolipin, and ceramide monohexoside), with minor constituents nearly absent.[33]

Marriott[34] has described the presence of a significant difference in the contents of plasma membranes from the yeast and mycelial forms of *Candida albicans* with the latter form being richer in carbohydrates. In addition, marked differences were also observed between the phospholipids, free and esterified sterols, and total fatty acids from the two forms of *C. albicans*.

Antifungal agents can disrupt the integrity of fungal cell membranes by either interrupting the proper interaction between the membrane sterols and phospholipids (polyene antibiotics) or by inhibiting the sterol biosynthesis (azole derivatives).[4,35]

29.3 MECHANISM OF ACTION OF POLYENE ANTIBIOTICS

The polyene antibiotics are a class of biologically active fungal metabolites isolated from various *Streptomyces* spp. Structurally, the polyene antibiotics represent macrolides with a large lactone ring containing between three and seven conjugated double bonds, and a sugar residue (most often mycosamine, but also perosamine) which is attached to the ring by a glycosidic bond.[25,36] Certain members of the heptaene subgroup (candicidin, ascosin, hamycin) contain an aromatic amine side chain, such as *p*-aminoacetophenone, which is alkali-sensitive; in other heptaene antibiotics (e.g., candimycin), the aromatic side chain is *N*-methylated.[36]

The conjugated polyene region of the lactone ring confers both rigidity and lipophilicity to the molecule, while the hydroxyl-containing region is conformationally flexible and hydrophilic. In general, the presence of sugar residue imparts basicity on the polyene molecule. However, because of the presence in the molecule of equal number of basic (hexosamine or aromatic side chain) and acidic (carboxyl) groups, some of the polyene antibiotics (amphotericin B, nystatin, candicidin) are amphoteric by nature. Other polyenes (filipin, fungichromin) contain no ionizable functions at all, and are therefore, nonpolar.[4]

The mechanism of action of the polyene antibiotics has been related to their ability to bind to membrane sterols resulting in the formation of transmembrane pores which disrupt the structural integrity of the cell membrane as seen by its increased permeability, the leakage of cytoplasmic contents, such as potassium cations, and ultimately the cell death.[36-38] In this regard, it is important to emphasize that the polyene antibiotics can interact with both fungal (ergosterol) and mammalian (cholesterol) sterols. However, at least in the case of the clinically important antibiotics (amphotericin B, nystatin), the affinity towards the fungal ergosterol has been higher.[39,40] It has been reported that both amphotericin B and nystatin did not affect the lipid biosynthesis *in vivo* at concentrations as high as 0.1 μM.[5]

A partial model explaining the formation of amphotericin B-cholesterol transmembrane pores has been suggested by Andreoli (Figure 29.1).[37] In this model, the aliphatic residues of the phospholipids are, at least partially, stabilized by London-van der Waals forces which assures their parallel alignment within the hydrophobic core of the bilayer. One fundamental functional characteristic of the membrane sterols is their ability to interact with the membrane phospholipids. By doing so, the sterols are able either to increase the order and rigidity of the relatively fluid phospholipid bilayers,[41-43] or to increase the fluidity and permeability of the tightly organized condensed phospholipid bilayers,[43-45] thus regulating the dissipative permeability of the membrane

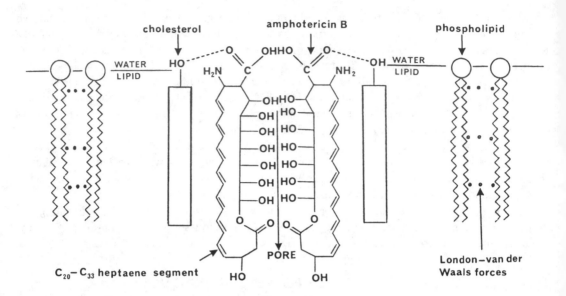

Figure 29.1 Partial model of amphotericin B-cholesterol pores (after Ref. 37).

and controlling the phase transition from condensed, gel-like crystalline arrays into fluid, liquid crystal structures.[37] During such transitions from crystalline to "melted" fluid states,[46-49] the mobility and ordering of the hydrocarbon chains in the membrane interior would be, respectively, increased and decreased.[37] In general, organized crystalline bilayer membranes are less permeable to water and solutes as compared to more fluid liquid crystal membranes.[50-54] The increased permeability of the more "fluid" bilayer membranes towards water and solutes is thought to be the result of molecular cavities or defects in the ordering of the hydrocarbon region of the membranes[55,56] caused, for example, by greater water content in the lipid lamelae[57] and shortening, branching, or unsaturation of phospholipid hydrocarbon residues.[50-52] In the context of the sterol-phospholipid interaction, the polyene antibiotics will act as a "counterfeit" phospholipid. The polyene molecule will position itself in such a manner that its C_{15} hydroxyl, C_{16} carboxyl, and C_{19} mycosamine amino groups will be situated at the membrane–water interface, whereas the C_1–C_{14} and C_{20}–C_{33} regions will be parallel to each other and within the membrane interior. Because of its hydrophobic nature, the C_{20}–C_{33} heptaene chain will also align itself along the cholesterol molecule in a hydrophobic environment, while the hydroxyl groups of the C_1–C_{14} moiety will face the aqueous interface along the inner side of the pore. The overall result of such an arrangement will be an increased fluidity and hydration of the pore interior approaching that of bulk water (Figure 29.1). As demonstrated by light microscopy, the formation of polyene-sterol pores will cause substantial morphologic changes in the fungal cell, as seen by marked granularity, loss of organelle definition, and ultimately cell death.[37]

Since the total length of the polyene-sterol complex approximates the length of the fatty acid and glycerol moieties of the phospholipid molecule, the complex will be sufficient to form only a "half pore" through the lipid bilayer. A conducting "full length" pore would need two "half pores" to join together.[36] "Half pores" may float independently in the lipid environment. Usually, a "full pore" would require between 5 and 10 polyene molecules.[58,59] It has been found that the diameter of each pore approximated that of a glucose molecule.[58-60] Furthermore, only an intact polyene molecule may participate in the construction of pore structures since either hydrolysis of the lactone ring of the antibiotic or saturation of its conjugated double bonds system would make pore formation theoretically impossible — so far, there has been no experimental evidence to demonstrate pore formation by such structurally modified polyene molecules.[59]

The structure of nystatin, another clinically useful polyene antibiotic, differs from that of amphotericin B in that its conjugated double bond system is interrupted by saturation leaving two separate tetraene and diene chromophores. Such double bond arrangements should allow the bending of an otherwise rigid conformation. A structure similar to the amphotericin B-cholesterol pore model has been proposed for the nystatin-sterol complex in lipid membrane bilayers.[59,61,62] Since the permeability characteristics of the nystatin-sterol pores closely matched those of an amphotericin B-sterol pore, it has been possible to form mixed pores when nystatin was added to one side of the lipid bilayer and amphotericin B to the other.[63]

In contrast to both amphotericin B and nystatin, the pentaene antibiotic filipin carries no ionizable groups or a sugar residue, and is therefore nonpolar. Instead, it contains a hydrophobic alkyl side chain adjacent to the hydrophilic hydroxylated portion of the molecule. These structural elements should make it possible for the construction of a filipin-sterol complex that is oriented parallel to the plane of the lipid bilayer — a radical departure from the distinctive perpendicular arrangement of the amphotericin B-cholesterol complex. Moreover, several of these parallel constructs may further join together to form aggregates. One of the sides of such aggregates will become hydrophobic by the presence of the pentaene chromophore, while the opposite side will be hydrophilic due to the polyol surface.[37] Two of these planar aggregates may then combine to produce a "sandwich"-like structure, which would have its hydrophilic regions facing each other towards the center, whereas the hydrophobic regions will be situated on the outside surface of the "sandwich" and in a position to interact with the membrane sterols. Even though such filipin-sterol complexes will bear no resemblance to the amphotericin B-cholesterol pores, they still should be able to disrupt the integrity of the lipid membrane structure by effectively removing sterols from the environment, thereby preventing sterol-phospholipid interaction.[64-66] Similarly to the amphotericin B-cholesterol complexing, the filipin-sterol interaction has been hydrophobic by nature.[65,66] It has also been observed that the lysis of lipid bilayers by filipin-sterol complexes was much faster and with no prior formation of pores.[67]

Experimental evidence has revealed that the major effect taking place immediately after treatment with polyene antibiotics has been the leakage of potassium cations. To replace their loss, a subsequent transfer of H^+ from the environment will follow.[68] The ensuing inflow of protons will cause acidification of the fungal cytoplasm — for example, the pH of the cell cytoplasm of *C. albicans* treated with a lethal dose of candicidin fell from 6.12 to 5.20.[68] Such drastic change in the cytoplasmic pH would lead, in turn, to an increase in the optical density and precipitation of cytoplasmic components.[69]

29.4   INHIBITION OF GLUCAN BIOSYNTHESIS

Two classes of antibiotics, papulacandins and echinocandins, are known to have exerted their antifungal activity by suppressing the β-glucan synthesis.[16,70] The echinocandins were found to inhibit the glucan synthase in a manner that did not compete with UDP-Glc.[16,70,71] Chemical modifications of echinocandins, including changes in the peptide core,[72] have produced analogs with significantly improved activity.

29.5   CELL WALL MANNOPROTEINS AS POTENTIAL TARGET
OF ANTIFUNGAL AGENTS

The sequence of events by which the manno-oligosaccharides are assembled, transferred to asparagine residues in proteins, and trimmed by glycosidases is very much the same in both yeast and mammalian cells, which makes it highly unlikely that selective inhibitors of this process would be successfully designed.[73,74] However, during their intracellular maturation, mannoproteins which are predetermined for the outer wall are coupled to glycosylphosphatidylinositol.[73,75] Once at the plasma membrane, they are separated from their membrane anchors, and attached to β-(1,3)-glucan. Because this process is unique to yeast cells and has nothing comparable in mammalian cells, it has been identified as a potentially selective target for antifungal action.[75]

The presumed activity of two classes of antifungal benzonaphthacene quinone antibiotics, benanomicins and pradimicins, appeared to involve complexing with the saccharide portions of cell-surface mannoproteins in a calcium-dependent fashion.

29.6   CHITIN BIOSYNTHESIS AS TARGET OF ANTIFUNGAL AGENTS

Chitin, which is a chemically unique component of the cell wall of most fungi pathogenic to humans, has been a potential target for antifungal agents because of its vital role as one of the major structural components of the cell wall.[70,76-78] There has been convincing evidence that the inhibition of chitin synthase enzymes by structural analogs of the substrate of chitin biosynthesis, UDP-N-acetylglucosamine, often suppressed fungal growth, and in some conditions, may cause even fungal death.[70,76]

Similarly to *Saccharomyces cerevisiae*, there are three chitin synthases (Chs1, Chs2, and Chs3) in *C. albicans*.[29-31] The physiologic function of each one of them has been defined by disrupting the relevant encoding genes *CHS1*, *CHS2*, and *CSD2(CAL2)*.[6,78]

One important aspect in designing effective chitin inhibitors has been to characterize those chitin synthase domains that may serve as potential targets of their action.[78] In this regard, Szaniszlo and Momany[79] have described within the highly conserved region of the *CHS* amplicons, a region which shared striking similarity with *Ara G*, a member of a gene family which encodes hydrophilic membrane components of the periplasmic permeases.[80] The latter have been shown to bind ATP and GTP, presumably as part of the active transport system. The region that the *CHS* homologs shared with *Ara G* is highly conserved among these permeases and is thought to define part of the ATP binding site. Furthermore, like the permeases, the *CHS* sequences also bear homology with the "Walker motifs" of adenylate cyclase,[81] which also defines ATP binding sites.[82] In adenylate kinase, the ATP is thought to nestle between an α-helix and β-sheet at the center of a classic Rossman nucleotide binding fold.[83]

Further studies have demonstrated that a predicted nucleotide binding fold in the *CHS* sequences potentially identifies a binding site for UDP-N-acetylglucosamine, the substrate for chitin biosynthesis.[78] The region of the "Walker motif" that aligns with the *CHS* sequences is thought to form the binding site for α- and β-phosphates rather than the γ-phosphate of ATP,[81] which is consistent with the binding of the UDP portion of the substrate. The eventual confirmation that this region is, indeed, the substrate binding domain for chitin biosynthesis would suggest that at least one common domain had been identified among most chitin synthases.[78] If so, this domain, in turn, would serve as a suitable action site for novel antifungal chitin inhibitors.

The polyoxins and nikkomycins, two classes of nucleoside-peptide antibiotics,[84,85] have been shown to be competitive inhibitors of chitin synthase with inhibition constants (K_i) ranging between 0.1 to 1.0 μM, which is two to three orders of magnitude lower than the Michaelis constant (K_m) of the UDP-GlcNAc substrate.[24] Furthermore, the nikkomycins have displayed synergistic activity with some azole antimycotics and glucan-synthase inhibitors.[70]

C. albicans and other pathogenic fungi have shown resistance to polyoxins mainly due to the poor transport of these antibiotics through the cell membrane.[11] Synthetic modifications aimed to improve the ability of these drugs to penetrate across the cell membrane have largely failed to produce any candidates of clinical value.[86,87]

The glucosamine-6-phosphate, which is necessary for chitin synthesis, is produced by the enzyme L-glutamine:fructose-6-phosphate amidotransferase. The latter is the target of bacilysin, a dipeptide antibiotic, also known as tetaine and bacillin. Bacilysin acts as a prodrug which is cleaved by intracellular peptidases to generate the bioactive epoxyamino acid anticapsin.[88] Another antibiotic,

A 19009 (N^3-fumaroyl-L-2,3,diaminopropanoyl-L-alanine) acted in a similar manner.[89] Both bacilysin and A 10009 were antagonized by glutamine and appeared to have nonselective activity as evidenced by their inhibition of both prokaryotic and eukaryotic forms of the amidotransferase.[6]

29.7 STEROL BIOSYNTHESIS AS TARGET OF ANTIFUNGAL AGENTS

The second major mode of action by which antifungal drugs exert their activity is through the inhibition of the fungal sterol biosynthesis.[4,90] Any impairment of the synthesis of cell membrane sterols will slow down normal fungal growth. Ergosterol is the major sterol component of the fungal cell membrane. Similarly to the mammalian cholesterol, ergosterol plays an important role in controlling membrane fluidity and integrity (a nonspecific function), as well as specifically regulating cell growth and proliferation.[91-94] While the nonspecific function requires large ("bulk") quantities of ergosterol, its specific control of membrane-associated processes should require only minute ("sparking") amounts of the sterol.[5] In general, antifungal agents which substantially (but not completely) inhibit the ergosterol biosynthesis are likely to affect also its nonspecific function resulting in suppressed cell growth as well.[5]

The biosynthesis of fungal ergosterol may be divided into four distinct stages: (1) formation of mevalonic acid; (2) polymerization of mevalonic acid into squalene; (3) cyclization to lanosterol; and (4) modification of lanosterol leading to ergosterol (Figure 29.2).

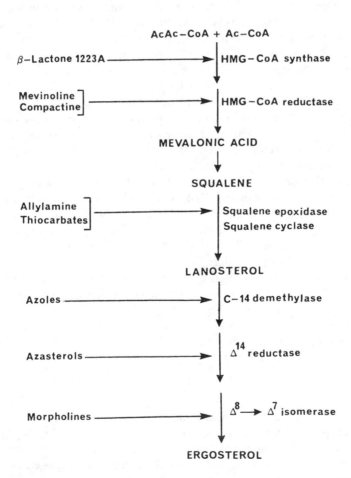

Figure 29.2 Biosynthesis of ergosterol, with potential sites of inhibition by antifungal agents (after Ref. 4).

Enzymes that control the first stage are mitochondrial, whereas those catalyzing the second stage are mainly cytosolic. Enzymes involved in the third and fourth stages are microsomal.[4,5,95] All four stages of the ergosterol biosynthesis may serve as potential targets for antifungal agents.

3-Hydroxy-3-methylglutaryl CoA synthase (HMG-CoA synthase) is the enzyme which activates the condensation of acetoacetyl-CoA with acetyl-CoA to generate 3-hydroxy-3-methyl-glutaryl CoA (HMG-CoA). Subsequent reduction of the carbonyl group of HMG-CoA produces mevalonic acid. The reduction is catalyzed by HMG-CoA reductase and, similarly to the cholesterol biosynthesis, it is the rate-limiting step of the biosynthesis of ergosterol.[96-98]

Sesquiterpenes, such as mevinolin and compactin, have been shown to suppress in a specific manner the activity of HMG-CoA reductase[99] — the inhibition was reversible and competitive with respect to HMG-CoA.[100,101] The latter finding comes as no surprise because of the existing structural similarity between the acid form of sesquiterpenes and HMG-CoA; experiments by Endo[102] have demonstrated that the affinity of HMG-CoA reductase for compactin was 10,000-fold higher than its affinity for the natural substrate HMG-CoA. Structure-activity relationship studies have indicated that the lactone ring of the sesquiterpenes is critical for activity; for example, the 5′-phosphono-compactin acid showed only one tenth of the potency of compactin.[102] So far, the enzyme-inhibiting activity of the sesquiterpenes has been of little clinical value due to their poor permeability into the fungal cells.[5]

The lactone antibiotic 1233A was reported to exert a potent and specific inhibition of HMG-CoA synthase without affecting the acetoacetyl-CoA thiolase or HMG-CoA reductase.[103] As with the case of sesquiterpenes, the poor permeability of lactone 1233A into the fungal cells significantly curtailed its therapeutic effect precluding any clinical application.[5]

The formation of squalene — the second stage of ergosterol biosynthesis, is carried out by tail-to-tail condensation of two farnesyl pyrophosphate molecules[104-107] with squalene synthase serving as the catalyst.[108] The oxidation of squalene into 2,3-oxidosqualene utilizes molecular oxygen with the help of squalene epoxidase. 2,3-Oxidosqualene, in turn, is cyclized into lanosterol. The enzyme involved in this cyclization, squalene cyclase,[108-110] showed optimal activity at low ionic strength.[111] Between squalene epoxidase and squalene cyclase, the two enzymes which control the formation of lanosterol, inhibition of squalene epoxidase is more preferable as antifungal drug target since accumulation of 2,3-oxidosqualene would be more damaging to the host cells than accumulation of squalene.[5,112] A number of allylamine (e.g., terbinafine, naftifine) and thiocarbamate (e.g., tolnaftate, tolciclate) derivatives were found to elicit antifungal activity by suppressing the activity of squalene epoxidase.[113-116] The IC_{50} values of these agents have been from <1.0 μM (terbinafine) to 100 μM (tolnaftate).[5] Furthermore, the allylamines also reduced the unsaturated-to-saturated fatty acid ratio and caused a shift from C_{18} to C_{16} *in vivo*.[5]

The conversion of lanosterol into ergosterol is rather complex and may involve the synthesis of as many as 13 different sterols as either end products or potential biosynthetic intermediates with lanosterol being the key precursor (Figure 29.3).[117-120]

Among the known *in vivo* enzymes participating in the lanosterol-ergosterol conversion,[121,122] the activities of three of them, C-14-demethylase, Δ^{14}-reductase, and Δ^8-Δ^7-isomerase have been the targets of numerous antifungal agents.

29.7.1 INHIBITION OF FUNGAL SQUALENE EPOXIDASE

The allylamines are a class of synthetic antifungal agents with topical and oral activity against a wide variety of pathogenic fungi, especially dermatophytes (*Trichophyton mentagro-phytes*).[123-127] Among the large number of analogs,[128,129] naftifine[130] and terbinafine[131] have been found to act by inhibiting in a specific and reversible manner the fungal ergosterol biosynthesis

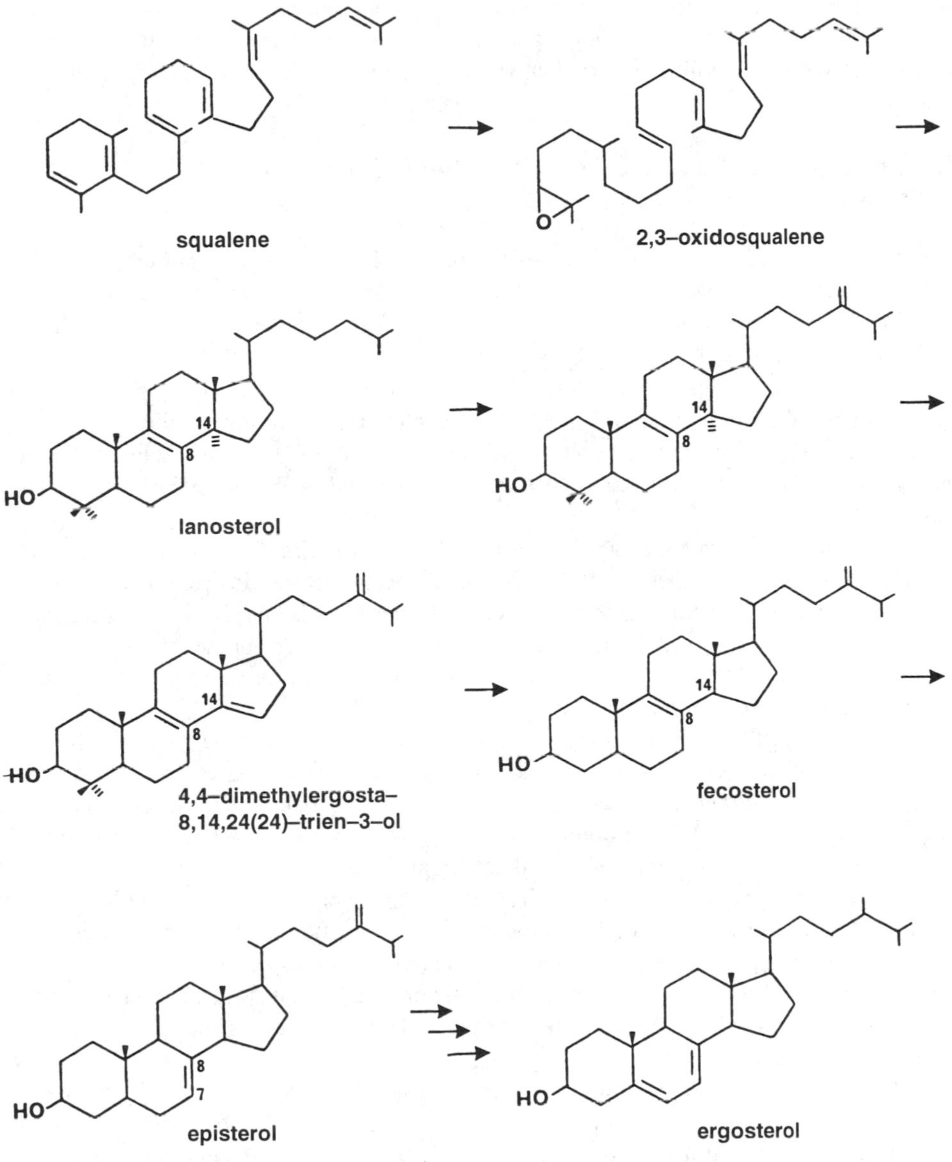

Figure 29.3 Biosynthetic conversion of squalene into ergosterol (after Ref. 4).

at the stage of squalene epoxidation.[127] Squalene epoxidase was characterized in microsomes of *C. albicans*[132] and *C. parapsilosis*[133] and found to require molecular oxygen, NADPH, and FAD for activity.

The epoxidation of squalene is as essential for the biosynthesis of mammalian cholesterol as that of ergosterol in fungi. However, both naftifine and terbinafine have displayed high selectivity in their action, with naftifine showing a very weak nonspecific inhibition of cholesterol biosynthesis (IC$_{50}$ >100 mg/l), and terbinafine causing weak but specific inhibition of incorporation (IC$_{50}$ = 30 mg/l).[127] It should also be noted that mammals are able to satisfy much of their cholesterol need from dietary sources, therefore making them not as sensitive as fungi.

While the molecular mechanism of inhibition by the allylamines is still not fully understood, one possible mode of action may lie outside the ergosterol biosynthesis pathway, such as allosteric interactions of the drugs with some regulatory site on the squalene epoxidase, such as a lipid-binding site.[127]

29.7.2   INHIBITION OF FUNGAL CYTOCHROME P-450-DEPENDENT 14α-STEROL DEMETHYLASE

The azole class of antimycotics have been invariably C-14α-demethylase inhibitors.[1,2,90,134,135] The oxidative 14α-demethylation of sterols is cytochrome P-450-dependent.[136] Its suppression by the azole antimycotics results from the binding of nitrogen from the heterocyclic portion of the azole molecule (e.g., imidazole, 1,2,4-triazole, pyridine, pyrimidine) to the heme iron of cytochrome P-450.[137-139] At therapeutic concentrations, the azole antimycotics have shown greater affinity for the fungal rather than mammalian P-450 14α-demethylase, resulting in the accumulation of 14α-methylated sterols (mainly lanosterol and 3,6-diol sterols). It is this selective effect that, depending on the fungal species, leads to the fungistatic and/or fungicidal activity of the azole derivatives.[134,135,140]

Extensive studies on enzyme purified from *S. cerevisiae* and *C. albicans* have shown that 14α-demethylase from both species shared the same spectral properties (oxidized Soret maxima at 417 nm and CO-reduced Soret maxima at 447).[141] There has been 62% amino acid identity of their nucleotide sequences, and when reconstituted into a model membrane system, both enzymes catalyzed the 14α-demethylation reaction; it was also found that the *C. albicans* gene can functionally replace the corresponding *S. cerevisiae* gene.[134,135,142]

First reported for two imidazole compounds, clotrimazole[143] and miconazole,[144,145] the inhibition of C-14-demethylation reaction is associated with profound morphologic and functional damage to the fungal cell membrane, such as loss of permeability to potassium cations and leakage of intracellular phosphorus-containing components.[146,147] At higher concentrations, clotrimazole and miconazole were found to be fungicidal by their action on the cell membrane; however, at lower doses both drugs were only fungistatic.[148,149] The newer azole derivatives (fluconazole, itraconazole) having a 1,2,4-triazole ring in place of imidazole, have been shown to possess better pharmacokinetic profiles resulting in more potent antifungal activity with lesser toxicity.[1]

Detailed spectrophotometric and reconstituted enzyme studies have shown that azole antifungals bind to 14α-demethylase with one-to-one stoichiometry. However, little is known about the structure of the enzyme-azole complex.

In addition to causing accumulation of methylated sterols, as demonstrated by the decrease in ergosterol-to-methylated sterol ratio, the azoles, in general, decreased the unsaturated-to-saturated fatty acid ratio and initiated a shift from C_{18} to C_{16} fatty acids *in vivo*.[5] Furthermore, stimulation of chitin synthase activity *in vivo* (likely the result of ergosterol depletion in the plasma membrane) has also been observed.[5]

A number of *N*-containing sterols were also found to elicit antifungal activity by suppressing ergosterol biosynthesis. For example, the 14-azasterol antibiotic A28522B was reported to inhibit the activity of $Δ^{14}$-reductase leading to accumulation of 8,14-diene sterol.[150] Another derivative, 23-azasterol was able to inhibit the 24-methylene-24(28) reductase in yeast fungi,[151] whereas some 25-azasterols were potent inhibitors of the C-24 methylation reaction in yeasts.[152] To date, however, none of the antifungal azasterols have found any clinical application.

Among other antimycotic agents suppressing ergosterol biosynthesis, some morpholine analogs (tridemorph, fenpropimorph) have been known primarily as agricultural fungicides active against powdery mildews.[153,154] In 1980, Kato et al.[155] provided evidence for the accumulation of fecosterol after treatment with tridemorph, suggesting inhibition of the $Δ^8$-$Δ^7$ isomerization reaction. Later, Kerkenaar et al.[156] observed that tridemorph also suppressed the $Δ^{14}$-reductase step. Such dual action by these morpholines may eventually lead to a lower incidence of drug resistance by fungi.[5] Subsequently, amorolfine, a structural analog of fenpropimorph, was found active against several fungal pathogens in humans.[157,158]

29.7.3 INHIBITION OF FUNGAL Δ^{14}-REDUCTASE AND Δ^8-Δ^7-ISOMERASE

Several morpholine derivatives, some of them known as agrofungicides (fenpropimorph), have been found to be highly efficacious against pathogenic fungi in mammals. One such compound, amorolfin, has shown potent topical activity against superficial mycoses (trichophytosis and vaginal candidiasis).[158,159] Based on the analysis of sterol biosynthesis pattern data, the targets of amorolfin and fenpropimorph were the Δ^{14}-reductase and Δ^8-Δ^7-isomerase,[160-165] the two enzymes involved in the bioconversion of lanosterol into ergosterol (Figure 29.3). These two enzymes have shown some similarities. Thus, it has been suggested that the Δ^8-Δ^7 isomerization reaction begins with Δ^8 hydrogenation,[165] which represents an NADPH/H$^+$-dependent reduction of the Δ^8-double bond — a reaction which shares analogy with the NADPD/H$^+$-dependent reduction of the Δ^{14}-double bond. It was further proposed that high-energy carbonium ion intermediates form at C-14 (for the reductase) and at C-8 (for the isomerase).[165,166] The N-alkylmorpholines, which at pH 7.4 form morpholinium ions, have shown electronic and structural similarities with these high-energy carbonium ion intermediates and may, therefore, display high affinity for the Δ^{14}-reductase and Δ^8-Δ^7-isomerase, thereby inhibiting their action.[158] It is interesting to note that the degree of morpholine-induced inhibition on the two enzymes varied depending on the configuration (*cis* or *trans*) and the entiomorphism (R or S) of the morpholines.[163]

In *C. albicans* (H$_{29}$ ATCC) and *Saccharomyces cerevisiae* (NCYC 739 high sterol strain), both amorolfine and fenpropimorph produced acummulation of equal amounts of two intermediate sterols, ignosterol and ergosta-8,14,22-trienol, along with 4,4-cholesta-8,14,24-trienol. The formation of ignosterol is initiated soon after exposure to morpholines (69% conversion at 4 h) at low noninhibitory concentrations, suggesting inhibition of sterol biosynthesis as their primary site of action.[158]

29.8 THE ROLE OF IRON IN FUNGAL METABOLISM

Nearly all living organisms will require elemental iron for proper discharge of their biochemical processes. However, despite its abundance in nature, the insolubility of environmental ferric ions has evoked the development of elaborate uptake mechanisms, some of which are subject to subversion as part of the competition between free-living organisms.[78] In pathogenic fungi, the several models existing for iron uptake[78] with potential therapeutic applications are discussed below.

29.8.1 REMOVAL OF IRON FROM ERYTHROCYTES

It has been suggested that yeasts such as *C. albicans* have been able to take iron directly from host erythrocytes utilizing reactions that involve the complement. Thus, fresh complement activated by the fungal cell wall through the alternative complement activation pathway is believed to be deposited on the membrane of nearby erythrocytes as iC3b. It is thought that the presence of this ligand would allow *Candida* to bind to the erythrocytes through the yeast's own complement receptor, thereby stimulating the production and/or release of fungal hemolysin that permits fungal access to hemoglobin.[167]

29.8.2 SECRETION OF CHELATORS

The secretion of chelators is the best understood microbial iron uptake system which involves the synthesis and excretion of siderophores (water-soluble, low-molecular-weight, ferric-binding compounds), and the elaboration of receptors for ferrated siderophores on the cell membrane.[78] Coprogen B, one such siderophore containing three hydroxamic acid groups, has been isolated by Burt[168] from spent *Histoplasma* culture medium and shown to facilitate growth at low inocula. Microorganisms which elaborate ferrihydroxamate receptors without secreting siderophores are believed to exploit the siderofores of other species, a phenomenon clinically manifested in the occurrence of zygomycosis in patients receiving metal chelation therapy with deferoxamine (a hydroxamate siderophore,[169] and iron-chelated vitamin for certain pathogenic zygomycetes[170]). Athough hydroxamate siderophores have not yet been detected in the supernatant of iron-starved cultures of *Cryptococcus neoformans*, ferric hydroxamate receptors may still exist in this species.[171-173]

A number of hydroxamic acid-containing antibiotics[174] have been found to inhibit iron uptake, and one such class, the neoenactins, are currently under development as antifungal agents.[175]

29.8.3 CITRATE OR TRANSFERIN-MEDIATED UPTAKE

In contrast to *Escherichia coli*, which possesses a system for the uptake of ferric citrate that can be induced in the presence of exogenous citrate, there has been no evidence to indicate either secretion of citrate or that a similar mechanism exists in *Cryptococcus*.[172] However, *Neisseria* spp. have a mechanism that provides for removing the ferric iron from unsaturated human transferrins found in blood and mucosal secretions.[78]

29.8.4 PLASMA MEMBRANE FERRIC REDUCTASES

Since the aerobic uptake of iron is a reductive process, higher plants and certain microorganisms use membrane ferric reductases as the base for their entire iron uptake mechanism.[78] Frequently, such systems seemed to be constitutive, to utilize NADH as an electron source, and to require flavine mononucleotide as co-factor.[176,177] This appeared to be the mechanism of iron uptake in *S. cerevisiae*, where it is accomplished by genetically distinct plasma membrane ferrireductase and Fe(II) transporter enzymes, and is regulated by the external concentration of iron.[178,179] The iron uptake has been inhibited by strong chelators of Fe(II), indicating that the reductive step was external to the plasma membrane. In *Cryptococcus*, both growth[173] and iron uptake[180] were suppressed by the ferrous chelator, bathyphenathroline disulfonate, suggesting that the ferrous ion must be reduced prior to its internalization.[78]

29.9 MOLECULAR APPROACHES TO NOVEL TARGETS FOR ANTIFUNGAL THERAPY

The recent advancement of molecular biology has opened the possibility to identify novel, unique, and fundamental targets that may be used for the development of new approaches for antifungal chemotherapy. For example, techniques applied at the molecular level, such as differential hybridization and differential display–polymerase chain reaction (PCR)-based cloning, have made it possible to define unique and vital cellular functions (e.g., virulence factors) which, if disrupted, will incapacitate the pathogen and make it vulnerable to the action of antifungal agents. Since many of the fungal genes encoding distinctive traits are likely to be regulated in response to either physical or environmental variables associated with the host environment (e.g., in tissue or in macrophages), the identification of genes regulated in this manner may define novel and useful approaches for antifungal therapy.[136]

29.9.1 CRYPTOCOCCAL DIPHENOL OXIDASE

The production of a melanin-like pigment by *Cryptococcus neoformans* was found to be dependent on the presence of various *o*- or *p*-diphenols or diaminobenzenes.[181] Melanogenesis is characteristic for various biological systems, whereby mono- and polyphenolic substrates are oxidized to their respective quinones, which in turn, undergo nonenzymatic polymerization to generate pigmented products.[136]

In *C. neoformans*, melanin production is thought to be a virulence factor since melanin-negative mutants lose their virulence. Alternatively, coreversion of the melanin phenotype was followed by restoration of virulence.[182] Physiologically, melanin is believed to protect the fungus by scavenging leukocytic antimicrobial oxidants as evidenced by some oxygen-sensitive mutants which also exhibited defective catechol oxidation.[183]

The diphenol oxidase enzyme is thought to be involved in the biosynthesis of fungal melanin. It has been purified and characterized as a laccase having wide specificity for polyaminobenzene and phenolic compounds.[184] The cloned cDNA of the diphenol oxidase gene (CNLAC1) showed an open reading frame of 2.3 kb encoding an amino acid sequence containing *N*-terminal.[155] The predicted amino acid sequence has very little homology with other proteins, as is typical of laccase enzymes.[185] However, within two regions of the proposed copper-binding sites, there was 66% amino acid identity compared to the consensus sequence from the phenoloxidase from *Coriolus hirsutus*, laccase from *Neurospora crassa* and human ceruloplasm.[185]

29.9.2 MyristoylCoA: Protein *N*-Myristoyltransferase

In *C. neoformans* and *C. albicans*, myristoylCoA:protein *N*-myristoyltransferase (NMT) catalyzes the cotranslational transfer of myristate (C14:0) from CoA to the *N*-terminal glycine of eukaryotic and viral proteins.[186] The enzyme's reaction is ordered B_iB_i.[187] MyristoylCoA was shown to bind to the apoenzyme to produce a high-affinity binary myristoylCoA:Nmt binary complex. Following linkage of C14:0 to the Gly residue of nascent substrates through an amide bond, CoA was released followed by myristoylpeptide.[136]

Preliminary data have suggested that the peptide substrate specificities of human and fungal (*C. neoformans*) NMTs have diverged more than their acylCoA substrate specificities.[136] To determine whether the NMT is essential for the growth and viability of *C. albicans* and *C. neoformans*, the conserved carboxyl-terminal Gly has been changed in *C. neoformans*(Gly_{487}) and *C. albicans*(Gly_{447}) NMTs to an Asp. The activities of the wild-type and mutant acyltransferases were compared and contrasted at 24°C and 37°C using the *Escherichia coli* co-expression system and Arf (ADP rybosylation factors) substrates. The results of these and other related experiments have demonstrated that NMT is required for the growth of *C. neoformans* and *C. albicans*, and therefore, may represent a target for the development of fungicidal drugs.[136]

29.9.3 Candida albicans *PHR1* Gene and its Role in Cell Wall Growth

Using differential hybridization screening, a number of *C. albicans* cDNA clones exhibiting differential expression during morphogenesis have been isolated.[188] One of these clones hybridized to a 1.9 kb mRNA that was regulated in response to the pH of the growth environment. The mRNA was absent in cells grown at acid pH, but abundant in cells grown at neutral pH, and its expression was unaffected by temperature. The corresponding gene was designated as *PHR1* (for "*pH*-Regulated").[136] pH-induced deletion of PHR1 seriously damaged the apical wall growth of *C. albicans* mutants, resulting in inability to elongate their hyphae or yeast morphologies. Given the potential involvement of hyphae formation in the pathogenesis of *C. albicans*, the product of the *PHR1* gene and/or the factors regulating its expression may serve as potential targets for antifungal therapy.[136]

29.9.4 Macrophage-Induced Genes of *Histoplasma capsulatum*

In the infected host, *H. capsulatum* circumvents the primary defense mechanism, mainly by macrophages, by regulating expression of specific genes and gene products. Using differential display reverse transcription-PCR technique[189] has allowed the identification of at least 50 genes induced after attachment to, and phagocytosis by, murine macrophages.[136] Interfering with the expression of this set of genes may greatly diminish the capacity of *H. capsulatum* to adapt to the new environmental conditions present in the macrophage, and thereby provide a novel approach to successfully prevent and treat *Histoplasma* and possibly other dimorphic fungal infections.

29.10   REFERENCES

1. Georgiev, V. St., *Antifungal Drugs*, (Ann. NY Acad. Sci., Vol. 544), The New York Academy of Sciences, New York, 1988.
2. Georgiev, V. St., Fungal infections and the search for novel antifungal agents, *Ann. NY Acad. Sci.*, 544, 1, 1988.
3. Kwon-Chung, K. J. and Bennett, J. E., *Medical Mycology*, Lea and Febiger, Philadelphia, 1992, 3.
4. Georgiev, V. St., Fungal cell envelope and mode of action of antimycotic drugs, in *Recent Progress in Antifungal Chemotherapy*, Yamaguchi, H., Kobayashi, G. S., and Takahashi, H., Eds., Marcel Dekker, New York, 1990, 11.
5. Georgopapadakou, N. H., Effects of drugs on lipids and membrane integrity of fungi, in *Perspectives in Antiinfective Therapy*, Jackson, G. G., Schlumberger, H. D., and Zeiler, H. Z., Eds., Friedr. Vieweg and Sohn, Braunschweig/Wiesbaden, 1989, 60.
6. Georgopapadakou, N. H. and Tkacz, J. S., The fungal cell wall as a drug target, *Trends Microbiol.*, 3, 98, 1995.
7. McGinnis, M. R., Introduction to mycology, in *Medical Microbiology*, 3rd ed., Baron, M., Ed., Churchill Livingstone, New York, 1991, 921.
8. Zlotnik, H., Fernandez, M. P., Bowers, B., and Cabib, E., *Saccharomyces cerevisiae* mannoproteins form external cell wall polymer that determines wall porosity, *J. Bacteriol.*, 159, 1018, 1984.
9. Arnold, W. N., Physical aspects of the yeast cell envelope, in *Yeast Cell Envelope: Biochemistry, Biophysics, Ultrastructure*, Arnold, W. N., Ed., CRC Press, Boca Raton, 1981, 25.
10. Arnold, W. N. and Garrison, R. G., Kinetic limitations in the trapping of nascent phosphate for cytochemical localization of yeast acid phosphatase, *Curr. Microbiol.*, 5, 57, 1981.
11. Cabib, E., Roberts, R., and Bowers, B., Synthesis of the yeast cell wall and its regulation, *Annu. Rev. Biochem.*, 51, 763, 1982.
12. Borgia, P. T. and Dodge, C. L., Characterization of *Aspergillus nidulans* mutants deficient in cell wall chitin or glucan, *J. Bacteriol.*, 174, 377, 1992.
13. Kurtz, M. B., Heath, I. B., Marrinan, J., Dreikorn, S., Onishi, J., and Douglas, C., Morphological effects of lipopeptides against *Aspergillus fumigatus* correlate with activities against $(1\rightarrow3)$-β-D-glucan synthase, *Antimicrob. Agents Chemother.*, 38, 1480, 1994.
14. James, P. G., Cherniak, R., Jones, R. G., and Stortz, C. A., Cell-wall glucans of *Cryptococcus neoformans* CAP 67, *Carbohydrate Res.*, 198, 23, 1990.
15. Mol, P. C., Park, H.-M., Mullins, J. T., and Cabib, E., A GTP-binding protein regulates the activity of $(1\rightarrow3)$-β-glucan synthase, an enzyme directly involved in yeast cell wall morphogenesis, *J. Biol. Chem.*, 269, 31267, 1994.
16. Tkacz, J. S., Glucan biosynthesis in fungi and its inhibition, in *Emerging Targets in Antibacterial and Antifungal Chemotherapy*, Sutcliffe, J. A. and Georgopapadakou, N. H., Eds., Chapman and Hall, New York, 1992, 495.
17. Kang, M. S. and Cabib, E., Regulation of fungal cell wall growth: a guanine nucleotide-binding proteinaceous component required for activity of $(1\rightarrow3)$-β-D-glucan synthase, *Proc. Natl. Acad. Sci. U.S.A.*, 83, 5808, 1986.
18. Shematek, E. M. and Cabib, E., Biosynthesis of the yeast cell wall. II. Regulation of β-$(1\rightarrow3)$glucan synthetase by ATP and GTP, *J. Biol. Chem.*, 255, 895, 1980.
19. Notario, V., Kawai, H., and Cabib, E., Interaction between yeast beta-$(1\rightarrow3)$glucan synthetase and activating phosphorylated compounds, *J. Biol. Chem.*, 257, 1902, 1982.
20. Ballou, C. E., Structure and biosynthesis of the mannan component of the yeast cell envelope, *Adv. Microb. Physiol.*, 14, 93, 1976.
21. Horisberger, M. and Volanthen, M., Location of mannan and chitin on thin sections of budding yeasts with gold markers, *Arch. Microbiol.*, 115, 1, 1977.

22. Molano, J., Bowers, B., and Cabib, E., Distribution of chitin in the yeast cell wall: an ultrastructural and chemical study, *J. Cell Biol.*, 85, 199, 1980.
23. Bulawa, C. E., Genetics and molecular biology of chitin synthesis in fungi, *Annu. Rev. Microbiol.*, 47, 505, 1993.
24. Cabib, E., The synthesis and degradation of chitin, *Adv. Enzymol.*, 59, 59, 1987.
25. Hilenski, L. L., Naider, F., and Becker, J. M., Polyoxin D inhibits colloidal gold-wheat germ agglutinin labelling of chitin in dimorphic forms of *Candida albicans*, *J. Gen. Microbiol.*, 132, 1441, 1986.
26. Davis, T. E., Jr., Domer, J. E., and Li, Y. T., Cell wall studies of *Histoplasma capsulatum* and *Blastomyces dermatitides* using autologous and heterologous enzymes, *Infect. Immun.*, 15, 978, 1977.
27. Wheat, R., Terai, T., Kiyomoto, A., Conant, N. F., Lowe, E. P., and Converse, J. L., Studies on the composition and structure of *Coccidioides immitis* cell walls, in *Coccidioidomycosis*, Ajello, A., Ed., University of Arizona Press, Tempe, 1967, 237.
28. Duran, A., Bowers, B., and Cabib, E., Chitin synthetase zymogen is attached to the yeast plasma membrane, *Proc. Natl. Acad. Sci. U.S.A.*, 72, 3952, 1975.
29. Au-Young, J. and Robbins, P. W., Isolation of a chitin synthase gene (*CHC1*) from *Candida albicans* by expression in *Saccharomyces cerevisiae*, *Mol. Microbiol.*, 4, 197, 1990.
30. Sudoh, M., Nagahashi, S., Doi, M., Ohta, A., Takagi, M., and Arisawa, M., Cloning of the chitin synthase 3 gene from *Candida albicans* and its expression during yeast-hyphal transition, *Mol. Gen. Genet.*, 241, 351, 1993.
31. Chen-Wu, J. L., Zwicker, J., Bowen, A. R., and Robbins, P. W., Expression of chitin synthase genes during yeast and hyphal growth phases of *Candida albicans*, *Mol. Microbiol.*, 6, 497, 1992.
32. Georgopapadakou, N. H., Chitin synthase as a chemotherapeutic target, in *Emerging Targets in Antibacterial and Antifungal Chemotherapy*, Sutcliffe, J. A. and Georgopapadakou, N. H., Eds., Chapman and Hall, New York, 1992, 476.
33. Kaneko, H., Hosodara, M., Tanaka, M., and Itoh, T., Lipid composition of 30 species of yeast, *Lipids*, 11, 837, 1976.
34. Marriott, M. S., Isolation and chemical characterization of plasma membranes from the yeast and mycelial forms of *Candida albicans*, *J. Gen. Microbiol.*, 86, 115, 1975.
35. Hamilton-Miller, J. M. T., Fungal sterols and the mode of action of polyene antibiotics, *Adv. Appl. Microbiol.*, 17, 109, 1977.
36. Hammond, S. M., Biological activity of polyene antibiotics, *Progr. Med. Chem.*, 14, 105, 1977.
37. Andreoli, T. E., On the anatomy of amphotericin B-cholestrol pores in lipid membranes, *Kidney Int.*, 4, 337, 1973.
38. Hammond, S. M., Lambert, P. A., and Kliger, B. N., The mode of action of polyene antibiotics: induced potassium leakage in *Candida albicans*, *J. Gen. Microbiol.*, 81, 325, 1974.
39. Teerlink, T., de Kruijff, B., and Demel, R. A., The action of pimaricin, etruscomycin, and amphotericin B on liposomes with varying sterol content, *Biochim. Biophys. Acta*, 599, 484, 1980.
40. Medoff, G., Kobayashi, G. S., Kwan, C. N., Schlessinger, D., and Venkov, P., Potentiation of rifampin and 5-fluorocytosine as antifungal antibiotics by amphotericin B, *Proc. Natl. Acad. Sci. U.S.A.*, 69, 196, 1972.
41. Ghosh, D., Williams, M. A., and Tinoco, J., The influence of lecithin structure on their monolayer behavior and interactions with cholesterol, *Biochim. Biophys. Acta*, 291, 351, 1973.
42. Boggs, J. M. and Hsia, J. C., Effect of cholesterol and water on the rigidity and order of phosphatidylcholine bilayers, *Biochim. Biophys. Acta*, 290, 32, 1972.
43. Marsh, D. and Smith, I. C. P., An interaction spin label study of the fluidizing and condensing effects of cholesterol on lecithin, *Biochim. Biophys. Acta*, 298, 133, 1973.
44. Bittman, R. and Blau, L., The phospholipid-cholesterol interaction: kinetics of water permeability in liposomes, *Biochemistry*, 11, 4831, 1972.
45. Lippert, J. L. and Peticolas, W. L., Laser Raman investigation of the effect of cholesterol on conformational changes in dipalmitoyl lecithin multilayers, *Proc. Natl. Acad. Sci. U.S.A.*, 68, 1572, 1971.
46. Steim, J. M., Tourtelotte, M. E., Reinert, J. C., McElhaney, R. N., and Rader, R. L., Calorimetric evidence for the liquid-crystalline state of lipids in a biomembrane, *Biochemistry*, 63, 104, 1969.
47. Phillips, M. C., Williams, R. M., and Chapman, D., Hydrocarbon chain motions in lipid liquid crystals, *Chem. Phys. Lipids*, 3, 234, 1969.

48. Melchior, D. L., Morowitz, H. J., Sturtevant, J. M., and Tsong, T. Y., Characterization of the plasma membrane of *Mycoplasma laidlawii*. VII. Phase transitions of membrane lipids, *Biochim. Biophys. Acta*, 219, 114, 1970.

49. Ashe, G. B. and Steim, J. M., Membrane transition in Gram-positive bacteria, *Biochim. Biophys. Acta*, 233, 810, 1971.

50. van Deenen, L. L. M., Permeability and topography of membranes, *Chem. Phys. Lipids*, 8, 366, 1972.

51. de Kruyff, B., de Greef, W. J., van Eyk, R. V. W., and van Deenen, L. L. M., The effect of different fatty acid and sterol composition on the erythritol flux through the cell membrane of *Acholeplasma laidlawii*, *Biochim. Biophys. Acta*, 298, 479, 1973.

52. McElhaney, R. N., de Gier, J., and van der Neut-Kok, E. C. M., The effect of alterations in fatty acid composition and cholesterol content on the nonelectrolyte permeability of *Acholeplasma laidlawii* B cells and derived liposomes, *Biochim. Biophys. Acta*, 298, 500, 1973.

53. Graziani, V. and Livne, A., Water permeability of bilayer lipid membranes: sterol-lipid interaction, *J. Membr. Biol.*, 7, 275, 1972.

54. Finkelstein, A. and Cass, A., Effect of cholesterol on the water permeability of thin lipid membranes, *Nature*, 216, 717, 1967.

55. Träuble, H., The movement of molecules across lipid membranes: a molecular theory, *J. Membr. Biol.*, 4, 193, 1971.

56. Sackman, E. and Träuble, H., Studies of the crystalline-liquid crystalline phase transition of lipid model membranes. I. Use of spin labels and optical probes as indicators of the phase transition, *J. Am. Chem. Soc.*, 94, 4482, 1972.

57. Luzzati, V., X-ray difraction studies of lipid-water systems, in *Biological Membranes: Physical Fact and Function*, Chapman, D., Ed., Academic Press, New York, 1968, 71.

58. de Kruijff, B., Geritsen, W. J., Oerlemans, A., Demel, R. A., and van Deenen, L. L. M., Polyene antibiotic-sterol interactions in membranes of *Acholeplasma laidlawii* cells and lecithin liposomes. I. Specificity of the membrane permeability changes induced by the polyene antibiotics, *Biochim. Biophys. Acta*, 339, 30, 1974.

59. Cass, A., Finkelstein, A., and Krepsi, V., The ion permeability induced in thin lipid membranes by the polyene antibiotics nystatin and amphotericin B, *J. Gen. Physiol.*, 56, 100, 1970.

60. Denis, V. W., Stead, N. W., and Andreoli, T. E., Molecular aspects of polyene- and sterol-dependent pore formation in thin lipid membranes, *J. Gen. Physiol.*, 55, 375, 1970.

61. de Kruijff, B. and Demel, R. A., Polyene antibiotic-sterol interactions in membranes of *Acholeplasma laidlawii* cells and lecithin liposomes. III. Molecular structure of the polyene antibiotic-cholesterol complexes, *Biochim. Biophys. Acta*, 339, 57, 1974.

62. Finkelstein, A. and Holz, R., Aqueous pores created in thin membranes by the polyene antibiotics nystatin and amphotericin B, in *Membranes*, Vol. 2, Eisenman, G., Ed., Marcell Dekker, New York, 1972, 377.

63. Kasumov, Kh., Liberman, E. A., Nenashev, V. A., and Yurkov, I. S., Study of cation selectivity of biomolecular membranes in the presence of nystatin and amphotericin B, *Biofizika*, 20, 62, 1975.

64. Norman, A. W., Demel, R. A., de Kruijff, B., Guerts van Kessel, W. S. M., and van Deenen, L. L. M., Studies on the biological properties of polyene antibiotics: comparison of other polyenes with filipin in their ability to interact specifically with sterol, *Biochim. Biophys. Acta*, 290, 1, 1972.

65. Norman, A. W., Demel, R. A., de Kruyff, B., and van Deenen, L. L. M., Studies on the biological properties of polyene antibiotics: evidence for the direct interaction of filipin with cholesterol, *J. Biol. Chem.*, 247, 1918, 1972.

66. de Kruijff, B., Geritsen, W. J., Oerlemans, A., van Dijk, P. W. M., Demel, R. A., and van Demel, L. L. M., Polyene antibiotic-sterol interactions in membranes of *Acholeplasma laidlawii* cells and lecithin liposomes: temperature dependence of the polyene antibiotic-sterol complex formation, *Biochim. Biophys. Acta*, 339, 44, 1974.

67. van Zutphen, H., van Deenen, L. L. M., and Kinsky, S. C., The action of polyene antibiotics on bilayer lipid membranes, *Biochem. Biophys. Res. Commun.*, 22, 393, 1966.

68. Hammond, S. M., Lambert, P. A., and Kliger, B. N., The mode of action of polyene antibiotics: induced entry of hydrogen ions as a consequence of polyene action on the cell membrane of *Candida albicans*, *J. Gen. Microbiol.*, 81, 331, 1974.

69. Hammond, S. M. and Kliger, B. N., Polyene resistant *C. albicans*: a proposed nutritional influence, *Microbios*, 13, 15, 1975.

70. Hector, R. F., Compounds active against cell walls of medically important fungi, *Clin. Microbiol. Rev.*, 6, 1, 1993.

71. Tang, J. and Parr, T. R., W-1 solubilization and kinetics of inhibition by cilofungin in *Candida albicans* $(1\rightarrow3)$-β-D-glucan synthase, *Antimicrob. Agents Chemother.*, 35, 99, 1991.

72. Bouffard, F. A., Zambias, R. A., Dropinski, J. F., Balkovec, J. M., Hammond, M. L., Abruzzo, G. K., Bartizal, K. F., Marrinan, J. A., Kurtz, M. B., McFadden, D. C., Nollstadt, K. H., Powles, M. A., and Schmatz, D. M., Synthesis and antifungal activity of novel cationic pneumocandin B_0 derivatives, *J. Med. Chem.*, 37, 222, 1994.

73. Herscovics, A. and Orlean, P., Glycoprotein biosynthesis in yeast, *FASEB J.*, 7, 540, 1993.

74. Moremen, K. W., Trimble, R. B., and Herscovics, A., Glycosidases of the asparagine-linked oligosaccharide processing pathway, *Glycobiology*, 4, 113, 1994.

75. de Nobel, H. and Lipke, P. N., Is there a role for GPIs in yeast cell-wall assembly? *Trends Cell. Biol.*, 4, 42, 1994.

76. Cabib, E., Differential inhibition of chitin synthetase 1 and synthetase 2 from *Saccharomyces cerevisiae* by polyoxin D and nikkomycins, *Antimicrob. Agents Chemother.*, 35, 170, 1991.

77. Cabib, E., Bowers, B., Sburlati, A., and Silverman, S. J., Fungal cell wall synthesis: the construction of a biological structure, *Microbiol. Sci.*, 5, 370, 1988.

78. Boyle, S. M., Szaniszlo, P. J., Nozawa, Y., Jacobson, E. S., and Cole, G. T., Potential molecular targets of metabolic pathways, *J. Med. Vet. Mycol.*, 32(Suppl. 1), 79, 1994.

79. Szaniszlo, P. J. and Momany, M., Chitin, chitin synthase and chitin synthase conserved region in *Wangiella dermatitidis*, in *Molecular Biology and its Application to Medical Mycology*, Maresca, B., Kobayashi, G. S., and Yamaguchi, H., Eds., NATO ASI Series, Vol. 69, Springer-Verlag, Berlin, 1993, 229.

80. Mimura, C. S., Holbrook, S. R., and Ames, G. F., Structural model of the nucleotide-binding conserved component of periplasmic permeases, *Proc. Natl. Acad. Sci. U.S.A.*, 88, 84, 1991.

81. Fry, D. C., Kuby, S. A., and Mildvan, A. S., ATP-binding site of adenylate kinase: mechanistic implications of its homology with *ras*-encoded p21, F_1-ATPase, and other nucleotide-binding proteins, *Proc. Natl. Acad. Sci. U.S.A.*, 83, 907, 1986.

82. Walker, J. E., Saraste, M., Runswick, M. J., and Gay, N. J., Distantly related sequences in the α- and β-subunits of ATP synthase, myosin, kinases and other ATP-requiring enzymes and a common nucleotide binding fold, *EMBO J.*, 1, 945, 1982.

83. Rossman, M. G., Liljas, A., Branden, C.-I., and Banaszak, L. J., Evolutionary and structural relationships among dehydrogenases, in *The Enzymes*, Vol. 11, Boyer, P. D., Ed., Academic Press, New York, 1975, 61.

84. Isono, K. and Suzuki, S., The polyoxins: pyrimidine nucleoside peptide antibiotics inhibiting fungal cell wall biosynthesis, *Heterocycles*, 13, 333, 1979.

85. Decker, H., Zähner, H., Heitsch, H., König, W. A., and Fiedler, H. P., Structure-activity relationships of the nikkomycins, *J. Gen. Microbiol.*, 137, 1805, 1991.

86. Gaughran, J. P., Lai, M. H., Kirsch, D. R., and Silverman, S. J., Nikkomycin Z is a specific inhibitor of *Saccharomyces cerivisiae* chitin synthase isozyme Chs3 *in vitro* and *in vivo*, *J. Bacteriol.*, 176, 5857, 1994.

87. Khare, R. K., Becker, J. M., and Naider, F. R., Synthesis and anticandidal properties of polyoxin L analogues containing alpha-amino fatty acids, *J. Med. Chem.*, 31, 650, 1988.

88. Chmara, H., Inhibition of glycosamine synthase by bacilysin and anticapsin, *J. Gen. Microbiol.*, 131, 265, 1985.

89. Milewski, S., Chmara, H., Andruszkiewicz, R., and Borowski, E., Synthetic derivatives of N^3-fumaroyl-L-2,3,-diamonopropanoic acid inactivate glycosamine synthetase from *Candida albicans*, *Biochim. Biophys. Acta*, 828, 247, 1985.

90. vanden Bossche, H., Marichal, P., Gorrens, J., Geerts, H., and Janssen, P. A. J., Basis for the search of new antifungal drugs, *Ann. NY Acad. Sci.*, 544, 191, 1988.

91. Rodriguez, R. J., Taylor, F. R., and Parks, L. W., A requirement for ergosterol to permit growth of yeast sterol auxotrophs on cholesterol, *Biochem. Biophys. Res. Commun.*, 106, 435, 1982.

92. Ramgopal, M. and Bloch, K., Multiple functions for sterol in *Saccharomyces cerevisiae*, *Proc. Natl. Acad. Sci. U.S.A.*, 80, 712, 1983.

93. Pinto, W. J., Lozano, R., Sekula, B. C., and Nes, W. R., Stereochemically distinct roles for sterol in *Saccharomyces cerevisiae*, *Biochem. Biophys. Res. Commun.*, 112, 47, 1983.
94. Rodriguez, R. J., Low, C., Bottema, C. D. K., and Parks, L. W., Multiple functions for sterols in *Saccharomyces cerivisiae*, *Biochim. Biophys. Acta*, 837, 336, 1985.
95. Nishino, T., Hata, S., Taketani, S., Yabusaki, Y., and Katsuki, H., Subcellular localization of the enzymes involved in the late stage of ergosterol biosynthesis in yeast, *J. Biochem.*, 89, 1391, 1981.
96. Boll, M., Lowel, M., Still, J., and Berndt, J., Sterol biosynthesis in yeast: 3-hydroxy-3-methylglutaryl-coenzyme A reductase as a regulatory enzyme, *Eur. J. Biochem.*, 54, 435, 1975.
97. Brodie, J. D., Wasson, G., and Porter, W., The participation of malonyl coenzyme A in the biosynthesis of mevalonic acid, *J. Biol. Chem.*, 238, 1294, 1963.
98. Clayton, R. B., Biosynthesis of sterols, steroids, and terpenoids. I. Biogenesis of cholesterol and the fundamental steps in terpenoid biosynthesis, *Q. Rev. Chem. Soc.*, 19, 168, 1965.
99. Endo, A., Kuroda, M., and Tsujita, Y., ML-236A, ML-236B, and ML-236C, new inhibitors of cholesterogenesis produced by *Penicillium citrinum*, *J. Antibiot.*, 29, 1346, 1976.
100. Endo, A., Kuroda, M., and Tanzawa, K., Competitive inhibition of 3-hydroxy-3-methylglutaryl coenzyme A reductase by ML-236A and ML-236B fungal metabolites, having hypocholesterolemic activity, *FEBS Lett.*, 72, 323, 1976.
101. Tanzawa, K. and Endo, A., Kinetic analysis of the reaction catalyzed by rat-liver 3-hydroxy-3-methylglutaryl-coenzyme-A reductase using two specific inhibitors, *Eur. J. Biochem.*, 98, 195, 1979.
102. Endo, A., Compactin (ML-236B) and related compounds as potential cholesterol-lowering agents that inhibit HMG-CoA reductase, *J. Med. Chem.*, 28, 401, 1985.
103. Onishi, J. C., Abbruzzo, G. K., Fromtling, R. A., Garrity, G. M., Milligan, J. A., Pelak, B. A., Rozdilsky, W., and Weissberger, B., Mode of action of β-lactone 1233A in *Candida albicans*, *Ann. NY Acad. Sci.*, 544, 230, 1988.
104. Altman, L. J., Kowerski, R. C., and Rilling, H. C., Synthesis and conversion of presqualene alcohol to squalene, *J. Am. Chem. Soc.*, 93, 1782, 1971.
105. Rilling, H. C., Poulter, C. D., Epstein, W. W., and Larsen, B., Studies on the mechanism of squalene biosynthesis: presqualene pyrophosphate, stereochemistry and a mechanism for its conversion to squalene, *J. Am. Chem. Soc.*, 93, 1783, 1971.
106. Popjak, G. and Cornforth, J. W., Substrate stereochemistry in squalene biosynthesis, *Biochem. J.*, 101, 553, 1966.
107. Amdur, B. H., Rilling, H. C., and Bloch, K., The enzymatic conversion of mevalonic acid to squalene, *J. Am. Chem. Soc.*, 79, 2646, 1957.
108. Lynen, F., Eggerer, H., Henning, V., and Kessel, I., Biosynthesis of terpenes. III. Farnesyl pyrophosphate and 3-methyl-3-buten-1-yl pyrophosphate, *Angew. Chem.*, 70, 738, 1958.
109. Shechter, I. and Bloch, K., Solubilization and purification of *trans*-farnesyl pyrophosphate-squalene synthetase, *J. Biol. Chem.*, 246, 7690, 1971.
110. Dean, P. D. G., Ortiz de Montellano, P. R., Bloch, K., and Corey, E. J., A soluble 2,3-oxidosqualene sterol cyclase, *J. Biol. Chem.*, 242, 3014, 1967.
111. Mercer, E. I. and Johnson, M. W., Cyclization of squalene 2,3-oxide to lanosterol in a cell-free system from *Phycomycetes blakesleeanus*, *Phytochemistry*, 8, 2329, 1969.
112. Shechter, I., Sweat, F. W., and Bloch, K., Comparative properties of 2,3-oxidosqualene-lanosterol cyclase from yeast and liver, *Biochim. Biophys. Acta*, 220, 463, 1970.
113. Paltauf, F., Daum, G., Zuder, G., Hogenauer, G., Schulz, G., and Seidl, G., Squalene and ergosterol biosynthesis in fungi treated with naftifine, a new antimycotic agent, *Biochim. Biophys. Acta*, 712, 268, 1982.
114. Ryder, N. S. and Dupont, M.-C., Inhibition of squalene epoxidase by allylamine antimycotic compounds, *Biochem. J.*, 230, 765, 1985.
115. Morita, T. and Nozawa, Y., Effects of antifungal agents on ergosterol biosynthesis in *Candida albicans* and *Trychophyton mentagrophytes*: differential inhibitory sites of naphthiomate and miconazole, *J. Invest. Dermatol.*, 85, 434, 1985.
116. Ryder, N. S., Frank, I., and Dupont, M.-C., Ergosterol biosynthesis inhibition by the thiocarbamate antifungal agents tolnaftate and tolciclate, *Antimicrob. Agents Chemother.*, 29, 858, 1986.
117. Weete, J. D., Sterols of the fungi: distribution and biosynthesis, *Phytochemistry*, 12, 1843, 1973.

118. Barton, D. H. R., Kempe, U. M., and Widdowson, D. A., Biosynthesis of steroids and terpenoids. VI. Sterols of yeast, *J. Chem. Soc. Perkin I*, 1, 513, 1972.

119. Barton, D. H. R., Corrie, J. E. T., Marshall, P. J., and Widdowson, D. A., Biosynthesis of terpenes and steroids. VII. Unified scheme for the biosynthesis of ergosterol in *Saccharomyces cerevisiae*, *Bioorg. Chem.*, 2, 363, 1973.

120. Barton, D. H. R., Corrie, J. E. T., Widdowson, D. A., Bard, M., and Woods, R. A., Biosynthesis of terpenes and steroids. IX. Sterols of mutant yeasts and their relation to the biosynthesis of ergosterol, *J. Chem. Soc. Chem. Commun.*, 30, 1974.

121. Rattray, J. B. M., Schibeci, A., and Kidby, D. K., Lipids of yeasts, *Bacteriol. Rev.*, 39, 197, 1975.

122. Gaylor, J. L., Enzymes of sterol biosynthesis, in *Biochemistry of Lipids*, Biochemistry Series One, Vol. 4, Goodwin, T. W., Ed., Butterworth, London, 1974, 1.

123. Georgopoulos, A., Petranyi, G., Mieth, H., and Drews, J., *In vitro* activity of naftifine, a new antifungal agent, *Antimicrob. Agents Chemother.*, 19, 386, 1981.

124. Petranyi, G., Georgopoulos, A., and Mieth, H., *In vivo* antimycotic activity of naftifine, *Antimicrob. Agents Chemother.*, 19, 390, 1981.

125. Petranyi, G., Ryder, N. S., and Stütz, A., Allylamine derivatives: new class of synthetic antifungal agents inhibiting fungal squalene epoxidase, *Science*, 224, 1239, 1984.

126. Petranyi, G., Meingassner, J. G., and Mieth, H., Antifungal activity of the allylamine derivative terbinafine *in vitro*, *Antimicrob. Agents Chemother.*, 31, 1365, 1987.

127. Ryder, N. S., Mechanism of action and biochemical selectivity of allylamine antimycotic agents, *Ann. NY Acad. Sci.*, 544, 208, 1988.

128. Stütz, A., Synthesis and structure-activity correlations within allylamine antimycotics, *Ann. NY Acad. Sci.*, 544, 46, 1988.

129. Stütz, A., Allylamine derivatives — a new class of active substances in antifungal chemotherapy, *Angew. Chem. Int. Ed. Engl.*, 26, 320, 1987.

130. Ryder, N. S., Seidl, G., and Troke, P. F., Effect of the antimycotic drug naftifine on growth of and sterol biosynthesis in *Candida albicans*, *Antimicrob. Agents Chemother.*, 25, 483, 1984.

131. Ryder, N. S., Specific inhibition of fungal sterol biosynthesis by SF 86,327, a new allylamine antimycotic agent, *Antimicrob. Agents Chemother.*, 27, 252, 1985.

132. Ryder, N. S. and Dupont, M. C., Properties of a particulate squalene epoxidase from *Candida albicans*, *Biochim. Biophys. Acta*, 794, 466, 1984.

133. Ryder, N. S. and Dupont, M. C., Inhibition of squalene epoxidase by allylamine antimycotic compounds: a comparative study of the fungal and mammalian enzymes, *Biochem. J.*, 230, 765, 1985.

134. Hitchcock, C. A., Cytochrome P-450-dependent 14-alpha-sterol demethylase of *Candida albicans* and its interaction with azole antifungals, *Biochem. Soc. Trans.*, 19, 782, 1991.

135. vanden Bossche, H. and Marichal, P., Is there a role for sterols and steroids in fungal growth and transition from yeast to hyphal-form and vice-versa? An overview, in *Recent Progress in Antifungal Chemotherapy*, Yamaguchi, H., Kobayashi, G. S., and Takahashi, H., Eds., Marcell Dekker, New York, 1991, 177.

136. Maresca, B., Bennett, J., Fonzi, W., Hitchcock, C. A., Lodge, J. K., and Williamson, P. R., Molecular approaches to identify novel targets for future development of antifungal agents, *J. Med. Vet. Mycol.*, 32(Suppl. 1), 287, 1994.

137. Baldwin, B. C., Fungicidal inhibitors of ergosterol biosynthesis, *Biochem. Soc. Trans.*, 11, 659, 1983.

138. Gadher, P., Mercer, E. I., Baldwin, B. C., and Wiggins, T. E., A comparison of potency of some fungicides as inhibitors of sterol 14-demethylation, *Pestic. Biochem. Physiol.*, 19, 1, 1983.

139. Wiggins, T. E. and Baldwin, B. C., Binding of azole fungicides related to diclobutrazol to cytochrome P-450, *Pestic. Sci.*, 15, 206, 1984.

140. Kelly, S. L., Quail, M. A., Rowe, M. A., and Kelly, D. F., Sterol 14α-demethylase: target of the azole antifungal agents, in *New Approaches for Antifungal Drugs*, Birkhauser, Boston, 1992, 155.

141. Kalb, V. F., Woods, C. W., Turi, T. G., Dey, C. R., Sutter, T. R., and Loper, J. C., Primary structure of the P450 lanosterol demethylase gene from *Saccharomyces cerivisiae*, *DNA*, 6, 529, 1987.

142. Lai, M. H. and Kirsch, D. R., Nucleotide sequence of cytochrome P450 LIA1 (lanosterol 14α-demethylase) from *Candida albicans*, *Nucl. Acids Res.*, 17, 804, 1989.

143. Buchenauer, H., Analogy in the mode of action of fluotrinazole and clotrimazole in *Ustilago avenae*, *Pestic. Biochem. Physiol.*, 8, 15, 1978.

144. vanden Bossche, H., Willemsen, G., Cools, W., Lauwers, W. F. J., and Le Jeune, L., Biochemical effects of miconazole on fungi. II. Inhibition of ergosterol biosynthesis by *Candida albicans, Chem.-Biol. Interact.*, 21, 59, 1978.

145. vanden Bossche, H., Willemsen, G., Cools, W., Lauwers, W. F. J., and Le Jeune, L., Inhibition of ergosterol biosynthesis in *Candida albicans* by miconazole, *Curr. Chemother.*, 3, 228, 1978.

146. Iwata, K., Yamaguchi, H., and Hiratani, T., Mode of action of clotrimazole, *Sabouraudia*, 11, 158, 1973.

147. De Nollin, S. and Borgers, M., Scanning electron microscopy of *Candida albicans* after *in vitro* treatment with miconazole, *Antimicrob. Agents Chemother.*, 7, 704, 1975.

148. Sud, I. J. and Feingold, D. S., Heterogeneity of action mechanisms among antimycotic imidazoles, *Antimicrob. Agents Chemother.*, 20, 71, 1981.

149. Sud, I. J. and Feingold, D. S., Mechanism of action of antimycotic imidazoles, *J. Invest. Dermatol.*, 76, 438, 1981.

150. Rodriguez, R. J. and Parks, L. W., Physiological response of *Saccharomyces cerevisiae* to 15-azasterol-mediated growth inhibition, *Antimicrob. Agents Chemother.*, 20, 184, 1981.

151. Pierce, H. D., Jr., Pierce, A. M., Srinivasan, R., Unrau, A. M., and Oehlschlager, A. C., Azasterol inhibitors in yeast: inhibition of 24-methylene sterol $\Delta^{24(28)}$ reductase and Δ^{24}-sterol methyltransferase of *Saccharomyces cerevisiae* by 23-azacholesterol, *Biochim. Biophys. Acta*, 529, 429, 1978.

152. Avruch, L., Fischer, S., Pierce, H. D., Jr., and Oehlschlager, A. C., The induced biosynthesis of 7-dehydrocholesterols in yeast: potential sources of new provitamin D_3 analogs, *Can. J. Biochem.*, 54, 657, 1975.

153. König, K. H., Pommer, E. H., and Sanne, W., *N*-Substituted tetrahydro-1,4-oxazines — a new class of fungicidal compounds, *Angew. Chem. Int. Ed. Engl.*, 4, 336, 1965.

154. Himmele, W. and Pommer, E. H., 3-Phenylpropylamines, a new class of systemic fungicides, *Angew. Chem. Int. Ed. Engl.*, 19, 184, 1980.

155. Kato, T., Shoami, M., and Kawase, Y., Comparison of tridemorph with buthiobate in antifungal mode of action, *J. Pestic. Sci.*, 5, 69, 1980.

156. Kerkenaar, A., Uchiyama, M., and Versluis, G. G., Specific effects of tridemorph on sterol biosynthesis in *Ustilago maydis, Pestic. Biochem. Physiol.*, 16, 97, 1981.

157. Polak, A., Antifungal activity *in vitro* of Ro 14,4767/002, a phenylpropyl-morpholine, *Sabouraudia*, 21, 205, 1983.

158. Polak, A., Mode of action of morpholine derivatives, *Ann. NY Acad. Sci.*, 544, 221, 1988.

159. Rhode, E., Zang, M., and Hartmann, D., Preliminary clinical experience with Ro 14,4767 (amorolfin) in superficial mycoses, in *Recent Trends in the Discovery, Development, and Evaluation of Antifungal Agents*, Fromtling, R. A., Ed., J. R. Prous, Barcelona, 1986, 575.

160. Kerkenaar, A., The mode of action of dimethylmorpholines, in *Recent Trends in the Discovery, Development, and Evaluation of Antifungal Agents*, Fromtling, R. A., Ed., J. R. Prous, Barcelona, 1986, 523.

161. Kerkenaar, A., Barug, D., and Kaars Supersteijn, A., On the antifungal mode of action of tridemorph, *Pestic. Biochem. Physiol.*, 12, 195, 1979.

162. Baloch, R. I., Mercer, E. I., Wiggins, T. E., and Baldwin, B. C., Inhibition of ergosterol biosynthesis in *Saccharomyces cerevisiae* and *Ustilago maydis* by tridemorph, fenpropimorph and fenpropidin, *Phytochemistry*, 23, 2219, 1984.

163. Baloch, R. I. and Mercer, E. I., Inhibition of Δ^8-Δ^7-isomerase and Δ^{14}-reductase by fenpropimorph, tridemorph, and fenpropidin in cell-free enzyme systems from *Saccharomyces cerevisiae*, *Phytochemistry*, 26, 663, 1987.

164. Kerkenaar, A., van Rossum, J. M., Versluis, G. G., and Marsman, J. W., Effect of fenpropimorph and imazalil on sterol biosynthesis in *Penicillium italicum, Pestic. Sci.*, 15, 177, 1984.

165. Benveniste, P., Bladoche, M., Costet, M.-F., and Ehrhard, A., Use of inhibitors of sterol biosynthesis to study plasmalemma structure and function, in *Annual Proceedings of the European Phytochemistry Society*, Vol. 24, Boudet, A. M., Allibert, G., Marigo, G., and Lea, P. J., Eds., Clarendon, Oxford, 1984, 283.

166. Rahier, A., Taton, M., Schmitt, P., Benveniste, O., Place, P., and Auding, C., Inhibition of Δ^8-Δ^7-sterol isomerase and cycloeucalenolobtusifoliol isomerase by *N*-benzyl-8-aza-4α,10-dimethyl-*trans*-decal-3β-ol, an analogue of carbocationic high-energy intermediate, *Phytochemistry*, 24, 1223, 1985.

167. Moors, M. A., Mannis, J., Buckley, H. R., and Mosser, H. R., A novel mechanism for the acquisition of iron by *Candida albicans*, *Proc. Conf. Candida and Candidiasis: Biology, Pathogenesis and Management*, American Society for Microbiology, Baltimore, March 25–28, 1993.

168. Burt, W. R., Identification of coprogen B and its breakdown products from *Histoplasma capsulatum*, *Infect. Immun.*, 35, 990, 1982.

169. Boelaert, J. R., Fenves, A. Z., and Coburn, J. W., Deferoxamine therapy and mycormycosis in dialysis patients: report of an international registry, *Am. J. Kidney Dis.*, 18, 660, 1991.

170. Boelaert, J. R., De Locht, M., van Cutsem, J., Kerrels, V., Cantinieaux, B., Verdonck, A., van Landuyt, H. W., and Schneider, Y.-J., Mycormycosis during deferoxamine therapy is a siderophore-mediated infection: *in vitro* and *in vivo* animal studies, *J. Clin. Invest.*, 91, 1979, 1993.

171. Halley, V., Boelaert, J. R., Dromer, F., and Schneider, Y.-J., *In vitro* effects of DFO and LI on *Cryptococcus neoformans*, *Proc. Conf. Iron and Iron Chelates*, Brugge, Nov. 5–6, Abstr. P20, 1993.

172. Jacobson, E. S. and Petro, M. J., Extracellular iron chelation in *Cryptococcus neoformans*, *J. Med. Vet. Mycol.*, 25, 415, 1987.

173. Jacobson, E. S. and Vartivarian, S. E., Iron assimilation in *Cryptococcus neoformans*, *J. Med. Vet. Mycol.*, 30, 443, 1992.

174. Neilands, J. B., Microbial iron compounds, *Annu. Rev. Biochem.*, 50, 715, 1989.

175. Okada, H., Yamamoto, K., Tsutano, S., Inouye, Y., Nakamura, S., and Furukawa, J., A new group of antibiotics, hydroxamic acid antibiotics. II. The structure of neoenactins NL_1 and NL_2, structure-activity relationship, *J. Antibiot.*, 42, 276, 1989.

176. Huyer, M. and Page, W. J., Ferric reductase activity in *Azetobacter vinelandii* and its inhibition by Zn^{2+}, *J. Bacteriol.*, 171, 4031, 1989.

177. Moody, M. D. and Dailey, H. A., Ferric iron reductase of *Rhodopseudomonas sphaeroides*, *J. Bacteriol.*, 163, 1120, 1985.

178. Dancis, A., Klausner, R. D., Hinnebusch, A. G., and Barriocanal, J. G., Genetic evidence that ferric reductase is required for iron uptake in *Saccharomyces cerevisiae*, *Mol. Cell. Biol.*, 10, 2294, 1990.

179. Eide, D., Davis-Kaplan, S., Jordan, I., Sipe, D., and Kaplan, J., Regulation of iron uptake in *Saccharomyces cerivisiae*: the ferrireductase and Fe(II) transporter are regulated independently, *J. Biol. Chem.*, 267, 20774, 1992.

180. Vartivarian, S. E., Coward, R. E., and Springs, H., Cryptococcal iron uptake, *Proc. 2nd Int. Conf. on Cryptococcus and Cryptococcosis*, Milan, Abstr. P1-7, 1993, p. 110.

181. Chaskes, S. and Tyndall, R. L., Pigment production by *Cryptococcus neoformans* and other *Cryptococcus* species from aminophenols and diaminobenzenes, *J. Clin. Microbiol.*, 7, 146, 1978.

182. Kwon-Chung, K. J., Polachek, I., and Popkin, T. J., Melanin-lacking mutants of *Cryptococcus neoformans* and their virulence for mice, *J. Bacteriol.*, 150, 1414, 1982.

183. Jacobson, E. S. and Emery, H. S., Catecholamine uptake, melanization, and oxygen toxicity in *Cryptococcus neoformans*, *J. Bacteriol.*, 173, 401, 1991.

184. Williamson, P. R., Biochemical and molecular characterization of the diphenol oxidase of *Cryptococcus neoformans*: identification as a laccase, *J. Bacteriol.*, 176, 656, 1994.

185. Kojima, Y., Tsukuda, Y., Kawai, Y., Tsukamoto, A., Sugiura, J., Sakaino, M., and Kita, Y., Cloning sequence analysis, and expression of ligninolytic phenoloxidase genes of the white-rot basidiomycete *Coriolus hirsutus*, *J. Biol. Chem.*, 265, 15224, 1990.

186. Rudnick, D. A., McWherter, C. A., Gokel, G. W., and Gordon, J. I., Myristoyl-CoA:protein *N*-myristoyltransferase, *Adv. Enzymol.*, 67, 375, 1993.

187. Rudnick, D. A., McWherter, C. A., Rocque, W. J., Lennon, P. J., Getman, D. P., and Gordon, J. I., Kinetic and structural evidence for a sequential ordered B_iB_i mechanism of catalysis by *Saccharomyces cerevisae* myristoyl-CoA:protein *N*-myristoyltransferase, *J. Biol. Chem.*, 266, 9732, 1991.

188. Birse, C. E., Irwin, M. Y., Fonzi, W. A., and Sypherd, P. S., Cloning and characterization of ECE1, a gene expressed in association with cell elongation of the dimorphic pathogen *Candida albicans*, *Infect. Immun.*, 61, 3648, 1993.

189. Bauer, D., Muller, H., Reich, J., Riedel, J., Ahrenkiel, V., Warthoe, V., and Strauss, M., Identification of differential expressed mRNA species by an improved dysplay technique (DDRT-PCR), *Nucleic Acids Res.*, 21, 4272, 1993.

30 Deuteromycota (Fungi Imperfecti)

The form-phylum Deuteromycota contains three form-classes: Blastomycetes, Coelomycetes, and Hyphomycetes.[1]

The form-class Blastomycetes represents a group of fungi with yeast-like somatic cells. They include two form-orders, Sporobolomycetales and Cryptococcales.[1,2] In terms of human diseases, the latter form-order is much more important. Cryptococcales is a heterogeneous group of asexual yeast fungi without ballistospore formation. Most of them are pathogenic to humans and some of the better known genera include *Candida*, *Cryptococcus*, *Rhodotorulla*, and *Malassezia*. The last three genera have basidiomycetous affinity and some of their members produce basidiomycete teleomorphs classified in the genera *Filobasidiella* (anamorph, *Cryptococcus neoformans*), *Filobasidium* (anamorphs, *C. uniguttulatus* and *C. albidus*), *Cystofilobasidium* (anamorph, *C. infirmo-miniatus*), and *Rhodosporidium* (anamorphs, *Rhodotorula glutinis* and *R. minuta*).

Under a more traditional classification, the Hyphomycetes was divided into two form-orders, Moniliales and Agonomycetales. Further, depending on the hyphal color and the presence or absence of sporodochia or synnemata, the form-order Moniliales was divided into four form-families: Moniliaceae, Dematiaceae, Tuberculariaceae, and Stilbellaceae. The better known family of Moniliaceae include *Aspergillus*, *Penicillium*, *Paecilomyces*, and *Fusarium*. The Dematiaceae include also a number of genera pathogenic to humans, such as *Phialophora*, *Exophiala*, *Curvularia*, *Bipolaris*, and *Cladosporidium*. The currently accepted concepts for classification of Hyphomycetes are not to divide them below the rank of class, and are based on the modes (thallic and blastic) of their conidial ontogeny.[1]

In the thallic mode of development, the somatic hyphal element is converted into conidium either by fragmentation at the septa (thallic-arthric) or by disarticulation of a portion (usually the tip) of the hypha (holothallic or thallic-solitary). *Geotrichum candidum*, *Coccidioides immitis*, and *Trichosporon beigelii* are among the pathogenic fungi producing thallic-arthric conidia. Representative fungi with thallic-solitary (holothallic) type of conidiogenesis include *Microsporum*, *Trychophyton*, and *Epidermophyton* spp.[3] Although the aleuriospore, a holothallic type of conidia, has been associated with *Histoplasma capsulatum* and *Blastomyces dermatitidis*, there has been no detailed conidial ontogeny study of these two species.[1]

In the blastic development, a conidiogenous cell or a fertile hypha will burst out to form a conidium. This process may be limited to a single occurrence resulting in a single terminal conidium (e.g., *Nigrospora*), or be repeated to form conidial chains (e.g., *Aspergillus* spp.) or spore balls (e.g., *Phialophora*). Furthermore, during the blastic development of conidia, the conidiogenous cells may proliferate (e.g., *Bipolaris specifer*, *Sporothrix schenkii*); cease extension growth and remain unchanged, as seen in *Fusarium*, *Aspergillus*, and *Cladosporidium*; or become progressively shorter as the result of successful conidial formation, such as in *Trichothecium roseum*.[1]

30.1   REFERENCES

1. Kwon-Chung, K. J. and Bennett, J. E., The fungi, in *Medical Mycology*, Lea and Febiger, Philadelphia, 1992, 3.
2. Kreger-van Rij, N. J. W., Ed., *The Yeasts: A Taxonomic Study*, 3rd ed., Elsevier, Amsterdam, 1984.
3. Galgoczy, J., Dermatophytes: conidium ontogeny and classification, *Acta Microbiol. Acad. Sci.*, 22, 105, 1975.

31 *Cryptococcus neoformans*

31.1 INTRODUCTION

The genus *Cryptococcus* belongs to the form-order Cryptococcales of the form-class Blastomycetes. *Cryptococcus neoformans* is a yeast-like fungus that is pathogenic to both animals and man. It was first isolated in 1894 by Busse[1] from a patient with osteomyelitis of the tibia. The fungus is a saprophitic organism which can be found in soil, on a variety of fruits, as well as in close association with pigeon nests.[2,3] There are two varieties of *C. neoformans*: *C. neoformans* var. *neoformans* and *C. neoformans* var. *gattii*. Each of these varieties, in turn, has two serotypes: A and D for var. *neoformans*, and B and C for var. *gattii*. In addition, there have been reports of human infections caused by two other *Cryptococcus* species: *C. albidus* and *C. laurentii*.

Morphologically, *C. neoformans* represents an encapsulated yeast which reproduces by budding. The cell can vary from 4.0 to 6.0 μm in diameter and is surrounded by a mucoid polysaccharide capsule that is 1.0 to 30 μm wide.[4] The capsule is resistant to washing by water and may be removed, but only partially, by acid hydrolysis. When grown on Sabouraud's medium or chocolate sugar, *C. neoformans* forms yellow-tan colonies within 4 to 7 d of inoculation.

Infection with *C. neoformans* is usually acquired by its inhalation. Although the fungus is common in pigeon feces, the birds are not clinically infected.[5] There is no human-to-human transmission of the disease observed.[4]

When injected to mice, *C. neoformans* may utilize creatinine as a nitrogen source to produce meningitis and hydrocephalus within 3 weeks.[4] While the fungus itself does not generate toxins and usually evokes a minimal inflammatory response in tissues, its large carbohydrate capsule is the major virulence factor by preventing ingestion by polymorphonuclear leukocytes.[6] Moreover, the presence of anticryptococcal antibody alone is not of primary importance[7] since complement is also needed for opsonization.[8] For example, a complement depletion observed during cryptococcemia[9] is thought responsible for the decrease in the survival rate following complications of cryptococcal infections.[4]

Cell-mediated immunity seems to provide the major defense against cryptococcal infections, leaving patients with compromised cell-mediated responses (lymphoma, leukemia, sarcoidosis, and those patients receiving corticosteroid therapy) more vulnerable and, therefore, more likely to develop a cryptococcal infection.[10-19] Experiments by Aguirre et al.[20] have demonstrated that both interferon-γ (IFN-γ) and tumor necrosis factor-α (TNF-α) were important factors in mediating acquired resistance to cryptococcal meningoencephalitis.

Cryptococcosis may develop as an acute, subacute, or chronic pulmonary, systemic, or meningeal mycosis. While the pulmonary form is usually transitory, mild, and often asymptomatic, the involvement of the central nervous system is manifested by subacute or chronic meningitis that in immunocompromised hosts could be life-threatening. During dissemination of the disease, skeletal and visceral lesions may occur. Nearly all of the immunocompromised patients are likely to develop disseminated cryptococcosis[21,22] with susceptibility to infection being reported for the skin,[23-26] bone,[27] prostate,[28] kidney,[29] eyes,[30,31] liver,[2-34] spleen,[35] adrenals,[35,36] lymph nodes,[24,34,37,38] and the gastrointestinal tract.[39] Although infrequently, deep cryptococcal infections of the breast have been reported.[40] Hypereosinophilia in disseminated disease has also been observed.[41]

Larsen et al.[42] have reported a persistent cryptococcal infection of the prostate in AIDS patients even after adequate therapy with amphotericin B alone or in combination with flucytosine; this observation suggests the possibility of the prostate serving as a sequestered reservoir of infection from which systemic relapse may occur. In this regard, cryptococcal prostatitis in a patient with Behcet's disease was also described.[43]

The coexistence of different diseases within the same lesion could be a distinct possibility in patients with HIV infection. In this context, there have been several reports of simultaneous Kaposi's sarcoma and cutaneous cryptococcosis occurring at the same site in a patient with AIDS.[44] Limbal nodules and multifocal choroidal lesions due to *C. neoformans* may also occur in AIDS patients.[45] Munoz-Peréz et al.[46] have described disseminated cryptococcosis presenting as molluscum-like lesions as the first manifestation of AIDS.

Molnar-Nadasdy et al.[47] have described a unique case of placental cryptococcosis in a pregnant mother with systemic lupus erythematosus and steroid treatment. Although there were no clinical or placental signs of transplacental infection, immunohistochemical labeling of villous stromal cells showed a conspicuously increased number of fetal macrophages.

In patients with AIDS, cryptococcal infections are often associated with high relapse rate and poor response to treatment.[48-52] Currently, cryptococcosis is considered to be one of the most life-threatening mycoses in patients with AIDS.[53-59] In addition to being a common opportunistic mycosis in adults, cryptococcosis complicating pediatric AIDS has also been well documented.[60]

In the majority of patients with normal immunity, cryptococcosis is confined to the lung or the hilar nodes[21,61-66] and will hardly require any antifungal therapy.[21,67,68] Occasionally, cryptococcal osteomyelitis has also been described in normal hosts.[69] Cutaneous cryptococcosis in the nonimmuno-compromised host is also a rare entity, and when it does occur, it presents with protean manifestations, making clinical diagnosis difficult.[70,71] One unusual case of progressive pulmonary disease in an immunocompetent patient presenting as a discrete endobronchial cryptococcoma has been reported by Emmons et al.;[59] Mahida et al.[72] also reported a patient with endobronchial cryptococcal obstruction. Cryptococcal meningitis with severe visual and hearing loss and radiculopathy was described in an immunocompetent patient,[73] as well as CNS cryptococcosis with multiple intraventricular cysts.[74] The development of adult respiratory distress syndrome (ARDS) (see Chapter 37, Section 37.5.4.3) caused by pulmonary cryptococcosis in an immunocompetent host has been reported.[75]

By far, cryptococcal meningitis is the most dangerous form of the disease. Since some patients with cryptococcal meningitis may be asymptomatic,[10,12,76-78] it is important that the cerebrospinal fluid (CSF) be examined whenever *C. neoformans* is isolated or detected from any site. The onset of cryptococcal meningitis is most likely to be insidious, but often it is acute in cases of severely immunocompromised hosts. In the latter case, if untreated, the infection is always fatal.[10,79-82]

Benard et al.[83] have described the case reports of two patients with immunodeficiency secondary to paracoccidioidomycosis and opportunistic cryptococcosis. Secondary immunodeficiency likely occurred as a consequence of the intestinal loss of proteins and lymphocytes associated with malabsorption syndrome due to obstructed lymphatic drainage — both patients had severe abdominal involvement during the acute paracoccidioidomycosis disease.[83]

Nelson et al.[84] found as valuable, a positive test for serum cryptococcal antigen in the diagnosis of cryptococcosis in AIDS patients, especially in cases where no evidence of cryptococcal infection on repeated CSF examination is observed.

31.2   STUDIES ON THERAPEUTICS

31.2.1   AMPHOTERICIN B

Graybill et al.[85] have investigated the effect of amphotericin B on cryptococcal infection in immuno-deficient mice. In congenitally athymic nude (nu/nu) and thymus-containing heterozygous (nu/X) mice infected intraperitoneally with *C. neoformans*, the disease progressed more rapidly in nu/nu mice than in the nu/X animals. When the nu/X mice were treated intraperitoneally with 6.0 mg/kg of amphotericin B administered every other day for a total of five doses, all mice survived what otherwise would have been a lethal dose of *C. neoformans*. Following treatment with amphotericin B, the survival rate was also prolonged in nu/nu mice given larger challenge, but they succumbed to cryptococcosis. These findings support the notion that an interaction between antifungal chemotherapy and thymus-dependent defense mechanisms does occur.[85]

Atkinson and Bindschadler[86] have studied the pharmacokinetics of intrathecally administered amphotericin B. A pharmacokinetic model was proposed based on the rate of elimination of the drug from cerebrospinal fluid. When given to patients with cryptococcal meningitis, the antibiotic was removed from the CSF by bulk flow through the arachnoid villi. Daily injection of 0.3 mg of the drug resulted in the continuous maintenance of amphotericin B concentrations that were fungistatic for *C. neoformans* but caused mild arachnoiditis.[86] Data obtained from autopsy have shown the highest concentrations of amphotericin B to be in the liver (as high as 41% of the total dose).[87] No evidence of drug metabolism was found and bioassays of tissue extracts indicated that the drug retained its biological activity.[87]

31.2.1.1 Lipid-Based Formulations of Amphotericin B

Lipid-based forms of amphotericin B (e.g., Abelcet®, AmBisome®), have been better tolerated and therefore given at much higher dose than the conventional antibiotic.[88-94]

Amphotericin B encapsulated in liposomes was used to control dissseminated cryptococcosis in mammals.[95] The liposomes were substantially sterol-free and consisted of dimyristoyl phosphatidylcholine and dimyristoyl phosphatidylglycerol in a 7:3 ratio; the content of amphotericin B was about 640 µg per 25 mg of lipid mixture.[95]

When compared to amphotericin B deoxycholate, liposome-encapsulated amphotericin B was found to be less toxic and more efficacious in BALB/c mice challenged with *C. neoformans*; the mice survived longer and had lower tissue counts of cryptococci.[96] *In vivo* experiments by Dromer et al.[97] have demonstrated that small doses of amphotericin B (0.12 mg/kg) intercalated into E1-bearing immunoliposomes when administered to mice increased the survival rate significantly longer than did mice given the same dose of amphotericin B alone or intercalated into nontargeted liposomes, or control immunoliposomes. It has been known from previous studies, that the immunoglobulin GI (IgGI) anti-*C. neoformans* serotype A monoclonal antibody (E1) was protective against experimental cryptococcosis in mice. The findings of Dromer et al.[97] may allow for a specific targeting of amphotericin B intercalated into immunoliposomes that bear E1, thus leading to improvement in the therapeutic index of the drug.[97] It should be also noted that a successful application of this type of therapy will require a prior knowledge of the antigenic type of the infecting organism.

Amphotericin B with deoxycholate (Fungizone®) and amphotericin B incorporated into mixed micelles (AmB-mixMs) comprised of egg lecithin with glycocholate, deoxycholate, or taurocholate were compared for efficacy in mice infected with *C. neoformans*.[91] When injected intravenously, the maximal tolerated dose of fungizone was 2.5 mg/kg. At doses of 80 and 100 mg/kg, the AmB-mixMs were nontoxic and more potent than the maximal tolerated dose of fungizone. However, when given at equivalent doses, fungizone was more active in treating murine cryptococcosis.[91]

Joly et al.[92] have studied the *in vitro* toxicity against renal tubular cells in primary culture, and *in vivo* therapeutic efficacy in experimental murine cryptococcosis of amphotericin B deoxycholate associated with 20% Intralipid[R] (ILd-AmB). The results have shown that when compared to a glucose solution of amphotericin B dissolved, the ILd-AmB was equally efficient but better tolerated by mice with experimental cryptococcosis. By allowing higher doses of amphotericin B to be infused, Intralipid enhanced the concentration of the antibiotic in the infected sites.

Kohno et al.[98] described a lipid emulsion of amphotericin B which reduced the toxicity of the antibiotic and showed therapeutic efficacy in treatment of murine cryptococcosis; mice treated with amphotericin B (0.8 mg/kg) died within 18 d, while those given an amphotericin B emulsion died within 26 d.

Bates et al.[99] have observed anaphylaxis due to liposomal amphotericin B (AmBisome).

31.2.1.2   Combinations of Amphotericin B With Other Drugs

Polak et al.[100] studied the combination of amphotericin B with ketoconazole in a mouse model of experimental cryptococcosis and found it additive and even slightly synergistic. Graybill et al.[101] also reported a synergistic effect for amphotericin B and ketoconazole in a murine model of disseminated cryptococcosis. In a study conducted by Perfect and Durack,[102] a combined treatment with amphotericin B and ketoconazole in steroid-treated rabbits with cryptococcal meningitis for 2 weeks, was as effective as amphotericin B-flucytosine combination.

At 100 d postinfection, there was an increase in the survival of immunosuppressed mice infected intranasally with *C. neoformans* and a decrease in the incidence of cryptococci in both lungs and brain, following combined treatment for 15 d with amphotericin B and ketoconazole.[103] However, when the therapy was extended to 30 d, there appeared to be antagonism towards the action of amphotericin B.[38]

Growth inhibition studies on encapsulated and nonencapsulated strains of *C. neoformans* at the minimum inhibitory concentration (MIC) values of amphotericin B and ketoconazole (alone, or in combination) showed a significant inhibition of the yeast over a 5-d period.[104]

Amphotericin B and itraconazole were administered to mice with experimental cryptococcosis at different ratios;[105] overall, the combinations were largely indifferent or even weakly antagonistic.

When compared to the effect of either drug administered alone, the combined amphotericin B-miconazole therapy showed neither additive nor antagonistic effect on the survival rate in a murine model of cryptococcosis.[106]

Fujita and Edwards[107] studied *in vitro* the activity of a combination of amphotericin B and rifampin (a semisynthetic tetracycline antibiotic) against seven strains of *C. neoformans* and found the two drugs to act synergistically in inhibiting and eradicating the yeast as measured by the checkboard microfiltration technique.

Lew et al.[108] have investigated *in vitro* the ability of minocycline (a tetracycline antibiotic) to enhance the potency of amphotericin B against *C. neoformans* using the time-killing technique. Synergism was observed at 4 h with eight of eight strains of the yeast; seven strains showed a ≥3-log reduction in colony count in 4 h, and all strains displayed the same reduction in 24 h at concentrations of amphotericin B of ≤0.4 µg/ml in the presence of minocycline.[109]

The activity of recombinant interferon-γ (rIFN-γ) in combination with amphotericin B in the treatment of experimental murine cryptococcosis was studied.[109] rIFN-γ alone at 10 µg injected intraperitoneally 18 h before, at, and 24 h after *C. neoformans* infection, significantly increased the survival and decreased the colony-forming unit (CFU) counts in the lungs compared with untreated mice. rIFN-γ association markedly increased the effect of a single dose of amphotericin B (0.25 mg/kg 24 h after infection) to prolong mouse survival and to reduce the CFU in the brain. This finding suggested that the use of exogenous IFN-γ may improve the effect of antifungal therapy against cryptococcosis.

31.2.1.3   Amphotericin B Esters

The methyl ester of amphotericin B was significantly less effective (lower therapeutic ratio) than the parent compound (given in colloidal dispersion with sodium deoxycholate) in the treatment of cryptococcal infection.[110] The intravenous LD_{50} value of amphotericin B methyl ester was 28.5 mg/kg.[110]

Structurally, compound SCH 28191 represents the methyl ester of D-ornithyl-amphotericin B. The therapeutic efficacy of SCH 28191 against experimental cryptococcal meningitis was compared with that of amphotericin B.[111] While SCH 28191 provided slightly higher concentrations in the serum, both drugs displayed similar elimination curves and equally poor penetration into the CSF. Overall, amphotericin B was much more active than SCH 28191 in treatment of cryptococcal meningitis in rabbits.[111]

31.2.2 5-Fluorocytosine

Shadomy et al.[112] have found *C. neoformans* highly susceptible to 5-fluorocytosine (5-FC, flucytosine) at concentrations far exceeding those of patients receiving daily doses of 100 mg/kg of the drug.

Poon et al.[113] studied the susceptibility *in vitro* of 5-FC against *C. neoformans* isolates from patients with AIDS. Within the achievable serum levels, 90% of the isolates were inhibited at concentrations of 32.0 mg/l; by comparison, the corresponding values for amphotericin B, ketoconazole, and miconazole were 1.0, 0.5, and 0.25 mg/l, respectively. The fungicidal concentrations of 5-FC, amphotericin B, ketoconazole, and miconazole (64.0, 4.0, 4.0, and 2.0 mg/l, respectively) for 90% of the isolates also exceeded their achievable therapeutic levels in CSF.[113]

In vivo experiments by Polak[114] have demonstrated that a triple combination of 5-fluorocytosine–amphotericin B–triazole was beneficial against cryptococcosis (but slightly antagonistic when used against *Aspergillus*).

31.2.3 Azole Derivatives

31.2.3.1 Miconazole

When tested in an experimental model of murine cryptococcosis, miconazole given subcutaneously or intraperitoneally, produced serum levels exceeding MIC for the challenged strain of *Cryptococcus*. However, the maximum tolerable dose of the drug did not increase the survival rate. When applied in combination with amphotericin B, miconazole produced neither additive nor antagonistic effect.[115] *In vivo* studies have also shown a delayed onset of activity for miconazole as compared to amphotericin B, as well as markedly reduced antifungal activity in the serum.[106]

As determined by Uchida and Yamaguchi,[116] the peak serum levels of miconazole when given intravenously at doses of 200 to 600 mg reached 1.0 to 1.6 µg/ml at the end of the infusion, followed by a rapid decrease (as much as 25%) after 7 to 8 h. Serum concentrations measured by high-pressure liquid chromatography (HPLC) tended to be higher, likely because this technique will detect not only free but also protein-bound miconazole.[117] In terms of body distribution, miconazole has been found largely in the adrenals, liver, lungs, and kidneys.[118] It easily enters the joint fluid and the aqueous fluid of the anterior chamber but not the spinal fluid.[117,119-122] Miconazole is usually rapidly metabolized in the liver and only 1% or less of its initial dose is excreted unchanged in the urine;[123] the excretion was not affected even by renal failure.[124]

A submicron emulsion of miconazole was stabilized by using a combination of three emulsifiers comprising phospholipids, poloxamer, and deoxycholic acid.[125] The latter was crucial for maintaining prolonged emulsion stability owing to its contribution to the elevated zeta potential of the emulsion. While the miconazole emulsion had an improved safety ratio and was well tolerated up to a dose of 0.6 ml injected intravenously to BALB/c mice, the drug therapeutic levels in the brain were below those required for complete eradication of *C. neoformans*.

31.2.3.2 Ketoconazole

When compared to other pathogenic fungi (especially dimorphic systemic pathogens), isolates of *C. neoformans* appeared to be less susceptible *in vitro* to ketoconazole, at least to drug concentrations of ≤1.56 μg/ml.[126] In this regard, it should be noted that *C. neoformans* grew best on modified yeast nitrogen base culture medium.[127] The nutritional adequacy of the culture medium is important because the antifungal activity of the drug may be inadvertently exaggerated by testing in a nutritionally suboptimal milieu.

Scanning and transmission electron microscopy performed on *C. neoformans* exposed *in vitro* for 48 h to different concentrations of ketoconazole have revealed surface changes, fatty degeneration of the cytoplasm, and lysis of subcellular organelles.[128]

The potency of ketoconazole was evaluated *in vivo* by Craven et al.[129] in a murine model of cryptococcosis. Although oral ketoconazole prolonged the survival of infected mice, most of them ultimately succumbed to the infection; ketoconazole dramatically reduced the cryptococcal count in the liver, but had minimal effect on the count in brain. Consequently, high levels of the drug were found in the lung, spleen, and heart muscle but not in the brain.[129]

A synergistic activity for a ketoconazole–trifluoperazine combination on the *in vitro* growth of *C. neoformans* was reported.[130] The optimal pH value of the medium was 7.0 to 7.6; at pH 5.0, the combination was antagonistic.[130]

Combination of ketoconazole and flucytosine, when tested in a mouse model of cryptococcal meningitis consistently produced superior results (as measured by the mortality rate and cryptococcal counts in the liver and brain) than either drug given alone.[131] By comparison, in the same model, combination of ketoconazole and amphotericin B did not show any additive effect.[122] However, Graybill et al.[101] presented evidence for synergism between the two drugs in an animal model of disseminated cryptococcosis. Aside for cryptococcosis, combinations of amphotericin B and ketoconazole were reported to be strongly antagonistic.[105,132]

31.2.3.3 Fluconazole

Fluconazole, a triazole-containing antimycotic, is one of the newer azole antimycotics approved in the U.S. for treatment of opportunistic fungal infections. The presence of a second triazole ring in its molecule, along with hydroxyl and difluorophenyl groups, resulted in a decreased lipophilicity (protein binding of only 12%) and increased metabolic stability.[133-135] In the body, fluconazole is cleared mainly by glomerular filtration, with over 80% of an oral dose being excreted unchanged in the urine.[135] Sanati et al.[136] have developed a microdilution method for measuring susceptibility of *C. neoformans* to fluconazole superior to the M27-P reference method currently accepted by the National Committee for Clinical Laboratory Standards; there have been some inherent problems with the M27-P method, including suboptimal growth of the organism in RPMI 1640 medium, a longer incubation, and a narrow range of MICs.

Fluconazole is water-soluble, and therefore, suitable for both oral and intravenous administration. The pharmacokinetic properties of the drug were similar after administration by either route. In the fasting state, the peak plasma levels were reached at 0.5 to 1.5 h postdosing. The bioavailability after oral ingestion was greater than 90%, with a plasma half-life of 25 to 30 h.[135] Oral or intravenous administration of fluconazole resulted in rapid distribution to various body fluids and tissues with high and sustained therapeutic concentrations; for example, in patients with fungal meningitis, the drug levels in the CSF during therapy reached over 80% of the corresponding serum levels.[135] In two patients with cryptococcal meningitis, the CSF levels of fluconazole were between 3.0 and 5.4 μg/ml 2 h after an oral dose of 50 mg daily, and between 7.9 and 9.0 μg/ml after an oral dose of 100 mg daily; both levels were in the same range as the plasma levels.[137] In rabbits, fluconazole was shown to penetrate the CSF, and although its levels were at least 50% of concurrent plasma levels,[138,139] the drug was still effective in eradicating cryptococcal meningitis.[140] Measurement of fluconazole concentrations in human serum and prostate tissue revealed a high correlation ($r = 0.783$) between serum (mean, 6.6 μg/ml) and tissue (mean, 1.9 μg/ml) fluconazole concentrations.[141]

Polak[105] investigated the effects of a combination of fluconazole and 5-fluorocytosine in a mouse model of cryptococcosis. While the combination was indifferent in this particular model, it was found to be synergistic in experimental candidiasis in mice. Bava and Negroni[142] also concluded that the association of flucytosine and fluconazole did not seem to be more effective than either drug administered alone. However, Allendoerfer et al.[143] studied the efficacy of fluconazole–flucytosine combination on cryptococcal meningitis in BALB/c athymic nu/nu mice. The treatment was initiated 24 h after the infection and continued for 10 to 14 d — the combined therapy markedly delayed mortality when compared to controls and single-drug regimens.

Using a murine cryptococcosis model, Correa et al.[144] have compared the efficacies of fluconazole and D0870, a new triazole antimycotic. While fluconazole prolonged the surival rate primarily in mice infected with isolates which were susceptible *in vitro*, D0870 prolonged the survival for all isolates except one, which was also resistant *in vitro* to both fluconazole and D0870.

31.2.3.4 Itraconazole

A lipophilic triazole derivative, itraconazole has a broad antifungal spectrum of activity, with most of the pathogenic fungi responding to concentrations of 100 ng/ml.[145] The lipophilicity of its molecule confers a pronounced tissue affinity, resulting in drug tissue levels that usually are substantially higher than the corresponding plasma levels — an important fact which must be taken into consideration when plasma measurements are being used to determine a therapeutic approach for systemic fungal infection. Reduced absorption of itraconazole may result because of concurrent chemotherapy or dramatic changes in the acid pH — use of antacids and/or H2-antagonists may lower the absorption of itraconazole although not very often in a clinically meaningful way.[145]

Graybill and Ahrens[146] have compared itraconazole with ketoconazole in the treatment of murine cryptococcosis. Whereas serum concentrations of itraconazole were lower than those of keto-conazole, they nevertheless were sustained for longer periods of time. The MIC values of itra-conazole were also lower, while the minimum fungicidal concentrations (MFC) of both drugs were similar. Furthermore, both itraconazole and ketoconazole prolonged equally the survival rate of mice after intraperitoneal or intracerebral challenge with *C. neoformans*. Neither drug sterilized brains of mice challenged intracerebrally, and tissue counts of *C. neoformans* were similar in mice treated with either of the drugs. Even though itraconazole was equipotent to ketoconazole, it did not offer any real therapeutic advantage either.[146] In another experiment,[147] 1 month after inoculation with *C. neoformans*, cats were treated daily with either ketoconazole (10 mg/kg) or itraconazole (10 mg/kg) for 3 months. During the treatment, the serum cryptococcal antigen titer progressively decreased in all cats, and animals treated with ketoconazole became anorectic and lost weight. By comparison, itraconazole-treated cats showed no side effects, although in one animal, cryptococcal organisms were found in the kidneys.[147]

Perfect et al.[140] have compared itraconazole with fluconazole in the treatment of cryptococcal meningitis in rabbits. Fluconazole easily crossed the blood-CSF barrier and active drug was eliminated in high concentrations in the urine; itraconazole, in turn, did not cross the blood-CSF barrier in any measurable amounts and its concentrations in the urine were variable. In spite of such pharmacokinetic differences, at the site of infection both drugs appeared to be equipotent against cryptococcal meningitis.[140] Combinations of itraconazole and fluconazole were also tested in progressive meningeal, generalized, and disseminated cryptococcosis in guinea pigs.[148]

Various combinations of itraconazole and flucytosine were investigated against experimental cryptococcosis in mice.[136] In general, the combinations were indifferent (but definitely synergistic or additive against experimental aspergillosis in mice).[133] Treatment of meningeal and disseminated cryptococcosis in neutropenic guinea pigs with itraconazole (5.0 mg/kg daily, orally for 35 d) and flucytosine (10 or 40 mg/kg daily, intraperitoneally for 35 d), resulted in 100% cure of cryptococcomas.[148]

Combinations of itraconazole and amphotericin B when tested against experimental crypto-coccosis in mice were mostly indifferent or in some cases even weakly antagonistic.[133] Itra-conazole–amphotericin B combinations were also examined for activity against meningeal and disseminated cryptococcosis in neutropenic guinea pigs.[148] The combinations consisting of 5.0 mg/kg itraconazole (given orally on a daily basis for 35 d) and 1.25 or 2.5 mg/kg amphotericin B (intraperitoneally, daily for 35 d) resulted in 100% cure of cryptococcomas.[148]

The efficacies of two different daily dosages of itraconazole (25 and 50 mg/kg) and the combination of flucytosine (75 mg/kg) with itraconazole (50 mg/kg) in the treatment of experimental cryptococcosis in hamsters, have shown that the 50-mg/kg dose of itraconazole was the most effective, with 70% of brain cultures becoming negative and 95% of treated animals surviving to the end of the study period. The itraconazole–flucytosine combination was less effective than monotherapy with each drug.[149]

31.2.3.5   Other Azole Antifungal Agents

When studied in mice with experimental cryptococcosis, clotrimazole displayed good therapeutic activity against both pulmonary and disseminated cryptococcosis, but had only a moderate potency against the hepatic form and no effect on cerebral cryptococcosis.[150] At daily doses of 100 or 150 mg/kg, clotrimazole was less effective against *C. neoformans* in mice than amphotericin B (1.0 mg/kg, twice daily).[150] However, when *C. neoformans* was tested for susceptibility, clotrimazole was more potent than amphotericin B and flucytosine at attainable serum concentrations of the three drugs of 2.0, 100, and 1.5 µg/ml, respectively.[151] Overall, clotrimazole was not very effective in systemic anticryptococcal therapy.[152] Its major toxicity was gastrointestinal intolerance that severely limited its oral use.[151]

Compound BAY n 7133 was evaluated in mice challenged with *C. neoformans*.[153] At high challenge doses, thymus-containing normal mice showed a prolonged survival rate following application of BAY n 7133. The drug did not protect athymic mice with severely deficient cell-mediated immunity; however, when low challenge doses were applied, BAY n 7133 did prolong the survival rate of athymic mice. In general, BAY n 7133 was less effective when compared to either ketoconazole or compound ICI 153,066 (another experimental triazole-containing antimy-cotic). Also, BAY n 7133 was less potent in mice challenged intracerebrally than in mice challenged intravenously.[154]

C. neoformans was found to be extremely sensitive *in vitro* to sulconazole nitrate;[153] the fungistatic activity of the drug was unchanged by the pH of the medium, inoculum size, or by the addition of human blood. When compared to clotrimazole, sulconazole was found to be superior.[155]

Wright et al.[156] have studied the pharmacokinetics and antifungal efficacy of BAY R 3783 in rabbits and compared the results with those obtained for fluconazole and itraconazole under similar conditions. At least two active metabolites, BAY U 3624 and BAY U 3625, were detected. The parent compound and its two metabolites did cross the blood-brain barrier, and the mean CSF level of BAY R 3783 was 30.5% of simultaneous serum levels. When tested *in vivo* against cryptococcal meningitis in immunosuppressed rabbits, BAY R 3783, fluconazole, and itraconazole were equally effective in reducing the yeast counts in the CSF at daily doses of 100 mg administered over a 10-d period.

31.2.4   Antibiotics Other Than Amphotericin B

Subcutaneous administration of cyclosporin A to normal and athymic nude mice prolonged the survival rate against pulmonary cryptococcosis but was ineffective against cryptococcal replication in the central nervous system.[157]

Three water-soluble pneumocandin analogs, L-733560, L-705589, and L-731373 (β-(1,3)-D-glucan inhibitors), when evaluated in a mouse model of disseminated cryptococcosis, were ineffective in reducing the number of CFU of *C. neoformans* in the brain and spleen at 10 mg/kg, while amphotericin B at 0.31 mg/kg sterilized the organs; in contrast, in mouse models of aspergillosis and disseminated candidiasis, all three derivatives showed significant antifungal activity comparable to that of amphotericin B.[158]

31.2.4.1 Hamycin

The antibiotic hamycin was isolated from *Streptomyces pimprina*. It contains a conjugated heptaene chain and is structurally related to amphotericin B. Hamycin was studied in mice with acute experimental infection of *C. neoformans*.[159] The drug was applied by gastric intubation for 28 d with daily dosages ranging from 12.5 to 250 mg/kg; amphotericin B was used as comparison. Although hamycin was 5- to 10-fold more active *in vitro* than amphotericin B, the latter proved to be both more potent and less toxic *in vivo*; at doses of 12.5 to 25.0 mg/kg, hamycin provided only slight protection against *C. neoformans*. It also caused death due to toxicity in over 50% of uninfected mice at daily doses exceeding 25 mg/kg.[159] In another study,[160] at daily doses of 20 mg/kg, hamycin was reported to protect mice with experimental cryptococcal infection.

In one case of cryptococcal meningitis, hamycin was given orally at daily doses of 2 to 50 mg/kg for a period of 11 weeks (a total of 183 g). The observed toxicity was minimal (gastrointestinal irritation), but no visible improvement was recorded either.[161]

31.2.4.2 Pradimicins

Pradimicin A is a novel benzo[*a*]naphthacenequinone antibiotic isolated from *Actinomadura hibisca* sp. nov. No. P157-2, and *A. verrucospora* subsp. *neobisca* sp. nov. No. R103-3.[162-164] The antibiotic elicited broad antifungal activity both *in vitro* and *in vivo*.[162] Two pradimicin derivatives, pradimicin FA-2 (a D-serine congener of pradimicin B)[165] and BMY-28864 (a water-soluble product of the reductive alkylation of pradimicin FA-2),[166] were also reported to elicit antifungal activities. In a comparative study,[164] BMY-28864, pradimicin A, amphotericin B, and ketoconazole showed MIC values against *C. neoformans* of 1.6, 1.6, 0.4, and 0.2 µg/ml, respectively. One derivative of pradimicin A, 17-epipradimicin A, however, did not exert any antifungal activity, strongly suggesting that a change in the stereochemistry of C-17 is critical for antifungal activity.[167]

In vivo experiments in ICR mice infected with a lethal inoculum of *C. neoformans* confirmed the anticryptococcal efficacy of pradimicin antibiotics.[164] Single intravenous administration of BMY-28864, pradimicin A, amphotericin B, and ketoconazole resulted in PD_{50} (protective dose) values of 11.0, 11.0, 0.36, and >100 mg/kg, respectively; when the drugs were applied twice daily for 5 consecutive days, the corresponding PD_{50} values for BMY-28864, pradimicin A, and amphotericin B were 2.8, 0.95, and 0.18 mg/kg, respectively.

The mode of action of the pradimicin antibiotics involved a facile Ca^{2+}-dependent binding to fungal cell surface mannans to form insoluble complexes and leakage of potassium.[164] This action appeared to be selective since human erythrocytes and various mammalian cells did not bind BMY-28864, and no potassium leakage or cell death in the presence of Ca^{2+} was observed.[164] Electron microscopic evidence revealed the presence of invagination and detachment of fungal cell membrane, nuclear membrane damage, delocalization of nuclei, and damaged microtubules indicating perturbation of cell membrane function.[164]

31.2.4.3 Benanomicins and Nikkomycins

Benanomicin A, another benzo[*a*]naphthacene antibiotic isolated from *Actinomadura* sp. MH193-16 F4,[168] was also found active against *C. neoformans*.[169] *In vitro*, benanomicin A showed MIC values of 1.25 to 5.0 µg/ml (geometric mean, 2.1 µg/ml); by comparison, the corresponding values for amphotericin B were 0.63 to 2.5 and 1.44 µg/ml. *In vivo*, mice were given an inoculum of *C. neoformans* (10^6 CFU/mouse) — the ED_{50} values for benanomicin A and amphotericin B were 18.0 and 1.8 to 7.5 mg/kg/d (subcutaneous administration).[169] Similarly to pradimicins, the mode of action of benanomicin A was related to Ca^{2+}-dependent binding to the fungal cell surface mannans with leakage of potassium that led to general perturbation of cell membrane function.[169]

C. neoformans showed poor susceptibility to inhibitors of fungal cell synthesis, such as nikkomycin X and Z (MIC = 125 and 250 µg/ml, respectively)[170] and cilofungin.[171]

31.2.5 MISCELLANEOUS ANTIFUNGAL AGENTS

Fukazawa et al.[172] examined the ability of a synthetic polyprenol derivative, dihydroheptaprenol (DHP), to enhance resistance to experimental cryptococcosis in mice. Animals that received repeatedly 100 mg/kg of DHP, at 4-d intervals for 6 weeks survived longer than controls. When injected daily for 3 d prior to infection, the drug enhanced protection against *C. neoformans* — the increased protection may be attributed to a DHP-induced increase in the number and function of peripheral blood neutrophils and elicitation of the C3 component of the complement and cytokines. The increased neutrophil production was mediated by colony-stimulating factor(s) generated in the serum of DHP-treated mice.

Compound RI-331 [(*S*)-2-amino-4-oxo-5-hydroxypentanoic acid] was found active against several pathogenic fungi including *C. neoformans*.[173] The mechanism of action of RI-331 was likely associated with inhibition of the fungal homoserine dehydrogenase activity during the biosynthesis of homoserine.

Trichothecin is a naturally occurring fused tricyclic lactone having a MIC value against *C. neoformans* of 0.5 µg/ml.[174] Whereas no mean effective dose could be ascertained when trichothecin was tested *in vivo* at doses of 0.1 to 50 µg/kg, its combination with amphotericin B was significantly beneficial to mice challenged intravenously with *C. neoformans*.[174]

The immunotherapeutic efficacy of recombinant granulocyte colony-stimulating factor in neutropenic mice infected with *C. neoformans* was studied.[175] While all controls died within 6 d after infection, mice injected subcutaneously 1 d postinfection with 30 to 240 µg/kg, once daily for 3 d, showed a markedly prolonged survival rate elicited by rG-CSF.

Conard and Lerner[176] and Gross et al.[177] have observed improvement in patients with crypto-coccal meningitis following treatment with transfer factor. Both studies, however, were limited in scope.

Chinese investigators[178] have described the use of garlic in the treatment of cryptococcal meningitis — 70% of the treated patients were claimed to be cured or experienced improvement.

31.2.5.1 Compound SCH 39304

The antifungal efficacy of compound SCH 39304 was studied in a murine model of crypto-coccosis.[179] The drug was given orally to BALB/c mice (nu/nu and nu/t) at daily doses of 1.0 to 60 mg/kg; it prolonged the survival at doses as low as 1.0 mg/kg. By comparison, oral fluconazole was ineffective at that dose regimen. Overall, at equal doses (administered either orally or intra-nasally), SCH 39304 was more potent than fluconazole in increasing the survival time, but less effective than amphotericin B.[179] The therapeutic efficacy of SCH 30304 and fluconazole was also evaluated against disseminated cryptococcosis in Wistar rats.[180] Both drugs were administered by gavage once daily at three doses (8.0, 16, and 32 mg/kg) beginning either 1 week postinfection (and lasting for 3 weeks), or prophylactically 3 d prior to infection and continuing for an additional 3 weeks. Measurement of CFUs was used to ascertain efficacy — overall, SCH 39304 was found to be the more effective drug in both regimens.[180]

Perfect et al.[181] examined the pharmacokinetics and *in vivo* activity of SCH 39304 in rabbits. The drug crossed the blood-brain barrier in the presence or absence of meningeal inflammation, reaching nearly 60% of the simultaneous concentrations in the serum. In the treatment of experimental cryptococcal meningitis, SCH 39304 was equally potent to fluconazole in reducing the yeast counts in the subarachnoid space.[181]

Combinations of amphotericin B (10 mg/kg) and SCH 39304 (given in a fairly narrow dose range) provided optimum protection when administered to BALB/c mice 1 d after cryptococcal meningitis was induced by intracerebral injection of *C. neoformans*. When compared to controls or animals receiving single-drug therapy, the majority of combinations applied showed additive effect and markedly prolonged the survival by reducing the yeast counts in tissues.[182]

31.3 HOST IMMUNE RESPONSE TO CRYPTOCOCCAL INFECTION

Studies on the role of the cytokine network and cellular interactions in the context of T cell-mediated inflammatory response in the lungs following infection by *C. neoformans*, have revealed that in a resistant strain of mice, moderately virulent cryptococci were progressively cleared from the lungs after week 1.[183] Furthermore, during the first 3 weeks of infection the T cells in the lungs resembled Th0 rather than Th1 cells. There have also been changes in the cytokine production, namely, increases in the alveolar levels of TNF-α and IL-6 at weeks 1 to 3 and the chemokines monocyte chemoattractant protein-1 at weeks 1 to 2, followed by macrophage inflammatory protein-1α and ENA-78 at week 3. Overall, the pulmonary inflammatory response to *C. neoformans* evolved over 5 weeks from granulocytic to mononuclear, suggesting a maturation to a Th1-type response by week 5.[183]

Assessment of the direct anticryptococcal activity of murine lymphocytes from both *C. neoformans*-immunized and control mice was the focus of a study conducted by Muth and Murphy.[184] At a 2:1 effector cell-to-cryptococcal target cell ratio, effector cell populations comprised of $\alpha\beta$ T cell receptor-positive T lymphocytes (98 to 99% CD3$^+$) from *C. neoformans*-immunized mice inhibited the growth of cryptococcal cells better than similar populations of lymphocytes from nonimmunized mice — vital staining of cryptococci after incubation with the T cell-enriched populations showed that the T lymphocytes killed the cryptococcal cells.

Macrophage colony-stimulating factor (M-CSF) injected subcutaneously at a dose of 2.5 mg/kg (4.75 $\times$ 10^6 U/kg) to CD-1 male mice was found to enhance significantly the fungistasis of bronchoalveolar macrophages against *C. neoformans*.[185] When M-CSF was given between 1 and 13 d prior to an *ex vivo* challenge with *C. neoformans*, fungistasis was increased compared with that induced by control bronchoalveolar macrophages — the maximum effect was seen by days 1 and 3 after the administration of M-CSF. These results provide a rationale for *in vivo* use of M-CSF to enhance resistance to infection with *C. neoformans*.

Granulocyte-macrophage colony-stimulating factor (GM-CSF) induced in a dose-dependent manner the anticryptococcal activity of alveolar macrophages *in vitro*.[186] In addition, the combination of GM-CSF and IFN-γ showed rapid and sustained anticryptococcal activity, unlike either cytokine alone.

Administration of exogenous recombinant tumor necrosis factor-α (rTNF-α) significantly prolonged the survival rate of mice infected intrathecally with *C. neoformans*.[187] These and other relevant findings, such as the production of TNF-α during the afferent phase of the immune response,[188] have suggested that endogenously released TNF-α may not only contribute to the elimination of the yeast but may also partly mediate the protective effect of IL-12.

Alveolar macrophages stimulated by IFN-α demonstrated reduced fungistasis for *C. neoformans* compared to controls (49% $\pm$ 15% vs. 75% $\pm$ 12%; mean % growth inhibition $\pm$ SD, $p < .001$).[189]

31.3.1 INTERLEUKIN-12

Kawakami et al.[190] have examined the role of interleukin-12 (IL-12) in host resistance to *C. neoformans* using a murine model of pulmonary and disseminated infection. Compared to untreated mice, which all died within 4 to 6 weeks because of uncontrollable multiplication of yeast cells in the lung and a cryptococcal dissemination to the brain and meningitis, IL-12 when administered from the day of tracheal infection for 7 d, induced a marked infiltration of inflammatory cells (mainly mononuclear cells) and significantly reduced the number of viable yeast cells in the lung. Furthermore, IL-12 suppressed brain dissemination, and significantly increased the survival rate of infected mice. In contrast, late administration of IL-12 commencing on day 7 after infection failed to protect the animals. In further experiments, early administration of IL-12 substantially increased the level of interferon-γ mRNA in the lungs of infected mice, while no detectable IFN-γ mRNA has been observed in untreated controls.[190]

In BALB/c mice infected with *C. neoformans*, subcutaneously injected IL-12 at 0.1 or 1.0 μg once daily, reduced the level of brain infection by approximately 10-fold ($p < .05$); at the same doses, IL-12 enhanced the efficacy of fluconazole (5.0 mg/kg daily) ($p < .05$).[191] In liver, both the efficacy of IL-12 alone (0.01 or 0.1 μg daily; $p < .05$) and enhancement of the efficacy of fluconazole ($p < .05$) were also present, whereas no efficacy of IL-12 was seen in spleens or lungs.

31.3.2 THE ROLE OF ANTIBODIES IN PROTECTION AGAINST *C. NEOFORMANS* INFECTION

C. neoformans as an encapsulated organism shares many similarities with other encapsulated bacteria, such as *S. pneumoniae* and *H. influenza*. However, while for the latter two pathogens antibody immunity has played an important protective role, the antibody immunity in protection against *C. neoformans* has been controversial.[192] For example, experiments with polyclonal sera have produced conflicting evidence for and against the importance of antibody immunity in host defense.

Nussbaum et al.[193] have examined whether in a mixture of protective (to *C. neoformans*) and nonprotective antibodies, the latter will block the activity of the protective MAbs since the antibody isotype and epitope specificity are important factors in ascertaining the ability to prolong survival in mice given a lethal *C. neoformans* infection. Three different nonprotective IgG3 MAbs to cryptococcal capsular polysaccharide were used to study the interaction between the IgG3 isotype and protective IgG1 and IgG2a MAbs in murine cryptococcal infection. One IgG3 MAb reduced the protective efficacy of an IgG1 with identical epitope specificity. A second IgG3 MAb with different epitope specificity also reduced the protection provided by the IgG1 MAb. Furthermore, the protective efficacy of an IgG2a MAb was also greatly reduced by still another IgG3 MAb. Overall, the results of these experiments represented the first report of blocking antibodies to a fungal pathogen, that may have implication for the development of vaccines and passive antibody therapy against *C. neoformans*. Taken together these findings revealed the existence of protective, nonprotective, and disease-enhanced MAbs, suggesting that the divergent results obtained with polyclonal preparations may be a result of the relative proportion of protective and nonprotective antibodies in immune sera.[192]

In related studies, experiments to determine the efficacy of the monoclonal antibody 2H1 (MAb 2H1) in combination with either amphotericin B or fluconazole[194] against *C. neoformans* infection have been carried out *in vitro* in the murine macrophage-like cell line J774.16, and *in vivo* in infected mice. MAb 2H1 was a potent opsonin of *C. neoformans*, known to bind to the capsular glucuronoxylomannan of *C. neoformans*, to prolong survival, and to decrease the fungal burden in experimental murine infection. *In vitro*, the combination of MAb 2H1 with either amphotericin B or fluconazole was more efficacious than either of these drugs given alone in reducing the number of CFU of *C. neoformans* cocultured with J774.16 cells. Furthermore, in combinations with fluconazole, glucuronoxylomannan-binding MAbs of the immunoglobulin M (IgM), IgG1, IgG2a, IgG2b, IgG3, and IgA isotypes were also effective in decreasing the numbers of CFU in *C. neoformans*-J774.16 cocultures. In A/JCr mice, the therapeutic effect of MAb 2H1 was primarily the result of a reduction in the number of CFU in the lung and the serum glucuronoxylomannan level, whereas fluconazole was most effective in decreasing the number of

CFU in the brain. Mice receiving combination therapy had lower numbers of CFU in the lung and serum glucuronoxylomannan levels than mice treated with fluconazole alone. Administration of MAb 2H1 with or without fluconazole had little or no effect on the number of CFU in the brain.[194]

31.4 EVOLUTION OF THERAPIES AND TREATMENT OF CRYPTOCOCCOSIS

The optimal therapeutic approaches for management of cryptococcal meningitis, especially in AIDS patients with underlying T cell dysfunction, and those with neoplasia or on corticosteroid therapy, are still not completely clear and need to be resolved in large comparative trials.[195,196] While fluconazole and itraconazole have been associated with response rates of 50% to 60%, amphotericin B is still the drug of choice for inducing a rapid clearance of the fungus, and therefore, a preferable option for initial therapy. Results from a recently completed large clinical trial (MSG 17/ACTG 159)[195] have indicated that initial treatment for 2 weeks with amphotericin B (0.7 mg/kg once daily), followed by triazole (fluconazole at 400 mg daily, or itraconazole at 400 mg daily) therapy for further 8 weeks resulted in a mortality rate of less than 8%, which is substantially lower than that of previous studies.[197]

Based on the results of a retrospective review of 30 consecutive AIDS patients with cryptococcal infection (median CD4+ count of 0.042×10^9 cells/l) given fluconazole at 400 mg daily, Nightingale[198] supported the use of fluconazole as initial therapy for AIDS-associated cryptococcosis in these patients. In fact, in the largest comparative study[199] there was no difference in the response rates associated with amphotericin B and fluconazole.

Studies by Haubrich et al.[200] have also shown that a high dose (800 mg daily) of fluconazole was well tolerated by HIV-infected patients and appeared effective primary therapy for cryptococcal disease in AIDS patients.

First-line fluconazole therapy (200 to 400 mg daily) has also been found effective and well tolerated in patients with AIDS-associated nonmeningeal cryptococcosis.[201]

The standard therapy of disseminated cryptococcosis, particularly of cerebral manifestations, is still amphotericin B–flucytosine combination.[58,196] The use of high-dose oral fluconazole for treatment of disseminated cryptococcosis has also been recommended.[202]

Disease relapses are frequent in AIDS patients (20% to 60%) if a long-term maintenance therapy is not applied promptly. In this regard, fluconazole at 200 mg daily has shown to be superior than itraconazole at the same dosage level.[195]

Fluconazole has also been used prophylactically.[203-205] At 200 to 400 mg daily, it reduced significantly the incidence of cryptococcosis (and mucosal candidiasis), especially in AIDS patients with CD4+ counts of less than 50 cells/mm^3.

31.4.1 AMPHOTERICIN B

Before the introduction of chemotherapy, 86% of all cases of cryptococcal infections associated with neurological involvement were fatal within 1 year of onset,[82] with death usually resulting from raised intracranial pressure producing cerebral compression. Amphotericin B, which has been in use to treat cryptococcosis since the 1950s, is still one of the most often applied therapeutic agents against this infection.[206] Thus, following the introduction of amphotericin B, cure rates as high as 85% have been reported.[207]

When given intravenously at daily doses of up to 1.0–1.5 mg/kg (or every other day), amphotericin B accounted for as high as 64% cure rate of patients with cryptococcal meningitis.[4] In AIDS patients with cryptococcal meningitis, continuing weekly infusions of amphotericin B after the standard course of therapy has been completed, apparently offered some degree of protection against relapse.[208]

A typical primary course of therapy may consist of amphothericin B given daily for at least 4 weeks with a total dose ranging from 1.60 to 2.76 g (mean 2.11 g), while a maintenance therapy would include treatment with 40 to 100 mg/week of amphotericin B ranging from 0.7 to 1.5 mg/kg body weight.[208] It should be emphasized that although a maintenance therapy with this antibiotic will not necessarily provide total protection against relapse of cryptococcosis in patients with AIDS, the weekly maintenance regimen with amphotericin B is still a recommended current practice that may be carried out indefinitely with AIDS patients who have survived their primary course of antifungal therapy.[209,210] However, the continued infusion of amphotericin B is not without a danger and may cause toxicity making it unacceptable to many patients.[208]

The total dose of the antibiotic administered during primary therapy may be highly variable — this, in addition to the requirement for maintenance therapy (which may become a life-long treatment), will make the end point of amphothericin B therapy not well defined. Thus, in one study[210] involving 48 cases of cryptococcosis complicating AIDS, the cumulative amphotericin B dosage administered to the time of clinical response (defervescence and resolution of symptoms in 48% of the patients) varied between 0.1 and 1.76 g; in the majority of patients, the clinical response was noted early in the treatment when the average cumulative dose was 0.4 g.[210]

In a study involving 31 consecutive AIDS patients with cryptococcal disease (28 with meningitis, and 3 with disseminated extrameningeal cryptococcosis), de Lalla et al.[211,213] have examined the efficacy and safety of a short-course primary treatment with a relatively high dose of amphotericin B[212] at 1.0 mg/kg daily for 14 d (26 patients also received flucytosine at 100 to 150 mg/kg daily, given either intravenously or orally), followed by maintenance therapy with fluconazole or itraconazole. Successful therapy was defined as the resolution of symptoms and negative cultures of CSF and/or blood 2 months after the initial diagnosis. The therapeutic regimen was successful in 29 (93.5%) of all 31 cases, and in 26 (92.8%) of the 28 cases of culture-proven or presumed cryptococcal meningitis; treatment failed in 2 patients.

A therapy comprising amphotericin B and flucytosine, if maintained over a period of 6 weeks, while showing a high rate of success, also required permanent relapse prevention.[55] With regard to prevention therapy, oral fluconazole can be very effective and is considered by some investigators to be the drug of choice.[55]

As reported by Zuger et al.[48] and Kovacs et al.,[49] in spite of antifungal medication, the mortality rate resulting from cryptococcal meningitis in AIDS patients has ranged from 17% to 35%, and was 25% in patients having persistently positive cultures.[49] By comparison, the relapse rate in non-AIDS patients was between 0% and 35%.[10,14,214]

Polsky et al.[215] have conducted a retrospective study evaluating the use of intraventricular application of amphotericin B in cases of cryptococcal meningitis in non-AIDS patients. Death during therapy occurred in only one of six patients who received intraventricular and systemic therapy, and in six of seven patients who received systemic therapy alone. No major adverse effects were reported with the intraventricular administration of the drug. However, the preliminary information in AIDS patients did not provide much encouragment since those patients who received intraventricular amphotericin B did not show any therapeutic benefits.[48,49] In addition, the treatment was often complicated by infection of the ventricular shunt and chemical arachnoiditis (consisting of fever, headache, and CSF pleocytosis) forcing the premature discontinuation of the intraventricular therapy.[48,49]

An earlier long-term study involving 31 patients with cryptococcal meningitis receiving intravenous amphotericin B (with half of the patients on intrathecal therapy as well) has shown an overall mortality rate of 45%, of which 39% was due to cryptococcal meningitis.[12] Roberts and Douglas[216] reported a successful amphotericin B therapy (with a total dose of 3.0 g) in one case of cryptococcal meningitis accompanied by cryptococcemia. In another study, Sapico[217] described the disappearance of a focal cryptococcal brain lesion following intravenous infusion of amphotericin B at gradually increasing doses (a total of 3.0 g), whereas Bastin et al.[218] applied the drug to cure a case of cryptococcal meningitis associated with polyradiculitis.

Although amphotericin B therapy greatly improved the prognosis of patients with cryptococcal meningitis, overall, there are still important clinical limitations associated with its use, including modest efficacy, nephrotoxicity, and the inconvenience of intravenous application.[219]

AmBisome®, a unilamellar liposomal formulation of amphotericin B, was used in the treatment of cryptococcal meningitis in three patients; clinical and mycological remission were observed in two of the patients, with the remaining one showing improvement.[220] Coker et al.[221] have described a successful treatment of cryptococcal meningitis with liposomal amphotericin B after failure of treatment with fluconazole and conventional amphotericin B. Schurmann et al.[222] investigated the safety and efficacy of liposomal amphotericin B in treating AIDS-associated disseminated cryptococcosis.

Japanese scientists[223,224] have described an unusual therapy of cryptococcal meningitis consisting of small doses of amphotericin B, a large dose of prednisolone, and a continuous removal of CSF.

An individual case of a patient with a solid intracranial cryptococcal granuloma in the motor cortex area was treated initially with intrathecal and intravenous amphotericin B; since no regression of the granuloma was observed, a subsequent gross total surgical excision was successfully performed.[225] There are several other reports of combined treatment of intracranial cryptococcal infection with surgery and systemic amphotericin B.[226-229]

Intrathecal administration of amphotericin B has been routinely performed by usage of subcutaneous CSF reservoir. The latter comprised a subcutaneous dome of siliconized rubber that can fit into a cranial burr hole with a catheter extending from the dome into a lateral cerebral ventricle.[214,230,231] Schonheyder et al.[232] observed some complications following intrathecal infusion of amphotericin B using the Rickham reservoir — mainly a persistent infection resulting from the presence of the reservoir.

A renal transplant recipient who was on immunosuppressive medication (prednisone, azathioprine) and with developed pulmonary cryptococcosis was successfully treated with intravenous amphotericin B.[233] In this regard, a Japanese study[234] indicated a poor prognosis of antifungal therapies for cryptococcal infections in renal transplant recipients; thus, only one of six patients survived following the graft. While amphotericin B was found most effective, its nephrotoxicity is always of prime concern in graft survival.

Shindo[235] has found amphotericin B superior to fluconazole, itraconazole, miconazole, and flucytosine (given in various combinations) in the treatment of one patient with cryptococcal meningitis and slight azotemia caused by hypertensive nephrosclerosis.

A diabetic patient with isolated adrenal cryptococcosis (characterized with fungal granuloma and poorly encapsulated pathogen) was treated successfully with surgery and medication with amphotericin B; after a 7-month follow-up period, there was no evidence of recurrence or dissemination.[236]

The use of intravenous amphotericin B in nine cases involving pulmonary cryptococcosis was also reported.[237]

Amphotericin B when used at cumulative doses of 189 to 551 mg, effectively decreased the systemic infections in patients with lymphocytic lymphoma and progranulocytic leukemia.[95] Fajardo[238] has reported the failure of topical amphotericin B to cure cutaneous cryptococcosis in a patient who previously had Hodgkin's disease in a cervical lymph node; the topical treatment comprised 3% amphotericin B ointment in a polyethylene and mineral oil gel base applied four times daily. In another case report, Kojima et al.[239] described a successful treatment by amphotericin B of acute lymphocytic leukemia complicated with a generalized cryptococcosis.

Mycotic endocarditis is a rare fungal infection.[240,241] Colmers et al.[2] described a successful therapy of *C. neoformans*-induced endocarditis manifesting fungemia with intravenous amphotericin B (a total dose of 1.58 g).

31.4.1.1 Toxicity of Amphotericin B

Toxicity studies included a follow-up evaluation of 53 patients treated with amphotericin B. The patients showed an increase in the blood urea nitrogen, acute and permanent nephrotoxicity (age- but not dose-dependent), and a transient reduction of the creatinine clearance during therapy.[242] The antibiotic has been also used in cases of pregnancy complicated with cryptococcosis and showing no clinical damage to the fetus.[243,244] Li and Lai[245] observed acute visual loss in a patient with systemic lupus erythematosus and cryptococcal meningitis who was receiving a test dose (1.0 mg) of intravenous amphotericin B; caution was recommended in using the anibiotic in cases of cryptococcal meningitis when a disease of the optic nerve is strongly suspected.

31.4.2 COMBINATIONS OF AMPHOTERICIN B WITH 5-FLUOROCYTOSINE AND OTHER DRUGS

Currently, the combination of amphotericin B and 5-fluorocytosine is one of the most frequently used for the treatment of cryptococcosis.[246] According to Armstrong,[247] therapy of invasive cryptococcosis should include daily doses of amphotericin B (1.0 mg/kg, intravenously) and oral flucytosine (100 mg/kg daily, divided in four doses) for a duration (or total dose) depending on the patient's response; maintenance therapy of fluconazole (200 mg daily) is often required and can be administered indefinitely.

Concerning the mechanism of combined amphotericin B–5-FC treatment, it is thought that amphotericin B at low doses would potentiate[248,249] the uptake of the flucytosine, thus facilitating a synergistic effect.[250]

In 1978, Jimbow et al.[251] reported an evaluation of the therapeutic effectiveness of amphotericin B and flucytosine, alone and in combination, in 28 patients with cryptococcal meningitis. The combined regimen (at 0.35 mg/kg amphotericin B daily, IV, and 150 mg/kg daily of oral flucytosine) was significantly more effective than either drug given alone, both in terms of toxicity and shorter duration of treatment.

Bennett et al.[252] have conducted a prospective, uncontrolled trial of 15 patients with cryptococcal meningitis to compare a combined therapy of intravenous amphotericin B and oral flucytosine (a 6-week trial) with amphotericin B given alone (a 10-week trial). Results showed that as compared to monotherapy with amphotericin B, the combination cured more patients, with fewer failures or relapses, more rapid sterilization of CSF ($p < .001$), and less nephrotoxicity ($p < .05$). The applied regimens were as follows: (1) combination therapy: 0.3 mg/kg of amphotericin B daily, IV, and 150 mg/kg of 5-FC daily, divided in 6-hourly oral doses; and (2) amphotericin B alone: 0.4 mg/kg daily, IV for 42 d, followed by 0.8 mg/kg every other day for 28 d.[252]

In order to reduce potential toxicity without compromising the efficacy, in a subsequent study, Dismukes et al.[50] conducted a multicenter, prospective, randomized clinical trial of 194 patients having cryptococcal meningitis. The trial was designed to compare the efficacy and toxicity of 4- vs. 6-week regimens (identical with those applied by Bennett et al.[252]) of combined amphotericin B–5-fluorocytosine therapy. Cure or improvement was observed in 75% of those patients who were treated for 4 weeks, and in 85% of those treated for 6 weeks, with relapse rates of 27% and 16%, respectively, and a similar incidence of toxicity (44% and 43%, respectively). Based on the results of the trial, the investigators recommended that the 4-week regimen be applied to patients having no neurological complications, underlying disease or immunosuppressive therapy; patients who do not meet these criteria should be receiving for at least 6 weeks the combined amphotericin B–5-fluorocytosine treatment.[50] Alternatively, MacGregor[253] suggested a modified therapy involving a relatively short course of amphotericin B treatment (3 to 4 weeks) combined with a longer course of 5-fluorocytosine medication. It was assumed that the period necessary for the pathogen to develop a resistance towards 5-FC has been early in the treatment when the cryptococcal population is in its peak; therefore, a short initial period of combined therapy (involving the use of amphotericin B) would be sufficient to reduce the cryptococcal population and thereby, the possibility of developing a resistance towards flucytosine. In turn, such a therapeutic regimen will allow for a more extended course of single 5-FC therapy and less of amphotericin B-induced toxicity.[253]

In an earlier study, Utz et al.[14] described the treatment of 15 patients with cryptococcal meningitis with a combination of low-dose intravenous amphotericin B (20 mg daily) and oral flucytosine (150 mg/kg daily) — 53% of the patients were reported cured with no relapse. Other reports have indicated that increasing the doses of the antibiotic to conventional levels (0.6 to 1.0 mg/kg daily) improved the cure rate of patients on a single amphotericin B therapy to 47%–58%; repeated courses of amphotericin B treatment increased the cure rate even further (61%–67%).[10,12,13]

A trial of 24 patients with cryptococcal meningitis using amphotericin B (1.0 mg/kg daily, IV) and oral flucytosine (150 mg/kg daily) was conducted by Schmutzhard and Vejajjiva.[254] None of the patients received corticosteroid therapy. The duration of treatment ranged from 56 to 104 d. Upon completion, none of the patients died. However, four patients had a relapse within 6 months; an overall relapse rate of 17% was observed in spite of the higher total dosage of amphotericin B and 5-FC and longer duration of therapy.

In addition to data already discussed, there have been reports from various groups which indicated that, in general, the difference between amphotericin B administered alone, or as part of combined therapy with flucytosine has not been statistically significant.[48,49,255] Furthermore, 5-fluorocytosine would be difficult to consider for AIDS patients because of its adverse bone marrow-suppressive[255,256] and gastrointestinal[50] effects, which often are superimposed on symptoms caused by the human immunodeficiency virus (HIV).[257,258] After reviewing the records of 106 patients with cryptococcal infections and AIDS (criteria considered included efficacy of treatment with amphotericin B alone or in combination with flucytosine, efficacy of suppressive therapy, prognostic clinical characteristics, and the course of nonmeningeal cryptococcosis), Chuck and Sande[259] have concluded that addition of flucytosine to amphotericin B neither enhanced survival nor prevented relapse, but long-term suppressive therapy appeared to be beneficial. Nevertheless, in a significant number of patients, the flucytosine medication had to be stopped because of cytopenia.[259,260]

Cryptococcal infections associated with the central nervous system can be manifested as focal granulomatous lesions which may contribute to increased mortality (often exceeding 50%). A case report of cerebral cryptococcoma linked to cryptococcal meningitis was treated successfully with a short course of intravenous amphotericin B and oral flucytosine.[261] The combined therapy consisted of 20 mg daily of amphotericin B and 150 mg/kg daily of 5-FC for a period of 6 weeks, after which the antibiotic was administered alone at a dose of 50 mg given every other day until a total dose of 2.16 g of the antibiotic had been dispensed. The observed side effects (parasthesia of the hands, edema of the ankles, increased serum creatinine level [168 mol/l], and a lowered serum potassium level [to 3.0 mmol/l]) were transitory.[261] One case of cryptococcal meningo-encephalitis, which developed after 9 years of corticosteroid therapy, was resolved successfully with amphotericin B and flucytosine (for 6 weeks) and with itraconazole (for another 8 weeks).[262]

Systemic treatment with amphotericin B and flucytosine led to resolution of choroidal infiltrates in two AIDS patients with optic edema and cryptococcal choroiditis.[263] Picon et al.[264] have successfully treated with amphotericin B and flucytosine an AIDS patient with cutaneous crypto-coccosis manifesting as molluscum contagiosum-like skin lesions.

Tobias et al.[265] reported the treatment of two patients with Hodgkin's disease and cryptococcal meningitis with amphotericin B and oral flucytosine; amphotericin B was administered intrathecally as well as by a rapid low-dose intravenous injection.

Watson et al.[266] described a long-term study (spanning over 11 years) that involved treatment of cryptococcal infection in renal transplant recipients on continued immunosuppressive therapy (prednisolone). The treatment of cryptococcosis, which consisted of combination amphotericin B

(0.3 to 0.5 mg/kg daily, IV) and/or oral flucytosine (150 mg/kg daily) led to cure in 10 of 11 patients. In order to preserve graft viability in those patients with stable renal function at the time of diagnosis, maintenance immunosuppressive therapy was continued throughout the antifungal medication.[266] Previous reports[16,267,268] suggested the need to reduce or even to discontinue the immunosuppressive therapy in order to achieve a cure of cryptococcal infection in cases of renal transplantation. Kong et al.[269] have treated cryptococcal meningitis in eight cases of renal transplant recipients with systemic lupus erythematosus. The therapy comprised amphotericin B and flucytosine; at the time of medication all patients were also receiving immunosuppressive therapy (steroids in association with either azathioprine or cyclosporine).[269] Kimura et al.[270] described the successful treatment of a case of systemic lupus erythematosus complicated with cryptococcal meningitis using combination amphotericin B and 5-fluorocytosine.

Pulmonary cryptococcosis with an early systemic spread was managed with combination amphotericin B, and flucytosine; following that, a rapid 1-h intravenous infusion of amphotericin B (30 mg) on alternative days was instituted as an outpatient maintenance therapy for a period of approximately 6 weeks.[271]

Cryptococcal osteomyelitis (manifested either as a single bone lesion or a systemic illness in addition to osteomyelitis), has been described on several occasions.[272-275] Poliner et al.[39] discussed a case of cryptococcal cervical vertebral osteomyelitis that was cured with oral 5-FC (150 mg/kg daily) and amphotericin B (0.3 mg/kg daily, IV) for 6 weeks with no evidence of systemic toxicity or relapse. In another case,[276] a patient who developed osteomyelitis of the skull due to cryptococcosis was successfully treated with amphotericin B and flucytosine.

An AIDS patient who presented with oral lesion of cryptococcosis (gingival ulceration) was successfully cured with amphotericin and flucytosine given over a 4-week period.[277]

Iida et al.[278] have described the successful treatment of a case of cryptococcal meningitis with combined amphotericin B–ketoconazole therapy. Echevarria et al.[279] reported a case of pulmonary cryptococcosis that was treated successfully with combination of amphotericin B and ketoconazole.

A "fungus ball" which developed in an inactive tuberculosis cavity was treated with infusion of amphotericin B (total dose of 2.4 g) and sodium iodide (total of 56 g over a 30-d period) directly into the cavity through an indwelling percutaneously inserted endobronchial catheter for a period of 3 months.[280] A marked improvement was observed without any complications caused by the use of the catheter.[280]

31.4.2.1   Toxicity of Amphotericin B–5-Fluorocytosine Combinations

In view of the existing toxicity of both amphotericin B and flucytosine (especially the negative effect of the latter on the bone marrow), medication of cryptococcal infections with combination of these two drugs should be considered wery carefully when severely immunocompromised patients (advanced state of AIDS) are involved. Thus, in a multicenter, prospective randomized trial[281] that lasted for either 4 or 6 weeks, the treatment with intravenous amphotericin B (0.3 mg/kg daily) and oral 5-fluorocytosine (150 mg/kg daily) of 194 patients with cryptococcal meningitis led to the development of one or more adverse side effects in 103 patients. The toxicity included azotemia (51 patients), renal tubular necrosis (2 patients), leukopenia (30 patients), thrombocytopenia (22 patients), diarrhea (26 patients), nausea/vomiting (10 patients), and hepatitis (13 patients). Overall, both the 4- and 6-week regimens were complicated by toxicity in 44% and 43% of the patients, respectively. In general, the observed side effects appeared during the first 2 weeks of therapy in 56%, and during the first 4 weeks in 87% of the patients.[281]

Shindo et al.[282] have observed, alongside improvement, the presence of granulocytopenia and thrombocytopenia in one patient given concomitantly amphotericin B and low-dose flucytosine (50 mg/kg daily); it was suggested that both side effects might have been the result of toxic reactions by flucytosine in the azotemic state caused by amphotericin B. In another example, Bryan and McFarland[283] have reported a fatal bone marrow aplasia in one patient with multiple myeloma and cryptococcal meningitis, following medication of the infection with combined amphotericin B and flucytosine (a total of 151 mg and 30.5 g, respectively). Although amphotericin B is considered beneficial in reducing the flucytosine toxicity on the bone marrow, again, caution should be in order with patients having hematologic malignancies and where a reduced marrow reserve is suspected.[284]

31.4.3 5-FLUOROCYTOSINE

In 1965, flucytosine was first introduced in the therapy of cryptococcosis.[136,284] The drug is effective orally and also readily absorbed. Over 90% of it is excreted in the urine within the first 48 h; the observed levels in the CSF were half those present in the plasma.[285,286]

Although encouraging, earlier studies on the clinical usefulness of 5-FC against cryptococcal infections were carried out only with a limited number of patients. For example, when 5-FC (100 mg/kg daily, given in four oral doses for 20 weeks) was applied to one patient following excision of multiple intracerebral supperative cryptococcal granulomas, the drug was well tolerated and the patient was apparently free of cryptococcal infection 1 year after the end of medication.[287] In addition, a rapid development of resistance towards 5-FC by *C. neoformans* is commonly observed.[288] This has been especially true for patients receiving less than 150 mg/kg daily of the drug at the onset of the infection when the cryptococcal population is at its peak.[288]

In order to administer flucytosine in cases when clinical and laboratory evidence of raised intracranial pressure were present, Stanton and Sanderson[289] recommended subcutaneous insertion of a ventriculostomy reservoir beneath the scalp. Such treatment is thought to provide a relatively painless route for CSF aspiration and to allow for large volumes of fluid to be removed without the risk of coning.

Lymphonodular cryptococcosis without clinical manifestations of lung and CNS involvement has been rarely observed.[290,291] In one case of developed cryptococcosis involving cervical, supraclavicular, and right tracheobronchial lymph nodes, therapy with oral flucytosine (30 mg/kg daily for 6 d, followed by 60 mg/kg daily for the next 8 d) resulted in a rapid improvement in overall general and local conditions.[291] Another case of disseminated lymphonodular cryptococcosis (supraclavicular, preauricular, posterior, cervical, axillary, and inguinal lymph nodes) was also found to respond well to therapy with oral flucytosine (500 mg given three times daily for 10 weeks).[292]

A diabetic patient with cryptococcal osteomyelitis of the ribs was successfully treated with curatage of the rib and administration of oral flucytosine (total of 284 g) on an outpatient basis.[293]

In the therapy of cryptococcal meningitis, 5-FC alone was found often inadequate for a successful treatment. According to one study,[294] only 30% cure rate was observed while relapses and failures resulting from development of drug resistance were common.[295-297] Currently, the combination of amphotericin B and 5-FC is recommended whenever cryptococcal infection with neurological involvement is diagnosed (see Section 31.4.2).

Utz et al.[298] have treated 15 patients with cryptococcosis with oral flucytosine (1.67 g daily, divided into four equal doses) for a period of 14 to 42 d. Three of the patients with pulmonary cryptococcosis improved upon medication and showed mycologically negative cultures from sputum specimens. In 9 of 11 patients with cryptococcal meningitis, improvement and inability to culture *C. neoformans* were also observed; during the follow-up period (as long as 13 months) relapse occurred in 4 of the 9 patients with cryptococcal meningitis.[298] In another study,[299] 15 cases of cryptococcal infection were treated with oral flucytosine. Failures associated with a drug-resistant *C. neoformans* occurred in 6 of 10 patients receiving 100 mg/kg daily. The mean drug concentrations in the serum and CSF were twofold higher in those patients given higher doses. Steer et al.[300] also reported a clinical trial of 17 patients having cryptococcal infection who responded well to medication with 5-fluorocytosine.

Flucytosine-associated toxicity included liver damage, transient thrombocytopenia, neutropenia, anemia, and eosinophilia.[301] In addition, pancytopenia and severe agranulocytosis were also reported.[302-304] The damage on bone marrow[295,305] (including a fatal marrow aplasia[305,306]) is by far the most severe adverse effect of 5-FC and should be addressed properly.

Philpot and Lo[307] reported the use of flucytosine in the treatment of cryptococcal meningitis in pregnancy without damage to the fetus.

31.4.3.1   Mechanism of Action of 5-Fluorocytosine and Drug Resistance

The combinations of 5-fluorocytosine with amphotericin B have been discussed in Section 31.4.2. The information discussed here is relevant to the mechanism of action of 5-FC in such combinations and the development of drug-resistant fungal strains of *Cryptococcus*.

Cryptococcus organisms were found to be highly sensitive to flucytosine with MICs ranging from 0.1 to 2.0 µg/ml; while *Candida* spp. were equally susceptible (MIC = 0.1 to 2.0 µg/ml), *Aspergillus* spp. were only moderately sensitive (MIC = 1.0 to 25 µg/ml).[308]

In the fungal cell, 5-fluorocytosine is converted to 5-fluorouracil, resulting in disruption of DNA synthesis and subsequent cell death. The mechanism of action of 5-fluorocytosine has been associated with its ability to promote the intracellular formation of 5-FDUMP, a known inhibitor of thymidylate synthetase, and the incorporation of 5-FUTP into RNA. It is important that uracil deaminase (a key enzyme involved in the antifungal mechanism of action of 5-fluorocytosine) is present in the fungal cell. Uracil deaminase is not found in mammalian cells.[309]

A single therapy with 5-FC may often lead to development of drug-resistant strains of *Cryptococcus*. Initially, only 1.8% of the strains tested were found to be naturally resistant. However, after a single therapy with 5-FC, their number had increased noticeably, ultimately compromising the therapeutic value of the drug.[309] Combinations of amphotericin B and 5-FC not only significantly reduced the number of drug-resistant fungi,[310,311] but have also proved synergistic in both *in vitro* and *in vivo* experiments.[312]

In two thoroughly randomized prospective clinical trials, combinations of flucytosine and amphotericin B have shown positive results, and also adverse side effects; azotemia, leukopenia, and thrombocytopenia were seen in as much as 44% of the cases.[308]

Following 5-fluorocytosine–amphotericin B medication, high concentrations of 5-FC (exceeding 100 µg/ml) have remained in patients over long periods of time. One reason for that has been the inherited nephrotoxicity of amphotericin B. Since the latter is excreted through the urine, any impairment of the kidney function caused by amphotericin B will increase the levels of 5-FC. Addition of sodium salts to the regimen is expected to lower the toxicity of amphotericin B.[114,313]

Currently, both mono- and combination therapies of cryptococcosis with 5-fluorocytosine have been recommended for clinical use. For example, in one therapeutic approach (mostly applied in Europe), the preferred treatment has been to use combinations: 5-fluorocytosine–amphotericin B,[314] 5-fluorocytosine–itraconazole,[315] or amphotericin B–fluconazole.[316] In the U.S., Chernoff and Sande[317] have suggested a single therapy with fluconazole to treat cryptococcal infections in patients with AIDS. An initial triple combination comprising flucytosine–fluconazole–amphotericin B (at daily doses of 200, 400, and 0.3 mg, respectively), followed by a maintenance daily therapy with 200 mg fluconazole, was also reported to be highly effective.[318]

31.4.4   Azole Derivatives

31.4.4.1   Miconazole

Graybill and Levine[119] have described an overall improvement in two patients with cryptococcal meningitis following therapy by intraventricularly administered miconazole (6.0 mg daily for 4 months). Both patients, however, benefited from prior treatment with amphotericin B–flucytosine combination and intravenous miconazole. In another study,[319] intraventricular infusion of miconazole to treat cryptococcal meningitis was also well received. Fukui et al.[320] treated successfully cryptococcal meningitis by intravenous (total of 90.6 g) and intrathecal (total of 505 mg) infusion of miconazole and continuous drainage to relieve the increased intracranial pressure.

In a report by Weinstein and Jacoby,[321] a case of cryptococcal meningitis and cerebral cryptococcoma failed to improve after combined medication with amphotericin B and 5-fluorocytosine. However, treatment with miconazole (400 mg, intravenously every 8 h for 8 weeks) was successful and led to disappearance of brain lesions; 5 years after the therapy, there was no evidence of relapse. Similarly, de Witt[322] described three cases of cryptococcal meningitis that showed clinical improvement following medication with miconazole; previous therapy with amphotericin-B-5-fluorocytosine combination, again, had failed. Miconazole was well tolerated when injected intravenously at daily doses between 3.8 and 5.5 g for 4 to 8 weeks; small amounts of the drug (totaling 55 to 505 mg) were also applied intrathecally.[322]

Ito[117] has reported 79% clinical cure for miconazole in the treatment of cryptococcosis, with mycological success rate of 50%; when classified by disease, the effective cure rate was 76% for meningeal cryptococcosis, 83% for pulmonary cryptococcosis, and 100% for cutaneous cryptococcosis.[117]

On a negative note, Sung et al.[323] reported the failure of miconazole (administered both intravenously and intrathecally) to cure one patient with cryptococcal meningitis and suffering from multiple other complications; a previous combined amphotericin B–flucytosine therapy had also been unsuccessful.[323] Deresinski et al.[324] have applied miconazole intravenously to two patients with cryptococcosis with inconclusive results and a clinical response that could not be evaluated.

One general regimen for miconazole therapy of cryptococcal meningitis that has been recommended[324] required an initial intravenous infusion of 30 mg/kg of the drug daily for 3 weeks; following that period, if the patient was still unresponsive, miconazole was applied into the CSF space at a dosage of 20 mg twice daily, then going to 20 mg every other day.

In one Japanese study,[117] deep-seated mycoses were treated with miconazole at an initial dose of 200 mg (dissolved in at least 200 ml of solvent medium) injected intravenously (by drip-infusion) over a 30- to 60-min period. If no side effects were observed, 200 to 400 mg of the drug were administered intravenously over 30 min, one to three times daily.

Because of many contradicting reports, the efficacy of miconazole in the therapy of cryptococcal meningitis is still very much in doubt. Since miconazole penetrates poorly into CSF when given systemically, the therapy of most cryptococcal infections associated with CNS involvement will eventually require intrathecal administration of flucytosine.[321,324-326] Controlled, randomized trials will be necessary to define unambiguously the usefulness of miconazole in the management of cryptococcal meningitis. In the treatment of pulmonary cryptococcosis, the efficacy of miconazole has also been very much in doubt.

A case of primary cutaneous cryptococcosis affecting the left forearm was treated with miconazole by alternating oral (1.0 g, three times daily for 4 d, and 1.0 g, three times daily for 2 weeks) and intravenous (1.0 g daily for 6 d, and 200 mg daily for 6 d) administration.[327] Another case of localized skin cryptococcosis showed improvement after systemic administration of miconazole.[328]

Other applications of miconazole included successful treatment of a patient with dermatomyositis who developed systemic cryptococcosis — the medication with miconazole was initiated (600 mg every 8 h intravenously for 4 weeks, followed by 750 mg orally, three times daily for 13 months).[329] Kaneko et al.[330] treated a case of primary pulmonary cryptococcosis with transbronchial injection of amphotericin B, in addition to intravenous administration of miconazole.

31.4.4.2 Ketoconazole

Granier et al.[331] reported successful therapy of localized cutaneous cryptococcosis in a renal allograft recipient receiving ketoconazole in conjunction with systemic steroids and azathioprine — ketoconazole was given orally at 400 mg daily for 6 months with no relapse or dissemination being observed.

Perfect et al.[332] have found ketoconazole ineffective in the treatment of cryptococcal meningitis following therapy with high doses. In a contradicting report,[333] however, a case of cryptococcal meningitis showed improvement after high doses of the drug were applied.

Karaffa et al.[334] initiated ketoconazole therapy in a patient with AIDS and disseminated cryptococcosis — the drug was applied at 400 mg daily but the patient, who continued to do well 5 months after the diagnosis, still had extremely high serum levels of cryptococcal antigen.

A case of granulomatous prostatitis induced by capsule-deficient cryptococcal infection was treated with combination of transurethral prostatectomy and ketoconazole.[154]

31.4.4.3 Fluconazole

Fluconazole has been extensively studied for its therapeutic efficacy against cryptococcosis,[335-340] especially against cryptococcal meningitis.[341-348]

Jones et al.[349] have conducted a clinical trial using oral fluconazole to treat 32 AIDS patients with cryptococcal meningitis. Of the 11 patients who received a daily primary therapy of 200 to 400 mg/kg of fluconazole, 67% had a favorable clinical response; in 87% of these cases, the CSF cultures were negative. In addition, fluconazole was used as a secondary therapy in 15 patients who were not responsive to amphotericin B (or amphotericin B–fluconazole combination); positive clinical and mycological responses were obtained in over 60% of the patients. As maintenance therapy, 26 patients received 100 to 200 mg/kg fluconazole daily; the relapse rate of cryptococcal meningitis was 3.2 cases per 1000 patient weeks (mean duration of 22 weeks of maintenance therapy).[349]

Dupont[350] has reported a study involving 16 patients with AIDS and cryptococcal meningitis treated with oral fluconazole. The majority of patients received an initial loading dose of 400 mg, followed by 200 mg daily for 2 months, then maintenance therapy of 100 mg daily. Eleven of 16 patients were clinically cured, concurrent with mycological clearance of all infected sites as well; 4 of 16 patients had clinical improvement but still showed positive CSF cultures; and 1 of 16 patients had clinical deterioration and died with positive CSF culture in spite of being switched to standard treatment.[350] This study, however, was not an open one, and the obtained results were not compared to standard therapy with amphotericin B–flucytosine.

Byrne and Wajszczuk[351] also described a successful use of 150 mg daily of fluconazole against cryptococcal meningitis in one patient with AIDS who had not responded well to initial therapy with amphotericin B.

In more extensive clinical trials, the therapeutic efficacy of fluconazole was compared to that of amphotericin B. In a randomized multicenter study[200] lasting for 10 weeks, intravenously injected amphotericin B was compared with oral fluconazole (200 mg daily) as primary therapies in AIDS patients with acute cryptococcal meningitis; amphotericin B was given either at a mean daily dose of 0.4 mg/kg, or at 0.5 mg/kg depending on patients' response ($p = .34$). The treatment was successful in 25 of 63 patients receiving amphotericin B (40%; 95% confidence interval, 26% to 53%) and in 44 of the 131 fluconazole recipients (34%; 95% confidence interval, 25% to 42%) ($p = .40$). There was no significant difference in the overall mortality rate between the two groups (amphotericin B vs. fluconazole, 14% and 18%, respectively; $p = .48$) — however, during the first 2 weeks of treatment, the mortality in the fluconazole group was higher (15% vs. 8%; $p = .25$). Treatment was considered successful when the patients had two consecutive negative CSF cultures by the end of the 10-week trial period. The median length of time to the first negative CSF culture was 42 d (95% confidence interval, 28% to 71%) for the amphotericin B group, and 64 d (95% confidence interval, 53% to 67%) for the fluconazole group ($p = .25$).[200]

In a recently completed retrospective clinical study, the efficacies of amphotericin B and fluconazole were evaluated in HIV-negative patients (organ transplant recipients, patients with neoplastic disease) with meningeal and extrameningeal cryptococcosis.[352] Patients with more severe infections (i.e., meningitis, neurological disorders, or higher level of antigen in CSF) were more frequently treated with amphotericin B. A cure rate of less than 70% was achieved regardless of the initial treatment and severity of infection. In general, a Cox regression analysis has shown that in patients older than 60 years, neoplastic disease, abnormal mental status, disseminated infection at the time of diagnosis, and therapeutic failure were independent predictors of death. Although fluconazole appeared to be equipotent to amphotericin B, only a prospective multicenter study would be sufficient to determine the best treatment regimen for cryptococcal infections in HIV-negative patients.[352]

In another randomized clinical trial of AIDS patients with cryptococcal meningitis, Larsen et al.[353] compared the therapeutic efficacies of fluconazole with a combination of amphotericin B and flucytosine. The all-male group was randomly assigned to either oral fluconazole (400 mg daily) for 10 weeks, or to amphotericin B (0.7 mg/kg daily) for 1 week, then three times weekly for 9 weeks combined with flucytosine (150 mg/kg daily, in four divided doses). Eight of 14 patients (57%) assigned to fluconazole failed to respond, compared to none of 6 patients assigned to amphotericin B plus flucytosine therapy. The mean duration of positive CSF cultures was 40.6 ± 5.4 d in patients receiving fluconazole, and 15.6 ± 6.6 d in those receiving amphotericin B plus flucytosine. Although such results show that combined amphotericin B–flucytosine medication may be superior to fluconazole in the treatment of cryptococcal meningitis in AIDS patients, the intravenous therapy of amphotericin B has been associated with frequent and often severe side effects compared to oral fluconazole given once daily. Further studies should provide the necessary information to determine the feasibility of the amphotericin B–flucytosine combination and the contribution of flucytosine.[354] According to a cost-minimization analysis conducted by Buxton et al.,[355] costs associated with the use of fluconazole as primary therapy will likely be significantly lower than those for amphotericin B, but similar (or slightly less) for a maintenance therapy.

A case of cryptococcal meningoencephalitis in a patient with Hodgkin's disease at third stage B became asymptomatic after 1 week of therapy with intravenous fluconazole (400 mg daily); 2 months later, all laboratory tests of CSF and blood specimens were negative.[356] Combination of amphotericin B (20 mg daily, IV) and flucytosine (2.5 g daily, IV) did not lead to any improvement.[356] Iacopino et al.[357] also used fluconazole to treat disseminated cryptococcosis in a patient with Hodgkin's disease.

Oral fluconazole (once daily at doses of 50 to 200 mg/kg) was applied to 20 AIDS patients having disseminated cryptococcosis.[358] All patients received amphotericin B as primary therapy before entry. Fluconazole medication was successfully maintained in nine patients for a median of 11 months; seven patients died (five of them did not have evidence of active cryptococcosis at the time of death), and two patients experienced a relapse. Fluconazole had to be discontinued in only one patient when thrombocytopenia developed, and then resolved when the drug was stopped.[358]

Bozzette et al.[359] have also evaluated maintenance therapy with fluconazole in a placebo-controlled, double-blind clinical trial of AIDS patients with cryptococcal meningitis. The drug was given at 100 mg daily in the first phase of the study, and 200 mg daily in the second phase. Following a clinically successful therapy with flucytosine, 19% of the enrolled patients presented a silent, persistent cryptococcal infection. However, there was no recurrent meningeal infection observed in those patients taking fluconazole (mean duration of follow-up, 164 d; $p = .03$), suggesting it as an effective alternative for maintenance therapy against cryptococcal infections.[359]

The suppressive efficacy of fluconazole in preventing relapse from cryptococcal meningitis in AIDS patients was corroborated by findings from a larger trial.[360] Two suppressive regimens were compared: fluconazole at daily oral doses of 200 mg (11 patients; 59%) vs. amphotericin B at 1.0 mg/kg per week (78 patients; 41%). The failure rate of the amphotericin B-treated group was markedly higher (33%; 26 of 78 patients) compared to only 8% of the fluconazole-receiving patients (9 of 11 patients).[360] A successful maintenance therapy of cryptococcosis with fluconazole was also described for 80 AIDS patients from Burundi.[361]

In an uncontrolled, open trial with a small number of AIDS patients with cryptococcosis, fluconazole was found to be effective in preventing relapses after the active disease was controlled with amphotericin B;[362] however, the drug was found not very effective at conventional doses (50 to 100 mg daily) usually applied for treatment of active cryptococcosis. Observed side effects of fluconazole included an increase in hepatic function test values in one patient, and seizures in another; in both cases fluconazole had to be discontinued.

C. neoformans-induced pleural empyema secondary to liver cirrhosis due to hepatitis C virus infection responded well to oral fluconazole.[363]

Retinitis resulting from disseminated cryptococcosis in a renal allograft recipient showed remarkable improvement following therapy with oral fluconazole.[364] Cryptococcal endophthalmitis is a rare disorder, nearly always diagnosed after enucleation or at postmortem examination. Custis et al.[365] have described a culture-positive cryptococcal endophthalmitis in a patient with chronic uveitis diagnosed by vitreous biopsy at the time of retinal detachment repair. The fungus, *Cryptococcus laurentii* was a previously unreported non-*neoformans* ocular pathogen. After a 5-month course of oral fluconazole, the patient was culture-negative; however, the visual declined to hand motions because of hyphema and hypotony.

Cases of cutaneous cryptococcosis are frequently diagnosed in AIDS patients, but they have only seldom been observed in other immunocompromised patients.[366-368] Vandersmissen et al.[366] have described the successful use of a 6-week course of oral fluconazole in two corticosteroid-treated HIV-negative patients who developed cutaneous cryptococcosis. In a relevant case,[369] cryptoccocal whitlow in an HIV-positive patient (unusual clinical presentation of cutaneous cryptococcosis never seen before in this population) was cured with fluconazole at 400 mg daily for 2 months, and 200 mg daily thereafter. Contrary to AIDS patients who need life-long antifungal maintenance therapy to prevent relapses, suppressive treatment may not be indicated for immunocompromised non-AIDS patients.[366]

Other reports describing successful use of oral fluconazole against cryptococcal infections, included laryngeal cryptococcosis,[370] neck mass resulting in lytic destruction of a portion of the cervical vertebrae,[371] and pulmonary cryptococcosis in non-AIDS patients (400 mg daily, for 10 to 12 weeks).[372]

After evaluation of 4048 patients who received fluconazole for at least 7 d, some of the undesirable side effects included nausea (3.7%), headache (1.9%), skin rash (1.8%), vomiting (1.7%), abdominal pain (1.7%), and diarrhea (1.5%).[135] Although adverse effects are more likely to occur in HIV-positive patients, their pattern remained essentially the same, with only 1.5% of patients having their medication discontinued because of side effects.[133] Fluconazole may also induce multiple hepatic abnormalities usually characterized by asymptomatic and reversible mild hepatic necrosis. However, Guillaume et al.[373] have described severe subacute liver damage occurring in an AIDS patient that may be related to prolonged fluconazole maintenance therapy for cryptococcosis — electron microscopic studies revealed the presence of unusual giant mitochondria with paracrystalline inclusions and enlarged smooth endoplasmic reticulum. All microscopic abnormalities were reversed after discontinuation of fluconazole. Alopecia appeared to be a common adverse effect associated with higher dose (400 mg daily) of fluconazole given for 2 months or longer; although sometimes severe, the effect is reversed by discontinuing fluconazole therapy or substantially reducing the daily dose.[374,375]

Drug interaction studies demonstrated that when fluconazole was administered in multiple daily doses of up to 400 mg, it did not produce noticeable effects on testosterone, estrogen, or the ACTH-stimulated cortisol concentrations.[135] Furthermore, there has been no drug interaction observed when fluconazole was administered (at daily doses of 100 mg or more) concomitantly with cyclosporin A to bone marrow transplant recipients (but not renal transplant patients).[135]

Failures of fluconazole in treatment of cryptococcal meningitis[376] and prostate cryptococcosis[377] have also been reported. For example, a 10-week regimen of fluconazole, if first given intravenously then orally, resulted in failure in 62% of patients (8 of 13).[378] However, when the drug was administered entirely by oral route, the failure rate was only 10% (5 of 17 patients).[379]

31.4.4.4 Itraconazole

Itraconazole, another recently developed triazole-containing antimycotic,[380] has been used in the treatment of AIDS patients with meningeal and/or additional neurological cryptococcosis at daily oral doses of 200 to 400 mg.[350] There was no report on the success rate of the treatment, but maintenance therapy with the drug (200 to 400 mg daily) was recommended to prevent relapses.

According to Van Cutsem and Cauwenbergh,[148] in patients with meningeal or pulmonary cryptococcosis, daily treatment with 200 mg itraconazole for 88 (median) or 139 (median) d produced global responses of 57% and 83% of patients, respectively, and negative mycological response in 51% and 50%, respectively; a similar study involving daily administration of 400 mg of itraconazole to both groups for 160 to 216 d (median; meningeal) and 160 d (median; pulmonary) resulted in global responses of 86% and 89%, respectively.[148]

Data from itraconazole treatment (200 mg daily) of three AIDS patients with disseminated cryptococcosis were reported by Viviani et al.[381] All patients received conventional therapy with amphotericin B prior to itraconazole. Within 1 month of treatment, suppression of clinical symptoms in two of the patients, and further improvement in the third, were observed. Although cultures became negative, two of the patients still had encapsulated yeast present in the CSF.[381] Long-term maintenance therapy with the drug (3.0 mg/kg) was recommended.[382]

The therapeutic efficacy of itraconazole has been examined in 33 patients with various manifestations of cryptococcosis (meningitis, cryptococcemia, cryptococcuria, osteomyelitis, pulmonary cryptococcosis, and soft-tissue cryptococcosis).[383] Thirty-two of the patients were immunocompromised, including 4 transplant recipients and 26 with AIDS. The treatment consisted of 200 mg oral itraconazole, two times daily. Results showed that cryptococcemia was abolished 100%. Furthermore, 65% of the patients with cryptococcal meningitis showed complete response (as manifested by clinical resolution and negative cultures), while 25% had partial response, and in 10% the treatment failed. In 71% of patients with AIDS who had meningitis and were treated with itraconazole as their sole therapy, the response was complete, whereas 21% responded partially, and the therapy failed in 7%. All patients who had pulmonary cryptococcosis, soft-tissue cryptococcosis, or osteomyelitis responded 100% to itraconazole therapy, compared to only 60% of patients with cryptococcuria. Since itraconazole hardly penetrated the CSF, the results for cryptococcal meningitis suggested that meningeal and parenchymal penetration were important in lowering the therapeutic efficacy.[383]

In another report,[384] oral itraconazole was successful in 28 patients with cryptococcal meningitis — 18 of them achieved complete response, including 16 of 24 patients with AIDS.

A clinical trial of five AIDS patients conducted by de Gans et al.[385] demonstrated a promise for itraconazole as maintenance therapy for cryptococcal meningitis. Each patient received initial treatment with amphotericin B (0.3 mg/kg daily, intravenously) and oral 5-fluorocytosine (150 mg/kg daily, every 6 h) for 6 to 8 weeks. In four of the patients, the titer of cryptococcal antigen in CSF declined. Two of the patients were still alive, respectively, 10 and 12 months after maintenance therapy with itraconazole had begun, with no toxic side effects from the drug.[385]

Batungwanayo et al.[386] have found itraconazole to be highly effective in the prevention of disseminated cryptococcal disease among HIV-positive Rwandan patients with primary pulmonary cryptococcosis.

Oral itraconazole at 100,[387] 200,[388] or 400 mg[389] once daily, was also used successfully in treatment of localized cutaneous cryptococcosis.[387] In another case of cutaneous cryptococcosis in a patient receiving immunosuppressive therapy, treatment with itraconazole resulted in lesion improvement after topical medication proved ineffective.[368]

Among the interactions of itraconazole with other drugs, it should be mentioned that its levels were decreased by rifampicin, phenytoin, and phenobarbital, while itraconazole increased the levels of cyclosporin A. Caution should be applied in patients receiving concomitant anticoagulants.[145]

31.5   *CRYPTOCOCCUS NEOFORMANS* VAR. *GATTII*

Before the rise of the AIDS epidemic, cryptococcal meningitis in the tropical and subtropical regions usually affected apparently immunocompetent persons, in contrast to those presenting in temperate climates, where infection was most often associated with immunosuppression.[390,391] Biotyping of clinical isolates showed that serotypes B and C characteristic for *C. neoformans* var. *gattii* were commonly identified in patients from the tropical and subtropical areas,[392-395] whereas serotypes A, D, and A/D of *C. neoformans* var. *neoformans* were found in predominantly temperate regions.[396] It seemed that the human disease caused by var. *gattii* had predilection for the respiratory and central nervous systems, and has been endemic for Australia,[397] Papua New Guinea,[391-395] Southern California, and parts of Africa, India, Southeast Asia, and Central and South America (Mexico, Brazil, and Paraguay).[396] Based on results of searches conducted in Australia, the eucalypt species *Eucalyptus camaldulensis* and *E. tereticornis* constituted, although circumstantially, are the only known environmental niche of *C. neoformans* var. *gattii*.[393,398-400] Comparison of a single Californian environmental isolate with three environmental isolates from Australia by karyotyping revealed that although genetically different the four isolates were related.[401,402]

The course of meningitis caused by the two different varieties of *C. neoformans* may differ,[403,404] with mortality rate in the tropics remaining particularly high.[391,395,405]

Treatment of *C. neoformans* var. *gattii*-associated meningitis has been most successful with amphotericin B (0.3 to 1.0 mg/kg daily, parenterally) and flucytosine (150 mg/kg daily, orally).[395]

31.6   *CRYPTOCOCCUS ALBIDUS*

Loison et al.[406] have described what appeared to be the first case of septicemia due to *C. albidus* in an HIV-positive patient. The yeast was sensitive *in vitro* to amphotericin B, fluconazole, miconazole, itraconazole, and 5-fluorocytosine. Although the infection was resolved initially with a 2-week treatment with oral fluconazole at 600 mg daily, followed by fluconazole prophylaxis, a relapse did occur, prompting change of the antifungal treatment to oral itraconazole (400 mg daily) — the patient died shortly thereafter from cardiovascular arrest.

C. albidus is a commonly isolated yeast from skin of healthy persons, as well as indoor or outdoor air.[407] The organism has also been isolated from blood specimens.[408,409] Although rarely, it has been the cause of meningitis,[410-412] lung abscess,[408,413] and empyema[414] in immunocompromised, but not HIV-positive patients.

31.7   *CRYPTOCOCCUS LAURENTII*

The natural habitat of *C. laurentii* and its prevalence in the environment have not been yet established. There have been no data about its isolation from normal respiratory flora either, although it would appear to be extraordinarily rare.[415,416] Vadkertiova and Slavikova[417] have isolated *C. laurentii* from water and sediment specimens. Together with another non-*neoformans* yeast (*C. albidus*), *C. laurentii* was shown to produce antibacterial toxins against *Pseudomonas fluorescens* and *Staphylococcus aureus*.[417,418]

In 1977, Damalam et al.[419] isolated *C. laurentii* on cultures and have demonstrated its presence in tissues on two separate biopsies from chronic granulomatous lesions of the leg and foot of a patient.

Lynch et al.[415] have also reported the first case of pulmonary infection caused by *C. laurentii* manifested as a lung abscess in a patient with dermatomyositis receiving corticosteroid therapy. The isolation of the yeast appeared to be consistent with an opportunistic infection (pulmonary infiltration with cavity formation developed in association with corticosteroid therapy), rather than saprophytic colonization. Treatment has been carried out successfully with a 6-week course of amphotericin B (total dose, 2.0 g). *In vitro*, the antibiotic showed a MIC value of 0.1 µg/ml against a clinical isolate. The latter was not susceptible to 5-fluorocytosine (MIC = 500 µg/ml), and there was no synergism between amphotericin B and 5-fluorocytosine.

C. laurentii has been diagnosed as the etiologic pathogen in a rare case of cryptococcal endophthalmitis cured successfully with oral fluconazole.[365]

The alkyl glycerol ether, *rac*-1-*O*-dodecylglycerol was shown to inhibit the growth of a number of *Candida* (*C. albicans*, *C. tropicalis*, and *C. parapsilosis*) and *Cryptococcus* (*C. neoformans*, *C. albidus*, and *C. laurentii*) yeasts, and was also strongly synergistic with amphotericin B.[421] Electron microscopic studies demonstrated that yeasts grown in the presence of dodecylglycerol had abnormal, severely damaged capsules. Although the mechanism of action of dodecylglycerol is presently not known, it did not act simply as a detergent, since sodium deoxycholate, a natural detergent, at comparable and higher concentrations, showed no activity against the yeasts. The lipid-soluble hydrophobic properties of amphotericin B appeared to be important for this synergistic effect, in that alkyl glycerol ethers could promote synergism with amphotericin B by potentially increasing the interaction between membrane-bound ergosterol and amphotericin B.[420]

31.8 REFERENCES

1. Busse, O., Über Parasitare zelleinschlusse und ihre Zuchtung, *Centralbl. Bakteriol.*, 16, 175, 1894.
2. Colmers, R. A., Irniger, W., and Steinberg, D. H., *Cryptococcus neoformans* endocarditis cured by amphotericin, *JAMA*, 199, 762, 1967.
3. Arasteh, K., Staib, F., Grosse, G., Futh, U., and L'Age, M., Cryptococcosis in HIV infection of man: an epidemiological and immunological indicator? *Zentralbl. Bakteriol.*, 284, 153, 1996.
4. Sabetta, J. R. and Andriole, V. T., Cryptococcal infection of the central nervous system, *Med. Clin. North Am.*, 69, 333, 1985.
5. Littman, M. C. and Walter, J. E., Cryptococcosis: current status, *Am. J. Med.*, 45, 922, 1968.
6. Diamond, R. D., Root, R. K., and Bennett, J. E., Factors influencing killing of *Cryptococcus neoformans* by human leukocytes *in vitro*, *J. Infect. Dis.*, 125, 367, 1972.
7. Diamond, R. D. and Bennett, J. E., Prognostic factors in cryptococcal meningitis: a study in 111 cases, *Ann. Intern. Med.*, 80, 176, 1974.
8. Diamond, R. D., May, J. E., Kane, M. A., Frank, M. M., and Bennett, J. E., The role of the classical and alternate complement pathways in host defense against *Cryptococcus neoformans* infection, *J. Immunol.*, 112, 2260, 1974.
9. Macher, A. M., Bennett, J. E., Gadek, J. E., and Frank, M. M., Complement depletion in cryptococcal sepsis, *J. Immunol.*, 120, 1686, 1978.
10. Butler, W. T., Alling, D. W., Spickard, A., and Utz, J. P., Diagnostic and prognostic value of clinical and laboratory findings in cryptococcal meningitis, *N. Engl. J. Med.*, 270, 59, 1964.
11. De Wytt, C. N., Dickson, P. L., and Holt, G. W., Cryptococcal meningitis: a review of 32 years' experience, *J. Neurol. Sci.*, 53, 283, 1982.
12. Sarosi, G. A., Parker, J. D., Doto, I. L., and Tosh, F. E., Amphotericin B in cryptococcal meningitis: long-term results of treatment, *Ann. Intern. Med.*, 71, 1079, 1969.
13. Spickard, A., Butler, W. T., Andriole, V., and Utz, J. P., The improved prognosis of cryptococcal meningitis with amphotericin B therapy, *Ann. Intern. Med.*, 58, 66, 1963.
14. Utz, J. P., Garriques, I. L., Sande, M. A., Warner, J. F., Mandell, G. L., McGehee, R. F., Duma, R. J., and Shadomy, S., Therapy of cryptococcosis with a combination of flucytosine and amphotericin B, *J. Infect. Dis.*, 132, 368, 1975.

15. Zimmerman, L. E. and Rappaport, H., Occurrence of cryptococcosis in patients with malignant disease of the reticuloendothelial system, *Am. J. Clin. Pathol.*, 24, 1050, 1954.
16. Perfect, J. R., Durack, D. T., and Gallis, H. A., Cryptococcemia, *Medicine (Baltimore)*, 62, 98, 1983.
17. Graybill, J. R. and Alford, R. H., Cell-mediated immunity in cryptococcosis, *Cell. Immunol.*, 14, 12, 1974.
18. Schimpff, S. C. and Bennett, J. E., Abnormalities in cell-mediated immunity in patients with *C. neoformans* infections, *J. Allergy Clin. Immunol.*, 55, 430, 1975.
19. Krick, J. A., Familial cryptococcal meningitis, *J. Infect. Dis.*, 143, 133, 1981.
20. Aguirre, K., Havell, E. A., Gibson, G. W., and Johnson, L. L., Role of tumor necrosis factor and gamma interferon in acquired resistance to *Cryptococcus neoformans* in the central nervous system of mice, *Infect. Immun.*, 63, 1725, 1995.
21. Kerkering, T. M., Duma, R. J., and Shadomy, S., The evolution of pulmonary cryptococcosis, *Ann. Intern. Med.*, 94, 611, 1981.
22. Reblin, T., Meyer, A., Albrecht, H., and Greten, H., Disseminated cryptococcosis in a patient with AIDS, *Mycoses*, 37, 275, 1994.
23. Sarosi, G. A., Silberfarb, P. M., and Tosh, F. E., Cutaneous cryptococcosis: a sentinel of disseminated disease, *Arch. Dermatol.*, 104, 1, 1971.
24. Srur, E., Misad, C., and Henriquez, A., Extrameningeal cryptococcosis in a patient with AIDS, *Rev. Med. Chil.*, 123, 1009, 1995.
25. Houston, S., Lipp, K., Cobian, L., and Sinnott, J. T., Skin rash in renal transplant recipients, *Hosp. Pract. (Off. Ed.)*, 30, 89, 1995.
26. Haight, D. O., Esperanza, L. E., Greene, J. N., Sandin, R. L., et al., Case report: cutaneous manifestations of cryptococcosis, *Am. J. Med. Sci.*, 308, 192, 1994.
27. Gosling, H. R. and Gilmer, W. S., Skeletal cryptococcosis: report of a case and review of the literature, *J. Bone Joint Surg.*, 38A, 660, 1956.
28. Hinchey, W. W. and Someren, A., Cryptococcal prostatis, *Am. J. Clin. Pathol.*, 75, 257, 1981.
29. Randal, R. E., Jr., Stacy, W. K., Prout, G. R., Jr., Madge, G. E., Shadomy, H. J., Shadomy, S., and Utz, J. P., Cryptococcal pyelonephritis, *N. Engl. J. Med.*, 279, 60, 1968.
30. Okun, E. and Butler, W. T., Ophthalmologic complications of cryptococcal meningitis, *Arch. Ophthalmol.*, 71, 52, 1964.
31. Weiss, C., Perry, I. H., and Shevky, M. C., Infections of the human eye with *Cryptococcus neoformans (Torula histolytica)*, *Arch. Ophthalmol.*, 39, 739, 1948.
32. Procknow, J. J., Benfield, J. R., Ripon, J. W., Diener, C. F., and Archer, F. L., Cryptococcal hepatitis presenting as a surgical emergency, *JAMA*, 191, 269, 1965.
33. Sabesin, S. M., Fallon, H. J., and Andriole, V. T., Hepatic failure as a manifestation of cryptococcosis, *Arch. Intern. Med.*, 111, 661, 1963.
34. Goenka, M. K., Mehta, S., Yachha, S., Nagi, B., Chakraborty, A., and Malik, A. K., Hepatic involvement culminating in cirrhosis in a child with disseminated cryptococcosis, *J. Clin. Gastroenterol.*, 20, 57, 1995.
35. Baker, R. D. and Haugen, R. K., Tissue damages and tissue diagnosis in cryptococcosis, *Am. J. Clin. Pathol.*, 25, 14, 1955.
36. Bowman, H. E. and Ritchey, J. O., Cryptococcosis (torulosis) involving brain, adrenal, and prostate, *J. Urol.*, 71, 373, 1954.
37. Voyles, G. O. and Beck, E. M., Systemic infection due to *Torula histolytica (C. hominis)*: report of four cases and review of the literature, *Arch. Intern. Med.*, 77, 504, 1946.
38. Zelman, S., O'Neil, H., and Plaut, A., Disseminated visceral torulosis without nervous system involvement, with clinical appearance of granulocytic leukemia, *Am. J. Med.*, 11, 568, 1951.
39. Poliner, J. R., Wilkins, E. B., and Fernald, G. W., Localized osseous cryptococcosis, *J. Pediatr.*, 94, 597, 1979.
40. Goldman, M. and Pottage, J. C., Jr., Cryptococcal infection of the breast, *Clin. Infect. Dis.*, 21, 1166, 1995.
41. Merwaha, R. K., Trehan, A., Jayashree, K., and Vasishta, R. K., Hypereosinophilia in disseminated cryptococcal disease, *Pediatr. Infect. Dis. J.*, 14, 1103, 1995.

42. Larsen, R. A., Bozzette, S., McCutchan, J. A., Chiu, J., Leal, M. A., Richman, D. D., and the California Collaborative Treatment Group, Persistent *Cryptococcus neoformans* infection of the prostate after successful treatment of meningitis, *Ann. Intern. Med.*, 111, 125, 1989.

43. Fuse, H., Ohkawa, M., Yamaguchi, K., Hirata, A., and Matsubara, F., Cryptococcal prostatitis in a patient with Behcet's disease treated with fluconazole, *Mycopathologia*, 130, 147, 1995.

44. Glassman, S. J. and Hale, M. J., Cutaneous cryptococcosis and Kaposi's sarcoma occurring in the same lesions in a patient with the acquired immunodeficiency syndrome, *Clin. Exp. Dermatol.*, 20, 480, 1995.

45. Muccioli, C., Belfort Junior, R., Neves, R., and Rao, N., Limbal and choroidal *Cryptococcus* infection in the acquired immunodeficiency syndrome, *Am. J. Ophthalmol.*, 120, 539, 1995.

46. Munoz-Peréz, M. A., Colmenero, M. A., Rodriguez-Pichardo, A., Rodriguez-Pinero, F. J., Rios, J. J., and Camacho, F., Disseminated cryptococcosis presenting as moluscum-like lesions as the first manifestation of AIDS, *Int. J. Dermatol.*, 35, 646, 1996.

47. Molnar-Nadasdy, G., Haesly, I., Reed, J., and Altshuler, G., Placental cryptococcosis in a mother with systemic lupus erythematosus, *Arch. Pathol. Lab. Med.*, 118, 757, 1994.

48. Zuger, A., Louie, E., Holzman, R. S., Simberkoff, M. S., and Rahal, J. J., Cryptococcal disease in patients with acquired immunodeficiency syndrome: diagnostic features and outcome of treatment, *Ann. Intern. Med.*, 104, 234, 1986.

49. Kovacs, J. A., Kovacs, A. A., Polis, M., Wright, W. C., Gill, V. J., Tuazon, C. U., Gelmann, E. P., Lane, H. C., Longfield, R., Overturf, G., Macher, A. M., Fauci, A. S., Parrills, J. E., Bennett, J. E., and Masur, H., Cryptococcosis in the acquired immunodeficiency syndrome, *Ann. Intern. Med.*, 103, 533, 1985.

50. Dismukes, W. E., Cloud, G., Gallis, H. A., Kerkering, T. M., Fisher, J. F., Gregg, C. R., Bowles, C. A., Shadomy, S., Stamm, A. M., Diasio, R. B., Kaufman, L., Soong, S.-J., Blackwelder, W. C., and the NIAID Mycoses Study Group, Treatment of cryptococcal meningitis with combination amphotericin B and flucytosine for four as compared with six weeks, *N. Engl. J. Med.*, 317, 334, 1987.

51. Eng, R. H. K., Bishburg, E., Smith, S. M., and Kapila, R., Cryptococcal infections in patients with acquired immune deficiency syndrome, *Am. J. Med.*, 81, 19, 1986.

52. Theunissen, A. W. J. and Zanen, H. C., Dertig petienten net een "verborgen" ziekte: cryptococcenmeningitis, *Ned. Tijdschr. Geneeskd.*, 131, 1123, 1987.

53. Castro Guardiola, A., Ocana Rivera, I., Gasser Laguna, I., Ruiz Camps, I., Planes Reig, A. M., Juste Sanchez, C., and Martinez Vazquez, J. M., 16 cases of infections by *Cryptococcus neoformans* in patients with AIDS, *Enferm. Infec. Microbiol. Clin.*, 9, 90, 1991.

54. Sugar, A. M., Overview: Cryptococcosis in the treatment of AIDS, *Mycopathologia*, 114, 153, 1991.

55. Fur, B., Cryptococcosis in AIDS: therapeutic concepts, *Mycoses*, 33(Suppl. 1), 55, 1990.

56. Kirchner, J. T., Opportunistic fungal infections in patients with HIV disease: combating cryptococcosis and histoplasmosis, *Postgrad. Med. J.*, 99, 209, 1996.

57. Mitchell, T. G. and Perfect, J. R., Cryptococcosis in the era of AIDS — 100 years after the discovery of *Cryptococcus neoformans*, *Clin. Microbiol. Rev.*, 8, 515, 1995.

58. Just-Nübling, G., Therapy of candidiasis and cryptococcosis in AIDS, *Mycoses*, 37(Suppl. 2), 56, 1994.

59. Emmons, W. W. III, Luchsinger, S., and Miller, L., Progressive pulmonary cryptococcosis in a patient who is immunocompetent, *South. Med. J.*, 88, 657, 1995.

60. Gonzalez, C. E., Shetty, D., Lewis, L. L., Mueller, B. U., Pizzo, P. A., and Walsh, T. J., Cryptococcosis in human immunodeficiency virus-infected children, *Pediatr. Infect. Dis. J.*, 15, 796, 1996.

61. Littman, M. L. and Zimmerman, L. E., *Cryptococcosis*, Grune and Stratton, New York, 1956.

62. Haugen, R. K. and Baker, R. D., The pulmonary lesions in cryptococcosis with special reference to subpleural nodules, *Am. J. Clin. Pathol.*, 24, 1381, 1954.

63. Talerman, A., Bradley, J. M., and Woodland, B., Cryptococcal lymphadenitis, *J. Med. Microbiol.*, 3, 633, 1970.

64. Salyer, W. R., Salyer, D. C., and Baker, R. D., Primary complex of *Cryptococcus* and pulmonary lymph nodes, *J. Infect. Dis.*, 130, 74, 1974.

65. Houk, V. N. and Moser, K. M., Pulmonary cryptococcosis: must all receive amphotericin B, *Ann. Intern. Med.*, 63, 583, 1965.

66. Campbell, G. D., Primary pulmonary cryptococcosis, *Am. Rev. Respir. Dis.*, 94, 236, 1966.

67. Duperval, R., Hermans, P. E., Brewer, N. S., and Roberts, G. D., Cryptococcosis with emphasis on the significance of isolation of *C. neoformans* from the respiratory tract, *Chest*, 72, 13, 1977.

68. Hammerman, K. J., Powell, K. E., and Christianson, C. S., Pulmonary cryptococcosis: clinical forms and treatment — CDC cooperative mycoses study, *Am. Rev. Respir. Dis.*, 108, 1116, 1973.

69. Gurevitz, O., Goldschmiedt-Reuven, A., Block, C., Kopolovic, J., Farfel, Z., and Hassin, D., *Cryptococcus neoformans* vertebral osteomyelitis, *J. Med. Vet. Mycol.*, 32, 315, 1994.

70. Anthony, S. A. and Anthony, S. J., Primary cutaneous cryptococcosis in nonimmunocompromised patients, *Cutis*, 56, 96, 1995.

71. Gordon, P. M., Ormerod, A. D., Harvey, G., Atkinson, P., and Best, P. V., Cutaneous cryptococcal infection without immunodeficiency, *Clin. Exp. Dermatol.*, 19, 181, 1994.

72. Mahida, P., Morar, R., Goolam Mohamed, A., Song, E., Tissandie, J. P., and Feldman, C., Cryptococcosis: an unusual cause of endobronchial obstruction, *Eur. Respir. J.*, 9, 837, 1996.

73. Schepelmann, K., Muller, F., and Dichgans, J., Cryptococcal meningitis with severe visual and hearing loss and radiculopathy in a patient without immunodeficiency, *Mycoses*, 36, 429, 1993.

74. Vender, J. R., Miller, D. M., Roth, T., Nair, S., and Reboli, A. C., Intraventricular cryptococcal cysts, *Am. J. Neuroradiol.*, 17, 110, 1996.

75. Yu, F. C., Perng, W. C., Wu, C. P., Shen, C. Y., and Lee, H. S., Adult respiratory distress syndrome caused by pulmonary cryptococcosis in an immunocompetent host: a case report, *Chung Hua I Hsueh Tsa Chih (Taipei)*, 52, 120, 1993.

76. Hellman, R. N., Hinrichs, J., Sicard, G., Hoover, R., Golden, P., and Hoffsten, P., Cryptococcal pyelonephritis and disseminated cryptococcosis in a renal transplant recipient, *Arch. Intern. Med.*, 141, 128, 1984.

77. Liss, H. P. and Rimland, D., Asymptomatic cryptococcal meningitis, *Am. Rev. Respir. Dis.*, 124, 88, 1981.

78. Tarala, R. A. and Smith, J. D., Cryptococcosis treated by rapid infusion of amphotericin B, *Br. Med. J.*, 281, 28, 1980.

79. Mosberg, W. H. and Arnold, J. G., Torulosis of the central nervous system: review of the literature and report of five cases, *Ann. Intern. Med.*, 32, 1153, 1950.

80. Beeson, P. B., Cryptococcal meningitis of nearly sixteen years' duration, *Arch. Intern. Med.*, 89, 797, 1952.

81. Campbell, G. D., Carrier, R. D., and Busey, J. F., Survival in untreated cryptococcal meningitis, *Neurology*, 31, 1154, 1981.

82. Carton, C. A. and Mount, L. A., Neurosurgical aspects of cryptococcosis, *J. Neurosurg.*, 8, 143, 1951.

83. Benard, G., Gryschek, R. C., Duarte, A. J., and Shakanai-Yasuda, M. A., Cryptococcosis as an opportunistic infection in immunodeficiency secondary to paracoccidioidomycosis, *Mycopathologia*, 133, 65, 1996.

84. Nelson, M. R., Bower, M., Smith, D., Reed, C., Shanson, D., and Gazzard, B., The value of serum cryptococcal antigen in the diagnosis of cryptococcal infection in patients infected with the human immunodeficiency virus, *J. Infect.*, 21, 175, 1990.

85. Graybill, J. R., Craven, P. C., Mitchell, L. F., and Drutz, D. J., Interaction of chemotherapy and immune defenses in experimental murine cryptococcosis, *Antimicrob. Agents Chemother.*, 14, 659, 1978.

86. Atkinson, A. J., Jr. and Bindschadler, D. D., Pharmacokinetics of intrathecally administered amphotericin B, *Am. Rev. Respir. Dis.*, 99, 917, 1969.

87. Christiansen, K. J., Bernard, E. M., Gold, J. W. M., and Armstrong, D., Distribution and activity of amphotericin B in humans, *J. Infect. Dis.*, 152, 1037, 1985.

88. Herbrecht, R., The changing epidemiology of fungal infections: are the lipid-forms of amphotericin B an advance? *Eur. J. Haematol.*, 57(Suppl.), 12, 1996.

89. Viviani, M. A., Rizzardini, G., Tortorano, A. M., Fasan, M., Capetti, A., Roverselli, A. M., Gringeri, A., and Suter, F., Lipid-based amphotericin B in the treatment of cryptococcosis, *Infection*, 22, 137, 1994.

90. Hay, R. J., Liposomal amphotericin B, AmBisome, *J. Infect.*, 28(Suppl. 1), 35, 1994.

91. Brajtburg, J., Elberg, S., Travis, S. J., and Kobayashi, G. S., Treatment of murine candidiasis and cryptococcosis with amphotericin B incorporated into egg lecithin-bile salt mixed micelles, *Antimicrob. Agents Chemother.*, 38, 294, 1994.

92. Joly, V., Farinotti, R., Saint-Julien, L., Cheron, M., Carbon, C., and Yeni, P., *In vitro* renal toxicity and *in vivo* therapeutic efficacy in experimental murine cryptococcosis of amphotericin B (Fungizone) associated with Intralipid, *Antimicrob. Agents Chemother.*, 38, 177, 1994.

93. Fernandez B. de Quiros, J., Telenti, M., Fernandez Castro, A., Mateos, V., and Arnaez Moral, E., Liposome amphotericin B in the treatment of deep mycoses in patients not severely immunosuppressed: an efficient alternative with low toxicity, *Med. Clin. (Barcelona)*, 101, 421, 1993.

94. Coker, R. J., Viviani, M., Gazzard, B. G., Du Pont, B., Pohle, H. D., Murphy, S. M., Atouguia, J., Champalimand, J. L., and Harris, J. R. W., Treatment of cryptococcosis with liposomal amphotericin B (AmBisome) in 23 patients with AIDS, *AIDS*, 7, 829, 1993.

95. Lopez-Berestein, G., Fainstein, V., Hersh, E. M., Hopfer, R. L., Juliano, R. L., Mehta, K., and Mehta, R., Treatment of disseminated fungal infections in mammals with liposome-encapsulated amphotericin B, U.S. Patent 4,663,167, 1987.

96. Graybill, J. R., Craven, P.C., Taylor, R. C., Williams, D. M., and Magee, W. E., Treatment of murine cryptococcosis with liposome-associated amphotericin B, *J. Infect. Dis.*, 145, 748, 1982.

97. Dromer, F., Barbet, J., Bolard, J., Charreire, J., and Yeni, P., Improvement of amphotericin B activity during experimental cryptococcosis by incorporation into specific immunoliposomes, *Antimicrob. Agents Chemother.*, 34, 2055, 1990.

98. Kohno, S., Hara, K., Murahashi, N., and Watanabe, T., Amphotericin B incorporated in lipid emulsion (lipid microsphere), in *Recent Progress in Antifungal Chemotherapy*, Yamaguchi, H., Kobayashi, G. S., and Takeuchi, H., Eds., Marcel Dekker, New York, 1992, 333.

99. Bates, C. M., Carey, P. B., and Hind, C. R., Anaphylaxis to liposomal amphotericin (AmBisome), *Genitourin. Med.*, 71, 414, 1995.

100. Polak, A., Scholer, H. J., and Wall, M., Combination therapy of experimental candidiasis, cryptococcosis and aspergillosis in mice, *Chemotherapy*, 28, 461, 1982.

101. Graybill, J. R., Williams, D. M., Van Cutsem, E., and Drutz, D. J., Combination therapy of experimental histoplasmosis and cryptococcosis with amphotericin B and ketoconazole, *Rev. Infect. Dis.*, 2, 551, 1980.

102. Perfect, J. R. and Durack, D. T., Treatment of experimental cryptococcal meningitis with amphotericin B, 5-fluorocytosine, and ketoconazole, *J. Infect. Dis.*, 146, 429, 1982.

103. Cohen, I. R., Sciutto, M. S., Brown, G. L., and Polk, H. C., Jr., Treatment of murine pulmonary cryptococcosis with ketoconazole and amphotericin B, *J. Infect. Dis.*, 149, 650, 1984.

104. Smith, D., McFadden, H. W., and Miller, N. G., Effect of ketoconazole and amphotericin B on encapsulated and nonencapsulated strains of *Cryptococcus neoformans*, *Antimicrob. Agents Chemother.*, 24, 851, 1983.

105. Polak, A., Combination therapy of experimental candidiasis, cryptococcosis, aspergillosis and wangiellosis in mice, *Chemotherapy*, 33, 381, 1987.

106. Graybill, J. R., Mitchell, L., and Levine, H. B., Treatment of experimental murine cryptococcosis: a comparison of miconazole and amphotericin B, *Antimicrob. Agents Chemother.*, 13, 277, 1978.

107. Fujita, N. K. and Edwards, J. E., Jr., Combined *in vitro* effect of amphotericin B and rifampin on *Cryptococcus neoformans*, *Antimicrob. Agents Chemother.*, 19, 196, 1981.

108. Lew, M. A., Beckett, K. M., and Levin, M. J., Combined activity of minocycline and amphotericin B *in vitro* against medically important yeast, *Antimicrob. Agents Chemother.*, 14, 465, 1978.

109. Joly, V., Saint-Julien, L., Carbon, C., and Yeni, P., *In vivo* activity of interferon-gamma in combination with amphotericin B in the treatment of experimental cryptococcosis, *J. Infect. Dis.*, 170, 1331, 1994.

110. Gadebush, H. H., Pansy, F., Klepner, C., and Schwind, R., Amphotericin B and amphotericin B methyl ester ascorbate. I. Chemotherapeutic activity against *Candida albicans*, *Cryptococcus neoformans*, and *Blastomyces dermatitidis* in mice, *J. Infect. Dis.*, 134, 423, 1976.

111. Perfect, J. R. and Durack, D. T., Comparison of amphotericin and *N*-D-ornithyl amphotericin B methyl ester in experimental cryptococcal meningitis and *Candida albicans* endocarditis with pyelonephritis, *Antimicrob. Agents Chemother.*, 28, 751, 1985.

112. Shadomy, S., Shadomy, H. J., McCay, J. A., and Utz, J. P., *In vitro* susceptibility of *Cryptococcosus neoformans* to amphotericin B, hamycin and 5-fluorocytosine, *Antimicrob. Agents Chemother.*, 452, 1968.

113. Poon, M., Cronin, D. C. III, Wormser, G. P., and Bottone, E. J., *In vitro* susceptibility of *Cryptococcus neoformans* isolates from patients with acquired immunodeficiency syndrome, *Arch. Pathol. Lab. Med.*, 112, 161, 1988.

114. Polak, A., Combination therapy for systemic mycosis, *Infection*, 17, 203, 1989.

115. Shadomy, S., Paxton, L., Espinel-Ingroff, H., and Shadomy, H. J., *In vitro* studies with miconazole and miconazole nitrate, *J. Antimicrob. Chemother.*, 3, 147, 1977.

116. Uchida, K. and Yamaguchi, H., Bioassay for miconazole and its levels in human body fluids, *Chemotherapy*, 32, 541, 1984.

117. Ito, A., Therapeutic results with miconazole in Japan, in *Recent Progress in Antifungal Chemotherapy*, Yamaguchi, H., Kobayashi, G. S., and Takeuchi, H., Eds., Marcel Dekker, New York, 1991, 183.

118. Kosuzume, H., Ishiguro, J., Tsuchiya, T., Kurita, M., and Ohnishi, H., Metabolic fate of miconazole (1), *Iyakuhin Kenkyu*, 7, 382, 1976.

119. Graybill, J. R. and Levine, H. B., Successful treatment of cryptococcal meningitis with intraventricular miconazole, *Arch. Intern. Med.*, 138, 814, 1978.

120. Stevens, D. A., Levine, H. B., and Deresinski, S. C., Miconazole in coccidioidomycosis. II. Therapeutic and pharmacologic studies in man, *Am. J. Med.*, 60, 191, 1976.

121. Deresinski, S. C., Galgiani, J. N., and Stevens, D. A., Miconazole treatment of human coccidioidomycosis: status report, in *Coccidioidomycosis, Current Clinical and Diagnostic Status*, Ajillo, L., Ed., Symposia Specialists, Miami, 1977, 267.

122. Hoeprich, P. D. and Goldstein, E., Miconazole therapy for coccidioidomycosis, *JAMA*, 230, 1153, 1974.

123. Brugmans, J., Systemic antifungal potential, safety, biotransport and transformation of miconazole nitrate, *Eur. J. Clin. Pharmacol.*, 5, 93, 1972.

124. Boelaert, J., Daneels, R., Landuyt, H. V., and Symoens, J., Miconazole plasma levels in healthy subjects and in patients with impaired renal function, in *Chemotherapy*, Williams, J. D. and Geddes, A. M., Eds., Plenum Press, New York, 1976, 165.

125. Levy, M. Y., Polacheck, I., Barenholz, Y., and Benita, S., Efficacy evaluation of a novel submicron miconazole emulsion in a murine cryptococcus model, *Pharm. Res.*, 12, 223, 1995.

126. Shadomy, S., White, S. C., Yu, H. P., Dismukes, W. E., and the NIAID Mycoses Study Group, Treatment of systemic mycoses with ketoconazole: *in vitro* susceptibilities of clinical isolates of systemic and pathogenic fungi to ketoconazole, *J. Infect. Dis.*, 152, 1249, 1985.

127. Hoeprich, P. D. and Merry, J. M., Influence of culture medium on susceptibility testing with BAY n 7133 and ketoconazole, *J. Clin. Microbiol.*, 24, 269, 1986.

128. Negroni de Bonvehi, M. B., Van de Ven, M., Borgers, M., and Negroni, R., Ultrastructural changes produced by ketoconazole in *Cryptococcus neoformans* and *Sporothrix schenckii*, *Clin. Res. Rev.*, 3, 5, 1983.

129. Craven, P. C., Graybill, J. R., and Jorgensen, J. H., Ketoconazole therapy of murine cryptococcal meningitis, *Am. Rev. Respir. Dis.*, 125, 696, 1982.

130. Ben-Gigi, G., Polacheck, I., and Eilam, Y., *In vitro* synergistic activity of ketoconazole with trifluoroperazine and with chlorpromazine against medically important yeasts, *Chemotherapy*, 34, 96, 1988.

131. Craven, P. C. and Graybill, J. R., Combination of oral flucytosine and ketoconazole as therapy for experimental cryptococcal meningitis, *J. Infect. Dis.*, 149, 584, 1984.

132. Schaffner, A. and Frick, P. G., The effect of ketoconazole on amphotericin B in a model of disseminated aspergillosis, *J. Infect. Dis.*, 151, 902, 1985.

133. Troke, P. F., Marriott, M. S., Richardson, K., and Tarbit, M. H., *In vitro* potency and *in vivo* activity of azoles, *Ann. NY Acad. Sci.*, 544, 284, 1988.

134. Richardson, K., Cooper, K., Marriott, M. S., Tarbit, M. H., Troke, P. F., and Whittle, P. J., Design and evaluation of systemically active agent, fluconazole, *Ann. NY Acad. Sci.*, 544, 4, 1988.

135. Feczko, J. M., Overview of fluconazole in *Recent Progress in Antifungal Chemotherapy*, Yamaguchi, H., Kobayashi, G. S., and Takahashi, H., Eds., Marcel Dekker, New York, 1992, 191.

136. Sanati, H., Messer, S. A., Pfaller, M., Witt, M., Larsen, R., Espinel-Ingroff, A., and Ghannoum, M., Multicenter evaluation of broth microdilution method for susceptibility testing of *Cryptococcus neoformans* against fluconazole, *J. Clin. Microbiol.*, 34, 1280, 1996.

137. van't Wout, J. W., de Graeff-Meeder, E. R., Paul, L. C., Kuis, W., and van Furth, R., Treatment of two cases of cryptococcal meningitis with fluconazole, *Scand. J. Infect. Dis.*, 20, 183, 1988.

138. Perfect, J. R. and Durack, D. T., Penetration of imidazoles and triazoles into cerebrospinal fluid of rabbits, *J. Antimicrob. Chemother.*, 16, 81, 1985.

139. Perfect, J. R., Fluconazole therapy for experimental cryptococcosis and candidiasis in the rabbit, *Rev. Infect. Dis.*, 12(Suppl. 3), S299, 1990.

140. Perfect, J. R., Savani, D. V., and Durack, D. T., Comparison of itraconazole and fluconazole in treatment of cryptoccocal meningitis and *Candida* pyelonephritis in rabbits, *Antimicrob. Agents Chemother.*, 29, 579, 1986.

141. Finley, R. W., Cleary, J. D., Goolsby, J., and Chapman, S. W., Fluconazole penetration into the human prostate, *Antimicrob. Agents Chemother.*, 39, 553, 1995.

142. Bava, A. J. and Negroni, R., Flucytosine plus fluconazole association in the treatment of a murine experimental model of cryptococcosis, *Rev. Inst. Med. Trop. Sao Paolo*, 36, 551, 1994.

143. Allendoerfer, R., Marquis, A. J., Rinaldi, M. G., and Graybill, J. R., Combined therapy with fluconazole and flucytosine in murine cryptococcal meningitis, *Antimicrob. Agents Chemother.*, 35, 726, 1991.

144. Correa, A. L., Velez, G., Albert, M., Luther, M., Rinaldi, M. G., and Graybill, J. R., Comparison of D0870 and fluconazole in the treatment of murine cryptococcal meningitis, *J. Med. Vet. Mycol.*, 33, 367, 1995.

145. Cauwenbergh, G., Pharmacokinetics of itraconazole, *Mycoses*, 37(Suppl. 2), 27, 1994.

146. Graybill, J. R. and Ahrens, J., R 51211 (itraconazole) therapy of murine cryptococcosis, *Sabouraudia*, 22, 445, 1984.

147. Medleau, L., Greene, C. E., and Rakich, P. M., Evaluation of ketoconazole and itraconazole for treatment of disseminated cryptococcosis in cats, *Am. J. Vet. Res.*, 51, 1454, 1990.

148. Van Cutsem, J. and Cauwenbergh, G., Results of itraconazole treatment in systemic mycoses in animals and man, in *Recent Progress in Antifungal Chemotherapy*, Yamaguchi, H., Kobayashi, G. S., and Takahashi, H., Eds., Marcel Dekker, New York, 1992, 203.

149. Iovannitti, C., Negroni, R., Bava, J., Finquelievich, J., and Kral, M., Itraconazole and flucytosine plus itraconazole combination in the treatment of experimental cryptococcosis in hamsters, *Mycoses*, 38, 449, 1995.

150. Plempel, M. and Bartmann, K., Therapeutic activity of clotrimazole (Bay b 5097) in experimental yeast infections, in *Yeast Yeast-Like Microorg. Med Sci.*, (Proceedings of the 2nd Int. Symp. Yeast), Iwata, K., Ed., Tokyo Press, Tokyo, 1976, 305.

151. Hoeprich, P. D. and Huston, A. C., Susceptibility of *Coccidioides immitis*, *Candida albicans* and *Cryptococcus neoformans* to amphotericin B, flucytosine and clotrimazole, *J. Infect. Dis.*, 132, 133, 1975.

152. Meinhof, W. and Gunther, D., Treatment of chronic mucocutaneous candidiasis of children (*Candida* granuloma) with clotrimazole, *Arch. Dermatol. Forsch.*, 242, 293, 1972.

153. Graybill, J. R., Kaster, S. R., and Drutz, D. L., Comparative activities of Bay n 7133, ICI 153,066, and ketoconazole in murine cryptococcosis, *Antimicrob. Agents Chemother.*, 24, 829, 1983.

154. Milchgrub, S., Visconti, E., and Avellini, J., Granulomatous prostatitis induced by capsule-deficient cryptococcal infection, *J. Urol.*, 143, 365, 1990.

155. Iwata, K. and Yamamoto, Y., Studies on antifungal activities of sulconazole nitrate. II. Influences of various factors on the antifungal activity, *Shinkin to Shinkinsho*, 25, 147, 1984.

156. Wright, K. A., Perfect, J. R., and Ritter, W., The pharmacokinetics of BAY R 3783 and its efficacy in the treatment of experimental cryptococcal meningitis, *J. Antimicrob. Chemother.*, 26, 387, 1990.

157. Mody, C. H., Toews, G. B., and Lipscomb, M. F., Treatment of murine cryptococcosis with cyclosporin A in normal and athymic mice, *Am. Rev. Respir. Dis.*, 139, 8, 1989.

158. Abruzzo, G. K., Flattery, A. M., Gill, C. J., Kong, L., Smith, J. G., Krupa, D., Pikounis, V. B., Kropp, H., and Bartizal, K., Evaluation of water-soluble pneumocandin analogs L-733560, L-705589, and L-731373 with mouse models of disseminated aspergillosis, candidiasis, and cryptococcosis, *Antimicrob. Agents Chemother.*, 39, 1077, 1995.

159. Shadomy, S., Shadomy, H. J., and Utz, J. P., *In vivo* susceptibility of *Cryptococcus neoformans* to hamycin, amphotericin B and 5-fluorocytosine, *Infect. Immun.*, 1, 128, 1970.

160. Thirumalachar, M. J., Sethna, S. B., Rahalkar, P. W., Wagle, A. P., and Subramanyan, A., *In vitro* activity of hamycin with reference to its *in vivo* effect in treatment of systemic mycosis, *Hindustan Antibiot. Bull.*, 14, 123, 1972.

161. Utz, J. P., Witorsch, P., Williams, T. W., Jr., Emmons, C. W., Shadomy, H. J., and Piggott, W., Hamycin: chemotherapeutic studies in systemic mycoses in man, *Am. Rev. Respir. Dis.*, 95, 506, 1967.

162. Oki, T., Konishi, M., Tomatsu, K., Tomita, K., Saitoh, K., Tsunikawa, W., Nishio, M., Miyaki, T., and Kawaguchi, H., Pradimicins, a novel class of potent antifungal antibiotics, *J. Antibiot.*, 41, 1701, 1988.

163. Tsunikawa, M., Nishio, M., Ohkuma, H., Tsuno, T., Konishi, M., Naito, T., Oki, T., and Kawaguchi, H., The structures of pradimicins A, B and C: a novel family of antifungal antibiotics, *J. Org. Chem.*, 54, 2532, 1989.

164. Oki, T., A new family of antibiotics: benzo[a]naphthacenequinones: a water-soluble pradimicin derivative, BMY-28864, in *Recent Progress in Antifungal Chemotherapy*, Yamaguchi, H., Kobayashi, G. S., and Takahashi, H., Eds., Marcel Dekker, New York, 1992, 381.

165. Sawada, Y., Hatori, M., Yamamoto, H., Nishio, M., Miyaki, T., and Oki, T., New antifungal antibiotics pradimicins FA-1 and FA-2: D-serine analogs of pradimicins A and C, *J. Antibiot.*, 43, 1223, 1990.

166. Oki, T., Kakushima, M., Nishio, M., Kamei, H., Hirano, M., Sawada, Y., and Konishi, M., Water-soluble pradimicin derivatives, synthesis and antifungal evaluation of *N,N*-dimethyl pradimicins, *J. Antibiot.*, 43, 1230, 1990.

167. Kakushima, M., Nishio, M., Numata, K., Konishi, M., and Oki, T., Effect of stereochemistry at the C-17 position on the antifungal activity of pradimicin A, *J. Antibiot.*, 43, 1028, 1990.

168. Takeuchi, T., Hara, T., Naganawa, H., Okada, M., Hamada, M., Umezawa, H., Gomi, S., Sezaki, M., and Kondo, S., New antifungal antibiotics, benanomicins A and B from an Actinomycete, *J. Antibiot.*, 41, 807, 1988.

169. Yamaguchi, H., Inouye, S., Orikasa, Y., Tohyama, H., Komuro, K., Gomi, S., Ohuchi, S., Matsumoto, T., Yamaguchi, M., Hiratani, T., Uchida, K., Ohsumi, Y., Kondo, S., and Takeuchi, T., A novel antifungal antibiotic, benanomicin A, in *Recent Progress in Antifungal Chemotherapy*, Yamaguchi, H., Kobayashi, G. S., and Takahashi, H., Eds., Marcel Dekker, New York, 1992, 393.

170. Hector, R. F., Zimmer, B. L., and Pappagianis, D., Inhibitors of cell wall synthesis, in *Recent Progress in Antifungal Chemotherapy*, Yamaguchi, H., Kobayashi, G. S., and Takahashi, H., Eds., Marcel Dekker, New York, 1992, 341.

171. Perfect, J. R., Cilofungin, in *Recent Progress in Antifungal Chemotherapy*, Yamaguchi, H., Kobayashi, G. S., and Takahashi, H., Eds., Marcel Dekker, New York, 1992, 355.

172. Fukazawa, Y., Kagaya, K., Yamada, T., Araki, S., Kimura, M., Sugihara, Y., and Kitoh, K., Enhancement of resistance to experimental candidiasis and cryptococcosis in mice by dihydroheptaprenol, a synthetic polyprenol derivative, in *Recent Progress in Antifungal Chemotherapy*, Yamaguchi, H., Kobayashi, G. S., and Takahashi, H., Eds., Marcel Dekker, New York, 1992, 283.

173. Yamaki, H., Yamaguchi, M., and Yamaguchi, H., RI-331 and other amino acid analogs, in *Recent Progress in Antifungal Chemotherapy*, Yamaguchi, H., Kobayashi, G. S., and Takahashi, H., Eds., Marcel Dekker, New York, 1992, 403.

174. Sneller, M. R., Hariri, A., Sorenson, W. G., and Larxh, H. W., Comparative study of trichothecin, amphotericin B, and 5-fluorocytosine against *Cryptococcus neoformans in vitro* and *in vivo*, *Antimicrob. Agents Chemother.*, 12, 390, 1977.

175. Yamamoto, Y., Uchida, K., Hasegawa, T., Friedman, H., Klein, T. W., and Yamaguchi, H., Recombinant G-CSF induces anti-*Candida albicans* activity in neutrophil cultures and protection in fungal infected mice, in *Recent Progress in Antifungal Chemotherapy*, Yamaguchi, H., Kobayashi, G. S., and Takahashi, H., Eds., Marcel Dekker, New York, 1992, 309.

176. Conard, R. and Lerner, W., The use of transfer factor in a patient with chronic cryptococcal meningitis, *Clin. Res.*, 21, 596, 1973.

177. Gross, P. A., Patel, C., and Spitler, L. E., Disseminated cryptococcosis treated with transfer factor, *JAMA*, 240, 2460, 1978.

178. Anonymous, Garlic in cryptococcal meningitis: a preliminary report of 21 cases, *Chin. Med. J.*, 93, 123, 1980.

179. Restrepo, B. I., Ahrens, J., and Graybill, J. R., Efficacy of SCH 39304 in murine cryptococcosis, *Antimicrob. Agents Chemother.*, 33, 1242, 1989.

180. Negroni, R., Costa, M. R., Finquelievich, J. L., Iovannitti, C., Agorio, I., Tiraboschi, I. N., and Loebenberg, D., Treatment of experimental cryptococcosis with SCH 39304 and fluconazole, *Antimicrob. Agents Chemother.*, 35, 1460, 1991.

181. Perfect, J. R., Wright, K. A., Hobbs, M. M., and Durack, D. T., Treatment of experimental cryptococcal meningitis and disseminated candidiasis with SCII 39304, *Antimicrob. Agents Chemother.*, 33, 1735, 1989.

182. Albert, M. M., Graybill, J. R., and Rinaldi, M. G., Treatment of murine cryptococcal meningitis with an SCH 39304-amphotericin B combination, *Antimicrob. Agents Chemother.*, 35, 1721, 1991.

183. Huffnagle, G. B., Role of cytokines in T cell immunity to a pulmonary *Cryptococcus neoformans* infection, *Biol. Signals*, 5, 215, 1996.

184. Muth, S. M. and Murphy, J. W., Direct anticryptococcal activity of lymphocytes from *Cryptococcus neoformans*-immunized mice, *Infect. Immun.*, 63, 1637, 1995.

185. Nassar, F., Brummer, E., and Stevens, D. A., Effect on *in vitro* macrophage colony-stimulating factor on fungistasis of bronchoalveolar and peritoneal macrophages against *Cryptococcus neoformans*, *Antimicrob. Agents Chemother.*, 38, 2162, 1994.

186. Chen, G. H., Curtis, J. L., Mody, C. H., Christensen, P. J., Armstrong, L. R., and Toews, G. B., Effect of granulocyte-macrophage colony-stimulating factor on rat alveolar macrophage anticryptococcal activity *in vitro*, *J. Immunol.*, 152, 724, 1994.

187. Kawakami, K., Qifeng, X., Tohyama, M., Qureshi, M. H., and Saito, A., Contribution of tumour necrosis factor-alpha (TNA-alpha) in host defence mechanism against *Cryptococcus neoformans*, *Clin. Exp. Immunol.*, 106, 468, 1996.

188. Huffnagle, G. B., Toews, G. B., Burdick, M. D., Boyd, M. B., McAllister, K. S., McDonald, R. A., Kunkel, S. L., and Strieter, R. M., Afferent phase production of TNF-alpha is required for the development of protective T cell immunity to *Cryptococcus neoformans*, *J. Immunol.*, 157, 4529, 1996.

189. Reardon, C. C., Kim, S. J., Wagner, R. P., and Kornfeld, H., Interferon-gamma reduces the capacity of human alveolar macrophages to inhibit growth of *Cryptococcus neoformans in vitro*, *Am. J. Respir. Cell. Mol. Biol.*, 15, 711, 1996.

190. Kawakami, K., Tohyama, M., Xie, Q., and Saito, A., IL-12 protects mice against pulmonary and disseminated infection caused by *Cryptococcus neoformans*, *Clin. Exp. Immunol.*, 104, 208, 1996.

191. Clemons, K. V., Brummer, E., and Stevens, D. A., Cytokine treatment of central nervous system infection: efficacy of interleukin-12 alone and synergy with conventional antifungal therapy in experimental cryptococcis, *Antimicrob. Agents Chemother.*, 38, 460, 1994.

192. Pirofski, L. A. and Casadevall, A., *Cryptococcus neoformans*: paradigm for the role of antibody immunity against fungi? *Zentralbl. Bakteriol.*, 284, 475, 1996.

193. Nussbaum, G., Yuan, R., Casadevall, A., and Scharff, M. D., Immunoglobulin G3 blocking antibodies to the fungal pathogen *Cryptococcus neoformans*, *J. Exp. Med.*, 183, 1905, 1996.

194. Mukherjee, J., Feldmesser, M., Scharff, M. D., and Casadevall, A., Monoclonal antibodies to *Cryptococcus neoformans* glucuronoxylomannan enhance fluconazole efficacy, *Antimicrob. Agents Chemother.*, 39, 1398, 1995 (see also *Antimicrobiol. Agents Chemother.*, 38, 580, 1994).

195. Powderly, W. G., Recent advances in the management of cryptococcal meningitis in patients with AIDS, *Clin. Infect. Dis.*, 22(Suppl. 2), S119, 1996.

196. Dismukes, W. E., Management of cryptococcosis, *Clin. Infect. Dis.*, 17(Suppl. 2), S507, 1993; (see also *Clin. Infect. Dis.*, 19, 975, 1994).

197. Van der Horst, C., Saag, M., Cloud, G., Hamill, R., Graybill, J., Sobel, J., Johnson, P., Tuazon, C., Kerkering, T., Fisher, J., Henderson, H., Stansell, J., Mildvan D., Riser, L., Schneider, D., Hafner, R., Thomas, C., Weisinger, B., Moskovitz, B., and the NIAID AIDS Clinical Trials Group and Mycoses Study Group, Randomized double blind comparison of amphotericin B (AMB) plus flucytosine to AMB alone (step 1) followed by a comparison of fluconazole to itraconazole (step 2) in the treatment of acute cryptococcal meningitis in patients with AIDS. I, *Proc. 35th Intersci. Conf. Antimicrob. Agents Chemother.*, American Society for Microbiology, Washington, D.C., Abstr. I216, 1995.

198. Nightingale, S. D., Initial therapy for acquired immunodeficiency syndrome-associated cryptococcosis with fluconazole, *Arch. Intern. Med.*, 13, 538, 1995.

199. Saag, M. S., Powderly, W. G., Cloud, G. A., Robinson, P., Grieco, M. H., Sharkey, P. K., Thompson, S. E., Sugar, A. M., Tuazon, C. U., Fisher, J. F., and the NIAID Mycoses Study Group and AIDS Clinical Trial Group, Comparison of amphotericin B with fluconazole in the treatment of acute AIDS-associated cryptococcal meningitis, *N. Engl. J. Med.*, 326, 83, 1992.

200. Haubrich, R. H., Haghighat, D., Bozzette, S. A., Tilles, J., and McCutchan, J. A., High-dose fluconazole for treatment of cryptococcal disease in patients with human immunodeficiency virus infection, *J. Infect. Dis.*, 170, 238, 1994.

201. Meyohas, M. C., Meynard, J. L., Bollens, D., Roux, P., Deluol, A. M., Poirot, J. L., Rozenbaum, W., Mayaud, C., Frottier, J., and Centre d'Informations et de Soins de l'Immunodeficience Humaine de l'Est Parisien, Treatment of non-meningeal cryptococcosis in patients with AIDS, *J. Infect.*, 33, 7, 1996.

202. Sitbon, O., Fourme, T., Bouree, P., Du Pasquier, L., and Salmeron, S., Successful treatment of disseminated cryptococcusis with high-dose oral fluconazole, *AIDS*, 7, 1685, 1993.

203. Ammassari, A., Linzalone, A., Murri, R., Marasca, G., Morace, G., and Antinori, A., Fluconazole for primary prophylaxis of AIDS-associated cryptococcosis: a case controlled study, *Scand. J. Infect. Dis.*, 27, 235, 1995.

204. Nelson, M. R., Fisher, M., Cartledge, J., Rogers, T., and Gazzard, B. G., The role of azoles in the treatment and prophylaxis of cryptococcal disease in HIV infection, *AIDS*, 8, 651, 1994 (see also *AIDS*, 9, 300, 1995).

205. Manfredi, R., Mastroianni, A., Coronado, O. V., and Chiodo, F., Fluconazole as prophylaxis against fungal infection in patients with advanced HIV infection, *Arch. Intern. Med.*, 157, 64, 1997

206. Georgiev, V. St., Opportunistic/nosocomial infections: treatment and developmental therapeutics. I. Cryptococcus, *Med. Res. Rev.*, 13, 493, 1993.

207. Emmons, C. W., Binford, C. H., and Utz, J. P., *Medical Mycology*, 2nd ed., Lea and Fabiger, Philadelphia, 1970, 190.

208. Zuger, A., Schuster, M., Simberkoff, M. S., Rahal, J. J., and Holzman, R. S., Maintenance amphotericin B for cryptococcal meningitis in the acquired immunodeficiency syndrome (AIDS), *Ann. Intern. Med.*, 109, 592, 1988.

209. Holmberg, K. and Meyer, R. D., Fungal infections in patients with AIDS and AIDS-related complex, *Scand. J. Infect. Dis.*, 18, 179, 1986.

210. Chechani, V. and Kamholz, S. L., Optimal therapy of cryptococcosis in patients with the acquired immunodeficiency syndrome, *NY State J. Med.*, 91, 292, 1991.

211. de Lalla, F., Pellizzer, G., Vaglia, A., Manfrin, V. et al., Amphotericin B as primary therapy for cryptococcosis in patients with AIDS: reliability of relatively high doses administered over a relatively short period, *Clin. Infect. Dis.*, 20, 263, 1995.

212. Churchill, D. and Coker, R., Amphotericin B as primary therapy for cryptococcosis in patients with AIDS: reliability of relatively high doses over a relatively short period, *Clin. Infect. Dis.*, 21, 1352, 1995.

213. de Lalla, F., Pellizzer, G., Vaglia, A., Manfrin, V., Franzetti, M., Fabris, P., and Stecca, C., Amphotericin B as primary therapy for cryptococcosis in patients with AIDS: reliability of relatively high doses over a relatively short period: a reply, *Clin. Infect. Dis.*, 21, 1353, 1995.

214. Diamond, R. D. and Bennett, J.E., A subcutaneous reservoir for intrathecal therapy of fungal meningitis, *N. Engl. J. Med.*, 288, 186, 1973.

215. Polsky, B., Depman, M. R., Gold, J. W. M., Galicich, J. H., and Armstrong, D., Intraventricular therapy of cryptococcal meningitis via a subcutaneous reservoir, *Am. J. Med.*, 81, 24, 1986.

216. Roberts, N. J. and Douglas, R. G., Cryptococcal meningitis: cure despite cryptococcemia, *Arch. Neurol.*, 35, 179, 1978.

217. Sapico, F. L., Disappearance of focal cryptococcal brain lesion on chemotherapy alone, *Lancet*, 1, 560, 1979.

218. Bastin, R., Vildé, J. L., Drouhet, E., and Carbon, C., Primary meningitis due to *Cryptococcus neoformans* associated with polyradiculitis: cure by amphotericin B, *Sem. Hop. Paris.*, 50, 337, 1974.

219. Sugar, A. M., Stern, J. J., and Dupont, B., Overview: treatment of cryptococcal meningitis, *Rev. Infect. Dis.*, 12(Suppl. 3), S338, 1990.

220. Hay, R. J., Use of Ambisome, liposomal amphotericin B, in systemic fungal infections: preliminary findings of a European multicenter study, in *Recent Progress in Antifungal Chemotherapy*, Yamaguchi, H., Kobayashi, G. S., and Takeuchi, H., Eds., Marcel Dekker, New York, 1992, 323.

221. Coker, R., Tomlinson, D., and Harris, J., Successful treatment of cryptococcal meningitis with liposomal amphotericin B after failure of treatment with fluconazole and conventional amphotericin B, *AIDS*, 5, 231, 1991.

222. Schurmann, D., de Matos Marques, B., Grunewald, T., Pohle, H. D., Hahn, H., and Ruf, B., Safety and efficacy of liposomal amphotericin B in treating AIDS-associated disseminated cryptococcosis, *J. Infect. Dis.*, 164, 620, 1991.

223. Ikemoto, H., Yashiro, M., Furugori, T., and Kudo, Y., Unusual treatment of cryptococcal meningitis successfully treated with a small amount of amphotericin B, a large amount of prednisolone, and continued removal of cerebrospinal fluid, *J. Antibiot.*, 20, 374, 1967.

224. Yashiro, M., Furugori, T., Kudo, Y., and Ikemoto, H., Cryptococcal meningitis successfully treated with amphotericin B, adrenal corticosteroid, and continuous removal of the cerebrospinal fluid, *Naika*, 20, 1155, 1967.

225. Brisman, R., Reid, R., and Harrington, G., Intracranial cryptococcal granuloma — amphotericin B and surgical excision, *Surg. Neurol.*, 1, 43, 1973.

226. Dillon, M. C. and Sealy, W. C., Surgical aspects of opportunistic fungus infection, *Lab. Invest.*, 11, 1231, 1962.

227. Reeves, D. C., Cryptococcic (*Torula*) granuloma of the skull, *J. Neurol.*, 27, 70, 1967.

228. Rish, B. L. and Meacham, W. F., Intracerebral cystic toruloma, *J. Neurosurg.*, 28, 603, 1968.

229. Vijayan, N., Bhatt, G. P., and Dreyfus, P. M., Intraventricular cryptococcal granuloma, *Neurology*, 21, 728, 1971.

230. Einstein, H. E., Brown, J. F., and Holmes, C. W., Some treatment aspects of coccidioidal meningitis, in *Progress Report of the VA-Armed Forces Coccidioidomycosis Study Group No. 7*, Salkin, D. and Huppet, M., Eds., California VA Hospital, San Francisco, 1969, 17.

231. Pappagianis, D., Meningitis in children, in *Progress Report of the VA-Armed Forces Coccidioidomycosis Study Group No. 8*, Salkin, D. and Huppet, M., Eds., California VA Hospital, San Francisco, 1969, 16.

232. Schonheyder, H., Thestrup-Pedersen, K., Esmann, V., and Stenderup, A., Cryptococcal meningitis: complications due to intrathecal treatment, *J. Infect. Dis.*, 12, 155, 1980.

233. Swenson, R. S., Kountz, S. L., Blank, N., and Merigan, T. C., Successful renal allograft in a patient with pulmonary cryptococcosis, *Arch. Intern. Med.*, 124, 502, 1969.

234. Oka, S., Sugimoto, H., and Shimada, K., Problems in the treatment of fungal infections after renal transplantation in Japan, in *Recent Progress in Antifungal Chemotherapy*, Yamaguchi, H., Kobayashi, G. S., and Takeuchi, H., Eds., Marcel Dekker, New York, 1992, 239.

235. Shindo, K., Treatment of cryptococcal meningitis with five antifungal drugs: the role of amphotericin B, *Drugs Exp. Clin. Res.*, 16, 327, 1991.

236. Liu, Y. C., Cheng, D. L., Liu, C. Y., Yen, M. Y., and Wang, R. S., Isolated cryptococcosis of the adrenal gland, *J. Intern. Med.*, 230, 285, 1991.

237. Perkins, W., Pulmonary cryptococcosis: report on the treatment of nine cases, *Dis. Chest*, 56, 398, 1969.

238. Fajardo, L. F., Failure of topical amphotericin B in cryptococcosis, *Ann. Intern. Med.*, 78, 777, 1973.

239. Kojima, T., Matsuzaki, M., Sano, M., Suzuki, H., Hino, Y., Nagura, E., and Saito, H., Acute lymphocytic leukemia, complicated with generalized cryptococcosis successfully treated by amphotericin B: a case report, *Rinsho Ketsueki*, 26, 217, 1985.

240. Lerner, P. I. and Weinstein, L., Infective endocarditis in the antibiotic era, *N. Engl. J. Med.*, 274, 388, 1966.

241. Lombardo, T. A., Rabson, A. D., and Dodge, H. T., Mycotic endocarditis: report of a case due to *Cryptococcus neoformans*, *Am. J. Med.*, 22, 664, 1957.

242. Miller, R. P. and Bates, J. H., Amphotericin B toxicity: a follow-up report of 53 patients, *Ann. Intern. Med.*, 71, 1089, 1969.

243. Ellincy, B. R., Amphotericin B usage in pregnancy complicated by cryptococcosis, *Am. J. Obstet. Gynecol.*, 115, 285, 1973.

244. Silberfarb, P. M., Sarosi, G. A., and Tosh, F. E., Cryptococcosis and pregnancy, *Am. J. Obstet. Gynecol.*, 112, 714, 1972.

245. Li, P. K. and Lai, K. N., Amphotericin B induced ocular toxicity in cryptococcal meningitis, *Br. J. Ophthalmol.*, 73, 397, 1989.

246. Kaminaga, Y., Shindo, K., Ito, A., and Iizuma, H., Mycological and clinical study of cryptococcosis in Yokohama City University Hospital during the period from 1965 to 1989, *Kansenshogaku Zasshi*, 65, 374, 1991.

247. Armstrong, D., Treatment of fungal infections in the immunocompromised host, in *Recent Progress in Antifungal Chemotherapy*, Yamaguchi, H., Kobayashi, S. G., and Takeuchi, H., Eds., Marcel Dekker, New York, 1992, 251.

248. Hackett, A. J., Sylvester, S. S., Joss, U. R., and Calvin, M., Synergistic effect of rifamycin derivatives and amphotericin B on viral transformation of a murine cell line, *Proc. Natl. Acad. Sci. U.S.A.*, 69, 3653, 1972.

249. Kuwano, M., Akiyama, S., Endo, H., and Kohga, M., Potentiation of fusidic acid and lentinan effects upon normal and transformed fibroblastic cells by amphotericin B, *Biochem. Biophys. Res. Commun.*, 49, 1241, 1972.

250. Medoff, G. and Kobayashi, G. S., Amphotericin B and 5-fluorocytosine, *J. Infect. Dis.*, 132, 489, 1975.

251. Jimbow, T., Tejima, Y., and Ikemoto, H., Comparison between 5-fluorocytosine, amphotericin B and the combined administration of these agents in the therapeutic effectiveness for cryptococcal meningitis, *Chemotherapy*, 24, 374, 1978.

252. Bennett, J. E., Dismukes, W. E., Duma, R. J., Medoff, G., Sande, M. A., Gallis, H., Leonard, J., Fields, B. T., Bradshaw, M., Haywood, H., McGee, Y. A., Cate, T. R., Cobbs, C. G., Warner, J. F., and Alling, D. W., A comparison of amphotericin B alone and combined with flucytosine in the treatment of cryptococcal meningitis, *N. Engl. J. Med.*, 301, 127, 1979.

253. MacGregor, R. R., Treatment of cryptococcal meningitis, *N. Engl. J. Med.*, 318, 380, 1988.

254. Schmutzhard, E. and Vejajjiva, A., Treatment of cryptococcal meningitis with high-dose, long-term combination amphotericin B and flucytosine, *Am. J. Med.*, 85, 737, 1988.

255. Sahai, J., Management of cryptococcal meningitis in patients with AIDS, *Clin. Pharmacy*, 7, 528, 1988.

256. Kauffman, C. A. and Frame, P. T., Bone marrow toxicity associated with 5-fluorocytosine therapy, *Antimicrob. Agents Chemother.*, 11, 244, 1977.

257. Donahue, R. E., Johnson, M. M., Zon, L. I., Clark, S. C., and Groopman, J. E., Suppression of *in vitro* haematopoiesis following human immunodeficiency virus infection, *Nature*, 326, 200, 1987.

258. Kotler, D. P., Gaetz, H. P., Lange, M., Klein, E. B., and Holt, P. R., Enteropathy associated with acquired immunodeficiency syndrome, *Ann. Intern. Med.*, 101, 421, 1984.

259. Chuck, S. L. and Sande, M. A., Infections with *Cryptococcus neoformans* in the acquired immuno-deficiency syndrome, *N. Engl. J. Med.*, 321, 794, 1989.

260. Dismukes, W. E., Treatment of systemic fungal diseases in patients with AIDS, in *Recent Progress in Antifungal Chemotherapy*, Yamaguchi, H., Kobayashi, G. S., and Takeuchi, H., Eds., Marcel Dekker, New York, 1992, 227.

261. Bayardelle, P., Giard, N., Maltais, R., Delorme, J., and Brazean, M., Success with amphotericin B and 5-fluorocytosine in treating cerebral cryptococcoma accompanying cryptococcal meningitis, *Can. Med. Assoc. J.*, 127, 732, 1982.

262. Koeleman, J. G., Rustemejer, C., Wijermans, P. W., and MacLaren, D. M., Cryptococcal meningo-encephalitis after prolonged corticosteroid therapy, *Neth. J. Med.*, 36, 242, 1990.

263. Carney, M. D., Combs, J. L., and Waschler, W., Cryptococcal choroiditis, *Retina*, 10, 27, 1990.

264. Picon, L., Vaillant, L., Duong, T., Lorette, G., Bacq, Y., Besnier, J.M., and Choutet, P., Cutaneous cryptococcosis resembling molluscum contagiosum: a first manifestation of AIDS, *Acta Derm. Venereol. (Stockholm)*, 69, 365, 1989.

265. Tobias, J. S., Wrigley, P. F. M., and Shaw, E., Combination antifungal therapy for cryptococcal meningitis, *Postgrad. Med. J.*, 52, 305, 1976.

266. Watson, A. J., Russell, R. P., Cabreja, R. F., Braverman, R., and Whelton, A., Cure of cryptococcal infection during continued immunosuppressive therapy, *Q. J. Med.*, 55, 169, 1985.

267. Gallis, H. A., Berman, R. A., Cate, T. R., Hamilton, J. D., Gunnels, J.C., and Stickel, D. L., Fungal infection following renal transplantation, *Arch. Intern. Med.*, 135, 1163, 1975.

268. Mills, S. A., Seigler, H. F., and Wolfe, W. G., The incidence and management of pulmonary mycosis in renal allograft patients, *Ann. Surg.*, 182, 617, 1975.

269. Kong, N. C., Sharriah, W., Morad, Z., Suleiman, A. B., and Wong, Y. H., Cryptococcosis in a renal unit, *Aust. NZ J. Med.*, 20, 645, 1990.

270. Kimura, K., Hatekayama, M., Miyagi, J., Takeda, A., Sumiya, M., Kano, S., Takaku, F., and Yamamoto, K., A case of systemic lupus erythematosus with cryptococcal meningitis successfully treated with amphotericin B and 5-FC, *Nipon Naika Gakkai Zasshi*, 75, 406, 1986.

271. Butler, W. P. and Kaufer, G. I., Primary cutaneous cryptococcosis successfully treated with outpatient amphotericin B and 5-fluorocytosine, *Nita*, 8, 295, 1985.

272. Woolfitt, R., Park, H. M., and Greene, M., Localized cryptococcal osteomyelitis, *Radiology*, 120, 290, 1976.

273. Nottebart, H. C., McGehee, R. F., and Utz, J. P., *Cryptococcus neoformans* osteomyelitis: case report of two patients, *Sabouraudia*, 12, 127, 1974.

274. Chand, K. and Lall, K. S., Cryptococcosis of the knee joint, *Acta Orthop. Scand.*, 47, 432, 1976.

275. Nathan, C. F., Cryptococcal osteomyelitis treated with 5-fluorocytosine, *Am. Rev. Respir. Dis.*, 110, 78, 1974.

276. Luhr, H. and Svane, S., Pulmonary pseudomotor caused by *Cryptococcus neoformans*, *Tidsskr. Nor. Laegeforen.*, 111, 3288, 1991.

277. Schmidt-Westhausen, A., Grunewald, T., Reihart, P. A., and Pohle, H. D., Oral cryptococcosis in a patient with AIDS: a case report, *Oral. Dis.*, 1, 77, 1995 (see also *Oral Dis.*, 1, 61, 1995).

278. Iida, Y., Maehara, K., Okamoto, Y., Mase, K., Uwamori, H., Yonezu, S., Takeuchi, J., Simojo, M., and Yasunaga, K., A case of cryptococcal meningitis treated by ketoconazole and amphotericin B combination therapy, *Kansenshogaku Zasshi*, 60, 189, 1986.

279. Echevarria, A., Pinzon, V., Toro, J., and Diaz Issacs, M., Pulmonary cryptococcosis, *Rev. Med. Panama*, 16, 50, 1991.

280. Aslam, P. A., Larkin, J., Eastridge, C. E., and Hughes, F. A., Endocavitary infusion through percutaneous endobronchial catheter, *Chest*, 57, 94, 1970.

281. Stamm, A. M., Diasio, R. B., Dismukes, W. E., Shadomy, S., Cloud, G. A., Bowles, C. A., Karam, G. H., Espinel-Ingroff, A., and the NIAID Mycoses Study Group, Toxicity of amphotericin B plus flucytosine in 194 patients with cryptococcal meningitis, *Am. J. Med.*, 83, 236, 1987.

282. Shindo, K., Mizuno, T., Matsumoto, Y., Hashimoto, Y., Matsumura, M., Ito, A., and Shionoiri, H., Granulocytopenia and thrombocytopenia associated with combination therapy of amphotericin B and low-dose flucytosine in a patient with cryptococcal meningitis, *DICP*, 23, 672, 1989.

283. Bryan, C. S. and McFarland, J. A., Cryptococcal meningitis: fatal marrow aplasia from combined therapy, *JAMA*, 239, 1068, 1978.

284. Tassel, D. and Madoff, M. A., Treatment of *Candida* sepsis and *Cryptococcosus* meningitis with 5-fluorocytosine: a new antifungal agent, *JAMA*, 260, 830, 1968.

285. Koechlin, B. A., Rubio, S., Palmer, S., Gabriel, T., and Duschinsky, R., The metabolism of 5-fluorocytosine-2[^{14}C] and cytosine[^{14}C] in the rat and the disposition of 5-fluorocytosine-2[^{14}C] in man, *Biochem. Pharmacol.*, 15, 435, 1966.

286. Shadomy, S., Further *in vitro* studies with 5-fluorocytosine, *Infect. Immun.*, 2, 484, 1970.

287. Roberts, M., Rinaudo, P. A., Tilton, R. C., and Vilinskas, J., Treatment of multiple intracerebral cryptococcal granulomas with 5-fluorocytosine, *J. Neurosurg.*, 37, 229, 1972.

288. Editorial, Cryptococcosis and 5-fluorocytosine, *Aust. NZ J. Med.*, 4, 296, 1974.

289. Stanton, K. G. and Sanderson, C. R., The treatment of systemic cryptococcosis with 5-fluorocytosine, *Aust. NZ J. Med.*, 4, 262, 1974.

290. Molaret, P., Reilly, J., and Bastin, R., La forme ganglionnaire localisee de la cryptococcose, *Lyon Med.*, 203, 71, 1960.

291. Tolentino, P. and Borrone, C., Multiple lymphonodular cryptococcosis, cured by 5-fluorocytosine, *Scand. J. Infect. Dis.*, 8, 61, 1976.

292. Fusner, J. E. and McClain, K. L., Disseminated lymphonodular cryptococcosis treated with 5-fluorocytosine, *J. Pediatr.*, 94, 599, 1979.

293. Nathan, C. F., Cryptococcal osteomyelitis treated with 5-fluorocytosine, *Am. Rev. Respir. Dis.*, 110, 78, 1974.

294. Sabetta, J. R. and Andriole, V. T., Cryptococcal infections in the central nervous system, *Med. Clin. North Am.*, 69, 334, 1985.

295. Block, E. R. and Bennett, J. E., Clinical and pharmacological studies with 5-fluorocytosine (5-FC), *Clin. Res.*, 20, 525, 1972.

296. Utz, J. P., Shadomy, S., McGehee, R. F., and Tynes, B. S., 5-Fluorocytosine: experience in patients with pulmonary and other forms of cryptococcosis, *Am. Rev. Respir. Dis.*, 99, 975, 1969.

297. Zylstra, W., Cryptococcosis and 5-fluorocytosine: comment, *Aust. NZ J. Med.*, 4, 296, 1974.

298. Utz, J. P., Tynes, B. S., Shadomy, H. J., Duma, R. J., Kannan, M. M., and Mason, D. N., 5-Fluorocytosine in human cryptococcosis, *Antimicrob. Agents Chemother.*, 344, 1968.
299. Shadomy, S., *In vitro* studies with 5-fluorocytosine, *Infect. Immun.*, 2, 484, 1970.
300. Steer, P. L., Marks, M. I., Klite, P. D., and Eickhoff, T. C., 5-Fluorocytosine, an oral antifungal compound: report on clinical and laboratory experience, *Ann. Intern. Med.*, 76, 15, 1972.
301. Vandevelle, A. G., Nauceri, A. A., and Johnson, J. E. III, 5-Fluorocytosine in the treatment of mycotic infections, *Ann. Intern. Med.*, 77, 43, 1972.
302. Fass, R. J. and Perkins, R. L., 5-Fluorocytosine in the treatment of cryptococcal and *Candida* mycoses, *Ann. Intern. Med.*, 74, 535, 1971.
303. Schlegel, R. J., Bernier, G. M., Bellanti, J. A., Maybee, D. A., Osborne, G. B., Stewart, J. L., Pearlman, D. S., Ouelette, J., and Biehusen, F. C., Severe candidiasis associated with thymic displasia, IgA deficiency and plasma antilymphocyte effects, *Pediatrics*, 45, 926, 1970.
304. McDonnell, F. I., Clunie, G. J. A., Petrie, J. J. G., and Rao, A., Experience with 5-fluorocytosine in a dialysis-transplant unit, *Aust. NZ J. Med.*, 3, 438, 1973.
305. Kauffman, C. A. and Frame, P. T., Bone marrow toxicity associated with 5-fluorocytosine therapy, *Antimicrob. Agents Chemother.*, 11, 244, 1977.
306. Bryan, C. S. and McFarland, J. A., Cryptococcal meningitis: fatal marrow aplasia from combined therapy, *JAMA,* 239, 1068, 1978.
307. Philpot, C. R. and Lo, D., Cryptococcal meningitis in pregnancy, *Med. J. Aust.*, 2, 1005, 1972.
308. Polak, A. and Scholer, H. J., Mode of action of 5-fluorocytosine, *Rev. Inst. Pasteur Lyon*, 13(2), 233, 1980.
309. Polak, A., 5-Fluorocytosine and its combination with other antifungal agents, in *Recent Developments in Antifungal Chemotherapy*, Yamaguchi, H., Kobayashi, G. H., and Takeuchi, H., Eds., Marcel Dekker, New York, 1992, 77.
310. Polak, A., Synergism of polyene antibiotics with 5-fluorocytosine, *Chemotherapy*, 24, 2, 1978.
311. Polak, A., Antifungal combination therapy in localized candidiasis, *Mycoses*, 33, 215, 1990.
312. Polak, A., Scholer, H. J., and Wall, M., Combination therapy of experimental candidiasis, cryptococcosis and aspergillosis in mice, *Chemotherapy*, 28, 461, 1982.
313. Heidemann, H., Jacqz, E., Ohnhaus, E., Ray, W., and Branch, R., The importance of Na loading on amphotericin B nephrotoxicity considering the combination with 5-fluorocytosine and ticarcillin [Rec. Adv. Chemother., Antimicrobial Section 3], in *Proc. 14th Int. Congr. Chemother. Kyoto*, 2628, 1987.
314. Staib, F., Roegler, G., Pruefer-Kraemer, L., Seibold, M., Eichenlaub, D., and Pohle, H. D., Disseminierte kryptokokkose bei zwei AIDS-patienten, *Dtsch. Med. Wochenschr.*, 111, 1061, 1986.
315. Viviani, M. A., Tortorano, A. M., Pagano, A., Vigevani, G. M., Gubertini, G., Cristina, S., Assaisso, M. L., Suter, F., Farina, C., Minetti, B., Faggian, G., Curetta, M., Di Fabrizio, N., and Vaglia, A., European experience with itraconazole in systemic mycoses, *J. Am. Acad. Dermatol.*, 23, 587, 1990.
316. Tozzi, V., Bordi, E., Glagani, S., Leoni, G. C., Narciso, P., Sette, P., and Visco, G., Fluconazole treatment of cryptococcosis in patients with acquired immunodeficiency syndrome, *Am. J. Med.*, 87, 353, 1989.
317. Chernoff, D. N. and Sande, M. A., Cryptococcal infections in patients with the acquired immunodeficiency syndrome (AIDS), *Proc. Int. Conf. AIDS*, Paris, Abstr. 543, 1986.
318. Just-Nübling, G., Laubenberger, C., Helm, E. B., Falk, S., and Stille, W., Diagnose, klinischer verlauf und behandlung der kryptokokken-meningitis bei AIDS patienten, *Forschg. Praxis*, 9, VI, 1990.
319. Nasu, S., Fukuoka, Y., Kumagai, Y., Okamoto, S., Sawae, Y., and Nagabuchi, S., A case of cryptococcal meningitis successfully treated with intraventricular infusion of miconazole, *Kensenshogaku Zasshi*, 56, 1230, 1982.
320. Fukui, K., Okamura, K., Watanabe, M., Nakamura, S., and Yamamoto, M., A case of cryptococcal meningitis successfully treated with miconazole and CSF drainage, *Kansenshogaku Zasshi*, 63, 649, 1989.
321. Weinstein, L. and Jacoby, I., Successful treatment of cerebral cryptococcoma and meningitis with miconazole, *Ann. Intern. Med.*, 93, 569, 1980.

322. de Witt, C. N., Cryptococcal meningitis: treatment of three patients with miconazole, *Med. J. Aust.*, 1, 525, 1981.
323. Sung, J. P., Grendale, J. G., and Levine, H. B., Intravenous and intrathecal miconazole therapy for systemic mycosis, *West. J. Med.*, 126, 5, 1977.
324. Deresinski, S. C., Lilly, R. B., Levine, H. B., Galgiani, J. N., and Stevens, D. A., Treatment of fungal meningitis with miconazole, *Arch. Intern. Med.*, 137, 1180, 1977.
325. Belle, W. E., Treatment of fungal infections of the central nervous system, *Ann. Neurol.*, 9, 417, 1981.
326. Sung, J. P., Campbell, G. D., and Grendahl, J. C., Miconazole therapy for fungal meningitis, *Arch. Neurol.*, 35, 443, 1978.
327. Bee, O. B., Tan, T., and Pang, R., A case of primary cutaneous cryptococcosis successfully treated with miconazole, *Arch. Dermatol.*, 117, 290, 1981.
328. Yamada, Y., Dekio, S., Jidoi, J., Yokogi, H., and Moriki, S., A case of cutaneous localized cryptococcosis, *Nippon Hifuka Gakkai Zasshi*, 100, 205, 1990.
329. Morgans, M. E., Thomas, M. E. M., and MacKenzie, D. W. R., Successful treatment of systemic cryptococcosis with miconazole, *Br. Med. J.*, 2, 100, 1979.
330. Kaneko, T., Noda, K., Sano, F., Nomura, I., Kameda, Y., and Iida, M., Primary pulmonary cryptococcosis treated with transbronchial injection of amphotericin B, *Nippon Kyobu Shikkan Gakkai Zasshi*, 27, 1534, 1989.
331. Granier, F., Kamitakis, J., Hermier, C., Zhu, Y. Y., and Thivolet, J., Localized cutaneous cryptococcosis successfully treated with ketoconazole, *J. Am. Acad. Dermatol.*, 16, 243, 1987.
332. Perfect, J. R., Durack, D. T., Hamilton, J. D., and Gallis, H. A., Failure of ketoconazole in cryptococcal meningitis, *JAMA*, 247, 3349, 1982.
333. Ogushi, F., Tamura, M., Ozaki, T., Kamei, T., Nakanishi, M., Shimada, H., Kawano, T., Yasuoka, S., and Tsubura, E., A case of cryptococcal meningitis improved in the treatment of high dose ketoconazole, *Kansenshogaku Zasshi*, 59, 405, 1985.
334. Karaffa, C. A., Rehm, S. J., and Keys, T. F., The acquired immunodeficiency syndrome and cryptococcosis, *Ann. Intern. Med.*, 104, 891, 1986.
335. Bernard, E., Carles, M., Toussaint-Gari, M., Fournier, J. P., and Dellamonica, P., Value of fluconazole in the treatment of systemic yeast infection, *Pathol. Biol. (Paris)*, 37, 690, 1989.
336. Shuttleworth, D., Philpot, C. M., and Knight, A. G., Cutaneous cryptococcosis: treatment with oral fluconazole, *Br. J. Dermatol.*, 120, 683, 1989.
337. Nakashima, M., The clinical study of fluconazole against pulmonary cryptococcosis and aspergillosis, and its pharmacokinetics in patients, *Jpn. J. Antibiot.*, 42, 127, 1989.
338. Mares, M., Sartori, M. T., Carretta, M., Bertaggia, A., and Girolami, A., Rhinophyma-like cryptococcal infection as an early manifestation of AIDS in a hemophilia B patient, *Acta Haematol.*, 84, 101, 1990.
339. Zalcman, G., Lechapt, E., Milleron, B., Denis, M., Mayaud, C., and Akoun, G., Pleuropulmonary cryptococcosis disclosing AIDS, *Rev. Pneumol. Clin.*, 47, 133, 1991.
340. Bozzette, S. A., Larsen, R. A., Chiu, J., Leal, M. A., Tilles, J. G., Richman, D. D., Leedom, J. M., and McCutchan, J. A., Fluconazole treatment of persistent *Cryptococcus neoformans* prostatic infection in AIDS, *Ann. Intern. Med.*, 115, 285, 1991.
341. Sugar, A. M., Overview: cryptococcosis in the treatment of AIDS, *Mycopathologia*, 114, 153, 1991.
342. Levesque, H., Alie-Legrand, M. C., Omnient, Y., Micaud, G., Lemeland, J. F., Gancel, A., and Courtois, H., *Cryptococcus neoformans* meningitis and cirrhosis: value of fluconazole, *Clin. Biol.*, 13, 942, 1989.
343. Michelone, G., Tacconi, F., Maccabruni, A., Lanzarini, P., Tinelli, M., and Dei Cas, A., Clinical and therapeutic profile of 3 cases of cryptococcal meningitis in patients with AIDS, *G. Ital. Chemoter.*, 36, 95, 1989.
344. Krisch, H. and Sarnow, E., Collection of cases in relation to clinical trials of fluconazole in Germany, *Mycoses*, 33(Suppl. 1), 14S, 1990.
345. Reents, S. B. and Powell, G., Fluconazole success after amphotericin B and flucytosine failure in cryptococcal meningitis, *DICP*, 24, 885, 1990.
346. Lindberg, J. and Edebo, L., Successful treatment of cryptococcal meningitis with fluconazole, *Lakartidningen*, 88, 2245, 1991.

347. Good, C. B. and Leeper, H. F., Profound papilledema due to cryptococcal meningitis in acquired immunodeficiency syndrome: successful treatment with fluconazole, *South. Med. J.*, 84, 394, 1991.

348. Dismukes, W. E., Treatment of systemic fungal diseases in patients with AIDS, in *Recent Progress in Antifungal Chemotherapy*, Yamaguchi, H., Kobayashi, G. S., and Takahashi, H., Eds., Marcel Dekker, New York, 1992, 227.

349. Jones, P. D., Marriott, D., and Speed, B. R., Efficacy of fluconazole in cryptoccocal meningitis, *Diagn. Microbiol. Infect. Dis.*, 12(Suppl. 4), 235S, 1989.

350. Dupont, B., Treatment of cryptococcal meningitis, in *Proc. Xth Congr. Int. Soc. Human Animal Mycol., Barcelona*, Torres-Rodriguez, J. M., Ed., J. R. Prous, 1988, 197.

351. Byrne, W. R. and Wajszczuk, C. P., Cryptococcal meningitis in the acquired immunodeficiency syndrome (AIDS): successful treatment with fluconazole after failure of amphotericin B, *Ann. Intern. Med.*, 108, 384, 1988.

352. Dromer, F., Mathoulin, S., Dupont, B., Brugiere, O., and Letenneur, L., Comparison of the efficacy of amphotericin B and fluconazole in the treatment of cryptococcosis in human immunodeficiency virus-negative patients: retrospective analysis of 83 cases, *Clin. Infect. Dis.*, 22(Suppl. 2), S154, 1996.

353. Larsen, R. A., Leal, M. A., and Chan, L. S., Fluconazole compared with amphotericin B plus flucytosine for cryptococcal meningitis in AIDS: a randomized trial, *Ann. Intern. Med.*, 113, 183, 1990.

354. Wong, R. D. and Goetz, M. B., Treatment of cryptococcal meningitis in AIDS, *J. Infect. Dis.*, 113, 992, 1990.

355. Buxton, M. J., Dubois, D. J., Turner, R. R., Sculpher, M. J., Robinson, P. A., and Searcy, C., Cost implications of alternative treatments for AIDS patients with cryptococcal meningitis: comparison of fluconazole and amphotericin-based therapies, *J. Infect.*, 23, 17, 1991.

356. Bolignano, G., Chindemi, G., and Criseo, G., Cryptococcal meningoencephalitis in a patient with Hodgkin's lymphoma: successful treatment with fluconazole, *Mycoses*, 34, 63, 1991.

357. Iacopino, P., Morabito, F., Martino, B., Bolignano, G., and Nobile, F., Fluconazole for disseminated cryptococcosis in a patient with Hodgkin's disease, *Haematologica*, 76, 260, 1991.

358. Sugar, A. M. and Saunders, C., Oral fluconazole as suppressive therapy of disseminated cryptococcosis in patients with acquired immunodeficiency syndrome, *Am. J. Med.*, 85, 481, 1988.

359. Bozzette, S. A., Larsen, R. A., Chiu, J., Leal, M. A., Jacobsen, J., Rothman, P., Robinson, P., Gilbert, G., McCutchan, J. A., Tilles, J., Leedom, J. M., Richman, D. D., and the California Collaborative Treatment Group, A placebo-controlled trial of maintenance therapy with fluconazole after treatment of cryptococcal meningitis in the acquired immunodeficiency syndrome, *N. Engl. J. Med.*, 324, 580, 1991.

360. Powderly, W., Saag, M., Cloud, G. et al., Fluconazole versus amphotericin B as maintenance therapy for prevention of relapse of AIDS-associated cryptococcal meningitis, *Proc. 30th Intersci. Conf. Antimicrob. Agents Chemother.*, American Society for Microbiology, Washington, D.C., Abstr. 1162, 1990.

361. Laroche, R., Deppner, M., Floch, J. J., Kadende, P., Goasguen, J., Sauniere, J. F., and Dupont, B., Cryptococcosis in Bujumbura, Burundi: apropos of 80 observed cases in 42 months, *Bull. Soc. Pathol. Exot. Fil.*, 83, 159, 1990.

362. Stern, J. J., Hartman, B. J., Sharkey, K., Rowland, V., Squires, K. E., Murray, H. W., and Graybill, J. R., Oral fluconazole therapy for patients with acquired immunodeficiency syndrome and cryptococcosis: experience with 22 patients, *Am. J. Med.*, 85, 477, 1988.

363. Sort, P., Morales, M., Gomez, J., Pares, A., and Rodes, J., Pleural empyema caused by *Cryptococcus neoformans* in a patient with liver cirrhosis, *Gastroenterol. Hepatol.*, 19, 302, 1996.

364. Agarwal, A., Gupta, A., Sakhuja, V., Talwar, P., Joshi, K., and Chugh, K. S., Retinitis following disseminated cryptococcosis in a renal allograft recipient: efficacy of oral fluconazole, *Acta Ophthalmol. (Copenhagen)*, 69, 402, 1991.

365. Custis, P. H., Haller, J. A., and de Juan, E., Jr., An unusual case of cryptococcal endophthalmitis, *Retina*, 15, 300, 1995.

366. Vandersmissen, G., Meuleman, L., Tits, G., Verhaeghe, A., and Peetermans, W. E., Cutaneous cryptococcosis in corticosteroid-treated patients without AIDS, *Acta Clin. Belg.*, 51, 111, 1996.

367. Halweg, H., Korzeniewska-Kosela, M., Podsiadlo, B., and Krakowka, P., A case of skin cryptococcosis in systemic lupus erythematosus, *Pneumonol. Pol.*, 58, 544, 1990.

368. Pineski, R., Mathurin, S. A., Ruffinengo, O., Alonso, H. O., and Corallini de Bracelenti, B., Cutaneous cryptococcosis in a patient receiving chronic immunosuppressive therepy, *Cutis*, 57, 229, 1996.

369. Verneuil, L., Dompmartin, A., Duhamel, C., Cren, P., Six, M., Le Maitre, M., Galateau, F., Moreau, A., and Leroy, D., Cryptococcal whitlow in a HIV-positive patient, *Ann. Dermatol. Venereol.*, 122, 688, 1995.

370. Kerchner, J. E., Ridley, M. B., and Greene, J. N., Laryngeal cryptococcus: treatment with oral fluconazole, *Arch. Otolaryngol. Head Neck Surg.*, 121, 1193, 1995.

371. Schmidt, D. M., Sercarz, J. A., Kevorkian, K. F., and Canalis, R. F., Cryptococcus presenting as a neck mass, *Ann. Otol. Rhinol. Laryngol.*, 104, 711, 1995.

372. Yew, W. W., Wong, P. C., Wong, C. F., Lee, J., and Chau, C. H., Oral fluconazole in the treatment of pulmonary cryptococcosis in non-AIDS patients, *Drugs Exp. Clin. Res.*, 22, 25, 1996.

373. Guillaume, M. P., De Prez, C., and Cogan, E., Subacute mitochondrial liver disease in a patient with AIDS: possible relationship to prolonged fluconazole administration, *Am. J. Gastroenterol.*, 91, 165, 1996.

374. Pappas, P. G., Kauffman, C. A., Perfect, J., Johnson, P. C., Mckinsey, D. S., Bamberger, D. M., Hamill, R., Sharkey, P. K., Chapman, S. W., and Sobel, J. D., Alopecia associated with fluconazole therapy, *Ann. Intern. Med.*, 123, 354, 1995 (see comment in *Ann. Intern. Med.*, 125, 153, 1996).

375. Weinroth, S. E., and Tuazon, C. U., Alopecia associated with fluconazole treatment, *Ann. Intern. Med.*, 119, 637, 1993.

376. Coker, R. J. and Harris, J. R., Failure of fluconazole treatment in cryptococcal meningitis despite adequate CSF levels, *J. Infect.*, 123, 101, 1991.

377. Bailly, M. P., Boibieux, A., Biron, F., Durieu, I., Piens, M. A., Peyramond, D., and Bertrand, J. L., Persistence of *Cryptococcus neoformans* in prostate: failure of fluconazole despite high doses, *J. Infect. Dis.*, 164, 435, 1991.

378. Pietroski, N., Buckley, R. M., Braffman, M. N., and Stern, J. J., Intravenous and oral fluconazole in treatment of acute cryptococcal meningitis in AIDS, *Proc. 30th Intersci. Conf. Antimicrob. Agents Chemother.*, American Society for Microbiology, Washington, D.C., Abstr. 576, 1990.

379. Squires, K., Rowland, V., Gassyuk, E. et al., Fluconazole as therapy for acute cryptococcal meningitis, *Proc. 30th Intersci. Conf. Antimicrob. Agents Chemother.*, American Society for Microbiology, Washington, D.C., Abstr. 573, 1990.

380. Georgiev, V. St., Opportunistic/nosocomial infections: treatment and developmental therapeutics. II. Cryptococcosis, *Med. Res. Rev.*, 13, 507, 1993.

381. Viviani, M. A., Tortorano, A. M., Giani, P. C., Arici, C., Goglio, A., Crocchiolo, P., and Almaviva, M., Itraconazole for cryptococcal infection in the acquired immunodeficiency syndrome, *Ann. Intern. Med.*, 106, 106, 1987.

382. Viviani, M. A., Tortorano, A. M., Langer, M., Almaviva, M., Negri, C., Cristina, S., Scoccia, S., De Maria, R., Fiocci, R., Ferrazzi, P., Coglio, A., Gavazzeni, G., Faggian, G., Rinaldi, R., and Cadrobbi, P., Experience with itraconazole in cryptococcosis and aspergillosis, *J. Infect.*, 18, 151, 1989.

383. Denning, D. W., Tucker, R. M., Hanson, L. H., Hamilton, J. R., and Stevens, D. A., Itraconazole therapy for cryptococcal meningitis and cryptococcosis, *Arch. Intern. Med.*, 149, 2301, 1989.

384. Denning, D. W., Tucker, R. M., Hanson, L. H., and Stevens, D. A., Itraconazole in opportunistic mycoses: cryptococcosis and aspergillosis, *J. Am. Acad. Dermatol.*, 3, 602, 1990.

385. de Gans, J., Eeftinck Schattenkerk, J. K. M., and van Ketel, R. J., Itraconazole as maintenance treatment for cryptococcal meningitis in the acquired immunodeficiency syndrome, *Br. Med. J.*, 296, 339, 1988.

386. Batungwanayo, J., Taelman, H., Bogaerts, J., Allen, S., Lukas, S., Kagame, A., Clerinx, J., Montané, J., Saraux, A., Mühlberger, F., and Van de Perre, P., Pulmonary cryptococcosis associated with HIV-1 infection in Rwanda: a retrospective study of 37 cases, *AIDS*, 8, 1271, 1994.

387. Sato, T., Koseki, S., Takahashi, S., and Maie, O., Localized cutaneous cryptococcosis successfully treated with itraconazole: review of medication in 18 cases reported in Japan, *Mycoses*, 33, 455, 1990.

388. Goh, C. L., Cutaneous cryptococcosis successfully treated with itraconazole, *Cutis*, 51, 377, 1993.

389. Bettoli, V., Virgili, A., Zampino, M. R., Bedetti, A., and Montanari, P., Cutaneous cryptococcosis in AIDS: successful treatment with itraconazole, *Mycoses*, 36, 433, 1993.

390. Lewis, J. L. and Rabinovich, S., The wide spectrum of cryptococcal infections, *Am. J. Med.*, 53, 315, 1972.

391. Lalloo, D., Fisher, D., Naraqi, S., Laurenson, I., Temu, P., Sinha, A., Saweri, A., and Mavo, B., Cryptococcal meningitis (*C. neoformans* var. *gattii*) leading to blindness in previously healthy Melanesian adults in Papua New Guinea, *Q. J. Med.*, 87, 343, 1994.

392. Currie, B., Vigus, T., Leach, G., and Dwyer, B., *Cryptococcus neoformans* var. *gattii*, *Lancet*, 336, 1442, 1990.

393. Laurenson, I. F., Naraqi, S., Howcroft, N., Burrows, I., and Saulei, S., Cryptococcal meningitis in Papua New Guinea: ecology and the role of eucalyptus, *Med. J. Aust.*, 158, 213, 1993.

394. Laurenson, I. F., Naraqi, S., Trevett, A., Lalloo, D., Nwokolo, N., Matuka, A., Ogunbanjo, B., Igo, J., and Tefurani, N., Cryptococcal investigations in Papua New Guinea, *Proc. 2nd Int. Conf. Cryptococcus and Cryptococcosis*, Milan, 1993, p. 114.

395. Laurenson, I. F., Trevett, A. J., Lalloo, D. G., Nwokolo, N., Naraqi, S., Black, J., Tefurani, N., Saweri, A., Mavo, B., Igo, J., and Warrell, D. A., Meningitis caused by *Cryptococcus neoformans* var. *gattii* and var. *neoformans* in Papua New Guinea, *Trans. R. Soc. Trop. Med. Hyg.*, 90, 57, 1996.

396. Kwon-Chung, K. J. and Bennett, J. E., Epidemiologic differences between the two varieties of *Cryptococcus neoformans*, *Am. J. Epidemiol.*, 120, 123, 1984.

397. Ellis, D. H., *Cryptococcus neoformans* var. *gattii* in Australia, *J. Clin. Microbiol.*, 25, 430, 1987.

398. Sorrell, T. C., Brownlee, A. G., Ruma, P., Malik, R., Pfeiffer, T. J., and Ellis, D. H., Natural environmental sources of *Cryptococcus neoformans* var. *gattii*, *J. Clin. Microbiol.*, 34, 1261, 1996.

399. Pfeiffer, T. J. and Ellis, D. H., Environmental isolation of *Cryptococcus neoformans* var. *gattii* from *Eucalyptus tereticornis*, *J. Med. Vet. Mycol.*, 30, 407, 1992.

400. Sorrell, T. C., Chen, S. C. A., Ruma, P., Meyer, W., Pfeiffer, T. J., Ellis, D. H., and Brownlee, A. G., Concordance of clinical and environmental isolates of *Cryptococcus neoformans* var. *gattii* by random amplification of polymorphic DNA analysis and PCR fingerprinting, *J. Clin. Microbiol.*, 34, 1253, 1996.

401. Kwon-Chung, K. J., Wickes, B. L., Stockman, L., Roberts, G. D., Ellis, D., and Howard, D. H., Virulence, serotype, and molecular characteristics of environmental strains of *Cryptococcus neoformans* var. *gattii*, *Infect. Immun.*, 60, 1869, 1992.

402. Varma, A., Swinne, D., Staib, F., Bennett, J. E., and Kwon-Chung, K. J., Diversity of DNA fingerprints in *Cryptococcus neoformans*, *J. Clin. Microbiol.*, 33, 1807, 1995.

403. Mitchell, D. H., Sorrell, T. C., Allworth, A. M., Heath, C. H., McGregor, A. R., Papanoum, K., Richards, M. J., and Gottlieb, T., Cryptococcal disease of the CNS in immunocompetent hosts: influence of cryptococcal variety on clinical manifestations and outcome, *Clin. Infect. Dis.*, 20, 611, 1995.

404. Speed, R. and Dunt, D., Clinical and host differences between the two varieties of *Cryptococcus neoformans*, *Clin. Infect. Dis.*, 21, 28, 1995.

405. Slobodnik, R. and Naraqi, S., Cryptococcal meningitis, in the Central Province of Papua New Guinea, *Papua New Guinea Med. J.*, 23, 111, 1980.

406. Loison, J., Bouchara, J. P., Gueho, E., de Gentile, L., Cimon, B., Chennebault, J. M., and Chabasse, D., First report of *Cryptococcus albidus* septicemia in an HIV patient, *J. Infect.*, 33, 139, 1996.

407. Gluck, J. L., Myers, J. P., and Pass, L. M., Cryptococcemia due to *Cryptococcus albidus*, *South. Med. J.*, 80, 511, 1987.

408. Gordon, M. A., Pulmonary cryptococcosis: a case due to *Cryptococcus albidus*, *Am. Rev. Respir. Dis.*, 106, 786, 1972.

409. Lin, S. R., Peng, C. E., Yung, S. A., and Yu, H. S., Isolation of *Cryptococcus albidus* var. *albidus* in patient with pemphigus foliaceous, *Kao-Hsiung I Hsueh Ko Hsueh Tsa Chih*, 5, 126, 1989.

410. Weiser, H. G., Zur frage der pathogenität der *Cryptococcus albidus*, *Schweiz. Med. Wochenschr.*, 103, 475, 1973.

411. da Cunha, T. and Lusins, J., *Cryptococcus albidus* meningitis, *South. Med. J.*, 66, 1230, 1973.

412. Mello, J. C., Srinivasan, S., Scott, M. L., and Raff, M. J., *Cryptococcus albidus* meningitis, *J. Infect.*, 2, 79, 1980.

413. Krumholz, R. A., Pulmonary cryptococcosis: a case due to *Cryptococcus albidus*, *Am. Rev. Respir. Dis.*, 105, 421, 1972.

414. Horowitz, I. D., Blumberg, E. A., and Krevolin, L., *Cryptococcus albidus* and mucormycosis empyema in a patient receiving hemodialysis, *South. Med. J.*, 86, 1070, 1993.

415. Lynch, J. P. III, Schaberg, D. R., Kissner, D. G., and Kauffman, C. A., *Cryptococcus laurentii* lung abscess, *Am. Rev. Respir. Dis.*, 123, 135, 1981.

416. Chander, J., Sapra, R. K., and Talwar, P., Incidence of cryptococcosis in and around Chandigarch, India during the period 1982–1991, *Mycoses*, 37, 23, 1994.

417. Vadkertiova, R. and Slavikova, E., Killer activity of yeasts isolated from the water environment, *Can. J. Microbiol.*, 41, 759, 1995.

418. McCormack, P. J., Wildman, H. G., and Jeffries, P., Production of antibacterial compounds by phylloplane-inhibiting yeasts and yeastlike fungi, *Appl. Environ. Microbiol.*, 60, 927, 1994.

419. Damalam, A., Yesudian, P., and Thambiah, A. S., Cutaneous infection by *Cryptococcus laurentii*, *Br. J. Dermatol.*, 97, 221, 1972.

420. Haynes, M. P., Buckley, H. R., Higgins, M. L., and Pieringer, R. A., Synergism between the antifungal agents amphotericin B and alkyl glycerol ethers, *Antimicrob. Agents Chemother.*, 38, 1523, 1994.

32   *Candida* spp.

32.1   INTRODUCTION

Candidiasis is an acute or chronic, superficial or disseminated mycosis caused by species of the genus *Candida*. The latter is a genus of nearly 200 yeast-like anamorphic (sexually imperfect) fungi (form-order Cryptococcales, form-class Blastomycetes), characterized by a polymorphic nature because of their ability to produce budding yeast cells (blastoconidia), mycelia, pseudomycelia, and blastospores.[1-3] Some *Candida* spp. have been found capable of mating, producing teleomorphic (sexually perfect) forms.

Although commonly part of the normal flora of the skin, mouth, intestinal tract, and vagina, *Candida* spp. are the etiologic agents of a variety of infections, including candidiasis, onychomycosis, tinea corporis, tinea pedis, vaginitis, and thrush. The fungus appears to have involved receptors (known as adhesins) for human fluid phase glycoproteins, such as fibronectin and immobilized basement membrane glycoproteins in order to establish itself in mucus-lined cavities. The *Candida* adhesins may be analogous or perhaps homologous to the human integrin receptors.[4]

Several conditions have been identified to favor the predominance of *Candida* spp. over normal microbial flora, namely, elimination of bacterial competition following oral or parenteral antibacterial therapy, the use of cimetidine or histamine-2 blockers, as well as the significant elevation of extracellular glucose concentrations in diabetic patients.[5-11] The reason for histamine antagonists to promote candidal growth is their ability to elevate the local pH, thereby creating an environment more conducive to fungal growth.

C. albicans is the most frequent etiologic agent of candidiasis capable of causing any of the clinical types of mycosis, and the leading cause of opportunistic fungal disease. In addition to *C. albicans*, *C. albicans* var. *stellatoidea*, *C. tropicalis*, *C. parapsilosis*, *C. krusei*, *C. lusitaniae*, and *C. guilliermondii* have been increasingly identified as causative agents of opportunistic infections in the immunocompromised host.[12,13] The advent of the AIDS pandemic and the widespread use of azole antimycotics (fluconazole) has contributed to a significant increase in *C. krusei* infections (even though this species is less virulent than *C. albicans*), particularly because of the high incidence of resistance of this yeast to fluconazole.[14]

All candidal yeasts generally grow well in aerobic conditions on both enriched and minimal media at pH range of 2.5 to 7.5 and temperatures of 20 to 39°C. The optimal temperature of the most virulent species, *C. albicans* and *C. tropicalis,* is about 37°C; at temperatures below 33°C, single-cell yeast morphology is predominant.

32.2   HUMAN CANDIDIASIS

Based on pathologic studies, three distinct forms of human candidiasis have been distinguished: superficial, locally invasive, and deep (systemic) mycoses.

Cases of superficial candidiasis are most commonly observed in lining surfaces (skin, oropharynx, gastrointestinal tract, and upper and lower respiratory tracts). Characteristic features include velvety appearance of the lesions, whereas the adjacent mucosal membrane appears dark red and moderately swollen; ulcerative or necrotic lesions indicate deeper tissue invasion.[15]

Among immunosuppressed patients, locally invasive candidiasis may present as pneumonia, cystitis, esophagitis, or pyelonephritis. Typically, it is characterized by fairly sharply defined ulcerations of the intestinal, respiratory, or genitourinary tracts.[15]

Systemic candidiasis is the most serious manifestation of the disease that can affect any organ, but most frequently it involves the heart, kidneys, liver, spleen, lung, and the brain. Usually, dissemination is defined as an invasive infection striking the parenchyma of two or more visceral organs, excluding the mucosa of the gastrointestinal, respiratory, or the genitourinary tract.[15-17] The most likely organ combination involved has been the gastrointestinal tract, liver, kidney, and the lung.[16]

Because of their decreased resistance to infection, patients at high risk of developing systemic candidiasis include immunocompromised patients, those with hematologic and solid malignancies, or on immunosuppressive therapy, and postoperative patients.[16,18-20] By some accounts,[21] *Candida* spp. are the seventh most common pathogen to cause nosocomial infections,[22] and the fifth most common cause of primary blood-stream infection.[23]

The most severe form of systemic candidiasis has been observed in leukemic patients and organ transplant recipients receiving immunosuppressive therapy (irradiation, corticosteroids, antineoplastic and antibacterial drugs).[24-26] The gastrointestinal tract is the most frequent source of systemic candidiasis in patients with hematologic malignancies and neutropenia.[25] Although it has been diagnosed,[16,18,27] ocular candidiasis is very rare.

32.2.1 CUTANEOUS CANDIDIASIS

C. albicans and *C. tropicalis* have been by far the most common species recovered from over 80% of clinical specimens from patients with cutaneous candidiasis.[28] While in healthy individuals, cutaneous candidiasis was rarely associated with serious sequelae,[29] in immunocompromised patients the infection was often recalcitrant and the morbidity far more extensive, leading even to bacterial superinfection. Cutaneous ulcerations of the lower extremities have been observed secondary to candidal invasion.[30] In another case, Patel et al.[31] have diagnosed candidal cellulitis as a complication of percutaneous endoscopic gastrostomy placement in a diabetic patient. *Candida*-induced thrombophlebitis and skin abscess formation have followed instrumentation.[32,33]

32.2.2 CHRONIC MUCOCUTANEOUS CANDIDIASIS

Chronic mucocutaneous candidiasis is manifested by persistent and recurrent infections of the skin, nails, and mucous membranes caused, in the overwhelming number of cases, by *C. albicans*.[34,35] Although the disease can be observed at any age, the growing populations of immunocompromised patients, especially those who are HIV-positive, are at greater risk of developing oropharyngeal and esophageal candidiasis.[36] In HIV-infected patients, oral candidiasis-affected tissues may become markedly erythematous with white or creamy plaques present.[37]

In general, all antifungal therapies do not correct the host factors that predispose to chronic candidiasis, and patients eventually relapse after antifungal treatment is terminated.[34]

The association of chronic mucocutaneous candidiasis with endocrine dysfunction, such as the candidiasis-endocrinopathy syndrome (CES) has been defined as a complex immune disorder in which autoimmunity is found besides selective impairment of cellular immunity and atrophy (agenesis, asplenia) of the spleen. Boni et al.[38] have reported one case of CES associated with alopecia areata; topical immunotherapy with diphenylcyclopropenone was unsuccessful.

32.2.3 ORAL AND ESOPHAGEAL CANDIDIASIS

Oral and esophageal candidiasis are common candidal infections occurring in all age groups.[39] The various types of oral candidiasis were classified by Lehner[40] to include acute pseudomembranous candidiasis, acute and chronic atrophic candidiasis, and chronic hyperplastic candidiasis, comprising *Candida* leukoplakia, the endocrine candidiasis syndrome, and chronic diffuse and chronic localized mucocutaneous candidiasis.[41] In spite of some objections,[42,43] the Lehner classification, after proper modifications to account for the spectrum of oral lesions in HIV-infected patients,[44,45] is being widely used.

Manifestations of esophageal candidiasis include dysphagia, retrosternal pain,[46-49] and odynophagia;[47,49] less common symptoms may include nausea, vomiting, and hematemesis,[49] as well as fever in some cases.[49-52]

32.2.4 LOWER GASTROINTESTINAL CANDIDIASIS

Although *Candida* spp. have been most frequently recovered from the oropharynx, on numerous occasions they have also been isolated from the gastrointestinal tract.[18,53-57] Some of the predisposing factors include age (infancy, elderly), mucocutaneous candidiasis, HIV infection, depressed phagocytic functions, diabetes, endocrinopathies, disruption of mucosal integrity, as well as some exogenous factors (treatment with antimicrobial or immunosuppressive agents, antacids, microbial synergy).[53] Even though the concentrations of *Candida* spp. are high, the presence of defense mechanisms (gastric acidity, peristalsis, local antibodies, secretion of antibacterial factors, and the endogenous flora) help to maintain microbial balance and to minimize the likelihood of candidal infections occurring in the GI tract under normal circumstances.[53] The optimal growth of *C. albicans* is at pH 7.4 and becomes completely inhibited at pH 4.5. Thus, any disruption of gastric acid secretion will increase the risk of fungal colonization.

After the esophagus, the stomach is the most common site of candidal infection. Other manifestations of GI involvement include intestinal candidiasis (enterocolitis of the small and large bowels), diarrheal syndromes, ischemic enteritis, liver and pancreatic involvement, cholecystitis, and candidiasis hypersensitivity syndrome[58-60] (also known as the "yeast connection").[53] Failure to define the candidiasis hypersensitivity syndrome more clearly have prompted some investigators[61] to deny its existence.

32.2.5 CHRONIC CANDIDIASIS SYNDROME

The chronic candidiasis syndrome, also known as "*Candida*-related complex" is intestinal infection thought to be the result of overgrowth of *C. albicans* in the gastrointestinal tract and secondarily in the genital organs.[62] Except for the recurrent flu-like symptoms, patients with chronic candidiasis syndrome have experienced many of the same symptoms observed in patients with the chronic fatigue syndrome (CFS). The positive response of a large number of patients with CFS to oral antimycotics and a diet for intestinal candidiasis has led to the suggestion that chronic intestinal candidiasis could be a causative factor in CFS.[62] In addition, some evidence that might corroborate the validity of this hypothesis include the finding that *C. albicans*-associated infections of mucous membranes caused suppression of T cell and natural killer (NK) cell functions; similar abnormalities have been observed in patients with CFS.

While immune dysfunction found in CFS has been considered to be the primary underlying causal factor of this disorder, normal functions of cytotoxic T lymphocytes, T helper cells, and NK cells can also prevent the reactivation of infections caused by the Epstein-Barr virus, cytomegalovirus, and other herpesviruses, which can all produce flu-like symptoms in the CFS.[62]

32.2.6 DISSEMINATED CANDIDIASIS

The term "hematogenous candidiasis" is used to identify all infections involving the bloodstream, thereby describing candidemia (with or without deep tissue invasion), disseminated infection (with or without candidemia), or both.[63]

In 1937, Bogden and Kessel[64] were the first to report disseminated candidiasis in an adult patient. In general, disseminated candidiasis is primarily diagnosed in immunocompromised and debilitated patients,[65] such as those with diabetes mellitus, pancreatitis, hepatic cirrhosis, hepatitis, systemic lupus erythematosus, uremia, inflammatory GI disease, aplastic anemia, severe trauma,[66-70] and organ transplant recipients.[71] When the infection is disseminated to multiple organs its prognosis is poor.[66] Dissemination may also involve a single organ resulting in endocarditis,[72] meningitis,[73] pneumonitis,[74] osteomyelitis, and pancreatitis.

C. albicans has been the most commonly identified species in hematogenous candidiasis, whereas *C. parapsilosis* and *C. glabrata* have been associated with fungemia.[65] *C. glabrata* also appeared to be more common in women, surgical patients, and those receiving parenteral alimentation.[75,76] *C. tropicalis* is also emerging as an important pathogen in hematogenous candidiasis.[77,78] Since it may be more virulent than *C. albicans*, *C. tropicalis* may be more likely to cause systemic infection, especially in immunocompromised hosts[79-82] (children with leukemia[83,84]). Among other *Candida* species, *C. krusei* has been reported to colonize patients receiving fluconazole as antifungal prophylaxis[85] (most likely due to fluconazole resistance), and *C. lusitaniae* which seems to affect immunocompromised patients, especially those with leukemia.[86,87]

Disseminated candidiasis is a serious infectious complication that may reach a mortality rate as high as 50%.[88]

Predisposing factors associated with candidal dissemination include broad-spectrum antibiotic, immunosuppressive, and corticosteroid therapies, prosthetic devices, and parenteral hyper-alimentation. Generalized immunosuppression leading to weakened host immune defense functions (such as neutropenia, and impaired neutrophil and T lymphocyte functions) as a result of organ transplantation, malignancies, AIDS, malnutrition, and prolonged postoperative therapeutic courses, have been critical for tissue invasion and dissemination of *Candida* spp.[89] Interestingly, AIDS patients who have low numbers of helper T lymphocytes while having frequent superficial infections, rarely develop hematogenous candidiasis.[65]

In a study by Bodey,[90] patients with acute leukemia who developed hematogenous candidiasis[91] spent more time with lymphopenia and received adrenal corticosteroids and antibiotics for longer periods than did patients who had localized candidiasis. The importance of prior bacterial infections as a contributing factor to the development of hematogenous candidiasis has also been emphasized.[18,92,93]

The frequency of disseminated candidiasis has been relatively high in liver transplant recipients.[94,95] Bone marrow transplant recipients are particularly susceptible to *Candida* infections because of the prolonged period of severe neutropenia lasting about 30 d after transplantation.[80,96] In a case-controlled study, Wey at al.[97] have determined a 38% attributable mortality rate from candidemia. Harvey and Myers[92] reported an overall mortality rate of 75% among patients with candidemia in a community hospital. Data collected in several studies[78,80,93,98-100] suggested that mortality rates among patients with candidemia varied depending on the underlying disease, and that not all of the deaths were due to the infection.

32.2.7 ENDOGENOUS CANDIDAL ENDOPHTHALMITIS

Contrary to exogenous candidal endophthalmitis, which is associated with either accidental or iatrogenic (postoperative) injury of the eye and inoculation of the pathogen from the environment, the endogenous (hematogenous) candidal endophthalmitis (HCE) results from hematogenous seeding of the eye corollary to dissemination.[101-103] However, some patients, such as heroin addicts, have been diagnosed with HCE without any evidence of candidal infection elsewere.[104-110]

The HCE lesions represent usually retinal and/or vitreal abscess containing a dense accumulation of inflammatory cells. The most frequent etiologic agent of HCE is *C. albicans* with very few cases caused by other *Candida* species (*C. parapsilosis, C. krusei, C. tropicalis*).[111-119] The reasons for the higher propensity of *C. albicans* for HCE[120,121] are still unknown.[101]

32.2.8 CANDIDAL INFECTION OF THE CENTRAL NERVOUS SYSTEM

Candida-associated infection of the central nervous system secondary to dissemination is not unusual and has been reported on numerous occasions.[101,122-126] Its occurrence has been especially common in cases of endocarditis.[127]

Among the various *Candida* spp., *C. albicans*,[126,128-131] *C. tropicalis*,[132,133] *C. lusitaniae*,[134,135] *C. parapsilosis*,[125,136] and *C. glabrata*[137] have been most frequently diagnosed as causative agents.

Similarly to other manifestations of disseminated candidiasis, predisposing factors for *Candida*-associated CNS involvement include immunosuppressive and antibiotic therapies, malignancies, neurosurgery or neurosurgical shunts, diabetes, hyperalimentation, alcoholism, chronic organ impairment (cirrhosis), intravenous drug use, and intravenous catheters.[101] In addition, candidal meningitis has been associated with immunodeficiency syndrome, such as severe combined immunodeficiency,[138] chronic mucocutaneous candidiasis,[139] chronic granulomatous disease,[128] and AIDS.[140]

Candida-associated mass lesions have been observed in the cerebral cortex,[126] cerebellum,[141] and the spinal cord.[142,143] Patients presented with aphasia, hemiparesis, focal seizure, papilledema,[126] nystagmus, ataxia,[141] and paralysis.[142,143]

The mortality rate for patients with candidal meningitis, especially after the introduction of the newer antimycotics[124] has been relatively low as compared to other forms of disseminated candidiasis.[101,129] By comparison, prognosis of patients with *Candida* brain abscess is usually poor.[101] Thus, only 1 of 16 patients with brain abscess or granuloma survived for more than 4 months after the diagnosis was made, whereas 18 of 27 patients with candidal meningitis survived.[126]

Chronic meningitis is an uncommon manifestation of candidiasis.[144] In general, the infection, which is characterized by headache, fever, and nuchal rigidity, can mimic tuberculosis, and the more common fungal meningitides, such as cryptococcosis.

32.2.9 CANDIDAL ENDOCARDITIS

Candida-associated endocarditis is a recognized but uncommon complication of disseminated infection.[145-147] Even patients with AIDS, who are frequently infected with *Candida* spp., rarely present with candidal endocarditis.

The aortic and mitral valves have been most often infected in native valve candidal endocarditis;[148-156] involvement of multiple valves has also been reported.[147,157] *C. albicans* is the most commonly isolated species, although drug addicts frequently have predilection for *C. parapsilosis*[158] and other *Candida* spp. (*C. guillermondi, C. krusei, C. stellatoidea, C. tropicalis,* and *C. glabrata*).

32.2.10 GENITAL CANDIDIASIS

C. albicans has been the most common yeast (85% to 90%) isolated from the vagina;[50,159,160] of the remaining species, *C. glabrata* and *C. tropicalis* have also been isolated.[159-161] One reason for the preponderance of *C. albicans* infections is its markedly higher ability to adhere to the vaginal epithelium (exfoliated vaginal and buccal epithelial cells) as compared to non-*albicans* species.[162] However, although still infrequent, non-*albicans Candida* infections are rising dramatically.[163]

Vulvovaginal candidiasis, which is a common infection reported worldwide, is the most frequent cause of acute vaginitis in tropical regions. In the U.S., *Candida* sp. is the second most common cause of vaginal infections, with bacterial vaginosis being the most common diagnostic entity.[164]

Vulvar pruritis, which is present virtually in all symptomatic patients, is the most frequent manifestation of vulvovaginal candidiasis.[50,165]

32.2.11 URINARY AND PERITONEAL CANDIDIASIS

Lower urinary tract candidal infections are very common, and may be community- or hospital (nosocomial)-acquired.[166] Among the predisposing factors, hospitalized patients with indwelling bladder catheters are at higher risk,[167-171] as well as patients with diabetes mellitus, those on broad-spectrum antibiotic therapy, immunosuppressed patients, and female patients.[172,173] In diabetic patients, the presence of single or multiple bezoars, or fungus balls, in the upper urinary tract have been observed; these symptoms may be associated with papillary necrosis.[174-178]

Jenks et al.[179] have reported an unusual case of *C. glabrata*-associated epididymo-orchitis in an 83-year-old diabetic patient with urinary outflow obstruction and previous bladder malignancy.

The upper urinary tract candidal infections[166] may be divided into primary infections (which develop by ascending route from the bladder), and secondary infections resulting from hematogenous spread of the fungus. The kidney, because of its high volume of blood, is one of the most commonly infected organs as a result of candidal dissemination. Chronically ill or immunosuppressed (often organ transplant recipients, and those receiving broad-spectrum antibiotic therapy) patients are at higher risk to develop renal fungus balls by *Candida* spp.[166]

32.2.12 RHEUMATOLOGIC INVOLVEMENT OF *CANDIDA* SPP.

Fungal arthritis due to *Candida* spp. infection is relatively rare and so far has been described in 45 cases.[180] The increased use of potent antibiotic and immunosuppressive therapies,[181] and especially the use of artificial joints, have been identified as the major predisposing factors to the infection. Weight-bearing joints, such as the knees (warm, tender, and swollen joints) have been more frequently affected.

Lasday and Jay[182] presented a case of candidal osteomyelitis in a patient with multiple risk factors for opportunistic infections.

32.2.13 NEONATAL CANDIDIASIS

Since 1966, when congenital and neonatal systemic candidiasis were first described,[183] it became an increasingly important nosocomial infection in very low-birth-weight neonates.[184-189] Dyke and Ott[190] have reported the presence of severe thrombocytopenia in extremely low-birth-weight infants with systemic candidiasis, which may be a useful indicator for this condition in such infants.

Total parenteral nutrition (TPN) has been reported to be a significant risk for neonatal candidiasis.[184,187,188,191] Prior therapy with antibiotics has been linked with candidemia.[184,187,192,193] In addition, the use of aminophylline, which decreases the candidicidal activity of neutrophils, and corticosteroids, which may change the bacterial flora or immune functions as immune modulators,[194] may increase the risk of neonatal candidiasis. Both aminophylline and the corticosteroids have been given to improve the respiratory status of premature infants.

Immunologic factors contributing to higher incidence of neonatal candidiasis include deficiency in the level of specific antibodies, and decreased concentrations of both classical and alternative complement pathway components,[195] as well as abnormalities in the functions (chemotaxis to the site of infection) of neutrophils and macrophages.[196] In addition, the T lymphocytes of neonates are naive and may fail to produce adequate concentrations of interferon (IFN)-γ when stimulated.[197,198]

The most common manifestation of neonatal oral candidiasis is thrush with or without a perineal rash.[186] In a small comparative study, infants with thrush treated with ketoconazole responded with better resolution of symptoms than those receiving nystatin, and with no apparent ketoconazole toxicity.[199]

In neonatal intensive care units, systemic candidiasis has been diagnosed in 1% to 3% of the infants, with blood being the most frequent site of isolation of the pathogen.[185,200]

Candida-associated obstructive uropathy caused by upper urinary tract fungal ball formation, although uncommon (only 35 cases described), is a well-recognized entity in neonates and infants. Premature birth, use of broad-spectrum antibiotics, prolonged hospital stay, and the use of intravascular catheters are predisposing factors. In addition, young age, small size, the presence of candidemia, and withholding antifungal therapy may be considered as poor prognostic factors contributing to a 35% mortality rate.[201] The use of intravenous amphotericin B and oral flucytosine has been the recommended treatment for this disorder.[201]

32.3 CANDIDAL INFECTIONS IN IMMUNOCOMPROMISED HOSTS

Virtually, all HIV-infected individuals with cutaneous candidiasis will harbor *C. albicans* as the pathogen, with *C. tropicalis* only rarely being diagnosed.[202] In patients with the AIDS-related complex (ARC), the observed perirectal pain and ulceration has often been associated with *C. albicans*. In female patients with HIV infection, candidal vaginitis is a recurring problem.

Oral candidiasis is the most common and usually the earliest opportunistic infection affecting HIV-positive patients.[203] It has been used as an initial manifestation of AIDS in all high-risk populations,[204] although by some accounts it is considered more prevalent in the homosexual HIV-infected population.[205]

If oral candidiasis is not treated, it may progress to candidal esophagitis.[206,207] In the HIV-infected persons, the latter may be presented with similar manifestations as herpes virus or cytomegalovirus disease, necessitating the use of esophagoscopy and biopsy to establish the diagnosis.

Hairy leukoplakia, which is a more imminent sign of impending AIDS should be differentiated from candidal infection by its reticulate, smooth plaque, typically found on the lateral side of the tongue which will not come off by scraping. Hairy leukoplakia is caused by the Epstein-Barr virus and will often carry herpes virus, papillomavirus, and candida as secondary invaders.[202]

As the CD4+ T helper cell population is progressively depleted, the development of systemic candidiasis in AIDS patients becomes increasingly likely.[202]

Invasive candidal infections remains also a major problem in transplant recipients. As in other groups of immunocompromised patients, empirical treatment with amphotericin B, as well as itraconazole and fluconazole, has increased the rates of survival.[208]

32.4 PATHOGENICITY OF *CANDIDA* SPP.

Together with *C. tropicalis*, *C. albicans* is considered to be the most virulent candidal species to humans. *C. albicans* is known with two serotypes, A and B.[209,210] While immunocompetent patients have equal likelihood of carrying either serotype A or B isolates, immunocompromised hosts, including those with AIDS, were twice as likely to be infected with serotype B.[211-213] In immunosuppressed patients, the incidence of disseminated candidiasis associated with more than one species was found to be less than 5%;[214] however, incidence ranging from 5% to 25% has been reported in other patient populations.[18,24]

C. lusitaniae infections, which have been associated with a high incidence of amphotericin B resistance, although still infrequent, have been serious enough to cause even death.[215-217]

One major factor contributing to *Candida* spp. virulence is their ability to persist on mucosal surfaces.[15,20,50,218,219] The strong adherence and persistence of *C. albicans* and *C. tropicalis* to epithelial cells or oral and vaginal mucosa have been closely correlated with their high pathogenicity.[218] In general, *C. albicans* has been found to adhere better to epithelial cells under conditions that facilitate germ tube formation.[220,221] Several different adherence mechanisms have been suggested.[222] Although the precise composition of candidal adherence molecules is still not clear, it is believed that they are surface glycoproteins such as mannoproteins,[223,224] and a lectin-like protein.[225] Fibronectin[226,227] and fibrin in the thrombi[220] have been suggested as host-cell receptors for *Candida* adhesins. Calderone and Braun[228] have provided evidence that the nature of the host immune receptors played a role in the adherence process.

Another factor involved in the pathogenesis of *Candida* is the secretion of enzymes, specifically proteinases and lipases, that enable the fungus to effectively compromise the integrity of host cell membranes and invade the tissues. Candidal proteinases (proteolytic and keratinolytic in nature) are capable of hydrolyzing peptide bonds[218] and have collagenolytic activity;[229] the phospholipases (demonstrated in *C. albicans*[230]) hydrolyze phosphoglycerides, whereas the lysophospholipases hydrolyze lysophosphoglycerides.[218]

Additional factors contributing to candidal pathogenicity include fungal cell surface hydrophobicity,[231-234] pH,[221] interference with the host immune functions (phagocytosis, complement activity, immune defenses),[20] fungal dimorphism (hyphal production) and phenotypic variability (switching), toxins, temperature, and synergism with other bacteria.[20,50,218,230,235]

Germ tube formation in the case of *C. albicans* has also been a factor[20,218] by directly penetrating the epithelial cell membrane, possibly with the help of phospholipase C or other hydrolytic enzymes.[236]

32.5 HOST IMMUNE DEFENSE AGAINST *CANDIDA ALBICANS*

While the stratified squamous epithelium of the skin is an effective barrier against microbial infections, and in particular *C. albicans*, the mucosal surfaces (mouth, gut, and the vagina) are much more vulnerable and become colonized by the fungus.[237,238] The interaction between *Candida* spp. and other bacteria is one very important environmental factor affecting the degree of candidal colonization of mucosal surfaces.[20,239-241]

Humoral immunity is less important in the defense against *Candida* spp. than phagocytes and cellular immune factors.[20,242] Sinha et al.[243] have demonstrated in B cell-deficient mice with experimental candidiasis that their cell-mediated responses were normal and B cell deficiency did not result in increased susceptibility to candidiasis.

Complement-deficient mice showed diminished resistance to *Candida* infections,[244] whereas in humans with hereditary C2 deficiency, the phagocytosis of *Candida* spp. has been flawed.[245] Further studies have shown that although complement in fresh serum was not directly candidicidal, it facilitated leukocyte chemotaxis towards the site of infection and enhanced the phagocytosis of *Candida* spp. by nonimmune-specific mechanisms.[246,247]

Studies by Caroline et al.[249] and Elin and Wolff[248] have shown that elevated serum levels of free unbound iron and transferrin stimulated the growth of *C. albicans*. While, in general, iron-deficient serum was inhibitory, it has been suggested that iron deficiency may predispose to oral candidiasis.[250] On the other hand, Vaughn and Weinberg[251] have found that copper may increase the virulence of *Candida* spp. in mice.

Phagocytosis carried out by neutrophils, eosinophils, monocytes, and other macrophage-like cells in the lung and reticuloendothelial system plays an important role in the immune defense response to *Candida* spp.[20] As reported by several groups, the high incidence of disseminated candidiasis in leukemic patients has been linked to neutropenia.[89,252-254]

It has been established that the candidicidal activity of neutrophils was associated with oxidative mechanisms involving interactions of hydrogen peroxide and myeloperoxidases, and possibly the release of lysosomal enzymes from specific granules.[255-257] A rise in the neutrophilic cytosolic calcium stimulated by opsonized and nonopsonized hyphae would trigger the respiratory burst with the response to nonopsonized hyphae being delayed.[258,259]

Another mechanism of neutrophil candidicidal activity involved the release by dying neutrophils of tumor necrosis factor (TNF),[260] a cytoplasmic cytokine which inhibits the fungal growth by competing for zinc[261] and defensins.[262] Drugs that inhibit neutrophil phagocytosis (such as antibiotics, corticosteroids, colchicine, and phenylbutazone) were found to reduce host resistance to *Candida* infections by negating the candidicidal activity of neutrophils.[256,263]

Other phagocytic cells, such as normal human peripheral blood monocytes, have been observed to phagocytose and kill *C. albicans in vitro* through myeloperoxidase involvement as well as other mechanisms when oxidative mechanisms were impaired.[264,265] Candidicidal activity was found also in rabbit alveolar and peritoneal macrophages;[266] human alveolar macrophages have been demonstrated to be phagocytic[267] and may be candidicidal.[268] Impairment of host monocyte-macrophage functions by corticosteroids,[269] or infections by parainfluenza I (Sendai) virus[270] or cytomegalovirus[241] led to increased susceptibility to candidal infections. On the other hand, macrophage-activating agents, such as Freund's adjuvant,[89] *Corynebacterium parvum*,[271] and muramyl dipeptide and its analogs,[272,273] have been shown to enhance host resistance to *Candida* infections *in vivo*, thereby leaving open the possibility for their clinical use as nonspecific enhancers of host resistance.[20]

In several studies,[274-278] the ability of macrophages to detect and destroy the yeast and hyphal forms of *Candida* have been demonstrated. In addition, macrophage colony-stimulating factor (M-CSF) was shown to increase the candidicidal activity of macrophages.[279]

A number of cytokines have also been implicated in the regulation of monocyte-macrophage anticandidal activities. Thus, IFN-γ was shown to augment the candidicidal ability of macrophages by improving superoxide anion generation and phagocytosis.[280] Furthermore, IFN-γ enhanced the cidal activity of alveolar macrophages and monocytes by inducing TNF and IL-1 secretion[281] and by augmenting the generation of proteinaceous substances by increasing the acidification of phagolysosomes.[282]

Leshem et al.[283] investigated the ability of IL-1, IL-2, IL-3, and GM-CSF to potentiate hematopoietic activity *in vitro* and *in vivo* in normal, immunosuppressed, and bone marrow transplanted mice against *C. albicans* infection. IL-1 alone or combined with other cytokines showed the best protective activity in normal and immunocompromised mice.

In an experimental trial,[284] recombinant granulocyte-macrophage colony-stimulating factor (GM-CSF) was shown to reduce the lung injury and mortality of naive (neutrophil-replete) and neutropenic rats during *Candida* sepsis. In addition, IL-3 and GM-CSF also regulated the activity of monocytes by pathways different from those of IFN-γ.[285] GM-CSF also increased the candidicidal activity of monocytes by enhancing superoxide anion secretion,[286] augmenting the number of mannose receptors on the surface of monocytes,[287] and by decreasing complement C3 factor production.[288]

Hill et al.[289] have demonstrated that treatment with GM-CSF significantly enhanced the survival of malnourished mice infected with *C. albicans* by stimulating the production of IL-6, superoxide anion, and nitric oxide in splenic macrophages, and decreasing IL-4 production from splenocytes.

Studies by Louie et al.[290] in a murine model of fatal disseminated candidiasis demonstrated that endogenously produced tumor necrosis factor (TNF)-α prolonged the survival of the infected host. Exogenous TNF-α and drugs that increase the endogenous production of TNF-α may prove useful adjuncts to azole antimycotics. Data by Netea et al.[291] have shown that pharmacologic inhibitors of TNF-α production (pentoxifylline, chlorpromazine, thalidomide) worsened the outcome in *C. albicans*-infected mice. Both TNF-α and IL-1β are the principal mediators of septic shock, and inhibition of TNF-α production may ameliorate the outcome in severe infections.

di Francesco et al.[292] have found that thymosin α1 (a thymus-derived immunostimulant) in combination with fluconazole promoted the recovery of normal NK cell activity and intracellular killing of *C. albicans* by polymorphonuclear leukocytes in morphine-immunosuppressed mice.

The role of cell-mediated immunity (CMI) against *Candida* infections has been the subject of extensive studies.[20] While there has been strong evidence that anticandidal protection correlated better with cellular rather than humoral immunity,[242,293] in particular, when immunity was associated with the passive transfer of immune lymphocytes but not with immune serum,[294] some investigators disagreed.[295,296] However, the mechanisms by which the lymphocytes may control *Candida* have been only partially defined. For example, Pearsall et al.[297] have shown that lymphokine-like substances released from antigen- or mutagen-activated lymphocytes were toxic to *C. albicans*, and Sen et al.[298] observed a protective effect against *Candida* infections of a human dialyzable leukocyte extract. In addition, IL-2-induced lymph node cells with functional and phenotypic characteristics similar to those of activated NK cells, have been shown to inhibit the growth of *C. albicans* hyphae.[299] However, NK cells themselves were unable to kill *Candida* yeast cells.[300]

One important confirmation of the role of cell-mediated immunity in resistance to *Candida* infection was the findings that specific defects in CMI observed in patients with chronic mucocutaneous candidiasis,[301-306] patients receiving immunosuppressive (corticosteroids) therapy,[307-309] and HIV-infected patients[310] failed to adequately protect the hosts against candidiasis.

32.5.1 Reconstitution of Defective Cell-Mediated Immunity

A number of studies have been conducted attempting to correct defects of cell-mediated immunity by either transplantation of bone marrow or thymic tissue,[311-314] or injections of thymic peptides,[315] with variable results.

C. albicans-specific transfer factor has also been used to treat chronic candidiasis.[316] Transfer factors are peptide molecules of approximately 5 kDA that are thought capable of "transferring" antigen-specific cell-mediated immunity from immune donors to nonimmune recipients.[317-319]

32.6 STUDIES ON THERAPEUTICS

32.6.1 Amphotericin B

Martino et al.[320] investigated prospectively the association between colonization with *Candida* spp., subsequent occurrence of invasive candidiasis, and empiric use of amphotericin B in 139 neutropenic patients with hematologic malignancies. The data showed that treatment with amphotericin B was required in 67% of patients colonized in multiple noncontiguous body sites (multicolonization) vs. 31% of patients colonized in single or contiguous sites (monocolonization), and in 21% of noncolonized patients (p = .0037 and 0.00026, respectively).

The clinical efficacy of intraluminal amphotericin B treatment of central venous catheter candidal infections in patients receiving parenteral nutrition at home was evaluated by Benoit et al.[321] Although the infection in the subcutaneously tunneled catheter was suppressed during treatment, the patients later relapsed.

The efficacy of escalating doses of liposomal amphotericin B (AmBisome) was examined in immunosuppressed (neutropenic) CF1 mice against hematogenous *C. lusitaniae* and *C. krusei* infections.[322] The mice were treated with daily doses of either 1.0 to 2.0 mg/kg of amphotericin B desoxycholate, escalating doses of liposomal amphotericin B (8.0 to 30.0 mg/kg) or left untreated. While higher doses of the liposomal formulation were equipotent to a standard dose of amphotericin B desoxycholate in prolonging survival, they were significantly more effective in reducing the fungal burden in the kidneys of animals infected with drug-susceptible strains of both *C. lusitaniae* and *C. krusei*.

The *in vitro* anticandidal activity, toxicity, blood residence time, and therapeutic efficacy of pegylated amphotericin B liposomes (PEG-AmB-LIP) were compared with those of laboratory-prepared nonpegylated amphotericin B liposomes (AmB-LIP; a formulation with a lipid composition the same as that in AmBisome), and commercially prepared AmBisome.[323] The *in vivo* evaluations were conducted in a model of systemic candidiasis in leukopenic mice at a dose of 5.0 mg/kg of amphotericin B; while PEG-AmB-LIP was completely effective, AmB-LIP was partially effective, and AmBisome was ineffective. At 11 mg/kg, AmB-LIP was still partially effective, whereas at 29 mg/kg AmBisome was completely effective.

In a recent report, Sivakumara et al.[324] have shown that a liposomal preparation of amphotericin B (AmBisome) failed to prevent development of *C. glabrata* fungemia in a patient with relapsed acute promyelocytic leukemia, whereas the conventional form of the antibiotic, at a much lower dose, rapidly controlled the fungemia. AmBisome was initially given at 150 mg daily, and the dose regimen increased 4 d later to 200 mg (3.0 mg/kg) daily. Due to continuing persistent candidemia and progression of pulmonary lesion, AmBisome was discontinued and conventional amphotericin B was reintroduced at a dose of 60 mg every other day leading to subsidence of candidemia within 5 d. In another study,[325] however, an 8-week course of liposomal amphotericin B led to a marked clinical improvement in a 4-year-old patient with acute lymphoblastic leukemia who developed hepatic candidiasis during the consolidation phase.

Atkinson at al.[326] have established a model of immunosuppressed mice to study and to compare the therapeutic efficacies of amphotericin B, fluconazole, and flucytosine and their combination against *C. glabrata* infections. After 5 d of treatment, amphotericin B was shown to be superior to both fluconazole and flucytosine used alone. Furthermore, the combination of fluconazole and flucytosine was also superior to either of the two agents given alone in reducing the fungal burden in kidney tissue in one isolate to *C. glabrata*. While high doses of fluconazole alone produced modest reductions in kidney counts, it did not reduce spleen tissue counts. In general, there was poor correlation between *in vitro* MIC values and the *in vivo* results.[326]

DU-6859a, an investigational fluoroquinoline agent with potent bactericidal activity, but itself inactive against *Candida* spp., when combined with amphotericin B, clearly enhanced the antibiotic's anticandidal activity in the *in vitro* microdilution assay.[327] In an *in vitro* time-kill study, combination of DU-6859a with amphotericin B in a concentration-dependent fashion significantly suppressed the regrowth of *C. albicans* as compared with amphotericin B alone. Furthermore, the combination prolonged the survival of *C. albicans*-infected mice by markedly reducing fungal load in the infected kidneys. A similar synergistic effect was also observed with the combination of DU-6859a and fluconazole.[327]

The activity of MS-8209, a new water-soluble nonester derivative of amphotericin B, has been examined in several murine models of systemic fungal infections.[328] Thus, against systemic candidiasis, MS-8209 at 15 mg/kg significantly increased the survival time compared to amphotericin B deoxycholate; both compounds were equally effective in reducing the colony-forming units (CFU) counts in the kidney.

32.6.2 FLUCONAZOLE

Mice infected with a series of fluconazole-susceptible and -nonsusceptible *Candida* strains were treated with varying doses of fluconazole beginning 1 d postinfection.[329] For all fluconazole-susceptible isolates, the drug was highly effective at <0.25 mg/kg (b.i.d.); to the contrary, against fluconazole-resistant isolates, fluconazole was ineffective at doses of 40 mg/kg or higher. These results indicated that although not very precise, *in vitro* susceptibility testing of *C. albicans* may be used to predict *in vivo* response to fluconazole.[329]

Antifungal combination therapy with G-CSF and fluconazole in a mouse model of experimental disseminated candidiasis has shown that although G-CSF had no direct activity, its combination with fluconazole extended the survival rate and reduced the renal tissue counts beyond those for fluconazole given alone.[330]

de Pauw et al.[88] studied the efficacy and toxicity of fluconazole in an open noncomparative trial involving 24 patients (9 of them with acute, and the remaining 15 with chronic disseminated, candidiasis). The drug was administered intravenously for the first 3 d at a dose of 200 mg b.i.d., followed by 200 mg twice daily orally until resolution of signs and symptoms or evident treatment failure. Clinical response was achieved in 67% of cases with acute disseminated disease and in 86% of cases of chronic disseminated candidiasis; the median duration of therapy was 15 d and 6 months, respectively. No apparent drug-related toxicity was observed.[88]

Gearhart[331] observed worsening of liver functions (elevation in aspartate aminotransferase, alanine aminotransferase, total bilirubin concentrations, as well as increased prothrombin time and activated partial thromboplastin time) in a patient with hepatitis when treated with fluconazole for candidiasis. After discontinuation of fluconazole treatment, the liver parameters returned to their normal baseline levels.

32.6.3 CLOTRIMAZOLE

In vitro studies to evaluate the effect of C. albicans infection and clotrimazole treatment on the vaginal microflora have been carried out by Ross et al.[332] Using a model simulating the healthy vaginal ecosystem (a mixed culture of Lactobacillus acidophylus, Staphylococcus epidermidis, Prevotella bivia, and group D Staphylococcus sp. grown in continuous culture in a chemically defined medium), the investigators have demonstrated that challenge of the model with C. albicans was followed by the development (within 24 h) of abnormal microbial populations. Treatment with clotrimazole (100 µg/ml) resulted in a decrease in C. albicans counts within 48 h. However, clotrimazole also altered other components of the vaginal microflora, which did not return to normal. Furthermore, addition of clotrimazole (100 µg/ml) to the model system in the absence of C. albicans also had deleterious effects on the components of the normal vaginal microflora resulting in an abnormal model by 24 h.[332]

32.6.4 COMPOUND D0870

A new triazole antimycotic, D0870, has been evaluated in vitro against 100 C. albicans strains isolated from the oral cavities of HIV-infected patients using a broth macrodilution assay.[333] Fifty of the isolates were fluconazole-susceptible (MIC = 4.0 µg/ml or less) and 50 were fluconazole-resistant (MIC = 8.0 µg/ml or higher). The results showed that while in 90% of all strains tested, the MIC values of D0870 were 0.5 µg/ml, the MIC values for fluconazole-susceptible strains were lower than those for the fluconazole-resistant isolates.[333] Results by Barchiesi et al.[334] were in agreement with these findings.

Atkinson et al.[335] used an immunosuppressed mouse model for disseminated C. glabrata infection to evaluate the efficacy of D0870 and compare its activity to those of amphotericin B, fluconazole, as well as their combinations. D0870 and fluconazole were administered orally at doses of 1.0 to 50 mg/kg (daily or on alternate days) and 100 mg/kg (b.i.d.), respectively; amphotericin B (3.0 mg/kg daily) was injected intraperitoneally. After a 5-d course, D0870 (at 5.0 mg/kg daily) significantly reduced the fungal counts in kidney and spleen tissues ($p < .05$), while amphotericin B was modestly effective; the combination of D0870 (25 mg/kg) and amphotericin B (3.0 mg/kg) was markedly more effective than either drug alone ($p < .01$). There were, however, three C. glabrata strains that showed resistance to D0870 (MIC = 4.0 µg/ml).[335]

32.6.5 COMPOUND SCH 39304

SCH 39304 is a new broad-spectrum triazole antifungal agent topically and orally active against C. albicans vaginal infections.[336] The drug represents a 50:50 mixture of two enantiomers, SCH 42427 and SCH 42426.

When compared to fluconazole in a hamster model, SCH 39304, when given orally at 1.6 mg/kg for 4 d, showed 100% cure rate and was fourfold more active than fluconazole. In addition, a single oral dose of 10 mg/kg of SCH 39304 also cured all hamsters. In topical intravaginal treatment for 8 d, SCH 39304 was again more active than fluconazole (twofold) with 100% cure rate at concentrations as low as 0.025%.[336]

The pharmacokinetic profile of SCH 39304 was investigated in 17 HIV-positive male patients.[337] Following the ingestion of a single daily dose of 200 mg for 16 d, wide intersubject variations in SCH 39304 plasma concentration-vs.-time profiles were observed on each study day. Drug absorption appeared to be slow with mean day 1 peak plasma concentrations of 1.2 µg/ml at 2.1 h (50 mg) and 3.9 µg/ml at 4 h (200 mg) after drug administration. The mean peak plasma concentrations of SCH 39304 on day 16 were 7.6 µg/ml at 4.3 h (50 mg) and 17.2 µg/ml at 3.2 h (200 mg) after drug administration.[337]

The efficacies of SCH 39304, fluconazole, and ketoconazole were compared against systemic *C. albicans* infection in mice.[338] In normal mice, SCH 39304 at 0.5 mg/kg (once daily, orally) was 3 and 200 times more active than fluconazole and ketoconazole, respectively. In immuno-compromised mice, SCH 39304 (1.3 mg/kg, once daily, orally) was 35 and >100 times more active than fluconazole and ketoconazole, respectively. Furthermore, SCH 39304 was equally effective after either oral or intravenous administration.

The *in vivo* and *in vitro* activities of SCH 39304, SCH 42426, and SCH 42427 have been investigated by Loebenberg et al.[339] SCH 42427 was twofold more potent *in vitro* than SCH 39304, while SCH 42426 was inactive. In systemic *C. albicans* in mice, SCH 42427 and SCH 39304 when given orally showed ED_{50} values of 0.47 and 0.62 mg/kg, respectively; the corresponding value of SCH 42426 was over 100 mg/kg. In *C. albicans* vaginal infection in hamsters, the ED_{50} values of SCH 42427, SCH 39304, and SCH 42426 were 3.5, 8.5, and 320 mg/kg, respectively. The results clearly indicated that enantiomer SCH 42427 was responsible for all of the antifungal activity observed with SCH 39304.[339]

32.6.6 SERTACONAZOLE

Sertaconazole, a new benzo[*b*]thiophene imidazole derivative was tested for efficacy in a randomized, parallel, double-blind clinical trial in patients with *C. albicans* superficial mycosis.[340] The drug, which was applied as either 1% or 2% cream for a period of 20 d, showed high efficacy in 19 of 20 patients with no relapse of infection occurring.

32.6.7 LANOCONAZOLE

The therapeutic activity of 1% cream and 1% solution of lanoconazole, a new imidazole antimycotic, has been examined in experimental cutaneous candidiasis in prednisolone-treated guinea pigs.[341] Once-a-day application of both lanoconazole formulations was found markedly superior to that of comparable formulations of bifonazole.

32.6.8 ALLYLAMINE DERIVATIVES

A number of allylamine antimycotics (terbinafine, amorolfine) have been shown to be orally and topically active against a broad range of dermatophyte, filamentous, dimorphic, and dematiaceous fungi, including candidal infections.[342,343] Amorolfine has shown a long retention time in the horny layer of the skin. In vaginal candidiasis, 0.1% amorolfine cleared the vagina of viable *Candida* cells in rats.[343]

32.6.9 [α-(1*H*-IMIDAZOL-1-YL)ARYLMETHYL]PYRROLES

A new class of 3-aryl-4-[α-(1*H*-imidazol-1-yl)arylmethyl]pyrrole derivatives have been described to possess potent anticandidal activity (*C. albicans* and other *Candida* spp.) both *in vitro* and *in vivo* (rabbit skin candidiasis). The most active congeners have shown MIC_{90} values comparable or twofold better than that of bifonazole and two to four times greater than those of miconazole and ketoconazole.[344]

32.6.10 ANTICANDIDAL LIPOPEPTIDES

WF11899A, -B, and -C, three novel water-soluble lipopeptides structurally related to the echinocandins, have been shown to exert potent anti-*C. albicans* activities in microbroth assay at concentrations of 0.004 to 0.03 μg/ml.[345] The 1,3-β-glucan synthase was inhibited by these compounds with IC_{50} concentrations of 0.7, 0.7, and 1.8 μg/ml for WF11899A, -B, and -C, respectively. However, the compounds also hemolysed mouse red blood cells *in vitro* at a concentration of 62 µg/ml.[345]

A new generation of semisynthetic amine derivatives of the natural product pneumocandin B_0 (L-688786)[346] has been developed.[347] These new lipopeptides have shown enhanced potencies and expanded spectrum of *in vivo* antifungal activity (specifically against *Candida* spp.[348-350] and *Pneumocystis carinii*[348,349,351]) compared to the parent pneumocandin B_0, as well as improved pharmacokinetic profiles in rodents and rhesus monkeys.[352] *In vivo* efficacies have been demonstrated in animal models of disseminated candidiasis,[349,350,353] and oropharyngeal and gastrointestinal candidiases.[354] Their fungicidal mode of action involves inhibition of the biosynthesis of the fungal cell wall 1,3-β-D-glucan. The latter, a critical nonmammalian structural component of the cell wall, provides structural integrity and osmotic stability to the wall. One of these analogs, L-733560, is a semisynthetic hybrid that has been derived from L-731373 and L-705589, two other derivatives of pneumocandin B_0. All three compounds, which represented water-soluble cyclic hexapeptides containing a fatty acyl side chain, were found to be 10- to 100-fold more potent inhibitors of 1,3-β-D-glucan biosynthesis than pneumocandin B_0.[348,350,355,356]

The efficacies of cilofungin (Ly121019), a semisynthetic lipopeptide, and amphotericin B in the treatment of disseminated candidiasis in normal and neutropenic mice have been investigated.[357] Doses of 25 or 35 mg/kg, given by intraperitoneal injection for 10 d produced survival rates of 83% and 90%, respectively. By comparison, intravenous amphotericin B at 1.0 mg/kg once daily elicited 93% survival. Granulocytopenic mice showed survival rates of 83% and 80% when treated with 25 or 35 mg/kg cilofungin for 10 d, compared with 43% survival rate in mice treated with 1.0 mg/kg of amphotericin B (p = .0030 and .0080, respectively). Cilofungin eradicated *C. albicans* from the kidney, spleens, and the livers of the surviving animals, with no apparent toxic side effects at any dosage regimens used.[357]

32.6.11 NIKKOMYCINS

The anticandidal activities of nikkomycins X and Z, two competitive inhibitors of fungal chitin synthetase, have been investigated both *in vitro* and *in vivo*.[358,359] Nikkomycin Z was shown to be a strong inhibitor of *C. albicans* chitin biosynthesis *in vitro* and *in vivo* in two different mouse infection models.[358] In addition, both nikkomycins acted synergistically with several azole antifungals against *C. albicans* isolates; however, no synergistic effects were demonstrated against *C. tropicalis*, *C. parapsilosis*, and *C. krusei*, although against the latter two species the results suggested an additive effect.[359] In a *C. albicans*-infected mouse model, nikkomycin Z (at single doses ranging from 5.0 to 50 mg/kg, given twice daily) was effective in delaying the onset of mortality but showed no dose-response effect.[359]

32.6.12 DRUG RESISTANCE OF CANDIDA SPP.

The incidence of invasive infections with *Candida* spp. has dramatically increased during the past several decades due to the overgrowing population of immunocompromised patients. Particularly in HIV-infected individuals, the yeast may develop resistance to fungistatic drugs as the result of altered species and the extensive use of azole antimycotics.[360] Thus, the emergence of fluconazole-resistant strains of *Candida* spp.[334,361,362] after its repeated use (at daily doses as high as 400–800 mg) for therapy of mucosal candidiasis (oropharyngeal, esophageal, and vaginal) has been reported in patients with HIV infection.[363-376] Amphotericin B is usually effective initially but requires parenteral administration. To circumvent fluconazole resistance, Dewsnup and Stevens[377] have used an oral formulation of amphotericin B to treat successfully two AIDS patients with oral thrush caused by fluconazole-resistant *C. glabrata* infection; improvement in both patients was noticed in less than 1 week, with eventual clearing and absence of side effects.

Several mechanisms of fluconazole resistance have been postulated, including reduced fungal cell wall permeability to azoles,[378] reduced sensitivity[379] or levels of target enzyme lanosterol 14α-demethylase, reduced sterol C5-6 saturase activity,[380] and the overproduction of target cytochrome P 450.[381] The variety of resistance mechanisms may account for the apparent occurrence of both azole cross-resistance and sole fluconazole resistance, both clinically and *in vitro*.[373]

Evidence reported by Venkateswarlu et al.[382] have suggested the presence of correlation between resistance to fluconazole in AIDS patients with mucosal candidiasis and the reduced (6- to 10-fold) intracellular accumulation of the drug. The observed resistance was not associated with a change in the target enzyme (sterol 14α-demethylase), as indicated by the equivalent levels of fluconazole inhibition of activity in extracts from all fungal isolates studied, or by mutations in sterol $\Delta^{5,6}$-desaturase as previously observed in *Saccharomyces cerevisiae* and *Ustilago maydis*.

St.-Germain et al.[383] have examined 255 *C. albicans* isolates collected from 93 HIV-infected patients and found very low incidence of resistance ($IC_{50} > 0.25$ mg/l) for either ketoconazole or itraconazole.

Resistance of *Candida* spp. to amphotericin B has been rare (see also the sections on *C. lusitaniae*, *C. rugosa*, and *C. guilliermondii* below).[384]

C. rugosa isolates from burn patients treated with topical nystatin were analyzed retrospectively and demonstrated resistance to nystatin and moderate susceptibility to amphotericin B and fluconazole.[385]

32.7 EVOLUTION OF THERAPIES AND TREATMENT OF CANDIDIASIS

32.7.1 CUTANEOUS CANDIDIASIS

The therapy of cutaneous candidiasis is best determined after evaluation of the location, the extent of involvement, and the immune status of the patient.[29] It could involve both topical and/or oral therapy. In case of immunocompromised patients, especially in extensive fungal involvement, systemic antimycotic therapy may be required. Both oral ketoconazole and fluconazole have been used, with the latter being preferred when treating resistant organisms.

In a double-blind, randomized study of 40 patients with culturally proven dermatophytosis (pityriasis versicolor) or cutaneous candidiasis, del Palacio et al.[386] compared the efficacy and tolerance of flutrimazole and bifonazole (both as 1% solutions applied once daily for 4 weeks). At the end of therapy, negative microscopy and cultures were recorded in 85% of the flutrimazole group and 65% in the bifonazole group. However, there was significant difference in the efficacy: 80% of the flutrimazole-treated patients received effective treatment, as compared to only 40% in the bifonazole group.

Topical antifungal therapy may be added in conjunction with systemic medication, or used alone in less extensive disease.[29] Topical nystatin and amphotericin B have not been effective against cutaneous candidiasis and have been largely supplanted by the more effective azole (ketoconazole, miconazole, clotrimazole, econazole) antimycotics.

In a multicenter, randomized, double-blind, double-dummy trial, Stengel et al.[387] compared the therapeutic activities of fluconazole and ketoconazole in the treatment of cutaneous candidiasis and dermatophytoses (tinea corporis, tinea cruris) lasting for 2 to 4 weeks. The patients received either fluconazole (150 mg once weekly, plus daily placebo), or ketoconazole (200 mg once daily plus weekly placebo for 2 to 6 weeks). The results have shown that both drug regimens were equally effective in terms of clinical and mycological cure rates, with fluconazole having the advantage of once-weekly oral administration that is not only more cost effective but also may improve patient compliance.[388]

32.7.2 CHRONIC MUCOCUTANEOUS CANDIDIASIS

Amphotericin B, which at one time was used exclusively in the treatment of chronic mucocutaneous candidiasis,[306] has been substituted by oral systemic azole antifungals. Polizzi et al.[389] have evaluated the clinical efficacy of a 16-month course of cimetidine (400 mg, t.i.d.) and zinc sulfate (200 mg, daily) in a patient with chronic mucocutaneous candidiasis. The favorable response was attributed to the immunopotentiating effect of the combined treatment.

32.7.3 ORAL AND ESOPHAGEAL CANDIDIASIS

In addition to oral systemic therapy, topical antimycotics, such as clotrimazole buccal troches, have been effective in the treatment of chronic oral candidiasis without developing evidence of drug resistance.[34] However, if no maintenance suppressive antifungal therapy is applied, nearly all patients with HIV and successfully treated esophageal candidiasis develop a recurrence, usually within 2 to 3 months.[390]

Initial treatment of oral and esophageal candidiasis should be focused on minimizing predisposing factors. Subsequent therapy would consist of either topical or systemic agents according to the clinical status of the patient (Table 32.1).[39,202,392] In HIV-infected patients, a recommended regimen consists of nystatin suspension (usually 5.0 ml of nystatin, four times daily) or clotrimazole trochet (four times daily), or both.[202] Although in the early stages of HIV infection this regimen is usually effective, candida recurrence is nearly a certainty and patients may have to be on this regimen continuously.[202] Encarnacion and Chin[391] have determined the salivary nystatin concentrations after administration of an osmotic-controlled release tablet for oral cavity therapy. The tablet was designed to deliver approximately 200,000 U of nystatin over 2-h dosing; the mean salivary drug concentrations, which consistently exceeded those produced by a pastille at the same time points, were 279 µg/ml, 654 µg/ml, and 532 µg/ml at 30, 60, and 120 min, respectively.

Systemic therapy is usually considered for immunocompromised patients (with granulocytopenia, or receiving immunosuppressive therapy) who are at high risk for dissemination, or for patients unresponsive to topical therapy.[39] In a prospective study in AIDS patients with esophageal

---

TABLE 32.1
Treatment of Oral and Esophageal Candidiasis

Drug	Dose
Topical	
Nystatin	0–30 ml (1–3,000,000 U), 4–5 times daily (swish and swallow)
Clotrimazole	1 troche (10 mg), 4–5 times daily
Systemic	
Ketoconazole	200–400 mg daily, orally[a]
Fluconazole	50–200 mg daily, orally
Itraconazole	100–200 mg daily, orally[b]
Amphotericin B	0.4–0.6 mg/kg daily, IV

[a] Proper gastric acidity is required for adequate absorption.

[b] Taken with food and proper gastric acidity to ensure adequate absorption.

Data from Refs. 39, 202, and 392.

candidiasis, Laine and Rabeneck[392] examined the clinical efficacy of fluconazole suspensions (200 mg loading dose followed by 100 mg, q.d.s.). The therapy, which was implemented for 2 weeks after symptom resolution, was successful in all 41 evaluable patients.

Newton et al.[393] have implemented weekly fluconazole therapy for the suppression of recurrent thrush in HIV-infected patients. However, Azon-Masoliver and Vilaplana[394] reported a case of an HIV-infected patient who developed a toxic epidermal necrolysis affecting over 70% of the body surface area and severe mucosal involvement after starting fluconazole for a recurrent oral trush with dysphagia.

In an open phase III clinical trial of 103 HIV-infected patients with oral candidiasis, therapy with oral fluconazole at 100 mg daily for 7 to 21 d, achieved clinical cure in 71% of patients and improvement in another 16%; mycological tests revealed elimination in 57% and reduction in colony counts in 23% of patients.[395] Just-Nübling et al.[396] conducted a randomized, open-label clinical trial of fluconazole as a prophylactic treatment for recurrent oral candidiasis in AIDS patients with CD4+ of less than 100 cells/mm^3. As compared to untreated controls, of the 58 evaluable patients who received fluconazole at either 50 or 100 mg daily (observation time: 137 to 215 d) prophylaxis significantly reduced the frequency of candidiasis relapse. The two fluconazole doses were equally effective.

In comparison with other drugs used to treat mucosal candidiasis in HIV-infected patients, fluconazole was found to be superior to nystatin, similar to itraconazole, and at least as effective as clotrimazole and ketoconazole.[397] Furthermore, in a study of AIDS patients with candidal esophagitis, fluconazole was shown to elicit a rapid clinical response that may necessitate only a 1-week course of empiric treatment for newly developed esophageal symptoms.[398]

In a multicenter, prospective, and randomized trial of 334 HIV-infected patients with oropharyngeal candidiasis, Pons et al.[399] have found a 2-week course of oral fluconazole (100 mg daily) and clotrimazole troches (10 mg orally five times daily) to be equally effective; the clinical response was statistically equivalent in both groups: 98% and 94% of fluconazole and clotrimazole recipients, respectively, were cured or improved. Furthermore, fluconazole was more effective in eliminating *C. albicans* from the oral flora (65% vs. 48%) and maintaining an asymptomatic state through 2 weeks of follow-up examination (82.3% vs. 50%).[399]

In patients undergoing chemotherapy or bone marrow transplant recipients, fluconazole as primary prophylaxis has shown greater clinical benefit than clotrimazole.

In a double-blind, randomized study of 102 HIV-infected patients with endoscopically diagnosed esophageal candidiasis, Barbaro and Di Lorenzo[400] have compared the therapeutic efficacies of orally given fluconazole and itraconazole. Two groups of 60 patients each received a 3-week course of either fluconazole (100 mg, b.i.d.) or itraconazole (100 mg, b.i.d.), and were monitored for another 2 months post-therapy. The results showed complete remission of endoscopic lesions in 45 patients (75%) from the fluconazole group and in 23 patients (38%) from the itraconazole group (*p* <.001); partial remission was achieved in 25% and 47% of patients from the fluconazole and itraconazole groups, respectively. In each group, the number of nonresponders was the same (9 patients; 15%). Complete clinical remission was observed in 47 patients (78%) in the fluconazole group and in 44 patients (73%) in the itraconazole group. Partial clinical remission was shown in 22% and 20% of the fluconazole and itraconazole groups, respectively, and no clinical response was observed in four patients (7%) from the itraconazole group. No apparent side effects were seen in patients of either treatment group. Overall, the results of this study demonstrated that fluconazole was significantly better than itraconazole in resolving endoscopic lesions, with both drugs nearly equipotent in eliciting complete clinical remission of esophageal candidiasis.[400] The same investigators[401] also compared the efficacies of fluconazole and flucytosine in a double-blind, placebo-controlled trial of 60 AIDS patients with endoscopically diagnosed esophageal candidiasis. Three randomly selected groups of 20 patients each received orally either fluconazole (3.0 mg/kg daily), flucytosine (100 mg/kg daily), or placebo. After 2 weeks of treatment, the placebo-receiving patients were double-blindly randomized to receive fluconazole (8 patients) or flucytosine (9 patients). The results at the end of 2 weeks showed that endoscopic cure was achieved in 13 patients (65%) of the fluconazole group vs. only 3 patients (15%) in the flucytosine group, whereas partial endoscopic cure was evident in 2 patients (10%) in the placebo-receiving group. Complete clinical remission was observed in 16 patients (80%) from the fluconazole group and 12 patients (60%) from the flucytosine group, while 6 patients from the placebo group presented with partial clinical remission. At the end of the follow-up period (5 week post-treatment) the numbers of patients showing endoscopic cure were 19 (70%) and 9 (33%) from the fluconazole- and flucytosine-treated groups, respectively; the corresponding numbers for patients achieving complete clinical remission were 21 (77.7%) in the fluconazole group, and 17 (63%) in the flucytosine group. Overall, while both fluconazole and flucytosine were safe and well tolerated by AIDS patients with esophageal candidiasis, fluconazole exhibited greater therapeutic efficacy than flucytosine, especially in the rate of endoscopic cure.[401]

Rodriguez-Tudela et al.[402] have demonstrated the presence of correlation between *in vitro* susceptibility (as determined in RPMI-2% glucose broth) and the clinical response to fluconazole and ketoconazole in AIDS patients with oropharyngeal or esophageal candidiasis.

In a double-blind trial in HIV-positive patients with oral and esophageal candidiasis, Smith et al.[403] have compared the efficacies of oral itraconazole (200 mg, once daily) and oral ketoconazole (200 mg, b.i.d.). The clinical responses at the end of the 4-week trial were equal for both drug regimens. In another study, de Repentigny et al.[404] also compared the potencies of itraconazole and ketoconazole in 128 HIV-infected patients. Both drugs were administered orally once daily at doses of 200 mg to 76 patients with oropharyngeal, and 16 patients with endoscopically proven esophageal candidiasis for 14 and 28 d, respectively. Although no significant differences in time to clearing infection was observed between the two regimens, time to relapse was greater and cumulative relapse rates were lower in patients treated with itraconazole as compared to ketoconazole.[404]

Capetti et al.[405] have treated resistant esophageal candidiasis in AIDS patients with GM-CSF. The latter was given consecutively for 10 d at 150 μg daily. Three of the four patients treated showed complete resolution of colonization within 7 d and one patient only partial regression over the treatment period. Scadden[406] has suggested that GM-CSF might play an important role in the treatment of HIV-positive patients by its ability to correct HIV-correlated or drug-induced neutropenia, and potentiating the monocyte-macrophage response[407] to fungal and mycobacterial infections.

Zingman[408] has reported resolution of refractory (fluconazole-resistant) AIDS-related mucosal candidiasis after initiation of retroviral therapy consisting of didanosine (125 mg, b.i.d.) and sequinavir (600 mg, t.i.d.).

32.7.4   SYSTEMIC CANDIDIASIS

Amphotericin B has been used extensively in the therapy of systemic candidiasis.[409] The antibiotic is given intravenously at 0.5 to 1.0 mg/kg.[410] Its drawbacks include extensive toxicity (renal toxicity, nausea, headache, neutropenia, as well as a general flu-like illness[202]) and prolonged hospitalization.

Miyata et al.[411] have applied successfully intrahepatic arterial infusion of amphotericin B (5.0 to 20 mg daily) using an inplantable drug delivery system (reservoir) to treat patients with acute myelocytic leukemia who developed intractable *Candida*-associated multiple liver abscesses.

Bowden et al.[412] applied a colloidal dispersion of amphotericin B (amphocil) in a phase I dose-escalation study of 75 marrow transplant recipients with invasive fungal infections (primarily *Aspergillus* or *Candida* spp.) to evaluate its toxicity, maximum tolerated dose, and clinical response. Escalating doses of 0.5 to 8.0 mg/kg in 0.5-mg/kg per patient increments were given up to 6 weeks. No infusion-related toxicity were observed in 32% of the patients, and no appreciable renal toxicity was observed at any dose level. The estimated maximum tolerated dose was 7.5 mg/kg as defined by rigors and chills, and hypotension. The complete or partial response rate across dose levels and infection types was 52%.[412] Caillot et al.[413] have also determined the efficacy and tolerance of a new amphotericin B lipid emulsion (Amb-OL) in 14 neutropenic patients with candidemia. The formulation consisting of the antibiotic diluted in a lipid solution for parenteral nutrition, was applied at a mean daily dosage of 1.18 mg/kg (range 0.73 to 1.55) for 22 d (range 6 to 62). Seven patients were cured, and six showed improvement.[413]

Studies on the tolerance of high doses of amphotericin B by infusion of a liposomal formulation in children with cancer showed that daily doses ranging from 1.0 to 6.0 mg/kg (median 3.0 mg/kg) and cumulative doses of 13 to 311 mg/kg (median 75 mg/kg) were tolerated well in terms of acute toxicity and duration of treatment.[414]

In a multicenter, prospective, and observational study involving 427 consecutive patients with candidemia, Nguyen et al.[415] assessed the efficacy of low- vs. high-dose amphotericin B, and fluconazole vs. amphotericin B, as well as the morbidity and mortality of *Candida* fungemia. The results showed a 34% mortality rate for patients with candidemia. The mortality rate for patients with catheter-related candidemia in whom the catheters were retained was significantly higher than that of patients having their catheters removed (41% vs. 21%, $p < .001$). Furthermore, there was no overall difference in mortality in patients treated with low-dose (total amphotericin B dose of 500 mg or less) (13%) as compared with those receiving high-dose amphotericin B (total dose of >500 mg) (15%); however, patients who received the low-dose regimen experienced fewer side effects (40% vs. 55%, $p = .03$). In addition of being as effective as amphotericin B, fluconazole also elicited fewer side effects than amphotericin B (12% and 44%, respectively, $p < .001$).[415]

Results from a randomized trial comparing fluconazole (400 mg daily, IV infusion for the first 7 d, then oral administration) with intravenous amphotericin B (0.5 to 0.6 mg/kg daily for the first week, then three times weekly) for the treatment of candidemia in 206 patients without neutropenia and no major immunodeficiency (most common diagnoses were renal failure, nonhematologic cancer, and gastrointestinal disease) revealed that the therapeutic efficacies of both drugs were not significantly different.[416] Even though fluconazole may be considered a safe alternative to amphotericin B in treating candidemia in non-neutropenic patients, a high risk of death is still present,[417,418] as well as some uncertainties with regard to duration of treatment, the need to initiate the therapy intravenously, the optimal timing to remove intravenous catheters, and the most proper medication of children.[419-421]

5-Fluorocytosine (5-FC) was also found to be beneficial in the treatment of systemic candidiasis,[422,423] although there may be the problem of drug resistance[424] and adverse myelosuppressive toxicity. *In vitro* and *in vivo* experiments showed that amphotericin B and 5-FC acted synergistically.[425,426]

Two azole derivatives, miconazole and ketoconazole, have also been shown effective in some cancer patients with disseminated candidiasis.[427,428]

32.7.4.1 Endogenous (Hematogenous) Candidal Endophthalmitis (HCE)

The recommended therapy for HCE is intravenous amphotericin B either alone or in combination with 5-FC. The latter combination should be considered in cases of either lesions threatening the macula, the presence of extensive intraocular inflammation, and/or when the inflammatory response is rapidly progressive.[101] Despite the low eye levels of amphotericin B,[101] its use apparently facilitated healing of HCE. Thus, Edwards et al.[429] have reported that in a group of 76 patients with HCE, the 7 patients who received 200 mg or more of intravenous amphotericin B had the highest rate of healing. The recommended minimal therapeutic dose of amphotericin B should be at least 200 mg. However, dose regimens of 1.0 to 1.5 g (if tolerated by the patient) should be used in cases of severe vitrous abscess formation, and if resolution did not occur rapidly.[101]

Combination of amphotericin B and rifampin has been used successfully in one patient (the two drugs acted synergistically in an *in vitro* system).[430]

The use of 5-FC alone has been rather limited and with marginal success (two of four patients responded, and two did not).[113,431]

Nomura and Ruskin[432] reported failure of fluconazole to prevent blinding from endophthalmitis secondary to candidal sepsis despite aggressive and lengthy therapy.

Miconazole failed to elicit favorable response in one patient with HCE,[433] whereas the clinical experience with fluconazole in human HCE has been rather limited[434] and its effect in a rabbit model of *C. albicans*-associated disseminated candidiasis and endophthalmitis was short-lived (24 d) and there was evidence that endophthalmitis actually worsened during the later stages of treatment with fluconazole.[435]

Intravitreal injection of antifungal agents as potential therapy for HCE has not been adequately supported either experimentally[431] or clinically.[108,436] In addition, the potential toxicity of intravitreal amphotericin B has been raised,[437] although in some studies,[431,438] 5.0- and 10-µg doses of intravitreal amphotericin B were reported safe in a rabbit model of exogenous candidal endophthalmitis. Furthermore, while intravitreally administered therapeutic doses of liposome-bound amphotericin B successfully eradicated *Candida* infection in rabbits with endophthalmitis, the treatment resulted in retinal damage to the eyes of all rabbits.[439]

Other therapeutic approaches for HCE include vitrectomy,[104,107,431] and laser therapy.[440]

32.7.4.2 Candidal Meningitis

For treatment of candidal meningitis, the recommended therapy consists of amphotericin B and 5-FC.[129,441] In one clinical trial,[441] 15 of 17 patients receiving this combination for 4 to 8 weeks improved or were cured, with the median time to sterilization of CFS cultures being 7 d. The addition of intrathecal amphotericin B facilitated the sterilization of CFS fluid.[442]

32.7.4.3 Candidal Endocarditis

Candida endocarditis has been nearly always fatal before the introduction of open heart surgery and amphotericin B therapy.[151,443-445] Currently, the recommended treatment of candidal endocarditis uniformly consists of combined medical and surgical interventions with systemic amphotericin B given before and after surgery.[145,150,446-455] However, neither the dose nor the duration of treatment with amphotericin B have been clearly established; rather, both are determined by the patient's tolerance of the drug.[145] Hallum and Williams[145] have recommended that in patients with no severe heart failure, a course of parenteral amphotericin B be implemented at approximately 500 mg before surgery and an additional 1.0 to 1.5 g after valvular replacement. In cases where the patient is in severe heart failure and fails to improve dramatically within 36 to 48 h after a full medical treatment for the heart failure, emergency valvular replacement may have to be carried out; in such cases, a dose regimen of 1.5 to 2.0 g of amphotericin B should be given after the cardiac surgery.[145]

5-Fluorocytosine has been used adjunctively in several patients with candidal endocarditis, with inconclusive results.[446,456]

At daily doses of 100 to 200 mg (3 mg/kg daily), fluconazole has also been used to treat *Candida* endocarditis.[457-459] In one of these studies,[458] the patient with *C. parapsilosis* complicating treatment for non-Hodgkin's lymphoma received a 3-month course of intravenous and oral fluconazole in addition to GM-CSF for persistent neutropenia. Furthermore, the therapeutic efficacy of fluconazole has been tested in a rabbit model of candidal endocarditis; at much higher doses (20 to 50 mg/kg given intraperitoneally), it successfully sterilized all *Candida* vegetations.[460]

Nishida et al.[461] have described a case of active valve infective endocarditis due to *C. glabrata* that was successfully treated by systemic administration of fluconazole. The drug was administered intravenously or orally at doses of 400 mg daily for 46 d.

32.7.4.4 Vulvovaginal Candidiasis

A number of agents have been used to treat acute candidal vaginitis. Among the polyene antifungals, nystatin cream and vaginal suppositories have been used for nearly three decades with approximately 75% to 80% rate of success.[462] Other polyenes, such as amphotericin B, meparteicin, and trichomycin appeared at least as effective as nystatin.[165] Several azole derivatives (butoconazole, clotrimazole, miconazole, econazole, fenticonazole, tioconazole, terconazole) when compared to the polyenes seemed to be more effective by achieving clinical and mycological cure rates in the range of 85% to 90%.[463,464]

In several clinical trials, shorter treatment courses or higher single-dose regimens have proven effective for most of the azole antimycotics against acute candidal vaginitis.[465,466] The higher dose resulted in the persistence of inhibitory drug concentrations for several days — for example, clotrimazole when given as 500-mg suppositories maintained measurable therapeutic concentrations for at least 2 to 3 d;[467] similar data are now available for miconazole.[468] In addition, single high-dosage therapy with clotrimazole was reported beneficial in pregnant women.[469]

Of the orally active azole derivatives, ketoconazole (at 400 mg daily, for 5 d), itraconazole (at either 200 mg daily for 3 d, or 400 mg on a single day), and fluconazole (150 mg single daily dose, or 150 mg once weekly for 3 weeks) have been shown to be highly effective in achieving clinical and mycological cure of acute candidal vaginitis.[470-473]

In an open, noncomparative study, Kukner et al.[474] have evaluated the efficacy of neo-penotran, a combination of metronidazole (500 mg) and miconazole nitrate (100 mg), in patients with candidal vaginitis. Each patient was treated with a neo-penotran pessary twice daily for 2 weeks; vaginitis was resolved in 84.4% of the cases.

A comparison of oral metronidazole (500 mg, b.i.d. for 1 week), 0.75% metronidazole vaginal gel (5 g, b.i.d. for 5 d), and 2% clindamycin vaginal cream (5 g, once daily for 1 week), have shown equivalent cure rates of vulvovaginal candidiasis.[475]

In a single-blind, randomized, controlled trial, the clinical efficacy of fluconazole (a single daily oral dose of 150 mg) was compared with that of clotrimazole (100-mg suppository given twice daily in the morning and at bedtime) in the treatment of vulvovaginal candidiasis over a 3-d period.[476] There was no significant difference between the two drugs regarding mycological cure 1 week after treatment (79.2% for fluconazole- and 80% for clotrimazole-treated groups); approximately 4 weeks after treatment, the corresponding cure rates were 60.4% and 66%, respectively. The toxic side effects were minimal.

Sobel et al.[477] conducted a randomized study of 151 patients with a history of recurrent vulvovaginal candidiasis to compare the efficacy of oral ketoconazole (400 mg daily for 2 weeks) with that of topical clotrimazole (100 mg daily as vaginal suppositories for 1 week). One week after the completion of therapy, clinical cure or improvement was observed in 86.4% of the ketoconazole- and 81.7% of clotrimazole-treated groups, with mycological response in 80.3% and 81.7%, respectively. However, in the absence of maintenance suppressive antifungal therapy, the clinical and mycologic failures in both groups were very high, reaching 52.5% and 62.6% for the ketoconazole and clotrimazole groups, respectively, thus necessitating the need for immediate initiation of maintenance therapy following an initial clinical improvement.[477]

Azzena and Vasoin[478] successfully treated candidal vulvovaginitis with itraconazole with a single daily oral dose of 200 mg for 3 d.

The management of recurrent and chronic vulvovaginal infections is more problematic, especially in immunocompromised hosts.[165] In the latter case, if there are underlying conditions (e.g., diabetes) and/or predisposing factors (corticosteroid or other immunosuppressive, or estrogen therapies), in general, recalcitrant candidal infection will require long-term maintenance suppressive prophylactic therapy.[479-481] Treatment with low-dose oral ketoconalzole (100 mg daily, for 6 months) has been described as effective.[479]

32.7.4.5 Urinary and Peritoneal Candidiasis

One of the recommended therapies of *Candida*-associated cystitis and candiduria is treatment with intravenous amphotericin B. Doses as high as 200 µg/ml have been reported to cause minimal toxicity.[482,483] The usual amphotericin B concentrations are in the 50- to 60-µg/ml range added to 1.0 l of 5% dextrose and water and infused at a rate of 40 ml/h.[483] Other drugs used to treat candidal cystitis include 5-fluorocytosine (5-FC) and azole (fluconazole[484]) antimycotics.[485] Since fungal resistance against 5-FC is likely to develop, combined therapy with amphotericin B may be beneficial.[174]

Strassner and Friesen[486] have shown that alkalinization of the urine (to adjust the pH to 7.0–7.5) with oral potassium-sodium-hydrogen citrate may provide a simple and effective method to treat candiduria in patients with an indwelling catheter. An additional advantage was the metaphylaxis and prophylaxis of renal stone formation in immobilized patients.

Since candiduria has emerged as a major therapeutic problem over the past 40 years, treatment by means of bladder irrigation with amphotericin B solutions has been widely used in clinical practice. However, some specific aspects of this procedure, such as drug concentrations and duration of treatment, and the benefit of continuous washing over instillation with cross-clamping (to allow "dwell-times"), have not been clearly defined by prospective, randomized, double-blind trials. In view of the current knowledge (based exclusively on anecdotal experiences), Sanford[487] has recommended that 200 to 300 ml of amphotericin B solution at optimal concentrations of 5.0 to 10 mg/l, should be administisistered by triple-lumen urethral catheter with cross-clamping for 60 to 90 min; because of potential uroepithelial damage, irrigation for no more than 2 d should be sufficient. However, some aspects of Sanford's recommended procedure have drawn criticism from a number of investigators.[488-491]

Treatment of catheter-associated candiduria with fluconazole irrigation (prepared as 1.0 mg/ml solution with normal saline) was effective and safe in eliminating the candiduria without changing the catheter.[492] Montenegro et al.[493] have treated candidal peritonitis with fluconazole with delayed removal of the peritoneal dialysis catheter.

Candidal pyelonephritis, which is one of the most common manifestations of upper urinary tract infections, may be life-threatening, and intravenous amphotericin B is the recommended therapy.[494-496] The recommended regimen usually commences with 10 mg of the antibiotic on the first day, and 25 mg daily on the subsequent 4 d.[166] Instillation of amphotericin B directly into the renal pelvis has been successful in several cases.[496-498]

The incidence of *Candida*-associated peritoneal infections have increased with *C. albicans* and *C. tropicalis* being the most frequent etiologic agents.[499] In addition to peritoneal dialysis,[500-507] imunosuppression and broad-spectrum antibiotic therapies are risk factors for the development of candidal peritonitis.[166]

In patients on peritoneal dialysis in whom the infection has been localized to the peritoneum, treatment with either intraperitoneal 5-FC or miconazole plus oral ketoconazole was reported to be well tolerated and effective.[499] In two other reports, treatment of patients on chronic ambulatory peritoneal dialysis (CAPD) included intraperitoneal lavage with 5-FC alone[508,509] or low-dose amphotericin B (2.0 to 4.0 µg/ml final concentration in dialysate fluid); in the latter case, although effective, this treatment may not only cause abdominal pain during instillation,[507,510] but may also preclude patients of continuing peritoneal dialysis.[166] The amphotericin B-associated abdominal pain may be dose-related since it occurs at doses of 4.0 µg/ml or higher. In addition, intraperitoneal amphotericin B has been linked with peritoneal fibrosis and adhesion.[500] Two patients who developed fungal peritonitis after receiving CAPD were successfully treated with intracatheter retention of amphotericin B (1.0 to 2.0 mg) and oral flucytosine or fluconazole (50 mg, b.i.d.) for 5 weeks; the catheter was not removed and efficient peritoneal permeability was maintained.[511]

Because of its ability to penetrate into the peritoneal fluid after oral administration,[512,513] fluconazole was found effective (100 to 200 mg daily, for 2 to 6 weeks) in the treatment of candidal peritonitis.[514,515]

Voss et al.[516] have reviewed the efficacy of fluconazole in the management of candidal urinary tract infections in several small studies (a total of 99 patients). The drug appeared to be of value in the treatment of both uncomplicated and complicated infections.

Corbella et al.[517] reported a case of *C. glabrata* upper urinary tract infection causing urethral obstruction which was successfully treated with intravenous fluconazole (200 mg daily) combined with ureteral catheterization; oral fluconazole at 200 mg daily was instituted as preventive maintenance therapy for 1 month post-treatment. However, Ansari et al.[518] cautioned about the possibility of failure to eradicate fluconazole in such settings due to either inherent resistance of *C. glabrata* to fluconazole[519,520] or development of resistance after prolonged therapy with the drug.[521,522]

In another therapeutic strategy,[523] a combination of intravenous or intraperitoneal administration of 5-fluorocytosine and oral fluconazole was also used.

32.7.4.6 Candidal Arthritis and Osteomyelitis

Amphotericin B has been the drug of choice for therapy of candidal arthritis. In cases of no response, the therapy was supplemented with either flucytosine or ketoconazole. Local candidal arthritis healed in all cases. However, candidal arthritis in an artificial joint resulted in all cases in removal of the prostheses.[180]

Lafont et al.[524] have described three patients with a history of intravenous heroin addiction who presented with indolent persistent lumbar pain revealing septic spondilodiscitis and vertebral osteomyelitis caused by *C. albicans*. Two of the patients were treated with intravenous amphotericin B, and the other with fluconazole, with excellent results.

Treatment of arthritis and osteomyelitis secondary to disseminated *C. tropicalis* infection in a premature infant with amphotericin B and oral flucytosine (25 mg/kg, four times daily) resulted in sterilization of the synovial fluid within 4 d. The intraarticular level of flucytosine (synovial fluid) was 39.6 μg/ml; corresponding serum level was 47.5 μg/ml.[525] In another case,[526] *C. lusitaniae* osteomyelitis in a premature infant was successfully resolved following therapy with flucytosine and fluconazole.

Tang[527] reported a case of a patient with candidal osteomyelitis who because of renal impairment was treated with fluconazole rather than amphotericin B; the patient made full recovery. However, fluconazole therapy failed to cure sternal osteomyelitis due to *C. albicans*.[528]

32.7.4.7 Neonatal Candidiasis

Disseminated neonatal candidiasis will necessitate the use of amphotericin B.[186,529] However, the toxicity may be a serious problem, as reported by Baley et al.,[530] who found 7 of 10 infants receiving amphotericin B with severe renal abnormalities manifested by oliguria or anuria and significant increase in blood urea nitrogen and creatinine at an average cumulative dose of 6.5 mg/kg; 6 infant deaths were attributed to amphotericin B-associated nephrotoxicity. In two neonatal studies,[531,532] after 1 week of amphotericin B treatment, the creatinine levels rose an average of 0.299 μg/dl but reversed to baseline levels after the end of therapy.

Aydin et al.[533] described three cases of candidal meningitis of low-birth-weight infants treated with amphotericin B. *C. albicans* was isolated from cerebrospinal fluid (CSF) cultures and treatment was instituted 1 to 4 weeks before the onset of candidiasis. Amphotericin B was administered intravenously at an initial daily dose of 0.25 mg/kg, which was later increased to 2.0 mg/kg daily. The side effects included a transient and mild elevation in hepatic enzyme concentration, and transient thrombocytopenia.[533] Delaplane et al.[531] found that in five infants the amphotericin B levels in the CSF were 40% to 50% of those in the serum; by comparison, in adults, the CSF concentrations were between 2% and 4% that of serum.[534]

A case of widespread cutaneous candidiasis in an infant with methylmalonic acidemia was treated successfully with liposomal amphotericin B (AmBisome).[535] Results from another study[536] have shown a high cure rate of invasive candidiasis in immunocompromised children following AmBisome therapy.

The management of obstructive uropathy in neonates and infants has been successfully carried out by treatment with intravenous amphotericin B and oral 5-fluorocytosine.[201]

It is recommended that therapy with amphotericin B in infants is started with 0.25 mg/kg diluted in 5% or 10% dextrose and infused over 2 to 4 h (test dose is usually not necessary), followed by daily increases of 0.25 mg/kg to achieve a daily dose from 0.5 mg/kg to 1.0 mg/kg.[186] In severe cases, dose increases have been carried out every 12 h; daily doses of up to 1.5 mg/kg in cases of persistent fungemia have been safely given.[537]

Lackner et al.[538] reported the use of liposomal amphotericin B (AmBisome) in the treatment of one low-birth-weight infant (1020 g) with disseminated candidiasis. The liposomal formulation was given intravenously at an initial daily dose of 1.5 mg/kg, which was later increased to 5.0 mg/kg daily with no severe side effects observed. After 1 week no fungal contamination was detected, and treatment was stopped after 26 d. However, based on their clinical experience with disseminated candidiasis in low-birth-weight infants, Pereira da Silva et al.[539] have recommended increasing the initial 1.0-mg/kg dose of AmBisome (given for 1 week) to a lower dose (1.25 mg/kg); after 1 week at a dose regimen of 1.25 mg/kg AmBisome, clinical improvement was evident.

5-Flucytosine (5-FC) is usually used as an adjunctive therapy with amphotericin B.[186] However, the need for it has been questioned.[187] Dose regimens may vary from 25 to 50 mg/kg (four times daily) to a single daily dosing of 50 or 100 mg/kg.[186]

Clarke and Davies[540] have found miconazole effective in the treatment of neonatal disseminated candidiasis at 4.0 mg/kg daily. Antagonism with amphotericin B has been reported.[541]

Fluconazole at daily doses of 1.0 to 16 mg/kg (mean 5.3 mg/kg daily) eliminated *Candida* colonization in low-birth-weight infants with no apparent toxicity.[542,543] The clinical and mycological responses reached 97% of the patients.[543] Marr et al.[544] reported successful treatment of candidal sepsis and meningitis in a very low-birth-weight infant using fluconazole and flucytosine. While fluconazole given alone failed in a case of an infant with candidal meningitis,[545] it was reported to be effective in resolving *C. albicans* septicemia when given orally to a premature low-birth-weight infant (5.0 mg/kg daily for 20 d).[546]

The therapeutic efficacy of oral itraconazole for disseminated candidiasis in low-birth-weight infants was discussed by Bhandari and Narang.[547]

32.8 CANDIDAL ONYCHOMYCOSIS

Onychomycosis is defined as fungal infection of the nail plate, caused by various species of the *Epidermophyton*, *Microsporum*, and *Trychophyton* families, including various dermatophytes, *Candida* spp., *Scopulariopsis brevicalis*, *Scytalidum*, *Fusarium*, *Penicillium*, *Aspergillus*, and *Acremonium* species, and *Pyranochaeta unguis-hominis* sp.[548] Usually, onychomycosis can affect both healthy and compromised nail plates, producing nails that are opaque, white, thickened, friable, and brittle.[549]

Clinically, onychomycosis infections are classified as superficial, distal and lateral, and proximal.[550,551] In the advanced stage of the disease, the whole plate may be affected, leading to total dystrophic onychomycosis.

32.8.1 CANDIDAL PARONYCHIA

Paronychium is an infection of the nail fold caused most often by *C. albicans*.[552,553] It is characterized by a swollen and distorted nail plate in which the fold retracts from it at the lunula. In addition to chronic infection which is common, proximal onychomycosis may develop secondary to *Candida* paranochia. Patients with paranochia often have some predisposing problem.[549]

32.8.2 CANDIDAL ONYCHOMYCOSIS

The most common pattern by which *Candida* infects the nail plate is secondary to a paronychium. However, in patients with chronic mucocutaneous candidiasis or immunodeficiencies, the nail plate and the surrounding tissues may be involved with a severe and hyperkeratotic candidiasis. In these patients, hyperkeratosis secondary to *Candida* invasion may also develop in skin adjacent to the nails.[549]

32.8.3 TREATMENT OF CANDIDAL ONYCHOMYCOSIS AND PARONYCHIA

In addition to identifying the etiologic agent, one important aspect of the therapy of onychomycosis is to define the range of nail disease and the extent of skin involvement if present. Since the penetration of most antifungal agents into the nail plate is variable and the rate of growth of toenails is one third to one half that of fingernails, therapy of the former with systemic antimycotics may last for 12 to 15 months, whereas fingernail infection may be cured in 6 months.[549] The use of chemical removal or surgical avulsion of the nail plate, although it may shorten considerably duration of therapy, has been limited, at least partially, because subsequent recurrences have been common.

Many topical antifungals, such as 28% tioconazole,[554,555] amorolfine,[556] cyclopiroxolamine,[557] bifonazole/urea, and tolnaftate may be applied directly to the nail, with variable results.

Amorolfine, a new morpholine analog, was found to confer antifungal activity by blocking the production of cell membrane ergosterol via the inhibition of at least two separate enzymes (14α-reductase and $\Delta^{7,8}$-isomerase) involved in fungal sterol biosynthesis.[558] Some preliminary data with topical amorolfine suggested that this allylamine antimycotic may be effective in some cases. Thus, in a multicenter study,[559] 456 patients with early nail infections (not affecting more than 80% of the nail surface area and not involving the nail bed) were treated twice weekly with 5% amorolfine nail lacquer for up to 6 months; 3 months after the end of therapy, the treatment produced a 54% clinical response.

Ketoconazole has broad-spectrum activity against most superficial fungal pathogens causing onychomycosis, including *Candida* spp.[560] In patients with chronic cutaneous candidiasis, ketoconazole did elicit a permanent remission of *Candida* onychomycosis.[561] On rare occasions, however, an idiosyncratic form of drug-induced hepatitis[556,562,563] has been associated with its use that appeared to be more prevalent in patients with onychomycosis.[564] The risk of hepatitis, even though rare, has limited to a large extent the use of ketoconazole in candidal onychomycosis.[549]

Studies with itraconazole have shown that this lipid-soluble drug was capable of penetrating into the nails and found there in measurable amounts within 2 weeks after the start of therapy and for a considerable period thereafter.[549] One implication of this finding is the possibility of shorter courses of drug therapies in treating onychomycosis. Itraconazole was found useful in patients with previously treatment-unresponsive dermatophytosis and *Candida* nail infections.[565]

Fluconazole, another triazole antimycotic has also been shown to have activity in superficial candidal infections,[564] as well as good penetrability into the nails, where detectable levels of the drug were found within 48 h of the beginning of treatment.[566]

Terbinafine, a member of the allylamine class of antifungal drugs, is confering activity by inhibiting the epoxidation of squalene, a step in the formation of ergosterol in the fungal cell membrane that occurs at an earlier stage than that inhibited by the azole antimycotics.[567] Although exerting a wide range of antifungal activity *in vitro*, *in vivo* terbinafine has been found useful only for dermatophytosis. In the treatment of onychomycosis, mycologic remission of infected fingernails was seen within 3 months of starting therapy.[568] In a placebo-controlled multicenter clinical trial, terbinafine at daily doses of 250 mg elicited 82% and 71% remission rates at 6-month follow-up examination of toenail and fingernail infections, respectively.[569] In a study carried out to examine the value of 6 vs. 12 vs. 24 weeks of treatment, the cure rates were 67%, 82%, and 85%, respectively.[570]

Griseofulvin is an orally applied antifungal antibiotic produced by *Penicillium griseofulvum*. It is active only against dermatophyte fungi by inhibiting the formation of intracellular microtubules, probably by direct effect on the structural protein tubulin. While, in general, griseofulvin is effective against fingernail infection, its activity against toenail onychomycosis is clearly unsatisfactory.[549]

Candida-associated nail dystrophy is best treated with oral itraconazole or ketoconazole, or chemical removal followed by local antifungal treatment.[549]

32.9   EMERGING *CANDIDA* SPP. INFECTIONS

More than 150 species of *Candida* have been idenfified, but only a dozen or so have been regarded as important pathogens in humans. Although single reports describing one or more cases of infection caused by unusual *Candida* species do not necessarily mark the emergence of a new yeast infection, at least some of these species may arise as potential human opportunistic pathogens, especially among immunocompromised hosts.[571]

Among the various emerging *Candida* spp. pathogenic to humans, *C. glabrata*,[529,572] *C. guilliermondii*,[573-575] *C. krusei*,[12,85] and *C. parapsilosis*[576] are the most frequently isolated. Other emerging pathogenic yeasts include *C. stellatoidea*,[18,577] *C. famata*,[578,579] *C. kefyr* (*C. pseudotropicalis*),[580] *C. lusitaniae*,[86,581,582] *C. norvegensis*,[583] *C. lipolytica*,[584] *C. rugosa*,[585-587] *C. utilis*,[588,589] *C. zeylanoides*,[590,591] *C. haemulonii*,[592] *C. humicola*,[593] *C. pintolopesii*,[594,595] *C. pulcherrima*,[596] and *C. viswanathii*.[597]

Concurrent isolation of more than one non-*albicans* species of *Candida* from blood cultures of patients with disseminated candidiasis, although rare, has been reported.[13] Given the increasing clinical significance of these yeasts in immunocompromised hosts and the difference in virulence, maximum caution should be applied to properly identify the emerging non-*C. albicans* species.

Some of the particular clinical and/or microbiological aspects of these less frequently encountered, but emerging, *Candida* infections will be reviewed in this section.

32.9.1   CANDIDA ZEYLANOIDES

In nature, *C. zeylanoides* has been isolated from fish.[598] Bialasiewicz et al.[599] have recovered *C. zeylanoides* from the oral cavity of children with retrogenic and other defects. The organism persisted despite the use of disinfectants and treatment with nystatin.

Meyer et al.[600] have indicated that *C. zeylanoides* did not grow at 37°C, an observation that has also been substantiated by the behavior of the American Type Culture Collection strains.

In several reports, *C. zeylanoides* has been isolated and identified as the causative agent of human disease. Liao et al.[601] have reported four cases of superficial *C. zeylanoides* mycosis presenting as tinea cruris which responded to treatment with ketoconazole. In addition, on several occasions, this yeast has been identified as the causative agent of onychomycosis.[602,603]

After Roberts[604] described the first case of *C. zeylanoides*-induced fungemia, two other accounts followed.[590,591] Bisbe et al.[590] have reported on an insulin-dependent diabetic who underwent kidney and pancreas transplantation and subsequently developed septic arthritis of the knee due to *C. zeylanoides*. The fungemia, which resulted from hematogenous spread of the organism to the synovium, responded to intravenous amphotericin B (total dose 1.0 g). A *C. zeylanoides* strain obtained by arthrocentesis was sensitive *in vitro* to amphotericin B, 5-fluorocytosine, miconazole, econazole, clotrimazole, and ketoconazole.[590] Next, Levenson et al.[591] described a patient with a long history of scleroderma and gastrointestinal malabsorption requiring total parenteral nutrition who was diagnosed with *C. zeylanoides* fungemia. While the patient responded to therapy with amphotericin B (total dose, 716 mg), on two subsequent admissions for episodes of fever, blood cultures yielded the same yeast that necessitated further treatment with amphotericin B. Antimicrobial susceptibility testing performed on three clinical isolates and one control strain has shown MIC values, at 48 h, of <0.13, 1.0 to 2.0, 4.0 to 8.0, and 0.173 to 0.5 µg/ml for 5-fluorocytosine, amphotericin B, fluconazole, and ketoconazole, respectively; in contrast, a fourth clinical isolate was resistant to 5-fluorocytosine and fluconazole with corresponding MIC values of >128 and 16 µg/ml, respectively.[591] Furthermore, the clinical isolates also differed from the description of Meyer et al.[600] by exhibiting luxuriant growth at 35°C and 37°C; however, the control strains did not grow at the elevated temperatures, but grew only at 30°C.

Recently, Whitby et al.[605] reported a case of *C. zeylanoides* endocarditis in an HIV-positive patient which developed in the absence of the usual risk factors for systemic candidiasis.

32.9.2 CANDIDA FAMATA

C. famata (formerly known as *Torulopsis candida*) is a saprophytic yeast which has been previously isolated from human skin[606-608] and mucosa[608,609] but regarded as a contaminant.[606] On Sabouraud dextrose agar, the yeast produced smooth, cream-colored colonies after 24 h of incubation at 30°C, which under microscopic examination revealed round-to-oval cells ranging in size from 3.7 to 5.0 by 2.7 to 4.7 µm.[578]

The first report of human *C. famata*-induced fungemia by Albaret et al.[610] did not provide any clinical or mycological description. Later, St.-Germain and Laverdière[578] described the first documented case of intravenous catheter-associated fungemia due to *C. famata* in a leukemic patient following allogeneic bone marrow transplantation. Both the intravascular cannula and the immunosuppressed status of the patient were believed to have played major roles as predisposing factors. To this end, Khan et al.[611] demonstrated the ability of *C. famata* to produce systemic disease in cortisone-treated mice, thus emphasizing the potential of this yeast to cause disease in immunosuppressed patients. Removal of the catheter and treatment with intravenous amphotericin B rapidly resolved the fungemia.[578]

Quindos et al.[612] have reported a fatal case of *C. famata*-induced peritonitis in a patient undergoing continuous ambulatory peritoneal dialysis who failed to respond to fluconazole therapy.

In another report,[613] *C. famata* was associated with endophthalmitis following extracapsular cataract extraction with implantation of a posterior chamber intraocular lens. The localized intraocular inflammation presented with symptoms virtually identical to *Propionibacterium acnes* infection. The infection was cured with oral flucytosine (2.0 g, four times daily for 6 weeks; then reduced to 1.0 g, four times daily because of toxicity).

When tested for antimicrobial susceptibility, a clinical isolate of *C. famata* showed MIC values of 0.08, 0.2, and 0.78 µg/ml for amphotericin B, flucytosine, and ketoconazole, respectively.[578]

32.9.3 CANDIDA KEFIR

C. kefir (also known as *C. pseudotropicalis*) has a comparatively restricted natural habitat. While the yeast has been isolated from cattle[614] and dairy products,[615] there have been no reports about its distribution in other mammals, primates, birds, or food products, or in nature.[614-616] However, *C. kefir* is a component of the human indigenous flora and although at significantly low levels (<1%) as compared to other *Candida* species, it has been found to colonize the oral cavity,[616-620] rectum and feces,[621] and the vagina.[621]

Hog asen et al.[622] have studied the ability of *C. kefir* to stimulate production of the complement components C3 and factor B by monocytes, and the release of GM-CSF. The monocyte responses elicited by a specific yeast species may be linked to its pathogenicity, and may also explain the predilection of some yeasts for particular underlying diseases. Compared to *C. albicans*, *C. tropicalis*, and *C. parapsilosis* (all three the most effective inducers of C3, factor B, and GM-CSF production), *C. kefir*, *C. famata*, and *C. guilliermondii* had only a moderate stimulatory effect on C3 production and did not affect either factor B or GM-CSF release.

Pawlik and Jodlowska[623] have studied the frequency of appearance of *C. kefir* strains, their diagnosis and susceptibility to drugs, as well as their importance in the pathogenesis of reproductive tract infections. Clinical symptoms were present in 47.8% of patients with *C. kefir* infections.

The susceptibility of *C. kefir* to fluconazole[624] and other azole antimycotics,[625] as well as two antibiotics (cilofungin[626] and the pneumocandin analog L-733,560[627]) have also been determined.

32.9.4 CANDIDA GLABRATA

C. glabrata (also known as *Torulospsis glabrata* and *Cryptococcus glabratus*) is a small, round yeast thought to be saprophytic in humans. Most commonly, *C. glabrata* is found as a commensal of the gastrointestinal tract, and incidently has been isolated from the oral cavity, skin, and urine cultures of healthy individuals.[76,628-631]

C. glabrata is primarily an opportunistic pathogen associated with high mortality rates ranging from 38% to 83%.[79,631,632] It has been frequently isolated from various secretions of hospitalized patients.[76] The underlying conditions most often associated with fungemia, bronchopneumonia, salpingitis, and urinary tract infections caused by *C. glabrata* included malignancies, diabetes mellitus, transplantation, and alcoholism.[76,631,633] This yeast could also become pathogenic under other conditions leading to altered host immune defenses, such as therapies with corticosteroids, immunosuppressive drugs, and broad-spectrum antibiotics or major surgery.[79,572]

Among the risk factors commonly associated with *C. glabrata* fungemia in neonates have been extreme prematurity, indwelling central lines (in the umbilical vessels or the vena cava), prolonged intubation, and excessive use of broad-spectrum antibiotics.[188,192,529,632,634]

The most common clinical manifestations of *C. glabrata* fungemia have been high fever and hypotension, resembling bacterial endotoxic shock.[635]

Therapy with amphotericin B has been the most preferred treatment modality for *C. glabrata* fungemia.[79,572] Multiple tests evaluating the sensitivity of the yeast to amphotericin B furnished MIC values ranging from 0.1 to 1.0 µg/ml.[79] In the presence of disseminated infection, the use of higher doses of amphotericin B (30 mg/kg) has been recommended.[634] Glick et al.[529] have reported a successful outcome of *C. glabrata* fungemia in a neonate patient following treatment with amphotericin B at 0.5 mg/kg daily for 5 d and then every other day for five more doses. Yet, Komshian et al.[78] found no statistical difference in mortality whether antifungal therapy was administered or not (55% and 69% mortality rates, respectively), although an early initiation of therapy may improve the response rate.[529] High mortality rates among neonates have also been reported.[632,636-638]

32.9.5 CANDIDA LUSITANIAE

C. lusitaniae was first described by van Uden and Buckley[639] as common commensal of the gastrointestinal tract of warm-blooded animals. In humans, it was recovered from a variety of clinical specimens, but most often from blood, urine, and the respiratory tract.[86,87,135,139,215,640-646] In view of these findings, the most likely portals of entry appeared to be the genitourinary and respiratory tracts or colonized indwelling intravascular catheters.

The identification of *C. lusitaniae*, especially in earlier reports,[215,580,647] has proven difficult because of misidentification with *C. parapsilosis*, *C. tropicalis*,[135,215,581,644,647] or even *Saccharomyces* spp.[86,87] The major differential characteristics of *C. lusitaniae* relate to the assimilation of cellobiose and fermentation of trehalose (both negative for *C. parapsilosis*).[215,644] In addition, the lack of growth on cycloheximide-containing medium, pink-appearing colonies on triphenyltetrazolium chloride agar, the assimilation of rhamnose, and the absence of maltose and sucrose fermentation served to distinguish *C. lusitaniae* from *C. tropicalis*.[215,648]

Pappagianis et al.[581] and Holzschu et al.[644] have reported the first documented case of opportunistic infection associated with *C. lusitaniae* in a patient with acute leukemia.

Although so far *C. lusitaniae* seems to be a rare opportunistic pathogen, it has been associated with serious and often fatal disease.[86,87,134,135,215,582,640-643,647] From the reported cases, immunocompromised patients with hematologic malignancies, bone marrow transplant recipients, and patients with central venous catheters or receiving immunosuppressive therapies (corticosteroids, broad-spectrum antibiotics) were at highest risk of developing infection.[86,87,215,582,640-642,647]

In vitro susceptibility testing of *C. lusitaniae* isolates conducted in several laboratories[134,135,582,643] has shown mean inhibitory concentrations of 0.1 to 0.4, 0.03 to 0.2/>160, and <0.03 µg/ml for amphotericin B, flucytosine, and ketoconazole, respectively. Ahearn and McGlohn,[649] while reviewing the susceptibilities of several *C. lusitaniae* isolates, have found that although the MIC values of amphotericin B fell within attainable serum levels, the minimal fungicidal concentrations were more than two dilutions greater. Based on their overall results, Ahearn and McGlohn concluded that flucytosine may be the drug of choice for *C. lusitaniae* infections.

In 1985, Pensler et al.[646] reported the first successful therapy of *C. lusitaniae*. Later, Blinkhorn et al.[86] also described two leukemic patients with *C. lusitaniae* fungemia who responded to treatment with amphotericin B.

However, developing resistance to amphotericin B seemed to be a major problem with *C. lusitaniae*.[581,647] Guinet et al.[215] have described the first case of a *C. lusitaniae* isolate resistant to amphotericin B before therapy. All of the reported fatal cases of *C. lusitaniae* fungemia were associated with such resistance,[215,641,642,644,647,650] suggesting that amphotericin B should not be used as a single therapeutic modality in the management of *C. lusitaniae*, especially with the possibility of developing drug resistance during treatment.[135,581,643] Flucytosine–ketoconazole was one combination which was successfully used by Yinnon et al.[582] to eradicate the yeast from the urinary tract of an infant; both drugs were given at daily oral doses of 75 mg/kg and 9.0 mg/kg (divided every 6 h), respectively. Thomas et al.[651] have reported that the addition of flucytosine to a therapeutic regimen consisting of amphotericin B, resulted in sterilization of the blood in what appeared to be a persistent *C. lusitaniae* fungemia. In contrast, Baker et al.[645] described a failure of flucytosine to control *C. lusitaniae* urinary tract infection which was eradicated with amphotericin B bladder irrigation.

Despite their widespread use, *Candida* spp. resistance to polyene antibiotics (e.g., amphotericin B, nystatin) has been relatively rare.[581,646,647,652-656] For this reason, the clearly observed resistance to amphotericin B by *C. lusitaniae*, although unusual (see also, *C. rugosa* and *C. guilliermondii* below), has not been entirely unexpected. It is well documented that resistance to polyenes is associated with alterations in fungal cell membrane sterols.[573,647,653-655,657,658]

After examining 1372 yeast isolates collected from 308 patients, Dick et al.[654] found the emergence of polyene resistance only in patients undergoing treatment for acute leukemia or in aplastic patients following bone marrow transplantation. In general, these patients experienced prolonged periods of hospitalization, granulocytopenia, therapy with cytotoxic drugs, and extended treatment with antibiotics. Both Pappagianis et al.[581] and Dick et al.[654] concluded that the use of cytotoxic drugs should be considered a contributing factor in the development of resistance to polyene antibiotics.

32.9.6 CANDIDA KRUSEI

Previously, *C. krusei* has been characterized as a less virulent pathogen in humans. This assumption was based on experimental data stemming from its decreased abilities to adhere to human mucosal epithelial cells *in vitro*,[659] and to elicit cell death in mouse kidney tissue culture.[660] In addition, Edwards et al.[661] have shown that higher inocula of *C. krusei*, compared to other *Candida* species, were required to establish infections in animal models.

Recently, however, there have been an increasing number of reports describing substantial virulence of this yeast in immunocompromised hosts.[85,662-665] In a study by Goldman et al.,[12] at the onset of *C. krusei* fungemia 85% of patients were neutropenic with neutrophil counts below 1000 cells/m³. This prevalence of neutropenia was significantly higher than the 40% previously reported for cancer patients with *C. albicans* fungemia and only slightly higher than the 70% prevalence of neutropenia reported for patients with *C. tropicalis* fungemia.[664] Furthermore, over 75% of the patients studied by Goldman et al. showed evidence of gastrointestinal mucosal barrier damage, mostly the result of cytotoxic chemotherapy or radiation. The gastrointestinal tract is believed to be an important portal of entry for *Candida* spp. into the blood stream,[77] and gastrointestinal mucosal breakdown has been reported to be a risk factor for both nosocomially acquired candidemia in nonleukemic patients,[666] and cancer patients sustaining damage to the GI mucosa from the presence of tumor infiltrates or directly from cytotoxic antitumor agents themselves.[667-669]

Goldman et al.[12] have found 69% of the evaluable patients with evidence of *C. krusei* colonization, which was in agreement with the results of Wey et al.,[670] who described colonization by *Candida* spp. to be a risk factor for candidemia. Merz et al.[663] reported that *C. krusei* colonized 12.4% of granulocytopenic patients undergoing chemotherapy for hematologic malignancies or bone marrow transplantation.

A common risk factor of patients with *C. krusei*-induced endophthalmitis was prolonged intravenous catheterization.[671]

Clinical manifestations of *C. krusei* most often include the development of cutaneous lesions (diffuse erythematous maculopapular eruption, erythematous macronodular skin lesions, skin nodules), myalgias, endophthalmitis,[12,671,672] and disseminated disease.[12,77,663,664,671,673-675] Gordon et al.[676] have described a case of an immunocompromised leukemic patient with well-localized intra-abdominal abscess caused by *C. krusei*, which disseminated when treated by surgical drainage. In another unusual case, Diggs et al.[677] reported on a fatal *C. krusei* muscle granulomata in a patient with acute lymphoblastic leukemia and granulocytopenia. Other rarely diagnosed *C. krusei* infections include infectious arthritis,[678,679] ureteral obstruction,[680] ocular infections (blepharo-conjunctivitis without retinitis),[681,682] and esophagitis.[683]

The overall mortality in patients with *C. krusei* fungemia may approach 50%, and if left untreated, the outcome has been nearly always fatal.[12]

Recommended treatment of *C. krusei* fungemia included amphotericin B alone (0.5 to 1.0 mg/kg daily) or in combination with flucytosine (at doses adequate to achieve levels of 30 to 60 μg/ml), as well as liposomal amphotericin B (2.6 mg/kg daily); adjunctive leukocyte transfusion has also been applied.[12,671,676]

Although the prophylactic use of fluconazole has contributed significantly to the decline in the number of disseminated infections caused by the more virulent *C. albicans* and *C. tropicalis*, in another disturbing trend, recent reports have focused attention on the emergence of fungemia caused by the less virulent but drug-resistant *C. krusei* in immunocompromised patients (such as bone marrow transplant recipients) treated prophylactically with fluconazole.[85,579,662,684-690] However, in several other reports of controlled trials,[663,689,691-693] the use of prophylactic fluconazole was not associated with increased incidence of *C. krusei* fungemia. There may be a host of other epidemiologic factors[689] that need to be considered in order to explain the different results seen at various centers. As compared to amphotericin B (MIC = 1.25 μg/ml[684]), fluconazole was consistently much less susceptible[579,694,695] (e.g., MIC = 25 μg/ml[684] or 32 μg/ml[685]). However, the MIC values themselves cannot imply resistance because the clinical efficacy of fluconazole is thought to be greater than that predicted by its minimum inhibitory concentration.[696] On the other hand, the use of animal models have suggested that *C. krusei* indeed displayed a high degree of resistance to fluconazole.[586] Moreover, a patient with acute monocytic leukemia and typhlitis (neutropenic enterocolitis) has developed *C. krusei* fungemia while receiving intravenous fluconazole given at 400 mg loading dose followed by 200 mg every 24 h (see also *Hansenula* spp. infections).[686]

32.9.7 CANDIDA RUGOSA

C. rugosa was originally isolated from human feces in 1917 by Anderson and named *Mycoderma rugosa*.[697] Later, it was found in bovine droppings, stale butter, seawater,[697] and implicated as a causative agent of bovine mastitis.[698,699]

In humans, *C. rugosa* has been reported to cause opportunistic infections, predominantly in immunocompromised patients.[385,585,587,700-702] In one case,[700] the patient was suffering from acute myelocytic leukemia and had disseminated infection with cutaneous lesions that yielded *C. rugosa*. Another patient had alcoholic cirrhosis and an intravenous catheter-associated fungemia.[701] Guymon et al.[702] and Dubé et al.[385] have reported frequent colonization by *C. rugosa* of seriously burned patients.

In an earlier report of intravenous catheter-associated *C. rugosa* fungemia, the patient was treated with intravenous amphotericin B (total dose, 500 mg) and made an uneventful recovery.[585] Another case of invasive *C. rugosa* disease in a pediatric cystic fibrosis patient with central venous catheter also responded completely to amphotericin B (at 10 mg/kg) and removal of the catheter.[587]

Susceptibility testing of one clinical *C. rugosa* isolate revealed inhibition of growth by 0.156, 0.39, and 0.4 µg/ml of amphotericin B, 5-fluorocytosine, and ketoconazole, respectively.[585] In a recent study,[385] *C. rugosa* isolates from patients in a burn unit showed resistance to nystatin (MIC = 18.5 µg/ml or higher at 24 h) and only moderate susceptibility to amphotericin B (MIC = 0.58 µg/ml at 24 h) and fluconazole (mean MIC = 4.44 µg/ml); ketoconazole uniformly inhibited all isolates at low to moderate concentrations (range, 0.012 to 0.2 µg/ml at 24 h). While yeast resistance to nystatin and amphotericin B has been linked,[654] subtle differences in the mechanism of action of these two polyene antibiotics may not always produce cross-resistance (see also, *C. lusitaniae* and *C. guilliermondii*).[385,658]

By comparison, of 18 yeast species isolated from infected bovine mammary glands, *C. rugosa* was the least susceptible of all species evaluated.[698] In another study, while none of 13 bovine mammary gland isolates was susceptible to a 9.6-µg amphotericin B disk and 45-µg fluorocytosine disk, and only 25% were inhibited by a 4.8-µg miconazole disk, 100% of the isolates were inhibited by a 1.0-µg ketoconazole disk.[703]

32.9.8 CANDIDA GUILLIERMONDII

C. guilliermondii is part of the normal fungal flora of the skin. While within the genus *Candida* it appeared to be the least pathogenic in experimental animal models,[704] *C. guilliermondii* has been occasionally associated with cases of endocarditis and septic arthritis.[705]

Dick et al.[573] have described a rare case of fatal disseminated candidiasis due to amphotericin B-resistant *C. guilliermondii*. The drug was given daily on days 11 through 24 and every other day on days 24 through 37 (total dose, 883 mg). The patient, with aplastic anemia, died after developing a progressive resistance to amphotericin B. The most disturbing aspect of this case was the emergence of resistance to amphotericin B during therapy by a seemingly weakly pathogenic yeast. The decrease and eventual loss of ergosterol with increasing amphotericin B resistance supported previous descriptions of the mechanism of resistance by *Candida* spp. to polyene antibiotics[647,653-655] (see also *C. lusitaniae* and *C. rugosa* above).

32.9.9 CANDIDA NORVEGENSIS

The occurrence in nature of *C. norvegensis* is largely unknown. On several occasions, however, this yeast has been isolated from clinical specimens.[649]

C. norvegensis formed yellowish grey colonies when cultured on Sabouraud maltose agar (pH 4.0) at 25°C and 37°C after 2 d, but produced no filaments in the serum tube test.[583]

Nielsen et al.[583] have reported a fatal case of invasive *C. norvegensis* fungemia related to CAPD peritonitis in a renal transplant recipient receiving immunosuppressive therapy with prednisone, cyclosporine, and azathioprine. Treatment with flucytosine and amphotericin B (in the peritoneal dialysis fluid) and intravenous amphotericin B failed to control the infection.

Results from susceptibility antifungal testing of one clinical isolate of *C. norvegensis* revealed sensitivity to amphotericin B and ketoconazole (MIC = 0.2 and 0.4 μg/ml, respectively) but not to flucytosine (MIC = 3.2 μg/ml). After 10 and 4 d, respectively, of flucytosine and amphotericin B therapy, another clinical isolate showed an increase in the MIC values to 0.8 μg/ml for amphotericin B, 12.5 μg/ml for flucytosine, and 1.0 μg/ml for ketoconazole.[583]

32.9.10 CANDIDA LIPOLYTICA

On Sabouraud glucose agar, *C. lipolytica* formed distinctive cerebriform, convoluted, whiter firm colonies. Blastoconidia, which generally developed only after several days of incubation, were found at the apices and less commonly along the length of the hyphae.[584]

C. lipolytica (Harrison) Diddens et Lodder is another yeast that has emerged as pathogenic to humans. Initially included in several large-case series,[706-709] only very few well-documented cases of *C. lipolytica*-induced fungemia have been published.[584,710] In general, the yeast was weakly pathogenic to humans, and most clearly associated with vascular catheter fungemia. There was no evidence of deep visceral infection, such as endophthalmitis, osteomyelitis, arthritis, or hepatic infection.[584,710] However, even after the removal of the infected catheters, the fungemia persisted.[584]

In vitro susceptibility testing of nine *C. lipolytica* isolates have rendered mean MIC values after 24 h of incubation of 0.660 (range, 0.313 to 1.25) and 0.22 (0.078 to 0.313) μg/ml for amphotericin B and ketoconazole, respectively.[584] A treatment regimen of amphotericin B at 0.5 mg/kg daily has been recommended.[584]

32.9.11 CANDIDA VISWANATHII

The major morphologic and biochemical characteristics of *C. viswanathii* include the absence of chlamydospore formation, and the ability to hydrolyze β-glucosides.[597] Although a preliminary study has demonstrated low pathogenicity in laboratory animals,[711] *C. viswanathii* was shown to be very pathogenic in cortisone-treated mice, where 5 of 10 animals died during 1 week, and 3 during the second week following intravenous challenge.[597]

In humans, *C. viswanathii* was first isolated in 1959 from the cerebrospinal fluid of a fatal case of meningitis in a pediatric patient.[712] Later, Sandhu and Randhawa[713] recovered the yeast in routine sputum cultures.

In a second report of human infection,[597] *C. viswanathii* was again isolated from the cerebrospinal fluid of a patient with meningitis who also died.

In addition to humans, *C. viswanathii* has also been isolated from gills of fish caught in the Indian Ocean[714] and from soil in South Africa,[639] which suggested a wide geographic distribution for this fungal species.

32.9.12 CANDIDA HAEMULONII

C. haemulonii (van Uden et Kolipinski) Meyer et Yarrow was isolated initially from the scales of the common grunt (*Haemulon scirius*) in the Atlantic Ocean.[715] In humans, Lavarde et al.[716] reported the first clinical isolation of *C. haemulonii* from the blood of a patient with an indwelling catheter who died from renal failure, after failing to respond to antifungal therapy with flucytosine and amphotericin B. Marjolet[717] has described an additional case of fungemia due to *C. haemulonii* in a cancer patient.

Results from a study by Gargeya et al.[592] confirmed the occurrence of *C. haemulonii* among clinical specimens, particularly isolations from feet and nails. All of the clinical isolates demonstrated extracellular proteolysis on casein agar but no hydrolysis of keratin (suspended in yeast carbon base agar), and no structures resembling conjugation tubes or ascospores were observed. The major phenotypic difference between *C. famata* and *C. haemulonii* was the absence of "capped cells" and the generally negative assimilation of raffinose by the latter.[592]

32.9.13 PICHIA JADINII (CANDIDA UTILIS)

When grown on Sabouraud dextrose agar medium, the colonies of *C. utilis* were smooth and cream colored. On cornmeal agar, the yeast produced the typically branched chains of cylindrical blastoconidia.[598]

Although still commonly referred to as *Candida utilis*, in 1979 this anamorphic yeast was determined by Kurtzman et al.[718] to be conspecific with the teleomorphic yeast *Hansenula jadinii* based on DNA reasssociation. Subsequently, *H. jadinii* was transferred to the genus *Pichia* by Kurtzman,[719] who considered the two genera to be synonymous through comparisons of deoxyribonucleic acid and relatedness. Later, the conspecificity of *C. utilis* and *H. jadinii* was corroborated by genomic studies carried out by Bougnoux et al.,[589] as well as phylogenetic relationships based on identical partial sequences of their 18S and 26S ribosomes.[720]

Furthermore, Kogan et al.[721] have investigated the structure of a cell-wall glucomannan from *C. utilis* and found that it differed from the cellular mannans of other *Candida* species in that the longer tetra- and pentasaccharide side chains were terminated with a glucosyl residue. This presence of nonreducing glucosyl groups at the ends of the side chains prevented *C. utilis* from cross-reacting in a double immunodiffusion test with other *Candida* species that possessed mannan antigens and to cross-react with *Hansenula* species with glucomannan antigens.

Only rarely, *C. utilis* has been isolated as a contaminant from clinical specimens (e.g., sputum, digestive tract, vaginal discharge).[722,723] When tested in immunosuppressed mice, *C. utilis* showed low pathogenicity.[724] Yet, the first case of opportunistic fungemia due to *C. utilis* was reported by Alsina et al.[588] in an AIDS patient with an indwelling catheter. Removal of the catheter and treatment with amphotericin B (0.5 mg/kg daily) and flucytosine cleared the infection.

Bougnoux et al.[589] have described a case of fungemia caused by *C. utilis* in a non-neutropenic, immunocompetent host. Treatment with intravenous amphotericin B (0.5 mg/kg every 2 d) for 26 d resolved the fungemia.

32.10 REFERENCES

1. Bodey, G. P., Ed., *Candidiasis: Pathogenesis, Diagnosis, and Treatment*, 2nd ed., Raven Press, New York, 1993.
2. Emmons, C. W., Binford, C. H., and Utz, J. P., *Medical Mycology*, 2nd ed., Lea and Febiger, Philadelphia, 1970, 167.
3. Barnett, J. A., Payne, R. W., and Yarrow, D., *Yeasts — Characteristics and Identification*, 2nd ed., Cambridge University Press, New York, 1991.
4. Klotz, S. A., Plasma and extracellular matrix proteins mediate in the fate of *Candida albicans* in the human host, *Med. Hypotheses*, 42, 328, 1994.
5. Nicholls, P. E. and Henry, K., Gastritis and cimetidine: a possible explanation, *Lancet*, 1, 1095, 1978.
6. Ruddell, W. S. J., Azon, A. T. R., Findlay, J. M., Bartholomew, B. A., and Hill, M. J., Effect of cimetidine on the gastric bacterial flora, *Lancet*, 1, 672, 1980.
7. Seelig, M. S., The role of antibiotics in the pathogenesis of Candida infections, *Am. J. Med.*, 40, 887, 1966.
8. Stark, F. R., Ninos, N., Hutton, J., Katz, R., and Butler, M., Candida peritonitis and cimetidine, *Lancet*, 2, 744, 1978

9. Triger, D. R., Goepel, J. R., Slater, D. N., and Underwood, J. C. W., Systemic candidiasis complicating acute hepatic failure in patients treated with cimetidine, *Lancet*, 2, 837, 1981.

10. McVay, L. V., Jr. and Sprunt, D. H., A study of moniliasis in aureomycin therapy, *Proc. Soc. Exp. Biol. Med.*, 78, 759, 1951.

11. Hughes, W. T., Kuhn, S., Chaudhary, S., Feldman, S., Verzosa, M., Aur, R. J. A., Pratt, C., and George, S. L., Successful chemoprophylaxis for Pneumocystis carinii pneumonia, *N. Engl. J. Med.*, 297, 1419, 1977.

12. Goldman, M., Pottage, J. C., Jr., and Weaver, D. C., *Candida krusei* fungemia: report of 4 cases and review of the literature, *Medicine (Baltimore)*, 72, 143, 1993.

13. Sandin, R. L., Meier, C. S., Crowder, M. L., and Greene, J. N., Concurrent isolation of *Candida krusei* and *Candida tropicalis* from multiple blood cultures in a patient with acute leukemia, *Arch. Pathol. Lab. Med.*, 117, 521, 1993.

14. Smaranayake, Y. H. and Samaranayake, L. P., *Candida krusei*: biology, epidemiology, pathogenicity and clinical manifestations of an emerging pathogen, *J. Med. Microbiol.*, 41, 295, 1994.

15. Rinaldi, M., Biology and pathogenicity of *Candida* species, in *Candidiasis: Pathogenesis, Diagnosis, and Treatment*, 2nd ed., Bodey, G. P., Ed., Raven Press, New York, 1993, 1.

16. Maksymiuk, A. W., Thongprasert, S., Hopfer, R., Luna, M. A., Fainstein, V., and Bodey, G. P., Systemic candidiasis in cancer patients, *Am. J. Med.*, 77, 20, 1984.

17. Myerowitz, R. L., Localized and disseminated candidiasis, in *The Pathology of Opportunistic Infections*, Myerowitz, R. L., Ed., Raven Press, New York, 1983, 95.

18. Myerowitz, R. L., Pazin, G. J., and Allen, C. M., Disseminated candidiasis: changes in incidence, underlying disease, and pathology, *Am. J. Clin. Pathol.*, 68, 29, 1977.

19. Gaines, J. D. and Remington, J. S., Disseminated candidiasis in the surgical patient, *Surgery*, 72, 730, 1972.

20. Vartivarian, S. and Smith, C. B., Pathogenesis, host resistance, and predisposing factors, in *Candidiasis: Pathogenesis, Diagnosis, and Treatment*, 2nd ed., Bodey, G. P., Ed., Raven Press, New York, 1993, 59.

21. Wade, J. C., Epidemiology of *Candida* infections, in *Candidiasis: Pathogenesis, Diagnosis, and Treatment*, 2nd ed., Bodey, G. P., Ed., Raven Press, New York, 1993, 85.

22. Schaberg, D. R., Culver, D. H., and Gaines, R. P., Major trends in the microbial etiology of nosocomial infection, *Am. J. Med.*, 91(S3B), 72S, 1991.

23. Banerjee, S. N., Emori, T. G., Culver, D. H., Gaynes, R. P., Jarvis, W., Horan, T., Edwards, J. R., Tolson, J., Henderson, T., and Martone, W. J., Secular trends in nosocomial primary blood-stream infections in the United States, 1980–1989, *Am. J. Med.*, 91(S3), 86S, 1991.

24. Stein, D. K. and Sugar, A. M., Fungal infections in the immunocompromised host, *Diagn. Microbiol. Infect. Dis.*, 12, 221S, 1989.

25. Luna, M. A. and Tortoledo, M. E., Histologic identification and pathologic patterns of disease caused by *Candida*, in *Candidiasis: Pathogenicity, Diagnosis, and Treatment*, 2nd ed., Bodey, G. P., Ed., Raven Press, New York, 1993, 21.

26. Mancher, A. M., De Vinatea, M., Tuur, S. M., and Amgritt, P., AIDS and the mycosis, *Infect. Dis. Clin. North Am.*, 2, 827, 1988.

27. Edwards, J. E., Foos, R. Y., Montgomerie, J. Z., and Guze, J. B., Ocular manifestations of *Candida* septicemia: review of 76 cases of hematogenous *Candida* endophthalmitis, *Medicine (Baltimore)*, 53, 47, 1974.

28. Kiehn, T. E., Edwards, F. F., and Armstrong, D., The prevalence of yeasts in clinical specimens from cancer patients, *Am. J. Clin. Pathol.*, 73, 518, 1980.

29. Hymes, S. R. and Duvic, M., Cutaneous candidiasis, in *Candidiasis: Pathogenesis, Diagnosis, and Treatment*, 2nd ed., Bodey, G. P., Ed., Raven Press, New York, 1993, 159.

30. Galimberti, K. L., Flores, V., Gonzales Ramos, M. C., and Villalba, L. I., Cutaneous ulcers due to Candida albicans in an immunocompromised patient — response to therapy with itraconazole, *Clin. Exp. Dermatol.*, 14, 295, 1989.

31. Patel, A. S., DeRidder, P. H., Alexander, T. J., Veneri, R. J., and Lauter, C. B., Candida cellulitis: a complication of percutaneous endoscopic gastrostomy, *Gastrointest. Endosc.*, 35, 571, 1989.

32. Mochizuki, T., Urabe, Y., Hirota, Y., Watanabe, S., and Shiino, A., A case of Candida albicans skin abscess associated with intravenous catheterization, *Dermatologica*, 177, 115, 1988.

33. Torres-Rojas, J. R., Stratton, C. W., Sanders, C. V., Horsman, T. A., Hawley, H. B., Dascomb, H. E., and Vial, L. J., Jr., Candidal suppurative peripheral thrombophlebitis, *Ann. Intern. Med.*, 96, 431, 1982.

34. Kirkpatrick, C. H., Chronic mucocutaneous candidiasis, in *Candidiasis: Pathogenesis, Diagnosis, and Treatment*, 2nd ed., Bodey, G. P., Ed., Raven Press, New York, 1993, 167.

35. Kirkpatrick, C. H., Rich, R. R., and Bennett, J. E., Chronic mucocutaneous candidiasis: model-building in cellular immunity, *Ann. Intern. Med.*, 74, 955, 1971.

36. Klein, R. S., Harris, C. A., Small, C. B., Moll, B., Lesser, M., and Freedland, G. H., Oral candidiasis in high-risk patients as the initial manifestation of the acquired immunodeficiency syndrome, *N. Engl. J. Med.*, 311, 354, 1984.

37. Greenspan, D. and Greenspan, J. S., Oral manifestations of HIV infections, *Dermatol. Clin. North Am.*, 9, 517, 1991.

38. Boni, R., Trueb, R. M., and Wuthrich, B., Alopecia areata in a patient with candidiasis-endocrinopathy syndrome: unsuccessful treatment trial with diphenylcyclopropenone, *Dermatology*, 191, 68, 1995.

39. Roseff, S. A. and Sugar, A. M., Oral and esophageal candidiasis, in *Candididiasis: Pathogenesis, Diagnosis, and Treatment*, 2nd ed., Bodey, G. P., Ed., Raven Press, New York, 1993, 185.

40. Lehner, T., Oral candidosis, *Dent. Practit.*, 17, 209, 1967.

41. Lehner, T., Chronic candidiasis, *Br. Dent. J.*, 116, 539, 1964.

42. Holmstrup, P. and Besserman, M., Clinical, therapeutic and pathogenic aspects of chronic oral multifocal candidosis, *Oral Surg.*, 56, 388, 1983.

43. Holmstrup, P. and Axell, T., Classification and clinical manifestations of oral yeast infections, *Acta Odontol. Scand.*, 48, 57, 1990.

44. Korting, H. C., Clinical spectrum of oral candidosis and its role in HIV-infected patients, *Mycoses*, 32(Suppl. 2), 23, 1989.

45. Samaranayake, L. P. and Holmstrup, P., Oral candidiasis and human immunodeficiency virus infection, *J. Oral Pathol. Med.*, 18, 554, 1989.

46. Holt, J. M., *Candida* infection of the esophagus, *Gut*, 9, 227, 1986.

47. Kodsi, B. E., Wickremesinghe, P. C., Kozinn, P. J., Iswara, K., and Goldberg, P. K., *Candida* esophagitis: a prospective study of 27 cases, *Gastroenterology*, 71, 715, 1976.

48. Eras, P., Goldstein, M. J., and Sherlock, P., *Candida* infection of the gastrointestinal tract, *Medicine (Baltimore)*, 51, 367, 1972.

49. Wheeler, R. R., Peacock, J. E., Cruz, J. M., and Richter, J. E., Esophagitis in the immunocompromised host: role of esophagoscopy in diagnosis, *Rev. Infect. Dis.*, 9, 88, 1987.

50. Odds, F. C., *Candida and Candidosis*, 2nd ed., Bailliere Tindall, London, 1988.

51. Haulk, A. A. and Sugar, A. M., *Candida* esophagitis, in *Advances in Internal Medicine*, Stollerman, G. H., Lamont, J. T., Leonard, J. J., and Siperstein, M. D., Eds., Mosby-Yearbook, St. Louis, 1991, 307.

52. Clotet, B., Grifol, M., Parra, O., Boix, J., Junca, J., Tor, J., and Foz, M., Asymptomatic esophageal candidiasis in the acquired-immunodeficiency syndrome-related complex, *Ann. Intern. Med.*, 105, 145, 1986.

53. Bodey, G. P. and Sobel, J. D., Lower gastrointestinal candidiasis, in *Candidiasis: Pathogenesis, Diagnosis, and Treatment*, 2nd ed., Bodey, G. P., Ed., Raven Press, New York, 1993, 205.

54. Gillespie, P. E., Green, P. H., Barrett, P. J., Riley, J. W., and Nagy, G. S., Gastric candidiasis, *Med. J. Aust.*, 1, 228, 1978.

55. Myerowitz, R. L., Gastrointestinal and disseminated candidiasis: an experimental model in the immunosuppressed rat, *Arch. Pathol. Lab. Med.*, 105(3), 138, 1981.

56. Richter, J. M., Jacoby, G. A., Schapiro, R. H., and Warshaw, A. L., Pancreatic abscess due to *Candida albicans*, *Ann. Intern. Med.*, 97, 221, 1982.

57. Schreiber, M., Black, L., Noaz, Z., Saulmon, S. T., Yogen, R., and Venezio, F. R., Gallbladder candidiasis in a leukemic child, *Am. J. Dis. Child*, 136, 462, 1982.

58. Crook, W. G., *The Yeast Connection. A Medical Breakthrough*, Vintage Books, New York, 1986.

59. Renfro, L., Feder, H. M., Lane, T. J., Manu, P., and Matthews, D. A., Yeast connection among 100 patients with chronic fatigue, *Am. J. Med.*, 86, 165, 1989.

60. Dismukes, W. E., Wade, J. S., Lee, J. Y., Dockery, B. K., and Hain, J. D., A randomized, double-blind trial of nystatin therapy for the candidiasis hypersensitivity syndrome, *N. Engl. J. Med.*, 323, 1717, 1990.

61. Anderson, J. A., Chai, H., Claman, H. N., Elliz, E. F., Fink, J. N., Kaplan, A. P., Lieberman, P. L., Pierson, W. E., Salvaggio, J. E., Sheffer, A. L., and Slavin, R. G., Candida hypersensitivity syndrome: position statement, *J. Allergy Clin. Immunol.*, 78, 271, 1986.

62. Cater, R. E. II, Chronic intestinal candidiasis as a possible etiological factor in the chronic fatigue syndrome, *Med. Hypotheses*, 44, 507, 1995.

63. Bodey, G. P., Anaissie, E. J., and Edwards, J. E., Jr., Definitions of Candida infections, in *Candidiasis: Pathogenesis, Diagnosis, and Treatment*, 2nd ed., Bodey, G. P., Ed., Raven Press, New York, 1993, 407.

64. Bogden, E. and Kessel, J., Monilial meningitis, *Arch. Pathol.*, 23, 909, 1937.

65. Bodey, G. P., Hematogenous and major organ candidiasis, in *Candidiasis: Pathogenesis, Diagnosis, and Treatment*, 2nd ed., Bodey, G. P., Ed., Raven Press, New York, 1993, 279.

66. Barrett, B., Volwiler, W., Kirby, W. M. M., and Jensen, C. R., Fatal systemic moniliasis following pancreatitis, *Arch. Intern. Med.*, 99, 209, 1957.

67. Dennis, D. L., Peterson, C. G., and Fletcher, W. S., Candida septicemia in the severely traumatized patient, *J. Trauma*, 8, 177, 1968.

68. Louria, D. B., Stiff, D. P., and Bennett, B., Disseminated moniliasis in the adult, *Medicine (Baltimore)*, 41, 307, 1962.

69. Pillay, V. K. G., Wilson, D. M., Ing, T. S., and Kark, R. M., Fungus infection in steroid-treated systemic lupus erythematosus, *JAMA*, 205, 261, 1968.

70. Jacobs, M. I., Magid, M. S., and Jarowski, C. I., Disseminated candidiasis: newer approaches to early recognition and treatment, *Arch. Dermatol.*, 116, 1277, 1980.

71. Briegel, J., Forst, H., Spill, B., Haas, A., Grabein, B., Haller, M., Kilger, E., Jauch, K. W., Maag, K., Ruckdeschel, G., and Peter, K., Risk factors for systemic fungal infections in liver transplant recipients, *Eur. J. Clin. Microbiol. Infect. Dis.*, 14, 375, 1995.

72. Andriole, V. T., Kraveta, H. M., and Roberts, W. E., Candida endocarditis, *Am. J. Med.*, 32, 251, 1962.

73. Bayer, A. S., Edwards, J. E., and Seidel, J. S., Candida meningitis, *Medicine (Baltimore)*, 55, 477, 1976.

74. Rosenbaum, R. B., Barber, J. V., and Stevens, D. A., *Candida albicans* pneumonia, *Am. Rev. Respir. Dis.*, 109, 373, 1974.

75. Horn, R., Wong, B., Kiehn, T., and Armstrong, D., Fungemia in a cancer hospital: changing frequency, earlier onset and results of therapy, *Rev. Infect. Dis.*, 7, 646, 1985.

76. Valdivieso, M., Luna, M., Bodey, G. P., Rodriguez, V., and Groschell, D., Fungemia due to Torulopsis glabrata in the compromised host, *Cancer*, 38, 1750, 1976.

77. Meunier-Carpentier, F., Kiehn, T. E., and Armstrong, D., Fungemia in the immunocompromised host, *Am. J. Med.*, 71, 363, 1981.

78. Komshian, S. V., Uwaydah, A. K., Sobel, J. D., and Crane, L. R., Fungemia caused by *Candida* species and *Torulopsis glabrata* in the hospitalized patient: frequency, characteristics and evaluation of factors influencing outcome, *Rev. Respir. Dis.*, 11, 379, 1989.

79. Sandford, G. R., Merz, W. G., Winegard, J. R., Charache, P., and Saral, R., The value of fungal surveillance cultures as predictors of systemic fungal infections, *J. Infect. Dis.*, 142, 503, 1980.

80. Verfaillie, C., Weisdorf, D., Haake, R., Hostetter, M., Mansay, N. K. C., and McGlave, P., Candida infections in bone marrow transplant recipients, *Bone Marrow Transplant.*, 8, 177, 1991.

81. Marina, N. W., Flynn, P. M., Rivera, G. K., and Hughes, W. T., *Candida tropicalis* and *Candida albicans* fungemia in children with leukemia, *Cancer*, 68, 594, 1991.

82. Winegard, J. R., Merz, W. G., and Saral, R., *Candida tropicalis*: a major pathogen in immunocompromised patients, *Ann. Intern. Med.*, 91, 539, 1979.

83. Flynn, P. M., Marina, N. M., Rivera, G. K., and Hughes, W. T., *Candida tropicalis* infections in children with leukemia, *Leuk. Lymphoma*, 10, 369, 1993.

84. Huang, J. L., Yang, C. P., and Hung, I. J., *Candida tropicalis* fungemia in children with leukemia and lymphoma, *Acta Paediatr.*, 34, 257, 1993.

85. Winegard, J. R., Merz, W. G., Rinaldi, M. G., Johnson, T. H., Karp, J. E., and Saral, R., Increase in *Candida krusei* infection among patients with bone marrow transplantation and neutropenia treated prophylactically with fluconazole, *N. Engl. J. Med.*, 325, 1274, 1991.

86. Blinkhorn, R. J., Adelstein, A., and Spagnuolo, P. J., Emergence of a new opportunistic pathogen, *Candida lusitaniae*, *J. Clin. Microbiol.*, 27, 236, 1989.

87. Hadfield, T. L., Smith, M. B., Winn, R. E., Rinaldi, M. G., and Guerra, C., Mycoses caused by *Candida lusitaniae*, *Rev. Infect. Dis.*, 9, 1006, 1987.

88. de Pauw, B. E., Raemaekers, J. M., Donnelly, J. P., Kullberg, B. J., and Meis, J. F., An open study on the safety and efficacy of fluconazole in the treatment of disseminated Candida infection in patients treated for hematologic malignancy, *Ann. Hematol.*, 70, 83, 1995.

89. Lehrer, R. I. and Cline, M. J., Leukocyte candidacidal activity and resistance to systemic candidiasis in patients with cancer, *Cancer*, 27, 1211, 1971.

90. Bodey, G. P., Fungal infections complicating acute leukemia, *J. Chron. Dis.*, 19, 667, 1966.

91. Bodey, G. P., The emergence of fungi as major hospital pathogens, *J. Hosp. Infect.*, 11(Suppl. A), 411, 1988.

92. Harvey, R. L. and Myers, J. P., Nosocomial fungemia in a large community teaching hospital, *Arch. Intern. Med.*, 147, 2117, 1987.

93. Burchard, K. W., Minor, L. B., Slotman, G. J., and Gann, D. S., Fungal sepsis in surgical patients, *Arch. Surg.*, 118, 217, 1983.

94. Schroter, G. P. J., Hoelscher, M., Putnam, C. W., Porter, K. A., and Starzl, T. E., Fungal infections after liver transplantation, *Ann. Surg.*, 186, 115, 1977.

95. Wajszczuk, C. P., Dummer, J. S., Ho, M., Van Thiel, D. H., Starzl, T. E., Iwatsuki, S., and Shaw, B., Fungal infections in liver transplant recipients, *Transplantation*, 49, 347, 1985.

96. Winston, D., Gale, R. P., Meyer, D. V., and Young, L. S., Infectious complications of human bone marrow transplantation, *Medicine (Baltimore)*, 58, 1, 1979.

97. Wey, S. B., Mori, M., Pfaller, M. A., Wollson, R. F., and Wenzel, R. P., Hospital-acquired candidemia: the attributable mortality and excess length of stay, *Arch. Intern. Med.*, 148, 2642, 1988.

98. Roberts, F. J., Geere, I. W., and Coldman, A., A three-year study of positive blood cultures, with emphasis on prognosis, *Rev. Infect. Dis.*, 12, 34, 1991.

99. Goodrich, J. M., Reed, E., Mori, M., Fisher, L. D., Skerrett, S., Dandliker, P. S., Klis, B., Counts, G. W., and Meyers, J. D., Clinical features and analysis of risk factors for invasive candidal infection after marrow transplantation, *J. Infect. Dis.*, 164, 731, 1991.

100. Marsh, P. K., Tally, F. P., Kellum, J., Callow, A., and Gorbach, S. L., Candida infections in surgical patients, *Ann. Surg.*, 198, 42, 1983.

101. Moyer, D. V. and Edwards, J. E., Jr., *Candida* endophthalmitis and central nervous system infection, in *Candidiasis: Pathogenesis, Diagnosis, and Treatment*, 2nd ed., Bodey, G. P., Ed., Raven Press, New York, 1993, 331.

102. Towler, H. M., Lightman, S., and Matheson, M., Candida endophthalmitis, *Br. J. Ophthalmol.*, 79, 1141, 1995.

103. Menezes, A. V., Sigesmund, D. A., Demajo, W. A., and Devenyi, R. G., Mortality of hospitalized patients with Candida endophthalmitis, *Arch. Intern. Med.*, 154, 2093, 1994.

104. Aguilar, G. L., Blumenkrantz, M. S., Egbert, P. R., and McCulley, J. P., Candida endophthalmitis after intravenous drug abuse, *Arch. Ophthalmol.*, 97, 96, 1979.

105. Getnick, R. A. and Rodriguez, M. M., Endogenous fungal endophthalmitis in a drug addict, *Am. J. Ophthalmol.*, 77, 680, 1974.

106. Horne, M. J., Ma, M. H., Taylor, R. F., Williams, R., and Zylstra, W., Candida endophthalmitis, *Med. J. Aust.*, 1, 170, 1975.

107. Snip, R. C. and Michels, R. G., Pars plana vitrectomy in the management of endogenous Candida endophthalmitis, *Am. J. Ophthalmol.*, 82, 699, 1976.

108. Stern, G. A., Fetkenhour, C. L., and O'Grady, R. B., Intravitreal amphotericin B treatment of Candida endophthalmitis, *Arch. Ophthalmol.*, 95, 89, 1977.

109. Stone, R. D., Irvine, A. R., and O'Connor, G. R., Candida endophthalmitis: report of an unusual case with isolation of the etiologic agent by vitreous biopsy, *Ann. Ophthalmol.*, 7, 757, 1975.

110. Vastine, D. W., Horsley, W., Guth, S. B., and Goldberg, M. F., Endogenous candida endophthalmitis associated with heroin use, *Arch. Ophthalmol.*, 94, 1805, 1976.

111. Hvidberg-Hansen, A., Endogenous mycotic retinopathy: report of a case, *Acta Ophthalmol.*, 50, 515, 1972.

112. Meyers, B. R., Lieberman, T. W., and Ferry, A. P., Candida endophthalmitis complicating candidemia, *Ann. Intern. Med.*, 79, 647, 1973.

113. Peyman, G. A., Vastine, D. W., and Meisels, H. I., The experimental and clinical use of intravitreal antibiotics to treat bacterial and fungal endophthalmitis, *Doc. Ophthalmol.*, 39, 183, 1975.

114. Rosen, R. and Friedman, A. H., Successfully treated postoperative Candida parakrusei endophthalmitis, *Am. J. Ophthalmol.*, 76, 574, 1973.

115. Sixbey, J. W. and Caplan, E. S., Candida parapsilosis endophthalmitis, *Ann. Intern. Med.*, 89, 1010, 1978.

116. Weinstein, A. J., Johnson, E. H., and Moellering, R. C., Jr., Candida endophthalmitis: a complication of candidemia, *Arch. Intern. Med.*, 132, 749, 1973.

117. Joshi, N. and Hamory, B. H., Endophthalmitis caused by non-albicans species of Candida, *Rev. Infect. Dis.*, 13, 281, 1991.

118. McQuillen, D. P., Zingman, B. S., Meunier, F., and Levitz, S. M., Invasive infections due to Candida krusei: report of fungemia that include cases of endophthalmitis, *Clin. Infect. Dis.*, 14, 472, 1992.

119. Cohen, M. and Montgomerie, J. Z., Hematogenous endophthalmitis due to *Candida tropicalis*: report of two cases and review, *Clin. Infect. Dis.*, 17, 270, 1993.

120. Edwards, J. E., Jr., Montgomerie, J. Z., Ishida, K., Morrison, J. O., and Guze, L. B., Experimental hematogenous endophthalmitis due to Candida: species variation in ocular pathogenicity, *J. Infect. Dis.*, 135, 294, 1977.

121. Jones, D. B., Chemotherapy of experimental endogenous Candida albicans endophthalmitis, *Trans. Am. Soc. Ophthalmol.*, 76, 846, 1980.

122. Parker, J. C., Jr., McCloskey, J. J., and Lee, R. S., The emergence of candidosis: the dominant postmortem cerebral mycosis, *Am. J. Clin. Pathol.*, 70, 31, 1978.

123. Lipton, S. A., Hickey, V. F., Morris, J. H., and Loscalzo, J., Candidal infection in the central nervous system, *Am. J. Med.*, 76, 101, 1984.

124. Buchs, S. and Pfister, P., Candida meningitis: course, prognosis, and mortality before and after introduction of the new antimycotics, *Mykosen*, 26, 73, 1982.

125. Coker, S. B. and Beltran, R. B., Candida meningitis: clinical and radiographic diagnosis, *Pediatr. Neurol.*, 4, 317, 1988.

126. Black, J. T., Cerebral candidiasis: case report of brain abscess secondary to Candida albicans, and review of the literature, *J. Neurol. Neurosurg. Psychiatr.*, 33, 864, 1970.

127. Parker, J. C., Jr., McCloskey, J. J., and Lee, R. S., Human cerebral candidosis — a postmortem evaluation of 19 patients, *Hum. Pathol.*, 12, 23, 1981.

128. Fleischman, J., Church, J. A., and Lehrer, R. I., Case report: primary Candida meningitis and chronic granulomatous disease, *Am. J. Med. Sci.*, 291, 334, 1986.

129. Chesney, P. J., Justman, R. A., and Bogdanowicz, W. M., Candida meningitis in newborn infants: a review and report of combined amphotericin B-flucytosine therapy, *Johns Hopkins Med. J.*, 142, 155, 1978.

130. Lilien, L. D., Ramamurthy, R. S., and Pildes, R. S., Candida albicans meningitis in premature neonates successfully treated with 5-flucytosine and amphotericin B: a case report and review of the literature, *Pediatrics*, 61, 57, 1978.

131. Edelson, R. N., McNatt, E. N., and Porro, R. S., Candida meningitis with cerebral arteritis, *NY State J. Med.*, 75, 900, 1975.

132. Chadwick, D. W., Hartley, E., and Mackinnon, D. M., Meningitis caused by Candida tropicalis, *Arch. Neurol.*, 37, 175, 1980.

133. Gelfand, M. S., Mcgee, Z. A., Kaiser, A. B., Tally, F. P., and Moses, J., Candidal meningitis following bacterial meningitis, *South. Med. J.*, 83, 567, 1990.

134. Leggiadro, R. J. and Collins, T., Postneurosurgical Candida lusitaniae meningitis, *Pediatr. Infect. Dis. J.*, 7, 368, 1988.

135. Sanchez, P. J. and Cooper, B. H., Candida lusitaniae: sepsis and meningitis in a neonate, *Pediatr. Infect. Dis. J.*, 6, 758, 1987.

136. Faix, R. G., Candida parapsilosis meningitis in a premature infant, *Pediatr. Infect. Dis. J.*, 2, 462, 1983.

137. Anhalt, E., Alvarez, J., and Berg, R., Candida glabrata meningitis, *South. Med. J.*, 79, 916, 1986.

138. Smego, R. A., Jr., Devoe, P. W., Sampson, H. A., Perfect, J. R., Wilfert, C. M., and Buckley, R. H., Candida meningitis in two children with severe combined immunodeficiency, *J. Pediatr.*, 104, 902, 1984.

139. Kauffman, C. A., Shea, M. J., and Frame, P. T., Invasive fungal infections in patients with chronic mucocutaneous candidiasis, *Arch. Intern. Med.*, 141, 1076, 1981.

140. Ehni, W. F. and Ellison, R. T. III, Spontaneous Candida albicans meningitis in a patient with the acquired immune deficiency syndrome, *Am. J. Med.*, 83, 806, 1987.

141. Ilgren, E. B., Westmorland, D., Adams, C. B. T., and Mitchell, R. G., Cerebellar mass caused by Candida species, *J. Neurosurg.*, 60, 428, 1984.

142. Kumar, S., Kaza, R. C., Tandon, A., and Nayar, M., Subdural spinal fungal granuloma due to Candida tropicalis, *J. Neurosurg.*, 50, 395, 1979.

143. Ho, K., Williams, A., Gronseth, G., and Aldrich, M., Spinal cord swelling and candidiasis, *Neuroradiology*, 24, 117, 1982.

144. Voice, R. A., Bradley, S. F., Sangeorzan, J. A., and Kauffman, C. A., Chronic candidal meningitis: an uncommon manifestation of candidiasis, *Clin. Infect. Dis.*, 19, 60, 1994.

145. Hallum, J. L. and Williams, T. W., Jr., *Candida* endocarditis, in *Candidiasis: Pathogenesis, Diagnosis, and Treatment*, 2nd ed., Bodey, G. P., Ed., Raven Press, New York, 1993, 357.

146. Han-Soeb, K., Weilbaecher, D. G., Lie, J. T., and Titus, J. L., Myocardial abscess, *Am. J. Clin. Pathol.*, 70, 18, 1977.

147. Walsh, T. J., Hutchins, G. M., Bulkley, B. H., and Mendelsohn, G., Fungal infections of the heart: analysis of 51 autopsy cases, *Am. J. Cardiol.*, 45, 357, 1979.

148. Drutz, D., The spectrum of fungal endocarditis, *Cal. Med.*, 115, 34, 1971.

149. Kaye, D., Change in the spectrum, diagnosis and management of bacterial and fungal endocarditis, *Med. Clin. North Am.*, 57, 941, 1973.

150. Lerner, P. I., Infective endocarditis: a review of selected topics, *Med. Clin. North Am.*, 58, 605, 1974.

151. Rubinstein, E., Noriega, E. R., Simberkoff, M. S., Holzman, R., and Rahal, J. J., Fungal endocarditis: analysis of 24 cases and review of the literature, *Medicine (Baltimore)*, 54, 331, 1975.

152. Norenberg, R. G., Sethi, G. K., Scott, S. M., and Takaro, T., Opportunistic endocarditis following open-heart surgery, *Ann. Thorac. Surg.*, 19, 592, 1975.

153. Premsingh, N., Kapila, R., Tecson, F., Smith, L. G., and Louria, D. B., Candida endocarditis in two patients, *Arch. Intern. Med.*, 136, 208, 1976.

154. Watanakunakorn, C., Infective endocarditis as a result of medical progress, *Am. J. Med.*, 64, 917, 1978.

155. Parker, J. C., The potentially lethal problem of cardiac candidosis, *Am. J. Clin. Pathol.*, 73, 356, 1979.

156. Atkinson, J. B. and Virmani, R., Infective endocarditis: changing trends and general approach for examination, *Hum. Pathol.*, 18, 603, 1987.

157. Harris, P. D., Yeoh, C. B., Breault, J., Meltzer, J., and Katz, S., Fungal endocarditis secondary to drug addiction, *J. Thorac. Cardiovasc. Surg.*, 63, 980, 1972.

158. Reisberg, B. E., Infective endocarditis in the narcotic addict, *Prog. Cardiovasc. Dis.*, 22, 193, 1979.

159. Oriel, J. D., Partridge, B. M., Denn, M. J., and Coleman, J. C., Genital yeast infections, *Br. Med. J.*, 4, 761, 1972.

160. Morton, R. S. and Rashid, S., Candidal vaginitis: natural history, predisposing factors and prevention, *Proc. R. Soc. Med.*, 70(Suppl. 4), 3, 1977.

161. Horowitz, B. J., Edelstein, S. W., and Lippman, L., *Candida tropicalis* vulvovaginitis, *Obstet. Gynecol.*, 66, 229, 1985.

162. King, R. D., Lee, J. C., and Morris, A. L., Adherence of *Candida albicans* and other candida species to mucosal epithelial cells, *Infect. Immun.*, 27, 667, 1980.

163. Kent, H. L., Epidemiology of vaginitis, *Am. J. Obstet. Gynecol.*, 165, 1168, 1991.

164. Centers for Disease Control, Non-reported sexually transmitted diseases, *Morbid. Mortal. Wkly. Rep.*, 28, 61, 1979.

165. Sobel, J. D., Genital candidiasis, in *Candidiasis: Pathogenesis, Diagnosis, and Treatment*, 2nd ed., Bodey, G. P., Ed., Raven Press, New York, 1993, 225.

166. Gentry, L. O. and Price, M. F., Urinary and peritoneal *Candida* infections, in *Candidiasis: Pathogenesis, Diagnosis, and Treatment*, 2nd ed., Bodey, G. P., Ed., Raven Press, New York, 1993, 249.

167. Turck, M., Goffce, B., and Petersdorf, R. G., The urethral catheter and urinary tract infection, *J. Urol.*, 88, 834, 1962.

168. Schaeffer, A. J. and Chmiel, J., Urethral meatal colonization in the catheter-associated bacteriuria, *J. Urol.*, 130, 1096, 1983.

169. Garibaldi, R. A., Burke, J. P., Britt, M. R., Miller, W. A., and Smith, C. B., Meatal colonization and catheter associated bacteriuria, *N. Engl. J. Med.*, 303, 316, 1980.
170. Daifuku, R. and Stamm, W., Association of rectal and urethral colonization with urinary tract infection in patients with indwelling catheters, *JAMA,* 252, 2028, 1984.
171. Hamory, B. H. and Wezel, R. P., Hospital-associated candiduria: predisposing factors and a review of the literature, *J. Urol.*, 120, 444, 1978.
172. Warren, J. W., Platt, R., Thomas, R. J., Rosner, B., and Kass, E. H., Antibiotic irrigation and catheter-associated urinary tract infection, *N. Engl. J. Med.*, 299, 570, 1978.
173. Platt, R., Polk, B. F., Murdock, B., and Rosner, B., Risk factors for nosocomial urinary tract infection, *Am. J. Epidemiol.*, 124, 977, 1986.
174. Dreetz, D. J. and Fetchick, R., Fungal infections of the urinary tract and kidney, in *Diseases of the Kidney*, Vol. 1, Schrier, R. W. and Gottschalk, C. W., Eds., Little, Brown, Boston, 1988, 1015.
175. McDonald, D. F. and Fagan, C. J., Fungus balls in the urinary bladder, *Am. J. Roentgenol.*, 114, 753, 1988.
176. Margolin, H. N., Fungus infection of the urinary tract, *Semin. Roentgenol.*, 6, 323, 1971.
177. Rovinescu, I., Belanger, P. M., and Lapalme, R., Monilial infection of the urinary bladder, *Urol. Int.*, 23, 428, 1968.
178. Schönebeck, J., Studies of Candida infection of the urinary tract and on the antimycotic drug 5-fluorocytosine, *Scand. J. Urol. Nephrol.* Suppl., 11, 35, 1972.
179. Jenks, P., Brown, J., Warnock, D., and Barnes, N., *Candida glabrata* epididymo-orchitis: an unusual infection rapidly cured with surgical and antifungal treatment, *J. Infect.*, 31, 71, 1995.
180. Hansen, B. L. and Andersen, K., Fungal arthritis, *Scand. J. Rheumatol.*, 24, 248, 1995.
181. Barbara, J. A., Clarkson, A. R., LaBrooy, J., McNeil, J. D., and Woodroffe, A. J., *Candida albicans* arthritis in a renal allograft recipient with an interaction between cyclosporin and fluconazole, *Nephrol. Dial. Transplant.*, 8, 263, 1993.
182. Lasday, S. D. and Jay, R. M., Candida osteomyelitis, *J. Foot Ankle Surg.*, 33, 173, 1994.
183. Dvorak, A. M. and Gavaller, P., Congenital systemic candidiasis: report of a case, *N. Engl. J. Med.*, 274, 540, 1966.
184. Baley, J. E., Kliegman, R. M., and Faranoff, A. A., Disseminated fungal infections in very low birth weight infants: clinical manifestations and epidemiology, *Pediatrics*, 73, 144, 1984.
185. Johnson, D. E., Thompson, T. R., Green, T. P., and Ferrieri, P., Systemic candidiasis in very low birth weight infants (<1500 grams), *Pediatrics*, 73, 138, 1984.
186. Hughes, P. A., Lepow, M. L., and Hill, H. R., Neonatal candidiasis, in *Candidiasis: Pathogenesis, Diagnosis, and Treatment*, 2nd ed., Bodey, G. P., Ed., Raven Press, New York, 1993, 261.
187. Butler, K. M., Rench, M. A., and Baker, C. J., Amphotericin B as a single agent in the treatment of systemic candidiasis in neonates, *Pediatr. Infect. Dis. J.*, 9, 51, 1990.
188. Faix, R. G., Kovarik, S. M., Shaw, T. R., and Johnson, R. V., Mucocutaneous and invasive candidiasis among very low birth weight (<1500 grams) infants in intensive care nurseries: a prospective study, *Pediatrics*, 83, 101, 1989.
189. Hagemen, J. R., Stenske, J., Keuler, H., and Randall, E., Candida colonization and infection in very low birth weight (VLBW) in the intensive care nursery (ICU), *Pediatr. Res.*, 19, 345A, 1985.
190. Dyke, M. P. and Ott, K., Severe thrombocytopenia in extremely low birth weight infants with systemic candidiasis, *J. Paediatr. Child Health*, 29, 298, 1993.
191. Boeckman, C. R. and Krill, C. E., Bacterial and fungal infections complicating parenteral alimentation in infants and children, *J. Pediatr. Surg.*, 5, 117, 1970.
192. Weese-Mayer, D. E., Fondriest, D. W., Brouillette, R. T., and Schulman, S. T., Risk factors associated with candidemia in the neonatal intensive care unit: a case-control study, *Pediatr. Infect. Dis. J.*, 6, 190, 1987.
193. Kotloff, K. L., Blackmon, L. R., Tenney, J. H., Rennels, M. B., and Morris, J. G., Nosocomial sepsis in the neonatal intensive care unit, *South. Med. J.*, 82, 699, 1989.
194. Bourne, H. R., Lehrer, R. I., Cline, M. J., and Melmon, K. L., Cyclic $3^1:5^1$-adenosine monophosphate in the human leukocyte: synthesis, degradation, and effects on neutrophil candidacidal activity, *J. Clin. Invest.*, 50, 920, 1971.
195. Gonzales, L. A. and Hill, H. R., The current status of intravenous gammaglobulin use in neonates, *Pediatr. Infect. Dis. J.*, 68, 315, 1989.

196. Hill, H. R., Biochemical, structural and functional abnormalities of polymorphonuclear leukocytes in the neonate, *Pediatr. Res.*, 22, 375, 1987.

197. Lewis, D. B., Yu, C. C., Meyer, J., English, B. K., Kahn, S. J., and Wilson, C. B., Cellular and molecular mechanisms for reduced interleukin 4 and interferon-gamma production by neonatal T cells, *J. Clin. Invest.*, 87, 194, 1991.

198. Hill, H. R., Augustine, N. H., and Jaffe, H. S., Human recombinant interferon-gamma enhances neonatal PMN activation and movement and increases free intracellular calcium, *J. Exp. Med.*, 173, 767, 1991.

199. Boon, J. M., Lafeber, H. N., 't Mannetje, A. H., van Olphen, A. H., Smeets, H. L., Toorman, J., and van der Vlist, G. J., Comparison of ketoconazole suspension and nystatin in the treatment of newborns and infants with oral candidosis, *Mycoses*, 32, 312, 1989.

200. Baley, J. E., Kliegman, R. M., Boxerbaum, B., and Faranoff, A. A., Fungal colonization in the very low birth weight infant, *Pediatrics*, 78, 225, 1986.

201. al-Rasheed, S. A., The management of fungal obstructive uropathy in neonates and infants, *Ann. Trop. Paediatr.*, 14, 169, 1994.

202. Green, B. I., Treatment of fungal infections in the human immunodeficiency virus-infected individual, in *Antifungal Drug Therapy: A Complete Guide For the Practitioner*, Jacobs, P. H. and Nall, L., Eds., Marcel Dekker, New York, 1990, 237.

203. Wilcox, C. M. and Karowe, M. W., Esophageal infections: etiology, diagnosis, and management, *Gastroenterologist*, 2, 188, 1994.

204. Selik, R. M., Starcher, E. T., and Curran, J. W., Opportunistic diseases reported in AIDS patients: frequencies, associations, and trends, *AIDS*, 1, 175, 1987.

205. Torssander, J., Morfeldt-Manson, L., Biberfeld, G., Karlsson, A., Putkonen, P. O., and Wasserman, J., Oral *Candida albicans* in HIV infection, *Scand. J. Infect. Dis.*, 19, 291, 1987.

206. Tavitian, A., Raufman, J. P., and Rosenthal, L. E., Oral candidiasis as a marker for esophageal candidiasis in the acquired immunodeficiency syndrome, *Ann. Intern. Med.*, 104, 54, 1986.

207. Pedersen, C., Gerstoft, J., Lindhardt, B. O., and Sindrup, J., Candida esophagitis associated with acute human immunodeficiency virus infection, *J. Infect. Dis.*, 156, 529, 1987.

208. Warnock, D. W., Fungal complications of transplantation: diagnosis, treatment and prevention, *J. Antimicrob. Chemother.*, 36(Suppl. B), 73, 1995.

209. Hasenclever, H. F. and Mitchell, W. O., Antigenic studies of candida. I. Observation of two antigenic groups in *Candida albicans*, *J. Bacteriol.*, 82, 570, 1961.

210. Hasenclever, H. F. and Mitchell, W. O., Antigenic studies of candida. III. Comparative pathogenicity of *Candida albicans* group A, group B, and *Candida stellatoidea*, *J. Bacteriol.*, 82, 578, 1961.

211. Brawner, D. L., Anderson, G. L., and Yuen, K. Y., Serotype prevalence of *Candida albicans* from blood culture isolates, *J. Clin. Microbiol.*, 30, 149, 1992.

212. Brawner, D. L. and Cutler, J. E., Oral *Candida albicans* isolates from nonhospitalized normal carriers, immunocompetent hospitalized patients, and immunocompromised patients with or without acquired immunodeficiency syndrome, *J. Clin. Microbiol.*, 27, 1335, 1989.

213. Odds, F. C., Schmid, J., and Soll, D. R., Epidemiology of *Candida* infections in AIDS, in *Mycoses in AIDS Patients: Proceedings of the 3rd Symposium, Topics in Mycology*, vanden Bossche, H., Mackenzie, D. W. R., Cauwenbergh, G., Van Cutsem, J., and Dupont, D., Eds., Plenum Press, London, 1990, 67.

214. Hopfer, R. L., Fainstein, V., Luna, G. P., and Bodey, G. P., Disseminated candidiasis caused by four different *Candida* species, *Arch. Pathol. Lab. Med.*, 105, 454, 1981.

215. Guinet, R., Chanas, J., Goullier, A., Bonnefoy, G., and Ambroise-Thomas, P., Fatal septicemia due to amphotericin B-resistant *Candida lusitaniae*, *J. Clin. Microbiol.*, 18, 443, 1983.

216. Merz, W. G., Khazan, U., Jabra-Rizk, M. A., Wu, L. C., Osterhout, G. J., and Lehmann, P. F., Strain delineation and epidemiology of Candida (clavispora) lusitaniae, *J. Clin. Microbiol.*, 30, 449, 1992.

217. Sanchez, V., Vazquez, J. A., Barth-Jones, D., Dembry, L., Sobel, J. D., and Zervos, M. J., Epidemiology of nosocomial acquisition of *Candida lusitaniae*, *J. Clin. Microbiol.*, 30, 3005, 1992.

218. Ruechel, R., Virulence factors of *Candida* species, in *Oral Candidiasis*, Samaranayake, L. P. and MacFarlane, T. W., Eds., Wright, London, 1990, 47.

219. Minagi, S., Miyake, Y., Inagaki, K., Tsuru, H., and Suginaka, H., Hydrophobic interaction in *Candida albicans* and *Candida tropicalis*: adherence to various denture base dental resin materials, *Infect. Immun.*, 47, 11, 1985.

220. Kimura, L. H. and Pearsall, N. N., Adherence of *Candida albicans* to human buccal epithelial cells, *Infect. Immun.*, 21, 64, 1978.

221. Sobel, J. D., Myers, P. G., Kaye, D., and Levison, M. E., Adherence of *Candida albicans* to human vaginal and buccal epithelial cells, *J. Infect. Dis.*, 14, 464, 1980.

222. Brawner, D. L., Smith, F. O., Mori, M., and Nonoyama, S., Adherence of *Candida albicans* to tissues from mice with genetic immunodeficiencies, *Infect. Immun.*, 59, 3069, 1991.

223. Sawyer, R. T., Horst, M. N., Garner, R. E., Hudson, J., Jenkins, P. R., and Richardson, A. L., Altered hepatic clearance and killing of *Candida albicans* in the isolated perfused mouse liver model, *Infect. Immun.*, 58, 2869, 1990.

224. Douglas, L. J., Adhesion of pathogenic *Candida* species to host surfaces, *Microbiol. Sci.*, 2, 243, 1985.

225. Critchley, I. A. and Douglas, L. J., Role of glycosides as epithelial cell receptors for *Candida albicans*, *J. Gen. Microbiol.*, 133, 637, 1987.

226. Skerl, K. G., Calderon, R. A., Segal, E., Sreevalsan, T., and Scheld, W. M., *In vitro* binding of *Candida albicans* yeast cells to human fibronectin, *Can. J. Microbiol.*, 30, 221, 1984.

227. Scheld, W. M., Strunk, R. W., Balian, G., and Calderone, R. A., Microbial adhesion to fibronectin *in vitro* correlates with production of endocarditis in rabbits, *Proc. Soc. Exp. Biol. Med.*, 180, 474, 1985.

228. Calderone, R. A. and Braun, P. C., Adherence and receptor relationships in *Candida albicans*, *Microbiol. Rev.*, 55, 1, 1991.

229. Kaminishi, H., Hagihara, Y., Hayashi, S., and Cho, T., Isolation and characterization of a collagenolytic enzyme produced by *Candida albicans*, *Infect. Immun.*, 53, 312, 1986.

230. Ghannoum, M. A. and Abu-Elteen, K. H., Pathogenicity determinants of *Candida*, *Mycoses*, 33, 265, 1990.

231. Hazen, K. C., Cell surface hydrophobicity of medically important fungi, especially *Candida* species, in *Microbial Cell Surface Hydrophobicity*, Doyle, R. J. and Rosenberg, M., Eds., American Society for Microbiology, Washington, D.C., 1990, 249.

232. Hazen, K. C., Plotkin, B. J., and Klimas, D. M., Influence of growth conditions on cell surface hydrophobicity of *Candida glabrata*, *Infect. Immun.*, 54, 269, 1986.

233. Hazen, B. W. and Hazen, K. C., Dynamic expression of cell surface hydrophobicity during initial yeast cell growth and before germ tube formation of *Candida albicans*, *Infect. Immun.*, 56, 2521, 1988.

234. Hazen, K. C., Lay, J. G., Hazen, B. W., Fu, R. C., and Murthy, S., Partial biochemical characterization of cell surface hydrophobicity and hydrophilicity of *Candida albicans*, *Infect. Immun.*, 58, 3469, 1990.

235. Cutler, J. E., Putative virulence factors of *Candida albicans*, *Annu. Rev. Microbiol.*, 45, 187, 1991.

236. Pugh, D. and Cawson, R. A., The cytochemical localization of phospholipase in *Candida albicans* infecting the chick chorio-allantoic membrane, *Sabouraudia*, 15, 29, 1977.

237. Gorbach, S. L., Nahas, L., Lerner, P. I., and Weinstein, L., Studies of intestinal microflora, *Gastroenterology*, 53, 845, 1967.

238. Krause, W., Matheis, H., and Wulf, K., Fungaemia and funguria after oral administration of *Candida albicans*, *Lancet*, 1, 598, 1969.

239. Carlson, E., Synergistic effect of *Candida albicans* and *Staphylococcus aureus* on mouse mortality, *Infect. Immun.*, 38, 921, 1982.

240. Isenberg, H. D., Pisano, M. A., Carito, S. L., and Berkman, J. I., Factors leading to overt monilial disease, *Antibiot. Chemother.*, 10, 353, 1960.

241. Hamilton, J. R., Overall, J. C., and Glasgow, L. A., Synergistic effect on mortality in mice with murine cytomegalovirus and *Pseudomonas aeruginosa*, *Staphylococcus aureus*, or *Candida albicans* infections, *Infect. Immun.*, 14, 982, 1976.

242. Kagaya, K., Shinoda, T., and Fukazawa, Y., Murine defense mechanism against *Candida albicans* infection. I, *Microbiol. Immunol.*, 25, 647, 1981.

243. Sinha, B. K., Prasad, S., and Monga, D. P., Studies of the role of B-cells in the resistance of mice to experimental candidiasis, *Zentrlbl. Bakteriol. Mikrobiol. Hyg. 1. Abt. Orinale A. Med. Mikrobiol. Infektionskrankheiten Parasitol.*, 266, 316, 1987.

244. Morelli, R. and Rosenberg, L. T., Role of complement during experimental Candida infection in mice, *Infect. Immun.*, 3, 521, 1971.

245. Meuwissen, H. J., Rhee, M. S., Rynes, R. I., and Pikering, R. J., Phagocytosis, chemoluminescence, and intracellular killing of fungi by phagocytes from subjects with deficiency of the second component of complement, *Int. Arch. Allergy Appl. Immunol.*, 68, 22, 1982.

246. Kagaya, K. and Fukazawa, Y., Murine defense mechanism against *Candida albicans* infection. II, *Microbiol. Immunol.*, 25, 807, 1981.

247. Morelli, R. and Rosenberg, L. T., The role of complement in the phagocytosis of *Candida albicans* by mouse peripheral blood leukocytes, *J. Immunol.*, 107, 476, 1971.

248. Elin, R. J. and Wolff, S. M., Effect of pH and iron concentration on growth of *Candida albicans* in human serum, *J. Infect. Dis.*, 127, 705, 1973.

249. Caroline, L., Rosner, R., and Kozinn, P., Elevated serum iron, low unbound transferrin and candidiasis in acute leukemia, *Blood*, 34, 441, 1969.

250. Sofaer, J. A., Holbrook, W. P., and Southam, J. C., Experimental oral infection with the yeast *Candida albicans* in mice with or without inherited iron-deficiency anaemia, *Arch. Oral Biol.*, 27, 497, 1982.

251. Vaughn, V. and Weinberg, E., *Candida albicans* dimorphism and virulence: role of copper, *Mycopathologia*, 64, 39, 1978.

252. Bodey, G. P., Fungal infections complicated acute leukemia, *J. Chron. Dis.*, 19, 667, 1966.

253. Young, R. C., Bennett, J. E., Geelhoed, G. W., and Levine, A. S., Fungemia with compromised host resistance, *Ann. Intern. Med.*, 80, 605, 1974.

254. DeGregorio, M. W., Lee, W. M. F., Linker, C. A., Jacobs, R. A., and Ries, C. A., Fungal infections in patients with acute leukemia, *Am. J. Med.*, 73, 543, 1982.

255. Diamond, R. D., Krzesicki, R., and Jao, W., Damage to pseudohyphal forms of *Candida albicans* by neutrophils in the absence of serum *in vitro*, *J. Clin. Invest.*, 61, 349, 1978.

256. Diamond, R. D. and Krzesicki, R., Mechanisms of attachment of neutrophils to *Candida albicans* pseudohyphae in the absence of serum, and of subsequent damage to pseudohyphae by microbicidal processes of neutrophils *in vitro*, *J. Clin. Invest.*, 61, 360, 1978.

257. Diamond, R. D., Clark, R. A., and Haudenschild, C. C., Damage to *Candida albicans* hyphae and pseudohyphae by the myeloperoxidase system and oxidative products of neutrophil metabolism *in vitro*, *J. Clin. Invest.*, 66, 908, 1980.

258. Levitz, S. M., Lyman, C. A., Murata, T., Sullivan, J. A., Mandell, G. I., and Diamond, R. D., Cytosolic calcium change in individual neutrophils stimulated by opsonized and unopsonized *Candida albicans* hyphae, *Infect. Immun.*, 55, 2783, 1987.

259. Lyman, C. A., Simmons, E. R., Melnick, D. A., and Diamond, R. D., Unopsonized *Candida albicans* hyphae stimulate a neutrophil respiratory burst and a cytosolic calcium flux without membrane depolarization, *J. Infect. Dis.*, 165, 770, 1987.

260. Djeu, J. Y., Tumor necrosis factor and *Candida albicans*, *Behring Inst. Mitt.*, 88, 222, 1991.

261. Sohnle, P. G., Collins-Lech, C., and Wiessner, J. H., The zinc-reversible antimicrobial activity of neutrophil lysates and abscess fluid supernatants, *J. Infect. Dis.*, 164, 137, 1991.

262. Lehrer, R. I., Ganz, T., Szklarek, D., and Selsted, M. E., Modulation of the *in vitro* candidacidal activity of human neutrophil defensins by target cell metabolism and divalent cations, *J. Clin. Invest.*, 81, 1829, 1988.

263. Leijh, P. C. J., Barselaar, M. T., and Furth, R., Kinetics of phagocytosis and intracellular killing of *Candida albicans* by human granulocytes and monocytes, *Infect. Immun.*, 17, 313, 1977.

264. Diamond, R. D. and Haudenschild, C. C., Monocyte-mediated serum-independent damage to hyphal and pseudohyphal forms of *Candida albicans in vitro*, *J. Clin. Invest.*, 67, 172, 1981.

265. Lehrer, R. I., The fungicidal mechanisms of human monocytes, *J. Clin. Invest.*, 55, 38, 1975.

266. Lehrer, R. I., Ferrari, L. G., Patterson-Delafield, J., and Norrell, T., Fungicidal activity of rabbit alveolar and peritoneal macrophages against *Candida albicans*, *Infect. Immun.*, 28, 1001, 1980.

267. Sordelii, D. O., Cassino, R. J. J., Macri, C. N., Kohan, M., Dillon, M. H., and Pivetta, O. H., Phagocytosis of *Candida albicans* by alveolar macrophages from patients with cystic fibrosis, *Clin. Immunol. Immunopathol.*, 22, 153, 1982.

268. Edwards, J. E., Lehrer, R. I., Stiehm, R. E., Fischer, T. J., and Young, L. S., Severe candidal infections: clinical perspective, immune mechanisms, and current concepts of therapy, *Ann. Intern. Med.*, 89, 91, 1978.

269. Balow, J. E. and Rosenthal, A. S., Corticosteroid suppression of macrophage inhibition factor, *J. Exp. Med.*, 137, 1031, 1973.

270. Jakab, G. J. and Warr, G. A., Immune-enhanced phagocytic dysfunction in pulmonary macrophages infected with parainfluenza I (Sendai) virus, *Am. Rev. Respir. Dis.*, 124, 575, 1981.

271. Sawyer, R. T., Moon, R. J., and Beneke, E. S., Trapping and killing of *Candida albicans* by *Corynebacterium parvum*-activated livers, *Infect. Immun.*, 32, 945, 1981.

272. Cummings, N. P., Pabst, M. J., and Johnston, R. B., Activation of macrophages for enhanced release of superoxide anion and greater killing of *Candida albicans*, *J. Exp. Med.*, 152, 1659, 1980.

273. Fraser-Smith, E. B., Waters, R. V., and Matthews, T. R., Correlation between *in vivo* anti-*Pseudomonas* and anti-*Candida* activities and clearance of carbon by reticuloendothelial system for various muramyl dipeptide analogs, using normal and immunosuppressed mice, *Infect. Immun.*, 35, 105, 1982.

274. Baccarini, M., Bistoni, F., and Lohmann-Matthes, M. L., Organ-associated macrophage precursor activity: isolation of candidacidal and tumoricidal effectors from the spleens of cyclophosphamide-treated mice, *J. Immunol.*, 136, 837, 1986.

275. Bistoni, F., Verducci, G., Perito, S., Vecchiarelli, A., Puccetti, P., Marconi, P., and Cassone, A., Immunomodulation by a low-virulence, agerminative variant of *Candida albicans*: further evidence for macrophage activation as one of the effector mechanisms of nonspecific anti-infectious protection, *J. Med. Vet. Mycol.*, 26, 285, 1988.

276. Vecchiarelli, A., Mazzolla, R., Farinelli, S., Cassone, A., and Bistoni, F., Immunomodulation by *Candida albicans*: crucial role of organ colonization and chronic infection with an attenuated agerminative protection, *J. Gen. Microbiol.*, 134, 2583, 1988.

277. Hashimoto, T., *In vitro* study of contact-mediated killing of *Candida albicans* hyphae by activated murine peritoneal macrophages in a serum-free medium, *Infect. Immun.*, 59, 3555, 1991.

278. Vecchiarelli, A., Todisco, T., Puliti, M., Dottorini, M., and Bistoni, F., Modulation of anti-Candida activity of human alveolar macrophages by interferon-gamma or interleukin-1 alpha, *Am. J. Respir. Cell. Mol. Biol.*. 1, 49, 1989.

279. Karbassi, A., Becker, J. M., Foster, J. S., and Moore, R. N., Enhanced killing of *Candida albicans* by murine macrophages treated with macrophage colony-stimulating factor: evidence for augmented expression of mannose receptors, *J. Immunol.*, 139, 417, 1987.

280. Redmond, H. P., Shou, J., Kelly, C. J., Leon, P., and Daly, J. M., Protein-calorie malnutrition impairs host defense against *Candida albicans*, *J. Surg. Res.*, 50, 552, 1991.

281. Vecchiarelli, A., Dottorini, M., Puliti, M., Todisco, T., Cenci, E., and Bistoni, F., Defective candidacidal activity of alveolar macrophages and peripheral blood monocytes from patients with chronic obstructive pulmonary disease, *Am. Rev. Respir. Dis.*, 143, 1049, 1991.

282. Watanabe, K., Kagaya, K., Tamada, T., and Fukuzawa, Y., Mechanism for candidacidal activity in macrophages activated by recombinant gamma interferon, *Infect. Immun.*, 59, 521, 1991.

283. Leshem, B., Dekel, R., Bercovier, H., Tchakirov, R., Polacheck, I., Zakay-Rones, Z., Schlesinger, M., and Kedar, E., Cytokine-induced resistance to microbial infections in normal, immunosuppressed and bone marrow transplanted mice, *Bone Marrow Transplant.*, 9, 471, 1992.

284. Lechner, A. J., Lamprech, K. E., Potthoff, L. H., Tredway, T. L., and Matuschak, G. M., Recombinant GM-CSF reduces lung injury and mortality during neutropenic *Candida* sepsis, *Am. J. Physiol.*, 266(Suppl. 1), L561, 1994.

285. Wang, M., Friedman, H., and Djeu, J. Y., Enhancement of human monocyte function against *Candida albicans* by the colony-stimulating factors (CSF): IL-3, granulocyte-macrophage CSF, and macrophage-CSF, *J. Immunol.*, 143, 671, 1989.

286. Smith, P. D., Lamerson, C. L., Banks, S. M., Saini, S. S., and Wahl, L. M., Granulocyte-macrophage colony-stimulating factor augments human monocyte fungicidal activity for *Candida albicans*, *J. Infect. Dis.*, 161, 999, 1990.

287. Calderone, R. and Sturtevant, J., Macrophage interactions with *Candida*, *Immunol. Ser.*, 60, 505, 1994.

288. Hogasen, A. K. and Abrahamsen, T. G., Increased C3 production in human monocytes after stimulation with *Candida albicans* is suppressed by granulocyte-macrophage colony-stimulating factor, *Infect. Immun.*, 61, 1779, 1993.

289. Hill, A. D., Naama, H., Shou, J., Calvano, S. E., and Daly, J. M., Antimicrobial effects of granulocyte-macrophage colony-stimulating factor in protein-energy malnutrition, *Arch. Surg.*, 130, 1273, 1995.

290. Louie, A., Baltch, A. L., Smith, R. P., Franke, M. A., Ritz, W. J., Singh, J. K., and Gordon, M. A., Fluconazole and amphotericin B antifungal therapies do not negate the protective effect of endogenous tumor necrosis factor in a murine model of fatal disseminated candidiasis, *J. Infect. Dis.*, 171, 406, 1995.

291. Netea, M. G., Blok, W. L., Kullberg, B. J., Bemelmans, M., Vogels, M. T., Buurman, W. A., and van der Meer, J. W., Pharmacologic inhibitors of tumor necrosis factor production exert differential effects in lethal endotoxemia and in infection with live microorganisms in mice, *J. Infect. Dis.*, 171, 393, 1995.

292. di Francesco, P., Gaziano, R., Casalinuovo, I. A., Belogi, L., Palamara, A. T., Favelli, C., and Garaci, E., Combined effect of fluconazole and thymosin alpha 1 on systemic candidiasis in mice immuno-suppressed by morphine treatments, *Clin. Exp. Immunol.*, 97, 347, 1994.

293. Hector, R. F., Domer, J. E., and Carrow, E. W., Immune responses to *Candida albicans* in genetically distinct mice, *Infect. Immun.*, 38, 1020, 1982.

294. Miyake, T., Takeyo, K., Nomoto, K., and Muraoka, J., Cellular elements in the resistance to Candida infection in mice: contribution of T lymphocytes and phagocytes at various stages of infection, *Microbiol. Immunol.*, 21, 703, 1977.

295. Pearsall, N. N., Adams, B. L., and Bunni, E., Immunologic responses to *Candida albicans*. III. Effects of passive transfer of lymphoid cells or serum on murine candidiasis, *J. Immunol.*, 120, 1176, 1978.

296. Hurtrel, F., LaGrange, P. H., and Michel, A., Absence of correlation between delayed type hyper-sensitivity and protection in experimental systemic candidiasis in immunized mice, *Infect. Immun.*, 31, 95, 1981.

297. Pearsall, N. N., Sundsmo, J. S., and Weiser, R. S., Lymphokine toxicity for yeast cells, *J. Immunol.*, 110, 1444, 1973.

298. Sen, P., Smith, K. J., Buse, M., Hsieh, H. C., Lavenhar, M. A., Lintz, D., and Luria, D. B., Modification of an experimental mouse Candida infection by human dialyzable leukocyte extract, *Sabouraudia*, 20, 85, 1982.

299. Beno, D. W. and Mathews, H. L., Growth inhibition of *Candida albicans* by interleukin-2-induced lymph node cells, *Cell. Immunol.*, 128, 89, 1990.

300. Zunino, S. J. and Hudig, D., Interactions between human natural killer (NK) lymphocytes and yeast cells: human NK cells do not kill *Candida albicans*, although *C. albicans* blocks NK lysis of K562 cells, *Infect. Immun.*, 56, 564, 1988.

301. Dwyer, J. M., Chronic mucocutaneous candidiasis, *Annu. Rev. Med.*, 32, 491, 1981.

302. Valdimarsson, H., Higgs, J. M., Wells, R. S., Yamamura, J., Hobbs, J. R., and Holt, P. J. L., Immune abnormalities associated with chronic mucocutaneous candidiasis, *Cell. Immunol.*, 6, 348, 1973.

303. Provost, T. T., Garrettson, L. K., Zeschke, R. H., Rose, N. R., and Tomasi, T. B., Combined immune deficiency, autoantibody formation, and mucocutaneous candidiasis, *Clin. Immunol. Immunopathol.*, 1, 429, 1973.

304. Kirkpatrick, C. H. and Windhorst, D. B., Mucocutaneous candidiasis and thymoma, *Am. J. Med.*, 66, 939, 1979.

305. Fundenberg, H. H., Spitler, L. E., and Levin, A. S., Treatment of immune deficiency, *Am. J. Pathol.*, 69, 529, 1972.

306. Kirkpatrick, C. H. and Smith, T. K., Chronic mucocutaneous candidiasis: immunologic and antibiotic therapy, *Ann. Intern. Med.*, 80, 310, 1974.

307. Rogers, T. J. and Balish, E., Immunity to *Candida albicans*, *Microbiol. Rev.*, 44, 660, 1980.

308. Louria, D. B., Stiff, D. P., and Bennett, B., Disseminated moniliasis in the adult, *Medicine (Baltimore)*, 41, 307, 1962.

309. Fauci, A. S., Dale, D. C., and Balow, J. E., Glucocorticosteroid therapy: mechanism of action and clinical considerations, *Ann. Intern. Med.*, 84, 304, 1976.

310. Quinti, I., Palma, C., Guerra, E. C., Gomez, M. J., Mezzaroma, I., Aiuti, F., and Cassone, A., Proliferative and cytotoxic responses to mannoproteins of *Candida albicans* by peripheral blood lymphocytes of HIV-infected subjects, *Clin. Exp. Immunol.*, 85, 485, 1991.

311. Cleveland, W. W., Fogel, B. J., Brown, W. T., and Kay, H. E. M., Foetal thymus transplant in a case of DiGeorge's syndrome, *Lancet*, 2, 1211, 1968.

312. Levy, R. L., Huang, S. W., Bach, M. L., Bach, F. H., Hong, R., Ammann, A. J., Bortin, M., and Kay, H. E. M., Thymic transplantation in a case of chronic mucocutaneous candidiasis, *Lancet*, 2, 898, 1971.

313. Kirkpatrick, C. H., Ottesen, E. A., Smith, T. K., Wells, S. A., and Burdick, J. F., Reconstitution of defective cellular immunity with foetal thymus and dialysable transfer factor: long term studies in a patient with chronic mucocutaneous candidiasis, *Clin. Exp. Immunol.*, 23, 414, 1976.

314. Ballow, M. and Hyman, L. R., Combination immunotherapy in chronic mucocutaneous candidiasis: synergism between transfer factor and fetal thymus tissue, *Clin. Immunol. Immunopathol.*, 8, 504, 1977.

315. Wara, D. W. and Ammann, A. J., Thymosin treatment of children with primary immunodeficiency disease, *Transplant. Proc.*, 10, 203, 1978.

316. Kirkpatrick, C. H. and Greenberg, L. E., Treatment of chronic mucocutaneous candidiasis with transfer factor, in *Immune Regulators in Transfer Factors*, Kahn, A., Kirkpatrick, C. H., and Hill, N. O., Eds., Academic Press, New York, 1979, 547.

317. Rozzo, S. J. and Kirkpatrick, C. H., Purification of transfer factors, *Mol. Immunol.*, 29, 167, 1992.

318. Kirkpatrick, C. H., Rich, R. R., and Smith, T. K., Effect of transfer factor on lymphocyte function in anergic patients, *J. Clin. Invest.*, 51, 2948, 1972.

319. Rozzo, S. J., Merryman, C. F., and Kirkpatrick, C. H., Murine transfer factor. IV. Studies with genetically regulated immune responses, *Cell. Immunol.*, 115, 130, 1988.

320. Martino, P., Girmenia, C., Micozzi, A., De Bernardis, F., Boccanera, M., and Cassone, A., Prospective study of Candida colonization, use of empiric amphotericin B and development of invasive mycosis in neutropenic patients, *Eur. J. Clin. Microbiol. Infect. Dis.*, 13, 797, 1994.

321. Benoit, J. L., Carandang, G., Sitrin, M., and Arnow, P. M., Intraluminal antibiotic treatment of central venous catheter infections in patients receiving parenteral nutrition at home, *Clin. Infect. Dis.*, 21, 1286, 1995.

322. Karyotakis, N. C. and Anaissie, E. J., Efficacy of escalating doses of liposomal amphotericin B (AmBisome) against hematogenous *Candida lusitaniae* and *Candida krusei* infection in neutropenic mice, *Antimicrob. Agents Chemother.*, 38, 2660, 1994.

323. van Etten, E. W., ten Kate, M. T., Stearne, L. E., and Bakker-Woudenberg, I. A., Amphotericin B liposomes with prolonged circulation in blood: *in vitro* antifungal activity, toxicity, and efficacy in systemic candidiasis in leukopenic mice, *Antimicrob. Agents Chemother.*, 39, 1954, 1995.

324. Sivakumara, M., Swann, R. A., Mitchell, V. E., Qureshi, H., and Wood, J. K., Therapeutic efficacy of AmBisome: a cautionary note, *Am. J. Hematol.*, 48, 208, 1995.

325. Sharland, M., Hay, R. J., and Davies, E. G., Liposomal amphotericin B in hepatic candidosis, *Arch. Dis. Child.*, 70, 546, 1994.

326. Atkinson, B. A., Bouthet, C., Bocanegra, R., Correa, A., Luther, M. F., and Graybill, J. R., Comparison of fluconazole, amphotericin B and flucytosine in treatment of a murine model of disseminated infection with *Candida glabrata* in immunocompromised mice, *J. Antimicrob. Chemother.*, 35, 631, 1995.

327. Nakajima, R., Kitamura, A., Someya, K., Tanaka, M., and Sato, K., *In vitro* and *in vivo* antifungal activities of DU-6859a, a fluoroquinolone, in combination with amphotericin B and fluconazole against pathogenic fungi, *Antimicrob. Agents Chemother.*, 39, 1517, 1995.

328. Saint-Julien, L., Joly, V., Seman, M., Carbon, C., and Yeni, P., Activity of MS-8209, a nonester amphotericin B derivative, in treatment of experimental systemic mycoses, *Antimicrob. Agents Chemother.*, 36, 2722, 1992.

329. Graybill, J. R., Najvar, K. L., Holmberg, J. D., Correa, A., and Luther, M. F., Fluconazole treatment of *Candida albicans* infection in mice: does *in vitro* susceptibility predict *in vivo* response? *Antimicrob. Agents Chemother.*, 39, 2197, 1995.

330. Graybill, J. R., Bocanegra, R., and Luther, M., Antifungal combination therapy with granulocyte colony-stimulating factor and fluconazole in experimental disseminated candidiasis, *Eur. J. Clin. Microbiol. Infect. Dis.*, 14, 700, 1995.

331. Gearhart, M. O., Worsening of liver function with fluconazole and review of azole antifungal hepatotoxicity, *Ann. Pharmacother.*, 28, 1177, 1994.

332. Ross, R. A., Lee, M. L., and Onderdonk, A. B., Effect of *Candida albicans* infection and clotrimazole treatment on vaginal microflora *in vitro*, *Obstet. Gynecol.*, 86, 925, 1995.

333. Barchiesi, F., Colombo, A. L., McGough, D. A., Fothergill, A. W., and Rinaldi, M. G., *In vitro* activity of a new antifungal triazole, DO870, against *Candida albicans* isolates from oral cavities of patients infected with human immunodeficiency virus, *Antimicrob. Agents Chemother.*, 38, 2553, 1994.

334. Barchiesi, F., Hollis, R. J., Del Poeta, M., McGough, D. A., Scalise, G., Rinaldi, M. G., and Pfaller, M. A., Transmission of fluconazole-resistant *Candida albicans* between patients with AIDS and oropharyngeal candidiasis documented by pulsed-field gel electrophoresis, *Clin. Infect. Dis.*, 21, 561, 1995.

335. Atkinson, B. A., Bocanegra, R., Colombo, A. L., and Graybill, J. R., Treatment of disseminated *Torulopsus glabrata* infection with DO870 and amphotericin B, *Antimicrob. Agents Chemother.*, 38, 1604, 1994.

336. Parmegiani, R. M., Loebenberg, D., Cacciapuoti, A., Antonacci, B., Norris, C., Menzel, F., Moss, L., Yarosh-Tomaine, T., Hare, R. S., and Miller, G. H., Sch 39304, a new antifungal agent: oral and topical treatment of vaginal and superficial infections, *J. Med. Vet. Mycol.*, 31, 239, 1993.

337. Hardin, T. C., Sharkey, P. K., Lam, Y. F., Wallace, J. F., Rinaldi, M. G., and Graybill, J. R., Pharmacokinetics of SCH-39304 in human immunodeficiency virus-infected patients following chronic oral dosing, *Antimicrob. Agents Chemother.*, 36, 2790, 1992.

338. Cacciapuoti, A., Loebenberg, D., Parmegiani, R., Antonacci, B., Norris, C., Moss, E. L., Jr., Menzel, F., Jr., Yarosh-Tomaine, T., Hare, R. S., and Miller, G. H., Comparison of SCH 39304, fluconazole, and ketoconazole for treatment of systemic infections in mice, *Antimicrob. Agents Chemother.*, 36, 64, 1992.

339. Loebenberg, D., Cacciapuoti, A., Parmegiani, R., Moss, E. L., Jr., Menzel, F., Jr., Antonacci, B., Norris, C., Yarosh-Tomaine, T., Hare, R. S., and Miller, G. H., *In vitro* and *in vivo* activities of SCH 42427, the active enantiomer of the antifungal agent SCH 39304, *Antimicrob. Agents Chemother.*, 36, 498, 1992.

340. Umbert, P., Nasarre, J., Bello, A., Herrero, E., Roset, P., Marquez, M., Torres, J., and Ortiz, J. A., Phase II study of the therapeutic efficacy and safety of the new antimycotic sertaconazole in the treatment of superficial mycoses caused by *Candida albicans*, *Arzneimit.-Forsch.*, 42(5A), 757, 1992.

341. Niwano, Y., Seo, A., Kanai, K., Hamaguchi, H., Uchida, K., and Yamaguchi, H., Therapeutic efficacy of lanoconazole, a new imidazole antimycotic agent, for experimental cutaneous candidiasis in guinea pigs, *Antimicrob. Agents Chemother.*, 38, 2204, 1994.

342. Balfour, J. A. and Faulds, D., Terbinafine: a review of its pharmacodynamic and pharmacokinetic properties, and therapeutic potential in superficial mycoses, *Drugs*, 43, 259, 1992 (published error appeared in *Drugs*, 43, 699, 1992).

343. Polak, A., Preclinical data and mode of action of amorolfine, *Dermatology*, 184(Suppl. 1), 3, 1992.

344. Artico, M., Di Santo, R., Costi, R., Massa, S., Retico, A., Artico, M., Apuzzo, G., Simonetti, G., and Strippoli, V., Antifungal agents. IX. 3-Aryl-4-[α-(1*H*-imidazol-1-yl)arylmethyl]pyrroles: a new class of potent anti-*Candida* agents, *J. Med. Chem.*, 38, 4223, 1995.

345. Iwamoto, T., Fujie, A., Nitta, K., Hashimoto, S., Okuhara, M., and Kohsaka, M., WF11899 A, B and C, novel antifungal polypeptides. II. Biological properties, *J. Antibiot.*, 47, 1092, 1994.

346. Bouffard, F. A., Zambias, R. A., Dropinski, J. F., Balkovec, J. M., Hammond, M. L., Abruzzo, G. K., Bartizal, K. F., Marrinan, J. A., Kurtz, M. B., McFadden, D. C., Nollstadt, K. H., Powles, M. A., and Schmatz, D. M., Synthesis and antifungal activity of novel cationic pneumocandin B₀ derivatives, *J. Med. Chem.*, 37, 222, 1994.

347. Bartizal, K., Scott, T., Abruzzo, G. K., Gill, C. J., Pacholok, C., Lynch, L., and Kropp, H., *In vitro* evaluation of the pneumocandin antifungal agent L-733560, a new water-soluble hybrid of L-705589 and L-731373, *Antimicrob. Agents Chemother.*, 39, 1070, 1995.

348. Bartizal, K., Abruzzo, G., and Schmatz, D., The pneumocandins: biological activity of the pneumocandins, in *Cutaneous Fungal Infections*, Rippon, J. and Fromtling, R. A., Eds., Marcell Dekker, New York, 1993, 421.

349. Bartizal, K., Abruzzo, G. K., Flattery, A. M., Gill, C. J., Smith, J. G., Lynch, L., Pacholok, C., Scott, P., Kong, L., Krupa, D., and Kropp, H., Anti-*Candida in vivo* efficacy of water soluble lipopeptides, L-705589, L-731373 and L-733560, *Proc. 33rd Intersci. Conf. Antimicrob. Agents Chemother.*, American Society for Microbiology, Washington, D.C., Abstr. 353, 1993, 184.

350. Bartizal, K., Abruzzo, G., Trainer, C., Krupa, D., Nollstadt, K., Schmatz, R., Schwartz, R., Hammond, M., Balkovec, J. M., and Vanmiddlesworth, F., *In vitro* antifungal activities and *in vivo* efficacies of 1,3-β-D-glucan synthesis inhibitors L-671329, L-646991, tetrahydroechinocandin B, and L-687781, a papulacandin, *Antimicrob. Agents Chemother.*, 36, 1648, 1992.

351. Schmatz, D., McFadden, D. C., Liberator, P., Anderson, J., and Powles, M. A., Evaluation of new semisynthetic pneumocandin against *Pneumocystis carinii* in the immunocompromised rat, *Proc. 33rd Intersci. Conf. Antimicrob. Agents Chemother.*, American Society for Microbiology, Washington, D.C., Abstr. 356, 1993, 184.

352. Hajdu, R., Thompson, R., White, K., Stark-Murphy, B., and Kropp, H., Comparative pharmacokinetics of three water-soluble analogues of the lipopeptide antifungal compound L-688786 in mice and rhesus, *Proc. 33rd Intersci. Conf. Antimicrob. Agents Chemother.*, American Society for Microbiology, Washington, D.C., Abstr. 357, 1993, 185.

353. Abruzzo, G. K., Flattery, A. M., Gill, C. J., Kong, L., Smith, J. G., Krupa, D., Pikounis, V. B., Kropp, H., and Bartizal, K., Evaluation of water-soluble pneumocandin analogs L-733560, L-705589, and L-731373 with mouse models of disseminated aspergillosis, candidiasis, and cryptococcosis, *Antimicrob. Agents Chemother.*, 39, 1077, 1995.

354. Flattery, A., Smith, J., Abruzzo, G., Gill, C., and Bartizal, K., Activity of lipopeptide prodrug L-693,989, nystatin, and amphotericin B in a new CD4+ T-cell deficient mouse model for oropharyngeal and gastrointestinal candidiasis, *Proc. 33rd Intersci. Conf. Antimicrob. Agents Chemother.*, American Society for Microbiology, Washington, D.C., Abstr. 1057, 1992, 286.

355. Pacholok, C., Lynch, L., Kropp, H., and Bartizal, K., *In vitro* evaluation of L-733560, a new water soluble lipopeptide hybrid of L-705589 and L-731373, *Proc. 33rd Intersci. Conf. Antimicrob. Agents Chemother.*, American Society for Microbiology, Washington, D.C., Abstr. 351, 1993, 184.

356. Kurtz, M. B., Douglas, C., Marrinan, J., Nollstadt, K., Onishi, J., Dreikorn, S., Milligan, J., Mandala, S., Thompson, J., Balkovec, J. M., Bouffard, F. A., Dropinski, J. F., Hammond, M. L., Zambias, R. A., Abruzzo, G., Bartizal, K., McManus, O. B., and Garcia, M. L., Increased antifungal activity of L-733560, a water soluble semi-synthetic pneumocandin, is due to enhanced inhibition of cell wall synthesis, *Antimicrob. Agents Chemother.*, 38, 2750, 1994.

357. Khardori, N., Nguyen, H., Stevens, L. C., Kalvakuntla, L., Rosenbaum, B., and Bodey, G. P., Comparative efficacies of cilofungin (Ly121019) and amphotericin B against disseminated *Candida albicans* infection in normal and granulocytopenic mice, *Antimicrob. Agents Chemother.*, 37, 729, 1993.

358. Chapman, T., Kinsman, O., and Houston, J., Chitin biosynthesis in *Candida albicans* grown *in vitro* and *in vivo* and its inhibition by nikkomycin Z, *Antimicrob. Agents Chemother.*, 36, 1909, 1992.

359. Hector, R. F. and Schaller, K., Positive interaction of nikkomycins and azoles against *Candida albicans in vitro* and *in vivo*, *Antimicrob. Agents Chemother.*, 36, 1284, 1992.

360. Kullberg, B. J. and Voss, A., The changing pattern of Candida infections: different species and increased resistance, *Belg. Tijdshr. Geneeskd.*, 140, 148, 1996.

361. Espinel-Ingroff, A., Rodriguez-Tudela, J. L., and Martinez-Suarez, J. V., Comparison of two alternative microdilution procedures with the National Committee for Clinical Laboratory Standards reference microdilution method M27-P for *in vitro* testing of fluconazole-resistant and -susceptible isolates of *Candida albicans*, *J. Clin. Microbiol.*, 33, 3154, 1995.

362. Essayag, S. M., Baily, G. G., Denning, D. W., and Burnie, J. F., Karyotyping of fluconazole-resistant yeast with phenotype reported as *Candida krusei* or *Candida inconspicua*, *Int. J. Syst. Bacteriol.*, 46, 35, 1996.

363. Ruhnke, M., Eigler, A., Tennagen, I., Geiseler, B., Engelmann, E., and Trautmann, M., Emergence of fluconazole-resistant strains of *Candida albicans* in patients with recurrent oropharyngeal candidosis and human immunodeficiency virus infection, *J. Clin. Microbiol.*, 32, 2092, 1994.

364. Laguna, F., Rodriguez-Tudela, J. L., and Enriquez, A., Fungemia due to fluconazole-resistant *Candida albicans* in a patient with AIDS, *Clin. Infect. Dis.*, 19, 542, 1994.

365. Powderly, W. G., Resistant candidiasis, *AIDS Res. Hum. Retroviruses*, 10, 925, 1994.

366. White, A. and Goetz, M. B., Azole-resistant *Candida albicans*: report of two cases of resistance to fluconazole and review, *Clin. Infect. Dis.*, 19, 687, 1994.

367. Newman, S. L., Flanigan, T. P., Fisher, A., Rinaldi, M. G., Stein, M., and Vigilante, K., Clinically significant mucosal candidiasis resistant to fluconazole treatment in patients with AIDS, *Clin. Infect. Dis.*, 19, 684, 1994.

368. Maenza, J. R., Keruly, J. C., Moore, R. D., Chaisson, R. E., Merz, W. G., and Gallant, J. E., Risk factors for fluconazole-resistant candidiasis in human immunodeficiency virus-infected patients, *J. Infect. Dis.*, 173, 219, 1996.

369. Chavanet, P., Lopez, J., Grappin, M., Bonnin, A., Duong, M., Waldner, A., Buisson, M., Camerlynck, P., and Portier, H., Cross-sectional study of the susceptibility of *Candida* isolates to antifungal drugs and *in vitro-in vivo* correlation in HIV-infected patients, *AIDS*, 8, 945, 1994.

370. Sangeorzan, J. A., Bradley, S. F., He, X., Zarins, L. T., Ridenour, G. L., Tiballi, R. N., and Kauffman, C. A., Epidemiology of oral candidiasis in HIV-infected patients: colonization, infection, treatment, and emergence of fluconazole resistance, *Am. J. Med.*, 97, 339, 1994.

371. Thomas-Greber, E., Korting, H. C., Bogner, J., and Goebel, F. D., Fluconazole-resistant oral candidosis in a repeatedly treated female AIDS patient, *Mycoses*, 37, 35, 1994.

372. Bart-Delabesse, E., Boiron, P., Carlotti, A., and Dupont, B., *Candida albicans* genotyping in studies with patients with AIDS developing resistance to fluconazole, *J. Clin. Microbiol.*, 31, 2933, 1993.

373. Baily, G. G., Perry, F. M., Denning, D. W., and Mandal, B. K., Fluconazole-resistant candidosis in an HIV cohort, *AIDS*, 8, 787, 1994.

374. Vuffray, A., Durussel, C., Boerlin, P., Boerlin-Petzold, F., Bille, J., Glauser, M. P., and Chave, J. P., Oropharyngeal candidiasis resistant to single-dose therapy with fluconazole in HIV-infected patients, *AIDS*, 8, 708, 1994.

375. Troillet, N., Durussel, C., Bille, J., Glauser, M. P., and Chave, J. P., Correlation between *in vitro* susceptibility of *Candida albicans* and fluconazole-resistant oropharyngeal candidiasis in HIV-infected patients, *Eur. J. Clin. Microbiol. Infect. Dis.*, 12, 911, 1993.

376. Boken, D. J., Swindells, S., and Rinaldi, M. G., Fluconazole-resistant *Candida albicans*, *Clin. Infect. Dis.*, 17, 1018, 1993.

377. Dewsnup, D. H. and Stevens, D. A., Efficacy of oral amphotericin B in AIDS patients with thrush clinically resistant to fluconazole, *J. Vet. Med. Mycol.*, 32, 389, 1994.

378. Ryley, J. F., Wilson, R. G., and Barrett-Bee, K. J., Azole resistance in *Candida albicans*, *J. Med. Vet. Mycol.*, 22, 53, 1984.

379. Hitchcock, C. A., Barrett-Bee, K. J., and Russell, N. J., Inhibition of 14α-sterol demethylase activity in *Candida albicans* Darlington does not correlate with resistance to azoles, *J. Vet. Med. Mycol.*, 25, 329, 1987.

380. Watson, P. F., Rose, M. E., Ellis, M. E., England, H., and Kelly, S. L., Defective sterol C5-6 desaturation and azole resistance: a new hypothesis for the mode of action of azole antifungals, *Biochem. Biophys. Res. Commun.*, 164, 1170, 1989.

381. vanden Bossche, H., Marichal, P., Odds, F. C., Le Jeune, L., and Coene, M.-C., Characterization of an azole resistant *Candida glabrata* isolate, *Antimicrob. Agents Chemother.*, 36, 2602, 1992.

382. Venkateswarlu, K., Denning, D. W., Manning, N. J., and Kelly, S. L., Resistance to fluconazole in *Candida albicans* from AIDS patients correlated with reduced accumulation of drug, *FEMS Microbiol. Lett.*, 131, 337, 1995.

383. St.-Germain, G., Dion, C., Espinel-Ingroff, A., Ratelle, J., and de Repentigny, L., Ketoconazole and itraconazole susceptibility of *Candida albicans* isolated from patients infected with HIV, *J. Antimicrob. Chemother.*, 36, 109, 1995.

384. Conly, J., Rennie, R., Johnson, J., Farah, S., and Hellman, L., Disseminated candidiasis due to amphotericin B-resistant *Candida albicans*, *J. Infect. Dis.*, 165, 761, 1992.

385. Dubé, M. P., Heseltine, P. N., Rinaldi, M. G., Evans, S., and Zawacki, B., Fungemia and colonization with nystatin-resistant *Candida rugosa* in a burn unit, *Clin. Infect. Dis.*, 18, 77, 1994.

386. del Palacio, A., Cuetara, S., Izquierdo, I., Videla, S., Delgadillo, J., Boncompte, E., and Rodriguez Noriega, A., A double-blind, randomized comparative trial: flutrimazole 1% solution versus bifonazole 1% solution once daily in dermatomycoses, *Mycoses*, 38, 395, 1995.

387. Stengel, F., Robles-Soto, M., Galimberti, R., and Suchil, P., Fluconazole versus ketoconazole in the treatment of dermatophytoses and cutaneous candidiasis, *Int. J. Dermatol.*, 33, 726, 1994.

388. Millikan, L. E. and Shrum, J. P., Systemic therapy for mycoses: changing targets and changing agents, *Int. J. Dermatol.*, 33, 701, 1994.

389. Polizzi, B., Origgi, L., Zuccaro, G., Matti, P., and Scorza, R., Case report: successful treatment with cimetidine and zinc sulphate in chronic mucocutaneous candidiasis, *Am. J. Med. Sci.*, 311, 189, 1996.

390. Laine, L., The natural history of esophageal candidiasis after successful treatment in patients with AIDS, *Gastroenterology*, 107, 744, 1994.

391. Encarnacion, M. and Chin, I., Salivary nystatin concentrations after administration of an osmotic controlled release tablet and a pastille, *Eur. J. Clin. Pharmacol.*, 46, 533, 1994.

392. Laine, L. and Rabeneck, L., Prospective study of fluconazole suspension for the treatment of esophageal candidiasis in patients with AIDS, *Aliment Pharmacol. Ther.*, 9, 553, 1995.

393. Newton, J. A., Jr., Tasker, S. A., Bone, W. D., Oldfield, E. C. III, Olson, P. E., Nguyen, M.-T., and Wallace, M. R., Weekly fluconazole for the suppression of recurrent thrush in HIV-seropositive patients: impact on the incidence of disseminated cryptococcal infection, *AIDS*, 9, 1286, 1995.

394. Azon-Masoliver, A. and Vilaplana, J., Fluconazole-induced toxic epidermal necrolysis in a patient with human immunodeficiency virus infection, *Dermatology*, 187, 268, 1993.

395. Plettenberg, A., Stoehr, A., Höffken, G., Bergs, C., Tschechne, B., Ruhnke, M., Heise, W., Dieckmann, S., and Meigel, W., Fluconazole therapy of oral candidiasis in HIV-infected patients: results of a multicentre study, *Infection*, 22, 118, 1994.

396. Just-Nübling, G., Gentschew, G., Meissner, K., Odewall, J., Staszewski, S., Helm, E. B., and Stille, W., Fluconazole prophylaxis or recurrent oral candidiasis in HIV-positive patients, *Eur. J. Clin. Microbiol. Infect. Dis.*, 10, 917, 1991.

397. Goa, K. L. and Barradell, L. B., Fluconazole: an update of its pharmacodynamic and pharmacokinetic properties and therapeutic use in major supeficial and systemic mycoses in immunocompromised patients, *Drugs*, 50, 658, 1995.

398. Wilcox, C. M., Short report: time course of clinical response with fluconazole for Candida oesophagitis in patients with AIDS, *Aliment. Pharmacol. Ther.*, 8, 347, 1994.

399. Pons, V., Greenspan, D., and Debruin, M., Therapy for oropharyngeal candidiasis in HIV-infected patients: a randomized, prospective multicenter study of oral fluconazole versus clotrimazole troches, *J. Acquir. Immun. Defic. Syndr.*, 6, 1311, 1993.

400. Barbaro, G. and Di Lorenzo, G., Comparison of therapeutic activity of fluconazole and itraconazole in the treatment of oesophageal candidiasis in AIDS patients: a double-blind, randomized, controlled clinical study, *Ital. J. Gastroenterol.*, 27, 175, 1995.

401. Barbaro, G., Barbarini, G., and Di Lorenzo, G., Fluconazole vs. flucytosine in the treatment of esophageal candidiasis in AIDS patients: a double-blind, placebo-controlled study, *Endoscopy*, 27, 377, 1995.

402. Rodriguez-Tudela, J. L., Martinez-Suarez, J. V., Dronda, F., Laguna, F., Chaves, F., and Valencia, E., Correlation of in-vitro susceptibility test results with clinical response: a study of azole therapy in AIDS patients, *J. Antimicrob. Chemother.*, 35, 793, 1995.

403. Smith, D. E., Midgley, J., Allan, M., Connolly, G. M., and Gazzard, B. G., Itraconazole versus ketoconazole in the treatment of oral and oesophageal candidiasis in patients infected with HIV, *AIDS*, 5, 1367, 1991.

404. de Repentigny, L., Ratelle, J., and the HIVIK Project group, Itraconazole vs. ketoconazole in HIV-positive patients with oropharyngeal and/or esophageal candidiasis, *Proc. 32nd Intersci. Conf. Antimicrob. Agents Chemother.*, American Society for Microbiology, Washington, D.C., Abstr. 1117, 1992.

405. Capetti, A., Bonfanti, P., Magni, C., and Milazzo, F., Employment of recombinant human granulocyte-macrophage colony stimulating factor in oesophageal candidiasis in AIDS patients, *AIDS*, 9, 1378, 1995.

406. Scadden, D. T., The use of GM-CSF in AIDS, *Infection*, 20(Suppl. 2), S103, 1992.

407. Jones, T. C., The effects of rHuGM-CSF on macrophage function, *Eur. J. Cancer*, 29A(Suppl. 3), S10, 1993.

408. Zingman, B. S., Resolution of refractory AIDS-related mucosal candidiasis after initiation of didanosine plus sequinavir, *N. Engl. J. Med.*, 334, 1674, 1996.

409. Bennett, J. E., Chemotherapy of systemic mycoses, *N. Engl. J. Med.*, 290, 30, 1974.

410. Borgers, M., vanden Bossche, H., and Cauwenbergh, G., The pharmacology of agents used in the treatment of pulmonary mycoses, *Clin. Chest Med.*, 7, 439, 1986.

411. Miyata, A., Honda, K., Fujita, M., and Kikuchi, T., Multiple Candida liver abscesses successfully treated by continuous intrahepatic arterial infusion of amphotericin B using a reservoir in a case with acute myelocytic leukemia (M2), *Rinsho Ketsueki*, 36, 1217, 1995.

412. Bowden, R. A., Cays, M., Gooley, T., Mamelok, R. D., and van Burik, J. A., Phase I study of amphotericin B colloidal dispersion for the treatment of invasive fungal infections after marrow transplant, *J. Infect. Dis.*, 173, 1208, 1996.

413. Caillot, D., Casasnovas, O., Solary, E., Chavanet, P., Bonnotte, B., Reny, G., Entezam, F., Lopez, J., Bonnin, A., and Guy, H., Efficacy and tolerance of an amphotericin B lipid (intralipid) emulsion in the treatment of candidaemia in neutropenic patients, *J. Antimicrob. Chemother.*, 31, 161, 1993.

414. Emminger, W., Graninger, W., Emminger-Schmidmeier, W., Zoubek, A., Pillwein, K., Susani, M., Wasserer, A., and Gadner, H., Tolerance of high doses of amphotericin B by infusion of a liposomal formulation in children with cancer, *Ann. Hematol.*, 68, 27, 1994.

415. Nguyen, M. H., Peacock, J. E., Jr., Tanner, D. C., Morris, A. J., Nguyen, M. L., Snydman, D. R., Wagener, M. M., and Yu, V. L., Therapeutic approaches in patients with candidemia: evaluation of a multicenter, prospective, observational study, *Arch. Intern. Med.*, 155, 2429, 1995.

416. Rex, J. H., Bennett, J. E., Sugar, A. M., Pappas, P. G., van der Horst, C. M., Edwards, J. E., Washburn, R. G., Scheld, W. M., Karchmer, A. W., Dine, A. P., Levenstein, M. J., and Webb, C. D., A randomized trial comparing fluconazole with amphotericin B for the treatment of candidemia in patients without neutropenia, *N. Engl. J. Med.*, 331, 1325, 1994.

417. Wey, S. B., Mori, M., Pfaller, M. A., Woolson, R. F., and Wenzel, R. P., Hospital-acquired candidemia: the attributable mortality and excess length of stay, *Arch. Intern. Med.*, 148, 2642, 1988.

418. Fraser, V. J., Jones, M., Dunkel, J., Storfer, S., Mcdoff, G., and Dunagan, W. C., Candidemia in a tertiary care hospital: epidemiology, risk factors, and predictors of mortality, *Clin. Infect. Dis.*, 15, 414, 1992.

419. Raad, I. I. and Bodey, G. P., Infectious complications of indwelling vascular catheters, *Clin. Infect. Dis.*, 15, 197, 1992.

420. Lecciones, J. A., Lee, J. W., Navarro, E. E., Witebsky, F. G., Marshall, D., Steinberg, S. M., Pizzo, P. A., and Walsh, T. J., Vascular catheter-associated fungemia in patients with cancer: analysis of 155 episodes, *Clin. Infect. Dis.*, 14, 875, 1992.

421. Meunier, F., Management of candidemia, *N. Engl. J. Med.*, 331, 1371, 1994.

422. Eilard, T., Alestig, K., and Wahlen, P., Treatment of disseminated candidiasis with 5-fluorocytosine, *J. Infect. Dis.*, 130, 155, 1974.

423. Vandevelde, A. G., Mauceri, A. A., and Johnson, J. E. III, 5-Fluorocytosine in the treatment of mycotic infections, *Ann. Intern. Med.*, 77, 1972.

424. Hoeprich, P. D., Ingraham, J. L., Kleker, E., and Winship, M. J., Development of resistance to 5-fluorocytosine in *Candida parapsilosis* during therapy, *J. Infect. Dis.*, 130, 112, 1974.

425. Montgomerie, J. Z., Edwards, J. E., and Guze, L. B., Synergism of amphotericin B and 5-fluorocytosine for *Candida* species, *J. Infect. Dis.*, 132, 82, 1975.

426. Rabinovich, S., Shaw, B. D., Bryant, T., and Donta, S. T., Effect of 5-fluorocytosine and amphotericin B on *Candida albicans* infection in mice, *J. Infect. Dis.*, 130, 28, 1974.

427. Fainstein, V., Bodey, G. P., Elting, L., Maksymiuk, A., Keating, M., and McCredie, K. B., Amphotericin B or ketoconazole therapy of fungal infections in neutropenic cancer patients, *Antimicrob. Agents Chemother.*, 31, 11, 1987.

428. Jordan, W. M., Bodey, G. P., Rodriguez, V., Ketchel, S. J., and Henney, J., Miconazole therapy for treatment of fungal infections in cancer patients, *Antimicrob. Agents Chemother.*, 16, 792, 1979.

429. Edwards, J. E., Jr., Foos, R. Y., Montgomerie, J. Z., and Guze, L. B., Ocular manifestations of Candida septicemia: review of seventy-six cases of hematogenous Candida endophthalmitis, *Medicine (Baltimore)*, 53, 47, 1974.

430. Lou, P., Kazdan, J., Bannatyne, R. M., and Cheung, R., Successful treatment of Candida endophthalmitis with a synergistic combination of amphotericin B and rifampin, *Am. J. Ophthalmol.* 83, 12, 1977.

431. Huang, K., Peyman, G. A., and McGetrick, J., Vitrectomy in experimental endophthalmitis. I. Fungal infection, *Ophthalmic Surg.*, 10, 84, 1979.

432. Nomura, J. and Ruskin, J., Failure of therapy with fluconazole for candidal endophthalmitis, *Clin. Infect. Dis.*, 17, 888, 1993.

433. Blumenkranz, M. S. and Stevens, D. A., Therapy of endogenous fungal endophthalmitis: miconazole or amphotericin B for coccidioidal and candidal infection, *Arch. Ophthalmol.*, 98, 1216, 1980.

434. Venditti, M., De Bernardis, F., Micozzi, A., Pontieri, E., Chirletti, P., Cassone, A., and Martino, P., Fluconazole treatment of catheter-related right-sided endocarditis caused by *Candida albicans* and associated with endophthalmitis and folliculitis, *Clin. Infect. Dis.*, 14, 422, 1992.

435. Filler, S. G., Crislip, M. A., Mayer, C. L., and Edwards, J. E., Jr., Comparison of fluconazole and amphotericin B for treatment of disseminated candidiasis and endophthalmitis in rabbits, *Antimicrob. Agents Chemother.*, 35, 288, 1991.

436. Perraut, L. E., Jr., Perraut, E., Bleiman, B., and Lyons, J., Successful treatment of *Candida albicans* endophthalmitis with intravitreal amphotericin B, *Arch. Ophthalmol.*, 99, 1565, 1981.

437. Souri, E. N. and Green, W. R., Intravitreal amphotericin B toxicity, *Am. J. Ophthalmol.*, 78, 77, 1974.

438. Axelrod, A. J. and Payman, G. A., Intravitreal amphotericin B treatment of experimental fungal endophthalmitis, *Am. J. Ophthalmol.*, 76, 584, 1973.

439. Liu, K. R., Peyman, G. A., and Khoobehi, B., Efficacy of liposome-bound amphotericin B for the treatment of experimental fungal endophthalmitis in rabbits, *Invest. Ophthalmol. Vis. Sci.*, 30, 1527, 1989.

440. Santos, R., de Buen, S., and Juarez, P., Experimental *Candida albicans* chorioretinitis treated by laser, *Am. J. Ophthalmol.*, 63, 440, 1967.

441. Smego, R. A., Jr., Perfect, J. R., and Durack, D. T., Combined therapy with amphotericin B and 5-fluorocytosine for Candida meningitis, *Rev. Infect. Dis.*, 6, 791, 1984.

442. Mohan Rao, H. K. and Myers, G. J., Candida meningitis in the newborn, *South. Med. J.*, 72, 1468, 1979.

443. Merchant, R. K., Louria, D. B., Geiseler, P. H., Edgcomb, J. H., and Utz, J. P., Fungal endocarditis: review of the literature and report of three cases, *Ann. Intern. Med.*, 48, 242, 1958.

444. Kay, J. H., Bernstein, S., Feinstein, D., and Biddle, M., Surgical cure of *Candida albicans* endocarditis with open heart surgery, *N. Engl. J. Med.*, 264, 907, 1961.

445. Kay, J. H., Bernstein, S., Tsuji, H. K., Redington, J. V., Milgram, M., and Brem, T., Surgical treatment of Candida endocarditis, *JAMA*, 203, 105, 1968.

446. Record, C. O., Skinner, J. M., Speight, P., and Speller, D. C. E., Candida endocarditis treated with 5-fluorocytosine, *Br. Med. J.*, 1, 262, 1971.

447. McRae, A. T., Pate, J. W., and Richardson, R. L., Aortic valve replacement for Candida endocarditis, *Chest*, 62, 757, 1972.

448. Fass, R. J. and Perkins, R. L., 5-Fluorocytosine in the treatment of cryptococcal and Candida mycoses, *Ann. Intern. Med.*, 74, 535, 1971.

449. Utley, J. R., Mills, J., Hutchinson, J. C., Edmunds, L. H., Sanderson, R. G., and Roe, B. B., Valve replacement for bacterial and fungal endocarditis, *Circulation*, 42-43(Suppl. 3), 42, 1973.

450. Utley, R. J., Mills, J., and Roe, B. B., Role of valve replacement in the treatment of fungal endocarditis, *J. Thorac. Cardiovasc. Surg.*, 69, 255, 1974.

451. Rubinstein, E., Noriega, E. R., Simberkoff, M. S., and Rahal, J. T., Tissue penetration of amphotericin B in Candida endocarditis, *Chest*, 66, 376, 1974.

452. Stinson, E. B., Griepp, R. B., Vostik, K., Copeland, J. G., and Shumway, N. E., Operative treatment of active endocarditis, *J. Thorac. Cardiovasc. Surg.*, 71, 659, 1975.

453. Rotheman, E. B. and Magovern, G. J., Two year cure of Candida infection of prosthetic mitral valve, *Postgrad. Med. J.*, 61, 237, 1977.

454. Richardson, J. V., Karp, R. B., Kirklin, J. W., and Dismukes, W. E., Treatment of infective endocarditis: a ten year comparative analysis, *Circulation*, 58, 589, 1978.

455. Stinson, E. B., Surgical treatment of infective endocarditis, *Prog. Cardiovasc. Res.*, 22, 145, 1979.

456. Montague, N. T. and Sugg, W. L., Candida endocarditis with femoral emboli, *J. Thorac. Cardiovasc. Surg.*, 67, 322, 1973.

457. Isalaska, B. J. and Stanbridge, T. N., Fluconazole in the treatment of candidal prosthetic valve endocarditis, *Br. Med. J.*, 297, 178, 1988.

458. Martino, P., Meloni, G., and Cassone, A., Candidal endocarditis and treatment with fluconazole and granulocyte-macrophage colony-stimulating factor, *Ann. Intern. Med.*, 112, 966, 1990.

459. Wells, C. J., Leech, G. J., Lever, A. M., and Wansbrough-Jones, M. H., Treatment of native valve Candida endocarditis with fluconazole, *J. Infect.*, 31, 233, 1995.

460. Longman, L. P., Hibbert, S. A., and Martin, M. V., Efficacy of fluconazole in prophylaxis and treatment of experimental Candida endocarditis, *Rev. Infect. Dis.*, 12(Suppl. 3), S294, 1990.

461. Nishida, T., Mayumi, H., Kawachi, Y., Tokunaga, S., Maruyama, Y., Nakashima, A., Yasui, H., and Tokunaga, K., The efficacy of fluconazole in treating prosthetic valve endocarditis caused by *Candida glabrata*: report of a case, *Surg. Today*, 24, 651, 1994.

462. Isaacs, J. H., Nystatin vaginal cream in monilial vaginitis, *Int. Med. J.*, 143, 240, 1973.
463. Droegemueller, W., Adamson, D. G., Brown, D., Cibley, L., Fleury, F., LePage, M. E., and Henzl, M., Three day treatment with butoconazole nitrate for vulvovaginal candididasis, *Obstet. Gynecol.*, 64, 530, 1984.
464. Corson, S. L., Kapikian, R. R., and Nehring, R., Terconazole and miconazole cream for treating vulvovaginal candidiasis: a comparison, *J. Reprod. Med.*, 36, 561, 1991.
465. Breuker, G., Jurczok, F., Naerts, M., Weinhold, E., and Krause, U., Single-dose therapy of vaginal mycoses with clotrimazole vaginal cream 10%, *Mykosen*, 29, 427, 1986.
466. Van der Meijden, W. I., Van der Hoek, J. C. S., Staal, H. J. M., Van Joost, T., and Stolz, E., Double-blind comparison of 200 mg ketoconazole oral tablets and 1200 mg micronazole vaginal capsule in the treatment of vaginal candidosis, *Eur. J. Obstet. Gynecol. Reprod. Biol.*, 22, 133, 1986.
467. Ritter, W., Pharmacokinetic fundamentals of vaginal treatment with clotrimazole, *Am. J. Obstet. Gynecol.*, 152, 945, 1985.
468. Odds, F. C. and MacDonald, F., Persistence of miconazole in vaginal secretions after single applications of the antifungal: implications for the treatment of vaginal candidosis, *Br. J. Vener. Dis.*, 57, 400, 1981.
469. Lindeque, B. G. and Van Niekerk, W. A., Treatment of vaginal candidiasis in pregnancy with a single clotrimazole 500 mg vaginal pessary, *S. Afr. Med. J.*, 65, 123, 1984.
470. Bingham, J. S., Single blind comparison of ketoconazole 200 mg oral tablets and clotrimazole 100 mg vaginal tablets and 1% cream in treating acute candidosis, *Br. J. Vener. Dis.*, 60, 175, 1984.
471. Cauwenbergh, G., Itraconazole: the first orally active antifungal for single-day treatment of vaginal candidosis, *Curr. Ther. Res.*, 41, 210, 1987.
472. Brammer, K. W., Treatment of vaginal candidiasis with a single oral dose of fluconazole, *Eur. J. Clin. Microbiol. Infect. Dis.*, 7, 364, 1988.
473. Frega, A., Gallo, G., Di Renzi, F., Stolfi, G., and Stentella, P., Persistent vulvovaginal candidiasis: systemic treatment with oral fluconazole, *Clin. Exp. Obstet. Gynecol.*, 21, 259, 1994.
474. Kukner, S., Ergin, T., Cicek, N., Ugur, M., Yesilyurt, H., and Gokmen, O., Treatment of vaginitis, *Int. J. Gynaecol. Obstet.*, 52, 43, 1996.
475. Ferris, D. G., Litaker, M. S., Woodward, L., Mathis, D., and Hendrich, J., Treatment of bacterial vaginosis: a comparison of oral metronidazole, metronidazole vaginal gel, and clindamycin vaginal cream, *J. Fam. Pract.*, 41, 443, 1995.
476. O-Prasertsawat, P. and Bourlert, A., Comparative study of fluconazole and clotrimazole for the treatment of vulvovaginal candidiasis, *Sex. Transm. Dis.*, 22, 228, 1995.
477. Sobel, J. D., Schmitt, C., Stein, G., Mummaw, N., Christensen, S., and Meriwether, C., Initial management of recurrent vulvovaginal candidiasis with oral ketoconazole and topical clotrimazole, *J. Reprod. Med.*, 39, 517, 1994.
478. Azzena, A. and Vasoin, F., Systemic treatment of recurrent candidal vulvovaginitis by itraconazole, *Clin. Exp. Obstet. Gynecol.*, 21, 59, 1994.
479. Sobel, J. D., Recurrent vulvovaginal candidiasis: a perspective study of the efficacy of maintenance ketoconazole therapy, *N. Engl. J. Med.*, 315, 1455, 1986.
480. Sobel, J. D., Management of recurrent vulvovaginal candidiasis with intermittent ketoconazole prophylaxis, *Obstet. Gynecol.*, 65, 123, 1985.
481. Davidson, F. and Mould, R. F., Recurrent genital candidosis in women and the effect of intermittent prophylactic treatment, *Br. J. Vener. Dis.*, 54, 176, 1978.
482. Nix, D. E., Durrence, C. W., and May, J. R., Amphotericin B bladder irrigation, *Drug Intell. Clin. Pharm.*, 19, 299, 1985.
483. Wise, G. J., Kozinn, P. J., and Goldberg, P., Amphotericin B as a urologic irrigant in the management of noninvasive candiduria, *J. Urol.*, 128, 82, 1982.
484. Nito, H., Clinical efficacy of fluconazole in urinary tract fungal infections, *Jpn. J. Antibiot.*, 42, 171, 1989.
485. Edwards, J. E., Jr., Candida species, in *Principles and Practice of Infectious Diseases*, Mandell, G. L., Douglas, R. G., Jr., and Bennett, J. E., Eds., Churchill Livingstone, New York, 1990, 1954.
486. Strassner, C. and Friesen, A., Therapy of candiduria by alkalinization of urine: oral treatment with potassium-sodium-hydrogen citrate, *Fortschr. Med.*, 113, 359, 1995.

487. Sanford, J. P., The enigma of candiduria: evolution of bladder irrigation with amphotericin B for management — from anecdote to dogma and a lesson from Machiavelli, *Clin. Infect. Dis.*, 16, 145, 1993.

488. Occhipinti, D. J., Schoonover, L. L., and Danziger, L. H., Bladder irrigation with amphotericin B for treatment of patients with candiduria, *Clin. Infect. Dis.*, 17, 812, 1993.

489. Sanford, J. P., Bladder irrigation with amphotericin B for treatment of patients with candiduria: a reply, *Clin. Infect. Dis.*, 17, 813, 1993.

490. Johnson, J. R., Should all catheterized patients with candiduria be treated? *Clin. Infect. Dis.*, 17, 814, 1993.

491. Sanford, J. P., Should all catheterized patients with candiduria be treated?: a reply, *Clin. Infect. Dis.*, 17, 814, 1993.

492. Simsek, U., Akinci, H., Oktay, B., Kavrama, I., and Ozyurt, M., Treatment of catheter-associated candiduria with fluconazole irrigation, *Br. J. Urol.*, 75, 75, 1995.

493. Montenegro, J., Aguirre, R., Gonzalez, O., Martinez, I., and Saracho, R., Fluconazole treatment of candida peritonitis with delayed removal of the peritoneal dialysis catheter, *Clin. Nephrol.*, 44, 60, 1995.

494. Cartwright, R. Y., Shaldon, C., and Hall, G. H., Urinary candidiasis after renal transplantation, *Br. Med. J.*, 2, 351, 1972.

495. Price, E., Webb, E. A., and Smith, B. A., Urinary tract candidiasis treated with amphotericin B, *Br. J. Urol.*, 98, 523, 1967.

496. Blum, J. A., Acute monilial pyohydronephrosis: report of a case successfully treated with amphotericin B, *J. Urol.*, 96, 614, 1966.

497. Cohen, G. H., Obstructive uropathology caused by urethral candidiasis, *J. Urol.*, 110, 285, 1973.

498. Gerle, R. D., Roentgenographic features of primary renal candidiasis: fungus ball of the renal pelvis and ureter, *Am. J. Roentgenol. Radium Ther. Nucl. Med.*, 119, 731, 1973.

499. Bayer, A. S., Blumenkranta, M. J., Mongomerie, J. Z., Galpin, J. E., Coburn, J. W., and Guze, L. B., *Candida* peritonitis: report of 22 cases and review of the English literature, *Am. J. Med.*, 61, 832, 1976.

500. Eisenberg, E. S., Leviton, I., and Soerio, R., Fungal peritonitis in patients receiving peritoneal dialysis: experience with 11 patients and review of the literature, *Rev. Infect. Dis.*, 8, 309, 1986.

501. Fabris, A., Biasioli, S., Borin, D., Brendolan, A., Chiaramonte, S., Feriani, M., Pisani, E., Ronco, C., and Lagrega, G., Fungal peritonitis in peritoneal dialysis: our experience and review of treatments, *Perit. Dial. Bull.*, 4, 75, 1984.

502. Johnson, R. J., Ramsey, P., Gallagher, N., and Ahmad, S., Fungal peritonitis in patients on peritoneal dialysis: incidence, clinical features and prognosis, *Am. J. Nephrol.*, 5, 169, 1985.

503. Benevent, D., Peyronnet, P., Lagarde, C., and Leroux-Robert, C., Fungal peritonitis in patients on continuous ambulatory peritoneal dialysis: three recoveries in 5 cases without catheter removal, *Nephron*, 41, 203, 1985.

504. Vergemezis, V., Papadopoulou, Z. L., Liamos, H., Belechri, A. M., Natscheh, T., Vergoulas, G., Antoniadou, R., Kilintzis, V., and Papadimitriou, M., Management of fungal peritonitis during continuous ambulatory peritoneal dialysis (CAPD), *Perit. Dial. Bull.*, 6, 17, 1986.

505. Tapson, J. S., Mansy, H., Freeman, R., and Wilkinson, R., The high morbidity of CAPD fungal peritonitis — description of 10 cases and review of treatment strategies, *Q. J. Med.*, 61, 1047, 1986.

506. Rubin, J., Kirchner, K., Walsh, D., Green, M., and Bower, J., Fungal peritonitis during continuous ambulatory peritoneal dialysis: a report of 17 cases, *Am. J. Kidney Dis.*, 10, 361, 1987.

507. Struijk, D. G., Krediet, R. T., Boeschoten, E. W., Rietra, P. J., and Arisz, L., Antifungal treatment of candida peritonitis in continuous ambulatory peritoneal dialysis patients, *Am. J. Kidney Dis.*, 9, 66, 1987.

508. Pocheville, M., Charpentier, B., Brocard, J. F., Benarbia, S., Hammouche, M., and Fries, D., Successful in situ treatment of fungal peritonitis during CAPD, *Nephron*, 37, 66, 1984.

509. Cecchin, E., De Marchi, S., Panarello, G., and Tesio, F., Chemotherapy and/or removal of the peritoneal catheter in the management of fungal peritonitis complicating CAPD? *Nephron*, 40, 251, 1985.

510. Arfania, D., Everett, E. D., Nolph, K. D., and Rubin, J., Uncommon causes of peritoneal dialysis, *Arch. Intern. Med.*, 141, 61, 1981.

511. Lee, S. H., Chiang, S. S., Hsieh, S. J., and Shen, H. M., Successful treatment of fungal peritonitis with intracatheter antifungal retention, *Adv. Perit. Dial.*, 11, 172, 1995.

512. Dismukes, W. E., Azole antifungal drugs: old and new, *Ann. Intern. Med.*, 109, 177, 1988.

513. Saag, M. S. and Dismukes, W. E., Azole antifungal agents: emphasis on new triazoles, *Antimicrob. Agents Chemother.*, 32, 1, 1988.

514. Levin, J., Bernard, D. B., Idelson, B. A., Farnham, H., Saunders, C., and Sugar, A. M., Fungal peritonitis complicating continuous ambulatory peritoneal dialysis: successful treatment with fluconazole, a new orally active antifungal agent, *Am. J. Med.*, 86, 825, 1989.

515. Corbella, X., Sirvent, J. M., and Carratala, J., Fluconazole treatment without catheter removal in Candida albicans peritonitis complicating peritoneal dialysis, *Am. J. Med.*, 90, 227, 1991.

516. Voss, A., Meis, J. F., and Hoogkamp-Korstanje, J. A., Fluconazole in the management of fungal urinary tract infections, *Infection*, 22, 247, 1994.

517. Corbella, X., Carratala, J., Castells, M., and Berlanga, B., Fluconazole treatment in Torulopsis glabrata upper urinary tract infection causing ureteral obstruction, *J. Urol.*, 147, 1116, 1992.

518. Ansari, S. H., Levin, M. H., and Lipshitz, S., Re: fluconazole treatment in Toluropsis glabrata upper urinary tract infection causing ureteral obstruction, *J. Urol.*, 154, 1870, 1995.

519. Dermoumi, H., *In vitro* susceptibility of yeast isolates from the blood to fluconazole and amphotericin B, *Chemotherapy*, 38, 112, 1992.

520. Morace, G., Manzara, S., and Dettori, G., *In vitro* susceptibility of 119 yeast isolates to fluconazole, 5-fluorocytosine, amphotericin B and ketoconazole, *Chemotherapy*, 37, 23, 1991.

521. Hitchcock, C. A., Pye, G. W., Troke, P. F., Johnson, E. M., and Warnock, D. W., Fluconazole resistance in Candida glabrata, *Antimicrob. Agents Chemother.*, 37, 1962, 1993.

522. Warnock, D. W., Burke, J., Cope, N. J., Johnson, E. M., von Fraunhofer, N. A., and Williams, E. W., Fluconazole resistance in Candida glabrata, *Lancet*, 2, 1310, 1988.

523. Michel, C., Courdavault, L., al Khayat, R., Viron, B., Roux, P., and Mignon, F., Fungal peritonitis in patients on peritoneal dialysis, *Am. J. Nephrol.*, 14, 113, 1994.

524. Lafont, A., Olivé, A., Gelman, M., Roca-Burniols, J., Cots, R., and Carbonell, J., *Candida albicans* spondylodiscitis and vertebral osteomyelitis in patients with intravenous heroin drug addiction: report of 3 new cases, *J. Rheumatol.*, 21, 953, 1994.

525. Weisse, M. E., Person, D. A., and Berkenbaugh, J. T., Jr., Treatment of Candida arthritis with fluconazole and amphotericin B, *J. Perinatol.*, 13, 402, 1993.

526. Oleinik, E. M., Della-Latta, P., Rinaldi, M. G., and Saiman, L., *Candida lusitaniae* osteomyelitis in a premature infant, *Am. J. Perinatol.*, 10, 313, 1993.

527. Tang, C., Successful treatment of *Candida albicans* osteomyelitis with fluconazole, *J. Infect.*, 26, 89, 1993.

528. Dan, M. and Priel, I., Failure of fluconazole therapy for sternal osteomyelitis, *Clin. Infect. Dis.*, 18, 126, 1994.

529. Glick, C., Graves, G. R., and Feldman, S., Neonatal fungemia and amphotericin B, *South. Med. J.*, 86, 1368, 1993.

530. Baley, J. E., Kliegman, R. M., and Faranoff, A. A., Disseminated fungal infections in very low birth weight infants: therapeutic toxicity, *Pediatrics*, 73, 153, 1984.

531. Delaplane, D., Wiringa, K. S., Shulman, S. F., and Yogev, R., Congenital mucocutaneous candidiasis following diagnostic amniocentesis, *Am. J. Obstet. Gynecol.*, 147, 342, 1983.

532. Starke, J. R., Mason, E., Kraner, W. G., and Kaplan, S. L., Pharmacokinetics of amphotericin B in infants and children, *J. Infect. Dis.*, 155, 766, 1987.

533. Aydin, M., Kucukoduk, S., Yalin, T., Cetinkaya, F., and Gurses, N., Amphotericin B in the treatment of candida meningitis in three neonates, *Turk. J. Pediatr.*, 37, 247, 1995.

534. Plak, A., Pharmacokinetics of amphotericin B and flucytosine, *Postgrad. Med. J.*, 55, 667, 1979.

535. Stöckler, S., Lackner, H., Ginter, G., Schwinger, W., Plecko, B., and Müller, W., Liposomal amphotericin B (AmBisome) for treatment of cutaneous widespread candidosia in an infant with methylmalonic acidaemia, *Eur. J. Pediatr.*, 152, 981, 1993.

536. Ringdén, O., Tollemar, J., Dahllof, G., and Tyden, G., High cure rate of invasive fungal infections in immunocompromised children using ambisome, *Transplant. Proc.*, 26, 175, 1994.

537. Butler, K. M. and Baker, C. J., *Candida*: an increasingly important pathogen in nursery, *Pediatr. Clin. North Am.*, 35, 543, 1988.

538. Lackner, H., Schwinger, W., Urban, C., Müller, W., Ritschl, E., Reiterer, F., Kuttnig-Haim, M., Urlesberger, B., and Hauer, C., Liposomal amphotericin B (AmBisome) for treatment of disseminated fungal infections in two infants of very low birth weight, *Pediatrics*, 89, 1259, 1992.

539. Pereira da Silva, L., Videira Amaral, J. M., and Cordeiro Ferreira, N., Which is the most appropriate dosage of liposomal amphotericin B (AmBisome) for the treatment of fungal infections in infants of very low birth weight? *Pediatrics*, 91, 1217, 1993.

540. Clarke, M. and Davies, D. P., Neonatal systemic candidiasis treated with miconazole, *Br. Med. J.*, 281, 354, 1980.

541. Dupont, B. and Drouet, E., *In vitro* synergy and antagonism of antifungal agents against yeast-like fungi, *Postgrad. Med. J.*, 55, 683, 1979.

542. Viscolli, C., Castagnola, E., Fioredda, F., Ciravegna, B., Barigone, G., and Terragna, A., Fluconazole in the treatment of candidiasis in immunocompromised children, *Antimicrob. Agents Chemother.*, 35, 365, 1991.

543. Fasano, C., O'Keeffe, J., and Gibbs, D., Fluconazole treatment of neonates and infants with severe fungal infections not treatable with conventional agents, *Eur. J. Clin. Microbiol. Infect. Dis.*, 13, 351, 1994.

544. Marr, B., Gross, S., Cunningham, C., and Weiner, L., Candidal sepsis and meningitis in a very-low-birth-weight infant successfully treated with fluconazole and flucytosine, *Clin. Infect. Dis.*, 19, 795, 1994.

545. Epelbaum, S., Laurent, C., Morin, G., Berquin, P., and Piussan, C., Failure of fluconazole treatment in Candida meningitis, *J. Pediatr.*, 123, 168, 1993.

546. Bode, S., Pedersen-Bjergaard, L., and Hjelt, K., *Candida albicans* septicemia in a premature infant successfully treated with oral fluconazole, *Scand. J. Infect. Dis.*, 24, 673, 1992.

547. Bhandari, V. and Narang, A., Oral itraconazole therapy for disseminated candidiasis in low birth weight infants, *J. Pediatr.*, 120(2 Part 1), 330, 1992.

548. Puntithalingham, E. and English, M. P., *Pyranochaeta unguis-hominis* sp. nov. on human toenails, *Trans. Br. Mycol. Soc.*, 64, 539, 1975.

549. Hay, R. J., Onychomycosis: agents of choice, *Dermatol. Clin.*, 11, 161, 1993.

550. Hay, R. J. and Baran, R., Fungal (onychomycosis) and other infections of the nail apparatus, in *Diseases of the Nails and Their Management*, Baran, R. and Dawber, R. P. R., Eds., Blackwell Scientific Publications, Oxford, 1986, 212.

551. Zaias, N., Onychomycosis, *Arch. Dermatol.*, 105, 263, 1972.

552. Frain-Bell, W., Chronic paronychia: short review of 590 cases, *Trans. St. Johns Hosp. Derm. Soc.*, 38, 29, 1957.

553. Barlow, A. J. E., Chattaway, F. W., Holgate, W. C., and Aldersley, T. A., Chronic paronychia, *Br. J. Dermatol.*, 82, 448, 1970.

554. Hay, R. J., Mackie, R. M., and Clayton, Y. M., Tioconazole (28%) nail solution: an open study of its efficacy in onychomycosis, *Clin. Exp. Dermatol.*, 10, 152, 1985.

555. Hay, R. J., Clayton, Y. M., and Moore, M. K., A comparison of tioconazole 28% nail solution versus base as an adjunct to oral griseofulvin in patients with onychomycosis, *Clin. Exp. Dermatol.*, 12, 175, 1987.

556. Polak, A., Mode of action of morpholine derivatives, *Ann. NY Acad. Sci.*, 544, 221, 1988.

557. Ceschin-Roques, C. G., Hanel, H., Pruja-Bougaret, S. M., Luc, J., Ven der Mander, J., and Michel, G., Cicloprox nail lacquer 8%: *in vivo* penetration into and through nails and *in vitro* effect on pig skin, *Skin Pharmacol.*, 4, 89, 1991.

558. Polak, A., Preclinical data and mode of action of amorolfine, *Dermatology*, 184(Suppl.), 3, 1992.

559. Reinel, D., Topical treatment of onychomycosis with amorolfine 5% nail lacqeur: comparative efficacy and tolerability of once and twice weekly use, *Dermatology*, 182(Suppl.), 21, 1992.

560. Botter, A. A., Detheir, F., Mertens, R. I. J., Morias, J., and Peremans, W., Skin and nail mycoses: treatment with ketoconazole, a new oral antimycotic agent, *Mykosen*, 22, 274, 1979.

561. Hay, R. J. and Clayton, Y. M., The treatment of patients with chronic mucocutaneous candidosis and *Candida* onychomycosis with ketoconazole, *Clin. Exp. Dermatol.*, 7, 155, 1982.

562. Strauss, J. S., Ketoconazole and the liver, *J. Am. Acad. Dermatol.*, 6, 546, 1982.

563. Tkach, J. R. and Rinaldi, M. G., Severe hepatitis associated with ketoconazole therapy for mucocutaneous candidosis, *Cutis*, 29, 482, 1982.

564. Fromtling, R. A., Overview of medically important antifungal azole derivatives, *Clin. Microbiol. Rev.*, 1, 187, 1988.
565. Hay, R. J., Clayton, Y. M., Moore, M. K., and Midgley, G., An evaluation of itraconazole in the management of onychomycosis, *Br. J. Dermatol.*, 119, 359, 1988.
566. Hay, R. J., New oral treatments for dermatophytosis, *Ann. NY Acad. Sci.*, 544, 580, 1988.
567. Petranyi, L. A., Meingassner, J. G., and Mieth, H., Antifungal activity of the allylamine derivative, terbinafine, *in vitro, Antimicrob. Agents Chemother.*, 31, 1365, 1987.
568. Goodfield, M. J. D., Rowell, N. R., Forster, R. A., Evans, E. G. V., and Raven, A., Treatment of dermatophyte infections of the finger or toe nails with terbinafine (SFG 86-327, lamisil) an orally active fungicidal agent, *Br. J. Dermatol.*, 121, 753, 1989.
569. Goodfield, M. J. D., Short duration therapy with terbinafine for dermatophyte onychomycosis: a multicentre study, *Br. J. Dermatol.*, 126(Suppl. 39), 33, 1992.
570. Schroeff, J. G., Cirkel, P. K. S., Crijns, M. B., Van Dijk, T. J. A., Govaert, F. J., Groencweg, D. A., Tazelaar, D. J., De Wit, R. F. E., and Wuite, J., A randomised treatment duration-finding study of terbinafine in onychomycosis, *Br. J. Dermatol.*, 126(Suppl. 39), 36, 1992.
571. Hazen, K. C., New and emerging yeast pathogens, *Clin. Microbiol. Rev.*, 8, 462, 1995.
572. Morris, J. T. and McAllister, C. K., Fungemia due to *Torulopsis glabrata, South. Med. J.*, 86, 356, 1993.
573. Dick, J. D., Rosengard, B. R., Merz, W. G., Stuart, R. K., Hutchins, G. M., and Saral, R., Fatal disseminated candidiasis due to amphotericin B-resistant *Candida guilliermondii, Ann. Intern. Med.*, 102, 67, 1985.
574. Booth, L. V., Collins, A. L., Lowes, J. A., and Radford, M., Skin rash associated with *Candida guilliermondii, Med. Pediatr. Oncol.*, 16, 295, 1988.
575. Gugnani, H. C., Okafor, B. C., Nzelibe, F., and Njoku-Obi, A. N., Etiological agents of otomycosis in Nigeria, *Mycoses*, 32, 224, 1989.
576. Piper, J. P., Rinaldi, M. G., and Winn, R. E., *Candida parapsilosis*: an emerging problem, *Infect. Dis. Newsl.*, 7, 49, 1988.
577. Myers, B. R., Lieberman, T. W., and Ferry, A. P., Candida endophthalmitis complicating candidemia, *Ann. Intern. Med.*, 79, 647, 1973.
578. St.-Germain, G. and M. Laverdière, M., *Torulopsis candida*, a new opportunistic pathogen, *J. Clin. Microbiol.*, 24, 884, 1986.
579. Price, M. F., LaRocco, M. T., and Gentry, L. O., Fluconazole susceptibilities of *Candida* species and distribution of species recovered from blood cultures over a 5-year period, *Antimicrob. Agents Chemother.*, 38, 1422, 1994.
580. Morgan, M. A., Wilkowske, C. J., and Roberts, G. D., *Candida pseudotropicalis* fungemia and invasive disease in an immunocompromised patient, *J. Clin. Microbiol.*, 20, 1006, 1984.
581. Pappagianis, D., Collins, M. S., Hector, R., and Remington, J., Development of resistance to amphotericin B in *Candida lusitaniae* infecting a human, *Antimicrob. Agents Chemother.*, 16, 123, 1979.
582. Yinnon, A. M., Woodin, K. A., and Powell, K. R., *Candida lusitaniae* infection in the newborn: case report and review of the literature, *Pediatr. Infect. Dis. J.*, 11, 878, 1992.
583. Nielsen, H., Stenderup, J., Bruun, B., and Ladefoged, J., *Candida norvegensis* peritonitis and invasive disease in a patient on continuous ambulatory peritoneal dialysis, *J. Clin. Microbiol.*, 28, 1664, 1990.
584. Walsh, T. J., Salkin, I. F., Dixon, D. M., and Hurd, N. J., Clinical, microbiological, and experimental animal studies of *Candida lipolytica, J. Clin. Microbiol.*, 27, 927, 1989.
585. Reinhardt, J. F., Ruane, P. J., Walker, L. J., and George, W. L., Intravenous catheter-associated fungemia due to *Candida rugosa, J. Clin. Microbiol.*, 22, 1056, 1985.
586. Fisher, M. A., Shueh-Hui, S., Haddad, J., and Tarry, W. F., Comparison of *in vivo* activity of fluconazole with that of amphotericin B against *Candida tropicalis, Candida glabrata*, and *Candida krusei, Antimicrob. Agents Chemother.*, 33, 1443, 1989.
587. Arisoy, E. S., Correa, A., Seilheimer, D. K., and Kaplan, S. L., *Candida rugosa* central venous catheter infection in a child, *Pediatr. Infect. Dis. J.*, 12, 961, 1993.
588. Alsina, A., Mason, M., Uphoff, R. A., Riggsby, W. S., Becker, J. M., and Murphy, D., Catheter-associated *Candida utilis* fungemia in a patient with acquired immunodeficiency syndrome: species verification with a molecular probe, *J. Clin. Microbiol.*, 26, 621, 1986.

589. Bougnoux, M.-E., Gueho, E., and Potocka, A.-C., Resolutive *Candida utilis* fungemia in a nonneutropenic patient, *J. Clin. Microbiol.*, 31, 1644, 1993.

590. Bisbe, J., Vilardell, J., Valls, M., Moreno, A., Brancos, M., and Andreu, J., Transient fungemia and candida arthritis due to *Candida zeylanoides*, *Eur. J. Clin. Microbiol.*, 6, 668, 1987.

591. Levenson, D., Pfaller, M. A., Smith, M. A., Hollis, R., Gerarden, T., Tucci, C. B., and Isenberg, H. D., *Candida zeylanoides*: another opportunistic yeast, *J. Clin. Microbiol.*, 29, 1689, 1991.

592. Gargeya, I. B., Pruitt, W. R., Meyer, S. A., and Ahearn, D. G., *Candida haemulonii* from clinical specimens in the USA, *J. Med. Vet. Mycol.*, 29, 335, 1991.

593. Al-Hedaithy, S. S. A., The medically important yeasts present in clinical specimens, *Ann. Saudi Med.*, 12, 57, 1992.

594. Anaissie, E., Bodey, G. P., Kantarjian, H., Ro, J., Vartivarian, S. E., Hopfer, R., Hoy, J., and Rolston, K., New spectrum of fungal infections in patients with cancer, *Rev. Infect. Dis.*, 11, 369, 1989.

595. Krogh, P., Holmstrup, P., Thorn, J. J., Vedtofte, P., and Pindborg, J. J., Yeast species and biotypes associated with oral leukoplakia and lichen planus, *Oral Surg. Oral Med. Oral Pathol.*, 63, 48, 1987.

596. Pospisil, L., The significance of *Candida pulcherrima* findings in human clinical specimens, *Mycoses*, 32, 581, 1989.

597. Sandhu, D. K., Sandhu, R. S., and Misra, V. C., Isolation of *Candida viswanathii* from cerebrospinal fluid, *Sabouraudia*, 14, 251, 1976.

598. Vazquez-Juarez, R., Ascencio, F., Andlid, T., Gustafson, L., and Wadstrom, T., The expression of potential colonization factors of yeasts isolated from fish during different growth conditions, *Can. J. Microbiol.*, 39, 1135, 1993.

599. Bialasiewicz, D., Kurnatowska, A., and Smiech-Slomkowska, G., Characteristics of fungi and attempts of their elimination from the oral cavity in children treated with orthodontic appliances, *Med. Dosw. Mikrobiol.*, 45, 389, 1993.

600. Meyer, S. A., Ahearn, D. G., and Yarrow, D., in *The Yeasts: A Taxonomic Study*, 3rd ed., Kreeger-van Rij, N. J. W., Ed., Elsevier, Amsterdam, 1984, 839.

601. Liao, W. Q., Li, Z. G., Guo, M., and Zhang, J. Z., *Candida zeylanoides* causing candidiasis as tinea cruris, *Chin. Med. J.*, 106, 542, 1993.

602. Rippon, J. W., Candidiasis and the pathogenic yeasts, in *Medical Mycology*, Rippon, J. W., Ed., W. B. Saunders, Philadelphia, 1982, 484.

603. Crosier, W. J., Two cases of onychomycosis due to *Candida zeylanoides*, *Australas. J. Dermatol.*, 34, 23, 1993.

604. Roberts, G., Detection of fungemia, *Infect. Dis. Newsl.*, 4, 18, 1985.

605. Whitby, S., Madu, E. C., and Bronze, M. S., Case report: *Candida zeylanoides*, infective endocarditis complicating infection with the human immunodeficiency virus, *Am. J. Med. Sci.*, 312, 138, 1996.

606. Cooper, B. H. and Silva-Hutner, M., Yeasts of medical importance, in *Manual of Clinical Microbiology*, 4th ed., Lennette, E. H., Balows, A., Hausler, W. J., Jr., and Shadomy, J., Eds., American Society for Microbiology, Washington, D.C., 1985, 526.

607. Badillet, G., Sené, S., Barnel, C., and Jung, C., Les levures du genre *Torulopsis* en dermatologie, *Bull. Soc. Fr. Mycol. Méd.*, 14, 235, 1985.

608. Barthe, J. and Barthe, M.-F., The ecology of *Torulopsis* in man, *Sabouraudia*, 11, 192, 1973.

609. De Closets, F. and Combescot, C., Étude de levures isolées de prélèvements pathologiques, *Bull. Soc. Fr. Mycol. Méd.*, 9, 9, 1980.

610. Albaret, S., Hoquet, P., Cavellat, J.-F., Delhumean, A., and Cavellat, M., Le traitement des septicémies a levures: ses limites, *Anasth. Analg. Reanim.*, 36, 13, 1979.

611. Khan, Z. V., Misra, V. C., Randhawa, H. S., and Damodaran, V. N., Pathogenicity of some ordinarily harmless yeast for cortisone-treated mice, *Sabouraudia*, 18, 319, 1980.

612. Quindos, G., Cabrera, F., Arilla, M. C., Burgos, A., Ortiz-Vigon, R., Canon, J. L., and Ponton, J., Fatal *Candida famata* peritonitis in a patient undergoing continuous ambulatory peritoneal dialysis who was treated with fluconazole, *Clin. Infect. Dis.*, 18, 658, 1994.

613. Rao, N. A., Nerenberg, A. V., and Forster, D. J., *Torulopsis candida* (*Candida famata*) endophthalmitis simulating *Propionibacterium acnes* syndrome, *Arch. Ophthalmol.*, 109, 1718, 1991.

614. Austwick, P. K. C., Pepin, G. A., Thompson, J. C., and Yarrow, D., *Candida albicans* and other yeasts associated with animal disease, in *Symposium on* Candida *Infections*, Winner, H. I. and Hurley, R., Eds., Livingstone Press, London, 1966, 89.

615. Gentles, J. C. and La Touche, C. J., Yeasts as human and animal pathogens, in *The Yeasts*, Vol. 1, Rose, A. H. and Harrison, J. S., Eds., Academic Press, London, 1969, 108.

616. Do Carmo-Sousa, L., Distribution of yeast in nature, in *The Yeasts*, Vol. 1, Rose, A. H. and Harrison, J. S., Eds., Academic Press, London, 1969, 79.

617. Russell, C. and Lay, K. M., Natural history of *Candida* species and yeasts in the oral cavities of infants, *Arch. Oral Biol.*, 18, 957, 1975.

618. Budtz, J., Stenderup, A., and Grabowski, M., An epidemiologic study of yeasts in elderly denture wearers, *Community Dent. Oral Epidemiol.*, 3, 115, 1975.

619. McKendrick, A. J., Wilson, M. I., and Main, D. M. G., Oral *Candida* and long-term tetracycline therapy, *Arch. Oral Biol.*, 12, 281, 1967.

620. Stenderup, A. and Pedersen, G. T., Yeast of human origin, *Acta Pathol. Microbiol. Scand.*, 54, 462, 1962.

621. Sonck, C. E. and Somersalo, O., The yeast flora of the anogenital region in diabetic girls, *Arch. Dermatol.*, 88, 846, 1963.

622. Hog asen, A. K., Abrahamsen, T. G., and Gaustad, P., Various *Candida* and *Torulopsis* species differ in their ability to induce the production of C3, factor B and granulocyte-macrophage colony-stimulating factor (GM-CSF) in human monocyte cultures, *J. Med. Microbiol.*, 42, 291, 1995.

623. Pawlik, B. and Jodlowska, V., The role of *Candida kefir* (*C. pseudotropicalis*) in reproductive tract infections, *Med. Dosw. Mikrobiol.*, 44, 83, 1992.

624. Yamaguchi, H., Uchida, K., Kawasaki, K., and Matsunaga, T., *In vitro* activity of fluconazole, a novel bistriazole antifungal agent, *Jpn. J. Antibiot.*, 42, 1, 1989.

625. Carrilo-Munoz, A. J., Tur, C., and Torres, J., In-vitro antifungal activity of sertaconazole, bifonazole, ketoconazole, and miconazole against yeasts of the *Candida* genus, *J. Antimicrob. Chemother.*, 37, 815, 1996.

626. Odds, F. C., Activity of cilofungin (LY-121,019) against *Candida* species *in vitro*, *J. Antimicrob. Chemother.*, 22, 891, 1988.

627. Vazquez, J. A., Lynch, M., and Sobel, J. D., *In vitro* activity of a new pneumocandin antifungal agent, L-733,560 against azole-susceptible and -resistant *Candida* and *Torulopsis* species, *Antimicrob. Agents Chemother.*, 39, 2689, 1995.

628. Marks, M., Langston, C., and Eickhoff, T., *Torulopsis glabrata* — an opportunistic pathogen in man, *N. Engl. J. Med.*, 283, 1131, 1970.

629. Hahn, H., Condie, F., and Bulger, R., Diagnosis of *Torulopsis glabrata* infection, *JAMA*, 203, 835, 1968.

630. Friedman, E., Blahut, R., and Bender, M., Hepatic abscesses and fungemia from *Torulopsis glabrata*, *J. Clin. Gastroenterol.*, 9, 711, 1987.

631. Connolly, J. and Mitas, J., *Torulopsis glabrata* fungemia in a diabetic patient, *South. Med. J.*, 83, 352, 1990.

632. Walter, E., Gingras, J., and McKinney, R., Systemic *Torulopsis glabrata* in a neonate, *South. Med. J.*, 83, 837, 1990.

633. Aisner, J., Schimpff, S., Sutherland, J., Young, V. M., and Wiernick, P. H., *Torulopsis glabrata* infections in patients with cancer, *Am. J. Med.*, 61, 23, 1976.

634. Butler, K. M., Rench, M. A., and Baker, C. J., Amphotericin B as a single agent in the treatment of systemic candidiasis in neonates, *Pediatr. Infect. Dis. J.*, 9, 51, 1990.

635. Pankey, G. and Daloviso, J., Fungemia caused by *Torulopsis glabrata*, *Medicine (Baltimore)*, 52, 395, 1973.

636. Baley, J. E., Kliegman, R. M., Annable, W. L., Dahms, B. B., and Fanaroff, A. A., *Torulopsis glabrata* sepsis appearing as necrotizing enterocolitis and endophthalmitis, *Am. J. Dis. Child.*, 138, 965, 1984.

637. Sander, C. H., Martin, J. N., Rogers, A. L., Barr, M., Jr., and Heidelberger, K. P., Perinatal infection with *Torulopsis glabrata*: a case associated with maternal sickle cell anemia, *Obstet. Gynecol.*, 61, 21S, 1983.

638. Quirke, P., Hwang, W. S., and Validen, C. C., Congenital *Torulopsis glabrata* infection in man, *Am. J. Clin. Pathol.*, 73, 137, 1980.

639. van Uden, N. and Buckley, H., *Candida* Berkhout, in *The Yeasts — A Taxonomic Study*, Lodder, J., Ed., North-Holland, Amsterdam, 1970, 893.

640. Bradsher, R. W., Transient fungemia due to *Candida lusitaniae*, *South. Med. J.*, 78, 626, 1985.

641. Libertin, C. R., Wilson, W. R., and Roberts, G. D., *Candida lusitaniae*: an opportunistic pathogen, *Diagn. Infect. Dis. J.*, 3, 69, 1985.

642. Merz, W. G., *Candida lusitaniae*: frequency of recovery, colonization, infection and amphotericin resistance, *J. Clin. Microbiol.*, 20, 1194, 1984.

643. Christenson, J. C., Guruswamy, A., Mukwaya, G., and Rettig, P. J., *Candida lusitaniae*: an emerging human pathogen, *Pediatr. Infect. Dis. J.*, 6, 755, 1987.

644. Holzschu, D. L., Presley, H. L., Miranda, M., and Phaff, H. J., Identification of *Candida lusitaniae* as an opportunistic yeast in humans, *J. Clin. Microbiol.*, 10, 202, 1979.

645. Baker, J. G., Nadler, H. L., Forgacs, P., and Kurtz, S. R., *Candida lusitaniae*: a new opportunistic pathogen of the urinary tract, *Diagn. Microbiol. Infect. Dis.*, 2, 145, 1984.

646. Pensler, M. I., Krawczyk, P., and LeBar, W. D., *Candida lusitaniae*, *Clin. Microbiol. Newsl.*, 7, 86, 1985.

647. Merz, W. G. and Sanford, G. R., Isolation and characteristics of a polyene-resistant variant of *Candida tropicalis*, *J. Clin. Microbiol.*, 9, 677, 1979.

648. Schlitzer, R. L. and Ahearn, D. G., Characterization of atypical *Candida tropicalis* and other uncommon clinical yeast isolates, *J. Clin. Microbiol.*, 15, 511, 1982.

649. Ahearn, D. G. and McGlohn, M. S., *In vitro* susceptibilities of sucrose-negative *Candida tropicalis*, *Candida lusitaniae*, and *Candida norvegensis* to amphotericin B, 5-fluorocytosine, miconazole, and ketoconazole, *J. Clin. Microbiol.*, 19, 412, 1984.

650. Bründel, K.-H., Zum problem der dermatomykosen bei bergleuten der grube, *Anna. Berufs-Dermatosen*, 25, 181, 1977.

651. Thomas, M. G., Parr, D. H., di Menna, M., and Lang, S. D. R., *Candida lusitaniae* septicemia: successful combination therapy, *Clin. Microbiol. Newsl.*, 7, 142, 1985.

652. Hamilton-Miller, J., Non-emergence of polyene-resistant yeasts: a hypothesis, *Microbios*, 10(Suppl. A), 91, 1974.

653. Safe, L., Safe, S., Subden, R., and Morris, D., Sterol content and polyene antibiotic resistance in isolates of *Candida krusei*, *Candida parakrusei*, and *Candida tropicalis*, *Can. J. Microbiol.*, 23, 398, 1977.

654. Dick, J. D., Merz, W. G., and Saral, R., Incidence of polyene-resistant yeasts recovered from clinical specimens, *Antimicrob. Agents Chemother.*, 18, 158, 1980.

655. Drutz, D. J. and Lehrer, R. I., Development of amphotericin B-resistant *Candida tropicalis* in a patient with defective leukocyte function, *Am. J. Med. Sci.*, 276, 77, 1978.

656. Bodenhoff, J., Resistance studies of *Candida albicans*, with special reference to two patients subjected to prolonged antibiotic treatment, *Odontol. Tidskr.*, 76, 279, 1968.

657. Hamilton-Miller, J. M. T., Chemistry and biology of the polyene macrolide antibiotics, *Bacteriol. Rev.*, 37, 166, 1973.

658. Woods, R. A., Nystatin-resistant mutants of yeast: alterations in sterol content, *J. Bacteriol.*, 108, 69, 1971.

659. King, R. D., Lee, J. C., and Morris, A. L., Adherence of *Candida albicans* and other *Candida* species to mucosal epithelial cells, *Infect. Immun.*, 27, 667, 1980.

660. Stanley, V. C. and Hurley, R., Growth of *Candida* species in cultures of mouse epithelial cells, *J. Pathol. Bacteriol.*, 94, 301, 1967.

661. Edwards, J. E., Jr., Montgomerie, J. Z., Ishida, K., Morrison, J. O., and Guze, L. B., Experimental hematogenous endophthalmitis due to *Candida*: species variation in ocular pathogenicity, *J. Infect. Dis.*, 135, 294, 1977.

662. Casasnovas, R.-O., Caillot, D., Solary, E., Bonotte, B., Chavanet, P., Bonin, A., Camerlynck, P., and Guy, H., Prophylactic fluconazole and *Candida krusei* infection, *N. Engl. J. Med.*, 326, 891, 1992.

663. Merz, W. G., Karp, J. E., Schron, D., and Saral, R., Increased incidence of fungemia caused by *Candida krusei*, *J. Clin. Microbiol.*, 24, 581, 1986.

664. Horn, R., Wong, B., Kiehn, T. E., and Armstrong, D., Fungemia in a cancer hospital: changing frequency, earlier onset, and results of therapy, *Rev. Infect. Dis.*, 7, 646, 1985.

665. Meunier, F., Aoun, M., and Bitar, N., Candidemia in immunocompromised patients, *Clin. Infect. Dis.*, 14, S120, 1992.

666. Bross, J., Talbot, G. H., Maislin, G., Hurvitz, S., and Strom, B. L., Risk factors for nosocomial candidemia: a case-control study in adults without leukemia, *Am. J. Med.*, 87, 614, 1989.

667. Slavin, R. E., Dias, M. A., and Saral, R., Cytosine arabinoside induced gastrointestinal toxic alterations in sequential chemotherapeutic protocols: a clinical-pathologic study of 33 patients, *Cancer*, 42, 1747, 1978.

668. Burke, P. J., Karp, J. E., Braine, H. G., and Vaughan, W. P., Timed sequential therapy of human leukemia based upon the response of leukemic cells to humoral growth factors, *Cancer Res.*, 37, 2138, 1977.

669. Burke, B. J., Vaughan, W. P., Karp, J. E., and Saylor, P. L., The correlation of maximal drug dose, tumor recruitment, and sequence timing with therapeutic advantage: schedule-dependent toxicity of cytosine arabinoside, *Med. Pediatr. Oncol.*, 1(Suppl.), 201, 1982.

670. Wey, S. B., Mori, M., Pfaller, M. A., Woolson, R. F., and Wenzel, R. P., Risk factors for hospital acquired candidemia: a matched case-control study, *Arch. Intern. Med.*, 149, 2349, 1989.

671. McQuillen, D. P., Zingman, B. S., Meunier, F., and Levitz, S. M., Invasive infections due to *Candida krusei*: report of ten cases of fungemia that include three cases of endophthalmitis, *Clin. Infect. Dis.*, 14, 472, 1992.

672. Rubinstein, E., Noriega, E. R., Simberkoff, M. S., Holzman, R., and Rahal, J. J., Jr., Fungal endocarditis: analysis of 24 cases and review of the literature, *Medicine (Baltimore)*, 54, 331, 1974.

673. Young, R. C., Bennett, J. E., Geelhoed, G. W., and Levine, A. S., Fungemia with compromised host resistance, *Ann. Intern. Med.*, 80, 605, 1974.

674. Jacobs, M. I., Magid, M. S., and Jarowski, C. I., Disseminated candidiasis: newer approaches to early recognition and treatment, *Arch. Dermatol.*, 116, 1277, 1980.

675. Rose, H. D. and Varkey, B., Deep mycotic infection in the hospitalized adult: a study of 132 patients, *Medicine (Baltimore)*, 54, 499, 1975.

676. Gordon, R. A., Simmons, B. P., Appelbaum, P. C., and Aber, R. C., Intra-abdominal abscess and fungemia caused by *Candida krusei*, *Arch. Intern. Med.*, 140, 1239, 1980.

677. Diggs, C. H., Eskenasy, G. M., Sutherland, J. C., and Wiernik, P. H., Fungal infection of muscle in acute leukemia, *Cancer*, 38, 1771, 1976.

678. Nguyen, V. Q. and Penn, R. L., *Candida krusei* infectious arthritis — a rare complication of neutropenia, *Am. J. Med.*, 83, 963, 1987.

679. Carcassi, A., Saletti, M., and Boschi, S., Artrite acuta da *Candida* — isolamento di *Candida krusei* in un eroinomane, *Minerva Med.*, 73, 2905, 1982.

680. Thomalla, J. V., Steidle, C. P., Leapman, S. B., and Filo, R. S., Ureteral obstruction of a renal allograft secondary to *Candida krusei*, *Transplant. Proc.*, 20, 551, 1988.

681. Segal, E., Romano, A., Eylan, E. et al., Isolation of *Candida tropicalis* from an orbital infection as a complication of maxillary osteomyelitis, *Infection*, 2, 111, 1974.

682. Segal, E., Romano, A., Eylan, E., and Stein, R., Experimental and clinical studies of 5-fluorocytosine activity in *Candida* ocular infections, *Chemotherapy*, 21, 358, 1975.

683. Mathieson, R. and Dutta, S. K., *Candida* esophagitis, *Dig. Dis. Sci.*, 28, 365, 1983.

684. Bugnardi, G. E., Savage, M. A., Coker, R., and Davis, S. G., Fluconazole and *Candida krusei* infections, *J. Hosp. Infect.*, 18, 326, 1991.

685. Case, C. P., MacGowan, A. P., Brown, N. M., Reeves, D. S., Whitehead, P., and Felmingham, D., Prophylactic oral fluconazole and *Candida* fungemia, *Lancet*, 337, 790, 1991.

686. NcIlroy, M. A., Failure of fluconazole to suppress fungemia in a patient with fever, neutropenia, and typhlitis, *J. Infect. Dis.*, 163, 420, 1991.

687. Persons, D. A., Laughlin, M., Tanner, D., Perfect, J., Gockerman, J. P., and Hathorn, J. W., Fluconazole and *Candida krusei* fungemia, *N. Engl. J. Med.*, 325, 1315, 1991.

688. Tam, J. Y., Blume, K. G., and Prober, C. G., Prophylactic fluconazole and *Candida krusei* infections: a reply, *N. Engl. J. Med.*, 326, 891, 1992.

689. Schuler, U. and Ehninger, G., Prophylactic fluconazole and *Candida krusei* infections: a reply, *N. Engl. J. Med.*, 326, 892, 1992.

690. Winston, D. J., Islam, Z., and Buell, D. N. for the Acute Leukemia Study Group, Fluconazole prophylaxis of fungal infections in acute leukemia patients: results of a placebo-controlled, double-blind, multicenter trial, *Proc. 31st Intersci. Conf. Antimicrob. Agents Chemother.*, American Society for Microbiology, Washington, D.C., 1991, 99.

691. Chandrasekar, P. H. and Gathy, C. for the Bone Marrow Transplantation Team, Reduction of candidal colonization with fluconazole in neutropenic cancer patients, *Proc. 31st Intersci. Conf. Antimicrob. Agents Chemother.*, American Society for Microbiology, Washington, D.C., 1991, 292.

692. Goodman, J., Beull, D., Gilbert, G. et al., Fluconazole prevents fungal infections in bone marrow transplantations: results of a placebo-controlled, double-blind, randomized, multi-center trial, *Proc. 31st Intersci. Conf. Antimicrob. Agents Chemother.*, American Society for Microbiology, Washington, D.C., 1991, 149.

693. Samonis, G., Rolston, K., Karl, C., Miller, P., and Bodey, G. P., Prophylaxis of oropharyngeal candidiasis with fluconazole, *Rev. Infect. Dis.*, 12(Suppl. 3), S369, 1990.

694. Morace, G., Manzara, S., and Dettori, G., *In vitro* susceptibility of 119 yeast isolates to fluconazole, 5-fluorocytosine, amphotericin B and ketoconazole, *Chemotherapy*, 37, 23, 1991.

695. Galgiani, J. N., Susceptibility of *Candida albicans* and other yeast to fluconazole: relation between *in vitro* and *in vivo* studies, *Rev. Infect. Dis.*, 12, S272, 1990.

696. Hay, R. J., Fluconazole, *J. Infect.*, 21, 1, 1990.

697. van Uden, N. and Buckley, H., *Candida rugosa* (Anderson) Duddens et Lodder, in *The Yeasts — A Taxonomic Study*, Lodder, J., Ed., North-Holland, Amsterdam, 1970, 1032.

698. Richard, J. L., McDonald, J. S., Fichtner, R. E., and Anderson, A. J., Identification of yeasts from infected bovine mammary glands and their experimental infectivity in cattle, *Am. J. Vet. Res.*, 41, 1991, 1980.

699. Dion, W. M. and Dukes, T. W., *Candida rugosa*: experimental mastitis in a dairy cow, *Sabouraudia*, 20, 95, 1982.

700. Sugar, A. M. and Stevens, D. A., *Candida rugosa* in immunocompromised infection: case reports, drug susceptibility and review of the literature, *Cancer*, 56, 318, 1985.

701. Reinhardt, J. F., Ruane, P. J., Walker, L. J., and George, W. L., Intravenous catheter-associated fungemia due to *Candida rugosa*, *J. Clin. Microbiol.*, 22, 1056, 1985.

702. Guymon, C. H., McManus, A. T., Mason, A. D., and McManus, W. F., Yeast colonization and infection in seriously burned patients, in *Proc. 91st Gen. Meet. Am. Soc. Microbiol.*, American Society for Microbiology, Washington, D.C., Abstr. L-38, 1991, 429.

703. McDonald, J. S., Richard, J. L., Anderson, A. J., and Fichtner, R. E., *In vitro* antimycotic sensitivity of yeasts isolated from infected bovine mammary glands, *Am. J. Vet. Res.*, 41, 1987, 1980.

704. Hurley, R. and Winner, H. I., Pathogenicity in the genus *Candida*, *Mycopathologia*, 24, 337, 1964.

705. Rippon, J. W., Candidiasis and the pathogenic yeasts, in *Medical Mycology: The Pathogenic Fungi and the Pathogenic Actinomycetes*, Rippon, J. W., Ed., W. B. Saunders, Philadelphia, 1982, 565.

706. Bille, J., Stockman, L., and Roberts, G. D., Detection of yeasts and filamentous fungi in blood cultures during a ten-year period (1972 to 1981), *J. Clin. Microbiol.*, 16, 968, 1982.

707. Hopfer, R. L., Orengo, A., Chesnut, S., and Wenglar, M., Radiometric detection of yeasts in blood cultures of cancer patients, *J. Clin. Microbiol.*, 12, 329, 1980.

708. Horn, R., Wong, B., Kiehn, T. E., and Armstrong, D., Fungemia in a cancer hospital: changing frequency, earlier onset, and results of therapy, *Rev. Infect. Dis.*, 7, 646, 1985.

709. Prevost, E. and Bannister, E., Detection of yeast septicemia by byphasic and radiometric methods, *J. Clin. Microbiol.*, 13, 655, 1981.

710. Wherspann, P. and Fullbrandt, U., *Yarrowia lipolytica* (Wickerham et al) van der Walt and von Arx isolated from a blood culture, *Mykosen*, 28, 217, 1985.

711. Sandhu, R. S., Randhawa, H. S., and Gupta, I. M., Pathogenicity of *Candida viswanathii* for laboratory animals: a preliminary study, *Sabouraudia*, 4, 37, 1965.

712. Viswanathan, R. and Randhawa, H. S., *Candida viswanathii* sp. nov., isolated from a case of meningitis, *Science Culture*, 25, 86, 1959.

713. Sandhu, R. S. and Randhawa, H. S., On the re-isolation and taxonomic study of *Candida viswanathii*, Viswanathan et Randhawa, *Mycopath. Mycol. Appl.*, 18, 179, 1962.

714. Fell, J. W. and Meyer Sally, A., Systematics of yeast species in the *Candida parapsilosis* group, *Mycopathol. Mycol. Appl.*, 32, 177, 1967.

715. van Uden, N. and Kolipinski, M. C., *Torulopsis haemulinii* nov. spec. a yeast from the Atlantic ocean, *Antonie van Leeuwenhoek*, 28, 78, 1962.

716. Lavarde, V., Daniel, F., Saez, H., Arnold, M., and Faguer, B., Peritonite mycosique a *Torulopsis haemulonii*, *Bul. Soc. Fr. Mycol. Méd.*, 13, 173, 1984.

717. Marjolet, M., *Torulopsis ernobii*, *Torulopsis haemulonii*: levures opportunistes chez l'immunodéprimé? *Bull. Soc. Fr. Mycol. Méd.*, 15, 143, 1986.

718. Kurtzman, C. P., Johnson, C. J., and Smiley, M. J., Determination of conspecificity of *Candida utilis* and *Hansenula jadinii* through DNA reassociation, *Mycologia*, 71, 844, 1979.

719. Kurtzman, C. P., Synonymy of the yeast genera *Hansenula* and *Pichia* demonstrated through comparisons of deoxyribonucleic acid and relatedness, *Antonie van Leeuwenhoek*, 50, 209, 1984.

720. Yamada, Y., Matsuda, M., and Mikata, K., The phylogenetic relationships of *Pichia jadinii*, formerly classified in the genus *Hansenula*, and related species based on the partial sequences of 18S and 26S ribosomal RNAs (*Saccharomycetaceae*), *Biosci. Biotechnol. Biochem.*, 59, 518, 1995.

721. Kogan, G., Sandula, J., and Simkovicova, V., Glucomannan from *Candida utilis*: structural investigation, *Folia Microbiol. (Praha)*, 38, 219, 1993.

722. Phaff, H. J., Biology of yeasts other than *Saccharomyces*, in *Biology of Industrial Microorganisms*, Demain, A. L. and Solomon, N. A., Eds., Benjamin Cummings, Menlo Park, CA, 1985, 537.

723. Viviani, M. A., Tortorano, A. M., Piazza, T., Bassi, F., Grioni, A., and Langer, M., Candidosis surveillance in intensive care unit patients, *Bull. Soc. Fr. Mycol. Méd.*, 15, 121, 1986.

724. Holzcshu, D. L., Chandler, F. W., Ajello, L., and Ahearn, D. G., Evaluation of industrial yeasts for pathogenicity, *Sabouraudia*, 17, 71, 1979.

33 *Malassezia (Pityrosporum)* spp.

33.1 INTRODUCTION

The genus *Malassezia* consists of two saprophytic yeast-like species, *M. furfur* and *M. pachyder-matitis*.[1,2] Both species, when grown under favorable conditions produce oval "yeast forms" with unipolar buds which then can reproduce asexually by budding repeatedly from the same pole of the parent cell, giving rise to a characteristic "collatette" at the bud site.[1,2]

M. furfur is a dimorphic, lipophilic yeast with requirement of fatty acids of C-12 to C-24 chain length. Its growth on most common mycologic media (e.g., Sabouraud dextrose agar) will require supplementation of sterile olive oil[3] or cow's milk.[4] *In vivo M. furfur* can presumably obtain such obligatory lipids from sebum and/or fatty acid of epidermal cell origin. It exists predominantly in the yeast form although it may also form characteristic filaments or abortive hyphae on the skin in tinea versicolor. The organism can produce filaments also *in vitro* during culture in 7% carbon dioxide or in the presence of cholesterol.[5] Leeming et al.[6] have found that the skin of both healthy and hospitalized neonates becomes colonized by *M. furfur* in the first 1 to 3 months of life.

M. furfur (synonymous with *Pityrosporum orbiculare* and *Pityrosporum ovale*)[7] is most commonly known to be the etiologic agent of tinea versicolor, a distinctive superficial dermatosis,[3,8] but also for causing deep-seated infections. The presence of *M. furfur* on the skin will trigger the production of IgA, IgG, and IgM antibodies. In addition, this yeast is also capable of activating the complement through the alternative and classical pathways.[9,10] However, specific deficiencies in either antibodies or complement fractions have not been associated with *M. furfur* infections.[2]

M. pachydermatitis is less fastidious, has no known filamentous form, and will grow on complex media without the addition of olive oil.[11,12] It is most often associated with dogs, where it produces otitis externa.[13,14] However, *M. pachydermatitis* has also been associated with cutaneous and systemic infections in humans.[15-20]

Wikler et al.[21] have studied the effect of ultraviolet (UV) light on *Malassezia* yeasts cultured from skin isolates. Immediately following irradiation by UV A (25, 50, and 75 J/cm²) and UV B (900 mJ/cm²) light dosages, electron microscopic studies have shown a significant or no yeast growth, and a moderate inhibition after irradiation with 250 mJ/cm² UV B. The growth inhibition was accompanied by ultrastructural degenerative alterations: clumping of ribosomes and lysis of nuclei. Furthermore, the content of vacuoles ("stacked material" amount) was diminished or the vacuoles were completely empty. The yeast cell walls, however, remained unchanged.[21]

33.2 EVOLUTION OF THERAPIES AND TREATMENT OF *MALASSEZIA* INFECTIONS

Malassezia spp. have been associated with several clinical conditions:[22] fungemia and systemic infections associated with high-lipid-content infusions, predominantly in neonates and young infants[23-26] but also in adults; folliculitis, most often observed in patients with the acquired immuno-deficiency syndrome and less commonly in patients with diabetes mellitus and/or receiving broad-spectrum antibiotic or steroid treatment;[27-30] seborrheic dermatitis;[29-39] and tinea versicolor,[29,30,40-42] a superficial dermatosis seen in healthy young individuals. *M. furfur*-induced papulopustular folliculitis[43] produces lesions closely resembling those of disseminated candidiasis and other fungal diseases.[1,2] Crozier and Wise[44] presented 10 cases of onychomycosis due to *M. furfur*.

Kroger et al.[45] presented laboratory and clinical evidence for a possible role of *M. furfur* in the pathophysiology of atopic eczema. Positive type 1 prick test reactions to *M. furfur* correlated with the intensity of eczematous skin lesions, and yeast extracts were found to increase IL-4, IL-10, and IgE synthesis in patients with atopic eczema. The data supported the hypothesis that *M. furfur* antigens may play a role in skin inflammation in at least a subgroup of patients with atopic eczema characterized by the presence of specific IgE antibodies to the organism. To this end, Bäck et al.[46] found that in the treatment of atopic dermatitis, the therapeutic response to ketoconazole (200 mg daily for 2 months and 200 mg twice weekly for an additional 3 months) correlated with a decrease in the serum *M. furfur*-specific IgE levels.

Malassezia has been known to frequently colonize the skin of normal and immunocompromised individuals, particularly in regions well supplied with sebaceous glands (scalp, chest, and the back).[47,48] The fact that skin colonization by *M. furfur* has its highest incidence in young adults (up to 93%) where the sebaceous glands are very active and the concentration of skin lipids is increased, correlated with the dependence of these organisms on an outside source of higher lipids.[12,23]

33.2.1 Fungemia and Systemic Disease

In 1981, the first case of *M. furfur* fungemia was reported in an infant receiving intravenous lipid therapy.[15] The introduction of intravenous lipid infusions appeared to have changed the epidemiology and pathogenesis of *M. furfur* infections from a predominantly superficial disease to a systemic mycosis diagnosed in neonates, young infants, and adults receiving intravenous alimentation, including lipid supplementation.[1,2,23,26,49-61] In a fatal case of solitary pyogenic liver abscess in a neonate, *M. furfur* has been grown from a central line culture and an echocardiogram revealed multiple pedunculated lesions.[62]

In several instances, however, patients developed the infection without receiving exogenous lipids. It may have been possible that endogenous lipids from the patient's blood, small amounts of residual lipids adherent to their catheter, or carbon sources from the catheter itself may provide adequate nutrition for the persistence of *Malassezia*.[1] In addition, some central venous catheters may also become colonized by *Malassezia* causing catheter-related infection.[23,26,63-68] *M. furfur* fungemia has been reported in a patient on chronic ambulatory peritoneal dialysis where the necessary lipids for yeast growth were presumably supplied in the form of cholesterol and triglycerides present in the dialysis fluid in the immediate postgrandial state.[69]

Neonates, especially premature, low-birth-weight infants, are at particular risk for *M. furfur* fungemia.[70-73] The role of antibody cell-mediated immunity and phagocytes against *M. furfur* is still not well understood. In adult patients receiving hyperalimentation, the infection has been associated with the presence of severe underlying diseases; however, fever has been the only common sign.[23,26,74]

At risk of developing *M. furfur* systemic infection also are cancer patients who have a long duration of hospitalization and who are receiving intravenous hyperalimentation through central venous catheters.[26,75,76]

M. furfur is known to cause severe illness in immunosuppressed patients (e.g., acute nonlymphocytic leukemia) receiving total parenteral nutrition.[60] Aoba et al.[77] have described an unusual case of meningitis due to *Malassezia* species masquerading as painful ophthalmoplegia. At the time of diagnosis, the patient was on prednisolone (30 mg daily) therapy that led to exacerbation of the neurological manifestations.

Treatment of *M. furfur* sepsis usually requires the removal of the catheter with or without antifungal chemotherapy.[1,2,23] In one report, cure was achieved with antifungal therapy and the catheter left in place.[78]

M. furfur was found susceptible to azole antimycotics *in vitro* with minimum inhibitory concentration (MIC) values of 0.4 to 1.5 and 0.25 to 0.4 µg/ml for miconazole and ketoconazole, respectively; moderately sensitive to amphotericin B (MIC = 0.3 to 2.5 µg/ml); and resistant to flucytosine (MIC = >100 µg/ml).[79] In another study involving *M. furfur*, Van Gerven and Odds[80] have evaluated the *in vitro* activity and *in vivo* efficacy of six imidazole derivatives. The most potent inhibitor *in vitro* was ketoconazole, with MIC value of 0.51 µg/ml, followed by bifonazole, miconazole, clotrimazole, flutrimazole, and sertaconazole with MIC values of 8.1, 14, 15, 16, and 52 µg/ml, respectively. Itraconazole was also found effective, with MIC value of 0.05 µg/ml, as compared to 0.1 and 12.5 to 25 µg/ml for ketoconazole and bifonazole, respectively.[81]

33.2.2 FOLLICULITIS

Malassazia (Pityrosporum) folliculitis was first described by Weary et al.[28] in 1969, and was established as a clinical and histopathological entity by Potter et al.[82] in 1973.

The clinical manifestations of *Malassezia* folliculitis is of particular importance to clinicians because of its potential for confusion with life-threatening fungal infections, such as candidiasis, torulopsis, sporotrichosis, and cryptococcosis.[1,2,43,83]

It is diagnosed predominantly in postadolescent patients as compared to acne vulgaris, which may superficially resemble *Malassezia* folliculitis but is found predominantly in adolescents.[2,61,84] In a study by Jacinto-Jamora et al.[85] *Malassezia* folliculitis was found to coexist with acne vulgaris in as many as 56% of the patients.

Malassezia folliculitis has also been diagnosed in many immunosuppressed patients with AIDS, diabetes mellitus, malignancies (leukemia, papillary adenocarcinoma), chronic renal failure, patients receiving broad-spectrum antibiotic or steroid chemotherapy, as well as in bone marrow transplant recipients.[86]

Circulating IgG antibodies against *M. furfur* were found to be present in higher titers in patients with *Malassezia* folliculitis than in patients with tinea versicolor or healthy controls.[87] In addition, the cellular immune response in skin lesions was more pronounced, and the cell infiltrates were larger than in tinea versicolor.[87]

The folliculitis may be intensely pruritic, with profound polymorphonuclear leukocyte infiltration present if the folicle wall had burst.[2,43,82] Budding yeasts have been numerous within the hair folicles but no hyphal or filamentous forms were present.[29] Skin lesions in disseminated candidiasis, which have been commonly found on the face as well as on the shoulders and chest,[43,74,88] have similar clinical manifestations but can be differentiated from that of *Malassezia* by yielding the responsible fungus when biopsy material is placed on standard fungal culture media, whereas tissue from *Malassezia* folliculitis will require lipid supplementation to the culture media for isolation of the yeast.[2]

Malassezia folliculitis may be treated successfully with topical or orally administered azole antifungals.[2] However, skin lesions associated with systemic candidal infections will require intravenous therapy with amphotericin B.

Topical treatment of *Malassezia* folliculitis usually involves the daily application of miconazole or clotrimazole cream for 2 to 3 weeks, 1% econazole nitrate solution, selenium sulfide shampoo, or 50% aqueous solutions of propylene glycol applied twice daily for 3 weeks.[27,84]

Oral therapy with ketoconazole has been carried out at daily doses of 200 mg for 2 to 3 weeks,[84,89] as well as a 2% shampoo applied twice weekly.[84]

Patients with AIDS may present with two types of folliculitis: chronic acneform folliculitis considered to be an early warning sign of AIDS,[90] and eosinophilic pustular folliculitis.[91-94] It has been known that *Malassezia* yeast may produce inflammation with eosinophilic reaction by activating the alternative complement pathway as well as through the free acids produced as a result of its lipase activity.[95]

M. furfur folliculitis in AIDS patients has been seen on the trunk and legs and has been highly resistant to any form of therapy.[50,88] Ferrandiz et al.[94] have reported on two AIDS patients with intensely pruritic pustular folliculitis associated with the presence of *Malassezia* yeasts in the hair follicles. Topical application of ketoconazole cream every night resolved the eruption and its attendant itch after 4 and 6 weeks, respectively.

After Finn et al.[96] described a distinctive follicular dermatosis in 45% of male patients with the Down's syndrome without discussing the possible etiology of this rash, speculations have been focused on the probable association of *Malassezia* as a causative agent. Kavanagh et al.[97] have reported on 10 male and 2 female patients with Down's syndrome with follicular rash consistent with *Malassezia* folliculitis who responded to a 2-week course of oral itraconazole treatment (100 mg daily). Even though a significant improvement in the papulopustular folliculitis, accompanied by a decrease in the skin *Malassezia* count was observed, relapse quickly occurred when treatment was ceased.

33.2.3 TINEA (PITYRIASIS) VERSICOLOR

Since the lipophilic *M. furfur* is keratinophilic, tinea versicolor is a scaling dermatosis occurring in the stratum corneum, and usually confined to small patches of skin on the trunk and shoulders of affected individuals.[1,2,42,98] It has been sometimes confused with other dermatologic disorders, such as pityriasis alba, secondary syphilis, and vitiligo. Aljabre and Sheikh[99] have presented a case with a penile involvement in pityriasis versicolor.

Predisposing factors of tinea versicolor include excessive sweating, malnutrition, chronic illness, immunosuppression, and a warm environment.[98]

Since tinea versicolor is the most superficial of all fungal infections (commonly seen on the head and neck as small oval or round hyper- or hypopigmented patches), its importance is primarily cosmetic.

Tinea versicolor, which is easily managed with daily topical medication with clotrimazole or miconazole creams or lotions, 50% aqueous solutions of propylene glycol (applied twice daily), as well as oral ketoconazole (200 mg daily), has also a high relapse rate.[41]

In an open, randomized trial, Galimberti et al.[100] treated 28 patients with pityriasis versicolor with oral itraconazole at 200 daily for either 5 or 7 d. Transmission and scanning electron microscopy have revealed that the 7-d course was more effective, with cytopathic changes resulting in intracellular necrosis being complete within 7 to 28 d.

A double-blind comparison of 2% ketoconazole cream and placebo resulted in clinical response of 98% and 28% of patients with tinea versicolor, respectively.[101] There was an overall 84% mycological cure rate for patients receiving ketoconazole vs. 10% of the placebo group. In addition, 75% of those responding to placebo relapsed within 8 weeks.

Faergemann[102] reported that fluconazole, at 400 mg (given as a single dose) may be effective to treat pityriasis versicolor. Fenticonazole (another imidazole agent) cream or lotion has also been used successfully.[103]

In addition to imidazole antimycotics, topical selenium sulfide, as 2.5% suspension, when applied for 12 h and repeated in 1 week has also been used to treat tinea versicolor.[1,2] In a comparative trial of itraconazole and selenium sulfide shampoo, 40 patients with tinea versicolor were randomly assigned to receive either oral itraconazole (200 mg once daily for 5 d) or 2.5% selenium sulfide shampoo (once daily application for 1 week).[104] At a follow-up examination 3 weeks after the end of treatment, the response rates to both regimens were almost analogous, but the oral administration was the patients' preference.

Topical sodium thiosulfate as 25% solution, tolnaftate, and halprogin have also been used.[98] Griseofulvin failed to cure tinea versicolor.[105]

Ciclopiroxolamine (2-pyridone antifungal) as 1% solution has been used in the treatment of tinea versicolor. Using scanning and emission electron microscopy, del Palacio Hernanz et al.[106] have described significant ultrastructural changes on the surface of yeasts and hyphae of *M. furfur*,

15 d after the start of therapy. Extensive internal damage (severe necrosis of the cytoplasm) was also noticed.

Because tinea versicolor has a high rate of recurrence (reaching 60% in the first year and 80% after 2 years), prophylactic treatment has also been recommended.[107]

33.2.4 SEBORRHEIC DERMATITIS

There has been a connection between seborrheic dermatitis and *M. furfur*.[38,39,108,109] The possibility of an abnormal immune response to the yeast as one explanation for the development of this clinical condition has been suggested.[38] It has been shown that *M. furfur* can evoke humoral and cellular immune reactions in an affected host,[110] as well as high antibody titers to *Malassezia* in dandruff.[111]

It is likely that *M. furfur* may have an indirect exacerbating effect mediated by immunologic mechanisms.[112] Thus, Sohnle et al.[9,10] have demonstrated that *M. furfur* can activate the complement by both the classical and alternative pathways. In addition, *M. furfur* can trigger the alternative pathway of complement fixation,[113] and can induce the leukocyte chemotaxis.[114] Activation of the alternative complement pathway by *M. furfur*, which does not require T cell function, may be one possible explanation for the inflammatory response.[38]

In patients with AIDS and AIDS-related complex who have been known to have greatly diminished T cell functions, a high incidence (as much as 80%[115]) of seborrheic dermatitis and dandruff has been reported.[36,115-119] Defects in delayed cutaneous hypersensitivity or a link with circulating immune complexes may explain such high incidence. Another relevant explanation may involve epidermal keratinocyte stimulation by either HIV or by lymphokines released by monocytes, or T cells infected by the virus.[120] A quantitative correlation between the number of yeast cells adherent to keratinocytes and the clinical severity of seborrheic dermatitis in AIDS patients[116] seemed to lend credence to a causative role for *M. furfur* in seborrheic dermatitis. However, these assumptions have not been confirmed by other studies[35] and may still be only circumstantial evidence.

A seborrheic dermatitis-like exanthema associated with AIDS has also been reported.[121]

In addition, patients with Parkinson's disease (a CNS disorder) have also shown predilection for seborrheic dermatitis.[122] A report[123] of unilateral seborrheic dermatitis after nerve injury further emphasized the potential role of neural involvement.[108]

Drugs with antipityrosporal activity have been used most often to treat seborrheic dermatitis.[120] Anti-inflammatory, antikeratolytic, and antiseptic properties have also been used but to a lesser extent.

Selenium sulfide, although classified by the U.S. Food and Drug Administration as an antikeratolytic agent, has been shown also to have antipityrosporal effect,[124] and as a 2.5% shampoo was used in cases of seborrheic dermatitis.[125]

Another antikeratolytic agent, zinc pyrithione (as 1% shampoo) was shown to affect the membrane transport, macromolecular synthesis, cell structure and functions of *M. furfur*[126] and has been used in seborrheic dermatitis.[127]

In several reports,[128-131] the topical use of lithium succinate in the treatment of seborrheic dermatitis has been described. The drug, which was applied as an ointment, although poorly sustained proved beneficial and was well tolerated. The assertion that lithium succinate acted as an anti-inflammatory agent[129] has been disputed[130] based on previous findings of *in vitro* and *in vivo* antipityrosporal activity.[132]

Corticosteroids have decreased pruritus, reduced the number of *M. furfur*, and produced clinical improvement in seborrheic dermatitis and dandruff.[120,133,134] However, in addition to high relapse rates, the prolonged use of corticosteroids may lead to undesirable side effects, such as atrophy, poor wound healing, purpura, and perioral dermatitis.[31]

Among other antikeratolytic and antiseptic agents, sulfur, coal tar, and salicylic acid have also been used.[120] Studies by Heng et al.[135] have established a correlation between the density of *M. furfur* with the clinical severity of seborrheic dermatitis both before and after therapy with a precipitated sulfur-salicyclic acid shampoo.

More than a dozen imidazole derivatives have been investigated for their activities against seborrheic dermatitis.[120,136] *In vitro* and *in vivo* experiments by Faergemann[137] have demonstrated that ketoconazole was the most effective of them against *M. furfur*, with MIC value of 0.01 mg/l. One reason for the observed high potency of ketoconazole may be due to its greater effects on 5-lipoxygenase and leukotriene B_4 production in the skin, thus suppressing inflammation more readily.[138] In albino guinea pigs involving three consecutive days of topical treatments, bifonazole 1% cream, clotrimazole 1% cream, flitrinazole 1% and 2% creams, ketoconazole 2% cream and shampoo, and miconazole 2% cream all reduced *M. furfur* dermatitis lesion severity below that of untreated control animals; sertaconazole 2% gel and cream showed no reduction in lesion severity below controls.[80]

Ford et al.[139] have used systemic ketoconazole (200 mg orally, once daily) for 4 weeks to treat seborrheic dermatitis, with good to excellent results. However, the systemic use of ketoconazole is not recommended since seborrheic dermatitis usually affects small body areas and is generally a chronic relapsing condition which will require long-term treatment. Because of its side effects (hepatotoxicity and effects on steroidal biosynthesis), long-term treatment with ketoconazole is unwarranted.

Subsequently, topical ketoconazole preparations (cream, shampoo, scalp gel formulations) have been developed.[140-146] On average, about 80% of patients who used ketoconazole 2% cream for 4 weeks (including in five double-blind clinical trials[143-145,147,148]) experienced good symptomatic improvement or clinical resolution. The therapeutic efficacy of ketoconazole 2% shampoo has also been investigated in several double-blind, placebo-controlled studies.[148-154] Good to excellent response of seborrheic dermatitis was seen in 90% of treated patients compared with a placebo response of about 30%; 1% ketoconazole shampoo elicited a comparative response in 80% of patients. Van Cutsem et al.[155] have found that ketoconazole possessed a high affinity for keratinous materials, with significant concentrations in hair maintained over several days. Ketoconazole 2% scalp gel has also been shown to be effective in treating seborrheic dermatitis and dandruff.[142]

Rapelanoro et al.[156] have described *M. furfur*-associated papulopustular eruption of the face of neonates. Treatment with ketoconazole 2% cream applied topically twice daily was effective in 1 week.

In several studies, however, topical treatment of seborrheic dermatitis with ketoconazole has been reported to elicit often only partial response; complete resolution was not universal.[147,148,157,158]

In addition to ketoconazole, bifonazole (1% cream or lotion),[118,136,159] fluconazole (2% shampoo),[160] fenticonazole,[161] and tioconazole (1% cream or lotion)[162] have also been investigated against *M. furfur*-associated seborrheic dermatitis. Massone et al.[118] reported an especially good response to 1% bifonazole cream among patients with lymphadenopathy syndrome/AIDS-related complex.

Overall, when applied topically, ketoconazole either as cream, shampoo, or gel was well tolerated after short- and long-term therapy.[163] Autoradiographic studies by Stippie et al.[164] have shown that ketoconazole did not penetrate beyond the epidermis.

Using a checkboard-style assay, Tucker et al.[165] studied *in vitro* and in patients the combined effects of azole antimycotics and other drugs against various yeasts, including the yeast phase of *M. furfur*. An itraconazole–rifampin combination was selected to correspond to that administered to two patients who in addition to AIDS and cryptococcosis suffered from active seborrheic dermatitis while receiving combination therapy with itraconazole and rifampin. The potential for drug interaction was characterized by calculation of the fractional inhibitory concentration (FIC) index, as previously described.[166,167] The FIC indices of the two *M. furfur* isolates showed indifference; that is, the absence of either synergy or antagonism. In one of the patients, the longstanding seborrheic dermatitis was resolved during treatment with itraconazole alone (found active *in vitro* against *M. furfur*[81,168,169]), then recurred during rifampin therapy, and disappeared when rifampin was stopped. In the second case, the seborrheic dermatitis, which was present before the itraconazole treatment, persisted during the rifampin therapy. Since there has been no synergy between itraconazole and rifampin *in vitro*, the progression of seborrhea or the lack of improvement in the two patients taking concurrently itraconazole and rifampin lent credence to an *in vitro*-clinical efficacy correlation.[165]

In a double-blind controlled study, 89% of patients with seborrheic dermatitis responded to 15% aqueous propylene glycol.[170]

33.3 REFERENCES

1. Teglia, O., Schloch, P. E., and Cunha, B. A, *Malassezia furfur* infections, *Infect. Control Hosp. Epidemiol.*, 12, 676, 1991.
2. Klotz, S. A., *Malassezia furfur*, *Infect. Dis. Clin. North Am.*, 3, 53, 1989.
3. Faergemann, J. and Frederiksson, T., Age, incidence of *Pityrosporum orbiculare* on human skin, *Acta Derm. Venereol.*, 60, 531, 1980.
4. Leeming, J. P. and Notman, F. H., Improved methods for isolation and enumeration of *Malassezia furfur* from human skin, *J. Clin. Microbiol.*, 25, 2017, 1987.
5. Faergemann, J., Aly, R., and Maibach, H. I., Growth and filament production of *Pityrosporum orbiculare* and *P. ovale* on human stratum corneum *in vitro*, *Acta Derm. Venereol.*, 63, 388, 1983.
6. Leeming, J. P., Sutton, T. M., and Fleming, P. J., Neonatal skin as a reservoir of *Malassezia* species, *Pediatr. Infect. Dis. J.*, 14, 719, 1995.
7. Yarrow, D. and Ahearn, D. G., *Malassezia* Baillon, in *The Yeasts; A Taxonomic Study*, Kreger-Van Rij, N. J. W., Ed., Elsevier, Amsterdam, 1984, 883.
8. Faergemann, J. and Fredericksson, T., Tinea versicolor: some new aspects on etiology, pathogenesis and treatment, *Int. J. Dermatol.*, 21, 8, 1981.
9. Sohnle, P. G. and Collins-Lech, C., Activation of complement by *Pityrosporum orbiculare*, *J. Invest. Dermatol.*, 80, 93, 1983.
10. Sohnle, P. G., Collins-Lech, C., and Hihta, K. E., Class-specific antibodies in young and aged humans against organisms producing superficial infections, *Br. J. Dermatol.*, 108, 69, 1983.
11. Marcon, M. J. and Powell, D. A., *Malassezia furfur*, *Clin. Microbiol. Newsl.*, 10, 41, 1988.
12. Powell, D. A., Hayes, J., Durrell, D. E., Miller, M., and Marcon, M. J., *Malassezia furfur* skin colonization in infants hospitalized in intensive care units, *J. Pediatr.*, 111, 217, 1987.
13. Nazzoro Porro, N. M., Passi, S., Caprill, E., Nazzaro, P., and Morpurgo, G., Growth requirements and lipid metabolism of *Pityrosporum orbilucare*, *J. Invest. Dermatol.*, 66, 178, 1976.
14. Abou-Kabal, M., Chastain, C. B., and Hogle, R. M., *Pityrosporum (pachydermatitis) canis* as a major cause of otitis externa in dogs, *Mykosen*, 22, 192, 1979.
15. Redline, R. W. and Dahms, B. B., *Malassezia* pulmonary vasculitis in an infant on long-term intralipid therapy, *N. Engl. J. Med.*, 305, 1395, 1981.
16. Guého, E., Simmons, R. B., Pruitt, W. R., Meyer, S. A., and Ahearn, D. G, Association of *Malassezia pachydermatitis* with systemic infections in humans, *J. Clin. Microbiol.*, 25, 1789, 1987.
17. Anaissie, E. J., Bodey, G. P., and Rinaldi, M., Emerging fungal pathogens, *Eur. J. Clin. Microbiol. Infect. Dis.*, 8, 323, 1989.
18. Larocco, M., Dorenbaum, A., Robinson, A., and Pickering, L. K., Recovery of *Malassezia pachydermatitis* from eight infants in a neonatal intensive care nursery: clinical and laboratory features, *Pediatr. Infect. Dis. J.*, 7, 398, 1988.
19. Mickelsen, P. A., Viano-Paulson, M. C., Stevens, D. A., and Diaz, P. S., Clinical and microbiological features of infection with *Malassezia pachydermatitis* in high-risk infants, *J. Infect. Dis.*, 157, 1163, 1988.
20. Welbel, S. F., McNeil, M. M., Pramanik, A., Silberman, R., Oberle, A. D., Midgley, G., Crow, S., and Jarvis, W. R., Nosocomial *Malassezia pachydermatitis* bloodstream infections in a neonatal intensive care unit, *Pediatr. Infect. Dis. J.*, 13, 104, 1994.
21. Wikler, J. R., Janssen, N., Bruynzeel, D. P., and Nieboer, C., The effect of UV-light on pityrosporum yeasts: ultrastructural changes and inhibition of growth, *Acta Derm. Venereol.*, 70, 69, 1990.

22. Guého, E., Faergemann, J., Lyman, C., and Anaissie, E. J., *Malassezia* and *Trichosporon*: two emerging pathogenic basidiomycetous yeast-like fungi, *J. Med. Vet. Mycol.*, 32(Suppl. 1), 367, 1994.

23. Marcon, M. J. and Powell, D. A., Epidemiology, diagnosis, and management of *M. furfur* systemic infection, *Diagn. Microbiol. Infect. Dis.*, 10, 161, 1987.

24. Roberts, W., *Pityrosporum orbiculare*: incidence and distribution on clinically normal skin, *Br. J. Dermatol.*, 81, 264, 1969.

25. Bell, L. M., Alpert, G., Slight, P. H. et al., Skin colonization of hospitalized and nonhospitalized infants with lipophilic yeast, *Proc. 25th Intersci. Conf. Antimicrob. Agents Chemother.*, American Society for Microbiology, Washington, D.C., Abstr. 519, 1985.

26. Dankner, W. M., Spector, S. A., Fierer, J., and Davis, C. E., *Malassezia* fungemia in neonates and adults: complication of hyperalimentation, *Rev. Infect. Dis.*, 9, 743, 1987.

27. Bäck, O., Faergemann, J., and Hörnquist, R., *Pityrosporum* folliculitis: a common disease of the young and middle-aged, *J. Am. Acad. Dermatol.*, 12, 56, 1985.

28. Weary, P. E., Russell, C. M., Butler, H. K., and Hsu, Y. T., Acneform eruption resulting from antibiotic administration, *Arch. Dermatol.*, 100, 179, 1969.

29. Faergemann, J., *Pityrosporum* infections, *J. Am. Acad. Dermatol.*, 31, S18, 1994.

30. Piérard, G. E., Piérard-Franchimont, C., and Ben Mosbah, T., Pityrosporiasis: pityriasis versicolor, folliculitis, pityrosporum, seborrheic dermatitis and pellicular status, *Rev. Med. Liege*, 44, 267, 1989.

31. Faergemann, J., Seborrhoeic dermatitis and *Pityrosporum orbiculare*: treatment of seborrhoeic dermatitis of the scalp with miconazole-hydrocortisone (Daktacort), miconazole and hydrocortisone, *Br. J. Dermatol.*, 114, 695, 1986.

32. Ford, G. P., Farr, P. M., Ive, F. A., and Shuster, S., The response of seborrhoeic dermatitis to ketoconazole, *Br. J. Dermatol.*, 111, 603, 1984.

33. Shuster, S., The aetiology of dandruff and the mode of action of therapeutic agents, *Br. J. Dermatol.*, 111, 235, 1984.

34. Janniger, C. K. and Schwartz, R. A., Seborrheic dermatitis, *Am. Fam. Physician*, 52, 149, 1995.

35. Bergbrant, I. M. and Faergemann, J., The role of *Pityrosporum ovale* in seborrheic dermatitis, *Semin. Dermatol.*, 9, 262, 1990.

36. Selden, S. T., Immune responses to *Pityrosporum orbiculare* and seborrheic dermatitis, *Am. Fam. Physician*, 53, 2278, 1996.

37. Piérard, G. E., Piérard-Franchimont, C., Van Cutsem, J., Rurangirwa, A., Hoppenbrouwers, M. L., and Schrooten, P., Ketoconazole 2% emulsion in the treatment of seborrheic dermatitis, *Int. J. Dermatol.*, 30, 806, 1991.

38. Bergbrant, I. M., Seborrhoeic dermatitis and *Pityrosporum* yeasts, *Curr. Top. Med. Mycol.*, 6, 95, 1995.

39. Faergemann, J., Jones, J. C., Hettler, O., and Loria, Y., *Pityrosporum ovale* (*Malassezia furfur*) as the causative agent of seborrhoeic dermatitis: new treatment options, *Br. J. Dermatol.*, 134(Suppl. 46), 12 (discussion 38), 1996.

40. Burke, R. C., Tinea versicolor: susceptibility factors and experimental infections in human beings, *J. Invest. Dermatol.*, 36, 389, 1961.

41. Savin, R., Diagnosis and treatment of tinea versicolor, *J. Fam. Pract.*, 43, 127, 1996.

42. McGinley, K. J., Lantis, L. R., and Marples, R. R., Microbiology of tinea versicolor, *Arch. Dermatol.*, 102, 168, 1970.

43. Klotz, S. A., Drutz, D. J., Huppert, M., and Johnson, J. E., *Pityrosporum* folliculitis: its potential for confusion with skin lesion of systemic candidiasis, *Arch. Intern. Med.*, 142, 2186, 1982.

44. Crozier, W. J. and Wise, K. A., Onychomycosis due to *Pityrosporum*, *Australas. J. Dermatol.*, 34, 109, 1993.

45. Kroger, S., Neuber, K., Gruseck, E., Ring, J., and Abeck, D., *Pityrosporum ovale* extracts increase interleukin-4, interleukin-10 and IgE synthesis in patients with atopic eczema, *Acta Derm. Venereol.*, 75, 357, 1995.

46. Bäck, O., Scheynius, A., and Johansson, S. G., Ketoconazole in atopic dermatitis: therapeutic response is correlated with decrease in serum IgE, *Arch. Dermatol.*, 287, 448, 1995.

47. Noble, W. C., *Microbiology of Human Skin*, 2nd ed., Lloyd-Luke, London, 1981, 17.

48. Slooff, W. C., Genus 6. *Pityrosporum* Sabouraud, in *The Yeasts: a Taxonomic Study*, 2nd ed., Lodder, J., Ed., North-Holland, Amsterdam, 1970, 1167.

49. Long, J. G. and Keyserling, H. L., Catheter-related infection in infants due to an unusual lipophilic yeast — *Malassezia furfur, Pediatrics,* 76, 896, 1985.
50. Redline, R. W., Redline, S. S., Boxerbaum, B., and Dahms, B. B., Systemic *Malassezia furfur* infection in patients receiving intralipid therapy, *Hum. Pathol.*, 16, 815, 1985.
51. Garcia, C. R., Johnston, B. L., Corvi, G., Walker, L. J., and George, W. L., Intravenous catheter-associated *Malassezia furfur* fungemia, *Am. J. Med.*, 83, 790, 1987.
52. Hassall, E., Ulich, T., and Ament, M. E., Pulmonary embolus and *Malassezia* pulmonary infection related to urokinaze therapy, *J. Pediatr.*, 102, 722, 1983.
53. Prober, C. G. and Ein, S. H., Systemic tinea versicolor or how far can furfur go? *Pediatr. Infect. Dis. J.*, 3, 592, 1984.
54. Brooks, R. and Brown, L., Systemic infection with *Malassezia furfur* in an adult receiving long-term hyperalimentation therapy, *J. Infect. Dis.*, 156, 410, 1987.
55. Dankner, W. M. and Spector, S. A., *Malassezia furfur* sepsis in neonates, *J. Pediatr.*, 107, 643, 1985.
56. Rinaldi, M. G., Emerging opportunists, *Infect. Dis. Clin. North Am.*, 3, 65, 1989.
57. Shparago, N. I., Bruno, P. P., and Bennett, J., Systemic *Malassezia furfur* infection in an adult receiving total parenteral nutrition, *J. Am. Osteopath. Assoc.*, 95, 375, 1995.
58. Bjerregaard-Andersen, H., Bengtsson, B., and Bogelund, L., Septicemia caused by *Malassezia furfur*, *Ugeskr. Laeger.*, 155, 2154, 1993.
59. Surmont, I., Gavilanes, A., Vandepitte, J., Devlieger, H., and Eggermont, E., *Malassezia furfur* fungaemia in infants receiving intravenous lipid emulsions: a rarity or just underestimated? *Eur. J. Pediatr.*, 148, 435, 1989.
60. Middleton, C. and Lowenthal, R. M., *Malassezia furfur* fungemia as a treatable cause of obscure fever in a leukemia patient receiving parenteral nutrition, *Aust. NZ J. Med.*, 17, 603, 1987.
61. Cuadra Oyanguren, J., Barbera Montesinos, E., Sanchez Carazo, J. L., and Aliaga Boniche, A., Folliculitis caused by *Pityrosporum*, *Med. Cutan. Ibero Lat. Am.*, 13, 357, 1985.
62. Doerr, C. A., Demmler, G. J., Garcia-Prats, J. A., and Brandt, M. L., Solitary pyogenic liver abscess in neonates: report of three cases and review of the literature, *Pediatr. Infect. Dis. J.*, 13, 64, 1994.
63. Alpert, G., Bell, L. M., and Campos, J. M., *Malassezia furfur* fungemia in infancy, *Clin. Pediatr.*, 26, 528, 1987.
64. Powell, D. A., Aungst, J., Snedden, S., Hansen, S., Hansen, N., and Brady, M., Broviac catheter-related *Malassezia furfur* sepsis in five infants receiving intravenous fat emulsions, *J. Pediatr.*, 105, 987, 1984.
65. Aschner, J. L., Punsalang, A., Jr., Maniscalco, W. M., and Menegus, M. A., Percutaneous central venous catheter colonization with *Malassezia furfur* incidence and clinical significance, *Pediatrics*, 80, 535, 1987.
66. Linaris, J., Sitges-Serra, A., Garau, J., Pérez, J. L., and Martin, R., Pathogenesis of catheter sepsis: a prospective study with quantitative and semi-quantitative cultures of catheter hub and segments, *J. Clin. Microbiol.*, 21, 357, 1985.
67. Powell, D. A., Marcon, M. J., Durrell, D. E., and Pfister, R. M., Scanning electron microscopy of *Malassezia furfur* attachment to broviac catheters, *Hum. Pathol.*, 18, 740, 1987.
68. Arnow, P. M. and Kushner, R., *Malassezia furfur* catheter infection cured with antibiotic lock therapy, *Am. J. Med.*, 90, 128, 1991 (correction: *Am. J. Med.*, 92, 582, 1992).
69. Wallace, M., Bagnall, H., Glen, D., and Averill, S., Isolation of lipophilic yeast in "sterile" peritonitis, *Lancet*, 2, 956, 1979.
70. Redline, R. W. and Barrett Dahms, B., *Malassezia* pulmonary vasculitis in an infant on long-term intralipid therapy, *N. Engl. J. Med.*, 305, 1395, 1981.
71. Shek, Y. H., Tucker, M. C., Viciana, A. L., Manz, H. J., and Connor, D. H., *Malassezia furfur*: disseminated infection in premature infants, *Am. J. Clin. Pathol.*, 92, 595, 1989.
72. Stuart, S. M. and Lane, A. T., *Candida* and *Malassezia* as nursery pathogens, *Semin. Dermatol.*, 11, 19, 1992.
73. Carey, B. E., *Malassezia furfur* infection in the NICU, *Neonatal Netw.*, 9, 19, 1991.
74. Brown, L. and Brooks, R., Systemic infection with *Malassezia furfur* in an adult receiving long-term hyperalimentation therapy, *J. Infect. Dis.*, 156, 410, 1987.
75. Samonia, G. and Bfaloukos, D., Fungal infections in cancer patients: an escalating problem, *In Vivo*, 6, 183, 1992.

76. Francis, P. and Walsh, T. J., Approaches to management of fungal infections in cancer patients, *Oncology*, 6, 133, 1992.
77. Aoba, S., Komiyama, A., and Hasegawa, O., Fungal meningites caused by *Malassezia* species masquerading as painful ophthalmoplegia, *Rinsho Shinkeigaku*, 33, 462, 1993.
78. Weiss, S. J., Schoch, P. E., and Cunha, B. A., *Malassezia furfur* fungemia associated with central venous catheter lipid emulsion infusion, *Heart Lung*, 20, 87, 1991.
79. Marcon, M. J., Durrell, D. E., Powell, D. A., and Buesching, W. J., In vitro activity of systemic antifungal agents against *Malassezia furfur*, *Antimicrob. Agents Chemother.*, 31, 951, 1987.
80. Van Gerven, F. and Odds, F. C., The anti-*Malassezia furfur* activity *in vitro* and in experimental dermatitis of six imidazole antifungal agents: bifonazole, clotrimazole, flutrimazole, ketoconazole, miconazole, and sertaconazole, *Mycoses*, 38, 398, 1995.
81. Nenoff, P. and Haustein, U. F., Effect of anti-seborrhea substances against *Pityrosporum ovale in vitro*, *Hautarzt*, 45, 464, 1994.
82. Potter, B. S., Burgeon, C. F., Jr., and Johnson, W. C., *Pityrosporum* folliculitis, *Arch. Dermatol.*, 107, 388, 1973.
83. Yohn, J. J., Lucas, J., and Camisa, C., *Malassezia* folliculitis in immunocompromised patients, *Cutis*, 25, 536, 1985.
84. Abdel-Razek, M., Fadaly, G., Abdel-Raheim, M., and Al-Morsy, F., Pityrosporum (*Malassezia*) folliculitis in Saudi Arabia — diagnosis and therapeutic trials, *Clin. Exp. Dermatol.*, 20, 406, 1995.
85. Jacinto-Jamora, S., Tamesis, J., and Katigbak, M. L., *Pityrosporum* folliculitis in the Philippines: diagnosis, prevalence, and management, *J. Am. Acad. Dermatol.*, 24, 693, 1991.
86. Bufill, J. A., Lum, L. G., Caya, J. G., Chitambar, C. R., Ritch, P. S., Anderson, T., and Ash, R. C., *Pityrosporum* folliculitis after bone marrow transplantation: clinical observations in five patients, *Ann. Intern. Med.*, 108, 560, 1988.
87. Faergemann, J., Johansson, S., and Bäck, O., An immunologic and cultural study of *Pityrosporum* folliculitis, *J. Am. Acad. Dermatol.*, 14, 429, 1986.
88. Dupont, B. and Drouhet, E., Cutaneous, ocular, and osteoarticular candidiasis in heroin addicts: new clinical and therapeutic aspects in 38 patients, *J. Infect. Dis.*, 152, 577, 1985.
89. Ford, G. P., Ive, F. A., and Midgley, G., *Pityrosporum* folliculitis and ketoconazole, *Br. J. Dermatol.*, 107, 691, 1982.
90. Muhlemann, M. F., Anderson, M. G., Paradinas, F. J., Key, P. R., Dawson, S. G., Evans, B. A., Murray-Lyon, I. M., and Cream, J. J., Early warning signs in AIDS and persistent generalized lymphadenopathy, *Br. J. Dermatol.*, 114, 419, 1986.
91. Soeprono, F. F. and Schinella, R. A., Eosinophilic pustular folliculitis in patients with acquired immunodeficiency syndrome, *J. Am. Acad. Dermatol.*, 14, 1020, 1986.
92. Buchness, M. R., Lim, H. W., Hatcher, V. A., Sanchez, M., and Soter, N. A., Eosinophilic pustular folliculitis in the acquired immunodeficiency syndrome: treatment with ultraviolet B phototherapy, *N. Engl. J. Med.*, 318, 1183, 1988.
93. Jenkins, D., Jr., Fisher, B. K., Chalvardjian, A., and Adam, P., Eosinophilic pustular folliculitis in a patient with AIDS, *Int. J. Dermatol.*, 27, 34, 1988.
94. Ferrandiz, C., Ribera, M., Barranco, J. C., Clotet, B., and Lorenzo, J. C., Eosinophilic pustular folliculitis in patients with acquired immunodeficiency syndrome, *Int. J. Dermatol.*, 31, 193, 1992.
95. Faergemann, J. and Mailbach, H. I., *Pityrosporum* yeasts: their role as pathogens, *Int. J. Dermatol.*, 23, 463, 1984.
96. Finn, O. A., Grant, P. W., McCallum, D. I., and Raffle, E. J., A singular dermatosis of mongols, *Arch. Dermatol.*, 114, 1493, 1978.
97. Kavanagh, G. M., Leeming, J. P., Marshman, G. M., Reynolds, N. J., and Burton, J. L., Folliculitis in Down's syndrome, *Br. J. Dermatol.*, 129, 696, 1993.
98. Rezabek, G. H. and Friedman, A. D., Superficial fungal infections of the skin: diagnosis and current treatment recommendations, *Drugs*, 43, 674, 1992.
99. Aljabre, S. H. and Sheikh, Y. H., Penile involvement in pityriasis versicolor, *Trop. Geogr. Med.*, 46, 184, 1994.
100. Galimberti, R. L., Villalba, I., Galarza, S., Raimondi, A., and Flores, V., Itraconazole in pityriasis versicolor: ultrastructural changes in *Malassezia furfur* produced during treatment, *Rev. Infect. Dis.*, 9(Suppl. 1), S134, 1987.

101. Savin, R. C. and Horwitz, S. N., Double-blind comparison of 2% ketoconazole cream and placebo in the treatment of tinea versicolor, *J. Am. Acad. Dermatol.*, 15, 500, 1986.

102. Faergemann, J., Treatment of pityriasis versicolor with a single dose of fluconazole, *Acta Derm. Venereol. (Stockholm)*, 72, 74, 1992.

103. Di Silverio, A., Mosca, M., Brandozzi, G., Vignoli, G. P., Gatti, M., Gabba, P., and Ubezio, S., Studio dell'efficacia del fenticonazolo su pazienti affetti da *Pityriasis versicolor*, *G. Ital. Dermatol. Venereol.*, 124, XLVII-IL, 1989.

104. del Palacio Hernanz, A., Delgado Vicente, S., Menendez Ramos, F., and Rodruguez-Noriega Belaustegui, A., Randomized comparative clinical trial of itraconazole and selenium sulfide shampoo for the treatment of pityriasis versicolor, *Rev. Infect. Dis.*, 9(Suppl. 1), S121, 1987.

105. Stein, D., Superficial fungal infections, *Pediatr. Clin. North Am.*, 30, 545, 1983.

106. del Palacio Hernanz, A., Guarro Artigas, J., Figueras Salvat, M. J., Esteban Moreno, J., and Lopez Gomez, S., Changes in fungal ultrastructure after short-course ciclopiroxolamine therapy in pityriasis versicolor, *Clin. Exp. Dermatol.*, 15, 95, 1990.

107. Faergemann, J., Pityriasis versicolor (tinea versicolor), in *Clinical Dermatology*, Vol. 3, Demis, D., Ed., Harper and Row, Philadelphia, 1986, 1.

108. Webster, G., Seborrheic dermatitis, *Int. J. Dermatol.*, 30, 843, 1991.

109. Macotela Ruiz, E., Lopez Martinez, R., Majorada, A., and Carmona Castanon, A., Pathogenic role of *Pityrosporum ovale* in dermatitis seborrheica and pityriasis versicolor, *Gac. Med. Mex.*, 123, 187, 1987.

110. Weary, P. E., *Pityrosporum ovale*: observations on some aspects of host-parasite interrelationships, *Arch. Dermatol.*, 98, 408, 1968.

111. Alexander, S., Loss of hair and dandruff, *Br. J. Dermatol.*, 79, 549, 1967.

112. Hay, R. J. and Midgley, G., Pathogenic mechanisms of *Pityrosporum* infection, in *Seborrhoeic Dermatitis and Dandruff — a Fungal Disease*, Shuster, S. and Blatchfold, N., Eds., International Congress and Symposium Series, No. 132, Royal Society of Medicine Services Ltd., London, 1988, 13.

113. Belew, P. W., Rosenberg, E. W., and Jennings, B. R., Activation of the alternative pathway of complement by *Malassezia ovalis* (*Pityrosporum ovale*), *Mycopathologia*, 70, 187, 1980.

114. Sohnle, P. G. and Collins-Lech, C., Analysis of the lymphocytic transformation response to *Pityrosporum orbiculare* in patients with tinea versicolor, *Clin. Exp. Immunol.*, 49, 559, 1982.

115. Mathes, B. M. and Douglass, M. C., Seborrheic dermatitis in patients with acquired immunodeficiency syndrome, *J. Am. Acad. Dermatol.*, 13, 947, 1985.

116. Groisser, D., Bottone, E. J., and Lebwohl, M., Association of *Pityrosporum orbiculare* (*Mallassezia furfur*) with seborrheic dermatitis in patients with acquired immunodeficiency syndrome, *J. Am. Acad. Dermatol.*, 20, 770, 1989.

117. Wishner, A. J., Teplitz, E. D., and Goodman, D. S., Pityrosporum, ketoconazole and seborrheic dermatitis, *J. Am. Acad. Dermatol.*, 17, 140, 1987.

118. Massone, L., Borghi, S., Pestarino, A., Piccini, R., Solari, G., Casini Lemmi, M., and Isola, V., Seborrheic dermatitis in otherwise healthy patients and in patients with lymphadenopathy syndrome/AIDS-related complex: treatment with 1% bifonazole cream, *Chemioterapia*, 7, 109, 1988.

119. Wishner, A. J., Teplitz, E. D., and Goodman, D. S., *Pityrosporum*, ketoconazole, and seborrheic dermatitis, *J. Am. Acad. Dermatol.*, 17, 140, 1987.

120. McGrath, J. and Murphy, G. M., The control of seborrheic dermatitis and dandruff by antipytirosporal drugs, *Drugs*, 41, 178, 1991.

121. Eisenstat, B. A. and Wormser, G. P., Seborrhoeic dermatitis and butterfly rash in AIDS, *N. Engl. J. Med.*, 311, 198, 1984.

122. Binder, R. L. and Jonclis, F. J., Seborrheic dermatitis in neurologic-induced parkinsonism, *Arch. Dermatol.*, 119, 473, 1983.

123. Bettley, F. R. and Martin, R. H., Unilateral seborrheic dermatitis following a nerve lesion, *Arch. Dermatol.*, 73, 110, 1956.

124. Butterfield, W., Sensitivities of *Pityrosporum* sp. to selected commercial shampoos, *Br. J. Dermatol.*, 116, 233, 1987.

125. Fredriksson, T., Controlled comparison of Clinitar shampoo and Selsun shampoo in the treatment of seborrheic dermatitis of the scalp, *Br. J. Clin. Pract.*, 39, 25, 1985.

126. Chandler, C. J. and Segel, I. H., Mechanism of the antimicrobial action of pyrithione: effects on membrane transport, ATP levels, and protein synthesis, *Antimicrob. Agents Chemother.*, 14, 60, 1978.

127. Marks, R., Pearse, A. D., and Walker, A. P., The effects of a shampoo containing the zinc pyrithione on the control of dandruff, *Br. J. Dermatol.*, 112, 415, 1985.
128. Boyle, J., Burton, J. L., and Faergemann, J., Use of topical lithium succcinate for seborrheic dermatitis, *Br. J. Med.*, 292, 28, 1986.
129. Cuelenaere, C., De Bersaques, J., and Kint, A., Use of topical lithium succinate in the treatment of seborrhoeic dermatitis, *Dermatology*, 184, 194, 1992.
130. Leeming, J. P., Use of topical lithium succinate in the treatment of seborrhoeic dermatitis, *Dermatology*, 187, 149, 1993.
131. Nenoff, P., Haustein, U. F., and Munzberger, C., *In vitro* activity of lithium succinate against *Malassezia furfur*, *Dermatology*, 190, 48, 1995.
132. Leeming, J. P. and Burton, J. L., Lithium succinate and seborrhoeic dermatitis: an antifungal mode of action? *Br. J. Dermatol.*, 122, 718, 1990.
133. Broberg, A. and Faergemann, J., Topical antimycotic treatment of atopic dermatitis in the head/neck area: a double-blind randomized study, *Acta Derm. Venereol.*, 75, 46, 1995.
134. Katsambas, A., Antoniou, C., Frangouli, E., Avgerinou, G., Michailidis, D., and Stratigos, J., A double-blind trial of treatment of seborrhoeic dermatitis with 2% ketoconazole cream compared with 1% hydrocortisone cream, *Br. J. Dermatol.*, 121, 353, 1989.
135. Heng, M. C. Y., Henderson, C. L., Barker, D. C., and Haberfelde, G., Correlation of *Pityrosporum ovale* density with clinical severity of seborrheic dermatitis as assessed by a simplified technique, *J. Am. Acad. Dermatol.*, 23, 82, 1990.
136. Sei, Y., Hamaguchi, T., Ninomiya, J., Nakabayashi, A., and Takiuchi, I., Seborrhoeic dermatitis: treatment with anti-mycotic agents, *J. Dermatol.*, 21, 334, 1994.
137. Faergemann, J., *In vitro* and *in vivo* activities of ketoconazole and itraconazole against *Pityrosporum ovale*, *Antimicrob. Agents Chemother.*, 26, 773, 1984.
138. Cauwenbergh, G., International experience with ketoconazole shampoo in the treatment of seborrhoeic dermatitis and dandruff, in *Seborrhoeic Dermatitis and Dandruff: a Fungal Disease*, Shuster, S. and Blatchford, N., Eds., International Congress and Symposium Series, Royal Society of Medicine Services, London, 1988, 35.
139. Ford, G. P., Farr, P. M., Ive, F. A., and Shuster, S., The response of seborrhoeic dermatitis to ketoconazole, *Br. J. Dermatol.*, 111, 603, 1984.
140. Farr, P. M. and Shuster, S., Treatment of seborrhoeic dermatitis with topical ketoconazole, *Lancet*, 2, 1271, 1984.
141. Bergsma, W. and Koster, M., Ketoconazole 2% cream in the treatment of seborrhoeic dermatitis, *2nd Int. Skin Therapy Symp.: Proc. Satellite Symp.*, Antwerp, Janssen Pharmaceutica, 1988, 49.
142. Peerbom-Wynia, J. D. R. and Koster, M., Treatment of seborrhoeic dermatitis, of the scalp and dandruff with ketoconazole 2% scalp gel, *2nd Int. Skin Therapy Symp.: Proc. Satellite Symp.*, Antwerp, Janssen Pharmaceutica, 1988, 51.
143. Guin, J. D., Double-blind comparison of 2% ketoconazole cream in the treatment of seborrhoeic dermatitis, *Clin. Res. Rep. R 41 400/139*, Janssen Pharmaceutica, 1985.
144. Rosenberg, E. W., Double-blind comparison of 2% ketoconazole cream in the treatment of seborrhoeic dermatitis, *Clin. Res. Rep. R 41 400/138*, Jenssen Pharmaceutica, 1985.
145. Whitmore, M. C., Double-blind comparison of 2% ketoconazole cream in the treatment of seborrhoeic dermatitis, *Clin. Res. Rep. R 41 400/136*, Jenssen Pharmaceutica, 1985.
146. Ive, F. A., An overview of experience with ketoconazole shampoo, *Br. J. Clin. Pract.*, 45, 279, 1991.
147. Skinner, R. B., Noah, P. W., Taylor, N. M., Zanolli, M. D., West, S., Guin, J. D., and Rosenberg, E. W., Double blind treatment of seborrheic dermatitis with 2% ketoconazole cream, *J. Am. Acad. Dermatol.*, 12, 852, 1985.
148. Green, C. A., Farr, P. M., and Shuster, S., Treatment of seborrheic dermatitis with ketoconazole. II. Response of seborrhoeic dermatitis of the face, scalp and trunk, *Br. J. Dermatol.*, 116, 217, 1987.
149. Carr, M. M., Pryce, D. M., and Ive, F. A., Treatment of seborrhoeic dermatitis with ketoconazole. I. Response of seborrhoeic dermatitis of the scalp to topical ketoconazole, *Br. J. Dermatol.*, 116, 213, 1987.
150. Hull, P. R. and Presbury, D. G. C., Ketoconazole in the treatment of seborrhoeic dermatitis: a double blind placebo controlled study, *Clin. Res. Rep. R 41 400/65*, Janssen Pharmaceutica, 1988.

151. Mertens, R., Vankeerberghen, R., and Van Lint, J., Ketoconazole 2% shampoo in the treatment of dandruff and for seborrhoeic dermatitis: a double-blind placebo controlled study, *Clin. Res. Rep. R 41 400/162*, Janssen Pharmaceutica, 1987.

152. Schrooten, P. and Cauwenbergh, G., Ketoconazole shampoo in the treatment of dandruff or seborrhoeic dermatitis: a double-blind placebo controlled study, *Clin. Res. Rep. R 41 400/157*, Janssen Pharmaceutica, 1986.

153. Thulliez, M., Cornelis, H., Schiettekatte, L., Vankeerberghen, R., Offermans, W. et al., Comparison of 4 concentrations of a ketoconazole shampoo with a placebo shampoo in dandruff and/or seborrhoeic dermatitis, *Clin. Res. Rep. R 41 400/161*, Janssen Pharmaceutica, 1987.

154. Van Derheyden, D., Cauwenbergh, G., Thulliez, M., Cornelis, H., Schiettekatte, L. et al., Ketoconazole shampoo in the treatment of dandruff and/or seborrhoeic dermatitis: a randomized double-blind placebo controlled comparison of different concentrations, *Clin. Res. Rep. R 41 400/163*, Janssen Pharmaceutica, 1987.

155. Van Cutsem, J., Van Gerven, F., Van Peer, A., Woestenborghs, R., Fransen, J. et al., Ketoconazole concentration in plasma and hair samples from volunteers after 8 weeks application of a ketoconazole 2% shampoo, *Clin. Res. Rep. R 41 400/152*, Janssen Pharmaceutica, 1986.

156. Rapelanoro, R., Mortureux, P., Couprie, B., Maleville, J., and Taieb, A., Neonatal *Malassezia furfur* pustulosis, *Arch. Dermatol.*, 132, 190, 1996.

157. Stratigos, J. D., Antoniou, C., Katsambas, A., Böhler, K., Fritsch, P., Schmölz, A., Michailidis, D., and De Beule, K., Ketoconazole 2% cream versus hydrocortisone 1% cream in the treatment of seborrheic dermatitis, *J. Am. Acad. Dermatol.*, 19, 85, 1988.

158. Ruiz-Maldonado, R., Lopez-Matinez, R., Perez-Chavarria, E. L., Rocio Castanon, I., and Tamayo, L., *Pityrosporum ovale* in infantile seborrheic dermatitis, *Pediatr. Dermatol.*, 6, 16, 1989.

159. Zienicke, H., Korting, H. C., Braun-Falco, O., Effendy, I., Hagedorn, M., Küchmeister, B., and Meisel, C., Comparative efficacy and safety of bifonazole 1% cream and the corresponding base preparation in the treatment of seborrhoeic dermatitis, *Mycoses*, 36, 325, 1993.

160. Rigopoulos, D., Katsambas, A., Antoniou, C., Theocharis, S., and Stratigos, J., Facial seborrheic dermatitis treated with fluconazole 2% shampoo, *Int. J. Dermatol.*, 33, 136, 1994.

161. Merlino, A., Malvano, L., Cervetti, O., and Forte, M., Role of *Malassezia furfur* in seborrheic dermatitis in adults and therapeutic efficacy of fenticonazole, *G. Ital. Dermatol. Venereol.*, 123, XXXVII, 1988.

162. Haustein, U. F., Seebacher, C., and Taube, K. M., Treatment of fungus infections of the skin with tioconazole (Mykontral), *Dermatol. Monatsschr.*, 175, 751, 1989.

163. Blatchford, N. R., The pharmacokinetics of ketoconazole 2% cream and shampoo, *2nd Int. Skin Therapy Symp.: Proc. Satellite Symp.*, Antwerp, Janssen Pharmaceutica, 1988, 46.

164. Stippie, P., Cauwenbergh, G., Van de Heyning-Meier, J., De Greef, H., and Borgers, M., An autoradiographic study of the penetration of a 2% ketoconazole formulation into human skin, *Adv. Ther.*, 4, 219, 1987.

165. Tucker, R. M., Denning, D. M., Hanson, L. H., Rinaldi, M. G., Graybill, J. R., Sharkey, P. K., Pappagianis, D., and Stevens, D. A., Interaction of azoles with rifampin, phenytoin, and carbamazepine: *in vitro* and clinical observations, *Clin. Infect. Dis.*, 14, 165, 1992.

166. Elion, G., Singer, S., and Hitchings, G., Antagonism of nucleic acid derivatives, *J. Biol. Chem.*, 208, 477, 1954.

167. Stevens, D. A. and Vo, P. T., Synergistic interaction of trimethoprim and sulfamethoxazole on *Paracoccidioides brasiliensis*, *Antimicrob. Agents Chemother.*, 21, 852, 1982.

168. Faergemann, J., *In vitro* and *in vivo* activities of ketoconazole and itraconazole against *Pityrosporum orbiculare*, *Antimicrob. Agents Chemother.*, 26, 773, 1984.

169. Faergemann, J., Activity of triazole derivatives against *Pityrosporum orbiculare in vitro* and *in vivo*, *Ann. NY Acad. Sci.*, 544, 348, 1988.

170. Faergemann, J., Propylene glycol in the treatment of seborrheic dermatitis of the scalp: a double-blind study, *Cutis*, 42, 69, 1988.

34 *Trichosporon beigelii*

34.1 INTRODUCTION

The genus *Trichosporon* represents a group of imperfect filamentous yeast fungi of the family Cryptococcaceae, order Monilialis, which are normal flora of the respiratory and digestive tracts of humans and animals. These basidiomycetous organisms have multilamellar cell walls and dolipores with or without parenthesomes.[1] The major species of the genus capable of causing invasive disease in humans is *T. beigelii* (formerly *T. cutaneum*).[2] Currently, however, the taxonomy of the genus *Trichosporon* is still controversial and the species *T. beigelii* has been proposed to comprise several different species.[1]

The yeasts grow rapidly on ordinary laboratory media, such as Sabouraud's dextrose agar (but is inhibited by cycloheximide) to produce cream-colored colonies that may develop radial furrows. Microscopic examination reveals the formation of rectangular or oval anthospores, blastospores, hyphae, pseudohyphae, and budding yeast cells.[2,3] Furthermore, *T. beigelii* may be identified by its abilities to assimilate glucose, galactose, sucrose, maltose, and lactose and to split arbutin.

T. beigelii (Kuchenmeister et Rabenhorst) Vuillemin is a common pathogen in humans and one of the causative agents of white piedra,[4,5] as well as of disseminated trichosporonosis in immuno-compromised hosts.[4,6-25] While its major habitat is soil, it may also be found as part of the normal flora of the human skin. Because *T. beigelii* and *Cryptococcus neoformans* share common antigens,[26] early immunodiagnosis of trichosporonosis by anticryptococcal latex-agglutination test of serum has been permitted.[27-29] However, the test may be negative in patients receiving amphotericin B.[9]

In immunocompromised patients, trichosporonosis is rapidly emerging as an opportunistic invasive fungal disease, with frequently fatal outcome (up to 64%[4]) especially in patients with hematologic malignancies.[6-9,27-29,30-50] Some non-neutropenic patients with trichosporonosis have been reported to experience mortality rates as high as 78%.[11] In addition, *Trichosporon* spp. have been diagnosed in endocarditis[10,12,15,17,18,51] and endophthalmitis[52] in immunocompetent hosts.

The most likely portals of entry for *Trichosporon* spp. are the alimentary tract and the lungs.[11] Indwelling catheters (Hickman catheters, central venous catheters, and peripheral venous cannulae), and intravenous injections can be other potential portals of entry.[9,12,14,53]

34.2 EVOLUTION OF THERAPIES AND TREATMENT OF TRICHOSPORONOSIS

As part of the normal flora of the human skin, *Trichosporon* spp. may cause benign cutaneous infections, known as white piedra, when the organisms penetrate the cells of the cuticle, forming whitish-yellow nodules on the hair follicles especially of the beard, axillary, and genital regions. Other supeficial infections due to *T. beigelii* include onychomycosis,[54] and possibly otomycosis.[55] Torssander et al.[56] have described anal colonization by *T. beigelii* in homosexual men, and white piedra of scrotal hair follicles. In the environment, *T. beigelii* has been implicated as the cause of hypersensitivity pneumonitis.[57,58]

In addition to superficial infections, *Trichosporon* spp. may cause deep and potentially life-threatening localized visceral or disseminated disease, usually in immunocompromised patients.[4]

The first noncutaneous infection by *Trichosporon* was described by Watson and Kallichurum[47] who isolated *T. beigelii* (*cutaneum*) from a brain abscess. Since then, serious systemic infections caused by *T. beigelii* have been reported to include the blood, liver, spleen, pulmonary system, CNS (meningitis),[25] endocardium (most often related to prosthetic valve surgery[15,39,52] or intravenous drug abuse[10]), kidney,[9,11,31,32,37,41,51] and the peritoneum.[9,11-14,53,59,60]

Trichosporonosis has been characterized by the presence of cutaneous lesions (discrete maculo-papular erythematous skin rash),[61] pulmonary and renal[31,32,37,48,51,62] involvement, peritonitis,[12,63-65] and chorioretinitis.[46] Disseminated trichosporonosis in granulocytopenic patients usually has a rapid onset of fever, fungemia, funguria, azotemia, pulmonary infiltrates, and cutaneous lesions with invasion of the kidney, lungs, skin, and other tissues.[66]

Immunocompromised patients, such as those with neoplastic disease (acute and chronic leukemia, multiple myeloma, solid tumors, aplastic anemia, and non-Hodgkin's lymphoma) have been at high risk to develop invasive trichosporonosis.[9,67-70] Other immunosuppressed conditions (solid organ[21,22,71] and bone marrow[24] transplantation, prosthetic valve surgery, chronic active hepatitis, intravenous drug abuse, and cataract extractions), have also been reported to be predisposing factors for trichosporonosis. Studies by Wong et al.[49] have demonstrated that trichosporonosis has been common among non-neutropenic patients with iron overload and hemochromatosis. Small clusters of infection have also been observed in low-birth-weight neonates.[72,73]

There have been three reports of trichosporonosis in HIV-positive individuals.[74-76] In two of these cases,[74,75] the patients had a bloodstream infection with *T. beigelii*. In the third case, the patient, who had chronic renal failure, developed peritonitis (with no evidence of disseminated disease) while on continuous ambulatory peritoneal dialysis (CAPD).[76]

In vitro antifungal susceptibility studies conducted by McBride et al.[77] have shown that *T. beigelii* has been consistently sensitive to miconazole, econazole, ketoconazole, clotrimazole, and amphotericin B. However, Walsh et al.[66] have demonstrated a pattern of resistance towards amphotericin B which may account for some cases of persistent trichosporon fungemia.[50] In other investigations, frequent resistance towards flucytosine has been demonstrated,[9,60,64] but some studies[32,78] have also suggested that *T. beigelii* was susceptible. In general, correlation between *in vitro* antifungal susceptibility and the clinical response is stil not clearly defined.[79] The response *in vivo* has been variable, with poor outcome reported, mainly in neutropenic patients, especially those who had failed to reestablish normal granulocyte counts.[60]

Even though amphotericin B has been widely used in the therapy of trichosporonosis,[6,9,30,63] its efficacy has not been clearly established because of the retrospective nature of most studies.[80] While successful amphotericin B therapy was achieved in most cases of patients recovering from myelo-suppression, those patients with persistent and profound neutropenia have failed to recover.[11] In granulocytopenic patients, intravenous therapy with amphotericin B may be initiated at 0.5 mg/kg daily. In cases of refractory trichosporonosis, the daily dose regimen may be increased to 1.0 mg/kg or perhaps even higher.[4] In addition to conventional amphotericin B, the therapeutic efficacies of liposomal amphotericin B and its deoxycholate have also been evaluated in experimental mouse trichosporonosis.[81] Liposome-encapsulated formulation may allow the administration of higher doses of amphotericin B with a reduced risk of nephrotoxicity.

Ujhelyi et al.[63] have successfully treated *T. beigelii* peritonitis with intravenous amphotericin B and removal of the peritoneal dialysis catheter. The initial dose of the antibiotic, 15 mg daily, was escalated over a 1-week period to 35 mg daily; 2 weeks later the dose was again escalated to 70 mg daily for a total dose of 1.0 g of amphotericin B. Flucytosine at a daily dose of 1.25 g (14 mg/kg), which was also added to the antifungal regimen was seemingly not beneficial because of drug resistance and had to be discontinued.[63] Antifungal susceptibility testing of *T. beigelii* isolated from the patients showed minimum inhibitory concentration (MIC) values of 0.08, >100,

0.07 to 0.15, and 10.0 µg/ml.[63] Other antifungal agents successfully used to treat *Trichosporon*-induced CAPD peritonitis included oral fluconazole, oral ketoconazole, and intravenous miconazole given for periods of 18 to 40 d; in some cases, however, the dialysis catheter had to be removed.[12,64,65]

Alballaa et al.[50] have described a fatal case of disseminated trichosporonosis due to *T. beigelii* in a patient with acute lymphocytic leukemia despite therapy with amphotericin B. However, the fatal outcome may have been the result of lack of recovery of bone marrow function rather than drug tolerance.[66] Amphotericin B was started at 0.5 mg/kg daily, then increased to 1.0 mg/kg daily; 5-fluorocytosine at a dose of 150 mg/kg daily was also added to the antifungal regimen. The susceptibility MIC values of a clinical isolate for amphotericin B, fluconazole, flucytosine, and miconazole were 0.78, >100, >100, and 1.56 µg/ml, respectively.[50]

Walsh et al.[66] have also reported two cases of disseminated *T. beigelii* infection with persistent fungemia which was refractory to amphotericin B; the MIC values of several clinical isolates for amphotericin B ranged from <0.14 to 1.16 µg/ml. It was postulated that inhibition alone, but not killing of resistant *T. beigelii* isolates, may be inadequate to cure trichosporonosis in granulocyto-penic patients, in whom there are no granulocytes to facilitate host clearance and in whom fungicidal activity is needed.[66]

In several reports,[44,46] 5-fluorocytosine has also been shown to be effective in the treatment of trichosporonosis.

Anaissie et al.[80] have studied the therapeutic efficacy of several azole antimycotics (fluconazole, miconazole, and SCH 39304) against trichosporonosis in patients with serious underlying disease (solid tumor and hematologic malignancies or immunosuppressive chemotherapy for liver transplantation), as well as in a murine model of disseminated disease. Fluconazole was found to be effective at the various dose regimens used (100 to 400 mg daily, or at 7.0 mg/kg, then 3.5 mg/kg). Miconazole was also found to be effective at daily doses of 1.2 g. SCH 39304 was given to a patient with acute lymphocytic leukemia who in addition to trichosporonosis also had disseminated aspergillosis; at daily doses of 200 mg given for 5 weeks, SCH 39304 eradicated trichosporonosis while evidence of aspergillosis was still present.

However, in one case of acute prosthetic valve endocarditis, fluconazole at daily doses of 400 mg failed to eradicate the fungus.[18]

A combination of intravenous miconazole (1.2 g) and oral norfloxacin (600 mg) even though effective had to be coupled with splenectomy in order to cure disseminated trichosporonosis in a patient with acute myelogenous leukemia.[23]

While ketoconazole was reported to be effective in a patient with a history of intravenous drug abuse,[14] it failed to elicit response in a case of *T. beigelii*-related aortic valve endocarditis where the patient experienced a relapse 6 months after treatment with 400 mg of ketoconazole daily.[15] In the latter case, amphotericin B (total of 250 mg) also failed to eradicate the pathogen.

Lowenthal et al.[19] have described a case of disseminated *T. beigelii* infection in a bone marrow transplant recipient who fully recovered following combination therapy comprising of amphotericin B, miconazole, and ketoconazole. Amphotericin B was administered intravenously for 6 d at a gradually increasing dose until it reached 20 mg. However, because of hepatic and renal toxicity, the patient was switched to intravenous miconazole (800 mg, t.i.d.) for 2 weeks, followed by oral ketoconazole at 200 mg daily for an additional 4 weeks on an outpatient basis.

Hajjeh and Blumberg[82] have described a case of bloodstream infection due to *T. beigelii* in a burn patient. A combination of amphotericin B (0.5 mg/kg daily; total of 1.2 g) and flucytosine (100 mg/kg daily) successfully treated the mycosis. Patients with severe thermal injuries (over 40% of total body surface area) are known to have depressed humoral and cellular immune responses. In particular, burn victims are known to have a transient defect in neutrophil function that can be a major predisposing factor to opportunistic infections.[83-85] In addition, unwarranted changes also occur in other immune functions, including increased T cell suppressor activity, decreased number and function of helper T cells, decreased IgG levels, and defects in the monocyte functions.[86]

34.3   *BLASTOSCHIZOMYCES CAPITATUS*

Trichosporon capitatum, long considered to be another pathogenic member of the genus *Trichosporon*, is now reclassified as *Blastoschizomyces capitatus*[87] (or *Geotrichum capitatum*[88]) based on photomicroscopic, cinematographic, and electron microscopic observations defining its "arthroconidia" as anneloconidia.[87] This new combination was established to accommodate two previous taxa, *Trichosporon capitatum* and *Blastoschizomyces pseudotrichosporon*[89] that were recognized to be conspecific.[87] In contrast to *T. capitatum*, *B. capitatus* consistently assimilates glucose but no other carbohydrates.

Since the deep infections caused by *T. beigelii* and *B. capitatus* appear similar both clinically and histopathologically, both will be described in this chapter for consistency with previous reports.[4]

Disseminated infections caused by *B. capitatus* have been rarely diagnosed and have involved immunocompromised patients.[90-99]

In vitro antifungal susceptibility testing has shown *B. capitatus* to be sensitive to amphotericin B, flucytosine, fluconazole, and various other azole antimycotics.[100,101]

In a case of chronic meningeal trichosporonosis in an allogeneic bone marrow recipient, oral fluconazole at 100 to 400 mg daily failed to eradicate *B. capitatus* after 11 months of treatment.[99] The patient was immunosuppressed while receiving corticosteroid and cyclosporin A chemotherapy for chronic graft-versus-host disease. A similar clinical presentation was reported in an acute leukemia patient infected with *T. beigelii*.[25]

Since eradication of *B. capitatus* in severely immunosuppressed patients has been difficult to achieve,[60] continuous suppressive antifungal therapy may be necessary, especially in CNS infections, as has been previously established for *Cryptococcus neoformans* meningitis.[102]

Recently, Sanz et al.[103] have reported three new cases of *B. capitatus* infection occurring in neutropenic patients with acute myeloblastic leukemia. All three patients were treated with amphotericin B, but only one survived after receiving a total of 1660 mg (1.3 mg/kg daily) over a 16-d period.

34.4   REFERENCES

1. Guého, E., Smith, M. T., de Hoog, G. S., Billon-Grand, G., Christen, R., and Batenburg-van der Vegte, W. H., Contributions to a revision of the genus *Trichosporon, Antonie van Leeuwenhoek*, 61, 289, 1992.
2. Kwon-Chung, K. J. and Bennett, J. E., *Medical Mycology*, Lea & Febiger, Philadelphia, 1992, 774.
3. McGinnis, M. R., *Laboratory Handbook of Medical Mycology*, Academic Press, San Diego, 1980, 399.
4. Walsh, T. J., Trichosporonosis, *Infect. Dis. Clin.*, 3, 43, 1989.
5. Kalter, D. C., Tschen, J. A., Cernoch, P. L., McBride, M. E., Speiber, J., Bruce, S., and Wolf, J. E., Jr., Genital white piedra: epidemiology, microbiology, and therapy, *J. Am. Acad. Dermatol.*, 14, 982, 1986.
6. Gardella, S., Nomdedeu, B., Bombi, J. A., Munoz, J., Puig de la Ballacasa, J., Pumarola, A., and Rozman, C., Fatal fungemia with arthritic involvement caused by *Trichosporon beigelii* in a bone marrow transplant recipient, *J. Infect. Dis.*, 151, 566, 1985.
7. Gold, J. W. M., Poston, W., Mertelsmann, R., Lange, M., Kiehn, T., Edwards, F., Bernard, E., Christiansen, K., and Armstrong, D., Systemic infection with *Trichosporon cutaneum* in a patient with acute leukemia: report of a case, *Cancer*, 48, 2163, 1981.
8. Yung, C. W., Hanauer, S. B., Freitzin, D., Rippon, J. W., Shapiro, C., and Gonzalez, M., Disseminated *Trichosporon beigelii (cutaneum)*, *Cancer*, 48, 2107, 1981.
9. Walsh, T. J., Newman, K. R., Moody, M., Wharton, R. C., and Wade, J. C., Trichosporonosis in patients with neoplastic disease, *Medicine (Baltimore)*, 65, 268, 1986.
10. Brahn, E. and Leonard, P. A., *Trichosporon cutaneum* endocarditis: a sequela of intravenous drug abuse, *Am. J. Clin. Pathol.*, 78, 792, 1982.
11. Hoy, J., Hsu, K. C., Rolston, K., Hopfer, R. L., Luna, M., and Bodey, G. P., *Trichosporon beigelii* infection: a review, *Rev. Infect. Dis.*, 8, 959, 1986.

12. Reinhart, H. H., Urbanski, D. M., Harrington, S. D., and Sobel, J. D., Prosthetic valve endocarditis caused by *Trichosporon beigelii*, *Am. J. Med.*, 84, 355, 1988.

13. Bhansali, J., Karanes, C., Palutke, W., Crane, L., Kiel, R., and Ratanatharathora, V., Successful treatment of disseminated *Trichosporon beigelii* (*cutaneum*) infection with associated splenic involvement, *Cancer*, 58, 1630, 1986.

14. Moreno, S., Buzon, L., and Sanchez-Sousa, A., *Trichosporon capitatum* fungemia and intravenous drug abuse, *Rev. Infect. Dis.*, 9, 1202, 1987.

15. Thomas, D., Mogahed, A., Leclerc, J. P., and Grosgogeat, M., Prosthetic valve endocarditis caused by *Trichosporon cutaneum*, *Int. J. Cardiol.*, 5, 83, 1984.

16. Anaissie, E., Bodey, G. P., Kantarjian, H., Ro, J., Vartivarian, S. E., Hopfer, R., Hoy, J., and Rolston, K., New spectrum of fungal infections in patients with cancer, *Rev. Infect. Dis.*, 11, 369, 1989.

17. Keay, S., Denning, D. W., and Stevens, D. A., Endocarditis due to *Trichosporon beigelii*: *in vitro* susceptibility of isolates and review, *Rev. Infect. Dis.*, 13, 383, 1991.

18. Martinez-Lacasa, J., Mana, J., Niubo, R., Rufi, G., Saez, A., and Fernandez-Nogues, F., Long-term survival of a patient with prosthetic valve endocarditis due to *Trichosporon beigelii*, *Eur. J. Clin. Microbiol.*, 10, 756, 1991.

19. Lowenthal, R. M., Atkinson, K., Challis, D. R., Tucker, R. G., and Biggs, J. C., Invasive *Trichosporon cutaneum* infection: an increasing problem in immunosuppressed patients, *Bone Marrow Transplant.*, 2, 321, 1987.

20. Martino, P., Venditti, M., Micozzi, A., Morace, G., Polonelli, L., Mantovani, M. P., Petti, M. C., Burgio, V. L., Santini, C., Serra, P., and Mandelli, F., *Blastoschizomyces capitatus*: an emerging cause of invasive fungal disease in leukemic patients, *Rev. Infect. Dis.*, 12, 570, 1990.

21. Murray-Leisure, K. A., Aber, R. C., Rowley, L. J., Applebaum, P. C., Wisman, C. B., Pennock, J. L., and Pierce, W. S., Disseminated *Trichosporon beigelii* (*cutaneum*) infection in an artificial heart recipient, *JAMA*, 256, 2995, 1986.

22. Ness, M. J., Markin, R. S., Wood, R. P., Shaw, B. W., and Woods, G. L., Disseminated *Trichosporon beigelii* infection after orthotopic liver transplantation, *Am. J. Clin. Pathol.*, 92, 119, 1989.

23. Ogata, K., Tanabe, Y., Iwakuri, K., Ito, T., Yamada, T., Dan, K., and Nomura, T., Two cases of disseminated *Trichosporon beigelii* infection treated with combination antifungal therapy, *Cancer*, 65, 2793, 1990.

24. Siegert, W., Henze, G., Wagner, J., Rodloff, A., Zimmermann, R., Malchus, R., Schwerdtfeger, R., Reichelt, A., Gräf, K., and Huhn, D., Invasive *Trichosporon cutaneum* (*beigelii*) infection in a patient with relapsed acute myeloid leukemia undergoing bone marrow transplantation, *Transplantation*, 46, 151, 1988.

25. Surmont, I., Vergauwen, B., Marcelis, L., Verbist, L., Verhoef, G., and Boogaerts, M., First report of chronic meningitis caused by *Trichosporon beigelii*, *Eur. J. Clin. Microbiol. Infect. Dis.*, 9, 226, 1990.

26. Seeliger, H. P. R. and Schroter, R., A serologic study on the antigenic relationship to the form genus *Trichosporon*, *Sabouraudia*, 2, 248, 1963.

27. Campbell, C. K., Payne, A. L., Teall, A. J., Brownell, A., and Mackenzie, D. W. R., Cryptococcal latex antigen test positive in patient with *Trichosporon beigelii*, *Lancet*, 2, 43, 1985.

28. McManus, E. J. and Jones, J. M., Detection of a *Trichosporon beigelii* antigen cross-reactive with *Cryptococcus neoformans* capsular polysaccharide in serum from a patient with disseminated *Trichosporon* infection, *J. Clin. Microbiol.*, 21, 681, 1985.

29. McManus, E. J., Bozdech, M. J., and Jones, J. M., Role of latex agglutination test for cryptococcal antigen in diagnosing disseminated infections with *Trichosporon beigelii*, *J. Infect. Dis.*, 151, 1167, 1985.

30. Reyes, C. V., Stanley, M. M., and Rippon, J. W., *Trichosporon beigelii* endocarditis as a complication of peritoneovenous shunt, *Hum. Pathol.*, 16, 857, 1985.

31. El-Ani, A. S. and Castillo, N. B., Disseminated infection with *Trichosporon beigelii*, *NY State Med. J.*, 84, 457, 1984.

32. Evans, H. L., Kletzel, M., Lawson, R. D., Frankel, L. S., and Hopfer, R. L., Systemic mycosis due to *Trichosporon cutaneum*: a report of two additional cases, *Cancer*, 45, 367, 1980.

33. Fainstein, V., Hopfer, R. L., Trier, P., and Bodey, G. P., Bone marrow cultures: their value in diagnosing fungal and mycobacterial infection in patients with cancer, *J. Infect. Dis.*, 144, 79, 1981.

34. Gordon, M. A., Systemic trichosporonosis: diagnosis by immunofluorescence, *Proc. Annu. Meet. Am. Soc. Microbiol.*, American Society for Microbiology, Washington, D.C., 1983, 396.

35. Hsu, K., Rolston, K., and Bodey, G. P., Trichosporon infection in cancer patients, *Proc. Annu. Meet. Am. Soc. Microbiol.*, American Society for Microbiology, Washington, D.C., 1985, 370.

36. Jameson, B., Carter, R. L., Watson, J. G., and Nay, R. J., An unexpected fungal infection in a patient with leukemia, *J. Clin. Pathol.*, 34, 267, 1981.

37. Kirmani, M., Tuazon, C. V., and Geelhoed, G. W., Disseminated trichosporon infection: occurrence in an immunosuppressed patient with chronic active hepatitis, *Arch. Intern. Med.*, 140, 277, 1980.

38. Libertin, C. R., Davies, N. J., Halper, J., Edson, R. S., and Roberto, G. D., Invasive disease caused by *Trichosporon beigelii*, *Mayo Clin. Proc.*, 58, 684, 1983.

39. Madharan, T., Eisses, J., and Quinn, E. L., Infections due to *Trichosporon cutaneum*, an uncommon systemic pathogen, *Henry Ford Hospital Med. J.*, 24, 27, 1976.

40. Manzella, J. P., Berman, I. J., and Jukrilea, M. L., *Trichosporon beigelli* fungemia and cutaneous dissemination, *Arch. Dermatol.*, 118, 343, 1982.

41. Rivera, R. and Cangir, A., *Trichosporon* sepsis and leukemia, *Cancer*, 36, 1106, 1975.

42. Saul, S. H., Khachatourian, T., Poorsattar, A., Myerowitz, R. L., Geyer, S. J., Pasculle, A. W., and Ho, M., Opportunistic trichosporon pneumonia: association with invasive aspergillosis, *Arch. Pathol. Lab. Med.*, 105, 456, 1981.

43. Singer, C., Kaplan, M. H., and Armstrong, D., Bacteremia and fungemia complicating neoplastic disease: a study of 364 cases, *Am. J. Med.*, 62, 731, 1977.

44. Steer, P. L., Marks, M. I., Klite, P. D., and Eickhoff, T. C., 5-Fluorocytosine: an oral antifungal compound. A report on clinical and laboratory experience, *Am. J. Med.*, 76, 15, 1971.

45. Taschdjian, C. L., Kozinn, P. J., and Toni, E. F., Opportunistic yeast infections, with special reference to candidiasis, *Ann. NY Acad. Sci.*, 174, 606, 1970.

46. Walsh, T. J., Orth, D. H., Shapiro, C. M., Levine, R. A., and Keller, J. L., Metastatic fungal chorioretinitis developing during trichosporon sepsis, *Ophthalmology*, 89, 152, 1982.

47. Watson, K. C. and Kallichurum, S., Brain abscess due to *Trichosporon cutaneum*, *J. Med. Microbiol.*, 3, 191, 1970.

48. Apaliski, S. J., Moore, M. D., Reiner, B. J., and Wald, E. R., Disseminated *Trichosporon beigelii* in an immunocompromised child, *Pediatr. Infect. Dis. J.*, 3, 451, 1984.

49. Wong, B., Bernard, E. M., Gold, J. W. M., and Armstrong, D., *Trichosporon* infection in three patients with leukemia: evidence for a permissive role for excess iron, *Proc. 22nd Intersci. Conf. Antimicrob. Agents Chemother.*, Abstr. 7, American Society for Microbiology, Washington, D.C., 1982.

50. Alballaa, S., Bryce, E. A., Roberts, F. J., and Sekhon, A., Fatal trichosporonosis is not related to tolerance to amphotericin B, *Mycoses*, 34, 317, 1991.

51. Marier, R., Zakhireh, B., Downs, J., Wynne, B., Hammond, G. L., and Andriole, V. T., *Trichosporon cutaneum* endocarditis, *Scand. J. Infect. Dis.*, 10, 255, 1978.

52. Sheikh, H. A., Mahgub, S., and Badi, K., Postoperative endophthalmitis due to *Trichosporon cutaneum*, *Br. J. Ophthalmol.*, 58, 591, 1974.

53. Finkelstein, R., Singer, P., and Lefler, E., Catheter-related fungemia caused by *Trichosporon beigelii* in nonneutropenic patients, *Am. J. Med.*, 86, 133, 1989.

54. Fusaro, R. M. and Miller, N. G., Onychomycosis caused by *Trichosporon beigelii* in the United States, *J. Am. Acad. Dermatol.*, 11, 747, 1984.

55. Reiersol, S., *Trichosporon cutaneum* isolated from a case of otomycosis, *Acta Otol. Microbiol. Scand.*, 37, 459, 1955.

56. Torssander, J., Carlsson, B., and van Krogh, G., *Trichosporon beigelii*: an increased occurrence in homosexual men, *Mykosen*, 28, 355, 1984.

57. Shimazu, K., Ando, M., Sakata, T., Yoshida, K., and Araki, S., Hypersensitivity pneumonitis induced by *Trichosporon cutaneum*, *Am. Rev. Respir. Dis.*, 130, 407, 1984.

58. Soda, K., Ando, M., Shimazu, K., Sakata, T., Yoshida, K., and Araki, S., Different classes of antibody activities to *Trichosporon cutaneum* antigen in summer-type hypersensitivity pneumonitis by enzyme-linked immunosorbent assay, *Am. Rev. Respir. Dis.*, 133, 83, 1986.

59. Korinek, J. K., Guarda, L. A., Bolivar, R., and Stroehlein, J. R., *Trichosporon* hepatitis, *Gastroenterology*, 85, 732, 1983.

60. Walling, D. M., McGraw, D. J., Merz, W. G., Karp, J. E., and Hutchins, G. M., Disseminated infection with *Trichosporon beigelii*, *Rev. Infect. Dis.*, 9, 1013, 1987.
61. Pierard, G. E., Read, D., Pierard-Franchimont, C., Lother, Y., Rurangirwa, A., and Arrese Estrada, J., Cutaneous manifestations in systemic trichosporonosis, *Clin. Exp. Dermatol.*, 17, 79, 1992.
62. Rose, H. D. and Kurup, V. P., Colonization of hospitalized patients with yeast-like organisms, *Sabouraudia*, 15, 251, 1977.
63. Ujhelyi, M. R., Raasch, R. H., van der Horst, C., and Mattern, W. D., Treatment of peritonitis due to *Curvularia* and *Trichosporon* with amphotericin B, *Rev. Infect. Dis.*, 12, 621, 1990.
64. Ahlmen, J., Edebo, L., Eriksson, C., Carlsson, L., and Torgersen, A. K., Fluconazole therapy for fungal peritonitis in continuous ambulatory peritoneal dialysis (CAPD): a case report, *Perit. Dial. Int.*, 9, 79, 1989.
65. Eisenberg, E. S., Leviton, I., and Soeiro, R., Fungal peritonitis in patients receiving peritoneal dialysis: experience with 11 patients and review of the literature, *Rev. Infect. Dis.*, 8, 309, 1986.
66. Walsh, T. J., Melcher, G. P., Rinaldi, M. G., Lecciones, J., McGough, D. A., Kelly, P., Lee, J., Callender, D., Rubin, M., and Pizzo, P. A., *Trichosporon beigelii*, an emerging pathogen resistant to amphotericin B, *J. Clin. Microbiol.*, 28, 1616, 1990.
67. Nasu, K., Akizuki, S., Yoshiyama, K., Kikuchi, H., Higuchi, Y., and Yamamoto, S., Disseminated *Trichosporon* infection: a case report and immunohistochemical study, *Arch. Pathol. Lab. Med.*, 118, 191, 1994.
68. Alegre, A., Algora, M., Penalver, M. A., Llanos, M. L., Pérez-Pons, C., Garcia Plaza, I., Lozano, M., and Padilla, B., Focal hepato-splenic mycosis caused by *Trichosporon beigelii* in a patient with acute leukemia, *Sangre*, 36, 311, 1991.
69. Yamauchi, K. and Sato, T., *Trichosporon beigelii* following busulfan-induced leucopenia, *Eur. Respir. J.*, 5, 594, 1992.
70. Fujishita, M., Kataoka, R., Kobayashi, M., and Miyoshi, I., Clinical features of 32 cases of fungal pneumonia, *Nippon Kyobu Shikkan Gakkai Zasshi*, 29, 420, 1991.
71. Mirza, S. H., Disseminated *Trichosporon beigelii* infection causing skin lesions in a renal transplant patient, *J. Infect.*, 27, 67, 1993.
72. Fisher, D. J., Christy, C., Spafford, P., Maniscalco, W. M., Hardy, D. J., and Graman, P. S., Neonatal *Trichosporon beigelii* infection: report of a cluster of cases in a neonatal intensive care unit, *Pediatr. Infect. Dis. J.*, 12, 149, 1993.
73. Giacoia, G. P., *Trichosporon beigelii*: a potential cause of sepsis in premature infants, *South. Med. J.*, 85, 1247, 1992.
74. Leaf, H. L. and Simberkoff, M. S., Invasive trichosporonosis in a patient with the acquired immuno-deficiency syndrome, *J. Infect. Dis.*, 160, 356, 1989.
75. Nahass, G. T., Rosenberg, S. P., Leonardi, C. L., and Penneys, N. S., Disseminated infection with *Trichosporon beigelii*: report of a case and review of the cutaneous and histologic manifestations, *Arch. Dermatol.*, 129, 1020, 1993.
76. Parsonnet, J., *Trichosporon beigelii* peritonitis, *South. Med. J.*, 82, 1062, 1989.
77. McBride, M. E., Kalter, D. C., and Wolf, J. E., Jr., Antifungal susceptibility testing of *Trichosporon beigelii* to imidazole compounds, *Can. J. Microbiol.*, 34, 850, 1988.
78. Hussain Qadri, S. M. H., Flournoy, D. J., Qadry, S. G. M., and Ramirez, E. G., Susceptibility of clinical isolates of yeasts to anti-fungal agents, *Mycopathologia*, 95, 183, 1986.
79. Galgiani, J. N., Antifungal susceptibility tests, *Antimicrob. Agents Chemother.*, 31, 1867, 1987.
80. Anaissie, E., Gokaslan, A., Hachem, R., Rubin, R., Griffin, G., Robinson, R., Sobel, J., and Bodey, G., Azole therapy for trichosporonosis: clinical evaluation of eight patients, experimental therapy for murine infection, and review, *Clin. Infect. Dis.*, 15, 781, 1992.
81. Anaissie, E. J., Hachem, R., Karyotakis, N. C., Gokaslan, A., Dignani, M. C., Stephens, L. C., and Tin-U, C. K., Comparative efficacies of amphotericin B, triazoles, and combination of both as experimental therapy for murine trichosporonosis, *Antimicrob. Agents Chemother.*, 38, 2541, 1994.
82. Hajjeh, R. A. and Blumberg, H. M., Bloodstream infection due to *Trichosporon beigelii* in a burn patient: case report and review of therapy, *Clin. Infect. Dis.*, 20, 913, 1995.
83. McCabe, W. P., Rebuck, J. W., Kelly, A P., Jr., and Ditmars, D. M., Jr., Leukocytic response as a monitor of immunodepression in burn patients, *Arch. Surg.*, 106, 155, 1973.

84. Alexander, J. W., Ogle, C. K., Stinnett, J. D., and Macmillan, B. G., A sequential, prospective analysis of immunologic abnormalities and infection following severe thermal injury, *Ann. Surg.*, 188, 808, 1978.

85. Yurt, R. W. and Shires, C. T., Burns, in *Principles and Practice of Infectious Diseases*, 3rd ed., Mandell, G. M., Douglas, R. G., Jr., and Bennett, J. E., Eds., Churchill Livingstone, New York, 1990, 830.

86. Shelby, J. and Merrell, S. W., *In vivo* monitoring of postburn immune response, *J. Trauma*, 27, 213, 1987.

87. Salkin, I. F., Gordon, M. A., Samsonoff, W. A., and Rieder, C. L., *Blastoschizomyces capitatus*, a new combination, *Mycotaxon*, 22, 375, 1985.

88. Guého, E., de Hoog, G. S., Smith, M. T., and Meyer, S. A., DNA relatedness, taxonomy and medical significance of *Geotrichum capitatum*, *J. Clin. Microbiol.*, 25, 1191, 1987.

89. Salkin, I. F., Gordon, M. A., Samsonoff, W. A., and Rieder, C. L., *Blastoschizomyces pseudo-trichosporon*, gen. et sp. nov., *Mycotaxon*, 14, 497, 1982.

90. Haupt, H. M., Merz, W. G., Beschorner, W. E., Vaughan, V. P., and Saral, R., Colonization and infection with *Trichosporon* species in the immunocompromised host, *J. Infect. Dis.*, 147, 199, 1983.

91. Oelz, O., Schaffner, A., Frick, P., and Schaer, G., *Trichosporon capitatum*: thrush-like oral infection, local invasion, fungemia, and metastatic abscess formation in a leukemic patient, *J. Infect.*, 6, 183, 1983.

92. Winston, D. J., Balsley, G. E., Rhodes, J., and Linné, S. R., Disseminated *Trichosporon capitatum* infection in an immunosuppressed host, *Arch. Intern. Med.*, 137, 1192, 1977.

93. Arnold, A. G., Gribbin, B., De Leval, M., Macartney, F., and Slack, M., *Trichosporon capitatum* causing recurrent fungal endocarditis, *Thorax*, 86, 478, 1981.

94. Ito, T., Ischikawa, Y., Fujii, R., Hattori, T., Konno, M., Kawakami, S., and Kosakai, M., Disseminated *Trichosporon capitatum* infection in a patient with acute leukemia, *Cancer*, 61, 585, 1988.

95. Baird, D. R., Harris, M., Menon, R., and Stoddart, R. W., Systemic infection with *Trichosporon capitatum* in two patients with acute leukaemia, *Eur. J. Clin. Microbiol. Infect. Dis.*, 4, 62, 1985.

96. Deicke, P. and Gemeinhardt, H., Embolisch-metastatische pilzenzephalitis durch *Trichosporon capitatum* nach infusions-therapie, *Dtsch. Gesundhitswesen*, 35, 673, 1980.

97. Wolff, M., Curran, Y., Bure, A., Legrand, P., Marche, C., Regnier, B., Drouhet, E., and Vachon, F., Septicemie mortelle a *Trichosporon* sp. chez 3 malades immunodeprimes, *Presse Med.*, 25, 1201, 1986.

98. Baird, D. R., Harris, M., Menon, R., and Stoddard, R. W., Systemic infection of *Trichosporon capitatum* in two patients with acute leukemia, *Eur. J. Clin. Microbiol.*, 4, 62, 1985.

99. Sicova-Mila, Z., Sufliarsky, J., and Krcméry, V., Jr., *Blastoschizomyces capitatus* fungemia in a compromised patient successfully treated with amphotericin, *J. Hosp. Infect.*, 40, 1131, 1992.

100. Girmenia, C., Micozzi, A., Venditti, M., Meloni, G., Iori, A. P., Bastianello, S., and Martino, P., Fluconazole treatment of *Blastoschizomyces capitatus* meningitis in an allogeneic bone marrow recipient, *Eur. J. Clin. Microbiol. Infect. Dis.*, 10, 752, 1991.

101. Venditti, M., Posteraro, B., Morace, G., and Martino, P., *In vitro* comparative activity of fluconazole and other antifungal agents against *Blastoschizomyces capitatus*, *J. Chemother.*, 3, 13, 1991.

102. Sugar, A. M. and Saunders, C., Oral fluconazole suppressive therapy of disseminated cryptococcosis in patients with acquired immunodeficiency syndrome, *Am. J. Med.*, 85, 481, 1988.

103. Sanz, M. A., Lopez, F., Martinez, M. L., Sanz, G. F., Martinez, Jesus, A., Martin, G., and Gobernado, M., Disseminated *Blastoschizomyces capitatus* infection in acute myeloblastic leukaemia, *Support. Care Cancer*, 4, 291, 1996.

35 *Rhodotorula* spp.

35.1 INTRODUCTION

Rhodotorula is a genus of imperfect pink-colored yeasts of the family Cryptococcaceae, subfamily Rhodotorulodae, which grows as a globose budding fungus.[1] One characteristic feature of these saprophyte organisms is the production of a coral red pigment. In addition, they do not assimilate inositol, have rudimentary or no pseudomycelia, and do not ferment conventional sugars.[2]

The genus contains eight species of which *R. rubra* (also known as *R. mucilaginosa*) is the most common one involved in human infections.[3,4] Other species of the genus that have been recovered from clinical isolates include *R. minuta* (reported also as *R. marina* and *R. pallida*), *R. aurantiaca*, *R. glutinis*, and *R. pilimanae*.[4] *Rhodotorula* spp. are common airborne fungi found in human skin, lungs, urine, and feces, particularly in patients with cancer[5,6] and other debilitating diseases. In addition, these organisms have been isolated from a number of other sources, including cheese and milk products, air, soil, and water. There have also been reports[7-9] of *R. rubra* pseudoepidemics caused by contamination of bronchoscopy equipment with the yeast.

Rhodotorula spp. have been an infrequent cause of human infections. However, with the rise of immunocompromised patients, the presence of such underlying conditions as endocarditis, diabetes, cancer (cervical, epidermoid and gastric carcinomas, acute lymphoblastic leukemia, melanoma), pulmonary disease, AIDS, and the presence of indwelling vascular access devices, may become predisposing factors for systemic disease, with mortality rates reaching 40% to 60%.[6,10-24]

35.2 EVOLUTION OF THERAPIES AND TREATMENT OF *RHODOTORULA* INFECTIONS

Although *Rhodotorula* spp. have been rarely known to cause human disease,[3,4,10,25] a number of cases where the infection was clearly opportunistic have been reported, mainly in cancer[5,6,26] and AIDS[20] patients, as peritonitis in patients undergoing continuous ambulatory peritoneal analysis (CAPD),[11,21,27-29] but also as meningitis,[30] endocarditis,[31] and ocular infections.[32-36]

Rhodotorula spp. were resistant to fluconazole,[6] miconazole,[6] and itraconazole[6,37] but susceptible to 5-fluorocytosine with minimum inhibitory concentrations (MICs) generally of less than 0.1 µg/ml. Thus, Kiehn et al.[6] have assessed nine clinical isolates of *Rhodotorula* for antifungal drug susceptibility and found MIC_{90} values of 1.6, 0.1, 0.8, 6.4, 3.2, >100, and <0.1 µg/ml for amphotericin B, amphotericin B–rifampin (10 µg/ml), ketoconazole, miconazole, itraconazole, fluconazole, and 5-fluorocytosine, respectively.

Results from reported cases of *Rhodotorula* spp. fungemia have shown the efficacy of amphotericin B to be about 40%.[15] 5-Fluorocytosine is currently the recommended choice of treatment for such conditions.[15] Thus, Naveh et al.[31] have used 5-fluorocytosine to successfully resolve a *Rhodotorula* associated endocarditis.

Donald et al.[38] have described a case of postoperative ventriculitis in an immunocompetent patient due to *R. rubra*. The patient fully responded to a therapeutic regimen consisting of oral flucytosine (2.0 g, four times daily, then reduced to 1.5 g, four times daily, because of vomiting) and intravenous amphotericin B. The latter was given first as a test dose of 1.0 mg, followed by 13.7 mg (0.3 mg/kg) on the first day, then 33 mg (0.6 mg/kg) on the second day, and increasing over the next 7 d to a maximum of 50 mg daily total dose. After 5 weeks, the intravenous therapy was discontinued and oral flucloxacillin (2.0 g, four times daily) was given with rifampicin for 5 additional weeks. The flucytosine therapy lasted for 12 weeks in total.[38]

The therapy of catheter-related *Rhodotorula* fungemia may or may not require the removal of the catheter in addition to antifungal chemotherapy. Because of the ability of host polymorpho-nuclear leukocytes to ingest and kill the pathogen,[10] in some patients, the removal of the catheter alone without antifungal chemotherapy has been sufficient to resolve the fungemia.[6] Kiehn et al.[6] have recommended that 0.7 mg/kg daily of amphotericin B be administered through all ports of the catheter for 2 weeks if the catheter is not removed and for 1 week if the catheter is removed.

Marinova et al.[15] have described a case of *Rhodotorula* spp. fungemia in an immuno-compromised pediatric patient secondary to neurosurgery. The infection was successfully treated with miconazole (600 mg daily) which was given for 6 d but then changed to intravenously administered 5-fluorocytosine (2.0 g daily for 3 weeks) because of unwarranted elevation of the liver enzyme levels.

A case of *R. minuta* central venous catheter infection with fungemia has been described in a patient with advanced AIDS, HIV nephropathy, end-stage renal disease requiring hemodialysis, and a permanent Quinton catheter in place for 6 months.[19] At the time of the fungemia, the patient was taking oral fluconazole (100 mg daily) for a previous episode of *Candida* esophagitis. The catheter-associated *Rhodotorula* fungemia was successfully treated intravenously with 455 mg total dose of amphotericin B (0.6 mg/kg daily) given over a 25-d period without the removal of the catheter.[19] In another case,[39] *R. minuta* was isolated from the blood of a pediatric patient with AIDS, CNS lymphoma, and systemic candidiasis; the patient died before antifungal therapy had started.

R. minuta systemic infection with liver abscesses and bone marrow involvement has been described in a leukemic patient who was successfully treated with 1.5 g total dose of amphotericin B and flucytosine.[40]

Guerra et al.[35] reported a case of deep keratomycosis due to *R. glutinis*. Although in this and other cases,[36] the infection was resolved by penetrating keratoplasty, these authors did not recommend it as a first procedure in the treatment of keratomycosis.[35] Rather, topical administration of pimaricin 5% or amphotericin B 0.15% would have been the more appropriate initial treatment and penetrating keratoplasty should be considered only after failure of the medical treatment.[41]

35.2.1 ANTIBIOTIC YM-47522

YM-47522 is a novel polyene amide ester antibiotic isolated from cultural broth of the *Bacillus* sp. YL-03709B.[42] *In vitro* testing of antifungal activity revealed an unusually potent activity against *R. acuta* (strain JCM1602) with MIC of 0.05 μg/ml; the corresponding values for amphotericin B and miconazole were 1.56 and 3.13 μg/ml. The activity against other *Rhodotorula* spp. (*R. aurantiaca*, *R. rubra*, and *R. bogoriensis*) was equally impressive, ranging between 0.05 and 0.1 μg/ml.[42]

35.3 REFERENCES

1. Phaff, H. J. and Ahern, D. G., *Rhodotorula* Harrison, in *The Yeasts*, 2nd ed., Lodder, J., Ed., North-Holland, Amsterdam, 1970, 1187.
2. Warren, N. G. and Shadomy, H. J., Yeasts of medical importance, in *Manual of Clinical Microbiology*, 5th ed., Balows, A., Hausler, W. J., Jr., Hermann, K. L., Isenberg, H. D., and Shadomy, H. J., Eds., American Society for Microbiology, Washington, D.C., 1991, 617.
3. Kwon-Chung, K. J. and Bennett, J. E., Infections due to *Trichosporon* and other miscellaneous yeast-like fungi, in *Medical Mycology*, Kwon-Chung, K. J. and Bennett, J. E., Eds., Lea & Febiger, Philadelphia, 1992, 768.

4. Jennings, A. E. and Bennett, J. E., The isolation of red yeast-like fungi in a diagnostic laboratory, *J. Med. Microbiol.*, 5, 391, 1972.

5. Kiehn, T. E., Edwards, F. F., and Armstrong, D., The prevalence of yeasts in clinical specimens from cancer patients, *Am. J. Clin. Pathol.*, 73, 518, 1980.

6. Kiehn, P., Gorey, E., Brown, A., Edwards, F., and Armstrong, D., Sepsis due to *Rhodotorula* related to use of indwelling central venous catheters, *Clin. Infect. Dis.*, 14, 841, 1992.

7. Hagan, M. E., Klotz, S. A., Bartholomew, W., Potter, L., and Nelson, M., A pseudoepidemic of *Rhodotorula rubra*: a marker for microbial contamination of the bronchoscope, *Infect. Control Hosp. Epidemiol.*, 16, 727, 1995.

8. Hoffmann, K. K., Weber, D. J., and Rutala, W. A., Pseudoepidemic of *Rhodotorula rubra* in patients undergoing fiberoptic bronchoscopy, *Infect. Control Hosp. Epidemiol.*, 10, 511, 1989.

9. Whitlock, W. L., Dietrich, R. A., Steimke, E. H., and Tenholder, M. F., *Rhodotorula rubra* contamination in fiberoptic bronchoscopy, *Chest*, 102, 1516, 1992.

10. Louria, D. B., Greenberg, S. M., and Molander, D. W., Fungemia caused by certain nonpathogenic strains of the family Cryptococcaceae, *N. Engl. J. Med.*, 263, 1281, 1960.

11. Benezra, D., Kiehn, T., Gold, J. W., Brown, A., Tubull, A. D. M., and Armstrong, D., Prospective study of infections in indwelling central venous catheters using quantitative blood cultures, *Am. J. Med.*, 85, 495, 1988.

12. Pinch, F. D., *Rhodotorula* septicemia, *Mayo Clin. Proc.*, 55, 258, 1980.

13. Shelburn, P. F. and Carey, J., *Rhodotorula* fungemia complicating staphylococcal endocarditis, *JAMA*, 180, 38, 1962.

14. Lauria, D. B., Blevins, A., Armstrong, G. D., Burdich, R., and Lieberman, P., Fungemia caused by "nonpathogenic" yeasts, *Arch. Intern. Med.*, 119, 247, 1967.

15. Marinova, I., Szabadosova, V., Brandeburova, O., and Krcméry, V., Jr., *Rhodotorula* spp. fungemia in an immunocompromised boy after neurosurgery successfully treated with miconazole and 5-fluorocytosine: case report and review of the literature, *Chemotherapy*, 40, 287, 1994.

16. Kiehn, T. E. and Armstrong, D., Changes in the spectrum of organisms causing bacteremia and fungemia in immunocompromised patients due to venous access devices, *Eur. J. Clin. Microbiol. Infect. Dis.*, 9, 869, 1990.

17. Anaissie, E., Bodey, G. P., Kantarjian, H., Ro, J., Vartivarian, S. E., Hopfer, R., Hoy, J., and Rolston, K., New spectrum of fungal infections in patients with cancer, *Rev. Infect. Dis.*, 11, 369, 1989.

18. Vartivarian, S. E., Anassie, E. J., and Bodey, G. P., Emerging fungal pathogens in immuno-compromising patients: classification, diagnosis, and management, *Clin. Infect. Dis.*, 17(Suppl. 2), S487, 1993.

19. Goldani, L. Z., Craven, D. E., and Sugar, A. M., Central venous catheter infection with *Rhodotorula minuta* in a patient with AIDS taking suppressive doses of fluconazole, *J. Med. Vet. Mycol.*, 33, 267, 1995.

20. Walsh, T. J., Gonzalez, C., Roilides, E., Mueller, B. U., Ali, N., Lewis, L. L., Whitcomb, T. O., Marshall, D. J., and Pizzo, P. A., Fungemia in children infected with the human immunodeficiency virus: new epidemiologic patterns, emerging pathogens, and improved outcome with antifungal therapy, *Clin. Infect. Dis.*, 20, 900, 1995.

21. Pennington, J. C. III, Hauer, K., and Miller, W., *Rhodotorula rubra* peritonitis in an HIV+ patient on CAPD, *Del. Med. J.*, 67, 184, 1995.

22. Sheu, M. J., Wang, C. C., Shi, W. J., and Chu, M. L., *Rhodotorula* septicemia: report of a case, *J. Formos. Med. Assoc.*, 93, 645, 1994.

23. Jiménez-Mejias, M. E., Ortiz Leyba, C., Jiménez Gonzalo, F. J., del Nozal, M., Campos, T., and Jiménez Jiménez, F. J., Fungemia caused by *Rhodotorula mucilaginosa* in relation to total parenteral nutrition, *Enferm. Infecc. Microbiol. Clin.*, 10, 543, 1992.

24. Samonis, G. and Bafaloukos, D., Fungal infections in cancer patients: an escalating problem, *In Vivo*, 6, 183, 1992.

25. Cogate, A., Deodhar, L., and Cogate, S., Hydrosalpinx due to *Rhodotorula glutinis*: a case report, *J. Postgrad. Med.*, 33, 34, 1987.

26. Paula, C. R., Sampaio, M. C. C., Birman, E. G., and Siqueira, A. M., Oral yeasts in patients with cancer of the mouth, before and during radiotherapy, *Mycopathologia*, 112, 119, 1990.

27. Eisenberg, E. S., Alpert, B. E., Weiss, R. A., Mittman, N., and Soeiro, R., *Rhodotorula rubra* peritonitis in patients undergoing continuous ambulatory peritoneal analysis, *Am. J. Med.*, 75, 349, 1983.

28. Johnson, R. I., Ramsey, P. G., Gallagher, P. G., and Ahmad, S., Fungal peritonitis in patients on peritoneal analysis: incidence, clinical features and prognosis, *Am. J. Nephrol.*, 5, 169, 1985.
29. Wong, V., Ross, L., Opas, L., and Lieberman, E., *Rhodotorula rubra* peritonitis in a child undergoing intermittent cycling peritoneal dialysis, *J. Infect. Dis.*, 157, 393, 1988.
30. Pore, R. S. and Chien, J., Meningitis caused by *Rhodotorula, Sabouraudia*, 14, 331, 1976.
31. Naveh, Y., Friedman, A., Merzbach, D., and Hashman, N., Endocarditis caused by *Rhodotorula* successfully treated with 5-fluorocytosine, *Br. Heart J.*, 37, 101, 1975.
32. Romano, A., Segal, E., and Ben-Tovim, T., Epithelial keratitis due to *Rhodotorula, Ophthalmologica*, 166, 353, 1973.
33. Francois, J. and Rijsselaere, M., Corneal infections by *Rhodotorula, ophthalmologica*, 178, 241, 1979.
34. Segal, E., Romano, A., Eylan, E. et al., *Rhodotorula rubra*, cause of eye infection, *Mykosen*, 18, 107, 1975.
35. Guerra, R., Cavallini, G. M., Longanesi, L., Casolari, C., Bertoli, G., Rivasi, F., and Fabio, U., *Rhodotorula glutinis* keratitis, *Int. Ophthalmol.*, 16, 187, 1992.
36. Casolari, C., Nanetti, A., Cavallini, G. M., Rivasi, F. et al., Keratomycosis with an unusual etiology (*Rhodotorula glutinis*): a case report, *Microbiologica*, 15, 83, 1992.
37. Otcenasek, M., The *in vitro* susceptibility of some mycotic agents to a new orally active triazole, itraconazole, *J. Hyg. Epidemiol. Microbiol. Immunol.*, 34, 129, 1990.
38. Donald, F. E., Sharp, J. F., Firth, J. L., Crowley, J. L., and Ispahani, P., *Rhodotorula rubra* ventriculitis, *J. Infect.*, 16, 187, 1988.
39. Leibovitz, E., Rigaud, M., Chandwani, S., Kaul, S., Greco, M. A., Pollack, H., Lawrence, R., Di John, D., Hanna, B., Krasinski, K. et al., Disseminated fungal infections in children infected with human immunodeficiency virus, *Pediatr. Infect. Dis. J.*, 10, 888, 1991.
40. Rusthoven, J. J., Feld, R., and Tuffnell, P. G., Systemic infection by *Rhodotorula* spp. in the immunocompromised host, *J. Infect.*, 8, 241, 1984.
41. Wood, T. O. and Williford, W., Treatment of keratomycosis with amphotericin B, *Am. J. Ophthalmol.*, 81, 847, 1976.
42. Shibazaki, M., Sugawara, T., Nagai, K., Shimizu, Y., Yamaguchi, H., and Suzuki, K., YM-47522, a novel antifungal antibiotic produced by *Bacillus* sp. I. Taxonomy, fermentation, isolation, and biological properties, *J. Antibiot.*, 49, 340, 1996.

36 Other Yeast-like Fungi

36.1 *HANSENULA* SPP.

36.1.1 Introduction

The genus *Hansenula* belongs to the class Ascomycetes, order Endomycetales, family Saccharomycetaceae. To date, only two species of this genus have been implicated in human disease: *H. anomala* and *H. polymorpha*.[1,4] *H. anomala*, by far the most common human pathogen of the two, is an ascosporogenous yeast that represents the perfect (sexual) stage of *Candida pelliculosa*.

H. anomala (also synonymous with *Pichia anomala*[5,6]) is a free-living organism that has been found in plants, fruit juices, soil, insects, and other organic material (as a contaminant in industrial and food fermentation), even soft drinks.[7] It is also part of the normal or transient flora of the human throat and alimentary tract.[8,9]

H. anomala grows well in a high-sugar medium.[10] On corn meal agar, *H. anomala* will produce spheroidal to elongate (2 to 4 by 2 to 6 μm) budding cells either singly, in pairs, or grouped in small clusters. After one week at 30°C, the yeast will form abundant branched pseudohyphae but not true hyphae. One very characteristic feature of *H. anomala* is the formation of one to four hat-shaped ascospores,[11] with the asci being dehiscent.[12] Furthermore, the yeast assimilates and ferments dextrose, maltose, sucrose, and galactose.[13]

The first infection caused by *H. anomala* has been described by Csillag et al.[14,15] in an infant who died from interstitial pneumonia. The yeast, which was isolated from the infant's aspirate, was later identified by Wang and Schwarz[1] as being *H. anomala*. In 1980, McGinnis et al.[4] described infected mediastinal lymph nodes due to *H. polymorpha* in a child with chronic granulomatous disease.

There have been several reports of isolation of *H. anomala* or *H. polymorpha* from blood cultures,[16] cerebrospinal fluid,[2,3,17-19] and hilar, posterior mediastinal, and paratracheal nodes,[4] and tissue.[12]

36.1.1.1 Yeast-Produced Killer Toxins and Pathogenicity

Similarly to other yeasts (e.g., *Candida glabrata*,[20] *C. albicans*,[21] *Cryptococcus neoformans*, and *Saccharomyces cerevisiae*),[20,22-33] *H. anomala* has been known for its ability to produce *in vitro*[5,34] the so-called "killer toxin," a glucoprotein factor capable of killing sensitive strains of the same species,[26] other eukaryotic organisms, and bacteria,[20,26,27] but resistant to the toxin produced by itself.[22] Furthermore, it has also been shown that *H. anomala* produced the killer toxin *in vivo* in the tissue of normal and immunosuppressed experimentally infected mice, suggesting that toxin production may be involved in the mechanism of yeast-associated infections. In addition, *Hansenula*, as is the case with *Candida*, has the ability to pass unharmed through the gastrointestinal tract of animals,[10] which under certain conditions may enable *Hansenula* to colonize the intestine and invade the mucosa as described.[12] The finding of tissue invasion by *H. anomala* should lend further support to this hypothesis.

Based on the very high frequency (over 70%[26]) of killer phenotype expression observed for *H. anomala* strains in nature, and the knowledge that toxins produced by enteric organisms can alter the secretory and absorptive intestinal processes,[35,36] Pettoello-Mantovani et al.[37] have studied the potential role of the killer toxin in the pathogenesis of *H. anomala*-induced enteritis by examining its effects on the intestinal fluid homeostasis and electrolyte balance of the proximal intestine in a rat model. The *H. anomala* toxin potentiated a significant secretion of water and electrolytes (Na^+, Cl^-, and K^+ transport), but no substantial change was observed when either heat-inactivated *H. anomala* killer toxin or control growth medium were tested. Histologic analysis showed ischemic degeneration of villi and sloughing of surface epithelium in 50% of active *H. anomala* killer toxin-perfused jejuna. The results obtained seemed compatible with the hypothesis that a killer toxin may play a role in the pathogenesis of *H. anomala*-induced enteritis.[37]

In contrast to its potential human pathogenicity, Polonelli et al.[38] have found that in experimental infections produced in guinea pigs, rabbits, and dogs, the *H. anomala* toxin may have curative effect against lesions similar to those observed in human seborrheic dermatitis and otitis externa after cutaneous application of cultures of *Malassezia furfur* and *M. pachydermatis*. The clinical recovery and the negative mycological test cultures of the infected animals were clearly associated with the topical treatment with the killer toxin.[38]

36.1.2 Evolution of Therapies and Treatment of *Hansenula* spp. Infections

Of the *Hansenula* spp. infections described so far, the majority involved fungemia[2,19,39,40] and indwelling catheters.[17,19,41-43] However, interstitial pneumonia,[15] infectious endocarditis,[3] urinary tract infection,[44] and oral mucosal infection,[45] have also been described.

The predisposing factors for infections by *Hansenula* have been similar to those for *Candida* species (humoral and cell-mediated immune deficiencies, surgery, central venous catheters, broad-spectrum antibiotic and corticosteroid therapies).[12,19,46] The administration of hyperalimentation through an infected central intravascular catheter has been a particularly important risk factor because of the propensity of *Hansenula* spp. for high-carbohydrate environments.[10,19] *H. anomala*, which is rarely described as a pathogen in humans, may be the cause of morbidity and mortality among immunocompromised and other severely ill patients, and infants.[1,2,12,14,17-19,47,48]

Eradication of *Hansenula* spp. has generally been achieved by treatment with amphotericin B at daily doses of 0.1 to 1.0 mg/kg.[39,40,42,46-49]

In a recent report, Kunova et al.[49] have described the successful use of intravenous amphotericin B (1.0 mg/kg daily; total dose, 1.725 g) in the treatment of *H. anomala* fungemia in a patient with acute myelogenous leukemia, after initial therapy with intravenous fluconazole (400 mg daily) failed to eradicate the yeast.

The aforementioned case corroborated the findings of two other studies.[46,50] Thus, Alter and Farley[46] have described a patient who developed *H. anomala* infection while receiving intravenous fluconazole therapy (6.0 mg/kg initially, followed by 4.0 mg/kg daily). Therapy with amphotericin B was initiated and maintained at a dose of 1.0 mg/kg daily (total cumulative dose, 15 mg/kg). The minimum inhibitory concentrations of a clinical isolate for amphotericin B, ketoconazole, 5-fluorocytosine, miconazole, and fluconazole were 0.8, 3.1, >100, 6.25, and 25 µg/ml, respectively, suggesting resistance of *H. anomala* to fluconazole.[46] In the other case,[50] the patient, who was immunocompetent, developed fungemia secondary to acute necrotizing pancreatitis. Daily treatment with 200 mg of fluconazole (amphotericin B was not given because of urinary excretion problems and elevated creatinine levels), failed to eradicate the yeast and the patient died.

It is thought that inhibition of the bacterial flora through the use of broad-spectrum antibiotics coupled with suppression of the more common fungal pathogens by use of fluconazole would permit natively resistant yeast species, such as *Hansenula*, to emerge as pathogens (see also *Candida krusei* in candidiasis). However, in an earlier report, Hirasaki et al.[41] reported the successful treatment of *H. anomala* fungemia in an adult cancer patient with intravenous fluconazole (200 mg daily; total dose, 3.0 g) given over 16 d, and removal of the central venous catheter. Yamada et al.[43] also reported that intravenous fluconazole (at 9.9 to 10 mg/kg daily) was efficacious in treating three cases of catheter-related *H. anomala* fungemia in children (coupled with removal of the catheter) even though in one of the cases the fungemia had developed while the patient was already receiving fluconazole. In a fourth case, however, fluconazole had failed and was replaced with miconazole (10 mg/kg daily) and flucytosine (120 mg/kg daily) which led to clinical improvement.

Murphy et al.[2] described an outbreak of infection and colonization with *H. anomala* in a neonatal intensive care unit, where 10% of all admissions were colonized with the yeast; clinical infections included fungemia and ventriculitis. Treatment, which was comprised of intravenous amphotericin B (initially at 100 µg/kg daily, later increased to 500 µg/kg daily) and flucytosine (initially given intravenously at 100 mg/kg daily and then enterally thereafter), lasted for 3 weeks. In another case, *H. anomala* fungemia in an infant with gastric and cardiac complications was treated successfully with a combination of amphotericin B (0.1 mg/kg, four times daily; total dose, 20 mg/kg) and flucytosine (100 mg daily).[40] However, Moses et al.[12] reported a case of an infant with invasive *H. anomala* disease who responded poorly to intravenous amphotericin B (1.0 mg/kg daily; total dose of 130 mg given over 31 d). The amphotericin B therapy was discontinued and oral ketoconazole was initiated at 5.0 mg/kg daily; the patient gradually defervesced and blood cultures became sterile after a 16-week therapy.[12]

Goss et al.[48] have reported the first case of *H. anomala* infection in a bone marrow transplant recipient. The patient was treated with intravenous amphotericin B (1.0 mg/kg daily; cumulative dose, 680 mg) for 24 d, followed by prophylactic oral fluconazole (400 mg daily) for one additional week during treatment with corticosteroids. In a first report of urinary tract infection due to *H. anomala*, the patient (kidney transplant recipient receiving treatment with immunosuppressive drugs) recovered spontaneously without antifungal therapy.[44]

In another case of transient *H. anomala* fungemia which resolved without treatment, the infection was associated with intravenous drug abuse in a patient with AIDS.[50] Nevertheless, a clinical isolate was susceptible to amphotericin B, 5-fluorocytosine, nystatin, ketoconazole, miconazole, and econazole with MIC values of 1.0, 0.062, 8.0, 2.0, 2.0, and 4.0 µg/ml.[51]

In one case, *H. anomala* was isolated from the oral mucosa of a patient with acute stomatitis who was successfully treated with a 2-week course of oral clotrimazole.[45]

The only clinical isolate of *H. polymorpha* tested for *in vitro* sensitivity to antifungal agents was susceptible to amphotericin B and miconazole (MIC values of 0.05 and 1.56 µg/ml, respectively), but resistant to 5-fluorocytosine (MIC >100 µg/ml).[4]

36.1.3 REFERENCES

1. Wang, C. J. K. and Schwarz, J., The etiology of interstitial pneumonia: identification as *Hansenula anomala* of a yeast isolated from lungs of infants, *Mycopathol. Mycol. Appl.*, 9, 299, 1958.
2. Murphy, N., Damijanovic, V., Hart, C. A., Buchanan, C. R., Whitaker, R., and Cooke, R. W., Infection and colonization of neonates by *Hansenula anomala*, *Lancet*, 1, 291, 1986.
3. Nohinek, B., Zee-Cheng, C. S., Barnes, W., Dall, L., and Gibbs, H. R., Infective endocarditis of a bicuspid aortic valve caused by *Hansenula anomala*, *Am. J. Med.*, 82, 165, 1987.
4. McGinnis, M. R., Walker, D. H., and Folds, J. D., *Hansenula polymorpha* infection in a child with granulomatous disease, *Arch. Pathol. Lab. Med.*, 104, 290, 1980.
5. Polonelli, L., Conti, S., Campani, L., Gerloni, M., Morace, G., and Chezzi, C., Differential toxinogenesis in the genus *Pichia* detected by an anti-yeast killer toxin monoclonal antibody, *Antonie van Leeuwenhoek*, 59, 139, 1991.
6. Yamada, Y., Maeda, K., and Mikata, K., The phylogenetic relationship of the hat-shaped ascospore-forming, nitrate-assimilating *Pichia* species, formerly classified in the genus *Hansenula* Sydow et Sydow, based on the partial sequences of 18S and 26 S ribosomal RNSs (Saccharomycetaceae), *Biosci. Biotechnol. Biochem.*, 58, 1245, 1994.

7. Sand, F. E. M. J. and van Grinsven, A. M., Comparison between the yeast flora of Middle Eastern and Western European soft drinks, *Antonie van Leeuwenhoek*, 42, 523, 1976.
8. MacKenzie, D. W. R., Yeasts from human sources, *Sabouraudia*, 1, 8, 1961.
9. Anderson, H. W., Yeast-like fungi of the human intestinal tract, *J. Infect. Dis.*, 21, 341, 1917.
10. Cook, A. H., Ed., *The Chemistry and Biology of Yeasts*, Academic Press, Orlando, FL, 1958.
11. Pavliak, V., Kogan, G., Slavikova, E., Sandula, J., and Masler, L., Immunochemical and structural analysis of the cell wall mannan as the basis of the taxonomic reidentification of a yeast strain, *J. Basic Microbiol.*, 30, 587, 1990.
12. Moses, A., Maayan, S., Shvil, Y., Dudin, A., Ariel, I., Thalji, A., and Polacheck, I., *Hansenula anomala* infections in children: from asymptomatic colonization to tissue invasion, *Pediatr. Infect. Dis. J.*, 10, 400, 1991.
13. Balows, A., Hausler, W. J., Herrmann, K. L., Isenberg, H. D., and Shadomy, H. J., Eds., *Manual of Clinical Microbiology*, 5th ed., American Society for Microbiology, Washington, D.C., 1991, 619.
14. Csillag, A., Brandstein, L., Faber, V., and Maczo, J., Adatok a koraszulottkori interstitialis pneumonia koroktanahoz, *Orv. Hetil.*, 94, 1303, 1953.
15. Csillag, A. and Brandstein, L., The role of *Blastomyces* in the aetiology of interstitial plasmocytic pneumonia of the premature infant, *Acta Microbiol. Hung.*, 2, 179, 1954.
16. Taylor, G. D., Buchanan-Chell, M., Kirkland, T., McKenzie, M., and Wiens, R., Trends and sources of nosocomial fungaemia, *Mycoses*, 37, 187, 1994.
17. Haron, E., Anaissie, E., Dumpy, F., McCredie, K., and Fainstein, V., *Hansenula anomala* fungemia, *Rev. Infect. Dis.*, 10, 1182, 1988.
18. Dickensheets, D. L., *Hansenula anomala* infection, *Rev. Infect. Dis.*, 11, 507, 1989.
19. Klein, A. S., Tortora, G. T., Malowitz, R., and Greene, W. H., *Hansenula anomala*: a new fungal pathogen: two cases and a review of the literature, *Arch. Intern. Med.*, 148, 1210, 1988.
20. Bussey, H. and Skipper, N., Membrane mediated killing of *Saccharomyces cerevisiae* by glycoproteins from *Torulopsis glabrata*, *J. Bacteriol.*, 124, 476, 1975.
21. Polonelli, L., Fanti, F., Conti, S., Campani, L. et al., Detection by immunofluorescent anti-idiotypic antibodies of yeast killer toxin cell wall receptors of *Candida albicans*, *J. Immunol. Methods*, 132, 205, 1990.
22. Gunge, N. and Sakaguchi, K., Intergenetic transfer of deoxyribonucleotic acid killer plasmids, pGK 11 and pGK 12, from *Kluyveromyces lactis* into *Saccharomyces cerevisiae* by cell fusion, *J. Bacteriol.*, 147, 155, 1981.
23. Bussey, H., Physiology of killer factor in yeast, *Adv. Microbiol. Physiol.*, 22, 93, 1981.
24. Tipper, D. J. and Bostian, K. A., Double-stranded ribonucleic acid killer systems in yeasts, *Microbiol. Rev.*, 48, 125, 1984.
25. Young, T. W., Killer yeasts, in *The Yeasts*, Vol. 2, Rose, A. H. and Harrison, J. S., Eds., Academic Press, New York, 1987, 131.
26. Rosini, G., The occurrence of killer characters in yeasts, *Can. J. Microbiol.*, 29, 1462, 1983.
27. Polonelli, L. and Morace, G., Reevaluation of the yeast killer phenomenon, *J. Clin. Microbiol.*, 24, 866, 1986.
28. Polonelli, L., Conti, S., Gerloni, M., Campani, L., Pettoello-Mantovani, M., and Morace, G., Production of yeast killer toxin in experimentally infected animals, *Mycopathologia*, 110, 169, 1990.
29. Hayman, G. T. and Bolen, P. L., Linear plasmids of *Pichia inositovora* are associated with a novel killer toxin activity, *Curr. Genet.*, 19, 389, 1991.
30. Wickner, R. B., Icho, T., Fujimura, T., and Winder, W. R., Expression of yeast L-A double-stranded RNA virus proteins produces derepressed replication: a *sky* phenocopy, *J. Virol.*, 65, 155, 1991.
31. Woods, D. R. and Bevan, E. A., Studies on the nature of the killer factor produced by *Saccharomyces cerevisiae*, *J. Gen. Microbiol.*, 81, 115, 1968.
32. Polonelli, L., Manzara, S., Conti, S., Dettori, G., Morace, G., and Chezzi, C., Serological study of yeast killer toxins by monoclonal antibodies, *Mycopathologia*, 108, 211, 1989.
33. Vadkertiova, R. and Slavikova, E., Killer activity of yeasts isolated from the water environment, *Can. J. Microbiol.*, 41, 759, 1995.
34. Polonelli, L. and Morace, G., Yeast killer toxin-like anti-idiotypic antibodies, *J. Clin. Microbiol.*, 26, 602, 1988.

35. Field, M., Rao, M. C., and Chang, E. B., Intestinal electrolyte transport and diarrheal disease. I, *N. Engl. J. Med.*, 321, 800, 1989.

36. Field, M., Rao, M. C., and Chang, E. B., Intestinal electrolyte transport and diarrheal disease. II, *N. Engl. J. Med.*, 321, 879, 1989.

37. Pettoello-Mantovani, M., Nocerino, A., Polonelli, L., Morace, G., Conti, S., Di Martino, L., De Ritis, G., Iafusco, M., and Guandalini, S., *Hansenula anomala* killer toxin induces secretion and severe acute injury in the rat intestine, *Gastroenterology*, 109, 1900, 1995.

38. Polonelli, L., Lorenzini, R., De Bernardis, F., and Morace, G., Potential therapeutic effect of yeast killer toxin, *Mycopathologia*, 96, 103, 1986.

39. Milstoc, M. and Siddiqui, N. A., Fungemia due to *Hansenula anomala*, *NY State J. Med.*, 86, 541, 1986.

40. Sekhon, A. S., Kowalewska-Grochowska, K., Garg, A. K., and Vaudry, W., *Hansenula anomala* fungemia in an infant with gastric and cardiac complications with a review of the literature, *Eur. J. Epidemiol.*, 8, 305, 1992.

41. Hirasaki, S., Ijuchi, T., Fujita, N., Araki, S., Gotoh, H., and Nakagawa, M., Fungemia caused by *Hansenula anomala*: successful treatment with fluconazole, *Intern. Med.*, 31, 622, 1992.

42. Munoz, P., Garcia Leoni, M. E., Berenguer, J., Bernaldo de Quiros, J. C., and Bouza, E., Catheter-related fungemia by *Hansenula anomala*, *Arch. Intern. Med.*, 149, 709, 1989.

43. Yamada, S., Maruoka, T., Nagai, K., Tsumura, N., Yamada, T., Sakata, Y., Tominaga, K., Motohiro, T., Kato, H., Makimura, K., and Yamaguchi, H., Catheter-related infections by *Hansenula anomala* in children, *Scand. J. Infect. Dis.*, 27, 85, 1995.

44. Qadri, S. M. H., Al Dayel, F., Strampfer, M. J., and Cunha, B. A., Urinary tract infection caused by *Hansenula anomala*, *Mycopathologia*, 104, 99, 1988.

45. Kostiala, I., Kostiala, A. A. I., Elonen, E., Valtonen, V. V., and Vuopio, P., Comparison of clotrimazole and chlorhexidine in the topical treatment of acute fungal stomatitis in patients with hematological malignancies, *Curr. Ther. Res. Clin. Exp.*, 31, 752, 1982.

46. Alter, S. J. and Farley, J., Development of *Hansenula anomala* infection in a child receiving fluconazole therapy, *Pediatr. Infect. Dis. J.*, 13, 158, 1994.

47. Lopez, F., Martin, M. L., and Paz y Sanz, M. A., Infeccion por *Hansenula anomala* en leucemia aguda, *Enferm. Infecc. Microbiol. Clin.*, 8, 363, 1990.

48. Goss, G., Grigg, A., Rathbone, P., and Slavin, M., *Hansenula anomala* infection after bone marrow transplantation, *Bone Marrow Transplant.*, 14, 995, 1994.

49. Kunova, A., Spanik, S., Kollar, T., Trupl, J., and Krcméry, V., Jr., Breakthrough fungemia due to *Hansenula anomala* in a leukemic patient successfully treated with amphotericin B, *Chemotherapy*, 42, 157, 1996.

50. Neumeister, B., Rockemann, M., and Marre, R., Fungaemia due to *Candida pelliculosa* in a case of acute pancreatitis, *Mycoses*, 35, 309, 1992.

51. Salesa, R., Burgos, A., Fernandez-Mazarrasa, C., Quindos, G., and Ponton, J., Transient fungaemia due to *Candida pelluculosa* in a patient with AIDS, *Mycoses*, 34, 327, 1991.

37 Fungi of the Order Moniliales

The order Moniliales (previously called Conidiosporales) is part of the Hyphomycetes, a class of Deuteromycota (Fungi Imperfecti) which comprises fungi with no pycnidium or acervulos. The conidia of Moniliales are usually borne directly on undifferentiated mycelia. It includes the families Cryptococcaceae, Moniliaceae, Dematiaceae, and Tuberculariaceae.

37.1 DEMATIACEAE: PHAEOHYPHOMYCOSIS AND CHROMOBLASTOMYCOSIS

37.1.1 INTRODUCTION

The dematiaceous fungal infections are caused by the so-called "black" (darkly pigmented) or dematiaceous fungi.[1,2] They are characterized by the dark pigmentation of the mycelial structure, and most of them do not have a recognized mode of sexual reproduction.[3] However, upon histopathologic or direct examination of pathologic material, in many cases only a few hyphae have been visibly pigmented and sometimes a specific melanin stain was necessary to detect the presence of the pigment.

The dematiaceous fungi are ubiquitous saprophytes in water, soil, and vegetation, and may be plant pathogens or airborne spores.

In addition to several human pathogens causing well-defined infections (sporotrichosis, onychomycosis, chromoblastomycosis, phaeohyphomycosis, fungal peritonitis), this group includes a significant number of ubiquitous environmental species, which may frequently contaminate the skin and occasionally become causative agents of opportunistic infections.

The dematiaceous fungi have become significant because of their broad spectrum of clinical features ranging in severity from superficial and mild to deep-seated, serious, and occasional fatal outcome. In general, these infections are best characterized by a concept based upon the combined clinical, pathologic, and mycologic relationships exhibited in these diseases. Another reason for their importance lies in the confusion surrounding the clinical nomenclature of diseases they represent, as well as the taxonomy of the various fungi classified as dematiaceous that show considerable pleomorphism both *in vitro* and *in vivo*.[4,5]

Currently, it is generally accepted that dematiaceous fungi produce three kinds of disease: phaeohyphomycosis, chromoblastomycosis, and mycetoma.

Over the years, terms such as chromomycosis, chromoblastomycosis, and phaeohyphomycosis have been applied to a variety of mycoses having distinctly different clinical, pathologic, and mycologic characteristics, thereby bringing misunderstanding, confusion, and lack of clarity and consistency in the terminology and conceptual basis for the entities known as chromoblastomycosis and phaeohyphomycosis.[6]

The term "chromoblastomycosis" was introduced by Terra et al.[7] in 1922 to discern a unique cutaneous fungal infection found in Brazil from the confusing clinical entity known as "dermatitis verrucosa". In 1935, Moore and de Almeida[8] proposed a new term "chromomycosis" as a replacement for the name "chromoblastomycosis" since they reasoned that the latter name has been misleading by implying that the etiologic agents grew as yeast in tissues. In the subsequent years, however, the term "chromomycosis" was inappropriately expanded from the original concept to include other mycoses caused by several different genera and species of dematiaceous fungi. To correct this problem and preserve the concept examplified by the term "chromoblastomycosis" as originally conceived, Ajello et al.[9] coined a companion name "phaeohyphomycosis" to describe all mycotic infections caused by "black" fungi which are clinically, pathologically, and mycologically distinct from classic chromoblastomycosis and black grain mycetomata.

The fundamental difference between chromoblastomycosis and phaeohyphomycosis lies in the tissue form represented by their respective etiological agents. That is, in chromoblastomycosis, the fungi are characterized as large, muriform, thick-walled dematiaceous cells produced by fungus detained between a yeast-like and hyphal form.[5] In phaeohyphomycosis, the fungi exist as dark-walled ("black"), septate hyphal elements, pseudohyphae, or as solitary cells that divide either by budding, by septation in only one plane, or in various combinations of these.

According to current understanding, clinical chromoblastomycosis encompasses chronic, localized infections of the cutaneous and subcutaneous tissues that contain sclerotic bodies and histologically demonstrate hyperkeratotic pseudoepitheliomatous hyperplasia with keratolytic microabscess formation in the epidermis.[6] In contrast, phaeohyphomycosis is a broader term describing a heterogeneous group of superficial, cutaneous and corneal, subcutaneous, and systemic mycoses that contain dematiaceous yeast-like cells, pseudohyphae-like elements, hyphae that may be short or elongated, regular, distorted to swollen in shape, or any combination of these forms in tissue.[6] The term "chromomycosis" has been rejected for mycoses caused by dematiaceous fungi.

37.1.1.1 *Bipolaris* spp., *Exserohilum* spp., and *Drechslera* spp.

In 1936, a fungus identified as a *Helminthosporium* sp. was diagnosed as the causative agent of granulomatous nasal infections in cattle.[10] Following this first case, a number of fungi classified as either *Helminthosporium* or *Drechslera* spp. were associated with numerous infections in both animals and humans.[11] The major reason for the ensuing confusion was the indiscriminate lumping together (in the interest of biosystematics) of various and seemingly unrelated species under the name *Helminthosporium*. In the following years, a number of investigators[12-17] have resolved the confusion by segregating the genera *Bipolaris*, *Drechslera*, and *Exserohilum* from the genus *Helminthosporium*.

The major mycological characteristics used to distinguish these species from each other include the conidial shape, septation, and size, hilar characteristics, the origin of the germ tube from the basal cell and, to a lesser extent, other conidial cells, and the sequence and location of the conidial septa.[1]

Thus, *Helminthosporium* species produce conidiophores characterized with parallel walls that bear their conidia in a pleurogenous manner; that is, the conidia is formed along the sides of the conidiophores. Since the latter will not continue to increase in length after a conidium is formed at its apex, the conidiophores of *Helminthosporium* spp. are considered determinate.[1] This feature of *Helminthosporium* sp. is the major difference from the genera *Bipolaris*, *Drechslera*, and *Exserohilum*.

In contrast to *Helminthosporium* spp., organisms of the genera *Bipolaris*, *Drechslera*, and *Exserohilum* produce conidiophores that grow in a sympodial manner and are characterized by continuing increase in length by forming a new growing point just below each new terminal conidium. Therefore, the conidiophores of these three genera are considered indeterminate in development.[1] Differentiation between them is based upon a combination of features that include morphological differences of conidia (shape, size, color, and number of septa),[17-20] the presence or absence of a protruding hilum (the scar at the base of the conidium which shows where it was attached to its conidiophore; in *Bipolaris*, *Drechslera*, and *Exserohilum*, the hilum is recognized through differences from the rest of the conidium in morphology, color, or combination of both), the contour of the basal portion of the conidium and its hilum, the point at which the germ tube originates from the basal cell and, to a lesser extent, the other cells of the conidium that produce germ tubes, and the sequence and location of the first three conidial septa.[1]

Although germination of conidia is an important feature in distinguishing the three genera, it is variable and must be considered in conjunction with other characteristics.[1] The *Bipolaris* spp. have fusoid, egg-shaped conidia germinating only from end cells. The *Drechslera* spp. have cylindric conidia germinating from all cells. The *Exserohilum* spp. have conidia with protuberant hila.[17]

Major species of the genus *Bipolaris* include *B. australiensis*, *B. hawaiiensis*, *B. maydis*, *B. melinidis*, and *B. spicifera* (often reported as *Drechslera spicifera*). Those of the genus *Drechslera* include *D. avenae*, and *D. dictyoides*. Among the species of genus *Exserohilum* are *E. longirostratum*, *E. holmii*, *E. mcginnisii*, *E. pedicellatum*, and *E. rostratum*. According to Leonard,[21] *E. halodes* and *E. rostratum* are synonymous.

The conidia produced by *Bipolaris* and *Exserohilum* species pathogenic to humans and animals are somewhat smaller than those produced by isolates from environmental and plant sources. It appears that only *B. australiensis*, *B. hawaiiensis*, *B. spicifera* (*D. spicifera*), *E. longirostratum*, *E. mcginnisii*, and *E. rostratum* have been confirmed as causative agents of phaeohyphomycosis.[1,22] No isolate of *Helminthosporium* (*sensu stricto*) has been convincingly documented to be an etiologic agent of phaeohyphomycosis in either humans or animals.[1] In addition, human infections reported to be caused by *Drechslera* species also represent instances in which the etiologic agents were either misidentified or classified according to an obsolete taxonomy.[1,22]

37.1.1.2 *Wangiella dermatitidis* and *Exophiala* spp.

W. dermatitidis is a dematiaceous yeast (synanamorph) fungus that is an important etiological agent of both cutaneous and subcutaneous, and visceral or systemic phaeohyphomycosis.[5,23] It was originally isolated by Kano[24] from human skin under the name *Hormiscium dermatitidis*. In subsequent studies, this organism was classified to several other taxonomically diverse genera, as *Fonsecaea*, *Hormodendrum*, and *Phialophora*.[5,25] Based on the ability of the Kano's species to develop phialidic conidiogenous cells that lacked distinct collarettes, McGinnis[26,27] accommodated *H. dermatitidis* Kano into a new nomenclatural neotype, *Wangiella dermatitidis*. However, de Hoog[28] disagreed with this classification and placed the fungus in the genus *Exophiala* Carmichael. Both McGinnis[26] and de Hoog[29,30] observed the pleomorphic nature of conidiogenesis of the Kano's isolate. It seems, however, that the Kano's organism is closer to *Wangiella* than *Exophiala* since both de Hoog and others[31] failed to study the neotype for this taxon. It is important to emphasize that existing nomenclatural types should be studied prior to reaching taxonomic decisions because they represent the permanently preserved element to which the name of the fungus is attached.[5,32]

37.1.1.3 *Alternaria* spp.

Alternaria is a genus of dematiaceous fungi found most commonly as soil saprophytes and plant pathogens. Some of the species have been etiologic agents of human phaeohyphomycosis, including *A. alternata*, *A. chartarum*, *A. chlamidospora*, *A. dianthicola*, *A. infectoria*, *A. stemphyloides*, and *A. tenuissima*, with *A. alternata* (Fr.) Keissler and *A. tenuissima* (Kunze ex Pers.) being the most pathogenic.[33] However, infections caused by *A. dianthicola* Neergaard[34] and *A. chlamydospora* Mouchacca[35] have also been reported.

Although *A. longipes* (Ellis & Evert.) Mason has been isolated from various regions of the world, it has been known mainly as the cause of brown spot lesions in tobacco.[36] Recently, it has been implicated as the agent of cutaneous phaeohyphomycosis in humans.[37] *A. longipes* is distinguished by its rather small conidia with smooth or slightly verruculose walls and a pale brown beak which rarely extends into secondary conidiophore. Morphologically, *A. longipes* is closely related to *A. infectans*, which differs by having conidia in strongly branched chains. The *A. infectans* conidia usually have only transverse septa and a very short apical beak which extends into a geniculate secondary conidiophore.[37]

37.1.1.4   *Curvularia* spp.

Curvularia spp. are saprobic dematiaceous molds that reside primarily in soil. Of the 40 species of the genus *Curvularia*, 7 have been reported to cause human infections: *C. brachyspora*,[38,39] *C. clavata*, *C. geniculata*,[40] *C. lunata*,[41] *C. lunata* var. *aeria*,[42] *C. pallescens*,[43,44] *C. senegalenses*,[45] and *C. verruculosa*.[46] *Curvularia* spp. produce rapidly growing brown to dark black-colored colonies, with branched, septate brown hyphae (2 to 5 μm thick). The conidiophores are darkly pigmented, usually solitary, may be branched or not, and are geniculate (zig-zag shaped). The multicelled conidia are further characterized by the presence of a typical "curved" appearance to a dark, larger central cell as contrasted with end cells.[47]

   Curvularia spp. are differentiated from other dematiaceous Hyphomycetes (e.g., *Bipolaris*) by their curved conidia and narrow septa.[1,48]

37.1.1.5   *Phialophora* spp.

Phialophora spp. represent a genus of dematiaceous fungi that contain eight species known as opportunistic pathogens in humans and animals.[29] Among the human pathogens, *P. bubakii*, *P. parasitica*, *P. repens*, *P. richardsiae*, and *P. verrucosa* have been reported to cause phaeohyphomycosis, endocarditis, keratitis, and onychomycosis.[9,49,50]

   Confusion also dominates the terminology of the *Phialophora* genus, since it too had another earlier generic name, *Fonsecaea*. The name *Phialophora* was adopted after Emmons et al.[51] showed that these species commonly produce spore-bearing structures called phialophores. *E. spinifera* was described in 1968 by Nielsen and Conant[52] as *Phialophora spinifera*. It was reclassified by McGinnis[53] into the genus *Exophiala* due to its ability to produce annelides on spine-like conidiophores. Although the fungus can also produce phialides with collarettes, they are unstable, thereby precluding the fungus to be classified in the genus *Phialophora* as originally proposed.

   P. richardsiae has been the cause of blueing of wood pulp.[54,55] It has also been isolated from a vessel surface at a noodle factory during a sanitation test,[56] as well as from food.[57] Although more commonly found in tropical and subtropical regions, *Phialophora* spp. are distributed worldwide and have been isolated on such diverse vegetable matter as plant debris, wood in saunas, and wasp nests.[58]

   The frequency of infections with *Phialophora* spp. is expected to rise with the increasing population of immunosuppressed patients.[59]

37.1.1.6   *Xylohypha bantiana*

The morphological characteristics of *Xylohypha bantiana* (previously designated as *Cladosporium trichoides* or *C. bantianum*) include darkly pigmented, branched septate hyphae in unstained tissue or routine H&E stain. At 37°C, *X. bantiana* produces brown to black velvety colonies within 7 d.[60] Unambiguous identification of this fungus has been based on culture and characteristic microscopic features.[60,61]

   X. bantiana has a wide geographical distribution in nature. Its conidia have been isolated from decaying vegetation, plants, and soil.[62,63] It appears that the infection is acquired through inhalation. Dixon et al.[64] have found that intranasal challenge by *X. bantiana* produced infection in cortisone-treated mice.

37.1.1.7 *Ochroconis (Dactylaria)* spp.

Ochroconis (Dactylaria) spp. are thermotolerant, dematiaceous fungi that are usually found in nature at ambient temperatures reaching 40 to 60°C.[65-71] They have been isolated from hot spring water, thermal soil, self-heated coal-waste piles,[72] coil spoil tips,[73] effluents from nuclear reactors,[74,75] and broiler house litter.[76] The geographic distribution of *Ochroconis* is widespread, with reports of its isolation from Europe,[70] the U.S.,[69-71,77-84] Japan,[82] Africa,[78] and Australia.[70]

Ochroconis (Dactylaria) spp. possess some unique features, such as the ability to trap nematodes[66] and amoebae[65] with an unusual "trapping ring". Other characteristic properties of these dematiaceous fungi include the production of several metabolites: dactariol,[85] dactalarin (an agent with antiprotozoal activity),[85] dactylfungins,[86] and a novel angiogenesis inhibitor.[87]

There appears to be a great deal of confusion about the taxonomy of these species. For example, over the years *Ochroconis gallopava* has been classified as *Dactylaria constricta* var. *gallopava*, *Ochroconis constricta*,[77,78,82] *Ochroconis gallopavum*,[77,78,82] *Ochroconis tshawytschae*,[78,82] *Scolecobasidium constrictum*,[71,78,82] *Scolecobasidium humicola*,[80,82] *Diplorhinotrichum gallopavum*,[80,82] *Heterosporium terrestre*,[88] and possibly *Scolecobasidium tshawytschae*.[82]

Originally, the fungus was classified as *Diplorhinotrichum gallopavum* by Georg et al.[80] Later, Bhatt and Kendrick[65] after examination proposed a new name, *Dactylarya gallopava*. In 1973, de Hoog and von Arx[89] assigned a new genus *Ochroconis* for most species formerly classified under the genus *Scolecobasidium* that produced one- to four-celled, pale olivaceous-brown, smooth or rough-walled, ellipsoidal, cylindrical, clavate to cuniform conidia; among these species, three of them (*O. gallopavum*, *O. humicola*, and *O. tschawytschae*) were pathogenic to both animals and humans.[29] However, because of the morphologic similarity of two-celled conidia produced by *O. gallopavum* and *Scolecobasidium constrictum*, these two species were reduced to varietal status under the names *Dactylaria constricta* var. *gallopava* and *Dactylaria constricta* var. *constricta*.[90,91] Since according to the International Commisssion on the Taxonomy of Fungi (ICTF),[92] the mode of secession of conidia in *Dactylaria* is schizolytic, and in *Ochroconis* the conidial secession is rhexolytic,[29,93] there may be justification for separating these two genera.[78]

37.1.1.8 *Hormonema dematioides* and *Aureobasidium pullulans*

Hormonema dematioides was first described in 1927 by Lagerberg et al.[94] It is a dematiaceous mold found throughout the world. The organism grows rapidly on Sabouraud dextrose agar at optimal temperature of 24°C to produce smooth black colonies in 1 to 2 weeks.[95] Furthermore, the fungus forms a light, slimy mass as a result of conidation. Its hyphae are initially colorless but soon turn to brown, becoming larger in width than in length, with longitudinal septa.

H. dematioides has been extremely hard to identify in tissue.[95] They are small and highly pleomorphic, yeast-like organisms that may or may not be pigmented in tissue. Since the lack of melanin in the yeast-like cells would lead to a negative Fontana-Masson staining (melanin-specific stain), this can make the task of their positive identification very difficult.

On a number of occasions *Hormonema* species have been confused mycologically with another dematiaceous fungi, *Aureobasidium* spp.[96,97] (especially *A. pullulans*[98]). However, they can still be differentiated because *Hormonema* spp. will form their conidia in basipetal succession from hyaline or dark hyphae in contrast to synchronously formed conidia in *Aureobasidium* spp.[96] The latter genus is also known to be pathogenic to humans.[3,98-105]

Hermanides-Nijhof[96] has classified the genus *Aureobasidium* based on the size and shape of conidia. The colonial morphology has been less important in their identification.

Aureobasidium pullulans (previously known as *Pullularia* and *Dematium*) is a saprobial conidial fungus which grows best at room temperature on nutrient or Sabouraud's agar, producing cream-colored, yeast-like mucoid colonies in 24 to 48 h. It is widely distributed in nature, predominantly in moist environments, and is unexacting in its nutritional requirements.[106,107]

37.1.1.9 *Cladosporium* spp.

Cladosporium spp. are among the most prevalent airborne fungal spores in temperate zones of the world.[108] Six species of the genus *Cladosporium* have been known to be pathogenic to humans: *C. carrionii*, *C. cladosporidiosis*, *C. devriesii*, *C. elatum*, *C. oxysporum*, and *C. sphaerospermum*.[109] In addition, two *Cladosporium* spp. seem to be major sources of allergenicity: *C. herbarum* and *C. cladosporioides*.[110]

37.1.1.10 Melanin Biosynthesis and Virulence of Phaeoid Pathogenic Fungi

The dark pigments of the vegetative mycellium of dematiaceous fungi are often called melanins regardless of their mode of biosynthesis or chemical structure.[5] Although their biosynthesis is usually facilitated by phenoloxidase enzymes, in *W. dermatitidis* it occurs in the pentaketide pathway within the fungal cell walls as evidenced by the isolation of 1,8-dihydroxynaphthalene (DHN), the immediate precursor of DHN-melanin.[111,112] Using the same tricyclazole-blocking approach and chemical analysis of intermediates, Taylor et al.[113] extended the concept of pentaketide DHN-melanin biosynthesis among human phaeoid pathogenic fungi to three other agents of phaeohyphomycosis, four agents of chromoblastomycosis, and one agent of pityriasis nigra.

Dixon et al.[114] and Geis and Szaniszlo[115] have studied the role that DHN-melanin might play in the survival of dematiaceous fungi in nature or during infections leading to phaeohyphomycosis. The data obtained suggested that in nature, DHN-melanin at the very least served to protect the fungus against the mutagenic effects of UV-irradiation, or the lytic effects of enzymes produced by competing environmental species. The presence of carotenoid pigments in the cell walls of these pathogens may also play a role in photoprotection from damage by UV irradiation.

The DHN-melanin biosynthesis is thought to be involved in the pathogenesis of a number of phytopathogenic fungi.[114] It may also be a factor in the pathogenesis of *W. dermatitidis*. Thus, Szaniszlo et al.[116] have found that the parasitic form of *W. dermatitidis* contained fivefold more melanin in its cell wall than the saprophytic form. In further studies, Geis et al.[111] and Dixon et al.[117,118] have compared the pathogenicity and virulence of wild-type and melanin-deficient (*mel3*) *W. dermatitidis* strains, and found a significant decrease in the virulence of the melanin-deficient mutants. Thus, in a mouse model, an inoculum of 3×10^7 cells/mouse of the melanized parental strain of *mel3* caused 100% mortality within 3 d, whereas *mel3* itself was essentially nonlethal for 3 weeks at the same inoculation concentration.[117] Additional support for the concept that DHN-melanin has been associated with the virulence of *W. dermatitidis* has been demonstrated by the finding that no essential difference existed between the mortality rates caused by the melanized wild-type strain and a temperature-sensitive morphological (*cdc*) mutant derived from it, even though both strains were markedly less virulent when nonmelanized.[119]

However, there has been no apparent correlation between the presence of melanin and *in vitro* antifungal susceptibility. In addition, there has been no evidence to support the hypothesis that if melanin is responsible for the drug resistance of dematiaceous fungi, than melanin-deficient strains should be more susceptible to antifungal agents than the melanin-rich wild-type strains.[120]

Although still at an early stage of research,[4,121,122] these findings may open the possibility for some melanin synthesis inhibitors, such as tricyclazole, to be used as therapeutic agents against *Wangiella* infections.[112] Thus, Polak and Dixon[123] have shown that when the wild strain of *W. dermatitidis* was considerably demelanized by treatment with tricyclazole prior to inoculation into mice, it was less virulent than its nontreated melanized controls. By comparison, when the melanin-deficient *mel3* strain was melanized by feeding with the DHN-melanin precursor scytalone, it was more virulent than its untreated control.

In cases of little or no hyphal pigmentation, melanin may be demonstrated by specific stains, such as the Fontana-Mason silver stain.[124]

37.1.2 PHAEOHYPHOMYCOSIS

In its broadest definition, phaeohyphomycosis encompasses a wide group of opportunistic infections variously referred to by different investigators as systemic chromoblastomycosis, subcutaneous chromoblastomycosis, cerebral chromoblastomycosis, hypodermomycosis, encephalomycosis, cystic chromomycosis, phaeomycotic cyst, keratochromomycosis, subcutaneous chromomycosis, cladosporiosis, cladosporoma, subcutaneous cystic granuloma, sporotrichosis (in part), phaeosporotrichose, cerebral dematiomycosis, cerebral chromycosis, and chromohyphomycosis — a confusing array of diseases[125] that underscores the important need for a consistent, unifying, and unambiguous terminology.[6]

Fungi of the genera *Bipolaris* and *Exserohilum* have been closely associated as etiologic agents of human phaeohyphomycosis.[1,6,22]

Other common etiologic agents of phaeohyphomycosis appear to be *Exophiala jeanselmei* and *Wangiella dermatitidis*.[5,24,126-159] Both species have been recovered from plant materials, wood, and soil. Fungi known to cause cerebral phaeohyphomycosis include *Xylohypha bantiana* (synonymous with *Cladosporium bantianum* and *C. trichoides*), *Phialophora pedrosoi*, and *W. dermatitidis*.[160,161]

Both normal and immunocompromised hosts (renal transplant recipients, patients with malignancies, and diabetes) can become infected, and often the clinical disease that follows is characterized by invasive fungal growth. The management of such patients can present formidable therapeutic problems, especially in immunocompromised hosts.[22,154] There were relatively very few cases of phaeohyphomycosis afflicting HIV-positive patients, mostly *Alternaria alternata* and *Exophiala jeanselmei*. Since HIV-induced immune deficiency affects predominantly the T cell population, the predominant mycoses in AIDS are those normally controlled by T lymphocytes. Primarily, granulocytes are involved in the control of fungi of hyalo- and phaeohyphomycosis and zigomycosis. Since those cell populations remain relatively intact, infections by these fungi have been rare and cannot be expected to rise significantly in variety and frequency in HIV-positive patients.[109]

In immunocompromised patients, the disease can disseminate through hematogenous spread with extensive vascular invasion and necrosis.[22] Other reported cases of disseminated disease include dysmyelopoietic syndrome and neutropenia concurrent with multiple skin nodules (acute vasculitis),[1,22,162] and aortic insufficiency due to *E. rostratum* vegetation.[163] An immunocompetent child has been diagnosed with *B. spicifera*-associated osteomyelitis of the femur and multiple brain abscesses.[164]

37.1.2.1 Evolution of Therapies and Treatment of Phaeohyphomycosis

Treatment of phaeohyphomycosis, which is usually carried out by surgery and antifungal chemotherapy, has been dificult and on many occasions frustrating. The outcome of treatment of phaeohyphomycosis may be influenced often by the immunocompetence of the host, the site of infection, and the extent of involvement.[22,109,165-168]

In general, therapy with amphotericin B has been disappointing because of the high rates of failure and frequent relapses.[22,166,169] The therapeutic efficacy of ketoconazole and miconazole has been equally ineffective. However, the efficacy of itraconazole was more encouraging.[154,165,169-172] Sharkey et al.[154] have recommended daily dosages ranging from 50 to 600 mg; daily doses greater than 200 mg have been given twice daily.

37.1.2.1.1 Bipolaris- and Exserohilum-associated infections
The last two decades have seen a dramatic increase in the frequency of phaeohyphomycosis caused by members of the genera *Bipolaris* Shoemaker and *Exserohilum* Leonard et Suggs.[1,11,22,94,164,173-182] In both immunocompetent and immunocompromised patients, infections associated with *B. australiensis*,[94] *B. hawaiiensis*,[174,176,179,181] *B. spicifera*,[11,22,164] *E. rostratum*,[173] *E. longirostratum*,[180]

and *E. mcginnisii*[182] have been recognized as causing sinusitis, pansinusitis, endocarditis, cutaneous infections, and osteomyelitis. The first fatal human infection of meningoencephalitis related to *B. hawaiiensis* was reported by Fueste et al.[176] in 1973. In addition, *B. hawaiiensis* has been implicated as the cause of nasal obstruction and bone destruction,[179] pulmonary infection,[181] sinusitis,[1] and granulomatous encephalitis.[179]

Bipolaris species, particularly *B. spicifica* and *B. hawaiiensis* are associated most frequently with infections of the lower and upper respiratory tract, specifically the paranasal sinuses.[22,164,183,184] While *Bipolaris*-induced sinusitis in immunocompetent hosts may be an insidiously progressive infection that may take months or even years to evolve, in immunocompromised patients the disease may be more rapidly invasive. On the other hand, *Bipolaris* spp. seldom cause cutaneous ulcers in immunocompromised hosts.[185-187] These molds have also been implicated as the cause of granulomatous encephalitis in immunocompetent hosts.[179] The fungi may also extend into the contiguous orbit with potential loss of vision.[165,183,188,189]

Therapy of *Bipolaris* infections depends upon the host and location of the infection.[109] In general, amphotericin B with or without 5-fluorocytosine is used in treatment of severely immunocompromised patients with sinusitis, pneumonia, or fungemia. Koshi et al.[175] have applied local excision of the crusted lesion followed by local application of 0.03% nystatin solution (four times daily in 2-ml aliquots) for 3 weeks to cure nasal phaeohyphomycosis caused by *B. hawaiiensis* in an immunocompromised patient.

Itraconazole has been used increasingly for treatment of *Bipolaris* infections in immunocompetent hosts as well as in immunocompromised patients with refractory infections.[154] Where feasible, surgical resection of lesions should be performed.[1,190]

In the experience of Burges et al.,[191] surgical debridement of an accessible focus of infection along with oral therapy with ketoconazole may provide adequate therapy of subcutaneous phaeohyphomycosis caused by *E. rostratum* in an immunocompetent patient.

In cases of disseminated phaeohyphomycosis, complete surgical debridement appeared to be important in the treatment of locally invasive disease.[22] In addition, amphotericin B may prove useful in these patients as seen in a patient with disseminated *B. spicifera* skin lesions who responded promptly to the antibiotic given at 50 mg per dose, 3 times weekly, for a total of 750 mg.[22] However, in another case of an immunosuppressed cardiac allograft recipient, *B. spicifica* involvement of the lung, pericardium, and the heart failed to respond to combination of amphotericin B and ketoconazole (800 mg daily).[22]

In a case of localized *E. rostratum* (reported as *D. rostrata*) osteomyelitis, the patient responded after multiple relapses over a 5-year period to surgical debridement and intravenous amphotericin B.[173] The ability of *Bipolaris* and *Exserohilum* spp. to penetrate the bone was demonstrated by this case, as well as in cases of bone invasion with disseminated disease[164] and sinusitis.[11,22,174]

In *Bipolaris*-induced meningoencephalitis, the onset of symptoms has been acute or subacute with polymorphonuclear or mononuclear pleocytosis of the cerebrospinal fluid.[22,161] It is believed that CNS involvement may result from fungal invasion through infected sinuses.[192] In one such case, a breast cancer patient with meningeal carcinomatosis and *Bipolaris* meningoencephalitis died after failing to respond to intravenous chloramphenicol following tentative diagnosis of bacterial meningitis.[22] In two other cases of *Bipolaris*-induced CNS infections,[176,193] one patient died without antifungal therapy and severe granulomatous and suppurative leptomeningitis with vasculitis.[176] In the second case,[193] the patient who showed granulomatous fungal encephalitis responded to combined therapy consisting of 5-fluorocytosine and amphotericin B (a total of 2.0 g). Albeit cured, the patient was left with neurologic sequalae (residual seizure disorder and personality change).[193] It should be noted, however, that in spite of its excellent CNS penetration, the therapeutic value of 5-fluorocytosine is uncertain because of the observed *in vitro* resistance by *Bipolaris* species.[194]

Although pathologic evidence of bone invasion in *Bipolaris/Exserohilum* sinusitis may not be always present, there has been frequent radiographic data suggesting invasive disease.[22] Allergic rhinitis may be a risk factor for the development of *Bipolaris* sinusitis. Whether the use of corticosteroids increases the risk of infection is still not known. Treatment has been by surgical debridement in addition to intravenous amphotericin B.[22] Surgical debridement alone was followed by a relapse.[164,174] Sinusitis has also been caused by dematiaceous fungi other than *Bipolaris*, including *Curvularia lunata*,[195] *Cladosporium*,[192] and *Alternaria*.[196,197] While complete surgical debridement seemed essential in the treatment of *Bipolaris/Exserohilum* sinusitis,[22,164] therapy with amphotericin B helped in preventing a relapse.[13]

Keratitis and corneal ulcers induced by *Bipolaris/Exserohilum* were related to *E. rostratum* (reported as *D. halodes*),[177] *B. spicifera*,[177,198] and "*Helminthosporium*" (most likely to be *Bipolaris* species).[194,199,200] In all cases, patients presented with eye pain following trauma to the eye; corneal ulceration and inflammation with varying degrees of visual deficit were also observed.[22] Topical amphotericin B,[194,198,199] pimaricin,[177,194] gentamicin,[177] 5-fluorocytosine (flucytosine),[22,194] nystatin/griseofulvin,[199] or tolnaftate[194] have been used to clear ulceration, occasionally after penetrating keratoplasty. In two cases, however, amphotericin B was apparently ineffective; in addition, intraocular amphotericin B caused severe local reaction and marginal efficacy against *Bipolaris*-associated keratitis.[22] On the other hand, pimaricin, a topical polyene antimycotic, has shown promise in treating fungal keratitis. Visual acuity following treatment varied from normal to near blindness.[22,198,200]

Allergic bronchopulmonary disease related to *Bipolaris/* "*Helminthosporium*" invasion has been reported to present with a syndrome very similar to that caused by *Aspergillus*: productive cough, bronchospasm, bronchiectasis, localized pulmonary infiltrates, eosinophilia, and elevated IgE level.[2,22,178,201-204] Clinical improvement was seen with surgical resection[178] or with corticosteroid therapy.[2,22,202-204]

37.1.2.1.2   Phaeohyphomycosis due to Wangiella dermatitidis and Exophiala spp.

The preponderance of the cases of *W. dermatitidis*-related phaeohyphomycosis came from Japan.[5,126,128-130,142,150,205] This geographical localization may indicate the existence of virulence differences among strains, genetically based immunological susceptibility, and propensity for environmental exposure.[109]

W. dermatitidis infections are usually chronic CNS or cutaneous disease. The manifestations of CNS infections are those of a local neurological deficit most often simulating a brain tumor or abscess.[109] Cutaneous lesions appear as chronic infections (usually without verrucoid hyperkeratosis),[158] as well as subcutaneous cysts.[23,143,206]

Several cases describing pulmonary phaeohyphomycosis have also been reported,[207] including one in a patient with cystic fibrosis.[208] The symptoms consisted of chronic pneumonia with cough, fever, and pulmonary infiltrates, occasionally accompanied by hemoptysis. In addition, *W. dermatitidis* has been implicated in lesions of the digestive tract[129] and the lymph nodes.[126,129,136,142] Hiruma et al.[150,205] have described a case of systemic *W. dermatitidis* disease in which the infection first appeared as swelling of the cervical lymph nodes, followed by development of lesions in various organs, including the common bile duct and the brain. Surgical debridement, and repeated antifungal therapy with intravenous (drip infusion) miconazole (600 mg daily), oral flucytosine (12 g daily), and intralesional, intravenous (a total dose of 600 mg over a 3-month period) and oral (4.8 to 7.2 g daily, with drug plasma level 1 year after the start of oral therapy at 0.140 µg/ml) amphotericin B, did not prevent the systemic infection from recurring and the patient died from respiratory failure.[205] While high oral doses of amphotericin B appeared to suppress fungal growth in the abdominal cavity, they were ineffective on the intracranial lesions.

Infections caused by *W. dermatitidis* have been notoriously resistant to antifungal therapy. Surgical excision is usually performed on small, localized cutaneous and subcutaneous lesions. However, when the infection is widespread, or deep-seated, visceral and disseminated, chemotherapy with amphotericin B, flucytosin, or combination of both drugs has been recommended. Among newer antimycotics, ketoconazole, fluconazole, itraconazole, and terbinafine have shown therapeutic promise.[156,209]

Pospisil et al.[156] have described a case of corneal phaeohyphomycosis in a patient with von Recklinghausen's disease and immunodeficiency (lower T lymphocyte count). Despite treatment with amphotericin B, the patient was left blind in one eye.

Exophiala spp. and E. jeanselmei (conspecific with Phialophora gougerotii),[210] in particular, have been reported to cause both subcutaneous phaeohyphomycosis[211-223] and mycetomas with increasing frequency,[224-229] especially among patients with immune deficiencies.[230-232] The pathogen generally penetrates the skin by a traumatic inoculation with contaminated splinters or slivers of wood or other organic material.[54,220]

In the majority of cases, E. jeanselmei-induced subcutaneous phaeohyphomycosis is characterized initially with solitary, discrete, asymptomatic, well-encapsulated subcutaneous nodules, and little involvement of the overlying epidermis.[6,220,233] Histologic changes include the formation of extensive granulation tissue with abscesses that may enlarge into the sinuses. The fungus can be found as aggregates situated mostly in the center of the abscesses.

Despite its occurrence in immunocompromised patients, E. jeanselmei-induced cutaneous and subcutaneous phaeohyphomycosis remains a generally localized disease, and surgical excision and antifungal therapy are usually curative. Moreover, human cerebral infections with Exophiala spp. were also reported, in particular with E. jeanselmei,[28,132] and one still unclassified species.[234] While there are no apparent predisposing factors in cerebral phaeohyphomycosis, defective host immunity coupled with an environmental source of the organism may be important in establishing CNS infections in humans. In addition, a case of pulmonary infection due to E. jeanselmei in a diabetic patient has also been described.[235]

Hachisuka et al.[236] have reported a case of E. jeanselmei-associated cutaneous phaeohypho-mycosis in a renal transplant recipient. 5-Fluorocytosine at a total daily dose of 50 mg/kg (in two equally divided oral doses) successfully led to gradual decrease of the lesion in size, which completely disappeared 6 months later. The serum concentration was 50.7 µg/ml 6 h after the administration of 2.0 g of the drug. Mauceri et al.[213] recommended a higher dosage of flucytosine (150 mg/kg daily) conditional on the patient's tolerance. In another case of postrenal transplantation cutaneous phaeohyphomycosis caused by E. jeanselmei, Sindhuphak et al.[237] used surgical excision and oral ketoconazole (200 to 400 mg daily) for 2 years to clear the lesions. South et al.[215] also recommended ketoconazole at 200 mg daily.

Recently, itraconazole has been increasingly applied in the treatment of subcutaneous E. jeanselmei phaeohyphomycosis.[238-240] In vitro susceptibility testing has shown the drug to be effective against Exophiala spp. at concentrations of 0.0001 to 0.015 µg/ml (E. jeanselmei),[239,241,242] 0.018 to 0.02 µg/ml (E. spinifera),[154,211] and 0.018 µg/ml (E. castellanii).[211] After initial surgical debridement, Whittle and Kominos[239] successfully applied a 4-month course of oral itraconazole (200 mg, b.i.d.) to treat subcutaneous E. jeanselmei phaeohyphomycosis; the initial treatment with amphotericin B was discontinued because of renal insufficiency.

Chuan and Wu[238] have used 200 mg daily of itraconazole for 2 months, combined with incision and drainage, to relieve the symptoms of subcutaneous phaeohyphomycosis in an elderly patient with systemic lupus erythematosus who was being treated with prednisone. This case was one of several reports of subcutaneous phaeohyphomycosis developing in immunosuppressed patients as a result of prolonged steroid treatment — while most often lesions would remain solitary, in the immunosuppressed patient they may enlarge with frank tissue invasion or disseminate with fatal outcome.[238] However, in another case, Schwinn et al.[240] had to cease treatment of E. jeanselmei phaehyphomycotic cyst with a 200-mg daily regimen of itraconazole after 6 weeks because of side effects (headache, gastrointestinal disorders, body weakness, and increasing liver enzyme levels). In general, response to itraconazole treatment was found to be higher in patients with a shorter duration of illness and with no previous treatment.[170]

An elderly non-insulin-dependent diabetic patient with *E. jeanselmei* pulmonary phaeohyphomycosis was treated successfully with oral ketoconazole (400 mg daily) for 5 months.[235]

Intralesional amphotericin B (30 to 50 mg weekly) was found to be helpful in the therapy of subcutaneous phaeohyphomycosis due to *E. moniliae*.[243]

E. spinifera can infect both animals[244] and humans.[52,211,245-249] The first case of human disease, reported by Rajam et al.,[249] involved a fatal infection in a child. In addition to cutaneous infection,[247] *E. spinifera* was identified as the etiologic agent of a systemic disease in a 9-year-old child.[248] With regard to treatment of human *E. spinifera* pheohyphomycosis, the outcome may be fatal. In two cases, one of nasal granuloma and the other of pustular lesion on the forearm, the infections were diagnosed early and were successfully treated by surgical excision alone.[211] Reported antifungal therapy involved a combined treatment of ketoconazole and flucytosine which was effective, as well as itraconazole alone (after treatment with amphotericin B, ketoconazole, and flucytosine failed to elicit any clinical improvement). Rinaldi[250] reported a case of a renal transplant recipient with recurrent subcutaneous nodules caused by *E. spinifera* who was successfully treated with repeated surgical excision of the lesions following failed attempt with antifungal chemotherapy. *In vitro* susceptibility testing has shown the pathogen being susceptible to amphotericin B (MIC = 0.14 µg/ml or less), flucytosine (MIC = 10.09 µg/ml or less), ketoconazole (MIC = 0.2 µg/ml), and itraconazole (MIC = 0.018 µg/ml or less).[211]

Gold et al.[211] reported the first case of prosthetic valve endocarditis due to *E. castellanii* that was managed with surgical debridement and valve replacement, and chemotherapy consisting of amphotericin B (total of 1.6 g) and flucytosine (250 mg, four times daily). After recurrence (bilateral psoas abscesses), surgical drainage was applied, followed by a 6-month course of amphotericin B (1.0 g total) and itraconazole (100 mg daily). Antifungal susceptibility testing showed that the organism was susceptible to amphotericin B (MIC = 0.58 µg/ml), flucytosine (MIC = 10.09 µg/ml or less), ketoconazole (MIC = 0.4 µg/ml), fluconazole (MIC = 2.5 µg/ml), and itraconazole (MIC = 0.018 µg/ml or less).

37.1.2.1.3 *Alternaria*-associated phaeohyphomycosis

From all of the isolated *Alternaria* spp., *A. alternata* has been the most frequent cause of disease in humans.[251-257] According to one compilation of data,[258] *Alternaria alternata* together with *Exophiala jeanselmei* were among the most common phaeoid fungi afflicting AIDS patients. *A. tenuissima* has been identified in nearly one third of the cases.[259-265] Other *Alternaria* spp. shown pathogenic to humans include *A. dianthicola*,[266] *A. chartarum*,[267] *A. stemphyloides*,[268] and *A. chlamydospora*.[257]

Alternaria spp. have been identified as the causative agents of various clinical conditions, including skin lesions,[253,259,269-274] hypersensitivity pneumonitis,[275] granulomatous lung disease,[276] allergic fungal sinusitis,[277,278] ocular infections,[279-282] peritonitis,[283] and osteomyelitis.[284,285]

Cutaneous alternariosis can no longer be considered a rare fungal infection.[253,259,269-274] Since 1933, when the first case was observed,[251] this mycosis has been well documented in numerous reports involving immunocompromised patients (those with Cushing's syndome, kidney, liver and bone marrow transplant recipients, with hematologic malignances, chronic polyarthritis, discoid lupus erythematosus with leukopenia, primitive pulmonary hypertension, and nephrotic syndrome),[51,251-254,256,262,269,286-298] although infections in immunocompetent individuals have also been recognized.[229,260,272,299] Cutaneous *Alternaria* infections have been distributed worldwide: the Mediterranean region (Spain, France, Greece) and nearly all other European countries,[256,260,263,287,292,300] India,[257] Taiwan,[301] Japan, and the U.S. Cutaneous alternariosis, which usually originates by a traumatic implantation of fungal spores, is relatively common in farmers.[37,292]

Clinical manifestations of cutaneous alternariosis include the presence of single or multiple, reddish brown, erythematous squamous, papulonodular, or frankly nodular lesions with smooth or heaped-up surfaces.[286] Male and Pehamberger[302] have classified cutaneous alternariosis into endogenous, exogenous, and dermatopathic. In the endogenous form, the infection very likely is initially transmitted by inhalation, followed by hematogenous spread to the skin where the fungus causes typical verruciform or granulomatous lesions. In exogenous cutaneous alternariosis, the organisms are inoculated by trauma. The dermatopathic condition develops when *Alternaria* secondarily colonizes preexisting lesions (e.g., steroid-treated facial eczema), in what appears to be nosoparasitism rather than genuine infection.

There have been numerous reports implicating corticosteroids as a major pathogenic factor in cutaneous alternariosis. Usually, corticosteroids are given as therapy for a subjacent internal disease,[251,252,254,256,269,286,287,292] or for other reasons,[251,255,263,291,293,301,303-305] or are produced as a manifestation of Cushing's disease.[273,294] In most instances, cutaneous alternariosis improved or healed after tapering of corticosteroid medication,[252,263,265,303,304,306] even without interruption of other chemotherapeutic regimens.[290] Richardson et al.[307] described one case of subcutaneous alternariosis of the foot in an immunocompromised patient on corticosteroid medication.

There have been several reports,[273,308-312] affiliating Cushing's syndrome with cutaneous alternariosis and other superficial mycoses.[313] The apparent cause of fungal infections in patients with Cushing's syndrome has been the immunosuppressive state of such patients due to the excessive endogenous glucocorticoid production associated with this syndrome, which serves as a predisposing factor.[273] Kasperlik-Zaluska and Bielunska[255] have described a case of successful resolution of an unusual *A. alternata* cutaneous infection in a patient with Cushing's syndrome related to mitotane medication. Because of the life-threatening signs of Cushing's syndrome, mitotane therapy (up to 6.0 g daily, for a total of 241 g over 5 weeks) was implemented in order to reduce the endogenous high level of cortisol secretion. Since mitotane is not an antifungal drug and direct anti-alternaria action would be highly unlikely, the resolution of alternariosis was attributed to the mitotane's inhibitory effect on steroidogenesis.[255] Guerin et al.[273] have described the successful use of ketoconazole in the treatment of a patient suffering from both the Cushing's syndrome and associated cutaneous alternariosis. Loli et al.[314] have found that ketoconazole elicited rapid reduction of plasma and urinary cortisol levels and regression of clinical and biological abnormalities of Cushing's syndrome. However, the place of ketoconazole in the therapy of Cushing's syndrome has not been well documented. Since ketoconazole does not remove the cause of increased corticotropin secretion, it cannot be considered as treatment of choice of the pituitary-dependent Cushing's disease. In addition, ketoconazole also failed when used for the treatment of Cushing's syndrome of peripheral origin.[315]

In general, ketoconazole, which has been widely used to treat cutaneous alternariosis, has shown mixed success. It failed to resolve cutaneous lesions despite topical and systemic therapy in an immunocompromised patient with thrombocytopenic purpura,[292] as well as in other cases,[262,289] but was reported to elicit positive responses in several other studies.[263,264,273,306] Bécherel et al.[316] used daily occlusive local ketoconazole therapy for 2 months to heal cutaneous alternariosis in a renal transplant recipient.

Amphotericin B (intralesional injections[259,301] and systemic[254,256,262]), miconazole,[317] and oral fluconazole[303] have also been reported to be sometimes effective.[33] Thus, Benedict et al.[270] have described three cases of cutaneous alternariosis following solid organ transplantation which were successfully treated with intravenous amphotericin B or oral ketoconazole. Shearer and Chandrasekar[318] used intravenous amphotericin B (at 10 mg/kg for a total of 305 mg) to resolve skin lesions and cure lymphadenitis in a bone marrow recipient; however, 10 d after discontinuation of therapy, the skin lesions reappeared and had to be surgically excised, followed by the additional administration of another 75 mg of amphotericin B.[318]

Combined drug therapies, such as oral erythromycin with topical miconazole, have also been applied.[286]

Recently, several cases of cutaneous alternariosis have been successfully resolved with the use of oral daily doses of 100 to 200 mg of itraconazole.[37,252,254,261,269,272,287,303] Thus, Duffill and Coley[252] have recommended 100-mg daily oral itraconazole to treat *A. alternata* cutaneous phaeohyphomycosis in an elderly patient on prednisone medication (60 mg daily) for a nephrotic syndrome; while the prednisone dosage was tapered, the rash cleared following the itraconazole treatment. Oral itraconazole (400 mg daily) was also used to treat multifocal cutaneous lesions due to *A. tenuissima*.[261]

Viviani et al.[286] have described cutaneous alternariosis caused by *A. tenuissima* in two patients with primitive myeloproliferative syndrome and lymphocytic lymphoma, respectively. Both cases were treated with a combination of surgical excision of lesions and therapy with ketoconazole at 200 mg, b.i.d. In the first case, because of low blood levels, the ketoconazole dosage had to be increased to 300 mg, b.i.d.; there was a disease relapse and dissemination, leading to a fatal outcome. In the second case, drug levels in the blood were sufficiently high (1.6 μg/ml on the ninth day, at 2 h after the administration); there was no relapse despite continued corticosteroid therapy to control the underlying lymphocytic lymphoma.

Gené et al.[37] have reported the first case of cutaneous phaeohyphomycosis due to *A. longipes* in a patient with underlying neoplastic disease. The patient was treated initially with oral ketoconazole (200 mg, b.i.d.) for 3 weeks with no response, and then with oral itraconazole (100 mg, b.i.d.). After 2 months of itraconazole therapy no new lesions had developed. *In vitro* antifungal susceptibility testing of the same *A. longipes* isolate has shown susceptibility to amphotericin B, ketoconazole, miconazole, and itraconazole, with MIC values of 0.29 to 0.58, 1.6, 2.5, and 0.24 μg/ml, respectively; the isolate was resistant to fluconazole (MIC = 40 μg/ml) and 5-fluorocytosine (MIC >322.75 μg/ml).[37]

Locally, invasive sinonasal *Alternaria* infections in several immunocompetent patients have been described.[196,197,284,285,319] Morrison and Weisdorf[320] described six cases of invasive sinonasal disease caused by *Alternaria* spp. that occurred in bone marrow transplant recipients. The infections which were localized to the sinonasal region with no evidence of disseminated disease, were either asymptomatic (three of six patients) or the symptoms were mild and nonspecific (fever, headache, increased nasal secretions, nasal pain, and mild epistaxis). All patients received surgical debridement as well as therapy with amphotericin B for 5 to 61 d (median, 27). The total dose of the drug varied from 181 mg (in one patient who died 5 d after diagnosis) to 2.64 g; excluding the former patient, the mean total dose of amphotericin B was 1.952 mg. In addition, two patients received flucytosine and rifampin; granulocyte transfusions were administered to four patients, for periods of 1, 3, 3, and 16 d. As a result of this combined therapy, the sinonasal alternariosis resolved in all surviving patients.[320] Invasive sinonasal alternariosis in patients with AIDS[168] and in neutropenic patients during therapy for hematologic malignancies has also been reported.[321,322]

A plant fungicide, imazalil, was used in the treatment of alternariosis involving the palate, nose, and sinuses, which was not responsive to conventional therapy.[323] The drug, which was used topically (instillation and irrigation) as well as orally (up to 1.2 g daily), arrested but did not cure the disease.

Ophthalmic infections associated with *Alternaria* spp. include blepharitis, conjunctivitis, keratomycosis, and endophthalmitis.[279,280,324-326] A case of chronic *A. alternata* endophthalmitis in a diabetic patient was completely resolved following treatment with systemic amphotericin B (up to 60 mg daily) and flucytosine (250 mg, four times daily) for 3 weeks, combined with cycloplegic eyedrops three times daily.[279] In another case, a deep *Alternaria* keratomycosis with intraocular extension was successfully treated with topical 1% miconazole and oral fluconazole (200 mg daily).[280]

37.1.2.1.4 Phaeohyphomycosis due to Curvularia spp.

C. lunata (first described as *Acrothecium lunata*[327]) has been identified as pathogenic to humans, causing infections that include endocarditis, brain abscess,[328] skin and subcutaneous lesions,[41] onychomycosis, keratitis, pneumonia, disseminated disease, mycetoma, allergic bronchopulmonary disease, and sinusitis. The first two cases of human disease due to *C. lunata* were mycetomas in Africa.[329,330]

Although disseminated *Curvularia* disease has been prevalent in immunocompromised patients, most cases of *C. lunata* sinusitis have been in immunocompetent hosts.[47,331-334]

Rinaldi et al.[47] have described five cases of *C. lunata* paranasal sinusitis in immunocompetent patients with no underlying debilitating disease. All patients were treated with surgery (debridement and aeration) alone and fully recovered. The results of antifungal susceptibility varied depending on the medium used for testing, with the exception of 5-fluorocytosine, to which all strains were resistant. The reported MIC values (at 24 h) were as follows: amphotericin B, 1.16 and 2.31 μg/ml; miconazole, 1.20 and 4.79 μg/ml; ketoconazole, 0.4 and >12.8 μg/ml; and 5-fluorocytosine, >322.75 μg/ml.[47]

In another case of phaeohyphomycotic sinusitis due to *C. lunata*, the treatment involved an initial extensive surgical debridement by Caldwell-Luc operation, followed immediately by daily chemotherapy with intravenous amphotericin B (gradual daily increases to 50 mg). In addition, the sinuses were irrigated with 10 mg of amphotericin B daily by a catheter placed at the time of surgery. The antifungal medication was tolerated well by the patient who received a total of 1.0 g of the antibiotic intravenously, and another 200 mg administered into the sinuses in a 3-week period. In this case, as well as with other *C. lunata* infections,[203,335,336] a peripheral eosinophilia was observed. In related reports involving *C. pallescens*,[44] *Drechslera hawaiiensis*,[203] and *Bipolaris spicifera* (a granulomatous encephalitis in which the cerebrospinal fluid contained 30% eosinophils),[193] the presence of eosinophilia has also been noticed. Whether or not the observed eosinophilia represented an inflammatory or hypersensitivity response to the fungus, or was indicative of an underlying allergic disorder remained speculative.[331]

Ismail et al.[336] have described an invasive *C. lunata*-associated pansinusitis presenting with extensive bone destruction and intracranial extension. The patient received numerous surgical procedures coupled with a 12-month course of antifungal therapy consisting of 4.0 g of intravenous amphotericin B and an 8-month course of 400 mg of oral ketoconazole daily.

Even though *C. pallescens* is commonly isolated from tropical regions of the world, infections by this species are very rare. Lampert et al.[44] were the first to describe a disseminated infection in an immunocompetent young adolescent patient — the lesions were initially detected in the lung but later metastasized into the brain. Inhalation of dirt was considered to be the most probable portal of entry, resulting in a primary pulmonary mycetoma with secondary cerebral metastasis. Treatment with amphotericin B and miconazole was described as moderately effective.[44] In another case, invasive cutaneous infection caused by *C. pallescens* was cured by combination of surgical excision and oral ketoconazole for 7 months.[337]

Allergic bronchopulmonary disease due to *C. senegalensis*, a rare saprophytic fungus, was described in an immunocompetent pediatric patient.[338] Prednisone therapy was initiated at a dose of 2.0 mg/kg (60 mg daily). The dose regimen was decreased to 20 mg daily on alternate days after 3 months, and subsequently tapered and discontinued after 6 months of therapy. The patient remained asymptomatic 5 years after completion of therapy.

A rare case of disseminated *C. lunata* disease involving infection of the lung and brain, as reported by de la Monte and Hutchins,[339] was successfully treated with intravenous amphotericin B (1.0 mg/kg daily, for a total of 3.4 g) for 6 weeks. However, in two subsequent reports, Pierce et al.[340,341] have elaborated on some additional therapeutic and clinical considerations involving the same case. Rather than 6 weeks, as initially reported by de la Monte and Hutchins,[339] the patient had a long and complicated treatment course lasting 30 months, during which a major clinical relapse occurred and 12.2 g of amphotericin B (total dose over 30 months) was given. In addition, immunologic studies have suggested that the infection was accompanied by an unexplained cell-mediated immune deficiency.[341] In three previously reported cases,[44,335,339] treatment of pulmonary and cerebral involvement of *Curvularia* was unsuccessful.

A pulmonary *Curvularia* infection in a profoundly immunosuppressed patient with mega-karyocytic leukemia was also successfully cured with amphotericin B.[342] The treatment consisted of initial surgical excision, followed by administration of 1.0 mg/kg of amphotericin B every other day for approximately 1 month; the therapy was then continued on an outpatient basis until a total dose of 2.5 g of amphotericin B was administered.

In another case involving an immunocompromised patient with granulocytic leukemia, *Curvularia* and *Alternaria* have been isolated from the nasal septum and tissue invasion was documented histologically.[321] The dual infection was managed without antifungal therapy (no evidence of distal organ involvement) following surgical excision of the nasal septum and spontaneous resolution of neutropenia.

Berlanga et al.[343] described successful treatment with liposomal amphotericin B of *Curvularia* infection which developed in a patient with acute promyelocytic leukemia (AML type M3 on FAB classification). The latter condition showed resistance to primary chemotherapy but responded to treatment with all-*trans*-retinoic acid (a differentiation inducer of promyelocytic blast).

Bryan et al.[344] described a patient who developed *C. lunata*-induced endocarditis on a Carpentier-Edwards porcine heterograft with clinical involvement of the ring of the aortic valve and the aortic root. Because curative surgery was considered to be extremely high risk, the patient was treated with terbinafine (an allylamine antimycotic) after initial therapy with amphotericin B and ketoconazole failed to eradicate the fungus. Terbinafine at doses of 125 mg, b.i.d. was administered for nearly 7 years without serious (hepatotoxicity) side effects. *In vitro*, a *C. lunata* isolate was susceptible to terbinafine with MIC value of 0.2 μg/ml.[345]

One recommended treatment of *Curvularia* keratitis consisted of topical miconazole every hour, daily subconjunctival injections of 5.0 mg of miconazole for 5 d, and oral ketoconazole (200 mg) once daily.[346] Topical and subconjunctival administration of miconazole produced good intraocular penetration both in humans[347] and a rabbit model.[348] Upon examination, the clinical differentiation between moniliaceous and dematiaceous keratomycoses can often be difficult; however, one helpful histologic distinction observed in dematiaceous (*C. lunata*) fungal keratitis has been the diffused brown pigmentation throughout the ulcer bed.[349]

Agrawal and Singh[43] reported the first case of cutaneous phaeohyphomycosis caused by *C. pallescens*. *In vitro* antifungal susceptibility testing showed that oxiconazole was the most active drug with MIC value of 0.001 μg/ml, followed by amorolfine (MIC = 3.0 μg/ml), and ketoconazole (MIC = 30 μg/ml); itraconazole was ineffective.[43] One case of *Curvularia*-associated persistent subcutaneous infection was also reported by Subramanyam et al.[350]

An invasive burn wound *Curvularia* infection was successfully treated with a 10-d course of amphotericin B (1.0 mg/kg daily).[351] Yau et al.[352] described a case of a neonate with congenital heart disease in whom a sternal wound infection caused by *C. lunata* developed following cardiac surgery.

37.1.2.1.5 Phaeohyphomycosis due to *Xylohypha bantiana* (*Cladosporium bantianum*)

X. bantiana is an infrequent but often fatal cause of infection of the central nervous system.[109,353] Clinical features of the infection include chronic headache, fever, and hemiparesis. Although pharmacological immunosuppression has not been considered to be an important predisposing factor, there has been evidence from patients with a history of systemic nocardiosis or facial phaeohyphomycosis caused by *Alternaria* spp. suggesting that some impairment of host immune responses may play a role as predisposing factor. Antifungal therapy did not significantly affect the outcome of infection with survival rates reaching only 35% in all patients, and 45% for all neurosurgically treated patients.[109] Surgical resection still remains the single most important treatment of patients with *X. bantiana*-induced CNS phaeohyphomycosis, especially in those with solitary encapsulated masses that may be completely resected. Multifocal or nonencapsulated masses have poor prognosis despite antifungal chemotherapy. The clinical resistance to antimycotic agents has been consistent with data from experimental murine *X. bantiana* infection, where resistance to antifungal therapy was also present.[353]

In 1952, Binford et al.[354] reported the first case of brain abscess caused by *X. bantiana*. While the neurotropism of this phaeoid fungus has been well documented,[354-362] its portal of entry has not been apparent. The multiplicity of CNS lesions, however, supports the concept of hematogenous spread.[355,363-365] The fungus showed remarkable affinity for glial tissue in both experimental animals and humans.[365] In several reports of CNS involvement, *Xylohypha* was isolated from systemic sites (skin, lung, ear, and paranasal sinus).[358,363,366-370] Kim et al.[371] have indicated that on occasion, the infection may be iatrogenic in nature. Buxi et al.[372] reported a case of unusual multiple, conglomerated brain abscesses due to *X. bantiana*, with unique neuroimaging features.

Cases of paranasal sinus, ear, and pulmonary infection have also been reported.[373,374]

The symptoms are largely nonspecific, with headache and papilledema being the most common.[60,354,364]

While brain abscesses caused by *X. bantiana* have been observed predominantly in immuno-competent hosts (mostly males),[358,375] one report of *X. bantiana* cerebral phaeohyphomycosis in a liver transplant recipient, as well as in several other cases[376-378] underscored the distinct possibility of immunocompromised patients being at higher risk of infection by this phaeoid mold.[373] Experimental models utilizing cortisone-treated mice seemed to support this concept.[64] Furthermore, cerebral *X. bantiana* infection has been associated with HIV infection, and listed as an indicator of the acquired immunodeficiency syndrome.[379]

Dixon and Polak[209] have conducted an *in vivo* study to assess drug activity against experimental infection of *X. bantiana* in mice. Overall, the best life-protecting activity was achieved with oral 5-fluorocytosine, with ED_{50} values ranging from 50 to 100 mg/kg; the corresponding values for amphotericin B (subcutaneous administration), oral fluconazole, and oral ketoconazole were 25 to 100, 50 to 100, and 200 mg/kg, respectively. Previously, Block et al.,[380] using a similar murine model of cladosporiosis, found survival values ranging from 40% to 100% depending on the fungal strain at 5 weeks after infection in mice given 800 mg/kg of 5-fluorocytosine. In addition to demonstrating differences in susceptibility to 5-fluorocytosine by different strains of *X. bantiana*, the same investigators also showed that individual strains displayed dose-related responses in mortality rates over a dosage range of 100 to 800 mg/kg.[380]

Treatment of cerebral phaeohyphomycosis due to *X. bantiana* has been largely unsuccessful, with survival not expected to exceed 1 year.[381] Surgical excision has been performed in the majority of cases although antifungal therapy with flucytosine has been used on several occasions.[60,378,382] Amphotericin B in combination with flucytosine also proved unsuccessful.[61]

However, aggressive antifungal chemotherapy with fluconazole (400 mg daily for 3 months) in combination with surgery resulted in good clinical and radiologic outcome of multiple intracranial *X. bantiana*-induced mass lesions.[365]

Borges et al.[376] have described one of several rare cases[355,383] of localized pulmonary involvement of *X. bantiana*. The patient had a history of steroid-treated inflammatory bowel disease. Surgical excision, which was curative, appeared to be the treatment of choice, since antifungal chemotherapy had little effect on the course of infection.

37.1.2.1.6   Phaeohyphomycosis due to Ochroconis gallopava

Ochroconis gallopava (synonymous with *Dactylaria constricta* var. *gallopava*) is the etiologic agent of a seldom diagnosed but potentially lethal pulmonary and disseminated infection in immunocompromised patients.[71,77] *Ochroconis* is not known to cause systemic disease in immuno-competent hosts. In all reported cases, the patients had underlying immune deficiencies.

Most likely, the pathogen's portal of entry is the respiratory tract.[71] In addition, this phaeoid fungus is known to cause CNS infection in experimental murine models.[384] As compared to CNS phaeohyphomycosis due to *X. bantiana* and *W. dermatitidis*, the *O. gallopava*-associated CNS involvement has the tendency for causing ventriculitis.[385] This preference may be also observed in immunocompromised patients. In view of the absence of reliable distinguishing histologic features between *O. gallopava*, *X. bantiana*, *W. dermatitidis*, and *Phialophora pedrosoi* (*Fonseca pedrosoi*),[385] a definitive identification of *O. gallopava* is important for timely therapy. Amphotericin B appears to be effective.[109]

Fukushiro et al.[82] have reported the first human infection caused by *O. gallopava* in a patient with an acute myeloblastic leukemia. A second disseminated fatal infection was described by Terreni et al.[77] Although rare, human CNS involvement of *Ochroconis* has been reported.[78,83,84,386]

Using a *Dactylaria constricta*-infected mouse model, Dixon and Polak[209] have found that *in vitro* susceptibility testing had no predictive value for *in vivo* activity. Of the compounds tested, flucytosine was the most effective (at doses of 25 to 100 mg/kg), followed by amphotericin B (5 to 10 mg/kg), fluconazole (25 to 100 mg/kg), and ketoconazole (100 mg/kg). Nevertheless, amphotericin B remains the drug of choice.

Kralovic and Rhodes[386] have described a case of cerebral phaeohyphomycosis in a liver transplant recipient in what appeared to be a nosocomially acquired infection. Treatment with amphotericin B (1.0 mg/kg) for 10 d, then itraconazole (400 mg daily) failed to resolve the infection and the patient died. In another fatal case of cerebral dactylariosis,[78] amphotericin B (0.5 mg/kg) and flucytosine (150 mg/kg) given for over 2 weeks also failed to elicit positive response. However, Vukmir et al.[83] have treated successfully cerebral dactylariosis in a liver transplant recipient using a combination of colloidal dispersion of amphotericin B (8.5 g total dose) and flucytosine for 4 weeks, followed by itraconazole (200 mg daily) for 1 year.

Mancini and McGinnis[71] used amphotericin B alone at a dosage of 0.7 mg/kg (total of 811 mg) to cure *Dactylaria*-induced pulmonary phaeohyphomycosis.

37.1.2.1.7   Phaeohyphomycosis associated with Phialophora spp.

Phialophora spp. have a worldwide distribution and are considered the etiologic agent of a broad spectrum of clinical infections ranging from superficial skin lesions to disseminated visceral involvement.[58,122,387-389] *Phialophora* appeared to have predilection for causing infection in debilitated and immunocompromised patients, such as those with hematologic malignancies, systemic lupus erythematosus, solid organ transplantion, chronic renal failure, diabetes mellitus, and corticosteroid therapy.[59,212,388,390-393] However, even in severely immunosuppressed patients *Phialophora* infections often tended to stay localized.[59,212,388,390,393] Using an experimental murine model of *P. verrucosa*, Gugnani et al.[394] have observed that although cortisone-treated mice had more extensive lesions as compared to normal controls, the infection was rarely fatal.

Infection usually occurs through traumatic skin inoculation with contaminated matter, with the majority of lesions occurring on the feet and legs of outdoor workers.[395,396]

The course of *Phialophora* phaeohyphomycosis is subacute to chronic, with lesions developing over months to years.[55] Pruritis, although an uncommon manifestation, has also been observed.[387] Satellite lesions may also occur through lymphatic spread and, occasionally, hematologic dissemination to muscle, brain, or other visceral organs may also occur.[389]

In vitro susceptibility studies[58,59,122,387-389,397,398] have shown that while most *Phialophora* spp. were resistant to miconazole and flucytosine, several species were resistant to amphotericin B and ketoconazole.[398]

Corrado et al.[399] and Weitzman et al.[400] have evaluated the susceptibilities of three *Phialophora* spp. (*P. parasitica*, *P. richardsiae*, and *P. repens*) against amphotericin B, flucytosine, miconazole, and ketoconazole. Their results showed that *P. parasitica* (12 isolates tested) did not vary much in its response to each drug; while the MIC values against miconazole (2.5 to 10 μg/ml) were most uniform, *P. parasitica* proved notably resistant to ketoconazole (the MICs for the majority of isolates were 40 μg/ml and over). The sensitivities of *P. richardsiae* (three clinical isolates) and *P. repens* (a single wood isolate) differed substantially from those of *P. parasitica*. These two species were very sensitive to amphotericin B, miconazole, and ketoconazole but resistant to flucytosine.[400]

For *P. richardsiae*, Ikai et al.[59] have demonstrated MIC values of 3.13, 3.13, and 1.56 µg/ml for ketoconazole, miconazole, and amphotericin B, respectively. In animal model studies, however, Dixon and Polak[209] have observed no correlation between *in vitro* susceptibility values and *in vivo* efficacy.

Treatment of both localized and systemic *Phialophora* infections has been difficult. Duggan et al.[401] have described an extensive cutaneous *P. verrucosa*-induced infection in an AIDS patient. The disease failed to respond to ketoconazole (400 mg daily) but regression of lesions was achieved with itraconazole (200 mg daily). In another case of *P. verrucosa*-induced infection, an immuno-suppressed patient presented with a subcutaneous phaeomycotic cyst involving the dorsum of the foot; the infection was treated with ketoconazole.[390]

In 1968, Schwartz and Emmons[54] have described the first case of human phaeohyphomycosis (a subcutaneous abscess) caused by *P. richardsiae*. Since then, the organism has been isolated from lesions of the subcutaneous tissues,[54,221,396,399] the lacrimal gland,[402] the olecranon bursa,[403] infected foot bone,[404] and from the prostate gland.[59] Ikai et al.[59] have described a case of subcutaneous phaeohyphomycosis on the dorsum of the foot associated with *P. richardsiae*. The patient was treated with oral flucytosine and topical injection of amphotericin B, in combination with surgical excision of the subcutaneous abscess; however, the lesion immediately recurred.

Singh et al.[397] have used topical clotrimazole cream twice daily for 15 d to cure cutaneous lesions due to *P. richardsiae*; *in vitro* susceptibility testing has shown an MIC value of 1.0 µg/ml (after 72 h) for clotrimazole against the same isolate. Amorolfine was the best drug against another clinical isolate of *P. richardsiae* with an MIC value of 0.1 µg/ml.[397]

A 3-month course of itraconazole completely resolved *P. richardsiae*-induced cutaneous lesions in a pharmacologically immnunosuppressed patient.[405]

37.1.2.1.8   Phaeohyphomycosis caused by Hormonema dermatioides

Coldiron et al.[95] have described a rare cutaneous phaeohyphomycosis associated with *Hormonema dermatioides* in an immunocompetent patient. The lesions were cured with oral ketoconazole at 200 mg, b.i.d. given for 12 weeks. Antifungal sensitivity measured at 24 h has demonstrated susceptibility to amphotericin B (MIC = 0.29 µg/ml), ketoconazole (MIC = 0.8 µg/ml), itraconazole (MIC = 0.15 µg/ml), and fluconazole (MIC = 20 µg/ml).[95]

37.1.2.1.9   Phaeohyphomycosis caused by Aureobasidium spp.

A. pullulans has been well recognized as the etiologic agent of hypersensitivity pneumonitis.[406-411] In addition, the mold has also been diagnosed as the cause of cutaneous[100,104,105] and corneal[101,412] phaeohyphomycosis. The organism is most likely to enter through the respiratory tract or inoculation of the skin.

Jones and Christensen[101] described a corneal ulcer due to *A. pullulans* which was cured following a 3-week course of topical 5% suspension of natamycin applied every hour; previous treatment with topical amphotericin B (2.5 mg/ml applied every 2 h for 5 d) failed to bring any improvement of the corneal thickness. Antifungal susceptibility testing of *A. pullulans* demonstrated sensitivity to amphotericin B, nystatin, natamycin, clotrimazole, and miconazole at concentrations of 1.5, 12.5, 1.5, 6.0, and 0.75 µg/ml; the fungus was resistant to 5-fluorocytosine (>50 µg/ml).[101]

An unusual *A. pullulans* infection of the jaw was reported by Koppang et al.[413] in an immuno-competent patient. The fungus, which filled an intraosseous cavity, was successfully treated with daily oral doses of 10 mg of flucytosine given for 30 d; bone regeneration was evident 6 months post-treatment.

Systemic infections with *A. pullulans* have also been reported. In one such case,[99] the pathogen was repeatedly isolated from blood cultures of a patient with acute myeloid leukemia. Treatment with amphotericin B (0.5 mg/kg daily; total 0.5 g) failed to eradicate the organism.

Salkin et al.[98] described an opportunistic visceral infection of the spleen due to *A. pullulans* in a patient with disseminated lymphoma. Although the portal of entry and mode of dissemination have been unclear, the patient's immunosuppression caused by the malignant lymphoproliferative disorder very likely allowed the secondary invasion of the fungus.

Krcméry et al.[103] have reported *A. mansoni*-induced meningitis in a leukemic patient in what appeared to be the first case of *Aureobasidium* spp. CNS involvement. Intravenous amphotericin B was administered for 44 d at a total dose of 2.2 g. On day 6, the frequency of symptoms decreased, and on day 10 the patient was without meningitis-associated symptomatology.

37.1.2.1.10 Phaeohyphomycosis Caused by Cladosporium spp.

Naim-ur-Rahman et al.[414] have reported a fatal case of multiple phaeohyphomycotic brain abscesses caused by *Cladosporium* spp. in an immunocompetent patient. The clinical course of the infection was characterized by spontaneous remissions and relapses despite continued chemotherapy with amphotericin B, flucytosine, and ketoconazole. Surgical intervention appeared to be the only treatment modality that seemed capable of prolonging the life of the patient or altering the course of the disease. An interesting transitory pulmonary phase of the phaeohyphomycosis resembling miliary tuberculosis was observed. The latter may help to explain the portal of entry and mode of fungal spread to the brain.[414]

In another case of fatal disseminated phaeohyphomycosis, *C. devriesii* was identified as the causative agent.[415]

Buiting et al.[416] treated successfully a *C. normodendrum*-associated foot mycetoma with curettage of fistulous ducts and administration of itraconazole.

37.1.2.2 Fungal Peritonitis in Continuous Ambulatory Peritoneal Dialysis (CAPD)

Continuous ambulatory peritoneal dialysis (CAPD), which has become a major therapeutic modality in the treatment of end-stage renal disease, is complicated primarily by catheter malfunction and acute peritonitis.[417] It has been estimated that nearly 100% of patients will experience at least one episode of peritonitis during the first 3 years of CAPD.[418] Among the opportunistic pathogens reported with increasing frequency as causes of peritonitis in CAPD patients, coagulative-negative staphylococcal bacteria have predominated. Although to a lesser extent (less than 5%), fungi have also been implicated in CAPD peritonitis,[419] with *Candida albicans* being the most common (as high as 36.4%) (see 32.7.4.5).[420] *Curvularia* spp. were also diagnosed as causative agents of peritonitis in CAPD patients,[421-424] as well as *Alternaria* species.[425]

Several cases of CAPD peritonitis caused by *Bipolaris* species have also been reported.[22,283,426,427] Manifestations include abdominal pain, and in some instances fever and cloudy peritoneal fluid.[22,283] The most commonly applied therapy involved catheter removal and intraperitoneal amphotericin B alone, or in combination with flucytosine[22] or ketoconazole;[426] intraperitoneal amphotericin B has also been applied.[22]

Intravenous amphotericin B was also used to treat these infections.[421,422] In one case described, the antibiotic dose has been escalated by 10 mg daily to reach 50 mg for a total of 1.0 g.[421] The results of antifungal susceptibility testing of *Curvularia* isolates from a patient with CAPD peritonitis have shown MIC values of 0.08, >100, 0.035 to 0.3, and 10 to >80 µg/ml for amphotericin B, flucytosine, itraconazole, and fluconazole, respectively.[421] In another case, *Aureobasidium pullulans*-associated peritonitis in a CAPD patient was successfully treated with catheter removal and a prolonged course of intravenous amphotericin B, allowing for the resumption of CAPD.[428] Pritchard and Muir[3] have also identified *Aureobasidium* spp. (*A. pullulans* and *A. melanogenum*) as causative agents of fungal peritonitis in CAPD patients.

In the absence of peritonitis, DeVault et al.[417] related a case of Tenckhoff catheter malfunction in a CAPD patient with a mechanical obstruction caused by colonization with *C. lunata*. Catheter removal alone was sufficient to eradicate the fungus since recurrence of colonization or peritonitis did not occur following the resumption of CAPD.

Several predisposing factors, such as antibiotic therapy,[419,429-432] immunosuppressive therapy, recent bacterial peritonitis, and the presence of bowel perforation,[429,431] may facilitate the development of fungal peritonitis. It has been estimated that between 55% and 100% of fungal peritoneal infections have been preceded by recent antibiotic use.[419,431,432]

Even though a number of effective chemotherapeutic regimens have been described, high morbidity and mortality of fungal peritonitis remained a problem.[419,430] Among the antifungal agents used successfully to treat CAPD fungal peritonitis, amphotericin B, flucytosine, econazole, miconazole, and ketoconazole have been considered to be the most effective.[424,425,429,433-436] However, other factors, such as route of administration (systemic or intravenous), dosage, duration of treatment, and the use of combination antifungal therapy seem to be important for successful clinical resolution of fungal peritonitis.[323]

As part of the clinical management of fungal peritonitis in CAPD patients, the early removal of the dialysis catheter in the opinion of many investigators has been critical for consistant therapeutic success.[396,429,430,432-434] Although in a number of cases reported[419,425,427,429,434-436] success has been achieved without removal of the catheter with the use of intraperitoneal antifungal therapy alone or in combination with systemic antifungal drugs, only about 50% of these patients returned to CAPD after the successful treatment of their peritonitis because of the development of multiple complications, such as relapse of infection, abscess formation, catheter obstruction, peritoneal adhesions, and fibrosis.[419,421,429,431]

37.1.2.3 Allergic Fungal Sinusitis

Allergic fungal sinusitis is a new clinical entity distinctly different from chronic sinusitis.[277,437] It is one of three forms of fungal sinusitis, the other two being mycetoma and invasive fungal sinusitis.

Allergic fungal sinusitis involving *Aspergillus* infection has been originally described in 1983 by Katzenstein et al.[438] The disease, which is characterized with pansinusitis and allergic mucinous infiltrates in all involved sinuses, is a combination of both type 1 (Gell and Coombs) or IgE-mediated and type 3 or immune complex-mediated immunologic reactions to the specific fungal antigens. The term "allergic fungal sinusitis" rather than the initial name "allergic *Aspergillus* sinusitis"[439-442] is now generally accepted since other fungal species besides *Aspergillus* (e.g., *Alternaria*, *Curvularia*, *Bipolaris*, *Exserohilum*, and *Drechslera*) have been shown to cause clinical conditions similar to that found originally with *Aspergillus* spp.[277,332-334,336,345,438,443-447]

The most pronounced clinical and pathologic features of allergic fungal sinusitis include atopic individuals with chronic refractory pansinusitis — typically young adults with history of recurrent nasal polyposis who underwent multiple surgical procedures and failed repeated medical treatments.[345,443] Upon histologic examination, the presence of a thick, eosinophil-containing, inspissated mucus within the involved paranasal sinus, defined as allergic mucin,[438] Charcot-Leyden crystals, and fungal hyphae (identified by silver stains), have been observed.[443,448]

Because of the limited number of cases reported, the treatment of allergic fungal sinusitis is still based on the theoretic analogy to allergic bronchopulmonary aspergillosis (ABPA).[449] Thus, by analogy[450] and because of high recurrence rates, allergic fungal sinusitis is treated with high-dose parenteral corticosteroids for 2 weeks, followed by an every-other-day regimen for 6 months, and finally tapered slowly for the remainder of the year.[438,448,451,452] Thus, one recommended dose regimen consisted of prednisone, 80 to 100 mg daily, tapered over several weeks to the lowest dose necessary to maintain a disease-free state, usually between 10 and 20 mg daily (but sometimes as low as 2 to 5 mg).[345] Another therapeutic approach that has been recommended involved surgical drainage and debridement through either external or intranasal intervention. However, a combination of these two therapeutic approaches may provide the optimum treatment for allergic fungal sinusitis; that is, wide surgical debridement and drainage of all involved sinuses, followed by parenteral corticosteroid therapy.[443]

Bartynski et al.[277] have reported two cases of allergic fungal sinusitis, one caused by *Curvularia lunata*, and the other by *Alternaria* spp. In the former case, after a thorough surgical debridement the patient was treated with antihistamines (terfenadine) and allergy immunotherapy injections; while the computerized tomography (CT) scan of the paranasal sinuses demonstrated diminished membrane thickening in the ethmoid sinuses, the frontal sinuses, the sphenoid sinus, and clearing of the maxillary antrum, the efficacy of allergy immunotherapy injections in the management of allergic fungal sinusitis remains to be defined. In the case of the *Alternaria*-induced allergic sinusitis, the patient underwent surgical debridement followed by nasal irrigations and intranasal beclomethasone therapy; 1 year postoperative, the patient remained disease-free.[277]

The pathophysiology of sinusitis produced by *Curvularia lunata* and *Drechslera* has been similar to the allergic fungal sinusitis as described by Katzenstein et al.[438,443] The presence of thick, brown, greasy material in the sinuses has been similar in both conditions, as were histologic findings consisting of plasma cells, eosinophils, mucin, and septate hyphae.[164,332-334,336,445] Although *Curvularia* and *Drechslera* sinusitis produced similar signs and symptoms, *Drechslera* sinusitis was somewhat more aggressive as manifested by cases of intracranial extension and by a higher recurrence rate.[334]

37.1.2.4 Fungal (Mold) Allergy and Immunotherapy

Although not directly associated with opportunistic infections, fungal (mold) sensitivity is a common clinical problem contributing significantly to the pathogenesis of asthma[453] and broncho-constriction.[454] Sampling studies have shown that fungal spores are common in the atmosphere, both in the indoor and outdoor environment.[455] The fungi that can be isolated from the air vary considerably, and some of them may be allergenic.[456]

Most common among the allergenic fungi are the various Deuteriomycetes (Imperfect fungi), *Aspergillus* spp., *Aurebasidium pullulans*, *Cladosporium* spp., *Curvularia lunata*, *Drechslera* spp., *Fusarium* spp., *Paecilomyces* spp., *Penicillium* spp., *Ascomycetes* spp., Zygomycetes, and Basidiomycetes.[455]

The prevalence of fungal sensitivity is not known. In some countries the prevalence of allergic inhalant diseases may reach as high as 15% to 20%, with more than 10% of patients being sensitized to fungal allergens.[457] A recent survey of skin test reactivity to common allergens conducted in the U.S.[110] has revealed that, for example, the *Alternaria* spp. sensitivity accounted for 3.6%, which was greater than animal dander sensitivity, but less than dust mite or pollen sensitivity.

Many fungal spores are less than 10 μm in size, which permits their penetration in the smaller airways of the lung.[457]

Controlled immunotherapy trials with fungal extracts have identified selected populations who may benefit from this type of therapy.[234,458-469]

37.1.3 Chromoblastomycosis

Chromoblastomycosis is a subcutaneous mycotic disease also caused by dematiaceous fungi.[1,470] Its most characteristic feature is the presence of verrucous nodules on the distal extremities. The terms phaeohyphomycosis and mycetoma (Madura foot) were created to delineate the other two mycoses caused by dematiaceous fungi but in which these pigmented sclerotic bodies were absent. In tissue, the sclerotic bodies (also called "copper pennies") are chestnut brown, cross-walled cells representing the tissue form of the fungus.[470] Initially, these sclerotic cells were thought to be budding yeasts, prompting the creating of the name "chromoblastomycosis".

Pedroso and Gomes[471] have been credited with the initial description of the causative agent of the disease as large, yellow, spherical bodies in tissue from a Brazilian patient with a nodular and ulcerated lower extremity lesion. However, the first cases of chromoblastomycosis in the literature were described in 1914 by Rudolph,[472] who consolidated clinical findings he observed also in patients from Brazil. Medlar[473] and Lane[474] have been credited for describing the first known etiologic agent of the disease, *Phialophora verrucosa*.

As stated in the beginning of this chapter, the nomenclature for chromoblastomycosis has been the subject of much controversy and change, with multiple names and etiologic agents being associated with this clinical condition.[1] The most common names used over the years to describe this disease include blastomycose nigra, figueira, dermatite verrucosa por *Phialophora verrucosa*, formigueiro, cutaneous chromoblastomycosis, cutaneous chromomycosis, dermatite verrucosa cromomicosica, dermatitis verrucosa blastomicotica, Pedrosso's disease, Fonseca's disease, Gome's disease, and Carrion's disease.[1,470]

While persons of all ages appear to be susceptible of developing chromoblastomycosis, the majority of them have been males between 30 and 50 years old. However, Campins and Scharyj,[475] who studied 34 Venezuelan patients, found that nearly half of them (15) were females. The lower male-to-female ratio was attributed, in part, to the fact that both sexes had worked together. The mycosis is believed not be contagious, with no known human-to-human transmission. Since the fungus is a saprophite growing in soil, decaying vegetation, and rotting wood (predominantly in tropical and subtropical regions), farm laborers make up the majority of those infected when trauma leads to inoculation of the pathogen.[1,470]

A number of other infections (blastomycosis, leprosy, leishmaniasis, tertiary syphilis, mossy foot, and tropical lymphagenitis) produce symptoms that can be confused with those of chromoblastomycosis, especially during its early development stages.[476]

In general, five fungi account for most of the infections: *Fonseceae compactum*, *Fonseceae pedrosoi*, *Phialophora verrucosa*, *Cladosporium carrionii*, and *Rhinocladiella aquaspersa*, with *F. pedrosoi* being most often isolated.[242] However, in Australia, *Cladosporium carrionii* has been the most common organism found.[1,470] *Cladosporium herbarum*-associated chromoblastomycosis has also been observed.[477]

37.1.3.1   *Fonsecaea compacta* Carrion

Fonsecaea compacta Carrion, 1940 (also synonymous with *Hormodendrum compactum*, *Phialophora compacta*, and *Rhinocladiella compacta*) is characterized by its slow growing (on potato dextrose agar), velvety to wooly, and olive to olivaceous to black-colored colonies that may produce up to four different types of conidiophores.[1] The diagnostic form consists of one-celled, pale brown, primary conidia which develop upon pegs at the apices of erect, dark, irregularly swollen (apices only) conidiophores.

37.1.3.2   *Fonseceae pedrosoi* (Brumpt) Negroni

Fonseceae pedrosoi (Brumpt) Negroni, 1936 (also synonymous with *Hormodendrum pedrosoi*, *Phialophora pedrosoi*, and *Rhinocladiella pedrosoi*) develops in a similar manner as *F. compacta*, except that the colonies grow faster and the primary conidia are larger in size.[1]

37.1.3.3   *Rhinocladiella aquaspersa* (Borelli) Schell, McGinnis et Borelli

Rhinocladiella aquaspersa (Borelli) Schell, McGinnis et Borelli, 1983 (originally described as *Acrotheca aquaspera*[478]) is the rarest agent associated with chromoblastomycosis.[1] The colonies are moderately rapid-growing, wooly, and dark olivaceous gray in color. This organism produces, as distinct from the vegetative hyphae, erect dematiaceous conidiophores that bear one-celled, thick-walled conidia arranged along and around the apices of the conidiophores.

37.1.3.4 *Phialophora verrucosa* Medlar

Phialophora verrucosa Medlar, 1915 is characterized by colonies that are rapid growing, spreading, wooly, flat with a raised center, and olivaceous gray in color.[1] The conidia are one-celled, ellipsoidal to oblong, hyaline to pale brown, and accumulate in balls at the apices of the collarettes.

37.1.3.5 *Cladosporium carrionii* Trejos

The colonies of *Cladosporium carrionii* Trejos, 1954, which are slow-growing on potato dextrose agar, are velvety with a raised center, and gray-green to olivacious gray in color.[1] Their conidiophores are erect, one-celled, ellipsoidal to oval, and form distinct, stable, and unique branched chains. Phialides having collarettes may occur in some isolates.[1]

37.1.3.6 Evolution of Therapies and Treatment of Chromoblastomycosis

The distinctive margins of the lesions and the development of satellite lesions that may often result from autoinoculation are two distinctive clinical features to be considered in differentiating chromoblastomycosis.[479] According to Carrion[476] there are five morphologic types of infection: nodular, tumorous, verricous, plaque, and cicatrical lesions. Major pathologic characteristics include pseudoepitheliomatous hyperplasia, dermal granulomas, intraepidermal microabscess formation, and fibrosis.[1] Although there is evidence[480] describing the spontaneous resolution of infection, in general, chromoblastomycosis is an indolent and progressively expanding disease.[1,470]

The infection is difficult to manage, with relapses, drug resistance, and partial cure being common.[1,470,481,482]

In the early stages of infection, wide and deep excision followed by grafting usually has been beneficial.[481,483] However, electrodesiccation and curettage should be avoided lymphatic spread and recurrence may be facilitated.[1] Carbon laser surgery has also been applied as an effective alternative over cold steel surgery.[484] Other physical therapeutic modalities used with some success in the treatment of chromoblastomycosis include Mohs' surgery, cryosurgery,[485] heat therapy,[486-488] and small pocket[489] and larger electric bed[486] warmers.

Antifungal therapy with amphotericin B, 5-fluorocytosine, ketoconazole, and thiabendazole (alone or in combinations) has been used with varying degrees of success in the treatment of chromoblastomycosis.[1,470,482] Amphotericin B has been applied both intralesionally and intravenously[490-492] but with limited success because of relatively high fungal resistance and the inability to achieve adequate fungicidal tissue concentrations. Although painful, direct local subcutaneous injections of amphotericin B (20 to 25 mg in 2% procaine) led to sloughing of the treated tissue with eventual healing.

The combined use of amphotericin B and 5-fluorocytosine appeared to be effective against chromoblastomycosis.[493] The recommended treatment consisted of amphotericin B given intravenously every other day, three times daily for 3 months (1.8 g total dose), along with 3 g of 5-fluorocytosine daily for 3 months (270 g total dose).

Treatment with 5-fluorocytosine at doses of 150 to 200 mg/kg (given in four doses) has been successful in providing rapid regression of lesions and symptoms as well as eradication of the organism.[494-497] The duration of therapy has been usually over 6 months. However, some resistance toward flucytosine has been reported.[495] Combination of flucytosine and clotrimazole was also reported effective.[498]

Although at 200 to 400 mg daily, ketoconazole was also found to be effective in clinical trials, leading to improvement and even cure in some instances,[499,500] it was not superior to flucytosine.

The combination of ketoconazole and 5-fluorocytosine has shown synergistic activity.[501]

In recent studies, itraconazole has been actively investigated in the treatment of chromo-blastomycosis.[482,502-505] In order to achieve clinical and mycological cure, itraconazole was used at daily doses of 200 to 400 mg (b.i.d.) for 6 to 12 months or longer.[482,504,505] In general, infections due to *C. carrionii* responded better to itraconazole therapy than those induced by *F. pedrosoi*. Thus, Yu[502] used oral itraconazole at 100 mg daily (total dose, 45.5 g) given over 15 months, to treat an unusually severe case of chromoblastomycosis due to *Cladosporium carrionii* unresponsive to flucytosine, miconazole, and ketoconazole. The patient had a complete clinical and mycological recovery without any side effects. Smith et al.[505] reported clinical and mycologic cure following a treatment regimen consisting of oral itraconazole solution (100 mg daily) for 6 months, then tablets (100 mg daily) for 12 months.

While Bayles[503] reported little progress in eight patients with chromoblastomycosis after treatment with itraconazole (100 mg daily), the combination of itraconazole and flucytosine (100 mg daily of each drug) proved to be synergistic in resolving the lesions. Furthermore, the addition of flucytosine appeared to enhance the response of *F. pedrosoi* to itraconazole.

The therapeutic value of fluconazole has also been investigated.[506-508] Yu and Gao[506] used fluconazole to treat a case of refractory *C. carrionii*-induced chromoblastomycotic lesions after ketoconazole, flucytosine, and miconazole medication failed because of drug resistance. Intravenous fluconazole was started at 400 mg for the first day, followed by 200 mg daily. After 30 d of treatment (total dose, 6.2 g), there was successful resolution of lesions; the patient remained on oral fluconazole maintenance therapy (50 mg daily) for 2 years.[506] Robertson et al.[507] also used fluconazole (200 to 400 mg daily) to achieve improvement of lesions after 56 d. However, in another study, only one of seven patients with chromoblastomycosis showed improvement after receiving fluconazole.[508]

Franco et al.[509] introduced saperconazole as another chemotherapeutic modality for treatment of chromoblastomycosis. After a 6- to 12-month course (median, 9 months) with oral saperconazole at 200 mg daily, there was no relapse at the 20-month follow-up examination among the seven patients treated.

Bayles[510] has found thiabendazole to be effective in less than 40% of patients when administered at 25 mg/kg daily (200 to 400 mg, b.i.d., and given with meals). The combination of thiabendazole with flucytosine also appeared to be very beneficial, at least, in cases reported in Natal, South Africa.[511]

Overall, itraconazole and 5-fluorocytosine, alone or in combination with amphotericin B, have provided the most active antimycotic chemotherapy. However, the combination of surgery, temperature manipulation, and antifungal chemotherpy seemed to be the most effective treatment of chromoblastomycosis.[1,470]

37.1.4 REFERENCES

1. McGinnis, M. R., Rinaldi, M. G., and Winn, R. E., Emerging agents of phaeohyphomycosis: pathogenic species of *Bipolaris* and *Exserohilum*, *J. Clin. Microbiol.*, 24, 250, 1986.
2. Halloran, T. J., Allergic bronchopulmonary helmintosporiosis, *Am. Rev. Respir. Dis.*, 128, 578, 1983.
3. Pritchard, R. C. and Muir, D. B., Black fungi: a survey of dematiaceous hyphomycetes from clinical specimens identified over a five year period in a reference laboratory, *Pathology*, 19, 281, 1987.
4. Matsumoto, T. and Ajello, L., Dematiaceous fungi potentially pathogenic to humans and lower animals, in *Handbook of Applied Mycology*, Vol. 2, Arora, D. K., Ajello, L., and Mukerji, K. G., Eds., Marcel Dekker, New York, 1991, 117.
5. Matsumoto, T., Matsuda, T., McGinnis, M. R., and Ajello, L., Clinical and mycological spectra of *Wangiella dermatitidis* infections, *Mycoses*, 36, 145, 1993.
6. McGinnis, M. R., Chromoblastomycosis and phaeohyphomycosis: new concepts, diagnosis, and mycology, *J. Am. Acad. Dermatol.*, 8, 1, 1983.
7. Terra, F., Torres, M., da Fonseca, O., and Area Leao, A. E., Novo typo de dermatite verrucosa mycose por *Acrotheca* com associacao de leishmaniosa, *Brasil-Med.*, 2, 363, 1922.

8. Moore, M. and de Almeida, F., Etiologic agents of chromoblastomycosis (chromoblastomycosis of Terra, Torres, Fonseca and Leao, 1922), of North and South America, *Rev. Biol. Med.*, 6, 94, 1935.
9. Ajello, L., Georg, L. K., Steigbigel, R. T., and Wang, C. J. K., A case of phaeohyphomycosis caused by a new species of *Phialophora*, *Mycologia*, 66, 490, 1974.
10. Davis, C. L. and Shorten, H. L., Granulomatous nasal swelling in a bovine, *J. Am. Vet. Med. Assoc.*, 89, 91, 1936
11. Rolston, K. V. I., Hopfer, R. L., and Larson, D. L., Infections caused by *Drechslera* species: case report and review of the literature, *Rev. Infect. Dis.*, 7, 525, 1985.
12. Ito, S., On some new ascigerous stages of the species of *Helminthosporium* parasitic on cereals, *Proc. Imp. Acad. (Tokyo)*, 6, 352, 1930.
13. Shoemaker, R. A., Nomenclature of *Drechslera* and *Bipolaris*, grass parasites segregated from "*Helminthosporium*", *Can. J. Bot.*, 37, 879, 1959.
14. Shoemaker, R. A., A pleomorphic parasite of cereal seeds, *Pyrenophora semeniperda*, *Can. J. Bot.*, 44, 1451, 1966.
15. Leonard, K. J. and Suggs, E. G., *Setosphaeria prolata*, the ascigerous state of *Exserohilum prolatum*, *Mycologia*, 66, 281, 1974.
16. Luttrell, E. S., Correlations between conidial and ascigerous state characters in *Pyrenophora*, *Cochliobolus*, and *Setosphaeria*, *Rev. Mycol. (Paris)*, 41, 271, 1977.
17. Alcorn, J. L., Generic concepts in *Drechslera*, *Bipolaris* and *Exserohilum*, *Mycotaxon*, 17, 1, 1983.
18. Kafi, A. and Tarr, S. A. J., Growth, sporulation and conidial characteristics of five graminicolous species of *Helminthosporium*. I. Effect of nutrients, *Trans. Br. Mycol. Soc.*, 49, 327, 1966.
19. Platt, H. W., Morrall, R. A. A., and Gruen, H. E., The effects of substrate, temperature, and photoperiod on conidiation of *Pyrenophora tritici-repentis*, *Can. J. Bot.*, 55, 254, 1977.
20. Tarr, S. A. J. and Kafi, A., Growth, sporulation and conidial characteristics of five graminicolous species of *Helminthosporium*. II. Effect of nitrogen and pH, *Trans. Br. Mycol. Soc.*, 51, 771, 1968.
21. Leonard, K. J., Synonymy of *Exserohilum halodes* with *E. rostratum*, and induction of the ascigerous state, *Setosphaeria rostrata*, *Mycologia*, 68, 402, 1976.
22. Adam, R. D., Paquin, M. L., Petersen, E. A., Saubolie, M. A., Rinaldi, M. G., Corcoran, J. G., Galgiani, J. N., and Sobonya, R. E., Phaeohyphomycosis caused by the fungal genera *Bipolaris* and *Exserohilum*: a report of 9 cases and review of the literature, *Medicine (Baltimore)*, 65, 203, 1986.
23. Matsumoto, T., Padhye, A. A., Ajello, L., Standard, P. G., and McGinnis, M. R., Critical review of human isolates of *Wangiella dermatitidis*, *Mycologia*, 76, 232, 1984.
24. Kano, K., Uber die chromoblastomykose durch einen noch nicht als pathogen beschriebenen pilz: *Hormiscium dermatitidis* n. sp., *Aichi Igakkai Zasshi*, 41, 1657, 1934.
25. Jotisankasa, V., Nielsen, H. S., Jr., and Conant, N. F., *Phialophora dermatitidis*, its morphology and biology, *Sabouraudia*, 8, 98, 1970.
26. McGinnis, M. R., *Wangiella*, a new genus to accommodate *Hormiscium dermatitidis*, *Mycotaxon*, 5, 353, 1977.
27. McGinnis, M. R., *Wangiella*, a correction, *Mycotaxon*, 6, 367, 1977,
28. de Hoog, G. S., *Rhinocladiella* and allied genera, in *Stud. Mycol.*, No. 15, Baarn: Centraalbureau voor Schimmelcultures, 1, 1977.
29. de Hoog, G. S., On the potentially pathogenic dematiaceous hyphomycetes, in *The Fungi Pathogenic for Humans and Animals*, Part A, Howard, D. H., Ed., Marcel Dekker, New York, 1982, 149.
30. de Hoog, G. S., The taxonomic structure of *Exophiala*, in *The Fungi Pathogenic for Humans and Animals*, Part B, Howard, D. H., Ed., Marcel Dekker, New York, 1985, 327.
31. Nishimura, K. and Miyaji, M., Studies on a saprophyte of *Exophiala dermatitidis* isolated from a humidifier, *Mycopathologia*, 77, 173, 1982.
32. Sigler, L. and Hawksworth, D. L., International Commission on the Taxonomy of Fungi (ICTF): code of practice for systemic mycologists, *Microbiol. Sci.*, 4, 83, 1987.
33. Badillet, G., Les alternarioses cutanées: revue de la littérature, *J. Mycol. Med.*, 118, 59, 1991.
34. Mitchell, A. J., Solomon, A. R., Beneke, E. S., and Anderson, S., Subcutaneous alternariosis, *J. Am. Acad. Dermatol.*, 8, 673, 1983.
35. Singh, S. M., Naidu, J., and Pouranik, M., Ungual and cutaneous phaeohyphomycosis caused by *Alternaria alternata* and *Alternaria chlamydospora*, *J. Med. Vet. Mycol.*, 28, 275, 1990.
36. Simmons, E. G., *Alternaria* themes and variations (1-6), *Mycotaxon*, 13, 16, 1981.

37. Gené, J., Azon-Masoliver, A., Guarro, J., Ballister, F., Pujol, I., Loovera, M., and Ferrer, C., Cutaneous phaeohyphomycosis caused by *Alternaria longipes* in an immunosuppressed patient, *J. Clin. Microbiol.*, 2774, 1995.

38. Barde, A. K. and Singh, S. M., A case of onychomycosis caused by *Curvularia lunata* (Wakker) Boedijn, *Mycosen*, 26, 311, 1983.

39. Harris, J. J. and Downham, T. F., Unusual fungal infections associated with immunologic hyper-reactivity, *Int. J. Dermatol.*, 17, 323, 1978.

40. Kaufman, S. M., *Curvularia* endocarditis following cardiac surgery, *Am. J. Clin. Pathol.*, 56, 466, 1971.

41. Grieshop, T. J., Yarbrough, D. III, and Farrar, W. E., Case report: phaeohyphomycosis due to *Curvularia lunata* involving skin and subcutaneous tissue after an explosion at a chemical plant, *Am. J. Med. Sci.*, 305, 387, 1993.

42. Rinaldi, M. G., Human *Curvularia* infections, *Diag. Microbiol. Infect. Dis.*, 6, 27, 1987.

43. Agrawal, A. and Singh, S. M., Two cases of cutaneous phaeohyphomycosis caused by *Curvalaria pallescens*, *Mycoses*, 38, 301, 1995.

44. Lampert, R. P., Hutto, J. H., Donnelly, W. H., and Shulman, S. T., Pulmonary and cerebral mycetoma caused by *Curvularia pallescens*, *J. Pediatr.*, 91, 603, 1977.

45. Travis, W. D., Unusual aspects of allergic bronchopulmonary fungal disease: report of two cases due to *Curvularia* associated with allergic fungal sinusitis, *Hum. Pathol.*, 22, 1240, 1991.

46. Kwon-Chung, K. J. and Bennett, J. E., in *Medical Mycology*, Kwon-Chung, K. J. and Bennett, J. E., Eds., Lea & Febiger, Philadelphia, 1992, 620.

47. Rinaldi, M. G., Phillips, P., Schwartz, J. G., Winn, R. E., Holt, G. R., Shagets, F. W., Elrod, J., Nishioka, G., and Aufdemorte, T. B., Human *Curvularia* infections: report of five cases and review of the literature, *Diagn. Microbiol. Infect. Dis.*, 6, 27, 1987.

48. McGinnis, M. R., Dematiaceous fungi, in *Manual of Clinical Microbiology*, 4th ed., Lennette, E. H., Balows, A., Hausler, W. J., Jr., and Shadomy, H. J., Eds., American Society for Microbiology, Washington, D.C., 1985, 561.

49. Singh, S. M. and Barde, A. K., Opportunistic infections of skin and nails by non-dermatophytic fungi, *Mykosen*, 29, 272, 1984.

50. Polak, F. M., Siverio, C., and Bresky, R. H., Corneal chromomycosis: double infection with *Phialophora verrucosa* (Medlar) and *Cladosporium cladosporioidis* (Fresenius), *Ann. Ophthalmol.*, 8, 139, 1976.

51. Emmons, C. W., Binford, C. B., and Utz, J. F., *Medical Mycology*, Lea & Febiger, Philadelphia, 1970, 347.

52. Nielsen, H. S. and Conant, N. F., A new human pathogenic *Phialophora*, *Sabouraudia*, 6, 228, 1968.

53. McGinnis, M. R., *Exophiala spinifera*, a new combination for *Phialophora spinifera*, *Mycotaxon*, 5, 337, 1977.

54. Schwartz, L. S. and Emmons, G. W., Subcutaneous cystic granuloma caused by a fungus of wood pulp (*Phialophora richardsiae*), *Am. J. Clin. Pathol.*, 49, 500, 1968.

55. Domsch, K. H., Grams, W., and Anderson, T. H., *Phialophora richardsiae*, in *Compendium of Soil Fungi*, Vol. 1, Domsch, K. H., Grams, W., and Anderson, T. H., Eds., Academic Press, London, 1980, 628.

56. Iwatsu, T. and Udagawa, S., Materials for the fungus flora of Japan, *Trans. Mycol. Soc. Jpn.*, 25, 389, 1984.

57. Ulloa, M. and Herrera, T., *Phialophora richardsiae*, un hongo causante de feosporotricosis en el hombre, aislado del pozol, *Rev. Latinoam. Microbiol.*, 15, 199, 1973.

58. Gezuele, E., Mackinnon, J. E., and Conti-Diaz, I. A., The frequent isolation of *Phialophora verrucosa* and *Phialophora pedrosoi* from natural sources, *Sabouraudia*, 10, 266, 1972.

59. Ikai, K., Tomono, H., and Watanabe, S., Phaeohyphomycosis caused by *Phialophora richardsiae*, *J. Am. Acad. Dermatol.*, 19, 478, 1988.

60. Palaoglu, S., Sav, A., Basak, T., Yalcinlar, Y., and Scheithauer, B. W., Cerebral phaeohyphomycosis, *Neurosurgery*, 33, 894, 1993.

61. Sekhon, A. S., Galbraith, J., Mielke, B. W., Garg, A. K., and Sheehan, G., Cerebral phaeohyphomycosis caused by *Xylohypha bantiana*, with a review of the literature, *Eur. J. Epidemiol.*, 8, 387, 1992.

62. Dixon, D. M., Shadomy, H. J., and Shadomy, S., Dematiaceous fungal pathogens isolated from nature, *Mycopathologica*, 70, 153, 1980.

63. Klite, P. D., Kelley, H. B., and Dierks, F. V., A new solid sampling technique for pathogenic fungi, *Am. J. Epidemiol.*, 81, 124, 1965.

64. Dixon, D. M., Merz, W. G., Elliott, H. L., and Macley, S., Experimental central nervous system phaeohyphomycosis following intranasal inoculation of *Xylohypha bantiana* in cortisone-treated mice, *Mycopathologia*, 100, 145, 1987.

65. Bhatt, G. C. and Kendrick, W. B., The generic concepts of *Diplorhinotrichum* and *Dactylaria*, and a new species of *Dactylaria* from soil, *Can. J. Bot.*, 46, 1253, 1968.

66. Rudek, W. T., The constriction of the trapping rings in *Dactylaria brochopaga*, *Mycopathologia*, 55, 193, 1975.

67. Ajello, L., McGinnis, M. R., and Camper, J., An outbreak of phaeohyphomycosis in rainbow trout caused by *Scolecobasidium humicola*, *Mycopathologia*, 62, 15, 1977.

68. Weitzman, I., Rosenthal, S. A., and Shupack, J. L., A comparison between *Dactylaria gallopava* and *Scolecobasidium humicola*: first report of an infection in a tortoise caused by *S. humicola*, *Sabouraudia/ J. Med. Vet. Mycol.*, 23, 287, 1985.

69. Ranck, F. M., Georg, L. K., and Wallace, D. H., Dactylariosis — a newly recognized fungus disease of chicken, *Avian Dis.*, 18, 4, 1974.

70. Randall, C. T., Owen, D. M., and Kirkpatrick, K. S., Encephalitis in broiler chickens caused by a hyphomycete resembling *Dactylaria gallopava*, *Avian Pathol.*, 10, 31, 1981.

71. Mancini, M. C. and McGinnis, M. R., *Dactylaria* infection of a human being: pulmonary disease in a heart transplant recipient, *J. Heart Lung Transplant.*, 11, 827, 1992.

72. Tansey, M. R. and Brock, T. D., *Dactylaria gallopava*, a cause of avian encephalitis, in hot spring effluents, thermal soils and self heated coal waste piles, *Nature*, 242, 202, 1973.

73. Sumner, J. L. and Evans, H. C., The fatty acid composition of *Dactylaria* and *Scolecobasidium*, *Can. J. Microbiol.*, 17, 7, 1971.

74. Tansey, M. R., Fliermans, C. B., and Kern, C. D., Aerosol dissemination of veterinary pathogenic and human opportunistic thermophilic fungi from thermal effluents of nuclear production reactors, *Mycopathologia*, 69, 91, 1979.

75. Rippon, J. W., Gerhold, R., and Heath, M., Thermophillic and thermotolerant fungi isolated from the thermal effluent of nuclear power generating reactors: dispersal of human opportunistic and veterinary pathogenic fungi, *Mycopathologia*, 70, 169, 1980.

76. Waldrup, D. W., Padhye, A. A., Ajello, L., and Ajello, M., Isolation of *Dactylaria gallopava* from broiler-house litter, *Avian Dis.*, 18, 445, 1974.

77. Terreni, A. A., Di Salvo, A. F., Baker, A. S., Crymes, W. B., Morris, P. R., and Dowd, A. H., Disseminated *Dactylaria gallopava* infection in a diabetic patient with chronic lymphocytic leukemia of the T-cell type, *Am. J. Clin. Pathol.*, 94, 104, 1990.

78. Sides, E. H. III, Benson, J. D., and Padhye, A. A., Phaeohyphomycosis brain abscess due to *Ochroconis gallopavum* in a patient with malignant lymphoma of a large cell type, *J. Med. Vet. Mycol.*, 29, 317, 1991.

79. Blalock, H. G., Georg, L. K., and Derieux, W. T., Encephalitis in turkey poults due to *Dactylaria* (*Diplorhinotrichum*) *gallopava* — a case report and its experimental reproduction, *Avian Dis.*, 7, 197, 1973.

80. Georg, L. K., Bierer, B. W., and Cooke, W. B., Encephalitis in turkey poults due to a new fungus species, *Sabouraudia*, 3, 239, 1964.

81. Padhye, A. A., Amster, R. L., Browning, M., and Ewing, E. P., Fatal encephalitis caused by *Ochroconis gallopavum* in a domestic cat (*Felis domesticus*), *J. Med. Vet. Mycol.*, 32, 141, 1994.

82. Fukushiro, K. R., Udagawa, S., Kawashima, Y., and Kawamura, Y., Subcutaneous abscesses caused by *Ochroconis gallopavum*, *J. Med. Vet. Mycol.*, 24, 175, 1986.

83. Vukmir, R. B., Kusne, S., Linden, P., Pasculle, W., Fothergill, A. W., Shaeffer, J., Nieto, J., Segal, R., Merhav, H., Martinez, A. J., and Rinaldi, M. G., Successful treatment of cerebral phaeohyphomycosis due to *Dactylaria gallopava* in a liver transplant recipient, *Clin. Infect. Dis.*, 19, 714, 1994.

84. Prevost-Smith, E., Hutton, N., Padhye, A. A., Upshur, J. K., and Van Bakel, A. B., Fatal phaeohyphomycosis infection due to *Dactylaria gallopava* and *Scedosporium prolificans* in a cardiac transplant patient, *Proc. 93rd Annu. Meet. Am. Soc. Microbiol.*, Abstr. F-35, American Society for Microbiology, Washington, D.C., 1993.

85. Becker, A. M., Richards, R. W., Schmalzl, K. J., and Yick, H. C., Metabolites of *Dactylaria lutea*: the structures of dactariol, and the antiprotozoal antibiotic dactylarin, *J. Antibiot.*, 31, 324, 1978.
86. Xaio, J., Kumazawa, S., Yoshikawa, N., Mikawa, T., and Sato, Y., Dactylfungins, novel antifungal antibiotics produced by *Dactylaria parvispora*, *J. Antibiot.*, 46, 48, 1993.
87. Otsuka, T., Shibata, T., Tsurumi, Y., Takase, S., Okuhara, M., Terano, H., Kohsaka, M., and Imanaka, H., A new angiogenesis inhibitor, FR-111142, *J. Antibiot.*, 45, 348, 1992.
88. Dixon, D. M., Walsh, T. J., Salkin, I. F., and Polak, A., *Dactylaria constricta*: another dematiaceous fungus with neotropic potential in mammals, *J. Med. Vet. Mycol.*, 25, 55, 1986.
89. de Hoog, G. S. and von Arx, J. A., Revision of *Scolecobasidium* and *Pleurophragmium*, *Kavaka*, 1, 55, 1973.
90. Dixon, D. M. and Salkin, I. F., Morphologic and physiologic studies of three dematiaceous pathogens, *J. Clin. Morphol.*, 24, 12, 1986.
91. Salkin, I. F. and Dixon, D. M., *Dactylaria constricta*: description of two varieties, *Mycotaxon*, 29, 377, 1987.
92. Cannon, P. F., Name changes in fungi of microbiological, industrial and medical importance. IV, *Mycopathologia*, 111, 75, 1990.
93. de Hoog, G. S., Taxonomy of *Dactylaria* complex, *Stud. Mycol.*, 26, 1, 1985.
94. Lagerberg, T., Lundberg, G., and Melin, E., Biological and practical research in pine and spruce, *Svenska Skogsv. For Tidskr.*, 25, 145, 1927.
95. Coldiron, B. M., Wiley, E. L., and Rinaldi, M. G., Cutaneous phaeohyphomycosis caused by a rare pathogen, *Hormonema dematioides*: successful treatment with ketoconazole, *J. Am. Acad. Dermatol.*, 23, 363, 1990.
96. Hermanides-Nijhof, E. J., *Aureobasidium* and allied genera, *Stud. Mycol.*, 15, 141, 1977.
97. de Hoog, G. S. and McGinnis, M. R., Ascomycetous black yeasts, *Stud. Mycol.*, 30, 187, 1987.
98. Salkin, I. F., Martinez, J. A., and Kemna, M. E., Opportunistic infection of the spleen caused by *Aureobasidium pullulans*, *J. Clin. Microbiol.*, 23, 828, 1986.
99. Kaczmarski, E. B., Liu Yin, J. A., Tooth, J. A., Love, E. M., and Delamore, I. W., Systemic infections with *Aureobasidium pullulans* in a leukemic patient, *J. Infect.*, 13, 289, 1986.
100. Vermeil, C., Gordeef, A., Leroux, M. J., Morin, O., and Bouc, M., Blastomycose cheloidienne a *Aureobasidium pullulans* (de Bary) Arnoud en Bretagne, *Mycopathol. Mycol. Appl.*, 43, 35, 1981.
101. Jones, F. R. and Christensen, G. R., *Pullaria* corneal ulcer, *Arch. Ophthalmol.*, 92, 529, 1974.
102. Akagi, M., Fujino, T., Hayashi, S. et al., A case of pulmonary infection caused by black yeast-like fungus, *Med. J. Osaka Univ.*, 8, 585, 1958.
103. Krcméry, V., Jr., Spanik, S., Danisovicova, Z., and Blahova, M., *Aureobasidium mansoni* meningitis in a leukemia patient successfully treated with amphotericin B, *Chemotherapy*, 40, 70, 1994.
104. Gordeef, A. and Leroux, M.-J., Peut-on parler, en Bretagne, d'une blastomycose cutanée possible a *Aureobasidium pullulans*. I. Etude clinique et anatomopathologique, *Bull. Soc. Fr. Mycol. Med.*, 16, 19, 1969.
105. Vermeil, C., Morin, O., and Bouc, M., Peut-on parler, en Bretagne, d'une blastomycose cutanée possible a *Aureobasidium pullulans*. II. Etude mycologique, *Bull. Soc. Fr. Mycol. Med.*, 16, 20, 1969.
106. Cole, G. T. and Kendrick, B., *Biology of the Conidial Fungi*, Vol. 2, Academic Press, New York, 1981, 121.
107. Cooke, W. B., An ecological life history of *Aureobasidium pullulans* (De Bary) Arnaud, *Mycopathol. Mycol. Appl.*, 12, 1, 1959.
108. Einarson, R. and Aukrust, L., Allergens of the fungi imperfect, *Clin. Rev. Allergy*, 10, 165, 1992.
109. Matsumoto, T., Ajello, L., Matsuda, T., Szaniszlo, P. J., and Walsh, T. J., Developments in hyalohyphomycosis and phaeohyphomycosis, *J. Med. Vet. Mycol.*, 32(Suppl. 1), 329, 1994.
110. Gergen, P. J., Turkeltaub, P. C., and Kovar, M. G., The prevalence of allergic skin test reactivity to eight common aeroallergens in the U.S. population: results from the second National Health and Nutrition Examination Survey, *J. Allergy Clin. Immunol.*, 80, 669, 1987.
111. Geis, P. A., Wheeler, M. H., and Szaniszlo, P. J., Pentaketide metabolites of melanin biosynthesis in the dematiaceous fungus *Wangiella dermatitidis*, *Arch. Microbiol.*, 137, 324, 1984.
112. Wheeler, M. H. and Stepanovic, R. D., Melanin biosynthesis and the metabolism of flaviolin and 3-hydroxyjuglone in *Wangiella dermatitidis*, *Arch. Microbiol.*, 142, 234, 1985.

113. Taylor, B. E., Wheeler, M. H., and Szaniszlo, P. J., Evidence for pentaketide melanin biosynthesis in dematiaceous human pathogenic fungi, *Mycologia*, 79, 320, 1987.

114. Dixon, D. M., Szaniszlo, P. J., and Polak, A., Dihydroxynaphthalene (DHN) melanin and its relationship with virulence in the early stages of phaeohyphomycosis, in *The Fungal Spore and Disease Initiation in Plants and Animals*, Cole, G. T. and Hoch, H. C., Eds., Plenum Press, New York, 1991, 297.

115. Geis, P. A. and Szaniszlo, P. J., Carotenoid pigments of the dematiaceous fungus *Wangiella dermatitidis*, *Mycologia*, 76, 268, 1984.

116. Szaniszlo, P. J., Geis, P. A., Jacobs, C. W., Cooper, C. R., and Harris, J. L., Cell wall changes associated with yeast-to-multicellular form conversion in *Wangiella dermatitidis*, in *Microbiology*, Vol. 83, Schlessinger, D., Ed., American Society for Microbiology, Washington, D.C., 1983, 239.

117. Dixon, D. M., Polak, A., and Szaniszlo, P. J., Pathogenicity and virulence of wild-type and melanin-deficient *Wangiella dermatitidis*, *J. Med. Vet. Mycol.*, 25, 97, 1987.

118. Dixon, D. M., Polak, A., and Conner, G. W., Mel mutants of *Wangiella dermatitidis* in mice: evaluation of multiple mouse and fungal strains, *J. Med. Vet. Mycol.*, 27, 335, 1989.

119. Dixon, D. M., Migliozzi, J., Cooper, C. R., Solis, O., Breslin, B. G., and Szaniszlo, P. J., Melanized and non-melanized multicellular-form mutants of *Wangiella dermatitidis* in mice: mortality and histopathology studies, *Mycoses*, 35, 17, 1992.

120. Polak, A. and Dixon, D. M., Loss of melanin in *Wangiella dermatitidis* does not result in greater susceptibility to antifungal agents, *Antimicrob. Agents Chemother.*, 33, 1639, 1989.

121. Polak, A., Melanin as a virulence factor in pathogenic fungi, *Mycoses*, 33, 215, 1989.

122. Dixon, D. M. and Polak-Wyss, A., The medically important dematiaceous fungi and their identification, *Mycoses*, 34, 1, 1991.

123. Polak, A. and Dixon, D. M., Pathogenicity of *Wangiella dermatitidis*, in *Dimorphic Fungi in Biology and Medicine*, vanden Bossche, H., Odds, F. C., and Kerridge, D., Eds., Plenum Press, New York, 1993, 307.

124. Matsumoto, T., Padhye, A. A., and Ajello, L., Medical significance of so- called black yeasts, *Eur. J. Epidemiol.*, 3, 87, 1987.

125. Zaias, N., Chromomycosis, *J. Cutan. Pathol.*, 5, 155, 1978.

126. Mizogami, I., Yamashita, K., Kawakami, I., and Matsumoto, I., On a case of chromoblastomycosis (or chromomycosis) originating in oropharynx, with special reference of the etiologic agent, *Pract. Otol.*, 52, 715, 1959.

127. Watanabe, S., Dematiaceous fungus infections, *Jpn. Med. J.*, 249, 31, 1961.

128. Shimazono, Y., Isaki, K., Torii, H., Otsuka, R., and Fukushiro, R., Brain abscess due to *Hormodendrum dermatitidis* (Kano) Conant, 1963: report of a case and review of the literature, *Folia Psych. Neurol. Jpn.*, 17, 80, 1963.

129. Sugawara, M., Sobajima, Y., and Tamura, H., A case of generalized chromoblastomycosis, *Acta Pathol. Jpn.*, 14, 239, 1964.

130. Takahashi, Y., Takahashi, S., Fukushi, G., and Kobayashi, K., A case in which a pathogenic dematiaceous fungus forming a yeast-like colony was isolated from the liver, *Jpn. J. Med. Mycol.*, 7, 42, 1966.

131. Hori, S., Sakurane, T., and Takagi, Y., A case of chromomycosis, *Jpn. J. Clin. Dermatol. Urol.*, 20, 1191, 1966.

132. Tsai, C. Y., Lu, Y. C., Wang, L. T., Hsu, T. L., and Sung, J. L., Systemic chromoblastomycosis due to *Hormodendrum dermatitidis* (Kano) Conant, *Am. J. Clin. Pathol.*, 46, 103, 1966.

133. Jen, T. M., Mycological study of *Hormodendrum dermatitidis* (*Fonsecaea dermatitidis*) isolated from the cervical lymph node of a Chinese in Taiwan (Formosa), China, *J. Formos. Med. Assoc.*, 65, 650, 1966.

134. Urabe, H., Yasumoto, K., and Nakashima, K., A case of chromoblastomycosis: probable involvement of central nervous system, *Jpn. J. Dermatol. Urol.*, 29, 1012, 1967.

135. Urabe, H., Nakama, T., and Nakahara, T., A case of chromoblastomycosis, *Jpn. J. Dermatol.*, 79, 775, 1969.

136. Hirayama, A., Takahashi, S., and Kasai, T., Chromomycosis of liver and brain, *Jpn. J. Med. Mycol.*, 12, 237, 1971.

137. Fujiwara, N., Mori, Y., Kamihata, S., Takami, T., Tsuru, K., and Mori, A., Six cases of chromomycosis, *Skin Res. (Osaka)*, 14, 297, 1972.

138. Saruta, T. and Nakamizo, Y., A case of chromomycosis, *Nishinihon J. Dermatol.*, 35, 9, 1973.

139. Harada, S., Ueda, T., and Kusunoki, T., Systemic chromomycosis, *J. Dermatol. (Tokyo)*, 3, 13, 1976.

140. Watanabe, S., Takigawa, M., and Aoshima, T., A case of chromomycosis, *Jpn. J. Med. Mycol.*, 16, 231, 1976.

141. Matsuzaki, O., Furuya, H., and Saruta, T., Chromomycosis in siblings, *Jpn. J. Med. Mycol.*, 17, 239, 1977.

142. Honbo, S., Kiryu, H., Nishio, K., and Urabe, H., Chromomycosis exclusively involving lymph nodes, *Jpn. J. Med. Mycol.*, 19, 47, 1978.

143. Hohl, P. E., Holly, H. P., Jr., Prevost, E., Ajello, L., and Padhye, A. A., *Wangiella dermatitidis* infections in humans: first documented case from the United States with review of the literature, *Rev. Infect. Dis.*, 5, 854, 1983.

144. Levenson, J. E., Gardner, S. K., Duffin, R. M., and Pettit, T. H., Dematiaceous fungal keratitis following penetrating keratoplasty, *Ophthal. Surg.*, 15, 578, 1984.

145. Takase, T., Chromomycosis due to *Exophiala dermatitidis*: report of a case with asteroid tissue forms, *Jpn. J. Med. Mycol.*, 26, 81, 1985.

146. Vartian, C. V., Shlaes, D. M., Padhye, A. A., and Ajello, L., *Wangiella dermatitidis* endocarditis in an intravenous drug user, *Am. J. Med.*, 78, 703, 1985.

147. Scott, J. W., Luckie, J., Pfister, W. C., Standard, P. G., Bohan, C. A., and Breazeale, R. D., Phaeohypho-mycotic cyst caused by *Wangiella dermatitidis*, *Mykosen*, 29, 243, 1986.

148. Cuce, L. C., Selebian, A., Porto, E., de Melo, N. T., and da Lacaz, C., Feo-hifomicose transplantada renal por *Exophiala dermatitidis* (Kano) de Hoog, 1977, *An. Bras. Dermatol.*, 61, 207, 1986.

149. Ventin, M., Ramirez, C., and Garau, J., *Exophiala dermatitidis* de Hoog from a vulvular aortal prothesis, *Mycopathologia*, 99, 45, 1987.

150. Hiruma, M., Yamachi, K., Shimizu, T., Ohata, H., and Kukita, J., Systemic *Exophiala dermatitidis* infection, *Jpn. J. Med. Mycol.*, 29, 24, 1988.

151. Collee, G., Verhoef, L. M. H., van't Wout, J. W., Van Brummelen, P., Eulderink, F., and Dijkmans, B. A. C., Tenosynovitis caused by *Exophiala mansonii* in an immunocompromised host, *Arthritis Rheum.*, 31, 1213, 1988.

152. Crosby, J. H., O'Quinn, M. H., Steele, J. C. H., and Rao, R. N., Fine-needle aspiration of subcutaneous phaeohyphomycosis caused by *Wangiella dermatitidis*, *Diag. Cytopathol.*, 5, 293, 1989.

153. Barenfanger, J., Ramirez, F., Tewari, R. P., and Eagleton, L., Pulmonary phaeohyphomycosis in a patient with hemoptysis, *Chest*, 95, 1158, 1989.

154. Sharkey, P. K., Graybill, J. R., Rinaldi, M. G., Stevens, D. A., Tucker, R. M., Peterie, J. D., Hoeprich, P. D., Greer, D. L., Frenkel, L., Counts, G. W., Goodrich, J., Zellner, S., Bradsher, R. W., van der Horst, C., Israel, K., Pankey, G. A., and Barranco, C. P., Itraconazole treatment of phaeohypho-mycosis, *J. Am. Acad. Dermatol.*, 23, 577, 1990.

155. Margo, C. E. and Fitzgerald, C. R., Postoperative endophthalmitis caused by *Wangiella dermatitidis*, *Am. J. Ophthalmol.*, 110, 322, 1990.

156. Pospisil, L., Skorkovska, S., and Moster, M., Corneal phaeohyphomycosis caused by *Wangiella dermatitidis*, *Ophthalmologica*, 201, 128, 1990.

157. Matsumoto, T., Matsuda, T., and McGinnis, M. R., A previously undescribed synanamorph of *Wangiella dermatitidis*, *J. Med. Vet. Mycol.*, 28, 437, 1990.

158. Matsumoto, T., Matsuda, T., Padhye, A. A., Standard, P. G., and Ajello, L., Fungal melanonychia: unusual phaeohyphomycosis caused by *Wangiella dermatitidis*, *Clin. Exp. Dermatol.*, 17, 83, 1992.

159. Kenney, R. T., Kwon-Chung, K. J., Waytes, A. T., Melnick, D. A., Pass, H. I., Merino, M. J., and Gallin, J. I., Successful treatment of systemic *Exophiala dermatitidis* infection in a patient with chronic granulomatous disease, *Clin. Infect. Dis.*, 14, 235, 1992.

160. Bennett, J. E., Bonner, H., Jennings, A. E., and Lopez, R. I., Chronic meningitis caused by *Cladosporium trichoides*, *Am. J. Clin. Pathol.*, 59, 398, 1973.

161. Salaki, J. S., Louria, D. B., and Chmel, H., Fungal and yeast infections of the central nervous system: a clinical view, *Medicine (Baltimore)*, 63, 108, 1984.

162. Estes, S. A., Merz, W. G., and Maxwell, L. G., Primary cutaneous phaeohyphomycosis caused by *Drechslera spicifera*, *Arch. Dermatol.*, 113, 813, 1977.

163. Drouhet, E. and Dupont, B., Laboratory and clinical assessment of ketoconazole in deep-seated mycoses, *Am. J. Med.*, 74(Suppl. 1B), 30, 1983.

164. Sobol, S. M., Love, R. G., Stutman, H. R., and Pysher, T. J., Phaeohyphomycosis of the maxilloethmoid sinus caused by *Drechslera spicifera*: a new fungal pathogen, *Laryngoscope*, 94, 620, 1984.
165. Maskin, S. L., Fetchick, R. J., Leone, C. R., Sharkey, P. K., and Rinaldi, M. G., *Bipolaris hawaiiensis*-caused phaeomycotic orbitopathy, *Ophthalmology*, 96, 175, 1989.
166. Washburn, R. G., Kennedy, D. W., Begley, M. G., Henderson, D. K., and Bennett, J. E., Chronic fungal sinusitis in apparently normal hosts, *Medicine (Baltimore)*, 67, 231, 1988.
167. Noel, S. B., Greer, D. L., Abadie, S. M., Zachary, J. A., and Pankey, G. A., Primary cutaneous phaeohyphomycosis, *J. Am. Acad. Dermatol.*, 18, 1023, 1988.
168. Wiest, P. M., Wiese, K., Jacobs, M. R., Morrissey, A. B., Abelson, T. I., Witt, W., and Lederman, M. M., *Alternaria* infection in a patient with the acquired immunodeficiency syndrome: case report and review of invasive *Alternaria* infections, *Rev. Infect. Dis.*, 9, 799, 1987.
169. Ganer, A., Arathoon, E., and Stevens, D. A., Initial experience in therapy for progressive mycoses with itraconazole, the first clinically studied triazole, *Rev. Infect. Dis.*, 9, 77, 1987.
170. Tucker, R. M., Williams, P. L., Arathoon, E. G., and Stevens, D. A., Treatment of mycoses with itraconazole, *Ann. NY Acad. Sci.*, 544, 451, 1988.
171. Frenkel, L., Kuhls, T. L., Nitta, K., Clancy, M., Howard, D. A., Ward, P., and Cherry, J. D., Recurrent *Bipolaris spicifera* following surgical and antifungal therapy, *Pediatr. Infect. Dis. J.*, 6, 1130, 1987.
172. Kotylo, P. K., Israel, K. S., Cohen, J. S., and Bartlett, M. S., Subcutaneous phaeohyphomycosis of the finger caused by *Exophiala spicifera*, *Am. J. Clin. Pathol.*, 91, 624, 1989.
173. Ajello, L., Iger, M., Wybel, R., and Vigil, F. J., *Drechslera rostrata* as an agent of phaeohyphomycosis, *Mycologia*, 72, 1094, 1980.
174. Young, C. N., Swart, J. G., Ackermann, D., and Davidge-Pitts, K., Nasal obstruction and bone erosion caused by *Drechslera hawaiiensis*, *J. Laryngol. Otol.*, 92, 137, 1978.
175. Koshi, G., Anandi, V., Kurien, M., Kirubakaran, M. G., Padhye, A. A., and Ajello, L., Nasal phaeohyphomycosis caused by *Bipolaris hawaiiensis*, *J. Med. Vet. Mycol.*, 25, 397, 1987.
176. Fuste, F. J., Ajello, L., Threlkeld, R., and Henry, J. E., Jr., *Drechslera hawaiiensis*: causative agent of a fatal fungal meningo-encephalitis, *Sabouraudia*, 11, 59, 1973.
177. Forster, R. K., Rebell, G., and Wilson, L. A., Dematiaceous fungal keratitis, *Br. J. Ophthalmol.*, 59, 372, 1975.
178. Dolan, C. T., Weed, L. A., and Dines, D. E., Bronchopulmonary helminthosporiosis, *Am. J. Clin. Pathol.*, 53, 235, 1970.
179. Morton, S. J., Midthun, K., and Merz, W. G., Granulomatous encephalitis by *Bipolaris hawaiiensis*, *Arch. Pathol. Lab. Med.*, 110, 1183, 1986.
180. Drouhet, E., Guilmet, D., Kouvalchouk, J. F., Chapman, A., Ziza, J. M., Laudet, J., and Brodaty, D., Premier cas humain de mycose a *Drechslera longirostrata*, *Nouv. Presse Med.*, 11, 3631, 1982.
181. Koenig, H., Warter, A., Bievre, C., De Waller, J., Weitzeblum, E., and Morand, G., Mycose pulmonaire a *Drechslera hawaiiensis*, *Bull. Soc. Fr. Mycol. Med.*, 13, 373, 1984.
182. Padhye, A. A., Ajello, L., Wieden, M. A., and Steinbronn, K. K., Phaeohyphomycosis of the nasal sinuses by a new species of *Exserohilum*, *J. Clin. Microbiol.*, 24, 245, 1986.
183. Antoine, G. A. and Raternik, M. H., *Bipolaris*, a serious new fungal pathogen of the paranasal sinus, *Otolaryngol. Head Neck Surg.*, 100, 158, 1989.
184. Merz, W. G., Karp, J. E., Hoagland, M., Jettgoheen, M., Junkins, J. M., and Hood, A. F., Diagnosis and successful treatment of fusariosis in the compromised host, *J. Infect. Dis.*, 158, 1046, 1988.
185. Costa, A. R., Porto, E., Tabuti, A. H., and da Lacaz, C., Subcutaneous phaeohyphomycosis caused by *Bipolaris hawaiiensis*: a case report, *Rev. Inst. Med. Trop. Sao Paolo*, 33, 74, 1991.
186. Jacobson, M., Galetta, S. L., Atlas, S. W., Curtis, M. T., and Wulc, A. W., *Bipolaris*-induced orbital cellulitis, *J. Clin. Neuro-Ophthalmol.*, 12, 250, 1992.
187. Straka, B. F., Cooper, P. H., and Body, B. A., Cutaneous *Bipolaris spicifera* infection, *Arch. Dermatol.*, 125, 1383, 1989.
188. Jay, W. M., Bradsher, R. W., Lemay, B., Snyderman, N., and Angtuago, E. J., Ocular involvement in mycotic sinusitis caused by *Bipolaris*, *Am. J. Ophthalmol.*, 105, 366, 1988.
189. Kershaw, P., Freeman, R., Templeton, D., DeGirolami, P. C., DeGirolami, U., Tarsy, D., Hoffman, S., Eliopoulos, G., and Karchmer, A. W., *Pseudallescheria boydii* infection of the central nervous system, *Arch. Neurol.*, 47, 468, 1990.

190. McGinnis, M. R., Campbell, G., Gourley, W. K., and Lucia, H. L., Phaeohyphomycosis caused by *Bipolaris spicifera*: an informative case, *Eur. J. Epidemiol.*, 8, 383, 1992.

191. Burges, G. E., Walls, C. T., and Maize, J. C., Subcutaneous phaeohyphomycosis caused by *Exserohilum rostratum* in an immunocompetent host, *Arch. Dermatol.*, 123, 1346, 1987.

192. Brown, J. W. III, Nadell, J., Sanders, C. V., and Sardenga, L., Brain abscess caused by *Cladosporium trichoides* (bantianum): a case with paranasal sinus involvement, *South. Med. J.*, 69, 1519, 1976.

193. Yoshimori, R. N., Moore, R. A., Itabashi, H. H., and Fujikawa, D. F., Phaeohyphomycosis of brain: granulomatous encephalitis caused by *Drechslera spicifera*, *Am. J. Clin. Pathol.*, 77, 363, 1982.

194. Krachmer, J. H., Anderson, R. L., Binder, P. S., Waring, G. O., Rousey, J. J., and Meeks, E. S., *Helminthosporium* corneal ulcers, *Am. J. Ophthalmol.*, 85, 666, 1978.

195. Berry, A. J., Kerkering, T. M., Giordano, A. M., and Chiacone, J., Phaeohyphomycotic sinusitis, *Pediatr. Infect. Dis.*, 3, 150, 1984.

196. Morgan, M. A., Wilson, W. R., Neel, H. B. III, and Roberts, G. D., Fungal sinusitis in healthy and immunocompromised individuals, *Am. J. Clin. Pathol.*, 82, 597, 1984.

197. Shugar, M. A., Montgomery, W. W., and Hyslop, N. E., Jr., *Alternaria* sinusitis, *Ann. Otol.*, 90, 251, 1981.

198. Zapater, R. C., Albesi, E. J., and Garcia, G. H., Mycotic keratitis by *Drechslera spicifera*, *Sabouraudia*, 13, 295, 1975.

199. Harris, R., Smith, R. E., Wood, T. R., and Biddle, M., *Helminthosporium* corneal ulcers, *Ann. Ophthalmol.*, 10, 729, 1978.

200. Chin, G. N., Corneal perforation due to *Helminthosporium* and *Mima polymorpha*, *Ann. Ophthalmol.*, 10, 607, 1978.

201. Matthiesson, A. M., Allergic bronchopulmonary disease caused by fungi other than *Aspergillus*, *Thorax*, 36, 719, 1981.

202. Glancy, J. J., Elder, J. L., and McAleer, R., Allergic bronchopulmonary fungal disease without clinical asthma, *Thorax*, 36, 345, 1981.

203. McAleer, R., Kroenert, D. B., Elder, J. L., and Froudist, J. H., Allergic bronchopulmonary disease caused by *Curvularia lunata* and *Drechslera hawaiiensis*, *Thorax*, 36, 338, 1981.

204. Hendrick, D. J., Ellithorpe, D. B., Lyon, F., Hattier, P., and Salvaggio, J. E., Allergic bronchopulmonary helminthosporiosis, *Am. Rev. Respir. Dis.*, 126, 935, 1982.

205. Hiruma, M., Kawada, A., Ohata, H., Ohnishi, Y., Takahashi, H., Yamazaki, M., Ishibashi, A., Hatsuse, K., Kakihara, M., and Yoshida, M., Systemic phaeohyphomycosis caused by *Exophiala dermatitidis*, *Mycoses*, 36, 1, 1993.

206. Scott, J. W., Luckie, J., Pfister, W. C., Padhye, A. A., Standard, P. G., Bohan, C. A., and Breazeale, R. D., Phaeohyphomycosis cyst caused by *Wangiella dermatitidis*, *Mykosen*, 29, 243, 1986.

207. Barenfanger, J., Ramirez, F., Tewari, R. P., and Eagleton, L., Pulmonary phaeohyphomycosis in a patient with hemoptysis, *Chest*, 95, 1158, 1989.

208. Haase, G., Skopnik, H., and Kusenbach, G., *Exophiala dermatitidis* infection in cystic fibrosis, *Lancet*, 336, 188, 1990.

209. Dixon, D. M. and Polak, A., *In vitro* and *in vivo* drug studies with three agents of central nervous system phaeohyphomycosis, *Chemotherapy*, 33, 129, 1987.

210. McGinnis, M. R. and Padhye, A. A., *Exophiala jeanselmei*, a new combination for *Phialophora jeanselmei*, *Myxotaxon*, 1, 341, 1977.

211. Gold, W. L., Vellend, H., Salit, I. E., Campbell, I., Summerbell, R., Rinaldi, M., and Simor, A. E., Successful treatment of systemic and local infections to *Exophiala* species, 19, 339, 1994.

212. Di Salvo, A. F. and Chew, W. H., *Phialophora gougerotii*: an opportunistic fungus in a patient treated with steroids, *Sabouraudia*, 6, 241, 1968.

213. Mauceri, A. A., Cullen, S. L., Vandevelde, A. G., and Johnson, J. E., Flucytosine: an effective oral treatment for chromomycosis, *Arch. Dermatol.*, 109, 873, 1974.

214. Kotrajaras, R. and Chongsathien, S., Subcutaneous chromomycotic abscesses caused by *Phialophora gougerotii*, *Int. J. Dermatol.*, 18, 150, 1979.

215. South, D. A., Brass, C., and Stevens, D. A., Chromoblastomycosis: treatment with ketoconazole, *Arch. Dermatol.*, 117, 311, 1981.

216. Monroe, P. W. and Floyd, W. E., Chromohyphomycosis of the hand due to *Exophiala jeanselmei* — case report and review, *J. Hand Surg.*, 6, 370, 1981.

217. Hironaga, M., Mochizuki, T., and Watanabe, S., Cutaneous phaeohyphomycosis of the sole caused by *Exophiala jeanselmei* and its susceptibility to amphotericin B, 5-FC and ketoconazole, *Mycopathologia*, 79, 101, 1982.

218. Lisi, P. and Caraffini, S., Imported skin disease — a case of subcutaneous chromomycosis caused by *Phialophora gougerotii*, *Int. J. Dermatol.*, 22, 180, 1983.

219. Bambirra, E. A., Miranda, D., Nogueira, A. M., and Barbosa, C. S. P., Phaeohyphomycotic cyst: a clinicopathologic study of the first four cases described from Brasil, *Am. J. Trop. Med. Hyg.*, 32, 794, 1983.

220. Ziefer, A. and Connor, D. H., Phaeomycotic cyst: a clinico-pathologic study of twenty five patients, *Am. J. Trop. Med. Hyg.*, 29, 901, 1980.

221. Guého, E., Bonnefoy, A., Luboinski, J., Petitt, J.-C., and de Hoog, G. S., Subcutaneous granuloma caused by *Phialophora richardsiae*: case report and review of the literature, *Mycoses*, 32, 219, 1989.

222. Sudduth, E. J., Crumbley, A. J. III, and Farrar, W. E., Phaeohyphomycosis due to *Exophiala* species: clinical spectrum of disease in humans, *Clin. Infect. Dis.*, 15, 639, 1992.

223. Sabbaga, E., Tedesco-Marchesi, L. M., Lacaz, C. da S., Cucé, L. C., Salebian, H., Heins-Vaccari, E. M., Sotto, M. N., Valente, N. Y., Porto, E., and Levy Neto, M., Subcutaneous phaeohyphomycosis due to *Exophiala jeanselmei*: report of 3 cases in patients with kidney transplants, *Rev. Inst. Med. Trop. Sao Paolo*, 36, 175, 1994.

224. Emmons, C. W., *Phialophora jeanselmei* comb. n. from mycetoma of the hand, *Arch. Pathol.*, 39, 364, 1945.

225. Nielsen, H. S., Conant, N. F., Weinberg, T. et al., Report of a mycetoma due to *Phialophora jeanselmei* and undescribed characteristics of the fungus, *Sabouraudia*, 6, 330, 1968.

226. Youngchaiyud, U., Thasnakorn, P., Chantarakul, N. et al., Maduromycosis of the hand due to *Phialophora jeanselmei*, *Southeast Asian J. Trop. Med. Public Health*, 3, 138, 1972.

227. Thammayya, A. and Sanyal, M., *Exophiala jeanselmei* causing mycetoma pedis in India, *Sabouraudia*, 18, 91, 1980.

228. Pupaibul, K., Sindhuphak, W., and Chindaporn, A., Mycetoma of the hand caused by *Phialophora jeanselmei*, *Mykosen*, 25, 321, 1981.

229. Lewis, G. M., Hopper, M. E., Sachs, W., Cormia, F. E., and Potelunas, C. B., Mycetoma-like chromoblastomycosis affecting the hand, *J. Invest. Dermatol.*, 10, 155, 1948.

230. Schnadig, V. J., Long, E. G., Washington, J. M., McNeely, M. C., and Troum, B. A., *Phialophora verrucosa*-induced subcutaneous phaehyphomycosis, *Arch. Cytol.*, 30, 425, 1986.

231. Zackheim, H. S., Halde, C., Goodman, R. S., Marchasin, S., and Buncke, H. J., Jr., Phaeohyphomycotic cyst of the skin caused by *Exophiala jeanselmei*, *J. Am. Acad. Dermatol.*, 12, 207, 1985.

232. Annessi, G., Cimitan, A., Zambruno, G., and DiSilverio, A., Cutaneous phaeohyphomycosis due to *Cladosporium cladosporioides*, *Mycoses*, 35, 243, 1992.

233. Ravisse, P. and Vindas, A. J. R., Les kystes mycosiques: etude histopathologique, *Bull. Soc. Pathol. Exot.*, 74, 46, 1981.

234. Tintelnot, K., de Hoog, G. S., Thomas, E., Steudel, W.-L., Huebner, K., and Seeliger, H. P. R., Cerebral phaeohyphomycosis caused by an *Exophiala* species, *Mycoses*, 34, 239, 1989.

235. Manian, F. A. and Brischetto, M. J., Pulmonary infection due to *Exophiala jeanselmei*: successful treatment with ketoconazole, *Clin. Infect. Dis.*, 16, 445, 1993.

236. Hachisuka, H., Matsumoto, T., Kusihara, M., Nomura, H., Nakano, S., and Sasai, Y., Cutaneous phaeohyphomycosis caused by *Exophiala jeanselmei* after renal transplantation, *Int. J. Dermatol.*, 29, 198, 1990.

237. Sindhuphak, W., MacDonald, E., Head, E., and Hudson, R. D., *Exophiala jeanselmei* infection in a postrenal transplant patient, *J. Am. Acad. Dermatol.*, 13, 877, 1985.

238. Chuan, M.-T. and Wu, M.-C., Subcutaneous phaeohyphomycosis caused by *Exophiala jeanselmei*: successful treatment with itraconazole, *Int. J. Dermatol.*, 34, 563, 1995.

239. Whittle, D. I. and Kominos, S., Use of itraconazole for treating subcutaneous phaeohyphomycosis caused by *Exophiala jeanselmei*, *Clin. Infect. Dis.*, 21, 1068, 1995.

240. Schwinn, A., Strohm, S., Helgenberger, M., Rank, C., and Bröcker, E.-B., Phaeohyphomycosis caused by *Exophiala jeanselmei* treated with itraconazole, *Mycoses*, 36, 445, 1993.

241. Van Cutsem, J., Van Gerven, F., and Janssen, P. A. J., Activity of orally, topically, and parenterally administered itraconazole in the treatment of superficial and deep mycoses: animal models, *Rev. Infect. Dis.*, 9(Suppl. 1), S15, 1987.

242. McGinnis, M. R. and Hilger, A. E., in *Laboratory Diagnosis of Infectious Diseases: Principle and Practice*, Balows, A., Hausler, W. J., Jr., and Lennette, E. H., Eds., Springer-Verlag, New York, 1988, 687.

243. Matsumoto, T., Nishimoto, K., Kimura, K., Padhye, A. A., Ajello, L., and McGinnis, M. R., Phaeohyphomycosis caused by *Exophilia moniliae*, *Sabouraudia*, 22, 17, 1984.

244. Kettlewell, P., McGinnis, M. R., and Wilkinson, G. T., Phaeohyphomycosis caused by *Exophiala spinifera* in two cats, *J. Med. Vet. Mycol.*, 27, 257, 1989.

245. Padhye, A. A., Ajello, L., Chandler, F. W., Banos, J. E., Hernandez-Perez, E., Llerena, J., and Linares, L. M., Phaeohyphomycosis in El Salvador caused by *Exophiala spinifera*, *Am. J. Trop. Med. Hyg.*, 32, 799, 1983.

246. Padhye, A. A., Kaplan, W., Neuman, M. A., Case, P., and Radcliffe, G. N., Subcutaneous phaeohyphomycosis caused by *Exophiala spinifera*, *J. Med. Vet. Mycol.*, 22, 493, 1984.

247. Lacaz, C. da S., Porto, E., de Andrade, J. G., and de Tellhes Filo, F., Feohifomicose disseminada por *Exophiala spinifera*, *An. Bras. Dermatol.*, 59, 238, 1984.

248. Dai, W. L., Ren, Z. F., Wen, J. Z., Liu, H. Y., Chen, R. E., Wang, D. L., Li, R. Y., and Wang, X. H., First case of systemic phaeohyphomycosis caused by *Exophiala spinifera* in China, *Chinese J. Dermatol.*, 20, 13, 1987.

249. Rajam, R. V., Kandhari, K. C., and Thirumalacher, M. J., Chromoblastomycosis caused by a yeast-like dematiaceous fungus, *Mycopathol. Mycol. Appl.*, 9, 5, 1958.

250. Rinaldi, M., Recurrent *Exophiala spinifera* diagnosed in a patient with a renal allograft, *Mycol. Observer*, 7, 1, 1987.

251. Chevrant-Breton, J., Boisseau-Lebreuil, M., Freour, E., Guiguen, G., Launois, B., and Guelfi, J., Les alternarioses cutanées humaines: a propos de 2 cas. Revie de la literature, *Ann. Dermatol. Venereol.*, 108, 653, 1981.

252. Duffill, M. B. and Coley, K. E., Cutaneous phaeohyphomycosis due to *Alternaria alternata* responding to itraconazole, *Clin. Exp. Dermatol.*, 18, 156, 1993.

253. Bang Pedersen, N., Mardh, P. A., Hallberg, T., and Jonsson, N., Cutaneous alternariosis, *Br. J. Dermatol.*, 94, 201, 1976.

254. Mirkin, L. D., *Alternaria alternata* infection of skin in a 6-year-old boy with aplastic anemia, *Pediatr. Pathol.*, 14, 757, 1994.

255. Kasperlik-Zaluska, A. A. and Bielunska, S., Effect of mitotane on *Alternaria alternata* infection in Cushing's syndrome, *Lancet*, 337, 53, 1991.

256. Rovira, M., Marin, P., Martin-Ortega, E., Montserrat, E., and Razman, L., *Alternaria* infection in a patient receiving chemotherapy for lymphoma, *Acta Haematol.*, 84, 98, 1990.

257. Singh, S. M., Naidu, J., and Pouranik, M., Ungual and cutaneous phaeohyphomycosis caused by *Alternaria alternata* and *Alternaria chlamydospora*, *J. Med. Vet. Mycol.*, 28, 275, 1990.

258. Ajello, L., Fungal infections in AIDS: a review, *L'Igiene Moderna*, 100, 288, 1993.

259. Iwatsu, T., Cutaneous alternariosis, *Arch. Dermatol.*, 124, 1822, 1988.

260. Di Silverio, A. and Sacchi, S., Cutaneous alternariosis: a rare chromoblastomycosis: report of a case, *Mycopathologia*, 95, 159, 1986.

261. Castanet, J., Lacour, J. P., Toussaint-Gary, M., Perrin, C., Rodot, S., and Ortonne, J. P., Infection cutanée pluri-focale a *Alternaria tenuissima*, 122, 115, 1995.

262. Bouthenet, M. F., Guyenne, C., Bonnin, A., Camerlynck, P., and Lambert, D., Cas pour diagnostic, *Ann. Dermatol. Venereol.*, 120, 169, 1993.

263. Panagiotidou, D., Kapetis, E., Chrysomallis, F. et al., Deux cas d'altérnariose cutanée an Gréce, *J. Mycol. Med.*, 1, 1, 1991.

264. Camenen, I., De Closets, F., Vaillant, L., De Muret, A., Pillette, M., Fouquet, B., and Lorette, G., Alternariose cutanée a *Alternaria tenuissima*, *Ann. Dermatol. Venereol.*, 115, 839, 1988.

265. Lulin, J., Lancien, G., Sandron, A. et al., Alternariose cutanée: a propos d'un nouveau cas, *Nouv. Dermatol.*, 9, 183, 1990.

266. Mitchell, A. J., Solomon, A. R., Beneke, E. S., and Anderson, T. F., Subcutaneous alternariosis, *J. Am. Acad. Dermatol.*, 8, 673, 1983.

267. Blanc, C., Lamey, B., and Lapalu, J., Alternariose cutanée chez, un transplante renal, *Bull. Soc. Fr. Mycol. Med.*, 13, 213, 1984.

268. Schillinger, F., Bressieux, J. M., Montagnac, R., and Hopfner, C., Les alternarioses humaines: analyse de la littérature a propos d'un cas personnel, *Semin. Hop. Paris*, 62, 1369, 1986.

269. Repiso, T., Martin, N., Huguet, P., Luelmo, J., Roca, M., Gonzalez-Castro, U., Margarit, C., and Castells, A., Cutaneous alternariosis in a liver transplant recipient, *Clin. Infect. Dis.*, 16, 729, 1993.

270. Benedict, L. M., Kusne, S., Torre-Cisneros, J., and Hunt, S. J., Primary cutaneous fungal infection after solid organ transplantation: report of five cases and review, *Clin. Infect. Dis.*, 15, 17, 1992.

271. Wätzig, V. and Schmidt, U., Primäre kutane granulomatöse alternariose, *Hautarzt.*, 40, 718, 1989.

272. Lanigan, A. W., Cutaneous *Alternaria* infection treated with itraconazole, *Br. J. Dermatol.*, 127, 39, 1992.

273. Guerin, V., Barbaud, A., Duquenne, M., Contet-Audonneau, N., Amiot, F., Ortega, F., and Hartemann, P., Cushing's disease and cutaneous alternariosis, *Arch. Intern. Med.*, 151, 1863, 1991.

274. Mardh, P. A. and Hallberg, T., *Alternaria alternata* as a cause of opportunistic fungal infection in man, *Scand. J. Infect. Dis. Suppl.*, 16, 36, 1978.

275. Schlueter, D. P., Fink, J. N., and Hensley, G. T., Wood-pulp workers' disease: a hypersensitivity pneumonia caused by *Alternaria*, *Ann. Intern. Med.*, 77, 907, 1972.

276. Lobritz, R. W., Roberts, T. H., Marrato, R. V., Carlton, P. K., and Thorp, D. J., Granulomatous pulmonary disease secondary to *Alternaria*, *JAMA*, 241, 596, 1979.

277. Bartynski, J. M., McCaffrey, T. V., and Frigas, E., Allergic fungal sinusitis secondary to dematiaceous fungi — *Curvularia lunata* and *Alternaria*, *Otolaryngol. Head Neck Surg.*, 103, 32, 1990.

278. Manning, S. C., Schaaefer, S. D., Close, L. G., and Vuich, F., Culture-positive allergic fungal sinusitis, *Arch. Otolaryngol. Head Neck Surg.*, 117, 174, 1991.

279. Rummelt, V., Ruprecht, K. W., Boltze, H. J., and Naumann, G. O. H., Chronic *Alternaria alternata* endophthalmitis following intraocular lens implantation, *Arch. Ophthalmol.*, 109, 178, 1991.

280. Chang, S.-W., Tsai, M.-W., and Hu, F.-R., Deep *Alternaria* keratomycosis with intraocular extension, *Am. J. Ophthalmol.*, 117, 544, 1994.

281. Simmons, R. B., Buffington, J. R., Ward, M., Wilson, L. A., and Ahearn, D. G., Morphology and ultrastructure of fungi in extended-wear soft contact lenses, *J. Clin. Microbiol.*, 24, 21, 1986.

282. Azar, P., Aquavella, J. V., and Smith, R. S., Keratomycosis due to an *Alternaria* species, *Am. J. Ophthalmol.*, 79, 881, 1975.

283. Moulsdale, M. T., Harper, J. M., and Thatcher, G. N., Fungal peritonitis: complication of continuous ambulatory peritoneal dialysis, *Med. J. Aust.*, 1, 88, 1981.

284. Garau, J., Diamond, R. D., Lagrotteria, L. V., and Kabins, S. A., *Alternaria* osteomyelitis, *Ann. Intern. Med.*, 86, 747, 1977.

285. Murtagh, J., Smith, J. W., and Mackowiak, P. A., Case report: *Alternaria* osteomyelitis: eight years of recurring disease requiring cyclic courses of amphotericin B for cure, *Am. J. Med. Sci.*, 293, 399, 1987.

286. Viviani, M. A., Tortorano, A. M., Laria, G., Giannetti, A., and Bignotti, G., Two cases of cutaneous alternariosis with a review of the literature, *Mycopathologia*, 96, 3, 1986.

287. Stenderup, J., Bruhn, M., Gadeberg, C., and Stenderup, A., Cutaneous alternariosis: case report, *Acta Pathol. Microbiol. Immunol. Scand.*, 95, 79, 1987.

288. Bourlond, A. and Alexandre, G., Dermal alternariosis in a kidney transplant recipient, *Dermatologica*, 168, 152, 1984.

289. Lévy-Klotz, B., Badillet, G., Cavelier-Balloy, B., Chemaly, P., Leverger, G., and Civatte, J., Alternariose cutanée au cours d'un SIDA, *Ann. Dermatol. Venereol.*, 112, 739, 1985.

290. Junkins, J. M., Beveridge, R. A., and Friedman, K. J., An unusual fungal infection in an immuno-compromised oncology patient: cutaneous alternariosis, *Arch. Dermatol.*, 124, 1421, 1988.

291. Sneeringer, R. M. and Haas, D. W., Cutaneous alternaria infection in a patient on chronic cortico-steroids, *J. Tenn. Med. Assoc.*, 83, 15, 1990.

292. Chaidemenos, G. Ch., Mourellou, O., Karakatsanis, G., Koussidou, T., Panagiotidou, D., and Kapetis, E., Cutaneous alternariosis in an immunocompromised patient, *Cutis*, 56, 145, 1995.

293. Machet, L., Machet, M.-C., Maillot, F., Cotty, F., Vaillant, L., and Lorette, G., Cutaneous alternariosis occurring in a patient treated with local intrarectal corticosteroids, *Acta Derm. Venereol. (Stockholm)*, 75, 328, 1995.

294. Quieffin, J., Milleron, B., Billet, S., Roux, P., Blanchet, P., and Akoun, G., Alternariose cutanée chez un malade atteint de corticosurrenalome malin metastase, *Presse Med.*, 19, 1462, 1990.
295. Meyers, J. D., Infection in bone marrow transplant recipients, *Am. J. Med.*, 81(Suppl. 1A), 27, 1986.
296. Aloi, F. G., Cervetti, O., and Forte, M., *Alternaria* mycosis in a kidney transplant patient, *G. Ital. Dermatol. Venereol.*, 122, 35, 1987.
297. Morrison, V. A., Haake, R. J., and Weisdorf, D. J., The spectrum of non-*Candida* fungal infections following bone marrow transplantation, *Medicine (Baltimore)*, 72, 78, 1993.
298. Morrison, V. A., Haake, R. J., and Weisdorf, D. J., Non-*Candida* fungal infections after bone marrow transplantation: risk factors and outcome, *Am. J. Med.*, 96, 497, 1994.
299. Galgóczy, J., Simon, G., and Valyi-Nagy, T., Case report: human cutaneous alternariosis, *Mycopathologia*, 92, 77, 1985.
300. Simal, E., Navarro, M., Rubio, M. C. et al., Sobre ub caso de alternariasis cutanea, *Actas Dermosifilogr.*, 77, 252, 1986.
301. Chen, H. C., Kao, H. F., Hsu, M. L., and Lee, J. Y., Cutaneous alternariosis in association with scabies or iatrogenic Cushing's syndrome, *J. Formos. Med. Assoc.*, 91, 462, 1992.
302. Male, D. and Pehamberger, H., Secondary cutaneous mycoses caused by *Alternaria* species, *Hautarzl.*, 37, 94, 1983.
303. Machet, M. C., Stephanov, E., Estève, E., De Closets, F., Barrabès, A., Thérizol-Ferly, M., Lebret, G., Grangeponte, M. C., and Vaillant, L., Alternariose cutanée survenant au cours de l'évolution d'un pemphigus traité, *Ann. Pathol.*, 14, 186, 1994.
304. Miegeville, M., Bureau, B., Morin, O., Berthello, J. M., and Prost, A., Nouveau cas d'alternariose cutanée chez un malade sous corticotherapie, *Bull. Soc. Fr. Mycol. Med.*, 18, 329, 1989.
305. Miegeville, M., Dutartre, H., Bureau, B., Lajat, Y., and Avranche, P., Nouveau cas d'alternariose cutanée chez un malade sous corticotherapie, *J. Mycol. Med.*, 1, 160, 1991.
306. Aznar, R., Marigil, J., Puig de la Bellacasa, J., Serrano, R., Lacasa, J., Ziad, F., and Velazquez, J., Cutaneous alternariosis responding to ketoconazole, *Lancet*, 1, 667, 1989.
307. Richardson, A. A., Agger, W. A., Ringstrom, J. B., and Kemnitz, M. J., Subcutaneous alternariosis of the foot in a patient on corticosteroids, *J. Am. Podiatr. Med. Assoc.*, 83, 472, 1993.
308. Del Palacio Hernanz, A., Conde-Zurita, J. M., Reyes Pecharroman, S., and Rodriguez Noriega, A., A case of *Alternaria alternata* (Fr) Keissler infection of the knee, *Clin. Exp. Dermatol.*, 8, 641, 1983.
309. Bourlond, A., Decroix, J., Dobbelaere, F., and Lissoir, A., Alternariose dermique, *Ann. Dermatol. Syphil.*, 101, 413, 1974.
310. Lucas Morante, T., Rotes Mas, I., Sabate de la Cruz, X., Bonin Lafuente, R., and Soler Ramon, J., Sindrome de Cushing con alternariosis cutanea, *Rev. Clin. Esp.*, 156, 133, 1980.
311. Verret, J. L., Gaborieau, F., Chabasse, D., Rohmer, V., Avenel, M., and Smulevici, A., Alternariose cutanée révélatrice d'une maladie de Cushing: un cas avec éetude ultrastructurale, *Ann. Dermatol. Venereol.*, 109, 841, 1982.
312. Male, O. and Pehamberger, H., Die kutane alternariose: fallberichte und literaturübersicht, *Mykosen*, 28, 278, 1985.
313. Findling, J. W., Tyrell, J. B., Aron, D. C., Fitzgerald, P. A., Young, C. W., and Sohne, P. G., Fungal infections in Cushing's syndrome, *Ann. Intern. Med.*, 95, 392, 1981.
314. Loli, P., Berselli, M. E., and Tagliaferri, M., Use of ketoconazole in the treatment of Cushing's syndrome, *J. Clin. Endocrinol. Metab.*, 63, 1365, 1986.
315. Diop, S. N., Warnet, A., Duet, M., Firmin, C., Mosse, A., and Lubetzki, J., Traitement prolongé de la maladie de Cushing par le kétoconazole: possibilité d'un échappement thérapeutique, *Presse Med.*, 18, 1325, 1989.
316. Bécherel, P.-A., Chosidow, O., and Francés, C., Cutaneous alternariosis after renal transplantation, *Ann. Intern. Med.*, 122, 71, 1995.
317. De Moragas, J. M., Prats, G., and Verger, G., Cutaneous alternariosis treated with miconazole, *Arch. Dermatol.*, 117, 292, 1981.
318. Shearer, C. and Chandrasekar, P. H., Cutaneous alternariosis and regional lymphadenitis during allogeneic BMT, *Bone Marrow Transplant.*, 11, 497, 1993.
319. Diaz, M., Puente, R., and Trevino, M. A., Response of long-running *Alternaria alternata* infection to fluconazole, *Lancet*, 336, 513, 1990.

320. Morrison, V. A. and Weisdorf, D. J., *Alternaria*: a sinonasal pathogen of immunocompromised hosts, *Clin. Infect. Dis.*, 16, 265, 1993.

321. Loveless, M. O., Winn, R. E., Campbell, M., and Jones, S. R., Mixed invasive infection with *Alternaria* species and *Curvularia* species, *Am. J. Clin. Pathol.*, 76, 491, 1981.

322. Body, B. A., Sabio, H., Oneson, R. H., Johnson, C. E., Kahn, J., and Hanna, M. D., *Alternaria* infection in a patient with acute lymphocytic leukemia, *Pediatr. Infect. Dis. J.*, 6, 418, 1987.

323. Stiller, R. L. and Stevens, D. A., Studies with a plant fungicide, imazalil, with vapor-phase activity, in the therapy of human alternariosis, *Mycopathologia*, 93, 169, 1986.

324. Chin, G. N., Hyndiuk, R. A., Kwasny, G. P., and Schultz, R. O., Keratomycosis in Wisconsin, *Am. J. Ophthalmol.*, 79, 121, 1975.

325. Wenkel, H., Rummelt, V., Knorr, H., and Naumann, G. O., Chronic postoperative endophthalmitis following cataract extraction and intraocular lens implantation: report on nine patients, *Ger. J. Ophthalmol.*, 2, 419, 1993.

326. Ando, N. and Takatori, K., Keratomycosis due to *Alternaria alternata* corneal transplant infection, *Mycopathologia*, 100, 17, 1987.

327. Parmalee, J. A., The identification of the *Curvalaria* parasite of gladiolus, *Mycologia*, 48, 558, 1956.

328. Friedman, A. D., Campos, J. M., Rorke, L. B., Bruce, D. E., and Arbeter, A. M., Fatal recurrent curvularia brain abscess, *J. Pediatr.*, 99, 413, 1981.

329. Baylet, J., Camain, R., and Segretain, G., Identification des agents des maduromycoses du Senegal et de la Mauritaine: description d'une espece nouvelle, *Bull. Soc. Path. Exot. Filiales*, 52, 448, 1959.

330. Mahgoub, E. S., Mycetomas caused by *Curvularia lunata*, *Madurella grisea*, *Aspergillus nidulans* and *Nocardia brasiliensis* in Sudan, *Sabouraudia*, 11, 179, 1973.

331. Berry, A. J., Kerkering, T. M., Giordano, A. M., and Chiancone, J., Phaeohyphomycotic sinusitis, *Pediatr. Infect. Dis. J.*, 3, 150, 1984.

332. Brummund, W., Kurup, V. P., Harris, G. J., Duncavage, J. A., and Arkins, J. A., Allergic sino-orbital mycosis: a clinical and immunologic study, *JAMA*, 256, 3249, 1986.

333. McMillan, R. H. III, Cooper, P. H., Body, B. A., and Mills, A. S., Allergic fungal sinusitis due to *Curvularia lunata*, *Hum. Pathol.*, 18, 960, 1987.

334. Killingsworth, S. M. and Wetmore, S. J., *Curvularia/Drechslera* sinusitis, *Laryngoscope*, 100, 932, 1990.

335. Rohwedder, J. J., Simmons, J. L., Colfer, H., and Gatmaitan, B., Disseminated *Culvularia lunata* infection in a football player, *Arch. Intern. Med.*, 139, 940, 1979.

336. Ismail, Y., Johnson, R. H., Wells, M. V., Pusavat, J., Douglas, K., and Arsura, E. L., Invasive sinusitis with intracranial extension caused by *Curvularia lunata*, *Arch. Intern. Med.*, 153, 1604, 1993.

337. Berg, D., Garcia, J. A., Schell, W. A., Perfect, J. R., and Murray, J. C., Cutaneous infection caused by *Curvularia pallescens*: a case report and review of the spectrum of disease, *J. Am. Acad. Dermatol.*, 32(2 part 2), 375, 1995.

338. Mroueh, S. and Spock, A., Allergic bronchopulmonary disease caused by *Curvularia* in a child, *Pediatr. Pulmonol.*, 12, 123, 1992.

339. de la Monte, S. M. and Hutchins, G. M., Disseminated curvularia infection, *Arch. Pathol. Lab. Med.*, 109, 872, 1985.

340. Pierce, N. F., Millan, J. C., and Bender, B. S., Disseminated *Curvularia* infection, *Arch. Pathol. Lab. Med.*, 110, 871, 1986.

341. Pierce, N. F., Millan, J. C., Bender, B. S., and Curtis, J. L., Disseminated *Curvularia* infection: additional therapeutic and clinical consideration with evidence of medical cure, *Arch. Pathol. Lab. Med.*, 110, 959, 1986.

342. Brubaker, L. H., Cure of *Curvularia* pneumonia by amphotericin B in a patient with megakaryotic leukemia, *Arch. Pathol. Lab. Med.*, 112, 1178, 1988.

343. Berlanga, J. J., Querol, S., Gallardo, D., Ferra, C., and Granena, A., Successful treatment of *Curvularia* sp. infection in a patient with primarily resistant acute promyelocytic leukemia, *Bone Marrow Transplant.*, 16, 617, 1995.

344. Bryan, C. S., Smith, C. W., Gerg, D. E., and Karp, R. B., *Curvularia lunata* endocarditis treated with terbinafine: case report, *Clin. Infect. Dis.*, 16, 30, 1993.

345. Corey, J. P., Allergic fungal sinusitis, *Otolaryngol. Clin. North Am.*, 25, 225, 1992.

346. Fitzsimons, R. and Peters, A. L., Miconazole and ketoconazole as a satisfactory first-line treatment for keratomycosis, *Am. J. Ophthalmol.*, 101, 605, 1986.

347. Foster, C. S., Miconazole therapy for keratomycosis, *Am. J. Ophthalmol.*, 91, 622, 1981.

348. Foster, C. S. and Stefanyszyn, M., Intraocular penetration of miconazole in rabbits, *Arch. Ophthalmol.*, 97, 1703, 1979.

349. Berger, S. T., Katsev, D. A., Mondino, B. J., and Pettit, T. H., Macroscopic pigmentation in a dematiaceous fungal keratitis, *Cornea*, 10, 272, 1991.

350. Subramanyam, V. R., Rath, C. C., Mishra, M., and Chhotrai, G. P., Subcutaneous infection due to *Curvularia* species, *Mycoses*, 36, 449, 1993.

351. Still, J. M., Jr., Law, E. J., Pereira, G. I., and Singletary, E., Invasive burn wound infection due to *Curvularia* species, *Burns*, 19, 77, 1993.

352. Yau, Y. C., de Nanassy, J., Summerbell, R. C., Matlow, A. G., and Richardson, S. E., Fungal sternal wound infection due to *Curvularia lanata* in a neonate with congenital heart disease: case report and review, *Clin. Infect. Dis.*, 19, 735, 1994.

353. Dixon, D. M., Walsh, T. J., Merz, W. G., and McGinnes, M. R., Infections due to *Xylohypha bantiana* (*Cladosporium trichoides*), *Rev. Infect. Dis.*, 11, 515, 1989.

354. Binford, C. H., Thompson, R. K., and Gorhan, M. E., Mycotic brain abscess due to *C. trichoides*, a new species: report of a case, *Am. J. Clin. Pathol.*, 22, 535, 1952.

355. Duque, O., Meningoencephalitis and brain abscess caused by *Cladosporium* and *Fonsecaea*: review of two cases and experimental studies, *Am. J. Clin. Pathol.*, 36, 505, 1961.

356. Felger, C. E. and Friedman, L., Experimental cerebral chromoblastomycosis, *J. Infect. Dis.*, 3, 1, 1962.

357. McGill, H. C. and Brueck, J. W., Brain abscess due to *Hormodendrum* species: report of third case, *Arch. Pathol.*, 62, 303, 1956.

358. Riley, O. and Mann, S. H., Brain abscess caused by *C. trichoides*: review of three cases and report of a fourth case, *Am. J. Clin. Pathol.*, 33, 525, 1960.

359. Segretain, G., Mariat, F., and Drouket, E., Sur *Cladosporium trichoides* isole d'une mycose cerebrale, *Ann. Inst. Pasteur*, 89, 465, 1955.

360. Desai, S. C., Bhatikar, M. L., and Mehta, R. S., Cerebral chromoblastomycosis due to *C. trichoides* (*bantianum*). II, *Neurol. India*, 14, 6, 1966.

361. Dereymaeker, A. and De Somer, P., Arachnoidite fibro-purulente cerebello-cervical due a une moissiure (*Cladosporium*), *Acta Neurol. Psychiatr. (Belgium)*, 55, 629, 1955.

362. Bobra, S. T., Mycotic abscess of the brain probably due to *Cladosporium trichoides*: report of the fifth case, *Can. Med. Assoc. J.*, 79, 657, 1958.

363. Horn, I. H., Wilanksy, D. L., Harland, A., and Blank, F., Neurogenic hypernatremia with mycotic brain granulomas due to *Cladosporium trichoides*, *Can. Med. Assoc. J.*, 83, 1314, 1960.

364. Sandhyamani, S., Bhatia, R., Mohopatra, L. N., and Roy, S., Cerebral cladosporiosis, *Surg. Neurol.*, 15, 431, 1981.

365. Türker, A., Altinörs, N., Aciduman, A., Demiralp, O., and Uluoglu, U., MPI findings and encouraging fluconazole treatment results of intracranial *Cladosporium trichoides* infection, *Infection*, 23, 60, 1995.

366. Barnola, J. and Ortega, A. A., *Cladosporium profunda*, *Mycopathol. Mycol. Appl.*, 15, 422, 1961.

367. Brown, J. W., Nadell, J., Sanders, C. V., and Sardenga, L., Brain abscess caused by *Cladosporium trichoides* (*bantianum*): a case with paranasal sinus involvement, *South. Med. J.*, 69, 1519, 1976.

368. Chrichlow, D. K., Enrile, F. T., and Memon, M. Y., Cerebellar abscess due to *Cladosporium trichoides* (*bantianum*): case report, *Am. J. Clin. Pathol.*, 60, 416, 1973.

369. King, A. B. and Collette, T. S., Brain abscess due to *Cladosporium trichoides*: report of the second case due to the organism, *Bull. Johns Hopkins Hosp.*, 91, 298, 1952.

370. Watson, K. C., Cerebral chromoblastomycosis, *J. Pathol. Bacteriol.*, 84, 233, 1962.

371. Kim, R. C., Hodge, C. D., Jr., Lamberson, H. V., Jr., and Weiner, L. B., Traumatic intracerebral implantation of *Cladosporium trichoides*, *Neurology*, 31, 1145, 1981.

372. Buxi, T. B., Prakash, K., Vohra, R., and Bhatia, D., Imaging in phaeohyphomycosis of the brain: case report, *Neuroradiology*, 38, 139, 1996.

373. Aldape, K. D., Fox, H. S., Roberts, J. P., Ascher, N. L., Lake, J. R., and Rowley, H. A., *Cladosporium trichoides* cerebral phaeohyphomycosis in a liver transplant recipient: report of a case, *Am. J. Clin. Pathol.*, 95, 499, 1991.

374. Wilson, E., Cerebral abscess caused by *Cladosporium bantiana*: case report, *Pathology*, 14, 91, 1982.
375. Goel, A., Satoskar, A., Desai, A. P., and Pandya, S. K., Brain abscess caused by *Cladosporium trichoides*, *Br. J. Neurosurg.*, 6, 591, 1992.
376. Borges, M. C., Warren, S., White, W., and Pellettiere, E. V., Pulmonary phaeohyphomycosis due to *Xylohypha bantiana*, *Arch. Pathol. Lab. Med.*, 115, 627, 1991.
377. Musella, R. A. and Collins, G. H., Cerebral chromoblastomycosis: case report, *J. Neurosurg.*, 35, 219, 1971.
378. Seaworth, B. J., Kwon-Chung, K. J., Hamilton, J. D., and Perfect, J. R., Brain abscess caused by a variety of *Cladosporium trichoides*, *Am. J. Clin. Pathol.*, 79, 747, 1983.
379. Ginzburg, H. M. and Macher, A. M., Clinical-pathological correlates of human immunodeficiency virus (HIV) infections: a conference summary, *Mod. Pathol.*, 1, 316, 1988.
380. Block, E. R., Jennings, A. E., and Bennett, J. E., Experimental therapy of cladosporiosis and sporotrichosis with 5-fluorocytosine, *Antimicrob. Agents Chemother.*, 3, 95, 1973.
381. Masini, T., Riviera, L., Capricci, E., and Arienta, C., Cerebral phaeohyphomycosis, *Clin. Neuropathol.*, 4, 246, 1985.
382. Middleton, F. G., Jurgenson, P. F., Utz, J. P., Shadomy, S., and Shadomy, H. J., Brain abscess caused by *C. trichoides*, *Arch. Intern. Med.*, 136, 444, 1976.
383. Limsila, T., Stiltnimankarn, T., and Prayad, T., Pulmonary *Cladosporium*: report of a case, *J. Med. Assoc. Thai*, 53, 586, 1970.
384. Dixon, D. M., Walsh, T. J., Salkin, I. F., and Polak, A., *Dactylaria constricta*: another dematiaceous fungus with neurotropic potential in mammals, *J. Med. Vet. Mycol.*, 25, 55, 1987.
385. Walsh, T. J., Dixon, D. M., Polak, A., and Salkin, I. F., Comparative histopathology of *Dactylaria constricta*, *Fonsecaea pedrosoi*, *Wangiella dermatitidis*, and *Xylohypha bantiana* in experimental phaeohyphomycosis of the central nervous system, *Mykosen*, 30, 215, 1987.
386. Kralovic, S. M. and Rhodes, J. C., Phaeohyphomycosis caused by *Dactylaria* (human dactylariosis): report of a case with review of the literature, *J. Infect.*, 31, 107, 1995.
387. Matsumoto, T. and Matsuda, T., Chromoblastomycosis and phaeohyphomycosis, *Semin. Dermatol.*, 4, 240, 1985.
388. Pitrak, D. L., Koneman, E. W., Estupinan, R. C., and Jackson, J., *Phialophora richardsiae* infection in humans, *Rev. Infect. Dis.*, 10, 1195, 1988.
389. Wong, P. K., Ching, W. T. W., Kwon-Chung, K. J., and Meyer, R. D., Disseminated *Phialophora parasitica* infection in humans: case report and review, *Rev. Infect. Dis.*, 11, 770, 1989.
390. Schnadig, V. J., Long, E. G., Washington, J. M., McNeely, M. C., and Troum, B. A., *Phialophora verrucosa*-induced subcutaneous phaeohyphomycosis, *Acta Cytol.*, 30, 425, 1986.
391. Ahmad, S., Johnson, R. J., Hillier, S., Shelton, W. R., and Rinaldi, M. G., Fungal peritonitis caused by *Lecythophora mutabilis*, *J. Clin. Microbiol.*, 22, 182, 1985.
392. Iwatsu, T. and Miyaji, M., Subcutaneous cystic granuloma caused by *Phialophora verrucosa*, *Mycopathologia*, 64, 165, 1977.
393. Fincher, R. M. E., Fisher, J. F., Padhye, A. A., Ajello, L., and Steele, J. C. H., Subcutaneous phaeo-hyphomycotic abscess caused by *Phialophora* parasitica in a renal allograft recipient, *J. Med. Vet. Mycol.*, 26, 311, 1988.
394. Gugnani, H. C., Obiefuna, M. N., and Ikerionwu, S. E., Studies on pathogenic dematiaceous fungi. II. Pathogenicity of *Fonsecaea pedrosoi* and *Phialophora verrucosa* for laboratory mice, *Mykosen*, 29, 505, 1986.
395. Rubin, H. A., Bruce, S., Rosen, T., and McBride, M. E., Evidence for percutaneous inoculation as the mode of transmission for chromoblastomycosis, *J. Am. Med. Dermatol.*, 25, 951, 1991.
396. Moskowitz, L. B., Cleary, T. J., McGinnis, M. R., and Thomson, C. B., *Phialophora richardsiae* in a lesion appearing as a giant cell tumor of the tendon sheath, *Arch. Pathol. Lab. Med.*, 107, 374, 1983.
397. Singh, S. M., Agrawal, A., Naidu, J., de Hoog, G. S., and Figueras, M. J., Cutaneous phacohyphomy-cosis caused by *Phialophora richardsiae* and the effect of topical clotrimazole in its treatment, *Antonie van Leeuwenhoek*, 61, 51, 1992.
398. Corrado, M. L., Kramer, M., Cummings, M., and Eng, R. H., Susceptibility of dematiaceous fungi to amphotericin B, miconazole, ketoconazole, flucytosine and rifampin alone or in combination, *Sabouraudia*, 20, 109, 1982.

399. Corrado, M. L., Weitzman, I., Stanek, A., Goetz, R., and Agyare, E., Subcutaneous infection with *Phialophora richardsiae* and its susceptibility to 5-fluorocytosine, amphotericin B and miconazole, *Sabouraudia*, 18, 97, 1980.

400. Weitzman, I., Gordon, M. A., Henderson, R. W., and Lapa, E. W., *Phialophora parasitica*, an emerging pathogen, *J. Med. Vet. Mycol.*, 22, 331, 1984.

401. Duggan, J. M., Wolf, M. D., and Kauffman, C. A., *Phialophora verrucosa* infection in an AIDS patient, *Mycoses*, 38, 215, 1995.

402. Listemann, H., Die kulturelle untersuchung eines tranensteines mit isolierung des pilzes *Phialophora richardsiae*, *Ernst Rodenwaldt Arch.*, 2, 45, 1975.

403. Torstrick, R. F., Harrison, K., Heckman, J. D., and Johnson, J. E., Chronic bursitis caused by *Phialophora richardsiae*, *J. Bone Joint Surg.*, 61, 772, 1979.

404. Yangco, B. G., TeStrake, D., and Okafor, J., *Phialophora richardsiae* isolated from infected human bone: morphological, physiological and antifungal susceptibility studies, *Mycopathologica*, 86, 103, 1981.

405. Tam, M. and Freeman, S., Phaeohyphomycosis due to *Phialophora richardsiae*, *Australas. J. Dermatol.*, 30, 37, 1989.

406. Torok, M., De Weck, A. L., and Scherrer, M., Allergic alveolitis as a result of mould on a bedroom wall, *Schweiz. Med. Wochenschr.*, 3, 924, 1981.

407. Kersten, W. and Hoek, G. T., Mould allergy, *Wien Med. Wochenschr.*, 130, 275, 1980.

408. Storms, W. W., Occupational hypersensitivity lung diseases, *J. Occup. Med.*, 20, 823, 1978.

409. Blyth, W., Grant, I. W., and Blackadder, E. S., Fungal antigen as a cause of sensitization and respiratory disease in Scottish maltworkers, *Clin. Allergy*, 7, 549, 1977.

410. Velcovsky, H. G. and Graubner, M., Allergic alveolitis following inhalation of mould spores from pot plant earth, *Dtsch. Med. Wochenschr.*, 106, 115, 1981.

411. Metzger, W. J., Patterson, R., Fink, J., Semerdjian, R., and Roberts, M., Sauna-takers' disease: hypersensitivity pneumonitis due to contaminated water in a home sauna, *JAMA*, 236, 2209, 1976.

412. Ashikaga, Ueber eine besondere neve art von keratomykosis, *Klin. MBL Augenheilk.*, 66, 934, 1921.

413. Koppang, H. S., Olsen, I., Stuge, U., and Sandven, P., *Aureobasidium* infection of the jaw, *J. Oral Pathol. Med.*, 20, 191, 1991.

414. Naim-ur-Rahman, el Sheikh Mahgoub, Abu Aisha, H., Laajam, M., Yaqoub, B., and Chagla, A. H., Cerebral phaeohyphomycosis, *Bull. Soc. Pathol. Exot. Filiales*, 80, 320, 1987.

415. Mitchell, D. M., Fitz-Henley, M., and Horner-Bryce, J., A case of disseminated phaeohyphomycosis caused by *Cladosporium devriesii*, *West Indian Med. J.*, 39, 118, 1990.

416. Buiting, A. G., Visser, L. G., Barge, R. M., and van't Wout, J. W., Mycetoma of the foot: a disease from the tropics, *Ned. Tijdschr. Geneeskd.*, 137, 1513, 1993.

417. DeVault, G. A., Brown, S. T. III, King, J. W., Fowler, M., and Oberle, A., Tenckhoff catheter obstruction resulting from invasion by *Curvularia lunata* in the absence of peritonitis, *Am. J. Kidney Dis.*, 6, 124, 1985.

418. Peterson, P. K., Matzke, G., and Keane, W. F., Current concepts in the management of peritonitis in patients undergoing continuous ambulatory peritoneal dialysis, *Rev. Infect. Dis.*, 9, 604, 1987.

419. Johnson, R. J., Ramsey, P. G., Gallagher, N., and Ahmad, S., Fungal peritonitis in patients on peritoneal dialysis: incidence, clinical features and prognosis, *Am. J. Nephrol.*, 5, 169, 1985.

420. Ahlmen, J., Edebo, L., Ericksson, C., Carlsson, L., and Torgersen, A. K., Fluconazole therapy for fungal peritonitis in continuous ambulatory peritoneal dialysis (CAPD): a case report, *Perit. Dial. Int.*, 9, 79, 1989.

421. Ujhelyi, M. R., Raasch, R. H., van der Horst, C. M., and Mattera, W. D., Treatment of peritonitis due to *Curvularia* and *Trichosporon* with amphotericin B, *Rev. Infect. Dis.*, 12, 621, 1990.

422. Lopes, J. O., Alves, S. H., Benevenga, J. P., Brauner, F. B., Castro, M. S., and Melchiors, E., *Curvularia lunata* peritonitis complicating peritoneal dialysis, *Mycopathologia*, 127, 65, 1994.

423. Brackett, R. W., Shenouda, A. N., Hawkins, S. S., and Brock, W. B., *Curvularia* infection complicating peritoneal dialysis, *South. Med. J.*, 81, 943, 1988.

424. Guarner, J., Del Rio, C., Williams, P., and McGowan, J. E., Fungal peritonitis caused by *Curvularia lunata* in a patient undergoing peritoneal dialysis, *Am. J. Med. Sci.*, 298, 320, 1989.

425. Buchanan, W. E., Quinn, M. J., and Hasbargen, J. A., Peritoneal catheter colonization with *Alternaria*: successful treatment with catheter preservation, *Perit. Dial. Int.*, 14, 91, 1994.

426. Kerr, C. M., Perfect, J. R., Craven, P. C., Jorgensen, J. H., Drutz, D. J., Shelburne, J. D., Gallis, H. A., and Gutman, R. A., Fungal peritonitis in patients with continuous ambulatory peritoneal dialysis, *Ann. Intern. Med.*, 99, 334, 1983.

427. O'Sullivan, F. X., Stuewe, B. R., Lynch, J. M., Brandsberg, J. W., Wiegmann, T. B., Patak, R. V., Barnes, W. G., and Hodges, G. R., Peritonitis due to *Drechslera spicifera* complicating continuous ambulatory peritoneal dialysis, *Ann. Intern. Med.*, 94, 213, 1981.

428. Clark, E. C., Silver, S. M., Hollick, G. E., and Rinaldi, M. G., Continuous ambulatory peritoneal dialysis complicated by *Aureobasidium pullulans* peritonitis, *Am. J. Nephrol.*, 15, 353, 1995.

429. Eisenberg, E. S., Leviton, I., and Soeiro, R., Fungal peritonitis in patients receiving peritoneal dialysis: experience with 11 patients and review of the literature, *Rev. Infect. Dis.*, 8, 309, 1986.

430. Tapson, J. S., Freeman, M. R., and Wilkinson, R., The high morbidity of CAPD fungal peritonitis — description of 10 cases and review of treatment strategies, *Q. J. Med.*, 61, 1047, 1986.

431. Struijk, D. G., Krediet, R. T., Boeschotcn, E. W., Rietra, P. J. G. M., and Arisz, L., Antifungal treatment of candida peritonitis in continuous ambulatory peritoneal dialysis patients, *Am. J. Kidney Dis.*, 9, 66, 1987.

432. Kerr, C. M., Perfect, J. R., Craven, P. C., Jorgensen, J. H., Drutz, D. J., Shelbourne, J. D., Gallis, H. A., and Gutman, R. A., Fungal peritonitis in patients on continuous ambulatory peritoneal dialysis, *Ann. Intern. Dis.*, 99, 334, 1983.

433. Ahmad, S., Johnson, R. J., Hillier, S., Shelton, W. R., and Rinaldi, M. G., Fungal peritonitis caused by *Lecythophora mutabilis*, *J. Clin. Microbiol.*, 22, 182, 1986.

434. Fabris, A., Biasioli, S., Chiaramonte, S., Feriani, M., Piacentini, I., Pisani, E., Ronco, C., Viviani, A., and LaGreca, G., An unusual form of *Fusarium verticillioides* peritonitis in a patient on chronic peritoneal dialysis, *Dialysis Transplant.*, 12, 644, 1983.

435. Cecchin, E., De Marchi, S., Panarello, G., Franceschin, A., Chiaradia, V., Santini, G., and Tesio, F., *Torulopsis glabrata* peritonitis complicating continuous peritoneal dialysis: successful management with oral 5-fluorocytosine, *Am. J. Kidney Dis.*, 4, 280, 1984.

436. Arfania, D., Everett, E. D., Nolph, K. D., and Rubin, J., Uncommon causes of peritonitis in patients undergoing peritoneal dialysis, *Arch. Intern. Dis.*, 141, 61, 1981.

437. Stammberger, H., Endoscopic surgery for mycotic and chronic recurring sinusitis, *Ann. Otol. Rhinol. Laryngol. Suppl.*, 119, 1, 1985.

438. Katzenstein, A. L. A., Sale, S. R., and Greenberger, P. A, Allergic *Aspergillus* sinusitis: a newly recognized form of sinusitis, *J. Allergy Clin. Immunol.*, 72, 89, 1983.

439. Jackson, I. T., Schmitt, E., and Carpenter, H. A., Allergic *Aspergillus* sinusitis, *Plast. Reconstr. Surg.*, 79, 804, 1987.

440. Haury, J. A., Rhinite pseudo-allergique sur *Aspegillose* sinnusale a propos d'un cas, *Rev. Méd. Suisee Romande*, 108, 613, 1988.

441. Goldstein, M. F., Atkins, P. C., Cogen, C., Kornstein, M. J., Levine, R. S., and Zweiman, B., Allergic *Aspergillus* sinusitis, *J. Allergy Clin. Immunol.*, 76, 515, 1985.

442. Phillip, G. and Keen, C. E., Allergic fungal sinusitis, *Histopathology*, 14, 22, 1989.

443. Waxman, J. E., Spector, J. G., Sale, S., and Katzenstein, A., Allergic *Aspergillus* sinusitis: concepts in diagnosis and treatment of a new clinical entity, *Laryngoscope*, 97, 261, 1987.

444. Goldstein, M. F., Atkins, P. C., Cogen, F. C., Kornstein, M. J., Levine, R. S., and Zweiman, B., Allergy grand rounds: allergic *Aspergillus* sinusitis, *J. Allergy Clin. Immunol.*, 75, 515, 1985.

445. Pratt, M. F. and Burnett, J. R., Fulminant *Drechslera* sinusitis in an immunocompetent host, *Laryngoscope*, 98, 1343, 1988.

446. Gourley, D. S., Whisman, B. A., Jorgensen, N. L., Martin, M. E., and Reid, M. J., Allergic *Bipolaris* sinusitis: clinical and immunopathologic characteristics, *J. Allergy Clin. Immunol.*, 85, 583, 1990.

447. Nishioka, G., Schwartz, J. G., Rinaldi, M. G., Aufdermorte, T. B., and Mackie, E., Fungal maxillary sinusitis caused by *Curvularia lunata*, *Arch. Otolaryngol. Head Neck Surg.*, 113, 665, 1987.

448. Corey, J. P., Romberger, C. F., and Shaw, G. Y., Fungal disease of the sinuses, *Otolaryngol. Head Neck Surg.*, 103, 1012, 1990.

449. Saffirstein, B., Allergic bronchopulmonary aspergillosis with obstruction of the upper respiratory tract, *Chest*, 70, 788, 1976.

450. Saffirstein, B., D'Souza, M., Simon, G., Tai, E. H.-C., and Pepys, J., Five year followup of allergic bronchopulmonary aspergillosis, *Am. Rev. Respir. Dis.*, 108, 450, 1973.

451. Ence, B. K., Gourley, D. S., Jorgensen, N. L. et al., Allergic fungal sinusitis, *Am. J. Rhinol.*, 4, 169, 1990.

452. Katzenstein, A. L. A., Sale, S. R., and Greenberger, P. A., Pathologic findings in allergic *Aspergillus* sinusitis: a newly recognized form of sinusitis, *Am. J. Surg. Pathol.*, 7, 439, 1983.

453. Gergen, P. J. and Turkeltaub, P. C., The association of individual allergen reactivity with respiratory disease in a national sample: data from the second National Health and Nutrition Survey, 1976–80 (NHANES II), *J. Allergy Clin. Immunol.*, 90, 579, 1992.

454. Licorish, K., Novey, H. S., Kozak, P., Fairshter, R. D., and Wilson, A. F., Role of *Alternaria* and *Penicillium* spores in the pathogenesis of asthma, *J. Allergy Clin. Immunol.*, 76, 819, 1985.

455. Bush, R. K., Fungal extracts in clinical practice, *Allergy Proc.*, 14, 385, 1993.

456. Bush, R. K. and Yunginger, J. W., Standardization of fungal allergens, *Clin. Rev. Allergy*, 5, 3, 1987.

457. Helbling, A., Reese, G., Horner, W. E., and Lehrer, S. B., Aktuelles zur pilzsporen-allergie, *Schweiz. Med. Wochenschr.*, 124, 885, 1994.

458. Malling, H.-J., Immunotherapy for mold allergy, *Clin. Rev. Allergy*, 10, 237, 1992.

459. Dhillon, M., Current status of mold immunotherapy, *Ann. Allergy*, 66, 385, 1991.

460. Bonifazi, F., Immunotherapy in pollen and mould asthma, *Monaldi Arch. Chest Dis.*, 49, 150, 1994.

461. Malling, H. J. and Stahl Skov, P., Diagnosis and immunotherapy of mould allergy. VIII. Qualitative and quantitative estimation of IgE in *Cladosporium* immunotherapy, *Allergy*, 43, 228, 1988.

462. Malling, H. J., Diagnosis and immunotherapy of mould allergy. IV. Relation between asthma symptoms, spore counts and diagnostic tests, *Allergy*, 41, 342, 1986.

463. Malling, H. J., Dreborg, S., and Weeke, B., Diagnosis and immunotherapy of mould allergy. III. Diagnosis of *Cladosporium* allergy by means of symptom score, bronchial provocation test, skin prick test, RAST, CRIE and histamine release, *Allergy*, 41, 57, 1986.

464. Malling, H. J. and Djurup, R., Diagnosis and immunotherapy of mould therapy. VII. IgG subclass response and relation to the clinical efficacy of immunotherapy with *Cladosporium*, *Allergy*, 43, 60, 1988.

465. Malling, H. J., Dreborg, S., and Weeke, B., Diagnosis and immunotherapy of mould allergy. VI. IgE-mediated parameters during a one-year placebo-controlled study of immunotherapy with *Cladosporium*, *Allergy*, 42, 305, 1987.

466. Ostergaard, P. A., Kaad, P. H., and Kristensen, T., A prospective study on the safety of immunotherapy in children with severe asthma, *Allergy*, 41, 588, 1986.

467. Karlsson, R., Agrell, B., Dreborg, S., Foucard, T., Kjellman, N.-I. M., Koivikko, A., and Einarsson, R., A double-blind, multicenter immunotherapy trial in children, using a purified and standardized *Cladosporium herbarum* preparation. II. *In vitro* studies, *Allergy*, 41, 141, 1986.

468. Dreborg, S., Agrell, B., Foucard, T., Kjellman, N.-I. M., Koivikko, A., and Nilsson, S., A double-blind, multicenter immunotherapy trial in children, using a purified and standardized *Cladosporium herbarum* preparation. I. Clinical results, *Allergy*, 41, 131, 1986.

469. Malling, H. J., Dreborg, S., and Weeke, B., Diagnosis and immunotherapy of mould allergy. V. Clinical efficacy and side effects of immunotherapy with *Cladosporium herbarum*, *Allergy*, 41, 507, 1986.

470. Milam, C. P. and Fenske, N. A., Chromoblastomycosis, *Dermatol. Clin. North Am.*, 7, 219, 1989.

471. Pedroso, A. and Gomes, J. M., Sobre quatro casos de dermatite verrucosa produzida pela *Phialophora verrucosa*, *Ann. Paulist Med. Ctr.*, 11, 53, 1920.

472. Rudolph, M., Uber die brasilianische "Figueira", *Arch. Schiffs Tropen-Hyg.*, 18, 498, 1914.

473. Medlar, E. M., A cutaneous infection caused by a new fungus, *Phialophora verrucosa*, with a study of the fungus, *J. Med. Res.*, 32, 507, 1915.

474. Lane, C. G., A cutaneous lesion caused by a new fungus (*Phialophora verrucosa*), *J. Cutan. Dis.*, 33, 840, 1915.

475. Campins, H. and Scharyj, M., Chromoblastomicosis comentarios sobre 24 casos, con estudio clinico, histologico y micologico, *Gac. Med. Caracas*, 61, 127, 1953.

476. Carrion, A. L., Chromoblastomycosis, *Ann. NY Acad. Sci.*, 50, 1255, 1985.

477. Boudghène-Stambouli, O. and Mérad-Boudia, A., Chromomycose: 2 observations, *Ann. Dermatol. Venereol.*, 121, 37, 1994.

478. Borelli, D., *Acrotheca aquaspersa* nova species de cromomicosis, *Acta Cient. Venez.*, 23, 193, 1972.

479. Al-Doury, Y., *Chromomycosis*, Mountain Press, Missoula, Montana, 1972, 1.

480. Nishimoto, K., Yoshimura, S., and Honma, K., Chromomycosis spontaneously healed, *Int. J. Dermatol.*, 23, 408, 1984.

481. Tuffanelli, L. and Milburn, P. B., Treatment of chromoblastomycosis, *J. Am. Acad. Dermatol.*, 23, 728, 1990.

482. Dai, W., Approach of nonoperative therapy in cutaneous chromomycosis, *Chin. J. Dermatol.*, 20, 160, 1987.

483. Kwon-Chung, K. J. and Bennett, J., *Medical Mycology*, Lea & Febiger, Philadelphia, 1992, 337.

484. Kuttner, B. J. and Siegle, R. J., Treatment of chromomycosis with a CO_2 laser, *J. Dermatol. Surg. Oncol.*, 12, 965, 1986.

485. Lubritz, R. R. and Spence, J. E., Chromoblastomycosis: cure by cryosurgery, *Int. J. Dermatol.*, 17, 830, 1978.

486. Tagami, H., Ginoza, M., Imaizumi, S., and Urano-Suehisa, S., Successful treatment of chromoblastomycosis with topical heat therapy, *J. Am. Acad. Dermatol.*, 10, 615, 1984.

487. Tagami, H., Ohi, M., Aoshima, T., Moriguchi, M., Suzuki, N., and Yamada, M., Topical heat therapy for cutaneous chromomycosis, *Arch. Dermatol.*, 115, 740, 1979.

488. Campbell, I. T., Reis, C., Faria, E., and Campbell, G. A. M., Chromomycose: traitement par thermothérapie, *Nouv. Dermatol.*, 10, 468, 1991.

489. Yanase, K. and Yamada, M., "Pocket-warmer" therapy of chromomycosis, *Arch. Dermatol.*, 114, 1035, 1978.

490. Clark, R. F., Chromoblastomycosis of the ear: successful intralesional therapy with amphotericin B, *Cutis*, 24, 326, 1979.

491. Costello, M. J., DeFeo, C. P., Jr., and Littman, M. L., Chromoblastomycosis treated with local infitration of amphotericin B solution, *Arch. Dermatol.*, 79, 184, 1959.

492. Whiting, D. A. and Cloete, G. N. P., Chemotherapy and conservative surgery in the treatment of chromoblastomycosis, *S. Afr. Med. J.*, 42, 883, 1968.

493. Bopp, C., Cura de cromoblastomicose por novo método de tratamento, *Med. Cutan. Iber. Lat. Am.*, 4, 883, 1976.

494. Lopes, C. F., Alvarenga, R. J., Cisalpino, E. O., Resende, M. A., and Oliveira, L. G., Six years' experience in treatment of chromomycosis with 5-fluorocytosine, *Int. J. Dermatol.*, 17, 414, 1978.

495. Oliveira, L. G., Rezende, M. A., Cisalpino, E. O., Figueiredo, Y. P., and Lopes, C. F., *In vitro* sensitivity to 5-fluorocytosine of strains isolated from patients under treatment for chromomycosis, *Int. J. Dermatol.*, 14, 141, 1975.

496. Uitto, J., Santa-Cruz, D. J., Eisen, A. Z., and Kobayashi, G. S., Chromomycosis successful treatment with 5-fluorocytosine, *J. Cutan. Pathol.*, 6, 77, 1979.

497. Yu, R. Y., A case of chromoblastomycosis successfully treated by 5-FC, *Chin. J. Dermatol.*, 13, 44, 1980.

498. Yu, R. Y., Two cases of chromoblastomycosis successfully treated by combined 5-FC, *Chin. J. Dermatol.*, 19, 35, 1986.

499. Cucé, L. C., Wroclawski, E. L., and Sampaio, S. A. P., Treatment of paracoccidioidomycosis, candidiasis, chromomycosis, lobomycosis, and mycetoma with ketoconazole, *Int. J. Dermatol.*, 19, 405, 1980.

500. Symoens, J., Moens, M., Dom, J., Scheijgrond, H., Dony, J., Schuermans, V., Legendre, R., and Finestine, N., An evaluation of two years of clinical experience with ketoconazole, *Rev. Infect. Dis.*, 2, 674, 1980.

501. Silber, J. G., Gombert, M. E., Green, K. M., and Shalita, A. R., Treatment of chromomycosis with ketoconazole and 5-fluorocytosine, *J. Am. Acad. Dermatol.*, 8, 236, 1983.

502. Yu, R., Successful treatment of chromoblastomycosis with itraconazole, *Mycoses*, 38, 79, 1995.

503. Bayles, M. A. H., Tropical mycoses, *Chemotherapy*, 38(Suppl. 1), 27, 1992.

504. Telles, F. Q., Rurimm, K. S., Fillus, J. N., Bordignon, G. F., Lameira, R. P., van Cutsem, J., and Cauwenbergh, G., Itraconazole in the treatment of chromoblastomycosis due to *Fonseceae pedrosoi*, *Int. J. Dermatol.*, 31, 805, 1992.

505. Smith, C. H., Barber, J. N. W. N., and Hay, R., A case of chromoblastomycosis responding to treatment with itraconazole, *Br. J. Dermatol.*, 128, 436, 1993.

506. Yu, R. Y. and Gao, L., Chromoblastomycosis successfully treated with fluconazole, *Int. J. Dermatol.*, 33, 716, 1994.

507. Robertson, P. A., Krirach, A. K., and Joseph, J. A., Fluconazole for life-threatening fungal infections in patients who cannot be treated with conventional antifungal agents, *Rev. Infect. Dis.*, 12(Suppl. 3), S349, 1990.

508. Diaz, M., Negroni, R., Montero-Gei, F., Castro, L. G. M., Sampaio, S. A. P., Borelli, D., Restrepo, A., Franco, L., Bran, J. L., Arathoon, E. G., Stevens, D. A., and the Fluconazole Pan-American Study Group, A Pan-American 5 year study of fluconazole therapy for deep mycoses in the immunocompetent host, *Clin. Infect. Dis.*, 14(Suppl. 1), S68, 1992.

509. Franco, L., Gomez, I., and Restrepo, A., Saperconazole in the treatment of systemic and subcutaneous mycoses, *Int. J. Dermatol.*, 31, 725, 1992.

510. Bayles, M. A. H., Chromomycosis treatment with thiabendazole, *Arch. Dermatol.*, 104, 476, 1971.

511. Bayles, M. A. H., Chromomycosis, *Baillieres Clin. Med. Commun. Dis.*, 4, 45, 1989.

37.2 GEOTRICHUM CANDIDUM

37.2.1 INTRODUCTION

Geotrichum is a genus of yeast-like imperfect fungi of the family Cryptococcaceae, order Moniliales. *Geotrichum candidum* Link 1809 is the etiologic agent of geotrichosis, a fungal disease that can affect the bronchi, lungs, mouth, or the intestinal tract, as well as become disseminated.

G. candidum is an ubiquitous saprophytic fungus found in fruits and decaying vegetables, soil, and diary products.[1] While some saprobic strains may produce lesions when introduced in experimental animals, it has been considered to have low virulence in humans.[2-5] However, the morbidity of geotrichosis may well be dependent on the degree of invasion and the immunologic status of the host.[6]

In the sputum, *G. candidum* was found to form septate branching hyphae 3 to 5 μm in diameter, and disassociated cells, which may be cylindrical, barrel-shaped, elliptical, or subspherical in shape.[1] The same general morphology has been observed also in culture. The hyphae, and particularly the lateral branches, may become septate. The arthrospores, which are mostly rectangular with rounded ends (measuring 4–6 μm to 8–12 μm in size), separate early by fragmentation of hyphae at the numerous septa; at times, the arthrospores may be spherical. On Sabouraud dextrose agar at 37°C, *G. candidum* formed creamy-white colonies consisting of hyphal elements and arthroconidia; blastoconidia were characteristically absent.[7]

In general, *G. candidum* has no proteolytic activity and will utilize only glucose and galactose, while other *Geotrichum* species and most *Trichosporon* species would utilize additional carbohydrates (lactose, maltose, sucrose).[8] Most *G. candidum* did not grow at 37°C.[1]

In humans, *G. candidum*, has been isolated as nonpathogenic organisms from conjunctiva,[9] tonsils, throat, tracheobronchial secretions, skin, rectal ulcers,[10] and feces.[11-14] The organism can also infiltrate into tissues.[6,7,15] Jagirdar et al.[7] have identified *G. candidum* as a tissue invasive pathogen in the terminal ileum of an immunocompromised patient with hairy cell leukemia.

G. candidum has been recognized as a saprophytic commensal most often involving the lungs in patients with cavitary pulmonary lessions.[2,12,16-18] While as an opportunistic pathogen it may produce infection in previously damaged lungs, it only rarely can assume the role of a primary pathogen causing respiratory illness in immunodeficient hosts.[2] The clinical features of pulmonary geotrichosis may be similar to, and difficult to distinguish from, those of an underlying disease. Thus, Thjötta and Urdal[19] found chest roentgenograms of patients with pulmonary geotrichosis similar to pulmonary tuberculosis. In addition, bronchopulmonary geotrichosis has been described in association with chronic bronchitis, emphysema, *Klebsiella* pneumonia, and atherosclerotic heart disease.[13,20] Most common symptoms include fever, chills, weight loss, productive cough, wheezing, fatigue, and anorexia.[13,20-25]

Geotrichial fungemia (septicemia) has been rare.[13,16,21,26,27] Bendove and Ashe[16] have described a case of septicemia in an elderly patient with advanced stage of diabetes mellitus.

G. candidum has been reported to cause local and disseminated disease, especially in immunocompromised patients.[7,28-30] Disseminated geotrichosis, which has been reported in leukemic patients with neutropenia,[6] can be misdiagnosed as aspergillosis, trichosporonosis, or candidiasis.[6,28,31]

37.2.2 Evolution of Therapies and Treatment of Geotrichosis

Generally, in otherwise normal patients, pulmonary geotrichosis is a mild disease. Earlier therapeutic modalities that have been reported to elicit a favorable response include long courses of potassium iodide,[11,13,16,20,25,29] colistine methionate,[17,24] and neomycin.[16]

Gugnani et al.[32] have used isoconazole nitrate to treat dermatomycosis due to *G. candidum*.

Hrdy et al.[18] have described a traumatic joint infection caused by *G. candidum* in an immunocompetent patient who responded to surgical debridement and oral antifungal therapy with ketoconazole at 200 mg daily.

In a case of *G. candidum*-associated peritonitis in a patient on continued ambulatory peritoneal dialysis (CAPD), the recommended therapy was oral flucytosine; intraperitoneal amphotericin B, which was co-administered initially at 5.0 mg/l, had to be discontinued because of severe abdominal pain.[30]

Kassamali et al.[6] have described a virulent and fatal disseminated infection in a neutropenic patient with acute leukemia who failed to respond to therapy with intravenous amphotericin B (total dose, 90 mg) and leukocyte transfusions. Histopathologic examination revealed extensive renal tissue invasion as evidenced by the presence of multiple kidney abscesses. However, in another case of an immunocompromised patient with acute lymphoblastic leukemia, the *G. candidum* septicemia was successfully treated with amphotericin B.[33]

In vitro susceptibility studies with a clinical isolate of *G. candidum* revealed a borderline sensitivity to ketoconazole and amphotericin B (minimum inhibitory concentration (MICs) = 3.2 and 0.58 μg/ml at 24 h) and resistance to fluconazole (MIC >80 μg/ml at 24 h).[18,34] In a previous study,[35] two strains of *G. candidum* were relatively resistant to ketoconazole but susceptible to both amphotericin B and miconazole. Earlier, Ghamande et al.[2] found *G. candidum* to be relatively resistant *in vitro* to amphotericin B (MIC = 14.0 μg/ml). Otcenasek[36] has reported a rather broad range of response of *G. candidum* to itraconazole (MIC = 0.045 to 3.12 μg/ml).

In view of the inconclusive results from sensitivity tests and the lack of clearly established relationship between *in vitro* susceptibility and clinical outcome, the MICs for *G. candidum* may not be relevant for antifungal therapy in clinical settings.

In several preliminary reports, a number of natural products have exhibited promising activity against *G. candidum*, which may serve as a basis for the development of new and more efficacious antifungal agents. Thus, nikkomycin Z, a new antibiotic capable of inhibiting chitin (a building block of the fungal cell wall) synthesis, suppressed the colony radial extension and hyphal density (swelling and bursting of hyphal apices) of *G. candidum*.[37] Fusapyrone and deoxyfusapyrone, two antifungal α-pyrones isolated from *Fusarium semitectum* Berk. and Rav. have shown strong inhibitory activity against *G. candidum* in disk diffusion assays.[38] Furthermore, an essential oil separated from the aerial parts of *Artemisia afra* Jacq. was also found to exert significant activity.[39]

37.2.3 References

1. Emmons, C. W., Binford, C. H., and Utz, J. P., *Medical Mycology*, 2nd ed., Lea and Febiger, Philadelphia, 1970, 183.
2. Ghamande, A. R., Landis, F. B., and Snider, G. L., Bronchial geotrichosis with fungemia complicating bronchogenic carcinoma, *Chest*, 59, 98, 1971.
3. Reeves, R. J., The incidence of bronchomycosis in the South, *Am. J. Roentgenol.*, 45, 513, 1941.

4. Kunstadter, R. H. and Milzer, A., Incidence of mycotic infection in children with acute respiratory tract disease, *Am. J. Dis. Child.*, 81, 306, 1951.

5. Goldman, S., Lipscomb, P. R., and Ulrich, J. A., *Geotrichum* tumefaction of the hand: report of a case, *J. Bone Joint Surg.*, 51, 587, 1969.

6. Kassamali, H., Anaissie, E., Ro, J., Rolston, K., Kantarjian, H., Fainstein, V., and Bodey, G. P., Disseminated *Geotrichum candidum* infection, *J. Clin. Microbiol.*, 25, 1782, 1987.

7. Jagirdar, J., Geller, S. A., and Bottone, E. J., *Geotrichum candidum* as a tissue invasive human pathogen, *Hum. Pathol.*, 12, 668, 1981.

8. Morenz, J., Geotrichosis, in *Human Infection with Fungi, Actinomycetes, and Algae*, Baker, R. D., Ed., Springer-Verlag, New York, 1971, 919.

9. Maestro, T., A new type of mycosis of the conjunctiva, *Ann. Ottal. Clin. Ocul.*, 66, 439, 1938.

10. Almeida, F. and Lacaz, C. S., Fungus of genus *Geotrichum* isolated from ulcerative lesions of the rectum, *Folia Clin. Biol.*, 12, 57, 1940.

11. Conant, N. F., Smith, D. T., Baker, R. D., Callaway, J. L., and Martin, D. S., *Manual of Clinical Mycology*, W. B. Saunders, Philadelphia, 1954.

12. Webster, B. H., Bronchopulmonary geotrichosis: a review with report of four cases, *Dis. Chest*, 35, 273, 1959.

13. Greer, A. E., Disseminating fungal disease of the lung, in *American Lecture Series*, Charles C. Thomas, Springfield, IL, 1962, 278.

14. Schnoor, T. G., The occurrence of Monilia in normal stools, *Am. J. Trop. Med.*, 163, 1939.

15. Chang, W. W. L. and Buerger, L., Disseminated geotrichosis, *Arch. Intern. Med.*, 89, 107, 1952.

16. Bendove, R. A. and Ashe, B. I., Geotrichum septicemia, *Arch. Intern. Med.*, 89, 107, 1952.

17. Ross, J. D., Reid, K. O. G., and Speirs, C. F., Bronchopulmonary geotrichosis with severe asthma, *Br. J. Med.*, 1, 1400, 1966.

18. Hrdy, D. B., Nassar, N. N., and Rinaldi, M. G., Traumatic joint infection due to *Geotrichum candidum*, *Clin. Infect. Dis.*, 20, 468, 1995.

19. Thjötta, T. and Urdal, K., A family endemic of *Geotrichosis pulmonum*, *Acta Pathol. Microbiol. Scand.*, 26, 673, 1949.

20. Minton, R., Young, R. V., and Shanbrom, E., Endobronchial geotrichosis, *Ann. Intern. Med.*, 40, 340, 1954.

21. Webster, B. H., Pulmonary geotrichosis, *Am. Rev. Tuberc.*, 76, 286, 1957.

22. Bell, D., Brodie, J., and Henderson, A., A case of pulmonary geotrichosis, *Br. J. Dis. Chest*, 56, 26, 1962.

23. Carmichael, J. W., *Geotrichum candidum*, *Mycologia*, 49, 820, 1957.

24. Brodie, J., Chambers, W., and Henderson, A., Use of colistin in a pulmonary mycosis, *Lancet*, 2, 300, 1962.

25. Nasser, W. K. and Daly, W. J., Bronchopulmonary geotrichosis, *J. Indiana Med. Assoc.*, 58, 1329, 1965.

26. Kaliski, S. R., Beene, M. L., and Mattman, L., Geotrichum in blood stream of an infant, *JAMA*, 148, 1207, 1952.

27. Sheehy, T. W., Honeycutt, B. K., and Spencer, J. T., *Geotrichum* septicemia, *JAMA*, 235, 1035, 1976.

28. Anaissie, E., Bodie, G. P., Kantarjian, H., Ro, J., Vartivarian, S. E., Hopfer, R., Hoy, J., and Rolston, K., A new spectrum of fungal infections in patients with cancer, *Rev. Infect. Dis.*, 11, 369, 1989.

29. Magalhães, O., Lung infection with *Neogetrichum pulmoneum*, *Rev. Med. Cir. Brasil*, 41, 263, 1933.

30. Hernandez Jaras, J., Martinez-Martinez, L., Gallego, J. L., Fernandez Fernandez, J., and Botella, J., *Geotrichum* sp. as an agent of peritonitis in continuous peritoneal dialysis (CAPD), *Clin. Nephrol.*, 28, 210, 1987.

31. Samonis, G. and Bafaloukos, D., Fungal infections in cancer patients: an escalating problem, *In Vivo*, 6, 183, 1992.

32. Gugnani, H. C., Akpata, L. E., Gugnani, M. K., and Srivastava, R., Isoconazole nitrate in the treatment of tropical dermatomycoses, *Mycoses*, 37, 39, 1994.

33. Ng, K. P., Soo-Hoo, T. S., Koh, M. T., and Kwan, P. W., Disseminated *Geotrichum* infection, *Med. J. Malaysia*, 49, 424, 1994.

34. Rex, J. H., Pfaller, M. A., Rinaldi, M. G., Polak, A., and Galgiani, J. N., Antifungal susceptibility testing, *Clin. Microbiol. Rev.*, 6, 267, 1993.

35. Bergan, T. and Vangdal, M., *In vivo* activity of antifungal agents against yeast species, *Chemotherapy*, 29, 104, 1983.

36. Otcenasek, M., The *in vitro* susceptibility of some mycotic agents to a new orally active triazole, itraconazole, *J. Hyg. Epidemiol. Microbiol. Immunol.*, 34, 129, 1990.

37. Tariq, V. N. and Devlin, P. L., Sensitivity of fungi to nikkomycin Z, *Fungal Genet. Biol.*, 20, 4, 1996.

38. Evidente, A., Conti, L., Altomare, C., Bottalico, A., Sindona, G., Segre, A. L., and Logrieco, A., Fusapyrone and deoxyfusapyrone, two antifungal alpha-pyrones from *Fusarium semitectum*, *Nat. Toxins*, 2, 4, 1994.

39. Gundidza, M., Antifungal activity of essential oil from *Artemisia afra* Jacq., *Cent. Afr. J. Med.*, 39, 140, 1993.

37.3   *HISTOPLASMA* SPP.

37.3.1   INTRODUCTION

The genus *Histoplasma* is a dimorphic fungus comprised of two pathogenic species, *H. falciminosum* (the causative agent of the equine disease) and *H. capsulatum* which causes the disease in humans. *H. capsulatum*, in turn, is divided into two variants, *H. capsulatum* var. *capsulatum*, and *H. capsulatum* var. *duboisii*.[1,2] *H. capsulatum* var. *capsulatum* is responsible for the classical or small form (in tissues, the yeast form reaches 2 to 4 μm in diameter) of histoplasmosis. It is endemic in various parts of the world (the U.S., the West Indies, Central and South America, Africa, India, and the Far East) with the exception of Europe, and presents with pulmonary and disseminated infection affecting largely the lungs, reticuloendothelial system, mucosal surfaces, and the skin.[3] In the U.S., the geographic distribution of *Histoplasma* covers large areas mainly along the Mississippi and Ohio River Valleys. Infection by *H. capsulatum* is carried out by airborne microconidia (spores) which are inhaled. After reaching the alveoli, the microconidia convert into the yeast phase at body temperature.

The second variant, *H. capsulatum* var. *duboisii* is the causative agent of the African or large form (in tissues, the yeast form is 12 to 20 μm in diameter) of histoplasmosis.[4] The two variants differ in their antigenic compositions.

The exposure to *H. capsulatum* var. *capsulatum*, which is found in soil where large numbers of birds and bats have roosted, is incidental but occasionally can be seen in populations that may come into contact with a common source of the fungus, such as bird droppings. The first case of histoplasmosis was described by Darling[5] in a patient residing in Panama.

37.3.2   STUDIES ON THERAPEUTICS

37.3.2.1   Amphotericin B

For more than two decades, amphotericin B has been the mainstay therapy for disseminated histoplasmosis. When used in doses of 35 to 40 mg/kg, in non-AIDS patients, cure has been achieved in nearly 90% of the cases.[6,7] However, the outcome in AIDS patients treated with amphotericin B has been much less successful, with high frequency of relapses.[8-14] McKinsey et al.[15] have conducted a long-term, open, nonrandomized pilot study of intermittent maintenance therapy with amphotericin B in HIV-infected patients. Of the 16 patients who completed the study, 7 received an initial intensive course of 1.0 g of the drug, followed by weekly injections of 50 to 80 mg until a cumulative dose of 2.0 g was attained; biweekly infusions of 50 to 80 mg were then continued indefinitely. The remaining 9 patients underwent an initial course of 2.0 g amphotericin B, followed by weekly infusions of 80 mg. At the median 14-month follow-up evaluation, 13 of 14 patients (93%) who did not die of other causes remained relapse-free; there were no apparent differences in the outcome between patients treated with weekly and those receiving biweekly maintenance therapy. The single relapse occurred in a patient who was treated with corticosteroids and was not on amphotericin B medication at the time of relapse.[15] In a follow-up long-term study including the original cohort and additional patients, McKinsey et al.[16] applied a maintenance therapy of amphotericin B to 46 AIDS patients with disseminated histoplasmosis, with an overall efficacy of 97%; no significant nephrotoxicity was observed and the serum creatinine levels did not exceed 2.0 mg/dl.

Because of its acute and chronic toxicities, amphotericin B may be of limited use in certain patient populations, such as neutropenic and immunodeficient patients.[17] However, liposome-encapsulated amphotericin B has shown decreased toxicity and enhanced efficacy in experimental candidiasis in both non-neutropenic[18-20] and neutropenic mice.[21,22] When administered over a 35-d period to a patient with AIDS complicated with Kaposi's sarcoma and disseminated histoplasmosis, a cumulative dose of 2136 mg of liposomal amphotericin B elicited only a partial response.[23] Sculier et al.[24] have also used liposomal amphotericin B to treat cancer patients with fungal infections.

Clark et al.[25] have developed a phospholipid complex (ABLC) of amphotericin B with dimyristoyl phosphatidylcholine and dimyristoyl phosphatidylglycerol, and evaluated its activity in murine histoplasmosis. When injected intravenously to normal and immunosuppressed mice infected with *H. capsulatum*, ABLC showed mean ED_{50} doses of 0.2 mg/kg and 0.7 mg/kg, respectively. One interesting observation was that while ABLC, ketoconazole, itraconazole, and fluconazole were all active against histoplasmosis in normal mice, in immunosuppressed mice only ABLC and Fungizone® (the desoxycholate formulation of amphotericin B) retained their efficacy, while the azole antimycotics showed significantly decreased therapeutic potentials.[25] Esterification of the carboxyl group of amphotericin B yielded a water-soluble methyl ester,[26] which was found to have much less toxicity than the parent compound.[27-29] The peak concentrations of amphotericin B methyl ester in the serum were 10 times higher than those of amphotericin B; however, its efficacy *in vivo* against *H. capsulatum* was somewhat weaker.[30-33] Neihart et al.[34] have described successful treatment of a patient with disseminated histoplasmosis with amphotericin B methyl ester. The drug (total dose, 8.533 g) was given for 2 months, and follow-up evaluations over a 6-year period showed no recurrence of disease.

37.3.2.2 Azole Derivatives

37.3.2.2.1   *Ketoconazole*

Even though ketoconazole was found to be effective in the therapy of progressive disseminated histoplasmosis in immunocompetent patients,[35] it is clearly inadequate in AIDS patients.[11,36]

Slama[37] reported positive response of seven immunocompetent patients with chronic cavitary histoplasmosis (a progressive pulmonary infection) treated with daily doses of 200 mg ketoconazole for 6 months; six of seven patients showed clinical cure and no serious side effects.

In a prospective, multicenter, randomized trial comparing low-dose (400 mg) with high-dose (800 mg) daily oral therapy with ketoconazole in the treatment of non-life-threatening, nonmeningeal forms of histoplasmosis, including chronic cavitary infections (n = 19) and localized or disseminated disease (n = 20), the overall success rate was 84% (treatment of 6 months or more) with both regimens showing similar efficacy.[38] However, other reports have been less optimistic.[39,40] For example, Quinones et al.[40] have reported that daily doses of 400 mg or 800 mg of ketoconazole given to four patients with chronic cavitary disease for 48 to 65 weeks, resulted in failure in two of the patients; the remaining two patients have had relapses even after prolonged treatment. Maintenance therapy with ketoconazole against relapses of histoplasmosis in AIDS patients has often been ineffective and is not recommended.[41,42]

37.3.2.2.2   *Fluconazole*

One advantage of fluconazole over other azole antimycotics is that it can be administered both orally and intravenously. Its pharmacokinetic properties include good penetration into the cerebrospinal fluid even in the absence of inflammation, and a prolonged half-life of about 25 h, allowing for once-daily administration.[43,44]

In a Pan-American 5-year study of fluconazole therapy for systemic mycoses in immuno-competent patients, the drug was found effective; all eight patients with histoplasmosis responded to daily doses of 200 to 400 mg.[45] However, as part of an open noncomparative trial, fluconazole at daily doses of 200 to 400 mg failed in the treatment of one patient with histoplamosis and underlying sarcoidosis.[46] Graybill[47] also reported failure of fluconazole to treat histoplasmosis; the patients had received 50 to 100 mg daily (a dosage now considered to be suboptimal for treatment of systemic mycoses).

In a study conducted by Sharkey-Mathis et al.,[48] ten patients with AIDS and histoplasmosis were treated with fluconazole at daily doses of 100, 400, or 800 mg/kg. The differences in outcome among the five patients receiving the 100-mg/kg dose (one remission, one improvement, and three failures) and the five patients receiving the two higher doses (two remissions and three failures) were negligible.

The activities of fluconazole and amphotericin B against histoplasmosis compared favorably in normal and immunosuppressed (leukopenic) mice.[49] The minimum inhibitory concentrations (MIC) were 16 to 250 μg/ml for fluconazole (given orally twice daily for six consecutive days), and 0.12 to 0.47 μg/ml for amphotericin B (intraperitoneal administration once every other day for a total of six doses).

37.3.2.2.3   Itraconazole

Because of its lipophilic nature, itraconazole is able to achieve high and persistent concentrations in tissues rather than in plasma.[50-52] This orally active triazole antimycotic was found to be very effective in the treatment of chronic cavitary histoplasmosis as well as in disseminated nonmeningeal infections. In two open noncomparative trials involving patients with chronic pulmonary disease and disseminated infections,[53,54] itraconazole was administered initially at 100 mg daily until a clinical cure was achieved, and then at 50 mg daily for another 4 to 6 months. Clinical cure or improvement was noted in nearly all patients.

In a multicentered noncomparative trial, Dismukes et al.[55] assessed the efficacy and toxicity of oral itraconazole in the treatment of nonmeningeal, non-life-threatening forms of histoplasmosis. The drug was given at daily doses of 200 to 400 mg for a median duration of 9 months; follow-up evaluations were conducted at 12.1 months. The success rate was 81% (30 of 37 treated patients); the success rate among patients treated for over 2 months was 86% (30 of 35). All failures occurred in patients with chronic cavitary pulmonary disease. The observed toxicity was minimal (mainly gastrointestinal disorders: nausea, vomiting, and/or diarrhea).

Itraconazole was also found effective in the treatment of disseminated histoplasmosis in HIV-infected patients.[48,56,57] In one of the studies, 12 patients received 400 mg of the drug daily; after a mean treatment lasting for 12 months, in 7 patients the disease was in remission, 2 patients showed clinical improvement, and 2 patients failed to respond.[48] In another trial,[56] 23 of 27 patients responded to itraconazole after 6 months of therapy.

Drugs which induce hepatic drug-metabolizing enzymes were found to accelerate the metabolism of itraconazole, leading to its therapeutic failure. In two reports,[58,59] the co-administration of rifampin (used to treat tuberculosis in AIDS patients) and itraconazole resulted in undetectable serum levels of itraconazole. After discontinuation of rifampin, the itraconazole levels in the serum were again measurable and concurrent with clinical improvement.[59]

37.3.2.2.4   Other triazole antimycotics

The activity of SCH 39304 (a triazole antifungal agent with improved pharmacokinetic profile) against *H. capsulatum* was investigated both *in vitro* and *in vivo*, and compared with those of fluconazole and amphotericin B.[60] In normal and leukopenic mice infected with the fungus, SCH 39304, given parenterally, compared favorably with amphotericin B in treating disseminated histoplasmosis, and was superior to fluconazole. As with other triazoles, the *in vitro* activity of SCH 39304 was not predictive of *in vivo* activity. Because of its unacceptable toxicity (hepato-carcinoma formation in animal models), SCH 39304 is no longer of clinical interest.[60]

Pappagianis et al.[61] have evaluated the activity of Bay R 3783, another triazole derivative, in murine models of systemic histoplasmosis. Bay R 3783 was administered via the alimentary tract at three dosages (2.5, 10, and 25 mg/kg) and compared with ketoconazole, fluconazole, and itraconazole (given at the same dose regimens) and amphotericin B (1.0 mg/kg, injected intraperitoneally). At the 25-mg/kg dose, itraconazole, Bay R 3783, and amphotericin B were able to prevent deaths completely through day 44, and were statistically superior to fluconazole (at 25 mg/kg); under the same conditions, ketoconazole was the least potent of all drugs. In a short-term organ load assay, all drugs exerted significant reduction in viable fungal cells in both livers and spleens, with amphotericin B being statistically more active than any of the azoles.

37.3.2.3 Nikkomycins X and Z

Nikkomycins X and Z, two antibiotics structurally similar to the polyoxins, have been shown to possess fungal chitin synthase-inhibiting activity.[62,63] At doses of 5.0 and 20 mg/kg, nikkomycin Z was found highly effective in preventing deaths in a murine model of systemic histoplasmosis.[64] However, the drug was less efficacious in short-term organ load experiments, although its dose-response effect was comparable to that of fluconazole.[64]

37.3.3 EVOLUTION OF THERAPIES AND TREATMENT OF HISTOPLASMOSIS

In immunocompetent individuals, most cases of acute disease are asymptomatic and patients do not seek medical treatment. Even when symptomatic, the disease is expected to resolve quickly and without treatment. However, in immunocompromised patients, or when the infecting aerosol is large, the histoplasmosis could disseminate and become potentially lethal if not treated.[65-67] Based on its severity, rate of progression, and histopathologic differences, progressive disseminated histoplasmosis may present as acute, subacute, or chronic.[12,68-72] In the immunocompromised population, approximately 66% suffer from chronic infection, whereas 22% and 12% present with the subacute and acute forms, respectively.[73]

In immunocompetent hosts with acute disease and ventilatory failure, the preferred medication has been amphotericin B given in cumulative doses of 0.5 to 1.0 g. Such treatment is effective and patients usually respond within 1 to 2 weeks (Table 37.1).

Since its introduction into clinical use, itraconazole has become the drug of choice for most types of histoplasmosis with the exception of meningeal, endocarditis, and life-threatening pulmonary and disseminated infections.[55] The recommended daily regimen is usually 200 mg; however, the dose may be increased to 400 mg (given twice daily) if the patient fails to respond after several weeks of therapy at the lower dose.

So far, chronic cavitary pulmonary histoplasmosis has probably been the most difficult condition to treat because of the significant underlying chronic obstructive pulmonary disease found in patients with this condition.[55,74]

In an immunocompromised host, histoplasmosis is potentially life-threatening, and ampho-tericin B remains the treatment of choice[65,67] (Table 37.2). Treatment of AIDS patients who do not suffer from acute infection or meningeal involvement may include an initial daily regimen of 600 mg of itraconazole (200 mg three times daily) for 3 d, followed by 200-mg doses given twice daily. After 12 weeks of treatment, a life-long maintenance therapy of 200 mg daily of itraconazole should be implemented.[66,67] In some cases, amphotericin B may become part of the entire treatment, or after being administered initially to most patients, therapy may be switched to itraconazole after a positive response is observed (cultures becoming negative for *H. capsulatum* concurrent with stable clinical condition).[66]

TABLE 37.1
Treatment of Histoplasmosis in Immunocompetent Hosts[a]

Indication	Treatment
Acute infection	Observation
Acute infection with ventilatory failure	Amphotericin B: 0.5–1.0 g, IV (until improvement noted)
Cavitary infection	Itraconazole: 200–400 mg daily for 6 months, orally; or ketoconazole: 400–800 mg daily for 6 months, orally; or amphotericin B: 35 mg/kg, total dose, IV
Progressive disseminated	Amphotericin B: 0.5–1.0 g, IV, until patient is stable, then itraconazole: 200–400 mg daily, orally, for 6 months; or amphotericin B: 40 mg/kg, IV, total dose

[a] Data taken from Sarosi and Davies,[65] and Dismukes et al.[55] Some of the recommended dose regimens may reflect the personal preferences of the authors, and therefore, remain controversial.

TABLE 37.2
Treatment of Histoplasmosis in Immunocompromised Hosts[a]

Indication	Treatment	
	Without AIDS	With AIDS
Acute infection	Amphotericin B: 0.5–1.0 g, IV, then itraconazole: 400 mg daily, orally for 6 months	Amphotericin B: 0.5–1.0 g, IV, then itraconazole: 400 mg daily for life
Acute infection with ventilatory failure	Amphotericin B: 1.0 g, IV; then itraconazole: 400 mg daily, orally, for 6 months, or amphotericin B: 40 mg/kg cumulative dose, IV	Amphotericin B: 0.5–1.0 g, IV; then itraconazole: 400 mg daily, orally, for life
Chronic cavitary infection	Itraconazole: 200–400 mg daily, orally, for 6–12 months	Amphotericin B: 0.5–1.0 g, IV; then itraconazole: 400 mg daily, orally, for life
Progressive disseminated	Amphotericin B: 1.0 g, IV; then itraconazole: 400 mg daily, orally, for 6 months, or amphotericin B: 40 mg/kg cumulative dose, IV	Amphotericin B: 1.0 g, IV; then itraconazole: 400 mg daily, orally, for life

[a] Data taken from Sarosi and Davies,[65] Dismukes et al.,[55] Kauffman,[66] Graybill,[47] and Drew.[121] Some of the recommended dose regimens may reflect the personal preferences of the authors, and therefore, remain controversial.

Hypercalcemia associated with disseminated histoplasmosis has been described in two reports.[75,76] This condition has also been observed with other granulomatous diseases, such as sarcoidosis,[77] tuberculosis,[78-80] chronic berylliosis,[81] and two disseminated mycoses: coccidioidomycosis[82] and candidiasis.[83] Administration of vitamin D and calcium supplements should be avoided,[76] since as described for other granulomatous diseases,[78,79,83-85] hypercalcemia in disseminated histoplasmosis could be aggravated by these two treatments. It has been postulated that extrarenal conversion of vitamin D to its active 1α,25-dihydroxy metabolite may be the cause of the hypercalcemic condition.[86-88] This increased conversion may take place within the granulomatous tissue itself[89] and the macrophages, in particular.[90] Whereas the withdrawal of vitamin D and calcium supplements would lower the serum calcium levels,[78,83,91] steroid therapy may also correct the hypercalcemia in granulomatous disease by decreasing the conversion of vitamin D to the pathogenic 1α,25-dihydroxy metabolite.[84,92]

Fungal peritonitis is a well-known risk in patients undergoing chronic ambulatory peritoneal dialysis.[93] In the treatment of one such case involving histoplasma infection, the patient responded favorably to a combined therapy of fluconazole (200 mg loading dose, then 100 mg daily), 5-fluorocytosine (50 mg/l were added to the dialysis fluid for 4 weeks), and amphotericin B (30 mg for 10 d).[94]

In recent years, the use of methotrexate sodium to treat severe rheumatoid arthritis and psoriasis has been steadily increasing.[95,96] In this context, with the escalating use of methotrexate medication, the incidence of opportunistic infections (varicella zoster,[97,98] *Pneumocystis carinii* pneumonia,[99-101] nocardiosis,[102] cryptococcosis,[103] and histoplasmosis[104]) in these patients has also been on the rise. By inactivating the dihydrofolate reductase and ultimately blocking the DNA and amino acid biosynthesis[105] in rapidly proliferating cells, methotrexate therapy would lead to impairment of the cell-mediated immunity even when given at lower doses, thereby predisposing patients to opportunistic infections. Witty et al.[104] reported three cases of disseminated histoplasmosis in patients receiving low-dose methotrexate for psoriasis. All patients responded favorably to amphotericin B (total dose in the 2.0 to 3.0 g range), with one exception where the patient required long-term suppressive therapy because of persistent *Histoplasma* antigenuria.

37.3.3.1 Histoplasmosis in AIDS Patients

Although not significantly different from the disease observed in non-HIV-infected individuals, disseminated histoplasmosis is a serious and potentially lethal infection in patients with AIDS. Wheat et al.[11] and others[12-15,106-109] have described a septicemia-like syndrome characterized by hypotension, renal and hepatic failure, respiratory insufficiency, and disseminated coagulopathy. Skin manifestations, which are seen in about 10% of cases, include pustular, follicular, maculopapular, and erythematous lesions with papulonecrotic centers.[12,108,110,111] Disseminated histoplasmosis may also present with pericarditis,[12] rhabdomyolysis,[11] pancreatitis,[11] chorioretinitis,[112] colonic masses,[12,14,113,114] mesenteric and omental nodules,[115] and thrombocytopenia.[116] CNS involvement in disseminated disease has also been reported (5% to 20% of patients),[12,14] including encephalopathy, meningitis, and focal parenchymal lesions of the brain.[11,14] AIDS patients with CNS complications did not respond well to treatment as compared to those with other forms of disseminated disease (61% to 71% mortality rate).[41,117]

Since in nearly half of the cases, AIDS patients will present with unexplained fever, accompanied by diffuse reticulonodular or interstitial pulmonary infiltrates,[9,11,12] misdiagnosis as miliary tuberculosis has been common in many such cases.[106] To this end, detection of *H. capsulatum* polysaccharide antigen (HPA) in the urine (90% to 96% of patients), blood (50% to 78%), and other body fluids showed promise as a rapid diagnostic tool for disseminated histoplasmosis.[118,119] The HPA levels decreased with amphotericin B treatment but recurred in both the urine and blood at the time of relapse.[118,120]

Because of the severe clinical presentation, as well as impaired cellular immune functions, AIDS patients may not always respond to treatment of histoplasmosis as well as other immunocompromised patients, and without life-long maintenance therapy the incidence of relapse has been an ever present possibility. Since none of the currently available drugs for histoplasmosis is curative, the emphasis of treatment has been shifting from cure to disease suppression with the least toxic, best tolerated, and most effective drug regimen.[48,121]

One therapy that is often recommended involves initial treatment with amphotericin B, followed by indefinite suppression with intermittent doses of amphotericin B or itraconazole.[15,16,41] Even though amphotericin B has been widely used, too often its toxicity and the discomfort due to the required intravenous or intrathecal administration were not well tolerated. In these cases, alternative therapies with azole antifungals, especially itraconazole, should be considered (Table 37.2).[48]

Furthermore, as anemia still remains one of the most common hematologic abnormalities associated with HIV infections,[122] one complication in AIDS patients receiving concomitant amphotericin B and zidovudine is that each of these drugs will also cause anemia, thus making multifactorial anemia a serious clinical condition in these patients. Decreased endogenous erythropoietin levels have been observed in all of the above settings.[123,124] In a small study, Lancaster et al.[125] demonstrated that multifactorial anemia in AIDS patients with disseminated histoplasmosis receiving concomitant amphotericin B and zidovudine regimens, can be corrected in some patients with the administration of recombinant human erythropoietin.

Itraconazole is also highly potent against histoplasmosis. It reaches high tissue concentrations, has prolonged drug clearance, and greater gastrointestinal tolerance than ketoconazole. However, its usefulness may be limited by acid-dependent absorption and limited cerebrospinal fluid (CSF) penetration.[53,126-130] When used in daily doses of 200 to 400 mg, itraconazole has shown clinical efficacy against pulmonary or disseminated infection in nearly 90% of patients without AIDS.[54,55,131] The British Society for Antimicrobial Chemotherapy Working Party has recommended the use of itraconazole at daily doses of 400 mg for 6 weeks as an alternative therapy to amphotericin B for induction therapy for histoplasmosis, as well as the drug of choice for maintenance treatment.[132] With regard to its toxicity, however, at the 400-mg daily dose regimen, the adverse side effects of itraconazole have been more pronounced than those with a comparable dose of fluconazole, and included increased hepatic aminotransferase levels (in 5% to 10% of patients). At daily doses of 600 mg or more, other side effects may emerge, such as adrenal insufficiency and reversible idiosyncratic hepatitis.

Fluconazole, another of the newer triazole antimycotics, is water-soluble, easily absorbed, and shows high CSF penetrability.[130,133,134] However, in spite of some favorable clinical outcomes reported in treating histoplasmosis in immunocompetent hosts,[45] the role of fluconazole as primary therapy of histoplasmosis in AIDS patients has been very limited. Nevertheless, on several occasions fluconazole was used successfuly for maintenance therapy in AIDS patients with disseminated histoplasmosis;[16,135,136] however, daily doses of less than 200 mg are considered inadequate.[47,137]

Ketoconazole has been inferior to both amphotericin B and the triazole antimycotics. It is generally ineffective, and should not be used as primary therapy for disseminated histoplasmosis in AIDS patients.[11,41,138,139] The ineffectiveness of ketoconazole may be the result of its poor absorption in AIDS patients caused by their high gastric pH,[140] as well as poor compliance associated with its gastrointestinal toxicity. However, there have been some positive results. Thus, Mello et al.[141] have reported a single case of an HIV-positive patient with localized tonsilar infection and cervical adenopathy caused by *H. capsulatum*, who responded favorably to a 400-mg daily dose of ketoconazole administered over a 12-month period. Given such positive clinical responses, oral ketoconazole treatment of HIV-positive patients with evidence of early, localized histoplasma infection may eventually be considered, but only if disseminated disease is not evident.[141]

Since there is consistently a high risk of relapse in AIDS patients with disseminated disease, life-long suppressive therapy is always warranted. After maintenance therapy is discontinued, the relapse rate among these patients was very high.[12,16,142] Even with chronic maintenance therapy with ketoconazole, the relapse rate was over 58%; by comparison, with amphotericin B the relapse rate was 19%.[15,41,42] In another study, maintenance therapy with amphotericin B led to even better results — the relapse rate was only 5% (median follow-up, over 12 months), with the amphotericin B doses ranging between 50 and 100 mg/kg administered weekly or every 2 weeks.[16]

Wheat et al.[143] have evaluated the efficacy of itraconazole in preventing relapse of histoplasmosis in 42 AIDS patients who had successfully completed induction therapy for disseminated histoplasmosis with amphotericin B (at least 15-mg/kg dose). The drug was found to be highly effective when given at 200-mg twice daily. Ninety-five percent remained relapse-free at follow-up evaluations for at least 52 weeks. Only three patients failed to respond: one patient had discontinued medication because of toxicity (hypokalemia), and the other two relapsed. The antigen clearance from blood and urine correlated with the itraconazole clinical efficacy.

Fluconazole at 400 mg daily has also been recommended for maintenance therapy.[144] However, Pottage and Sha[145] reported a case of an HIV-positive patient with cryptococcosis who developed histoplasmosis while receiving suppressive fluconazole therapy for cryptococcal meningitis. The patient was treated successfully with amphotericin B, then switched to fluconazole (200 mg daily, orally) when he developed histoplasmosis. After being treated with amphotericin B for a second time, and again switched back to oral fluconazole (400 mg daily), the patient once more developed histoplasmosis.

37.3.3.2 Histoplasmosis in Transplant Recipients

Although not very frequently, progressive disseminated histoplasmosis has been diagnosed in patients from both endemic and nonendemic areas.[73] In 1983, Wheat et al.[146] described two large outbreaks of histoplasmosis in renal allograft recipients with incidence of infection reaching 2.1%. During a 4-year period, Davies et al.[147] reported five cases of progressive disseminated disease in approximately 1300 renal transplant recipients. In general, the disease may follow a primary infection, or be a reactivation of previous infection due, to a large extent, to the immunosuppressive effects of antirejection therapy.[147] Often, protracted fever and skin lesions are the most frequent symptoms of disseminated disease. CNS involvement, although occasionally seen in AIDS patients, is relatively rare in transplant recipients.[73]

Before the introduction of the azole antimycotics, amphotericin B was used for treatment of disseminated histoplasmosis in transplant recipients. Sarosi et al.[7] have suggested a regimen of 40 mg/kg for a cumulative dose of 2.0 to 2.5 g. However, because of its substantial toxicity, amphotericin B is not appropriate for renal allograft recipients and should be used with caution. Goetz and Jones[148] reported a case of disseminated histoplasmosis in a renal allograft recipient who was treated successfully with a short course of intravenous amphotericin B coupled with oral ketoconazole and rifampin, followed by prolonged therapy with ketoconazole alone. The addition of rifampin was believed to increase the survival rate of nonimmunocompromised hosts against disseminated histoplasmosis when given in combination with amphotericin B, as demonstrated in murine histoplasmosis;[149] in nude mice, however, this combination not only did not offer any advantage over amphotericin B given alone, but may possibly be deleterious.[150] In another combination, ketoconazole when given concomitantly with cyclosporin A (an immunosuppressive drug used in antirejection therapy) could adversely inhibit its metabolism resulting in unacceptable cyclosporin A-associated renal toxicity.[151]

37.3.3.3 Skin Manifestations of Histoplasmosis

Skin manifestations of histoplasmosis are part of the disseminated infection, and have been observed in 4% to 10% of the population,[12,68,152,153] including HIV-infected patients.[154-156] In the latter cases, the preferred therapy has been with intravenous amphotericin B.[155]

Cutaneous lesions may appear on the head, trunk, or the extremities,[68,152,153,157-163] and will present as macules, papules, nodules, indurated plaques that ulcerate, purpura, abscesses, impetigo, eczematous or exfoliative dermatitis, cellulitis, or panniculitis.[153] In AIDS patients, some unusual skin manifestations, such as macular, blanching rashes, and papulonecrotic lesions, have also been observed.[164-166] In acute and subacute disseminated infections, the usual manifestations are indurated plaques that may develop as punched-out ulcers. Erythema nodosum and erythema multiforme have been observed as hypersensitivity reactions in acute pulmonary histoplasmosis.[157] Perianal ulcers, although rare, have also been described.[160,167] In one such case, the patient was treated with daily infusion of 0.4 mg/kg amphotericin B. After gradual clinical improvement, the ulcer healed completely after a total dose of 570 mg of amphotericin B.[167]

Navarro et al.[166] have reported an unusual case of an immunosuppressed patient with systemic lupus erythematosus and disseminated histoplasmosis who presented with generalized cutaneous papulonodular lesions, which had evolved into vesicles with central necrosis that resembled molluscum contagiosum with an indurated erythematous halo. The patient was treated with intravenous amphotericin B (0.5 mg/kg daily) and oral 5-fluorocytosine (50 mg/kg daily). Since the clinical course was complicated by intractable hemolytic anemia (treated with prednisone, 20 mg daily), the 5-fluorocytosine was discontinued and ketoconazole therapy (400 mg daily) instituted for 14 months; the dosage of amphotericin B was increased to 1.0 mg/kg daily for a total cumulative dose of 3.0 g. In another case,[156] an HIV-infected patient with disseminated histoplasmosis who presented with ulcerated verrucous plaque localized above the upper lip, has been successfully treated with oral ketoconazole (400 mg daily) for 6 weeks; the ketoconazole regimen was continued as a maintenance therapy. The possibility of human-to-human transmission of histoplasmosis has been postulated.[156]

37.3.3.4 Gastrointestinal Histoplasmosis

While gastrointestinal involvement in disseminated histoplasmosis is not common, its manifestations may be serious, such as perforation of the small intestines or the presence of large colonic polyps. Whereas gastrointestinal invasion is most likely due to hematogenous dissemination, direct penetration of tissue may also occur. Because of its abundant lymphoid tissue, the ileocecal site has been most frequently involved.

Cimponeriu et al.[168] reported two cases of HIV-infected patients with gastrointestinal histoplasmosis, in which the radiographic and endoscopic mass lesions of the colon mimicked cancer; both patients were treated successfully with amphotericin B, followed by suppressive itraconazole therapy. In another report,[169] two HIV-infected patients with hemophilia A presented with hematochezia secondary to gastrointestinal infection with *H. capsulatum*. The patients responded to amphotericin B therapy, followed by itraconazole, with no recurrence of bleeding.

Graham et al.[170] described two cases of AIDS patients with colonic structures secondary to histoplasmosis. Both patients were successfully treated with intravenous amphotericin B (each receiving a total dose of 2.0 g), followed by maintenance therapy with amphotericin B. Earlier, there were two reports[113,171] of AIDS patients diagnosed with the same condition, as well as another two reports[172,173] of histoplasmosis-induced colonic structures in non-AIDS patients.

Cappell and Manzione[174] described a patient with hyperglobulinemia E-recurrent infection (Job's syndrome) who developed colonic histoplasmosis and was successfully treated with 600-mg daily doses of ketoconazole for 2 months. This report extends previous findings,[175-177] indicating that patients with Job's syndrome may be at higher risk of developing opportunistic fungal infections, including histoplasmosis.

37.3.3.5 Orofacial Manifestations of Histoplasmosis

Orofacial manifestations in histoplasmosis have been observed most frequently in disseminated disease,[68,178-180] although some patients with pulmonary histoplasmosis may also present with oral lesions.[181,182] The most commonly affected sites in the upper aerodigestive tract are the tongue, palate, buccal mucosa or gingiva, and the larynx.[183] Generally, orofacial histoplasmosis appears as indurated ulcers or exophytic lesions and are often difficult to distinguish from carcinoma, sarcoidosis, tuberculosis, and other mycoses.[184] Rare cases have been reported with antral involvement[185] and invasion of the mandible.[186] In disseminated disease, oral lesions have been seen, especially in HIV-infected patients,[187-192] and in those with Hodgkin's lymphoma.[193]

Oropharyngeal ulcers have also been observed in 14% to 17% of patients with gastrointestinal histoplasmosis.[175,194] In two reported studies,[68,195] between 42% and 66% of patients with disseminated histoplasmosis presented with oropharyngeal disease, and 15% to 24% will have laryngeal lesions. Although in most clinical settings laryngeal manifestations are associated with disseminated disease, there have been cases where the laryngeal lesions were believed to be primary.[196-204]

Hiltbrand and McGuirt[181] described a successful treatment of granulomatous lesions in the upper aerodigestive tract of a patient with chronic disseminated histoplasmosis with amphotericin B (2.0 g cumulative dose given over 4 months). In two other reports,[205,206] histoplasmosis of the larynx was successfully cured with ketoconazole (200 mg three times daily, for 3 months, and 400 mg daily for 11 weeks, respectively).

Metronidazole and fluconazole have also been used to treat localized oral histoplasmosis in a patient with HIV infection.[190]

37.3.3.6   Ocular Histoplasmosis

Feman and Tilford[207] have estimated that nearly 100 patients are diagnosed each year with ocular histoplasmosis. In a retrospective study by Simmons and Matthews,[208] ocular histoplasmosis has been prevalent in 47% of cases of posterior uveitis reported in the Mississippi River Valley, an endemic area of the disease. However, intraocular tumors associated with disseminated histoplasmosis have been rare.[209-211]

The infection is usually manifested by a syndrome consisting of multiple, peripheral, well-demarcated, atrophic-appearing lesions, peripapillary pigmentary lesions, and a macular diskiform lesion.[207] Ophthalmic lesions of this type are difficult to cure, although Feman et al.[211] reported one case where the lesion responded to intravenous amphotericin B (total dose of 1026 mg administered over a 32-d period) and topical drops of atropine and prednisolone acetate. The amphotericin B therapy was discontinued and treatment continued with oral ketoconazole for 9 additional months when the lesion appeared to be flat and atrophic.

37.3.3.7   Rheumatic Manifestations of Histoplasmosis

Rheumatic manifestations of histoplasmosis have been uncommon.[212] Cases of arthritis and arthralgias have been diagnosed occasionally in the knee, ankle, wrist, and fingers.[213-224] Polyarticular joint infections were observed in several outbreaks of primary acute histoplasmosis[213-217] (6.3% of patients in one epidemic[213]). With a few exceptions, radiographic evaluation of involved joints did not show erosive lesions.[212] In spite of the high incidence of bone marrow seeding in disseminated histoplasmosis, focal bone involvement, tenosynovitis, and arthritis have been rarely reported.[213,218-220]

Darouiche et al.[212] have described a patient with solitary monoarticular histoplasmosis of the knee which was successfully treated with oral fluconazole (200 mg daily for 9 months) without requiring surgical intervention. In previously reported cases[222-224] of solitary articular histoplasmosis of the wrist, resolution of infection was achieved by surgical excision, followed by intravenous amphotericin B (total doses ranging from 1.0 to 3.5 g) therapy.

Carpal tunnel syndrome due to *H. capsulatum* infection has been reported on several occasions.[222-227] This syndrome, commonly attributed to entrapment neuropathy of the median nerve at the wrist[228] and best known to be the result of work-related injuries,[229] may also be caused by various disorders, such as trauma, rheumatoid arthritis, gout, myxedema, acromegaly, pregnancy, amyloidosis, and infections.[230-233] Mascola and Rickman[225] have described a case of recurrent carpal tunnel syndrome caused by histoplasma infection which was resolved successfully by surgical intervention and subsequent therapy with ketoconazole (400 mg daily) for 6 months. In two of the previously reported cases,[222,227] in addition to surgery, treatment with amphotericin B (total doses of 3.5 and 1.0 g, respectively) was also applied.

37.3.3.8   Mediastinal Histoplasmosis

Sclerosing (fibrosing) mediastinitis is a condition of acute or chronic inflammation resulting in progressive fibrosis within the mediastinum.[234-239] It is a process of relentless proliferation of fibrous tissue that produces encroachment, entrapment, and eventual compression of mediastinal structures, such as the superior vena cava,[240] the azygos, innominate, and pulmonary veins,[241] the pulmonary arteries,[242] and the esophagus and trachea.[243,244] Mediastinal fibrosis may be caused by a variety of pathogens, including *H. capsulatum*.[245-250] The recognition that mediastinal fibrosis may be associated with an underlying disease, such as fungal infection, has markedly improved the management of this difficult to treat condition, and reduced the necessity of surgical decompression of entrapped organs. Thus, Urchel et al.[239] successfully managed sclerosing mediastinitis in six patients with underlying disseminated histoplasmosis with 400-mg daily oral ketoconazole regimens.

Coss et al.[251] described a case of esophageal fistula complicating mediastinal histoplasmosis; the patient was successfully treated with amphotericin B (35 mg/kg administered over a 4-month period). Esophageal involvement in patients with disseminated histoplasmosis is most likely due to hematogenous spread from a primary pulmonary infection.[252] In two previous reports, Jenkins et al.,[253] and Sarosi and Davies[254] also used amphotericin B to treat patients with dysphagia secondary to histoplasmosis.

A number of investigators[255-258] still recommend surgical management of complications arising from mediastinal histoplasmosis because of lack of evidence to demonstrate active infection.[271] In addition, surgical intervention is favored over amphotericin B therapy because of several other factors, namely (1) poor growth characteristics of *H. capsulatum* in the mediastinum, (2) the necessity for pathologic diagnosis of mediastinal masses, (3) the toxicity of amphotericin B, and (4) the potential prophylactic benefit of surgical excision of mediastinal granuloma to prevent fibrosis.[251] To this end, Cameron et al.[259] have suggested the following criteria for nonoperative treatment of esophageal complications: (1) esophageal disruptions confined within the mediastinum, or between the mediastinum and the visceral lung pleura, (2) drainage of the cavity back into the esophagus, (3) minimal symptoms, and (4) minimal signs of clinical sepsis.

Heart involvement due to disseminated histoplasmosis may present with endocarditis or endarteritis.[68,260-275] Disseminated histoplasmosis is reported to be the third leading cause of fungal endocarditis.[276] Histoplasmic endocarditis can affect not only normal cardiac valves but also grossly abnormal structures, such as diseased or prosthetic valves[264,270,273,274] and cardiac tumors.[260] In addition, infection of atheroma and aneurysms in great vessels and vascular drafts has been reported.[35,260]

The recommended therapy for histoplasmic endocarditis is a combination of valve replacement and amphotericin B. Thus, Wilmshurst et al.[277] reported a case of histoplasmic endocarditis on a stenosed aortic valve presenting as dysphagia and weight loss. The patient was treated with intravenous amphotericin B (gradually increasing dose regimens to a maximum of 50 mg daily), beginning 4 d prior to aortic valve replacement; amphotericin B therapy was discontinued 50 d later because of excessive renal toxicity (total dose of 2.55 g), and oral itraconazole (400 mg daily) was instituted for the next 17 months. In another report, however, Kanawaty et al.[275] described the first case of successful nonsurgical treatment of histoplasmic endocarditis involving a bioprosthetic valve using amphotericin B; a total dose of 4.0 g of the drug was infused via a Hickman catheter. Derby et al.[278] also treated a patient with endocarditis complicated with major arterial embolism with amphotericin B and without surgical intervention — the patient survived after receiving 4.8 g (total dose) of the drug. There have been several other reports[68,263,265-267,272] of histoplasmic endocarditis therapy consisting of amphotericin B alone and without surgical involvement.

37.3.3.9 Pulmonary Histoplasmosis and Pleural Effusions

Chronic pulmonary histoplasmosis usually occurs in patients with preexisting lung disease, such as emphysema and chronic bronchitis. The occurrence of pleural effusions associated with histoplasmosis is rarely seen (incidence rate of 0% to 6%).[279-287] In pediatric patients,[288-290] pleural effusion is sometimes diagnosed with concomitant pericarditis.[291] After reviewing the cases of 32 children with acute pulmonary histoplasmosis, Kakos and Kilman[287] found no evidence of pleural effusion. It is not unusual for pleural fluid of patients with histoplasmosis to demonstrate eosinophilia (up to 17%),[292-295] which in the majority of cases has been described as idiopathic.[296]

While, in general, pleural fluid cultures failed to grow the fungus, an exception was reported by Marshall et al.,[297] who were able to grow *H. capsulatum* from a pleural fluid of an AIDS patient. The failure to grow fungus from the pleural fluid of patients with histoplasmosis may support one of the proposed etiologies for the effusion, that it is the result of antigen diffusing from the granulomatous foci located near the pleural space.[294]

For chronic pulmonary histoplasmosis, treatment with amphotericin B has been recommended for patients with progressive, disseminated disease, especially in immunocompromised hosts.[55] The management of pleural effusion would largely depend on the severity of the symptoms.[298] In symptomatic patients with a large pleural effusion, thoracentesis may be indicated to relieve symptoms and eliminate some of the other causes of pleural effusion.[288-291]

37.3.3.10 Central Nervous System Involvement

Although infrequent among patients with disseminated histoplasmosis, CNS involvement has been seen in 10% to 20%, and as high as 50% of immunocompromised hosts.[299-309] According to Shapiro et al.,[300] it can present as miliary or solitary granulomas of the brain, focal or diffuse cerebritis, or histoplasmic meningitis. In the latter case, diagnosis may often be difficult since *H. capsulatum* is not readily grown from cerebrospinal fluid (CSF) samples and serology could be misleading.[307] In spite of the high incidence of meningeal histoplasmosis in both chronic and subacute disease, associated hydrocephalus has seldom been reported.[303,305,308]

Amphotericin B is widely used as therapy, but recurrence of infection is frequently observed.[14,310] In one report,[311] CNS histoplasmosis was cured in 61% of patients receiving at least 30 mg/kg of amphotericin B, as compared to 33% of those treated with lower doses. The higher dose regimens may be needed to overcome the poor penetration of the drug into CSF even in the presence of active meningitis.[312]

In AIDS patients, CNS histoplasmosis commonly presents as meningitis, single or multiple abscesses, or granulomas.[14] Tiraboschi et al.[313] treated one patient with chronic CNS histoplasmosis and hydrocephalus with oral fluconazole (200 mg daily for 6 weeks; then 100 mg daily as maintenance therapy), after amphotericin B (20 mg/kg) failed to sterilize the CSF and reinfection resulted in recurrence of the hydrocephalus. Even though fluconazole easily penetrated the CSF and successfully sterilized it, transverse myelopathy still persisted, and shunting was needed to control the hydrocephalus.[313]

Kelly et al.[314] described a case of disseminated histoplasmosis presenting with multifocal cerebritis and intramedullary spinal histoplasmoma which was successfully treated with amphotericin B resulting in nearly complete symptomatic recovery. In one previous report,[315] chronic administration of prednisone (as therapy for unrelated conditions) to a patient with spinal histoplasmosis was thought to have been the reason for the patient's relapse. Surgical intervention alone has also been used successfully to treat spinal histoplasmosis.[216,317]

37.3.3.11 Childhood Histoplasmosis

Butler et al.[318] have reviewed the clinical presentation and treatment of histoplasmosis among children hospitalized over a 21-year period (1968–1988), in the Vanderbilt University Children's

Hospital, serving an area in middle Tennessee with a high prevalence of endemic histoplasmosis. Of the 35 patients diagnosed with the disease, 83% (n = 29) had pulmonary/mediastinal infection, 14% (n = 5) had disseminated disease, and one patient (3%) had primary cutaneous histoplasmosis. While 80% (n = 28) of the patients did not receive specific antifungal chemotherapy, five patients (14%) were treated with amphotericin B, one patient (3%) with ketoconazole, and one patient received an initial course of amphotericin B, followed by oral ketoconazole. Follow-up evaluations ranged from 1 month to 15 years (mean, 30.1 months); persistency of symptoms existed in six patients, and two patients died of complications (disseminated pulmonary infection, and cardiopulmonary compromise due to mediastinal fibrosis, respectively).[318] This survey, as well as other findings, have shown that mediastinal fibrosis, although refractory to treatment, is relatively rare in children less than 10 years old and will generally resolve spontaneously without residual damage.[319,320] Histoplasmic pericarditis has been a more frequent manifestation in children than adults.[291,318,321]

Another somewhat puzzling and still unexplained fact that came out of the Vanderbilt study[318] as well as from other groups,[68,322] was the apparently reduced incidence of pediatric disseminated histoplasmosis after 1970. Cases of primary cutaneous histoplasmosis among children are highly unusual and very rare.[318,323]

Rescorla et al.[324] have described a case of an otherwise normal child with acute obstruction of the common bile duct caused by histoplasmic lymphadenitis of the peripancreatic lymph nodes. The lymphadenitis was probably the result of duodenal ulcerations caused by histoplasmosis. The patient was treated with amphotericin B (1.0 mg/kg over 24 h) for 38 d; prednisone was started at a dose of 2.0 mg/kg over 24 h for the first 7 d, 1.0 mg/kg over 24 h for the ensuing 7 d, and tapered slowly thereafter. Two weeks after the regimen was initiated, the abdominal computerized tomographic scan showed complete resolution of mass. The rationale to employ a short course of steroids (prednisone) was to provide more rapid relief of the ductal obstruction and eventually to prevent later fibrotic changes to the duct.[324]

37.3.4 Host Immune Defense Against Histoplasmosis

Within 24 h of exposure, inhaled fungal microconidia would trigger an early nonimmune response by fungicidal neutrophils. It is, however, the cell-mediated immune response that is largely responsible for defense against histoplasmosis. A vigorous cell-mediated immune response will usually begin to develop 10 to 21 d after the primary exposure. Development of specific cell-mediated immune response in immunocompetent hosts will frequently result in granuloma formation and containment of the pathogen. Therefore, without massive inhalational exposure, fungal virulence is generally low in immunocompetent patients.[8,9,11,121,325] However, reactivation of infection may occur, especially in immunocompromised patients. Macrophages will accumulate and attach to the pathogen through interaction with adherence-promoting proteins.[326] The mechanism(s) by which the histoplasmal yeasts manage to survive and proliferate inside the macrophages is still not well understood. However, it is known that phagocytosis of the yeasts by human monocytes/macrophages would stimulate the respiratory burst[326-328] and the phagolysosomal fusion.[329] Even so, the ingested yeasts are still capable of multiplying within the phagolysosomes.[330-332]

Lane et al.[333] have investigated the interaction of murine peritoneal macrophages with histoplasma yeasts and found that the acquisition of intracellular iron may be important for the fungal survival. In spite of its ubiquity in mammalian cells, the amount of free iron is very limited. It has been suggested that one mechanism by which interferon-γ-activated mouse peritoneal macrophages and interferon-γ–lipopolysaccharide-activated murine splenic macrophages[334] may suppress the intracellular growth of *H. capsulatum* is by downregulating murine transferrin receptors, thereby restricting the availability of intracellular iron.[334] The fact that most of the available iron is located intracellularly makes it difficult to be acquired by extracellular pathogens.

In addition, the small amount of iron which is in the body fluids is bound by high-affinity glycoproteins, such as transferin and lactoferrin.[335] By restricting infective microbial growth through deprivation of iron, these high-affinity iron-binding host proteins may, in fact, be able to provide a nonspecific nutritional immunity.[336-338] For example, addition of unsaturated transferrin to culture medium was found to suppress the growth of *H. capsulatum*,[339] as well as other fungi (*Candida* sp.[340,341] and *Cryptococcus neoformans*[342]). Furthermore, Lane et al.[333] have demonstrated that in a co-culture of histoplasma-infected murine peritoneal macrophages, the presence of deferoxamine (an iron chelator) inhibited the intracellular growth of yeasts in a concentration-dependent manner, and that this effect was reversed by iron-saturated transferin (holotransferrin) but not by iron-free transferrin (apotransferrin).

The issue whether interferon-γ-stimulated human macrophages will suppress the intracellular growth of histoplasma yeasts is still not clearly resolved. One report[343] suggesting that such inhibition takes place was contradicted by two other studies.[330,332] However, chloroquine, which prevents release of iron from transferrin by raising endocytic and lysosomal pH values, did induce the killing of *H. capsulatum* by human macrophages.[344] Thus, at doses of 40 to 120 mg/kg, given intraperitoneally for 6 d to histoplasma-infected C57BL/6 mice, chloroquine significantly reduced the fungal growth in a dose-dependent manner.[344] The drug not only markedly decreased the number of organisms in the spleen and liver of infected mice, but also provided protection from a lethal inoculum of *H. capsulatum*. These findings demonstrated that iron is still critical for the survival and multiplication of histoplasma yeasts in human macrophages, and chloroquine (as well as, hydroxychloroquine, or other lysosomotropic agents that increase the intraphagosomal pH values) may be effective in the treatment of active histoplasmosis or to prevent relapses of the disease. This mechanism of action, which was also confirmed to be the case with other intracellular pathogens (*Legionella pneumophila*, *M. tuberculosis*, *Listeria*, and *Trypanosoma cruzi*) requiring iron for multiplication,[345-349] while not acting directly on the invading pathogen, may help the host's capacity to destroy it by restricting the availability of iron, and therefore, may reduce the likelihood of microorganisms becoming drug resistant.[344]

Wheat et al.[350] have reported several cases of systemic salmonellosis in patients with disseminated histoplasmosis. While generalized defects of the cellular immunity could have predisposed these patients to both histoplasmosis and salmonellosis, it has been postulated that histoplasma yeast parasitization of the macrophages ("macrophage blockade") would certainly impair their ability to resist other invasive intracellular pathogens, thus becoming, at least in part, a predisposing factor to systemic *Salmonella* infections.[350,351]

37.3.5 REFERENCES

1. Kwong-Chung, K. J., Sexual stage of *Histoplasma capsulatum*, *Science*, 177, 368, 1972.
2. Schwartz, J., *Histoplasmosis*, Praeger, New York, 1981.
3. Hay, R. J., Histoplasmosis, *Semin. Dermatol.*, 12, 310, 1993.
4. Williams, A. O., Lawson, E. A., and Lucas, A. O., African histoplasmosis due to *Histoplasma duboisii*, *Arch. Pathol.*, 92, 306, 1971.
5. Darling, S. T. A., A protozoan general infection: Histoplasma capsulatum producing pseudotubercles in the lungs and focal necrosis in the liver, spleen and lymph nodes, *JAMA*, 46, 1283, 1906.
6. Reddy, P., Gorelick, D. F., Brasher, C. A., and Larsh, H., Progressive disseminated histoplasmosis as seen in adults, *Am. J. Med.*, 48, 629, 1970.
7. Sarosi, G. A., Voth, D. W., Dahl, B. A., Doto, I. L., and Tosh, F. E., Disseminated histoplasmosis: results of long-term follow-up, *Ann. Intern. Med.*, 75, 511, 1971.
8. Bonner, J. R., Alexander, W. J., Dismukes, W. E., App, W., Griffin, F. M., Little, R., and Shin, M. S., Disseminated histoplasmosis in patients with the acquired immune deficiency syndrome, *Arch. Intern. Med.*, 144, 2178, 1984
9. Wheat, L. J. and Small, C. B., Disseminated histoplasmosis in AIDS, *Arch. Intern. Med.*, 144, 2147, 1984.

10. Wheat, L. J., Ketoconazole therapy for AIDS patients with disseminated histoplasmosis, *Arch. Intern. Med.*, 145, 2272, 1985.

11. Wheat, L. J., Slama, T. G., and Zeckel, M. L., Histoplasmosis in the acquired immune deficiency syndrome, *Am. J. Med.*, 78, 203, 1985.

12. Johnson, P. C., Khardori, N., Najjar, A. F., Butt, F., Mansell, P. W., and Sarosi, G. A., Progressive disseminated histoplasmosis in patients with acquired immunodeficiency syndrome, *Am. J. Med.*, 85, 152, 1988.

13. Salzman, S. H., Smith, R. L., and Aranda, C. P., Histoplasmosis in patients at risk for acquired immunodeficiency syndrome in a nonendemic setting, *Chest*, 93, 916, 1988.

14. Anaissie, E., Fainstein, V., Samo, T., Bodey, G. P., and Sarosi, G. A., Central nervous system histoplasmosis; an unappreciated complication of the acquired immunodeficiency syndrome, *Am. J. Med.*, 84, 215, 1988.

15. McKinsey, D. S., Gupta, M. R., Riddler, S. A., Driks, M. R., Smith, D. L., and Kurtin, P. J., Long-term amphotericin B therapy for disseminated histoplasmosis in patients with the acquired immuno-deficiency syndrome (AIDS), *Ann. Intern. Med.*, 111, 655, 1989.

16. McKinsey, D. S., Gupta, M. R., Driks, M. R., Smith, D. L., and O'Connor, M., Histoplasmosis in patients with AIDS: efficacy of maintenance amphotericin B therapy, *Am. J. Med.*, 92, 225, 1992.

17. Bodey, G. P., Infectious complications in cancer patients, *Curr. Probl. Cancer*, 1, 1, 1977.

18. Juliano, R., Lopez-Berestein, G., Mehta, R., Hopfer, R., Mehta, K., and Kasi, L., Pharmacokinetic and therapeutic consequences of liposomal drug delivery: fluorodeoxyuridine and amphotericin B as examples, *Biol. Cell.*, 47, 39, 1983.

19. Lopez-Berestein, G., Mehta, R., Hopfer, R. L., Mills, K., Kasi, L., Mehta, K., Fainstein, V., Luna, M., Hersh, E. M., and Juliano, R., Treatment and prophylaxis of disseminated infection due to *Candida albicans* in mice with liposome-encapsulated amphotericin B, *J. Infect. Dis.*, 147, 939, 1983.

20. Lopez-Berestein, G., Mehta, R., Hopfer, R., Mehta, K., Hersh, E. M., and Juliano, R. L., Effects of sterols on the therapeutic efficacy of liposomal-amphotericin B in murine candidiasis, *Cancer Drug Delivery*, 1, 37, 1983.

21. Lopez-Berestein, G., Hopfer, R. L., Mehta, R., Mehta, K., Hersh, E. M., and Juliano, R. L., Prophylaxis of *Candida albicans* infections in neutropenic mice with liposome-encapsulated amphotericin B, *Antimicrob. Agents Chemother.*, 25, 366, 1984.

22. Lopez-Berestein, G., Hopfer, R., Mehta, R., Mehta, K., Hersh, E. M., and Juliano, R. L., Treatment of disseminated candidiasis in neutropenic mice with liposome-encapsulated amphotericin B, *J. Infect. Dis.*, 3, 278,1984.

23. Lopez-Berestein, G., Fainstein, V., Hopfer, R., Mehta, K., Sullivan, M. P., Keating, M., Rosenblum, M. G., Mehta, R., Luna, M., Hersh, E. M., Reuben, J., Juliano, R. L., and Bodey, G. P., Liposomal amphotericin B for the treatment of systemic fungal infections in patients with cancer: a preliminary study, *J. Infect. Dis.*, 151, 704, 1985.

24. Sculier, J.-P., Coune, A., Meunier, F., Brassinne, C., Laduron, C., Hollaert, C., Collette, N., Heymans, C., and Klastersky, J., Pilot study of amphotericin B entrapped in sonicated liposomes in cancer patients with fungal infections, *Eur. J. Cancer Clin. Oncol.*, 24, 527, 1988.

25. Clark, J. M., Whitney, R. R., Olsen, S. J., George, R. J., Swerdel, M. R., Kunselman, L., and Bonner, D. P., Amphotericin B lipid complex therapy of experimental fungal infections in mice, *Antimicrob. Agents Chemother.*, 35, 615, 1991.

26. Schaffner, C. P. and Mechlinski, W., Polyene macrolide derivatives. II. Physical-chemical properties of polyene macrolide esters and their water soluble salts, *J. Antibiot.*, 25, 259, 1972.

27. Keim, G. R., Poutsiaka, J. W., Kirpan, J., and Keysser, C. H., Amphotericin B methyl ester hydro-chloride and amphotericin B: comparative acute toxicity, *Science*, 179, 584, 1973.

28. Keim, G. R., Sibley, P. L., Yoon, Y. H., Kulesza, J. S., Zaidi, I. H., Miller, M. M., and Poutsiaka, J. W., Comparative toxicological studies of amphotericin B methyl ester and amphotericin B in mice, rats and dogs, *Antimicrob. Agents Chemother.*, 10, 687, 1976.

29. Lawrence, R. M. and Hoeprich, P. D., Comparison of amphotericin B and amphotericin B methyl ester: efficacy in murine coccidioidomycosis and toxicity, *J. Infect. Dis.*, 133, 168, 1976.

30. Bonner, D. P., Tewari, R. P., Solotorovsky, M., Mechlinski, W., and Schaffner, C. P., Comparative chemotherapeutic activity of amphotericin B and amphotericin B methyl ester, *Antimicrob. Agents Chemother.*, 7, 724, 1975.

31. Howarth, W. R., Tewari, R. P., and Solotorovsky, M., Comparative *in vivo* antifungal activity of amphotericin B and amphotericin B methyl ester, *Antimicrob. Agents Chemother.*, 7, 58, 1975.

32. Gadebush, H. H., Pansy, F., Klepner, C., and Schwind, R., Amphotericin B and amphotericin B methyl ester ascorbate. I. Chemotherapeutic activity against *Candida albicans, Cryptococcus neoformans* and *Blastomyces dermatitidis* in mice, *J. Infect. Dis.*, 134, 423, 1976.

33. Houston, A. C. and Hoeprich, P. D., Comparative susceptibility of four kinds of pathogenic fungi to amphotericin B and amphotericin B methyl ester, *Antimicrob. Agents Chemother.*, 13, 905, 1978.

34. Neihart, R. E., Hinthorn, D. R., Hoeprich, P. D., and Liu, C., Successful treatment of progressive disseminated histoplasmosis with amphotericin B methyl ester, *Diagn. Microbiol. Infect.*, 12, 17, 1989.

35. Hawkins, S. S., Gregory, D. W., and Alford, R. H., Progressive disseminated histoplasmosis: favorable response to ketoconazole, *Ann. Intern. Med.*, 95, 446, 1981.

36. Glatt, A. E., Chirgwin, K., and Landesman, S. H., Treatment of infections associated with human immunodeficiency virus, *N. Engl. J. Med.*, 318, 1439, 1988.

37. Slama, T. G., Treatment of disseminated and progressive cavitary histoplasmosis with ketoconazole, *Am. J. Med.*, 74, 70, 1983.

38. Dismukes, W. E., Cloud, G., Bowles, C., Sarosi, G. A., Gregg, C. R., Chapman, S. W., Scheld, W. M., Farr, B., Gallis, H. A., Marier, R. L., Karam, G. H., Bennett, J. E., Kauffman, C. A., Medoff, G., Stevens, D. A., Kaplowitz, L. G., Black, J. R., Roselle, G. A., Pankey, G. A., Kerkering, T. M., Fisher, J. F., Graybill, J. R., and Shadomy, S., Treatment of blastomycosis and histoplasmosis with ketoconazole: results of a prospective, randomized clinical trial, *Ann. Intern. Med.*, 103, 861, 1985.

39. Wheat, J. L., Wass, J., Norton, J., Kohler, R. B., and French, M. L. V., Cavitary histoplasmosis occurring during two large urban outbreaks, *Medicine (Baltimore)*, 63, 201, 1984.

40. Quinones, C. A., Reuben, A. G., Hamill, R. J., Musher, D. M., Gorin, A. B., and Sarosi, G. A., Chronic cavitary histoplasmosis: failure of oral treatment with ketoconazole, *Chest*, 95, 914, 1989.

41. Wheat, L. J., Connolly-Stringfield, P. A., Baker, R. L., Curfman, M. F., Eads, M. E., Israel, K. S., Norris, S. A., Webb, D. H., and Zeckel, M. L., Disseminated histoplasmosis in the acquired immunodeficiency syndrome: clinical findings, diagnosis, and review of the literature, *Medicine (Baltimore)*, 69, 361, 1990.

42. Nightingale, S. D., Parks, J. M., Pounders, S. M., Burns, D. K., Reynolds, J., and Hernandez, J. A., Disseminated histoplasmosis in patients with AIDS, *South. Med. J.*, 83, 624, 1990.

43. Humphrey, M. J., Jevons, S., and Tarbit, M. H., Pharmacokinetic evaluation of UK-49,858, a metabolically stable triazole antifungal drug, in animals and humans, *Antimicrob. Agents Chemother.*, 28, 648, 1985.

44. Arndt, C. A., Walsh, T. J., McCully, C. L., Balis, F. M., Pizzo, P. A., and Poplac, D. G., Fluconazole penetration into cerebrospinal fluid: implications for treating fungal infections of the central nervous system, *J. Infect. Dis.*, 157, 178, 1988.

45. Diaz, M., Negroni, R., Montoro-Gei, F., Castro, L. G. M., Sampaio, S. A. P., Borelli, D., Restrepo, A., Franco, L., Bran, J. L., Arathoon, E. G., Stevens, D. A., and the Fluconazole Pan-American Study Group, A Pan-American 5-year study of fluconazole therapy for deep mycoses in the immunocompetent host, *Clin. Infect. Dis.*, 14(Suppl. 1), S68, 1992.

46. Milatovic, D. and Voss, A., Efficacy of fluconazole in the treatment of systemic fungal infections, *Eur. J. Clin. Microbiol. Infect. Dis.*, 11, 395, 1992.

47. Graybill, J. R., Histoplasmosis and AIDS, *J. Infect. Dis.*, 158, 623, 1988.

48. Sharkey-Mathis, P. K., Velez, J., Fetchick, R., and Graybill, J. R., Histoplasmosis in the acquired immunodeficiency syndrome (AIDS): treatment with itraconazole and fluconazole, *J. Acquir. Immune Defic. Syndr.*, 6, 809, 1993.

49. Kobayashi, G. S., Travis, S. J., and Medoff, G., Comparison of fluconazole and amphotericin B in treatment of histoplasmosis in normal and immunosuppressed mice, *Rev. Infect. Dis.*, 12(Suppl. 3), S291, 1990.

50. Grant, S. M. and Clissold, S. P., Itraconazole: a review of its pharmacodynamic and pharmacokinetic properties, and therapeutic use in superficial and systemic mycoses, *Drugs*, 37, 310, 1989.

51. Odds, F. C., Itraconazole — a new oral antifungal agent with a very broad spectrum of activity in superficial and systemic mycoses, *J. Dermatol. Sci.*, 5, 65, 1993.

52. Zuckerman, J. M. and Tunkel, A. R., Itraconazole: a new triazole antifungal agent, *Infect. Control Hosp. Epidemiol.*, 15, 397, 1994.

53. Negroni, R., Palmieri, O., Koren, F., Tiraboschi, I. N., and Galimberti, R. L., Oral treatment of paracoccidioidomycosis and histoplasmosis with itraconazole in humans, *Rev. Infect. Dis.*, 9(Suppl. 1), S47, 1987.

54. Negroni, R., Robles, A. M., Arechavala, A., and Taborda, A., Itraconazole in human histoplasmosis, *Mycoses*, 32, 123, 1989.

55. Dismukes, W. E., Bradsher, R. W., Cloud, G. C., Kauffman, C. A., Chapman, S. W., George, R. B., Stevens, D. A., Girard, W. M., Saag, M. S., Bowles-Patton, C, and the NIAID Mycoses Study Group, Itraconazole therapy for blastomycosis and histoplasmosis, *Am. J. Med.*, 93, 489, 1992.

56. Negroni, R., Taborda, A., Robles, A. M., and Arechavala, A., Itraconazole in the treatment of histoplasmosis associated with AIDS, *Mycoses*, 35, 281, 1992.

57. Kell, P. D., Smith, D. E., Barton, S. E., Midgley, J., Samarasinghe, P. L., and Gazzard, B. G., Disseminated histoplasmosis in an AIDS patient treated with itraconazole, *Genitourin. Med.*, 67, 342, 1991.

58. Tucker, R. M., Denning, D. W., Hanson, L. H., Rinaldi, M. G., Graybill, J. R., Sharkey, P. K., Pappagianis, D., and Stevens, D. A., Interaction of azoles with rifampin, phenytoin, and carbamazepine: *in vitro* and clinical observations, *Clin. Infect. Dis.*, 14, 165, 1992.

59. Drayton, J., Dickinson, G., and Rinaldi, M. G., Coadministration of rifampin and itraconazole leads to undetectable levels of serum itraconazole, *Clin. Infect. Dis.*, 18, 266, 1994.

60. Kobayashi, G. S., Travis, S. J., Rinaldi, M. G., and Medoff, G., *In vitro* and *in vivo* activities of Sch 39304, fluconazole, and amphotericin B against *H. capsulatum*, *Antimicrob. Agents Chemother.*, 34, 524, 1990.

61. Pappagianis, D., Zimmer, B. L., Theodoropoulos, G., Plempel, M., and Hector, R. F., Therapeutic effect of the triazole Bay R 3783 in mouse models of coccidioidomycosis, blastomycosis, and histoplasmosis, *Antimicrob. Agents Chemother.*, 34, 1132, 1990.

62. Dahn, U., Hagenmaier, H., Hohne, H., Konig, W. A., Wolf, G., and Zahner, H., Nikkomycin, ein neuer hemmstoff der chitin-synthase bei pilzen, *Arch. Mikrobiol.*, 107, 143, 1976.

63. Brillinger, G. U., Metabolic products of microorganisms. 181. Chitin synthase from fungi, a test model for substances with insecticidal properties, *Arch. Microbiol.*, 121, 71, 1979.

64. Hector, R. F., Zimmer, B. L., and Pappagianis, D., Evaluation of nikkomycin X and Z in murine models of coccidioidomycosis, histoplasmosis, and blastomycosis, *Antimicrob. Agents Chemother.*, 34, 587, 1990.

65. Sarosi, G. A. and Davies, S. F., Concise review for primary-care physicians: therapy for fungal infections, *Mayo Clin. Proc.*, 69, 1111, 1994.

66. Kauffman, C. A., Newer developments in therapy for endemic mycoses, *Clin. Infect. Dis.*, 19(Suppl. 1), S28, 1994.

67. Wheat, L. J., Histoplasmosis — diagnosis and treatment, *Infect. Dis. Clin. Prac.*, 1, 277, 1992.

68. Goodwin, R. A., Shapiro, J. L., Thurman, G. H., Thurman, S. S., and Des Prez, R. M., Disseminated histoplasmosis: clinical and pathological correlations, *Medicine (Baltimore)*, 59, 1, 1980.

69. Goodwin, R. A., Jr. and Des Prez, R. M., Histoplasmosis, *Am. Rev. Respir. Dis.*, 117, 929, 1987.

70. Davies, S. F., Khau, M., and Sarosi, G. A., Disseminated histoplasmosis in immunologically suppressed patients, *Am. J. Med.*, 65, 923, 1978.

71. Wheat, L. J., Slama, T. G., Norton, J. A., Kohler, R. B., Eitzen, H. E., French, M. L., and Sathapatayavongs, B., Risk factors for disseminated and fatal histoplasmosis, *Ann. Intern. Dis.*, 96, 159, 1982.

72. Loyd, J. E., Des Prez, R. M., and Goodwin, R. A., *Histoplasma capsulatum*, in *Principles and Practice of Infectious Disease*, Mandell, G. L., Douglas, K. G., and Bennett, J. L., Eds., Churchill-Livingstone, New York, 1985, 1989.

73. Zeluff, B. J., Fungal pneumonia in transplant recipients, *Semin. Respir. Infect.*, 5, 80, 1990.

74. Goodwin, R. A., Owens, F. T., Snell, J. D., Hubbard, W. W., Buchanan, R. D., Terry, R. T., and Des Prez, R., Chronic pulmonary histoplasmosis, *Medicine (Baltimore)*, 55, 413, 1976.

75. Walker, J. V., Baran, D., Yakuk, N., and Freeman, R. B., Histoplasmosis with hypercalcemia, renal failure, and pulmonary necrosis, *JAMA*, 237, 1350, 1977.

76. Murray, J. J. and Heim, C. R., Hypercalcemia in disseminated histoplasmosis: aggravation by vitamin D, *Am. J. Med.*, 78, 881, 1985.

77. Goldstein, R. A., Israel, H. L., Becker, K. L., and Moore, C. F., The infrequency of hypercalcemia in sarcoidosis, *Am. J. Med.*, 51, 21, 1970.

78. Shai, F., Baker, R. K., Addrizzo, J. R., and Wallach, S., Hypercalcemia in mycobacterial infection, *J. Clin. Endocrinol. Metab.*, 34, 251, 1972.

79. Abbasi, A. A., Chemplavi, J. K., Farah, S., Muller, B. F., and Arnstein, A. R., Hypercalcemia in active pulmonary tuberculosis, *Ann. Intern. Med.*, 90, 324, 1979.

80. Need, A. G., Phillips, P. J., Chiu, F. T. S., and Prisk, H. M., Hypercalcemia associated with tuberculosis, *Br. Med. J.*, 280, 831, 1980.

81. Stoekle, J. D., Hardy, H. L., and Weber, A. L., Chronic beryllium disease: long-term follow-up of sixty cases and selective review of the literature, *Am. J. Med.*, 46, 545, 1969.

82. Lee, J. C., Catanzaro, A., Parthemore, J. G., Roach, B., and Deftos, L. J., Hypercalcemia in disseminated coccidioidomycosis, *N. Engl. J. Med.*, 297, 431, 1977.

83. Kantarjian, H. M., Saad, M. F., Esteg, E. H., Sellin, R. V., and Samaan, N. A., Hypercalcemia in disseminated candidiasis, *Am. J. Med.*, 74, 721, 1983.

84. Bell, N. H., Stern, P. H., Pantzer, E., Sinha, T. K., and DeLuca, H. F., Evidence that increased circulating 1α,25-dihydroxyvitamin D is the probable cause for abnormal calcium metabolism in sarcoidosis, *J. Clin. Invest.*, 64, 218, 1979.

85. Stern, P. H., DeOlazzabal, J., and Bell, N. H., Evidence for abnormal regulation of circulating 1α,25-dihydroxyvitamin D in patients with sarcoidosis and normal calcium metabolism, *J. Clin. Invest.*, 66, 852, 1980.

86. Zimmerman, J., Holick, M. F., and Silver, J., Normocalcemia in a hypoparathyroid patient with sarcoidosis: evidence for parathyroid-hormone-independent synthesis of 1,25-dihydroxyvitamin D, *Ann. Intern. Med.*, 98, 338, 1983.

87. Barbour, G. L., Coburn, J. W., Slatopolsky, E., Norman, A. W., and Horst, R. L., Hypercalcemia in an anephric patient with sarcoidosis: evidence for extrarenal generation of 1,25-dihydroxyvitamin D, *N. Engl. J. Med.*, 305, 440, 1981.

88. Maeska, J. K., Batuman, V., Pablo, N. C., and Shakamuri, S., Elevated 1,25-dihydroxyvitamin D levels: occurrence with sarcoidosis with end-stage renal disease, *Arch. Intern. Med.*, 142, 1206, 1982.

89. Mason, R. S., Frankel, T., Yuk-Luen, C., Lissner, D., and Posen, S., Vitamin D conversion by sarcoid lymph node homogenate, *Ann. Intern. Med.*, 100, 59, 1984.

90. Adams, J. S., Sharman, O. P., Gacad, M. A., and Singer, F. R., Metabolism of 25-hydroxyvitamin D₃ by cultured pulmonary alveolar macrophages in sarcoidosis, *J. Clin. Invest.*, 72, 1856, 1983.

91. Anderson, J., Dent, C. E., Harper, C., and Philpot, G. R., Effect of cortisone on calcium metabolism in sarcoidosis with hypercalcemia, *Lancet*, 2, 720, 1954.

92. Zerwekh, J. E., Pak, C. Y. C., Kaplan, R. A., McGuire, J. L., Upchurch, K., Breslau, N., and Johnson, R., Jr., Pathogenic role of 1α,25-dihydroxyvitamin D in sarcoidosis and absorptive hypercalciuria: different response to prednisolone therapy, *J. Clin. Endocrinol. Metab.*, 51, 381, 1980.

93. Cheng, I. J. P., Fang, G. X., Chan, T. M., Chan, P. C. K., and Chan, M. K., Fungal peritonitis complicating peritoneal dialysis: report of 27 cases and review of treatment, *Q. J. Med.*, 265, 407, 1989.

94. Lim, W., Chau, S. P., Chan, P. C. K., and Cheng, I. K. P., *Histoplasma capsulatum* infection associated with continuous ambulatory peritoneal dialysis, *J. Infect.*, 22, 179, 1991.

95. Weinstein, G. D., Methotrexate, *Ann. Intern. Med.*, 86, 199, 1977.

96. Wilkens, R. F. and Watson, M. A., Methotrexate: a perspective of its use in the treatment of rheumatic disease, *J. Lab. Clin. Med.*, 100, 314, 1982.

97. Groff, G. D., Shenberger, K. N., Wilke, W. S., and Taylor, T. H., Low-dose oral methotrexate in rheumatoid arthritis: an uncontrolled trial and review of the literature, *Semin. Arthritis Rheum.*, 12, 333, 1983.

98. Weinstein, A., Marlowe, S., Korn, J., and Farouhar, F., Low-dose methotrexate treatment of rheumatoid arthritis, *Am. J. Med.*, 79, 331, 1985.

99. Perruquet, J. L., Harrington, T. M., and Davis, D. E., *Pneumocystis carinii* pneumonia following methotrexate therapy for rheumatoid arthritis, *Arthritis Rheum.*, 26, 1291, 1983.

100. Wallis, P. J. W., Ryatt, K. S., and Constable, T. J., *Pneumocystis carinii* pneumonia complicating low dose methotrexate treatment for psoriatic arthropathy, *Ann. Rheum. Dis.*, 48, 247, 1989.

101. Leff, R. L., Case, J. P., and McKenzie, R., Rheumatoid arthritis, methotrexate therapy, and pneumocystis pneumonia, *Ann. Intern. Med.*, 112, 716, 1990.

102. Keegan, J. M. and Byrd, J. W., Nocardiosis associated with low dose methotrexate for rheumatoid arthritis, *J. Rheumatol.*, 15, 1585, 1988.

103. Altz-Smith, M., Kendall, L. G., Jr., and Stamm, A. M., Cryptococcosis associated with low-dose methotrexate for arthritis, *Am. J. Med.*, 83, 179, 1987.

104. Witty, L. A., Steiner, F., Curfman, M., Webb, D., and Wheat, L. J., Disseminated histoplasmosis in patients receiving low-dose methotrexate therapy for psoriasis, *Arch. Dermatol.*, 128, 91, 1992.

105. Jolivet, J., Cowan, K., Curt, G., Clendeninn, N., and Chabner, B., The pharmacology and clinical use of methotrexate, *N. Engl. J. Med.*, 309, 1094, 1983.

106. Huang, D. T., McGarry, T., Cooper, S., Saunders, R., and Andavolu, R., Disseminated histoplasmosis in the acquired immunodeficiency syndrome, *Arch. Intern. Med.*, 147, 1181, 1987.

107. Kaur, J. and Myers, A. M., Homosexuality, steroid therapy, and histoplasmosis, *Ann. Intern. Med.*, 99, 567, 1983.

108. Kalter, D. C., Tschen, J. A., and Klima, M., Maculopapular rash in a patient with acquired immuno-deficiency syndrome, *Arch. Dermatol.*, 121, 1455, 1985.

109. Dietrich, P. Y., Pugin, P., Regamey, C., and Bille, J., Disseminated histoplasmsosis and AIDS in Switzerland, *Lancet*, 2, 752, 1986.

110. Johnson, P. C., Sarosi, G. A., Septimus, E. J., and Satterwhite, T. K., Progressive disseminated histoplasmosis in patients with the acquired immune deficiency syndrome: a report of 12 cases and a literature review, *Semin. Respir. Infect.*, 1, 1, 1986.

111. Hazelhurst, J. A. and Vismer, H. F., Histoplasmosis presenting with unusual skin lesions in acquired immunodeficiency syndrome (AIDS), *Br. J. Dermatol.*, 113, 345, 1985.

112. Macher, B. E., Rodriguez, M. M., Kaplan, W., Pistole, M. C., McKittrick, A., Lawrinson, W. E., and Reichert, C. M., Disseminated bilateral chorioretinitis due to *Histoplasma capsulatum* in a patient with the acquired immunodeficiency syndrome, *Ophthalmology*, 92, 1159, 1985.

113. Haggerty, C. M., Britton, M. C., Dorman, J. M., and Marzoni, F. A., Jr., Gastrointestinal histoplasmosis in the acquired immunodeficiency syndrome, *West. J. Med.*, 143, 244, 1985.

114. Johnson, P. C. and Sarosi, G. A., AIDS and progressive disseminated histoplasmosis, *JAMA*, 258, 202, 1987.

115. Alterman, D. D. and Cho, K. C., Histoplasmosis involving the omentum in an AIDS patient, *J. Comput. Assist. Tomogr.*, 12, 664, 1988.

116. Pasternak, J. and Bolivar, R., Bone marrow examination and culture in the diagnosis of acquired immunodeficiency syndrome (AIDS), *Arch. Intern. Med.*, 143, 1495, 1983.

117. Wheat, L. J. and Batteriger, B. E., Histoplasmosis, *Handbook Clin. Neurol.*, 8, 437, 1988.

118. Wheat, L. J., Kohler, R. B., and Tewari, R. P., Diagnosis of disseminated histoplasmosis by detection of *Histoplasma capsulatum* antigen in serum and urine specimens, *N. Engl. J. Med.*, 314, 83, 1986.

119. Wheat, L. J., Connolly-Stringfield, P., Kohler, R. B., Frame, P. T., and Gupta, M. R., *Histoplasma capsulatum* polysaccharide antigen detection in diagnosis and management of disseminated histo-plasmosis in patients with acquired immunodeficiency syndrome, *Am. J. Med.*, 87, 396, 1989.

120. Wheat, L. J., Connolly-Stringfield, P., Blair, R., Connolly, K., Garringer, T., Katz, B. P., and Gupta, M., Effect of successful treatment with amphotericin B on *Histoplasma capsulatum* variety *capsulatum* polysaccharide antigen levels in patients with AIDS and histoplasmosis, *Am. J. Med.*, 92, 153, 1992.

121. Drew, R. H., Pharmacotherapy of disseminated histoplasmosis in patients with AIDS, *Ann. Pharmacother.*, 27, 1510, 1993.

122. Zon, L. I., Arkin, C., and Groopman, J. E., Haematologic manifestations of the human immune deficiency virus (HIV), *Br. J. Haematol.*, 66, 251, 1987.

123. Spivak, J. L., Barnes, D. C., Fuchs, E., and Quinn, T. C., Serum immunoreactive erythropoietin in HIV-infected patients, *JAMA*, 261, 3104, 1989.

124. Lin, A. C., Galdwasser, E., Bernard, E. M., and Chapman, S. W., Amphotericin B blunts erythropoietin response to anemia, *J. Infect. Dis.*, 161, 348, 1990.

125. Lancaster, D. J., Palte, S., and Ray, D., Recombinant human erythropoietin in the treatment of anemia in AIDS patients receiving concomitant amphotericin B and zidovudine, *J. Acquir. Immune Defic. Syndr.*, 6, 533, 1993.

126. Cauteren, H., Heykants, J., Decoster, R., and Cauwenberg, G., Itraconazole: pharmacologic studies in animals and humans, *Rev. Infect. Dis.*, 9(Suppl. 1), S43, 1987.

127. Hay, R. J., Dupont, B., and Graybill, J. R., First international symposium on itraconazole: a summary, *Rev. Infect. Dis.*, 9(Suppl. 1), S1, 1987.

128. Van Cutsem, J., Van Gerven, F., and Janssen, P. A. J., Activity of orally, topically, and parenterally administered itraconazole in the treatment of superficial and deep mycosis: animal models, *Rev. Infect. Dis.*, 9(Suppl. 1), S15, 1987.

129. Ganer, A., Arathoon, E., and Stevens, D. A., Initial experience in therapy for progressive mycoses with itraconazole, the first clinically studied triazole, *Rev. Infect. Dis.*, 9(Suppl. 1), S77, 1987.

130. Saag, M. S. and Dismukes, W. E., Azole antifungal agents: emphasis on new triazoles, *Antimicrob. Agents Chemother.*, 32, 1, 1988.

131. Tucker, R. M., Williams, P. L., Arathoon, E. G., and Stevens, D. A., Treatment of mycoses with itraconazole, *Ann. NY Acad. Sci.*, 544, 51, 1988.

132. British Society for Antimicrobial Chemotherapy Working Party, Antifungal chemotherapy in patients with acquired immunodeficiency syndrome, *Lancet*, 340, 648, 1992.

133. Baptist, S. J., Montana, J. B., Arden, S. B., Leon, L., and Dutel, M., Disseminated histoplasmosis in a man with AIDS, *NY State J. Med.*, 11, 664, 1985.

134. Humphrey, M. J., Jevon, S., and Tarbit, M. H., Pharmacokinetic evaluation of UK 49,858, a metabolically stable triazole antifungal drug, in animals and humans, *Antimicrob. Agents Chemother.*, 28, 648, 1985.

135. Smith, E., Franzmann, M., and Mathiesen, L. R., Disseminated histoplasmosis in Danish patients with AIDS, *Scand. J. Infect. Dis.*, 21, 573, 1989.

136. Graybill, J. R., Future directions of antifungal chemotherapy, *Clin. Infect. Dis.*, 14(Suppl. 1), S170, 1992.

137. Norris, S., McKinsey, D., Lancaster, D., and Wheat, J., Retrospective evaluation of fluconazole maintenance therapy for disseminated histoplasmosis in AIDS, *Proc. 32nd Intersci. Conf. Antimicrob. Agents Chemother.*, Anaheim, Abstr. 1207, American Society for Microbiology, Washington, D.C., 1992.

138. Jones, P. G., Cohen, R. L., Batts, D. H., and Silva, J., Jr., Disseminated histoplasmosis, invasive pulmonary aspergillosis, and other opportunistic infections in a homosexual patient with acquired immune deficiency syndrome, *Sex. Transm. Dis.*, 10, 202, 1983.

139. Salzman, S. H., Smith, R. L., and Aranda, C. P., Histoplasmosis in patients at risk for the acquired immunodeficiency syndrome in a nonendemic area, *Chest*, 93, 916, 1988.

140. Lake-Bakaar, G., Winston, T., Lake-Bakaar, D., Gupta, N., Beidas, S., Elsakr, M., and Straus, E., Gastropathy and ketoconazole malabsorption in the acquired immunodeficiency syndrome (AIDS), *Ann. Intern. Med.*, 109, 471, 1988.

141. Mello, K. A., Wheat, L. J., Lis, R., Donnelly, B., and Skolnik, P. R., Ketoconazole-responsive tonsilar infection due to *Histoplasma capsulatum* in an HIV-1-seropositive individual, *AIDS*, 5, 908, 1991.

142. Rawlinson, W. D., Packham, D. R., Gardner, F. J., and MacLeod, C., Histoplasmosis in the acquired immunodeficiency syndrome (AIDS), *Aust. NZ J. Med.*, 19, 707, 1989.

143. Wheat, J., Hafner, R., Wulfsohn, M., Spencer, P., Squires, K., Powderly, W., Wong, B., Rinaldi, M., Saag, M., Hamill, R., Murphy, R., Connolly-Stringfeld, P., Briggs, N., Owens, S., and the NIAID Clinical Trials and Mycoses Study Group, Prevention of relapse of histoplasmosis with itraconazole in patients with the acquired immunodeficiency syndrome, *Ann. Intern. Med.*, 118, 610, 1993.

144. Stansell, J. J. D., Pulmonary fungal infections in HIV-infected persons, *Semin. Respir. Infect.*, 8, 116, 1993.

145. Pottage, J. C., Jr. and Sha, B. E., Development of histoplasmosis in a human immunodeficiency virus-infected patient receiving fluconazole, *J. Infect. Dis.*, 164, 622, 1991.

146. Wheat, L. J., Smith, E. J., Sathapatayavongs, B., Batteiger, B., Filo, R. S., Leapman, S. B., and French, M. V., Histoplasmosis in renal allograft recipients: two large urban outbreaks, *Arch. Intern. Med.*, 143, 703, 1983.

147. Davies, S. F., Sarosi, G. A., Peterson, P. K., Khan, M., Howard, R. J., Simmons, R. L., and Najarian, J. S., Disseminated histoplasmosis in renal transplant recipients, *Am. J. Surg.*, 137, 686, 1979.

148. Goetz, M. B. and Jones, J. M., Combined ketoconazole and amphotericin B treatment of acute disseminated histoplasmosis in a renal allograft recipient, *South. Med. J.*, 78, 1368, 1985.

149. Kitahara, M., Kobayashi, G. S., and Medoff, G., Enhanced efficacy of amphotericin B and rifampicin combined treatment of murine histoplasmosis and blastomycosis, *J. Infect. Dis.*, 133, 663, 1976.

150. Williams, D. M., Graybill, J. R., and Drutz, D. J., Experimental chemotherapy of histoplasmosis in nude mice, *Am. Rev. Respir. Dis.*, 120, 837, 1979.

151. Ferguson, R. M., Sutherland, D. E. R., Simmons, R. L., and Najarian, J. S., Ketoconazole, cyclosporin metabolism, and renal transplantation, *Lancet*, 2, 882, 1982.

152. Studdard, J., Sneed, W. F., Taylor, J. R., Jr., and Campbell, G. D., Cutaneous histoplasmosis, *Am. Rev. Respir. Dis.*, 113, 689, 1976.

153. Dijkstra, J. W. E., Histoplasmosis, *Dermatol. Clin.*, 7, 251, 1989.

154. Cohen, P. R., Bank, D. E., Silvers, D. N., and Grosmann, M. E., Cutaneous lesions of disseminated histoplasmosis in human immunodeficiency virus- infected patients, *J. Am. Acad. Dermatol.*, 23, 422, 1990.

155. Machado, A. A., Branco Coelho, I. C., Ferreira Roselino, A. M., Simao Trad, E., Fernando de Castro Figueiredo, J., Martinez, R., and Carlos de Costa, J., Histoplasmosis in individuals with acquired immunodeficiency syndrome (AIDS): report of six cases with cutaneous-mucosal involvement, *Mycopathologia*, 115, 13, 1991.

156. Cohen, P. R., Held, J. L., Grossman, M. E., Ross, M. J., and Silvers, D. N., Disseminated histoplasmosis as an ulcerated verrucous plaque in a human immunodeficiency virus-infected man: report of a case possibly involving human-to-human transmission of histoplasmosis, *Int. J. Dermatol.*, 30, 104, 1991.

157. Madeiros, D. A., Marty, S. D., and Tosh, F. E., Erythema nodosum and erythema multiforme as clinical manifestations of histoplasmosis in a community outbreak, *N. Engl. J. Med.*, 274, 415, 1966.

158. Miller, H. E., Keddie, F. M., Johnstone, H. G., and Bostick, W. L., Histoplasmosis: cutaneous and membranous lesions, mycologic and pathologic observations, *Arch. Derm. Syphilol.*, 56, 715, 1947.

159. Farr, B., Beacham, B. E., and Stuk, N. O., Cutaneous histoplasmosis after renal transplantation, *South. Med. J.*, 74, 636, 1981.

160. Washburn, R. G. and Bennett, J. E., Reversal of adrenal glucocorticoid dysfunction in a patient with disseminated histoplasmosis, *Ann. Intern. Med.*, 110, 86, 1989.

161. Daman, L. A., Hashimoto, K., Kaplan, R. J., and Trent, M. G., Disseminated histoplasmosis in an immunosuppressed patient, *South. Med. J.*, 70, 355, 1977.

162. Abildgaard, W. H., Hargrove, R. H., and Kalivas, J., *Histoplasma* penicilitis, *Arch. Dermatol.*, 121, 914, 1985.

163. Johnson, C. A., Tang, C. K., and Tiji, R. M., Histoplasmosis of skin and lymph node and chronic lymphocytic leukemia, *Arch. Dermatol.*, 115, 336, 1979.

164. Strong, R. P., Study of some tropical ulcerations of skin with particular reference to their etiology, *Philippines J. Sci.*, 7, 91, 1986.

165. King, R. W., Kraikitpanich, S., and Lindeman, R. D., Subcutaneous nodules caused by *Histoplasma capsulatum*, *Ann. Intern. Med.*, 86, 586, 1977.

166. Navarro, E. E., Tupasi, T. E., Verallo, V. M., Romero, R. C., and Tuazon, C. U., Disseminated histoplasmosis with unusual cutaneous lesions in a patient from the Philippines, *Am. J. Trop. Med. Hyg.*, 46, 141, 1992.

167. Recondo, G., Sella, A., Ro, J. Y., Dexeus, F. H., Amato, R., and Kilbourn, R., Perianal ulcer in disseminated histoplasmosis, *South. Med. J.*, 84, 931, 1991.

168. Cimponeriu, D., LoPresti, P., Lavelanet, M., Roistacher, K., Remigio, P., Marfatia, S., and Glatt, A. E., Gastrointestinal histoplasmosis in HIV infection: two cases of colonic pseudocancer and review of the literature, *Am. J. Gastroenterol.*, 89, 129, 1994.

169. Becherer, P. R., Sokol-Anderson, M., Joist, J. H., and Milligan, T., Gastrointestinal histoplasmosis presenting as hematochezia in human immunodeficiency virus-infected hemophilic patients, *Am. J. Hematol.*, 47, 229, 1994.

170. Graham, B. D., McKinsey, D. S., Driks, M. R., and Smith, D. L., Colonic histoplasmosis in acquired immunodeficiency syndrome. Report of two cases, *Dis. Colon Rectum*, 34, 185, 1991.

171. Keelan, C. and Imbert, M., Colonic histoplasmosis simulating Crohn's disease in a patient with AIDS, *Bol. Asoc. Med. P. R.*, 80, 248, 1988.

172. United States Public Health Service Cooperative Mycoses Study, Course and prognosis of untreated histoplasmosis, *JAMA*, 177, 292, 1961.

173. Haws, C. C., Long, R. F., and Caplan, G. E., Histoplasmosis capsulatum as a cause of ileocolitis, *Am. J. Roentgenol.*, 128, 692, 1977.

174. Cappell, M. S. and Manzione, N. C., Recurrent colonic histoplasmosis after standard therapy with amphotericin B in a patient with Job's syndrome, *Am. J. Gastroenterol.*, 86, 119, 1991.

175. Cappell, M. S., Mandell, M., Grimes, M. M., and Neu, H. C. Gastrointestinal histoplasmosis, *Dig. Dis. Sci.*, 33, 353, 1988.

176. Hutto, J. O., Bryan, C. S., Greene, F. L., White, C. J., and Gallin, J. I., Cryptococcosis of the colon resembling Crohn's disease in a patient with the hyperimmunoglubulinemia E-recurrent infection (Job's syndrome), *Gastroenterology*, 94, 808, 1988.

177. Albert-Florr, J. J. and Granda, A., Ileocecal histoplasmosis mimicking Crohn's disease in a patient with Job's syndrome, *Digestion*, 33, 176, 1986.

178. Miller, R. L., Gould, A. R., Skolnick, J. L., and Epstein, W. M., Localized oral histoplasmosis, *Oral Surg. Oral Med. Oral Pathol.*, 53, 367, 1982.

179. Hupp, J. R., Layne, J. M., and Glickman, R. S., Solitary palatal ulcer, *J. Oral Maxillofac. Surg.*, 43, 365, 1985.

180. Zain, R. B. and Ling, K. C., Oral and laryngeal histoplasmosis in a patient with Addison's disease, *Ann. Dent.*, 47, 31, 1988.

181. Hiltbrand, J. B. and McGuirt, W. F., Orophayngeal histoplasmosis, *South. Med. J.*, 83, 227, 1990.

182. Cobb, C. M., Schultz, R. E., Brewer, J. H., and Dunlap, C. L., Chronic pulmonary histoplasmosis with an oral lesion, *Oral Surg. Oral Med. Oral Pathol.*, 67, 73, 1989.

183. Donovan, J. O. and Wood, M. D., Histoplasmosis of the larynx, *Laryngoscope*, 94, 206, 1984.

184. Scully, C. and Paes de Almeida, O., Orofacial manifestations of the systemic mycoses, *J. Oral Pathol. Med.*, 21, 289, 1992.

185. Toth, B. B. and Frame, B. B., Oral histoplasmosis: diagnostic complications and treatment, *Oral Surg. Oral Med. Oral Pathol.*, 55, 597, 1983.

186. Dobleman, T. J., Scher, N., Goldman, M., and Doot, S., Invasive histoplasmosis of the mandible, *Head Neck Surg.*, 11, 81, 1989.

187. Fowler, C. B., Nelson, J. F., Henley, D. W., and Smith, B. R., Acquired immune deficiency syndrome presenting as a palatal perforation, *Oral Surg. Oral Med. Oral Pathol.*, 67, 313, 1989.

188. Huber, M. A., Hall, E. H., and Rathbun, W. A., The role of the dentist in diagnosing infection in the AIDS patient, *Milit. Med.*, 154, 315, 1989.

189. Oda, D., McDougal, L., Fritsche, T., and Worthington, P., Oral histoplasmosis as a presenting disease in acquired immunodeficiency syndrome, *Oral Surg. Oral Med. Oral Pathol.*, 70, 631, 1990.

190. Swindells, S., Durham, T., Jahansson, S. L., and Kaufman, L., Oral histoplasmosis in a patient infected with HIV, *Oral Surg. Oral Med. Oral Pathol.*, 77, 126, 1994.

191. Cohen, P. R., Oral histoplasmosis in HIV-infected patients, *Oral Surg. Oral Med. Oral Pathol.*, 78, 277, 1994.

192. Heinic, G. S., Greenspan, D. S., MacPhail, L. A., Schiodt, M., Miyasaki, S. H., Kaufman, L., and Greenspan, J. S., Oral *Histoplasma capsulatum* infection in association with HIV infection: a case report, *J. Oral Pathol Med.*, 21, 85, 1992.

193. De Boom, G. W., Rhyne, R. R., and Correll, R. W., Multiple, painful oral ulcerations in a patient with Hodgkin's disease, *JADA*, 113, 807, 1986.

194. Miller, D. P. and Everett, E. D., Gastrointestinal histoplasmosis, *J. Clin. Gastroenterol.*, 1, 233, 1979.

195. Smith, J. W. and Utz, J. P., Progressive disseminated histoplasmosis: a prospective study of 26 patients, *Ann. Intern. Med.*, 75, 557, 1972.

196. Dean, L. W., Histoplasmosis of the larynx, *Arch. Otolaryngol. Head Neck Surg.*, 36, 390, 1942.

197. Van Pernis, P. A., Benson, M. E., and Holinger, P. H., Case reports: laryngeal and systemic histoplasmosis (Darling), *Ann. Intern. Med.*, 18, 384, 1943.

198. Parkes, M. and Burtoff, S., Histoplasmosis of the larynx: report of a case, *Med. Ann. D. C.*, 18, 641, 1949.

199. Roberts, S. E. and Forman, F. S., Histoplasmosis — a deficiency disease: report of two cases with laryngeal involvement, *Ann. Otol. Rhinol. Laryngol.*, 59, 809, 1950.

200. Hulse, W. F., Laryngeal histoplasmosis, *Arch. Otolaryngol. Head Neck Surg.*, 54, 65, 1951.

201. Hutchinson, H. E., Laryngeal histoplasmosis simulating carcinoma, *J. Pathol. Bacteriol.*, 64, 309, 1952.

202. Burton, C. T. and Wallenborn, P. A., Histoplasmosis of the larynx, *Va. Med. Month.*, 80, 665, 1953.

203. Withers, B. T., Pappas, J. J., and Erickson, E. E., Histoplasmosis primary in the larynx, *Arch. Otolaryngol. Head Neck Surg.*, 77, 26, 1963.

204. Demaldent, J. E., Gentilini, M., Amat, C., and Manach, Y., A propos d'un cas d'histoplasmose laryngée, *Ann. Otolaryngol. Chir. Cervicofac.*, 95, 287, 1978.

205. Sataloff, R. T., Wilborn, A., Prestipino, A., Hawkshaw, M., Heuer, R. J., and Cohn, J., Histoplasmosis of the larynx, *Am. J. Otolaryngol.*, 14, 199, 1993.

206. Fletcher, S. M. and Prussin, A. J., Histoplasmosis of the larynx treated with ketoconazole: a case report, *Otolaryngol. Head Neck Surg.*, 103, 813, 1990.

207. Feman, S. S. and Tilford, R. H., Ocular findings in patients with histoplasmosis, *JAMA*, 253, 2534, 1985.

208. Simmons, C. A. and Matthews, D., Prevalence of uveitis: a retrospective study, *J. Am. Optom. Assoc.*, 64, 386, 1993.

209. Maumenee, A. E., Clinical entities in uveitis, *Am. J. Ophthalmol.*, 69, 1, 1970.

210. Weingeist, T. A. and Watzke, R. C., Ocular involvement by *Histoplasma capsulatum*, *Int. Ophthalmol. Clin.*, 23, 33, 1983.

211. Feman, S. S., Pritchett, P., Johns, K., Weistrich, D. J., and Salmon, W. D., Intraocular tumor from disseminated histoplasmosis, *South. Med. J.*, 84, 780, 1991.

212. Darouiche, R. O., Cadle, R. M., Zenon, G. J., Weinert, M. F., Hamill, R. J., and Lidsky, M. D., Articular histoplasmosis, *J. Rheumatol.*, 19, 1991, 1992.

213. Rosenthal, J., Brandt, K. D., Wheat, L. J., and Slama, T. G., Rheumatologic manifestations of histoplasmosis in the recent Indianapolis epidemic, *Arthritis Rheum.*, 26, 1065, 1983.

214. Friedman, S. J., Black, J. L., and Duffy, J., Histoplasmosis presenting as erythema multiforme and polyarthritis, *Cutis*, 34, 396, 1984.

215. Thornberry, D. K., Wheat, L. J., Brandt, K. D., and Rosenthal, J., Histoplasmosis presenting with joint pain and hilar adenopathy: pseudosarcoidosis, *Arthritis Rheum.*, 25, 1396, 1982.

216. Wheat, L. J., Slama, T. G., Eitzen, H. E., Kohler, R. B., French, M. L. V., and Biesecker, J. L., A large urban outbreak of histoplasmosis: clinical features, *Ann. Intern. Med.*, 94, 331, 1981.

217. Class, R. N. and Cascio, F. S., Histoplasmosis presenting as acute polyarthritis, *N. Engl. J. Med.*, 287, 1133, 1972.

218. Pfaller, M. A., Kyriakos, M., Week, P. M., and Kobayashi, G. S., Disseminated histoplasmosis presenting as an acute tenosynovitis, *Diagn. Microbiol. Infect. Dis.*, 3, 251, 1985.

219. Jones, P. G., Rolston, K., and Hopfer, R. L., Septic arthritis due to *Histoplasma capsulatum* in a leukaemic patient, *Ann. Rheum. Dis.*, 44, 128, 1985.

220. Van der Schee, A. C., Dinkla, B. A., and Festen, J. J., Gonarthritis as only manifestation of chronic disseminated histoplasmosis, *Clin. Rheumatol.*, 9, 92, 1990.

221. Key, J. A. and Large, A. M., Histoplasmosis of the knee, *J. Bone Joint Surg.*, 24, 281, 1942.

222. Omer, G. E., Jr., Lockwook, R. S., and Travis, L. O., Histoplasmosis involving the carpal joint: a case report, *J. Bone Joint Surg.*, 45A, 1699, 1963.

223. Perlman, R., Jubelirer, R. A., and Schwarz, J., Histoplasmosis of the common palmar tendon sheath, *J. Bone Joint Surg.*, 54A, 676, 1972.

224. Strayer, D. S., Gutwein, M. B., Herbold, D., and Bresilier, R., Histoplasmosis presenting as the carpal tunnel syndrome, *Am. J. Surg.*, 141, 286, 1981.

225. Mascola, J. R. and Rickman, L. S., Infectious causes of carpal tunel syndrome: case report and review, *Rev. Infect. Dis.*, 13, 911, 1991.

226. Vanek, J. and Schwarz, J., The gamut of histoplasmosis, *Am. J. Med.*, 50, 89, 1971.

227. Randall, G., Smith, P. W., Korbitz, B., and Owen, D. R., Carpal tunnel syndrome caused by *Mycobacterium fortuitum* and *Histoplasma capsulatum*: report of two cases, *J. Neurosurg.*, 56, 299, 1982.

228. Phalen, G. S., The carpal-tunnel syndrome. Seventeen years' experience in diagnosis and treatment of six hundred fifty-four hands, *J. Bone Joint Surg.*, 48A, 211, 1966.

229. Baker, E. L. and Ehrenberg, R. L., Preventing the work-related carpal tunnel syndrome: physician reporting and diagnostic criteria, *Ann. Intern. Med.*, 112, 317, 1990.

230. Nakano, K. K., Entrapment neuropathies, in *Textbook of Rheumatoplogy*, 3rd ed., Kelley, W. N., Harris, E. D., Jr., Ruddy, S., and Sledge, C. B., Eds., W. B. Saunders, Philadelphia, 1989, 1845.

231. Biundo, J. J., Regional rheumatic pain syndromes, in *Primer on the Rheumatic Diseases*, Arthritis Foundation, Atlanta, 1988, 263.

232. Klofkorn, R. W. and Steigerwald, J. C., Carpal tunnel syndrome as the initial manifestation of tuberculosis, *Am. J. Med.*, 60, 583, 1976.

233. Inglis, A. E., Straub, L. R., and Williams, C. S., Median nerve neuropathy at the wrist, *Clin. Orthop.*, 83, 48, 1972.

234. Dines, D. E., Bernatz, P. E., and Pairolero, P. C., Mediastinal granuloma and fibrosing mediastinitis, *Chest*, 75, 320, 1979.

235. Engleman, P., Liebow, A. A., Gmelich, J., and Friedman, P. J., Pulmonary hyalinizing granuloma, *Am. Rev. Respir. Dis.*, 115, 997, 1977.

236. Hewlett, T. H., Steer, A., and Thomas, D. E., Progressive fibrosing mediastinitis, *Ann. Thorac. Surg.*, 2, 345, 1966.

237. Light, A. M., Idiopathic fibrosis of mediastinum as discussion of three cases and a review of the literature, *Am. J. Clin. Pathol.*, 31, 78, 1978.

238. Schonengerdt, C. B., Suyemoto, R., and Main, F. B., Granulomatosis and fibrosing mediastinitis: a review and analysis of 180 cases, *J. Thorac. Cardiovasc. Surg.*, 57, 365, 1979.

239. Urchel, H. C., Jr., Razzuk, M. A., Netto, G. J., Disiere, J., and Chung, S. Y., Sclerosing mediastinitis: improved management with histoplasmosis titer and ketoconazole, *Ann. Thorac. Surg.*, 50, 215, 1990.

240. Doty, D. B., Bypass of superior vena cava, *J. Thorac. Cardiovasc. Surg.*, 83, 3326, 1982.

241. Arnett, E. N., Bacos, J. M., Marsh, H. B., Savage, D. D., Fulmer, J. D., and Roberts, W. C., Fibrosing mediastinitis causing pulmonary arterial hypertension without pulmonary venous hypertension, *Am. J. Med.*, 63, 634, 1977.

242. Trinkle, J. K., Fibrous mediastinitis presenting as mitral stenosis, *J. Thorac. Cardiovasc. Surg.*, 62, 161, 1970.

243. James, E. C., Harris, S. S., and Dillenburg, C. J., Tracheal stenosis: an unusual presenting complication of idiopathic fibrosing mediastinitis, *J. Thorac. Cardiovasc. Surg.*, 80, 410, 1980.

244. Zajtchuk, R., Strevey, T. E., Heydorn, W. H., and Treasure, R. L., Mediastinal histoplasmosis, *J. Thorac. Cardiovasc. Surg.*, 66, 300, 1973.

245. Ahmad, M., Weinstein, A. J., Hughes, J. A., and Cosgrove, D. E., Granulomatous mediastinitis due to aspergillus flavors in a nonimmunosuppressed patient, *Am. J. Med.*, 70, 887, 1981.

246. Drutz, D. J. and Catanzaro, A., Coccidioidomycosis, *Am. Rev. Respir. Dis.*, 117, 559, 1978.

247. Goodwin, R. A., Nickell, J. A., and Des Prez, R., Mediastinal fibrosis complicating healed primary histoplasmosis and tuberculosis, *Medicine (Baltimore)*, 51, 227, 1972.

248. Leong, A. S. Y., Granulomatous mediastinitis due to *Rhisopos* species, *Am. J. Clin. Pathol.*, 70, 103, 1978.

249. Stead, W. W. and Bates, J. H., Tuberculosis, in *Harrison's Principles of Internal Medicine*, 10th ed., Petersdorf, R. G. et al., Eds., McGraw-Hill, New York, 1983, 1021.

250. Yacoub, M. H. and Thompson, V. C., Chronic idiopathic pulmonary hilar fibrosis, *Thorax*, 26, 365, 1971.

251. Coss, K. C., Wheat, L. J., Conces, D. J., Brashear, R. E., and Hull, M. T., Esophageal fistula complicating mediastinal histoplasmosis: response to amphotericin B, *Am. J. Med.*, 83, 343, 1987.

252. Lee, J. H., Newman, D. A., and Welsh, J. D., Disseminated histoplasmosis presenting with esophageal symptomatology, *Dig. Dis.*, 22, 831, 1977.

253. Jenkins, D. W., Fisk, D. E., and Byrd, R. B., Mediastinal histoplasmosis with esophageal abscess, *Gastroenterology*, 70, 109, 1976.

254. Sarosi, G. A. and Davies, S. F., Gastrointestinal involvement in histoplasmosis, *Pract. Gastroenterol.*, 8, 19, 1984.

255. Goodwin, R. A., Loyd, J. E., and Des Prez, R. M., Histoplasmosis in normal hosts, *Medicine (Baltimore)*, 60, 231, 1981.

256. Gilliland, M. D., Scott, L. D., and Walker, W. E., Esophageal obstruction caused by mediastinal histoplasmosis: beneficial results of operation, *Surgery*, 95, 59, 1984.

257. Schneider, R. P. and Edwards, W., Histoplasmosis presenting as an esophageal tumor, *Gastrointest. Endosc.*, 23, 158, 1977.

258. Dines, D. E., Payne, W. S., Bernatz, P. E., and Pairolero, P. C., Mediastinal granuloma and fibrosing mediastinitis, *Chest*, 75, 320, 1979.

259. Cameron, J. L., Kieffer, R. F., and Hendrix, T. R., Selective nonoperative management of contained intrathoracic disruptions, *Ann. Thorac. Surg.*, 27, 404, 1979.

260. Bradsher, R. W., Wickre, C. G., Savage, A, M., Harstone, W. E., and Alford, R. H., *Histoplasmu capsulatum* endocarditis cured by amphotericin B combined with surgery, *Chest*, 78, 791, 1980.

261. Haust, M. D., Wlodek, G. K., and Parker, J. O., Histoplasma endocarditis, *Am. J. Med.*, 32, 460, 1962.

262. Gerber, H. J., Schoonmaker, F. W., and Vazquez, M. D., Chronic meningitis associated with *Histoplasma* endocarditis, *N. Engl. J. Med.*, 275, 74, 1966.

263. Hartley, R. A., Remsberg, J. R. S., and Sinaly, N. P., Histoplasma endocarditis, *Arch. Int. Med.*, 119, 527, 1967.

264. Weaver, D. K., Batsakis, J. G., Nishiyama, R. H., and Arbor, A., Histoplasma endocarditis, *Arch. Surg.*, 96, 19, 1968.

265. Segal, C., Wheeler, C. G., and Tompsett, R., Histoplasma endocarditis cured with amphotericin, *N. Engl. J. Med.*, 28, 206, 1969.

266. Matthay, R. A., Levin, D. C., Wicks, A. B., and Ellis, J. H., Jr., Disseminated histoplasmosis involving an aortofemoral prosthetic graft, *JAMA*, 235, 1478, 1976.

267. Canlas, M. S. and Dillon, M. L., Jr., *Histoplasma capsulatum* endocarditis: report of a case following heart surgery, *Angiology*, 28, 454, 1977.

268. Olive, T., Lagier, A., Dumas, O., Bidart, J. M., and Bernard, P. M., Histoplasmose generalisée avec localosation laryngée et endocaroite, *Nouv. Presse Med.*, 7, 2262, 1978.

269. Rogers, E. W., Weyman, A. E., Noble, R. J., and Bruins, S. C., Left atrial myxoma infected with *Histoplasma capsulatum*, *Am. J. Med.*, 64, 683, 1978.

270. Alexander, W. J., Mowry, R. W., Cobbs, C. G., and Dismukes, W. E., Prosthetic valve endocarditis caused by *Histoplasma capsulatum*, *JAMA*, 242, 1399, 1979.

271. Waterhouse, G., Burney, D. P., and Prager, R. L., *Histoplasma capsulatum*: endocarditis requiring aortic valve replacement for aortic insufficiency, *South. Med. J.*, 73, 683, 1980.

272. Blair, T. P., Waugh, R. A., Pollack, M., Ashworth, H. E., Young, N. A., Anderson, S. E., and Bem, T. P., *Histoplasma capsulatum* endocarditis, *Am. Heart J.*, 99, 783, 1980.

273. Gaynes, R. P., Gardner, P., and Causey, W., Prosthetic valve endocarditis caused by *Histoplasma capsulatum*, *Arch. Int. Med.*, 141, 1533, 1981.

274. Svirbely, J. R., Ayers, L. W., and Buesching, W. J., Filamentous *Histoplasma capsulatum* endocarditis involving mitral and aortic valve porcine bioprostheses, *Arch. Pathol. Lab. Med.*, 109, 273, 1985.

275. Kanawaty, D. S., Stalker, J. B., and Munt, P. W., Nonsurgical treatment of histoplasma endocarditis involving a bioprosthetic valve, *Chest*, 99, 253, 1991.

276. Weinstein, L., Pathogenesis of infectious endocarditis, in *Heart Disease: A Textbook of Cardiovascular Medicine*, 3rd ed., Braunwald, E., Ed., W. B. Saunders, Philadelphia, 1988, 1093.

277. Wilmshurst, P. T., Venn, G. E., and Eykyn, S. J., Histoplasma endocarditis on a stenosed aortic valve presenting as dysphagia and weight loss, *Br. Heart J.*, 70, 565, 1993.

278. Derby, B. M., Coolidge, K., and Rogers, D. E., *Histoplasma capsulatum* endocarditis with major arterial embolism, *Arch. Intern. Med.*, 110, 101, 1962.

279. Curr, F. J. and Wier, J. A., Histoplasmosis, a review of one-hundred consecutively hospitalized patients, *Am. Rev. Respir. Dis.*, 77, 749, 1958.

280. Rubin, H., Furcolow, M. L., Yates, J. L., and Brasher, C. A., The course and prognosis of histoplasmosis, *Am. J. Med.*, 27, 278, 1959.

281. Baum, G. L. and Schwartz, J., Chronic pulmonary histoplasmosis, *Am. J. Med.*, 33, 873, 1962.

282. Palayew, M. J., Frank, H., and Sedlezsky, I., Histoplasmosis: our experience of seventy cases with follow-up study, *J. Can. Assoc. Radiol.*, 17, 142, 1966.

283. Brodsky, A. L., Gregg, M. B., Loewenstein, M. S., Kaufman, L., and Mallison, G. F., Outbreak of histoplasmosis associated with the 1970 Earth Day activities, *Am. J. Med.*, 54, 333, 1973.

284. Ward, J. L., Weeks, M., Allen, D., Hutcheson, R. H., Jr., Anderson, R., Fraser, D. W., Kaufman, L., Ajello, L., and Spickard, A., Acute histoplasmosis: clinical, epidemiologic and serologic findings of an outbreak associated with exposure to a fallen tree, *Am. J. Med.*, 66, 587, 1979.

285. Straus, S. E. and Jacobsen, E. S., The spectrum of histoplasmosis in a general hospital: a review of 55 cases diagnosed at Barnes Hospital between 1966 and 1977, *Am. J. Med. Sci.*, 279, 147, 1980.

286. Gustafson, T. L., Kaufman, L., Weeks, R., Ajello, L., Hutcheson, R. H., Jr., Wiener, S. L., Lamhe, D. W,, Jr., Sayvetz, T. A., and Schaffner, W., Outbreak of acute pulmonary histoplasmosis in members of a wagon train, *Am. J. Med.*, 71, 759, 1981.

287. Kakos, G. S. and Kilman, J. W., Symptomatic histoplasmosis in children, *Ann. Thorac. Surg.*, 15, 622, 1973.

288. Weissblith, M., Pleural effusion in histoplasmosis, *J. Pediatr.*, 88, 894, 1976.

289. Ericsson, C. D., Pickering, L. K., and Salmon, G. W., Pleural effusion in histoplasmosis, *J. Pediatr.*, 90, 327, 1977.

290. Brickman, H. F., Pleural effusion in histoplasmosis, *J. Pediatr.*, 90, 327, 1977.

291. Picardi, J. L., Kauffman, C. A., Schwarz, J., Holmes, J. C., Phair, J. P., and Fowler, N. O., Pericarditis caused by *Histoplasma capsulatum*, *Am. J. Cardiol.*, 37, 82, 1976.

292. Schub, H. M., Spivey, C. G., and Baird, G. D., Pleural involvement in histoplasmosis, *Am. Rev. Respir. Dis.*, 94, 225, 1966.

293. Brewer, P. L. and Himmelwright, J. P., Pleural effusion due to infection with *Histoplasma capsulatum*, *Chest*, 58, 76, 1970.

294. Swinburne, A. J., Fedullo, A. J., Wahl, G. W., and Fernand, B., Histoplasmoma, pleural fibrosis, and slowly enlarging pleural effusion in an asymptomatic patient, *Am. Rev. Respir. Dis.*, 135, 502, 1987.

295. Downey, E. F., Asymptomatic pleural effusion in histoplasmosis: case report, *Milit. Med.*, 147, 218, 1982.

296. Adelman, M., Albelda, S. M., Gottlieb, J., and Hoponik, E. F., Diagnostic utility of pleural fluid eosinophilia, *Am. J. Med.*, 77, 915, 1984.

297. Marshall, B. C., Cox, J. K., Carroll, K. C., and Morrison, R. E., Case report: histoplasmosis as a cause of pleural effusion in the acquired immunodeficiency syndrome, *Am. J. Med. Sci.*, 300, 98, 1990.

298. Quasney, M. W. and Leggiadro, R. J., Pleural effusion associated with histoplasmosis, *Pediatr. Infect. Dis. J.*, 12, 415, 1993.

299. Schultz, D. M., Histoplasmosis of the central nervous system, *JAMA*, 151, 549, 1953.

300. Shapiro, J. L., Lux, J. J., and Scrofkin, B. E., Histoplasmosis of the central nervous system, *Am. J. Pathol.*, 31, 319, 1955.

301. Cooper, R. A. and Goldstein, E., Histoplasmosis of the central nervous system: report of two cases and review of the literature, *Am. J. Med.*, 35, 45, 1963.

302. Ramseyer, J. C., Baker, R. N., and Tomiyasu, U., Ventriculovenous shunt in the treatment of obstructive hydrocephalus due to coccidioidomycotic meningitis, *Neurology*, 16, 701, 1966.

303. Fetter, B. F., Klintworth, G. K., and Hendry, W. S., *Mycoses of the Central Nervous System*, Williams & Wilkins, Baltimore, 1967.

304. Gelfand, J. A. and Bennett, J. E., Active histoplasma meningitis of 22 years duration, *JAMA*, 233, 1294, 1975.

305. Enarson, D. A., Keys, T. F., and Onofrio, B. M., Central nervous system histoplasmosis with obstructive hydrocephalus, *Am. J. Med.*, 64, 895, 1978.

306. Laurence, R. M. and Goldstein, E., Histoplasmosis, in *Infections of the Nervous System. Part III. Handbook of Clinical Neurology*, Vol. 35, Vinken, P. J. and Bruyn, G. W., Eds., North-Holland, Amsterdam, 1978, 503.

307. Jacobson, E. S. and Straus, S. E., Reevaluation of diagnostic histoplasma serologies, *Am. J. Med. Sci.*, 281, 143, 1981.

308. Young, R. P., Gede, G., and Grinnell, V., Surgical treatment for fungal infections of the central nervous system, *J. Neurosurg.*, 63, 371, 1985.

309. Snyder, C. H. and White, R. S., Successful treatment of histoplasma meningitis with amphotercin B, *J. Pediatr.*, 58, 554, 1961.

310. Kauffman, C. A., Israel, K. S., Smith, V. W., and White, A. C., Histoplasmosis in immunosuppressed patients, *Am. J. Med.*, 64, 923, 1978.

311. Wheat, L. J., Batteiger, B. E., and Sathapatayavongs, B., *Histoplasma capsulatum* infection of the central nervous system, *Medicine (Baltimore)*, 69, 244, 1990.

312. Louria, D. B., Some aspects of the absorption, distribution and excretion of amphotericin B in man, *Antimicrob. Agents Chemother.*, 5, 295, 1958.

313. Tiraboschi, I., Casas Parera, I., Pikielny, R., Scattini, G., and Micheli, F., Chronic *Histoplasma capsulatum* infection of the central nervous system successfully treated with fluconazole, *Eur. Neurol.*, 32, 70, 1992.

314. Kelly, D. R., Smith, C. D., and McQuillen, M. P., Successful medical treatment of a spinal histoplasmoma, *J. Neuroimag.*, 4, 327, 1994.

315. Tan, V., Wilkins, P., Badve, S., Coppen, M., Lucas, S., Hay, R., and Schon, F., Histoplasmosis of the central nervous system, *J. Neurol. Neurosurg. Psychiatry*, 55, 619, 1992.

316. Voelker, J. L., Muller, J., and Worth, R. M., Intramedullary spinal *Histoplasma* granuloma: case report, *J. Neurosurg.*, 70, 959, 1989.

317. Bazan, C. and New, P. Z., Intramedullary spinal histoplasmosis: efficacy of gadolinium enhancement, *Neuroradiology*, 33, 190, 1991.

318. Butler, J. C., Heller, R., and Wright, P. F., Histoplasmosis during childhood, *South. Med. J.*, 87, 476, 1994.

319. Loyd, J. E., Tillman, B. F., Atkinson, J. B., and Des Prez, R. M., Mediastinal fibrosis complicating histoplasmosis, *Medicine (Baltimore)*, 67, 295, 1988.

320. Prager, R. L., Burney, D. P., Waterhouse, G., and Bender, H. W., Jr., Pulmonary, mediastinal, and cardiac presentations of histoplasmosis, *Ann. Thorac. Surg.*, 30, 385, 1980.

321. Wheat, L. J., Stein, L., Corya, B. C., Wass, J. L., Norton, J. A., Grider, K., Slama, T. G., French, M. L., and Kohler, R. B., Pericarditis as a manifestation of histoplasmosis during two large urban outbreaks, *Medicine (Baltimore)*, 62, 110, 1983.

322. Leggiadro, R. J., Barrett, F. F., and Hughes, W. T., Disseminated histoplasmosis of infancy, *Pediatr. Infect. Dis. J.*, 7, 799, 1988.

323. Weinberg, G. A., Kleiman, M. B., Grosfeld, J. L., Weber, T. R., and Wheat, L. J., Unusual manifestations of histoplasmosis in childhood, *Pediatrics*, 72, 99, 1983.

324. Rescorla, F. J., Kleiman, M. B., and Grosfeld, J. L., Obstruction of the common bile duct in histoplasmosis, *Pediatr. Infect. Dis. J.*, 13, 1017, 1994.

325. Spitzer, E. D., Keath, E. J., Travis, S. J., Painter, A. A., Kobayashi, G. B., and Medoff, G., Temperature-sensitive variants of *Histoplasma capsulatum* isolates from patients with acquired immunodeficiency syndrome, *J. Infect. Dis.*, 162, 258, 1990.

326. Bullock, W. E. and Wright, S. D., Role of the adherence-promoting receptors, CR3, LFA-1, and p150,95, in binding of *Histoplasma capsulatum* by human macrophages, *J. Exp. Med.*, 165, 195, 1987.

327. Newman, S. L., Bucher, C., Rhodes, J., and Bullock, W. E., Phagocytosis of *Histoplasma capsulatum* yeasts and microconidia by human cultured macrophages and alveolar macrophages: cellular cytoskeleton requirement for attachment and ingestion, *J. Clin. Invest.*, 85, 223, 1990.

328. Schnur, R. A. and Newman, S. L., The respiratory burst response to *Histoplasma capsulatum* by human neutrophils: evidence for intracellular trapping of superoxide anion, *J. Immunol.*, 144, 4765, 1990.

329. Newman, S. L., Gootee, L., Morris, R., and Bullock, W. E., Digestion of *Histoplasma capsulatum* yeasts by human macrophages, *J. Immunol.* 149, 574, 1992.

330. Fleischmann, J., Wu-Hsieh, B., and Howard, D. H., The intracellular fate of *Histoplasma capsulatum* in human macrophages is unaffected by recombinant human interferon-γ, *J. Infect. Dis.*, 161, 143, 1990.

331. Newman, S. L., Gootee, L., Bucher, C., and Bullock, W. E., Inhibition of intracellular growth of *Histoplasma capsulatum* yeast cells by cytokine-activated human monocytes and macrophages, *Infect. Immun.*, 59, 737, 1991.

332. Newman, S. L. and Gootee, L., Colony-stimulating factors activate human macrophages to inhibit the intracellular growth of *Histoplasma capsulatum* yeasts, *Infect. Immun.*, 60, 4593, 1992.

333. Lane, T. E., Wu-Hsieh, B. A., and Howard, D. H., Iron limitation and the gamma-interferon-mediated antihistoplasma state of murine macrophages, *Infect. Immun.*, 59, 2274, 1991.

334. Lane, T. E., Wu-Hsieh, B. A., and Howard, D. H., Gamma interferon cooperates with lipopolysaccharide to activate mouse splenic macrophages to an antihistoplasma state, *Infect. Immun.*, 61, 1468, 1993.

335. Aisen, P. and Leibman, A., Lactoferrin and transferrin: a comparative study, *Biochim. Biophys. Acta*, 257, 314, 1972.

336. Finkelstein, R. A., Sciortino, C. V., and McIntosh, M. A., Role of iron in microbe-host interactions, *Rev. Infect. Dis.*, 5, S759, 1983.

337. Weinberg, E. D., Iron withholding: a defense against infection and neoplasia, *Physiol. Rev.*, 64, 65, 1984.

338. Litwin, C. M. and Calderwood, S. B., Role of iron in regulation of virulence genes, *Clin. Microbiol. Rev.*, 6, 137, 1993.

339. Sutcliffe, M. C., Savage, A. M., and Alford, R. H., Transferrin-dependent growth inhibition of yeast-phase *Histoplasma capsulatum* by human serum and lymph, *J. Infect. Dis.*, 142, 209, 1980.

340. Caroline, L., Taschdjian, C. L., Kozinn, P. J., and Schade, A. L., Reversal of serum fungistasis by addition of iron, *J. Invest. Dermatol.*, 42, 415, 1964.

341. Otto, V. and Howard, D. H., Further studies on the intracellular behaviour of *Torulopsis glabrata*, *Infect. Immun.*, 14, 433, 1976.

342. Hendry, A. T. and Bakerspigel, A., Factors affecting serum inhibited growth of *Candida albicans* and *Cryptococcus neoformans*, *Sabouraudia*, 7, 219, 1969.

343. Brummer, E., Kurita, N., Yoshida, S., Nishimura, K., and Miyaji, M., Killing of *Histoplasma capsulatum* by γ-interferon-activated human monocyte-derived macrophages: evidence for a superoxide anion-dependent mechanism, *J. Med. Microbiol.*, 35, 29, 1991.

344. Newman, S. L., Gootee, L., Brunner, G., and Deepe, G. S., Jr., Chloroquine induces human macrophage killing of *Histoplasma capsulatum* by limiting the availability of intracellular iron and is therapeutic in a murine model of histoplasmosis, *J. Clin. Invest.*, 93, 1422, 1994.

345. Byrd, T. F. and Horwitz, M. A., Chloroquine inhibits the intracellular multiplication of *Legionella pneumophila* by limiting the availability of iron: a potential new mechanism for the therapeutic effect of chloroquine against intracellular pathogens, *J. Clin. Invest.*, 88, 351, 1991.

346. Crowle, A. J. and May, M. H., Inhibition of tubercle bacilli in cultured human macrophages by chloroquine used alone and in combination with streptomycin, izoniazid, pyrazinamide, and two metabolites of vitamin D_3, *Antimicrob. Agents Chemother.*, 34, 2217, 1990.

347. Alford, C. E., King, T. E., Jr., and Campbell, P. A., Role of transferrin receptors, and iron in macrophage listericidal activity, *J. Exp. Med.*, 174, 459, 1991.

348. Loo, V. G. and Lalonde, R. G., Role of iron in intracellular growth of *Trypanozoma cruzi*, *Infect. Immun.*, 45, 726, 1984.

349. Lalonde, R. G. and Holbein, B. E., Role of iron in *Trypanozoma cruzi* infection of mice, *J. Clin. Invest.*, 73, 470, 1984.

350. Wheat, L. J., Rubin, R. H., Harris, N., Smith, E. J., Tewari, R., Chaudhary, S., Lascari, A., Mandell, W., Garvey, G., and Goldberg, D., Systemic salmonellosis in patients with disseminated histoplasmosis, *Arch. Intern. Med.*, 147, 561, 1987.

351. Kimberlin, C. L., Hariri, A. R., Hempel, H. O., and Goodman, N. L., Interactions between *Histoplasma capsulatum* and macrophages from normal and treated mice: comparison of the mycelial and yeast phases in alveolar and peritoneal macrophages, *Infect. Immunol.*, 34, 6, 1981.

37.4 AFRICAN HISTOPLASMOSIS

37.4.1 INTRODUCTION

The African histoplasmosis, caused by the dimorphic fungus *Histoplasma capsulatum* var. *duboisii*, has been limited largely to Central and Western Africa (especially Nigeria), and some other localized areas (the province of Natal in South Africa).[1-4] The yeast stage is relatively large and can reach sizes of 10 to 15 μm. Although occasional budding forms may be seen, hyphae are not present. The fungus is isolated from the soil and no animal source has been identified. Infections are believed to occur secondary to traumatic inoculation into the skin.[2]

The African histoplasmosis has several manifestations that are seldom seen with *H. capsulatum* var. *capsulatum*.[5] The lung does not usually contain clinically detectable lesions, although miliary infiltrates[6] and nodular lesions[7] have been occasionally described. The most common manifestations occur in bone and skin.[8,9]

Bone lesions, which tend to multiply, are particularly common in the rib, vertebra, femur, humeris, tibia, skull, and wrist.[9] Subcutaneous abscess from an underlying bone lesion has been one of the three cutaneous manifestations of this mycosis; the other two being subcutaneous granulomata and nodular lesions.[10]

37.4.2 MANAGEMENT OF AFRICAN HISTOPLAMOSIS AND EVOLUTION OF THERAPIES

The treatment of the disease is usually difficult and success is achieved only when therapy is initated early in the infection. The histologic appearance of the affected skin is characterized by epidermal atrophy with granulomatous infiltrate within the dermis, as well as acute and chronic infiltrates. Dissemination could affect the subcutis, muscles, the reticuloendothelial system, mucous membranes, lungs, and the bone.[2] Cutaneous lesions may be manifested as either multiple painless or pruritic papules and nodules anywhere on the body surface. In the chronic form, the disease affects the mucous membranes and the gastrointestinal tract and is manifested by ulcerations of the nose, mouth, anus, and genitalia. Bone involvement is often seen, especially in the femur and vertebrae. In progressive disease, the reticuloendothelial system is also affected, resulting in enlargement of the liver and the lymph nodes. Dissemination occurs largely by the hematogenous route. However, contrary to infections caused by *Histoplasma capsulatum* var. *capsulatum*, pulmonary involvement in African histoplasmosis is not common and occurs only in disseminated disease.[2]

For years, intravenous amphotericin B has been considered the drug of choice in treating the disease.[11] However, it is not always curative and its toxicity may become very serious by causing irreversible renal damage in some patients.

Oral ketoconazole is less toxic and seems to be of therapeutic value. Thus, Mabey and Hay[12] treated five patients (three children with disseminated disease, and two adults with localized cutaneous lesions) with ketoconazole at daily doses ranging from 5 to 15 mg/kg, depending on age and clinical conditions; in some cases amphotericin B was also used. Both patients with the cutaneous disease responded to treatment; of the three children with disseminated disease, one responded well, one responded initially but had a relapse, and one child did not respond to therapy.[4]

After its recent introduction into the clinic, itraconazole has been used successfully in the treatment of several cases of African histoplasmosis. Dupont and Drouhet[13] reported a case in which a patient, after falling repeatedly into relapses following treatments with amphotericin B and ketoconazole, was given oral itraconazole at daily doses of 100 mg for 6 months. The patient remained well at 9 months post-therapy. In another case,[14] the patient had no recurrence after itraconazole medication at a 2-year follow-up examination. Bayles[1] reported on a case presented with papular lesions resembling molluscum contagiosum, lymphadenopathy, and pulmonary and bone marrow involvement. The initial therapy included 100 mg daily of itraconazole for 3 months, increasing it afterwards to 200 mg daily for another 9 months; the patient was free from skin lesions 3 years later; however, the lung condition showed little change.

Localized orbital histoplasmosis due to *H. capsulatum* var. *duboisii* was successfully cured with two tablets daily of septrin (a combination of 80 mg trimethoprim and 400 mg sulfamethoxazole per tablet) and surgical drainage of the orbit.[15] Three previous reports[16-18] have also indicated a complete or partial response of histoplasmosis to septrin alone or in combination with amphotericin B. The mechanism of action by which sulfamethoxazole and trimethoprim exterted their effects on histoplasma is not clearly understood.

Abrucio Neto et al.[19] described a case of African histoplasmosis diagnosed in Brazil. The patient, an immigrant from Angola, had cutaneous lesions that were successfully treated with 100 mg daily of itraconazole for 52 d; no recurrent skin lesions were observed during the 10-month follow-up period. Earlier, Oddo et al.[20] reported the first case of *Histoplasma duboisii* in South America. Again, the patient lived in Africa before moving to Chile.

37.4.3 REFERENCES

1. Bayles, M. A. H., Tropical mycoses, *Chemotherapy*, 38(Suppl. 1), 27, 1992.
2. Gross, M. L. and Millikan, L. E., Deep fungal infections in the tropics, *Dermatol. Clin.*, 12, 695, 1994.
3. Vanbreuseghem, R., Reflexions sur l'histoplasmose africaine at l'histoplasmose americaine, *Mykosen*, 25, 171, 1982.
4. Williams, A. O., Lawson, E. A., and Lucas, A. O., African histoplasmosis due to *Histoplasma duboisii*, *Arch. Pathol.*, 92, 306, 1971.
5. Kwon-Chung, K. J. and Bennett, J. E., *Medical Mycology*, Lea and Febiger, Philadelphia, 1992, 487.

6. Dupont, B., Drouhet, E., and Lapresle, C., Histoplasmosis généralisée a *Histoplasma duboisii*, *Nouv. Presse Med.*, 3, 1005, 1974.

7. Seeliger, H. P. R., Kracht, J., and Bikfalvi, A., Grosszellige (afrikanische) histoplasmamykose der lunge, *Dtsch. Med. Wochenschr.*, 105, 609, 1980.

8. Cockshott, W. P. and Lucas, A. O., *Histoplasma duboisii*, *Q. J. Med.*, 33, 223, 1964.

9. Williams, A. O., Lawson, E. A., and Lucas, A. O., African histoplasmosis due to *Histoplasma duboisii*, *Arch. Pathol.*, 92, 306, 1971.

10. Lucas, A. O., Cutaneous manifestations of African histoplasmosis, *Br. J. Dermatol.*, 82, 435, 1970.

11. Dupont, B., Lortholary, O., Datry, A. et al., Imported histoplasmosis due to H. duboisii in France (1968–1994). *Proc. 36th Intersci. Conf. Antimicrob. Agents Chemother.*, American Society for Microbiology, Washington, D.C., Abstr. K58, 1996, 260.

12. Mabey, D. C. W. and Hay, R. J., Further studies on the treatment of African histoplasmosis with ketoconazole, *Trans. R. Soc. Trop. Med. Hyg.*, 83, 560, 1989.

13. Dupont, B. and Drouhet, E., Early experience with itraconazole *in vitro* and in patients: pharmaco-kinetic studies and clinical results, *Rev. Infect. Dis.*, 9(Suppl. 1), S71, 1987.

14. Drouhet, E., African histoplasmosis, *Baillieres Clin. Trop. Med. Commun. Dis.*, 4, 89, 1989.

15. Ajayi, B. G. K., Osuntokun, B., Olurin, O., Kale, O. O., and Junaid, T. A., Orbital histoplasmosis due to *Histoplasma capsulatum* var. *duboisii*: successful treatment with septrin, *J. Trop. Med. Hyg.*, 89, 179, 1986.

16. MacLeod, W. M., Treatment of histoplasmosis, *Lancet*, 2, 363, 1970.

17. Brown, K. G. E., Molesworth, B. D., Boerrigter, F. G. G., and Tozer, R. A., Disseminated histoplasmosis duboisii in Malawi: partial response to sulphonamide/trimethoprim combination, *East Afr. Med. J.*, 51, 584, 1974.

18. Egere, J. U., Gugnani, H. C., Okoro, A. N., and Suseelan, A. V., African histoplasmosis in Eastern Nigeria: report of two culturally proven cases treated with septrin and amphotericin B, *J. Trop. Med. Hyg.*, 81, 225, 1978.

19. Abrucio Neto, L., Takahashi, M. D. F., Salebian, A., and Cuce, L. C., African histoplasmosis: report of the first case in Brasil and treatment with itraconazole, *Rev. Inst. Med. Trop. Sao Paolo*, 35, 295, 1993.

20. Oddo, D., Etchart, M., and Thompson, L., *Histoplasma duboisii* (African histoplasmosis). An African case reported from Chile with ultrastructural study, *Pathol. Res. Pract.*, 186, 514, 1990.

37.5   *BLASTOMYCES DERMATITIDIS*

37.5.1   INTRODUCTION

Blastomycosis (Gilchrist's disease) was first described by Gilchrist as a protozoan infection in 1894.[1,2] However, in 1896, Gilchrist and Stokes[3] identified the pathogen as a fungus, which they named *Blastomyces dermatitidis*. Two years later, the disease was successfully transferred by inoculation of material from a human lesion to a dog.[4] Later, other cases of blastomycosis were reported by physicians, mainly from the Chicago area, and their keen interest in this mycosis led to its recognition at one time as the "Chicago disease."

Blastomycosis was originally believed to be endemic to North and Central America (the U.S., Canada, Mexico, and Central America) until 1952, when a case was reported from Tunisia in which the pathogen was identified as *Scopulariopsis americana*, a synonym of *B. dermatitidis*.[5,6] Later, other cases of blastomycosis in Africa, South America, and Asia followed.[7-13]

In 1968, McDonough and Lewis[14] discovered the ascomycetous state (*Ajellomyces dermatitidis*) of *B. dermatitidis* and provided a method for testing further the identity of fungi from North American and African blastomycosis. The exact incidence and epidemiology of blastomycosis is not well understood, mainly because of the lack of a reliable immunologic marker from previous infections.

Blastomyces (Ajellomyces) dermatitidis is a dimorphic fungus which can grow in mammalian tissues as budding cells (yeast phase), and in cultures as a dry, white mold (mycelial form) bearing spherical or ovoid conidia (arthrospores), 2 to 10 μm in diameter.[15-17] The fungal growth can be maintained also *in vitro* by incubation at 37°C on blood agar. The arthrospores represent the infectious particles of the parasite.[18] Inhalation of these conidia results in primary infection in the lungs where they convert into the yeast phase.[19] In tissues, the fungus represents a nearly spherical cell, 8 to 15 μm (rarely up to 30 μm) in diameter, with a thick wall (0.5 to 0.75 μm).[16] It reproduces by budding, and the typical bud is characterized by its large size, attachment to the parent cell by a persistent wall, and a wide pore (4 to 5 μm) between the bud and the parent cell.[16] The persistence of the bud attachment and the tendency of the parent cell to continue budding, frequently result in the so-called "multiple budding", a characteristic small cluster of cells having an additional bud protruding from the parent cell near the point of attachment of the first bud.[16]

In North America, blastomycosis is most frequently found in the regions of the Mississippi and Ohio River valleys, and the upper midwestern states and Canadian provinces bordering the Great Lakes and the Saint Laurence River.[20-23] It appears that soil with a high organic content and low pH value may facilitate growth of the fungus. The proximity of water also appears to promote the growth of *B. dermatitidis*.[24-27] Although isolation of the fungus from natural soil was found to be difficult,[28,29] Klein et al.[22,26] have reported the isolation, on two separate occasions, of *B. dermatitidis* from soil in association with an epidemic of the infection.

Blastomycosis is generally considered to be a soil-borne infection. In humans, *B. dermatitidis* causes a mixed pyogenic and granulomatous disease.[30] The fungus has also been found in dogs,[31] cats, and other mammals,[32,33] where the prevalence and incidence of infection, especially in dogs and other mammals, has been similar to that in humans,[34,35] and may be relevant to the correct diagnosis of human disease.[31,36]

The major route of human infection is most likely through the respiratory tract rather than the skin.[16,37,38] When organs other than lungs are affected by the fungus, it has been nearly always by dissemination from a primary lesion in the lung.[39] Skin injuries caused by bites of infected dogs have been reported to result in cutaneous blastomycosis.[40] Sexual transmission of blastomycosis has been described at least on two occasions.[41,42] Pulmonary blastomycosis in pregnant women has also been reported.[43-48] It is not unexpected that in such cases, the severity of infection may increase due to a depressed state of cell-mediated immunity likely to occur during pregnancy.[49] Intrauterine transmission to the fetus is very rarely observed.[48,50] Person-to-person aerial transmission of the infection has never been reported.

In immunocompetent patients, blastomycosis will most likely produce clinical manifestations ranging from asymptomatic to mild influenza-like or atypical pneumonia syndrome,[24,51] or a rapidly progressive respiratory or systemic illness.[23] The long-term carriage of the organism also presents the potential for reactivation following the initial exposure.[52]

In immunocompromised hosts, however, the disease may be life-threatening and has been described in renal,[53-58] heart,[57] and bone marrow[57] transplant recipients receiving corticosteroids,[59,60] and patients with underlying hematologic malignancies or solid tumors.[60,61] In some earlier reports, the mortality rate from systemic blastomycosis was estimated to be between 70% and 80%,[62] and as high as 90%.[63]

Presently, three clinical types of blastomycosis are most commonly described: pulmonary, disseminated, and cutaneous.[64]

Pulmonary blastomycosis is usually a chronic or subacute illness resembling tuberculosis rather than bacterial pneumonia.[65] The initial signs of primary pulmonary blastomycosis include a mild respiratory infection that progresses with dry cough, pleuritic pain, hoarsenes, and low grade fever. After the initial acute phase or after reactivation, pulmonary blastomycosis may become chronic. The pathogen is known to remain viable for long periods of time and may reactivate several years after the initial illness.[66] Ehni[52] has reported reactivation of infection with immunosuppression which occurred even 40 years after exposure to the fungus in an endemic area.

Clinical manifestations of pulmonary blastomycosis may be limited to acute primary pneumonia that may eventually resolve with or without treatment.[51] In spite of spontaneous resolution of pneumonia, in many instances endogenous reactivation of blastomycosis is possible,[67,68] with some pulmonary infections known to progress to a chronic form, with or without extrapulmonary dissemination. Chronic infection usually follows the course of a granulomatous lung disease without distinction; symptoms include anorexia, weight loss, malaise, low-grade fever, and cough with mucopurulent or blood-tinged sputum.[36]

A wide range of radiologic presentations of pulmonary blastomycosis have been described, with consolidation, fibronodular disease, cavitary lesions, miliary disease all noted by various investigators and in various proportions.[69-73] Massive pleural effusions and endobronchial lesions, although unlikely occurrences, have also been observed,[69] as well as circumscribed solid breast masses in female patients.[74,75]

Serious complications from blastomycosis that have been observed include adult respiratory distress syndrome (ARDS)[46,76-80] and CNS disease.[81,82] ARDS is an unusual and often lethal complication of blastomycosis in which survival is highly dependent on early diagnosis and therapy.[46]

In disseminated blastomycosis, the fungus usually infiltrates the skin, the oronasal mucosa and subcutaneous tissues, and the respiratory, osseous, genitourinary, and central nervous systems.[30,36,75,83-88] Involvement of the upper extremity has been very rare.[89] Bergman et al.[90] have described a rare case of primary blastomycosis of the hand that progressed to severe soft tissue destruction and significant loss of hand function. In contrast to paracoccidioidomycosis, the gastrointestinal tract is rarely involved in blastomycosis.[16]

In the head and neck, the most common sites of blastomycosis are the larynx, and the oral and nasal cavities.[91-95] Other areas that may be affected include the thyroid gland,[95,96] parotid gland,[97] mandible, and the maxilla.[98,99] Infection of the paranasal sinuses is extremely rare.[100] Ocular involvement includes the eyelid,[101-108] conjunctivae,[109] cornea,[102,110] and orbits.[103] There have also been cases of intraocular blastomycosis,[111-116] including choroidal disease.[117-122]

After pulmonary and skin involvement, bone lesions have been reported to be the third most common location of blastomycosis.[123-126] As many as 60% of all patients with disseminated blastomycosis present with skeletal infections.[29,127] Bone lesions may occur in vertebral bodies,[84,128] ribs, skull, facial and long bones, as well as small bones.[123] They often present as an area of inflammation and prominent osteolysis with sharp borders dividing involved and uninvolved bone.[129,130] Arthritis, which has been observed in about 8% of patients with systemic blastomycosis,[131] is usually monoarticular and most frequently associated with the knee, ankle, or elbow.[29,62,123] Acute blastomycotic arthritis may take place with or without articular bone lesions. Usually the diagnosis is made by isolating the organism from the synovial fluid.

Genitourinary infection is the fourth most common manifestation of blastomycosis after involvement of the lungs, skin, and bones. In males, the disease has been reported to present exclusively as either prostatitis or epididymo-orchitis.[83,86] Female genital blastomycosis reported presented as tubo-ovarian abscesses,[132-134] or ovarian tumor.[85]

Neuzil et al.[135] have described the first case of invasive extrapulmonary thoracic disease due to *B. dermatitidis* presenting as brachial plexopathy. In another previously unrecognized complication of blastomycotic infection, Lagerstrom et al.[136] reported a female patient with superior vena cava syndrome secondary to blastomycosis.

While isolated CNS blastomycosis seldom occurs, CNS involvement is seen in about 10% of cases of disseminated disease and then it is usually a late manifestation.[29,82,137-142]

A case of Addison's disease caused by adrenal blastomycosis has been reported by Rimondi et al.[143]

Because of the organism's isolated habitat, so far blastomycosis in HIV-infected patients has been relatively rare.[144-149] Severe immunodeficiency was indicated by the CD4+ counts — by one account,[148] 85% of HIV-infected patients with blastomycosis had CD4+ of <200 cells/mm^3, and a mortality rate of 54%. In a multicenter retrospective survey, Pappas et al.[150] described various clinical, demographic, radiographic, diagnostic, and therapeutic aspects of blastomycosis in 15 patients with AIDS. Two major patterns of the disease have emerged: localized pulmonary involvement (seven patients) and disseminated (extrapulmonary) blastomycosis (eight patients); in 40% of the patients studied there was central nervous system (CNS) involvement. Delayed hypersensitivity and granuloma formation (both associated with T cell functions) play an important role in the control of the infection in immunocompromised hosts.[60,144]

Winquist et al.[151] have described a case of reactivation and dissemination of blastomycosis complicating Hodgkin's disease.

Involvement of the mononuclear phagocyte system has also been observed. Granulomas and abscesses of the spleen and liver caused by *B. dermatitidis* are rarely found and then only in widely disseminated disease.[152] The most common sites of urogenital involvement are the prostate, epididymis, and testis; clinical manifestations include dysuria, pyuria, and hematuria.[16] However, the female genitourinary tract is seldom affected.

Cutaneous lesions may appear shortly or up to several years after the signs and symptoms of the initial respiratory infection have subsided.[38] In general, most cutaneous lesions are the result of hematogenous spread from a pulmonary or other visceral lesion to a localized subcutaneous or cutaneous site.[16,153] However, frequently, patients have been diagnosed with clear-cut cutaneous blastomycosis who have no antecedent respiratory symptoms.[38]

37.5.1.1 African Blastomycosis

Results from several reports have shown the existence of both macro- and microscopic differences between *B. dermatitidis* strains isolated from North American and African patients.[154] Initially described in the early 1950s,[5,6] cases of African blastomycosis have been described with increasing incidence.[155-157]

The capacity of *B. dermatitidis* to change its morphology from the mycelial form into a yeast-like form has been clearly documented — on histopathologic examination, *B. dermatitidis* is almost always found only in the yeast-like form.[19] One of the major differences observed between the North American and African strains was that in the latter, the conversion of the mycelial (hyphal) into the yeast-like phase (M-Y conversion) achieved after 5 to 6 d of incubation at 37°C in Columbia ANC culture medium, was only partial. It was rather mycelial modification presented with marked swelling of the hyphae and a few budding yeast-like cells.[154,157,158] Vermeil et al.[159] demonstrated the lack of the sexual form in African *B. dermatitidis* strains and the loss of M-Y conversion in the older strains, confirming the suggestion of McGinnis[160] that total transformation is not necessary to classify a strain such as *B. dermatitidis*. However, with regard to clinical and immunologic characteristics, Vanbreuseghem et al.[161] proposed that there may be two different species involved. Since significant genetic diversity among clinical isolates of *B. dermatitidis* has been observed,[162] this may also underscore a similar environmental diversification.

Baily et al.[163] have reviewed some of the clinical features, diagnosis, and treatment of blastomycosis in Africa.

37.5.2 Role of Host Immune Response Against *Blastomyces dermatitidis*

Inasmuch as antibodies to the fungus have been documented, they play little apparent role in the host defense against the pathogen.[164] Until now, the role of humoral response against human blastomycosis has not been fully evaluated because of the absence of a suitably active and specific antigen. Contrary to humoral immunity, however, cellular immunity is considered to be a major factor in preventing progressive disease caused by slow-growing, pathogenic fungi, such as *B. dermatitidis*.[37] Bradsher and Pappas[165] have used enzyme immunoassay to detect specific antibodies in human blastomycosis.

Alveolar macrophages constitute the first line of defense against blastomycosis through phagocytosis of inhaled spores. Although murine alveolar macrophages showed modest *in vitro* phagocytic activity with regard to the inhibition of yeast cells in culture,[166] resident peritoneal macrophages have been reported to engulf and kill yeast cells.[167,168] This may explain why some persons were not infected while exposed to the fungus during an epidemic. With the development of immunity, inflammatory reactions occur initially as a suppurative response consisting of polymorphonuclear leukocytes followed by influx of monocyte-derived macrophages.[83]

For dimorphic fungi, such as *B. dermatitidis*, the transition from mycelial to yeast phase is required for virulence. Such transition usually takes place in the host where higher temperatures exist. Although the trigger mechanism for transition seemingly involves elevation of ambient temperature, the biochemical events responsible for this event have not been clearly established.[169-171] However, if the fungus is incapable of completing the transition and converting into yeast-phase, growth will cease and infection will be aborted.[167,172-174] Because the fungal mycelium is unlikely to initiate infection, the interaction between conidia and host phagocytes is becoming increasingly important for the understanding of the pathogenesis of blastomycosis.

Sugar and Picard[167] have studied the role of host defense mechanisms against *B. dermatitidis* and in particular, the ability of murine bronchoalveolar macrophages and hydrogen peroxide to interfere with the transition of *B. dermatitidis* conidia into the yeast form at 37°C, as well as conditions under which phase transition could be dissociated from the ability of fungal conidia to germinate. These investigators found that bronchoalveolar macrophages incubated with conidia inhibited phase transition after 4 h, although the conidia were not killed under the conditions used, and maintained their ability to germinate. Germination, however, may be irrelevant because dimorphic fungi do not form hyphae at temperatures present in mammalian cells.[167] The finding that catalase was unable to reverse the macrophage-induced inhibition of phase transition suggested that nonoxidative mechanisms may be involved *in vivo*. Hydrogen peroxide in relatively high concentrations also suppressed the transition of conidia into yeast — its effect appeared to be irreversible. Since the effective fungistatic concentrations of H_2O_2 are thought to be much higher than those obtainable *in vivo*, its physiologic role as a mediator of macrophage activity remains unclear.

There has been synergy between itraconazole and macrophages in killing *B. dermatitidis* ATCC 26199 in 72-h assays.[175] Thus, fungistatic concentrations of itraconazole (0.01 µg/ml) (which restricted growth 55% as compared to controls) when co-cultured with macrophages resulted in fungicidal activity, as evidenced by 85% killing of the fungus. The observed synergy occurred even when itraconazole was added after the macrophages had surrounded the pathogen. However, there was no synergy when lymph node lymphocytes were used in place of macrophages. Fungistatic concentrations of ketoconazole under the same conditions were not synergistic.

It has been postulated that lymphokine production for macrophage activation is important for host defense against blastomycosis.[176] *In vitro* and *in vivo* experiments have demonstrated that murine pulmonary macrophages showed enhanced fungicidal activity against *B. dermatitidis* following treatment with IFN-γ or lymphokines.[177,178] Thus, macrophages from mice given intravenously 10^5 or 4×10^5 of IFN-γ had their fungicidal activity increased by 29% and 37.5%, respectively.[178] *In vivo* activation of peripheral blood polymorphonuclear neutrophils by IFN-γ also resulted in enhanced *in vitro* fungicidal activity against *B. dermatitidis*. The activation was dose-dependent but transitory, with maximal enhancing effect observed at the highest dose tested (250,000 U).[179] The reported findings may suggest a therapeutic role for IFN-γ against blastomycosis and other opportunistic fungal infections by activation of macrophages and polymorphonuclear neutrophils to enhance the immune defenses of the host.[179]

Brummer et al.[180] have found that elevated serum IgE levels are associated with progressive pulmonary murine blastomycosis. During acute progressive pulmonary blastomycosis in naive mice and low-grade chronic infection in immunized mice, the IgE serum levels correlated directly with interleukin (IL-4) (but inversely with IFN-γ) production. Furthermore, resistance and cure of the infection correlated with the ability of the lymph node and spleen cells to make proliferative responses to antigen. Successful treatment of the infection with SCH 39304 reduced the lymphokine production to background levels but sensitized the lymphocytes for proliferative responses to the antigen.[180]

Abuodeh et al.[181] have studied the role of different *B. dermatitidis* soluble antigenic preparations in the induction and detection of delayed-type hypersensitivity and other cell-mediated responses, such as phagocytic activity of peritoneal macrophages and lymphoproliferation.

37.5.2.1 Role of Cell-Surface Antigens of *B. dermatitidis* in Host-Pathogen Interactions

A 120-kDa glycoprotein antigen (WI-1), profusely expressed on *B. dermatitidis* yeasts, has been determined as the target of cellular and humoral immune responses in human infection,[182-184] as well as in radioimmunoassay serological procedures to diagnose blastomycosis.[185] Klein et al.[184] have found that one 25-amino acid repeat of WI-1 displayed an immunodominant B cell epitope, and that the carboxyl terminus of the molecule has an architecture that may promote fungal yeast adhesion to host cells or extracellular matrix proteins. WI-1 was found to contain a large amount of cystein (85 residues) and aromatic amino acids, but no detectable carbohydrates.[186] In contrast, A antigen (the only *Blastomyces* antigen commercially available), which had a molecular mass of 135 kDa, contained 37% carbohydrates. The A antigen shared with WI-1 the 25-amino acid repeat.[186,187] The latter represents the principal site of antibody recognition on both antigens. A major 98-kDa extracellular protein antigen, which was found to be highly reactive with serum antibodies from patients with blastomycosis, has been shown to be almost identical with the WI-1 antigen.[188]

Studies on the role of the *B. dermatitidis* cell-surface antigen WI-1 in host-pathogen interactions led to the hypothesis that similarly to the *Yersinia pseudotuberculosis* surface adhesin, invasin (a 103-kDa protein product of the *inv* locus), WI-1 may act as a virulence determinant that can direct attachment and penetration of the fungus into mammalian phagocytic and nonphagocytic cells. It is known that *Yersinia* invasin can bind the very late antigen (VLA) family of integrin cell-adhesion molecules, which express the same β_1 chain.[189,190] There has been structural similarity between the 25-amino acid tandem repeat of WI-1 and the *Yersinia* invasin,[191] with most of the analogy confined within the integrin-binding domain of invasin.[192] Further analysis of WI-1 has shown that a cystein-rich nonrepetitive sequence near the carboxyl terminus was similar to the epidermal growth factor (EGF)-like domains. The latter have been frequently identified in proteins that mediate cell-cell or cell-extracellular matrix interactions.[193] Taken together, the data have strongly suggested that WI-1 is organized into at least three domains: (1) an amino-terminal hydrophobic domain, which may insert WI-1 into the yeast-cell membrane; (2) an EGF-like domain at the carboxyl terminus, which may allow the yeast cell to bind to the extracellular matrix; and (3) a 25-amino acid "invasin-like" repeat, which constitutes much of the core of the protein, but which is predicted to occur at the surface of the molecule. With its adhesion-promoting capability, this invasin-like repeat may foster attachment of the yeast cell to host cells and tissues.[187]

These and other findings[194,195] may further advance the understanding of the molecular pathogenesis of blastomycosis[187] and provide new immunotherapeutic approaches for treatment of blastomycosis.

37.5.3 STUDIES ON THERAPEUTICS

37.5.3.1 Azole Derivatives

When tested *in vitro*, ketoconazole was found to be inhibitory towards *B. dermatitidis* at concentrations of ≤3.8 μmol/l.[196] The concentration of ketoconazole in the cerebrospinal fluid (CSF) was noted to average between 3% and 5% of serum levels. Average 4- to 6-h peak serum levels after 400- and 800-mg daily doses of ketoconazole have been determined to be 6.8 and 9.4 µg/ml, respectively.[197]

Itraconazole, when given orally to mice at daily doses of 50 to 150 mg/kg, was protective against lethal infection of *B. dermatitidis*. Although the infection was not sterilized, itraconazole was three times more potent than ketoconazole.[198]

Fluconazole is a new orally active triazole antifungal agent effective against systemic mycoses. The drug is metabolically stable with prolonged half-life and unusual pharmacologic properties, including low protein binding, urinary excretion of unchanged drug, and penetration into CSF.[199,200] When compared with ketoconazole against *B. dermatitidis in vitro*, fluconazole showed MIC value of 6.0 µg/ml; the corresponding value for ketoconazole was 0.08 µg/ml.[201] In a mouse model of pulmonary blastomycosis against the same virulent strain of *B. dermatitidis* ATCC 26199 (80% lethal dose challenge), ketoconazole at 100 mg/kg daily prolonged the survival rate ($p < .01$); by comparison, at 10 mg/kg daily, fluconazole exerted significantly better activity than ketoconazole at 100 mg/kg ($p < .01$). While the best therapeutic regimen for fluconazole was established to be at 100 mg/kg daily (tolerated for 3 weeks without evident toxicity), even at that dosage in the mouse model studied, fluconazole did not provide cure: the survival rate at 100 mg/kg was 40% — statistically not different ($p > .05$) from that in controls (20%) at the end of the experiment.[201] Nevertheless, during the 3-week treatment period and 2 months of follow-up observation, fluconazole was over 10 times more potent (on a milligram per kilogram basis) than ketoconazole in prolonging life against pulmonary blastomycosis.

The pharmacokinetics of fluconazole after a daily dose of 100 mg/kg showed a peak level at 1 h, a slow elimination phase, and serum concentrations exceeding the MIC for the challenge organism for a prolonged period.[201]

Compound SCH 39304 is a fluorinated triazole antimycotic with broad-spectrum activity.[202-204] Sugar et al.[205] compared the antifungal properties of SCH 39304 to those of fluconazole and amphotericin B in a model of experimental murine pulmonary blastomycosis. BALB/cByJ mice were challenged with *B. dermatitidis* ATCC 26199 and treated with either oral SCH 39304 or fluconazole, or intraperitoneal amphotericin B. A dose-response protective effect was observed with SCH 39304 at daily doses of 5.0 to 100 mg/kg. While both 5.0 mg/kg of SCH 39304 daily and 100 mg/kg of fluconazole daily effectively suppressed the fungal growth, the two drugs were unable to decrease the number of yeasts recovered from the lungs; on the other hand, the two highest doses of SCH 39304 (50 and 100 mg/kg daily) significantly reduced the colony counts during the treatment period. However, once therapy has been ceased, the fungal growth resumed, and by the end of the experiment, colony counts equaled or exceeded the original inoculum size.[205] Overall, in the model studied, SCH 39304 was 20 times more effective than fluconazole at daily doses of 100 mg/kg given for 4 weeks, with survival rate approaching that seen with amphotericin B; in fact, the colony counts in lungs recovered from mice treated with SCH 39304 were similar to those from mice treated with amphotericin B.[205] In another set of experiments, SCH 39304 was tested *in vivo* for activity against acute and established murine pulmonary blastomycosis and was compared with ketoconazole and fluconazole in a model of acute infection.[206] In order to simulate the clinical treatment of the common form of human blastomycosis, treatment of infected mice was withheld until they became sick and had an established pulmonary blastomycosis. In acute blastomycosis, SCH 39304 at doses of 25 and 50 mg/kg produced 100% survival for 30 d after the 20-d treatment; however, only 33% of the mice were cleared of infection. At 2.0 mg/kg daily, SCH 39304 showed potency similar to those of ketoconazole at 100 mg/kg daily, and 10 mg/kg of fluconazole daily. In a model of established blastomycosis used to evaluate long-term treatment of very sick or moribund mice, daily doses of 50 mg/kg of SCH 39304 protected animals against death with a 96% cumulative 8-week survival. It was noted that strong humoral and cellular immune responses to *B. dermatitidis* that had developed during the last 2 weeks of therapy may have contributed to the clearance of pathogen from the lungs of mice.[206] Overall, in acute blastomycosis, SCH 39304 was found to be superior on a milligram per kilogram basis to both ketoconazole and fluconazole, while in the long-term treatment of more severe blastomycosis the drug was curative.[206] The MIC values of SCH 39304, ketoconazole, and fluconazole against *B. dermatitidis* in broth cultures were 1.6, 0.6, and 6.0 µg/kg, respectively.[206] Due to its high toxicity, SCH 39304 is no longer studied.

Compound ICI 195,739, another novel orally active triazole derivative, was 50 times as potent as ketoconazole in the therapy of pulmonary blastomycosis.[207] *In vitro* susceptibility studies against a virulent strain of *B. dermatitidis* ATCC 26199 showed MIC and minimal fungicidal concentration (MFC) values of 0.25 and 0.5 µg/ml; the corresponding values for ketoconazole were 0.78 and 0.78 µg/ml. The drug produced clinical cure and completely eradicated residual infection when tested in BALB/cByJIMR mice[208] infected with the same virulent strain. None of the animals treated with ICI 195,739 at 10, 50, and 100 mg/kg daily died during the 60-d observation period, a result significantly superior to that obtained for treatment groups receiving 100 mg/kg of ketoconazole daily or 2.0 mg/kg of ICI 195,739 daily. Furthermore, none of the animals receiving daily doses of 50 or 100 mg/kg ICI 195,739 showed overt sign of drug toxicity.[207]

The pharmacokinetics of ICI 195,739 after a single 50-mg dose and in the steady state (50 mg daily) showed a prolonged half-life (>12 h) and a peak level of 17.6 µg/ml at 12 h post-dosage. In the steady state, a trough level of 19.5 µg/ml occurred at 4 h, and a peak level of 21.0 µg/ml at 8 h; the half-life was markedly prolonged (well over 48 h).[207] As compared with ketoconazole, ICI 195,739 not only provided complete protection from mortality in the murine model studied, but also showed fungicidal activity against *B. dermatitidis in vivo*, with no evidence of the infection after an extended follow-up period.[207]

The therapeutic effect against murine blastomycosis of Bay R 3783, a novel orally active triazole derivative, was investigated by Pappagianis et al.[209] Previously the drug was found effective *in vitro* against two other dimorphic fungi, *Coccidioides immitis*[210] and *Histoplasma capsulatum*.[211] *In vitro*, against the yeast phase of *B. dermatitidis*, the MIC value for Bay R 3783 was 0.5 µg/ml (read at 96 h); by comparison, the corresponding values for itraconazole, ketoconazole, fluconazole, and amphotericin B were <0.003, 0.012, 4.0, and 0.125 µg/ml, respectively.[209]

In a mouse model of blastomycosis where treatment was not started until the first death had occurred at day 6, 25 mg/kg of each Bay R 3783, ketoconazole, fluconazole, and itraconazole, given orally, were compared with amphotericin B (administered at 1.0 mg/kg once daily) for a total of 10 d.[209] Although initially, both Bay R 3783 and amphotericin B appeared to be less potent than itraconazole, all mice in the itraconazole group ultimately died. While the response to Bay R 3783 at 25 mg/kg was not statistically superior to 1.0 mg/kg of amphotericin B ($p = .5$), it was superior to that of itraconazole ($p = .04$); neither ketoconazole nor fluconazole at the dosages studied caused any delay in deaths. When a short-term organ load assay (with the lungs cultured as the target organ) involving the four azole antimycotics (at 25 mg/kg) and amphotericin B (at 1.0 mg/kg once daily) was carried out in the same mouse model, Bay R 3783 produced a statistically superior response to infection with *B. dermatitidis* as compared with any of the other drugs. A limited study of the pharmacokinetics of Bay R 3783 at a dose of 25 mg/kg was also carried out; the compound showed a peak concentration of 0.75 µg/ml at 30 min.[209]

Against pulmonary blastomycosis, 2 weeks of therapy with Bay R 3783 (25 mg/kg) was as effective in preventing deaths as that of 1.0 mg/kg of amphotericin B. In general, in the assays and dosages studied, Bay R 3783 was more efficient against *B. dermatitidis* than ketoconazole, itraconazole, and fluconazole. However, by adjusting the doses for any of the azoles tested, it may still be possible to increase the efficacy of all these drugs within a range of safe dosages.[209] For example, at higher daily doses (50 and 150 mg/kg), itraconazole showed efficacy against 60% and 75% lethal dose challenges with *B. dermatitidis*;[209] also, in a murine model of blastomycosis, all mice infected with 60 colony-forming units of the organism and treated with 160 mg of ketoconazole survived.[212]

The novel triazole derivative D0870 was evaluated for activity against *B. dermatitidis in vitro* and in a murine model of pulmonary blastomycosis.[213] The MIC and MFC values of D0870 were 0.048 and 0.097 µg/ml. *In vivo*, the compound was nearly 100-fold more potent than fluconazole when given once daily. Thus, at both 1.0 or 10 mg/kg (administered once daily) and 10 or 100 mg/kg given every other day, D0870 prolonged survival over fluconazole given once daily at 100 mg/kg. Although more potent, D0870 was also more toxic than fluconazole. For example, at 100 mg/kg administered once daily D0870 was lethally toxic, whereas at the same dose fluconazole was not.

The *in vitro* and *in vivo* activities of SCH 56592, a novel triazole analog with broad antifungal activity,[213-216] have been investigated by Sugar and Liu.[217] The *in vitro* activity of SCH 56592 against 12 *B. dermatitidis* isolates was compared to that of amphotericin B, itraconazole, and fluconazole. SCH 56592 was the most active of all four compounds, showing MIC_{90} and MFC values of 0.06 µg/ml and 4.0 µg/ml, respectively. Results from the treatment of *B. dermatitidis*-infected mice with three different doses of SCH 56592 (25, 5.0, and 1.0 mg/kg), amphotericin B (1.0 mg/kg), or itraconazole (150 mg/kg) confirmed the potent activity of SCH 56592 — survival was prolonged at each dose of SHC 56592, and sterilization of the lungs occurred in the high-dose group, but not in the groups treated with itraconazole or fluconazole.[217]

The *in vitro* activity of another new broad-spectrum triazole derivative, SCH 51048, against 13 isolates of *B. dermatitidis* was also evaluated.[218] In a murine model of acute pulmonary blastomycosis, the activity of SCH 51048 was comparable with that of amphotericin B, and at least 30 times more potent than that of itraconazole.[218]

37.5.3.2   Fungal Chitin Synthase Inhibitors

Cell walls of the majority of pathogenic fungi contain chitin, a polymeric polysaccharide $C_{30}H_{50}O_{19}N_4$ not found in mammalian cells.[219] On hydrolysis, chitin yields a linear homopolymer of β-(1→4)-2-acetamido-2-deoxy-D-glucose. In some dimorphic fungi (*B. dermatitidis* and *H. capsulatum*), chitin may constitute as much as 10% to 20% of the content of their cell walls.[220-226] Compounds that interfere with the biosynthesis of chitin would, therefore, inhibit the growth of fungal cells and be of interest as potential antifungal agents.[227-229] Indeed, a number of polyoxin antibiotics, structurally similar to UDP-*N*-acetylglucosamine (the substrate of chitin synthase), were found to be active *in vitro* against *Candida* spp.,[229-232] as well as some dimorphic fungi.[233,234] The nikkomycins, a group of antibiotics structurally related to polyoxins, were also effective as competitive inhibitors of chitin synthase.[227,235] Hector et al.[235] evaluated the antiblastomycotic activity of nikkomycins X and Z both *in vitro* and against systemic murine pulmonary blastomycosis. MIC values of 8.0 and 30 µg/ml (read at 96 h) were observed for nikkomycins X and Z, respectively. In the mouse model, however, nikkomycin Z was the more potent agent. Its activity at 20 mg/kg (given b.i.d.) was compared with that of four azoles (ketoconazole, fluconazole, itraconazole, and Bay R 3783) and amphotericin B (given at 1.0 mg/kg, four times daily); the therapy was commenced when the first death had occurred at day 6. The nikkomycin Z-treated mice had the fewest deaths, with no deaths occurring after day 8; however, the survival curves were not statistically superior to those from Bay R 3783- and amphotericin B-treated groups. Furthermore, in a short-term organ load experiment, when three doses of nikkomycin Z (5.0, 20, and 50 mg/kg) were compared with the four azoles and amphotericin B, the lowest dose of nikkomycin Z tested (5.0 mg/kg) was as active as amphotericin B at 1.0 mg/kg, and the most active azole (Bay R 3783) at 25 mg/kg. The 50-mg/kg nikkomycin Z dose sterilized the lungs of most animals.[235]

Pharmacokinetic studies have shown that after a 100-mg/kg dose injected intravenously, the initial serum concentration (320 µg/ml) of nikkomycin Z was rapidly eliminated, with a half-life of approximately 10 to 15 min.[235] Results from oral administration of 100 mg/kg, however, suggested that nikkomycin Z is absorbed slowly, with a peak concentration of 10 µg/ml occurring approximately 45 min after administration; the half-life appeared to be nearly 1 h. Toxicity studies in mice following daily oral administration of 100 and 400 mg/kg doses of the antibiotic for 28 d showed no visible damage except for increased incidence of gliosis in the brain of mice receiving the higher dose. Animals not sacrificed were held an additional 60 d for observation and no outward differences were apparent.[235]

37.5.4 EVOLUTION OF THERAPIES AND TREATMENT OF BLASTOMYCOSIS

2-Hydroxystilbamidine (given intravenously) was the first therapeutic agent that was effective and reduced mortality from blastomycosis.[36,236] The total dose applied ranged between 12 and 16 g.[236] Although it still may be useful in a few cases, 2-hydroxystilbamidine is now seldom used and is of historical interest only. While it showed less toxicity than amphotericin B, 2-hydroxystilbamidine was also less effective; as compared to ketoconazole, it was also less effective, but more toxic.

The toxicity of 2-hydroxystilbamidine is more likely to cause liver damage rather than the renal impairment associated with amphotericin B. Therefore, it is important that serum potassium levels are monitored closely. 2-Hydroxystilbamidine must be administered intravenously at recommended daily doses in adults of 225 mg and a total dose not exceeding 12 to 15 g.[236]

37.5.4.1 Amphotericin B

Since its introduction in 1956, amphotericin B has been the mainstay for treatment of various systemic mycoses. It is active against all types of blastomycosis, and dose regimens of 1.5 to 2.0 g should be adequate, especially in immunocompetent patients, and cases involving pulmonary blastomycosis with diffuse infiltrates and severe hypoxemia (a total cumulative dose of 500 to 1000 mg) (Table 37.3).[237]

For treatment of meningeal blastomycosis, amphotericin B is the treatment of choice.[82,95,100,121,137,139,238-247] Also, amphotericin B should be used preferentially in patients with ARDS because of its quick onset of action;[46,76] up to 2.0 g total dose of the antibiotic has been recommended.[46,248] Clinical response towards the drug was between 66% and 93% depending on total dose and duration of treatment.[238,244,249,250]

The antibiotic is always administered intravenously with a total dose ranging from 25 to 35 mg/kg (as much as 2.5 g).[93,248] Although intraventricular administration of amphotericin B has not been adequately evaluated, it may be useful in patients with obstructive hydrocephalus and rapid deterioration, or whenever the response to intravenous amphotericin B is unsatisfactory.[248]

Lewis et al.[118] and Gottlieb et al.[121] have cured disseminated choroidal blastomycosis after treatment with 2.0 of intravenous amphotericin B. Lopez et al.[115] have used amphotericin B (0.5 mg/kg; total, 1260 mg) as primary systemic therapy combined with subconjunctival injections of miconazole (0.5 mg/0.5 ml) to treat intraocular blastomycosis.

Albert et al.[251] have described a very unusual pediatric case of infection of the forearm synovium presenting as a soft tissue mass without bone or skin involvement — the patient was treated successfully with surgical debridement of the mass combined with amphotericin B (0.7 mg/kg daily, IV) for 6 weeks, followed by oral itraconazole (100 mg, b.i.d.) for another 12 weeks.

Relapse of blastomycosis following treatment with amphotericin B has been rare and appeared to be dose-dependent.[244,252,253] In the majority of cases, relapse was observed shortly after completion of amphotericin B therapy,[95] although in some patients, relapse occurred as long as 9 years after the treatment.[5,83]

In spite of its clinical efficacy, the use of amphotericin B is limited because of serious side effects,[254] such as azotemia (71%), anemia (53%), anorexia, nausea and vomiting (53%), fever and chills (49%), hypokalemia (37%), and thrombophlebitis (19%) (Table 37.4).[15] The toxicity of the antibiotic may become severe enough to require cessation of therapy. Some of the side effects of

TABLE 37.3

Recommended Therapies of Blastomycosis Infections (Single-Drug Regimens and Combinations)

Drug or Combination	Dose Regimen (Route of Administration)	Clinical Type	Duration of Therapy	Refs.
Amphotericin B	Total dose of 2.0 g (IV)	Chronic pulmonary;[a] extrapulmonary nonmeningeal;[a] paranasal sinuses; choroidal	Until cure	100, 121, 237
	50 mg weekly (IV), total dose of 2.0–3.0 g (IV)	Meningeal; [b,c] acute[b]	Prolonged	247
Ketoconazole	400–800 mg daily (orally)	Acute[a] Chronic pulmonary[a] Extrapulmonary nonmeningeal[a]	6 months 6 months 6 months	273, 274
Itraconazole	200–400 mg daily (orally)	Acute[d] Chronic pulmonary[a] Meningeal[b] Extrapulmonary nonmeningeal[a]	6 months 6 months Prolonged 6 months	30, 83, 85, 247, 299
	In children: 5–7 mg/kg (maximum: 200 mg daily) (orally)[e]	Pulmonary		305
Fluconazole	200–400 daily (orally)	Nonmeningeal; non-life-threatening	6.7 months (mean)	311
Amphotericin B Ketoconazole Itraconazole	500–1,000 mg (IV)[f] 400–800 mg daily (orally) 400 mg daily (orally)	Acute with ventilatory failure	Primary 6 months 6 months	237
Amphotericin B Itraconazole	500–1,000 mg (IV)[g] 400 mg daily (orally)[b]	Acute Acute with ventilatory failure Chronic pulmonary or extrapulmonary nonmeningeal	Primary 6 months	247

[a] In immunocompetent patients.

[b] In immunocompromised patients.

[c] In cases of immunocompetent hosts, a total cumulative dose of 2.0–3.0 g is recommended.[247]

[d] In immunocompetent patients (however, with greater toxicity compared to itraconazole).

[e] In low-birth-weight infants and children with fungal infections (disseminated candidiasis and aspergillosis, or chronic granulomatous disease), doses of 5.0–10 mg/kg of itraconazole have been used safely.[302-304]

[f] Amphotericin B is administered until patients's condition is stable, followed by either ketoconazole or itraconazole for a minimum of 6 additional months to complete therapy.

[g] In non-AIDS immunocompromised patients, the primary therapy is with amphotericin, then itraconazole for 6 months; in AIDS patients, the follow-up treatment with itraconazole is for life.

TABLE 37.4
Toxic Side Effects of Drugs Used to Treat Blastomycosis

Drug	Toxicity	Symptoms	Refs.
Amphotericin B	Dose-dependent	Nephrotoxicity (urinary abnormalities, hyposthenuria, azotemia, hypokalemia, nephrocalcinosis), normocytic, normochromic anemia (decreased erythropoietin levels and erythrocyte counts)	255
	Idiosyncratic	Flushing, rash, anaphylactic shock, acute liver failure, thrombocytopenia, vertigo, generalized pain, grand mal convulsion, ventricular fibrillation, cardiac arrest, fever (in nearly all patients), chill (in nearly all patients)	
Ketoconazole		Nausea, vomiting, diarrhea, pruritis, rash, increased alkaline phosphatase, hyperlipidemia, inhibition of gonadal and adrenal steroid synthesis	286
Itraconazole		Asymptomatic liver function abnormalities, increased blood levels of urea nitrogen and serum levels of transaminase	286, 306
Fluconazole		Nausea, headache, skin rash, vomiting, abdominal pain, diarrhea, hepatotoxicity, elevated serum transaminase levels, leukopenia, thrombocytopenia, reversible alopecia	287, 388, 311
Miconazole		Phlebitis, pruritis, nausea, fever, chill, rash, vomiting, anemia, decreased hematocrit (normoblastic hypoplasia), hyponatremia, anaphylaxis, ventricular tachycardia	286

amphotericin B may be minimized by pretreatment of the patient with antihistamines, antipyretics, and antiemetics, but these drugs should never be mixed with the antibiotic.[36]

In order to limit unwarranted toxicity,[255] amphotericin B has been either chemically modified (e.g., methyl ester formation),[256-259] or intercalated into lipid-based carriers, such as liposome encapsulation.[260-270] Clemons and Stevens[271,272] have compared the efficacies of amphotericin B lipid complex and a micellar amphotericin B-deoxycholate suspension (Fungizone®) against blastomycosis in a CD-1 mouse model. The lipid complex was a preparation of dimyristoyl phosphatidyl choline and dimyristoyl phosphatidyl glycerol (in a 7:3 molar ratio) containing 33 mol% of amphotericin B; the average particle size was 1.6 to 6.0 μm. The MIC (broth dilution) and MFC of Fungizone® against *B. dermatitidis* ATCC 26199 were 0.5 and 1.0 μg/ml; the corresponding values for the lipid complex were 0.25 and 1.0 μg/ml. All doses of each form prolonged survival (p <.05 to .001). Fungizone® showed higher potency at doses of 0.8 mg/kg. However, the lipid complex of amphotericin B showed an overt toxicity at doses of 12.8 mg/kg and was superior (p <.001) to Fungizone® given at 2.0 mg/kg (a toxic dose).[271]

37.5.4.2   Azole Derivatives

37.5.4.2.1   Ketoconazole

While amphotericin B is used predominantly in patients who are acutely ill or imunocompromised, or when CNS involvement has been diagnosed,[273] since 1985, ketoconazole has been the primary therapy for all but the most severe cases of human blastomycosis.[59,83,87,274-280] It was less effective in immunocompromised than immunocompetent patients.[54,281]

The mechanism of action of ketoconazole involves interaction with cytochrome P-450 enzymes, which results in reduced levels of ergosterol, a major building block of the fungal cell membrane.[282,283] Because ketoconazole competes with cyclosporin A for metabolism in the hepatic cytochrome P-450 system, there were some unpredictable elevated levels of cyclosporin A in some patients on immunosuppressive therapy.[281]

Ketoconazole, which has the advantages of oral administration and lesser toxicity than most azole antimycotics, was shown to be effective against acute symptomatic blastomycosis. In clinical trials conducted by the NIAID Mycoses Study Group, of the 80 patients involved in the study, 89% were cured with a recommended dose regimen of 400 to 800 mg daily given for an average of 6 months (Table 37.3).[274] Serum levels of the drug ranged from 3.32 to 6.2 µg/ml 2 h after an oral dose of 400 or 800 mg.[274,275,284] At the lower dose of 400 mg daily, the relapse or primary failure rate is about 10%.[59,274] Although it is difficult to predict which patients will develop a relapse, those with genitourinary involvement are more prone to do so, likely due to the lower concentration of ketoconazole in the urine and prostate.[274] When the high-dose (800 mg daily) regimen is applied for at least 6 months, the failure rate is negligible. However, adverse side effects such as anorexia, nausea, or vomiting (29.1%), menstrual irregularities (16.2%), rash (9.7%), pruritis (9.7%), impotence or decreased libido (8.3%), gynecomastia (7.2%), and hepatic dysfunction (2.9%) may also occur (Table 37.4).[59,274,283,285-288] The most severe toxicity of ketoconazole so far reported is hepatocellular damage; however, it has been very rarely observed.[289]

There have been several studies[59,82,290] of patients who developed CNS blastomycosis while receiving ketoconazole. The patients who initially did not have CNS symptoms, were treated for cutaneous and pulmonary blastomycosis that responded to ketoconazole. However, because of the poor ability of ketoconazole to penetrate the blood-brain barrier, it is possible that the therapeutic failure of the drug might have been caused by initially unrecognized CNS infection. Once diagnosed, CNS blastomycosis has been successfully treated with amphotericin B.[82] Since the rate of asymptomatic CNS blastomycosis may be substantial (3% to 10%,[137,139,242] and as high as 24%[38]), lumbar puncture or even cranial computed tomography have been recommended for all patients with disseminated blastomycosis before therapy with ketoconazole.[290] Such initial evaluation may also be important because systemic asymptomatic blastomycosis is more frequent than was previously thought.[197] Furthermore, blastomycomas, which are a common form of involvement when the CNS is infected by *B. dermatitidis,* may have a long asymptomatic phase.[291] Recently, Klein and Jones[182] described a radioimmunoassay for antibodies to the 120-kDa *B. dermatitides* surface immunoprotein that may also prove useful in detecting early CNS involvement.

Hii et al.[55] described the successful use of high-dose ketoconazole in a renal transplant recipient with pulmonary blastomycosis and evidence of systemic dissemination. The drug was given orally at 400 mg twice daily; random measuring produced ketoconazole levels of 3.22 and 4.56 µmol/l. Initiation of cyclosporine therapy was contraindicated because of its excessive nephrotoxicity.[292] Following the termination of ketoconazole medication, a relapse prompted the reinstitution of low-dose ketoconazole as chronic suppressive therapy.[55]

Miliary blastomycosis in an HIV-positive patient with insulin-dependent diabetes mellitus was successfully treated with 800-mg daily doses of ketoconazole; follow-up at 3 months showed complete clinical and radiologic resolution of the infection.[144]

A recent communication by Nouira et al.[293] described the successful use of ketoconazole in the treatment of one case of cutaneopulmonary blastomycosis which is weakly endemic in Tunisia.

Despite its therapeutic activity, a number of reports[54,59,60,280,294,295] have indicated failures of ketoconazole to treat blastomycosis, including early (primary) failure as well as late (post-treatment) relapse, mainly due to poor patient compliance or early termination of therapy,[59,274,275,294] altered host immunity,[54] altered drug absorption,[81] and drug interactions.[296] Hebert et al.[81] described an unusual case of an otherwise healthy patient with pulmonary blastomycosis, in which therapy with oral ketoconazole resulted in failure with dissemination following a prolonged (5-month) and apparently effective initial response to 400 mg daily of the drug.

37.5.4.2.2   Itraconazole

Itraconazole is a new triazole antifungal agent with a broad spectrum of activity against superficial and systemic mycosis. Like other azole antimycotics, its mechanism of action involves the impairment of ergosterol biosynthesis resulting in damage of the permeability and other functions of the fungal cell wall.[297]

In preclinical studies, itraconazole, when given orally to mice at daily doses of 50 to 150 mg/kg, was protective against lethal infection of *B. dermatitidis*. Although the infection was not sterilized, itraconazole was found to be three times more potent than ketoconazole.[198]

At daily doses of 200 mg given to 42 patients (including 13 patients who had either progression of disease while on ketoconazole medication, or a relapse following cure of blastomycosis with ketoconazole), all treated patients had a rapid initial response to the drug.[83] In the first documented case of blastomycosis in Namibia, a 42-year-old man was successfully treated with itraconazole.[298]

A 3-week course of oral itraconazole monotherapy (200 mg, once daily) elicited good clinical response (apyrexia and resolution of ascites) in a female patient with genital blastomycosis that presented as an ovarian tumor.[85]

In a multicenter, prospective, nonrandomized, open clinical trial involving 48 patients with blastomycosis, itraconazole was administered at daily doses ranging between 200 and 400 mg.[299] Patients receiving other systemic antifungal therapy were excluded. The observed success rate was 90% (43 of 48 patients); when patients were treated for more than 2 months, the success rate was 95% (38 of 40). The median duration of a successful therapy was determined at 6.2 months; the median duration of post-treatment evaluation for successfully treated patients was 11.9 months.

So far, results have shown good absorption and effective oral activity of itraconazole in the treatment of nonmeningeal, non-life-threatening blastomycosis (Table 37.3).[30,83,85,175,247,283,299-305] Its major advantage over ketoconazole was the lower rate of endocrinopathic toxicity (Table 37.4).[175,283,306] Based on its efficacy and the absence of serious adverse side effects following prolonged treatment, itraconazole should replace amphotericin B as the drug of choice for therapy of acute non-life-threatening or chronic blastomycosis (Table 37.3).[30,237,247,305,307]

37.5.4.2.3 Fluconazole

While an ongoing evaluation of fluconazole for treatment of nonacute blastomycosis is underway at daily doses of 200 to 400 mg, at least for now, it appears that the drug is not very effective in the management of blastomycosis.[283] For example, in a small number of patients, fluconazole at daily doses of 50 mg did not cure blastomycosis. It is possible, however, that this unsatisfactory result may be due to dose inadequacy rather than to deficiency of the drug.[37]

However, Pearson et al.[308] described two cases of systemic blastomycosis that were successfully treated with fluconazole. One case involved infection of the respiratory tract and presumably the CNS, whereas the second case consisted only of pulmonary blastomycosis. Both patients received oral fluconazole given at 200 mg twice daily for 6 and 9 months, respectively. The two patients had complete resolution of the disease and stayed asymptomatic for more than 6 months after completion of therapy.

Taillan et al.[309] reported an unusual case of blastomycosis in the brain stem. The abscess was successfully treated with a combination of fluconazole and flucytosine.[310]

In a recently completed multicenter, randomized, open-label pilot study,[311] two daily oral doses (200 and 400 mg) of fluconazole were found to be only moderately effective for the treatment of non-life-threatening, nonmeningeal blastomycosis — the treatment was successful in 15 of 23 evaluable patients (65%), including 8 of 16 patients (63%) who received the 200-mg dose, and 7 of 10 (70%) patients treated with the 400-mg dose. The toxicity of the drug was minimal — rash, diarrhea, constipation, stomach cramps, mildly elevated liver function tests, and reversible alopecia[288] were each seen in one patient, and nausea was seen in four patients (Table 37.4).[311] Overall, fluconazole appeared to be less effective than itraconazole for the treatment of blastomycosis.

37.5.4.2.4   Miconazole

Miconazole is an intravenously administered azole antimycotic with activity against *B. dermatitidis*. However, because of its adverse side effects, adequate trials have not been carried out.[83]

37.5.4.3   Treatment of Adult Respiratory Distress Syndrome (ARDS) Secondary to Blastomycosis

One unusual, and if left untreated, potentially very dangerous, even fatal, complication of blastomycosis is the adult respiratory distress syndrome (ARDS).[8,46,78-80,312-321] It is the pulmonary manifestation of a diffuse microcirculatory injury that results in exudation of a protein-rich fluid into the pulmonary interstitium and alveolary spaces.[322] Pulmonary fibroproliferation is one of the leading causes of death in patients with late ARDS. However, its course may be reversed after therapy with high doses of corticosteroids (HDC). Results from large, prospective clinical investigations have indicated that a short course (48 h or less) of HDC therapy had no benefit when applied at the onset of ARDS.[323-327] However, HDC therapy has been reported effective if initiated in late-stage or chronic ARDS.[322,328-336] Thus, Meduri et al.[322] reported that prolonged treatment of nine patients with late ARDS with HDC, given intravenously, resulted in a marked and rapid improvement in the lung injury score ($p <.003$ at 5 d). An initial bolus dose of 2.0 mg/kg of methylprednisolone sodium succinate was followed by 2.0 to 3.0 mg/kg doses at 6-h intervals; the dose was tapered based on the patient's pulmonary physiologic response. Most complications of the HDC therapy were infections (*P. aeruginosa, P. maltophilia*); all patients had received gastrointestinal prophylaxis with intravenous ranitidine. Because of the immunosuppressive activity and impairment of wound healing of HDC, caution should be applied when considering such a therapy, especially in immunocompromised patients.[246]

Describing a case of overwhelming pulmonary blastomycosis associated with ARDS, Meyer et al.[320] recommended aggressive therapy in which the dose of amphotericin B should be increased as rapidly as possible — within 24 to 48 h — to a daily maintenance dose of 0.7 to 1.0 mg/kg (or a maximum of 70 mg). Because of the life-threatening potential of ARDS, amphotericin B should still remain as primary therapy for this condition.

37.5.5   REFERENCES

1. Gilchrist, T. C., Protozoan dermatitis, *J. Cutan. Dis.*, 12, 496, 1894.
2. Gilchrist, T. C., A case of blastomycetic dermatitis in man, *Johns Hopkins Hosp. Rep.*, 1, 269, 1896.
3. Gilchrist, T. C. and Stokes, W. R., The presence of oidium in the tissues of a case of pseudo-lupus vulgaris, *Johns Hopkins Hosp. Rep.*, 7, 129, 1896.
4. Gilchrist, T. C. and Stokes, W. R., A case of pseudolupus caused by blastomyces, *J. Exp. Med.*, 3, 53, 1898.
5. Broc, R. and Haddad, N., Tumeur bronchique a *Scopulariopsis americana*, determination precoce d'une maladie de Gilchrist, *Bul. Mem. Soc. Med. Hop. Paris*, 68, 679, 1952.
6. Vermeil, C., Gordeeff, A., and Haddad, N., Sur un cas Tunisien de mycose generalisee mortelle, *Ann. Inst. Pasteur*, 86, 636, 1954.
7. Bhagwandeen, S. B., North American blastomycosis in Zambia, *Am. J. Trop. Med.*, 23, 231, 1974.
8. Campos Magalhaes, M., Drouhet, E., and Destombes, P., Premier cas de blastomycose a *Blastomyces dermatitidis* observe au Mozambique, *Bul. Soc. Pathol. Exot. Fil.*, 61, 210, 1968.
9. Drouhet, E., Enjalbert, L., Planques, J., Bollinelli, R., Moreau, G., and Sabatier, A., A propos d'un cas de blastomycose a localisations multiples chez un Francais d'origine Tunisienne, *Bul. Soc. Pathol. Exot. Fil.*, 61, 202, 1968.
10. Emmons, C. W., Murray, I. G., Lurie, H. I., King, M. H., Tulloch, J. A., and Connor, D. H., North American blastomycosis: two autochthonous cases from Africa, *Sabouraudia*, 3, 306, 1964.

11. Fragoyannis, S., VanWyk, G., and Debeer, M., North American blastomycosis in South Africa, *S. Afr. Med. J.*, 51, 169, 1977.

12. Gatti, F., Renoirte, R., and Vandepitte, J., Premier cas de blastomycose nord-americaine observee au Congo (Leopoldville), *Ann. Soc. Belge Med. Trop.*, 44, 1057, 1964.

13. Rippon, J. W., *Medical Mycology*, W. B. Saunders, Philadelphia, 1988, 438.

14. McDonough, E. S. and Lewis, A. L., The ascigerous stage of *Blastomyces dermatitidis*, *Mycologia*, 60, 76, 1968.

15. Conant, N. F. and Howell, A., Similarity of the fungi causing South American blastomycosis (paracoccidial granuloma) and North American blastomycosis (Gilchrist's disease), *J. Invest. Dermatol.*, 5, 353, 1942.

16. Emmons, C. W., Binford, C.H., and Utz, J. P., *Medical Mycology*, Lea and Febiger, Philadelphia, 1970, 309.

17. Hawley, C. and Felson, B., Roentgen aspects of intrathoracic blastomycosis, *Am. J. Roentgenol.*, 75, 751, 1956.

18. Garrison, R. G. and Boyd, K. S., Role of the conidium in dimorphism of *Blastomyces dermatitidis*, *Mycopathologia*, 64, 29, 1978.

19. Mirra, S. S., Trombley, I. K., and Miles, M. L., Blastomycoma of the cerebellum: an ultrastructural study, *Acta Neuropathol.*, 50, 109, 1990.

20. Kane, J., Righter, J., Krajden, S., and Lester, R. S., Blastomycosis: a new endemic region in Canada, *Can. Med. Assoc. J.*, 129, 728, 1983.

21. Kepron, N. W., Schoemperlen, C. B., Hershfield, E. S., Zylak, C.J., and Cherniack, R. M., North American blastomycosis in Central Canada: a review of 36 cases, *Can. Med. Assoc. J.*, 106, 243, 1972.

22. Klein, B. S., Vergeront, J. M., DiSalvo, A. F., Kaufman, L., and Davis, J. P., Two outbreaks of blastomycosis along rivers in Wisconsin: isolation of *Blastomyces dermatitidis* from riverbank soil and evidence of its transmission along waterways, *Am. Rev. Respir. Dis.*, 136, 1333, 1987.

23. Sarosi, G. A. and Davies, S. F., Blastomycosis, *Compr. Ther.*, 12, 31, 1986.

24. Bradsher, R. W., Systemic fungal infections: diagnosis and treatment. I. Blastomycosis, *Infect. Dis. Clin. North Am.*, 2, 877, 1988.

25. Dismukes, W. E., Blastomycosis: leave it to beaver, *N. Engl. J. Med.*, 314, 575, 1986.

26. Klein, B. S., Vergeront, J. M., Weeks, R. J., Kumar, U. N., Mathai, G., Varkey, B., Kaufman, L., Bradsher, R. W., Stoebing, J. F., Davis, J. P., and the Investigation Team, Isolation of *Blastomyces dermatitidis* in soil associated with a large outbreak of blastomycosis in Wisconsin, *N. Engl. J. Med.*, 314, 529, 1986.

27. McDonough, E. S., Wisniewski, T. R., Penn, L. A., Chan, D. M., and McNamara, W. J., Preliminary studies on conidial liberation of *Blastomyces dermatitidis* and *Histoplasma capsulatum*, *Sabouraudia*, 14, 199, 1976.

28. Denton, J. F., McDonough, E. S., Ajello, L., and Ausherman R. J., Isolation of *Blastomyces dermatitidis* from soil, *Science*, 133, 1126, 1961.

29. Tenenbaum, M. J., Greenspan, J., and Kerkering, T. M., Blastomycosis, *Crit. Rev. Microbiol.*, 9, 139, 1982.

30. Bradsher, R. W., Histoplasmosis and blastomycosis, *Clin. Infect. Dis.*, 22(Suppl. 2), S102, 1996.

31. Sarosi, G. A., Eckman, M. R., Davies, S. R., and Laskey, W. K., Canine blastomycosis as a harbinger of human disease, *Ann. Intern. Med.*, 91, 733, 1979.

32. McDonough, E. S. and Kuzma, J. F., Epidemiological studies on blastomycosis in the state of Wisconsin, *Sabouraudia*, 18, 173, 1980.

33. Sarosi, G. A. and Serstock, D. S., Isolation of *Blastomyces dermatitidis* from pigeon manure, *Am. Rev. Respir. Dis.*, 114, 1179, 1976.

34. Armstrong, C. W., Jenkins, S. R., Kaufman, L., Kerkering, T. M., Rouse, B. S., and Miller, G. B., Jr., Common-source outbreak of blastomycosis in hunters and their dogs, *J. Infect. Dis.*, 155, 568, 1987.

35. Furcolow, M. L., Chick, E. W., Busey, J. D., and Menges, R. W., Prevalence and incidence studies of human and canine blastomycosis. I. Cases in the United States, 1885–1968, *Am. Rev. Respir. Dis.*, 102, 60, 1970.

36. Steck, W. D., Blastomycosis, *Dermatol. Clin.*, 7, 241, 1989.

37. Bradsher, R. W., Blastomycosis. Fungal infections of the lung: update 1989, *Semin. Respir. Infect.*, 5, 105, 1989.
38. Schwartz, J. and Baum, G. L., Blastomycosis, *Am. J. Clin. Pathol.*, 21, 999, 1951.
39. Schwartz, J. and Salfelder, K., Blastomycosis: a review of 152 cases, *Curr. Topics. Pathol.*, 65, 165, 1977.
40. Jaspers, R. H., Transmission of *Blastomyces* from animals to man, *J. Am. Vet. Med. Assoc.*, 164, 8, 1974.
41. Craig, M. W., Davey, W. N., and Green, R. A., Conjugal blastomycosis, *Am. Rev. Respir. Dis.*, 102, 86, 1970.
42. Farber, E. R., Leahy, M. S., and Meadows, T. R., Endometrial blastomycosis acquired by sexual contact, *Obstet. Gynecol.*, 32, 195, 1968.
43. Daniel, L. and Salit, I. E., Blastomycosis during pregnancy, *Can. Med. Assoc. J.*, 131, 759, 1984.
44. Hager, H., Welt, S. I., Cardasis, J. P., and Alvarez, S., Disseminated blastomycosis in a pregnant woman successfully treated with amphotericin B: a case report, *J. Reprod. Med.*, 33, 485, 1988.
45. Ismail, M. A. and Lerner, S. A., Disseminated blastomycosis in a pregnant woman: a review of amphotericin B usage during pregnancy, *Am. Rev. Respir. Dis.*, 126, 350, 1982.
46. MacDonald, D. and Alguire, P. C., Adult respiratory distress syndrome due to blastomycosis during pregnancy, *Chest*, 98, 1527, 1990.
47. Neiberg, A. D., Mavromatis, F., Dyke, J., and Fayyad, A., *Blastomycosis dermatitidis* treated during pregnancy: a case report, *Am. J. Obstet. Gynecol.*, 128, 911, 1977.
48. Watts, E. A., Gard, P. D., and Tuthill, S. W., First reported case of intrauterine transmission of blastomycosis, *Pediatr. Infect. Dis. J.*, 2, 308, 1983.
49. Weinberg, E. D., Pregnancy-associated depression of cell-mediated immunity, *Rev. Infect. Dis.*, 6, 814, 1984.
50. Maxson, S., Miller, S. F., Tryka, F., and Schutze, G. E., Perinatal blastomycosis: a review, *Pediatr. Infect. Dis. J.*, 11, 760, 1992.
51. Sarosi, G. A., Hammerman, K. J., Tosh, F. E., and Kronenberg, R. S., Clinical features of acute pulmonary blastomycosis, *N. Engl. J. Med.*, 290, 540, 1974.
52. Ehni, W., Endogenous reactivation in blastomycosis, *Am. J. Med.*, 86, 831, 1989.
53. Butka, B. J., Bennett, S.R., and Johnson, A. C., Disseminated inoculation blastomycosis in a renal transplant recipient, *Am. Rev. Respir. Dis.*, 130, 1180, 1984.
54. Greene, N. B., Baughman, R. P., Kim, C. K., and Roselle, G. A., Failure of ketoconazole in an immunosuppressed patient with pulmonary blastomycosis, *Chest*, 88, 640, 1985.
55. Hii, J. H., Legault, L., DeVeber, G., and Vas, S. I., Successful treatment of systemic blastomycosis with high-dose ketoconazole in a renal transplant recipient, *Am. J. Kidney Dis.*, 15, 595, 1990.
56. Pechan, W. B., Novick, A. C., Lalli, A., and Gephardt, G., Pulmonary nodules in a renal recipient, *J. Urol.*, 124, 111, 1980.
57. Serody, J. S., Mill, M. R., Detterbeck, F. C., Harris, D. T., and Cohen, M. S., Blastomycosis in transplant recipients: report of a case and review, *Clin. Infect. Dis.*, 16, 54, 1993.
58. Winkler, S., Stanek, G., Hübsch, P., Willinger, B., Susani, S., Rosenkranz, A. R., and Pohanka, E., Pneumonia due to *Blastomyces dermatitidis*, in an European renal transplant recipient, *Nephrol. Dial. Transplant.*, 11, 1376, 1996.
59. Bradsher, R. W., Rice, D. C., and Abernathy, R. S., Ketoconazole therapy for endemic blastomycosis, *Ann. Intern. Med.*, 103, 872, 1985.
60. Recht, L. D., Davies, S. F., Eckman, M. R., and Sarosi, G. A., Blastomycosis in immunosuppressed patients, *Am. Rev. Respir. Dis.*, 125, 359, 1982.
61. Hasan, F. M., Jarrah, T., and Nassar, V., The association of adenocarcinoma in the lung and blastomycosis from an unusual geographic location, *Br. J. Dis. Chest*, 72, 242, 1978.
62. Bayer, A. S., Scott, V. J., and Guze, L. B., Fungal arthritis. IV. Blastomycotic arthritis, *Semin. Arthritis Rheum.*, 9, 145, 1979.
63. Logsdon, M. T. and Jones, H. E., North American blastomycosis: a review, *Cutis*, 24, 524, 1979.
64. Georgiev, V. St., Treatment and experimental therapeutics of blastomycosis, *Int. J. Antimicrob. Agents*, 6, 1, 1995.
65. Davies, S. F. and Sarosi, G. A., Blastomycosis, *Eur. J. Clin. Microbiol. Infect. Dis.*, 8, 474, 1989.
66. Laskey, W. and Sarosi, G.A., Endogenous activation in blastomycosis, *Ann. Intern. Med.*, 88, 50, 1978.

67. Recht, L. D., Phillips, J. R., Eckman, M. R., and Sarosi, G. A., Self-limited blastomycosis: a report of 13 cases, *Am. Rev. Respir. Dis.*, 120, 1109, 1979.
68. Sarosi, G. A., Davies, S. F., and Phillips, J. R., Self-limited blastomycosis: a report of 39 cases, *Semin. Respir. Infect.*, 1, 40, 1986.
69. Failla, P. J., Cerise, F. P., Karam, G. H., and Summer, W. R., Blastomycosis: pulmonary and pleural manifestations, *South. Med. J.*, 88, 405, 1995.
70. Sheflin, J. R., Campbell, J. A., and Thompson, G. P., Pulmonary blastomycosis: findings on chest radiographs in 63 patients, *Am. J. Roentgenol.*, 154, 1177, 1990.
71. Cush, R., Light, R. W., and George, R. B., Clinical and roentgenographic manifestations of acute and chronic blastomycosis, *Chest*, 69, 345, 1976.
72. Rabinowitz, J. G., Busch, J., and Buttram, W. R., Pulmonary manifestations of blastomycosis, *Radiology*, 120, 25, 1976.
73. Halvorsen, R. A., Duncan, J. D., Merten, D. E., Gallis, H. A., and Putman, C. E., Pulmonary blastomycosis: radiologic manifestations, *Radiology*, 150, 1, 1984.
74. Propeck, P. A. and Scanlan, K. A., Blastomycosis of the breast, *Am. J. Roentgenol.*, 166, 726, 1996.
75. Seymour, E. Q., Blastomycosis of the breast, *Am. J. Roentgenol.*, 139, 822, 1982.
76. Evans, M. E., Haynes, J. B., Atkinson, J. B., Delvaux, T. C., Jr., and Kaiser, A. B., *Blastomyces dermatitidis* and the adult respiratory distress syndrome: case report and review of the literature, *Am. Rev. Respir. Dis.*, 126, 1099, 1982.
77. Lockridge, R. S., Jr. and Glauser, F. L., Adult respiratory distress syndrome secondary to diffuse pulmonary blastomycoses, *South. Med. J.*, 72, 235, 1979.
78. Skillrud, D. M. and Douglass, W. W., Survival in adult respiratory distress syndrome caused by blastomycosis infection, *Mayo Clin. Proc.*, 60, 266, 1985.
79. Thiele, J. S., Buechner, H. A., and Deshotels, S. J., Jr., Blastomycosis and the adult respiratory distress syndrome, *J. Louis. State Med. Soc.*, 136, 38, 1984.
80. Unger, J. M., Peters, M. E., and Hinke, M. L., Chest case of the day, *Am. J. Roentgenol.*, 146, 1080, 1986.
81. Hebert, C. A., King, J. W., and George, J. B., Late dissemination of pulmonary blastomycosis during ketoconazole therapy, *Chest*, 95, 240, 1989.
82. Pitrak, D. L. and Andersen, B. R., Cerebral blastomycoma after ketoconazole therapy for respiratory tract blastomycosis, *Am. J. Med.*, 86, 713, 1989.
83. Bradsher, R. W., Blastomycosis, *Clin. Infect. Dis.*, 14(Suppl. 1), S82, 1992.
84. Güler, N., Palanduz, A., Önes, Ü., Öztürk, A., Somer, A., Salman, N., and Yalcin, I., Progressive vertebral blastomycosis mimicking tuberculosis, *Pediatr. Infect. Dis. J.*, 14, 816, 1995.
85. Mouzin, E. L. and Beilke, M. A., Female genital blastomycosis: case report and review, *Clin. Infect. Dis.*, 22, 718, 1996.
86. Blackard, C. E. and Berman, H. J., Genitourinary blastomycosis: a report of three cases, *J. Urol.*, 88, 94, 1962.
87. Witsell, D. L., Yarbrough, W. G., Garrett, C. G., and Weissler, M. C., Treatment of isolated laryngeal blastomycosis with ketoconazole, *N.C. Med. J.*, 55, 588, 1994.
88. Reder, P. and Neel, H., Blastomycosis in otolaryngology: review of a large series, *Laryngoscope*, 103, 53, 1993.
89. Monsanto, E. H., Johnston, A. D., and Dick, H. M., Isolated blastomycotic osteomyelitis: a case stimulating a malignant tumor of the distal radius, *J. Hand Surg.*, 11A, 896, 1986.
90. Bergman, B. A., Brown, R. E., and Khardori, N., Blastomycosis infection of the hand, *Ann. Plast. Surg.*, 33, 330, 1994.
91. Dennis, F. L., Blastomycosis of the upper respiratory tract, with report of a case primary in the larynx, *Ann. Otol. Rhinol. Laryngol.*, 27, 571, 1981.
92. Dumich, P. S. and Neel, H. B., Blastomycosis of the larynx, *Laryngoscope*, 74, 1266, 1983.
93. Mikaelian, A. J., Varkey, B., and Grossman, T. W., Blastomycosis of the head and neck, *Otolaryngol. Head Neck Surg.*, 101, 489, 1989.
94. New, G. B., Blastomycosis of the tongue, *JAMA*, 68, 186, 1971.
95. Witorsch, P. and Utz, J. P., North American blastomycosis: a study of 40 patients, *Medicine (Baltimore)*, 47, 169, 1968.

96. Busey, J. F., Baker, R., Birch, L., Buechner, H., Chick, E. W., Justice, F. K., Matthews, J. H., McDearman, S., Pickar, D. N., Sutliff, W. D., Walkup, H. E., and Zimmerman, S., Blastomycosis Cooperative Study of the Veterans Administration: blastomycosis — a review of 198 collected cases in Veterans Administration Hospitals, *Am. Rev. Respir. Dis.*, 89, 659, 1974.

97. Green, R., Blastomycosis of the lung and parotid gland: case report, *Milit. Med.*, 141, 100, 1976.

98. Bell, W. A., Gamble, J., and Garrington, G. E., North American blastomycosis with oral lesions, *Oral Surg.*, 28, 914, 1969.

99. Rose, H. D. and Gingrass, D. S., Localized oral blastomycosis mimicking actinomycosis, *Oral Surg. Oral Med. Oral Pathol.*, 54, 12, 1982.

100. Witzig, R. S., Quimosing, E. M., Campbell, W. L., Greer, D. L., and Clark, R. A., *Blastomyces dermatitidis* infection of the paranasal sinuses, *Clin. Infect. Dis.*, 18, 267, 1994.

101. Wood, C. A., Blastomycosis of the ocular structures, especially of the eyelids, *Ann. Ophthalmol.*, 13, 92, 1904.

102. McKee, S. H., Blastomycosis of the cornea: with a review of reported cases of blastomycosis of the eye, *Int. Clin.*, 3, 50, 1926.

103. Vida, L. and Moel, S. A., Systemic North American blastomycosis with orbital movement, *Am. J. Ophthalmol.*, 77, 240, 1974.

104. Bartley, G. B., Blastomycosis of the eyelid, *Ophthalmology*, 102, 2020, 1995.

105. Mohney, B., G., Blastomycosis of the eyelid, *Ophthalmology*, 103, 544, 1996.

106. Bartley, G. B., Blastomycosis of the eyelid: author's reply, *Ophthalmology*, 103, 544, 1996.

107. Barr, C. C. and Gamel, J. W., Blastomycosis of the eyelid, *Arch. Ophthalmol.*, 104, 96, 1986.

108. Bongiomo, F. J., Leavell, U. W., and Wirtschafter, J. D., The black dot sign and North American blastomycosis, *Am. J. Ophthalmol.*, 78, 145, 1974.

109. Theodoridis, E. and Koutrolikos, D., Blastomycosis of the conjunctiva, *Am. J. Ophthalmol.*, 33, 535, 1950.

110. Rodrigues, M. M., Laibson, P., and Kaplan, W., Exogenous mycotic keratitis caused by *Blastomyces dermatitidis*, *Am. J. Ophthalmol.*, 75, 782, 1973.

111. Churchill, T. and Stober, A, M., A case of systemic blastomycosis, *Arch. Intern. Med.*, 13, 568, 1914.

112. Schwartz, V. J., Intraocular blastomycosis, *Arch. Ophthalmol.*, 5, 581, 1931.

113. Moore, J. T., Blastomycosis: with report of a case dying from abscess of the brain, *Surg. Gynecol. Obstet.*, 31, 590, 1920.

114. Green, W. R., Uveal tract, in *Ophthalmic Pathology: An Atlas and Textbook*, Vol. 3, 3rd ed., Spencer, W. H., Ed., W. B. Saunders, Philadelphia, 1986, 1891.

115. Lopez, R., Mason, J. O., Parker, J. S., and Pappas, P. G., Intraocular blastomycosis: case report and review, *Clin. Infect. Dis.*, 18, 805, 1994.

116. Cassady, J. V., Uveal blastomycosis, *Arch. Ophthalmol.*, 35, 84, 1946.

117. Bond, W. I., Sanders, C. V., Joffe, L., and Franklin, R. M., Presumed blastomycosis endophthalmitis, *Ann. Ophthalmol.*, 14, 1183, 1982.

118. Lewis, H., Aaberg, T. M., Fary, D. R., and Stevens, T. S., Latent disseminated blastomycosis with choroidal involvement, *Arch. Ophthalmol.*, 106, 527, 1988.

119. Safneck, J. R., Hogg, G. R., and Napier, L. B., Endophthalmitis due to *Blastomyces dermatitidis*: case report and review of the literature, *Ophthalmology*, 97, 212, 1990.

120. Sinskey, R. M. and Anderson, W. B., Miliary blastomycosis with metastatic spread to the posterior uvea of both eyes, *Arch. Ophthalmol.*, 54, 602, 1955.

121. Gottlieb, J. L., McAllister, I. L., Guttman, F. A., and Vine, A. K., Choroidal blastomycosis: a report of two cases, *Retina*, 15, 248, 1995.

122. Font, R. L., Spaulding, A. G., and Green, W. R., Endogenous mycotic panophthalmitis caused by *Blastomyces dermatitidis*: report of a case and review of literature, *Arch. Ophthalmol.*, 77, 217, 1967.

123. Colonna, P. C. and Gucker, T. III, Blastomycosis of the skeletal system: a summary of sixty-seven recorded cases and a case report, *J. Bone Joint Surg.*, 26, 322, 1944.

124. MacDonald, P. R., Black, G. B., and MacKenzie, R., Orthopaedic manifestations of blastomycosis, *J. Bone Joint Surg.*, 72(A), 860, 1990.

125. Moore, R. M. and Green, N. E., Blastomycosis of bone: a report of six cases, *J. Bone Joint Surg.*, 7, 1, 1986.

126. Dee, P. M., Chest case of the day: disseminated pulmonary blastomycosis, *Am. J. Roentgenol.*, 167, 234, 1996.

127. Bassett, F. H. III and Tindall, J. P., Blastomycosis of bone, *South. Med. J.*, 65, 547, 1972.

128. Hardjasudarma, M., Willis, B., Black-Payne, C., and Edwards, R., Pediatric spinal blastomycosis: case report, *Neurosurgery*, 37, 534, 1995.

129. Chick, E. W., North American blastomycosis, in *Human Infection with Fungi, Actinomycetes, and Algae*, Baker, R. D., Ed., Springer-Verlag, New York, 1971, 30.

130. Gelman, M. I. and Everts, C. S., Blastomycotic dactylitis, *Radiology*, 107, 331, 1973.

131. George, A. L., Jr., Hays, J. T., and Graham, B. S., Blastomycosis presenting as monoarticular arthritis: the role of synovial fluid cytology, *Arthritis Rheumatol.*, 28, 516, 1985.

132. Hamblen, E. C., Baker, R. D., and Martin, D. S., Blastomycosis of the female reproductive tract: with report of a case, *Am. J. Obstet. Gynecol.*, 30, 345, 1935.

133. Murray, J. J., Clark, C. A., Lands, R. H., Heim, C. R., and Burnett, L. S., Reactivation blastomycosis presenting as a tuboovarian abscess, *Obstet. Gynecol.*, 64, 828, 1984.

134. Farber, E. R., Leahy, M. S., and Meadows, T. R., Endometrial blastomycosis acquired by sexual contact, *Obstet. Gynecol.*, 32, 195, 1968.

135. Neuzil, K. M., Mitchell, H. C., Loyd, J. E., Lagerstrom, C. F., Hammon, J. W., Jr., and Graham, B. S., Extrapulmonary thoracic disease caused by *Blastomyces dermatitidis*, *Chest*, 106, 1885, 1994.

136. Lagerstrom, C. F., Mitchell, H. G., Graham, B. S., and Hammon, J. H., Chronic fibrosing mediastinitis and superior vena caval obstruction from blastomycosis, *Ann. Thorac. Surg.*, 54, 764, 1992.

137. Buchner, H. A. and Clawson, C. M., Blastomycosis of the central nervous system. II. A report of nine cases from the Veteran Administration Cooperative Study, *Am. Rev. Respir. Dis.*, 95, 820, 1967.

138. Fetter, B. F., Klintworth, G. K., and Hendry, W. S., *Mycoses of the Central Nervous System*, Williams & Wilkins, Baltimore, 1978, 38.

139. Gonyea, E. F., The spectrum of primary blastomycosis meningitis: a review of central nervous system blastomycosis, *Ann. Neurol.*, 3, 26, 1978.

140. Morgan, D., Young, R. F., Chow, A. W., Mehringer, C. M., and Itabashi, H., Recurrent intracerebral blastomycotic granuloma: diagnosis and treatment, *Neurosurgery*, 4, 319, 1979.

141. Roos, K. L., Bryan, J. P., Maggio, W. W., Jane, J. A., and Scheld, W. M., Intracranial blastomycoma, *Medicine (Baltimore)*, 66, 224, 1987.

142. Treseler, C. B. and Sugar, A. M., Fungal meningitis, *Infect. Dis. Clin. North Am.*, 4, 789, 1990.

143. Rimondi, A. P., Bianchini, E., Barucchello, G., and Panzavolta, R., Addison's disease caused by adrenal blastomycosis: a case report with fine needle aspiration (FNA) cytology, *Cytopathology*, 6, 277, 1995.

144. Herd, A. M., Greenfield, S. B., Thompson, W. S., and Brunham, R. C., Miliary blastomycosis and HIV infection, *Can. Med. Assoc. J.*, 143, 1329, 1990.

145. Kitchen, L. W., Clark, R. A., Hoadley, D. J., Wisniewski, T. L., Janney, F. A., and Greer, D. L., Concurrent pulmonary *Blastomyces dermatitidis* and *Mycobacterium tuberculosis* infection in an HIV-1 seropositive man, *J. Infect. Dis.*, 160, 911, 1989.

146. Ludmerer, K. M. and Kissane, J. M., Deterioration and death in a 30-year old male with AIDS (clinical conference), *Am. J. Med.*, 100, 571, 1996.

147. Srinath, L., Ahkee, S., Huang, A., Raff, M. J., and Ramirez, J. A., Acute miliary blastomycosis in an AIDS patient, *J. Ky. Med. Assoc.*, 92, 450, 1994.

148. Witzig, R. S., Hoadley, D. J., Greer, D. L., Abriola, K. P., and Hernandez, R. L., Blastomycosis and human immunodeficiency virus: three new cases and review, *South. Med. J.*, 87, 715, 1994.

149. Nelson, M. R., Barton, S. E., Hawkins, D. A., and Gazzard, B. G., Blastomycosis in an HIV antibody positive male in the UK, *Int. J. STD AIDS*, 4, 176, 1993.

150. Pappas, P. G., Pottage, J. C., Powderly, W. G., Fraser, V. J., Stratton, C. W., McKenzie, S., Tapper, M. L., Chmel, H., Bonebrake, F. C., Blum, R., Shafer, R. W., King, C., and Dismukes, W. E., Blastomycosis in patients with the acquired immunodeficiency syndrome, *Ann. Intern. Med.*, 116, 847, 1992.

151. Winquist, E. W., Walmsley, S. L., and Barinstein, N. L., Reactivation and dissemination of blastomycosis complicating Hodgkin's disease: a case report and review of the literature, *Am. J. Hematol.*, 43, 129, 1993.

152. Dubuisson, R. L. and Jones, T. B., Splenic abscess due to blastomycosis: scintigraphic, sonographic, and CT evaluation, *Am. J. Roentgenol.*, 140, 66, 1983.

153. Barr, C. C. and Gamel, J. W., Blastomycosis of the eyelid, *Arch. Ophthalmol.*, 104, 96, 1986.

154. Mercantini, R., Marsella, R., Moretto, D., Mercantini, P., Balus, L., Mastroianni, A., and Ferraro, C., Macroscopic and microscopic characteristics of an African *Blastomyces dermatitidis* strain, *Mycoses*, 38, 477, 1995.

155. Cohen, L. M., Golitz, L. E., and Wilson, M. L., Widespread papulae and nodules in an Ugandan man with acquired immunodeficiency syndrome: African blastomycosis, *Arch. Dermatol.*, 132, 821, 1996.

156. Raftopoulos, C., Flament-Duvant, J., Coremans-Pelseneer, J., and Noterman, J., Intracerebellar blastomycosis abscess in an African man, *Clin. Neurol. Neurosurg.*, 88, 209, 1986.

157. Frean, J. A., Carman, W. F., Crewe-Brown, H.-H., Culligan, G. A., and Young, C. N., *Blastomyces dermatitidis* infections in the RSA, *S. Afr. Med. J.*, 76, 13, 1989.

158. Lombardi, G., Padhye, A. A., and Ajello, L., *In vitro* conversion of African isolates of *Blastomyces dermatitidis* to their yeast form, *Mycoses*, 31, 447, 1988.

159. Vermeil, C., Morin, O., Miegeville, M., Marjolet, M., and Gordeeff, A., Maladie de Gilchrist et taxonomie fongique: un épineux problème, *Bull. Soc. Pathol. Exit.*, 74, 27, 1981.

160. McGinnis, M. R., *Laboratory Handbook of Medical Mycology*, Academic Press, New York, 1980, 479.

161. Vanbreuseghem, R., De Vroey, Ch., and Takashio, M., *Practical Guide to Medical and Veterinary Mycology*, Masson, Paris, 1978, 28.

162. Yates-Siilata, K. E., Sander, D. M., and Keath, E. J., Genetic diversity in clinical isolates of the dimorphic fungus *Blastomyces dermatitidis* detected by a PCR-based random amplified polymorphic DNA assay, *J. Clin. Microbiol.*, 33, 2171, 1995.

163. Baily, G. G., Robertson, V. J., Neill, P., Garrido, P., and Levy, L. F., Blastomycosis in Africa: clinical features, diagnosis, and treatment, *Rev. Infect. Dis.*, 13, 1005, 1991.

164. Zeluff, B. J., Fungal pneumonia in transplant recipients, *Semin. Respir. Infect.*, 5, 80, 1990.

165. Bradsher, R. W. and Pappas, P. G., Detection of specific antibodies in human blastomycosis by enzyme immunoassay, *South. Med. J.*, 88, 1256, 1995.

166. Bradsher, R. W., Balk, R. A., and Jacobs, R. F., Growth inhibition of *Blastomyces dermatitidis* in alveolar and peripheral macrophages from patients with blastomycosis, *Am. Rev. Respir. Dis.*, 135, 412, 1987.

167. Sugar, A. M. and Picard, M., Macrophage- and oxidant-mediated inhibition of the ability of live *Blastomyces dermatitidis* conidia to transform to the pathogenic yeast phase: implications for the pathogenesis of dimorphic fungal infections, *J. Infect. Dis.*, 163, 371, 1991.

168. Brummer, E., Morozumi, P. A., and Stevens, D. A., Macrophages and fungi: *in vitro* effects of method of macrophage induction, activation by different stimuli, and soluble factors on *Blastomyces*, *J. Reticuloendothel. Soc.*, 28, 507, 1980.

169. Levine, S. and Ordal, Z. L., Factors influencing the morphology of *Blastomyces dermatitidis*, *J. Bacteriol.*, 52, 687, 1946.

170. Medoff, G., Painter, A., and Kobayashi, G. S., Mycelial-to-yeast-phase transitions of the dimorphic fungi *Blastomyces dermatitidis* and *Paracoccidioides brasiliensis*, *J. Bacteriol.*, 169, 4055, 1987.

171. Paris, S. and Garrison, R. G., Cyclic adenosine 3′,5′-monophosphate (c-AMP) as a factor in phase morphogenesis of *Blastomyces dermatitidis*, *Mykosen*, 27, 340, 1984.

172. Medoff, G., Kobayashi, G. S., Painter, A., and Travis, S., Morphogenesis and pathogenicity of *Histoplasma capsulatum*, *Infect. Immun.*, 55, 1355, 1987.

173. Medoff, G., Maresca, B., Lambowitz, A. M., Kobayashi, G., Painter, A., Sacco, M., and Carratu, L., Correlation between pathogenicity and temperature sensitivity in different strains of *Histoplasma capsulatum*, *J. Clin. Invest.*, 78, 1638, 1986.

174. Medoff, G., Sacco, M., Maresca, B., Schlessinger, D., Painter, A., Kobayashi, G. S., and Carratu, L., Irreversible blockade of the mycelial-to-yeast phase transition of *Histoplasma capsulatum*, *Science*, 231, 476, 1986.

175. Brummer, E., Bhagavathula, P. R., Hanson, L. H., and Stevens, D. A., Synergy of itraconazole with macrophages in killing *Blastomyces dermatitidis*, *Antimicrob. Agents Chemother.*, 36, 2487, 1992.

176. Brummer, E. C., Morrison, C. J., and Stevens, D. A., Recombinant and natural gamma-interferon activation of macrophages *in vitro*: different dose requirements for induction of killing activity against phagocytizable and nonphagocytizable fungi, *Infect. Immun.*, 49, 724, 1985.

177. Brummer, E. and Stevens, D. A., Activation of pulmonary macrophages for fungicidal activity by gamma-interferon or lymphokines, *Clin. Exp. Immunol.*, 70, 520, 1987.

178. Brummer, E., Hanson, L. H., Restrepo, A., and Stevens, D.A., *In vivo* and *in vitro* activation of pulmonary macrophages by IFN-γ for enhanced killing of *Paracoccidioides brasiliensis* or *Blastomyces dermatitidis*, *J. Immunol.*, 140, 2786, 1988.

179. Morrison, C. J., Brummer, E., and Stevens, D. A., *In vivo* activation of peripheral blood polymorpho-nuclear neutrophils by gamma interferon results in enhanced fungal killing, *Infect. Immun.*, 57, 2953, 1989.

180. Brummer, E., Hanson, L. H., and Stevens, D. A., IL-4, IgE, and interferon-γ production in pulmonary blastomycosis: comparison in mice untreated, immunized, or treated with an antifungal (SCH 39304), *Cell. Immunol.*, 149, 258, 1993.

181. Abuodeh, R. O., Winston, V., and Scalarone, G. M., Induction and detection of cell-mediated reactions with different *Blastomyces dermatitidis* antigenic preparations, *Mycoses*, 39, 85, 1996.

182. Klein, B. S. and Jones, J. M., Isolation, purification, and radio labeling of a novel 120-kD surface protein on *Blastomyces dermatitidis* yeasts to detect antibody in infected patients, *J. Clin. Invest.*, 85, 152, 1990.

183. Klein, B. S., Sondel, P. M., and Jones, J. M., WI-1, a novel 120-kilodalton surface protein on *Blastomyces dermatitidis* yeast cells, is a target antigen of cell-mediated immunity in human blasto-mycosis, *Infect. Immun.*, 60, 4291, 1992.

184. Klein, B. S., Hogan, L. H., and Jones, J. M., Immunologic recognition of a 25-amino acid repeat arrayed in tandem on a major antigen of *Blastomyces dermatitidis*, *J. Clin. Invest.*, 92, 330, 1993.

185. Soufleris, A. J., Klein, B. S., Courtney, B. T., Proctor, M. E., and Jones, J. M., Utility of anti-WI-1 serological testing in the diagnosis of blastomycosis in Wisconsin residents, *Clin. Infect. Dis.*, 19, 87, 1994.

186. Klein, B. S. and Jones, J. M., Purification and characterization of the major antigen WI-1 from *Blastomyces dermatitidis* yeasts and immunological comparison with A antigen, *Infect. Immun.*, 62, 3890, 1994.

187. Klein, B. S. and Newman, S. L., Role of cell-surface molecule of *Blastomyces dermatitidis* in host-pathogen interactions, *Trends Microbiol.*, 4, 246, 1996.

188. Hurst, S. F. and Kaufman, L., Western immunoblot analysis and serologic characterization of *Blastomyces dermatitidis* yeast extracellular antigens, *J. Clin. Microbiol.*, 30, 3043, 1992.

189. Isberg, R. R., Discrimination between intracellular uptake and surface adhesion of bacterial pathogens, *Science*, 252, 934, 1991.

190. Isberg, R. R. and Leong, J. M., Multiple beta I chain integrins are receptors for invasin, a protein that promotes bacterial penetration into mammalian cells, *Cell*, 60, 861, 1990.

191. Hogan, L. H., Josvai, S., and Klein, B. S., Genomic cloning, characterization, and functional analysis of the major surface adhesin WI-1 on *Blastomyces dermatitidis* yeasts, *J. Biol. Chem.*, 270, 30725, 1995.

192. Leong, J. M., Fournier, R. S., and Isberg, R. R., Identification of the integrin binding domain of the *Yersinia pseudotuberculosis* invasin protein, *EMBO J.*, 9, 1979, 1990.

193. Appella, E., Weber, I. T., and Blasi, F., Structure and function of epidermal growth factor-like regions in proteins, *FEBS Lett.*, 231, 1, 1988.

194. Williams, J. E., Moser, S. A., Turner, S. H., and Standard, P. G., Development of pulmonary infection in mice inoculated with *Blastomyces dermatitidis* conidia, *Am. J. Respir. Crit. Care Med.*, 149, 500, 1994.

195. Bradsher, R. W., Macrophages and *Blastomyces dermatitidis*, *Immunol. Ser.*, 60, 553, 1993.

196. Dixon, D., Shadomy, S., Shadomy, H. J., Espinel-Ingroff, A., and Kerkering, T. M., Comparison of the *in vitro* antifungal activities of miconazole and a new imidazole R 41,400, *J. Infect. Dis.*, 138, 245, 1978.

197. Sugar, A. M., Alsip, S. G., Galgiani, J. N., Graybill, J. R., Dismukes, W. E., Cloud, G. A., Craven, P. C., and Stevens, D. A., Pharmacology and toxicity of high dose ketoconazole, *Antimicrob. Agents Chemother.*, 31, 1874, 1987.

198. Arathoon, E. G., Brummer, E., and Stevens, D. A., Efficacy of itraconazole in blastomycosis in a murine model and comparison with ketoconazole, *Mycoses*, 32(Suppl. 1), 109, 1989.

199. Humphrey, M. J., Jevons, S., and Tarbit, M. H., Pharmacokinetic evaluation of UK-49,858, a metabolically stable triazole antifungal drug, in animals and humans, *Antimicrob. Agents Chemother.*, 28, 648, 1984.

200. Tucker, R. M., Williams, P. L., Arathoon, E. G., Levine, B. E., Hartstein, A. I., Hanson, L. H., and Stevens, D. A., Pharmacokinetics of fluconazole in cerebrospinal fluid and serum in human coccidioidal meningitis, *Antimicrob. Agents Chemother.*, 32, 369, 1988.

201. Stevens, D. A., Brummer, E., McEwen, J. G., and Perlman, A. M., Comparison of fluconazole and ketoconazole in experimental murine blastomycosis, *Rev. Infect. Dis.*, 12(Suppl.), 304, 1990.

202. McIntyre, K. A. and Galgiani, J. N., *In vitro* susceptibilities of yeast to a new antifungal triazole, SCH 39304: effects of test conditions and relation to *in vivo* efficacy, *Antimicrob. Agents Chemother.*, 33, 1095, 1989.

203. Perfect, J. R., Wright, K. A., Hobbs, M. M., and Durack, D.T., Treatment of experimental cryptococcal meningitis and disseminated candidiasis with SCH 39304, *Antimicrob. Agents Chemother.*, 33, 1735, 1989.

204. Restrepo, B. I., Ahrens, J., and Graybill, J. R., Efficacy of SCH 39304 in murine cryptococcosis, *Antimicrob. Agents Chemother.*, 33, 1242, 1989.

205. Sugar, A. M., Picard, M., and Noble, L., Treatment of murine pulmonary blastomycosis with SCH 39304, a new triazole antifungal agents, *Antimicrob. Agents Chemother.*, 34, 896, 1990.

206. Brummer, E., Hanson, L. H., and Stevens, D. A., SCH 39304 in the treatment of acute or established murine pulmonary blastomycosis, *Antimicrob. Agents Chemother.*, 35, 788, 1991.

207. Tucker, R. M., Hanson, L. H., Brummer, E., and Stevens, D. A., Activity of ICI 195,739, a new oral triazole, compared with that of ketoconazole in the therapy of experimental murine blastomycoses, *Antimicrob. Agents Chemother.*, 33, 573, 1989.

208. Harvey, R. P., Schmid, E. S., Carrington, C. C., and Stevens, D. A., Mouse model of pulmonary blastomycosis: utility, simplicity and quantitative parameters, *Am. Rev. Respir. Dis.*, 117, 695, 1978.

209. Pappagianis, D., Zimmer, B. L., Theodoropoulos, G., Plempel, M., and Hector, R. F., Therapeutic effect of the triazole Bay R 3783 in mouse models of coccidioidomycosis, blastomycosis, and histoplasmosis, *Antimicrob. Agents Chemother.*, 34, 1132, 1990.

210. Hector, R. F., Zimmer, B. L., and Pappagianis, D., Microtiter method for MIC testing with spherule-endospore-phase *Coccidioides immitis*, *J. Clin. Microbiol.*, 26, 2667, 1988.

211. Polak, A. and Dixon, D. M., Fungistatic and fungicidal effects of amphotericin B, ketoconazole and fluconazole (UK 49,858) against *Histoplasma capsulatum in vitro* and *in vivo*, *Mykosen*, 30, 186, 1987.

212. Harvey, R. P., Isenberg, R. A., and Stevens, D. A., Molecular modifications of imidazole compounds: studies of activity and synergy *in vitro* and in pharmacology and therapy of blastomycosis in a mouse model, *Rev. Infect. Dis.*, 2, 559, 1980.

213. Clemons, K. V., Hanson, L. H., and Stevens, D. A., Activities of triazole D0870 *in vitro* and against murine blastomycosis, *Antimicrob. Agents Chemother.*, 37, 1177, 1993.

214. Galgiani, J. N., Lewis, M. L., and Peng, T., *In vitro* studies of a new azole antifungal drug, SCH 56592, *Proc. 25th Intersci. Conf. Antimicrob. Agents Chemother.*, American Society for Microbiology, Washington, D.C., Abstr. F63, 1995.

215. Parmegianni, R., Cacciapuotti, A., Loebenberg, D., Antonacci, B., Norris, C., Yarosh-Tomaine, T., Michalski, M., Hare, R. S., and Miller, G. H., *In vitro* activity of SCH 56592, a new antifungal agent, *Proc. 35th Intersci. Conf. Antimicrob. Agents Chemother.*, American Society for Microbiology, Washington, D.C., Abstr. F62, 1995.

216. Perfect, J. R. and Schell, W. A., *In vitro* efficacy of the azole, SCH 56592, compared to amphotericin B, fluconazole, and itraconazole versus *Cryptococcus neoformans*, *Proc. 35th Intersci. Conf. Antimicrob. Agents Chemother.*, American Society for Microbiology, Washington, D.C., Abstr. F64, 1995.

217. Sugar, A. M. and Liu, X.-P., *In vitro* and *in vivo* activities of SCH 56592 against *Blastomyces dermatitidis*, *Antimicrob. Agents Chemother.*, 40, 1314, 1996.

218. Sugar, A. M. and Picard, M., Treatment of murine pulmonary blastomycosis with SCH 51048, a broad-spectrum triazole antifungal agent, *Antimicrob. Agents Chemother.*, 39, 996, 1995.

219. Cabib, E., The synthesis and degradation of chitin, *Adv. Enzymol. Relat. Areas Mol. Biol.*, 59, 59, 1988.

220. Davis, T. E., Jr., Domer, J. E., and Li, Y. T., Cell wall studies of *Histoplasma capsulatum* and *Blastomyces dermatitidis* using homologous enzymes, *Infect. Immun.*, 15, 978, 1977.

221. Domer, J. E., Monosaccharide and chitin content of cell walls of *Histoplasma capsulatum* and *Blastomyces dermatitidis*, *J. Bacteriol.*, 107, 870, 1971.

222. Domer, J. E., Hamilton, J. G., and Harkin, J. C., Comparative study of the cell walls of the yeast-like and mycelial phases of *Histoplasma capsulatum*, *J. Bacteriol.*, 94, 466, 1967.

223. Kanetsuma, F., Carbonell, L. M., Gil, F., and Azuma, I., Chemical and ultrastructural studies on the cell walls of *Histoplasma capsulatum*, *Mycopathol. Mycol. Appl.*, 54, 1, 1974.

224. Reiss, E., Serial enzymatic hydrolysis of cell walls of two serotypes of yeast-form *Histoplasma capsulatum* with α(1→3)glucanase, β(1→3)glucanase, pronase, and chitinase, *Infect. Immun.*, 16, 181, 1977.

225. Tronchin, G., Poulain, D., Herbaut, J., and Biguet, J., Localization of chitin in the cell wall of *Candida albicans* by means of wheat germ agglutinin: fluorescence and ultrastructural values, *Eur. J. Cell Biol.*, 26, 121, 1981.

226. Wheat, R. W., Tritschler, C., Connant, N. F., and Lowe, E. P., Comparison of *Coccidioides immitis* arthrospore, mycelium, and spherule cell walls, and influence of growth medium on mycelial cell wall composition, *Infect. Immun.*, 17, 91, 1977.

227. Brillinger, G. U., Metabolic products of microorganisms. 181.Chitin synthase from fungi, a test model for substances with insecticidal properties, *Arch. Microbiol.*, 121, 71, 1979.

228. Dahn, U., Hagenmaier, H., Hohne, H., Konig, W. A., Wolf, G., and Zahner, H., Nikkomycin, ein neuer hemmstoff der chitin-synthase bei pilzen, *Arch. Mikrobiol.*, 170, 143, 1976.

229. Gooday, B. W., Biosynthesis of the fungal cell — mechanism and implications, *J. Gen. Microbiol.*, 99, 1, 1977.

230. Becker, J. M., Covert, N. L., Shenbagmurthi, P., and Steinfeld, A. S., Polyoxin D inhibits the growth of zoopathogenic fungi, *Antimicrob. Agents Chemother.*, 23, 926, 1979.

231. McCarthy, P. J., Troke, P. F., and Gull, K., Mechanism of action of nikkomycin and the peptide transport system of *Candida albicans*, *J. Gen. Microbiol.*, 131, 775, 1985.

232. Yadan, J.-C., Gonneau, M., Sarthou, P., and Le Goffic, F., Sensitivity of nikkomycin Z in *Candida albicans*: role of peptide permeases, *J. Bacteriol.*, 160, 884, 1984.

233. Cooper, C. R., Harris, J. L., Jacobs, C. W., and Szaniszlo, P. J., Effects of polyoxin AL on cellular development in *Wangiella dermatitidis*, *Exp. Mycol.*, 8, 349, 1984.

234. Hector, R. F. and Pappagianis, D., Inhibition of chitin synthesis in the cell wall of *Coccidioides immitis* by polyoxin D, *J. Bacteriol.*, 154, 488, 1983.

235. Hector, R. F., Zimmer, B. L., and Pappagianis, D., Evaluation of nikkomycin X and Z in murine models of coccidioidomycosis, histoplasmosis, and blastomycosis, *Antimicrob. Agents Chemother.*, 34, 587, 1990.

236. Schoenbach, E. B. and Greenspan, E. M., The pharmacology, mode of action and therapeutic potentialities of stilbamidine, pentamidine, propamidine and other aromatic diamidines, *Medicine (Baltimore)*, 27, 327, 1948.

237. Sarosi, G. A. and Davies, S. F., Therapy for fungal infections, *Mayo Clin. Proc.*, 69, 1111, 1994.

238. Busey, J. F., Blastomycosis. III. A comparative study of 2-hydroxystilbamide and amphotericin B therapy, *Am. Rev. Respir. Dis.*, 105, 812, 1972.

239. Carmody, E. J. and Tappen, W., Blastomycosis meningitis: report of a case successfully treated with amphotericin B, *Ann. Intern. Med.*, 51, 139, 1959.

240. Kravitz, G. R., Davies, S. F., Eckman, M. R., and Sarosi, G. A., Chronic blastomycotic meningitis, *Am. J. Med.*, 71, 501, 1981.

241. Larkin, J. C., Young, J. M., and Sutliff, W. D., Clinicopathologic conference: systemic blastomycosis involving urinary tract and skin, *J. Tenn. Med. Assoc.*, 66, 1141, 1973.

242. Lockwood, W. R., Allison, F., Batson, B. E., and Busey, J. F., The treatment of North American blastomycosis, ten years' experience, *Am. Rev. Respir. Dis.*, 100, 314, 1969.

243. Loudon, R. G. and Lawson, R. A., Systemic blastomycosis: recurrent neurological relapse in a case treated with amphotericin B, *Ann. Intern. Med.*, 55, 139, 1961.

244. Parker, J. D., Doto, I. L., and Tosh, F. E., A decade of experience with blastomycosis and its treatment with amphotericin B, *Am. Rev. Respir. Dis.*, 99, 895, 1969.

245. Rainey, R. L. and Harris, T. R., Disseminated blastomycosis with meningeal involvement, *Arch. Intern. Med.*, 117, 744, 1966.

246. Seaburg, J. H. and Dascomb, H. E., Results of the treatment of systemic mycosis, *JAMA*, 188, 509, 1964.

247. Pappas, P. G., Threlkeld, M. G., Bedsole, G. D., Cleveland, K. O., Gelfand, M. S., and Desmukes, W. E., Blastomycosis in immunocompromised patients, *Medicine (Baltimore)*, 72, 311, 1993.

248. Johnson, P. and Sarosi, G., Current therapy of major fungal diseases of the lung, *Infect. Dis. Clin. North Am.*, 5, 635, 1991.

249. Furcolow, M. C., Watson, K. A., Tisdall, O. F., Julian, W. A., Saliba, N. A., and Balows, A., Some factors affecting survival in systemic blastomycosis, *Dis. Chest*, 54, 285, 1968.

250. Phillips, J. R., Jones, S., Adamson, J. S., and Abernathy, R. S., Long-term follow-up of 101 patients with blastomycosis, *Am. Rev. Respir. Dis.*, 105, 1006, 1972.

251. Albert, M. C., Zachary, S. V., and Alter, S., Blastomycosis of the forearm synovium in a child, *Clin. Orthop.*, 317, 223, 1995.

252. Bradsher, R. W., Martin, M. R., Wilkes, T. D., Waltman, C., and Bolyard, K., Unusual presentations of blastomycosis: ten case summaries, *Infect. Med.*, 7, 10, 1990.

253. Sarosi, G. A. and Davies, S. F., Blastomycosis: state of the art, *Am. Rev. Respir. Dis.*, 120, 911, 1979.

254. Gallis, H. A., Drew, R. H., and Pickard, W. W., Amphotericin B: 30 years of clinical experience, *Rev. Infect. Dis.*, 12, 308, 1990.

255. Georgiev, V. St., Treatment and developmental therapeutics in aspergillosis. I. Amphotericin B and its derivatives, *Respiration*, 59, 291, 1992.

256. Ellis, W. G., Sobel, R. A., and Nielsen, S. L., Leukoencephalopathy in patients treated with amphotericin B methyl ester, *J. Infect. Dis.*, 146, 125, 1982.

257. Graybill, J. R. and Kaster, S. R., Experimental murine aspergillosis: comparison of amphotericin B and a new polyene antifungal drug, SCH 28191, *Am. Rev. Respir. Dis.*, 129, 292, 1984.

258. Hoeprich, P. D., Amphotericin B methyl ester and leukoencephalopathy: the other side of the coin, *J. Infect. Dis.*, 146, 173, 1982.

259. Lawrence, R. M. and Hoeprich, P. D., Comparison of amphotericin B and amphotericin B methyl ester: efficacy in murine coccidioidomycosis and toxicity, *J. Infect. Dis.*, 133, 168, 1976.

260. Graybill, J. R., Craven, P. C., Taylor, R. L., Williams, D. M., and Magee, W. E., Treatment of murine cryptococcosis with liposome-associated amphotericin B, *J. Infect. Dis.*, 145, 748, 1982.

261. Hopfer, R. L., Mills, K., Mehta, R., Lopez-Berestein, G., Fainstein, V., and Juliano, R. L., *In vitro* antifungal activities of amphotericin B and liposome-encapsulated amphotericin B, *Antimicrob. Agents Chemother.*, 25, 387, 1984.

262. Lopez-Berestein, G., Liposomes as carriers of antifungal drugs, *Ann. NY Acad. Sci.*, 544, 590, 1988.

263. Lopez-Berestein, G., Bodey, G. P., Fainstein, V., Keating, M., Frankel, L. S., Zeluff, B., Gentry, L., and Mehta, K., Treatment of systemic fungal infections with liposomal amphotericin B, *Arch. Intern. Med.*, 149, 2533, 1989.

264. Patterson, T. F., Miniter, P., Dijkstra, J., Szoka, F., Ryan, J. L., and Andriole, V. T., Treatment of experimental invasive aspergillosis with novel amphotericin B/cholesterol-sulfate complexes, *J. Infect. Dis.*, 159, 717, 1989.

265. Shirhoda, A., Lopez-Berestein, G., Holbert, J. M., and Luna, M. A., Hepatosplenic fungal infection: CT and pathologic evaluation after treatment with liposomal amphotericin B, *Radiology*, 159, 349, 1986.

266. Szoka, F. C., Mulholland, D., and Barza, M., Effect of lipid composition and liposome size on toxicity and *in vitro* fungicidal activity of liposome-intercalated amphotericin B, *Antimicrob. Agents Chemother.*, 31, 421, 1987.

267. Taylor, R. L., Williams, D. M., Craven, P. C., Graybill, J. R., Drutz, D. J., and Magee, W. E., Amphotericin B in liposomes: a novel therapy for histoplasmosis, *Am. Rev. Respir. Dis.*, 125, 610, 1982.

268. Tremblay, C., Barza, M., Fiore, C., and Szoka, F., Efficacy of liposome-intercalated amphotericin B in the treatment of systemic candidiasis in mice, *Antimicrob. Agents Chemother.*, 26, 170, 1984.

269. Weber, R. S. and Lopez-Berestein, G., Treatment of invasive *Aspergillus* sinusitis with liposomal-amphotericin B, *Laryngoscope*, 97, 937, 1987.

270. Wiebe, V. J. and DeGregorio, M. W., Liposome-encapsulated amphotericin B: a promising new treatment for disseminated fungal infections, *Rev. Infect. Dis.*, 10, 1097, 1988.

271. Clemons, K. V. and Stevens, D. A., Comparative efficacies of amphotericin B lipid complex and amphotericin B deoxycholate suspension against murine blastomycosis, *Antimicrob. Agents Chemother.*, 35, 2144, 1991.

272. Clemons, K. V. and Stevens, D. A., Therapeutic efficacy of a liposomal formulation of amphotericin B (AmBisome) against murine blastomycosis, *J. Antimicrob. Chemother.*, 32, 465, 1993.

273. Saag, M. S. and Dismukes, W. E., Treatment of histoplasmosis and blastomycosis, *Chest*, 93, 848, 1988.

274. Dismukes, W. E., Cloud, G., Bowles, C., Sarosi, G. A., Gregg, C. R., Chapman, S. W., Scheld, W. M., Farr, B., Gallis, H. A., Marier, R. L., Karam, G. H., Bennett, J. E., Kauffman, C. A., Medoff, G., Stevens, D. A., Kaplowitz, L. G., Black, J. R., Roselle, G. A., Pankey, G. A., Kerkering, T. M., Fisher, J. F., Graybill, J. R., and Shadomy, S., Treatment of blastomycosis and histoplasmosis with ketoconazole: results of a prospective, randomized clinical trial, *Ann. Intern. Med.*, 103, 861, 1985.

275. Dismukes, W. E., Stamm, A. M., Graybill, J. R., Craven, P. C., Stevens, D. A., Stiller, R. L., Sarosi, G. A., Medoff, G., Gregg, C. R., Gallis, H. A., Fields, B. T., Jr., Marier, R. L., Kerkering, T. A., Kaplowitz, L. G., Cloud, G., Bowles, C., and Shadomy, C., Treatment of systemic mycoses with ketoconazole: emphasis on toxicity and clinical response in 52 patients, *Ann. Intern. Med.*, 98, 13, 1983.

276. Graybill, J. R. and Drutz, D. J., Ketoconazole: a major innovation for treatment of fungal disease, *Ann. Intern. Med.*, 93, 921, 1980.

277. Reynolds, R. J. and Burford, J. G., Blastomycosis, in: *Conn's Current Therapy*, Rakel, R. E., Ed., W. B. Saunders, Philadelphia, 1987, 921.

278. Ahasan, H. A., Rahman, K. M., Chowdhury, M. A., Azhar, M. A., and Rafiqueuddin, A. K., Pulmonary blastomycosis, *Trop. Doct.*, 25, 83, 1995.

279. Hudson, C. P. and Callen, J. P., Systemic blastomycosis treated with ketoconazole, *Arch. Dermatol.*, 120, 536, 1984.

280. McManus, E. J. and Jones, J. M., The use of ketoconazole in the treatment of blastomycosis, *Am. Rev. Respir. Dis.*, 133, 141, 1986.

281. Ferguson, R. M., Sutherland, D. E. R., Simmons, R. L., and Najarian, J. S., Ketoconazole, cyclosporin metabolism, and renal transplantation, *Lancet*, 2, 882, 1982.

282. Abernathy, R. S., Amphotericin therapy of North American blastomycosis, *Antimicrob. Agents Chemother.*, 3, 208, 1967.

283. Saag, M. S. and Desmukes, W. E., Azole antifungal agents: emphasis on new triazoles, *Antimicrob. Agents Chemother.*, 32, 1, 1988.

284. Daneshmend, T. K., Warnock, D. W., Turner, A., and Roberts, C. J. C., Pharmacokinetics of ketoconazole in normal subjects, *J. Antimicrob. Chemother.*, 8, 299, 1981.

285. Pont, A., Graybill, J. R., Craven, P. C., Galgiani, J. N., Dismukes, W. E., Reitz, R. E., and Stevens, D. A., High-dose ketoconazole therapy and adrenal and testicular function in humans, *Arch. Intern. Med.*, 144, 2150, 1984.

286. Georgiev, V. St., Treatment and developmental therapeutics in aspergillosis. II. Azoles and other antifungal drugs, *Respiration*, 59, 303, 1992.

287. Georgiev, V. St., Opportunistic/nosocomial infections: treatment and developmental therapeutics. II. Cryptococcosis, *Med. Res. Rev.*, 13, 507, 1993.

288. Pappas, P. G., Kauffman, C. A., Perfect, J., Johnson, P. C., Mckinsey, D. S., Bamberger, D. M., Hamill, R., Sharkey, P. K., Chapman, S. W., and Sobel, J. D., Alopecia associated with fluconazole therapy, *Ann. Intern. Med.*, 123, 354, 1995 (see comment in *Ann. Intern. Med.*, 125, 153, 1996).

289. Lewis, J. H., Zimmerman, H. J., Benson, G. D., and Ishak, K. G., Hepatic injury associated with ketoconazole therapy, *Gastroenterology*, 86, 503, 1984.

290. Yancey, R. W., Jr., Perlino, C. A., and Kaufman, L., Asymptomatic blastomycosis of the central nervous system with progression in patients given ketoconazole therapy: a report of two cases, *J. Infect. Dis.*, 164, 807, 1991.

291. Turner, S., Kaufman, L., and Jalbert, M., Diagnostic assessment of an enzyme-linked immunosorbent assay for human and canine blastomycosis, *J. Clin. Microbiol.*, 23, 294, 1986.

292. Kahan, B. D., Cyclosporine nephrotoxicity: pathogenesis, prophylaxis, therapy and prognosis, *Am. J. Kidney Dis.*, 8, 323, 1986.

293. Nouira, R., Denguezli, M., Skhiri, S., Belajouzac, C., Ben Said, M., Jarray, M., and Jamaa, B., Cutaneopulmonary blastomycosis, *Ann. Dermatol. Venereol.*, 121, 180, 1994.

294. Thiele, J. S., Bueckner, H. A., and Cook, E. W., Failure of ketoconazole in two patients with blastomycosis, *Am. Rev. Respir. Dis.*, 128, 763, 1983.

295. Serneels, R. A., Marshall, G. S., Wampler, J., Miller, D., and Adams, G., Pulmonary sequestration with primary blastomycosis: failure of ketoconazole therapy after resection, *Chest*, 103, 1291, 1993.

296. Abadie-Kemmerly, S., Pankey, G. A., and Dalvisio, J. R., Failure of ketoconazole treatment of *Blastomyces dermatitidis* due to interaction of isoniazid and rifampin, *Ann. Intern. Med.*, 106, 844, 1988.

297. Zuckerman, J. M. and Tunkel, A. R., Itraconazole: a new triazole antifungal agent, *Infect. Control Hosp. Epidemiol.*, 15, 397, 1994.

298. Jordaan, H. F., Blastomycosis in Namibia — report of a case successfully treated with itraconazole, *Clin. Exp. Dermatol.*, 14, 347, 1989.

299. Dismukes, W. E., Bradsher, R. W., Cloud, G. C., Kauffman, C. A., Chapman, S. W., George, R. B., Stevens, D. A., Girard, W. M., Saag, M. S., Bowles-Patton, C., and the NIAID Mycoses Study Group, Itraconazole therapy for blastomycosis and histoplasmosis, *Am. J. Med.*, 93, 489, 1992.

300. Van Cauteren, H. J., Heykants, J., De Coster, R., and Cauwenbergh, G., Itraconazole: pharmacologic studies in animals and humans, *Rev. Infect. Dis.*, 9(Suppl.), 43, 1987.

301. Kauffman, C. A., Newer developments in therapy for endemic mycosis, *Clin. Infect. Dis.*, 19(Suppl. 1), S28, 1994.

302. Neijens, H. J., Frenkel, J., de Muinck Keiser-Schrama, S. M. P. F., Dzoljic-Danilovic, G., Meradji, M., and Dongen, J. J. M., Invasive aspergillus infection in chronic granulomatous disease: treatment with itraconazole, *J. Pediatr.*, 115, 1016, 1989.

303. Bhandari, V. and Narang, A., Oral itraconazole therapy for disseminated candidiasis in low birth weight infants, *J. Pediatr.*, 120, 330, 1992.

304. Mony, R., Veber, F., Blanche, S., Donadieu, J., Brauner, R., Levron, J.-C., Griscelli, C., and Fischer, S., Long-term itraconazole prophylaxis against aspergillus infections in thirty-two patients with chronic granulomatous disease, *J. Pediatr.*, 125, 998, 1994.

305. Schutze, G. E., Hickerson, S. L., Fortin, E. M., Schellhase, D. E., Darville, T., Gubbins, P. O., and Jacobs, R. F., Blastomycosis in children, *Clin. Infect. Dis.*, 22, 496, 1996.

306. Dismukes, W. E., Azole antifungal drugs: old and new, *Ann. Intern. Med.*, 109, 177, 1988.

307. Bayles, M. A., Tropical mycoses, *Chemotherapy*, 38(Suppl. 1), 27, 1992.

308. Pearson, G. J., Chin, T. W., and Fong, I. W., Case report: treatment of blastomycosis with fluconazole, *Am. J. Med. Sci.*, 303, 313, 1992.

309. Taillan, B., Ferrari, E., Cosnefroy, J. Y., Gari-Toussaint, M., Michiels, J. F., Paquis, P., Lefichoux, Y., and Dujardin, P., Blastomycosis localized in the brain stem, *Presse Med.*, 21, 207, 1992.

310. Taillan, B., Ferrari, E., Cosnefroy, J. Y., Gari-Toussaint, M., Michiels, J. F., Paquis, P., Lefichoux, Y., and Dujardin, P., Favourable outcome of blastomycosis of the brain stem with fluconazole and flucytosine treatment, *Ann. Med. Interne (Paris)*, 24, 71, 1992.

311. Pappas, P. G., Bradsher, R. W., Chapman, S. W., Kauffman, C. A., Dine, A., Cloud, G. A., Dismukes, W. E., and the NIAID Mycoses Study Group, Treatment of blastomycosis with fluconazole: a pilot study, *Clin. Infect. Dis.*, 20, 267, 1995.

312. Craft, P. P., A case report of disseminated blastomycosis and adult respiratory distress syndrome, *J. Family Pract.*, 40, 597, 1995.

313. Recht, L. D., Davies, S. F., Eckman, M. R., and Sarosi, G. A., Blastomycosis in immunosuppressed patients, *Am. Rev. Respir. Dis.*, 125, 359, 1982.

314. Atkinson, J. B. and Curley, T. L., Pulmonary blastomycosis: filamentous forms in an immuno-compromised patient with fulminating respiratory failure, *Hum. Pathol.*, 14, 186, 1983.

315. Griffith, J. E. and Campbell, G. D., Acute miliary blastomycosis presenting as fulminating respiratory failure, *Chest*, 75, 630, 1979.

316. Lockridge, R. S. and Glauser, F. L., Adult respiratory distress syndrome secondary to diffuse pulmonary blastomycosis, *South. Med. J.*, 72, 23, 1979.

317. Palmer, P. E. and McFadden, S. W., Blastomycosis, *N. Engl. J. Med.*, 279, 979, 1968.

318. Onal, E., Lopata, M., and Lourenco, R. V., Disseminated pulmonary blastomycosis in an immuno-suppressed patient, *Am. Rev. Respir. Dis.*, 113, 83, 1976.

319. Arvanitakis, C., Sen, S. K., and Magnin, G. E., Fulminating fatal pneumonia due to blastomycosis, *Am. Rev. Respir. Dis.*, 105, 827, 1972.

320. Meyer, K. C., McManus, E. J., and Maki, D. G., Overwhelming pulmonary blastomycosis associated with the adult respiratory distress syndrome, *N. Engl. J. Med.*, 329, 1231, 1993.

321. Renston, J. P., Morgan, J., and Dimarco, A. F., Disseminated miliary blastomycosis leading to acute respiratory failure in an urban setting, *Chest*, 101, 1463, 1992.

322. Meduri, G. U., Belenchia, J. M., Estes, R. J., Wunderink, R. G., El Torky, M., and Leeper, K. V., Jr., Fibroproliferative phase of ARDS: clinical findings and effects of corticosteroids, *Chest*, 4, 943, 1991.

323. Bone, R. C., Fisher, C. J., Jr., Clemmer, T. P., Slotman, G. J., and Metz, C. A., Early methylprednisolone treatment for septic syndrome and the adult respiratory distress syndrome, *Chest*, 92, 1032, 1987.

324. Bernard, G. R., Luce, J. M., Sprung, C. L., Rinaldo, J. E., Tate, R. M., Sibbald, W. J., Kariman, K., Higgins, S., Bradley, R., Metz, C. A., Harris, T. R., and Brigham, K., High-dose corticosteroids in patients with the adult respiratory distress syndrome, *N. Engl. J. Med.*, 317, 1565, 1987.

325. Weigelt, J. A., Norcross, J. F., Broman, K. R., and Snyder, W. H., Early steroid therapy for respiratory failure, *Arch. Surg.*, 120, 536, 1985.

326. Veterans Administration Systemic Sepsis Cooperative Study Group, Effect of high-dose glucocorticoid therapy on mortality in patients with clinical signs of systemic sepsis, *N. Engl. J. Med.*, 317, 659, 1987.

327. Luce, J. M., Montgomery, A. B., Marks, J. D., Turner, J., Metz, C. A., and Murray, J. F., Ineffectiveness of high-dose methylprednisolone in preventing parenchymal lung injury and improving mortality in patients with septic shock, *Am. Rev. Respir. Dis.*, 138, 62, 1988.

328. Mittermayer, C. H., Hassenstein, J., and Riede, U. N., Is shock-induced lung fibrosis reversible? A report on recovery from "Shock-lung", *Pathol. Res. Pract.*, 162, 73, 1978.

329. Passamonte, P. M., Martinez, A. J., and Singh, A., Pulmonary gallium concentration in the adult respiratory distress syndrome, *Chest*, 85, 828, 1984.

330. Ashbaugh, D. G. and Maier, R. V., Idiopathic pulmonary fibrosis in adult respiratory distress syndrome, *Arch. Surg.*, 120, 530, 1985.

331. Hooper, R. G. and Kearl, R. A., Established ARDS treated with a sustained course of adrenocortical steroids, *Chest*, 97, 138, 1990.

332. Hooper, R. G. and Kearl, R. A., Treatment of established ARDS — steroids, antibiotics, and antifungal therapy, *Chest*, 100, 137S, 1991.

333. Suter, P. M., ARDS treated with sustained adrenocortical steroids, *Chest*, 98, 1310, 1990.

334. Ho, S. L., Lewis, G. A., and Young, D. W., Recovery from adult respiratory distress syndrome after high dose corticosteroids, *Intensive Care Med.*, 17, 241, 1991.

335. Meduri, G. U. and Chinn, A., Fibroproliferation in late adult respiratory distress syndrome: pathophysiology, clinical and laboratory manifestations, and response to corticosteroid rescue treatment, *Chest*, 105(Suppl.), 127S, 1994.

336. Meduri, G. U., Chinn, A. J., Leeper, K. V., Wunderink, R. G., Tolley, E., Winer-Muram, H. T., Khare, V., and El Torky, M., Corticosteroid rescue treatment of progressive fibroproliferation in late ARDS: patterns of response and predictors of outcome, *Chest*, 105, 1516, 1994.

37.6 *ASPERGILLUS* SPP.

37.6.1 INTRODUCTION

Aspergillosis may develop as a granulomatous, necrotizing, and cavitary disease that frequently affects the lungs, but may also disseminate to other organs as well.[1] The causative agents of the disease are fungi belonging to the genus *Aspergillus*. In 1856, Virchow, and then in 1897, Renon[2] were the first to describe several identifiable cases of aspergillosis in humans, related to occupational exposure. While aspergillosis is more frequent in older people, it may occur in other age groups as well, including childhood.[3] In addition to *A. fumigatus*, *A. flavus*,[4-14] *A. niger*,[4,15-18] *A. glaucus*,[19] *A. nidulans*,[4,19] *A. versicolor*,[8] *A. terreus*,[20-24] *A. candidus*,[24,25] *A. chevalieri*,[26] and *A. ustus*[27] have also been identified as causative agents of human aspergillosis. Yamamoto et al.[6] have reported a case of allergic bronchopulmonary aspergillosis (ABPA) caused by *A. fumigatus*, in which the patient during antifungal therapy with fluconazole developed infection with *A. flavus*.

Although the majority of *Aspergillus* spp. are exosaprophitic, some are known to invade tissues of both animals and humans, with the most common pathogen being *A. fumigatus*.[28-30] The latter, when grown on glucose-neopeptone agar rapidly produces white colonies that quickly change to gray-green color with formation of conidia. The conidiophores are 2 to 8 μm wide, reaching in length between 300 and 500 μm and expanding at the top into a dome-shaped vesicle 20 to 30 μm in diameter. Phialides, which are borne only on the upper half or two third of the vesicle, produce spores directly without secondary phialides.[1] In lung tissues, *A. fumigatus* grows in the form of richly branched and often dichotomous hyphae. Although the fungus generates endotoxins, the latter are not considered important for the pathology of the disease.

The adhesion of *A. fumigatus* to the extracellular matrix protein laminin has been demonstrated.[31-33] To this end, Tronchin et al.[31] have investigated the expression of laminin-binding receptors during swelling of *A. fumigatus* conidia, a step leading to germination and subsequent colonization of tissues. Scanning electron microscopy revealed the presence of high levels of laminin-binding receptors distributed over the external rodlet layer of the resting conidia. Analysis by sodium dodecyl sulfate-polyacrylamide gel electrophoresis (SDS-PAGE) and ligand blotting with laminin identified in a cell wall extract a major 72-kDa cell wall surface glycoprotein which recognized and bound to basement membrane laminin.[31] In a separate study, Gil et al.[33] identified one 37-kDa polypeptide which specifically interacted with laminin.

Data by DeHart et al.[34] suggested that an early event following inhalation of *A. fumigatus* conidia may be its binding to pneumocytes, followed by hyphal penetration of the epithelial cell layer. In a related study, Bromley and Donaldson[32] have used A549 pulmonary epithelial cells and purified basement membrane proteins to investigate the ability of *A. fumigatus* spores to bind to pulmonary cells and basement membrane proteins in the asthmatic lung, and the mechanisms involved in this susceptibility. Spores bound specifically to extracellular matrix components laid down by the A549 cells, and pretreatment of the extracellular matrix proteins with H_2O_2 (25 to 80 μM) enhanced spore binding by approximately one third. They also bound specifically and in a saturable manner to purified fibrinogen, fibronectin, laminin, type I and type IV collagens.[32,33] Furthermore, preinculation of spores with Arg-Gly-Asp tripeptide (RGD; 50 to 200 μg/ml) inhibited binding to fibronectin and type I collagen by 50%. The results of the study suggested that the presence of activated epithelial cells and the exposure of basement membrane that occurs in asthma, together with oxidant stress, may facilitate the colonization of the asthmatic lung by *A. fumigatus*, and that the RGD sequence may be involved in spore binding to some of the host cell extracellular matrix proteins.[32,33]

Sutton et al.[35] have found that pretreatment of normally resistant mice with a single injection of a sublethal dose of gliotoxin, an immunosuppressive fungal metabolite produced by the majority of strains of *A. fumigatus* exacerbated significantly the pathogenesis of invasive aspergillosis. Animals infected with a non-gliotoxin producing strain survived substantially longer than those infected with a gliotoxin-producing strain.[35]

In immunocompetent hosts the *Aspergillus* infection usually results in the development of allergic conditions such as asthma or ABPA. In general, normal hosts will rarely develop invasive aspergillosis.[36-38] The latter is, however, the primary manifestation in immunocompromised patients. Major predisposing factors include prolonged neutropenia,[39] bone marrow and solid organ transplantation[21,40-56] (lung recipients in particular[57-61]), chronic administration of adrenal corticosteroids, the insertion of prosthetic devices, indwelling catheters,[62] and tissue damage due to prior infection or trauma. Invasive aspergillosis is also becoming an increasingly reported complication in AIDS patients.[63-67] There have also been reports of invasive aspergillosis in patients in intensive care units,[68,69] in particular those with chronic respiratory failure.[70]

The most common way of infection is through the respiratory tract, resulting in pneumonia followed by sinusitis. However, the pathogen may penetrate across all natural barriers, including cartilage, bone, and the blood vessels where it may cause thrombosis and infarction.[71] *Aspergillus* spores may proliferate extensively in hospital ventilation systems[71] — airborne *Aspergillus* spp. related to air filter change was associated with fatal invasive aspergillosis in two mechanically ventilated patients.[72]

Pulmonary aspergillosis may express itself in several forms,[73] including (1) invasive pulmonary aspergillosis; (2) allergic bronchopulmonary aspergillosis (ABPA); (3) extrinsic alveolitis; and (4) saprophitic aspergillosis.

The first form, invasive pulmonary aspergillosis (IPA),[74] which has been closely (but not always) associated with immunocompromised hosts,[75] is produced by a direct invasion of *A. fumigatus* into the pulmonary parenchyma and vasculature causing necrotizing pulmonary vasculitis with hemorrhagic infarction.[76] In severe cases, formation of cavities and mycetomas may also take place.[77] The chronic necrotizing pulmonary aspergillosis, an indolent clinical variant of the invasive form, which has also been seen in immunocompromised hosts, resembles chronic pulmonary tuberculosis.[77]

While IPA has also been documented in immunocompetent hosts,[78-81] the vast majority of cases occur in immunocompromised patients, especially those with hematologic malignancies,[82-88] organ transplant recipients[68,89,90] and patients in advanced stages of acquired immune deficiency syndrome (AIDS).[91] Such predisposing factors as short-term[92] or high-dose steroid therapy, cytotoxic chemotherapy, and leukopenia associated with marrow-ablative chemotherapy or myelophthisic marrow replacement may significantly increase the incidence of infection.[82,93] With regard to corticosteroid chemotherapy, it is thought that steroids inhibit the fusion of lysosomal membranes of type II pneumophagocytes with the spores of *Aspergillus* after ingestion, thereby allowing for intracellular *Aspergillus* germination.[76] High doses of inhalation corticosteroids may also be involved in suppressing the T cell response locally.[94] In 10% to 25% of patients with IPA, extrapulmonary dissemination was found at autopsy[82,83] — the organs most often affected were the gastrointestinal tract, heart, liver, spleen, kidney, and the thyroid.

Semi-invasive pulmonary aspergillosis is also an identifiable entity. It is characterized by a slowly progressive course, with impairment of local pulmonary defense mechanisms and/or a mild systemic immunosuppression.[95]

Allergic bronchopulmonary aspergillosis (ABPA) is considered to be the clinical manifestation of a variety of immunologic reactions relevant to the presence of fungus in the bronchial tree.[77,96] The course of disease may be either spontaneous[97] or chronic. In its chronic form, ABPA may cause bronchiectasis,[78] which in turn, may result in the development of aspergilloma.[98,99] First described by Hinson et al.,[100] ABPA is characterized mainly by bronchospasms, pulmonary infiltrates, eosinophilia, and immunologic evidence of allergy (precipitating serum antibodies and elevation of serum IgE levels) to *Aspergillus* spp. antigen.[98] Egan et al.[101] have reported the first cases of ABPA (associated with systemic eosinophilia) in lung allograft recipients, whereas Meyer and Kirsten[102] have diagnosed ABPA during a life-threatening asthma exacerbation. Nosocomial outbreaks of ABPA, which have been linked to elevated spore counts in ventilation systems[103] or associated with hospital reconstruction,[104] have also been reported.

The basic underlying pathologic process in ABPA is a hypersensitivity reaction toward the presence of fungus in the bronchial tree since tissue invasion by the pathogen is not thought to occur.[98] ABPA is estimated to occur in 1% to 2% of patients with asthma involving hypersensitivity to *Aspergillus* species.[105] It appears that both type I (immediate) and type III (antigen-antibody, immune complexes) hypersensitivity reactions have been involved in the pathophysiologic mechanism of ABPA leading to chronic lung changes such as fibrosis, bronchiectasis, lung contraction, and lobar shrinkage.[98] A potential role for type IV cell-mediated (delayed) hypersensitivity reaction was also suggested. *In vitro* lymphocyte transformation to *Aspergillus* antigen in patients with ABPA has been demonstrated,[106] and the presence of parenchymal granulomata and mononuclear cellular infiltration have been seen in lung histopathology.[107] In addition, alternate pathway complement activation may also be involved in the inflammatory response to ABPA.[108]

ABPA is a serious complication in patients with cystic fibrosis and may be difficult to diagnose.[109] Merchant et al.[110] have used the fourfold rise in total IgE (particularly over 500 IU/ml) as a strong indicator of ABPA in children with cystic fibrosis.

Although all of the forms of pulmonary aspergillosis are characterized by specific clinical, radiologic, and pathologic manifestations, it may be common in a disease state that one form may overlap with another condition, such as mucoid impaction, eosinophilic pneumonia, bronchocentric granulomatosis, "farmer's lung," and asthma.[111] Moreover, more than one form of the disease may be manifested at the same time (for example, IPA complicating ABPA).[112,113] To further complicate matters, a limited invasion may take place and be viewed as a noninvasive form of aspergillosis. After consideration of all of the existing possibilities, the compartmentalization of the different types of pulmonary aspergillosis into one exclusive form of the disease may indeed be complex and very difficult to accomplish.

Bronchial stump aspergillosis (BSA), an *Aspergillus* infection of bronchial granulation tissue surrounding endobronchial suture threads, is a very rare variant of localized suppurative bronchial aspergillosis.[114]

Although the lungs are the major portal of entry, invasion by *Aspergillus* may also occur through the paranasal sinuses, nose, palate, gastrointestinal tract, or skin.[115,116] Furthermore, the hematogenous spread shows no marked tissue tropism, and many different viscera (brain, kidneys, liver, thyroid, heart, intestines, esophagus, stomach, larynx) may have lesions.[82,117,118] In the immunocompromised patients, lesions contain hyphae within the blood vessels producing infarction, edema, and hemorrhage.[115] Infection may also spread by contiguity. *Aspergillus*-associated osteomyelitis, although rare, has also been described,[12] with the spine being most often affected;[8,119] it can be induced hematogenously, by contiguity, or by direct inoculation.[119]

Mazzoni et al.[120] have described a case of apparently primary lymph node granulomatous aspergillosis. A survey of cases of primary aspergillosis has shown that granulomatous instead of exudative inflammation patterns have been observed in histologic sections only when neither major nor minor predisposing factors have been detected in the clinical history of the patients.[120]

Cases describing *A. fumigatus* pneumonia in patients with systemic lupus erythematosus (an autoimmune disorder that has seldom been associated with *Aspergillus* infections[121]) have also been reported.[121-123] In one such case, Nenoff et al.[122] have described a patient with systemic lupus erythematosus who had been treated by antibiotics and high-dose corticosteroids (a primary risk factor), and developed a fatal peracute disseminated *A. fumigatus* disease involving the central nervous system. The typical clinical presentation has been fever and cough in patients with systemic lupus erythematosus and invasive aspergillosis previously treated with corticosteroids, immunosuppressive drugs, and broad-spectrum antibiotics.[121]

Aspergillus peritonitis may also become a complication of continuous ambulatory peritoneal dialysis (CAPD).[124-126] In another case of infection involving an indwelling device, Girmenia et al.[127] described intravenous catheter-related cutaneous aspergillosis and *A. fumigatus* fungemia in an HIV-positive patient with Burkitt-cell acute lymphocytic leukemia who developed pulmonary aspergillosis with a rapidly fatal outcome despite recovery from neutropenia and improvement of the underlying malignancy. The unusual severity and rapid spread of the infection, despite normal neutrophil count and prompt antifungal therapy, underscored the risk of catheter-related cutaneous aspergillosis leading to severe deep-seated infection in immunocompromised patients.[127]

It is important to note that aspergillosis and mucormycosis,[128,129] two types of opportunistic fungal pneumonia, may often be clumped together because of their frequent occurrence in patients with leukemia and lymphoma and because they often invade vascular structures.[130] However, a number of characteristic radiographic abnormalities should facilitate an appropriate diagnosis and therapy.[130]

Tuberculosis is thought to be often associated with aspergillosis.[131,132] Furthermore, patients having chronic fibrosing pulmonary sarcoidosis would frequently develop cystic degeneration of the upper lobes as manifested by cysts and cavities.[133] Such preexisting parenchymal cavities are frequently the targets of *Aspergillus* colonization and proliferation resulting in formation of pulmonary aspergilloma.[134] Fatal hemorrhage from such aspergillomas is considered to be the second most common cause of death in sarcoidosis.[133,135]

A. niger is one of several fungi implicated in otomycosis, a condition manifested by ear irritation, pruritis, and impairment of hearing.[1] The pathogen may invade the ear canal following another infection such as facial dermatophytosis.[1]

It is not unusual for patients with *Aspergillus*-induced infections to remain asymptomatic with regard to lesion formation.[77] The most common symptom is hemoptysis which has been observed in 50% to 85% of the patients.[136] While the presence of precipitating antibodies to *Aspergillus* in the serum is found in virtually all immunocompetent patients,[137] in those with immune abnormalities, the presence of such antibodies may be an exception.[77] Therefore, chest roentgenograms should remain the single most important method of diagnosing pulmonary aspergillosis.

37.6.2 HOST IMMUNE RESPONSE TO ASPERGILLOSIS

Quantitative and qualitative defects in phagocytic activity render patients particularly susceptible to aspergillosis.[82,138-145] The major host defenses against *Aspergillus* spp. are the pulmonary alveolar macrophages and peripheral blood polymorphonuclear and mononuclear phagocytes.[146] Macrophages have been shown to make up the first line of defense by ingesting and exterminating inhaled conidia of *Aspergillus*, thereby preventing their germination to hyphae.[147-149] If fungal hyphae are produced, then the second line of defense, the circulating phagocytes, will damage and destroy hyphae by secreting microbicidal oxidative and nonoxidative metabolites.[147,149,150] The role of various cytokines on the phagocytic host defense against *Aspergillus* has only recently begun to be defined.[151-156]

The role of cytokine production by CD4[+] T helper cells and the effects of cytokine administration or neutralization on the course and outcome of aspergillosis have been investigated in a murine model of invasive disease.[157] Patterns of susceptibilities and resistance to infection were obtained with different strains of mice injected with different inocula of *A. fumigatus* conidia. The results have shown that mice that survived the primary infection also resisted a subsequent lethal infection which was associated with production of interferon-γ (IFN-γ) by CD4[+] T splenocytes. Furthermore, impaired neutrophil antifungal activity, observed in susceptible mice, was concomitant with a predominant production of IL-4 by CD4[+] splenocytes. In these mice, exogenous administration of IL-12 failed to induce any resistance to infection; to the contrary, treatment with soluble IL-4 receptor cured over 70% of the mice from primary infection and resulted in the onset of acquired resistance to a subsequent lethal infection. Taken together, these findings indicated that in murine invasive aspergillosis, production of IL-4 by the CD4[+] T cells may be one major factor discerning susceptibility and resistance to infection.[157]

Roilides et al.[138] have examined the effects of human IL-10 on the antifungal activity of monocytes from healthy adult subjects against *A. fumigatus* after incubation with IL-10 (2 to 20 ng/ml) at 37°C for 2 to 4 d. The pretreated monocytes exerted approximately 40% suppression of superoxide anion (O^{2-}) production in response to FMLP (a synthetic tripeptide) ($p < .003$). Furthermore, IL-10 (20 ng/ml)-pretreated monocytes exhibited 55% to 98% decrease of damage by *Aspergillus* hyphae after 2 to 4 d of exposure ($p < .04$). Overall, the IL-10 suppressed the oxidative burst and antifungal activity of monocytes against *A. fumigatus* hyphae, but increased their phagocytic activity, suggesting a potential role for IL-10 in the pathogenesis of invasive aspergillosis.

In the context of host immune defense against *Aspergillus* infections, Hamilton et al.[158] have studied the expression of Cu,Zn superoxide dismutase (SOD) by the fungus using a polyclonal antibody against the purified enzyme. Immunoelectron microscopy confirmed that the SOD was present within the hyphal cell wall, although there was also labeling in the cytoplasm. Evidence was presented that SOD may protect *Aspergillus* against oxidants produced by the host's immune effector cells and that the enzyme is available to perform its antioxidant function within the cell wall.[158]

Slight et al.[159] have isolated and partially characterized a small (<10 kDa) protein produced by *A. fumigatus* that was capable of inhibiting the macrophage respiratory burst and allowing the fungus to colonize the lung. The protein, a heat-stable toxin which is released from the surface of fungal spores, suppressed the release of superoxide anion by inhibiting the assembly of the macrophage NADPH-oxidase complex. Furthermore, fractions of the <10-kDa toxin also inhibited the spreading of alveolar macrophages, confirming an additional effect on macrophages that led to loss of adherence or impairment of cytoskeletal function. Overall, by its ability to diffuse rapidly into the lung lining fluid and diminish the macrophage respiratory burst, the surface toxin may be an important factor in the pathogenesis of aspergillosis.

Studying another aspect of host immune defense against aspergillosis, Overdijk et al.[160] have demonstrated the presence of chitinase activity in human serum and postulated about the possible role that mammalian chitinases may play as a defense mechanism against chitin-containing pathogens. Using a guinea pig model, these investigators have shown that upon infection with *A. fumigatus*, the serum chitinase activity levels in the circulation of pathogen-free guinea pig increased in a size-of-inoculum- and time-dependent manner. Antifungal therapy diminished the increase in chitinase activity, which was of guinea pig origin. The activity of three other enzymes of lysosomal origin (α-mannosidase, β-galactosidase, and β-glycosidase) did not increase.[160]

37.6.3 Studies on Therapeutics

37.6.3.1 Amphotericin B

The polyene antibiotic amphotericin B, when applied *in vitro*, completely inhibited the growth of *A. fumigatus* at a concentration of 0.5 µg/ml.[161] It suppressed both the exogenous and endogenous respiration and glycolysis of the fungus, as well as the assimilation of various intermediates from the glycolysis and tricarboxylic acid cycles. The minimum inhibitory concentration (MIC) value of amphotericin B against *A. fumigatus* was 0.81 µg/ml as reported by Redig and Duke.[162]

In four avian species the pharmacokinetics of amphotericin B against 11 isolates of *A. fumigatus* were studied following oral, intravenous, and intrathecal administrations.[162] It was found that inhibitory concentrations of the drug were observed only 2 and 6 h postadministration in birds receiving three doses of 1.5 mg/kg at 2-h intervals. In humans, however, the pharmacokinetics of amphotericin B are still not very well understood.[93]

Amphotericin B (1.5 mg/kg daily, IV) was found superior to fluconazole (60 mg/kg twice daily) in immunosuppressed, temporarily leukopenic rabbits with invasive aspergillosis. Both drugs, however, decreased or eliminated circulating *Aspergillus* antigen and improved the survival rate.[163]

37.6.3.1.1   Liposome-encapsulated amphothericin B

Liposome-encapsulated amphotericin B has shown reduced kidney toxicity and has been used successfully in treating aspergillosis.[164] Ahmad et al.[165,166] have developed a model system for aspergillosis in BALB/c mice to evaluate the therapeutic efficacy of amphotericin B. The antibiotic was most effective when intercalated into liposomes comprised of egg phosphatidyl-choline, phosphatidylethanolamine, and cholesterol in a molar ratio of 6:1:3. Compared to other formulations, amphotericin B when intercalated into mannose-grafted liposomes, was more effective.[167] Weber and Lopez-Berestein[168] described amphotericin B incorporated into multi-lamellar vesicles consisting of dimyristoyl phosphatidylcholine and dimyristoyl phosphatidyl-glycerol in a 7:3 ratio.

A pharmacokinetically distinctive unilamelar vesicle formulation of liposomal amphotericin B (5.0 mg/kg daily, IV) was compared with high-dose conventional amphotericin B desoxycholate (1.0 mg/kg, IV) in a model of pulmonary aspergillosis in persistently granulocytopenic rabbits.[169] The liposomal formulation was more effective in preventing nephrotoxicity, increasing survival, reducing the number of viable organisms, and decreasing tissue injury due to *Aspergillus*.

The efficacy of AmBisome® (a liposome-encapsulated amphotericin B) when compared with that of Fungizone® (amphotericin B deoxycholate; see below) in a rat model of unilateral, pulmonary aspergillosis, has shown the liposomal formulation to be more effective in reducing dissemination even when given in relatively low dosage.[170]

The prophylactic use of AmBisome was compared with the nonliposomal amphotericin B (Fungizone) in a murine model of pulmonary aspergillosis.[171] While both formulations prolonged survival of mice, AmBisome was conclusively superior to Fungizone in clearing the pathogen from the lungs (80% and 0%, respectively) of mice challenged with 10^7 A. *fumigatus* spores.

Encapsulation of amphotericin B in tuftsin-bearing liposomes greatly increased its efficacy in treatment of murine aspergillosis.[172] Furthermore, the efficacy of amphotericin B was markedly increased by pretreating the animals with drug-free tuftsin-bearing liposomes. The results of the study have indicated that macrophage activation can substantially enhance the therapeutic efficacy of the antibiotic.

37.6.3.1.2 Lipid-based amphotericin B complexes

An immunosuppressed rabbit model of invasive aspergillosis was used to evaluate a novel micellar preparation of deoxycholate and cholesterol sulfate complexed to amphotericin B.[173] The acute LD_{50} values of amphotericin B–deoxycholate and amphotericin B–cholesterol sulfate complexes were 5.1 and 20 mg/kg, respectively. Further comparison of these complexes showed that amphotericin B–deoxycholate when injected intravenously at 1.5 mg/kg was more effective in sterilizing the liver and kidney than the amphotericin B–cholesterol sulfate complex at 1.5 to 4.5 mg/kg, IV; however, infection persisted in the lungs of all rabbits treated at these dose regimens. Overall, although less potent than amphotericin B–deoxycholate, the amphotericin B–cholesterol sulfate complex, nevertheless, showed a fourfold decrease in acute lethality that improved significantly the therapeutic index of amphotericin B.[173]

The therapeutic efficacy and safety of amphotericin B colloidal dispersion (1.0, 5.0, and 10 mg/kg daily) for the treatment of invasive pulmonary aspergillosis in persistently granulocytopenic rabbits has also been investigated.[174] The treatment consisted of intravenous administration of either the colloidal dispersion or a conventional desoxycholate formulation of amphotericin B (1.0 mg/kg daily). Only the 5.0- and 10-mg/kg doses proved to be of therapeutic value as evidenced by the significant reduction in the tissue burden of A. *fumigatus* (colony-sorting units per gram of tissue). As determined by survival rates, the 5.0-mg/kg dose of colloidal dispersion was more effective than amphotericin B desoxycholate and the 10-mg/kg dose (which also happened to be more nephrotoxic).[174]

37.6.3.1.3 Combinations of amphotericin B with other antifungal agents

Combinations of amphotericin B and itraconazole were administered to mice with experimental aspergillosis in a variety of ratios;[175] the combinations were found to be mostly indifferent.

Schaffner and Frick[176] have studied the effect of a combined treatment of amphotericin B and ketoconazole in a model of disseminated aspergillosis. The neutropenic mice were challenged intravenously with a lethal dose of conidia from two strains of A. *fumigatus*. Results from the study indicated the presence of antagonistic effect of ketoconazole on the activity of amphotericin B; for example, pretreatment with ketoconazole for 48 h completely abolished the protective effect of subsequent therapy with amphotericin B whether ketoconazole therapy was stopped or not. Ketoconazole when given alone had no effect on the survival rate.[176] These findings would make prophylaxis with ketoconazole prior to amphotericin B therapy highly undesirable, especially for patients at high risk of developing invasive opportunistic fungal infections.

Synergistic activity of amphotericin B and rifampin was found both *in vitro* and *in vivo*. Often rifampin (at an approximately 600 mg daily dose) is added to amphotericin B in the treatment of adult patients; however, there are no controlled clinical data to corroborate the beneficial effect of rifampin.[177] Various combinations of amphotericin B and tetracycline antibiotics (tetracycline, doxycycline, minocycline) have been studied for activity against A. *fumigatus*.[178] Synergistic activity of amphotericin B and minocycline was observed in each of five isolates; time-kill curves showed eradication of A. *fumigatus* at concentrations of amphotericin B that were four- to eightfold lower in the presence of 5 or 15 µg/ml of minocycline than with amphotericin B alone.[178]

37.6.3.2   Amphotericin B Esters

Ungerminated conidia of *A. fumigatus* were insensitive to amphotericin B methyl ester at concentrations of over 50 µg/ml, but rapidly became sensitive to 1.0–2.0 µg/ml of the drug during the initial stages of germination.[179]

Both amphotericin B and compound SCH 28191 (the D-ornithyl-methyl ester of amphotericin B) showed similar *in vitro* activity against *A. fumigatus* isolate.[180] In a model of experimental murine aspergillosis, the two drugs exhibited similar potency in prolonging the survival rate after intravenous challenge with conidia of *A. fumigatus* when administered 24 h after the challenge, or when treatment was delayed until mice were moribund.[180] Overall, SCH 28191 appeared to be as effective as amphotericin B in the therapy of murine aspergillosis.

37.6.3.3   Miscellaneous Antibiotics

37.6.3.3.1   Polyene antibiotics

Nystatin, hamycin, natamycin, and ambruticin are all naturally occurring antibiotics that have been scrutinized for activity against *Aspergillus*-induced infections. The published reports have been limited in scope and mostly describe preclinical experiments, in addition to treatment of a few individual cases of aspergillosis. Therefore, the knowledge about their therapeutic efficacy remains uncertain and very much confined within the development stage.[181]

In vitro experiments have demonstrated that the susceptibility of *Aspergillus* strains to nystatin was less pronounced when compared to *Candida* strains.[182] Nevertheless, at a concentration of 100 µg/ml, nystatin completely abolished the growth of three isolates of *Aspergillus*.[183] When tested *in vivo*, nystatin was found active in chickens infected with *A. fumigatus* after administration of aerosol, but inactive when mixed in feed or drinking water.[184] However, earlier reports indicated that nystatin was effective in treatment of pulmonary aspergillosis when applied both orally[185] and as aerosol.[186]

Vedder and Schorr[187] have reported a reversal and clearing of infection following oral and aerosol nystatin therapy to a child with extensive pulmonary aspergillosis with multiple metastatic skin lesions. Inhalation therapy of bronchopulmonary aspergillosis comprising nystatin, brilliant green, and natamycin has been also described.[188] Gemeinhardt and Schuttmann[189,190] and Krakowka et al.[191] have managed successful treatment of pulmonary aspergillosis with nystatin.

Two other polyene antibiotics, natamycin (by inhalation or intrabronchial instillation)[192] and hamycin (by oral administration),[193] were used in the therapy of bronchopulmonary aspergillosis.

Hamycin, when incorporated into liposomes containing phosphatidylcholine and phosphatidic acid, showed reduced toxicity and enhanced antifungal activity in experimental aspergillosis in BALB/c mice.[194] The incorporation of cholesterol into the liposomes further reduced the toxicity of hamycin in a dose-dependent manner. Thus, the LD_{50} of hamycin incorporated in liposomes consisting of phosphatidylcholine–cholesterol–phosphatidic acid (in molar ratio of 4:5:1) was 2.8 mg/kg, whereas the corresponding value in phosphatidylcholine–phosphatidic acid liposomes (in a molar ration of 9:1) was 0.35 mg/kg. Overall, the liposome formulations of hamycin (both with or without cholesterol) effectively reduced the fungal load in the lungs, liver, spleen, and the kidney of mice.[194]

The activity of ambruticin was investigated *in vitro* by using a modification of the ICS agar dilution technique; the antibiotic showed potency which compared favorably to that of amphotericin B when assayed against *A. fumigatus*.[195]

37.6.3.3.2   Benzo[a]naphthacenequinone antibiotics

Pradimicin A, a novel benzo[*a*]naphthacenequinone antibiotic, was isolated from *Actinomadura hibisca* sp. nov. No. P157-2, and *Actinomadura verrucosospora* subsp. *neohibisca* sp. nov. No. R103-3.[196,197] Reductive alkylation of pradimicin FA-1 (the D-serine congener of pradimicin A) with $NaBH_4CN$ and formaldehyde produced the water-soluble derivative BMY-28864 (solubility >20 mg/ml).[198] The D-amino acid moiety of the pradimicins was shown to be important in confering antifungal activity. Also, the change in the stereochemistry of C-17 carbon of the pradimicin A to 17-epipradimicin A, resulted in complete loss of antifungal activity.[199]

In vitro studies that compared the activities of BMY-28864, pradimicin A, amphotericin B, and ketoconazole against A. fumigatus have shown MIC values of 3.1, 1.6, 1.6, and 3.1 µg/ml, respectively.[200] Furthermore, comparative in vivo studies in immunocompromised mice against Aspergillus lung infection showed PD_{50} (protective dose by 50% after single intravenous injection) values for BMY-28864, pradimicin A, amphotericin B, and ketoconazole of 36, 16, 0.28, and 45 mg/kg, respectively. The acute toxicities (expressed by LD_{50} values) for BMY-28864, pradimicin A, and amphotericin B were >600, 120, and 4.5 mg/kg, respectively.[200]

The mode of action of pradimicins involved a Ca^{2+}-dependent binding to fungal cell surface mannans to provide insoluble complexes and leakage of potassium. There was no binding of BMY-28864 to human erythrocytes and various mammalian cells even in the presence of a large amount of calcium ions. Electron microscopic evidence has shown significant perturbation of the fungal cell membrane functions expressed as invagination and detachment of cell membrane, nuclear membrane damage, delocalization of nuclei, and damaged microtubules.[200]

The pharmacokinetics of pradimicins were investigated in male ddY mice.[200] After intravenous administration of 20 mg/kg, the plasma concentrations of BMY-28864 and pradimicin A declined with a half-life of about 10 min and 2.6 h, respectively. Excellent urinary recovery (92% of the initial dose after 24 h) and a favorable tissue distribution were observed for BMY-28864, while pradimicin A showed a characteristic kidney accumulation and poor urinary recovery (42% of the initial dose after 24 h); high concentrations of pradimicin A were retained in the kidney for 24 h. Both compounds displayed metabolic stability with no metabolites being detected in the tissues, urine, or the plasma of mice receiving 100 mg/kg each of pradimicin A or BMY-28864.[200]

Furumai et al.[201] have reported the isolation of two new pradimicins, T1 and T2, which were found to exhibit potent activity against systemic aspergillosis in mice.

Benanomicin A, another novel benzo[a]naphthacene antibiotic, was isolated from Actinomadura sp. MH193-16F4.[202-204] When tested in vitro, benanomicin A exerted inhibitory activity against A. fumigatus with a geometric mean MIC value of 7.59 µg/ml; by comparison, the same value for amphotericin B was 3.79 µg/ml.[205] In vivo experiments showed activity in mice inoculated intravenously with A. fumigatus (10^6 colony-forming units (CFU)/mouse); the corresponding ED_{50} values for benanomicin A, amphotericin B, and fluconazole were 56, 0.042, and >50 mg/kg (once daily, IV), respectively.[205] After a single dosing of benanomicin A (20 mg/kg, IV) was administered to rats, mice, and dogs, plasma half-life values were 2.26, 1.85, and 2.13 h, respectively.[205] The antibiotic was excreted mainly through the kidney in rats and dogs with urinary excretion ratio of 70% (24 h) and 68.2% (5%), respectively. The mode of action of benanomicin A was similar to that of pradimicin A[206] — it caused perturbation of the fungal cell membrane.[205]

The overall toxicity of benanomicin A was low, and the drug was tolerated well in animals given intravenously at as much as 600 mg/kg.[205]

37.6.3.3.3   Nikkomycins and cilofungin

Because of its unique nature, the cell wall of eukaryotic fungi serves to differentiate them from host cells.[207] Accordingly, the chemistry and morphology of the fungal cell wall became the target of intensive investigations directed at the discovery of novel antimycotic drugs with mechanism of action involving the inhibition of two critical cell wall functions: the chitin and β-glucan synthesis. In the process, a number of naturally occurring or semisynthetic antibiotics have been identified as inhibitors of either chitin synthesis (polyoxins, nikkomycins),[208] or β-glucan synthesis (echinocandin B, aculeacins, papulacandin, cilofungin).[209] The antifungal potency of both groups of antibiotics was demonstrated in a number of in vivo assays.[208,210] Recently, various combinations of these drugs have been studied for their ability to complement each other's antifungal activity. It is known that in some pathogenic fungi, the structure of their cell wall will change during the life cycle.[207] Furthermore, inhibition of β-glucan synthesis may also result in an increased production of chitin.[211] These and other findings[212] have indicated that combinations of chitin synthesis inhibitors (such as nikkomycins) with β-glucan synthesis inhibitors (cilofungin, papulacandin) may exert a synergistic antifungal activity. Indeed, several reports[211,213] have confirmed such possibility. Perfect et al.[214] evaluated the synergistic effect of nikkomycin Z and cilofungin against diverse dimorphic fungi, including *A. fumigatus*. In these studies, cilofungin alone suppressed the filamentous growth of *A. fumigatus* at 125 μg/ml, while nikkomycin Z alone was inactive even when tested up to 4000 μg/ml; however, combinations of the two antibiotics were synergistic, with a FIC index of 0.07.[214]

Denning and Stevens[215] have compared the activity of cilofungin and amphotericin B given alone and in combination in immunocompetent mice with aspergillosis. While cilofungin was equipotent to amphotericin B in preventing death and eradicating the cerebral aspergillosis, it did not sterilize the kidneys. Combination of the two drugs, however, caused higher rate of mortality than either of them administered alone (p = .003 and .054, respectively).

The *A. fumigatus* β-(1,3)-D-glucan synthase inhibiting activity of cilofungin was examined by Beaulieu et al.[216] and compared with that of papulacandin A, echinocandin B, and aculeacin A — all four antibiotics were effective at 1.0 μg/ml (40% to 71% inhibition); at this dose, amphotericin B, fluconazole, ketoconazole, and nikkomycin were all ineffective.

37.6.3.3.4   Pneumocandins

The pneumocandins are semisynthetic water-soluble analogs of echinocandin, showing inhibiting activity on the β-(1,3)-D-glucan biosynthesis.

Kurtz et al.[217] have evaluated the therapeutic efficacies of several pneumocandin derivatives in a rat model of pulmonary aspergillosis. When inoculated with 10^6 conidia of *A. fumigatus* H11-20, the rats developed a progressive, rapidly fatal bronchopneumonia. Intraperitoneal administration of L-693,989, L-731,373, and L-733,560 at 5.0 mg/kg effectively delayed mortality. In a separate experiment, aerosol of L-693,989 (5.0 mg/kg) when administered 2 h before infection also delayed mortality, with 8 of 10 rats surviving for 7 d, whereas only 2 of 10 controls survived.

The activities of L-733,560, L-705,589, and L-731,373 were tested in a mouse model of disseminated aspergillosis.[218] L-733,560 and L-705,589 were effective in markedly prolonging the survival of DBA/2N mice challenged intravenously with *A. fumigatus* conidia, and comparable to amphotericin B (MIC_{90} = 0.48, 0.12, and 0.36 for L-733,560, L-705,589, and amphotericin B, respectively).

37.6.3.4   Azole Derivatives

In addition to amphotericin B and a number of other antibiotics, the therapeutic efficacy of various azole derivatives against aspergillosis has also been the subject of intensive research efforts at both preclinical and clinical levels.

Some basic characteristics of various azole antimycotics used in the treatment of aspergillosis are presented in Table 37.5. It is useful to point out that the actual MIC values of different antifungal agents is quite likely to be influenced by the type of medium used in the *in vitro* assay.[219] Moreover, changes in the pH values of the medium may also change the observed activity of the drug.[220] Thus, in the case of ketoconazole, its potency was markedly reduced at pH 5.6 as compared to pH 7.2; miconazole, on the other hand, was less affected by changes in the pH values, having been marginally more active at pH 5.6.[220]

37.6.3.4.1   Clotrimazole

Twice daily oral administration of 10 mg/kg of clotrimazole to mice with experimental aspergillosis beginning on the day of inoculation, caused ultrastructural changes in the cell membrane, nuclear

TABLE 37.5
Azole Antimycotics in the Treatment of Aspergillosis

Azole	MIC, μg/ml	Indication (Route of Administration)	Side Effects	Refs.
Clotrimazole	1.0	Pulmonary aspergillosis (oral)	Gastrointestinal, dysuria	353, 354, 358, 449
Miconazole	3.48	Pulmonary aspergillosis/hemoptysis (intracavitary instillation)	Phlebitis, pruritis, nausea, fever, chill, rash, vomiting, anemia, decreased hematocrit (normoblastic hypoplasia), hyponatremia; anaphylaxis, ventricular tachycardia	223, 356, 365, 450
Ketoconazole	7.0	Chronic *Aspergillus* sinusitis (oral), keratitis (topical)	Nausea, vomiting, diarrhea, pruritis, rash, increased alkaline phosphatase, hyperlipidemia; inhibition of gonadal and adrenal steroid synthesis	368, 449, 451–453
Itraconazole	≥0.07	Invasive aspergillosis, aspergilloma, allergic bronchopulmonary aspergillosis, chronic necrotizing pulmonary aspergillosis	Superficial mycoses: nausea, headache, pyrosis, dysuria. Systemic mycosis: asymptomatic liver function abnormalities, increased blood levels of urea nitrogen and serum levels of transaminase	351, 382, 383, 392–394, 436, 454
BAY n 7133		Murine aspergillosis (oral)		237
Enilconazole	0.1–1.0	Avian aspergillosis (fumigation)	Emesis, salivation, loss of body weight, decreased serum calcium, increased serum alkaline phosphatase	455
Oxiconazole	10.0	*A. terreus*-induced keratitis (subconjunctival)		247
Saperconazole	0.1–1.0	Murine aspergillosis (oral, intravenous, intraperitoneal)	No side effects observed	248
SCH 39304		Murine pulmonary aspergillosis (oral)		251
SM-9164		Murine aspergillosis (oral, intravenous)		251
BAY R 3783		Murine pulmonary aspergillosis		255

membrane, mitochondria, and cytoplasm of the fungus in the kidney.[221] The effect led in 4 d to complete disintegration of all cytoplasmic structures and ultimately to plasmolysis; the uninfected kidney tissue was not affected by clotrimazole.[221] Plempel et al.[222] reported that orally administered clotrimazole was systemically effective against *Aspergillus* spp.

37.6.3.4.2 Miconazole

When tested *in vitro* against *A. fumigatus*, miconazole showed a MIC value of 3.48 μg/ml.[223] Hoeprich and Huston[224] found that *in vitro* the activity of miconazole was influenced adversely by two complex undefined media (Sabouraud's glucose and brain-heart infusion agar), but not when synthetic amino acid medium or fungal and modified yeast-nitrogen base were used.

The use of intra-arterial and intramammary injection of miconazole against *A. fumigatus*-induced bovine mastitis was reported.[225]

37.6.3.4.3   Ketoconazole

Oral ketoconazole (5.0 mg/kg, every 12 h) given over a period of 2 to 18 weeks, was found similar in potency to thiabendazole in the treatment of canine nasal aspergillosis.[226]

In a rabbit model,[227] neither oral nor topical ketoconazole alone was effective against *A. fumigatus*-induced keratitis. However, when ketoconazole (either oral or topical administration) was used in conjunction with natamycin, it appeared to augment the sterilization of the fungus in this model of experimental keratitis.[227]

37.6.3.4.4   Fluconazole

The antifungal potency of fluconazole was evaluated in an immunosuppressed temporarily leukopenic rabbit model of invasive aspergillosis.[228] The treatment was commenced at 24 h after a lethal challenge with daily doses of 60 or 120 mg/kg, and compared with amphotericin B (1.5 mg/kg daily). Fluconazole reduced the mortality rate, and at the 120-mg dose, it diminished the tissue burden of *A. fumigatus* by 10- to 100-fold in the liver, kidney, and lungs. However, when compared with amphotericin B, it was less effective in sterilizing tissues. In general, fluconazole was more efficacious when applied as early treatment or prophylaxis of experimental invasive aspergillosis.[228] O'Day[229] studied the efficacy of orally administered fluconazole in a Dutch-belted rabbit model of *A. fumigatus*-induced keratomycosis, and found the drug to produce excellent corneal penetration resulting in significant therapeutic effect.

37.6.3.4.5   Itraconazole

When tested *in vivo* in IRC mice with experimental aspergillosis, itraconazole prolonged the survival rate only after intravenous administration; it was inactive when given intranasally.[230] The blood levels of itraconazole were found to be usually low (0.3 mg/l approximately 5 h after the administration of a single 200-mg dose); however, following repeated dosing, higher concentrations (0.5 to 0.6 mg/l) may be achieved.[231] Compared to ketoconazole, itraconazole had a much longer elimination half-life (8 and 20 to 30 h, respectively). While tissue levels of the drug greatly exceeded serum concentrations, its penetration into the cerebrospinal fluid was poor. Furthermore, itraconazole was extensively metabolized in the liver resulting in the formation of a large number of inactive metabolites which were excreted largely through the bile and urine; fecal excretion accounted for only 3% to 18% of the drug.[231] Itraconazole was less toxic than ketoconazole especially on the steroid biosynthesis.[232] In one more finding, its serum concentrations were reduced by a concomitant administration of rifampin.

Combinations of itraconazole with 5-fluorocytosine (5-FC) were synergistic when tested in experimental aspergillosis in mice.[233] In the same model, the combination with amphotericin B was indifferent and even antagonistic.[233] Shaw et al.[234] reported evidence about the possible interaction of itraconazole with cyclosporin A.

Berenguer et al.[235] used a rabbit model of invasive aspergillosis to compare the efficacy of itraconazole with that of amphotericin B and its interaction with cyclosporin A, as well as to determine the correlation between therapeutic response and itraconazole concentrations in plasma. While both drugs were efficacious at the doses given (40 mg/kg orally for itraconazole, and 1.0 mg/kg intravenously for amphotericin B), amphotericin B was superior in reducing the tissue burden ($\log_{10}$ CFU per gram) of *A. fumigatus* ($p < .05$) and the number of pulmonary lesions ($p < .01$). There was considerable variation in the near-peak concentrations of itraconazole in plasma (median, 4.15 µg/ml; range, <0.5 to 16.8 µg/ml) and a strong inverse correlation between the concentrations of itraconazole in plasma and the tissue burden of *A. fumigatus*. An inhibitory sigmoid maximum-effect model predicted the presence of significant pharmacodynamic relationship (r = 0.87; p <.001) between itraconazole concentrations in plasma and antifungal activity as a function of the tissue burden of *A. fumigatus* — plasma levels of over 6.0 µg/ml were associated with a substantially greater antifungal activity; any levels below 6.0 µg/ml were associated with rapidly declining antifungal effect. When compared with amphotericin B, itraconazole caused a twofold elevation of cyclosporin A levels (p <.01), but was less nephrotoxic (p <.01).[235]

The efficacy of an itraconazole–cyclodextrin solution against *A. fumigatus* was also assessed in an immunosuppressed, temporarily leukopenic rabbit model of invasive aspergillosis and compared with that of amphotericin B. Daily doses of 20 and 40 mg/kg increased survival rate as compared with that in controls. In addition, the 40-mg/kg daily dose also eradicated *A. fumigatus* from tissues and was as effective as amphotericin B.[236]

37.6.3.4.6   Other azole derivatives

Several other azole derivatives have also been studied for activity against *A. fumigatus*. One such compound, the triazole-containing antimycotic BAY n 7133 was tested in a murine model of aspergillosis — 1 d after BALB/c mice were challenged intravenously or by intranasal route with conidia of *A. fumigatus*, BAY n 7133 was applied orally; the drug easily penetrated all tissues investigated.[237] There was evidence of an accelerated inactivation of the drug following prolonged therapy. In general, BAY n 7133 extended the survival rate of the infected mice by reducing the counts of *A. fumigatus* in the lungs.[237]

In vitro exposure of *A. fumigatus* to 50 µg of econazole[238,239] for 24 h resulted in the formation of Ca-containing precipitates on mitochondria, vacuoles, and collapsed membrane.[240] Econazole impaired the cell permeability and energy metabolism of the fungus. When compared to amphotericin B, econazole was equipotent in activity and showed higher stability, higher solubility, and wider range between MIC and host cytotoxic concentrations.[241] However, when evaluated *in vivo* in experimental aspergillosis in mice, econazole exerted only slight effect with a minimal life-prolonging dose of 100 mg/kg.[242]

At concentrations of 0.1 to 1.0 µg/ml, enilconazole completely inhibited *in vitro Aspergillus* spp., and at higher doses it was fungicidal against *A. fumigatus* when used both in hanging-drop and lying-drop suspensions.[243] *In vivo* experiments have demonstrated that fumigation of 1-d-old chickens infected with various inoculum sizes of airborne spores of *A. fumigatus* (which causes high rates of mortality and morbidity) with enilconazole smoke pellets was highly successful in preventing mortality, reducing morbidity, and neutralizing growth inhibition of infected chickens with no side effects observed.[244] A single spray of enilconazole at a dosage of 1.5 g per 10 m² of housing ground, reduced significantly the mortality of broiler chicks with aspergillosis.[245] Sharp et al.[246] have used enilconazole (10 mg/kg, b.i.d., for 7 to 14 d) to treat successfully canine nasal aspergillosis. The drug was administered topically through tubes surgically implanted into the nasal chambers.

Subconjunctival oxiconazole therapy exerted complete cure of experimental keratitis caused by *A. terreus* in immunocompromised albino rabbits.[247] When tested *in vitro* against *A. terreus* by the agar dilution technique, oxiconazole and ketoconazole showed MIC values of 10 and 3.0 µg/ml, respectively.[247]

Saperconazole (R 66905) is a novel broad-spectrum fluorinated triazole antimycotic with potent *in vitro* activity against *Aspergillus* spp. — at concentrations of 0.1 and 1.0 µg/ml, the drug completely inhibited the development of, respectively, 80.3% and 99.6% of 279 strains of the fungus.[248] The efficacy of the drug was also tested in normal and immunocompromised guinea pigs infected intravenously with *A. fumigatus*. Saperconazole after being administered either orally, intravenously, or intraperitoneally, was compared to intraperitoneal amphotericin B; medication was applied once daily for 2 weeks. The activity of the drug was not altered in the immunocompromised animals and was, in general, superior to that of amphotericin B, as well as free of side effects.[248] Experiments conducted in pigeons confirmed the systemic activity of saperconazole.[248] Hanson et al.[249] have examined the efficacy of saperconazole in a murine model of systemic aspergillosis. The drug, which was dissolved in hydroxypropyl-β-cyclodextrin, was given orally twice daily for 11 d, beginning 1 d postinfection, at 50, 100, or 200 mg/kg. Each saperconazole regimen prolonged survival compared with untreated controls ($p < .01$), and was superior to amphotericin B therapy ($p < .01$). The 200-mg/kg dose reduced the number of CFUs of aspergillosis in kidneys more than 1000-fold as compared to untreated animals ($p < .001$).

The potency of the triazole derivative SCH 39304 against pulmonary aspergillosis was compared to that of amphotericin B and fluconazole in a model of corticoid-immunosuppressed mice; all three drugs were given orally, 1 d after the challenge.[250] At doses of 5.0 mg/kg or higher, SCH 39304 markedly prolonged the survival rate, as did amphotericin B at 3.0 mg/kg; by comparison, fluconazole did not significantly prolong the survival at doses of 15 or 30 mg/kg.[250] Compound SM-9164, an R,R-enantiomer of SCH 39304, was found superior to the latter in its water solubility and therapeutic index.[251] SM-9164 was administered orally or intravenously to mice with experimental aspergillosis, and was compared to amphotericin B — the drug was less efficient when treatment was commenced on day 0 (ED_{50} values of 8.2 and 0.27 µg/ml, respectively; IV); however, when treatment was started on day 1, amphotericin B was inactive even at the maximum nonlethal dose of 2.5 mg/kg (IV), while SM-9164 showed the ED_{50} value at 8.5 mg/kg (IV).[251] Because of its unacceptable toxicity SCH 39304 has been withdrawn from clinical studies.

SCH 51048, another triazole antimycotic was evaluated in a murine model of pulmonary aspergillosis at doses ranging from 5.0 to 50 mg/kg.[252] Mortality was significantly delayed by SCH 51048 in mice treated with doses of 5.0 mg or higher as compared to controls ($p < .05$). Also, both SCH 51048 and SCH 39304 at higher doses (30 and 50 mg/kg) reduced the number of viable *A. fumigatus* in lung tissue ($p < .05$).[252]

The therapeutic efficacy of D0870, a novel triazole antifungal compound (the mycologically active R-enantiomer of ICI 195,739), was compared with that of conventional amphotericin B and itraconazole in two murine models of invasive aspergillosis: a systemic nonimmunocompromised mouse model, and a temporarily neutropenic mouse respiratory model.[253] In the nonimmunocompromised mouse model, D0870 at 25 mg/kg, b.i.d., was slightly inferior to intraperitoneal amphotericin B (at 3.3 mg/kg) and oral itraconazole (5.0 to 50 mg/kg daily, or twice daily) with regard to mortality rates (median survival of 20 d for the three groups; $p = .03$). However, D0870, at 25 mg/kg, b.i.d., was inferior to amphotericin B (but not itraconazole) with respect to renal culture ($p = .01$) and brain culture ($p = .0001$) results. In the neutropenic mouse model, D0870 at 50 mg/kg daily was superior to amphotericin B, itraconazole, and controls with regard to mortality; however, a second experiment with a higher inoculum has shown that neither of the three drugs was effective in that model. The *in vitro* potency and *in vivo* efficacy of D0870 was also compared to those of fluconazole.[254] In both normal and immunosuppressed mouse models of systemic aspergillosis, D0870 was, respectively, 2- to 7-fold and 3- to 89-fold more effective than fluconazole. Furthermore, in immunocompromised mice, the therapeutic efficacy of D0870 was nearly equivalent to that in normal mice, whereas the activity of fluconazole was 5- to 50-fold lower than that in normal mice.[254]

Similarly to itraconazole, the triazole antimycotic BAY R 3783 was found effective in a rodent model of pulmonary aspergillosis.[255]

ER-30346 is a novel orally active triazole derivatives with a broad spectrum of potent antifungal activity.[256,257] The MIC_{90} of ER-30346 against *A. fumigatus* was 0.39 µg/ml.[256] Against systemic aspergillosis in mice, ER-30346 proved superior to itraconazole and amphotericin B,[256] and in experimental murine models of pulmonary aspergillosis, ER-30346 reduced significantly the numbers of CFUs in the lungs as compared to controls ($p < .05$).[257]

37.6.3.5   Miscellaneous Antifungal Compounds

When tested *in vitro* against *A. fumigatus* at concentrations of 100 µg/ml, 5-fluorocytosine caused abnormal behavior of the nuclei and lipidification of the mitochondria.[240] The drug was incorporated to a moderate degree into the fungal DNA. This latter finding may be an important factor in determining whether the activity of flucytosine is fungistatic (*A. fumigatus* and *Cryptococcus neoformans*) or fungicidal (*Candida* spp.).[258,259] In this regard, exogenously supplied purines, pyrimidines, and some of their nucleoside analogs are known for their ability to antagonize the fungistatic activity of 5-fluorocytosine.[260,261] At doses of 100 µ*M* neither allopurinol nor oxypurinol altered the MIC values of 5-FC against 18 pathogenic fungal isolates.[261] Watanabe et al.[262] reported the successful treatment of one patient with pulmonary aspergillosis by intracavitary infusion of 5-FC. The toxic side effects of 5-FC included nausea, vomiting, hepatotoxicity, and bone marrow depression.[263]

Treatment of individual cases, although lacking the convincing evidence of large-scale multicenter clinical trials, may still provide useful information about the antifungal activity of various agents. In one such example, Fernandez[264] has reported the successful and quick control of life-threatening pulmonary hemorrhage by intracavitary infusion of aminocaproic acid to a patient with pulmonary aspergillosis having hemoptysis.

In an earlier study,[265] stilbamidine (a stilbene derivative with antiprotozoal activity) when administered by parenteral injection was shown to cure a patient with bronchopulmonary aspergillosis.

Dimethyldithiocarbamate significantly attenuated lesion scores and inhibited the rate of isolation of *A. fumigatus* in trials using 5- and 10-week-old white leghorn chickens.[266]

Butenafine hydrochloride was reported to show excellent *in vitro* activity against *A. fumigatus*.[267] Terbinafine, on the other hand, was found ineffective when tested in a rat model of pulmonary aspergillosis.[268]

37.6.3.5.1   *Granulocyte colony-stimulating and granulocyte-macrophage colony-stimulating factors*

The granulocyte colony-stimulating factor (G-CSF) is known to play an important role in inducing hemopoietic cells to proliferate and differentiate into neutrophils.[269,270] When administered to neutropenic animals, G-CSF restored to normal the levels of neutrophils in the blood.[271,272] Experiments conducted by Yamamoto et al.[269] have demonstrated the ability of G-CSF to protect neutropenic mice from systemic infections caused by *Candida* and *Aspergillus* spp. When mice were treated once daily with either 15, 30, 60, or 120 µg/ml of G-CSF for 3 d before infection, and two daily doses postinfection, the hemopoietic factor prolonged the survival rate of *Aspergillus*-infected mice.[269]

In order to improve the functional activity of neutrophils, macrophages, and monocytes and therefore the efficacy of amphotericin B, Anaissie and Bodey[273] conducted a pilot study using granulocyte-macrophage colony-stimulating factor (GM-CSF) together with amphotericin B. A neutrophil count of less than 100 was required for patient inclusion, as well as serum creatinine levels of less than 3 mg/dl. The regimen included daily administration of amphotericin B at 1.0 mg/kg (as a 4-h infusion for a minimum of 1.0 g) until all signs and symptoms of infection were resolved; GM-CSF was used at 400 µg/m² daily (as a 24-h continuous infusion) and was given for 2 to 6 weeks depending on the response of the neutrophil count. The patients were evaluated at 6 weeks, and whenever possible at 6 months post-treatment. Of the two reported cases of disseminated aspergillosis, one responded only partially, while the other one was a failure — however, there had been a complete response in one case of pulmonary candidiasis, and one case of disseminated candidiasis.[273]

37.6.4 EVOLUTION OF THERAPIES AND TREATMENT OF ASPERGILLOSIS

Since the first report by Gerstl et al.,[274] surgical resection of lesions is one major option for therapy of aspergillomas.[275-278] However, drug therapy of *Aspergillus* infections[279,280] has been steadily increasing over the years, especially in those cases where other underlying pulmonary conditions (severe chronic obtrusive lung diseases, emphysema, pulmonary fibrosis, and bilateral aspergilloma) may be severe enough to preclude surgical intervention.

The clinical aspects and treatment outcomes of 72 cases of *Aspergillus* sinusitis analyzed over a 14-year period revealed 60 cases of primary type and 12 cases of secondary type, with the maxillary and ethmoid sinuses most commonly affected in both types.[281] Surgery was performed in most cases, among which four patients received chemotherapy after surgery with amphotericin B with or without flucytosine. In a single case report, Parker et al.[282] have described aspergillosis of the sphenoid sinus and associated osteomyelitis of the skull base presenting as a pituitary mass. A postoperative ^{67}Ga imaging showed intense uptake in the sphenoid sinus, which resolved after treatment with amphotericin B.

Sinusitis due to *Aspergillus* infection is also more frequently seen in HIV-positive patients.[283] Despite aggressive surgical intervention and systemic antifungal therapy, the prognosis of this invasive infection in these patients is poor.

When considering large-scale clinical trials relative to treatments of individual cases, it should be well understood that multicenter clinical therapy involving a significant number of patients is by far the better choice for a study, since it will not only furnish the necessary information and clinical experience to put into focus the therapeutic efficacy of experimental anti-infectious drugs, but also because it will provide viewpoint and directions necessary for future research. In this context, clinical reports describing treatments of limited numbers of patients or individual cases, when well documented, may serve the useful purpose of shedding light on the antifungal activity of various agents which may otherwise go unnoticed by those involved in drug research and development. In general, however, because of its limited scope, such information, even when valuable, should be viewed with caution in evaluating the therapeutic efficacy of a drug.

37.6.4.1 Amphotericin B

Even though for the last 30 years or so, amphotericin B has remained the drug of choice for treatment of aspergillosis (Table 37.6),[279] the drug has not been very effective in immuno-compromised patients and its dosage regimens in neutropenic patients are thought to be not very well defined.[93] In a recent study,[284] only 26% of cancer patients with aspergillosis when treated with amphotericin B survived their infections, and no patient with persistent neutropenia (<1000 neutrophils/mm^3) survived the infection. It should be emphasized that for the successful treatment of *Aspergillus* pneumonia in immunocompromised patients (even during profound neutropenia), early initiation of amphotericin B therapy is critical[285,286] — without prompt intervention, this condition is frequently fatal, especially when an underlying malignancy does not remit or a bone-marrow recovery does not occur.[287,288]

A survey[289] of antifungal and surgical treatment of invasive aspergillosis involving 2121 published cases has shown that the mortality from pulmonary aspergillosis in bone marrow transplant recipients exceeded 94% regardless of the therapy applied; a similar mortality rate has been attributed to cerebral aspergillosis in all hosts. On average, the rate of response to amphotericin B has been 55%. The antibiotic, when administered at a daily dose of 1.0 mg/kg in combination with 5-fluorocytosine to neutropenic patients with pulmonary aspergillosis who had not received a bone marrow transplant, lowered the mortality rate; however, relapses were common.

As therapy, the surgical resection of pulmonary tissue in cases of massive hemoptysis associated with pulmonary aspergilloma causes high morbidity and mortality in patients with inadequate pulmonary reserve.[77,135,290,291] An alternative therapy in such cases is provided by amphotericin B.

TABLE 37.6
Treatment of *Aspergillus* Infections with Amphotericin B

Infection	Route of Administration
Pulmonary aspergillosis	Intravenous
	Direct intracavitary instillation
	Transthoracic injection
	Paste
	Endobronchial instillation
	Aerosol
Sinonasal aspergillosis	Intravenous; Liposome-encapsulated
Aspergillus-induced endophthalmitis	Intravitreous; Intravenous
Aspergillus-induced peritonitis	Intraperitoneal
Aspergillus-induced empyema/bronchopleural fistula	Intrapleural

For example, Shapiro et al.[292] reported the case of successful treatment of four patients with acute hemoptysis by a percutaneously placed catheter and intracavitary infusion of amphotericin B (total of 500 mg); *N*-acetylcysteine was also given in order to facilitate the dissolution of the fungus ball and to help clearing debris, and on one occasion, the instillation of aminocaproic acid was also utilized. Cochrane et al.[293] also used intracavitary amphotericin B to treat aspergilloma and recurrent hemoptysis. Intracavitary instillation of amphotericin B (delivered by a flexible fiberoptic bronchoscope) had a beneficial effect on a patient with chronic necrotizing pulmonary aspergillosis (an indolent locally invasive form of *Aspergillus* infection).[294]

A case of primary aspergilloma was treated with a total dose of 950 mg of amphotericin B over a period of 32 d; upon completion of therapy, the fungal mass was reported to resolve.[295]

Fisher et al.[75] described a clinical study involving patients with invasive aspergillosis (with the majority of them having neutropenia and hematologic neoplasms as underlying disease) lasting for over 5 years — the therapy comprised amphotericin B (181 to 1363 mg; mean 717.2 mg) and when necessary pneumonectomy or lobectomy. In another report,[286] two patients with *Aspergillus* pneumonia and hematologic neoplasia were successfully treated with amphotericin B (total of 1.8 to 2.0 g) for a period of 2 months.

Invasive sinonasal aspergillosis is a severe and frequently fatal infection in immuno-compromised patients with hematologic malignancies.[168] It may result in bone erosion and extension into soft tissues of the cheek and orbit with facial pain and soft tissue edema; intracranial extension, if it occurs, may be fatal.[296] Further complications include dissemination to noncontiguous structures (sinus, lung, viscera, and brain) leading to 50%–80% mortality rate in immunocompromised patients.[75,297] Several cases of sinonasal aspergillosis that were managed by intravenous administration of amphotericin B in combination with surgery (Caldwell-Luc operation and antrostomy) in the invasive variety of the disease, have been reported.[296] An immunocompromised patient with acute lymphoblastic leukemia who presented initially with aspergillosis of the nasopharynx, responded rapidly to medication with amphotericin B.[298] Kusumoto et al.[299] discussed the use of intravenous amphotericin B combined with local lavage of amphotericin B in the treatment of aspergillosis of the maxillary sinus.

In a single case report, Ho et al.[300] described *Aspergillus*-induced endophthalmitis after a penetrating injury and primary repair of a scleral wound. Vitrectomy combined with intravitreous and intravenous amphotericin B (40 to 50 mg/kg daily) therapy for 34 d (total of 1560 mg) resulted in the preservation of useful vision in what appears to be the first successfully treated case of exogenous *Aspergillus* endophthalmitis. A case of localized aspergilloma of the eyelid responded to injections of amphotericin B directly into the lid granuloma.[301] Harris and Mill[302] used conservative debridement and local amphotericin B irrigation to treat orbital aspergillosis in a patient on long-term immunosuppressive therapy. Endogenous *A. flavus*-induced endophthalmitis in association with severe periodontitis has been reported by Matsuo et al.[9]

Stereotactic drainage of a bilateral *Aspergillus* brain abscess (craniotomy) combined with amphotericin B medication was applied to achieve long-term survival in four of five patients.[303] A case of non-Hodgkin's lymphoma complicated with invasive CNS aspergillosis was treated with amphotericin B.[304]

Peritonitis is the most commonly observed complication of continuous ambulatory (or cycling) peritoneal dialysis.[305] Although the majority of infections are caused by Gram-positive bacteria, cases of peritonitis secondary to fungi have been on the increase — in one such report,[306] as many as 15% of all cases were fungus-related. All reported incidences were also fatal.[305] An individual case of successfully treated *Aspergillus*-related peritonitis in a child undergoing continuous cycling dialysis involved intraperitoneal administration of amphotericin B; the antibiotic was mixed in dialysate (1.0 mg/l of dialysate) in order to preserve the peritoneal dialysis therapy. In another case of *A. fumigatus*-associated peritonitis related to CAPD, the treatment consisted of removal of the catheter and intravenous administration of amphotericin B, followed by oral itraconazole.[124]

Skorodin et al.[307] presented a case of mixed empyema with bronchopleural fistula due to *Mycobacterium tuberculosis*, *A. fumigatus*, and *A. flavus*, which was resolved by administration of antituberculosis drugs and intrapleural amphotericin B (total of 575 mg) over a 4-week period.

Conneally et al.[308] described the administration of nebulized amphotericin B (twice daily over a 12-month period) as prophylaxis against invasive aspergillosis in granulocytopenic patients. The results, which were compared to historical controls (11.4% incidence of those at risks), suggested that since commencing prophylaxis, no cases of invasive aspergillosis had occurred.[308]

Aspergillus-associated laryngotracheobronchitis presenting as stridor in a patient with peripheral T cell lymphoma responded to systemic treatment with amphotericin B.[309]

The toxicity of amphotericin B ranges from acute (idiosyncratic or dose-related) to chronic (Table 37.7).[93,285] Usually, when the creatinine levels exceed 3.0 to 3.5 mg/dl, amphotericin B therapy should be ceased for several days and then reinstated at a lower dose. Premedication with acetaminophen and the addition of hydrocortisone sodium succinate (25 to 50 mg) to the infusion solution has been reported to reduce some of the toxicity of the antibiotic.[285]

TABLE 37.7
Toxicities of Amphotericin B

Dose-dependent
  Nephrotoxicity (urinary abnormalities, hyposthenuria, azotemia, hypokalemia, nephrocalcinosis)
  Normocytic, normochromic anemia (decreased erythropoietin levels and erythrocyte counts)

Idiosyncratic
  Flushing, generalized pain, rash, *grand mal* convulsion, anaphylactic shock, ventricular
  fibrillation, acute liver failure, cardiac arrest, thrombocytopenia, fever (in nearly all patients),
  vertigo, chill (in nearly all patients)

37.6.4.1.1   Liposome-encapsulated and lipid-based formulations of amphotericin B

The therapeutic effect of AmBisome® (a unilamellar liposomal formulation of amphotericin B) in systemic fungal infections was evaluated in a European multicenter study.[310] The patients tested either had failed to respond to or tolerate alternatives, or who were in acute renal failure. Although preliminary, one important finding of the study was that, in general, the liposomal amphotericin B did not display serious toxicity such as renal tubular damage, and that patients were able to tolerate doses of amphotericin B which significantly exceeded those used in conventional formulations. The reported cases of aspergillosis showed that 25% of the patients recovered clinically, another 25% were rated as clinically improved, while the remaining 50% were considered as clinical failures; the mycological efficacy of AmBisome® resulted in 25% of patients being cured, 50% still having persistent cultures, and the remaining 25% not evaluated.[310]

In another study, AmBisome® was used to treat immunocompromised pediatric patients with invasive aspergillosis and candidiasis at a mean cumulative dose of 1.8 ± 1.3 g (± SD) and for a median of 19 d — side effects were minimal and in those children treated for at least 1 week, the overall cure rate was 86%.[311]

Weber and Lopez-Berestein[168] have also demonstrated that amphotericin B when encapsulated in liposomes[312] may become an effective and less toxic alternative to conventional amphotericin B therapy in patients with sinonasal aspergillosis who failed to respond to amphotericin B alone. In the reported trial, in six of seven patients an underlying hematologic malignancy or aplastic anemia was also present. The initial dose of liposomal amphotericin B was 0.4 mg/kg (in sodium chloride suspension), administered intravenously over 10 min; depending upon the patient's tolerance, the dose was gradually increased to 2 mg/kg daily for 3 weeks (median dose 1.4 g; total of 280 to 4000 mg). The results showed that five of the patients were complete responders (four of them remained neutropenic throughout the therapy), with the response being rapid and leading to resolution of symptoms occurring within 4 to 5 d. Two of the patients did not respond. No severe renal or CNS toxicity was observed.[168] Liposomal amphotericin B (AmBisome®) was also used in the treatment of five pediatric patients with malignancies who developed invasive pulmonary aspergillosis during chemotherapy-induced neutropenia.[313] In addition to liposomal amphotericin B, the patients also received G-CSF. Liposomal amphotericin B was well tolerated in patients receiving high doses of the antibiotic, such as those undergoing bone marrow or peripheral blood stem cell transplantation.[44] However, the use of liposomal amphotericin B to treat *A. fumigatus* infection in three lung transplant recipients, although successful, was not free of undesired side effects and nephrotoxicity as suggested by previous results.[60]

A. flavus colonization of the renal pelvis and upper ureter of a patient with concomitant urinary schistosomiasis was successfully treated with liposomal amphotericin B.[7]

A patient with asthma, bronchopulmonary aspergillosis, pulmonary thromboembolic disease, and pulmonary hypertension who developed *A. fumigatus* empyema complicating pneumothorax and had failed to respond to intravenous and intrapleutal amphotericin B, improved promptly after changing treatment to nebulized liposomal amphotericin B and oral itraconazole.[314]

Hospenthal et al.[85] have described the successful use of amphotericin B lipid complex in the treatment of invasive pulmonary aspergillosis complicating prolonged treatment-related neutropenia in acute myelogenous leukemia.

Mendicute et al.[315] have treated three patients with *Aspergillus* keratomycosis with collagen shields impregnated with amphotericin B (0.50%) for 2 h at 25°C before application. The shields (replaced daily) were used in conjunction with amphotericin B (0.25%) eye drops, which were applied every 2 h. The collagen shields, as prepared, delivered adequate concentration of amphotericin B to the cornea and increased its tolerance.

The clinical response and safety (toxicity profile and maximum tolerated dose) of amphotericin B colloidal dispersion (Amphocil®) was evaluated in a phase I dose-escalation trial in 75 bone marrow transplant patients with invasive fungal infection primarily due to *Aspergillus* and *Candida*.[42] Escalating doses of 0.5 to 8.0 mg/kg in 0.5-mg/kg/patient increments were given up to 6 weeks. There has been no infusion-related toxicities in 32% of patients; 52% had grade 2 and 5% had grade 3 toxicity. No appreciable renal toxicity was observed at any dose level. The estimated maximum tolerated dose was 7.5 mg/kg, defined by rigors and chills, and hypotension in three of five patients receiving 8.0 mg/kg of the drug.[42]

37.6.4.1.2   Routes of administration

For treatment of pulmonary aspergillosis, amphotericin B may be applied by one of several routes (Table 37.6). Intravenous administration, although often used in earlier trials, is being viewed with reservation.[133] For example, Hammerman et al.,[316] when treating 71 patients with saprophitic pulmonary aspergillosis with intravenous amphotericin B, found that such treatment was no more advantageous than a pulmonary toilet regimen. This finding was corroborated by other researchers as well,[134,317] although in several reports[318-320] successful therapy involving intravenous administration of amphotericin B has been described.

Direct intracavitary instillation of amphotericin B is usually accomplished by repeated transthoracic injections into the cavity. The drug is instilled in liquid form, but the use of a paste has also been recommended.[321] The drawbacks of intracavitary administration have included poor patient tolerance (development of fever), risk of pneumothorax, and relapse of infection in the cavity.[77] However, Hargis et al.[322] reported clinical improvement and stabilization in cases where a large dose of amphotericin B (500 mg) was instilled by intracavitary route in 50% dextrose in water. In general, however, endobronchial instillation of antifungal drugs had minimal success[323,324] and the possibility of relapse.[77]

Giron et al.[325] have reported 30 cases of percutaneous treatment of symptomatic pulmonary aspergilloma by injection of amphotericin B paste in patients who were not considered to be operable because of severe respiratory failure. The preparation of the paste and the type of percutaneous injection were aimed at obtaining a complete filling of the cavity and creating anaerobic environment for the fungus. Shirai et al.[326] and Furuse et al.[327] have also performed percutaneous instillation of amphotericin B to treat pulmonary aspergilloma.

In a rat model of pregressive pulmonary aspergillosis (characterized by hyphal broncho-pneumonia), amphotericin B was administered as an aerosol (1.6 mg/kg given 2 d before infection).[328] The application resulted in a markedly delayed mortality of the rats as compared to controls. When the same dose of aerosolized amphotericin B was administered as a treatment (1.6 mg/kg given 24 h after infection, and then daily for 6 d), it was found effective — 8 of 10 rats survived for 7 d, compared to only 1 of 10 controls. The colony counts in lung homogenates obtained 24 h after the infection showed an 80-fold reduction in the number of viable spores in rats which received 6.4-mg/kg doses of aerosolized amphotericin B 2 d prior to infection.[328] Studies on the pharmacokinetics showed that 48 h after the administration of aerosolized amphotericin B at a single dose of 1.6 or 3.2 mg/kg, the mean lung concentrations of the antibiotic were 2.79 and 5.22 µg/ml, respectively. The beneficial action of aerosolized amphotericin B was likely due not only to its ability to kill inhaled spores but also to delay the progression of pulmonary aspergillosis by inhibiting mycelial proliferation.[328] In humans, pulmonary deposition of amphotericin B could also be achieved by using commercially available nebulizers — inhalations were well tolerated with little systemic absorption of the drug.[329]

Cahill et al.[330] reported a successful palliative treatment of *A. fumigatus* orbital mass in a patient with AIDS by direct injection of amphotericin B into the abscess cavity. This case of intraorbital administration was suggested as an alternative to surgical debridement.

A case of erythroleukemia associated with lung aspergilloma was successfully treated with continuous drip infusion of amphotericin B, which allowed for maintaining high lung tissue drug levels.[331]

37.6.4.1.3   Combinations of amphotericin B with other drugs

In addition to therapy with amphotericin B alone, a number of combinations with other drugs, especially 5-fluorocytosine[332-336] have also been used to treat *Aspergillus* infections (Table 37.8).

While IPA occurs exclusively in severely immunocompromised patients, it is an increasingly recognized condition in apparently immunocompetent hosts. In the latter case, some potential risk factors (fibrotic lung disease, corticosteroid therapy, influenza, or psittacosis infection) may be

TABLE 37.8
Combinations of Amphotericin B with Other Drugs

Combination	Indication
Amphothericin B (intravenous)/5-FC (oral)	Invasive pulmonary aspergillosis
Amphotericin B (intravenous)/rifampin (oral)	Disseminated aspergillosis-chronic granulomatous disease
	Invasive pulmonary aspergillosis
Amphotericin B/tetracyclines	*In vitro* assay
Amphotericin B/nystatin (intrapleural instillation)	Pleural aspergillosis
Amphotericin B/itraconazole	Invasive CNS aspergillosis

present. If not treated early, the prognosis of IPA remains poor for both immunocompromised and immunocompetent patients.[81] Rodenhuis et al.[81] reported a case of successful therapy of IPA in an immunocompetent patient by applying systemic treatment with amphotericin B and 5-fluorocytosine together with inhalation of aerosolized amphotericin B. Apparently, the combination of the two drugs[337] acted locally, while the inhalation of amphotericin B helped to prevent continuing reinfection with 5-fluorocytosine-resistant strains of *Aspergillus*. Spiteri et al.[338] also described a case of successful recovery of an immunocompetent patient with primary IPA (but no other detectable lung damage or underlying systemic disease) using a combination of intravenous amphotericin B (initially 15 mg daily, increasing to 50 mg daily after 4 d) and oral 5-fluorocytosine (200 mg/kg daily; total dose of 3 g daily, every 6 h); the therapy lasted for 8 weeks.

Henze et al.[339] have described a case of developed pulmonary and cerebral aspergillosis in an immunosuppressed patient who received antineoplastic treatment for CNS relapse of acute lymphoblastic leukemia. The combination therapy of intravenous amphotericin B (total dosage exceeded 500 mg) and oral flucytosine (100 to 150 mg/kg), which was supported by natamycin inhalations, resulted in complete regression of pulmonary infiltrates after treatment for 53 d. Some enlargement of the cerebral lesion was observed, but no viable organisms were present in the completely resected abscess after 4-week treatment preceding neurosurgery.[339]

In one report of *Aspergillus*-associated pneumonia, combination therapy of intravenous amphotericin B (total of 1.3 g) and oral flucytosine (1.5 to 2.0 g, given four times daily) produced a rapid improvement and total eradication of the disease;[340] the amphotericin B therapy was stopped after 2 months, while 5-fluorocytosine administration was continued alone at a dosage of 2.0 g (four times daily) for another 3 months.

Bogner et al.[335] described successful treatment of *Aspergillus*-induced endocarditis with amphotericin B–flucytosine combination. The therapy commenced with daily intravenous injections of amphotericin B (increasing to 50 mg) combined with 1.5 g daily of oral 5-fluorocytosine; a total of 1.1 g of amphotericin B and 41.5 g of 5-FC were given over a 5-week period. A gradual decrease in symptoms and valve vegetation was observed.

In patients with acute leukemia, invasive *Aspergillus* rhinosinusitis may develop as a potentially lethal complication of chemotherapy-induced neutropenia. In the majority of cases, the causative agent is *A. flavus*. Talbot et al.[336] have recommended early treatment with aggressive surgery, high-dose amphotericin B, and 5-fluorocytosine; white blood cell transfusions may also be beneficial, particularly in cases of bone marrow recovery.

In view of the existing toxicity of both amphotericin B and flucytosine (especially the negative effect of the latter on the bone marrow), treatment of aspergillosis in terminally ill AIDS patients with combination amphotericin B–flucytosine should be applied with extreme caution. In addition, some of the gastrointestinal side effects of 5-FC may often superimpose on symptoms caused by the human immunodeficiency virus.[341,342]

In children with chronic granulomatous disease (CGD; an underlying immune disorder), therapy of disseminated aspergillosis with amphotericin B alone was only marginally effective and granulocyte transformations or a surgical excision was often required.[343-345] Corrado et al.[346] and Lizzarin and Capsoni[343] have recommended the combined use of rifampin and amphotericin B to manage disseminated aspergillosis in children with CGD. The therapy comprised intravenous amphotericin B (0.7 mg/kg daily) and oral rifampin (20 mg/kg daily) for 11 weeks; hypokalemia was the only adverse side effect observed.[343]

A combination of rifampin and amphotericin B was successfully used in the therapy of one immunosuppressed patient (acute leukemia) with IPA; the patient received rifampin (600 mg daily for 3 weeks) and a total dose of 1.8 g of amphotericin B.[347] Another case of pulmonary aspergillosis in a patient with acute leukemia that was managed by amphotericin B–rifampin, has also been reported.[348]

Colp and Cook[349] have described successful treatment of a patient with bronchopleural fistula and pleural aspergilloma by intrapleural instillation of amphotericin B (total of 750 mg over a 1-month period) and nystatin, followed by creation of an Eloesser flap for long-term drainage of the pleural space. In another example, a combination of amphotericin B and nystatin was applied topically for the treatment of aspergilloma;[321] the two antibiotics were used as a paste administered by intracavitary needling and instillation. It is thought that the paste covered the surface of the fungus ball and impaired the air supply coming to the pathogen.[321]

A patient with chronic necrotizing pulmonary aspergillosis complicated by a residual tuberculous cavity was treated successfully with oral itraconazole (200 mg daily) and inhaled amphotericin B (10 mg, four times daily). The serum concentration of amphotericin B was 0.09 μg/ml, which was equal to the level achieved after daily oral administration of 2.4 g of the antibiotic.[350]

In another successful application, liposomal amphotericin B and oral itraconazole were combined with surgical excision of abscesses to cure invasive aspergillosis of the central nervous system in an immunosuppressed pediatric patient with acute lymphatic leukemia and multiple *Aspergillus* brain abscesses.[351]

Maesaki et al.[352] have described a case of pulmonary aspergilloma which responded with complete disappearance of the fungus ball on chest computerized tomography (CT) scan after combination therapy of intravenous urinastatin (100,000 units) and intracavitary injection of amphotericin B.

37.6.4.2   Azole Derivatives

So far, published reports have indicated that the therapeutic efficacy of some of the azole antimycotics, such as clotrimazole, miconazole, and ketoconazole against various forms of aspergillosis is highly questionable. The observed lack of consistent antifungal effect coupled with the absence of large-scale clinical trials to prove otherwise have virtually precluded their use in treatment of aspergillosis.

37.6.4.2.1   *Clotrimazole*

In one clinical case, Evans et al.[353] described the successful management of pulmonary aspergillosis in a child by using systemic therapy with clotrimazole at daily doses of 70 mg/kg for 45 d; previously, inhalation of nystatin (120,000 units daily) and cephalexin (750 mg daily), and irrigation of the pleural space with nystatin suspension (500,000 units) for 6 d failed to cure the disease. During therapy, clotrimazole was tolerated well.[353]

In a contradictory report, Milne[354] revealed the lack of mycologic and clinical improvement in four patients with bronchopulmonary aspergillosis treated with daily doses of 100 mg/kg clotrimazole for up to 3 months. The observed maximum serum concentration of the drug was

0.17 µg/ml, while the MIC against *A. fumigatus* isolates was 1.0 µg/ml — this finding may be one reason for the lower therapeutic efficacy of clotrimazole.

Clinical experience from continuing oral administration of clotrimazole has shown an enhanced drug metabolism occurring after approximately 2 weeks of medication.[355] This inability to sustain adequate blood concentrations has proved to be a problem[356] for the systemic use of clotrimazole against various mycoses, including bronchopulmonary aspergillosis.[357]

Oral clotrimazole (60 mg/kg daily for 127 d) had no beneficial effect on paranasal aspergilloma as reported by Mahgub;[358] the drug also caused gastrointestinal side effects and disuria.[358]

Corneal infections caused by *A. fumigatus* are difficult to control especially in cases when hypopyon is present. Jones et al.[359] described as successful the treatment of two such cases by using a combined therapy of topical (1% solution in arachis oil) and oral clotrimazole.

37.6.4.2.2 Miconazole

Although miconazole can be administered orally, it requires high doses (1.0 g) to achieve adequate blood concentrations of 1.16 mg/l at 2 to 4 h post-administration.[360] A more useful approach would be to inject the drug intravenously at 50 mg/kg every 8 h.[356]

Miconazole usually will not penetrate the urine, cerebrospinal fluid (CSF), or the joints in high concentrations. Its serum levels were determined by bioassay after intravenous injection of 200 to 600 mg to patients with deep-seated mycoses — peak concentrations of 1.0 to 1.6 µg/ml were reached at the end of the administration, followed by a rapid decrease of 25% (or less) after 7 to 8 h.[361,362] When the serum levels were determined by high-pressure liquid chromatography (HPLC), the observed values tended to be higher than those determined by the bioassay, likely because the HPLC technique would measure not only the free but also the protein-bound miconazole.[361]

Intrapleural administration of miconazole led only to partial improvement in a case of *Aspergillus*-induced empyema with bronchopleural fistula — for the complete treatment, lobectomy and decortication were also performed.[363]

In another clinical application, parenteral miconazole was found to be very useful in the treatment of deep-seated aspergillosis of the respiratory tract.[364] Hamamoto et al.[365] have tried intracavitary infusion of miconazole to cure a patient with pulmonary aspergillosis and recurrent hemoptysis (accompanied with tuberculosis and diabetes), who did not respond to surgical excision. Miconazole, which was infused through a catheter in eight treatments for a total of 50 mg, initiated lysis of the fungal ball.

A case of chronic necrotizing pulmonary aspergillosis effectively treated with miconazole inhalation was reported by Maeda.[366]

Clinical studies in Japan[361] on the therapeutic efficacy of miconazole showed an 84% cure rate for pulmonary aspergillosis and 83% for pulmonary aspergilloma.

37.6.4.2.3 Ketoconazole

Ketoconazole was the first azole antimycotic able to produce sustainable therapeutic concentrations after oral administration.[367] Even though ketoconazole did not penetrate the CSF and urine, it still managed to produce high recovery rates in various mycoses.[356]

Farquhar et al.[368] treated a case of chronic sinusitis attributed to *A. fumigatus* with oral ketoconazole (200 mg daily for 2 months) with positive response.

Topical ketoconazole (2%) was used in the therapy of corneal infection induced by *A. flavus*; the drug, which was applied every 2 h for 17 d, healed the lesions completely.[369] Singh et al.[370] have found oral ketoconazole effective in experimental corneal ulcer induced by injecting intralamellary spore suspension of *A. fumigatus* into the eye of previously immunosuppressed albino and black wild rabbits; a partial response, followed by relapse were observed. O'Day et al.[371] described a case of deep corneal abscess caused by *Aspergillus* spp. which was successfully controlled by a combined corticosteroid-antifungal (amphotericin B, nystatin) medication, followed by penetrating keratoplasty.

Coriglione et al.[372] have described the first case of mycotic keratitis caused by *Neosartorya fischeri* var. *fischeri*, the teleomorph of *Aspergillus fischerianus*; ketoconazole failed to cure the infection.

37.6.4.2.4   Fluconazole

Oral fluconazole is a well-absorbed antimycotic, with over 70% of the administered dose detected in the serum.[373] The drug also penetrated the peritoneum and CSF in concentrations reaching those found in the serum.

A short-term (15 d) treatment of *A. fumigatus*-induced pneumonia in a previously healthy patient with fluconazole produced clinical cure and regression of infiltrates.[374] Oral fluconazole was given to six patients with chronic pulmonary aspergillosis once daily at 400 mg for periods ranging from 23 to 110 d (70 d on average); a marked contraction of the fungus ball was evidenced in only two patients.[375] Furthermore, successive fluconazole therapy at daily doses of 50, 100, and 400 mg for periods of 4, 6, and 4 weeks, failed to cure two cases of pulmonary aspergillosis.[376]

When administered to cancer patients in high doses, neurologic toxicity by fluconazole was noticed only at daily doses of 2.0 g. The drug was well tolerated at total daily doses of up to 1.6 g (average steady-state peak plasma concentration of 74.4 mg/l).[377]

In a survey of the clinical efficacy and safety of fluconazole involving 34 hospitals, the overall success rate in treatment of pulmonary aspergillosis was 50% (33 of 66 patients).[378]

37.6.4.2.5   Itraconazole

Itraconazole, a newly developed triazole-containing azole antimycotic, is a highly lipophilic substance which, similarly to ketoconazole, is absorbed much better with food. It is poorly soluble in aqueous solutions and produces low serum concentrations (200 to 300 ng/ml after a single 100-mg dose) 2 h after administration. The drug was avidly bound to plasma proteins,[379] and penetrated the urine and CSF at low concentrations. Furthermore, Niwa et al.[380] have observed high concentrations of itraconazole in a case of pulmonary aspergillosis with aspergilloma — the drug when given at 100 mg daily produced plasma concentrations of 249 ng/ml; the concentrations in lung specimens and aspergilloma specimens obtained by thoractomy were 81 ng/g and 837 ng/g, respectively. These high concentrations may be explained with the increased itraconazole levels in purulent fluid, its ability to enter easily the aspergilloma through the root at the cavity wall, and the ability of itraconazole to dissolve in lipid derived from destroyed fungus.[380]

The activity of itraconazole is directed at the fungal cell periphery and cytoplasmic vacuoles in which lipid-like vesicles will assemble.[381] Drug-induced changes in the fungal cell are usually manifested by a marked increase in the cell volume, impaired cell division, and/or abortive hyphal outgrowth. Complete inhibition of the hyphal growth of *A. fumigatus* by itraconazole was achieved at concentrations of ≥ 0.07 μg/ml (10^{-7} *M*).[382]

In a clinical trial conducted by Viviani et al.,[383] 9 of 35 patients with invasive aspergillosis when given itraconazole at doses of 100 to 400 mg were reported cured and another 12 patients showed marked improvement. The same investigators also found that a prolonged medication with itraconazole resulted in remission in 8 of 10 patients.[383] In general, positive responses to treatment of invasive aspergillosis in immunocompromised patients (with leukemia, lymphoma, and heart transplant recipients) were achieved by using relatively high doses of itraconazole (5 mg/kg or no less than 4 mg/kg) at least during the first 60 d of therapy.[383] This information makes it noteworthy to stress the difficulties encountered in evaluating a drug's antifungal efficacy because of the varying clinical characteristics of the infection and the changing immunological status of patients. During therapy, itraconazole was well tolerated and serious side effects have not, so far, been encountered.[231] Kreisel[384] has also recommended mean daily doses of 400 mg itraconazole for treatment of invasive aspergillosis.

The therapeutic efficacy of itraconazole was also evaluated in several studies involving a limited number of patients with pulmonary aspergillosis.[385-389] For example, itraconazole at daily oral doses of 100 to 200 mg was administered over a 5- to 20-month period to four patients with pulmonary aspergillosis.[387] Improvement (as evidenced by computerized tomography, chest roentgenograms, as well as symptomatic) was noticeable in two of the patients. Kramer et al.[388] have observed several cases of deep mucosal ulceration caused by invasive *Aspergillus*-induced tracheobronchitis in patients who received heart-lung and lung transplants — oral therapy with itraconazole was successful in five of six patients. A rare case of chronic pulmonary aspergillosis invading the thoracic wall responded well to itraconazole.[389]

Itraconazole, given once daily (200 to 400 mg) was applied to 49 patients having pulmonary aspergilloma, chronic necrotizing pulmonary aspergillosis and invasive aspergillosis. Overall, the drug showed more efficacy against the invasive and chronic necrotizing pulmonary aspergillosis; in aspergilloma it could be useful in inoperable cases.[390] A case of itraconazole (100 mg daily)-induced hypokalemia (serum potassium level at day 57, 2.33 mEq/l) with pulmonary aspergilloma has been reported — 31 d after discontinuation of therapy, the serum potassium level reached 3.57 mEq/l.[391]

Although surgical removal of endobronchial suture probably constitutes the key therapy for bronchial stump aspergillosis (BSA), Noppen et al.[114] have found oral itraconazole beneficial in effecting clinical, histologic, and microbiologic improvement in three patients with BSA.

A historical comparison of prophylactic treatment of neutropenic patients with itraconazole and ketoconazole has been summarized by Tricot et al.[392] Of the 52 neutropenic patients receiving ketoconazole, 36.5% developed aspergillosis as compared with only 11.5% of the population (a total of 45 patients) receiving prophylactic itraconazole. The drug, at 200 mg daily for 2 to 5 months, cleared the infection or led to a marked improvement in immunocompetent patients with pulmonary aspergillosis.[393]

In another trial conducted by Denning et al.,[394] data were presented on the itraconazole therapy of 21 patients with invasive aspergillosis. Itraconazole was given orally, with 18 of the patients receiving 400 mg daily and the remaining 3, 100 to 200 mg daily; 12 of 15 evaluable patients responded to the treatment. Furthermore, 8 of the responders were immunocompromised (either with neutropenia or renal transplant recipients). The reported side effects of itraconazole were minimal.[394]

In a number of reports,[395-398] itraconazole was found effective in the treatment of *Aspergillus* infections in patients with chronic granulomatous disease. Treatment of one such infection with oral itraconazole at 16 mg/kg led to significant clinical improvement and nearly complete disappearance of intracerebral lesions.[395] The observed toxicity was confined to transient elevation of the alkaline phosphatase and γ-glutamyl transferase.[395] Itraconazole showed better efficacy than either amphotericin B given alone,[397] or combination of amphotericin B and flucytosine.[398] In the latter case, the failure was attributed to cytochrome B deficiency; using itraconazole instead led to considerable improvement in a short period of time.[398]

Aspergillus spp. rarely can cause mycetomata. Witzig et al.[5] have described a patient with diabetes and nephrotic syndrome with *A. flavus* mycetoma of the back, with the development of epidural abscess, diskitis, and vertebral osteomyelitis — decompressive laminectomy and a 14-month course with itraconazole led to clinical cure.

There have been several other examples of clinical application of itraconazole involving individual cases. Thus, the drug was used to stabilize a case of sino-orbital aspergillosis after therapy with miconazole had failed.[399] In a similar report, oral itraconazole was used successfully to treat sino-orbital aspergillosis in an immunocompetent patient after two attempts with traditional therapeutic modalities (surgical debridement and intravenous amphotericin B) had failed.[400] Rowe-Jones and Freedman[401] have successfully treated three cases of destructive sphenoid aspergillosis (two of which had intracranial extension) with surgery and adjuvant itraconazole therapy.

A patient with systemic lupus erythematosus who developed pneumonia caused by *A. fumigatus* rapidly responded to oral itraconazole at 200 mg given twice daily.[123]

Impens et al.[402] described medication with oral itraconazole as an alternative to surgical intervention for the treatment of aspergilloma in a case of necrotic small cell lung cancer. A successful itraconazole therapy of aspergillosis in a cardiac transplant patient has been reported.[403] A deep traumatic keratomycosis with anterior chamber involvement due to *A. fumigatus* infection responded well to oral itraconazole and topical amphotericin B; apparently, itraconazole was able to penetrate both into the deeper layers of the cornea and the anterior chamber.[404] An *A. flavus*-induced onychomycosis was also successfully treated with oral itraconazole.[405]

Sanchez et al.[406] have described a patient with chronic asthma who presented with cerebral abscesses due to *A. fumigatus* after being treated with corticosteroids — therapy with high-dose itraconazole (800 mg daily for 5 months, followed by 400 mg daily for an additional 4.5 months) resulted in complete resolution of all lesions. The use of high-dose itraconazole may prove beneficial for high-risk patients with cerebral aspergillosis for whom conventional therapy had failed.

Other reports involved the clinical use of itraconazole in cases of *Aspergillus* spondylo-discitis.[11,407-409] It included a patient with *A. fumigatus*-induced spondylodiscitis who after lumbar surgery was treated successfully with itraconazole in combination with surgical debridement of the disc space.[407] Early recognition of this condition in immunocompromised hosts combined with itraconazole treatment alone (mean dose, 350 mg daily)[11] or in combination promises to be effective therapy. In another case, a patient with a long-standing ankylosing spondylitis who developed chronic necrotizing pulmonary aspergillosis also responded to medication with itraconazole.[410]

According to Van Cutsem and Cauwenbergh,[411] data from the treatment of 251 evaluable patients with various manifestations of aspergillosis (allergic, aspergilloma, pulmonary, invasive pulmonary, disseminated) receiving a median daily oral dose of 200 mg itraconazole over a period of 91 d (median), have shown a global response between 46% (disseminated aspergillosis) and 74% (allergic aspergillosis), and negative mycology ranging between 25% (disseminated aspergillosis) and 76% (pulmonary aspergillosis). One of the reasons which may explain the observed efficacy of itraconazole in treatment of aspergillosis is its good penetration into tissues and its low MIC value for *Aspergillus*.

Franco et al.[47] have reported a case of *Aspergillus* arthritis of the shoulder in a renal transplant recipient who failed to respond to a single therapy with itraconazole — after initial clinical and roentgenologic improvements, the patient relapsed with a fatal neurologic involvement taking place.

Concomitant administration of itraconazole and digoxin resulted in interaction leading to a statistically significant increase in the half-life of digoxin which necessitated reduction of the digoxin dose by nearly 60% — monitoring the digoxin serum levels may have to be considered and nonspecific gastrointestinal symptoms should be examined carefully since such symptoms may indicate early digoxin toxicity.[412]

37.6.4.3   Terbinafine

Schiraldi et al.[413,414] have evaluated on a compassionate basis the clinical efficacy of terbinafine, a new allylamine antimycotic, in three immunocompetent patients affected by lower respiratory tract aspergillosis (one chronic empyema, and two chronic necrotizing aspergillosis) and not responsive to conventional antifungal therapies. The patients received terbinafine at daily doses ranging from 5.0 to 15 mg/kg according to their clinical status, for 3 to 5 months depending on the clinical course of the disease and compliance.[413] At completion of therapy, one patient showed a negative anti-*A. fumigatus* precipitin together with eradication of the pathogen from the pleural cavity, which allowed a successful intrathoracic myo-omento-mammoplasty. In the other two patients, the fungus was also eradicated, the anti-*A. fumigatus* immunoprecipitins decreased, and clinical and radiologic findings significantly improved.

37.6.4.4 Sodium (Potassium) Iodide Therapy of Aspergilloma

Oral administration of 24 to 30 g of potassium iodide to two patients with pulmonary aspergilloma was found to be therapeutically effective.[415] However, the presence of electrolytic imbalance (hypokalemia, elevation of serum carbon dioxide content, hyponatremia, hypocalcemia, and hypophosphatemia) resulting from the ingestion of large doses of iodide should preclude any casual approach to such treatment.

Ramirez[416] described as successful the therapy of two patients with symptomatic pulmonary aspergilloma by repeated endobronchial administration of amphotericin B and sodium iodide (total of 580 and 1200 mg, respectively) for periods of 29 d and 3 months, respectively. In another case, 2% aqueous sodium iodide (total of 30 g for 29 d) was initiated 2 months after treatment with amphotericin B was completed.[416] The results suggested a more effective iodide therapy than amphotericin B in the management of pulmonary aspergilloma.[416]

Adelson and Malcolm[417] also described as successful the treatment of mycetoma in one patient by applying percutaneous catheter for endocavitary instillation of sodium iodide; in this particular case, surgical excision was not recommended since the aspergilloma was superimposed on sarcoidosis.

37.6.4.5 Therapy of Allergic Bronchopulmonary Aspergillosis (ABPA)

Early diagnosis and treatment of allergic bronchopulmonary aspergillosis (ABPA) is essential since inflammatory damage to the airways may be significantly reduced through the use of corticosteroids. If ABPA is left untreated, bronchiectasis causing permanent anatomic alteration of the airways may develop.[418] Successful therapy of ABPA is typically associated with a decline in total serum IgE.

Chronic uncontrolled ABPA is well known to cause extensive lung destruction as a result of type III immune response to *Aspergillus* antigen in the airways. Consequently, the reduction of antigen by antifungal therapy may lead to containment of lung damage, thereby limiting the progression of the disease. Shale et al.[419] conducted a 1-year trial using ketoconazole in 10 patients with ABPA. The medication included 400 mg daily of the drug or placebo given orally in a double-blind fashion. In the treated group (six patients), concentrations of serum IgG specific for *A. fumigatus* were reduced significantly (mean change of 42%); by comparison, the remaining four patients who received placebo showed no meaningful change in their serum IgG concentrations (mean change of 10%).

In recent years, corticosteroid therapy of ABPA has emerged as the more successful approach for management of this condition. It is generally accepted that corticosteroids such as prednisolone and triamcinolone would likely act by suppressing the allergic inflammatory reactions and by decreasing the sputum production, thus making the bronchus less vulnerable to further fungal colonization.[420-422] For instance, when prednisolone was given at daily doses of ≥7.5 mg, it reduced the number of cases of recurrent consolidation.[422] The inhalation of corticosteroids is considered to be less efficient because of the presence of mucus plugging and obstruction, two common symptoms of ABPA.[423]

Corticosteroid drugs have been also applied to patients with symptoms of *Aspergillus* allergy (or classic ABPA) coexisting with aspergilloma.[424] A combination of ABPA with aspergilloma was treated with prednisolone with considerable improvement.[425] Davies and Somner[426] used prednisolone therapy to treat two cases of pulmonary aspergilloma following the failure of antibiotics and brilliant green to cure the disease. Since in both patients the reduction in purulent sputum was significant, it was postulated that prednisolone acted on a type III or an Arthus-type immune response involving antibody-antigen reaction in the cavity wall. While Arthus reaction is commonly associated with ABPA, experimental evidence by Stevens et al.[427] lent support to the notion that in patients with aspergilloma, type III immune response may develop in the absence of clinical type I allergy.

Slavin et al.[428] treated two patients with ABPA with combination of oral corticosteroids and inhalation of amphotericin B. The therapy resulted in significant improvement as manifested by the clearing of pulmonary infiltrates, decrease in eosinophilia, weight gain, increase in vital capacity, negative sputum culture of *Aspergillus*, and the disappearance of precipitating antibody.

Recently, itraconazole was studied for its efficacy against ABPA.[385] Twice daily administration of 200 mg of the drug to patients for periods ranging from 1 to 6 months (mean 3.9 months) led, in general, to improvement of the pulmonary function with mean forced expiratory volume (FEV) increasing from 1.43 to 1.77 l/s, and mean forced vital capacity (FVC) increasing from 2.3 to 2.9 l in those treated for 2 months or longer. The mean steady-state serum concentration of itraconazole was 5.1 μg/ml.[385]

Currently, for treatment of ABPA the inhalation of aerosolized amphotericin B,[429] nystatin,[430] natamycin,[431] or clotrimazole[432] has seen rather limited use because of frequent relapses that require repeated applications.[433] Radha and Viswanathan[434] described the treatment of seven patients with ABPA with hamycin, a polyene antibiotic isolated from *Streptomyces pimprina thirum*. The drug, which was administered at a dose of 25 mg, four times daily for 10 d, was reported efficacious and led to a marked alleviation of subjective symptoms and absence of fungus in the sputum.

In order to assess the steroid paring potential of natamycin, Currie et al.[435] conducted a controlled double-blind trial of 20 patients with ABPA. The patients, already on a maintenance oral therapy with corticosteroids, were given 5.0 mg of natamycin or placebo by nebulizer twice daily for 1 year; standardized reductions in the corticosteroid dosage were undertaken every 5 weeks unless clinically contraindicated. The results showed no evidence of beneficial effect for natamycin.

Among other forms of treatment of ABPA,[436] immunotherapy through intradermal hypo-sensitization has had little success.[421] Similarly, medication with sodium chromoglycate, while ameliorating asthmatic symptoms, did not prevent recurrence in episodes of pulmonary infiltration of the fungal pathogen.[422]

37.6.4.6   Therapy of Aspergillus-Induced Otomycosis

Of all *Aspergillus* spp., *A. niger* has been most commonly associated with *Aspergillus*-induced otitis externa. The latter condition is characterized with ear pain and hearing loss due to canal occlusion.[437,438] In addition, the external ear canal may also contain a black mass of moldy growth.

Local therapy of otomycosis may include the use of cresylate, alcohol, nystatin, amphotericin B, thymol, and gentian violet. Bezjak and Arya[439] treated five patients with topical nystatin ointment for 3 to 4 weeks, with clinical cure seen in three patients. In another case report,[440] dusting with nystatin powder (in combination with boric acid) was applied three times weekly for at least 3 weeks.

Iodochlorhydroxyquine (as a powder) was found to be very effective when applied by insufflation into the infected auditory canal after removal of fungal growth; the treatment was followed by a regimen involving thrice daily application of 3% iodochlorhydroxyquine lotion in the ear canal for 1 week.[441] A combination of iodochlorhydroxyquine (1% in propylene glycol) with the corticosteroid flumethazone (0.02%) was also used to treat *Aspergillus*-induced otomycosis.[442]

According to Than et al.,[443] 10% 5-fluorocytosine ointment was most effective in treating *Aspergillus* otitis externa. Previously, Schoneback and Zakrisson[444] and Youssef and Abdou[445] have described the topical application of 5-fluorocytosine ointment as effective in treating otomycosis caused by *A. niger* — as many as 60% of all patients were reported cured.

Amphotericin B was found by McGonigle and Jillson[441] to be a useful alternative in the therapy of *Aspergillus* otomycosis when applied topically as 3% solution (a three-drop dose). With other antibiotics such as oxytetracycline-polymyxin itic, complete cure of otomycosis was registered in 70% of the treated cases.[437]

The use of nitrofungin and clotrimazole in combination with 1% decamine ointment in the treatment of *A. niger*-induced otomycosis, has been described.[446] Molina Utrilla et al.[447] have compared the efficacy of iodine-povidone, clotrimazole, and ciclopiroxolamine in the treatment of *Aspergillus*-induced otomycosis.

A. flavus, an unusual cause of malignant otitis, was identified in pure culture of tissue from two patients in which histologic examination revealed branching septate hyphae invading the temporal bone.[10] Treatment with amphotericin B, followed by a more protracted course of itraconazole, resulted in an apparent cure.

A case of *A. terreus*-induced chronic bilateral suppurative otitis media presenting with otorrheoa, itching, mild deafness, heaviness in the ear, and otalgia, has been reported by Tiwari et al.[20] — the infection responded well to topical ketoconazole therapy.

37.6.4.7 Therapy of *Aspergillus*-Induced Onychomycosis

In addition to dermatophytes and yeast fungi, *A. niger* and *A. fumigatus* were among several other pathogens (*Scopulariopsis brevicaulis*, *Hendersonula toruloidea*) implicated in human onychomycosis. Ulbricht and Worz[448] used topical 8% ciclopirox nail lacquer for a maximum of 6 months to achieve mycologic cure.

37.6.5 *ASPERGILLUS CHEVALIERI*

Naidu and Singh[26] have described the first three cases of cutaneous aspergillosis caused by *Aspergillus chevalieri*, a new opportunistic pathogen of human disease. The observed lesions were erythematous and hyperkeratotic with vesicopapular eruptions and scaling. Histopathologic examination revealed a granulomatous reaction showing polymorphonuclear leukocytes around the fungal hyphae, which were broad, septate, branched, and aggregated in the epidermal area.

In vitro, after 48 h of incubation, amphotericin B, 5-fluorocytosine, ketoconazole, oxiconazole, and the allylamine derivative, amorolfine, showed MIC values against a clinical isolate of *A. chevalieri* of 0.1, 0.1, 1.0, 0.1, and 0.3 μg/ml, respectively.[26]

37.6.6 REFERENCES

1. Emmons, C. W., Binford, C. H., and Utz, J. P., *Medical Mycology*, 2nd ed., Lea and Febiger, Philadelphia, 256. 1970,
2. Renon, L., *Etude Sur l'Aspergillose Chez Les Animaux et Chex l'Home*, Masson, Paris, 1897.
3. Evans, E. G. V., Watson, D. A., and Matthews, N. R., Pulmonary aspergilloma in a child treated with clotrimazole, *Br. Med. J.*, 4, 599, 1971.
4. McCarthy, D. S. and Pepys, J., Pulmonary aspergilloma: clinical immunology, *Clin. Allergy*, 3, 57, 1973.
5. Witzig, R. S., Greer, D. L., and Hyslop, N. E., Jr., *Aspergillus flavus* mycetoma and epidural abscess successfully treated with itraconazole, *J. Med. Vet. Mycol.*, 34, 133, 1996.
6. Yamamoto, K., Abe, M., Inoue, Y., Yokoyama, A. et al., Development of infection with *Aspergillus flavus* in a woman being treated for allergic pulmonary aspergillosis caused by *Aspergillus fumigatus*, *Nippon Kyobu Shikkan Gakkai Zasshi*, 33, 1099, 1995.
7. Khan, Z. U., Gopalakrishnan, G., al-Awadi, K., Gupta, R. K., Moussa, S. A., Chugh, T. D., and Krajci, D., Renal aspergilloma due to *Aspergillus flavus*, *Clin. Infect. Dis.*, 21, 210, 1995.
8. Liu, Z., Hou, T., Shen, Q., Liao, W., and Xu, H., Osteomyelitis of sacral spine caused by *Aspergillus versicolor* with neurologic defects, *Chin. Med. J.*, 108, 472, 1995.
9. Matsuo, T., Nakagawa, H., and Matsuo, N., Endogenous *Aspergillus* endophthalmitis associated with periodontitis, *Ophthalmologica*, 209, 109, 1995.
10. Gordon, G. and Giddings, N. A., Invasive otitis externa due to *Aspergillus* species: case report and review, *Clin. Infect. Dis.*, 19, 866, 1994.

11. Cortet, B., Richard, R., Deprez, X., Lucet, L., Flipo, R. M., Le Loet, X., Duquesnoy, B., and Delcambre, B., Aspergillus spondylodiscitis: successful conservative treatment in 9 cases, *J. Rheumatol.*, 21, 1287, 1994.

12. Hovi, L., Saarinen, U. M., Donner, U., and Lindqvist, C., Opportunistic osteomyelitis in the jaws of children on immunosuppressive chemotherapy, *J. Pediatr. Hematol. Oncol.*, 18, 90, 1996.

13. Estes, S. A., Hendricks, A. A., and Merz, W. G., Primary cutaneous aspergillosis, *J. Am. Acad. Dermatol.*, 3, 397, 1980.

14. Prystowsky, S. D., Yogelstein, B., and Ettinger, D. S., Invasive aspergillosis, *N. Engl. J. Med.*, 295, 655, 1976.

15. Lonneux, M., Nolard, N., Philippart, I., Henkinbrant, A., Hamels, J., Fastrez, J., and d'Odermont, J. P., A case of lymphocytic pneumonitis, myositis, and arthritis associated with exposure to *Aspergillus niger*, *J. Allergy Clin. Immunol.*, 95, 1047, 1995.

16. Niki, Y., Hashiguchi, K., Tamada, S., Yoshida, K. et al., A case of *Aspergillus niger* pneumonia cured with an early diagnosis, *Kansenshogaku Zasshi*, 68, 788, 1994.

17. English, M. P., Invasion of the skin by filamentous nondermatophyte fungi, *Br. J. Dermatol.*, 80, 282, 1968.

18. Leyden, J. J., Infection in the immunocompromised hosts, *Arch. Dermatol.*, 121, 855, 1985.

19. Weizman, I., Saprophytic molds as agents of cutaneous and subcutaneous infection in the immunocompromised host, *Arch. Dermatol.*, 122, 1161, 1986.

20. Tiwari, S., Singh, S. M., and Jain, S., Chronic bilateral suppurative otitis media caused by *Aspergillus terreus*, *Mycoses*, 38, 297, 1995.

21. Goldberg, S. L., Geha, D. J., Marshall, W. F., Inwards, D. J., and Hoagland, H. C., Successful treatment of simultaneous pulmonary *Pseudallescheria boydii* and *Aspergillus terreus* infection with oral itraconazole, *Clin. Infect. Dis.*, 16, 803, 1993.

22. Suscelan, A. V., Gugnani, H. C., and Ujukwu, J. O., Primary cutaneous aspergillosis due to *Aspergillus terreus*, *Arch. Dermatol.*, 112, 1468, 1976.

23. Sukroongreung, S. and Thakernogpol, S., Abnormal form of *Aspergillus terreus* isolated from mycotic abscesses, *Mycopathologia*, 91, 47, 1985.

24. Naidu, J., Singh, S. M., and Pouranik, M., Cutaneous aspergillosis due to *Aspergillus terreus* and *Aspergillus candidus*, *Biome*, 5, 101, 1992.

25. Fragner, P. and Kubickova, V., Onychomykoza vyvolna *Aspergillus candidus*, *Dermatologica*, 49, 322, 1974.

26. Naidu, J. and Singh, S. M., *Aspergillus chevalieri* (Mangin) Thom and Church: a new opportunistic pathogen of human cutaneous aspergillosis, *Mycoses*, 37, 271, 1994.

27. Stiller, M. J., Teperman, L., Rosenthal S. A., Riordan, A., Potter, J., Shupack, J. L., and Gordon, M. A., Primary cutaneous infection by *Aspergillus ustus* in a 62-year-old liver transplant recipient, *J. Am. Acad. Dermatol.*, 31, 344, 1994.

28. Jordan, F. T. W., Diseases of poultry, *Br. Vet.*, 137, 545, 1981.

29. Rippon, J. W., Ed., *Medical Mycology: The Pathogenic Fungi and the Pathogenic Actinomycetes*, W. B. Saunders, Philadelphia, 1982, 565.

30. Scholer, H. J., Chemotherapie der Aspergillenkrankheiten der Lunge, *Mykosen*, 26, 173, 1983.

31. Tronchin, G., Esnault, K., Renier, G., Filmon, R. et al., Expression and identification of a laminin-binding protein in *Aspergillus fumigatus* conidia, *Infect. Immun.*, 65, 9, 1997.

32. Bromley, I. M. and Donaldson, K., Binding of *Aspergillus fumigatus* spores to lung epithelial cells and basement membrane proteins: relevance to the asthmatic lung, *Thorax*, 51, 1203, 1996.

33. Gil, M. L., Penalver, M. C., Lopez-Ribot, J. L., O'Connor, J. E., and Martinez, J. P., Binding of extracellular matrix proteins to *Aspergillus fumigatus* conidia, *Infect. Immun.*, 64, 5239, 1996.

34. DeHart, D. J., Agwu, D. E., Julian, N. C., and Washburn, R. G., Binding and germination of *Aspergillus fumigatus* conidia on cultured A549 pneumocytes, *J. Infect. Dis.*, 175, 146, 1997.

35. Sutton, P., Waring, P., and Mullbacher, A., Exacerbation of invasive aspergillosis by the immunosuppressive fungal metabolite, gliotoxin, *Immunol. Cell. Biol.*, 74, 318, 1996.

36. Sugimura, S., Yoshida, K., Oba, H., Hashiguchi, K., Nakajima, M., Moriya, O., Okimoto, N., Niki, Y., and Soejima, R., Two cases of invasive pulmonary aspergillosis in non-immunocompromised hosts, *Nippon Kyobu Shikkan Gakkai Zasshi*, 32, 1032, 1994.

37. Muller, M., Fallen, H., and Zoller, I., Pulmonary aspergillosis in an immunocompetent female patient, *Dtsch. Med. Wochenschr.*, 119, 760, 1994 (see also *Dtsch. Med. Wochenschr.*, 119, 1716, 1994).
38. Valluri, S., Moorthy, R. S., Liggett, P. E., and Rao, N. A., Endogeneous *Aspergillus* endophthalmitis in an immunocompetent individual, *Int. Ophthalmol.*, 17, 131, 1993.
39. Nucci, M., Pulcheri, W., Bacha, P. C., Spector, N., Cainby, M. J., Costa, R. O., and de Oliveira, H. P., Amphotericin B followed by itraconazole in the treatment of disseminated fungal infections in neutropenic patients, *Mycoses*, 37, 433, 1994.
40. Hadley, S. and Karchmer, A. W., Fungal infections in solid organ transplant recipients, *Infect. Dis. Clin. North Am.*, 9, 1045, 1995.
41. Marks, W. H., Florence, L., Lieberman, J., Chapman, P., Howard, D., Roberts, P., and Perkinson, D., Successfully treated invasive pulmonary aspergillosis associated with smoking marijuana in a renal transplant recipient, *Transplantation*, 61, 1771, 1996.
42. Bowden, R. A., Cays, M., Gooley, T., Mamelok, R. D., and van Burik, J. A., Phase I study of amphotericin B colloidal dispersion for the treatment of invasive fungal infections after marrow transplant, *J. Infect. Dis.*, 173, 1208, 1996.
43. Warnock, D. W., Fungal complications of transplantation: diagnosis, treatment and prevention, *J. Antimicrob. Chemother.*, 36(Suppl. B), 73, 1995.
44. Kruger, W., Stockschläder, M., Rüssmann, B., Berger, C., Hoffknecht, M., Sobottka, I., Kohlschütter, B., Kroschke, G., Kröger, N., Horstmann, M., Kabisch, H., and Zander, A. R., Experience with liposomal amphotericin B in 60 patients undergoing high-dose therapy and bone marrow or peripheral blood stem cell transplantation, *Br. J. Haematol.*, 91, 684, 1995.
45. Choi, S. S., Milmoe, G. J., Dinndorf, P. A., and Quinones, R. R., Invasive *Aspergillus* sinusitis in pediatric bone marrow transplant patient: evaluation and management, *Arch. Otolaryngol. Head Neck Surg.*, 121, 1188, 1995.
46. Cassuto-Viguier, E., Mondain, J. R., Van Elslande, L., Bendini, J. C., Gaid, H., Franco, M., and Gari-Toussaint, M., Fatal outcome of *Aspergillus fumigatus* arthritis in a renal transplant recipient, *Transplant. Proc.*, 27, 2461, 1995.
47. Franco, M., Van Elslande, L., Robino, C., Gari-Toussaint, M., Bendini, C., Barillon, D., Mondain, J. R., Bracco, J., Padovani, B., and Cassuto-Viguier, E., Aspergillus arthritis of the shoulder in a renal transplant recipient: failure of itraconazole therapy, *Rev. Rhum. Engl. Ed.*, 62, 215, 1995.
48. Hagensee, M. E., Bauwens, J. E., Kjos, B., and Bowden, R. A., Brain abscess following marrow transplantation: experience at the Fred Hutchinson Cancer Research Center, 1984–1992, *Clin. Infect. Dis.*, 19, 402, 1994.
49. Collins, L. A., Samore, M. H., Roberts, M. S., Luzzati, R., Jenkins, R. L., Lewis, W. D., and Karchmer, A. W., Risk factors for invasive fungal infections complicating orthotopic liver transplantation, *J. Infect. Dis.*, 170, 644, 1994.
50. Wang, S. S., Chu, S. H., Lee, Y. C., Chang, S. C., and Yang, P. C., Successful treatment of invasive pulmonary aspergillosis, *Transplant. Proc.*, 26, 2329, 1994.
51. Saah, D., Drakos, P. E., Elidan, J., Braverman, I., Or, R., and Nagler, A., Rhinocerebral aspergillosis in patients undergoing bone marrow transplantation, *Ann. Otol. Rhinol. Laryngol.*, 103, 306, 1994.
52. O'Donnell, M. R., Schmidt, G. M., Tegmeier, B. R., Faucett, C., Fahey, J. L., Ito, J., Nademanee, A., Niland, J., Parker, P., Smith, E. P., Snyder, D. S., Stein, A. S., Blume, K. G., and Forman, S. J., Prediction of systemic fungal infection in allogeneic marrow recipients: impact of amphotericin prophylaxis in high-risk patients, *J. Clin. Oncol.*, 12, 827, 1994.
53. McWhinney, P. H., Kibbler, C. C., Hamon, M. D., Smith, O. P., Gandhi, L., Berger, L. A., Walesby, R. K., Hoffbrand, A. V., and Prentice, H. C., Progress in the diagnosis and management of aspergillosis in bone marrow transplantation: 13 years' experience, *Clin. Infect. Dis.*, 17, 397, 1993.
54. Holt, R. I., Kwan, J. T., Sefton, A. M., and Cunningham, J., Successful treatment of concomitant pulmonary nocardiosis and aspergillosis in an immunocompromised renal patient, *Eur. J. Clin. Microbiol. Infect. Dis.*, 12, 110, 1993.
55. Paya, C. V., Fungal infections in solid-organ transplantations, *Clin. Infect. Dis.*, 16, 677, 1993.
56. Monteforte, J. S. and Wood, C. A., Pneumonia caused by *Nocardia nova* and *Aspergillus fumigatus* after cardiac transplantation, *Eur. J. Clin. Microbiol. Infect. Dis.*, 12, 112, 1993.

57. Yeldandi, V., Laghi, F., McCabe, M. A., Larson, R., O'Keefe, P., Husain, A., Montoya, A., and Garrity, E. R., Jr., Aspergillus and lung transplantation, *J. Heart Lung Transplant.*, 14, 883, 1995.
58. Tomee, J. F., Mannes, G. P., van der Bij, W., van der Werf, T. S., Deboer, W. J., Koeter, G. H., and Kauffman, H. F., Serodiagnosis and monitoring of *Aspergillus* infections after lung transplantation, *Ann. Intern. Med.*, 125, 197, 1996.
59. Heurlin, N., Bergstrom, S. E., Winiarski, J., Ringdén, O., Ljungman, P., Lönnqvist, B., and Andersson, J., Fungal pneumonia: the predominant lung infection causing death in children undergoing bone marrow transplantation, *Acta Paediatr.*, 85, 168, 1996.
60. Mannes, G. P., van der Bij, W., and de Boer, W. J., Liposomal amphotericin B in three lung transplant recipients, *J. Heart Lung Transplant.*, 14, 781, 1995.
61. Flume, P. A., Egan, T. M., Paradowski, L. J., Detterbeck, F. C., Thompson, J. T., and Yankaskas, J. R., Infectious complications of lung transplantation: impact of cystic fibrosis, *Am. J. Respir. Crit. Care Med.*, 149, 1601, 1994.
62. Berner, R., Sauter, S., Michalski, Y., and Niemeyer, C. M., Central venous catheter infection by *Aspergillus fumigatus* in a patient with B-type non-Hodgkin lymphoma, *Med. Pediatr. Oncol.*, 27, 202, 1996.
63. Meyohas, M. C., Roux, P., Poirot, J. L., Meynard, J. L., and Frottier, J., Aspergillosis in acquired immunodeficiency syndrome, *Pathol. Biol. (Paris)*, 42, 647, 1994.
64. Keating, J. J., Rogers, T., Petrou, M., Cartledge, J. D., Woodrow, D., Nelson, M., Hawkins, D. A., and Gazzard, B. G., Management of pulmonary aspergillosis in AIDS: an emerging clinical problem, *J. Clin. Pathol.*, 47, 805, 1994.
65. Libanore, M., Pastore, A., Frasconi, P. C., Rossi, M. R., Bedetti, A., Sighinolfi, L., and Ghinelli, F., Invasive multiple sinusitis by *Aspergillus fumigatus* in a patient with AIDS, *Int. J. STD AIDS*, 5, 293, 1994.
66. Tumbarello, M., Ventura, G., Caldarola, G., Morace, G., Cauda, R., and Ortona, L., An emerging opportunistic infection in HIV patients: a retrospective analysis of 11 cases of pulmonary aspergillosis, *Eur. J. Epidemiol.*, 9, 638, 1993.
67. Lortholary, O., Meyohas, M. C., Dupont, B., Cadranel, J., Salmon-Ceron, D., Peyramond, D., Simonin, D., and Centre d'Informations et de Soins de l'Immunodéficience Humain de l'Est Parisien, for the French Cooperative Study Group on Aspergillosis in AIDS, Invasive aspergillosis in patients with acquired immunodeficiency syndrome: report of 33 cases, *Am. J. Med.*, 95, 177, 1993.
68. Le Conte, P., Blanloeil, Y., Germaud, P., Morin, O., and Moreau, P., Invasive aspergillosis in intensive care, *Ann. Fr. Anesth. Reanim.*, 14, 198, 1995 (see also *Ann. Fr. Anesth. Reanim.*, 14, 454, 1995).
69. Blanloeil, Y., Francois, T., Germaud, P., Le Conte, P., Morin, O., Michel, P., Levron, J. C., and Dixneuf, B., Invasive aspergillosis in surgical intensive care patients, *Ann. Fr. Anesth. Reanim.*, 12, 379, 1993.
70. Pouchelon, E., Murris-Espin, M., Didier, A., Rouquet, R. M., Carré, P., Carré, A. M., and Léophonte, P., Invasive pulmonary aspergillosis in 4 patients with acute decompensation of chronic respiratory insufficiency, *Rev. Mal. Respir.*, 10, 325, 1993.
71. Bodey, G. P. and Vartivarian, S., Aspergillosis, *Eur. J. Clin. Microbiol. Infect.*, 8, 413, 1989.
72. Pittet, D., Huguenin, T., Dharan, S., Sztajzel-Boissard, J., Ducel, G., Thorens, J.-B., Auckenthaler, R., and Chevrolet, J.-C., Unusual cause of lethal pulmonary aspergillosis in patients with chronic obstructive pulmonary disease, *Am. J. Respir. Crit. Care Med.*, 154, 541, 1996.
73. Logan, P. M. and Muller, N. L., High-resolution computed tomography and pathologic findings in pulmonary aspergillosis: a pictorial essay, *Can. Assoc. Radiol. J.*, 47, 444, 1996.
74. Morin, O. and Germaud, P., Invasive pulmonary aspergillosis, *Rev. Prat.*, 39, 1669, 1989.
75. Fisher, B. D., Armstrong, D., Yu, B., and Gold, J. W. M., Invasive aspergillosis: progress in early diagnosis and treatment, *Am. J. Med.*, 71, 571, 1981.
76. Herbert, P. A. and Bayer, A. S., Fungal pneumonia. IV. Invasive pulmonary aspergillosis, *Chest*, 80, 220, 1981.
77. Glimp, R. A. and Bayer, A. S., Pulmonary aspergilloma: diagnostic and therapeutic consideration, *Arch. Intern. Med.*, 143, 303, 1983.
78. Hunt, W., Broders, A. C., Jr., Stinson, J. C., and Carabasi, R. J., Primary pulmonary aspergillosis with invasion of the mediastinal contents and lymph nodes, *Am. Rev. Respir. Dis.*, 83, 886, 1961.
79. Fischer, J. J. and Walker, D. H., Invasive pulmonary aspergillosis associated with influenza, *JAMA*, 241, 1493, 1979.

80. Emmons, R. W., Able, M. E., Tenenberg, D. J., and Schachter, J., Fatal pulmonary psittacosis and aspergillosis — case report of dual infection, *Arch. Intern. Med.*, 140, 697, 1980.

81. Rodenhuis, S., Beaumont, F., Kauffman, H. F., and Sluiter, H. J., Invasive pulmonary aspergillosis in a nonimmunosuppressed patient: successful management with systemic amphotericin and flucytosine and inhaled amphotericin, *Thorax*, 39, 78, 1984.

82. Young, R. C., Bennett, J. E., Vogel, C. L., Carbone, P. P., and DeVita, V. T., *Aspergillus* — the spectrum of the disease in 98 patients, *Medicine (Baltimore)*, 49, 107, 1970.

83. Meyer, R. D., Young, L. S., Armstrong, D., and Yu, B., Aspergillosis complicating neoplastic disease, *Am. J. Med.*, 54, 6, 1973.

84. Merino, J. M., Diaz, M. A., Ramirez, M., Ruano, D., and Madero, L., Complicated pulmonary aspergillosis with pneumothorax and pneumopericardium in a child with acute lymphoblastic leukemia, *Pediatr. Hematol. Oncol.*, 12, 195, 1995.

85. Hospenthal, D. R., Byrd, J. C., and Weiss, R. B., Successful treatment of invasive aspergillosis complicating prolonged treatment-related neutropenia in acute myelogenous leukemia with amphotericin B lipid complex, *Med. Pediatr. Oncol.*, 25, 119, 1995.

86. Caillot, D., Durand, C., Casasnovas, O., Couaillier, J. F., Bernard, A., Buisson, M., Solary, E., Brachet, A., Cuisenier, B., Bonnin, A., Debuche, V., De Montaignac, A., Magnin, G., Arnoult, L., Petrella, T., and Guy, H., Invasive pulmonary aspergillosis in neutropenic patients. Analysis of a series of 36 cases: contribution of thoracic scanners and itraconazole, *Ann. Med. Interne (Paris)*, 146, 84, 1995.

87. von Eiff, M., Zuhlsdorf, M., Roos, N., Hesse, M., Schulten, R., and van de Loo, J., Pulmonary fungal infections in patients with hematological malignancies — diagnostic approaches, *Ann. Hematol.*, 70, 135, 1995.

88. Hernandez, J. M., Martin-Sanchez, A. M., de Arriba, F., Caballero, M. D., and San Miguel, J. F., Invasive aspergillosis in patients with malignant hemopathies: usefulness of direct and serologic diagnosis, *Sangre (Barcelona)*, 38, 283, 1993.

89. Burton, J. R., Zachery, J. B., Bessin, R., Rathbun, H. K., Greenough, W. B. III, Sterioff, S., Wright, J. R., Slavin, R. E., and Williams, G. M., Aspergillosis in four renal transplant recipients — diagnosis and effective treatment with amphotericin B, *Ann. Intern. Med.*, 77, 383, 1982.

90. Stinson, E. B., Bieber, C. P., Griepp, R. B., Clark, D. A., Shumway, N.E., and Remington, J. S., Infectious complications after cardiac transplantation in man, *Ann. Intern. Med.*, 74, 22, 1971.

91. Armstrong, D., Life-threatening opportunistic fungal infections in patients with the acquired immunodeficiency syndrome, *Ann. NY Acad. Sci.*, 544, 443, 1988.

92. Conesa, D., Rello, J., Valles, J., Mariscal, D., and Ferreres, J. C., Invasive aspergillosis: a life-threatening complication of short-term treatment, *Ann. Pharmacother.*, 29, 1235, 1995.

93. Bodey, G. P., Fungal infections in cancer patients, *Ann. NY Acad. Sci.*, 544, 431, 1988.

94. Smeenk, F. W., Klinkhamer, P. J., Breed, W., Jansz, A. R., and Jansveld, C. A., Opportunistic lung infections in patients with chronic obstructive lung disease: a side effect of inhalation corticosteroids? *Ned. Tijdschr. Geneeskd.*, 140, 94, 1996.

95. Milesi-Lecat, A. M., Aumaitre, O., Deusebis, T., Kaufman, P., Tridon, A., Cambon, M., and Marcheuix, J.-C., Semi-invasive diffuse pulmonary aspergillosis with antineutrophil cytoplasmic antibodies: 2 cases, *Ann. Med. Interne (Paris)*, 145, 140, 1994.

96. Zhaoming, W. and Lockey, R. P., A review of allergic bronchopulmonary aspergillosis, *J. Investig. Allergol. Clin. Immunol.*, 6, 144, 1996.

97. Rothe, T. B. and Radvila, A., Spontaneous course of allergic bronchopulmonary aspergillosis, *Schweiz. Med. Wochenschr.*, 124, 1895, 1994.

98. Glimp, R. A. and Bayer, A. S., Fungal pneumonias. III. Allergic bronchopulmonary aspergillosis, *Chest*, 80, 85, 1981.

99. Safirstein, B. H., Aspergilloma consequent to allergic bronchopulmonary aspergillosis, *Am. Rev. Respir. Dis.*, 108, 940, 1983.

100. Hinson, K. F. W., Moon, A. J., and Plummer, N. S., Bronchopulmonary aspergillosis, *Thorax*, 7, 317, 1952.

101. Egan, J. J., Yonan, N., Carroll, K. B., Delraniya, A. K., Webb, A. K., and Woodcock, A. A., Allergic bronchopulmonary aspergillosis in lung allograft recipients, *Eur. Respir. J.*, 9, 169, 1996.

102. Meyer, A. and Kirsten, D., Diagnosis of ABPA during a life-threatening asthma attack, *Pneumologie*, 50, 428, 1996.

103. Rose, H. and Hirsch, S. R., Filtering hospital air decreases *Aspergillus* spore counts, *Am. Rev. Respir. Dis.*, 114, 511, 1979.

104. Sessa, A., Meroni, M., Battini, G., Pitingolo, F., Giordano, F., Marks, M., and Casella, P., Nosocomial outbreak of *Aspergillus fumigatus* infection among patients in a renal unit? *Nephrol. Dial. Transplant.*, 11, 1322, 1996.

105. Krasnick, J., Greenberger, P. A., Roberts, M., and Patterson, R., Allergic bronchopulmonary aspergillosis: serologic update for 1995, *J. Clin. Lab. Immunol.*, 46, 137, 1995.

106. Rosenberg, M., Patterson, R., and Mintzer, R., Clinical and immunologic criteria for the diagnosis of allergic bronchopulmonary aspergillosis, *Ann. Intern. Med.*, 86, 405, 1977.

107. Chan-Yeung, M., Chase, W. H., Trapp, W., and Grzybowski, S., Allergic bronchopulmonary aspergillosis: clinical and pathologic study of three cases, *Chest*, 59, 33, 1971.

108. Marx, J. J., Jr. and Flaherty, D. K., Activation of the complement sequence by extracts of bacteria and fungi associated with hypersensitivity pneumonitis, *J. Allergy Clin. Immunol.*, 57, 328, 1976.

109. Mroueh, S. and Spock, A., Allergic bronchopulmonary aspergillosis in patients with cystic fibrosis, *Chest*, 105, 32, 1994 (see also *Chest*, 107, 883, 1995).

110. Merchant, J. L., Warner, J. O., and Bush, A., Rise in total IgE as an indicator of allergic bronchopulmonary aspergillosis in cystic fibrosis, *Thorax*, 49, 1002, 1994.

111. Greene, R., The pulmonary aspergilloses: three distinct entities or a spectrum of disease, *Radiology*, 140, 527, 1981.

112. Ganassini, A. and Cazzadori, A., Invasive pulmonary aspergillosis complicating allergic bronchopulmonary aspergillosis, *Respir. Med.*, 89, 143, 1995.

113. Shah, A., Bhagat, R., Panchal, N., Jaggi, O. P., and Khan, Z. U., Allergic bronchopulmonary aspergillosis with middle lobe syndrome and allergic *Aspergillus* sinusitis, *Eur. Respir. J.*, 6, 917, 1993.

114. Noppen, M., Claes, I., Maillet, B., Meysman, M., Monsieur, I., and Vincken, W., Three cases of bronchial stump aspergillosis: unusual clinical presentations and beneficial effect of oral itraconazole, *Eur. Respir. J.*, 8, 477, 1995.

115. Kwon-Chung, K. J. and Bennett, J. E., *Medical Mycology*, Lea and Febiger, Philadelphia, 1992, 217.

116. de Aquino, M. Z., Brasciner, A., Cristofani, L. M., Maluf, P. T., Odone Filho, V., Marques, H. H. de S., Heins-Vaccari, E. M., Lacaz, C. da S., and de Mello, N. T., Aspergillosis in immunocompromised children with acute myeloid leukemia and bone marrow aplasia: report of two cases, *Rev. Inst. Med. Trop. Sao Paolo*, 36, 465, 1994.

117. Nong, H., Li, J., and Huang, G., Aspergillosis of the larynx, *Chung Hua Erh Pi Yen Hou Ko Tsa Chih*, 30, 111, 1995.

118. Viale, P., Di Matteo, A., Sisti, M., Voltolini, F., Paties, C., and Alberici, F., Isolated kidney localization of invasive aspergillosis in a patient with AIDS, *Scand. J. Infect. Dis.*, 26, 767, 1994.

119. D'Hoore, K. and Hoogmartens, M., Vertebral aspergillosis: a case report and review of the literature, *Acta Orthop. Belg.*, 59, 306, 1993.

120. Mazzoni, A., Ferrarese, M., Manfredi, R., Facchini, A., Sturani, C., and Nanetti, A., Primary lymph node invasive aspergillosis, *Infection*, 24, 37, 1996.

121. Gonzalez-Crespo, M. R. and Gomez-Reino, J. J., Invasive aspergillosis in systemic lupus erythematosus, *Semin. Arthritis Rheum.*, 24, 304, 1995.

122. Nenoff, P., Horn, L.-C., Mierzwa, M., Leonhardt, R., Wiedenback, H., Lehmann, I., and Haustein, U.-F., Peracute disseminated fatal *Aspergillus fumigatus* sepsis as a complication of corticoid-treated systemic lupus erythematosus, *Mycoses*, 38, 467, 1995.

123. Collazos, J., Martinez, E., Flores, M., and Mayo, J., Aspergillus pneumonia successfully treated with itraconazole in a patient with systemic lupus erythematosus, *Clin. Invest.*, 72, 920, 1994.

124. Tanis, B. C., Verburgh, C. A., van't Wout, J. W., and van der Pijl, J. W., Aspergillus peritonitis in peritoneal dialysis: case report and a review of the literature, *Nephrol. Dial. Transplant.*, 10, 1240, 1995 (see also *Nephrol. Dial. Transplant.*, 10, 1124, 1995).

125. Miles, A. M. and Barth, R. H., Aspergillus peritonitis: therapy, survival, and return to peritoneal dialysis, *Am. J. Kidney Dis.*, 26, 80, 1995.

126. Nguyen, M. H. and Muder, R. R., Aspergillus peritonitis in a continuous ambulatory peritoneal dialysis patient: case report and review of the literature, *Diagn. Microbiol. Infect. Dis.*, 20, 99, 1994.

127. Girmenia, C., Gastaldi, R., and Martino, P., Catheter-related cutaneous aspergillosis complicated by fungemia and fatal pulmonary infection in an HIV-positive patient with acute lymphocytic leukemia, *Eur. J. Clin. Microbiol. Infect. Dis.*, 14, 524, 1995.

128. Baker, R. D., Pulmonary mucormycosis, *Am. J. Pathol.*, 32, 287, 1956.

129. Jurgens Mestre, A., Martinez Vecina, V., Peiro Cabrera, G., Dreier Spickernagel, A. et al., *Acta Otorrinolaringol. Esp.*, 45, 117, 1994.

130. Libshitz, H. I. and Pagani, J. J., Aspergillosis and mucormycosis: two types of opportunistic fungal pneumonia, *Radiology*, 140, 301, 1981.

131. British Thoracic and Tuberculosis Association, Aspergilloma and residual cavities: the result of a resurvey, *Tubercle*, 51, 227, 1970.

132. Kueh, Y. K., Chionh, S. B., Ti, T. Y., Tan, W. C., and Lee, Y. S., Tuberculosis and invasive pulmonary aspergillosis in a young woman with a myelodysplastic syndrome, *Singapore Med. J.*, 36, 107, 1995.

133. Freundlich, I. M., Libshitz, H. I., Glassman, L. M., and Israel, H. L., Sarcoidosis: typical and atypical thoracic manifestations and complications, *Clin. Radiol.*, 21, 376, 1970.

134. Israel, H. L. and Ostrow, A., Sarcoidosis and aspergillosis, *Am. J. Med.*, 47, 243, 1969.

135. Israel, H. L., Lenchner, G. S., and Atkinson, G. W., Sarcoidosis and aspergilloma: the role of surgery, *Chest*, 82, 430, 1982.

136. Flye, M. W. and Scaly, W. C., Pulmonary aspergilloma: a report of its occurrence in two patients with cyanotic heart disease, *Ann. Thorac. Surg.*, 20, 196, 1975.

137. Longbottom, J. L., Pepys, J., and Clive, F. T., Diagnostic precipitin test in *Aspergillus* pulmonary mycetoma, *Lancet*, 1, 588, 1964.

138. Roilides, E., Dimitriadou, A., Kadiltsoglou, I., Sein, T., Karpouzas, J., Pizzo, P. A., and Walsh, T. J., IL-10 exerts suppressive and enhancing effects on antifungal activity of mononuclear phagocytes against *Aspergillus fumigatus*, *J. Immunol.*, 158, 322, 1997.

139. Walsh, T. J., Invasive aspergillosis in patients with neoplastic diseases, *Semin. Respir. Infect.*, 5, 111, 1990.

140. Cohen, M. S., Isturiz, R. E., Malech, H. L., Root, R. K., Wilfert, C. M., Gutman, L., and Buckley, R. H., Fungal infection in chronic granulomatous disease: the importance of the phagocyte in defense against fungi, *Am. J. Med.*, 71, 59, 1981.

141. Denning, D. W., Follansbee, S. E., Scolaro, M., Norris, S., Edelstein, H., and Stevens, D. A., Pulmonary aspergillosis in the acquired immunodeficiency syndrome, *N. Engl. J. Med.*, 324, 654, 1991.

142. Rowen, J. L., Correa, A. G., Sokol, D. M., Hawkins, H. K., Levy, M. L., and Edwards, M. S., Invasive aspergillosis in neonates: report of five cases and literature review, *Pediatr. Infect. Dis. J.*, 11, 576, 1992.

143. Weinberger, M., Elattar, I., Marshall, D., Steinberg, S. M., Redner, R. L., Young, N. S., and Pizzo, P. A., Patterns of infection in patients with aplastic anemia and the emergence of *Aspergillus* as a major cause of death, *Medicine (Baltimore)*, 71, 24, 1992.

144. Brooks, R. G., Hofflin, J. M., Jamieson, S. W., Stinson, E. B., and Remington, J. S., Infectious complications in heart-lung transplant recipients, *Am. J. Med.*, 79, 412, 1985.

145. Morrison, V. A., Haake, R. J., and Weisdorf, D. J., The spectrum of non-*Candida* fungal infections following bone marrow transplantation, *Medicine (Baltimore)*, 72, 78, 1993.

146. Waldorf, A. R. and Diamond, R. D., Aspergillosis and mucormycosis, in *Immunology of the Fungal Disease*, Cox, R. A. Ed., CRC Press, Boca Raton, 1989, 29.

147. Schaffner, A., Douglas, H., and Braude, A., Selective protection against conidia by mononuclear and mycelia by polymononuclear phagocytes in resistance to *Aspergillus*: observations on these two lines of defense *in vivo* and *in vitro* with human and mouse phagocytes, *J. Clin. Invest.*, 69, 617, 1982.

148. Waldorf, A. R., Levitz, S., and Diamond, R. D., *In vivo* bronchoalveolar macrophage defense against *Rhizopus oryzae* and *Aspergillus fumigatus*, *J. Infect. Dis.*, 150, 752, 1984.

149. Levitz, S., Selsted, M. E., Ganz, T., Lehrer, R. I., and Diamond, R. D., *In vitro* killing of spores and hyphae of *Aspergillus oryzae* by rabbit neutrophil cationic peptides and bronchoalveolar macrophages, *J. Infect. Dis.*, 154, 483, 1986.

150. Diamond, R. D., Krzesicki, R., Epstein, B., and Jao, W., Damage to hyphal forms of fungi by human leukocytes *in vitro*: a possible host defense mechanism in aspergillosis and mucormycosis, *Am. J. Pathol.*, 91, 313, 1978.

151. Polak-Wyss, A., Protective effect of human granulocyte colony-stimulating factor on *Cryptococcus* and *Aspergillus* infections in normal and immunosuppressed mice, *Mycoses*, 34, 205, 1991.

152. Rex, J. H., Bennett, J. E., Gallin, J. I., Malech, H. L., Decarlo, E. S., and Melnick, D. A., *In vivo* interferon-γ therapy augments the *in vitro* ability of chronic granulomatous disease neutrophils to damage *Aspergillus* hyphae, *J. Infect. Dis.*, 163, 849, 1991.

153. Roilides, E., Holmes, A., Blake, C., Venzon, D., Pizzo, P. A., and Walsh, T. J., Antifungal activity of elutriated human monocytes against *Aspergillus fumigatus* hyphae: enhancement by granulocyte-macrophage colony-stimulating factor and interferon-γ, *J. Infect. Dis.*, 170, 894, 1994.

154. Roilides, E., Sein, T., Holmes, A., Blake, C., Pizzo, P. A., and Walsh, T. J., Effects of macrophage colony-stimulating factor on antifungal activity of mononuclear phagocytes against *Aspergillus fumigatus*, *J. Infect. Dis.*, 172, 1028, 1995.

155. Roilides, E., Uhlig, K., Venzon, D., Pizzo, P. A., and Walsh, T. J., Granulocyte colony-stimulating factor and interferon-γ enhance the oxidative responses and the damage caused by human neutrophils to *Aspergillus fumigatus* hyphae *in vitro*, *Infect. Immun.*, 61, 1185, 1993.

156. Walsh, T., Gonzalez, C., Lyman, C., Lee, S., Del Guercio, C., Gehrt, A., Sein, T., Roilides, E., Schafele, R., Francesconi, A., and Pizzo, P., Human recombinant macrophage colony-stimulating factor augments pulmonary host defense against *Aspergillus fumigatus*, *Proc. Annu. Meet. Am. Soc. Microbiol.*, American Society for Microbiology, Washington, D.C., Abstr. F-27, 1994, 593.

157. Cenci, E., Perito, S., Enssle, K. H., Mosci, P. et al., Th1 and Th2 cytokines in mice with invasive aspergillosis, *Infect. Immun.*, 65, 564, 1997.

158. Hamilton, A. J., Holdom, M. D., and Jeavons, L., Expression of the Cu,Zn superoxide dismutase of *Aspergillus fumigatus* as determined by immunochemistry and immunoelectron microscopy, *FEMS Immunol. Med. Microbiol.*, 14, 95, 1996.

159. Slight, J., Nicholson, W. J., Mitchell, C. G., Pouilly, N., Beswick, P. H., Seaton, A., and Donaldson, K., Inhibition of the alveolar macrophage oxidative burst by a diffusible component from the surface of the spores of the fungus *Aspergillus fumigatus*, *Thorax*, 51, 389, 1996.

160. Overdijk, B., Van Steijn, G. J., and Odds, F. C., Chitinase levels in guinea pig blood are increased after systemic infection with *Aspergillus fumigatus*, *Glycobiology*, 6, 627, 1996.

161. Sandhu, D. K., Effect of amphotericin B on the metabolism of *Aspergillus fumigatus*, *Mycopathologia*, 69, 23, 1979.

162. Redig, P. T. and Duke, G. E., Comparative pharmacokinetics of antifungal drugs in domestic turkeys, red-tailed hawks, broad-winged hawks, and great-horned owls, *Avian Dis.*, 29, 649, 1985.

163. Patterson, T. F., Miniter, P., and Andriole, V. T., Efficacy of fluconazole in experimental invasive aspergillosis, *Rev. Infect. Dis.*, 12(Suppl. 3), S281, 1990.

164. Katz, N. M., Pierce, P. F., Anzeck, R. A., Visner, M. S., Canter, H. G., Foegh, M. L., Pearle, D. L., Tracy, C., and Rahman, A., Liposomal amphotericin B for treatment of pulmonary aspergillosis in a heart transplant patient, *J. Heart Transplant.*, 9, 14, 1990.

165. Ahmad, I., Sarkar, A. K., and Bachhawat, B. K., Liposomal amphotericin B as a therapeutic measure to control experimental aspergillosis in BALB/c mice, *Indian J. Biochem. Biophys.*, 271, 370, 1990.

166. Ahmad, I., Sarkar, A. K., and Bachhawat, B. K., Liposomal amphotericin B in the control of experimental aspergillosis in mice. I. Relative therapeutic efficacy of free and liposomal amphotericin B, *Indian J. Biochem. Biophys.*, 26, 351, 1989.

167. Ahmad, I., Sarkar, A. K., and Bachhawat, B. K., Design of liposomes to improve delivery of amphotericin B in the treatment of aspergillosis, *Mol. Cell. Biochem.*, 91, 85, 1989.

168. Weber, R. S. and Lopez-Berestein, G., Treatment of invasive aspergillosis sinusitis with liposomal-amphotericin B, *Laryngoscope*, 97, 937, 1987.

169. Francis, P., Lee, J. W., Hoffman, A., Peter, J., Francesconi, A., Bacher, J., Shelhamer, J., Pizzo, P. A., and Walsh, T. J., Efficacy of unilamellar liposomal amphotericin B in treatment of pulmonary aspergillosis in persistently granulocytopenic rabbits: the potential role of bronchoalveolar D-mannitol and serum galactomannan as markers of infection, *J. Infect. Dis.*, 169, 356, 1994.

170. Leenders, A. C., de Marie, S., ten Kate, M. T., Bakker-Woudenberg, I. A., and Verbrugh, H. A., Liposomal amphotericin B (AmBisome) reduces dissemination of infection as compared with amphotericin B deoxycholate (Fungizone) in a rat model of pulmonary aspergillosis, *J. Antimicrob. Chemother.*, 38, 215, 1996.

171. Allen, S. D., Sorensen, K. N., Nejdl, M. J., Durrant, C., and Proffit, R. T., Prophylactic efficacy of aerosolized liposomal (AmBisome) and non-liposomal (Fungizone) amphotericin B in murine pulmonary aspergillosis, *J. Antimicrob. Chemother.*, 34, 1001, 1994.

172. Owais, M., Ahmed, I., Krishnakumar, B., Jain, R. K., Bachhawat, B. K., and Gupta, C. M., Tuftsin-bearing liposomes as drug vehicles in the treatment of experimental aspergillosis, *FEBS Lett.*, 326, 56, 1993.

173. Patterson, T. F., Miniter, P., Dijkstra, J., Szoka, F. C., Jr., Ryan, J. L., and Andriole, V. T., Treatment of experimental invasive aspergillosis with novel amphotericin B/cholesterol sulfate complexes, *J. Infect. Dis.*, 159, 717, 1989.

174. Allende, M. C., Lee, J. W., Francis, P., Garrett, K., Dollengerg, H., Berenguer, J., Lyman, C. A., Pizzo, P. A., and Walsh, T. J., Dose-dependent antifungal activity and nephrotoxicity of amphotericin B colloidal dispersion in experimental pulmonary aspergillosis, *Antimicrob. Agents Chemother.*, 38, 518, 1994.

175. Polak, A., Combination therapy of experimental candidiasis, cryptococcosis, aspergillosis and wangiellosis in mice, *Chemotherapy*, 33, 381, 1987.

176. Schaffner, A. and Frick, P. G., The effect of ketoconazole on amphotericin B in a model of disseminated aspergillosis, *J. Infect. Dis.*, 151, 902, 1985.

177. Armstrong, D., Treatment of fungal infections in the immunocompromised host, in *Recent Progress in Antifungal Chemotherapy*, Yamaguchi, H., Kobayashi, G. S., and Takahashi, H., Eds., Marcel Dekker, New York, 1992, 251.

178. Hughes, C. E., Harris, C., Peterson, L. R., and Gerding, D. N., Enhancement of the *in vitro* activity of amphotericin B against *Aspergillus* spp. by tetracycline analogs, *Antimicrob. Agents Chemother.*, 26, 837, 1984.

179. Russell, N. J., Kerridge, D., and Gale, E. F., Polyene sensitivity during germination of conidia of *Aspergillus fumigatus*, *J. Gen. Microbiol.*, 87, 351, 1975.

180. Graybill, J. R. and Kaster, S. R., Experimental murine aspergillosis: comparison of amphotericin B and a new polyene antifungal drug SCH 28191, *Am. Rev. Respir. Dis.*, 129, 292, 1984.

181. Hector, R. F., Compounds active against cell walls of medically important fungi, *Clin. Microbiol. Rev.*, 6, 1, 1993.

182. Golaescu, M., Voiculescu, M., and Burcea, H., Comparative susceptibility to nystatin, clotrimazole, and amphotericin B of 116 strains of pathogenic fungi: therapeutic implications, in Siegenthaler, *Current Chemotherapy*, Vol. 1, Proc. 10th Int. Congr. Chemother., Washington, W. and Luethy, R., Eds., American Society for Microbiology, Washington, D.C., 1978, 224.

183. Mohr, J. A., McKown, B. A., and Muchmore, H. G., Susceptibility of *Aspergillus* to steroids, amphotericin B and nystatin, *Am. Rev. Respir. Dis.*, 103, 283, 1971.

184. Ziger, K., Application of antimycotics in the therapy of experimental aspergillosis in chickens, *Vet. Arch.*, 41, 320, 1971.

185. Antinelli, J., Mathey, J., Herve, J., Cournot, L., and Chollet, M., Aspergillome bronchique: traitement prolonge par la mycostatine: guerison, *Bull. Mem. Soc. Med. Hop. Paris.*, 75, 564, 1959.

186. Gero, S. and Szekely, J., Pulmonary moniliasis treated with nystatin aerosol, *Lancet*, 1, 1229, 1958.

187. Vedder, J. S. and Schorr, W. F., Primary disseminated pulmonary aspergillosis with metastatic skin nodules: successful treatment with inhalation nystatin therapy, *JAMA*, 209, 1191, 1969.

188. McCarthy, D. S. and Robertson, D. G., Antifungal agents in bronchopulmonary aspergillosis, *Lancet*, 1, 1089, 1968.

189. Gemeinhardt, H. and Schuttmann, C., Acute pulmonary aspergillosis caused by *Aspergillus fumigatus* and successful treatment with nystatin, *Mycosen*, 8, 158, 1965.

190. Schuttmann, C. and Gemeinhardt, H., Acute lung aspergillosis and successful treatment with nystatin, *Z. Tuberk. Erkr. Thoraxorg.*, 124, 369, 1965.

191. Krakowka, P., Traczyk, K., Walczak, J., Halweg, H., Elsner, Z., and Pawlick, L., Local treatment of aspergilloma of the lung with a paste containing nystatin or amphotericin B, *Tubercle*, 51, 184, 1970.

192. Henderson, A. H. and Pearson, J. E. G., Treatment of bronchopulmonary aspergillosis with observation on the use of natamycin, *Thorax*, 23, 519, 1968.

193. Shende, G. Y., Padhye, A. A., and Thirumalachar, M. J., A case of bronchopulmonary aspergillosis treated with oral hamycin, *Hindustan Antibiot. Bull.*, 9, 229, 1967.

194. Moonis, M., Ahmad, I., and Bachhawat, B. K., Liposomal hamycin in the control of experimental aspergillosis in mice: effect of phosphatidic acid with and without cholesterol, *J. Antimicrob. Chemother.*, 31, 569, 1993.

195. Shadomy, S., Dixon, D. M., Espinel-Ingroff, A., Wagner, G. E., Yu, H. P., and Shadomy, H. J., *In vitro* studies with ambruticin, a new antifungal antibiotic, *Antimicrob. Agents Chemother.*, 14, 99, 1978.

196. Oki, T., Konishi, M., Tomatsu, K., Tomita, K., Saitoh, K., Tsunakawa, M., Nishio, M., Miyaki, T., and Kawaguchi, H., Pradimicins, a novel class of potent antifungal antibiotics, *J. Antibiot.*, 41, 1701, 1988.

197. Tsunukawa, M., Nishio, M., Ohkuma, H., Tsuno, T., Konishi, M., Naito, T., Oki, T., and Kawaguchi, H., The structures of pradimicin A, B and C: a novel family of antifungal antibiotics, *J. Org. Chem.*, 54, 2532, 1989.

198. Oki, T., Kakushima, M., Nishio, M., Kamei, H., Hirano, M., Sawada, Y., and Konishi, M., Water-soluble pradimicin derivatives, synthesis and antifungal evaluation of *N,N*-dimethyl pradimicins, *J. Antibiot.*, 43, 1230, 1990.

199. Kakushima, M., Nishio, M., Numata, K., Konishi, M., and Oki, T., Effect of stereochemistry at the C-17 position on the antifungal activity of pradimicin A, *J. Antibiot.*, 43, 1028, 1990.

200. Oki, T., A new family of antibiotics: benzo[*a*]naphthacenequinones: a water-soluble pradimicin derivative, BMY-28864, in *Recent Progress in Antifungal Chemotherapy*, Yamaguchi, H., Kobayashi, G. S., and Takahashi, H., Eds., Marcel Dekker, New York, 1992, 381.

201. Furumai, T., Hasegawa, T., Kakushima, M., Suzuki, K., Yamamoto, H., Yamamoto, S., Hirano, M., and Oki, T., Pradimicins T1 and T2, new antifungal antibiotics produced by an actinomycete. I. Taxonomy, production, isolation, physicochemical and biological properties, *J. Antibiot.*, 46, 589, 1993.

202. Takeuchi, T., Hara, T., Naganawa, H., Okada, M., Hamada, M., Umezawa, H., Gomi, S., Sezaki, M., and Kondo, S., New antifungal antibiotics, benanomicins A and B from an Actinomycete, *J. Antibiot.*, 41, 807, 1988.

203. Gomi, S., Sezaki, M., Kondo, S., Hara, T., Naganawa, H., and Takeuchi, T., The structures of new antifungal antibiotics, benanomicins A and B, *J. Antibiot.*, 41, 1019, 1988.

204. Gomi, S., Sezaki, M., Hamada, M., Kondo, S., and Takeuchi, T., Biosynthesis of benanomicins, *J. Antibiot.*, 42, 1145, 1989.

205. Yamaguchi, H., Inouye, S., Orisaka, Y., Tohyama, H., Komuro, K., Gomi, S., Ohuchi, S., Tatsumoto, T., Yamaguchi, M., Hiratani, T., Uchida, K., Ohsumi, Y., Kondo, S., and Takeuchi, T., A novel antifungal antibiotic, benanomicin A, in *Recent Progress in Antifungal Chemotherapy*, Yamaguchi, H., Kobayashi, G. S., and Takahashi, H., Eds., Marcel Dekker, New York, 1992, 393.

206. Sawada, Y., Numata, K., Murakami, T., Tanimichi, H., Yamamoto, S., and Oki, T., Calcium-dependent anticandidal action of pradimicin A, *J. Antibiot.*, 43, 715, 1990.

207. Bartnicki-Garcia, S., Cell wall chemistry, morphogenesis, and taxonomy of fungi, *Annu. Rev. Microbiol.*, 22, 87, 1968.

208. Hector, R. F., Zimmer, B. L., and Pappagianis, D., Evaluation of nikkomycins X and Z in murine models of coccidioidomycosis, histoplasmosis and blastomycosis, *Antimicrob. Agents Chemother.*, 34, 587, 1990.

209. Pfaller, M., Riley, J., and Koerner, T., Effects of cilofungin (LY 121019) on carbohydrate and sterol composition of *Candida albicans*, *Eur. J. Clin. Microbiol. Infect. Dis.*, 8, 1067, 1989.

210. Gordee, R. S., Zeckner, D. J., Ellis, L. F., Thakkar, A. L., and Howard, L. C., *In vitro* and *in vivo* anti-*Candida* activity and toxicology of LY 121019, *J. Antibiot.*, 37, 1054, 1984.

211. Hector, R. F. and Braun, P. C., Synergistic action of nikkomycins X and Z with papulacandin B on whole cells and regenerating protoplasts of *Candida albicans*, *Antimicrob. Agents Chemother.*, 29, 389, 1986.

212. Hector, R. F. and Pappagianis, D., Inhibition of chitin synthesis in the cell wall of *Coccidioides immitis* by polyoxin D, *J. Bacteriol.*, 154, 488, 1983.

213. Pfauer, M., Gordee, R., Gerarden, T., Yu, M., and Wenzel, R., Fungicidal activity of cilofungin (LY 121019) alone and in combination with anticapsin or other antifungal agents, *Eur. J. Clin. Microbiol. Infect. Dis.*, 8, 564, 1989.

214. Perfect, J. R., Wright, K. A., and Hector, R. F., Synergistic interaction of nikkomycin and cilofungin against diverse fungi, in *Recent Progress of Antifungal Chemotherapy*, Yamaguchi, H., Kobayashi, G. S., and Takahashi, H., Eds., Marcel Dekker, New York, 1992, 369.

215. Denning, D. W. and Stevens, D. A., Efficacy of cilofungin alone and in combination with amphotericin B in a murine model of disseminated aspergillosis, *Antimicrob. Agents Chemother.*, 35, 1329, 1991.

216. Beaulieu, D., Tang, J., Zeckner, D. J., and Parr, T. R., Jr., Correlation of cilofungin *in vivo* efficacy with its activity against *Aspergillus fumigatus* (1,3)-β-D-glucan synthase, *FEMS Microbiol. Lett.*, 108, 133, 1993.

217. Kurtz, M. B., Bernard, E. M., Edwards, F. F., Marrinan, J. A., Dropinski, J., Douglas, C. M., and Armstrong, D., Aerosol and parenteral pneumocandins are effective in a rat model of pulmonary aspergillosis, *Antimicrob. Agents Chemother.*, 39, 1784, 1995.

218. Abruzzo, G. K., Flattery, A. M., Gill, C. J., Kong, L., Smith, J. G., Krupa, D., Pilounis, V. B., Kropp, H., and Bartizal, K., Evaluation of water-soluble pneumocandin analogs L-733560, L-705589, and L-731373 with mouse models of disseminated aspergillosis, candidiasis, and cryptococcosis, *Antimicrob. Agents Chemother.*, 39, 1077, 1995.

219. Doern, G. V., Tubert, T. A., Chapin, K., and Rinaldi, M. G., Effect of medium composition on results of microbroth dilution antifungal susceptibility testing of yeasts, *J. Clin. Microbiol.*, 24, 507, 1986.

220. Ellis, D., Jarvinen, A., and Hansman, D., Effect of pH on *in vitro* antifungal sensitivity testing, in *Recent Advances in Chemotherapy*, Proc. 14th Int. Congr. Chemother. (Antimicrob. Sect. 3), Ishigami, J., Ed., University of Tokyo Press, Tokyo, 1985, 2554.

221. Voigt, W. H., The effect of clotrimazole (canisten) on the ultrastructure of molds (*Aspergillus fumigatus*) in infected animals, *Mykosen*, 19, 345, 1976.

222. Plempel, M., Bartmann, K., Buchell, K. H., and Regel, E., Experimental study of a new orally effective broad spectrum antimycotic agent, *Dtsch. Med. Wochenschr.*, 94, 1356, 1969.

223. Dixon, D., Wagner, G. E., Shadomy, S., and Shadomy, H. J., *In vitro* comparison of the antifungal activities of R 34,000, miconazole and amphotericin B, *Chemotherapy*, 24, 364, 1978.

224. Hoeprich, P. D. and Huston, A. C., Effect of culture media on the antifungal activity of miconazole and amphotericin B methyl ester, *J. Infect. Dis.*, 134, 336, 1976.

225. Katamoto, H. and Shimada, Y., Intra-arterial and intramammary injection of miconazole for bovine mastitis caused by *Aspergillus fumigatus*, *Br. Vet. J.*, 146, 354, 1990.

226. Sharp, N. J. and Sullivan, M., Use of ketoconazole in the treatment of canine nasal aspergillosis, *J. Am. Vet. Med. Assoc.*, 194, 782, 1989.

227. Komadina, T. G., Wilkes, T. D. I., Shock, J. P., Ulmer, W. C., Jackson, J., and Bradsher, R. W., Treatment of *Aspergillus fumigatus* keratitis in rabbits with oral and topical ketoconazole, *Am. J. Ophthalmol.*, 99, 476, 1985.

228. Patterson, T. F., George, D., Miniter, P., and Andriole, V. T., The role of fluconazole in the early treatment and prophylaxis of experimental invasive aspergillosis, *J. Infect. Dis.*, 164, 575, 1991.

229. O'Day, D. M., Orally administered antifungal therapy for experimental keratomycosis, *Trans. Am. Ophthalmol. Soc.*, 88, 685, 1990.

230. Graybill, J. R. and Ahrens, J., Itraconazole treatment of murine aspergillosis, *Sabouraudia*, 23, 219, 1985.

231. Warnock, D. W., Itraconazole and fluconazole: new drugs for deep fungal infection, *J. Antimicrob. Chemother.*, 24, 275, 1989.

232. Phillips, P., Graybill, J. R., Fetchick, R., and Dunn, J. F., Adrenal response to corticotropin during therapy with itraconazole, *Antimicrob. Agents Chemother.*, 31, 647, 1987.

233. Polak, A., Combination therapy of experimental candidiosis, cryptococcosis, aspergillosis and wangielosis in mice, *Chemotherapy*, 33, 381, 1987.

234. Shaw, M. A., Gumbleton, M., and Nicholls, P. J., Interaction of cyclosporin and itraconazole, *Lancet*, 2, 637, 1987.

235. Berenguer, J., Ali, N. M., Allende, M. C., Lee, J., Garrett, K., Battaglia, S., Piscitelli, S. C., Rinaldi, M. G., Pizzo, P. A., and Walsh, T. J., Itraconazole for experimental pulmonary aspergillosis: comparison with amphotericin B, interaction with cyclosporin A, and correlation between therapeutic response and itraconazole concentrations in plasma, *Antimicrob. Agents Chemother.*, 38, 1303, 1994.

236. Patterson, T. F., Fothergill, A. W., and Rinaldi, M. G., Efficacy of itraconazole solution in a rabbit model of invasive aspergillosis, *Antimicrob. Agents Chemother.*, 37, 2307, 1993.

237. Graybill, J. R., Kaster, S. R., and Drutz, D. J., Treatment of experimental murine aspergillosis with BAY n 7133, *J. Infect. Dis.*, 148, 898, 1983.

238. Thienpont, D., Van Cutsem, J., Van Nueten, J. M., Niemegeers, C. J. E., and Marsboom, R., Biological and toxicological properties of econazole, a broad-spectrum antimycotic, *Arzneimit.-Forsch.*, 25, 224, 1975.

239. Heel, R. C., Brogden, R. N., Speight, T. M., and Avery, G. S., Econazole: a review of its antifungal activity and therapeutic efficacy, *Drugs*, 16, 177, 1978.

240. De Nollin, S., Jacob, W., Garrevoet, T., Van Daele, A., and Dockx, P., Influence of econazole and 5-fluorocytosine on the ultrastructure of *Aspergillus fumigatus* and the cytochemical localization of calcium ions as measured by laser macroprobe mass analysis, *Sabouraudia*, 21, 287, 1983.

241. Wyler, R., Murback, A., and Moehl, H., An imidazole derivative (econazole) as an antifungal agent in cell culture systems, *In Vitro*, 15, 745, 1979.

242. Schoer, G., Kayser, F. H., and Dupont, M. C., Antimicrobial activity of econazole and miconazole *in vitro* and in experimental candidiasis and aspergillosis, *Chemotherapy*, 22, 211, 1976.

243. Van Cutsem, J., Van Gerven, F., and Janssen, P. A. J., *In vitro* activity of enilconazole against *Aspergillus* spp. and its fungicidal efficacy in a smoke generator against *Aspergillus fumigatus*, *Mykosen*, 31, 143, 1988.

244. Van Cutsem, J., Antifungal activity of enilconazole on experimental aspergillosis in chickens, *Avian Dis.*, 27, 36, 1983.

245. Redmann, T. and Schildger, B., Therapeutic use of enilconazole in broiler chicks with aspergillosis, *Dtsch. Tierarztl. Wochenschr.*, 96, 15, 1989.

246. Sharp, N. J., Sullivan, M., Harvey, C. E., and Webb, T., Treatment of canine nasal aspergillosis with enilconazole, *J. Vet. Intern. Med.*, 7, 40, 1993.

247. Singh, S. M., Sharma, S., and Chatterjee, P. K., Clinical and experimental mycotic keratitis caused by *Aspergillus terreus* and the effect of subconjunctival oxiconazole treatment in the animal model, *Mycopathologia*, 112, 127, 1990.

248. Van Cutsem, J., Van Gerven, F., and Janssen, P. A., Oral and parenteral therapy with saperconazole (R 66905) of invasive aspergillosis in normal and immunocompromised animals, *Antimicrob. Agents Chemother.*, 33, 2063, 1989.

249. Hanson, L. H., Clemons, K. V., Denning, D. W., and Stevens, D. A., Efficacy of oral saperconazole in systemic murine aspergillosis, *J. Med. Vet. Mycol.*, 33, 311, 1995.

250. Defaveri, J., Salazar, M. H., Rinaldi, M. G., and Graybill, J. R., Pulmonary aspergillosis in mice: treatment with a new triazole SCH 39304, *Am. Rev. Respir. Dis.*, 142, 512, 1990.

251. Tanio, T., Ohashi, N., Saji, I., and Fukusawa, M., SM-9164, an active enantiomer of SM-8668 (SCH 39304): oral and parenteral activity in systemic fungal infection models, in *Recent Progress in Antifungal Chemotherapy*, Yamaguchi, H., Kobayashi, G. S., and Takahashi, H., Eds., Marcel Dekker, New York, 1992, 473.

252. Allendoerfer, R., Loebenberg, D., Rinaldi, M. G., and Graybill, J. R., Evaluation of SCH 51048 in an experimental model of pulmonary aspergillosis, *Antimicrob. Agents Chemother.*, 39, 1345, 1995.

253. Denning, D. W., Hall, L., Jackson, M., and Hollis, S., Efficacy of D0870 compared with those of itraconazole and amphotericin B in two murine models of invasive aspergillosis, *Antimicrob. Agents Chemother.*, 39, 1809, 1995.

254. Yamada, H., Tsuda, T., Watanabe, T., Ohashi, M., Murakami, K., and Mochizuki, H., *In vitro* and *in vivo* antifungal activities of D0870, a new triazole agent, *Antimicrob. Agents Chemother.*, 37, 2412, 1993.

255. Hector, R. F. and Yee, E., Evaluation of BAY R 3783 in rodent models of superficial and systemic candidiasis, meningeal cryptococcosis, and pulmonary aspergillosis, *Antimicrob. Agents Chemother.*, 34, 448, 1990.

256. Hata, K., Kimura, J., Miki, J., Miki, H., Toyosawa, T., Nakamura, T., and Katsu, K., *In vitro* and *in vivo* antifungal activities of ER-30346, a novel oral triazole with broad antifungal spectrum, *Antimicrob. Agents Chemother.*, 40, 2237, 1996.

257. Hata, K., Kimura, J., Miki, H., Toyosawa, T., Moriyama, M., and Katsu, K., Efficacy of ER-30346, a novel oral triazole antifungal agent, in experimental models of aspergillosis, candidiasis, and cryptococcosis, *Antimicrob. Agents Chemother.*, 40, 2243, 1996.

258. Polak, A., Wain, W. H., and Scholer, H. J., Mode of action of 5-fluorocytosine (5-FC) in *Aspergillus fumigatus*, *Excerpta Med.*, 480, 269, 1980.

259. Wagner, G. and Shadomy, S., Mode of action of flucytosine in *Aspergillus* species, in *Chemotherapy*, Proc 9th Int. Congr. Chemother., Vol. 3, Williams, J. D. and Geddes, A. M., Eds., Plenum Press, New York, 1976, 211.

260. Wagner, G. E. and Shadomy, S., Effects of purines and pyrimidines on the fungistatic activity of 5-fluorocytosine in *Aspergillus* sp., *Antimicrob. Agents Chemother.*, 11, 229, 1977.

261. Kerkering, T. M., Schwartz, P. M., Espinel-Ingroff, A., Turek, P. J., and Diasio, R. B., 5-Fluorocytosine susceptibility of pathogenic fungi in the presence of allopurinol: potential for improving the therapeutic index of 5-fluorocytosine, *Antimicrob. Agents Chemother.*, 24, 448, 1983.

262. Watanabe, K., Hibino, A., Izumi, A., Mori, T., and Ikemoto, H., A case of pulmonary aspergilloma cured by intracavitary infusion of 5-fluorocytosine (5-FC), *Jpn. J. Med. Mycol.*, 21, 95, 1980.

263. Pizzo, P. A., Infectious complications in the child with cancer. II. Management of specific infectious organisms, *J. Pediatr.*, 98, 513, 1981.

264. Fernandez, N. A., Intracavitary aminocaproic acid for massive pulmonary hemorrhage, *Chest*, 85, 839, 1984.

265. Stevenson, J. G. and Reid, J. M., Bronchopulmonary aspergillosis: report of case, *Br. Med. J.*, 1, 985, 1957.

266. Delap, S. K., Skeeles, J. K., Beasley, J. N., Kreider, D. L., Whitfill, C. E., Houghten, G. E., Walker, E. M., Jr., Cannon, D. J., and Earls, P. L., *In vivo* studies with dimethyldithiocarbamate, a possible new antimicrobial for use against *Aspergillus fumigatus* in poultry, *Avian Dis.*, 33, 497, 1989.

267. Fukushiro, R., Urabe, H., Kagawa, S., Watanabe, S., Takahashi, H., Takahashi, S., and Nakajima, H., Butenafine hydrochloride, a new antifungal agent: clinical and experimental study, in *Recent Progress in Antifungal Chemotherapy*, Yamaguchi, H., Kobayashi, G. S., and Takahashi, H., Eds., Marcel Dekker, New York, 1992, 147.

268. Schmitt, H. J., Andrade, J., Edwards, F., Niki, Y., Bernard, E., and Armstrong, D., Inactivity of terbinafine in a rat model of pulmonary aspergillosis, *Eur. J. Clin. Microbiol. Infect. Dis.*, 9, 832, 1990.

269. Yamamoto, Y., Uchida, K., Hasegawa, T., Friedman, H., Klein, T. W., and Yamaguchi, H., Recombinant G-CSF induces anti-*Candida albicans* activity in neutrophil cultures and protection in fungal infected mice, in *Recent Progress in Antifungal Chemotherapy*, Yamaguchi, H., Kobayashi, G. S., and Takahashi, H., Eds., Marcell Dekker, New York, 1992, 309.

270. Metcalf, D., The molecular biology and functions of the granulocyte-macrophage colony-stimulating factors, *Blood*, 67, 257, 1986.

271. Welte, K., Bonilla, M. A., Gillion, A. P., Boone, T. C., Potter, G. K., Gabrilove, J. L., Moore, M. A. S., O'Reilly, R. J., and Souza, L. M., Recombinant human granulocyte colony-stimulating factor: effect on hematopoiesis in normal and cyclophosphamide-treated primates, *J. Exp. Med.*, 165, 941, 1987.

272. Tamura, M., Hattori, K., Nomura, H., Oheda, M., Kubota, N., Imazeki, I., Ono, M., Ueyama, Y., Nagata, S., Shirafuji, N., and Asano, S., Induction of neutrophilic granulocytosis in mice by administration of purified human native granulocyte colony-stimulating factor (G-CSF), *Biochem. Biophys. Res. Commun.*, 142, 454, 1987.

273. Anaissie, E. and Bodey, G. P., Granulocyte-macrophage colony-stimulating factor with amphotericin B for the treatment of disseminated fungal infections in neutropenic cancer patients, in *Recent Progress in Antifungal Chemotherapy*, Yamaguchi, H., Kobayashi, G. S., and Takahashi, H., Eds., Marcel Dekker, New York, 1992, 305.

274. Gerstl, B., Weidmen, W. H., and Newmann, A. V., Pulmonary aspergillosis: report of two cases, *Ann. Intern. Med.*, 28, 662, 1948.

275. Klossek, J. M., Peloquin, L., Fourcroy, P. J., Ferrie, J. C., and Fontanel, J. P., Aspergillomas of the sphenoid sinus: a series of 10 cases treated by endoscopic sinus surgery, *Rhinology*, 34, 179, 1996.

276. Klossek, J. M., Serrano, E., Peloquin, L., Percodani, J., Fontanel, J.-P., and Pessey, J.-J., Functional endoscopic sinus surgery and 109 mycetomas of paranasal sinuses, *Laryngoscope*, 107, 112, 1997.

277. Klinjongol, C., Chanyasawath, S., Pakdirat, B., and Pakdirat, P., One-stage surgical treatment of pulmonary aspergilloma with cavernostomy and muscle transposition flap: a case report, *J. Med. Assoc. Thai.*, 78, 692, 1995.

278. Robinson, L. A., Reed, B. C., Galbraith, T. A., Alonso, A., Moulton, A. L., and Fleming, W. H., Pulmonary resection for invasive *Aspergillus* infections in immunocompromised patients, *J. Thorac. Cardiovasc. Surg.*, 109, 1182, 1995.

279. Georgiev, V. St., Treatment and developmental therapeutics in aspergillosis. 1. Amphotericin and its derivatives, *Respiration*, 59, 291, 1992.

280. Georgiev, V. St., Treatment and developmental therapeutics in aspergillosis. 2. Azoles and other antifungal drugs, *Respiration*, 59, 303, 1992.
281. Min, Y. G., Kim, H. S., Kang, M. K., and Han, M. H., Aspergillus sinusitis: clinical aspects and treatment outcomes, *Otolaryngol. Head Neck Surg.*, 115, 49, 1996.
282. Parker, K. M., Nicholson, J. K., Cezayirli, R. C., and Biggs, P. J., Aspergillosis of the sphenoid sinus: presentation as a pituitary mass and postoperative gallium-67 imaging, *Surg. Neurol.*, 45, 354, 1996.
283. Teh, W., Matti, B. S., Marisiddaiah, H., and Minamoto, G. Y., Aspergillus sinusitis in patients with AIDS: report of three cases and review, *Clin. Infect. Dis.*, 21, 529, 1995.
284. Maksymiuk, A. W., Thongprasert, S., Hopfer, R., Luna, M., Fainstein, V., and Bodey, G. P., Systemic candidiasis in cancer patients, *Am. J. Med.*, 77(4D), 20, 1984.
285. Aisner, J., Schimpff, S. C., and Wiernik, P. H., Treatment of invasive aspergillosis: relation of early diagnosis and treatment to response, *Ann. Intern. Med.*, 86, 539, 1977.
286. Pennington, J. E., Successful treatment of *Aspergillus* pneumonia in hematologic neoplasia, *N. Engl. J. Med.*, 295, 426, 1976.
287. Pizzo, P. A., Infectious complications in the child with cancer. I. Pathophysiology of the compromised host and the initial evaluation and management of the febrile cancer patient, *J. Pediatr.*, 98, 341, 1981.
288. Pizzo, P. A., Infectious complications in the child with cancer. II. Management of specific infectious organisms, *J. Pediatr.*, 98, 513, 1981.
289. Denning, D. W. and Stevens, D. A., Antifungal and surgical treatment of invasive aspergillosis: review of 2,121 published cases, *Rev. Infect. Dis.*, 12, 1147, 1990.
290. Jewkes, J., Kay, P. H., Paneth, M., and Citron, K. M., Pulmonary aspergilloma: analysis of prognosis in relation to haemoptysis and survey of treatment, *Thorax*, 38, 572, 1983.
291. Pagano, L., Ricci, P., Nosari, A., Tonso, A., Buelli, M., Montillo, M., Cudillo, L., Canacchi, A., Savignana, C., Melillo, L., Chierichini, A., Marra, R., Bucaneve, G., Leone, G., Del Favero, A., and the Ginema Infection Program, Fatal haemoptysis in pulmonary filamentous mycosis: an under-devaluated cause of death in patients with acute leukaemia in haematological complete remission: a retrospective study and review of the literature, *Br. J. Haematol.*, 89, 500, 1995.
292. Shapiro, M. J., Albelda, S. M., Mayock, R. L., and McLean, G. K., Severe hemoptysis associated with pulmonary aspergilloma: percutaneous intracavitary treatment, *Chest*, 94, 1255, 1988.
293. Cochrane, L. J., Morano, J. U., Norman, J. R., and Mansel, J. K., Use of intracavitary amphotericin B in a patient with aspergilloma and recurrent hemoptysis, *Am. J. Med.*, 90, 654, 1991.
294. Bennett, M. R., Weinbaum, D. L., and Fiehler, P. C., Chronic necrotizing pulmonary aspergillosis treated by endobronchial amphotericin B, *South. Med. J.*, 83, 829, 1990.
295. Rodriguez, V., Bardwil, J. M., and Bodey, G. P., Primary aspergilloma cured with amphotericin B, *South. Med. J.*, 64, 396, 1971.
296. Bahadur, S., Kacker, S. K., D'Souza, B., and Chopra, P., Paranasal sinus aspergillosis, *J. Laryngol. Otol.*, 97, 836, 1983.
297. Schwartz, R. S., Macintosh, F. R., Schrier, S. L., and Greenberg, P. L., Multivariate analysis of factors associated with invasive fungal disease during remission induction therapy for acute myelogenous leukemia, *Cancer*, 53, 411, 1984.
298. Lashley, P. M., Callender, D. P., Graham, A. C., Gopwani, H., and Garriques, S., Aspergillosis in a patient with acute lymphoblastic leukaemia, *West Indian Med. J.*, 40, 37, 1991.
299. Kusumoto, S., Matsuda, A., Fukuda, M., Jinnai, I., Bessho, M., Saito, M., and Hirashima, K., Aspergillosis of the maxillary sinus in a patient with Ph1 positive acute lymphoblastic leukemia: a case report, *Rinsho Ketsueki*, 31, 1512, 1990.
300. Ho, P. C., Tolentino, F. I., and Baker, A. S., Successful treatment of exogenous aspergillus endophthalmitis: a case report, *Br. J. Ophthalmol.*, 68, 412, 1984.
301. Harrell, E. R., Wolter, J. R., and Gutow, R. F., Localized aspergilloma of the eyelid: treatment with local amphotericin B, *Arch. Ophthalmol.*, 76, 322, 1966.
302. Harris, G. L. and Mill, B. R., Orbital aspergillosis: conservative debridement and local amphotericin irrigation, *Ophthal. Plast. Reconstr. Surg.*, 5, 207, 1989.
303. Goodman, M. L. and Coffey, R. J., Stereotactic drainage of *Aspergillus* brain abscess with long-term survival: case report and review, *Neurosurgery*, 24, 96, 1989.
304. Shuper, A., Levitsky, H. I., and Cornblath, D. R., Early invasive CNS aspergillosis: an easily missed diagnosis, *Neuroradiology*, 33, 183, 1991.

305. Kravitz, S. P. and Berry, P. L., Successful treatment of *Aspergillus* peritonitis in a child undergoing continuous cycling peritoneal dialysis, *Arch. Intern. Med.*, 146, 2061, 1986.

306. Kerr, C., Perfect, J., Craven, P., Jorgensen, J. H., Drutz, D. J., Shelburne, J. J., Gallis, H. A., and Gutman, R. A., Fungal peritonitis in patients of continuous ambulatory peritoneal dialysis, *Ann. Intern. Med.*, 99, 334, 1983.

307. Skorodin, M. S., Gergans, G. A., Zvetina, J. R., and Siever, J. R., Xenon-133 evidence of bronchopleural fistula healing during treatment of mixed aspergillosis and tuberculosis empyema, *J. Nucl. Med.*, 23, 688, 1982.

308. Conneally, E., Cafferkey, M. T., Daly, P. A., Keana, C. T., and McCann, S. R., Nebulized amphotericin B as prophylaxis against invasive aspergillosis in granulocytopenic patients, *Bone Marrow Transplant.*, 5, 403, 1990.

309. Kuo, P. H., Lee, L. N., Yang, P. C., Chen, Y. C., and Luh, K. T., Aspergillus laryngotracheobronchitis presenting as stridor in a patient with peripheral T cell lymphoma, *Thorax*, 51, 869, 1996.

310. Hay, R. J., Use of ambisome, liposomal amphotericin B, in systemic fungal infections: preliminary findings of a European multicenter study, in *Recent Progress in Antifungal Chemotherapy*, Yamaguchi, H., Kobayashi, G. S., and Takahashi, H., Eds., Marcel Dekker, New York, 1992, 323.

311. Ringdén, O. and Tollemar, J., Liposomal amphotericin B (AmBisome) treatment of invasive fungal infections in immunocompromised children, *Mycoses*, 36, 187, 1993.

312. Mehta, R., Lopez-Berestein, G., Hopfer, R., Mills, K., and Juliano, R. L., Liposomal amphotericin B is toxic to fungal cells but not to mammalian cells, *Biochem. Biophys. Acta*, 770, 230, 1984.

313. Dornbusch, H. J., Urban, C. E., Pinter, H., Ginter, G., Fotter, R., Becker, H., Miorini, T., and Berghold, C., Treatment of invasive pulmonary aspergillosis in severely neutropenic children with malignant disorders using liposomal amphotericin B (AmBisome), granulocyte colony-stimulating factor, and surgery: report of five cases, *Pediatr. Hematol. Oncol.*, 12, 577, 1995.

314. Purcell, I. F. and Corris, P. A., Use of nebulised liposomal amphotericin B in the treatment of *Aspergillus fumigatus* empyema, *Thorax*, 50, 1321, 1995.

315. Mendicute, J., Ondarra, A., Eder, F., Ostolaza, J. I. et al., The use of collagen shields impregnated with amphotericin B to treat *aspergillosis* keratomycosis, *CLAO J.*, 21, 252, 1995.

316. Hammerman, K. J., Sarosi, G. A., and Tosh, F. E., Amphotericin B in the treatment of saprophytic forms of pulmonary aspergillosis, *Am. Rev. Respir. Dis.*, 109, 57, 1974.

317. Kilman, J. W., Ahn, C., Andrews, N. C., and Klassen, K., Surgery for pulmonary aspergillosis, *J. Thorac. Cardiovasc. Surg.*, 57, 642, 1969.

318. Reddy, P. A., Christianson, C. S., Brasher, C. A., Larsh, H., and Sutaria, M., Comparison of treated and untreated pulmonary aspergilloma: an analysis of 16 cases, *Am. Rev. Respir. Dis.*, 101, 928, 1970.

319. Peer, E. T., Case of aspergillosis treated with amphotericin B, *Dis. Chest*, 38, 222, 1960.

320. Tabeta, H. and Moriya, T., A case of chronic necrotizing pulmonary aspergillosis in which intravenous infusion of amphotericin B was effective, *Nippon Kyobu Shikkan Gakkai Zasshi*, 33, 342, 1995.

321. Krakowka, P., Traczyk, K., Walczak, J., Halweg, H., Elsner, Z., and Pawlicka, L., Local treatment of aspergilloma of the lung with a paste containing nystatin and amphotericin B, *Tubercle*, 51, 184, 1970.

322. Hargis, J. L., Bone, R. C., Stewart, J., Rector, N., and Hiller, F. C., Intracavitary amphotericin B in the treatment of symptomatic pulmonary aspergillosis, *Am. J. Med.*, 68, 389, 1980.

323. Henderson, A. H. and Pearson, J. E. G., Treatment of bronchopulmonary aspergillosis with observation on the use of natamycin, *Thorax*, 23, 519, 1968.

324. Ramirez, R. J., Pulmonary aspergillosis, *N. Engl. J. Med.*, 271, 1281, 1964.

325. Giron, J., Poey, C., Fajadet, P., Sans, N. et al., Palliative percutaneous treatment under x-ray computed tomographic control of inoperable pulmonary aspergilloma: apropos of 30 cases, *Rev. Mal. Respir.*, 12, 593, 1995.

326. Shirai, T., Taniguchi, M., Imokawa, S., Sugiura, W., Sato, A., and Genma, H., Usefulness of percutaneous instillation of antifungal agents for pulmonary aspergilloma, *Kekkaku*, 70, 9, 1995.

327. Furuse, F., Nakanishi, Y., Kotoh, H., Inoue, H. et al., Percutaneous intracavitary treatment of pulmonary aspergilloma — clinical efficacy and prognosis, *Nippon Kyobu Shikkan Gakkai Zasshi*, 32, 538, 1994.

328. Schmitt, H. J., Bernard, E. M., Haeuser, M., and Armstrong, D., Aerosol amphotericin B is effective for prophylaxis and therapy in a rat model of pulmonary aspergillosis, *Antimicrob. Agents Chemother.*, 32, 1676, 1988.

329. Beyer, J., Schwartz, S., Barzen, G., Risse, G., Dullenkopf, K., Weyer, C, and Siegert, W., Use of amphotericin B aerosols for the prevention of pulmonary aspergillosis, *Infection*, 22, 143, 1994.

330. Cahill, K. V., Hogan, C. D., Koletar, S. L., and Gersman, M., Intraorbital injection of amphotericin B for palliative treatment of *Aspergillus* orbital abscess, *Ophthal. Plast. Reconstr. Surg.*, 10, 276, 1994.

331. Inai, K., Ueda, T., Kagawa, D., Iwasaki, H., and Nakamura, T., A case of erythroleukemia associated with lung aspergilloma successfully treated with continuous drip infusion of amphotericin B, *Kansenshogaku Zasshi*, 69, 602, 1995.

332. Gevender, S., Rajoo, R., Goga, I. E., and Charles, R. W., Aspergillus osteomyelitis of the spine, *Spine*, 16, 746, 1991.

333. Yokoyama, S., Taniguchi, H., Kondo, Y., Matsumoto, K., and Okada, A., A case of bronchopulmonary aspergillosis recurring in a residual tuberculosis cavity, *Kekkaku*, 64, 579, 1989.

334. Saral, R., *Candida* and *Aspergillus* infections in immunocompromised patients: an overview, *Rev. Infect. Dis.*, 13, 487, 1991.

335. Bogner, J. R., Luftl, S., Middeke, M., and Spengel, F., Successful drug therapy in *Aspergillus* endocarditis, *Dtsch. Med. Wochenschr.*, 115, 1833, 1990.

336. Talbot, G. H., Huang, A., and Provencher, M., Invasive aspergillus rhinosinusitis in patients with acute leukemia, *Rev. Infect. Dis.*, 13, 219, 1991.

337. Shadomy, S., Wagner, G., Espinel-Ingroff, A., and Davis, B. A., *In vitro* studies with combinations of 5-fluorocytosine and amphotericin B, *Antimicrob. Agents Chemother.*, 8, 117, 1975.

338. Spiteri, M. A., McCall, J., and Clarke, S. W., Successful management of primary invasive pulmonary aspergillosis, *Br. J. Dis. Chest*, 80, 297, 1986.

339. Henze, G., Aldenhoff, P., Stephani, U., Grosse, G., Kazner, E., and Staib, F., Successful treatment of pulmonary and cerebral aspergillosis in an immunosuppressed child, *Eur. J. Pediatr.*, 138, 263, 1982.

340. Codish, S. D., Tobias, J. S., and Hannigan, M., Combined amphotericin B-flucytosine therapy in *Aspergillus* pneumonia, *JAMA*, 241, 2418, 1979.

341. Donahue, R. E., Johnson, M. M., Zon, L. I., Clark, S. C., and Groopman, J. E., Suppression of *in vitro* haematopoiesis following human immunodeficiency virus infection, *Nature*, 326, 200, 1987.

342. Kotler, D. P., Gaetz, H. P., Lange, M., Klein, E. B., and Holt, P. R., Enteropathy associated with acquired immunodeficiency syndrome, *Ann. Intern. Med.*, 101, 421, 1984.

343. Lazzarin, A. and Capsoni, F., Disseminated aspergillosis, *Am. J. Dis. Child.*, 136, 136, 1982.

344. Raubitschek, A. A., Levin, A. S., Stites, D. P., Phillips, J. C., and Ahonkhai, V. I., Normal granulocyte infusion therapy for aspergillosis in chronic granulomatous disease, *Pediatrics*, 51, 230, 1973.

345. Elgefors, B., Haugstvedt, S., Brorsson, J. E., and Esbjorner, E., Disseminated aspergillosis treated with amphotericin B and surgery in a boy with chronic granulomatous disease, *Infection*, 8, 174, 1980.

346. Corrado, M. L., Cleri, D., Fikrig, S. M., Shaw, E. B., and Fudenberg, H. H., Aspergillosis in chronic granulomatous disease: therapeutic consideration, *Am. J. Dis. Child.*, 134, 1092, 1980.

347. Beyt, B. E., Jr., Cannon, R. O. III, and Tuteur, P. G., Successful treatment of invasive pulmonary aspergillosis in the immunocompromised host, *South. Med. J.*, 71, 1164, 1978.

348. Ribner, B., Keusch, G. T., Hanna, B. A., and Perloff, M., Combination amphotericin B-rifampin therapy for pulmonary aspergillosis in a leukemic patient, *Chest*, 70, 681, 1976.

349. Colp, C. R. and Cook, W. A., Successful treatment of pleural aspergillosis and bronchopleural fistula, *Chest*, 68, 96, 1975.

350. Sato, A., Nakatani, K., Matsushita, Y., Matsuo, H. et al., Chronic necrotizing pulmonary aspergillosis treated with itraconazole and inhaled amphotericin B, *Nippon Kyobu Shikkan Gakkai Zasshi*, 33, 1141, 1995.

351. Coleman, J. M., Hogg, G. G., Rosenfeld, J. V., and Waters, K. D., Invasive central nervous system aspergillosis: cure with liposomal amphotericin B, itraconazole, and radical surgery — case report and review of the literature, *Neurosurgery*, 36, 858, 1995.

352. Maesaki, S., Kohno, S., Tanaka, K., Miyazaki, H., Mitsutake, K., Miyazaki, T., Tomomo, K., Kaku, M., Koga, H., and Hara, K., A case of pulmonary aspergilloma successfully treated with combination therapy of intracavitary injection of amphotericin B and intravenous administration of urinastatin, *Nippon Kyobu Shikkan Gakkai Zasshi*, 31, 1327, 1993.

353. Evans, E. G. V., Watson, D. A., and Mattews, N. R., Pulmonary aspergilloma in a child treated with clotrimazole, *Br. Med. J.*, 4, 599, 1971.

354. Milne, L. J. R., Mycological studies in the use of clotrimazole in bronchopulmonary aspergillosis and neonatal and vaginal candidiasis, *Postgrad. Med. J.*, 50(Suppl. 1), 20, 1974.

355. Holt, R. J. and Newman, R. L., Laboratory assessment of the antimycotic drug clotrimazole, *J. Clin. Pathol.*, 25, 1089, 1972.

356. Hay, R. J., Historical perspectives and projected needs for systemic azole antifungals, in *Recent Progress in Antifungal Chemotherapy*, Yamaguchi, H., Kobayashi, G. S., and Takahashi, H., Eds., Marcel Dekker, New York, 1992, 173.

357. Crompton, G. K. and Milne, L. J., Treatment of bronchopulmonary aspergillosis with clotrimazole, *Br. J. Dis. Chest*, 67, 301, 1973.

358. Mahgub, E. S., Laboratory and clinical experience with clotrimazole (BAY b 5097), *Sabouraudia*, 10, 212, 1972.

359. Jones, B. R., Richards, A. B., and Clayton, Y. M., Clotrimazole in the treatment of ocular infection by *Aspergillus fumigatus*, *Postgrad. Med. J.*, 50(Suppl. 1), 39, 1974.

360. Bolaert, J., Daneels, R., Van Landuyt, H., and Symoens, J., Miconazole plasma levels in healthy subjects and in patients with impaired renal function, *Chemotherapy*, 6, 165, 1976.

361. Ito, A., Therapeutic results with miconazole in Japan, in *Recent Progress in Antifungal Chemotherapy*, Yamaguchi, H., Kobayashi, G. S., and Takahashi, H., Eds., Marcel Dekker, New York, 1992, 183.

362. Uchida, K. and Yamaguchi, H., Bioassay for miconazole and its levels in human body fluids, *Chemotherapy*, 32, 541, 1984.

363. Mukae, H., Iwamoto, M., Tagawa, H., Mori, N., Ishino, T., Yamada, H., Komori, K., Kohno, S., Yamaguchi, K., Hirota, M. et al., A case of *Aspergillus* empyema with bronchopleural fistula, *Nippon Kyobu Shikkan Gakkai Zasshi*, 28, 1482, 1990.

364. Watanabe, A., Ohizumi, K., Motomiya, M., Takeuchi, K., Yoshida, T., Ida, S., Miura, Y., Nishioka, K., Tanno, Y., Takishima, T. et al., Therapeutic efficacy of miconazole on deep-seated fungal infections in the respiratory tract system, *Jpn. J. Antibiot.*, 43, 1392, 1990.

365. Hamamoto, T., Watanabe, K., and Ikemoto, H., Endobronchial miconazole for pulmonary aspergilloma, *Ann. Intern. Med.*, 98, 1030, 1983.

366. Maeda, T., A case of chronic necrotizing pulmonary aspergillosis effectively treated with miconazole inhalation, *Nippon Kyobu Shikkan Gakkai Zasshi*, 32, 168, 1994.

367. Huang, Y. C., Colaizzi, J. L., Bierman, R. H., Woestenborghs, R., and Heykants, J., Pharmacokinetics and dose proportionality of ketoconazole in normal volunteers, *Antimicrob. Agents Chemother.*, 30, 206, 1986.

368. Farquhar, D. L., Munro, J. F., Milne, J. R., and Piris, J., Ketoconazole and fungal sinusitis, *Scott. Med. J.*, 29, 192, 1984.

369. Torres, M. A., Mohamed, J., Cavazos-Adame, H., and Martinez, L. A., Topical ketoconazole for fungal keratitis, *Am. J. Ophthalmol.*, 100, 293, 1985.

370. Singh, S. M., Khan, R., Sharma, S., and Chatterjee, P. K., Clinical and experimental mycotic corneal ulcer caused by *Aspergillus fumigatus* and the effect of oral ketoconazole in the treatment, *Mycopathologia*, 106, 133, 1989.

371. O'Day, D. M., Moore, T. E., Jr., and Aronson, S. B., Deep fungal corneal abscess: combined corticosteroid therapy, *Arch. Ophthalomol.*, 86, 414, 1971.

372. Coriglione, G., Stella, G., Gafa, L., Spata, G., Oliveri, S., Padhye, A. A., and Ajiello, L., *Neosartorya fischeri* var. *fischeri* (Wehmer) Malloch and Cain 1972 (anamorph: *Aspergillus fischerianus* Samson and Gams 1985) as a cause of mycotic keratitis, *Eur. J. Epidemiol.*, 6, 382, 1990.

373. Humphrey, M. J., Jevons, S., and Tarbit, M. H., Pharmacokinetic evaluation of UK 49,858, a metabolically stable triazole antifungal in animals and humans, *Antimicrob. Agents Chemother.*, 28, 648, 1985.

374. Onist, P. and Tauris, P., Short-term curative treatment of *Aspergillus fumigatus* pneumonia with fluconazole, *Scand. J. Infect. Dis.*, 22, 749, 1990.

375. Yoneda, R., A clinical study of fluconazole in pulmonary aspergillosis, *Jpn. J. Antibiot.*, 42, 40, 1989.

376. Nakashima, M., The clinical study of fluconazole against pulmonary mycosis: effects of fluconazole on pulmonary cryptococcosis and aspergillosis, and its pharmacokinetics in patients, *Jpn. J. Antibiot.*, 42, 127, 1989.

377. Anaissie, E. J., Kontoyiannis, D. P., Hule, C., Vartivarian, S. E., Karl, C., Prince, R. A., Bosso, J., and Bodey, G. P., Safety, plasma concentrations, and efficacy of high-dose fluconazole in invasive mold infections, *J. Infect. Dis.*, 172, 599, 1995.

378. Takamoto, M., Ishibashi, T., Shinoda, A., Nakanishi, Y., Nomoto, K., Yoshida, M., Watanabe, K., Miyahara, T., Oizumi, K., Ichikawa, Y. et al., A clinical study on fluconazole against pulmonary mycosis associated with respiratory diseases, *Jpn. J. Antibiot.*, 47, 1145, 1994 (correction in *Jpn. J. Antibiot.*, 48, 162, 1995).

379. Heykants, J., Van Peer, A., Van de Velde, V., Van Rooy, P., Meuldermans, W., Lavrijsen, K., Woestenborghs, R., Van Cutsem, J., and Cauwenbergh, G., The clinical pharmacokinetics of itraconazole: an overview, *Mycoses*, 32(Suppl. 1), 67, 1989.

380. Niwa, H., Yamakawa, Y., Kondo, K., Kiriyama, M. et al., A high concentration of itraconazole in an aspergilloma, *Nippon Kyobu Shikkan Gakkai Zasshi*, 34, 67, 1996.

381. Borgers, M. and Van de Ven, M. A., Degenerative changes in fungi after itraconazole treatment, *Rev. Infect. Dis.*, 9(Suppl. 1), S33, 1987.

382. Van Cutsem, J., Van Gerven, F., Van de Ven, M. A., Borgers, M., and Janssen, P. A. J., Itraconazole, a new triazole that is orally active against aspergillosis, *Antimicrob. Agents Chemother.*, 26, 527, 1984.

383. Viviani, M. A., Tortorano, A. M., Langer, M., Almaviva, M., Negri, C., Cristina, S., Scoccia, S., De Maria, R., Fiocchi, R., Ferrazzi, P., Goglio, A., Gavazzeni, G., Faggiani, G., Rinaldi, R., and Cadrobbi, P., Experience with itraconazole in cryptococcosis and aspergillosis, *J. Infect.*, 18, 151, 1989.

384. Kreisel, W., Therapy of invasive aspergillosis with itraconazole: our own experiences and review of the literature, *Mycoses*, 37(Suppl. 2), 42, 1994.

385. Denning, D. W., Van Wye, J. E., Lewiston, N. J., and Stevens, D. A., Adjunctive therapy of allergic bronchopulmonary aspergillosis with itraconazole, *Chest*, 100, 813, 1991.

386. Niimi, T., Kajita, M., and Saito, H., Necrotizing bronchial aspergillosis in a patient receiving neoadjuvant chemotherapy for non-small cell lung carcinoma, *Chest*, 100, 277, 1991.

387. Kamei, K., Kohno, N., Tabeta, H., Honda, A., Unno, H., Nagao, K., Kuriyama, T., Yamaguchi, T., and Miyaji, H., The treatment of pulmonary aspergilloma with itraconazole, *Kansenshogaku Zasshi*, 65, 808, 1991.

388. Kramer, M. R., Denning, D. W., Marshall, S. E., Ross, D. J., Berry, G., Lewiston, N. J., Stevens, D. A., and Theodore, J., Ulcerative tracheobronchitis after lung transplantation: a new form of invasive aspergillosis, *Am. Rev. Respir. Dis.*, 144, 552, 1991.

389. Milleron, B., Roger, V., Roux, P., Lebreton, C., Koeger, A., Dupont, B., and Akoun, G., Semi-invasive aspergillosis with involvement of the thoracic wall cured by itraconazole, *Rev. Pneumol. Clin.*, 46, 175, 1990.

390. Dupont, B., Itraconazole therapy in aspergillosis: study in 49 patients, *J. Am. Acad. Dermatol.*, 23, 607, 1990.

391. Yamamoto, T., Suzuki, K., Yamakoshi, M., Tamamoto, T., and Ariga, K., A case of itraconazole-induced hypokalemia with pulmonary aspergilloma, *Kansenshogaku Zasshi*, 69, 1413, 1995.

392. Tricot, G., Joosten, E., Boogaerts, M. A., Vande Pitte, J., and Cauwenbergh, G., Ketoconazole versus itraconazole for antifungal prophylaxis in patients with severe granulocytopenia: preliminary results of two nonrandomized studies, *Rev. Infect. Dis.*, 9(Suppl. 1), S94, 1987.

393. Dupont, B. and Drouhet, E., Early experience with itraconazole *in vitro* and in patients: pharmacokinetic studies and clinical results, *Rev. Infect. Dis.*, 9(Suppl. 1), S71, 1987.

394. Denning, D. W., Tucker, R. M., Hanson, L. H., and Stevens, D. A., Treatment of invasive aspergillosis with itraconazole, *Am. J. Med.*, 86, 791, 1989.

395. Kloss, S., Schuster, A., Schroten, H., Lamprecht, J., and Wahn, V., Control of proven pulmonary and suspected CNS aspergillus infection with itraconazole in a patient with chronic granulomatous disease, *Eur. J. Pediatr.*, 150, 483, 1991.

396. Neijens, H. J., Frenkel, J., de Muinck Keiser-Schrama, S. M., Dzoljic-Danilovic, G., Meradji, M., and van Dongen, J. J., Invasive *Aspergillus* infection in chronic granulomatous disease: treatment with itraconazole, *J. Pediatr.*, 115, 1016, 1989.

397. van't Wout, J. W., Raven, E. J., and van der Meer, J. M., Treatment of invasive aspergillosis with itraconazole in a patient with chronic granulomatous disease, *J. Infect.*, 20, 147, 1990.

398. Lamprecht, J., Kuhn, A. G., and Sauer, S., Aspergillus mastoiditis in infected granulomatosis — a case report, *Laryngorhinootologia*, 69, 341, 1990.

399. Gresenguet, G., Belec, L., Testat, J., Lesbordes, J. L., Dupont, B., and Georges, A. J., Pseudotumoral naso-sinusal aspergillosis stabilized by itraconazole, *Med. Trop. (Mars.)*, 49, 73, 1989.

400. Massry, G. G., Hornblass, A., and Harrison, W., Itraconazole in the treatment of orbital aspergillosis, *Ophthalmology*, 103, 1467, 1996.

401. Rowe-Jones, J. M. and Freedman, A. R., Adjuvant itraconazole in the treatment of destructive sphenoid aspergillosis, *Rhinology*, 32, 203, 1994.

402. Impens, N., De Greve, J., De Beule, K., Meysman, M., De Beuckelaere, S., and Schandevyi, W., Oral treatment with itraconazole of aspergilloma in cavitary lung cancer, *Eur. Respir. Dis.*, 3, 837, 1990.

403. De Laurenzi, A., Aspergillosis in a cardiac transplant patient successfully treated with itraconazole, *Clin. Transplant.*, 321, 1989.

404. Villard, C., Lacroix, C., Rabot, M. H., Rovira, J. C., and Jacquemin, J. L., Severe *Aspergillus* keratomycosis treated with itraconazole per os, *J. Fr. Ophthalmol.*, 12, 323, 1989.

405. Scher, R. K. and Barnett, J. M., Successful treatment of *Aspergillus flavus* onychomycosis with oral itraconazole, *J. Am. Acad. Dermatol.*, 23, 749, 1990.

406. Sanchez, C., Mauri, E., Dalmau, D., Quintana, S., Aparicio, A., and Garau, J., Treatment of cerebral aspergillosis with itraconazole: do high doses improve the prognosis? *Clin. Infect. Dis.*, 21, 1485, 1995.

407. Peters-Christodoulou, M. N., de Beer, F. C., Bots, G. T., Ottenhoff, T. M., Thomson, J., and van't Hout, J. W., Treatment of postoperative *Aspergillus fumigatus* spondylodiscitis with itraconazole, *Scand. J. Infect. Dis.*, 23, 373, 1991.

408. Richard, R., Lucet, L., Mejjad, O., Daragon, A., Le Loet, X., Tully, H., Lemeland, J. F., and Leroy, J., Aspergillus spondylodiscitis: apropos of 3 cases, *Rev. Rhum. Ed. Fr.*, 60, 45, 1993.

409. Cortet, B., Deprez, X., Triki, R., Savage, C., Flipo, R. M., Duquesnoy, B., and Delcambre, B., Aspergillus spondylodiscitis: apropos of 5 cases, *Rev. Rhum. Ed. Fr.*, 60, 37, 1993.

410. Elliott, J. A., Milne, L. J., and Cumming, D., Chronic necrotizing pulmonary aspergillosis treated with itraconazole, *Thorax*, 44, 820, 1989.

411. Van Cutsem, J. and Cauwenbergh, G., Results of itraconazole treatment in systemic mycoses in animals and man, in *Recent Progress in Antifungal Chemotherapy*, Yamaguchi, H., Kobayashi, G. S., and Takahashi, H., Eds., Marcel Dekker, New York, 1992, 203.

412. Sachs, M. K., Blanchard, L. M., and Green, P. J., Interaction of itraconazole and digoxin, *Clin. Infect. Dis.*, 16, 400, 1993 (see also *Clin. Infect. Dis.*, 18, 259, 1994).

413. Schiraldi, G. F., Lo Cicero, S. L., Colombo, M. D., Rossato, D., Ferrarese, M., and Soresi, E., Refractory pulmonary aspergillosis: compassionate trial with terbinafine, *Br. J. Dermatol.*, 134(Suppl. 46), 25, 1996.

414. Schiraldi, G. F., Colombo, M. D., Harari, S., Lo Cicero, S., Ziglio, G., Ferrarese, M., Rossato, D., and Soresi, E., Terbinafine in the treatment of non-immunocompromised compassionate cases of bronchopulmonary aspergillosis, *Mycoses*, 39, 5, 1996.

415. Utz, J. P., German, J. L., Louria, D. B., Emmons, C. W., and Bartter, F. C., Pulmonary aspergillosis with cavitation: iodide therapy associated with unusual electrolyte imbalance, *N. Engl. J. Med.*, 260, 264, 1959.

416. Ramirez, R. J., Pulmonary aspergilloma, *N. Engl. J. Med.*, 271, 1281, 1964.

417. Adelson, H. T. and Malcolm, J. A., Endocavitary treatment of pulmonary mycetomas, *Am. Rev. Respir. Dis.*, 98, 87, 1968.

418. Greenberger, P. A., Diagnosis and management of allergic bronchopulmonary aspergillosis, *Allergy Proc.*, 15, 335, 1994.

419. Shale, D. J., Faux, J. A., and Lane, D. J., Trial of ketoconazole in non- invasive pulmonary aspergillosis, *Thorax*, 42, 26, 1987.

420. Rosenberg, M., Patterson, R., and Mintzer, R., Clinical and immunologic criteria for the diagnosis of allergic bronchopulmonary aspergillosis, *Ann. Intern. Med.*, 86, 405, 1977.

421. McCarthy, D. S. and Pepys, J., Allergic bronchopulmonary aspergillosis: clinical immunology. I. Clinical features, *Clin. Allergy*, 1, 261, 1971.

422. Safirstein, B. H., D'Souza, M., Simon, G., Tai, E. H.-C., and Pepys, J., Five-year follow-up of allergic bronchopulmonary aspergillosis, *Am. Rev. Respir. Dis.*, 108, 450, 1973.

423. Pingleton, W. W., Hiller, F. C., Bone, R. C., Kerby, G. R., and Ruth, W. E., Treatment of allergic aspergillosis with triamcinolone acetonide aerosol, *Chest*, 71, 782, 1977.

424. Glimp, R. A. and Bayer, A. S., Pulmonary aspergilloma: diagnosis and therapeutic consideration, *Arch. Intern. Med.*, 143, 303, 1983.

425. Shah, A., Khan, Z. U., Chaturvedi, S., Ramchandran, S., Randhawa, H. S., and Jaggi, O. P., Allergic bronchopulmonary aspergillosis with coexistent aspergilloma: a long-term follow up, *J. Asthma*, 26, 109, 1989.

426. Davies, D. and Somner, A. R., Pulmonary aspergilloma treated with corticosteroids, *Thorax*, 27, 156, 1972.

427. Stevens, E. A. M., Hilvering, C., and Orrie, N. G. M., Inhalation experiments with extracts of *Aspergillus fumigatus* on patients with allergic aspergillosis and aspergilloma, *Thorax*, 25, 11, 1970.

428. Slavin, R. G., Million, L., and Cherry, J., Allergic bronchopulmonary aspergillosis: characterization of antibodies and results of treatment, *J. Allergy*, 46, 150, 1970.

429. Slavin, R. G., Stanczyk, D. J., Lonigro, A. J., and Broun, G. O., Allergic bronchopulmonary aspergillosis — a North American rarity, *Am. J. Med.*, 47, 306, 1969.

430. Stark, J. E., Allergic pulmonary aspergillosis successfully treated with inhalation of nystatin, *Dis. Chest*, 51, 96, 1967.

431. Henderson, A. H. and Pearson, J. E. G., Treatment of bronchopulmonary aspergillosis with observation on the use of natamycin, *Thorax*, 23, 519, 1968.

432. Crompton, G. K. and Milne, L. J. R., Treatment of bronchopulmonary aspergillosis with clotrimazole, *Br. J. Dis. Chest*, 67, 301, 1973.

433. Patterson, T. F., Kirkpatrick, W. R., White, M., Hiemenz, J. W., Wingard, J. R., Rinaldi, M. G., Dupont, B., Stevens, D. A., and Graybill, J. R., *Proc. 36th Intersci. Conf. Antimicrob. Agents Chemother.*, American Society for Microbiology, Washington, D.C., Abstr. LM38, 1996.

434. Radha, T. G. and Viswanathan, R., Allergic bronchopulmonary aspergillosis, *Respiration*, 36, 104, 1978.

435. Currie, D. C., Lueck, C., Milburn, H. J., Harvey, C., Longbottom, J. L., Darbyshire, J. H., Nunn, A. J., and Cole, P. J., Controlled trial of natamycin in the treatment of allergic bronchopulmonary aspergillosis, *Thorax*, 45, 447, 1990.

436. Lebeau, B., Pelloux, H., Pinel, C., Michallet, M., Gout, J. P., Pison, C., Delormas, P., Bru, J. P., Brion, J. P., Ambroise-Thomas, P., and Grillo, R., Itraconazole in the treatment of aspergillosis: a study of 16 cases, *Mycoses*, 37, 171, 1994.

437. Lopez, L. and Evans, R. P., Drug therapy of aspergillosis otitis externa, *Otolaryngol. Head Neck Surg.*, 88, 649, 1980.

438. Lohoue Petmy, J., Bengono Toure, G., and Founda Onana, A., A study of otomycoses in Yaounde, *Rev. Laryngol. Otol. Rhinol. (Bord.)*, 117, 119, 1996.

439. Bezjak, V. and Arya, O. P., Otomycosis due to *Aspergillus niger*, *East Afr. Med. J.*, 47, 247, 1970.

440. Gregson, A. E. W. and LeTouche, C. J., The significance of mytotic infection in the etiology of otitis externa, *J. Laryngol. Otol.*, 75, 167, 1961.

441. McGonigle, J. J. and Jillson, O. F., Otomycosis: an entity, *Arch. Dermatol.*, 95, 45, 1967.

442. Bear, V. D., Otitis externa: immediate and long-term results with flumethasone pivalate/iodochlorhydroxyquine ear drugs, *Med. J. Aust.*, 1, 273, 1969.

443. Than, K. M., Naing, K. S., and Min, M., Otomycosis in Burma, and its treatment, *Am. J. Trop. Med. Hyg.*, 29, 620, 1980.

444. Schoneback, J. and Zakrisson, J. E., Topical 5-fluorocytosine therapy in otomycosis, *J. Laryngol. Otol.*, 88, 227, 1974.

445. Youssef, Y. A. and Abdou, M. H., Studies on fungus infection of the external ear. II. On the chemotherapy of otomycosis, *J. Laryngol. Otol.*, 81, 1005, 1967.

446. Pavlenko, S. A., Otomycosis in the Kuznetsk region and organization of medical services for this group of population, *Vestn. Otorinolaringol.*, 70, 1990.

447. Molina Utrilla, R., Lao Luque, J., Perello Scherdel, E., Companyo Hermo, C., and Casamitjana Claramunt, F., Otomycosis: case reports of 18 months in the General University Hospital of the Valle de Hebron in Barcelona, *An. Otorrinolaringol. Ibero Am.*, 21, 255, 1994.

448. Ulbricht, H. and Worz, K., Therapy with ciclopirox lacquer of onychomycoses caused by molds, *Mycoses*, 37(Suppl. 1), 97, 1994.

449. Tettenborn, D., Akute toxizitat und lokale vertraglichkeit von clotrimazole, *Arzneimit.-Forsch.*, 22, 1272, 1972.

450. Heel, R. C., Brogden, R. N., Pakes, G. E., Speight, T. M., and Avery, G. S., Miconazole: a preliminary review of its therapeutic efficacy in systemic fungal infections, *Drugs*, 19, 7, 1980.

451. Maryniak, D. M., Mullen, G. B., Allen, S. D., Mitchell, J. T., Kinsolving, C. R., and Georgiev, V. St., Studies on antifungal agents, *in vitro* activity of novel *cis*-5-alkoxy (or acyloxy)alkyl-3-phenyl-3-(1*H*-imidazol-1-ylmethyl)-2-methylisoxazolidine derivatives, *Arzneimit.-Forsch.*, 40, 95, 1990.

452. Heel, R.C., Brogden, R. N., Carmine, A., Morley, P. A., Speight, T. M., and Avery, G. S., Ketoconazole: a review of its therapeutic efficacy in superficial and systemic fungal infections, *Drugs*, 23, 1, 1982.

453. Sonino, N., The use of ketoconazole as an inhibitor of steroid production, *N. Engl. J. Med.*, 317, 812, 1987.

454. Cauwenbergh, G., De Doncker, P., Stoops, K., De Dier, A. M., Goyvaaerts, H., and Schuermans, V., Itraconazole in the treatment of human mycoses: review of three years of clinical experience, *Rev. Infect. Dis.*, 9(Suppl. 1), S146, 1987.

455. Thienpont, D., Van Cutsem, J., Van Cauteren, H., and Marsboom, R., The biological and toxicological properties of imazalil, *Arzneimit.-Forsch.*, 31, 309, 1981.

37.7 *COCCIDIOIDES IMMITIS*

37.7.1 INTRODUCTION

Coccidioidomycosis is a systemic fungal infection generally considered to be endemic to localized areas of the Western Hemisphere, in the so-called "Lower Sonoran Life Zone" (the semiarid section of the southwestern U.S. and Mexico), and Central and South America.[1,2] As recent reports have suggested, however, because of increased exposure to the pathogen, mainly because of expanded travel and tourism to endemic areas, coccidioidomycosis has been diagnosed in various other parts of the U.S. and the world.[3-9]

The causative agent of the disease, *Coccidioides immitis,* was originally described in the Chaco region of Paraguay. It represents a dimorphic fungus that has its mycelial form (saprobic phase) in the soil, and the parasitic phase in humans and other mammals.[10] Infection with *C. immitis* is usually caused by inhalation of airborne fungal arthroconidia. Cutaneous inoculation, in which the skin is directly infected with *C. immitis,* may be another route of coccidioidal infection.[11-14] Even though it is seen as a remote possibility, contracting coccidioidomycosis by exposure to contaminated material such as cotton grown in endemic areas, has also been reported.[15] Kohn et al.[16] have reported a case of acute disseminated coccidioidomycosis which they postulated was the result of inhalation of tissue-phase endospores aerosolized during the course of dissection.

After it enters the tissues, the fungus converts into its spherule state which reproduces by endosporulation. After infection, the incubation period lasts between 1 and 3 weeks. A mild bronchopneumonia ensues, followed by the development of granulomatous disease.[17]

Although in the immunocompetent host, the majority of infections are asymptomatic, in a number of cases the disease is manifested with a subacute influenza-like transient illness characterized by fatigue, cough, chest pain, sore throat, and headache, which usually resolves spontaneously.[18]

In immunocompromised patients, however, coccidioidomycosis can lead to serious complications because of dissemination. With the increase of cancer chemotherapy, organ and bone marrow transplantations, the use of corticosteroids, and the advent of the AIDS pandemic, the incidence of coccidioidomycosis resulting from reactivation of dormant infections has been on the rise. Other predisposition factors for dissemination of the disease include pregnancy, especially during the third trimester and the peripartum period,[2,19] Hodgkin's disease,[20] some genetic factors, such as race and ethnic background (Filipino, African-American, Hispanic, Native American, and oriental extraction),[21-26] and specific blood groups and histocompatibility types.[27,28]

Even though neonatal coccidioidomycosis has been reported,[29,30] infants of infected mothers are usually uninfected.[2] With the exception of pregnant women, disseminated coccidioidomycosis in males seems to be more prevalent than in women.[1,14] Age is probably a risk factor only in infants, young children, and adults over 50 years of age.[25,31-35] Diabetics may also be at high risk. Although there is no strong evidence to demonstrate a higher rate of dissemination in diabetics than in nondiabetics, the rate of pulmonary complications among diabetic patients is definitely higher.[36,37] If not treated, disseminated coccidioidomycosis is often life-threatening, especially in immuno-compromised hosts.

Pulmonary complications resulting from coccidioidomycosis may include adult respiratory distress syndrome (ARDS), formation of cavities and nodules, and empyema. Extrapulmonary dissemination of infection include skin lesions, abscesses, arthritis, osteomyelitis, and meningitis;[2] the latter is one of the most serious complication of coccidioidomycosis. In addition, coccidioidal infection can be observed in the thyroid,[38] eye,[39,40] sella turcica,[41] larynx,[42-44] external ear,[45,46] liver,[47,48] intestinal tract,[49] peritoneum,[50,51] prosthetic grafts of the femoral artery,[52] placenta during pregnancy,[53] and the female genital tract,[54,55] as well as various urogenital disorders.[56-59]

37.7.2 STUDIES ON THERAPEUTICS

37.7.2.1 Amphotericin B

For many years, amphotericin B has been the cornerstone of anticoccidioidal chemotherapy, especially in disseminated disease. The goal of the long-accepted intrathecal therapy of meningeal coccidioidomycosis with amphotericin B has been to reach a dose of 0.5 mg (injected three times weekly) until clinical and/or cerebrospinal fluid remission is achieved, and then to gradually taper this regimen over the following weeks or months.[60,61] In an attempt to completely eradicate the pathogen and reduce the likelihood of life-long suppressing chemotherapy, Labadie and Hamilton[62] introduced a high-dose regimen of intrathecal amphotericin B. In the trial they conducted, 11 patients with coccidioidal meningitis were given intrathecally high individual doses (1.0 to 1.5 mg) of the antibiotic mixed with 25 to 50 mg of hydrocortisone (aimed to ameliorate some of the side effects of amphotericin B) with the goal of achieving a dose of 12 mg per month for at least two consecutive months. The clinical results indicated that intrathecal ampho-tericin B when injected thrice weekly at a high-dose rate of 0.75 mg (or greater), not only promptly reached a monthly level of 20 mg, but also was associated with significantly enhanced survival rates (91%, as compared to earlier studies citing 51% to 70% survival rates for similar therapies).[62]

37.7.2.1.1   Liposome-encapsulated and lipid complexes of amphotericin B

There have been numerous attempts to reduce the unwarranted side effects of amphothericin B by intercalating its molecule into lipid-based carriers to form liposomes or lipid complexes.[63-70] The liposome-encapsulated amphotericin B and amphotericin B cholesteryl sulfate preparations were found to be less nephrotoxic, thereby allowing for the administration of higher doses of the drug. In a study by Clemons and Stevens,[71] the activities of two preparations of amphotericin B (conventional amphotericin B as deoxycholate suspension, and a lipid-based amphotericin B complex) have been tested in a murine model of coccidioidomycosis. Although at equal nontoxic concentrations the conventional amphotericin B was more effective than its lipid complex in reducing the colony-forming units (CFU), and about threefold more active on a milligram per kilogram basis, the lipid complex was ≥10-fold less toxic and, therefore, could be given at higher curative doses.[71] Allendoerfer et al.[72] have described similar results; in addition, they also compared the amphotericin B lipid complex with the new triazole antimycotic SCH 39304 and found the latter to be more efficacious. Another amphotericin B lipid-based complex, the colloidal dispersion of cholesteryl sulfate and amphotericin B in a 1:1 ratio, was compared to conventional amphotericin B in an acute murine model of coccidioidomycosis.[73] Again, while the conventional amphotericin B was reported to be three to four times more effective against *C. immitis* on a milligram per kilogram basis, it was also >5- to ≥8-fold more toxic.

Overall, the reduction of acute and chronic toxicities displayed by amphotericin B lipid complexes have shown an increased therapeutic index.

37.7.2.2 Azole Derivatives

37.7.2.2.1 Ketoconazole

Since the early 1980s, the antifungal activity of ketoconazole has been the subject of numerous investigations.[74-80] The oral route of administration and the significantly less toxic side effects have been two major advantages of ketoconazole over amphotericin B, and for a period of time its use to treat subacute and chronic nonmeningeal coccidioidal infections seemed appropriate.[80] Galgiani et al.[81] compared the antifungal efficacies and toxicities of 400- and 800-mg doses given daily to 112 patients with progressive pulmonary, skeletal, or soft tissue coccidioidal infections; during the therapy, if the clinical response was unsatisfactory, the protocol allowed for treatment with higher doses (as high as 1.2 or 1.6 g daily). While the observed success rates were similar for both the 400-mg and 800-mg dose regimens (23.2% and 32.1%, respectively; $p = .29$), the relapses among patients completing successful courses of therapy were more frequent in those receiving medication higher than 400 mg. The results of the trial demonstrated no real advantage of using higher doses of ketoconazole than the currently recommended 400-mg daily regimen.[81] The previously reported[74-79] greater efficacy of ketoconazole than the one observed by Galgiani et al.[81] was attributed to differences in the scoring systems used to assess the patient responses. The toxicity of ketoconazole was reversible and included nausea and vomiting (50%), gynecomastia (21%), decreased libido (13%), alopecia (8%), elevated liver function tests (5%), pruritus (5%), and rash (4%). The gastrointestinal and endocrinologic side effects were dose-dependent and increased at daily doses over 800 mg. The cumulative percent toxicity requiring discontinuation of therapy was 6%, 17%, 23%, and 56% for the 400-, 800-, 1200-, and 1600-mg doses, respectively, suggested that the maximum tolerable dose of ketoconazole is 800 mg daily.[82] Impairment of the steroid hormone biosynthesis (especially the production of testosterone and cortisol) by ketoconazole is a potentially serious side effect in adults,[83-85] as well as in children.[86,87]

Britton et al.[88] have studied the adrenal response in children receiving high doses (10 to 23 mg/kg daily) of oral ketoconazole for systemic coccidioidomycosis. The drug did impair the production of cortisol and aldosterone by partially interfering with the 11-β-hydroxylase step of the steroid hormone biosynthesis. However, there was no clinical evidence of adrenal insufficiency, and none of the children required adrenal steroid replacement therapy during acute illness or surgery.[88]

37.7.2.2.2 Fluconazole

Fluconazole is a water-soluble triazole antimycotic that exhibits significant cerebrospinal fluid (CSF) penetration and potent anticoccidioidal activity.

Catanzaro et al.[89] have conducted an open trial using fluconazole at daily doses of 50 or 100 mg to treat 14 patients with persistent coccidioidomycosis for a mean period of 13 ± 7 months. Only four patients were asymptomatic after cessation of therapy. Because of the low dosage regimens, the recurrence of chronic infection was significant. Evans et al.[90] have also reported a case in which fluconazole, at daily doses of 200 to 400 mg, failed to cure pulmonary coccidioidomycosis and to prevent dissemination to the skin and bone.

In a 5-year Pan-American study,[91] involving 88 immunocompetent patients with systemic mycoses (16 of them with coccidioidomycosis), the daily entry doses of fluconazole were raised from 100 to 400 mg, and increased during therapy to as much as 2.4 g daily. Fourteen of the 16 patients responded, including 10 patients with chronic pulmonary disease, 3 with meningitis, 2 with skin disease, and 1 with mediastinal disease. The majority of the responders (n = 10) received daily doses of 400 mg, one patient received 100 mg daily, and three patients were given the 600-mg dose because of slow or incomplete response. Only three of the responders relapsed, including the patient treated with the 100-mg dose.[91]

A common sequela of chronic coccidioidal meningitis is the obstruction of the flow of CSF.[92] Given the poor penetration of amphotericin B into CSF[93] and its considerable toxicity, fluconazole with its excellent CSF penetration has emerged as a very attractive alternative for treatment of coccidioidal meningitis. The activity of fluconazole in this condition has been evaluated by several groups. Tucker et al.[94] have administered fluconazole at daily doses of 50 to 400 mg to 18 patients for a mean of 9.8 months. Ten (67%) of 15 evaluable patients responded, 1 patient showed partial response, and 4 (27%) did not respond to therapy. Drug toxicity at the 400-mg daily dose remained minimal throughout the trial.[94] In a trial conducted by the NIAID Mycoses Study Group,[95] fluconazole was given to 50 consecutive patients with coccidioidal meningitis, of which 47 (94%) were evaluable. The drug was administered orally at 400 mg daily for up to 4 years in responding patients. Thirty-seven (79%) patients have responded to the treatment; the remaining 10 failed to respond. Most of the improvement occurred within 4 to 8 months after the therapy was initiated. However, given the seriousness of this condition, an increased dose of fluconazole (or instituting intrathecal therapy with amphotericin B) may still be required in some patients.[95]

Kostiuk et al.[96] investigated the penetration of fluconazole into a neck abscess caused by *C. immitis*. The drug was given intravenously at a daily dose of 800 mg and concurrently with surgical drainage of the abcsess. Five hours after administration, the level of fluconazole in the abscess fluid reached 28.4 mg/l.

Lee et al.[97] have described multiple anomalies in an infant born to a woman who received oral fluconazole during pregnancy. Although the reported findings were consistent with the Antley-Bixler syndrome (a genetic disorder), possible teratogenic effects of fluconazole could not be excluded.[97]

37.7.2.2.3   Itraconazole

Itraconazole, a new orally active triazole antimycotic, has demonstrated a broad spectrum of activity, mild toxicities, and a favorable pharmacokinetic profile.[98]

Tucker et al.[99] have reported beneficial clinical and laboratory response in 42 (72%) of 58 assessable cases of patients with nonmeningeal coccidioidomycosis. The dose regimens, which varied between 50 and 400 mg daily for a median duration of 10 months, showed minimal toxicity. Nonresponders were mostly patients who failed earlier therapy and most often had pulmonary disease; no patient failed when receiving itraconazole as initial therapy.[99] In another study, Graybill et al.[100] treated 47 evaluable patients with nonmeningeal coccidioidomycosis (osteoarticular, chronic pulmonary, and skin and soft tissue infections) with oral itraconazole at daily doses of 100 to 400 mg for periods of up to 39 months. Results showed a remission rate of 57% (n = 25), clinical failures in 16 patients (36%), and 1 patient (7%) who developed drug intolerance. After therapy for 1 year with a 400-mg daily dose of itraconazole, Diaz et al.[101] reported excellent or very good responses in 94% of 16 patients suffering from pulmonary coccidioidomycosis.

The efficacy of itraconazole against refractory coccidioidal meningitis was studied in a prospective, nonrandomized open trial of 10 patients given 300- to 400-mg dose regimens for a median duration of 10 months.[102] Of the eight evaluable patients, five received itraconazole as the sole treatment, and four have responded with minimal toxicity.

When administered at the commonly accepted 400-mg daily dose, the observed adverse effects of itraconazole were generally mild (mostly, nausea and vomiting, edema, rash, diarrhea, decreased libido, pruritis, and chills and fever).[100] However, when given at higher daily doses (e.g., 600 mg), itraconazole may cause symptomatic hypoadrenalism.[103] In one case of pruritic rash related to itraconazole, subsequent desensitization was successfully carried out.[104]

37.7.2.2.4   Other triazole antimycotics

SCH 39304 is a new orally effective triazole antimycotic showing excellent *in vitro* activity,[105] similar to that of itraconazole, and increased CSF penetration[106] comparable to that of fluconazole. In a murine model of coccidioidal meningitis, SCH 39304 was compared with itraconazole and fluconazole at oral doses of 1.0, 5.0, 10, and 30 mg/kg (for each drug) for 30 d. At equivalent doses, SCH 39304 was found to be more effective than any of the other two triazoles. It significantly prolonged the survival rate even at the lowest applied dose of 1.0 mg/kg.[107]

In a comparative study in murine disseminated coccidioidomycosis, Clemons et al.[108] found SCH 39304 to be between 5- and 10-fold more active than fluconazole. Furthermore, when SCH 39304 and its two isomers, RR 42427 and SS 42426, were compared for activity in murine coccidioidal meningitis, isomer RR 42427 was by far the most effective — at least 50 times more active than SS 42426, and approximately 5 times more potent than SCH 39304.[109]

Results from a clinical trial involving 54 patients with progressive nonmeningeal coccidioidomycosis (chronic pulmonary, bone and joint, and skin and soft tissue infections) treated with SCH 39304 have shown the cumulative overall response rates at 4, 8, and 12 months to be 7%, 36%, and 66%, respectively. The 12-month response rates by disease manifestations were 77% (pulmonary), 62% (skin and soft tissue), and 31% (bone and joints). Toxicities occurred in 24 patients (44%) and were characterized as mild (mainly, nausea and vomiting, dry lips, headache, and rash).[110] However, the apparent carcinogenicity of SCH 39304 following long-term therapy in rats appears to diminish its clinical significance.

A new triazole derivative, Bay R 3783, was compared in several murine models of coccidioidomycosis with ketoconazole, itraconazole, and fluconazole at 2.5, 10, and 25 mg/kg (given via the alimentary tract), and with amphotericin B, (administered intraperitoneally at 1.0 mg/kg).[111] In a pulmonary model of coccidioidomycosis, Bay R 3783, fluconazole, and itraconazole were essentially equipotent and more active than ketoconazole in protecting mice against death; however, they were inferior to amphotericin B, which completely prevented deaths through day 60. In a meningoencephalitis model of coccidioidomycosis, Bay R 3783, itraconazole, and fluconazole (all applied at 25 mg/kg), and amphotericin B prevented death only during therapy, with mortalities ensuing thereafter. Further experiments included a short-term organ load assay conducted by using the pulmonary model. In this assay, drugs were administered for 5 d, after which the lungs were removed after a 48-h washout period for quantitative cultures. Bay R 3783 and amphotericin B were found superior to the other azoles, eliciting a 5-log reduction in the number of CFU; ketoconazole was ineffective at the doses used. The overall data showed Bay R 3783 as comparable to itraconazole and fluconazole at doses of up to 25 mg/kg, and superior to ketoconazole, but inferior to 1.0 mg of intraperitoneal amphotericin B.[111]

Compound D0870 is an enantiomer of the previously studied ICI 195,739, a bis-triazole antifungal agent which was found active against experimental blastomycosis and candidiasis.[112,113] In a systemic model of murine coccidioidomycosis, D0870 at oral doses of 10 mg/kg daily or 100 mg/kg every other day, cured 20% or 30% of mice of residual infection, respectively, and was superior to 100-mg daily dose of fluconazole ($p < .001$). Overall, D0870 was 10-fold more active than fluconazole.[114]

The anticoccidioidal potency of another triazole derivative, SDZ89-485, was compared with that of fluconazole in experimental murine coccidioidomycosis.[115] Both drugs completely inhibited fungal growth when administered at 50 mg/kg twice daily; however, only SDZ89-485 was fully inhibitory at doses of 5.0 mg/kg (b.i.d.). Even though because of its better water solublity, fluconazole achieved higher peak levels in the blood sooner, SDZ89-485 was the more effective drug in the treatment of experimental systemic coccidioidomycosis in mice.[115] It is conceivable that due to its lipophilic nature, SDZ89-485 may associate with lipoproteins;[115] the resulting complexes, in turn, could be taken up by macrophages via a receptor-mediated endocytosis.[116] If such events were to take place, the antifungal activity of SDZ89-485 would be enhanced in a manner analogous to that of the liposome-encapsulated amphotericin B.[117]

37.7.2.3 Novel Antifungal Antibiotics

Nikkomycins X and Z, two antibiotics structurally related to the polyoxins, have been shown to act as competitive inhibitors of fungal chitin synthase.[118,119] Hector et al.[120] have investigated the antifungal properties of nikkomycins X and Z in several mouse models of coccidioidomycosis. At the three dose regimens studied, nikkomycin Z was more active than nikkomycin X. Thus, at oral doses of 20 and 50 mg/kg (b.i.d.) nikkomycin Z provided complete protection; in the 5-mg/kg dose group, the incidence of death was slightly higher than the one observed in the 50-mg/kg group. In short-term organ load experiments with the pulmonary model of coccidioidomycosis, nikkomycin Z was compared to fluconazole and Bay R 3783. The results demonstrated that (1) at 50 mg/kg (b.i.d.), nikkomycin Z was equipotent to a 25-mg/kg (b.i.d.) dose of Bay R 3783 in eradicating nearly all of *C. immitis* from the lungs, but was superior to fluconazole (2.5 mg/kg, b.i.d.); and (2) that nikkomycin Z was more effective when applied twice daily, very likely because of its short half-life. A model of meningiocerebral coccidioidomycosis was used to evaluate the ability of nikkomycin Z to penetrate into the CNS. In these experiments, the effect of a 50-mg/kg (b.i.d.) dose of nikkomycin Z was compared with that of 25-mg/kg (four times daily) dose of Bay R 3783 for a period of 3 weeks; data showed the survival curves of the two treatment groups to be not statistically significant.[120]

Cilofungin is an antifungal antibiotic which exerts its activity by inhibiting the fungal glucan synthase. Galgiani et al.[121] have found that cilofungin was able to suppress the mycelial growth of *C. immitis*, most likely by reducing the incorporation of *N*-acetylglucosamine. Data from light and electron microscopic studies have indicated delays in the development of the outer hyphal wall. When *C. immitis* was grown under conditions facilitating spherule growth, the activity of cilofungin dramatically decreased. Further evaluation in a model of murine coccidioidomycosis did not show efficacy.[121]

37.7.3 EVOLUTION OF THERAPIES AND TREATMENT OF COCCIDIOIDOMYCOSIS

The way therapeutic strategies and treatment of coccidioidomycosis have been determined depended to a large extent on the seriousness of infection after complete evaluation, and the immune status of the patient. In the majority of cases, patients with uncomplicated acute pulmonary coccidioido-mycosis or asymptomatic coccidioidal lung nodules may recover without treatment. However, immediate therapy is required in immunocompromised patients (especially those with AIDS) to prevent morbidity (e.g., destroyed joints) and mortality due to hypoxemia, dissemination, or meningitis.[2,14,122] Patients with severe primary pulmonary infections having a prolonged fever or prostration, persistent adenopathy, or extensive or progressive coccidioidomycotic pneumonia should also be treated, as well as the very young or the very old, patients with diabetes, and those with underlying malignancies or concurrent lung diseases.[2] Persistent thin-walled cavities are commonly observed in acute pulmonary infections. Treatment of such cavities is strongly advised when they begin to enlarge or when symptoms, such as productive cough and/or hemoptysis begin to develop.[122,123]

For years, intravenous amphotericin B has been the most efficacious drug for treating coccidioidomycosis in patients with extensive and rapidly progressive primary disease and at risk of developing dissemination, or in those already having disseminated disease. After their introduc-tion into the clinic, the oral azole antimycotics (ketoconazole, fluconazole, and most recently itraconazole) have been used extensively to treat less severe cases of the disease (Table 37.9).[26,122,124]

Because of the potential seriousness of its side effects, amphotericin B should always be applied with caution, especially in severely ill patients. In general, a total dose of 1.0 to 2.0 g of the antibiotic may be used in an attempt to prevent dissemination; the drug is given in 50-mg increments as either once-daily or thrice-weekly infusions administered over 1 to 2 hours. In cases of meningeal infection, amphotericin B should be administered by direct lumbar or protracted intracisternal injection, or by using ventricular or the cisternal Ommaya reservoir;[125] the average tolerated dose is 0.5 mg.[26]

Currently, treatment with fluconazole (400 to 800 mg daily) is recommended to prevent disease progression in high-risk patients with acute coccidioidomycosis, and in cases of meningeal

TABLE 37.9
Treatment of Coccidioidomycosis in the Immunocompetent Host

Indication	Clinical Stage	Treatment
Acute infection		
Low risk for dissemination		None
High risk for dissemination	Rapid progression	Amphotericin B: 1.5–2.0 g total dose, IV
	Slow progression	Fluconazole: 400–800 mg daily for 6–12 months, orally
Thin-walled cavity	Symptomatic, enlarging	Fluconazole: 400 mg daily for 6 months, orally; or resection
	High risk	Fluconazole: 400 mg daily for 6 months, orally; or resection
Ruptured cavity with empyema and pneumothorax		Amphotericin B: 1.5–2.5 g total dose, IV
Rapidly progressive miliary		Amphotericin B: 2.0–3.0 g total dose, IV
Meningeal infection	Patient awake	Fluconazole: 400–600 mg daily for 1 year or longer, orally
	Patient confused	Amphotericin B: 2.0–3.0 g (systemically + intracisternally 3× weekly until cultures negative, then decreased frequency); with improvement: fluconazole (400–800 mg daily, orally, for 1 year or longer)

Data taken from Sarosi and Davies,[122] Einstein and Johnson,[26] and Johnson and Sarosi.[124] Some of the recommended dose regimens may reflect the personal preferences of the authors, and therefore, may remain controversial.

infection.[26,122,126] Ketoconazole has been used orally in mild to moderate but stable infections at doses of 400 mg daily from 3 months to several years.[26] The recommended dose regimen for itraconazole in patients with nonmeningeal coccidioidomycosis is 100 mg daily given for periods up to 39 months.[100]

37.7.3.1 Coccidioidomycosis in Immunocompromised Hosts and AIDS Patients

Among the various opportunistic mycoses, infections caused by *C. immitis* have become a distinct possibility in patients who live in or travelled to endemic areas of the disease. If the infection is not treated immediately, the underlying immunodeficiencies associated with AIDS account for its high morbidity and mortality rate in those patients. Because of the sustained immune depression characteristic of AIDS, a complete eradication of the disease, even after a prolonged treatment, is virtually impossible with the currently available chemotherapeutics. Diffuse pulmonary infections and coccidioidal meningitis remain the most common and most dangerous manifestations of disseminated coccidioidomycosis in AIDS. Thus, in cases of diffuse pulmonary coccidioidomycosis, the mortality rate in HIV-infected patients within 1 month of diagnosis may reach as high as 70%, and at this point, it is not clear whether treatment will alter disease outcome.[127] It is highly recommended that a life-long therapy for such patients is initiated as soon as the CD4+ lymphocyte count becomes less than 200 cells/µl. One major management strategy would be to control the initial infection as effectively as possible, followed by indefinite suppressive chemotherapy aimed to prevent relapse (Table 37.10).[128] The initial therapy, especially in diffuse pulmonary disease and coccidioidal meningitis, should include treatment with amphotericin B. The recommended daily regimens vary between 0.5 and 1.0 mg/kg (usually between 40 and 60 mg daily for adults).[128]

For meningeal coccidioidal infections, amphotericin B is administered repeatedly into the cerebrospinal space and the treatment may last for months or even years. In this regard, the less toxic oral fluconazole has emerged as an attractive alternative to intrathecal therapy with

TABLE 37.10

Treatment of Coccidioidomycosis in Immunocompromised Hosts

Indication	Clinical Stage	Treatment	
		Without AIDS	With AIDS
Acute infection			
	Rapid progression	Amphotericin B: 1.5–2.0 g total dose, IV	Amphotericin B: 1.0-2.0 g; then, 400-800 mg for life, orally
	Slow progression	Fluconazole: 400 mg daily for 6–12 months, orally	Fluconazole: 800 mg daily for life, orally
Thin-walled cavity		Fluconazole: 400-800 mg daily for 6–12 months, orally	Fluconazole: 400–800 mg daily for life, orally
Ruptured cavity with empyema and pneumothorax		Amphotericin B: 1.5–2.0 g total dose, IV; then fluconazole (400–800 mg daily for 1 year), orally	Amphotericin B: 2.0–3.0 g total dose, IV; then fluconazole for life, orally
Rapidly progressive miliary		Amphotericin B: 2.0–3.0 g total dose, IV	Amphotericin B: 2.0–3.0 g total dose, IV; then fluconazole for life, orally
Meningeal infection	Patient awake	Fluconazole: 400–800 mg daily, orally, likely for life	Fluconazole: 400–800 mg orally for life; or amphotericin B 2.0–3.0 g (systemically + intracisternally 3× weekly); once awake and cultures negative: fluconazole (400–800 mg, orally, for life)
	Patient confused	Amphotericin B: 2.0–3.0 g total dose (systemically + intracisternally 3× weekly until cultures negative; then, fluconazole: 400–800 mg for life)	

Data taken from Sarosi and Davies,[122] and Johnson and Sarosi,[124] Some of the recommended dose regimens may reflect the personal preferences of the authors, and therefore, may remain controversial.

amphotericin B. Also, oral therapy (400 mg daily) with fluconazole and itraconazole should be considered for other forms of disseminated disease when the patient is clinically stable.[127] Both fluconazole and itraconazole are recommended for long-term suppressive chemotherapy usually at daily doses of 400 mg. Zar and Fernandez[129] reported failure of a 400-mg daily maintenance dose of oral ketoconazole to prevent recurrence of infection in an AIDS patient. For patients who did not respond to or could not tolerate azole therapy, treatment with amphotericin B should be considered.[127]

In one of many complications with AIDS patients, it is not uncommon to have concurrent pulmonary infections with *C. immitis* and *Pneumocystis carinii*.[130,131] In such cases, the diagnosis of *C. immitis* could be delayed or missed. In cases of *P. carinii* pneumonia (PCP), AIDS patients are often treated in the early stage of the infection with a combination of anti-PCP agents (trimethoprim-sulfamethoxazole) and adjuvant corticosteroids.[132-135] However, the use of corticosteroids in patients with PCP concurrent with coccidioidal pneumonia may be too risky in this setting since corticosteroids have been previously associated with severe, disseminated progression of coccidioidomycosis in patients without HIV disease.[136] Mahaffey et al.[137] reported two cases of concurrent pulmonary coccidioidomycosis and PCP in which the coccidioidal infection was not immediately recognized and the patients received trimethoprim-sulfamethoxazole medication combined with oral prednisone (40 mg daily); in both patients, the therapy led to clinical worsening associated with the development of a reticulonodular pulmonary infiltrate. Such distinct nodular pattern is visible on chest roentgenograms — because it is uncommon for PCP, the nodular pattern should be used as a diagnostic tool for coccidioidomycosis.[137]

37.7.3.2 Cutaneous Manifestations

Cutaneous manifestations have been observed in nearly half of all symptomatic infections involving *C. immitis*.[1,123,138,139] In addition, virtually all cases of dissemination involved the development of morphologically highly variable skin lesions.[140] There are three distinct cutaneous patterns of coccidioidal skin manifestations: toxic erythema, erythema nodosum, and erythema multiforme.

Although possible, primary cutaneous coccidioidomycosis, a skin infection acquired percutaneously has been very rarely observed (1% to 2% of total cases).[1] Its entry route is similar to other subcutaneous mycoses and results in a primary complex resembling that of tuberculosis (lymphangeitis and adenitis). In patients who are predisposed or are immunodeficient, a granulomatous lesion is established that is similar in appearance to verrucous tuberculosis, or the infection may follow the route of the regional lymph nodes as in lymphangitine sporotrichosis.[141-143]

Facial lesions are commonly observed and may carry the risk of a greater CNS involvement.[144] In an earlier report, Newland and Komisar[145] presented a case in which a slowly enlarging supraclavicular mass with cutaneous extension was the only evidence of disseminated coccidioidal infection — therapy with parenteral amphotericin B proved to be effective. Lavalle et al.[146] described mycologicual and clinical cure of a large coccidioidal forehead lesion 2 months after amphotericin B therapy was instituted.

One strategy that could be pursued in treatment of disseminated coccidioidomycosis involving the skin is to achieve clinical stabilization with either amphotericin B or some of the newer azole antimycotics, followed by a longer term of suppressive therapy if needed to reduce the likelihood of relapse.[1,147] To this end, Bonifaz et al.[143] reported a successful treatment of a patient with primary cutaneous coccidioidomycosis with itraconazole, given at a daily dose of 200 mg (b.i.d.) for 5 months.

37.7.3.3 Coccidioidomycosis in Pregnancy and Early Infancy

Pregnant women are at high risk for coccidioidal infections.[148] The dissemination rate is 40 to 100 times that of the general population and reaches its peak during the second and third trimesters. After the first cases of disseminated coccidioidomycosis in pregnant women were reported back in the 1940s,[149-151] it has become a major cause of mortality, ranging between 20% and 60%.[20,152] The increased risk of dissemination is likely a consequence of the relative immunosuppression observed in women during pregnancy, as well as the agonistic effect of 17-β-estradiol and progesterone in the serum of pregnant women on coccidial growth.[153,154] Reactivation or exacerbation of a chronic low-grade infection during pregnancy has been reported in patients previously treated for disseminated disease; in both reported cases the patients have been insulin-dependent diabetics.[155,156]

Disseminated coccidioidomycosis in early infancy has been relatively rare.[157-161] So far, in cases of neonatal coccidioidomycosis, there has been no evidence presented of transplacental infection.[157] Golden et al.[162] have described a case of *C. immitis* disseminated chorioretinis in a 7-week-old infant. Therapy involved gradually increasing dosages of intravenous amphotericin B until a daily maintenance dose of 1.0 mg/kg was reached. An additional 50-mg/kg course of amphotericin B was administered over a 3.5-month period; follow-up examinations at 4.5 and 6.5 months revealed no further change in the retinal lesion.[162]

In over 100 cases of coccidioidomycosis in pregnant women reported so far,[148] over half of them have been cases of disseminated infections which were treated with intravenous amphotericin B with favorable maternal and neonatal outcomes.[155,163-168] Recommended dose regimens begin with a test dose of 1.0 mg, followed by sequential dose increases of 5 to 10 mg every other day to reach a total dose of 50 mg every other day (maximum dose of 0.5 to 1.5 mg/kg every other day).[148] In case of emergency, following the 1.0-mg test dose, a 25-mg dose can be administered with subsequent rapid increases to the desired dosage.[148] During chemotherapy, the effects of amphotericin B should be monitored by weekly tests on electrolytes, hematocrit, and the renal function (blood urea nitrogen and creatinine). Decreased creatinine levels indicate an early nephrotoxicity.[169]

37.7.3.4   Coccidioidomycosis in Transplant Recipients

While primary coccidioidal infections are acquired in endemic areas, in immunocompromised hosts reactivation of the disease can develop months or even years later.[162] In cases when organ transplantations are needed, the question has been raised whether they should be even considered in endemic areas for coccidioidomycosis.[170,171] Since endogenous reactivation is a distinct possibility, caution should be applied for patients with a history of symptomatic coccidioidomycosis before transplant surgery is deliberated, especially in cases where extrapulmonary infections have been involved. To this end, Hall et al.[172] have proposed that before any transplantation surgery is performed, certain markers relevant to this problem should be examined. First in order will be the measurement of coccidioidal serum antibodies in patients with any endemic exposure. Patients having had previous history of coccidioidal pulmonary infections or with reactive coccidioidal serologies may benefit from receiving antifungal chemotherapy following the surgery. In addition, serologic surveillance and antifungal therapy should be considered during periods of increased immunosuppression which may occur during the treatment of rejection episodes.[172]

37.7.3.4.1   Cardiac transplant recipients

In cardiac transplant recipients, coccidioidal infections, even though seldom, have been reported.[170,172-175] Similarly, coccidioidomycosis of the myocardium has also been very rarely observed.[176] However, in patients on immunosuppressive therapy (either a two-drug regimen of prednisone–azathioprine or prednisone–cyclosporin A, or the triple-drug regimen of cyclosporin A–prednisone–azathioprine), the likelihood of primary or recurrent mycoses with higher rate of dissemination and mortality should not be underestimated. Therefore, screening for exposure to *C. immitis* before cardiac transplantation is performed would be important.

Hall et al.[177] have conducted a retrospective analysis of 199 patients who underwent transplantation in Arizona during a 6-year period. The data showed that in an endemic area, the incidents of coccidioidomycosis among heart transplant recipients accounted for only 4.5% of the population. In cases of either past medical history or positive serology, 200 mg of oral ketoconazole was applied twice daily beginning immediately after transplantation and maintained indefinitely. Vartivarian et al.[174] have described a case of reactivated disseminated coccidioidomycosis in an orthotopic cardiac transplant recipient, presented with invasion of the cardiac graft. The patient, who received immunosuppressive medication but not antifungal therapy, died. At the time of transplantation it was not known that coccidioidomycosis was apparently acquired by the patient during a brief visit to an endemic area several years prior to the transplant surgery.

In all earlier reports (before the introduction of the newer triazole antimycotics), the postoperative antifungal chemotherapy in the presence of prior clinical history of primary coccidioidal pneumonia or detectable coccidioidal serum antibodies at the time of surgery, consisted mainly of ketoconazole (200 mg daily), or amphotericin B (100 mg given to a child over a 4-month period); no relapses have been observed at follow-up monitoring.[172] Even so, the more effective fluconazole and itraconazole should be considered first for controlling recurrence of infection.

37.7.3.4.2   Renal transplant recipients

Although systemic fungal infection has been frequently diagnosed in renal allograft recipients subjected to immunosuppressive therapy,[178,179] cases of disseminated coccidioidomycosis, because of the endemic nature of the disease, have been rare.[180-185] However, if not treated, like in other transplant recipients, such infections usually have a high mortality rate. According to Cohen et al.,[180] predisposing factors for disseminated coccidioidomycosis in renal transplant recipients living in Arizona, included gender (males have been found to be at higher risk than females), and blood group (either B or AB, or a combination of both). Dissemination was manifested with pneumonia (59%), arthritis (24%), meningitis (12%), and pyelonephritis (6%). However, these conclusions should be viewed with caution since the study involved a limited number of patients and was conducted in only one localized endemic area. Amphotericin B (total dose of 1.5 to 2.7 g) was used to treat the pulmonary dissemination; the results were disappointing since relapse occurred in all patients treated. Ketoconazole was also used as an alternative.[180]

Chandler et al.[186] have described a case of disseminated coccidioidomycosis with choroiditis in which an apparent healed focus of pulmonary infection was reactivated after treatment with corticosteroids and immunosupressive therapy after renal transplantation. The following treatment with systemic polymyxin, methicillin, amphotericin B, and gentamicin sulfate proved unsuccessful and the patient died.

37.7.3.4.3   Liver transplant recipients

Disseminated fungal infections in recipients of liver allografts have a particularly poor prognosis.[187-192] Disseminated *C. immitis* infection was first diagnosed in a liver transplant recipient in 1990.[193] The reported case was unusual since the infection was not clinically suspected until the spherules of the pathogen were fortuitously detected in a percutaneous liver biopsy. Therapy with amphotericin B proved unsuccessful and the patient died.

37.7.3.4.4   Bone marrow transplant recipients

Riley et al.[194] reported three cases of coccidioidomycosis (one pulmonary and two disseminated) in allogeneic bone marrow transplant recipients. All three patients had been in an endemic area for *C. immitis* prior to the bone marrow transplantation. The treatment consisted mainly of intravenous amphotericin B. Both patients with disseminated infection died; the patient with localized pulmonary disease survived. One major impediment in managing coccidioidomycosis in bone marrow transplant recipients is the difficulty in diagnosing the infection. In treating such cases, one recommendation made was to reduce immunosuppressive medication as much as possible in order to allow for increased doses of amphotericin B.[194] The question whether itraconazole, high doses of fluconazole, or liposomal amphothericin B would be most efficacious in these patients is still not resolved.[194]

37.7.3.5   Ocular Coccidioidomycosis

Although relatively rare, ocular coccidioidomycosis has been diagnosed not only in patients with progressive disseminated illness but also in patients with very little or no systemic involvement.[195] Usually it is confined to the anterior segment and adnexa.[196] In general, the ocular dissemination of coccidioidomycosis is presented as either (1) extraorbital disease, involving the optic nerve and cranial nerve lesions; (2) extraocular disease, manifested as nonspecific phlyctenular conjunctivitis, episcleritis, scleritis, and fungal granulomata of the lids and orbit; or (3) intraocular disease, manifested as anterior uveitis (iris and ciliary body) or posterior uveitis (choroid), or both, as well as occasional retinal and vitreous manifestations.[195]

It has been reported,[197 200] that initial therapy with topical and systemic corticosteroids led to improvement in the ocular lesions. However, further evidence has suggested that continuation of such therapy may, in fact, exacerbate the ocular inflammation or as the corticosteroids were being tapered to cause progressive destruction of the eye.[186,198-200]

Since its introduction into the clinic in 1955 and in the subsequent years, amphotericin B has been used extensively in the therapy of ocular coccidioidomycosis.[195,201] The antibiotic can be used topically to treat external ocular infection as aqueous suspension at concentrations of 1 to 5 mg/ml, instilled one drop every 30 min; however, severe local irritations may frequently occur with its topical use.[202] When injected intravenously, amphotericin B has shown poor intraocular penetration unless used in large doses which, in turn, would increase its hepato- and nephrotoxicity. In the therapy of corneal ulcers and endophthalmitis, the antibiotic may be used by conjunctival and subconjunctival routes in doses ranging from 0.75 to 5.0 mg in a 1.0 ml aqueous suspension.[202,203] In the latter route, the injection is painful and may cause yellowing of the conjunctiva with a nodular formation.[204]

In treating a case of macular coccidioidomycosis, Lamer et al.[205] used amphotericin B in daily doses ranging from 20 to 50 mg given for 1 month; by the end of the period the lesion was cicatricial. It is important to mention that macular dissemination in coccidioidomycosis differs from that in histoplasmosis both funduscopically and angiographically.[205,206]

Miconazole has also been utilized to treat ocular coccidioidomycosis. Blumenkranz and Stevens[201] have found that at doses of 400 to 1000 mg, given three times daily for a period of 1 month, miconazole was ineffective in preventing the development of new lesions. In fact, new retinal lesions had developed, which were later reversed with the institution of amphotericin B therapy. Overall, in the reported study, miconazole was inferior to amphotericin B in the treatment of intraocular fungal infection.[201]

37.7.3.6   Acute Respiratory Failure

Acute respiratory failure in coccidioidomycosis is a rather serious complication occurring usually in the setting of a disseminated illness.[184,207-223] In the majority of cases there was one or more predisposing factors for disseminated illness.

In 1972, Knapp et al.[224] described a patient with primary pulmonary coccidioidomycosis who developed acute respiratory failure. Recently, two more such cases caused by primary pulmonary coccidioidomycosis have been described.[225] The acute failure is believed to be the consequence of an intense exposure to arthrospore-laden dust and massive inoculation with the pathogen. The proliferating fungus and the associated immune-mediated response would have caused the resulting lung injury.[226,227] Both patients survived after treatment with intravenous amphotericin B (total doses, 2.8 and 2.0 g, respectively); oral ketoconazole was also administered to one of the patients.[225]

37.7.3.7   Coccidioidal Peritonitis and Gastrointestinal Dissemination

Peritonitis is a rare complication of disseminated pulmonary coccidioidomycosis,[215,228-230] which is likely to occur by hematogenous dissemination at the time of the primary pulmonary infection.[230] Jamidar et al.[51] have described an HIV-positive patient with a very rare AIDS-defining peritoneal coccidioidomycosis. The patient, who presented with ascites, low serum-ascites albumin gradient, and laparoscopy showing peritoneal implants that grew *C. immitis*, was discharged after 2 weeks of amphotericin B therapy with a greatly reduced amount of ascites; 6 months later, the patient remained afebrile with no clinically detectable ascites.

So far, excluding autopsy series, only 15 cases of coccidioidal peritonitis have been reported,[49,228,230-232] and only 1 of these occurred in an AIDS patient who had a history of alcohol-induced cirrhosis, portal hypertension, and secondary hypersplenism.[51]

Amphotericin B was used widely for treatment of coccidioidal peritonitis even when there was no evidence for additional sites of dissemination. On the negative side, a lack of peritoneal clearance in a patient with fungal peritonitis given amphotericin B systemically has been reported.[233] However, the dose regimen of amphotericin B still remains largely empiric and is dependent upon the overall clinical response, sequential serologies, and the immunological status of patients.[49,234]

C. immitis is commonly believed not to spread into the gastrointestinal tract, with the possible exception of some widely disseminated terminal stages of the disease. However, Weisman et al.[49]

reported a unique case of gastrointestinal dissemination where histologic and culture evidence was presented to demonstrate invasion of the pathogen into chylous ascites, the mesentery, as well as into the entire length of the small bowel. As with the case of coccidioidal peritonitis, the gastrointestinal infiltration was the likely result of an initial hematogenous dissemination. The initial treatment of the patient consisted of intravenous amphotericin B (total dose, 4.25 g); in spite of the observed progressive clinical improvement, there has been recurrence of the disease. Following persistent renal toxicity, the amphotericin B medication was ceased and oral ketoconazole was instituted for 1 month at 400 mg daily, followed by increased dosage for an additional month. Both drugs failed, and stools continued to be positive for *C. immitis*. Next, itraconazole therapy was initiated. Repeat endoscopy 3 months after initiation of itraconazole showed nearly total resolution of the intraluminal duodenal disease, and stabilization in the patient's clinical condition with minimal persistent ascites.[19]

37.7.3.8 Coccidioidal Infections of Bones and Joints

Coccidioidomycosis involving the bones and joints is a very common occurrence during dissemination. Sometimes referred to as "desert rheumatism," it is reportedly present in 10% to 50% of cases involving extrathoracic infection.[235-238] The most affected sites of bone involvement include the ends of the long bones and bony prominences, as well as the spine and pelvis. However, diagnosis and treatment may pose difficult problems. Data from a retrospective study involving 24 patients with 44 separate skeletal lesions caused by *C. immitis* showed that a successful outcome was more likely to occur in those patients treated by a combination of chemotherapy and surgical intervention, rather than chemotherapy alone.[239-245] Patients with a complement fixation serum antibody titer ratio of 1:128 or less were more likely to fail chemotherapy alone ($p < .01$).[245] There have been earlier studies done before the availability of the newer generation of triazole antimycotics, with treatment regimens consisting of intravenous amphotericin B (total dose, 3.0 to 4.9 g[246]) or oral ketoconazole (400 to 800 mg daily for a minimum of several months).[247] Both drugs have been shown to produce detectable levels in the joints.[247,248] Synovial infection was more likely to improve as a result of ketoconazole medication than osteomyelitis.[247]

Buckley and Burkus[249] have presented a case of coccidioidal osteomyelitis of a tarsal bone which was successfully treated with local surgical debridement followed by long-term treatment with ketoconazole.

37.7.3.9 Genitourinary Coccidioidomycosis

Genitourinary involvement is commonly observed in disseminated coccidioidomycosis. Autopsy results have shown renal involvement in as many as 60% of patients suffering from disseminated infection.[215,229] Although less frequently, other sites of coccidioidal involvement include the kidney, adrenal, prostate, scrotal content, psoas, and the retroperitoneum.[215,219]

37.7.3.9.1 Coccidioidomycosis of the prostate

A number of clinically diagnosed cases of coccidioidal dissemination in the prostate have been described.[229,250-257] Earlier treatment included intravenous amphotericin B or ketoconazole.[250,252,255,256] Surgical procedures (transuretral resection[252,255,256]) have also been part of the therapy. The clinical outcome was dependent on the presence or absence of other sites of dissemination. While dissemination confined within the prostate gland had good prognosis for recovery, in general, the presence of extragenital dissemination was associated with high mortality rate.[257]

37.7.3.9.2 Infection of intrascrotal contents with or without prostatic involvement

Coccidioidal infection of the scrotal contents have been reported on numerous occasions.[251,253,258-266] The most common manifestations have been the development of a scrotal mass representing either granuloma or an abscess in the epididymus, and the presence of a sinus tract. In the most earlier reports, treatment was usually surgical, with only one patient treated with a combination of surgery and intravenous amphotericin B.[266]

37.7.3.9.3   Bladder involvement

Bladder involvement is a very rare manifestation of systemic coccidioidomycosis.[59] In a rather uncommon case, Weinberg et al.[267] found the mycelial phase of the fungus in the bladder. The patient was treated with ketoconazole and showed no clinical symptoms 1 year after the therapy. In another case report, Kuntze et al.[59] treated one patient with 2.0 g of amphotericin B followed by 200 mg of oral ketoconazole every morning for 1 year; at the 4-year follow-up examination, the patient was still asymptomatic.

37.7.3.9.4   Other coccidioidal genitourinary involvement

Infection of the female reproductive organs is also a rare manifestation of systemic coccidioido-mycosis.[59,268] It may be presented as pelvic inflammatory disease, pelvic mass, infertility, abdominal pain, hypermenorrhea, or vaginal discharge. The disease is usually associated with coccidioidal peritonitis. In earlier reported cases, the recommended therapy has been combination of surgical excision and systemic therapy.[269,270]

37.7.3.10   Coccidioidal Infection of Arterial Prosthesis

Schwartz et al.[271] have reported a case of disseminated coccidioidomycosis involving bilateral infection of femoral arterial prosthetic grafts and miliary pulmonary disease. Although the occurrence of vasculitis complicating coccidioidal meningitis has been previously reported,[272] what made this case highly unusual is that for the first time arterial involvement (whether native or prosthetic) of *C. immitis* was described in sites remote from the CNS. In the ensuing systemic chemotherapy (coupled with repeated percutaneous aspiration of the perivascular fluid collections), the patient failed to respond to ketoconazole and was intolerant to amphotericin B. However, treatment with oral fluconazole (200 to 400 mg daily for 9 months) led to clinical resolution; a life-long maintenance therapy with fluconazole (400-mg daily dose) was also instituted.[271]

37.7.4   Host Immune Response Against Coccidioidomycosis

Histologic evidence by Echols et al.[273] has demonstrated the presence of neutrophils and eosinophils at the sites of coccidioidal lesions in acute inflammation. However, with the advance of spherule maturation, the inhibition of fungal arthroconidia by neutrophils will progressively diminish with virtually no beneficial effect observed in the later stages of fungal growth.[274-276] As compared to other fungi which produce between 1 and 20 daughter cells, a coccidioidal spherule is capable of generating hundreds of endospores deposited in large packets. Concurrently, a fibrilar material is released that inhibits polymorphonuclear access to the emerging endospores.[277] Certain structural characteristics of the outer hyphal wall layer of the arthroconidia,[278] and a fungal proteinase capable of digesting antibodies[279,280] may also be contributing factors in increasing the resistance of coccidioidal spherules to neutrophil ingestion. Consequently, while the acute inflammatory response may slow fungal proliferation, in general, it is not adequate to confine or delay disease progression.[2]

Petkus and Baum[281] have found that human natural killer cells were also effective in inhibiting young spherules and endospores of *C. immitis*. Other host defense factors capable of killing arthroconidia include peripheral blood mononuclear cells.[282,283] Based on these and other findings, Galgiani[2] raised the interesting possibility that enhancement of such T cell-independent cellular defenses by immune response modifiers may effectively eradicate early coccidioidal infections, conceivably without the help of T cells. If found effective, such a therapeutic strategy would certainly benefit patients with AIDS and other patients whose T lymphocyte functions are deficient.

The role of T lymphocyte immunity to coccidioidomycosis has been studied by a number of investigators both *in vitro* and *in vivo*. Beaman et al.[284] have demonstrated that adoptive transfer of splenic lymphocytes from vaccinated mice were able to protect recipient mice from lethal coccidioidal infections. In another set of experiments by the same group, interferon-γ and other cytokines derived from splenic lymphocytes increased the phagosome-lysosome fusion and killing of coccidiodal endospores by macrophages *in vitro*.[285] When recombinant interferon-γ was used, it produced the same effect in both murine peritoneal macrophages and human blood monocytes.[286,287]

Recent reports from a number of laboratories[288-295] have provided convincing evidence that in humans, cell-mediated immune response will develop to naturally acquired coccidioidomycosis. The mechanisms regulating such response are still not well understood although studies by Cox et al.[296] have shown that certain specificities in the class of antibodies (immunoglobulin E) involved in the immune response to coccidioidomycosis did correlate with differences in the clinical progression of the disease.

Kong et al.[297] attempted to develop a vaccine against coccidioidomycosis using killed spherules in mice. The vaccine was effective only in limiting the spread, but not in preventing infection.

37.7.5 REFERENCES

1. Hobbs, E. R., Coccidioidomycosis, *Dermatol. Clin.*, 7, 227, 1989.
2. Galgiani, J. N., Coccidioidomycosis, *West. J. Med.*, 159, 153, 1993.
3. Hughes, C. V. and Kvale, P. A., Pleural effusion in Michigan caused by *Coccidioides immitis* after travel to an endemic area, *Henry Ford Hosp. Med. J.*, 37, 47, 1989.
4. Babycos, P. B. and Hoda, S. A., A fatal case of disseminated coccidioidomycosis in Louisiana, *J. La. State Med. Soc.*, 142, 24, 1990.
5. Taylor, G. D., Boettger, D. W., Miedzinski, L. J., and Tyrrell, D. L. J., Coccidioidal meningitis acquired during holidays in Arizona, *Can. Med. Assoc. J.*, 142, 1388, 1990.
6. Sekhon, A. S., Isaac-Renton, J., Dixon, J. M., Stein, L., and Sims, H. V., Review of human and animal cases of coccidioidomycosis diagnosed in Canada, *Mycopathologia*, 113, 1, 1991.
7. Ito, H., Itaoka, T., Onuki, T., Yokoyama, N., and Nitta, S., A case of pulmonary coccidioidomycosis, *Nippon Kyobu Geka Gakkai Zasshi*, 39, 1222, 1991.
8. Cayce, W. R., Cases from the aerospace medicine residents' teaching file — case #47: primary pulmonary coccidioidomycosis, *Aviat. Space Environ. Med.*, 62, 1200, 1991.
9. Lefler, E., Weiler-Ravell, D., Merzbach, D., Ben-Izhak, O., and Best, L. A., Traveler's coccidioidomycosis: case report of pulmonary infection diagnosed in Israel, *J. Clin. Microbiol.*, 30, 1304, 1992.
10. Sun, S. H. and Huppert, M. A., A cytological study of morphogenesis in *Coccidioides immitis*, *Sabouraudia*, 14, 185, 1976.
11. Levan, N. E. and Huntington, R. W., Jr., Primary cutaneous coccidioidomycosis in agricultural workers, *Arch. Dermatol.*, 92, 215, 1965.
12. Winn, W. A., Primary cutaneous coccidioidomycosis — reevaluation of its potentiality based on study of three new cases, *Arch. Dermatol.*, 92, 221, 1965.
13. O'Brien, J. J. and Gilsdorf, J. R., Primary cutaneous coccidioidomycosis in childhood, *Pediatr. Infect. Dis. J.*, 5, 485, 1986.
14. Bronnimann, D. A. and Galgiani, J. N., Coccidioidomycosis, *Eur. J. Clin. Microbiol. Infect. Dis.*, 8, 466, 1989.
15. Gehlbach, S. H., Hamilton, J. D., and Conant, N. F., Coccidioidomycosis: an occupational disease in cotton mill workers, *Arch. Int. Med.*, 131, 254, 1973.
16. Kohn, G. J., Linne, S. R., Smith, C. M., and Hoeprich, P. D., Acquisition of coccidioidomycosis at necropsy by inhalation of coccidioidal endospores, *Diagn. Microbiol. Infect. Dis.*, 15, 527, 1992.
17. Fraser, R. G., Pare, P. J. A., Pare, P. D., and Genereux, G. P., *Diagnosis of Diseases of the Chest*, Vol. 2, 3rd ed., W. B. Saunders, Philadelphia, 1989.
18. Yozwiak, M. L., Lundergan, L. L., Kerrick, S. S., and Galgiani, J. N., Symptoms and routine laboratory abnormalities associated with coccidioidomycosis, *West. J. Med.*, 149, 419, 1988.

19. Peterson, C. M., Schuppert, K., Kelly, P. C., and Pappagianis, D., Coccidioidomycosis and pregnancy, *Obstet. Gynecol. Surv.*, 48, 149, 1993.
20. Deresinski, S. C. and Stevens, D. A., Coccidioidomycosis in compromised hosts — experience at Stanford University Hospital, *Medicine (Baltimore)*, 54, 377, 1974.
21. Gifford, M. A., Buss, W. C., Douds, R. J., Miller, H. E., and Tupper, R. B., Data on coccidioides fungus infection: Kern County, Bakersfield, Calif., *Kern County Dept. Public Health Annual Report*, 1936, 39.
22. Huppert, M., Racism in coccidioidomycosis? *Am. Rev. Respir. Dis.*, 118, 797, 1978.
23. Pappagianis, D., Lindsay, S., Beall, S., and Williams, P., Ethnic background and the clinical course of coccidioidomycosis, *Am. Rev. Respir. Dis.*, 120, 959, 1979.
24. Williams, P. L., Sable, D. L., Mendez, P., and Smyth, L. T., Symptomatic coccidioidomycosis following a severe natural dust storm, *Chest*, 76, 566, 1979.
25. Johnson, W. M., Racial factors in coccidioidomycosis: mortality experience in Arizona: a review of the literature, *Ariz. Med.*, 39, 18, 1982.
26. Einstein, H. E. and Johnson, R. H., Coccidioidomycosis: new aspects of epidemiology and therapy, *Clin. Infect. Dis.*, 16, 349, 1993.
27. Deresinski, S. C., Pappagianis, D., and Stevens, D. A., Association of ABO blood group and outcome of coccidioidal infection, *Sabouraudia*, 17, 261, 1979.
28. Cohen, I. M., Galgiani, J. N., Potter, D., and Ogden, D. A., Coccidioidomycosis in renal replacement therapy, *Arch. Intern. Med.*, 142, 489, 1982.
29. Shafai, T., Neonatal coccidioidomycosis in premature twins, *Am. J. Dis. Child.*, 132, 634, 1978.
30. Bernstein, D. I., Tipton, J. R., Schott, S. F., and Cherry, J. D., Coccidioidomycosis in a neonate: maternal-infant transmission, *J. Pediatr.*, 99, 752, 1981.
31. Willet, F. M. and Weiss, A., Coccidioidomycosis in southern California: report of a new endemic area with a review of 100 cases, *Ann. Intern. Med.*, 23, 349, 1945.
32. Lonky, S. A., Catanzaro, A., Moser, K. M., and Einstein, H., Acute coccidioidal pleural effusion, *Am. Rev. Respir. Dis.*, 114, 681, 1976.
33. Bronnimann, D. A., Adam, R. D., Galgiani, J. N., Habib, M. P., Petersen, E. A., Porter, B., and Bloom, J. W., Coccidioidomycosis in the acquired immunodeficiency syndrome, *Ann. Intern. Med.*, 106, 372, 1987.
34. Bouza, E., Dreyer, J. S., Hewitt, W. L., and Meyer, R. D., Coccidioidal meningitis, *Medicine (Baltimore)*, 60, 139, 1981.
35. Bloom, J. W., Camilli, A. E., and Barbee, R. A., Disseminated coccidioidomycosis: a ten-year experience, in *Coccidioidomycosis*, Einstein, H. E. and Catanzaro, A., Eds., The National Foundation of Infectious Diseases, Washington, D.C., 1985, 369.
36. Einstein, H. E., Chia, J. K. S., and Meyer, R. D., Pulmonary infiltrate and pleural effusion in a diabetic man, *Clin. Infect. Dis.*, 14, 955, 1992.
37. Salkin, D. and Said, A., Reinfection with coccidioidomycosis, *Clin. Infect. Dis.*, 17, 1066, 1993.
38. Loeb, J. M., Livermore, B. M., and Wofsy, D., Coccidioidomycosis of the thyroid, *Ann. Intern. Med.*, 91, 409, 1979.
39. Rodenbiker, H. T. and Ganley, J. P., Ocular coccidioidomycosis, *Surv. Ophthalmol.*, 24, 263, 1980.
40. Moorthy, R. S., Rao, N. A., Sidikaro, Y., and Foos, R. Y., Coccidioidomycosis iridocyclitis, *Ophthalmology*, 101, 1923, 1994.
41. Scanarini, M., Rotillo, A., Rigobello, L., Pomes, A., Parenti, A., and Alessio, L., Primary intrasellar coccidioidomycosis simulating a pituitary adenoma, *Neurosurgery*, 28, 748, 1991.
42. Ward, P. H., Berci, G., Morledge, D., and Schwartz H., Coccidioidomycosis of the larynx in infants and adults, *Ann. Otol. Rhinol. Laryngol.*, 86, 655, 1977.
43. Hajare, S., Rakusan, T. A., Kalia, A., and Strunk, C. L., Laryngeal coccidioidomycosis causing airway obstruction, *Pediatr. Infect. Dis. J.*, 8, 54, 1989.
44. Boyle, J. O., Coulthard, S. W., and Mandel, R. M., Laryngeal involvement in disseminated coccidioido-mycosis, *Arch. Otolaryngol. Head Neck Surg.*, 117, 433, 1991.
45. Harvey, R. P., Pappagianis, D., Cochran, J., and Stevens, D. A., Otomycosis due to coccidioidomycosis, *Arch. Intern. Med.*, 138, 1434, 1978.
46. Busch, R. F., Coccidioidomycosis of the external ear, *Otolaryngol. Head Neck Surgery*, 107, 491, 1992.

47. Craig, J. R., Hillberg, R. H., and Balchum, O. J., Disseminated coccidioidomycosis — diagnosis by biopsy of liver, *West. J. Med.*, 122, 171, 1975.
48. Howard, P. F. and Smith, J. W., Diagnosis of disseminated coccidioidomycosis by liver biopsy, *Arch. Intern. Med.*, 143, 1335, 1983.
49. Weisman, I. M., Moreno, A. J., Parker, A. L., Sippo, W. C., and Liles, W. J., Gastrointestinal dissemination of coccidioidomycosis, *Am. J. Gastroenterol.*, 81, 589, 1986.
50. Ampel, N. M., White, J. D., Varanasi, U. R., Larwood, T. R., Van Wyck, D. B., and Galgiani, J. N., Coccidioidal peritonitis associated with ambulatory peritoneal dialysis, *Am. J. Kidney Dis.*, 11, 512, 1988.
51. Jamidar, P. A., Campbell, D. R., Fishback, J. L., and Klotz S. A., Peritoneal coccidioidomycosis associated with human immunodeficiency virus infection, *Gastroenterology*, 102, 1054, 1992.
52. Schwartz, D. N., Fihn, S. D., and Miller, R. A., Infection of an arterial prosthesis as the presenting manifestation of disseminated coccidioidomycosis: control of disease with fluconazole, *Clin. Infect. Dis.*, 16, 486, 1993.
53. McCaffree, M. A., Altshuler, G., and Benirschke, K., Placental coccidioidomycosis without fetal disease, *Arch. Pathol. Lab. Med.*, 102, 512, 1978.
54. Bylund, D. J., Nanfro, J. J., and Marsh, W. L., Jr., Coccidioidomycosis of the female genital tract, *Arch. Pathol. Lab. Med.*, 110, 232, 1986.
55. Saw, E. C., Smale, L. E., Einstein, H., and Huntington, R. W., Jr., Female genital coccidioidomycosis, *Obstet. Gynecol.*, 45, 199, 1975.
56. Conner, W. T., Drach, G. W., and Bucher, W. C., Jr., Genitourinary aspects of disseminated coccidioidomycosis, *J. Urol.*, 113, 82, 1975.
57. Frangos, D. N. and Nyberg, L. M., Jr., Genitourinary fungal infections, *West. Med. J.*, 79, 455, 1986.
58. Dunne, W. M., Jr., Ziebert, A. P., Donahoe, L. W., and Standard, P., Unexpected laboratory diagnosis of latent urogenital coccidioidomycosis in a nonendemic area, *Arch. Pathol. Lab. Med.*, 110, 236, 1986.
59. Kuntze, J. R., Herman, M. H., and Evans, S. G., Genitourinary coccidioidomycosis, *J. Urol.*, 140, 370, 1988.
60. Einstein, H. E., Holeman, C. W., Jr., Sandigde, L. L., and Holden, D. H., Coccidioidal meningitis: the use of amphotericin B in treatment, *Calif. Med.*, 94, 339, 1961.
61. Winn, W. A., The treatment of coccidioidal meningitis, *Calif. Med.*, 101, 78, 1964.
62. Labadie, E. L. and Hamilton, R. H., Survival improvement in coccidioidal meningitis by high-dose intrathecal amphotericin B, *Arch. Intern. Med.*, 146, 2013, 1986.
63. Graybill, J. R., Craven, P. C., Taylor, R. L., Williams, D. M., and Magee, W. E., Treatment of murine cryptococcosis with liposome-associated amphotericin B, *J. Infect. Dis.*, 145, 748, 1982.
64. Taylor, R. L., Williams, D. M., Craven, P. C., Graybill, P. C., Drutz, D. J, and Magee, W. E., Amphotericin B in liposomes: a novel therapy for histoplasmosis, *Am. Rev. Respir. Dis.*, 125, 610, 1982.
65. Tremblay, C., Barza, M., Fiore, C., and Szoka, F., Efficacy of liposome-intercalated amphotericin B in the treatment of systemic candidiasis in mice, *Antimicrob. Agents Chemother.*, 26, 170, 1984.
66. Shirkhoda, A., Lopez-Berestein, G., Holbert, J. M., and Luna, M. A., Hepatosplenic fungal infection: CT and pathologic evaluation after treatment with liposomal amphotericin B, *Radiology*, 159, 349, 1986.
67. Lopez-Berestein, G., Liposomes as carriers of antifungal drugs, *Ann. NY Acad. Sci.*, 544, 590, 1988.
68. Lopez-Berestein, G., Bodey, G. P., Fainstein, V., Keating, M., Frankel, L. S., Zeluff, B., Gentry, L., and Mehta, K., Treatment of systemic fungal infections with liposomal amphotericin B, *Arch. Intern. Med.*, 149, 2533, 1989.
69. Patterson, T. F., Miniter, P., Dijkstra, J., Szoka, F. C., Ryan, J. L., and Andriole, V. T., Treatment of experimental invasive aspergillosis with novel amphotericin B/cholesterol sulfate complexes, *J. Infect. Dis.*, 159, 717, 1989.
70. Clark, J. M., Whitney, R. R., Olsen, S. J., George, R. J., Swerdel, M. R., Kunselman, L., and Bonner, D. P., Amphotericin B lipid complex therapy of experimental fungal infections in mice, *Antimicrob. Agents Chemother.*, 35, 615, 1991.
71. Clemons, K. V. and Stevens, D. A., Efficacies of amphotericin B complex (ABLC) and conventional amphotericin B against murine coccidioidomycosis, *J. Antimicrob. Chemother.*, 30, 353, 1992.

72. Allendoerfer, R., Yates, R. R., Sun, S. H., and Graybill, J. R., Comparison of amphotericin B lipid complex with amphotericin B and SCH 39304 in the treatment of murine coccidioidal meningitis, *J. Med. Vet. Mycol.*, 30, 377, 1992.

73. Clemons, K. V. and Stevens, D. A., Comparative efficacy of amphotericin B colloidal dispersion and amphotericin B deoxycholate suspension in treatment of murine coccidioidomycosis, *Antimicrob. Agents Chemother.*, 35, 1829, 1991.

74. Catanzaro, A., Einstein, H., Levine, H. B., Ross, J. B., Schillaci, R., Fierer, J., and Friedman, P. J., Ketoconazole for treatment of disseminated coccidioidomycosis, *Ann. Intern. Med.*, 96, 436, 1982.

75. Ross, J. B., Levine, H. B., Catanzaro, A., Einstein, H., Schillaci, R., and Friedman, P. J., Ketoconazole for treatment of chronic pulmonary coccidioidomycosis, *Ann. Intern. Med.*, 96, 440, 1982.

76. Defelice, R., Galgiani, J. N., Campbell, S. C., Palpant, S. D., Friedman, B. A., Dodge, R. A., Weinberg, M. G., Lincoln, L. J., Tennican, P. O., and Barbee, R. A., Ketoconazole treatment of non-primary coccidioidomycosis. Evaluation of 60 patients during three years of study, *Am. J. Med.*, 72, 681, 1982.

77. Graybill, J. R., Craven, P. C., Donovan, W., and Matthew, E. B., Ketoconazole therapy for systemic fungal infections: inadequacy of standard dosage regimens, *Am. Rev. Respir. Dis.*, 126, 171, 1982.

78. Dismukes, W. E., Stamm, A. M., Graybill, J. R., Craven, P. C., Stevens, D. A., Stiller, R. C., Sarosi, G. A., Medoff, G., Gregg, C. R., Gallia, H. A., Fields, B. T., Jr., Marier, R. L., Kerkering, T. A., Kaplowitz, L. G., Cloud, G., Bowles, C., and Shadomy, S., Treatment of systemic mycoses with ketoconazole: emphasis on toxicity and clinical response in 52 patients, *Ann. Intern. Med.*, 98, 13, 1983.

79. Stevens, D. A., Stiller, R. L., Williams, P. L., and Sugar, A. M., Experience with ketoconazole in three major manifestations of progressive coccidioidomycosis, *Am. J. Med.*, 74(Suppl.), 58, 1983.

80. Galgiani, J. N., Ketoconazole in the treatment of coccidioidomycosis, *Drugs*, 26, 355, 1983.

81. Galgiani, J. N., Stevens, D. A., Graybill, J. R., Dismukes, W. E., Cloud, G. A., and the NIAID Mycoses Study Group, Ketoconazole therapy of progressive coccidioidomycosis: comparison of 400- and 800-mg doses and observations at higher doses, *Am. J. Med.*, 84, 603, 1988.

82. Sugar, A. M., Alsip, S. G., Galgiani, J. N., Graybill, J. R., Dismukes, W. E., Cloud, G. A., Craven, P. C., and Stevens, D. A., Pharmacology and toxicity of high-dose ketoconazole, *Antimicrob. Agents Chemother.*, 31, 1874, 1987.

83. DeCoster, R., Caers, I., Coene, M. C., Amery, W., Beerens, D., and Haelterman, C., Effects of high dose ketoconazole therapy on the main plasma testicular and adrenal steroids in previously untreated prostatic cancer patients, *Clin. Endocrinol.*, 24, 657, 1986.

84. Pont, A., Williams, P., Loose, D. E., Feldman, D., Reitz, R. E., Bochra, C., and Stevens, D. A., Ketoconazole blocks adrenal steroid synthesis, *Ann. Intern. Med.*, 97, 370, 1982.

85. Heyns, W., Drochmans, A., Van der Schuren, A., and Verhoeven, G., Endocrine effects of high-dose ketoconazole therapy in advanced prostatic cancer, *Acta Endocrinol.*, 110, 276, 1985.

86. Holland, F. J., Fishman, L., Bailey, J. D., and Fazekas, A. T. A., Ketoconazole in the management of precocious puberty not responsive to LHRH-analog therapy, *N. Engl. J. Med.*, 312, 1023, 1985.

87. Feuillan, P., Poth, M., Reilly, W., Bright, G., Loriaux, L., and Chrousos, G., Ketoconazole treatment of type 1 autoimmune polyglandular syndrome: effects of pituitary-adrenal axis, *J. Pediatr.*, 109, 363, 1986.

88. Britton, H., Shehab, Z., Lightner, E., New, M., and Chow, D., Adrenal response in children receiving high doses of ketoconazole for systemic coccidioidomycosis, *J. Pediatr.*, 112, 488, 1988.

89. Catanzaro, A., Fierer, J., and Friedman, P. J., Fluconazole in the treatment of persistent coccidioido-mycosis, *Chest*, 97, 666, 1990.

90. Evans, T. G., Mayer, J., Cohen, S., Classen, D., and Carroll, K., Fluconazole failure in the treatment of invasive mycoses, *J. Infect. Dis.*, 164, 1232, 1991.

91. Diaz, M., Negroni, R., Montero-Gei, F., Castro, L. G. M., Sampaio, S. A. P., Borelli, D., Restrepo, A., Franco, L., Bran, J. L., Arathoon, E. G., Stevens, D. A., and the Fluconazole Pan-American Study Group, A Pan-American 5-year study of fluconazole therapy for deep mycoses in the immunocompetent host, *Clin. Infect. Dis.*, 14(Suppl. 1), S68, 1992.

92. Kelly, P. C., Coccidioidal meningitis, in *Coccidioidomycosis: A text*, Stevens, D. A., Ed., Plenum Medical Books, New York, 1980, 163.

93. Tucker, R. M., Williams, P. L., Arathoon, E. G., Levine, B. E., Hartstein, A. I., Hanson, L. H., and Stevens, D. A., Pharmacokinetics of fluconazole in cerebrospinal fluid and serum in human coccidioidal meningitis, *Antimicrob. Agents Chemother.*, 32, 369, 1988.

94. Tucker, R. M., Galgiani, J. N., Denning, D. W., Hanson, L. H., Graybill, J. R., Sharkey, K., Eckman, M. R., Salemi, C., Libke, R., Klein, R. A., and Stevens, D. A., Treatment of coccidioidal meningitis with fluconazole, *Rev. Infect. Dis.*, 12(Suppl. 3), S380, 1990.

95. Galgiani, J. N., Catanzaro, A., Cloud, G. A., Higgs, J., Friedman, B. A., Larsen, R. A., Graybill, J. R., and the NIAID Mycoses Study Group, Fluconazole therapy for coccidioidal meningitis, *Ann. Intern. Med.*, 119, 28, 1993.

96. Kostiuk, K. A., Pons, V. G., and Guglielmo, B. J., Penetration of fluconazole into abscess fluid, *J. Antimicrob. Chemother.*, 34, 603, 1994.

97. Lee, B. E., Feinberg, M., Abraham, J. J., and Murthy, A. R. K., Congenital malformations in an infant born to a woman treated with fluconazole, *Pediatr. Infect. Dis. J.*, 11, 1062, 1992.

98. Grant, S. M. and Clissold, S. P., Itraconazole: a review of its pharmacodynamic and pharmacokinetic properties, and therapeutic use in superficial and systemic mycoses, *Drugs*, 37, 310, 1989.

99. Tucker, R. M., Denning, D. W., Arathoon, E. G., Rinaldi, M. G., and Stevens, D. A., Itraconazole therapy for nonmeningeal coccidioidomycosis: clinical and laboratory observations, *J. Am. Acad. Dermatol.*, 23, 593, 1990.

100. Graybill, J. R., Stevens, D. A., Galgiani, J. N., Dismukes, W. E., Cloud, G. A., and the NIAID Mycoses Study Group, Itraconazole treatment of coccidioidomycosis, *Am. J. Med.*, 89, 282, 1990.

101. Diaz, M., Puente, R., de Hoyos, L. A., and Cruz, S., Itraconazole in the treatment of coccidioidomycosis, *Chest*, 100, 682, 1991.

102. Tucker, R. M., Denning, D. W., Dupont, B., and Stevens, D. A., Itraconazole therapy for chronic coccidioidal meningitis, *Ann. Intern. Med.*, 112, 108, 1990.

103. Sharkey, P. K., Rinaldi, M. G., Lerner, C. J., Fetchick, R. J., Dunn, J. F., and Graybill, J. R., High dose itraconazole in the treatment of severe mycoses, *Proc. 28th Intersci. Conf. Antimicrob. Agents Chemother.*, American Society for Microbiology, Washington, D.C., 1988, 575.

104. Bittleman, D. B., Stapleton, J., and Casale, T. B., Report of successful desensitization to itraconazole, *J. Allergy Clin. Immunol.*, 94, 270, 1994.

105. McIntyre, K. A. and Galgiani, J. N., *In vitro* susceptibilities of yeast to a new antifungal triazole, SCH 39304: effects of test conditions and relation to *in vivo* efficacy, *Antimicrob. Agents Chemother.*, 33, 1095, 1989.

106. Lee, J. A., Lin, C., Loebenberg, D., Rubin, M., Pizzo, P. A., and Walsh, T. J., Pharmacokinetics and tissue penetration of Sch 39304 in granulocytopenic and non-granulocytopenic rabbits, *Antimicrob. Agents Chemother.*, 33, 1932, 1989.

107. Defaveri, J., Sun, S. H., and Graybill, J. R., Treatment of murine coccidioidal meningitis with SCH 39304, *Antimicrob. Agents Chemother.*, 34, 663, 1990.

108. Clemons, K. V., Hanson, L. H., Perlman, A. M., and Stevens, D. A., Efficacy of SCH 39304 and fluconazole in a murine model of disseminated coccidioidomycosis, *Antimicrob. Agents Chemother.*, 34, 928, 1990.

109. Allendoerfer, R., Yates, R. R., Marquis, A. J., Loebenberg, D., Rinaldi, M. G., and Graybill, J. R., Comparison of SCH 39304 and its isomers, RR 42427 and SS 42426, for the treatment of murine cryptococcal and coccidioidal meningitis, *Antimicrob. Agents Chemother.*, 36, 217, 1992.

110. Hostetler, J. S., Catanzaro, A., Stevens, D. A., Graybill, J. R., Sharkey, P. K., Larsen, R. A., Tucker, R. M., Al-Haidary, A. D., Rinaldi, M. G., Cloud, G. A., and Galgiani, J. N., Treatment of coccidioidomycosis with SCH 39304, *J. Med. Vet. Mycol.*, 32, 105, 1994.

111. Pappagianis, D., Zimmer, B. L., Theodoropoulos, G., Plempel, M., and Hector, R. F., Therapeutic effect of the triazole Bay R 3783 in mouse models of coccidioidomycosis, blastomycosis, and histoplasmosis, *Antimicrob. Agents Chemother.*, 34, 1132, 1990.

112. Ryley, J. F., McGregor, S., and Wilson, R. G., Activity of ICI 195,739 — a novel orally active bis-triazole in rodent models of fungal and protozoal infections, *Ann. NY Acad. Sci.*, 544, 310, 1988.

113. Tucker, R. M., Hanson, L. H., Brummer, E., and Stevens, D. A., Activity of ICI 195,739, a new oral triazole, compared with that of ketoconazole in the therapy of experimental murine blastomycosis, *Antimicrob. Agents Chemother.*, 33, 573, 1989.

114. Clemons, K. V. and Stevens, D. A., Utility of the triazole D0870 in the treatment of experimental systemic coccidioidomycosis, *J. Med. Vet. Mycol.*, 32, 323, 1994.

115. Fierer, J., Kirkland, T., and Finley, F., Comparison of fluconazole and SDZ89-485 for therapy of experimental murine coccidioidomycosis, *Antimicrob. Agents Chemother.*, 34, 13, 1990.

116. Brown, M. S. and Goldstein, J. L., Lipoprotein metabolism in the macrophage: implications for cholesterol deposition in atherosclerosis, *Annu. Rev. Biochem.*, 52, 223, 1983.

117. Patterson, T. F., Miniter, P., Dijkstra, J., Szoka, F. C., Jr., Ryan, L., and Andriole, V. T., Treatment of experimental invasive aspergillosis with novel amphotericin B/cholesterol sulfate complexes, *J. Infect. Dis.*, 159, 717, 1989.

118. Brillinger, G. U., Metabolic products of microorganisms. 181. Chitin synthase from fungi, a test model for substances with insecticidal properties, *Arch. Microbiol.*, 121, 71, 1979.

119. Dahn, U., Hagenmayer, H., Hohne, H., Konig, W. A., Wolf, G., and Zahner, H., Nikkomycin, ein neuer hemmstoff der chitin-synthase bei pilzen, *Arch. Mikrobiol.*, 107, 143, 1976.

120. Hector, R. F., Zimmer, B. L., and Pappagianis, D., Evaluation of nikkomycins X and Z in murine models of coccidioidomycosis, histoplasmosis, and blastomycosis, *Antimicrob. Agents Chemother.*, 34, 587, 1990.

121. Galgiani, J. N., Sun, S. H., Clemons, K. V., and Stevens, D. A., Activity of cilofungin against *Coccidioides immitis*: differential *in vitro* effects on mycelia and spherules correlated with *in vivo* studies, *J. Infect. Dis.*, 162, 944, 1990.

122. Sarosi, G. A. and Davies, S. F., Concise review for primary-care physicians. Therapy for fungal infections, *Mayo Clin. Proc.*, 69, 1111, 1994.

123. Werner, S. B., Pappagianis, D., Heindl, I., and Mickel, A., An epidemic of coccidioidomycosis among archeology students in Northern California, *N. Engl. J. Med.*, 286, 507, 1972.

124. Johnson, P. and Sarosi, G., Current therapy of major fungal diseases of the lung, *Infect. Dis. Clin. North Am.*, 5, 635, 1991.

125. LaPage, E., Using a ventricular reservoir to instill amphotericin B, *J. Neurosci. Nurs.*, 25, 212, 1993.

126. American Thoracic Society, Treatment of fungal infection, *Am. Rev. Respir. Dis.*, 120, 1393, 1979.

127. McNeil, M. M. and Ampel, N. M., Opportunistic coccidioidomycosis in patients infected with human immunodeficiency virus: prevention issues and priorities, *Clin. Infect. Dis.*, 21(Suppl. 1), S111, 1995.

128. British Society For Antimicrobial Chemotherapy Working Party, Antifungal chemotherapy in patients with acquired immunodeficiency syndrome, *Lancet*, 340, 648, 1992.

129. Zar, F. A. and Fernandez, M., Failure of ketoconazole maintenance therapy for disseminated coccidioidomycosis in AIDS, *J. Infect. Dis.*, 164, 824, 1991.

130. Bronnimann, D. A., Adam, R. D., Galgiani, J. N., Habib, M. P., Petersen, E. A., Porter, B., and Bloom, J. W., Coccidioidomycosis in the immunodeficiency syndrome, *Ann. Intern. Med.*, 106, 372, 1987.

131. Fish, D. G., Ampel, N. M., Galgiani, J. N., Dols, C. L., Kelly, P. C., Johnson, C. H., Pappagianis, D., Edwards, J. E., Wasserman, R. B., Clark, R. J., Antoniskis, D., Larsen, R. A., Englender, S. J., and Petersen, E. A., Coccidioidomycosis during human immunodeficiency virus infection: a review of 77 patients, *Medicine (Baltimore)*, 69, 384, 1990.

132. Bozzette, S. A., Sattler, F. R., Chiu, J., Wu, A. W., Gluckstein, D., Kemper, C., Bartok, A., Niosi, J., Abramson, I., Coffman, J., Hughlett, C., Loya, R., Cassens, B., Akil, B., Meng, T.-C., Boylen, C. T., Nielsen, D., Richman, D. D., Tilles, J. G., Leedom, J., McCutchan, J. A., and the California Collaborative Treatment Group, A controlled trial of early adjunctive treatment with corticosteroids for *Pneumocystis carinii* pneumonia in the acquired immunodeficiency syndrome, *N. Engl. J. Med.*, 323, 1451, 1990.

133. Gagnon, S., Boota, A. M., Fischl, M. A., Baier, H., Kirksey, O. W., and La Voie, L., Corticosteroids as adjunctive therapy for severe *Pneumocystis carinii* in the acquired immunodeficiency syndrome: a double-blind, placebo-controlled trial, *N. Engl. J. Med.*, 323, 1444, 1990.

134. MacFadden, D. K., Edelson, J. D., Hyland, R. H., Rodriguez, C. H., Innouye, T., and Rebuck, A. S., Corticosteroids as adjunctive therapy in treatment of *Pneumocystis carinii* pneumonia in patients with acquired immunodeficiency syndrome, *Lancet*, 1, 1477, 1987.

135. Montaner, J. S., Lawson, L. M., Levitt, N., Belzberg, H., Schechter, M. T., and Ruedy, J., Corticosteroids prevent early deterioration in patients with moderately severe *Pneumocystis carinii* pneumonia and the acquired immunodeficiency syndrome (AIDS), *Ann. Intern. Med.*, 113, 14, 1990.

136. Ampel, N. M., Ryan, K. J., Carry, P. J., Wieden, M. A., and Schifman, R. B., Fungemia due to *Coccidioides immitis*: an analysis of 16 episodes in 15 patients and a review of the literature, *Medicine (Baltimore)*, 65, 312, 1986.

137. Mahaffey, K. W., Hippenmeyer, C. L., Mandel, R., and Ampel, N. M., Unrecognized coccidioidomycosis complicating *Pneumocystis carinii* pneumonia in patients infected with the human immunodeficiency virus and treated with corticosteroids, *Arch. Intern. Med.*, 153, 1496, 1993.

138. Harvey, W. C. and Greendyke, W. H., Skin lesions in acute coccidioidomycosis, *Am. Fam. Physician*, 2, 81, 1970.

139. Lundergan, L. L., Kerrick, S. S., and Galgiani, J. N., Coccidioidomycosis at a university outpatient clinic: a clinical description, in *Coccidioidomycosis: Proceedings of the 4th International Conference on Coccidioidomycosis*, San Diego, 1984, National Federation of Infectious Diseases, Washington, D.C., 1985, 47.

140. Huntington, R. W., Jr., Coccidioidomycosis — a great imitator disease, *Arch. Pathol. Lab. Med.*, 110, 182, 1986.

141. Bonifaz, A., Coccidioidomycosis, in *Micologia Medica Basica*, Mendez, C., Ed., Mexico, D. F., 1991, 215.

142. Rippon, J. W., Coccidioidomycosis, in *Medical Mycology*, 3rd ed., W. B. Saunders, Philadelphia, 1988, 433.

143. Bonifaz, A., Saul, A., Galindo, J., and Andrade, R., Primary cutaneous coccidioidomycosis treated with itraconazole, *Int. J. Dermatol.*, 33, 720, 1994.

144. Meyer, R. D., Cutaneous and mucosal manifestations of the deep mycotic infections, *Acta Derm. Venereol. (Stockholm)*, 121(Suppl.), 52, 1986.

145. Newland, Y. and Komisar, A., Coccidioidomycosis of the head and neck, *Ear Nose Throat J.*, 65, 55, 60.

146. Lavalle, P., Suchil, P., De Ovando, F., and Reynoso, S., Itraconazole for deep mycosis: preliminary experience in Mexico, *Rev. Infect. Dis.*, 9(Suppl. 1), S64, 1987.

147. Drutz, D. J., Amphotericin B in the treatment of coccidioidomycosis, *Drugs*, 26, 337, 1983.

148. Peterson, C. M., Schuppert, K., Kelly, P.C., and Pappagianis, D., Coccidioidomycosis and pregnancy, *Obstet. Gynecol.*, 48, 149, 1993.

149. Farness, O. J., Coccidioidomycosis, *JAMA*, 116, 1749, 1941.

150. Mendenhall, J. C., Black, W. C., and Pottz, G. E., Progressive (disseminated) coccidioidomycosis during pregnancy, *Rocky Mountain Med. J.*, 45, 472, 1948.

151. Smale, L. E. and Birsner, J. W., Maternal deaths from coccidioidomycosis, *JAMA*, 140, 1152, 1949 (correction, *JAMA*, 141, 212, 1949).

152. Pappagianis, S., Epidemiology of coccidioidomycosis, in *Coccidioidomycosis: A Text*, Stevens, D. A., Ed., Plenum Medical, New York, 1980, 80.

153. Drutz, D. J., Huppert, M., Sun, S. H., and McGuire, W. L., Human sex hormones stimulate the growth and maturation of *Coccidioides immitis*, *Infect. Immunol.*, 32, 897, 1981.

154. Powell, B. L., Drutz, D. J., Huppert, M., and Sun, S. H., Relationship of progesterone and estradiol-binding proteins in *Coccidioides immitis* to coccidioidal dissemination in pregnancy, *Infect. Immunol.*, 40, 478, 1983.

155. Walker, M. P. R., Brody, C. Z., and Resnick, R., Reactivation of coccidioidomycosis in pregnancy, *Obstet. Gynecol.*, 79, 815, 1992.

156. Mongan, E. S., Acute disseminated coccidioidomycosis, *Am. J. Med.*, 24, 820, 1958.

157. Stark, R. P., Does transplacental spread of coccidioidomycosis occur? Report of a neonatal fatality and review of the literature, *Arch. Pathol. Lab. Med.*, 105, 347, 1981.

158. Townsend, T. E. and McKey, R. W., Coccidioidomycosis in children, *Am. J. Dis. Child.*, 86, 51, 1953.

159. Hyatt, H. W., Coccidioidomycosis in a 3-week-old infant, *Am. J. Dis. Child.*, 105, 93, 1963.

160. Bernstein, O. I., Tipton, J. R., Schott, S. F., and Cherry, J. D., Coccidioidomycosis in a neonate: maternal-fetal transmission, *J. Pediatr.*, 99, 752, 1981.

161. Cohen, R., Coccidioidomycosis: case studies in children, *Arch. Pediatr.*, 66, 241, 1949.

162. Golden, S. E., Morgan, C. M., Bartley, D. L., and Campo, R. V., Disseminated coccidioidomycosis with chorioretinitis in early infancy, *Pediatr. Infect. Dis. J.*, 5, 272, 1986.

163. Sanford, W. G., Rasch, J. R., and Stonehill, R. B., A therapeutic dilemma: the treatment of disseminated coccidioidomycosis with amphotericin B, *Ann. Intern. Med.*, 56, 533, 1962.

164. Hadsall, F. J. and Acquarelli, M. J., Disseminated coccidioidomycosis presenting as facial granulomas in pregnancy: a report of two cases and a review of the literature, *Laryngoscope*, 83, 51, 1973.

165. McCoy, M. J., Ellenberg, J. F., and Killam, A. P., Coccidioidomycosis complicating pregnancy, *Am. J. Obstet. Gynecol.*, 140, 739, 1980.

166. Peterson, C. M., Johnson, S. L., Kelly, J. V., and Kelly, P. C., Coccidioidal meningitis and pregnancy: a case report, *Obstet. Gynecol.*, 73, 835, 1989.

167. Catanzaro, A., Pulmonary mycosis in pregnant women, *Chest*, 86, 155, 1984.

168. Wack, E. E., Ampel, N. M., and Galgiani, J. N., Coccidioidomycosis during pregnancy, *Chest*, 94, 376, 1988.

169. Stevens, D. A., Chemotherapy of coccidioidomycosis, in *Coccidioidomycosis: A Text*, Stevens, D. A., Ed., Plenum Medical, New York, 1980, 253.

170. Zeluff, B. J., Fungal pneumonia in transplant recipients, *Semin. Respir. Infect.*, 5, 80, 1990.

171. Peterson, P. K., Pulmonary mycosis in organ transplant recipients, in *Fungal Diseases of the Lung*, Sarosi, G. A. and Davies, S. F., Eds., Grune and Stratton, Orlando, 1986, 283.

172. Hall, K. A., Copeland, J. G., Zukoski, C. F., Sethi, G. K., and Galgiani, J. N., Markers of coccidioidomycosis before cardiac or renal transplantation and the risk of recurrent infection, *Transplantation*, 55, 1422, 1993.

173. Britt, R. H., Enzmann, D. R., and Remington, J. S., Intracranial infection in cardiac transplant recipients, *Ann. Neurol.*, 9, 107, 1981.

174. Vartivarian, S. E., Coudron, P. E., and Markowitz, S. M., Disseminated coccidioidomycosis: unusual manifestations in a cardiac transplantation patient, *Am. J. Med.*, 83, 949, 1987.

175. Calhoun, D. D. L., Galgiani, J. N., Zukoski, C., and Copeland, J. G., Coccidioidomycosis in recent renal or cardiac transplant recipients, in *Coccidioidomycosis: Proceedings of the 4th Int. Conf. Coccidioidomycosis*, National Foundation for Infectious Diseases, Washington, D.C., 1985, 312.

176. Stevens, D. A., Coccidioides immitis, in *Principles and Practice of Infectious Diseases*, Mandell, G. L., Douglas, R. G., and Bennett, J. E., Eds., John Wiley & Sons, New York, 1985, 1485.

177. Hall, K. A., Sethi, G. K., Rosado, L. J., Martinez, J. D., Huston, C. L., and Copeland, J. G., Coccidioidomycosis and heart transplantation, *J. Heart Lung Transplant.*, 12, 525, 1993.

178. Rifkind, D., Marchioro, T. L., Schneck, S. A., and Hill, R. B., Jr., Systemic fungal infections complicating renal transplantation and immunosuppressive therapy, *Am. J. Med.*, 43, 28, 1967.

179. Tolkoff-Rubin, N. E. and Rubin, R. H., Opportunistic fungal and bacterial infection in the renal transplant recipient, *J. Am. Soc. Nephrol.*, 2(Suppl. 3), S264, 1992.

180. Cohen, I. M., Galgiani, J. N., Potter, D., and Ogden, D. A., Coccidioidomycosis in renal therapy, *Arch. Intern. Med.*, 142, 489, 1982.

181. Seltzer, J., Broaddus, V. C., Jacobs, R., and Golden, J. A., Reactivation of coccidioides infection, *West. J. Med.*, 145, 96, 1986.

182. Hart, P. D., Russell, E., and Remington, J. S., The compromised host and infection. II. Deep fungal infection, *J. Infect. Dis.*, 120, 169, 1969.

183. Schroter, G. P. J., Bakshanden, K., Husberg, B. S., and Weil, R., Coccidioidomycosis and renal transplantation, *Transplantation*, 23, 485, 1977.

184. Deresinski, S. C. and Stevens, D. A., Coccidioidomycosis in compromised hosts, *Medicine (Baltimore)*, 54, 377, 1974.

185. Murphy, M., Drash, A. L., and Donnelly, W. H., Disseminated coccidioidomycosis associated with immunosuppressive therapy following renal transplantation, *Pediatrics*, 48, 144, 1971.

186. Chandler, J. W., Kalina, R. E., and Milan, D. F., Coccidioidal choroiditis following renal transplantation, *Am. J. Ophthalmol.*, 74, 1080, 1972.

187. Colonna, J. O., Winston, D. J., Brill, J. E., Goldstein, L. I., Hoff, M. P., Hiatt, J. R., Quinones-Baldrich, W., Ramming, K. P., and Busuttil, R. W., Infectious complications in liver transplant recipients, *Arch. Surg.*, 123, 360, 1988.

188. Dummer, S. J., Hardy, A., Poorsattar, A., and Ho, M., Early infections in kidney, heart and liver transplant recipients on cyclosporine, *Transplantation*, 36, 259, 1983.

189. Ho, M., Wajszczuk, C. P., Hardy, A., Dummer, J. S., Starzl, T. E., Hakala, T. R., and Bahnson, H. T., Infections in kidney, heart, and liver transplant recipients on cyclosporine, *Transplant. Proc.*, 15(Suppl. 1), 2768, 1983.

190. Kusne, S., Dummer, J. S., Singh, N., Iwatsuki, S., Makowka, L., Esquivel, C., Tzakis, H. G., Starzl, T. E., and Ho, M., Infections after liver transplantation: an analysis of 101 consecutive cases, *Medicine (Baltimore)*, 67, 132, 1988.

191. Schroter, G. P. J., Hoelscher, M., Putnam, C. W., Porter, K. A., and Starzl, T. E., Fungus infections after liver transplantation, *Ann. Surg.*, 186, 115, 1977.

192. Wajszczuk, C. P., Dummer, J. S., Ho, M., Van Thiel, D., Starzl, T. E., Iwatsuki, S., and Shaw, B., Jr., Fungal infections in liver transplant recipients, *Transplantation*, 40, 347, 1985.

193. Dodd, L. G. and Nelson, S. D., Disseminated coccidioidomycosis detected by percutaneous liver biopsy in a liver transplant recipient, *Am. J. Clin. Pathol.*, 93, 141, 1990.

194. Riley, D. K., Galgiani, J. N., O'Donnell, M. R., Ito, J. I., Beatty, P. G., and Evans, T. G., Coccidioidomycosis in bone marrow transplant recipients, *Transplantation*, 56, 1531, 1993.

195. Rodenbiker, H. T. and Ganley, J. P., Ocular coccidioidomycosis, *Surv. Ophthalmol.*, 24, 263, 1980.

196. Blumenkranz, M. S. and Stevens, D. A., Endogenous coccidioidal endophthalmitis, *J. Ophthalmol.*, 87, 974, 1980.

197. Brown, W. C., Kellenberger, R. E., and Hudson, K. E., Granulomatous uveitis associated with disseminated coccidioidomycosis, *Am. J. Ophthalmol.*, 45, 102, 1958.

198. Cutler, J. E., Binder, P. S., Paul, T. O., and Beamis, J. F., Metastatic coccidioidal endophthalmitis, *Arch. Ophthalmol.*, 96, 689, 1978.

199. Hagele, A. J., Evans, D. J., and Larwood, T. R., Primary endophthalmic coccidioidomycosis: report of a case of exogenous primary coccidioidomycosis of the eye diagnosed prior to enucleation, in *Coccidioidomycosis*, Ajello, L., Ed., University of Arizona Press, Tucson, 1967, 37.

200. Petitt, T. H., Learn, R. N., and Foos, R. Y., Intraocular coccidioidomycosis, *Arch. Ophthalmol.*, 77, 655, 1967.

201. Blumenkranz, M. S. and Stevens, D. A., Therapy of endogenous fungal endophthalmitis: miconazole or amphotericin B for coccidioidal and candidal infection, *Arch. Ophthalmol.*, 98, 1216, 1980.

202. American Medical Association Department of Drugs, *American Medical Association Drug Evaluations*, PSG Publishing, Littleton, MA, 1977, 824.

203. Allen, H. F., Amphotericin B and exogenous mycotic endophthalmitis after cataract extraction, *Arch. Ophthalmol.*, 88, 640, 1972.

204. Bell, R. W. and Ritchey, M. C., Subconjunctival nodules after amphotericin B injection, *Arch. Ophthalmol.*, 90, 402, 1973.

205. Lamer, L., Paquin, F., Lorange, G., Bayardelle, P., and Ojeimi, G., Macular coccidioidomycosis, *Can. J. Ophthalmol.*, 17, 121, 1982.

206. Alexander, P. B. and Coodley, E. L., Disseminated coccidioidomycosis with intraocular involvement, *Am. J. Ophthalmol.*, 64, 283, 1967.

207. Bayer, A. S., Yoshikawa, T. T., Galpin, J. E., and Guze, L. R., Unusual syndromes of coccidioidomycosis: diagnostic and therapeutic considerations, *Medicine (Baltimore)*, 55, 131, 1976.

208. Harris, R. E., Coccidioidomycosis complicating pregnancy. Report of 3 cases and review of the literature, *Obstet. Gynecol.*, 28, 400, 1966.

209. Andersen, F. C. and Cuckian, J. C., Systemic lupus erythematosus associated with fatal pulmonary coccidioidomycosis, *Tex. Rep. Biol. Med.*, 26, 94, 1968.

210. Berry, C. Z., Goldberg, L. C., and Shepard, W. L., Systemic lupus erythematosus complicated by coccidioidomycosis, *JAMA*, 206, 1083, 1968.

211. Conger, J., Farrell, T., and Douglas, S., Lupus nephritis complicated by fatal disseminated coccidioidomycosis, *Calif. Med.*, 118, 60, 1973.

212. Hileman, W. T., Disseminated coccidioidomycosis occurrence in a patient receiving steroid therapy for rheumatoid arthritis: a case report, *Ariz. Med.*, 20, 268, 1963.

213. Farness, O. J., Some unusual aspects of coccidioidomycosis, in *Coccidioidomycosis*, Ajello, L., Ed., University of Arizona Press, Tucson, 1967, 23.

214. Winn, W. R., Finegold, S. M., and Huntington, R. W., Coccidioidomycosis with fungemia, in *Coccidioidomycosis*, Ajello, L., Ed., University of Arizona Press, Tucson, 1967, 93.

215. Huntington, R. W., Waldmann, W. J., Sargent, J. A., O'Connell, H., Wybel, R., and Croll, D., Pathological and clinical observations on 142 cases of fatal coccidioidomycosis with necropsy, in *Coccidioidomycosis*, Ajello, L., Ed., University of Arizona Press, Tucson, 1967, 143.

216. Castellot, J. J., Creveling, R. L., and Pitts, F. W., Fatal miliary coccidioidomycosis complicating prolonged prednisone therapy in a patient with myelofibrosis, *Ann. Intern. Med.*, 52, 254, 1960.

217. Johnson, W. M., Coccidioidomycosis mortality in Arizona, in *Coccidioidomycosis. Current Clinical and Diagnostic Status*, Ajello, L., Ed., Symposia Specialists, Miami, 1977, 33.

218. Rowland, V. S., Westfall, R. E., and Hinchcliffe, W. A., Fatal coccidioidomycosis: analysis of host factors, in *Coccidioidomycosis. Current Clinical and Diagnostic Status*, Ajello, L., Ed., Symposia Specialists, Miami, 1977, 91.

219. Huntington, R. W., Acute fatal coccidioidal pneumonia, in *Coccidioidomycosis. Current Clinical and Diagnostic Status*, Ajello, L., Ed., Symposia Specialists, Miami, 1977, 127.

220. Rowland, V. S., Westfall, R. E., Hinchcliffe, W. A., and Jarrett, P. B., Acute respiratory failure in miliary coccidioidomycosis, in *Coccidioidomycosis. Current Clinical and Diagnostic Status*, Ajello, L., Ed., Symposia Specialists, Miami, 1977, 139.

221. Allen, W. G., Olsen, G. N., and Yergin, B. M., Disseminated coccidioidomycosis respiratory failure presenting in Florida, *J. Fla. Med. Assoc.*, 68, 356, 1981.

222. Johnson, W. M. and Gall, E. P., Fatal coccidioidomycosis in collagen vascular disease, *J. Rheumatol.*, 10, 79, 1983.

223. Land, C. A., Dorn, G. L., and Hill, J. M., The isolation of disseminated *Coccidioides immitis* by an improved blood culture technique, in *Coccidioidomycosis. Current Clinical and Diagnostic Status*, Ajello, L., Ed., Symposia Specialists, Miami, 1977, 19.

224. Knapp, W. A., Seeley, T. T., and Reuben, E. H., Fatal coccidioidomycosis: report of two cases, *Calif. Med.*, 116, 86, 1972.

225. Larsen, R. A., Jacobson, J. A., Morris, A. H., and Benowitz, B. A., Acute respiratory failure caused by primary pulmonary coccidioidomycosis: two case reports and a review of the literature, *Am. Rev. Respir. Dis.*, 131, 797, 1985.

226. Drutz, D. J. and Huppert, M., Coccidioidomycosis: factors affecting the host parasite interaction, *J. Infect. Dis.*, 147, 372, 1983.

227. Huppert, M., Sun, S. H., Gleason-Jordan, I., and Vukovich, K. R., Lung weights parallels disease severity in experimental coccidioidomycosis, *Infect. Immun.*, 14, 1356, 1976.

228. Ruddock, J. C. and Hope, R. B., Coccidioidal peritoneoscopy, *JAMA*, 113, 2054, 1939.

229. Forbus, W. and Bestebreurtje, A. M., Coccidioidomycosis study of 95 cases of disseminated type with special reference to the pathogenesis of disease, *Milit. Surg.*, 99, 653, 1946.

230. Saw, E. C., Shields, S. J., Comer, T. P., and Huntington, R. W., Jr., Granulomatous peritonitis due to *Coccidioides immitis*, *Arch. Surg.*, 108, 369, 1974.

231. Crum, R. B., Peritoneal coccidioidomycosis, *Arch. Surg.*, 78, 91, 1959.

232. Chen, K. T. K., Coccidioidal peritonitis, *Am. J. Clin. Pathol.*, 80, 514, 1983.

233. Muther, R. S. and Bennett, W. M., Peritoneal clearance of amphotericin B and 5-fluorocytosine, *West. J. Med.*, 133, 157, 1980.

234. Einstein, H., Coccidioidomycosis, *Basic Respir. Dis.*, 9, 1, 1980.

235. Drutz, D. J. and Catanzaro, A., Coccidioidomycosis. I, *Am. Rev. Respir. Dis.*, 117, 559, 1978.

236. Drutz, D. J. and Catanzaro, A., Coccidioidomycosis. II, *Am. Rev. Respir. Dis.*, 117, 727, 1978.

237. Resnick, D. and Niwayama, G., *Diagnosis of Bone and Joint Disorders*, W. B. Saunders, Philadelphia, 1988.

238. Bernreuter, W. K., Coccidioidomycosis of bone: a sequela of desert rheumatism, *Arthritis Rheum.*, 32, 1608, 1989.

239. Bisla, R. S. and Taber, T. H., Coccidioidomycosis of bone and joints, *Clin. Orthop.*, 121, 196, 1976.

240. Rettig, A. C., Evanski, Waugh, P. M., and Prietto, C. A., Coccidioidal synovitis of the knee, a report of four cases and review of the literature, *Clin. Orthop.*, 132, 187, 1978.

241. Stein, S. R., Leukens, C. A., Jr., and Bagg, R. J., Treatment of coccidioidomycosis infection of bone with local amphotericin B suction — irrigation, report of a case, *Clin. Orthop.*, 108, 161, 1975.

242. Winter, W. G., Jr., Larson, R. K., Honeggar, M. M., Jacobsen, D. T., Pappagianis, D. T., and Huntington, R. W., Jr., Coccidioidal arthritis and its treatment — 1975, *J. Bone Joint Surg.*, 57A, 1152, 1975.

243. Winter, W. G., Jr., Larson, R. K., Zettas, J. P., and Libke, R., Coccidioidal spondylitis, *J. Bone Joint Surg.*, 60A, 240, 1978.

244. Thorpe, C. D. and Spout, H. J., Coccidioidal osteomyelitis in a child's finger, *J. Bone Joint Surg.*, 67A, 330, 1985.

245. Bried, J. M. and Galgiani, J. N., *Coccidioides immitis* infections in bones and joints, *Clin. Orthop. Relat. Res.*, 311, 235, 1986.

246. Mitlar, R. P. and Bates, J. H., Amphotericin B toxicity. A follow-up report of 53 patients, *Ann. Intern. Med.*, 71, 1089, 1969.

247. Galgiani, J. N., Ketoconazole in the treatment of coccidioidomycosis, *Drugs*, 26, 355, 1983.

248. Noyes, F. R., McCabe, J. D., and Fekety, F. R., Jr., Acute candida arthritis. Report of a case and use of amphotericin B, *J. Bone Joint Surg.*, 55A, 169, 1973.

249. Buckley, S. L. and Burkus, J. K., Coccidioidomycosis of the first cuneiform: successful treatment utilizing local debridement and long-term ketoconazole therapy, *Foot Ankle*, 6, 300, 1986.

250. Gritti, E. J., Cook, F. E., Jr., and Spencer, H. B., Coccidioidomycosis granuloma of the prostate: a rare manifestation of the disseminated disease, *J. Urol.*, 89, 249, 1963.

251. Weitzner, S., Coccidioidomycosis of prostate and epididymis, *Southwest. Med. J.*, 49, 67, 1968.

252. Bellin, H. J. and Bhagavan, S., Coccidioidomycosis of the prostate gland, *Arch. Pathol.*, 96, 114, 1973.

253. Gottesman, J. E., Coccidioidomycosis of prostate and epididymis with urethrocutaneous fistula, *Urology*, 4, 311, 1974.

254. Petersen, E. A., Friedman, B. A., Growder, E. D., and Rifkind, D., Coccidioidouria: clinical significance, *Ann. Intern. Med.*, 85, 34, 1976.

255. Sung, J. P., Sun, S. S. Y., and Crutchlow, P. F., Coccidioidomycosis of the prostate gland and its therapy, *J. Urol.*, 121, 127, 1979.

256. Price, M. J., Lewis, E. L., and Carmalt, J. E., Coccidioidomycosis of prostate gland, *Urology*, 19, 653, 1982.

257. Chen, K. T. K. and Schiff, J. J., Coccidioidomycosis of the prostate, *Urology*, 25, 82, 1985.

258. Weyrauch, H. M., Normand, F. W., and Bassett, J. B., Coccidioidomycosis of the genital tract, *Calif. Med.*, 72, 465, 1950.

259. Rohn, J. G., Davilla, J. C., and Gibson, T. E., Urogenital aspects of coccidioidomycosis: review of the literature and report of two cases, *J. Urol.*, 65, 660, 1951.

260. Amromin, G. and Blumenfeld, C. M., Coccidioidomycosis of the epididymis: a report of two cases, *Calif. Med.*, 78, 136, 1953.

261. Pace, J. M., Coccidioidomycosis of the epididymis, *South. Med. J.*, 48, 259, 1955.

262. Bodner, H., Howard, A. H., and Kaplan, J. H., Coccidioidomycosis of the spermatic cord; roentgen therapy: report of a case, *J. Int. Coll. Surg.*, 36, 530, 1959.

263. Stewart, B. G., Epididymitis and prostatitis due to coccidioidomycosis: a case report with 5-year follow up, *J. Urol.*, 91, 280, 1964.

264. Cheng, S. F., Bilateral coccidioidal epididymitis, *Urology*, 3, 362, 1974.

265. Conner, W. T., Drach, G. W., and Bucher, W. C., Jr., Genitourinary aspects of disseminated coccidioidomycosis, *J. Urol.*, 113, 82, 1975.

266. Chen, K. T. K., Coccidioidomycosis of the epididymis, *J. Urol.*, 130, 978, 1983.

267. Weinberg, M. G., Galgiani, J. N., Switzer, R. W., and Vega, E., Coccidioidomycosis of the urinary bladder, in *Coccidioidomycosis*, Einstein, H. E. and Catanzaro, A., Eds., The National Foundation for Infectious Diseases, Washington, D.C., 1985, 355.

268. Salgia, K., Bhatia, L., Rajashekaraiah, K. R., Zangan, M., Hariharan, S., and Kallick, C. A., Coccidioidomycosis of the uterus, *South. Med. J.*, 75, 614, 1982.

269. Saw, E. C., Smale, L. E., Einstein, H., and Huntington, R. W., Jr., Female genital coccidioidomycosis, *Obstet. Gynecol.*, 45, 199, 1975.

270. Parker, P. and Adcock, L. L., Pelvic coccidioidomycosis, *Obstet. Gynecol. Surv.*, 36, 225, 1981.

271. Schwartz, D. N., Fihn, S. D., and Miller, R. A., Infection of an arterial prosthesis as the presenting manifestation of disseminated coccidioidomycosis: control of disease with fluconazole, *Clin. Infect. Dis.*, 16, 486, 1993.

272. Williams, P. L., Johnson, R., Pappagianis, D., Einstein, H., Slager, U., Koster, F. T., Eron, J. J., Morrison, J., Aguet, J., and River, M. E., Vasculitic and encephalitic complications associated with *Coccidioides immitis* infection of the central nervous system in humans: report of 10 cases and review, *Clin. Infect. Dis.*, 14, 673, 1992.

273. Echols, R. M., Palmer, D. L., and Long, G. W., Tissue eosinophilia in human coccidioidomycosis, *Rev. Infect. Dis.*, 4, 656, 1982.

274. Drutz, D. J. and Huppert, M., Coccidioidomycosis: factors affecting the host-parasite interaction, *J. Infect. Dis.*, 147, 372, 1983.

275. Galgiani, J. N., Payne, C. M., and Jones, J. F., Human polymorphonuclear leukocyte inhibition of incorporation of chitin precursors into mycelia of *Coccidioides immitis*, *J. Infect. Dis.*, 149, 404, 1984.

276. Galgiani, J. N., Inhibition of different phases of *Coccidioides immitis* by human neutrophiles or hydrogen peroxide, *J. Infect. Dis.*, 153, 217, 1986.

277. Drutz, D. J. and Huppert, M., Coccidioidomycosis: factors affecting the host-parasite interaction, *J. Infect. Dis.*, 147, 372, 1983.

278. Frey, C. L. and Drutz, D. J., Influence of fungal surface components on the interaction of *Coccidioides immitis* fractions which are antigenic for immune T lymphocytes, *Infect. Immun.*, 59, 3952, 1991.

279. Cole, G. T., Zhu, S., Pan, S., Yuan, L., Kruse, D., and Sun, S. H., Isolation of antigens with proteolytic activity from *Coccidioides immitis*, *Infect. Immun.*, 57, 1524, 1989.

280. Yuan, L. and Cole, G. T., Isolation and characterization of an extracellular proteinase of *Coccidioides immitis*, *Infect. Immun.*, 55, 1970, 1987.

281. Petkus, A. F. and Baum, L. L., Natural killer cell inhibition of young spherules and endospores of *Coccidioides immites*, *J. Immunol.*, 139, 3107, 1987.

282. Ampel, N. M., Bejarano, G. C., and Galgiani, J. N., Killing of *Coccidioides immitis* by human peripheral blood mononuclear cells, *Infect. Immun.*, 60, 4200, 1992.

283. Ampel, N. M. and Galgiani, J. N., Interaction of human peripheral blood mononuclear cells with *Coccidioides immitis* arthroconidia, *Cell. Immunol.*, 133, 253, 1991.

284. Beaman, L., Pappagianis, D., and Benjamini, E., Mechanisms of resistance to infection with *Coccidioides immitis* in mice, *Infect. Immun.*, 23, 681, 1979.

285. Beaman, L., Benjamini, E., and Pappagianis, D., Activation of macrophages by lymphokines: enhancement of phagosome-lysosome fusion and killing of *Coccidioides immitis*, *Infect. Immun.*, 39, 1201, 1983.

286. Beaman, L., Effects of recombinant gamma interferon and tumor necrosis factor on *in vitro* interactions of human mononuclear phagocytes with *Coccidioides immitis*, *Infect. Immun.*, 59, 4227, 1991.

287. Beaman, L., Fungicidal activation of murine macrophages by recombinant gamma interferon, *Infect. Immun.*, 55, 2951, 1987.

288. Cox, R. A. and Vivas, J. R., Spectrum of *in vivo* and *in vitro* cell-mediated immune responses in coccidioidomycosis, *Cell. Immunol.*, 31, 130, 1977.

289. Cox, R. A., Vivas, J. R., Gross, A., Lecara, G., Miller, E., and Brummer, E., *In vivo* and *in vitro* cell-mediated responses in coccidioidomycosis. I. Immunologic responses of persons with primary, asymptomatic infections, *Am. Rev. Respir. Dis.*, 114, 937, 1976.

290. Cole, G. T., Seshan, K. R., Franco, M., Bukownik, E., Sun, S. H., and Hearn, V. M., Isolation and morphology of an immunoreactive outer wall fraction produced by spherules of *Coccidioides immitis*, *Infect. Immun.*, 56, 2686, 1988.

291. Cole, G. T., Kirkland, T. N., Franco, M., Zhu, S., Yuan, L., Sun, S. H., and Hearn, V. M., Immunoreactivity of a surface wall fraction produced by spherules of *Coccidioides immitis*, *Infect. Immun.*, 56, 2695, 1988.

292. Deresinski, S. C., Levine, H. B., and Stevens, D. A., Soluble antigens of mycelia and spherules in the *in vitro* detection of immunity to *Coccidioides immitis*, *Infect. Immun.*, 10, 700, 1974.

293. Catanzaro, A., Spitler, L. E., and Moser, K. M., Cellular immune response in coccidioidomycosis, *Cell. Immunol.*, 15, 360, 1975.

294. Barbee, R. A. and Hicks, M. J., Clinical usefulness of lymphocyte transformation in patients with coccidioidomycosis, *Chest*, 93, 1003, 1988.

295. Ampel, N. M., Bejarano, G. C., Salas, S. D, and Galgiani, J. N., *In vitro* assessment of cellular immunity in human coccidioidomycosis: relationship between dermal hypersensitivity, lymphocyte transformation, and lymphokine production by peripheral blood mononuclear cells from healthy adults, *J. Infect. Dis.*, 165, 710, 1992.

296. Cox, R. A., Baker, B. S, and Stevens, D. A., Specificity of immunoglobulin E in coccidioidomycosis and correlation with disease involvement, *Infect. Immun.*, 37, 609, 1982.

297. Kong, Y. M., Levine, H. B., Madin, S. H., and Smith, C. E., Fungal multiplication and histopathologic changes in vaccinated mice infected with *Coccidoides immitis*. I, *Immunology*, 92, 779, 1964.

37.8 *PARACOCCIDIOIDES BRASILIENSIS*

37.8.1 INTRODUCTION

Paracoccidioidomycosis is a systemic mycosis characterized by primary pulmonary lesions with dissemination to many visceral organs. Secondary lesions appear frequently as ulcerative granulomas of the buccal and nasal mucosa with extension to the skin, lymph nodes, adrenals, and by generalized lymphangitis.[1] The disease may often become severe and even fatal, especially in immunocompromised patients, such as those with AIDS.[2-5] In addition, subclinical infections have been documented in healthy individuals living in regions where the disease is endemic, namely the countries of Central and South America (most often in Brazil, Venezuela, and Colombia, as well as in Ecuador, Uruguay, and Argentina but not in the Guyanas, Surinam, and Chile).[5-12] Only one case (in Trinidad[13]) has been reported in the Caribbean islands.

The etiologic agent of paracoccidioidomycosis is a dimorphic fungus, *Paracoccidioides brasiliensis,* which propagates as a yeast at body temperature and as mycelium at lower temperatures. Mycelia, chlamidospores, and probably conidia, may grow in the soil, in water, and on plants at ambient temperatures, and are believed to be the infectious forms of the pathogen.[12,14] In humans, the fungus exists in the yeast phase, while the natural habitat of the saprobic phase is presently unknown.[14] The fungal colonies in the yeast phase are soft, wrinkled, and cream colored. The most characteristic feature of the yeast is the pilot's wheel appearance where multiple budding mother cells are surrounded by various peripheral daughter cells.[15]

In addition to α- and β-1,3-glucans and galactomannan found in both the yeast and mycelium phases, both phases also produce soluble antigens, including glycoproteins and proteins with enzymatic activity.[16] Among the three major glycoproteins (72,000, 55,000, and 43,000 molecular weights), the 43-kDa glycoprotein is the one universally recognized by sera from all patients with paracoccidioidomycosis. Mendes-Giannini et al.[17,18] have studied the humoral response of patients with paracoccidioidomycosis and found that all of them produced antibodies to the 43-kDa glycoprotein, thus making this antigen important for diagnostic value as well as for modulation of the host immune response.

With regard to *P. brasiliensis* dimorphism, the mycelium-to-yeast transformation requires a strict control of the glucan biosynthesis[19-21] since, *in vivo*, the α-1,3-glucan is the main polysaccharide within the yeast wall, with only traces of β-1,3-glucan.[5,10] In contrast, β-1,3-glucan is the only polysaccharide present in the mycelial form.[22-24] Two antifungal agents, itraconazole and amphotericin B, are known to elicit structural changes in the yeast and mycelial phases of *P. brasiliensis*. At concentrations of 0.07 ng/ml, itraconazole prevented reproduction of yeast cells and induced necrosis of the mycelial cells.[25] On the other hand, amphotericin B induced marked changes in the lipid composition of the yeast cells which resulted in decreased amounts of total lipids, steroids, and some fatty acids.[26]

Another factor which can influence the mycelium-to-yeast transformation as well as the conidium-to-yeast transformation is the host hormonal milieu. Female sex hormones have been found to influence the progression of paracoccidioidal infection towards overt disease, thus changing fungal behavior and pathogenicity. Restrepo et al.[27] have demonstrated that β-estradiol specifically inhibited the transformation of mycelium into the yeast form by affecting fungal cytosolic protein expression, which presumably is being mediated via a specific binding protein-ligand complex.[28-32]

Different strains of *P. brasiliensis* show a great variation in antigenicity and virulence. The portal of entry of the fungus, while still not firmly defined, is believed to involve inhalation of airborne propagules producing primary pulmonary lymph node complex as well as acute pulmonary disease. Hematogenous spread to other organs may also take place at the same time.[11] In recent years, some unusual localizations of *P. brasiliensis* in the host have been reported, including the peripheral nervous system presenting extracranial involvement of the XIIth nerve and the recurrent laryngeal branch of the Xth nerve (Tapia's syndrome),[33] and intraspinal cord and cerebral paracoccidioidomycosis.[34]

Blotta et al.[35] have described a case of placental involvement of juvenile-type paracoccidioidomycosis. The disease predated pregnancy, and although the infant was delivered with no evidence of infection, microscopic examination of the placenta showed numerous *P. brasiliensis* yeast organisms in the intervillous space enmeshed in a macrophagic-phagocytic reaction, with damage (necrosis) of the trophoblast layer. The immunologic evaluation of the patient at the 8th month of pregnancy showed depressed functional tests for cellular immunity even though the number of immunocompetent cells was normal.[35]

Paracoccidioidomycosis most often affects adults between 30 and 60 years of age, and is rarely observed in children (3%) and young adults (10%). It occurs more frequently in males than in females, with an overall ratio in endemic regions of 13:1;[5] this ratio is even larger (150:1) in Colombia, Ecuador, and Argentina.[36] A strong argument supporting the importance of female hormonal influences in paracoccidioidomycosis was the finding that there was no sex prevalence in children with overt disease.[37-40]

Two distinct clinical forms of paracoccidioidomycosis are currently defined: the acute (subacute) juvenile form (3% to 5% of all cases), and the chronic adult form (over 90% of patients). The chronic form is predominantly manifested with mucocutaneous lesions. Furthermore, depending on the evolution and localization of lesions, the chronic form may also be manifested with uni- or multifocal developments.[41] The juvenile form is usually more severe, with rapid progression, and involvement of the reticuloendothelial system (spleen, liver, lymph nodes, and bone marrow).[5,42-45] In children, it is characterized with high morbidity and mortality, which is probably related to an antigen-specific immunodeficiency.[46]

In both clinical forms, the cell-mediated immune responses are abnormal, and the lack of specific therapy is often associated with high mortality rate.[39,47-49] Remission is frequently related to extensive pulmonary fibrosis.[50-52] The fibrotic sequelae may still persist even after successful therapy.[52,53]

While oropharyngeal paracoccidioidomycosis may be fairly common as first presentation of the disease (although with relatively small number of reports[52-60] in support), cases of oral lesions caused by *P. brasiliensis* have been extremely rare and, so far, associated only with patients who have lived in or visited Brazil, Paraguay, or Venezuela.[18,61-68] One case of submandibular lymph node paracoccidioidomycosis has been diagnosed in an HIV-infected patient.[69]

The most common sites of oral disease affected have been the alveolar and gingival mucosa, and the palate.[18,62-68] The infection, which often remains subclinical or localized, may occasionally disseminate.[70]

37.8.2   HOST IMMUNE RESPONSE TO PARACOCCIDIOIDOMYCOSIS

In a murine model of chronic disseminated paracoccidioidomycosis, Castaneda et al.[71] have found that the immune responses to *P. brasiliensis* mimicked those of the chronic human disease. Furthermore, the same authors[72] studied the regulation of cellular immunity during the course of chronic murine disseminated paracoccidioidomycosis, and demonstrated that disease progression was associated with the development of T cell suppressor activity for the proliferative responses to concanavalin A by the peripheral blood lymphocytes, and that the delayed-type hypersensitivity responses to antigen were suppressed by the administration of serum with specific high titer antibodies.

In general, there is a strong correlation between inhibition of cell-mediated immune responses and the acute progressive form of paracoccidioidomycosis,[73-76] especially in the disseminated form of the disease.[75] It is thought that the fungal infection is primarily responsible for the impairment of cell-mediated immunity which, in turn, will contribute to disease progression.[5] The observed reversal in cell-mediated immunity functions after successful antifungal therapy lent credence to this hypothesis.[76,77] Factors associated with impairment of cell-mediated immunity that have been studied, included unidentified host-produced inhibitory factors in human plasma,[76,78] circulating immune complexes,[79-83] and imbalance in T cell subsets.[84,85]

Singer-Vermes et al.[86] have studied in an experimental murine model of paracoccidioidomycosis the relationships between disease dissemination, and humoral and cellular immune responses. The fungal load in the most affected organs correlated with the antibody titers and was inversely correlated with the intensity of the delayed-type hypersensitivity (DTH) reaction. The pattern of immune responses in the murine infection mimicked that of human disease, in which high specific antibody levels and suppressed DTH reaction are found in the multifocal and severe forms of the disease.

Gimenez et al.[87] have examined skin biopsy samples from infected patients and observed both significant reduction in the number, and morphological changes of Langerhans cells as compared to healthy controls, suggesting a possible inhibition of cell-mediated immunity by paracoccidioides at antigen-presenting level.

Moscardi-Bacchi et al.[88] have found that monocytes and monocyte-derived macrophages enhanced the intracellular replication of ingested *P. brasiliensis*; similar findings were also made microscopically.[89] However, following activation by interferon-γ (300 U/ml for 3 d), the monocyte-derived macrophages inhibited the intracellular replication of the ingested fungus. These findings suggested that lymphokines such as interferon-γ (IFN-γ) may play an important role in human resistance to *P. brasiliensis*.[89-91] For example, *in vitro* studies of murine peritoneal macrophages and *P. brasiliensis* have demonstrated increased killing of *P. brasiliensis* by treatment of macrophages with either lymphokines[91] or recombinant IFN-γ.[90] These effects were reversed with the addition of anti-IFN-γ; a similar finding was achieved with murine pulmonary macrophages.[92] The regulation of IFN-γ production by murine T helper CD4+ cells in systemic fungal infections may be due, at least in part, to the dichotomous relationship between Th1 and Th2 T helper cell subsets. These subsets are differentiated by the different roles they play in the cytokine production.[93,94] Whereas murine Th1 cells have been shown to produce IFN-γ and interleukin (IL)-2, and to mediate the delayed-type hypersensitivity, the Th2 cells were involved in the production of IL-4, IL-5, IL-6, and IL-10. Because of their promotion in the production of IL-4, Th2 cells have been defined as potent stimulators of B cell activity and inducers of antibody production, especially of IgE and IgG1.[95] Hostetler et al.[96] have investigated the possible roles of anti-IL-4 and IFN-γ as immunomodulators of murine *P. brasiliensis* infection and found that anti-IL-4 treatment of the acute phase of the disease resulted in an enhancement of host resistance to infection which correlated with decreased IgE serum levels.

Silva and Figueiredo[97] have observed significantly increased levels of tumor necrosis factor-α (TNF-α) in patients with paracoccidioidomycosis suggesting that it may play a role in the host defense mechanism, especially in regulating the production of IFN-γ or some other cytokines critical for the host defense against *P. brasiliensis*.

As compared to controls, significantly lower cytotoxic activity of circulating natural killer (NK) cells recovered from *P. brasiliensis*-infected patients (both treated and untreated), has also been observed.[98] Since Jimenez and Murphy[99] have found that murine NK cells were able to inhibit *in vitro* the growth of *P. brasiliensis*, disturbance in the immune effector functions of these cells may be an important factor in the host resistance against *P. brasiliensis*.

Hyporeactive proliferative responses of patient's peripheral blood lymphocytes (PBLs) to *P. brasiliensis* antigens or mitogens has been another immunologic reaction reported in several studies.[75,76,78,100,101]

Since changes in the ratio of CD4+ (T helper-inducer) and CD8+ (T suppressor-cytotoxic) cells has been considered indicative for impaired cellular immunity, a possible relationship between the suppressed cell-mediated immune responses and reduced CD4[+]/CD8[+] T cell ratios observed in patients with paracoccidioidomycosis, has been investigated.[85] In patients with the acute form of the disease these ratios were clearly reduced (mean, 1.2; range, 0.7 to 1.5; n = 15) as compared to controls (mean, 1.9; range, 1.5 to 2.4; n = 26); however, in patients with the chronic disease the association of reduced CD4[+]/CD8[+] ratios was not as clear cut (only 29 of 45 patients had ratios below 1.5).[85] Abnormalities in the CD4[+]/CD8[+] ratios were also found in cells recovered from bronchoalveolar lavage fluid of patients with paracoccidioidomycosis.[102]

Restrepo[103] has established that some of the fungal cell wall polysaccharides may activate the CD8[+] suppressor T lymphocytes leading to inhibition of the homologous and heterologous immune responses.

In another study, Rezkallah-Iwasso et al.[104] reported that patients with active paracoccidioidomycosis had a decreased number of T cells expressing IL-2 receptors.

Earlier studies of patients with paracoccidioidomycosis have revealed no hindrance of antibody production but rather a hyperactive humoral immunity as evidenced by the increased serum levels of IgG, IgE, and IgA, which is indicative of a polyclonal activation of the system.[105] This increment in antibody production may be due at least in part to the pathogenicity of the fungal strain. As demonstrated by Singer-Vermes et al.,[106] in B10.A mice, intermediate and slightly virulent *P. brasiliensis* strains induced weak IgG antibody production, whereas the most virulent isolates induced strong specific humoral response.

Studies on human histocompatibility complexes (HLA antigens) in paracoccidioidomycosis have produced different correlations.[12] The HLA-A9, HLA-B13, and HLA-B40 histocompatibility antigens have been commonly described in infected patients. The A9 antigen was especially prevalent in the unifocal pulmonary form, whereas the B40 antigen was associated with both the uni- and multifocal form, suggesting a genetic influence on the susceptibility and the development of the various clinical forms of paracoccidioidomycosis. To this end, de Restrepo et al.[107] have demonstrated the association of HLA-A9 and HLA-B13 in Colombian patients with the disease, whereas a preferential correlation with HLA-B13 was described in Venezuelan patients.[108] Furthermore, Lacerda et al.[109] have found in 83 Brazilian patients with paracoccidioidomycosis the presence of HLA-B40 at significantly higher level than in controls. Results by de Messias et al.[110] demonstrated that MHC class III products, especially the nonexpressed C4B allele (C4B:Q0), were also markedly elevated in comparison with controls, and associated with both the chronic uni- and multifocal forms, and thereby in a position to influence the course of disease. Taken together, all these findings underscored the involvement of the HLA system in the genetic susceptibility to paracoccidioidomycosis as well as the importance of ethnic variability in this association.[12]

Munk et al.[111] have shown that during reactivation of paracoccidioidomycosis, the classical complement system was activated as evidenced by the presence of circulating C4d component.

37.8.3 PARACOCCIDIOIDOMYCOSIS IN THE IMMUNOCOMPROMISED HOST

In one experimental study in rats, malignancy was shown to result in disseminated paracoccidioidomycosis.[112] In various reported cases of patients with compromised immune functions (organ transplant recipients,[113] cancer chemotherapy,[114] AIDS[115-117]), infection with *P. brasiliensis* or reactivation of latent paracoccidioidomycosis remained a threat, especially in areas of disease endemicity.[113,114,118-121] After the spread of the AIDS epidemic, the incidence of HIV-positive and AIDS cases in regions endemic for *P. brasiliensis* has been studied. However, in Brazil, the reported number of AIDS patients with paracoccidioidomycosis has been surprisingly small (by some estimates only seven cases).[69,115-117,122,123] All seven but one of these patients were adult males (mean age 37), and all presented the acute and subacute juvenile form of the disease (not regularly observed in patients older than 25 years). In addition, all patients had multifocal involvement, with the reticuloendothelial system being implicated in six of seven patients. One possible explanation for the low incidence of paracoccidioidomycosis among AIDS patients was the lack of exposure and that AIDS has been a predominantly urban disease, whereas paracoccidioidomycosis occurs mainly in rural areas.[124] While the reported findings did not clear whether AIDS should be considered a predisposing factor for reactivation of latent paracoccidioidomycosis or acquisition of primary disease, in non-AIDS patients the juvenile form of paracoccidioidomycosis has been associated with a marked decrease in cell-mediated immunity.[41]

Shikanai-Yasuda et al.[125] described four patients who have developed immunodeficiency secondary to juvenile paracoccidioidomycosis probably due to enteric protein loss and/or malabsorption and malnutrition.[126-128] Several concurrent infections (*Campilobacter foetus* sepsis, and *Shigella flexneri* and *Staphylococcus* infections) have been diagnosed, thus underscoring the possibility of associated infections to occur even after clinical and serological remission of paracoccidioidomycosis.

37.8.4 Evolution of Therapies and Treatment of Paracoccidioidomycosis

Until 1940, the year sulfamidopyridine was introduced,[129] paracoccidioidomycosis was considered to be an incurable disease. Subsequently, other sulfonamide drugs were used, and sulfadiazine, which was shown to be effective in over 60% of patients,[130] is occasionally still used.[131] Based on their elimination rate and activity, there are two defined types of sulfonamide drugs: rapidly eliminated drugs (e.g., sulfadiazine), and slowly eliminated drugs (e.g., sulfamethoxypyridazine).[11] The sulfonamides are administered orally (usually sulfadiazine every 6 h, and sulfamethoxy-pyridazine every 12 h) at daily doses of 3.0 to 5.0 g for rapidly eliminated drugs and 1.0 g for slowly eliminated drugs.[132] Blood levels of 50 mg/l should be maintained.[120,133]

Benard et al.[116] have treated successfully an AIDS patient initially with sulfadiazine (6.0 g daily for 4 months) followed by ketoconazole (400 mg daily for another 4 months); a maintenance dose of sulfadoxine (1.0 g daily) was instituted afterwards. A significant improvement of abnormalities was observed at the end of 3 months, with the pulmonary infiltrate, respiratory symptoms, cutaneous rash, and the hepatomegaly all dissolved.

In spite of their low cost and relatively low toxicity (occasional crystaluria with hematuria),[130,132] the sulfonamides have two significant drawbacks: long periods of treatment required (up to 5 years), and the significant rate of relapse.[131,134] In addition, there is also the possibility of fungal resistance to sulfonamides,[135] especially after early discontinuation of therapy.[120]

The use of trimethoprim–sulfonamide combinations has been recommended as an alternative to sulfonamides in patients with sulfadiazine-resistant isolates.[136,137] Cotrimazine (trimethoprim–sulfadiazine) was reported useful in the treatment of cerebral paracoccidioidomycosis since both drugs could penetrate the cerebrospinal blood barrier well.[137] Barraviera et al.[138] evaluated the acetylator phenotype (genetic factors linked to liver metabolism), renal function, and serum sulfadiazine levels in patients with paracoccidioidomycosis treated with cotrimazine; approximately 95% of patients had adequate sulfadiazine levels (over 40 µg/ml) with the highest levels measured in those qualified as slow acetylators.

Another combination, trimethoprim–sulfamethoxazole (co-trimoxazole) has also been used in the treatment of paracoccidioidomycosis.[11,139] The therapeutic efficacy of co-trimoxazole appeared to be similar to that of other sulfonamides; however, it may be used in patients with sulfonamide-resistant paracoccidioidomycosis. The usual dose of co-trimoxazole is one tablet, twice daily, for 12 months.[11]

Amphotericin B was introduced in the therapy of paracoccidioidomycosis in 1958 and immediately proved to be more effective than the sulfonamides.[47,132,140,141] Following amphotericin B treatment, remission has been observed in 50% to 60% of patients. Amphotericin B is administered intravenously at an initial daily dose of 0.2 mg/kg, then increasing the dosage to up to 0.8 mg/kg daily until a total dose of 1.5 tp 2.0 g is reached. The relapse rate following amphotericin B therapy has also been relatively high — in as many as 18% of patients.[47,134,142] In addition, the unwarranted toxicity of the antibiotic and difficulties with its administration require physician supervision which is not always available in areas of endemicity.[5] It is usually recommended that after amphotericin B treatment, a prolonged oral sulfonamide therapy be implemented to maintain remission under control.[47,131,134,143] Bakos et al.[115] successfully used a 3-week course of amphotericin B (total, 3.0 g) to treat disseminated paracoccidioidomycosis with skin lesions in a patient with AIDS.

Shikanai-Yasuda et al.[144] have reported a rare case of severe juvenile paracoccidioidomycosis manifested as cholestatic jaundice, lymph node enlargement, and an unusual form of polyserositis associated with portal hypertension secondary to schistosomiasis, as well as bacteremias caused by *Escherichia coli* and *Staphylococcus aureus* and post-transfusional hepatitis C. The patient was treated with amphotericin B (reaching a total dose of 2.0 g), followed by maintenance therapy with itraconazole for 1 year; the hepatosplenic schistosomiasis was treated with oxamniquine.[144]

The introduction of the orally administered azole antimycotics, especially ketoconazole[53,145] and itraconazole, not only has improved the prognosis but also facilitated the therapy of paracoccidioidomycosis.[5,132]

Miconazole was the first azole antifungal drug used in the treatment of paracoccidioido-mycosis.[146,147] In clinical trials involving 40 patients, the drug was administered intravenously at daily doses of 600 mg, or orally at daily doses of 3.0 g. Remission was observed in 25 patients, improvement in 11, and no changes in 2 patients. Side effects (which prompted discontinuation of therapy in 2 patients) included mainly diarrhea and venous thrombosis, and less frequently anemia, purpura, pruritis, and tachycardia.

Intravenous econazole was also used successfully in four cases of paracoccidioidomycosis at daily doses of 600 mg; oral administration was also applied at daily doses of 1.0 g. The duration of therapy was 6 to 12 months.[146]

Treatment with ketoconazole at daily doses of 200 to 400 mg for 1 year or less resulted in disease remission in more than 90% of cases.[5,11,148] Most external lesions resolved within 3 to 6 months concurrent with gradual clearing of lung lesions;[53,145] however, fibrosis was unaffected by therapy.[51,149] The relapse rate 3 years after therapy was ceased remained relatively low (11%) as compared to earlier therapies.[132,150] One requirement for proper ketoconazole treatment is the maintenance of acidic gastric pH in order for the drug to be properly absorbed.

The side effects of ketoconazole included gastrointestinal and endocrine (gynecomastia, decreased libido) disorders.[53,145] In addition, patients on ketoconazole therapy had decreased activity of antioxidant enzymes (glucose 6-phosphate dehydrogenase, glutathione reductase),[151] necessitating close monitoring of patients with erythrocyte enzyme abnormalities during treatment with ketoconazole. In patients with concurrent tuberculosis receiving rifampin,[132] the ketoconazole levels became markedly reduced and their monitoring has been recommended.[5]

Currently, the drug of choice for the treatment of paracoccidioidomycosis is itracona-zole.[5,11,148,152] Its higher activity allows for both shorter duration of therapy (6 months) and lower daily doses (100 mg) but as is the case with ketoconazole,[53] itraconazole did not arrest the progression of paracoccidioidic fibrotic sequalae.[52] Since itraconazole showed low toxicity (it did not interfere with the endocrine metabolism[52,153]) and relapses occurred at a lower level (3% to 5%) than with ketoconazole,[153,154] it has been recommended in the treatment of cases of the severe juvenile form of paracoccidioidomycosis.[45] As with ketoconazole, itraconazole requires an acid pH for its proper absorption. Consequently, antacids and β-blockers have been contraindicated during therapy.[153]

Among the other triazole antifungals, fluconazole and sapeconazole have been studied extensively for their efficacy against paracoccidioidomycosis. Diaz et al.[155] have reported fluconazole to be highly active because its water solubility allowed for rapid penetration into the fluid compartments of the patient, as well as for parenteral administration. In another study,[147] fluconazole was used in 37 patients at daily doses of 200 to 400 mg for at least 6 months. Significant clinical improvement was observed in 34 patients; however, one sudden death also occurred. Co-trimoxazole therapy as a means to prevent relapses following fluconazole treatment has been recommended.[147]

Saperconazole when used orally at 100 mg daily elicited prompt responses, resolution of symptoms, and healing of mucocutaneous lesions in less than 2 months; X-ray alterations also improved early (3 to 6 months).[156]

The currently used therapies of paracoccidioidomycosis are summarized in Table 37.11.[5,11]

TABLE 37.11
Currently Used Therapies for Paracoccidioidomycosis

Drug	Daily Dose	Duration of Therapy	Relapse Rate (in %)
Sulfonamides[a]			
Sulfadiazine	3.0–5.0 g (adults)	3–5 years	35
	0.2 g/kg (children)		
Sulfamethoxypyridazine	500 mg		
Amphotericin B[b]	0.5–0.75 mg (total dose: 1.5–2.0 g)	3–4 months	38
Ketoconazole[a]	200 mg	6–12 months	11
Itraconazole[a]	100 mg	3–6 months	3.5

[a]Oral administration.

[b]Intravenous dose per treatment. Sulfonamide therapy is recommended to follow amphotericin B treatment.

37.8.4.1 Adrenocortical Dysfunction in Paracoccidioidomycosis and Azole Therapy

The adrenal glands are important target organs for *P. brasiliensis*,[157-165] with the development of adrenal lesions contributing to the severity of symptoms. Autopsy results have demonstrated adrenal involvement in 80% to 95% of patients.[157-160] In nonfatal cases, adrenal involvement has been diagnosed in as many as 48% of patients.[166-170]

The spectrum of manifestations evolved from overt Addison's syndrome to diminished functional reserve;[166-169,171] Del Negro et al.[167] have found significant hypoadrenalism in as many as 44% such cases. In another study,[162] a high percentage of patients with paracoccidioidomycosis presented with increased plasma renin activity, reduced aldosterone response to ACTH or to postural stimulation, as well as with low or subnormal plasma dehydroepiandrosterone sulfate (DHEA-S) levels.

Patients treated with ketoconazole seemed to manage less well in terms of adrenal function compared to controls — in one such study,[161] 44% had a decreased adrenal reserve. It is well known that ketoconazole can adversely affect the adrenal steroid biosynthesis by lowering serum cortisol levels and blunting the response of corticotropin infusion.[172,173] In addition, ketoconazole suppressed the testosterone biosynthesis and lowered its concentrations,[173-175] largely as the result of selective inhibition of the mitochondrial P-450-mediated enzyme synthesis.[176-178] While ketoconazole also displaced dihydrotestosterone and estradiol from sex hormone-binding globulins, it did not affect the cortisol binding to serum proteins.[178] It should also be noted that the ketoconazole effects on the steroid biosynthesis are dose-dependent and reversible 8 to 16 h after discontinuation of therapy.

Francesconi do Valle et al.[163] have questioned the concept of irreversibility of the adrenal function damage in paracoccidioidomycosis and the necessity to initiate replacement corticoid therapy for the rest of the patient's life. These investigators reported that following specific ketoconazole or sulfonamide therapy (1 to 2 years), patients with adrenal insufficiency experienced complete recovery of adrenal function.

37.8.4.2   Structural Alterations by Antifungal Drugs on *P. brasiliensis*

Ultrastructural studies of the yeast and mycelial phases of *P. brasiliensis* have revealed that both ketoconazole and itraconazole inflicted changes on the fungal cell wall and intracellular vacuoles.[25,179,180]

Following exposure to ajoene, a garlic-derived compound, the cytoplasmic membrane of *P. brasiliensis* has shown structural alterations.[181-183] Similarly to azoles, the yeast phase was more susceptible (90% inhibition at a concentration of 50 mM) than the mycelium phase (60% inhibition at the same concentration). The mechanism of action of ajoene probably involves inhibition of the fungal sulfhydryl metabolism.[181]

The antibiotics papulacandin B and cilofungin, two inhibitors of fungal cell wall β-1,3-glucan biosynthesis, have been tested *in vitro* against *P. brasiliensis*. The results have demonstrated that although papulacandin B did not affect the morphology and growth of the yeast phase, it did inhibit mycelial growth and the yeast-to-mycelium transformation.[22] Cilofungin, on the other hand, was ineffective in inhibiting the growth of *P. brasiliensis*.[184] In both cases, it may be assumed that the lack of activity against the yeast stage was largely due to the predominant presence of α-1,3-glucan in its cell wall.

37.8.5   REFERENCES

1. Emmons, C. W., Binford, C. H., and Utz, J. P., *Medical Mycology*, 2nd ed., Lea and Febiger, Philadelphia, 1970, 330.
2. Goldani, L. Z. and Sugar, A. M., Paracoccidioidomycosis and AIDS: an overview, *Clin. Infect. Dis.*, 21, 1275, 1995.
3. Marques, S. A., Conterno, L. O., Sgarbi, L. P., Villagra, A. M., Sabongi, V. P. G., Bagatin, E., and Goncalves, V. L. C., Paracoccidioidomycosis associated with acquired immunodeficiency syndrome: report of seven cases, *Rev. Inst. Med. Trop. Sao Paolo*, 37, 261, 1995.
4. de Lima, M. A., Silva-Vergara, M. L., Demachki, S., and dos Santos, J. A., Paracoccidioidomycosis in a patient with human immunodeficiency virus: a necropsy case, *Rev. Soc. Bras. Med. Trop.*, 28, 279, 1995.
5. Brummer, E., Castaneda, E., and Restrepo, A., Paracoccidioidomycosis: an update, *Clin. Microbiol. Rev.*, 6, 89, 1993.
6. Londero, A. T. and Melo, I. S., Paracoccidioidomicose (Blastomicose Sul-Americana, Doenca de Lutz-Splendore-Almeida), *J. Bras. Med.*, 55, 96, 1988.
7. Sugar, A. M., Paracoccidioidomycosis, *Infect. Dis. Clin. North Am.*, 2, 913, 1988.
8. Franco, M., Mendes, R. P., Moscardi-Bacchi, M., and Montenegro, M. R., Paracoccidioidomycosis, *Bailliere's Clin. Trop. Med. Commun.*, 4, 185, 1989.
9. Restrepo, A., *Paracoccidioides brasiliensis*, in *Principles and Practice of Infectious Diseases*, Mandell, G. L. D., Douglas, G. R., and Bennett, J. E., Eds., Churchill Livingstone, London, 1990, 2021.
10. San-Blas, G., Restrepo, A., Stevens, D. A., San-Blas, F., Puccia, R., Travassos, L. R., Figueroa, J. I., Hamilton, A. J., Bartholomew, M. A., Harada, T., Fenelon, L., and Hay, R. J., Paracoccidioidomycosis, *J. Med. Vet. Mycol.*, 30(Suppl. 1), 59, 1992.
11. Negroni, R., Paracoccidioidomycosis (South American blastomycosis, Lutz's mycosis), *Int. J. Dermatol.*, 32, 847, 1993.
12. San-Blas, G., Paracoccidioidomycosis and its etiologic agent *Paracoccidioides brasiliensis*, *J. Med. Vet. Mycol.*, 31, 99, 1993.

13. Janky, N., Raju, G. C., and Barrow, S., Paracoccidioidomycosis in Trinidad, *Trop. Geogr. Med.*, 39, 83, 1987.

14. Restrepo, A., The ecology of *Paracoccidioides brasiliensis*: a puzzle still unsolved, *Sabouraudia/J. Med. Vet. Mycol.*, 23, 323, 1985.

15. Angulo-Ortega, A. and Pollak, L., Paracoccidioidomycosis, in *The Pathological Anatomy of the Mycoses. Human Infections with Fungi, Actinomycetes and Algeae*, Baker, R. D., Ed., Springer-Verlag, Berlin, 1971, 507.

16. Yarzabal, L., Composicion antigenica de *Paracoccidioides brasiliensis*, in *Paracoccidioidomicose*, Del Negro, G., Lacaz, C. S., and Fiorillo, A. M., Eds., S. A. Servier, EDUSP, Sao Paolo, Brazil, 1982, 59.

17. Mendes-Giannini, M. J. S., Bueno, J. P., Shikanai-Yasuda, M. A., Ferreira, A. W., and Masuda, A., Detection of the 43,000-molecular-weight glycoprotein in sera of patients with paracoccidioidomycosis, *J. Clin. Microbiol.*, 27, 2842, 1989.

18. Sposto, M. R., Mendes-Giannini, M. J., Moraes, R. A., Branco, F. C., and Scully, C., Paracoccidioidomycosis manifesting as oral lesions: clinical, cytological and serological investigation, *J. Oral Pathol. Med.*, 23, 85, 1994.

19. Kanetsuma, F., Carbonell, L. M., Azuma, I., and Yamamura, Y., Biochemical studies on the thermal dimorphism of *Paracoccidioides brasiliensis*, *J. Bacteriol.*, 110, 208, 1972.

20. Kanetsuma, F., Carbonell, L. M., Moreno, R. E., and Rodriguez, J., Cell wall composition of the yeast and mycelial forms of *Paracoccidioides brasiliensis*, *J. Bacteriol.*, 97, 1036, 1969.

21. San-Blas, F. and San-Blas, G., *Paracoccidioides brasiliensis*, in *Fungal Dimorphism*, Szaniszlo, P. J., Ed., Plenum Press, New York, 1985, 93.

22. Davilla, T., San-Blas, G., and San-Blas, F., Effect of papulocandin B on glucan synthesis in *Paracoccidioides brasiliensis*, *J. Med. Vet. Mycol.*, 24, 193, 1986.

23. San-Blas, G., Molecular aspects of dimorphism, in *Handbook of Applied Mycology: Humans, Animals, and Insects. Fungi Pathogenic to Humans*, Arora, D. K., Ajello, A., and Mukerjii, K. G., Eds., Marcel Dekker, New York, 1991, 459.

24. San-Blas, G., San-Blas, F., Rodriguez, L. E., and Castro, C. J., A model of dimorphism in pathogenic fungi: *Paracoccidioides brasiliensis*, *Acta Cient. Venz.*, 38, 202, 1987.

25. Borgers, M. and Van den Ven, M. A., Degenerative changes in fungi after itraconazole treatment, *Rev. Infect. Dis.*, 9(Suppl. 1), S33, 1987.

26. Hamdon, J. S. and Resende, M. A., Lipid composition and effect of amphotericin B on yeast cells of *Paracoccidioides brasiliensis*, *Mycopathologia*, 102, 97, 1988.

27. Restrepo, A., Salazar, M. E., Cano, L. E., Stover, E. P., Feldman, D., and Stevens, D. A., Estrogens inhibit mycelium-to-yeast transformation in the fungus *Paracoccidioides brasiliensis*: implication for resistance of females to paracoccidioidomycosis, *Infect. Immun.*, 46, 346, 1984.

28. Clemons, K. V., Feldman, D., and Stevens, D. A., Influence of estradiol on protein expression and methionine utilization during morphogenesis of *Paracoccidioides brasiliensis*, *J. Gen. Microbiol.*, 135, 1607, 1989.

29. Clemons, K. V. and Stevens, D. A., Interaction of mammalian esteroid hormones with *Paracoccidioides brasileinsis*: estradiol receptor binding and mediation of cellular functions, *Interciencia (Venezuela)*, 15, 206, 1990.

30. Clemons, K. V. and Stevens, D. A., A model for the study of hormonal influences in the morphogenesis of eucaryotic cells, *Proc. XIth Int. Symp. Human Animal Mycol. (ISHAM)* Montreal, Canada, Abstr. S18.1, 1991, 41.

31. Loose, D. S., Stover, E. P., Restrepo, A., Stevens, D. A., and Feldman, D., Estradiol binds to a receptorlike cytosol protein and initiates a biological response in *Paracoccidioides brasiliensis*, *Proc. Natl. Acad. Sci. U.S.A.*, 80, 7659, 1983.

32. Stover, E. P., Schar, G., Clemons, K. V., Stevens, D. A., and Feldman, D., Estradiol-binding proteins from mycelial and yeast-form cultures of *Paracoccidioides brasiliensis*, *Infect. Immun.*, 51, 199, 1986.

33. De-Freitas, M. R., Nascimento, O. J., and Chimelli, L., Tapia's syndrome caused by *Paracoccidioides brasiliensis*, *J. Neurol. Sci.*, 103, 179, 1991.

34. Morat-Fernandez, R. N., Beraldo, P. S. S., Masini, M., and Costa, P. H. C., Paracoccidioidomycose de localizacao intramedular e cerebral, *Arq. Neuro-Psiquitria*, 49, 192, 1991.

35. Blotta, M. H. S. L., Altemani, A. M., Amaral, E., Silva, L. J., and Camargo, Z. P., Placental involvement in paracoccidioidomycosis, *J. Med. Vet. Mycol.*, 31, 249, 1993.
36. Borelli, D., Prevalence of systemic mycoses in Latin America, *Proc. Int. Mycoses*, Publ. 205, Pan American Health Organization, Washington, D.C., p. 28.
37. Greer, D. L. and Restrepo, A., La epidemiologia de la paracoccidioidomicosis, *Bol. Of. Sanit. Panam.*, 83, 428, 1977.
38. Londero, A. T. and Melo, I. S., Paracoccidioidomycosis in childhood: a critical review, *Myco-pathologia*, 82, 49, 1983.
39. Londero, A. T. and Ramos, C. D., Paracoccidioidomicose: estudo clinico-micologico de 260 casos observados no interior do Estado do Rio Grande do Sul, *J. Pneumol. (Brasil)*, 16, 129, 1990.
40. Marques, S. A., Franco, M., Mendes, R. P., Silva, N. C. A., Bacilli, C., Curcelli, E. D., Feracin, A. C. M., Oliveira, C. S., Tagliarini, J. V., and Dillon, N. L., Aspectos epidemiologicos da paracoccidioidomicose na area endemica de Botucatu (Sao Paolo-Brasil), *Rev. Inst. Med. Trop. Sao Paolo*, 25, 87, 1983.
41. Franco, M., Host-parasite relationships in paracoccidioidomycosis, *J. Med. Vet. Mycol.*, 25, 5, 1987.
42. Franco, M. F., Montenegro, R. G., Mendes, R. P., Marcos, S. A., Dillon, N. L., and Mota, N. G. S., Paracoccidioidomycosis: a recently proposed classification of its clinical forms, *Rev. Soc. Bras. Med. Trop.*, 20, 129, 1987.
43. Giraldo, R., Restrepo, A., Gutierrez, F., Robledo, M., Londono, F., Hernandez, H., Sierra, F., and Calle, G., Pathogenesis of paracoccidioidomycosis: a model based on the study of 46 patients, *Mycopathologia*, 58, 63, 1976.
44. Montenegro, M. R. G., Formas clinicas de paracoccidioidomicose, *Rev. Inst. Med. Trop. Sao Paolo*, 28, 203, 1986.
45. Ochoa, M. T., Franco, L., and Restrepo, A., Caracteristicas de la paracoccidioidomicosis infantil: informe de cuatro casos, *Medicina U.P.B. (Madelin)*, 10, 97, 1991.
46. Benard, G., Orii, N. M., Marques, H. H. S., Mendonca, M., Aquino, M. Z., Campeas, A. E., Del Negro, G. B., Durandy, A., and Duarte, A. J. S., Severe acute paracoccidioidomycosis in children, *Pediatr. Infect. Dis. J.*, 13, 510, 1994.
47. Dillon, N. L., Sampaio, S. A. P., Habermann, M. C., Marques, S. A., Lastoria, J. C., Stolff, H. O., Silva, N. C. A., and Curi, P. R., Delayed results of treatment of paracoccidioidomycosis with amphotericin B plus sulfonamides versus amphotericin B alone, *Rev. Inst. Med. Trop. Sao Paolo*, 28, 265, 1986.
48. Lacaz, C. S., Porto, E., and Martins, J. E. C., Paracoccidioidomicose, in *Micologia Médica*, 8th ed., Servier Editora, Sao Paolo, Brazil, 1991, 248.
49. Terra, G. M. F., Rios-Goncalvez, A. J., Londero, A. T., Braga, M. P., Ourivuri, A. L., Mesquita, C. C., Marinho, J. C. A., Ervilha, L. M., Vieira, A. R. M., Deker-Mader, S., and Duarte, D. M. A., Paracoccidioidomicose em criancas ABP, *Arq. Bras. Med.*, 65, 8, 1991.
50. Campos, E. P., Padovani, C. R., and Cataneo, A. M. J., Paracoccidioidomicose: estudo radiologico e pulmonar de 58 casos, *Rev. Inst. Med. Trop. Sao Paolo*, 33, 267, 1991.
51. Guitierez, F., Silva, M., Pelaez, F., Gomez, I., and Restrepo, A., The radiological appearances of pulmonary paracoccidioidomycosis and the effect of ketoconazole therapy, *J. Pneumol. (Brasil)*, 11, 1, 1985.
52. Naranjo, M. S., Trujillo, M., Munera, M. I., Restrepo, P., Gomez, I., and Restrepo, A., Treatment of paracoccidioidomycosis with itraconazole, *J. Med. Vet. Mycol.*, 28, 67, 1990.
53. Restrepo, A., Gomez, I., Cano, E., Arango, M. D., Gutierrez, F., Sanin, A. S., and Robledo, M. A., Treatment of paracoccidioidomycosis with ketoconazole: a 3-year experience, *Am. J. Med.*, 78, 48, 1985.
54. Salman, L. and Sheppard, S. M., South American blastomycosis, *Oral Surg. Oral Med. Oral Pathol.*, 15, 671, 1962.
55. Pan American Health Organization, Paracoccidioidomycosis, Pan American Health Organization, Washington, D.C., 1972.
56. Murray, H. W., Littman, M. L., and Roberts, R. B., Disseminated paracoccidioidomycosis (South American blastomycosis) in the United States, *Am. J. Med.*, 56, 209, 1974.
57. Londero, A. T., Ramos, C. D., and Lopes, J. O. S., Progressive pulmonary paracoccidioidomycosis: a study of 34 cases observed in Rio Grande do Sul (Brazil), *Mycopathologia*, 63, 53, 1978.

58. de Almeida, O. P., Jorge, J., Scully, C., and Bozzo, L., Oral manifestations of paracoccidioidomycosis (South American blastomycosis), *Oral Surg. Oral Med. Oral Pathol.*, 72, 430, 1991.

59. Lazow, S. K., Seldin, R. D., and Solomon, M. P., South American blastomycosis of the maxilla: report of a case, *J. Oral Maxillofac. Surg.*, 48, 68, 1990.

60. Kwon-Chung, K. J. and Bennett, J. E., Paracoccidioidomycosis, in *Medical Mycology*, Lea and Febiger, Philadelphia, 1992, 594.

61. Lutz, A., Uma micose pseudococcidica localizada na boca e observada no Brazil: contribuicao ao conhencimento das hyphoblastomycoses americanas, *Bras. Med.*, 16, 151, 1908.

62. Salman, L. and Shepard, S. M., South American blastomycosis, *Oral Surg. Oral Med. Oral Pathol.*, 15, 671, 1962.

63. Joseph, E. A., Mare, A., and Irving, W. R., Oral South American blastomycosis in the USA, *Oral Surg. Oral. Med. Oral Med. Pathol.*, 21, 732, 1966.

64. Limongelli, W. A., Rothstein, S. S., Smith, L. G., and Clark, M. S., Disseminated South American blastomycosis (paracoccidioidomycosis): report of case, *J. Oral Surg.*, 36, 625, 1978.

65. Beckers, H., Seeliger, H., Gerber, H. G., and Motter, D., Manifestation einer system-mykose (Paracoccidioides brasiliensis) in der mundhole, *Dtsch. Z. Mund. Kiefer Gesichtschir.*, 12, 283, 1988.

66. Lazow, S. K., Seldin, R. D., and Solomon, M. P., South American blastomycosis of the maxilla: report of a case, *J. Oral Maxillofac. Surg.*, 48, 68, 1990.

67. Almeida, O. D. P., Jorge, J., Scully, C., and Bozzo, L., Oral manifestations of paracoccidioidomycosis (South American blastomycosis), *Oral Surg. Oral Med. Oral Pathol.*, 72, 430, 1991.

68. Sposto, M. R., Scully, C., de Almeida, O. P., Jorge, J., Graner, E., and Bozzo, L., Oral paracoccidioidomycosis: a study of 36 South American patients, *Oral Surg. Oral Med. Oral Pathol.*, 75, 461, 1993.

69. Goldani, L. Z., Coelho, I. C., Machado, A. A., and Martinez, R., Paracoccidioidomycosis and AIDS, *Scand. J. Infect. Dis.*, 23, 393, 1991.

70. Restrepo, A., Robledo, M., Gutierrez, F., San Clemente, M., Castaneda, E., and Calle, G., Paracoccidioidomycosis (South American blastomycosis): a study of 39 cases observed in Medellin, Colombia, *Am. J. Trop. Med. Hyg.*, 19, 68, 1970.

71. Castaneda, E., Brummer, E., Pappagianis, D., and Stevens, D. A., Impairment of cellular but not humoral immune responses in chronic pulmonary and disseminated paracoccidioidomycosis in mice, *Infect. Immun.*, 56, 1771, 1981.

72. Castaneda, E., Brummer, E., Pappagianis, D., and Stevens, D. A., Regulation of immune responses by T suppressor cells and by serum in chronic paracoccidioidomycosis, *Cell. Immunol.*, 117, 1, 1988.

73. Mendes, E. and Raphael, A., Impaired delayed hypersensitivity in patients with South American blastomycosis, *J. Allergy*, 47, 17, 1971.

74. Mendes, N. F., Musatti, C. C., Leao, R. C., Mendes, E., and Naspitz, C. K., Lymphocyte cultures and skin allograft survival in patients with South American blastomycosis, *J. Allergy Clin. Immunol.*, 48, 17, 1971.

75. Mota, N. G. S., Rezkallah-Iwasso, M. T., Peracoli, M. T. S., Audi, R. C., Mendes, R. P., Marcondes, J., Marques, S. A., Dillon, N. L., and Franco, M., Correlation between cell-mediated immunity and clinical forms of paracoccidioidomycosis, *Trans. R. Soc. Trop. Med. Hyg.*, 79, 765, 1985.

76. Restrepo, A., Restrepo, M., Restrepo, F., Aristizabal, L. H., Monkada, L. H., and Vélez, H., Immune responses in paracoccidioidomycosis: a controlled study of 16 patients before and after treatment, *Sabouraudia*, 16, 151, 1978.

77. Mok, P. W. Y. and Greer, D. L., Cell-mediated immune responses in patients with paracoccidioidomycosis, *Clin. Exp. Immunol.*, 28, 89, 1977.

78. Musatti, C. C., Rezkallah-Iwasso, M. T., Mendes, E., and Mendes, N. F., *In vivo* and *in vitro* evaluation of cell-mediated immunity in patients with paracoccidioidomycosis, *Cell. Immunol.*, 24, 365, 1976.

79. Arango, M., Oropeza, F., Anderson, O., Contreras, C., Bianco, M., and Yarzabal, L., Circulating immune complexes and *in vitro* reactivity in paracoccidioidomycosis, *Mycopathologia*, 79, 153, 1982.

80. Chequer-Bou-Habib, D., Daniel-Ribeiro, C., Banic, D. M., Francescone do Valle, A. C., and Galvao-Castro, B., Polyclonal B cell activation in paracoccidioidomycosis, *Mycopathologia*, 108, 89, 1989.

81. Chequer-Bou-Habib, D., Ferreira-da-Cruz, M. F., Oliveira-Neto, M. P., and Galvao-Castro, B., The possible role of circulating immune complexes in paracoccidioidomycosis, *Braz. J. Med. Biol. Res. Braz. Biol.*, 22, 205, 1989.

82. Silva, M. R., Campos, D. S., Taboada, D. C., Soares, G. H., Brascher, H. M., Vargens-Netto, J. R., Cruz, M. Q., Labarthe, N. V., Rocha, G. L., and Lima, A. O., Imunologia da paracoccidioidomicose, *An. Bras. Dermatol.*, 56, 227, 1981.

83. Chequer-Bou-Habib, D., Ferreira-da-Cruz, M., and Galvao-Castro, B., Immunosuppressive effect of paracoccidioidomycosis sera on the proliferative response of normal mononuclear cells: identification of a *Paracoccidioides brasiliensis* 34-kDa polypeptide in circulating immune complexes, *Mycopathologia*, 119, 65, 1992.

84. Moscardi-Bacchi, M., Soares, A., Mendes, R., Marques, S., and Franco, M., In situ localization of T lymphocyte subsets in human paracoccidioidomycosis, *J. Med. Vet. Mycol.*, 27, 149, 1989.

85. Mota, N. G. S., Peracoli, M. T. S., Mendes, R., Gattass, C. R., Marques, S. A., Soares, A. M. V. C., Izatto, I. C., and Rezkallah-Iwasso, M. T., Mononuclear cell subsets in patients with different clinical forms of paracoccidioidomycosis, *J. Med. Vet. Mycol.*, 26, 105, 1988.

86. Singer-Vermes, L. M., Caldeira, C. B., Burger, E., and Calich, V. L. G., Experimental murine paracoccidioidomycosis: relationship among the dissemination of the infection, humoral and cellular immune responses, *Clin. Exp. Immunol.*, 94, 75, 1993.

87. Gimenez, M. F., Tausk, F., Gimenez, M. M., and Gigli, I., Langerhans' cells in paracoccidioidomycosis, *Arch. Dermatol.*, 123, 479, 1987.

88. Moscardi-Bacchi, M., Brummer, E., and Stevens, D. A., Enhancement of *Paracoccidioides brasiliensis* multiplication by human monocytes or macrophages: inhibition by activated monocytes or macrophages, *Proc. 90th Annu. Meet. Am. Soc. Microbiol.*, American Society for Microbiology, Washington, D.C., Abstr. F-100, 1990, 425.

89. Brummer, E., Sun, S. H., Harrison, J. L., Perlman, A. M., Philpott, D. E., and Stevens, D. A., Ultrastructure of phagocytosed *Paracoccidioides brasiliensis* in nonactivated or activated macrophages, *Infect. Immun.*, 58, 2628, 1990.

90. Brummer, E., Hanson, L. H., and Stevens, D. A., Gamma-interferon activation of macrophages for killing of *Paracoccidioides brasiliensis* and evidence for nonoxidative mechanisms, *Int. J. Immunopharmacol.*, 10, 945, 1988.

91. Brummer, E., Hanson, L. H., Restrepo, A., and Stevens, D. A., Intracellular multiplication of *Paracoccidioides brasiliensis* in macrophages: killing and restriction of multiplication by activated macrophages, *Infect. Immun.*, 57, 2289, 1989.

92. Brummer, E., Hanson, L. H., Restrepo, A., and Stevens, D. A., *In vivo* and *in vitro* activation of pulmonary macrophages by gamma-interferon for enhanced killing of *Paracoccidioides brasiliensis* or *Blastomyces dermatitidis*, *J. Immunol.*, 40, 2786, 1988.

93. Mosmann, T. R., Cherwinski, H., Bond, M. W., Geidlin, M. A., and Coffman, R. L., Two types of murine helper T-cell clone. I. Definition according to profiles of lymphokine activities and secreted proteins, *J. Immunol.*, 136, 2348, 1986.

94. Georgiev, V. St. and Albright, J. F., Cytokines and their role as growth factors and in regulation of immune responses, *Ann. NY Acad. Sci.*, 685, 584, 1993.

95. Coffman, R. L., Seymour, B. W., Lebman, D. A., Hiraki, D. D., Christiansen, J. A., Shrader, B., Cherwinski, H. M., Savelkoul, H. F. J., Finkelman, F. D., Bond, M., and Mosmann, T. R., The role of helper T cell products in mouse B cell differentiation and isotype regulation, *Immunol. Rev.*, 102, 5, 1988.

96. Hostetler, J. S., Brummer, E., Coffman, R. L., and Stevens, D. A., Effect of anti-IL-4, interferon-gamma and an antifungal triazole (SCH 42427) in paracoccidioidomycosis: correlation of IgE levels and outcome, *Clin. Exp. Immunol.*, 94, 11, 1993.

97. Silva, C. L. and Figueiredo, F., Tumor necrosis factor in paracoccidioidomycosis patients, *J. Infect. Dis.*, 164, 1033, 1991.

98. Peracoli, M. T. S., Soares, A. M. V. C., Mendes, R. P., Marques, S. A., Pereira, P. C. M., and Rezkallah-Iwasso, M. T., Studies of natural killer cells in patients with paracoccidioidomycosis, *J. Med. Vet. Mycol.*, 29, 373, 1991.

99. Jimenez, B. E. and Murphy, J. W., *In vitro* effects of natural killer cells against *Paracoccidioides brasiliensis* yeast phase, *Infect. Immun.*, 46, 552, 1984.

100. Da Costa, J. C., Pagnano, P. M. G., Bechelli, L. M., Fiorillo, A. M., and Liina Filho, E. C., Lymphocyte transformation test in patients with paracoccidioidomycosis, *Mycopathologia*, 84, 55, 1983.

101. Bava, A. J., Mistchenko, A. S., Palacios, M. F., Esteves, M. E., Tiraboschi, N. I., Sen, L., Negroni, R., and Diez, R. A., Lymphocyte subpopulations and cytokine production in paracoccidioidomycosis patients, *Microbiol. Immunol.*, 35, 167, 1991.

102. Tapia, F. J., Goihman-Yahr, M., Caceres-Dittmar, G., Altieri, E., Gross, A., Isturiz, G., Rosquete, R., Viloria, N., Avila-Millan, E., Carrasquero, M., Borges, N. S., de Fernandez, B. P., Rothenberg, A., Albornoz, M. B., Pereira, J., de Gomez, M. H., San Martin, B., de Roman, A., and Bretana, A., Leukocyte immunophenotypes in broncholaveolar lavage and peripheral blood of paracoccidioidomycosis, sarcoidosis and silicosis, *Histol. Histopathol.*, 6, 395, 1991.

103. Restrepo, M. A., Immune responses to *Paracoccidioides brasiliensis* in human and animal hosts, *Curr. Top. Med. Mycol.*, 2, 239, 1988.

104. Rezkallah-Iwasso, M. T., Peracoli, M. T. S., Mendes, R. P., Guastale, H., Barraviera, B., Marques, S. A., and Soares, A. M. V. C., Defective expression of interleukin-2 (IL-2) receptors in patients with paracoccidioidomycosis, *Resumenes IV Encuentro Internacional Sobre Paracoccidioidomicosis*, Caracas, Venezuela, Abstr. I-21, 1989.

105. Arango, M. and Yarzabal, L., T-cell dysfunction and hyperimmunoglobulinemia E in paracoccidioidomycosis, *Mycopathologia*, 79, 115, 1982.

106. Singer-Vermes, L. M., Burger, E., Franco, M. F., Di Bacchi, M. M., Mendes-Giannini, M. J., and Calich, V. L., Evaluation of the pathogenicity and immunogenicity of seven *Paracoccidioides brasiliensis* isolates in susceptible inbred mice, *J. Med. Vet. Mycol.*, 27, 71, 1989.

107. de Restrepo, F. M., Restrepo, M., and Restrepo, A., Blood groups and HLA antigens in paracoccidioidomycosis, *Sabouraudia*, 21, 35, 1983.

108. Gonzalez, N. M., Albornoz, M., Rios, R., and Prado, L., Paracoccidioidomycosis y sui relacion con el sistema HLA. II. Encontro sobre paracoccidioidomicose, Brasil, Resumos adicionais, 1983.

109. Lacerda, G. B., Arce-Gomez, B., and Telles, F. Q., Increased frequency of HLA-B40 in patients with paracoccidioidomycosis, *J. Med. Vet. Mycol.*, 26, 253, 1988.

110. de Messias, I. J. T., Reis, A., Brenden, M., Queiroz-Telles, F., and Mauff, G., Association of major histocompatibility complex class III complement components C2, BF, and C4 with Brazilian paracoccidioidomycosis, *Compl. Inflamm.*, 8, 288, 1991.

111. Munk, M. E., Kajdacsy-Balla, A., Del Negro, G., Cuce, L. C., and Dias da Silva, W., Activation of human complement system in paracoccidioidomycosis, *J. Med. Vet. Mycol.*, 30, 317, 1992.

112. Teixeira, G. A., Kerr, I. B., Miranda, J. L., Machado Filho, J., and Oliveira, C. A. B., Blastomicose experimental no rat: evolucao da doenca experimental em animais implantados com sarcoma de Yoshida, *Hospital (Rio de Janeiro)*, 75, 505, 1969.

113. Sugar, A. M., Restrepo, A., and Stevens, D. A., Paracoccidioidomycosis in the immunocompromised host: report of a case and review of the literature, *Am. Rev. Respir. Dis.*, 129, 340, 1984.

114. Severo, L. C., Londero, A. T., Geyer, G. R., and Porto, N. S., Acute pulmonary paracoccidioidomycosis in an immunosuppressed patient, *Mycopathologia*, 68, 171, 1979.

115. Bakos, L., Kronfeld, M., Hampe, S., Castro, I., and Zampese, M., Disseminated paracoccidioidomycosis with skin lesions in a patient with acquired immunodeficiency syndrome, *J. Am. Acad. Dermatol.*, 20, 854, 1989.

116. Benard, G., Bueno, J. P., Yamashiro-Kanashiro, E. H., Shikanai-Yasuda, M. A., Del Negro, G. M. B., Melo, N. R., Sato, M. N., Amoto Neto, V., Shiroma, M., and Durate, A. J., Paracoccidioidomycosis in a patient with HIV infection: immunological studies, *Trans. R. Soc. Trop. Med. Hyg.*, 84, 151, 1990.

117. Goldani, L. Z., Martinez, R., Landell, G. A. M., Machado, A. A., and Coutinho, V., Paracoccidioidomycosis in a patient with acquired immunodeficiency syndrome, *Mycopathologia*, 105, 71, 1989.

118. Bodey, G. P., Infections in cancer patients, *Cancer Treat. Rev.*, 2, 89, 1975.

119. Rutala, P. G. and Smith, J. W., Coccidioidomycosis in potentially compromised hosts: the effect of immunosuppressive therapy in dissemination, *Am. J. Med. Sci.*, 275, 283, 1978.

120. Machado Filho, R. and Miranda, J. L., Consideracoes relativas a blastomicose sul-americana: evolucao, resultados consecutivos, *Hospital (Rio de Janeiro)*, 61, 375, 1961.

121. Rappoport, A., Santos, I. C., Andrade-Sobrinho, J., Faccio, C. H., and Menucelli, R., Importancia da blastomicose sul-americana no diagnostico con as neoplasias malignas de cabeca e pescoso, *Rev. Bras. Cab. Pesc.*, 1, 13, 1974.

122. Hadad, D. J., Pires, M. F. C., Petry, T. C., Orozco, S. F. B., Melham, M. S. C., Paes, R. A. P., and Gianini, M. J. M., *Paracoccidioides brasiliensis* isolated from blood in an AIDS patients, *Proc. XIth Congr. Int. Soc. Human Animal Mycol. (ISHAM)*, Montreal, Canada, Abstr. PS2.104, 1991, 116.

123. Pedro, R., Aoki, F. H., Boccato, R. S., Branchini, M. L., Goncales, F. L., Jr., Papaiordanou, P. M. de O., and Ramos, M. de C., Paracoccidioidomicose e infeccao pelo virus da immunodeficiencia humana, *Rev. Inst. Med. Trop. Sao Paolo*, 31, 119, 1989.

124. Lacaz, C. S., Ueda, M., Del Negro, G., Souza, A. M. C., Garcia, M. A., Rodriguez, E. G., Lirio, V. C., and Del Negro, G., Pesquisa de anticorpos HIV-1 em pacientes com paracoccidioidomicose ativa, *An. Bras. Dermatol.*, 65, 105, 1990.

125. Shikanai-Yasuda, M. A., Cotrim Segurado, A. A., Pereira Pinto, W., Nicodemo, A. C., Sato, M., Duarte, A. J. S., Del Negro, G. B., Hutzler, R. U., Shiroma, M., and Neto, V. A., Immunodeficiency secondary to juvenile paracoccidioidomycosis: associated infections, *Mycopathologia*, 120, 23, 1992.

126. Andrade, D. R., Hutzler, R. U., Carvalho, S. A., Rosenthal, C., Carvalho, M. A. B., and Ferreira, J. M., Hipoproteinemia em pacientes com paracoccidioidomicose do tubo digestivo e sistema linfatico abdominal, *Rev. Hosp. Clin. Fac. Med. Sao Paolo*, 31, 174, 1976.

127. Laudanna, A. A., Betarello, A., Van Bellen, B., and Kieffer, J., South American blastomycosis as a cause of malabsorption and protein-losing enteropathy, *Arq. Gastroent. Sao Paolo*, 12, 195, 1975.

128. Troncon, L. E. A., Martinez, R., Meneghelli, U. G., Oliveira, R. B., and Iazzigi, N., Perda intestinal de proteinas na paracoccidioidomocose, *Rev. Hosp. Clin. Fac. Med. Sao Paolo*, 36, 172, 1982.

129. Ribeiro, O. D., Nova terapeutica para blastomicose, *Publ. Med.*, 12, 36, 1940.

130. Borelli, D., Terapia de la paracoccidioidomicosis, valor actual de los antiguas tratamientos, *Rev. Argent. Micol. Suppl.*, 13, 1987.

131. Del Negro, G., Tratamiento de paracoccidioidomicose, *Rev. Assoc. Med. Bras.*, 20, 231, 1974.

132. Restrepo, A., Paracoccidioidomycosis (South American blastomycosis), in *Antifungal Drug Therapy: a Complete Guide to the Practitioner*, Jacobs, P. H. and Nall, L., Eds., Marcel Dekker, New York, 1990, 181.

133. Machado Filho, J. and Miranda, J. L., Consideracoes relativas a 238 casos consecutivos de blastomicose sulamericana: contribuicao para o seu estudo epidemiologico, *Hospital (Rio de Janeiro)*, 55, 721, 1959.

134. Borelli, D., Terapia de la paracoccidioidomicosis: valor actual de los tratamientos, *Rev. Argent. Micol. Suppl.*, 13, 1987.

135. Restrepo, A. and Arango, M. D., *In vitro* susceptibility testing of *Paracoccidioides brasiliensis* to sulfonamides, *J. Clin. Microbiol.*, 18, 190, 1980.

136. Lopez, C. F. and Armond, S., Ensaio terapeutico en casos sulforesistentes de blastomicose sul-americana, *Hospital (Rio de Janeiro)*, 73, 253, 1967.

137. Barraviera, B., Mendes, R. P., Machado, J. M., Pereira, P. C. M., Souza, M. J., and Meira, D. A., Evaluation of treatment of paracoccidioidomycosis with cotrimazine (combination of sulfadiazine and trimethoprim): preliminary report, *Rev. Inst. Med. Trop. Sao Paolo*, 31, 53, 1989.

138. Barraviera, B., Pereira, P. C. M., Mendes, R. P., Machado, J. M., Lima, C. R. G., and Meira, D. A., Evaluation of acetylator phenotype, renal function and serum sulfadiazine levels in patients with paracoccidioidomycosis treated with cotrimazine (a combination of sulfadiazine and trimethoprim), *Mycopathologia*, 108, 107, 1989.

139. Mercano, C. and Negroni, R., Paracoccidioidomicosis: aspectos terapeuticos, *Interciencia (Venezuela)*, 15, 227, 1990.

140. Lacaz, C. S. and Sampaio, S. A. P., Tratamento de blastomicose sulamericana com anfotericina B: resultados preliminares, *Rev. Paulista Med.*, 52, 443, 1958.

141. Campos, E. V., Sartori, J. C., Hetch, M. L., and Franco, M. F., Clinical and serologic features of 47 patients with paracoccidioidomycosis treated by amphotericin B, *Rev. Inst. Med. Trop. Sao Paolo*, 26, 179, 1984.

142. Dillon, N. L. and Marques, S. A., Vantagens e desvantagens da amfotericina B no tratamento da paracoccidioidomicose, *An. Bras. Dermatol.*, 65, 226, 1990.

143. Benard, G., Neves, C. P., Gryschek, R. C. B., and Duarte, A. J. S., Severe juvenile type paracoccidioidomycosis in an adult, *J. Med. Vet. Mycol.*, 33, 67, 1994.

144. Shikanai-Yasuda, M. A., Benard, G., Duarte, M. I. S., Leite, O. H. M., Eira, M., and Mendes-Giannini, M. J. S., Polyserositis in a patient with acute paracoccidioidomycosis and hepatosplenic schistosomiasis, *Mycopathologia*, 130, 75, 1995.

145. del Negro, G., Tratamento, controle de cura, profilaxia, in *Paracoccidioidomicose: Blastomicose Sul-Americana*, del Negro, G., Lacaz, C. de S., and Fiorillo, A. M., Eds., Sarvier, Sao Paolo, 1982, 271.

146. Negroni, R., Azole derivatives in the treatment of paracoccidioidomycosis, *Ann. NY Acad. Sci.*, 544, 497, 1988.

147. Negroni, R., Azoles in the treatment of paracoccidioidomycosis, in *Fungal Dimorphism*, Janssen Research Foundation, University of Cambridge, England, 1992, 105.

148. Negroni, R., Estado actual del empleo del ketoconazol en paracoccidioidomicosis (ketoconazol: 6 anos despues), *Rev. Argent. Micol.*, 1(Suppl.), 21, 1987.

149. Restrepo, A., Gomez, I., Cano, L. E., Arango, M. D., and Robledo, M. A., Post-therapy status of paracoccidioidomycosis patients treated with ketoconazole, *Am. J. Med.*, 78, 53, 1985.

150. Robledo, M. A., Gomez, I., Gutierrez, F., Cano, L. E., and Restrepo, A., Evaluacion a largo plazo de pacientes con paracoccidioidomicosis tratados con ketoconazol, *Acta Med. Colomb.*, 10, 155, 1985.

151. Barraviera, B., Mendes, R., Pereira, P. C. M., Machado, J. M., Curi, P. R., and Meira, D. A., Measurement of glucose 6-phosphate dehydrogenase and glutathione reductase activity in patients with paracoccidioidomycosis treated with ketoconazole, *Mycopathologia*, 104, 87, 1988.

152. Restrepo, A., Gomez, I., Robledo, J., Patino, M. M., and Cano, L. E., Itraconazole in the treatment of paracoccidioidomycosis: a preliminary report, *Rev. Infect. Dis.*, 9, 851, 1987.

153. Negroni, R., Robles, A. M., Arechavala, A., and Tiraboschi, I. N., Resultados del tratamiento con itraconazol por via oral en la paracoccidioidomicosis, *Rev. Argent. Micol. Suppl.*, 27, 1987.

154. Munera, M. I., Naranjo, M. S., Gomez, I., and Restrepo, A., Seguimiento post-terapia de pacientes con paracoccidioidomicosis tratados con itraconazol, *Medicina U.P.B. (Medellin)*, 8, 33, 1989.

155. Diaz, M., Negroni, R., Montero-Gei, F., Castro, L. G. M., Sampaio, S. A. P., Borelli, D., Restrepo, A., Franco, L., Bran, J. L., Arathoon, E. G., and Stevens, D. A., A Pan American 5-year study of fluconazole therapy for deep mycoses in the immunocompetent host, *Clin. Infect. Dis.*, 14(Suppl.), S68, 1992.

156. Franco, L., Gomez, I., and Restrepo, A., Treatment of subcutaneous and systemic mycoses with a new orally-administered triazole, saperconazole R-66905, *Int. J. Dermatol.*, 31, 725, 1992.

157. Angelo-Ortega, A. and Polak, L., Paracoccidioidomycosis, in *The Pathological Anatomy of the Mycosis*, Baker, R. D., Ed., Springer-Verlag, Berlin, 1970, 507.

158. Brass, K., Observaciones sobre la anatomia patologica, patogenesis y evolucion de la paracoccidioidomicosis, *Mycopathologia*, 37, 119, 1969.

159. Salfelder, K., Doehnert, G., and Doehnert, H. D., Paracoccidioidomycosis: anatomic study with complete autopsies, *Virchows Arch. Pathol. Anat.*, 348, 51, 1969.

160. Pena, C. E., Deep mycotic infections in Colombia: a clinico-pathologic study of 102 patients, *Am. J. Clin. Pathol.*, 47, 505, 1967.

161. Abad, A., Gomez, P., Velez, P., and Restrepo, A., Adrenal function in paracoccidioidomycosis: a prospective study in patients before and after ketoconazole therapy, *Infection*, 14, 22, 1986.

162. Moreira, A. C., Martinez, R., Castro, M., and Elias, L. L. K., Adrenocortical dysfunction in paracoccidioidomycosis: comparison between plasma β-lipotrophin/adrenocorticotrophin levels and adrenocortical tests, *Clin. Endocrinol.*, 36, 545, 1992.

163. Francesconi do Valle, A. C., Cotrim, M. R., Cuba, G. J., Wanke, B., and Tendrich, M., Recovery of adrenal function after treatment of paracoccidioidomycosis, *Am. J. Trop. Med. Hyg.*, 48, 626, 1993.

164. Tendrich, M., Wanke, B., Vaisman, M., Pedrosa, P. N., Santos, M. C. F., Guimaraes, M. M., and Cordeiro, J. G. H., Funcao da cortex adrenal em pacientes com paracoccidioidomicose: estudo atraves da dosagem radioimunologica do ACTH plasmatico, *Arq. Bras. Med.*, 61, 223, 1987.

165. Colombo, A. L., Estudo prospectivo da avaliacao funcional do cortex adrenal em pacientes com paracoccidioidomicose, *MA Thesis Sao Paolo*, Escola Paulista de Medicina, 1, 1989.

166. Del Negro, G., Wajchenberg, B. L., Pereira, V. G., Schneider, J., Ulhoa-Cintra, A. B., Assis, L. M., and Sampaio, S. A., Addison's disease associated with South American blastomycosis, *Ann. Intern. Med.*, 58, 189, 1961.

167. Del Negro, G., Melo, E. H. L., Rodbard, P., Melo, M. R., Layton, J., and Washslicht-Rodbard, H., Limited adrenal reserve in paracoccidioidomycosis: cortisol and aldosterone responses to 1-24 ACTH, *Clin. Endocrinol.*, 13, 553, 1980.

168. Costa, V. R., Mendes, T. I. A., and Scherman, J., Sindrome de Addison asociado a blastomicose sulamericana: a presentaceo de tres casos, *Rev. Bras. Med.*, 29, 224, 1978.

169. Marsiglia, I. and Pinto, J., Adrenal cortisol insufficiency associated with paracoccidioidomycosis (South American blastomycosis): report of four cases, *J. Clin. Endocrinol. Metabol.*, 26, 1109, 1966.

170. Torres, C. M., Duarte, E., Guimaraes, J. P., and Moreira, L. F., Destructive lesions of the adrenal gland in South American blastomycosis (Lutz disease), *Am. J. Pathol.*, 28, 145, 1952.

171. Osa, S. R., Peterson, R. E., and Roberts, R. E., Recovery of adrenal reserve following treatment of disseminated South American blastomycosis, *Am. J. Med.*, 71, 298, 1981.

172. Pont, A., Williams, P. L., Loose, D. S., Feldman, D., Reitz, R. E., Bochra, C., and Stevens, D. A., Ketoconazole blocks adrenal steroid synthesis, *Ann. Intern. Med.*, 97, 370, 1982.

173. Pont, A., Graybill, J. R., Craven, P. C., Galgiani, J. N., Dismukes, W. E., Reitz, R. E., and Stevens, D. A., High dose ketoconazole therapy and adrenal and testicular function in humans, *Arch. Intern. Med.*, 144, 2150, 1984.

174. Schurmeyerth, T. H. and Nieschlag, E., Effect of ketoconazole and other imidazole fungicides on testosterone biosynthesis, *Acta Endocrinol.*, 105, 275, 1982.

175. Pont, A., Williams, P. L., Azhar, S., Reitz, R. E., Bochra, C., Smith, E. R., and Stevens, D. A., Ketoconazole blocks testosterone synthesis, *Arch. Intern. Med.*, 142, 2137, 1982.

176. Kowal, L., The effect of ketoconazole on steroidogenesis in cultured mouse adrenal cortex tumor cells, *Endocrinology*, 112, 1541, 1983.

177. Loose, D. S., Kan, P. B., Hirst, M. A., Marcus, R. A., and Feldman, D., Ketoconazole blocks adrenal steroidogenesis by inhibiting cytochrome P 450-dependent enzymes, *J. Clin. Invest.*, 71, 1495, 1983.

178. Santen, R. J., vanden Bossche, H., Symoens, J., Brugmans, J., and De Coster, R., Site of action of low dose ketoconazole on androgen biosynthesis in men, *J. Clin. Endocrinol. Metabol.*, 57, 732, 1983.

179. Grosso, D. A., Boyden, T. W., Pamenter, R. X., Johnson, D. G., Stevens, D. A., and Galgiani, N. J., Ketoconazole inhibition of testicular secretion of testosterone and displacement of steroid hormones from serum transport proteins, *Antimicrob. Agents Chemother.*, 23, 207, 1983.

180. Borgers, M., Changes in fungal ultrastructure after itraconazole treatment, in *Recent Trends in the Discovery, Development and Evaluation of Antifungal Agents*, Fromtling, R. A., Ed., J. R. Prous, Barcelona, 1987, 193.

181. vanden Bossche, H., Mode of action of pyridine, pyrimidine, and azole antifungals, in *Sterol Biosynthesis Inhibitors*, Berg, D. and Plempel, M., Eds., Ellis Horwood, Chichester, 1988, 79.

182. San-Blas, G., San-Blas, F., Gil, F., Marino, L., and Apitz-Castro, R., Inhibition of growth of the dimorphic fungus *Paracoccidioides brasiliensis* by ajoene, *Antimicrob. Agents Chemother.*, 33, 1641, 1989.

183. San-Blas, G., San-Blas, F., and Marino, L., Ajoene, a component of garlic (*Allium sativum*), affects growth and dimorphism in *Paracoccidioides brasiliensis*, in *Recent Progress in Antifungal Chemotherapy*, Yamaguchi, H., Kobayashi, G. S., and Takahashi, H., Eds., Marcel Dekker, New York, 1991, 513.

184. Yoshida, S., Kasuga, S., Hayashi, N., Ushiroguchi, T., Matsuura, H., and Nkagawa, S., Antifungal activity of ajoene derived from garlic, *Appl. Environ. Microbiol.*, 53, 615, 1987.

185. Hanson, L. H. and Stevens, D. A., Evaluation of cilofungin, a lipopeptide antifungal agent, *in vitro* against fungi isolated from clinical specimens, *Antimicrob. Agents Chemother.*, 33, 1391, 1989.

37.9 HYALOHYPHOMYCOSIS

37.9.1 INTRODUCTION

The emerging filamentous fungal pathogens have been separated into two global disease entities: one with septate, hyaline hyphal tissue forms (hyalohyphomycosis), and the other with phaeoid, septate hyphal invasive forms (phaeohyphomycosis).[1-4]

The basic hyphal tissue form of the molds associated with hyalohyphomycosis consists of branched or unbranched hyaline, light-colored, hyphal elements without pigment in their cells.

The hyaline molds have been classified into phyla Deuteromycota, Ascomycota (namely, *Aphanoascus fulvescens* and *Pseudallescheria boydii*), or Basidiomycota (*Coprinus cinereum* and *Schizophyllum comune*).[3] The pathogenic species of the hyaline genera *Aspergillus*, *Penicillium*, and the phylum Zygomycota have been excluded from the umbrella term "hyalohyphomycosis" since they represent well-established mycosis (aspergillosis, penicilliosis, and zygomycosis). In addition, the zygomycetes would also have been excluded because their hyphae (both in tissue and culture) are aseptate.[3] Among the molds currently recognized as agents of hyalohyphomycosis, *Acremonium* spp., *Aphanoascus fulvescens*, *Coprinus cinereum*, *Fusarium* spp., *Paecilomyces* spp., *Pseudallescheria boydii*, *Scedosporium* spp., and *Schizophyllum commune*, are the most important human pathogens.[3,5]

37.9.1.1   *Scedosporium* spp.

The genus *Scedosporium* has been linked to a number of infections associated with two species: *Scedosporium prolificans* (*S. inflatum*), and the pleomorphic *Pseudallescheria boydii* (term used to distinguish the fungus when it is in the sexual [perfect or teleomorph] state, and synonymous with *Petriellidium boydii* and *Allescheria boydii*), or *S. apiospermum* (term used to identify the fungus in its asexual [imperfect or anamorph] state, and synonymous with *Monosporium apiospermum*).[6] The *Graphium* anamorph is another asexual conidiation of *P. boydii*. The teleomorph stage (*P. boydii*) consists of ascocarps (cleistothecia) that develop from a coil ascogonia.

Histopathologically, the hyphae of *P. boydii* may be difficult to distinguish from those of *Aspergillus*. However, some distinct features do exist. Thus, while both species may contain thin-walled vesicles, the hyphae of *P. boydii* are slightly narrower (2.0 to 5.0 µm) and do not branch regularly as compared to those of *Aspergillus*.[7] In addition, both fungi show proclivity for angioinvasion.

Results of taxonomic studies by Guého and de Hoog[8] have demonstrated that *S. inflatum* and *Lomentospora prolificans* were conspecific by means of DNA/DNA homologies. Since the specific name *prolificans* has priority according to the practice of botanical nomenclature, the name *Scedosporium prolificans* (Malloch and Salkin) Guého and de Hoog, has been suggested for the new combination. However, the change of name of this filamentous fungus is currently being disputed.[9] *S. prolificans* produces conidia in small groups on distinctive basally swollen, flask-shaped annellides. The conidia are single-celled, hyaline to pale brown, ovoid to pyriform (3.0 to 5.0 µm in size), and have smooth thin walls.[10-13] The organism, which is usually found in soil,[14] can be differentiated from *Scedosporium apiospermum* by its inability to grow on media containing cycloheximide.[10,15]

37.9.1.2   *Fusarium* spp.

The genus *Fusarium* represents hyaline filamentous, nondermatophyte fungi, which belong to the class Deuteromycetes of the order Moniliales. They are commonly found in soil and on subterranean and aerial vegetation parts, plant debris, and other organic substrates,[16-19] and have been frequently associated with diseases in plants causing spoilage of stored grains.[16] *Fusarium* spp. also produce potent mycotoxins[20-26] which, when ingested with contaminated grain cereals, may cause serious illness in humans.[27]

For many years, the taxonomy of *Fusarium* species has been complicated and controversial — at one time comprising more than 1000 species, varieties, and forms classified on the basis of superficial observations, with little or no regard for the cultural characteristics of these organisms.[28,29] In general, *Fusarium* spp. may produce three types of spores: macroconidia, microconidia, and chlamydospores.[19,30,31] The morphology of the macroconidia is the key characteristic for description of individual species and for the genus *Fusarium*, in general. While some species will propagate all three types of spores, other species do not.[28]

Fusarium spp. grow rapidly on all fungal media free of cycloheximide.[32,33] Microscopic examination reveals the characteristic fusoid macroconidia. The mature macroconidia are also called phragmospores (according to the Saccardoan classification).[34] The presence of fusoid macroconidia with a foot cell bearing some type of heel, has been accepted as the most definitive characteristic of the genus. It distinguishes *Fusarium* from *Acremonium*, the genus it most closely resembles.[16] In general, species identification of *Fusarium* has been difficult to accomplish because of the remarkable ability of these fungi for rapid change in their morphology and colony color.

Morphologically, the growth of *Fusarium* spp. may resemble that of an *Acremonium* species. Furthermore, in tissue, *Fusarium* spp. very often are difficult to differentiate from other hyaline filamentous fungi, including *Aspergillus* species, since all of them display dichotomously angularly branched septate hyphae.[35] The most distinctive feature of *F. moniliforme* (conspecific with *Oospora verticillioides*[36,37]) has been the formation of macroconidia in chains.[28] The latter is used to distinguish *F. moniliforme* from other medically important *Fusarium* species.[32]

Among the *Fusarium* spp. pathogenic to humans, in addition to *F. moniliforme*, *F. solani*, and *F. oxysporum*, *F. sporotrichoides*, *F. poae*, *F. dimerum*, *F. roseum*, and *F. nivale* have been most frequently isolated.[35,38]

37.9.2 EVOLUTION OF THERAPIES AND TREATMENT OF HYALOHYPHOMYCOSIS

Although hyalohyphomycosis is becoming increasingly an opportunistic infection among immunocompromised patients, it is only several molds (*Fusarium moniliforme*, *P. boydii*, and *S. commune*) that can afflict HIV-positive individuals.[39,40] Granulocytes, which are primarily involved in the control of the pathogens of hyalohyphomycosis, are relatively intact in patients with AIDS, and that may be one reason for the fewer cases of hyalo- and phaeohyphomycosis in the HIV-positive population.[3]

37.9.2.1 Pseudallescheriasis and *Scedosporium apiospermum* Infections

Pseudallescheria boydii has been found to be the causative agent of white grain mycetoma, pneumonia, or disseminated disease.[41-58] Other infections due to *P. boydii* include meningitis,[59-63] septicemia,[64] otomycosis,[65,66] prostatitis,[55] osteomyelitis and arthritis,[67-70] invasion of the conjunctiva, lacrimal glands, or the eyelids, corneal ulcers and endophthalmitis,[71] endocarditis,[54,72,73] and abscesses in the brain, kidney, thyroid,[74,75] prostate,[76] and the myocardium.[77] The infection has also been seen in patients with Cushing's disease,[67,78] renal failure,[79] and leukemia.[59,67,71,74,80-85] Over the years, there have been numerous reports of *P. boydii*-associated sinusitis in both immunocompetent and immunocompromised hosts,[80,81,86-91] ranging from chronic noninvasive form[86,92] and superficial invasion[88] to intracranial extension.[80]

Presently, *P. boydii* is recognized as an important cause of opportunistic infections in immunocompromised patients.[58,71] Central nervous system involvement was reported on several occasions presenting either as meningitis[59,60-63] or brain abscesses,[44,48,50,52,59,71,74,80,82,84,85,93,94] including a unique case of fungoma (fungus ball) in the brain of a patient with acute myelogenous leukemia.[95] In most cases, brain abscesses were the consequence of hematogenous dissemination of *P. boydii* from another site,[59,74,80,82,93,94] although in some instances[48,71,84,85] only brain involvement has been identified. Histopathologic studies have shown abscess formation in which necrotic brain tissue is being infiltrated by fungal hyphae. The observed extensive necrosis was in large part due to the propensity of *P. boydii* for blood vessel invasion,[94] resulting in thrombosis and infarction.

In nearly all reported cases, the prognosis of *P. boydii* brain abscess has been extremely poor, resulting in the patient's death. Of the very few reported survivors, two were children treated with either amphotericin B or miconazole and complete surgical removal of the abscess,[84,95] and one adult immunocompetent patient who developed the disease as a complication of infected central venous catheter.[50] In the latter case, a 2-month course with the recommended intraventricular dose of miconazole (20 mg; 10 mg/ml) applied every 72 h and a surgical removal of the abscess led to the recovery; intrathecal or intraventricular therapy is considered to be necessary because of the poor penetration of the drug into the cerebrospinal fluid.

Fessler and Brown[96] described *P. boydii* infection of the superior sagittal sinus in a patient with history of diabetes mellitus, chronic pancreatitis, and alcoholism, in what appeared to be the first reported case of hematogenous dissemination of this fungus that originated from the vascular structures into the CNS tissues. In addition to surgery, treatment with intravenous miconazole (500 mg, t.i.d.) for 55 d decreased the edema and the enhancement along the anterior aspect of the sagittal sinus.

Phillips et al.[97] have reported the first case of chronic granulomatous disease complicated by disseminated pseudallescheriasis. Clinical response occurred after prolonged therapy with intravenous miconazole (30 mg/kg divided into three daily doses) in association with recombinant interferon-γ (0.05 mg/m^2, three times weekly). The latter has been used as an immunoadjuvant in the management of patients with chronic granulomatous disease who have infections refractory to standard antimicrobial therapy.[98]

In a case of disseminated cutaneous *P. boydii* infection, a persistently neutropenic patient with acute myelogenic leukemia failed to respond to liposomal amphotericin B at a daily dose of 5.0 mg/kg; the patient died as a result of overwhelming fungal infection.[99] In contrast, a *P. boydii*-induced soft tissue infection of the foot of an elderly patient with newly diagnosed acute myelomonocytic leukemia responded well to treatment with intravenous amphotericin B despite being resistant *in vitro* to the antibiotic.[100] Surgical debridement combined with itraconazole therapy was also reported to resolve successfully maduromycosis of the foot of an immunocompromised patient with acute myelocytic leukemia.[101]

Pulmonary infection is thought to originate with inhalation of *P. boydii* ascospores.[71] The disease course may vary from relatively benign noninvasive to destructive tissue invasion, with most patients presenting with either allergic bronchopulmonary colonization, fungus ball (petriellidioma), or invasive pulmonary disease.[55-57,102] Pulmonary infections due to *P. boydii* have been seldom diagnosed in immunocompetent hosts.[77,102] In one such case,[102] an immunocompetent patient with a history of chronic lung disease had developed invasive pulmonary pseudallescheriasis with extension to the adjacent bone, probably by acquiring *P. boydii* via pulmonary colonization — the treatment consisted of amphotericin B therapy at a dose of 0.5 mg/kg daily. The minimum inhibitory concentration (MIC) values of amphotericin B, ketoconazole, and fluconazole for a clinical *P. boydii* isolate were 3.2, 6.4, and 100 µg/ml, respectively.[102]

In patients with chronic cystic or cavitary lung diseases (tuberculosis, sarcoidosis, bronchiectasis), the common course of pulmonary pseudallescheriasis has been that of a prolonged indolent disease. Fulminant, invasive lung infection usually occurred in immunocompromised patients, such as those with malignancies (colon carcinoma, melanoma, leukemia), rheumatoid arthritis, sarcoidosis, or on corticosteroid and antibiotic therapies, thus confirming the opportunistic nature of the organism.[56]

In patients with localized pulmonary disease, surgical excision has been widely implemented. In addition, the pulmonary infection also appeared to respond to antifungal therapy with azole antimycotics. Seale and Hudson[56] reported one such case of invasive pulmonary infection which was successfully treated with intravenous miconazole (300 mg, t.i.d.) for 30 d. Oral ketoconazole was also shown to be useful in the management of necrotizing pneumonia in a normal host.[77] However, Gumbart[103] reported a fatal *P. boydii* lung infection developed in a bone marrow transplant recipient while on prophylactic ketoconazole therapy at 400 mg daily.

Goldberg et al.[104] have described a rare case of simultaneous invasive pulmonary infection by *P. boydii* and *Aspergillus terrei* in a bone marrow transplant recipient who was successfully treated with a combination of surgical debridement and oral itraconazole (200 mg, b.i.d.) given for 2 months; initially, the patient was treated intravenously with a combination of amphotericin B (1.0 mg/kg daily) and miconazole (800 mg, t.i.d.); maintenance therapy with itraconazole (200 mg, b.i.d.) was also instituted. Antifungal susceptibility studies performed with a pulmonary *P. boydii* isolate showed MIC values of 0.39, 0.05, 5.0, and 0.018 µg/ml for ketoconazole, miconazole, fluconazole, and itraconazole, respectively.[104]

In another case, a patient with acute myeloblastic leukemia who during consolidation chemotherapy developed lobar pneumonia due to *S. apiospermum*, had the lobar infiltrate cleared with high doses of itraconazole (600 mg daily) after treatment with amphotericin B (1.0 mg/kg daily) had failed.[105,106]

Since *P. boydii* has frequently shown resistance to amphotericin B and flucytosine,[107-109] the management of pulmonary infections in patients with leukemia may often be complicated and even fatal. To this end, oral ketoconazole (400 mg daily) given for 8 weeks resolved *P. boydii* lung abscess in a leukemic patient despite a hematologic relapse and repeated episodes of granulo-cytopenia.[108] Although the susceptibility of *P. boydii* to miconazole[82] and ketoconazole[110] has been well documented, strains resistant to both drugs have been reported.[44]

Whereas most invasive pseudallescheriasis infections have occurred in immunocompromised hosts, Hung et al.[102] described a case of an immunocompetent patient with invasive pulmonary pseudallescheriasis and subsequent contiguous extension to the ribs and spine.

Sphenoidal or maxillary sinusitis has been predominant[8,88,91,93,111] and management has been mainly through surgical intervention.[91,92] Two cases of *P. boydii* infections in AIDS patients have been reported.[112,113] In one of them, the patient had a rapidly progressive native-valve endocarditis due to the anamorph form *S. apiospermum*,[112] while the other case involved renal and pulmonary dissemination caused by *P. boydii*.[113]

Ophthalmic infections involving *P. boydii* involved endophthalmitis,[45,48,114-118] keratitis,[119-126] lacrimal gland, and orbital infections.[71] Several well-documented occurrences of endophthalmitis secondary to *P. boydii*, all diagnosed in immunosuppressed patients, underscored the opportunistic nature of this fungus.[45,51,114-116,125] Glassman et al.[114] have described a patient with long history of diabetes mellitus who suffered *P. boydii*-induced endophthalmitis following cataract extraction and postoperative corticosteroid therapy. The infection was successfully treated with amphotericin B eyedrops (4.0 mg/ml) given every hour.[114] The first instance of endogenous *P. boydii* endophthalmitis that occurred in a patient with lupus erythemathosus and on immunosuppressive medication was reported by Lutwick et al.[82] Despite a partial vitrectomy coupled with intravitreal instillation of amphothericin B, followed by systemic therapy with intravenous miconazole, an enucleation of the globe was eventually required.[82]

In another case, a bilateral *P. boydii* endophthalmitis was diagnosed in a renal transplant recipient also on immunosuppressive therapy.[45] Bilateral vitrectomy with initial intravitreal amphotericin B, followed by systemic therapy with miconazole elicited only a poor clinical response, requiring enucleation of one eye, in spite of intravitreal miconazole therapy on the other eye; the patient died from brain abscess.[45] In two cases described by Pfeifer et al.,[51] intravitreal instillation of amphotericin B or miconazole was combined with systemic treatment with oral fluconazole (400 mg every 48 h). However, because therapeutic levels of fluconazole in the eye were difficult to achieve (the vitreous drug concentration reaching only 55% of the serum drug level), the fungus could not be eradicated.

Postoperative *P. boydii* endophthalmitis was successfully managed with a combination of vitrectomy, corneoscleral resection, and a patch graft, in addition to intraocular, topical, and oral antifungal medication with ketoconazole (200 mg, t.i.d.) for 10 weeks.[117]

Ruben[127] described what is believed to be the first case of *P. boydii* keratitis effectively treated with topical miconazole. In contrast, Bloom et al.[124] have reported failure in a case of *P. boydii* keratitis after using a regimen consisting of 1% miconazole drops (every hour), oral itraconazole (200 mg daily), and a subconjunctival injection of miconazole (0.5 ml of 10 mg/ml solution). Following the lack of clinical improvement, the oral systemic therapy was changed to intravenous miconazole (600 mg, t.i.d.) to no avail, and the eye had to be eventually eviscerated. Corticosteroids, either topical or systemic, have been recognized as aggravating fungal keratitis and should be avoided.[125]

Several occurrences of severe *P. boydii* corneoscleritis secondary to β-irradiation-induced scleral necrosis following pterygium excision[119,120] are discussed together with similar cases of *Scedosporium prolificans* corneoscleral infections (see Section 37.9.2.2).

Mycetoma (also known as the Madura foot, from the city of Madurai, India where it was first described and for its predilection for the feet[128]), is a chronic suppurative fungal infection of the extremities that has been associated among other etiologic agents (Eumycetoma, Actinomycetoma, and Botryomycosis), also with *P. boydii*. Mycetoma most often has been observed in tropical and hot temperate zones where it could be endemic (India, Central and South America, and parts of Africa). In the U.S., the highest incidence of mycetoma has been in the southeast region, but it has also been reported as far north as New England and Canada.[128-130] Mycetoma is characterized by extensive tissue erosion, formation of draining fistulas, and the presence of white grains.[52,131]

In several studies, oral ketoconazole has been used to treat *P. boydii* mycetoma.[110,129,130,132,133] In one such case, an initial dose of 200 mg, b.i.d., was ineffective and had to be increased to 400 mg, b.i.d., before a significant improvement was noticed.[129] Sheftel et al.[130] used *en bloc* resection and oral ketoconazole (600 mg daily for 8 d, then 400 mg daily for the remainder of a 4-month course) to treat an unusual nontraumatic presentation of *P. boydii* soft tissue abscess without draining sinus tracts. Aubock et al.[133] have described a case of mycetoma of the lower leg with bone involvement which after an initial favorable response could not be controlled with conventional therapy with ketoconazole (200 mg, b.i.d.) and ultimately necessitated amputation.

Pether et al.[134] have described a case of acute pyogenic *P. boydii* foot infection treated sequentially with intravenous miconazole (600 mg, t.i.d.) and oral itraconazole (200 mg daily).

P. boydii-associated arthritis and osteomyelitis have also been reported.[135-140] Ginter et al.[70] have described a case of *P. boydii*-associated severe chronic arthritis which although without grains had resulted in complete destruction of the cartilaginous surface. This case has been one of several similar reports describing post-traumatic arthritis of the knee joint caused by *P. boydii* in which the presence of fistulas was variable and grains remained absent.[68,141-143] The cases of *P. boydii*-produced arthritis have been remarkably similar to focal infections caused by *Scedosporium prolificans*, which has also the tendency to affect cartilage and joint areas and does not produce any fungal grains either.[15]

Since *P. boidii* has been almost invariably resistant to amphotericin B, therapy with azole antimycotics has been the most beneficial. Thus, in the aforementioned case by Ginter et al.,[70] the combination of miconazole and itraconazole was successful — miconazole was injected intravenously at 600 mg daily for the first 12 d, followed by 1.2 g of miconazole and 400 mg itraconazole (both given orally) for a further 4 weeks; then, itraconazole monotherapy at 200 mg was administered orally for the next 3 months.[70] Treatment with itraconazole was also reported successful in two other cases of osteoarthritis.[142,143]

The *in vitro* susceptibility of *P. boydii* to miconazole has shown MIC values in the range of ≤0.8 to 1.0 mg/ml.[144] The recommended daily dose of miconazole, which depended on the severity and localization of the infection and the general condition of the patient, has been between 10 and 30 mg/kg.[70]

Ketoconazole at 200 mg, b.i.d. has been largely ineffective in treating *P. boydii* osteomyelitis.[68,135]

Hung and Norwood[68] have described an interesting case of *P. boydii*-induced osteomyelitis in an immunocompetent patient who presented with no cutaneous or subcutaneous infection. Since osteomyelitis has been known to occur usually only after the soft tissue has been extensively involved,[145] this case (an insidious onset and an indolent course, basically symptom-free for the first 5 years) should illustrate the possibility that after trauma and deep laceration, deep fungal infections can occur without cutaneous manifestations.

A highly unusual *P. boydii*-related mycetoma of the scalp and osteomyelitis of the skull after craniotomy has been reported by Fernandez-Guerrero et al.[69] The patient was cured by wide resection of the involved bone alone and without antifungal therapy. A postcraniotomy wound infection due to *P. boydii* was effectively treated with intravenous miconazole.[146]

One consequence of Cushing's syndrome is the diminished capability of the host immune defense to resist a variety of infections (postoperative wound and pyogenic cutaneous infections, streptococcal sepsis, pneumonia, superficial cutaneous and mucosal fungal infections)[147] and *Pneumocystis carinii* pneumonia.[148] In this regard, Ansari et al.[67] have also reported a case of *P. boydii*-induced arthritis and osteomyelitis associated with Cushing's syndrome. The pathogen was successfully eradicated only after a combination therapy consisting of surgical debridement, long-term ketoconazole treatment (initially at 400 mg daily, then increased to 600 mg daily), and control of the endogenous hypercortisol production. The latter occurrence has been related to a marked increase in susceptibility to infections, especially those requiring cell-mediated immune defense.[147-149] There have been several studies aimed at elucidating the mechanism by which cortico-steroids exert their immunomodulating effect. Fauci et al.[150] have established that human peripheral blood lymphocytes are capable of expressing glucocorticoid receptors, and lymphopenia with selective affinity for T cells is one well-known effect of corticosteroids. Furthermore, the corticosteroids can also reduce accumulation of inflammatory cells at sites of inflammation, and inhibit cutaneous delayed hypersensitivity reactions by decreasing the recruitment of macrophages,[151] as well as curtail the ability of lymphokines to recruit the cells necessary for expression of cellular immunity.[151] Most importantly, the latter has been essential for effective defense against fungal infections.[67]

37.9.2.2 *Scedosporium prolificans (S. inflatum)* Infections

Scedosporium prolificans is an emerging pathogen associated with localized soft tissue and bone infections in immunocompetent hosts (most likely from traumatic inoculation), but frequently fatal disseminated infections in immunocompromised patients.[10,11,152-157]

In 1984, Malloch and Salkin[158] described the first case of infection caused by *S. prolificans* (*S. inflatum*). One likely portal of entry has been by penetrating trauma to the affected site[15] since most infections have been seen as localized infection of bone, joints, or soft tissues.[8,10,159,160]

Among immunocompromised patients, where dissemination is a distinct possibility,[161] the incidence of infections has been on the increase.[9-11,152-158,162-164] In this context, Summerbell et al.[14] have discussed the isolation of *S. prolificans* from hospital environment (potted plants) and its pathogenic potential as a nosocomial infection.

Diagnosis of disseminated disease due to *Scedosporium prolificans* is difficult to attain since its spectrum and symptoms strongly resemble those of pseudallescheriasis.[10,157] For example, cases of arthritis caused by *S. prolificans* and *P. boydii* have been nearly indistinguishable, even with mixed infection in the knee by both species being reported.[165] In view of the extreme drug tolerance by *S. prolificans*, early positive culture identification of the pathogen should be very essential. Furthermore, initial infections by *S. prolificans* may resemble pulmonary aspergillosis. Moreover, patients with disseminated disease may also present with fever, muscle tenderness, and papular cutaneous lesions, similar to those observed in acute hematogenous disseminated candidiasis.[3]

Despite antifungal therapy, the prognosis of disseminated *S. prolificans* infection is generally poor.[11,152-154,156,157,162-164] Farag et al.[152] and Wise et al.[11] have reported two fatal infections in immunocompromised patients, despite intravenous treatment in one of the cases[11] initially with amphotericin B (20 mg daily; increased to 30 mg daily), then with miconazole (600 mg, four times daily; increased to 800 mg, four times daily), and intravenous amphotericin B and flucytosine, in the second case.[152] Nielsen et al.[163] described another fatal outcome of disseminated *S. prolificans* infection in an immunocompromised patient where the clinical course was very similar to that of disseminated coccidioidomycosis, and the pathogen was resistant to amphotericin B (given intravenously initially at 1.0 mg/kg every 48 h; then increased to 1.4 mg/kg every 48 h, and flucytosine added to the therapeutic regimen).

The major reason *S. prolificans* infections in immunocompromised patients have been very difficult to treat is that, contrary to *S. apiospermum,* this organism has been nearly always resistant to azole antimycotics (miconazole, itraconazole) and even amphotericin B.[11,154,160] *In vitro* antifungal susceptibility studies have also shown *S. prolificans* to be repeatedly resistant to amphotericin B, miconazole, and ketoconazole.[10,11,15,166] In one of the studies,[9] the MIC values against amphotericin B, flucytosine, miconazole, ketoconazole, and itraconazole were ≥ 3.12, ≥ 3.12, 100, 100, and ≥ 100 µg/ml, respectively. These findings have been reflected in clinical settings where in the majority of serious cases of *S. prolificans* infections, treatment with amphotericin B has been unsuccessful.[10,15,154,156,160] Wilson et al.[15] suggested adjunctive topical or intra-articular administration of amphotericin B when the infections are localized.

There has been some anecdotal evidence that ketoconazole was effective in cases of chronic, recurrent osteomyelitis caused by *S. prolificans*.[15,160]

In view of the largely unsuccessful antifungal chemotherapy, it appears that adequate debridement should be considered immediately.[15,160]

As an ocular pathogen, *S. prolificans* has been documented as the causative agent of metastatic endophthalmitis that required enucleation.[157] Furthermore, Sullivan et al.[167] and Moriarty et al.[119,120] have reported the development of *S. prolificans* sclerokeratitis in the setting of late scleral necrosis complicating pterygium surgery with adjunctive β-irradiation. Therapy with oral ketoconazole at 200 mg daily was unsuccessful and led to enucleation of the eye.[167] In view of these and other reports, infective scleritis complicating scleral avascular necrosis following pterygium surgery[168-171] has become an increasingly recognized occurrence.[172]

37.9.2.3 *Fusarium* spp. Infections

A systemic infection caused by ingestion of *Fusarium*-contaminated cereals was first reported in 1913 in Russia,[173] and again at the end of World War II, when as many as 1 million people may have been poisoned by infected grain.[174] The disease, known as the alimentary toxic aleukia in Russia,[173,174] and as akakabi-byo in Japan,[175] is characterized by initial gastrointestinal symptoms and weakness that culminate in aplastic anemia and death if ingestion of *Fusarium*-contaminated grain persists.[28,176] The disease results from the effects of fusarial mycotoxins and not from a systemic fungal infection.[21,22,173] While in Russia, the alimentary toxic aleukia has been commonly due to *F. sporotrichioides* and *F. poae,*[176] in Japan the causative agent has been *F. graminearum* and less often *F. nivale, F. poae,* and *F. oxysporum.*[175] Currently, *F. moniliforme* is the *Fusarium* species most often associated with basic human and animal dietary staples, such as corn,[24,177] and consequently most studied for the mycotoxins (moniliformins, fusarins, and fumonisins) it produces.[28]

The increased use of immunosuppressive therapies, cytotoxic drugs in cancer patients, and the widespread use of antibiotics have resulted in increased incidence of newly recognized opportunistic pathogens, such as the *Fusarium* species.[4,34,35,178-181] In recent years, *Fusarium* spp. have emerged as important pathogens in community-acquired and nosocomial hyalohyphomycoses. Disseminated infections when they occurred have been predominantly in immunocompromised patients,[182] such as those with hematologic malignancies,[32,34-36,179,180,183-196] organ transplant recipients,[33,197] with chronic infectious mononucleosis syndrome,[198] and burn victims.[38,199,200]

Fusarium spp. have been reported to cause skin infections (necrotic, ecthyma gangrenosum-like or nodular lesions, or mycetomas),[36,179,180,182,183,194,197,201-207] osteomyelitis,[208] septic arthritis,[209] extensive interdigital infection,[210] cystitis,[211] peritonitis,[212-214] brain abscess,[198,199] invasive sinonasal disease,[207,215-217] myocarditis,[218] endocarditis,[219] and ocular infections.[220-233] In diabetic patients, leg ulcers may allow this common soil saprophite to become imbedded in the subcutaneous tissue.[234] Fungemia has been variable, ranging from 11% to 50% in small series of disseminated infections;[36,179] catheter-related fungemia has also been reported.[182] In some geographic regions of the world, especially the Western hemisphere, *Fusarium* (especially *F. solani*) has been the most common cause of keratomycosis.[224,235-245]

The portal of entry of *Fusarium* spp. is postulated to be the paranasal sinuses through inhalation of aerosolized conidia,[36] or through breaks of integumentary barriers, particularly in patients with *Fusarium*-associated onychomycosis.[4]

In the interaction of the immune system with *Fusarium* spp., the granulocytes and macrophages play essential roles in the defense against this pathogen. Thus, macrophages can inhibit the germination of conidia and the growth of hyphae, whereas granulocytes suppress the hyphal growth.[28]

While invasive fusarial infections most frequently develop in patients with granulocytopenia, they seldom complicate HIV infections.[226,246] In neutropenic patients, the manifestations of *Fusarium* infections include fever, severe myalgia, maculonodular cutaneous lesions, fungemia, and occasionally pulmonary infiltrates.[34,195,247,248] Myoken et al.[192] have described an oral *F. moniliforme* infection in a granulocytopenic patient with acute myelogenous leukemia who developed necrotic ulceration of the gingiva, extending to the alveolar bone, but free of any active systemic lesions.

The therapy and outcome of *Fusarium* infections were dependent on the degree of invasion of the pathogen, and the status of the host. Superficial *Fusarium* infections usually respond to local treatment. However, there have often been cases refractory to antifungal therapy as evidenced from experimental animal models[249] and humans, particulary in granulocytopenic patients.[34]

The prognosis in immunosuppressed patients with disseminated fusariosis is extremely poor. With very few exceptions,[178] the outcome was fatal for most patients, especially those with leukemia.[34,193,194,250] The treatment modalities recommended have included amphotericin B, flucytosine, rifampin, granulocyte transfusions, and local surgical debridement.[179,180,197,251] In general, the therapeutic efficacy of amphotericin B (1.2 mg/kg daily; 40 mg daily), fluconazole, and itraconazole in invasive fusarial infections in immunosuppressed hosts has been rather limited.[194,252] However, Cofrancesco et al.[248] and Viviani et al.[253] have used liposomal amphotericin B (AmBisome®) at 3.0 mg/kg daily (total dose 3.85 g) to successfully eradicate *Fusarium* infection in a neutropenic patient with acute lymphoblastic leukemia; the initial treatment was with conventional amphotericin B (0.7 to 1.0 mg/kg daily; total dose 1.63 g). There has been a complete regression of the pulmonary lesion.

Of the newer triazoles, SCH 39309 and D0870 have shown *in vivo* activity against *Fusarium* spp.[35] However, because of unacceptable toxicity, SCH 39309 (also found active against invasive human fusariosis) is no longer being developed.[35,254]

The first disseminated *Fusarium* infection was described in a child with acute lymphocytic leukemia by Cho et al.[184] Dissemination to the eye occurred hematogenously following initial colonization in the primary lesion. Treatment consisted of intravenous amphotericin B — the initial dose of 0.1 mg/kg was gradually increased within 1 week to 1.0 mg/kg daily; the patient was maintained on this dose for a total of 8 weeks. In addition, amphotericin B solution (1.0 mg/ml) was applied topically to the involved eye. In spite of the gradual improvement of skin and eye lesions, seizure activity and mental confusion remained unchanged and the patient died. The amphotericin B blood levels at 24 and 48 h were 0.59 and 0.24 µg/ml. *In vitro* amphotericin B sensitivity tests indicated a MIC of 3.0 µg/ml.[184]

Venditti et al.[183] presented two cases of invasive *F. solani* infection in immunosuppressed patients with acute myelomonocytic and myelogenous leukemia, respectively; neither patient had an intravascular catheter in place. The first patient, despite continued treatment with systemic amphotericin B (total 4.5 g) and 5-fluorocytosine (180 mg/kg daily; total 720 g) and progressive improvement of skin lesions and myalgias, died in the setting of persistent granulocytopenia. The outcome was also fatal for the second patient, who despite systemic therapy with amphotericin B (total 2.66 g) continued to show profound and persistent granulocytopenia. Both patients experienced an insidious loss of vision that culminated in blindness in the first patient, apparently from hematogenous spread of *F. solani* to the eye[183] (also suggested by previous observations[184,222]).

Earlier studies have established a relationship between the degree of leukopenia and the presence of infection in patients with acute leukemia[255-258] and various types of agranulocytosis.[259-261] Bodey et al.[185] have studied the quantitative relationships between circulating leukocytes and infection in patients with acute leukemia.[262] The data showed that the incidence of infections in these patients decreased with increasing levels of circulating granulocytes and lymphocytes — a critical level was established for granulocytes (1500 cells/mm^3) above which there was no further decrease in the incidence of infection. Since the risk of developing fungal infections is higher with increasing duration of granulocytopenia, recovery from granulocytopenia seems to be an important factor in survival after *Fusarium* infection in leukemic patients.[263-265]

Gutmann et al.[186] have described a fatal case of systemic fusariosis in a patient with a myasthenic-like syndrome (Eaton-Lambert syndrome) and aplastic anemia. The Eaton-Lambert syndrome is characterized by proximal muscle weakness resulting from the blockade of the acetylcholine release from nerve terminals at the neuromuscular junction.[266] The systemic granulomatous infection caused by *F. oxysporum* was similar in many respects to alimentary toxic aleukia, although it was complicated by the therapeutic use of guanidine, a drug also known to cause bone marrow suppression. The fact that other microbial derivatives produced a similar defect of acetylcholine release as seen in the Eaton-Lambert syndrome (e.g., neomycin, a *Streptomyces fradiae* metabolite) and bone marrow suppression (e.g., chloramphenicol, derived from *S. venezuelae*), lent further support to the hypothesis that *Fusarium* mycotoxins may be one cause of the Eaton-Lambert syndrome as well as aplastic anemia, as observed in this case.[186]

A disseminated *F. moniliforme* infection was described in a granulocytopenic patient with malignant lymphoma who was treated with cytotoxic drugs and corticosteroids.[32] The patient died following progressive renal and respiratory failure with diffuse alveolar infiltrates, massive gastrointestinal bleeding, and hypothermia. Steinberg et al.[198] have described a patient with *F. oxysporum* brain abscess who developed meningitis. The outcome was fatal despite treatment with amphotericin B: an initial loading dose of 0.75 mg/kg was followed by 1.0 mg/kg daily; next, after the abscess was aspirated, an Ommaya reservoir was placed to deliver intraventricular amphotericin B (0.1 mg every other day, then increased to 0.5 mg daily). In another case, a patient with B-type lymphoblastic lymphoma who underwent a bone marrow transplantation and aggressive chemotherapy, developed a *Fusarium* onychomycosis[267] of the great toenail.[268] Septicemic fungal dissemination followed a lymphoma relapse resulting in a fulminant and fatal disease despite the institution of amphotericin B therapy.

Spielberger et al.[269] have reported as safe and life-saving the combined use of amphotericin B, granulocyte transfusions, and granulocyte-macrophage colony-stimulating factor (GM-CSF) in a pancytopenic patient with disseminated fusariosis. Also, a disseminated *F. proliferatum*-associated fusariosis in a patient with acute lymphocytic leukemia responded to an early, aggressive treatment consisting of granulocyte transfusion combined with chemotherapy comprising amphotericin B, ketoconazole, rifampin, and griseofulvin.[196] Yet in another study, Hennequin et al.[270] have used high doses of amphotericin B (1.5 mg/kg daily), flucytosine (200 mg/kg daily), and granulocyte colony-stimulating factor (G-CSF) as adjuvant therapy, to treat disseminated cutaneous fusariosis in a neutropenic child — the lesions progressively diminished and disappeared after 15 d.

Even though a number of investigators have used successfully similar therapeutic regimens (high-dose amphotericin B, granulocyte transfusions, and intravenously administered GM-CSF) to treat other mycoses (*Candida albicans*-induced skin lesions, pulmonary aspergillosis),[271-273] the benefit of granulocyte transfusions in the therapy of fungal infections still remains controversial.[274,275] Granulocyte transfusions when given during amphotericin B treatment of invasive fungal infections in granulocytopenic patients have raised concern about pulmonary complications from leukostasis.[276,277] The GM-CSF, which has been used to shorten the duration of granulocytopenia following chemotherapy-induced myelosuppression, also has the ability to activate neutrophils and to increase the cytotoxicity of macrophages,[278,279] as well as to impair neutrophil chemotaxis.[280,281]

Engelhard et al.[282] have described a disseminated visceral fusariosis in a patient with T-type acute lymphoblastic leukemia who responded completely to amphotericin B–phospholipid complex (dimyristoyl phosphatidylcholine and dimyristoyl phosphatidylglycerol in a 7:3 ratio) administered at daily doses of 1.0 to 4.0 mg/kg (total dose 4.2 g). Wolff and Ramphal[283] also used a lipid complex of amphotericin B (0.5 mg/kg daily; total 11.89 g) to resolve disseminated cutaneous infection in a neutropenic patient with acute myelogenous leukemia. Of the various lipid complexes, amphotericin B desoxycholate has been the most widely used in neutropenic patients. However, the infusion of amphotericin B desoxycholate has often been poorly tolerated, and toxic effects were common. The toxicity has limited the maximum tolerable dose of amphotericin B desoxycholate to 0.7–1.5 mg/kg daily, which in turn, may be suboptimal for clinical success in the treatment of some filamentous fungal infections.[283]

Krulder et al.[190] have reported a patient with lymphoblastic non-Hodgkin's lymphoma who acquired a systemic *F. nygamai* infection during the granulocytopenic phase of cytostatic treatment. The patient survived after hematologic recovery and treatment with intravenous amphotericin B (total dose 543 mg).

The prognosis of *F. moniliforme* fungemia in children with neuroblastoma has been generally poor.[284] However, in one case,[285] treatment with amphotericin B at 1.0 mg/kg daily (total 132 mg; 11 mg/kg) administered over 2 weeks resulted in rapid defervescence without any localization of the infection.

Fusarium infections are being increasingly reported in immunocompromised patients (acute leukemia or solid tumors) with indwelling central venous catheters.[191,195,286] A combined therapeutic modality consisting of removal of the catheter and amphotericin B therapy has usually produced excellent response.[191] The first case of a Port-a-cath-related disseminated fusariosis in an HIV-infected patient was presented by Eljaschewitsch et al.[246] Treatment with liposomal amphotericin B (AmBisome®) at a daily dose of 2.0 mg/kg for 2 weeks was successful.

In another first occurrence, Mohammedi et al.[218] described disseminated *F. oxysporum* infection presenting with fungal myocarditis. Despite antifungal therapy and hematologic recovery, the patient died of cardiogenic shock, with the myocardial involvement clearly contributing to the fatal outcome.

Fusarium spp. have been recognized as one of the most common pathogens associated with fungal keratitis.[224,228,230,233,235-245,287-289] Cases of keratitis in contact lens wearers have also been increasing in numbers.[28,240,290-293]

While several *Fusarium* species (*F. episphaeria, F. dimerum, F. moniliforme, F. nivale, F. oxysporum,* and *F. solani*) can induce keratomycosis, *F. solani* has been the most prevalent pathogen of eye infections. *Fusaria* corneal ulcers when diagnosed early and treatment started immediately, have shown good prognosis for recovery.[224] Superficial fungal keratitis may be treated easily, but a scar will often remain — a leukoma of variable size that would diminish vision. In several reports,[281,294-297] *Fusarium* keratitis has been successfully treated with pimaricin (natamycin) as 5% suspension[230] or unguent[298] with 0.001% dexamethasone and 2% potassium iodide,[296,299] applied topically every 2 h until infection subsides. Donnenfeld et al.[289] reported a *Fusarium*-induced corneal perforation associated with corneal hydrops and contact lens wear in keratoconus.

Rowsey et al.[223] have described a patient with *F. oxysporum* endophthalmitis which responded to a combination treatment of vitrectomy, intravitreal and intravenous amphotericin B, and oral flucytosine. In order to prevent retinal necrosis, it was recommended that intravitreal amphotericin B (5.0 μg) is injected slowly into the midvitreous with a needle bevel toward the lens in a 0.1-ml volume.[223] With a vitreous volume of 4.0 ml, a central vitreous concentration of possibly 1.5 μg/ml of amphotericin B would be expected, which will be much higher than that available to the vitreous via the intravenous route alone.[300]

Patients with *Fusarium* keratitis have been known to develop endophthalmitis by direct extension from the corneal ulcer. However, Lieberman et al.[222] have reported a case of an immunocompetent host in which *Fusarium* endophthalmitis developed without apparent primary corneal involvement, suggesting an endogenous origin (hematogenous spread following inhalation of fungal spores) of the infection. There have been a number of reports of endogenous endophthalmitis, which has been increasingly recognized in susceptible individuals.[226,227,229,231,301,302] For example, a bilateral endogenous *Fusarium* endophthalmitis was diagnosed in a patient with AIDS and cytomegalovirus endophthalmitis — histopathologic examination showed a severe necrotizing acute and granulomatous reaction, with numerous fungal elements in the retina and uveal tract.[226] Despite intravitreous (two injections of 15 μg) and systemic (cumulative dose of 770 mg) treatment with amphotericin B and fluconazole therapy, the patient's endophthalmitis and mental status worsened and he died from disseminated fungal infection of the brain, lung, kidney, thyroid, and lymph nodes.[226] Disruption of the blood-retinal barriers from angiopathic causes related to AIDS or concurrent cytomegalovirus retinitis may have contributed to the retinal involvement.[303]

In another case,[227] an intravenous drug abuser who developed unilateral retinal infiltrates and retinal vasculopathy was successfully treated by a combination of pars plana vitrectomy and intravitreal and intravenous amphotericin B.

Fusarium-induced peritonitis associated with continuous ambulatory peritoneal dialysis (CAPD) has been reported on several occasions.[212-214,304] Successful treatment usually involved therapy with intravenous amphotericin B coupled with removal of the catheter.[212,214]

In another case of successful use of intravenous amphotericin B, an 8-week course of the antibiotic (total dose of 1.76 g) was combined with repeated aspirations to resolve septic arthritis (finger joint infection) due to *F. solani*.[209]

Kurien et al.[217] have described the first known cases of *F. solani* infections of the maxillary sinus with granuloma and oro-antral fistula in two immunocompetent hosts. Both patients responded to oral ketoconazole (200 mg daily) for 3 weeks followed by a Caldwell-Luc operation. Ketoconazole was continued for 2 months postoperatively. Successful use of oral ketoconazole has also been reported by Landau et al.[305] in a patient with leg ulcers due to *F. oxysporum*, by Baudraz-Rosselet et al.[205] in a patient with foot mycetoma, and by Ooi et al.[206] in the treatment of granuloma annulare-like skin lesion due to *F. roseum*.

A case of *Fusarium* eumycetoma that lasted for 18 years improved significantly after 6 months of oral itraconazole therapy (the initial dose of 100 mg daily was increased to 200 mg after 2 months).[306]

37.9.2.4 Non-*Candida* Mycoses After Solid Organ and Bone Marrow Transplantations

Fungal infections in solid organ and bone marrow transplant recipients continue to be a major cause of morbidity and mortality in these patients.[9,54,63,104,156,178,307-313] The high incidence of mycoses has been related to multiple factors, such as prolonged granulocytopenia, broad-spectrum antimicrobial therapy known to permit fungal colonization and disrupt normal mucosal barriers, radiotherapy, and the use of central venous access devices. In addition, graft-versus-host disease (GVHD) and impaired cell-mediated immunity due to primary disease or its therapy have also contributed to the high frequency of fungal infections among these patients, especially after bone marrow transplantation.[178,307] Thus, neutrophil dysfunction has been characterized after bone marrow transplantation in patients with and without GVHD.[314] Treatment of GVHD, usually with prednisone and/or azathioprine, has been known to increase the degree of immunosuppression, thereby contributing to the neutrophil disorder. The latter, coupled with impairment of the lymphocyte functions after bone marrow transplantation,[315] would create optimal host environment for the acquisition of fungal infections and their dissemination from sites that are only surface-colonized.[197]

Historically, *Candida* spp. have been the most frequently isolated fungi, followed by *Aspergillus* spp.[316-320] However, other less common fungal pathogens, such as *Pseudollescheria boydii*, *Scedosporium prolificans*, *Fusarium* spp., *Alternaria, Curvularia, Penicillium, Mucor, Histoplasma*, *Malassezia, Phialophora, Rhodotorula, Acremonium, Trichosporon, Moraxella*, and *Torulopsis*, have emerged as invasive opportunistic agents in patients who underwent transplantation surgery.[9,33,41,54,104,156,178,180,197,263,307,308,310-312,321-327]

To determine the incidence, risk factors, and outcome of non-*Candida* fungal infections in the bone marrow transplant population, Morrison et al.[178,307] have studied a consecutive series of 1186 patients during the period 1974–1989. The risk factors were analyzed with regard to clinical characteristics, such as age, sex, primary disease process, type of transplant, recipient cytomegalovirus serostatus, time to engraftment, and the presence of GVHD. The results of the study have shown that 10% of the patients (123 of 1186) developed a non-*Candida* fungal infection within 180 days of transplant surgery. The majority of infections (85%) occurred in allogeneic recipients, and 58% of patients were infected prior to white blood cell engraftment. Among the various non-*Candida* fungal pathogens, *Aspergillus* spp. were the most common isolates (70%), followed by *Fusarium* spp. (8%), and *Alternaria* spp. (5%). The percentages of single organ (or site) and disseminated infections were similar (47% and 44%, respectively), whereas fungemia was observed in only 9% of patients. One of the discouraging statistics has been the mortality rate — only 17% of patients survived, with 68% of deaths related to the fungal infection. Furthermore, in 83% of those patients who died from fungal infections, the death was caused by a non-*Candida* fungus. Limited infections, such as fungemia, had the best clinical outcome, followed by infections of a single organ, whereas disseminated infections were nearly all fatal. Among the different non-*Candida* species, *Aspergillus, Fusarium,* and *Scedosporium prolificans* have been the more virulent, more invasive, and therefore, highly likely to cause disseminated and fatal infections.[156,178,307] Fungi that have the tendency to cause either localized infections (*Alternaria*) or isolated fungemia without disseminated disease (*Acremonium* spp., *Penicillium, Malassezia, Moraxella*) were associated with a better outcome.[178,307]

By invariate analysis, the allogeneic transplant, positive recipient cytomegalovirus (CMV) serostatus, delayed engraftment, and the recipient of greater than or equal to 18 years, were identified as the major risk factors for non-*Candida* fungal infections.[178,307] The increased occurrence of opportunistic mycoses in the allogeneic bone marrow transplant population was likely related to the more intense preparative regimen and the more profound immunosuppressive effect of allografting. The increased risk among CMV-seropositive patients of developing deep mycoses stemmed from the CMV-induced suppression of both cell-mediated and humoral immune responses.[328,329] In addition, ongoing CMV infections may also disrupt normal integumentary barriers, such as the gastrointestinal and respiratory tracts, thus predisposing to invasive superinfections with colonizing fungi.[307]

Disseminated disease due to *Scedosporium prolificans* after bone marrow transplantation has also been described.[103,330] Recently, *S. prolificans* has been implicated in the fatal outcome of two cases, one after a bone marrow transplantation[156] and the other after a single-lung transplantation.[9] In the first case, the patient with acute myeloblastic leukemia underwent autologous bone marrow transplantation. The fungal infection had developed during the severe neutropenia resulting from the conditioning preceding the marrow transplantation. The conditioning regimen included, in addition to busulfan and cyclophosphamide, also prophylaxis with oral fluconazole (100 mg daily). The *S. prolificans* isolate was resistant to amphotericin B, flucytosine, ketoconazole, and fluconazole with MIC values of 64, ≥128, 64, and 8.0 µg/ml, respectively.[156] In the second case, the patient received a single lung transplant.[9] Prophylactic anti-infective therapy with antibiotics (ticarcillin plus clavulanic acid and pefloxacin), acyclovir, and amphotericin B (0.3 mg/kg daily, IV) for 15 d, and postoperative treatment with intravenous amphotericin B (1.0 mg/kg daily) failed to thwart the fungal infection.[9] In a separate case of fatal *S. prolificans* disease, the patient, who received a kidney transplant, first developed a locally invasive infection that subsequently disseminated to the pleura.[159,160]

Opportunistic *Pseudallescheria boydii* infections have also been associated with several deaths after solid organ transplantions.[54,63,304] In one case of fatal orthotopic liver transplantion, the patient developed *P. boydii* endocarditis of the pulmonic valve.[54] To a large extent, pulmonic valve endocarditis has been identified with either congenital heart disease,[331] indwelling catheters (especially pulmonary artery catheters[332]), or in intravenous drug users (most often with a right-sided endocarditis of the tricuspid valve).[331] What made this case highly unusual was that at autopsy the patient was found to have a vegetation on the pulmonic valve in addition to a septal abscess presented as endocardial mass along the left side of the septum, a rather unique association of pulmonic valve endocarditis with myocardial septal abscess.[54] Previously, *P. boydii* has been reported as the cause of infection in one liver transplant patient who acquired the infection nosocomially.[49]

Alsip and Cobbs[63] have described a fatal *P. boydii* infection which disseminated to the central nervous system after cardiac transplant surgery — meningitis was the primary CNS manifestation, with no evidence of brain abscess. Amphotericin B, given both intravenously (20 mg daily) and intraventricularly (1.0 mg administered during ventriculostomy), and miconazole (600 mg, t.i.d.) failed to control the disseminated disease.

A mycotic aneurysm and visceral infection due to *Scedosporium apiospermum* in a kidney transplant patient was described by Ben Hamida et al.[308] Sequential therapy with intravenous fluconazole (400 mg daily) and intravenous miconazole (1.2 g daily) was unsuccessful and the patient died.

However, oral itraconazole was successful in the treatment of concurrent pulmonary *P. boydii* and *Aspergillus terreus* infections in a bone marrow transplant recipient (see the preceding section).[104]

Robertson et al.[311] have described a patient who developed disseminated *Fusarium* infection with a secondary fungal endophthalmitis after an autologous bone marrow transplant for acute myeloid leukemia. The fusariosis was successfully eradicated after neutrophil recovery by a prolonged systemic administration of amphotericin B combined with aggressive local therapy, including enucleation of the affected eye. In another case of disseminated *Fusarium* disease in a bone marrow transplant recipient, the infection caused by *F. proliferatum* was successfully treated with a combination of rifampin and amphotericin B which acted in a synergistic manner to elicit a complete remission of infection although the neutrophil counts remained below 0.25×10^9 cells/l.[263]

Nucci et al.[313] have studied the efficacy and safety of itraconazole in combination with amphotericin B to treat fungal infections (pulmonary aspergilloma, *Aspergillus fumigatus* sinusitis, fusariosis, and disseminated candidiasis) in neutropenic patients after bone marrow transplant recovery.

In general, non-*Candida* fungal infections remain a substantial cause for morbidity and mortality among patients undergoing solid organ or bone marrow transplantations.[197] In prevention of systemic aspergillosis, itraconazole at 200 mg daily has been effective only when adequate serum concentrations have been achieved.[323] None of the currently available oral antimycotics provides effective prophylaxis against *Fusarium*, *Pseudallescheria*, *Trichosporon*, and *Torulopsis*.[323] Therefore, early diagnosis, antifungal therapy, and transplant regimens incurring a shorter period of neutropenia may help to reduce the incidence and clinical impact of non-*Candida* infections.

37.9.2.4.1 *Pharmacokinetic interactions of cyclosporin A with azole antimycotics*

Cyclosporin A, which is widely used in transplantaion surgeries to prevent organ rejections,[333] has frequently produced serious side effects as well as pharmacokinetic interactions with various antimicrobial agents, resulting in unwarranted changes of cyclosporin A blood concentrations that may often lead to either organ rejection or increase of toxicity.[334-340] Since the metabolic degradation of cyclosporin A is carried out primarily via the hepatic P-450 mixed function oxidase system,[341] cyclosporin A interactions with other drugs that involve modulation of the cytochrome P-450 system may significantly alter the clinical course after the transplantation surgery.[334] Thus, rifampin was found to accelerate the metabolism of cyclosporin A by inducing the P-450 system,[342] leading to decrease in its blood levels[337] and eventually to organ rejection. Cimetidine[343] and ketoconazole,[334,338,339,344,345] on the other hand, were shown to inhibit the P-450 system, thereby increasing cyclosporin A concentrations and consequently enhancing its nephrotoxicity secondary to a reduced elimination.

In addition to inhibiting cytochrome P-450 enzymes, azole antimycotics such as clotrimazole, miconazole, and ketoconazole have also been found to induce certain hepatic cytochrome P-450 isoenzymes (P-450p, P-450b/e, P-450c/d, P-450j)[346] as evidenced by studies conducted in both animal models and humans.[330,346-353] The results have shown that different azole drugs interacted with various cytochrome P-450 isoenzymes in different ways. For example, while the glucocorticoid and aromatic hydrocarbon-responsive P-450p and P-450c/d isoenzymes, respectively, were induced by clotrimazole, miconazole, and ketoconazole, the phenobarbital-responsive P-450b/e isoenzyme was induced by clotrimazole and miconazole, but not ketoconazole. Also, the ethanol-responsive P-450j isoenzyme while moderately induced by ketoconazole was not affected by either clotrimazole or miconazole.[346]

When administered simultaneously to heart and lung transplant recipients, itraconazole interacted with cyclosporin A by raising its levels;[354] however, the results from *in vitro*[330] and *in vivo*[355] experiments were inconclusive and would not have predicted the results in humans.

Horton et al.[334] have studied the interaction of cyclosporin A with the experimental triazole antimycotic agent SCH 39304.[254] Although elevated cyclosporin A levels were noticed at the end of the first course of SCH 39304 (days 119 through 122), they probably resulted from the increase in cyclosporin A dosage to 240 mg daily for days 112 to 118; it was unlikely that SCH 39304 had a delayed inhibitory effect on the metabolism of cyclosporin A. In this context, the principle of competitive hepatic enzyme inhibition affirms that when a drug competitively inhibits the hepatic metabolism of another drug, an increase in the serum concentration of the inhibited drug should occur shortly after therapy is instituted, provided that the inhibitory agent reaches an effective inhibitory concentration.[256] However, there have been no previous increases in the cyclosporin A concentrations during the first course of treatment with SCH 39309 that could not be attributed to increases in the doses of cyclosporin A.[334]

Contrary to other azoles, the interaction of fluconazole with cyclosporin A produced conflicting results.[357-362] Thus, while data from some studies suggested increased cyclosporin A concentrations with or without nephrotoxicity,[360-362] others have indicated the absence of pharmacokinetic interaction between the two drugs.[334,357-359] In the studies indicating the presence of fluconazole-cyclosporin A interaction, fluconazole was used at higher doses. A fluconazole-cyclosporin A interaction, therefore, might have been a dose-dependent phenomenon.[334] In addition, fluconazole has a large distribution volume and long elimination half-life (22 h)[363] which would allow its serum concentrations to accumulate over time. Another explanation for the contradictory results evaluating azole-cyclosporin A interactions may be the presence of interindividual variations in the hepatic metabolism of patients where some individuals may be more likely to either induce or inhibit certain cytochrome P-450 isoenzymes by the azole antimycotics.[334]

37.9.3 REFERENCES

1. Mishra, S. K., Ajello, L., Ahearn, D. G., Burge, H. A., Kurup, V. P., Pierson, D. L., Price, D. L., Samson, R. A., Sandhu, R. S., Shelton, B., Simmons, R. B., and Switzer, K. F., Environmental mycology and its importance to public health, *J. Med. Vet. Mycol.*, 30(Suppl. 1), 287, 1992.

2. Ajello, L., Hyalohyphomycosis and phaeohyphomycosis: two global disease entities of public health importance, *Eur. J. Epidemiol.*, 2, 243, 1986.
3. Matsumoto, T., Ajello, L., Matsuda, T., Szaniszlo, P. J., and Walsh, T. J., Developments in hyalohyphomycosis and phaeohyphomycosis, *J. Med. Vet. Mycol.*, 32(Suppl. 1), 329, 1994.
4. Vartivarian, S. E., Anaissie, E. J., and Bodey, G. P., Emerging fungal pathogens in immunocompromised patients: classification, diagnosis, and management, *Clin. Infect. Dis.*, 17(Suppl. 2), S487, 1993.
5. Kwon-Chung, K. J. and Bennett, J. E., Infections due to miscellaneous fungi, in *Medical Mycology*, Lea and Febiger, Philadelphia, 1992, 733.
6. Kwon-Chung, K. J. and Bennett, J. E., Pseudallescheriasis and scedosporium infections (allescheriosis, allescheriasis, petriellidiosis, monosporiosis, scedosporiosis), in *Medical Mycology*, Lea and Febiger, Philadelphia, 1992, 678.
7. Meyer, R. D., Gaultier, C. R., Yamashita, J. T., Babapour, R., Pitchon, H. E., and Wolfe, P. R., Fungal sinusitis in patients with AIDS: report of 4 cases and review of the literature, *Medicine (Baltimore)*, 73, 69, 1994.
8. Guého, E. and de Hoog, G. S., Taxonomy of the medical species of *Pseudallescheria* and *Scedosporium*, *J. Mycol. Med.*, 118, 3, 1991.
9. Rabodonirina, M., Paulus, S., Thevenet, F., Loire, R., Guého, E., Bastien, O., Mornex, J. F., Celard, M., and Piens, M. A., Disseminated *Scedosporium prolificans* (*S. inflatum*) infection after single-lung transplantation, *Clin. Infect. Dis.*, 19, 138, 1994.
10. Salkin, I. F., McGinnis, M. R., Dykstra, M. J., and Rinaldi, M. G., *Scedosporium inflatum*, an emerging pathogen, *J. Clin. Microbiol.*, 26, 498, 1988.
11. Wise, K. A., Speed, B. R., Ellis, D. H., and Andrew, J. H., Two fatal infections in immunocompromised patients caused by *Scedosporium inflatum*, *Pathology*, 25, 187, 1993.
12. Dykstra, M. J., Salkin, I. F., and McGinnis, M. R., An ultrastructural comparison of conidiogenesis in *Scedosporium apiospermum*, *Scedosporium inflatum* and *Scopulariopsis brumptii*, *Mycologia*, 81, 896, 1989.
13. Dixon, D. M. and Polak-Wyss, A., The medically important dematiaceous fungi and their identification, *Mycoses*, 34, 1, 1991.
14. Summerbell, R. C., Krajden, S., and Kane, J., Potted plants in hospitals as reservoirs of pathogenic fungi, *Mycopathologia*, 106, 13, 1989.
15. Wilson, C. M., O'Rourke, E. J., McGinnis, M. R., and Salkin, I. F., *Scedosporium inflatum*: clinical spectrum of a newly recognized pathogen, *J. Infect. Dis.*, 161, 102, 1990.
16. Booth, C., The genus *Fusarium*, Kew, Surrey, England, Commonwealth Mycological Institute, 1971.
17. Burgess, L. W., General ecology of the fusaria, in *Fusarium: Diseases, Biology, and Taxonomy*, Nelson. P. E., Toussoun, T. A., and Cook, R. J., Eds., Pennsylvania State University Press, University Park, 1981, 225.
18. Gordon, W. L., The occurrence of *Fusarium* species in Canada. VI. Taxonomy and habitats of *Fusarium* species from tropical and temperate regions, *Can. J. Bot.*, 38, 643, 1960.
19. Wollenweber, H. W. and Reinking, O. A., *Die Fusarien, ihre Beschreibung, Schadwirkung und Bekämpfung*, Paul Parey, Berlin, 1935.
20. Louria, D. B., Smith, J. K., and Finkel, G. C., Mycotoxins other than aflatoxins: tumor-producing potential and possible relation to human disease, *Ann. NY Acad. Sci.*, 174, 583, 1970.
21. Austwick, P. K. C., Mycotoxins, *Br. Med. Bull.*, 31, 222, 1975.
22. Wogan, G. N., Mycotoxins, *Annu. Rev. Pharmacol.*, 15, 437, 1975.
23. Trenholm, H. L., Prelusky, D. B., Young, J. C., and Miller, J. D., A practical guide to the prevention of *Fusarium* mycotoxins in grains and animal feedstuffs, *Arch. Environ. Contam. Toxicol.*, 18, 443, 1989.
24. Marasas, W. F. O., Nelson, P. E., and Toussoun, T. A., *Toxigenic Fusarium Species: Identity and Mycotoxicology*, Pennsylvania State University Press, University Park, 1984.
25. Matsuoka, Y. and Kubota, K., Characteristics of inflammation induced by fusarenon-X, a trichothecene mycotoxin from *Fusarium* species, *Toxicol. Appl. Pharmacol.*, 91, 333, 1987.
26. Kurobane, I., Zaita, N., and Fukuda, A., New metabolites of *Fusarium martii* related to dihydrofusarubin, *J. Antibiot.*, 39, 205, 1986.
27. Marasas, W. F. O. and Nelson, P. E., *Mycotoxicology: Introduction to the Mycology, Toxicology, and Pathology of Naturally Occurring Mycotoxicoses in Animals and Man*, Pennsylvania State Univerisy Press, University Park, 1987.

28. Nelson, P. E., Dignani, M. C., and Anaissie, E. J., Taxonomy, biology, and clinical aspects of *Fusarium* species, *Clin. Microbiol. Rev.*, 7, 479, 1994.

29. Toussoun, T. A. and Nelson, P. E., Variation and speculation in the fusaria, *Annu. Rev. Phytopathol.*, 13, 71, 1975.

30. Nelson, P. E., Toussoun, T. A., and Marasas, W. F. O., Fusarium *Species: An Illustrated Manual For Identification*, Pennsylvania State University Press, University Park, 1983.

31. Burgess, L. W., Liddell, C. M., and Summerell, B. A., *Laboratory Manual For* Fusarium *Research*, 2nd ed., University of Sydney, Australia, 1988.

32. Young, N. A., Kwon-Chung, K. J., Kubota, T. T., Jennings, A. E., and Fisher, R. I., Disseminated infection by *Fusarium moniliforme* during treatment for malignant lymphoma, *Clin. Microbiol.*, 7, 589, 1978.

33. Mutton, K. J., Lucas, T. J., and Harkness, J. L., Disseminated *Fusarium* species, *Med. J. Aust.*, 2, 624, 1980.

34. Anaissie, E., Kantarjian, H., Jones, P., Barlogie, B., Luna, M., Lopez-Berestein, G., and Bodey, G., *Fusarium*: a newly recognized fungal pathogen in immunosuppressed patients, *Cancer*, 57, 2141, 1986.

35. Matsumoto, T., Ajello, L., Matsuda, T., Szaniszlo, P. J., and Walsh, T. J., Developments in the hyalohyphomycosis and phaeohyphomycosis, *J. Med. Vet. Mycol.*, 32(Suppl. 1), 329, 1994.

36. Anaissie, E., Kantarjian, H., Ro, J., Hopfer, R., Rolston, K., Fainstein, V., and Bodey, G., The emerging role of *Fusarium* infections in patients with cancer, *Medicine (Baltimore)*, 62, 77, 1988.

37. Nirenberg, H., Untersuchungen über die morphologische und biologische differenzierung der *Fusarium, Section Liseola - Biolog. Bundesant. Land-und Forstw., Berlin-Dahlem*, 169, 1, 1976.

38. Wheeler, M. S., McGinnis, M. R., Schell, W. A., and Walker, D. H., *Fusarium* infection in burned patients, *Am. J. Clin. Pathol.*, 75, 304, 1981.

39. Ajello, L., Fungal infections in AIDS: a review, *L'Igiene Moderna*, 100, 288, 1993.

40. Rosenthal, J., Katz, R., Du Bois, D. B., Morrissey, A., and Machicao, A., Chronic maxillary sinusitis associated with the mushroom *Schizophylum commune* in a patient with AIDS, *Clin. Infect. Dis.*, 14, 46, 1992.

41. Anaissie, E., Bodey, G. P., Kantarjian, H., Ro, J., Vartivarian, S. E., Hopfer, R., Hoy, J., and Rolston, K., New spectrum of fungal infections in patients with cancer, *Rev. Infect. Dis.*, 11, 369, 1989.

42. Berenguer, J., Diaz-Mediavilla, J., Urra, D., and Munoz, P., Central nervous system infection caused by *Pseudallescheria boydii*: case report and review, *Rev. Infect. Dis.*, 11, 890, 1989.

43. Cooper, C. R. and Salkin, I. F., Pseudallescheriasis, in *Fungal Infections and Immune Responses*, Murphy, J. W., Friedman, H., and Bendinelli, M., Eds., Plenum Press, New York, 1993, 335.

44. Fisher, J. F., Shadomy, S., Teabaut, J. R., Woodward, J., Michaels, G. E., Newman, M. A., White, E., Cook, P., Seagraves, A., Yaghmai, F., and Rissing, J. P., Near drowning complicated by brain abscess due to *Petriellidium boydii*, *Arch. Neurol.*, 39, 511, 1982.

45. Caya, J. G., Farmer, S. G., Williams, G. A., Franson, T. R., Komorowski, R. A., and Kies, J. C., Bilateral *Pseudaschelleria boydii* endophthalmitis in an immunocompromised patient, *Wisconsin Med. J.*, 87, 11, 1988.

46. Hainer, J. W., Ostrow, J. H., and Mackenzie, D. W. R., Pulmonary monosporiosis: report of a case with precipitating antibody, *Chest*, 66, 601, 1974.

47. Kershaw, P., Freeman, R., Templeton, D., DeGirolami, P. C., DeGirolami, U., Tarsy, D., Hoffman, S., Eliopoulos, G., and Karchmer, A. W., *Pseudallescheria boydii* infection of the central nervous system, *Arch. Neurol.* 47, 468, 1990.

48. Yoo, D., Lee, W. H. S., and Kwon-Chung, K. J., Brain abscesses due to *Pseudallescheria boydii* association with primary non-Hodgkin's lymphoma of the central nervous system: a case report and literature review, *Rev. Infect. Dis.*, 7, 272, 1985.

49. Patterson, T. F., Andriole, V. T., Zervos, M. J., Therasse, D., and Kauffman, C. A., The epidemiology of pseudallescheriasis complicating transplantation: nosocomial and community-acquired infection, *Mycoses*, 33, 297, 1990.

50. Peréz, R. E., Smith, M., McClendon, J., Kim, J., and Eugenio, N., *Psedallescheria boydii* brain abscess: complication of an intravenous catheter, *Am. J. Med.*, 84, 359, 1988.

51. Pfeifer, J. D., Grand, M. G., Thomas, M. A., Berger, A. R., Lucarelli, M. J., and Smith, M. E., Endogenous *Pseudallescheria boydii* endophthalmitis: clinicopathologic findings in two cases, *Arch. Ophthalmol.*, 109, 1714, 1992.

52. Rippon, J. W., Pseudallescheriasis, in *Medical Mycology. The Pathogenic Fungi and the Pathogenic Actinomycetes*, 3rd ed., Rippon, J. W., Ed., W. B. Saunders, Philadelphia, 1988, 651.

53. Travis, L. B., Roberts, G. D., and Wilson, W. R., Clinical significance of *Pseudallescheria boydii*: a review of 10 years' experience, *Mayo Clin. Proc.*, 60, 531, 1985.

54. Welty, F. K., McLeod, G. X., Ezratty, C., Healy, R. W., and Karchmer, A. W., *Pseudallescheria boydii* endocarditis of the pulmonic valve in a liver transplant recipient, *Clin. Infect. Dis.*, 15, 858, 1992.

55. Arnett, J. C. and Hatch, H. B., Pulmonary allescheriasis, *Arch. Intern. Med.*, 135, 1250, 1975.

56. Seale, P. and Hudson, J. A., Successful medical treatment of pulmonary petriellidiosis, *South. Med. J.*, 78, 473, 1985.

57. McCarthy, D. S., Longbottom, J. L., Riddell, R. W., and Batten, J. C., Pulmonary mycetoma due to *Allescheria boydii*, *Am. Rev. Respir. Dis.*, 100, 213, 1969.

58. Guyotat, D., Piens, M. A., Bouvier, R., and Fiere, D., A case of disseminated *Scedosporium apiospermum* infection after bone marrow transplantation, *Mykosen*, 30, 151, 1987.

59. Forno, L. S. and Billingham, M. E., *Allescheria boydii* infection of the brain, *Pathology*, 106, 195, 1972.

60. Aronson, S. M., Benham, R., and Wolf, A., Maduromycosis of the central nervous system, *J. Neuropathol. Exp. Neurol.*, 12, 158, 1953.

61. Benham, R. and Georg, L. K., *Allescheria boydii*, causative agent in a case of meningitis, *J. Invest. Dermatol.*, 10, 99, 1948.

62. Selby, R., Pachymeningitis secondary to *Allerschia boydii*, *J. Neurosurg.*, 36, 225, 1972.

63. Alsip, S. G. and Cobbs, C. G., *Pseudallescheria boydii* infection of the central nervous system in a cardiac transplant recipient, *South. Med. J.*, 79, 383, 1986.

64. Creitz, J. and Harris, H. W., Isolation of *Allescheria boydii* from spitum, *Am. Rev. Tuberc.*, 71, 126, 1955.

65. Travis, R. E., Ulrich, E. W., and Phillips, S., Pulmonary allescheriasis, *Ann. Intern. Med.*, 54, 151, 1961.

66. Blank, F. and Stuart, E. A., *Monosporium apiospermum sacc.* 1911 associated with otomycosis, *Can. Med. Assoc. J.*, 72, 601, 1955.

67. Ansari, R. A., Hindson, D. A., Stevens, D. A., and Kloss, J. G., *Pseudallescheria boydii* arthritis and osteomyelitis in a patient with Cushing's disease, *South. Med. J.*, 80, 90, 1987.

68. Hung, L. H. Y. and Norwood, L. A., Osteomyelitis due to *Pseudallescheria boydii*, *South. Med. J.*, 86, 231, 1993.

69. Fernandez-Guerrero, M. L., Barnés, P. R., and Alés, J. M., Postcraniotomy mycetoma of the scalp and osteomyelitis due to *Pseudallescheria boydii*, *J. Infect. Dis.*, 156, 855, 1987.

70. Ginter, G., de Hoog, G. S., Pschaid, A., Fellinger, M., Bogiatzis, A., Berghold, C., Reich, E.-M., and Odds, F. C., Arthritis without grains caused by *Pseudallescheria boydii*, *Mycoses*, 38, 369, 1995.

71. Winston, D. J., Jordan, M. C., and Rhodes, J., *Allescheria boydii*: infections in the immunosuppressed host, *Am. J. Med.*, 63, 830, 1977.

72. Davis, W. A., Isner, J. M., Bracey, A. W., Roberts, W. C., and Garagusi, V. F., Disseminated *Petriellidium boydii* and pacemaker endocarditis, *Am. J. Med.*, 69, 929, 1980.

73. Ogihara, A., Chino, M., Yoshino, H., Nishikawa, K., Nara, M., Miyashita, M., Takenaka, N., and Nishimura, K., A case of prosthetic valve endocarditis due to *Scedosporium apiospermum*, *Nippon Naika Gakkai Zasshi*, 78, 432, 1989.

74. Rosen, F., Deck, J. H. N., and Rewcastle, N. B., *Allescheria boydii* unique systemic dissemination to thyroid and brain, *Can. Med. Assoc. J.*, 93, 1125, 1965.

75. de Ment, S. H., Smith, R. R., Karp, J. E., and Merz, W. G., Pulmonary, cardiac and thyroid involvement in disseminated *Pseudallescheria boydii*, *Arch. Pathol. Lab. Med.*, 108, 859, 1984.

76. Meyer, E. and Herrold, R. D., *Allescheria boydii* isolated from a patient with chronic prostatitis, *Am. J. Clin. Pathol.*, 35, 155, 1961.

77. Saadah, H. A. and Dixon, T., *Petriellidium boydii* (*Allescheria boydii*) necrotizing pneumonia in a normal host, *JAMA*, 245, 605, 1981.

78. Collignon, P. J., Macleod, C., and Packham, D. R., Miconazole therapy in *Pseudallescheria boydii* infection, *Australas. J. Dermatol.*, 26, 129, 1985.

79. Lichtman, D. M., Johnson, D. C., Mack, G. R., and Lack, E. E., Maduromycosis (*Allescheria boydii*) infection of the hand, *J. Bone Joint Surg. Am.*, 60, 546, 1978.

80. Bryan, C. S., DiSalvo, A. F., Kaufman, L., Kaplan, W., Brill, A. H., and Abbott, D. C., *Petriellidium boydii* infection of the sphenoid sinus, *Am. J. Clin. Pathol.*, 74, 846, 1980.

81. Schiess, R. J., Coscia, M. F., and McClellan, G. A., *Petriellidium boydii* pachymeningitis treated with miconazole and ketoconazole, *Neurosurgery*, 14, 220, 1984.

82. Lutwick, L. I., Galgiani, J. N., Johnson, R. H., and Stevens, D. A., Visceral fungal infections due to *Petriellidium boydii*, *Am. J. Med.*, 61, 632, 1976.

83. Shin, L. Y. and Lee, N., Disseminated petriellidiosis (allescheriasis) in a patient with refractory acute lymphoblastic leukemia, *J. Clin. Pathol.*, 37, 78, 1984.

84. Bell, W. E. and Myers, M. G., *Allescheria (Petriellidium) boydii* brain abscess in a child with leukemia, *Arch. Neurol.*, 35, 386, 1978.

85. Fry, V. G. and Young, C. N., A rare fungal brain abscess in an uncompromised host, *Surg. Neurol.*, 15, 446, 1981.

86. Agamanolis, D. P., Kalwinsky, D. K., Krill, C. E., Jr., Dasu, S., Halasa, B., and Galloway, P. G., *Fusarium* meningoencephalitis in a child with acute leukemia, *Neuropediatrics*, 22, 110, 1991.

87. Gluckman, S. J., Ries, K., and Abrutyn, E., *Allescheria (Petriellidium) boydii* sinusitis in a compromised host, *J. Clin. Microbiol.*, 5, 481, 1977.

88. Mader, J. T., Ream, R. S., and Heath, P. W., *Petriellidium boydii (Allescheria boydii)* sphenoidal sinusitis, *JAMA*, 239, 2368, 1978.

89. Morgan, M. A., Wilson, W. R., Neel, H. B. III, and Roberts, G. D., Fungal sinusitis in healthy and immunocompromised individuals, *Am. J. Clin. Pathol.*, 82, 597, 1984.

90. Salitan, M. L., Lawson, W., Som, P. M., Bottone, E. J., and Biller, H. F., Pseudallescheria sinusitis with itracranial extension in a nonimmunocompromised host, *Otolaryngol. Head Neck Surg.*, 102, 745, 1990.

91. Winn, R. E., Ramsey, P. D., McDonald, J. C., and Dunlop, K. J., Maxillary sinusitis from *Pseudallescheria boydii*, *Arch. Otolaryngol.*, 109, 123, 1983.

92. Washburn, R. G., Kennedy, D. W., Begley, M. G., Henderson, D. K., and Bennett, J. E., Chronic fungal sinusitis in apparently normal hosts, *Medicine (Baltimore)*, 67, 231, 1988.

93. Dubeau, F., Roy, L. E., Allard, J., Laverdiere, M., Rousseau, S., Duplantis, F., Boileau, J., and Lachapelle, J., Brain abscess due to *Petriellidium boydii*, *Can. J. Neurol. Sci.*, 11, 395, 1984.

94. Walker, D. H., Adamec, T., and Krigman, M., Disseminated petriellidiosis (allescheriosis), *Arch. Pathol. Lab. Med.*, 102, 158, 1978.

95. Anderson, R. L., Carroll, T. F., Harvey, R. T., and Myers, M. G., *Petriellidium (Allescheria) boydii* orbital and brain abscess treated with intravenous miconazole, *Am. J. Ophthalmol.*, 97, 771, 1984.

96. Fessler, R. G. and Brown, F. D., Superior sagittal sinus infection with *Petriellidium boydii*: case report, *Neurosurgery*, 24, 604, 1989.

97. Phillips, P., Forbes, J. C., and Speert, D. P., Disseminated infection with *Pseudallescheria boydii* in a patient with chronic granulomatous disease: response to gamma-interferon plus antifungal chemotherapy, *Pediatr. Infect. Dis. J.*, 10, 536, 1991.

98. The International Chronic Granulomatous Disease Cooperative Study Group, A controlled trial of interferon gamma to prevent infection in chronic granulomatous disease, *N. Engl. J. Med.*, 324, 509, 1991.

99. Bernstein, E. F., Schuster, M. G., Stieritz, D. D., Heuman, P. C., and Uitto, J., Disseminated cutaneous *Psedallescheria boydii*, *Br. J. Dermatol.*, 132, 456, 1995.

100. Cunningham, R. and Mitchell, D. C., Amphotericin B responsive *Scedosporium apiospermum* in a patient with acute myeloid leukaemia, *J. Clin. Pathol.*, 49, 93, 1996.

101. Ruxin, T. A., Steck, W. D., Helm, T. N., Bergfeld, W. F., and Bolwell, B. J., *Pseudallescheria boydii* in an immunocompromised host: successful treatment with debridement and itraconazole, *Arch. Dermatol.*, 132, 382, 1996.

102. Hung, C. C., Chang, S. C., Yang, P. C., and Hsieh, W. C., Invasive pulmonary pseudallescheriasis with direct invasion of the thoracic spine in an immunocompetent patient, *Eur. J. Clin. Microbiol. Infect. Dis.*, 13, 749, 1994.

103. Gumbart, C. H., *Pseudallescheria boydii* infection after bone marrow transplantation, *Ann. Intern. Med.*, 99, 193, 1983.

104. Goldberg, S. L., Geha, D. J., Marshall, W. F., Inwards, D. J., and Hoagland, H. C., Successful treatment of simultaneous pulmonary *Pseudallescheria boydii* and *Aspergillus terreus* infection with oral itraconazole, *Clin. Infect. Dis.*, 16, 803, 1993.

105. Nomdedéu, J., Brunet, S., Martino, R., Altés, A., Ausina, V., and Domingo-Albos, A., Successful treatment of pneumonia due to *Scedosporium apiospermum* with itraconazole: case report, *Clin. Infect. Dis.*, 16, 731, 1993.

106. Martino, R., Nomdedéu, J., Altés, A., Sureda, A., Brunet, S., Martinez, C., and Domingo-Albos, A., Successful bone marrow transplantation in patients with previous invasive fungal infections: report of four cases, *Bone Marrow Transplant.*, 13, 265, 1994.

107. Walsh, M., White, L., Atkinson, K., and Enno, A., Fungal *Pseudallescheria boydii* lung infiltrates unresponsive to amphotericin B in leukaemic patients, *Aust. NZ J. Med.*, 22, 265, 1992.

108. Mesnard, R., Lamy, T., Dauriac, C., and Le Prise, P.-Y., Lung abscess due to *Pseudallescheria boydii* in the course of acute leukaemia, *Acta Haematol.*, 87, 78, 1992.

109. Smith, A. G., Crain, S. M., Dejongh, C., Thomas, G. M., and Vigorito, R. D., Systemic pseudalle-scheriasis in a patient with acute myelocytic leukaemia, *Mycopathologia*, 90, 219, 1985.

110. Galgiani, J. N., Stevens, D. A., Graybill, J. R., Stevens, D. L., Tillinghast, A. J., and Levine, H. B., *Pseudallescheria boydii* infections treated with ketoconazole, *Chest*, 86, 219, 1984.

111. Hecht, R. and Montgomerie, J. Z., Maxillary sinus infection with *Allescheria boydii* (*Petriellidium boydii*), *Johns Hopkins Med. J.*, 142, 107, 1978.

112. Raffanti, S. P., Fyfe, B., Carreiro, S., Sharp, S. E., Hyman, B. A., and Ratzan, K. R., Native valve endocarditis due to *Pseudallescheria boydii* in a patient with AIDS: case report and review, *Rev. Infect. Dis.*, 12, 993, 1990.

113. Scherr, G. R., Evans, S. G., Kiyabu, M. T., and Klatt, E. C., *Pseudallescheria boydii* infection in the acquired immunodeficiency syndrome, *Arch. Pathol. Lab. Med.*, 116, 535, 1992.

114. Glassman, M. I., Henkind, P., and Alture-Werber, E., *Monosporium apiospermum* endophthalmitis, *Am. J. Ophthalmol.*, 76, 821, 1973.

115. Stern, R. M., Zakov, Z. N., Meisler, D. M., Hall, G. S., and Martin, A., Endogenous *Pseudallescheria boydii* endophthalmitis: a clinicopathologic report, *Cleveland Clin. Q.*, 53, 197, 1986.

116. Meadow, W. L., Tripple, M. A., and Rippon, J. W., Endophthalmitis caused by *Pseudallescheria boydii*, *Am. J. Dis. Child.*, 135, 378, 1981.

117. Bouchard, C. S., Chaco, B., Cupples, H. P., Cavanagh, H. D., and Mathers, W. D., Surgical treatment for a case of postoperative *Pseudallescheria boydii* endophthalmitis, *Ophthal. Surg.*, 22, 98, 1991.

118. Stern, R. M., Zakov, Z. N., Meisler, D. M., Hall, G. S., and Martin, A., Endogenous *Pseudallescheria boydii* endophthalmitis: a clinicopathologic report, *Cleve. Clin. Q.*, 53, 197, 1986.

119. Moriarty, A. P., Crawford, G. J., McAllister, I. L., and Constable, I. J., Severe corneoscleral infection: a complication of beta irradiation scleral necrosis following pterygium excision, *Arch. Ophthalmol.*, 111, 947, 1993.

120. Moriarty, A. P., Crawford, G. J., McAllister, I. L., and Constable, I. J., Fungal corneoscleritis complicating beta-irradiation-induced scleral necrosis following pterygium excision, *Eye*, 7, 525, 1993.

121. Gordon, M. A., Valloton, W. W., and Groffead, G. S., Corneal sclerosis: a case of keratomycosis treated successfully with nystatin and amphotericin B, *Arch. Ophthalmol.*, 62, 758, 1959.

122. Matsuzaki, O., Ocular infection with a fungus from rice leaf, *Jpn. J. Med. Mycol.*, 10, 239, 1969.

123. Zapater, R. C. and Albesi, E. J., Corneal monosporiosis, *Ophthalmologica*, 178, 142, 1979.

124. Bloom, P. A., Laidlaw, D. A. H., Easty, D. L., and Warnock, D. W., Treatment failure in a case of fungal keratitis caused by *Pseudallescheria boydii*, *Br. J. Ophthalmol.*, 76, 367, 1992.

125. Ksiazek, S. M., Morris, D. A., Mandelbaum, S., and Rosenbaum, P. S., Fungal panophthalmitis secondary to *Scedosporium apiospermum* (*Pseudallescheria boydii*) keratitis, *Am. J. Ophthalmol.*, 118, 532, 1994.

126. Legeais, J. M., Blanc, V., Basset, D., D'Hermies, F., Harrabi, S., Frau, E., Goichot, L., Renard, G., and Pouliquen, Y., Severe keratomycosis: diagnosis and treatment, *J. Fr. Ophthalmol.*, 17, 568, 1994.

127. Ruben, S., *Pseudallescheria boydii* keratitis, *Acta Ophthalmol. (Copenhagen)*, 69, 684, 1991.

128. Burns, E. L., Moss, E. S., and Brueck, J. W., Mycetoma pedis in the United States and Canada: with a report of three cases originating in Louisiana, *Am. J. Clin. Pathol.*, 15, 35, 1945.

129. Stierstorfer, M. B., Schartz, B. K., McGuire, J. B., and Miller, A. C., *Pseudallescheria boydii* mycetoma in Northern New England, *Int. J. Dermatol.*, 27, 383, 1988.

130. Sheftel, T. G., Mader, J. T., and Cierny, G., *Pseudallescheria boydii* soft tissue abscess, *Clin. Orthop.*, 215, 212, 1987.

131. Ajello, L., The isolation of *Allescheria boydii* Shear, an etiologic agent of mycetoma, from soil, *Am. J. Trop. Med. Hyg.*, 1, 227, 1952.

132. Drouhet, E. and Dupont, B., Chronic mucocutaneous candidiasis and other superficial and systemic mycoses successfully treated with ketoconazole, *Rev. Infect. Dis.*, 2, 606, 1980.

133. Aubock, J., Pichler, E., and Fritsch, P., Mycetoma caused by *Petriellidium boydii*: treatment with ketoconazole, *Hautarzt.*, 36, 453, 1985.

134. Pether, J. V. S., Jones, W., Greatorex, F. B., and Bunting, W., Acute pyogenic *Pseudallescheria boydii* foot infection sequentially treated with miconazole and itraconazole, *J. Infect.*, 25, 335, 1992.

135. Dellestable, F., Kures, L., Mainard, D., Pere, P., and Gaucher, A., Fungal arthritis due to *Pseudallescheria boydii* (*Scedosporium apiospermum*), *J. Rheumatol.*, 21, 766, 1994.

136. Hayden, G., Lapp, C., and Loda, F., Arthritis caused by *Monosporium apiospermum* treated with intra-articular amphotericin B, *Am. J. Dis. Child.*, 131, 927, 1977.

137. Kemp, H. B. S., Bedford, A. F., and Fincham, W. J., *Petriellidium boydii* infection of the knee: a case report, *Skeletal Radiol.*, 9, 114, 1982.

138. Dirschl, D. R. and Henderson, R. C., Patellar overgrowth after infection of the knee, *J. Bone Joint Surg.*, 73A, 940, 1991.

139. Halpern, A. A., Nagel, D. A., and Schurman, D. J., *Allescheria boydii* osteomyelitis following multiple steroid injections and surgery, *Clin. Orthop.*, 126, 232, 1977.

140. Gener, F. A., Kustimur, S., Sultan, N., and Sever, A., Fungus-induced arthritis caused by *Scedosporium apiospermum* (*Pseudallescheria boydii*), *Z. Rheumatol.*, 50, 219, 1991.

141. Gener, F. A., Kustimur, S., Sultan, N., and Sever, A., Uber eine pilz-induzierte arthritis durch *Scedosporium apiospermum* (*Pseudallescheria boydii*), *Zeitschr. Rheumatol.*, 50, 219, 1991.

142. Piper, J. P., Golden, J., Brown, D., Broestler, J., and Grant, D., Successful treatment of *Scedosporium apiospermum* suppurative arthritis with itraconazole, *Pediatr. Infect. Dis. J.*, 9, 674, 1990.

143. Chatté, G., Boibieux, A., Bailly, M. P. et al., Osteoarthrite du genou a *Scedosporium apiospermum*: succès de l'itraconazole, *J. Mycol. Méd.*, 3, 111, 1993.

144. Van Cutsem, J. M. and Thienpont, D., Miconazole, a broad-spectrum antimycotic agent with antibacterial activity, *Chemotherapy*, 17, 391, 1972.

145. McCall, R. E., Maduromycosis "*Allescheria boydii*" septic arthritis of the knee: a case report, *Orthopedics*, 4, 1144, 1981.

146. Lazarus, H. S., Myers, J. P., and Brocker, R. J., Post-craniotomy wound infection caused by *Pseudallescheria boydii*: case report, *J. Neurosurg.*, 64, 153, 1986.

147. Findling, J. W., Tyrell, J. B., Aron, D. C., Fitzgerald, P. A., Young, C. W., and Sohnle, P. G., Fungal infections in Cushing's syndrome, *Ann. Intern. Med.*, 95, 392, 1981.

148. Anthony, L. B. and Greco, F. A., *Pneumocystis carinii* pneumonia: a complication of Cushing's syndrome, *Ann. Intern. Med.*, 94, 488, 1981.

149. Plotz, C. M., Knowlton, A. I., and Ragan, C., The natural history of Cushing's syndrome, *Am. J. Med.*, 13, 597, 1952.

150. Fauci, A. S., Dale, D. C., and Balow, J. E., Glucocorticosteroid therapy: mechanism of action and clinical consideration, *Ann. Intern. Med.*, 84, 304, 1976.

151. Balow, J. E. and Rosenthal, A. S., Glucocorticoid suppression of macrophage migration inhibitory factor, *J. Exp. Med.*, 137, 1031, 1973.

152. Farag, S. S., Firkin, F. C., Andrew, J. H., Lee, C. S., and Ellis, D. H., Fatal disseminated *Scedosporium inflatum* infection in a neutropenic immunocompromised patient, *J. Infect.*, 25, 201, 1992.

153. Guarro, J., Gaztelurrutia, L., Marin, J., and Barcena, J., *Scedosporium inflatum*, a new pathogenic fungus, *Enfermed. Infec. Microbiol. Clin.*, 9, 557, 1991.

154. Marin, J., Sanz, M. A., Sanz, G. F., Guarro, J., Martinez, M. L., Prieto, M., Guého, E., and Menezo, J. L., Disseminated *Scedosporium inflatum* infection in a patient with acute myeloblastic leukemia, *Eur. J. Clin. Microbiol. Infect. Dis.*, 10, 759, 1991.

155. Rosenthal, S. A., Weitzman, I., Salkin, I. F., and Kemna, M., Fungal sepsis caused by *Scedosporium inflatum*, *Mycol. Observer*, 9, 1, 1989.

156. Salesa, R., Burgos, A., Ondiviela, R., Richard, C., Quindos, G., and Ponton, J., Fatal disseminated infection by *Scedosporium inflatum* after bone marrow transplantation, *Scand. J. Infect. Dis.*, 25, 389, 1993.

157. Wood, G. M., McCormack, J. G., Muir, D. B., Ellis, D. H., Ridley, M. F., Pritchard, R., and Harrison, M., Clinical features of human infection with *Scedosporium inflatum*, *Clin. Infect. Dis.*, 14, 1027, 1992.
158. Malloch, D. and Salkin, I. F., A new species of *Scedosporium* associated with osteomyelitis in humans, *Mycotaxon*, 21, 247, 1984.
159. Toy, E. C., Rinaldi, M. G., Savitch, C. B., and Leibovitch, E. R., Endocarditis and hip arthritis associated with *Scedosporium inflatum*, *South. Med. J.*, 83, 957, 1990.
160. Malekzadeh, M., Overturf, G. D., Auerbach, S. B., Wong, L., and Hirsch, M., Chronic, recurrent osteomyelitis caused by *Scedosporium inflatum*, *Pediatr. Infect. Dis. J.*, 9, 357, 1990.
161. Sparrow, S. A., Hallam, L. A., Wild, B. E., and Baker, D. L., *Scedosporium inflatum*: first case report of disseminated infection and review of the literature, *Pediatr. Hematol. Oncol.*, 9, 293, 1992.
162. Tapia, M., Richard, C., Baro, J., Salesa, R., Fogols, J., Zurbano, F., and Zubizarreta, A., *Scedosporium inflatum* infection in immunocompromised haematological patients, *Br. J. Haematol.*, 87, 212, 1994.
163. Nielsen, K., Lang, H., Shum, A. C., Woodruff, K., and Cherry, J. D., Disseminated *Scedosporium prolificans* infection in an immunocompromised adolescent, *Pediatr. Infect. Dis. J.*, 12, 882, 1993.
164. Spielberger, R. T., Tegtmeier, B. R., O'Donnell, M. R., and Ito, J. I., Fatal *Scedosporium prolificans* (*S. inflatum*) fungemia following allogeneic bone marrow transplantation: report of a case in the United States, *Clin. Infect. Dis.*, 21, 1067, 1995.
165. Wild, B. E., Clemens, B. S., Holt, M. J. G., Gray, A., and Gatus, B. J., Successful treatment of *Scedosporium inflatum* and *Scedosporium apiospermum* osteomyelitis in 2 children, *Proc. XIIth ISHAM Congress*, Adelaide, Abstr. D 38, 1994.
166. Gordon, M. A., Lapa, E. W., and Passero, P. G., Improved method for azole antifungal susceptibility testing, *J. Clin. Microbiol.*, 26, 1874, 1988.
167. Sullivan, L. J., Snibson, G., Joseph, C., and Taylor, H. R., *Scedosporium prolificans* sclerokeratitis, *Aust. NZ J. Ophthalmol.*, 22, 207, 1994.
168. Levine, D. J., Scleral complications following beta irradiation, *Arch. Ophthalmol.*, 112, 1016, 1994.
169. MacKenzie, F. D., Hirst, L. W., Kynarston, B., and Bain, C., Recurrence rate and complications after beta irradiation for pterygia, *Ophthalmology*, 98, 1776, 1991.
170. Alfonso, E., Surgical intervention in infectious keratoscleritis, *Arch. Ophthalmol.*, 112, 1017, 1994.
171. Levine, D. J., Beta irradiation of pterygium, *Ophthalmology*, 99, 841, 1992.
172. Farrell, P. L. R. and Smith, R. E., Bacterial corneoscleritis complicating pterygium excision, *Am. J. Ophthalmol.*, 107, 515, 1989.
173. Mayer, C. F., Endemic panmyelotoxicosis in the Russian grain belt. I. The clinical aspects of alimentary toxic aleukia (ATA): a comprehensive review, *Milit. Surg.*, 1, 173, 1953.
174. Marshall, E., The Soviet elephant grass theory, *Science*, 217, 2, 1982.
175. Saito, M. and Tatsuno, T., Toxins of *Fusarium nivale*, in *Microbial Toxins: Algal and Fungal Toxins*, Vol. 7, Kadis, S., Ciegler, A., and Ajl, S., Eds., Academic Press, New York, 1971, 293.
176. Joffe, A. Z., Alimentary toxic aleukia, in *Microbial Toxins: Algal and Fungal Toxins*, Vol. 7, Kadis, S., Ciegler, A., and Ajl, S., Eds., Academic Press, New York, 1971, 139.
177. Nelson, P. E., Taxonomy and biology of *Fusarium moniliforme*, *Mycopathologia*, 117, 29, 1992.
178. Morrison, V. A., Haake, R. J., and Weisdorf, D. J., The spectrum of non-*Candida* fungal infection following bone marrow transplantation, *Medicine (Baltimore)*, 72, 78, 1993.
179. Merz, W. G., Karp, J. E., Hoagland, M., Jettgoheen, M., Junkins, J. M., and Hood, A. F., Diagnosis and successful treatment of fusariosis in the compromised host, *J. Infect. Dis.*, 158, 1046, 1988.
180. Minor, R. L., Pfaller, M. A., Gingrich, R. D., and Burns, L. J., Disseminated *Fusarium* infections in patients following bone marrow transplantation, *Bone Marrow Transplant.*, 4, 653, 1989.
181. Guarro, J. and Gene, J., Opportunistic fusarial infections in humans, *Eur. J. Clin. Microbiol. Infect. Dis.*, 14, 741, 1995.
182. Richardson, S. E., Bannatyne, R. M., Summerbell, R. C., Milliken, J., Gold, R., and Weitzman, S. S., Disseminated fusarial infection in the immunocompromised host, *Rev. Infect. Dis.*, 10, 1171, 1988.
183. Venditti, M., Micozzi, A., Gentile, G., Polonelli, L., Morace, G., Bianco, P., Avvisati, G., Papa, G., and Martino, P., Invasive *Fusarium solani* infections in patients with acute leukemia, *Rev. Infect. Dis.*, 10, 653, 1988.
184. Cho, C. T., Vats, T. S., Lowman, J. T., Brandsberg, J. W., and Tosh, F. E., *Fusarium solani* infection during treatment for acute leukemia, *J. Pediatr.*, 83, 1028, 1973.

185. Bodey, G. P., Buckley, M., Sathe, Y. S., and Freireich, E. J., Quantitative relationships between circulating leukocytes and infection in patients with acute leukemia, *Ann. Intern. Med.*, 64, 328, 1966.
186. Gutmann, L., Chou, S. M., and Pore, R. S., Fusariosis, myasthenic syndrome, and aplastic anemia, *Neurology*, 25, 922, 1975.
187. Schneller, F. R., Gulati, S. C., Cunningham, I. B., O'Reilly, R. J., Schmitt, H. J., and Clarkson, B. D., *Fusarium* infections in patients with hematologic malignancies, *Leuk. Res.*, 14, 961, 1990.
188. Krcméry, V., Jr., Kunova, E., Jesenska, Z., Trupl, J. et al., Invasive mold infections in cancer patients: 5 years' experience with *Aspergillus*, *Mucor*, *Fusarium* and *Acremonium* infections, *Support Care Cancer*, 4, 39, 1996.
189. Chevalet, P., Tiab, M., Miegeville, M., Milpied, N. et al., Fusaria infection in patients with neutropenia: a propos of 3 cases, *Rev. Med. Interne*, 17, 474, 1996.
190. Krulder, J. W., Brimicombe, R. W., Wijermans, P. W., and Gams, W., Systemic *Fusarium nygamai* infection in a patient with lymphoblastic non-Hodgkin's lymphoma, *Mycoses*, 39, 121, 1996.
191. Velasco, E., Martins, C. A., and Nucci, M., Successful treatment of catheter-related fusarial infection in immunocompromised children, *Eur. J. Clin. Microbiol. Infect. Dis.*, 14, 697, 1995.
192. Myoken, Y., Sugata, T., Kyo, T., and Fujihara, M., Oral *Fusarium* infection in a granulocytopenic patient with acute myelogenous leukemia: a case report, *J. Oral Pathol. Med.*, 24, 237, 1995.
193. Rabodonirina, M., Piens, M. A., Monier, M. F., Guého, E., Fière, D., and Mojon, M., *Fusarium* infections in immunocompromised patients: case reports and literature review, *Eur. J. Clin. Microbiol. Infect. Dis.*, 13, 152, 1994.
194. Caux, F., Aractingi, S., Baurmann, H., Reygagne, P., Dombret, H., Romand, S., and Dubertret, L., *Fusarium solani* cutaneous infection in a neutropenic patient, *Dermatology*, 186, 232, 1993.
195. Nucci, M., Spector, N., Lucena, S., Bacha, P. C., Pulcheri, W., Lamosa, A., Derossi, A., Caiuby, M. J., Macieira, J., and Oliveira, H. P., Three cases of infection with *Fusarium* species in neutropenic patients, *Eur. J. Clin. Microbiol. Infect. Dis.*, 11, 1160, 1992.
196. Helm, T. N., Longworth, D. L., Hall, G. S., Bolwell, B. J., Fernandez, B., and Tonecki, K., Case report and review of resolved fusariosis, *J. Am. Acad. Dermatol.*, 23(2 part 2), 393, 1990.
197. Blazar, B. R., Hurd, D. D., Snover, D. C., Alexander, J. W., and McGlave, P. B., Invasive Fusarium infections in bone marrow transplant recipients, *Am. J. Med.*, 77, 645, 1984.
198. Steinberg, G. K., Britt, R. H., Enzmann, D. R., Finlay, J. L., and Arvin, A. M., *Fusarium* brain abscess: case report, *J. Neurosurg.*, 56, 598, 1983.
199. Abramowsky, C. R., Quinn, D., Bradford, W. D., and Conant, N. F., *J. Pediatr.*, 84, 561, 1974.
200. Becker, W. K., Cioffi, W. G., Jr., McManus, A. T., Kim, S. H., McManus, W. F., Mason, A. D., and Pruitt, B. A., Jr., Fungal burn wound infection: a 10-year experience, *Arch. Surg.*, 126, 44, 1991.
201. Benjamin, R. P., Callaway, J. L., Conant, N. F., and Durham, N. C., Facial granuloma associated with *Fusarium* infection, *Arch. Dermatol.*, 101, 598, 1970.
202. English, M. P., Invasion of the skin by non-dermatophyte filamentous fungi, *Br. J. Dermatol.*, 80, 282, 1968.
203. Destombes, P., Mariat, F., Rosati, L., and Segretain, G., Les mycétomes en Somalie — conclusions d'une enquéte menée de 1959 a 1964, *Acta Trop.*, 34, 355, 1977.
204. Peloux, Y. and Segretain, G., Mycetoma a *Fusarium*, *Bull. Fr. Mycol. Méd.*, 21, 31, 1966.
205. Baudraz-Rosselet, F., Monod, M., Borradori, L., Ginalsky, J. M., Vion, B., Boccard, C., and Frenk, E., Mycetoma of the foot due to *Fusarium* sp. treated with oral ketoconazole, *Dermatology*, 184, 303, 1992.
206. Ooi, S. P., Chen, T. T., Huang, T. H., Chang, H. S., and Hsieh, H. Y., Granuloma annulare-like skin lesion due to *Fusarium roseum*: therapy with ketoconazole, *Arch. Dermatol.*, 123, 167, 1987.
207. Attapattu, M. C. and Anandakrishnan, C., Extensive subcutaneous hyphomycosis caused by *F. oxysporum*, *J. Med. Vet. Mycol.*, 24, 105, 1986.
208. Bourguignon, R. L., Walsh, A. F., Flynn, J. C., Bare, C., and Spinos, E., *Fusarium* species osteomyelitis, *J. Bone Joint Surg.*, 58A, 722, 1976.
209. Jakle, C., Leek, J. C., Olson, D. A., and Robbins, D. L., Septic arthritis due to *Fusarium solani*, *J. Rheumatol.*, 10, 151, 1983.
210. Harris, J. J. and Downham, T. G., Unusual fungal infections associated with immunologic hyporeactivity, *Int. J. Dermatol.*, 17, 323, 1978.
211. Lazarus, J. A. and Schwartz, L. H., Infection of urinary bladder with an unusual fungus strain: *Fusarium*, *Urol. Cutan. Rev.*, 52, 185, 1948.

212. Kerr, C. M., Perfect, J. R., Craven, P. C., Jorgensen, J. H., Drutz, D. J., Shelburne, J. D., Gallis, H. A., and Gutman, R. A., Fungal peritonitis in patients on continuous ambulatory peritoneal dialysis, *Ann. Intern. Med.*, 99, 334, 1983.

213. Young, J. B., Ahmed-Jushuf, I. H., Brownjohn, A. M., Parsons, F. M., Foulkes, S. J., and Evans, E. G., Opportunistic peritonitis in continuous ambulatory peritoneal dialysis, *Clin. Nephrol.*, 22, 268, 1984.

214. Flynn, J. T., Meislich, D., Kaiser, B. A., Polinsky, M. S., and Baluarte, H. J., *Fusarium* peritonitis in a child on peritoneal dialysis: case report and review of the literature, *Perit. Dial. Int.*, 16, 52, 1996.

215. Valenstein, P. and Schell, W. A., Primary intranasal *Fusarium* infection: potential for confusion with rhinocerebral zygomycosis, *Arch. Pathol. Lab. Med.*, 110, 751, 1986.

216. Becelli, R., Sassano, P., Liberatore, G. M., Arcese, W., and Mengarelli, A., Surgical and local treatment in a case of fungal sinusitis in a patient with bone marrow aplasia, *Minerva Stomatol.*, 44, 171, 1995.

217. Kurien, M., Anandi, V., Raman, R., and Brahmadathan, K. N., Maxillary sinus fusariosis in immunocompetent hosts, *J. Laryngol. Otol.*, 106, 733, 1992.

218. Mohammedi, I., Gachot, B., Grossin, M., Marche, C., Grossin, M., Marche, C., Wolff, M., and Vachon, F., Overwhelming myocarditis due to *Fusarium oxysporum* following bone marrow transplantation, *Scand. J. Infect. Dis.*, 27, 643, 1995.

219. Hsu, C. M., Lee, P. I., Chen, J. M., Huang, L. M., Wu, M.-H., Chiu, I.-S., and Lee, C.-Y., Fatal *Fusarium* endocarditis complicated by hemolytic anemia and thrombocytopenia in an infant, *Pediatr. Infect. Dis. J.*, 13, 1146, 1994.

220. Forster, R. K., Zachary, I. G., Cottingham, A. J., and Norton, E. W. D., Further observations on the diagnosis, cause, and treatment of endophthalmitis, *Am. J. Ophthalmol.*, 81, 52, 1976.

221. Guss, R. B., Koenig, S., de la Pena, W., Marx, M., and Kaufman, H. E., Endophthalmitis after penetrating keratoplasty, *Am. J. Ophthalmol.*, 95, 651, 1983.

222. Lieberman, T. W., Ferry, A. P., and Bottone, E. J., *Fusarium solani* endophthalmitis without primary corneal involvement, *Am. J. Ophthalmol.*, 88, 764, 1979.

223. Rowsey, J. J., Acers, T. E., Smith, D. L., Mohr, J. A., Newson, D. L., and Rodriguez, J., *Fusarium oxysporum* endophthalmitis, *Arch. Ophthalmol.*, 97, 103, 1979.

224. Zapater, R. C. and Arrechea, A., Mycotic keratitis by *Fusarium*, *Ophthalmologica*, 170, 1, 1975.

225. Mohr, J. A., Nichols, N. B., Jones, J. H., Cherry, P., and Shaver, R. P., Fungal endophthalmitis, *South. Med. J.*, 66, 685, 1973.

226. Glasgow, B. J., Engstrom, R. E., Jr., Holland, G. N., Kreiger, A. E., and Wool, M. G., Bilateral endogenous *Fusarium* endophthalmitis associated with acquired immunodeficiency syndrome, *Arch. Ophthalmol.*, 114, 873, 1996.

227. Gabriele, P. and Hutchins, R. K., *Fusarium* endophthalmitis in an intravenous drug abuser, *Am. J. Ophthalmol.*, 122, 119, 1996.

228. Freidank, H., Hyalohyphomycoses due to *Fusarium* spp. — two case reports and review of the literature, *Mycoses*, 38, 69, 1995.

229. Louie, T., el Baba, F., Shulman, M., and Jimenez-Lucho, V., Endogenous endophthalmitis due to *Fusarium*: case report and review, *Clin. Infect. Dis.*, 18, 585, 1994.

230. Rosa, R. H., Jr., Miller, D., and Alfonso, E. C., The changing spectrum of fungal keratitis in South Florida, *Ophthalmology*, 101, 1005, 1994.

231. Comhaire-Poutchinian, Y., Berthe-Bonnet, S., Grek, V., and Cremer, V., Endophthalmitis due to *Fusarium*: an uncommon cause, *Bull. Soc. Belge Ophthalmol.*, 239, 75, 1990.

232. Vajpayee, R. B., Gupta, S. K., Bareja, U., and Kishore, K., Ocular atopy and mycotic keratitis, *Ann. Ophthalmol.*, 22, 369, 1990.

233. Duran, J. A., Malvar, A., Pereiro, M., and Pereiro, M., *Fusarium moniliforme* keratitis, *Acta Ophthalmol. (Copenhagen)*, 67, 710, 1989.

234. English, M. P., Observations on strains of *Fusarium solani*, *F. oxysporum*, *Candida parapsilosis* from ulcerated legs, *Sabouraudia*, 10, 35, 1972.

235. Foster, R. K., The diagnosis and management of keratomycosis. I. Cause and diagnosis, *Arch. Ophthalmol.*, 93, 975, 1975.

236. Garcia, N. P., Ascani, E., and Zapater, R., Queratomicosis por *Fusarium dimerum*, *Arch. Oftalmol. Buenos Aires*, 47, 332, 1972.

237. Gugnani, H. C., Talwar, R. S., Njoku-Obi, A. N. U., and Kodilinye, H. C., Mycotic keratitis in Nigeria: a study of 21 cases, *Br. J. Ophthalmol.*, 60, 607, 1976.

238. Jones, B. R., Principles in the management of oculomycosis, *Am. J. Ophthalmol.*, 79, 719, 1975.

239. Jones, D. B., Forster, R. K., and Rebell, G., *Fusarium solani* keratitis treated with natamycin (pimaricin): eighteen consecutive cases, *Arch. Ohthalmol.*, 88, 147, 1972.

240. Jones, D. B., Sexton, R., and Rebell, G., Mycotic keratitis in South Florida: a review of thirty-nine cases, *Trans. Ophthalmol. Soc. U.K.*, 89, 781, 1970.

241. Polack, F. M., Kaufman, E., and Newmark, E., Keratomycosis: medical and surgical management, *Arch. Ophthalmol.*, 85, 410, 1971.

242. Singh, G. and Malik, S. R. K., Therapeutic keratoplasty in fungal corneal ulcers, *Br. J. Ophthalmol.*, 56, 41, 1972.

243. Torres, M. A., Mohamed, J., Cavazos-Adame, H., and Martinez, L. A., Topical ketoconazole for fungal keratitis, *Am. J. Ophthalmol.*, 100, 293, 1985.

244. Zapater, R. C., de Arrachea, A., and Guevara, V. H., Queratomicosis por *Fusarium dimerum*, *Sabouraudia*, 10, 274, 1972.

245. Zapater, R. C., Brunzini, M. A., Albesi, E. J., and Silicarto, C. A., El genero *Fusarium* como agente etiologico de micosis oculares: presentacion de 7 casos, *Arch. Oftalmol. Buenos Aires*, 51, 279, 1976.

246. Eljaschewitsch, J., Sandfort, J., Tintelnot, K., Horbach, I., and Ruf, B., Port-a-cath-related *Fusarium oxysporum* infection in an HIV-infected patient: treatment with liposomal amphotericin B, *Mycoses*, 39, 115, 1996.

247. Viscoli, C., Castagnola, E., Moroni, C., Garaventa, A., Manno, G., and Savioli, C., Infection with *Fusarium* species in two children with neuroblastoma, *Eur. J. Clin. Microbiol. Infect. Dis.*, 9, 773, 1990.

248. Cofrancesco, E., Boschetti, C., Viviani, M. A., Bargiggia, C., Tortorano, H. M., Cortellaro, M., and Zanussi, C., Efficacy of liposomal amphotericin B (AmBisome) in the eradication of *Fusarium* infection in a leukemic patient, *Haematologica*, 77, 280, 1992.

249. Legrand, C., Anaissie, E., Hashem, R., Nelson, P., Bodey, G. P., and Ro, J., Experimental fusarial hyalohyphomycosis in a murine model, *J. Infect. Dis.*, 164, 944, 1991.

250. Bushelman, S. J., Callen, J. P., Roth, D. N., and Cohen, L. M., Disseminated *Fusarium solani* infection, *J. Am. Acad. Dermatol.*, 32, 346, 1995.

251. Lupinetti, F. M., Giller, R. H., and Trigg, M. E., Operative treatment of *Fusarium* fungal infection of the lung, *Ann. Thorac. Surg.*, 49, 991, 1990.

252. Anaissie, E. J., Kontoyiannis, D. P., Huls, C., Vartivarian, S. E., Karl, C., Prince, R. A., Bosso, J., and Bodey, G. P., Safety, plasma concentrations, and efficacy of high-dose fluconazole in invasive mold infections, *J. Infect. Dis.*, 172, 599, 1995.

253. Viviani, M. A., Cofrancesco, E., Boschetti, C., Tortorano, A. M., and Cortellaro, M., Eradication of *Fusarium* infection in a leukopenic patient treated with liposomal amphotericin B, *Mycoses*, 34, 255, 1991.

254. Graybill, J. R., New antifungal agents, *Eur. J. Clin. Microbiol. Infect. Dis.*, 8, 402, 1989.

255. Miller, S. P. and Shanbrom, E., Infectious syndromes of leukemias and lymphomas, *Am. J. Med. Sci.*, 246, 420, 1963.

256. Silver, R. T., Beal, G. A., Schneiderman, M. A., and McCullough, N. B., The role of the mature neutrophil in bacterial infections in acute leukemia, *Blood*, 12, 814, 1957.

257. Baker, R. D., Leukopenia and therapy in leukemia as factors predisposing to fatal mycoses: mucormycosis, aspergillosis, and cryptococcosis, *Am. J. Clin. Pathol.*, 37, 358, 1962.

258. Francis, P. and Walsh, T. J., Approaches to management of fungal infections in cancer patients, *Oncology (Huntingt.)*, 6, 133, 1992.

259. Browne, E. A. and Marcus, A. J., Chronic idiopathic neutropenia, *N. Engl. J. Med.*, 262, 795, 1960.

260. Kostman, R., Infantile genetic agranulocytosis, *Acta Paediatr. (Stockholm)*, 45(Suppl. 105), 1, 1956.

261. Spaet, T. H. and Dameshek, W., Chronic hypoplastic neutropenia, *Am. J. Med.*, 13, 35, 1952.

262. Hersh, E. M., Bodey, G. P., Nies, B. A., and Freireich, E. J., The causes of death in acute leukemia: a study of 414 patients from 1954–1963, *JAMA,* 193, 105, 1965.

263. Barrios, N. J., Kirkpatrick, D. V., Murciano, A., Stine, K., Van Dyke, R. B., and Humbert, J. R., Successful treatment of disseminated *Fusarium* infection in an immunocompromised child, *Am. J. Pediatr. Hematol. Oncol.*, 12, 319, 1990.

264. Merz, W. A., Karp, J. E., Hoagland, M., Jett-Goheen, M., Junkins, J. M., and Hood, A. F., Diagnosis and successful treatment of fusariosis in the compromised host, *J. Infect. Dis.*, 158, 1046, 1988.

265. Chaulk, C. P., Smith, P. W., Feagler, J. R., Verdirame, J., and Commers, J. R., Fungemia due to *Fusarium solani* in an immunocompromised child, *Pediatr. Infect. Dis. J.*, 5, 363, 1986.

266. Lambert, E. H. and Elmqvist, D., Quantal components of end-plate potentials in the myasthenic syndrome, *Ann. NY Acad. Sci.*, 183, 183, 1971.

267. Dordain-Bigot, M. L., Baran, R., Baixench, M. T., and Bazex, J., *Fusarium* onychomycosis, *Ann. Dermatol. Venereol.*, 123, 191, 1996.

268. Arrese, J. E., Pierard-Franchimont, C., and Pierrard, G. E., Fatal hyalohyphomycosis following *Fusarium* onychomycosis in an immunocompromised patient, *Am. J. Dermatol.*, 18, 196, 1996.

269. Spielberger, R. T., Falleroni, M. J., Coene, A. J., and Larsen, R. A., Concomitant amphotericin B therapy, granulocyte transfusions, and GM-CSF administration for disseminated infection with *Fusarium* in a granulocytopenic patient, *Clin. Infect. Dis.*, 16, 528, 1993.

270. Hennequin, C., Benkerrou, M., Gaillard, J. L., Blanche, S., and Fraitag, S., Role of granulocyte colony-stimulating factor in the management of infection with *Fusarium oxysporum* in a neutropenic child, *Clin. Infect. Dis.*, 18, 490, 1994.

271. Montgomery, B., Bianco, J. A., Jacobsen, A., and Singer, J. W., Localization of transfused neutrophils to site of infection during treatment with recombinant human granulocyte-macrophage colony-stimulating factor and pentoxifylline, *Blood*, 78, 533, 1991.

272. Anaissie, E., Wong, E., Bodey, G. P., O'Brien, S., Gutterman, J., and Vadhan, S., Granulocyte-macrophage colony-stimulating factor plus amphotericin B for disseminated mycoses in neutropenic cancer patients, *Proc. 29th Intersci. Conf. Antimicrob. Agents Chemother.*, American Society for Microbiology, Washington, D.C., Abstr. 73, 1989.

273. Groll, A., Renz, S., Gerein, V., Schwabe, D., Katschan, G., Schneider, M., Hübner, K., and Kornhuber, B., Fatal haemoptysis associated with invasive pulmonary aspergillosis treated with high-dose amphotericin B and granulocyte-macrophage colony-stimulating factor (GM-CSF), *Mycoses*, 35, 67, 1992.

274. McCullough, J., Granulocyte transfusion, in *Neoplastic Diseases of the Blood*, Wiernik, P. H., Canellos, G. P., Kyle, R. A., and Schiffer, C. A., Eds., Churchill Livingstone, New York, 1991, 899.

275. Patoux-Pibouin, M., Couatarmanach, A., Le Gall, F., Bergeron, C., De Bièvre, C., Guiguen, C., and Chevrant-Breton, J., Fusariose a *Fusarium solani* chez un adolescent leucémique, *Ann. Dermatol. Venereol.*, 119, 377, 1992.

276. Wright, D. G., Robichaud, K. J., Pizzo, P. A., and Deisseroth, A. B., Lethal pulmonary reactions associated with the combined use of amphotericin B and leukocyte transfusion, *N. Engl. J. Med.*, 304, 1185, 1981.

277. Dana, B. W., Durie, B. G. M., White, R. F., and Huestis, D. W., Concomitant administration of granulocyte transfusions and amphotericin B in neutropenic patients: absence of significant pulmonary toxicity, *Blood*, 57, 90, 1981.

278. Kaplan, S. S., Zdziarski, U. E., Basford, R. E., Wing, E., and Shadduck, R. K., Effect of *in vivo* recombinant granulocyte-macrophage colony stimulating factor on peripheral blood granulocyte functions, *Clin. Res.*, 36, 566, 1988.

279. Wing, E. J., Magee, D. M., Kaplan, S. S., and Shadduck, R. K., Stimulation of human monocytes by recombinant human granulocyte-macrophage colony stimulating factor in patients with refractory metastatic carcinoma, *Clin. Res.*, 36, 422, 1988.

280. Peters, W. P., Stuart, A., Affronti, M. L., Kim, C. S., and Coleman, R. E., Neutrophil migration is defective during recombinant human granulocyte-macrophage colony stimulating factor infusion after autologous bone marrow transplantation in humans, *Blood*, 72, 1310, 1988.

281. Addison, I. E., Johnson, B., Devereux, S., Goldstone, A. H., and Linch, D. C., Granulocyte-macrophage colony-stimulating factor may inhibit neutrophil migration *in vitro*, *Clin. Exp. Immunol.*, 76, 149, 1989.

282. Engelhard, D., Eldor, A., Polacheck, I., Hardan, I., Ben-Yahuda, D., Amselem, S., Salkin, I. F., Lopez-Berenstein, G., Sacks, T., Rachmilewitz, E. A., and Barenholz, Y., Disseminated visceral fusariosis treated with amphotericin B-phospholipid complex, *Leuk. Lymphoma*, 9, 385, 1993.

283. Wolff, M. A. and Ramphal, R., Use of amphotericin B lipid complex for treatment of disseminated cutaneous fusarium infection in a neutropenic patient, *Clin. Infect. Dis.*, 20, 1568, 1995.

284. Viscoli, C., Castagnola, E., Moroni, C., Garaventa, A., Manno, G., and Savioli, C., Infection with *Fusarium* species in two children with neuroblastoma, *Eur. J. Clin. Microbiol. Infect. Dis.*, 9, 773, 1990.

285. Castagnola, E., Garaventa, A., Conte, M., Barretta, A., Faggi, E., and Viscoli, C., Survival after fungemia due to *Fusarium moniliforme* in a child with neuroblastoma, *Eur. J. Clin. Microbiol. Infect. Dis.*, 12, 308, 1993.

286. Raad, I. and Hachem, R., Treatment of central venous catheter-related fungemia due to *Fusarium oxysporum*, *Clin. Infect. Dis.*, 20, 709, 1995.

287. Forster, R. K. and Rebell, G., Animal model of *Fusarium solani* keratitis, *Am. J. Ophthalmol.*, 79, 510, 1975.

288. Rihova, E., Havlikova, M., Boguszakova, J., and Pitrova, S., Keratomycoses, *Cesk. Slov. Oftalmol.*, 52, 164, 1996.

289. Donnenfeld, E. D., Schrier, A., Perry, H. D., Ingraham, H. J., Lasonde, R., Epstein, A., and Farber, B., Infectious keratitis with corneal perforation associated with corneal hydrops and contact lens wear in keratoconus, *Br. J. Ophthalmol.*, 80, 409, 1996.

290. Wilhelmus, K. R., Robinson, N. M., Font, R. A., Hamill, M. B., and Jones, D. B., Fungal keratitis in contact lens wearers, *Am. J. Ophthalmol.*, 106, 708, 1988.

291. Donzis, P. B., Mondino, B. J., Weissman, B. A., and Bruckner, D. A., Microbial contamination of contact lens care systems, *Am. J. Ophthalmol.*, 104, 325, 1987.

292. Simmons, R. B., Buffington, J. R., Ward, M., Wilson, L. A., and Ahearn, D. G., Morphology and ultrastructure of fungi in extended-wear soft contact lenses, *J. Clin. Microbiol.*, 24, 21, 1986.

293. Strelow, S. A., Kent, H. D., Eagle, R. C., Jr., and Cohen, E. J., A case of soft contact lens related *Fusarium solani* keratitis, *Contact Lens Assoc. Ophthalmol. J.*, 18, 125, 1992.

294. Francois, J. and De Vos, E., Traitement des mycoses oculaires par la pimaricine, *Bull. Soc. Belge Ophthalmol.*, 195, 97, 1962.

295. Newmark, E., Ellison, A. C., and Kaufman, H. E., Pimaricin therapy of *Cephalosporium* and *Fusarium* keratitis, *Am. J. Ophthalmol.*, 69, 458, 1970.

296. Newmark, E., Ellison, A. C., and Kaufman, H. E., Combined pimaricin and dexamethasone therapy of keratomycosis, *Am. J. Ophthalmol.*, 71, 718, 1971.

297. Rippon, J. W., Mycotic infections of the eye: diagnosis and treatment, *Ophthalmol. Digest*, 34, 18, 1972.

298. Ellison, A. C., Newmark, E., and Kaufman, H. E., Chemotherapy of experimental keratomycosis, *Am. J. Ophthalmol.*, 68, 812, 1969.

299. Ellison, A. C. and Newmark, E., Potassium iodide in mycotic keratitis, *Am. J. Ophthalmol.*, 69, 126, 1970.

300. Green, W. R., Bennett, J. E., and Goos, R. D., Ocular penetration of amphotericin B: a report of laboratory studies and a case report of postsurgical *Cephalosporium* endophthalmitis, *Arch. Ophthalmol.*, 73, 769, 1965.

301. Patel, A. S., Hemady, R. K., Rodrigues, M., Rajagopalan, S., and Elman, M. J., Endogenous *Fusarium* endophthalmitis in a patient wuth acute lymphocytic leukemia, *Am. J. Ophthalmol.*, 117, 363, 1994.

302. Pflugfelder, S. C., Flynn, H. W., Jr., Zwickey, T. A., Forster, R. K., Tsiligianni, A., Culbertson, W. W., and Mandelbaum, S., Exogenous fungal endophthalmitis, *Ophthalmology*, 95, 19, 1988.

303. Glasgow, B. J. and Weisberger, A. K., A quantitative and cartographic study of retinal micro-vasculopathy in acquired immunodeficiency syndrome, *Am. J. Ophthalmol.*, 118, 46, 1994.

304. Chiaradia, V., Schinella, D., Pascoli, L., Tesio, F., and Santini, G. F., *Fusarium* peritonitis in peritoneal dialysis: report of two cases, *Microbiologica*, 13, 77, 1990.

305. Landau, M., Srebrnik, A., Wolf, R., Bashi, E., and Brenner, S., Systemic ketoconazole treatment for *Fusarium* leg ulcers, *Int. J. Dermatol.*, 31, 511, 1992.

306. Resnik, B. I. and Burdick, A. E., Improvement of eumycetoma with itraconazole, *J. Am. Acad. Dermatol.*, 33, 917, 1995.

307. Morrison, V. A., Haake, R. J., and Weisdorf, D. J., Non-*Candida* fungal infection: risk factors and outcome, *Am. J. Med.*, 96, 497, 1994.

308. Ben Hamida, M., Bedrossian, J., Pruna, A., Fouqueray, B., Metivier, F., and Idatte, J. M., Fungal mycotic aneurysms and visceral infection due to *Scedosporium apiospermum* in a kidney transplant patient, *Transplant. Proc.*, 25, 2290, 1993.

309. Lupinetti, F. M., Behrendt, D. M., Giller, R. H., Trigg, M. E., and de Alarcon, P., Pulmonary resection for fungal infection in children undergoing bone marrow transplantation, *J. Thorac. Cardiovasc. Surg.*, 104, 684, 1992.

310. Gamis, A. S., Gudnason, T., Giebink, G. S., and Ramsay, N. K., Disseminated infection with *Fusarium* in recipients of bone marrow transplants, *Rev. Infect. Dis.*, 13, 1077, 1991.

311. Robertson, M. J., Socinski, M. A., Soiffer, R. J., Finberg, R. W., Wilson, C., Anderson, K. C., Bosserman, L., Sang, D. N., Salkin, I. F., and Ritz, J., Successful treatment of disseminated *Fusarium* infection after autologous bone marrow transplantation for acute myeloid leukemia, *Bone Marrow Transplant.*, 8, 143, 1991.

312. Mowbray, D. N., Paller, A. S., Nelson, P. E., and Kaplan, R. L., Disseminated *Fusarium solani* infection with cutaneous nodules in a bone marrow transplant patient, *Int. J. Dermatol.*, 27, 698, 1988.

313. Nucci, M., Pulcheri, W., Bacha, P. C., Spector, N., Cainby, M. J., Costa, R. O., and de Oliveira, H. P., Amphotericin B followed by itraconazole in the treatment of disseminated fungal infections in neutropenic patients, *Mycoses*, 37, 433, 1994.

314. Clark, R. A., Johnson, F. L., Klebanoff, S. J., and Thomas, E. D., Defective neutrophil chemotaxis in bone marrow transplant patients, *J. Clin. Invest.*, 58, 22, 1976.

315. Witherspoon, R., Lum, L., Storb, R., and Thomas, E. D., Transplant-related immune deficiency in man, in *Recent Advances in Bone Marrow Transplantation*, Gale, R. P., Ed., Alan R. Liss, New York, 1983, 473.

316. Meyers, J. D., Infection in recipients of bone marrow transplants, in *Current Clinical Topics in Infectious Diseases*, Remington, J. S. and Swartz, M. N., Eds., McGraw-Hill, New York, 1985, 262.

317. Tollemar, J., Ringdén, O., Boström, L., Nilsson, B., and Sundberg, B., Variables predicting deep fungal infections in bone marrow transplant recipients, *Bone Marrow Transplant.*, 4, 635, 1989.

318. Tollemar, J., Ringdén, O., Aschan, J., and Sundberg, B., Which bone marrow transplant recipients are at risk of acquiring life-threatening fungal infections? *Transplant. Proc.*, 22, 208, 1990.

319. Pirsch, J. D. and Maki, D. G., Infectious complications in adults with bone marrow transplantation and T-cell depletion of donor marrow, *Ann. Intern. Med.*, 104, 619, 1986.

320. Kusne, S., Dummer, J. S., Singh, N., Iwatsuki, S., Makowka, L., Esquivel, C., Tzakis, A. G., Starzl, T. E., and Ho, M., Infections after liver transplantation: an analysis of 101 consecutive cases, *Medicine (Baltimore)*, 67, 132, 1988.

321. Anaissie, E. J., Bodey, G. P., and Rinaldi, M. G., Emerging fungal pathogens, *Eur. J. Clin. Microbiol. Infect. Dis.*, 8, 323, 1989.

322. Anaissie, E. J., Opportunistic mycoses in the immunocompromised host: experience of a cancer center and review, *Clin. Infect. Dis.*, 14, 543, 1992.

323. Denning, D. W., Donnelly, J. P., Hellreigel, K. P., Ito, J., Martino, P., and van't Wout, J. W., Antifungal prophylaxis during neutropenia or allogeneic bone marrow transplantation: what is the state of the art? *Chemotherapy*, 38(Suppl. 1), 43, 1992.

324. Ellis, M. E., Clink, H., Younge, D., and Hainau, B., Successful combined surgical and medical treatment of fusarium infection after bone marrow transplantation, *Scand. J. Infect. Dis.*, 26, 225, 1994.

325. Drakos, P. E., Nagler, A., Or, R., Naparstek, E., Kapelushnik, J., Engelhard, D., Rahav, G., Ne'emean, D., and Slavin, S., Invasive fungal sinusitis in patients undergoing bone marrow transplantation, *Bone Marrow Transplant.*, 12, 203, 1993.

326. Meyers, J. D., Fungal infections in bone marrow transplant patients, *Semin. Oncol.*, 17, 10, 1990.

327. June, C. H., Beatty, P. G., Shulman, H. M., and Rinaldi, M. G., Disseminated *Fusarium moniliforme* infection after allogeneic marrow transplantation, *South. Med. J.*, 79, 513, 1986.

328. Paulin, T., Ringdén, O., and Nilsson, B., Immunological recovery after bone marrow transplantation: role of age, graft-versus-host disease, prednisolone treatment and infections, *Bone Marrow Transplant.*, 1, 317, 1987.

329. Howard, R. J. and Najarian, J. S., Cytomegalovirus-induced immune suppression. I. Humoral immunity, *Clin. Exp. Immunol.*, 18, 109, 1974.

330. Lavrijsen, K., Van Houdt, J., Thijs, D., Meuldermans, W., and Heykants, J., Interaction of miconazole, ketoconazole and itraconazole with rat-liver microsomes, *Xenobiotica*, 17, 45, 1987.

331. Cassling, R. S., Rogler, W. C., and McManus, B. M., Isolated pulmonic valve infective endocarditis: a diagnostically elusive entity, *Am. Heart J.*, 109, 558, 1985.

332. Rowley, K. M., Clubb, K. S., Smith, G. J. W., and Cabin, H. S., Right-sided infective endocarditis as a consequence of flow-directed pulmonary-artery catheterization, *N. Engl. J. Med.*, 311, 1152, 1984.

333. Keown, P. A., Stiller, C. R., Laupacis, A. L., Howson, W., Coles, R., Stawecki, M., Koegler, J., Carruthers, G., McKenzie, N., and Sinclear, N. R., The effects and side effects of cyclosporine: relationship to drug pharmacokinetics, *Transplant. Proc.*, 24, 659, 1982.

334. Horton, C. M., Freeman, C. D., Nolan, P. E., Jr., and Copeland, J. G. III, Cyclosporine interaction with miconazole and other azole-antimycotics: a case report and review of the literature, *J. Heart Lung Transplant.*, 11, 1127, 1992.

335. Yee, G. C. and McGuire, T. R., Pharmacokinetic drug interactions with cyclosporin. I, *Clin. Pharmacokinet.*, 19, 319, 1990.

336. Yee, G. C. and McGuire, T. R., Pharmacokinetic drug interactions with cyclosporin. II, *Clin. Pharmacokinet.*, 19, 400, 1990.

337. Cassidy, M. J., Van Zyl-Smit, R., Pascoe, M. D., Swanepoel, C. R., and Jacobson, J. E., Effect of rifampicin on cyclosporin A blood levels in a renal transplant recipient, *Nephron*, 41, 207, 1985.

338. Gumbleton, M., Brown, J. E., Hawksworth, G., and Whiting, P. H., The possible relationship between hepatic drug metabolism and ketoconazole enhancement of cyclosporine nephrotoxicity, *Transplantation*, 40, 454, 1985.

339. Shepard, J. H., Canafax, D. M., Simmons, R. L., and Najarian, J. S., Cyclosporine-ketoconazole: a potentially dangerous drug-drug interaction, *Clin. Pharmacol.*, 5, 468, 1986.

340. Sands, M. and Brown, R. B., Interactions of cyclosporine and antimicrobial agents, *Rev. Infect. Dis.*, 11, 691, 1989.

341. Maurer, G., Metabolism of cyclosporine, *Transplant. Proc.*, 27, 19, 1985.

342. Doble, N., Shaw, R., Rowland-Hill, C., Lush, M., Warnock, D. W., and Keal, E. E., Pharmacokinetic study of the interaction between rifampin and ketoconazole, *J. Antimicrob. Chemother.*, 21, 633, 1988.

343. Smith, S. R. and Kendall, M. J., Ranitidine versus cimetidine: a comparison of their potential to cause clinically important drug interactions, *Clin. Pharmacokinet.*, 15, 44, 1988.

344. Butman, S. M., Wild, J., Nolan, P., Fagan, T. C., Finley, P. R., Hicks, M. J., Mackie, M. J., and Copeland, J. G. III, Prospective study of the safety and financial benefit of ketoconazole as adjunctive therapy to cyclosporine after heart transplantation, *J. Heart Lung Transplant.*, 10, 351, 1991.

345. First, M. R., Weiskittel, P., Alexander, J. W., Schroeder, T. J., Myre, S. A., and Pesce, A. J., Concomittant administration of cyclosporin and ketoconazole in renal transplant recipients, *Lancet*, 2, 1198, 1989.

346. Hostetler, K. A., Wrighton, S. A., Molowa, D. T., Thomas, P. E., Levin, W., and Guzelian, P. S., Coinduction of multiple hepatic cytochrome P-450 proteins and their mRNAs in rats treated with imidazole antimycotic agents, *Mol. Pharmacol.*, 35, 279, 1989.

347. Sheets, J. J. and Mason, J. I., Ketoconazole: a potent inhibitor of cytochrome P-450-dependent drug metabolism in rat liver, *Drug Metab. Dispos.*, 12, 603, 1984.

348. Blyden, G. T., Abernethy, D. R., and Greenblatt, D. J., Ketoconazole does not impair antipyrine clearance in humans, *Int. J. Clin. Pharmacol. Ther. Toxicol.*, 24, 225, 1986.

349. Daneshmend, T. K., Warnock, D. W., Ene, M. D., Johnson, E. M., Parker, G., Richardson, M. D., and Roberts, C. J., Multiple dose pharmacokinetics in man, *J. Antimicrob. Chemother.*, 12, 185, 1983.

350. Meredith, C. G., Maldonado, A. L., and Speeg, K. V., The effect of ketoconazole on hepatic oxidative drug metabolism in the rat *in vivo* and *in vitro*, *Drug Metab. Dispos.*, 13, 156, 1985.

351. La Delfa, I., Zhu, Q. M., Mo, Z., and Blaschke, T. F., Fluconazole is a potent inhibitor of antipyrine metabolism *in vivo* in mice, *Drug Metab. Dispos.*, 17, 49, 1989.

352. Pasanen, M., Taskinen, T., Iscan, M., Sotaniemi, E. A., Kairaluoma, M., and Peikonen, O., Inhibition of human hepatic and placental xenobiotic monooxygenases by imidazole antimycotics, *Biochem. Pharmacol.*, 37, 3861, 1988.

353. Hajek, K. K., Cook, N. I., and Novak, R. F., Mechanism of inhibition of microsomal drug metabolism by imidazole, *J. Pharmacol. Exp. Ther.*, 223, 97, 1982.

354. Kramer, M. R., Marshall, S. E., Denning, D. W., Keogh, A. M., Tucker, R. M., Galgiani, J. N., Lewiston, N. J., Stevens, D. A., and Theodore, J., Cyclosporine and itraconazole interaction in heart and lung transplant recipients, *Ann. Intern. Med.*, 113, 327, 1990.

355. Damanhouri, Z., Gumbleton, M., Nicholls, P. J., and Shaw, M. A., In-vivo effects of itraconazole on hepatic mixed-function oxidase, *J. Antimicrob. Chemother.*, 21, 187, 1988.

356. Powell, J. R. and Cate, E. W., Induction and inhibition of drug metabolism, *Applied Pharmacokinetics: Principles of Therapeutic Drug Monitoring*, Evans, W. E., Schentag, J. J., and Jusko, W. J., Eds., Applied Therapeutics, Spokane, WA, 1986, 139.

357. Sugar, A. M., Saunders, C., Idelson, B. A., and Bernard, D. B., Interaction of fluconazole and cyclosporine, *Ann. Intern. Med.*, 110, 844, 1989.

358. Collignon, P., Hurley, B., and Mitchell, D., Interaction of fluconazole with cyclosporin, *Lancet*, 333, 1262, 1989.

359. Graves, N. M., Matas, A. J., Hiligoss, D. M., and Canafax, D. M., Fluconazole/cyclosporine interaction, *Clin. Pharmacol. Ther.*, 47, 208, 1990.

360. Ehninger, G., Jeschonek, K., Schuler, U., and Krüger, H. U., Interaction of fluconazole with cyclosporin, *Lancet*, 334, 104, 1989.

361. Conti, D. J., Tolkoff-Rubin, N. E., Baker, G. P., Jr., Doran, M., Cosimi, A. B., Delmonico, F., Auchincloss, H., Jr., Russell, P. S., and Rubin, R. H., Successful treatment of invasive fungal infection with fluconazole in organ transplant recipients, *Transplantation*, 48, 692, 1989.

362. Krüger, H. U., Schuler, U., Zimmerman, R., and Ehninger, G., Absence of significant interaction of fluconazole with cyclosporin, *J. Antimicrob. Chemother.*, 24, 781, 1989.

363. Humphrey, M. J., Javons, S., and Trabit, M. H., Pharmacokinetic evaluation of UK-49,858, a metabolically stable triazole antifungal drug, in animals and humans, *Antimicrob. Agents Chemother.*, 28, 648, 1985.

37.10 *PENICILLIUM MARNEFFEI*

37.10.1 INTRODUCTION

Fungi of the genus *Penicillium* are widely distributed in nature and presently, several hundred species have been identified.[1,2] Nevertheless, infections in humans caused by these fungi have been seldom described.[3-6] Among the species pathogenic to humans, *P. citrinum*, *P. commune*, *P. crustaceum*, *P. expansum*, *P. glaucum*, and *P. spinulosum* were reported to cause infections in the urinary tract,[7,8] lung,[9-11] brain,[11,12] ear and sinus,[13] cornea,[14] and the heart.[15-17] *P. notatum* was reported as the causative agent of a chronic infection of the paranasal sinuses.[18] *P. marneffei* is by far the most pathogenic of all *Penicillium* spp.[19] It has been diagnosed with increasing frequency as an invasive and life-threatening infection in both immunocompetent and immunocompromised hosts, especially in patients with HIV infection.[19-37]

P. marneffei is the only thermally dimorphic species in the genus *Penicillium*.[2,4,20,38,39] It grows in mycelial form at 25°C and as short hyphal elements in pulmonary cavities. In agar medium, the fungus produces a fast-growing, grayish floccose colony with diffusable red pigment.[23] *P. marneffei* proliferates within histiocytes, distending them. The latter, in turn, proliferate to accommodate the increasing number of fungi but appear to offer no resistance to proliferating *P. marneffei*. In necrotic tissues, some of these organisms may be seen clumped together to retain the counter of the previously viable histiocytes that contained them.[23]

P. marneffei was first described in 1956 when it infected and killed a bamboo rat (*Rhizomys sinensis*) in Vietnam.[20,40,41] In China, apparently healthy *R. pruinosus* have been reported as carriers of the fungus,[38,42] and in Thailand an additional bamboo rat host, *Cannomys badius* has been identified.[24,36]

In 1973, Di Salvo et al.[22] reported the first human infection caused by *P. marneffei*. Nearly all cases have been diagnosed in patients who lived or traveled to Southeast Asia (Thailand, Vietnam, Hong Kong, Indonesia, and Southestern China) where *P. marneffei* is endemic.[19,23,36,37,43-47]

Infection with *P. marneffei* (also known as *penicilliosis marneffei*[24,48]) has been reported to affect both immunocompetent[19,23,24,37,45,49-53] and immunocompromised[19,21,47,54] hosts. With the advance of the AIDS pandemic, penicilliosis marneffei has emerged as an AIDS-defining opportunistic infection in HIV-infected persons,[55] especially in Southeast Asia.[25-31,33-37,46,56-65]

In addition to HIV infection, patients at increased risk include those with lymphoproliferative disorders,[22] bronchiectasis and tuberculosis,[48] autoimmune disorders, and patients receiving corticosteroid therapy.[24]

In two reports,[66,67] *Penicillium* species have been identified as the etiologic agent of peritonitis in patients receiving continuous ambulatory peritoneal dialysis (CAPD). Fungal colonies were observed on the inner surface of the CAPD catheter. Cases of *Penicillium* spp. causing endophthalmitis have been rare.[68,69]

Although the precise manner of transmission of *P. marneffei* infection is not well understood, it is surmised that the fungus is either inhaled or ingested.[19,38] It is generally believed that outdoors is the major source of airborne fungal spores. However, during the course of monitoring airborne fungal spores in a bone marrow transplant hospital unit, Streifel et al.[70] have reported a prolonged and marked increase in *P. marneffei* spore levels in air samples — because filamentous fungi proliferate in decaying organic debris,[71] it was not surprising that the fungal source was ultimately traced to rotting wood in a cabinet under a sink with leaking pipework. Furthermore, *Penicillium* spp. were found to contaminate intravenous fluids, dialysis fluids, blood bank materials,[72] as well as irrigating solutions used during cataract surgery.[73]

Most often, penicilliosis affects the reticuloendothelial system, causing deep-seated infections that can be focal or disseminated.[37] One case of a localized, superficial human infection has also been described.[41]

Penicilliosis marneffei is usually disseminated and progressive and frequently starts suddenly with chills, persistent fever, painful cough, and pleurisy.[19,46,74] In HIV-positive patients, the disease is often manifested with fever, weight loss, and anemia, lymphadenopathy and hepatomegaly, and pulmonary symptoms; oropharyngeal and genital lesions (ulcers and papules), diarrhea, splenomegaly, and pericarditis have been reported to be less frequent.[19,37] Fungemia is present in the majority of cases.[75]

The fungus has been isolated from numerous organs, including lung, liver, intestine, lymph nodes, tonsil, skin,[26] bone marrow,[26] kidney,[75] bone and joints,[62] and the pericardium.[45] Contrary to histoplasmosis, in penicilliosis adrenal involvement has been rare.[76]

Hepatosplenomegaly, which is caused by diffuse micro-abscesses not visible on computerized tomography (CT), has been often observed in children.[19,63] Mucocutaneous involvement is also a common feature.[19,32,37] Usually cutaneous manifestations are presented as generalized small papules, crusted or necrotic papules, chronic ulcers, molluscum contagiosum-like umbillicated papules,[25,30,47] abscesses, and cutaneous nodules.[77]

Three forms of invasive pulmonary penicilliosis have been described: a subacute to chronic form,[78,79] a more acute and rapidly progressive form,[78,80] and an invasive pulmonary penicilliosis caused by *P. marneffei*.[81]

Histologic examination of immunocompromised patients has demonstrated the presence of an anergic and necrotizing reaction characterized by a diffuse infiltration of histiocytes saturated with proliferating yeast-like cells.[21] Granulomatous and suppurative reaction patterns may also be observed.[21,23,33]

Since some clinical and histologic appearances of penicilliosis marneffei may strongly resemble several invasive infectious diseases, it has often been misdiagnosed in the past as tuberculosis (e.g., suppurative lymphadenopathy[49]), histoplasmosis, or cryptococcosis.[19,23,24,37,43,44,48,49] *Histoplasma capsulatum* and *P. marneffei,* by being thermally dimorphic fungi that proliferate within histiocytes, have shown morphologic resemblance during their intrahistiocytic proliferation.[23]

Cases of *P. marneffei* osteomyelitis are often misdiagnosed as tuberculosis[24,45] and have high mortality rates even with antifungal treatment.[24,45,49,50] Chan and Woo[82] have described an unusual case in which the patient was afibrile and had no lymphadenopathy but presented with multiple and well-delineated lytic bone lesions.

For definitive diagnosis the pathogen must be isolated on standard mycologic culture media and histologic examination of tissue specimens should be carried out.[19,37]

37.10.2 EVOLUTION OF THERAPIES AND TREATMENT OF PENICILLIOSIS MARNEFFEI

When diagnosis is made promptly and therapy is instituted immediately, penicilliosis marneffei can be cured.[19] The duration of the illness may vary between 2 months and 3 years, with an average of 10 to 11 months, but if left untreated it may become fatal.[23]

Nystatin was the first therapeutic agent tried successfully in bamboo rats.[41] However, because of its poor systemic absorption[83] it is doubtful that oral nystatin would be effective in humans.

In spite of its relatively moderate *in vitro* activity,[86] intravenous amphotericin B alone (50 mg for 10 d to 8 weeks)[18,24,26,37,61,67,76,84] or in combination with oral 5-fluorocytosine, fluconazole, and/or ketoconazole[24,25,29,45,47,85] has been most beneficial in the treatment of penicilliosis marneffei.[30,36,37]

Gelfand et al.[81] have treated successfully a case of invasive pulmonary penicilliosis marneffei with intravenous amphothericin B at 50 mg given every other day, for a total dose of 1.3 g over a period of 8 weeks. Heath et al.[76] also treated a case of disseminated penicilliosis marneffei with amphotericin B (only 25 mg daily because of deteriorating renal functions; total dose, 500 mg) for 3 weeks, and maintenance therapy with oral itraconazole (200 mg, b.i.d.) for 3 months.

Relapses within 6 months after the end of amphotericin B therapy have been reported.[26,30] Azole antifungals (ketoconazole, fluconazole, and particularly itraconazole) because of lesser toxicities may be considered as first-line maintenance therapy.[25,26,30,36,37,57-59,86,87]

Swan et al.[69] have reported a rare case of *Penicillium* species causing endophthalmitis after parenteral drug abuse. The patient was treated with intravenous amphotericin B (total of 510 mg over a 24-d period) and oral flucytosine (150 mg/kg daily, but discontinued after 12 d because of worsening renal function). A similar dose regimen of amphotericin B (total dose 1.4 g, IV) and flucytosine (150 mg/kg daily) given over a 20-d period led to a complete resolution of symptoms in an HIV-positive patient with penicilliosis marneffei.[36] Afterwards, maintenance therapy with itraconazole was instituted at daily doses of 400 mg during the first month, followed by 200 mg thereafter.[36]

Peto et al.[25] have treated successfully an HIV-positive patient with intravenous amphotericin B (1.56 g total dose given over a 22-d period) and oral ketoconazole (200 mg, b.i.d.); the patient continued to receive ketoconazole (200 mg daily) as maintenance therapy. In another report, Sekhon et al.[88] described a patient with pulmonary penicilliosis marneffei who responded well to a regimen of amphotericin B (total dose, 1.5 g over a 5-month period) and ketoconazole (200 mg daily for 5 months; total dose, approximately 30 g).

A *P. marneffei*-induced retropharyngeal abscess, an unusual case of upper airway obstruction, was treated with amphotericin B (0.35 mg/kg daily, IV) and oral fluconazole (400 mg daily). After 6 weeks of treatment, the fever subsided, the cervical lymph nodes receded, and the osteolytic lesions responded with gradual radiographic resolution.[89]

Therapy with oral fluconazole alone (100 mg, b.i.d.) for 2 weeks was successful in resolving a case of disseminated penicilliosis marneffei with cutaneous lesions in an HIV-infected patient.[77]

The successful use of ketoconazole (200 mg, b.i.d. for 2 months)[56] and itraconazole (200 mg, b.i.d. for 7 months)[30] has also been reported.

In a prospective study of HIV-infected children with disseminated penicilliosis marneffei, early diagnosis and appropriate antifungal therapy (amphotericin B, fluconazole, or ketoconazole) reduced the mortality rate to 18%.[63]

37.10.3 REFERENCES

1. Raper, K. B. and Thom, C., *A Manual of the Penicillia*, Williams & Wilkins, Baltimore, 1949.
2. Ramirez, C., *Manual and Atlas of the Penicillia*, Elsevier Biomedical Press, New York, 1982.
3. Emmons, C. W., Binford, C. H., Utz, J. P., and Kwon-Chung, K. J., *Medical Mycology*, 3rd ed., Lea & Fabiger, Philadelphia, 1977.
4. Chandler, F. W., Kaplan, W., and Ajello, L., *Penicillium marneffei* (figures 509–513), in *Color Atlas and Text of the Histopathology of Mycotic Diseases*, Year Book Medical Publishers, Chicago, 1980, 103.
5. Rippon, J. W., *Medical Mycology: the Pathogenic Fungi and the Pathogenic Actinomycetes*, 2nd ed., W. B. Saunders, Philadelphia, 1982.
6. Schwarz, J., The diagnosis of deep mycoses by morphologic methods, *Hum. Pathol.*, 13, 519, 1982.
7. Chute, A. L., An infection of the bladder with *Penicillium glaucum*, *Boston Med. Surg. J.*, 164, 420, 1911.
8. Gillium, J. S., Jr. and Vest, S. A., Penicillium infection of the urinary tract, *J. Urol.*, 65, 484, 1951.
9. Nussbaum, R. and Benedek, T., Pneumonomycosis penicillina, eine gewerbekrankheit zum kapitel der lungengeschwülste, *Beitr. Klin. Tuberk.*, 67, 756, 1927.
10. Lacaz, C. da S., Consideracoes sobre um caso di peniciliose pulmonar, *O Hosp. Rio de Janeiro*, 15, 327, 1939.
11. Huang, S. N. and Harris, L. S., Acute disseminated penicilliosis: report of a case and review of pertinent literature, *Am. J. Clin. Pathol.*, 39, 167, 1963.
12. Polyanskiy, L. N., A case of otogenic abscess of the temporal lobe of the brain caused by *Penicillium*, *Zh. Ushnykh Nosovykh Gorlovykh Boleznei (Kiev)*, 15, 138, 1938.
13. Smyth, G. D. L., Fungal infection in otology, *Br. J. Dermatol.*, 76, 425, 1964.
14. Eschete, M. L., King, J. W., West, B. C., and Oberle, A., *Penicillium chrysogenum* endophthalmitis: first reported case, *Mycopathologia*, 74, 125, 1981.
15. Hall, W. J. III, Penicillium endocarditis following open heart surgery and prosthetic valve insertion, *Am. Heart J.*, 87, 501, 1974.
16. Upshaw, C. B., Jr., Penicillium endocarditis of aortic valve prosthesis, *J. Thorac. Cardiovasc. Surg.*, 68, 428, 1974.
17. DelRossi, A. J., Morse, D., Spagna, P. M., and Lemole, G. M., Successful management of penicillium endocarditis, *J. Thorac. Cardiovasc. Surg.*, 80, 945, 1980.
18. Nouri, M. E., Penicillinose der nasennebenhöhlen, *Laryng. Rhinol. Otol. (Stuttgart)*, 65, 420, 1986.
19. Deng, Z., Ribas, J. L., Gibson, D. W., and Connor, D. H., Infections caused by *Penicillium marneffei* in China and Southest Asia: review of eighteen published cases and report of four more Chinese cases, *Rev. Infect. Dis.*, 10, 640, 1988.
20. Segretain, G., Description d'une nouvelle espéce de penicillium: *Penicillium marneffei* n. sp., *Bull. Soc. Mycol. France*, 75, 412, 1959.
21. Borradori, L., Schmit, J.-C., Stetzkowski, M., Dussoix, P., Saurat, J.-H., and Filthuth, I., *Penicilliosis marneffei* infection in AIDS, *J. Am. Acad. Dermatol.*, 31, 843, 1994.
22. Di Salvo, A. F., Fickling, A. M., and Ajello, L., Infection caused by *Penicillium marneffei*: description of first natural infection in man, *Am. J. Clin. Pathol.*, 60, 259, 1973.
23. Deng, Z. and Connor, D. H., Progressive disseminated penicilliosis caused by *Penicillium marneffei*: report of eight cases and differentiation of the causative organism from *Histoplasma capsulatum*, *Am. J. Clin. Pathol.*, 84, 323, 1985.
24. Jayanetra, P., Nitiyanant, P., Ajello, L., Padhye, A. A., Lolekha, S., Atichartakarn, V., Vathesatogit, P., Sathaphatayavongs, B., and Prajaktam, R., Penicilliosis marneffei in Thailand: report of five human cases, *Am. J. Trop. Med. Hyg.*, 33, 637, 1984.
25. Peto, T. E. A., Bull, R., Millard, P. R., Mackenzie, D. W. R., Campbell, C. K., Haines, M. E., and Mitchell, R. G., Systemic mycosis due to *Penicillium marneffei* in a patient with antibody to human immunodeficiency virus, *J. Infect.*, 16, 285, 1988.
26. Piehl, M. R., Kaplan, R. L., and Haber, M. H., Disseminated penicilliosis in a patient with acquired immunodeficiency syndrome, *Arch. Pathol. Lab. Med.*, 112, 1262, 1988.
27. Ancelle, T., Dupouy-Camet, J., Pujol, F., Nassif, X., Ferradini, L., and Lapierre, J., Un cas de pénicilliose disséminée a *Penicillium marneffei* chez un malade atteint de SIDA, *Bull. Soc. Fr. Mycol. Méd.*, 17, 73, 1988.

28. Sathapatoyavongs, B., Damrongkitchaiporn, S., Saengditha, P., Kiatboonsri, S., and Jayanetra, P., Disseminated penicilliosis associated with HIV infection, *J. Infect.*, 19, 84, 1989.

29. Hulshof, C. M. J., van Zanten, R. A. A., Sluiters, J. F., Van der Ende, M. B., Samson, R. S., Zondevan, P. E., and Wagenvoon, J. H. T., *Penicillium marneffei* infection in an AIDS patient, *Eur. J. Clin. Microbiol. Infect. Dis.*, 9, 370, 1990.

30. Supparatpinyo, K., Chiewchanvit, S., Hirunsri, P., Uthammachai, C., Nelson, K. E., and Sirisanthana, T., *Penicillium marneffei* infection in patients infected with the human immunodeficiency virus, *Clin. Infect. Dis.*, 14, 871, 1992.

31. Tsang, D. N. C., Li, P. C. K., Tsui, M. S., Lau, Y. T., Ma, K. F., and Yeoh, E. K., *Penicillium marneffei*: another pathogen to consider in patients infected with human immunodeficiency virus, *Rev. Infect. Dis.*, 13, 766, 1991.

32. Chiewchanvit, S., Mahanupab, P., Hirunsri, P., and Vanittanakom, N., Cutaneous manifestations of disseminated *Penicillium marneffei* mycosis in five HIV-infected patients, *Mycoses*, 34, 245, 1991.

33. Tsui, W. M. S., Ma, K. F., and Tsang, D. N. C., Disseminated *Penicillium marneffei* infection in HIV-infected subject, *Histopathology*, 20, 287, 1992.

34. Jones, P. D. and See, J., *Penicillium marneffei* infection in patients infected with human immuno-deficiency virus: late presentation in an area of nonendemicity, *Clin. Infect. Dis.*, 15, 744, 1992.

35. Li, P. C. K., Tsui, M. S., and Ma, K. F., *Penicillium marneffei*: indicator disease for AIDS in East Asia, *AIDS*, 6, 240, 1992.

36. Viviani, M. A., Tortorano, A. M., Rizzardini, G., Quirino, T., Kaufman, L., Padhye, A. A., and Ajello, L., Treatment and serological studies of an Italian case of penicilliosis marneffei contracted in Thailand by a drug addict infected with the human immunodeficiency virus, *Eur. J. Epidemiol.*, 9, 79, 1993.

37. Hilmarsdottir, I., Meynard, J. L., Rogeaux, O., Guermonprez, G., Datry, A., Katlama, C., Brücker, G., Coutellier, A., Danis, M., and Gentilini, M., Disseminated *Penicillium marneffei* infection associated with human immunodeficiency virus and a review of 35 published cases, *J. Acquir. Immune Defic. Syndr.*, 6, 466, 1993.

38. Deng, Z. L., Yun, M., and Ajello, L., Human penicilliosis marneffei and its relations to the bamboo rat (*Rhizomys pruinosus*), *J. Med. Vet. Mycol.*, 24, 383, 1986.

39. Garrison, R. G. and Boyd, K. S., Dimorphism of *Penicillium marneffei* as observed by electron microscopy, *Can. J. Microbiol.*, 19, 1305, 1973.

40. Capponi, M., Sureau, P., and Segretain, G., Pénicilliose de *Rhyzomys sinensis*, *Bull. Soc. Pathol. Exot.*, 49, 418, 1956.

41. Segretain, G., *Penicillium marneffei* n. sp., agent d'une mycose du système réticulo-endothélial, *Mycopathol. Mycol. Appl.*, 11, 327, 1959.

42. Deng, Z. L., The relationship between human penicilliosis and the bamboo rat, *Guangxi Yixueyuan Xuebao*, 2, 1, 1985.

43. Deng, Z. L., Four cases of histoplasmosis in Guangxi, *Guangxi Yi Xue*, 5, 20, 1980.

44. Li, Z. S., Deng, Z. L., Li, E. J., Wei, Z. G., Yue, C. Y., and Wei, X. G., Histoplasmosis in South Guangxi (clinicopathological aspects of five cases), *Chung Hua I Hsueh Tsa Chih*, 62, 267, 1982.

45. So, S. Y., Chau, P. Y., Jones, B. M., Wu, P. C., Pun, K. K., Lam, W. K., and Lawton, J. W. M., A case of invasive penicilliosis in Hong Kong with immunologic evaluation, *Am. Rev. Respir. Dis.*, 131, 662, 1985.

46. Supparatpinyo, K., Khamwan, C., Baosoung, V., Nelson, K. E., and Sirisanthana, T., Disseminated *Penicillium marneffei* infection in Southeast Asia, *Lancet*, 344, 110, 1994.

47. Kok, I., Veenstra, J., Rietra, P. J. G. M., Dirks-Go, S., Blaauwgeers, J. L. G., and Weigel, H. M., Disseminated *Penicillium marneffei* infection as an imported disease in HIV-1 infected patients: description of two new cases and a review of the literature, *Neth. J. Med.*, 44, 18, 1994.

48. Pautler, K. B., Padhye, A. A., and Ajello, L., Imported penicilliosis marneffei in the United States: report of a second human infection, *J. Med. Vet. Mycol.*, 22, 433, 1984.

49. Yuen, W. C., Chan, Y. F., Loke, S. L., Seto, W. H., Poon, G. P., and Wong, K. K., Chronic lymphadenopathy caused by *Penicillium marneffei*: a condition mimicking tuberculosis lympho-denopathy, *Br. J. Surg.*, 73, 1007, 1986.

50. Tsang, D. N. C., Chan, J. K. C., Lau, Y. T., Lim, W., Tse, C. H., and Chan, N. K., *Penicillium marneffei* infection: an underdiagnosed disease? *Histopathology*, 13, 311, 1988.

51. Chan, J. K. C., Tsang, D. N. C., and Wong, D. K. K., *Penicillium marneffei* in bronchoalveolar lavage fluid, *Acta Cytol.*, 33, 523, 1989.

52. Chan, Y. and Chow, T. C., Ultrastructural observations on *Penicillium marneffei* in natural human infection, *Ultrastruct. Pathol.*, 14, 439, 1990.

53. Di Salvo, A. F., *Penicillium marneffei* infection: a follow-up, *Am. J. Clin. Pathol.*, 91, 507, 1989.

54. Rogers, A. L. and Kennedy, M. J., Opportunistic hyaline hyphomycetes, in *Manual of Clinical Microbiology*, 5th ed., Balows, A., Hausler, W. J., Jr., Herrmann, K. L., Isenberg, H. D., and Shadomy, H. J., Eds., American Society for Microbiology, Washington, D.C., 1991, 659.

55. Dupont, B., Denning, D. W., Marriott, D., Sugar, A., Viviani, M. A., and Sirisanthana, T., Mycoses in AIDS patients, *J. Med. Vet. Mycol.*, 32, 65, 1994.

56. Romana, C. A., Stern, M., Chovin, S., Drouhet, E., and Pays, J. F., Penicilliose pulmonaire a *Penicillium marneffei* chez un patient atteint d'un syndrome immunodeficitaire acquis: deuxième cas francais, *Bull. Soc. Fr. Mycol. Med.*, 18, 311, 1989.

57. Coen, M., Viviani, M. A., Rizzardini, G., Tortorano, A. M., Bonaccorso, C., and Quirino, T., Disseminated infection due to *Penicillium marneffei* in an HIV positive patient, *Proc. 5th Int. Conf. AIDS*, Ottawa, Abstr. MBP 94, 1989.

58. De Truchis, P., Bounioux, M. E., Roussi, J., Paraire, F., Nordmann, P., and Dournon, E., Septicémie a *Penicillium marneffei* au cours du SIDA, *Proc. 11th Interdisc. Meet. Anti-Infect. Chemother., Paris*, Société de Pathologie Infectieuse de Langue Francaise, Abstr. 35/C4, 1991.

59. Kok, I., Boot, H., Rietra, P. G. J. M., and Weigel, H. M., Successful treatment of *Penicillium marneffei* infection, *3rd Eur. Conf. Clinical Aspects and Treatment HIV Infection, Paris*, The European Network for the Treatment of AIDS, Abstr. 180, 1992.

60. Jones, P. D. and See, J., *Penicillium marneffei* infection in patients infected with human immunodeficiency virus: late presentation in an area of nonendemicity, *Clin. Infect. Dis.*, 15, 744, 1992.

61. Kronauer, Ch. M., Schär, G., Barben, M., and Bühler, H., Die HIV-assoziierte penicillium-marneffei-infektion, *Schweiz. Med. Wochenschr.*, 123, 385, 1993.

62. Sirisanthana, V. and Sirisanthana, T., *Penicillium marneffei* infection in children infected with human immunodeficiency virus, *Pediatr. Infect. Dis. J.*, 12, 1021, 1993.

63. Sirisanthana, V. and Sirisanthana, T., Disseminated *Penicillium marneffei* infection in human immunodeficiency virus-infected children, *Pediatr. Infect. Dis. J.*, 14, 935, 1995.

64. Stern, M., Romana, C. A., Chovin, S., Drouhet, E., Danel, C., and Pays, J. F., Pénicilliose pulmonaire a *Penicillium marneffei* chez un malade atteint d'un syndrome immunodeficitaire acquis, *Presse Med.*, 18, 2087, 1989.

65. Viviani, M. A. and Tortorano, A. M., Unusual mycoses in AIDS patients, in *Mycoses in AIDS Patients*, vanden Bossche, H. et al., Eds., Plenum Press, New York, 1990, 147.

66. Pearson, J. G., McKinney, T. D., and Stone, W. J., *Penicillium* peritonitis in a CAPD patient, *Perit. Dial. Bull.*, 3, 20, 1983.

67. Fahhoum, J. and Gelfand, M. S., Peritonitis due to *Penicillium* sp. in a patient receiving continuous ambulatory peritoneal dialysis, *South. Med. J.*, 89, 87, 1996.

68. Hirst, L. W., Thomas, J. V., and Green, W. R., Endophthalmitis, in *Principles and Practice of Infectious Diseases*, 2nd ed., Mandell, R. L., Douglas, R. G., Jr., and Bennett, J. E., Eds., John Wiley & Sons, New York, 1985, 760.

69. Swan, S. K., Wagner, R. A., Myers, J. P., and Cinelli, A. B., Mycotic endophthalmitis caused by *Penicillium* sp. after parenteral drug abuse, *Am. J. Ophthalmol.*, 100, 408, 1985.

70. Streifel, A. J., Stevens, P. P., and Rhame, F. S., In-hospital source of airborne *Penicillium* species spores, *J. Clin. Microbiol.*, 25, 1, 1987.

71. Aisner, J., Schimpff, S. C., Bennett, J. E., Young, V. M., and Wiernik, P. H., *Aspergillus* infections in cancer patients: association with fireproofing materials in a new hospital, *JAMA*, 235, 411, 1976.

72. Daisy, J. A., Abrutyn, E. A., and MacGregor, R. R., Inadvertent administration of intravenous fluids contaminated with fungi, *Ann. Intern. Med.*, 91, 563, 1979.

73. Samples, J. R., Contamination of irrigating solution used for cataract surgery, *Ophthalmic Surg.*, 1, 66, 1984.

74. McGinnis, M. R., Progressive disseminated penicilliosis caused by *Penicillium marneffei* — unfortunate omission, *Am. J. Clin. Pathol.*, 85, 529, 1986.

75. Deng, Z., Ribas, J., Gibson, D. W., and Connor, D. H., Infections caused by *Penicillium marneffei* in China and south east Asia: review of eighteen published cases and report of four more Chinese cases, *Rev. Infect. Dis.*, 10, 640, 1988.

76. Heath, T. C. B., Patel, A., Fisher, D., Bowden, F. J., and Currie, B., Disseminated *Penicillium marneffei*: presenting illness of advanced HIV infection; a clinicopathological review, illustrated by a case report, *Pathology*, 27, 101, 1995.

77. Liu, M.-T., Wong, C.-K., and Fung, C.-P., Disseminated *Penicillium marneffei* infection with cutaneous lesions in an HIV-positive patient, *Br. J. Dermatol.*, 131, 280, 1994.

78. Huang, S. N. and Harris, L. S., Acute disseminated penicilliosis, *Am. J. Clin. Pathol.*, 39, 167, 1963.

79. Maddoux, G. L., Mohr, J. A., and Muchmore, H. G., Pulmonary penicilliosis, *J. Okla. State Med. Assoc.*, 65, 418, 1972.

80. Shamberger, R. C., Weinstein, H. J., Grier, H. E., and Levey, R. H., The surgical management of fungal pulmonary infections in children with acute myelogenous leukemia, *J. Pediatr. Surg.*, 6, 840, 1985.

81. Gelfand, M. S., Cole, F. H., and Baskin, R. C., Invasive pulmonary penicilliosis successful therapy with amphotericin B, *South. Med. J.*, 83, 701, 1990.

82. Chan, Y.-F. and Woo, K. C., *Penicillium marneffei* osteomyelitis, *J. Bone Joint Surg.*, 72-B, 500, 1990.

83. Bennett, J. E., Antifungal agents, in *Principles and Practice of Infectious Diseases*, 2nd ed., Mandell, G. L., Douglas, R. G., and Bennett, J. E., Eds., John Wiley & Sons, New York, 1985, 263.

84. Kang, X. M., Penicilliosis marneffei: report of a case and review of literatures, *Chung Hua Chieh Ho Ho Hu Hsi Tsa Chih*, 15, 336, 1992.

85. Ancelle, T., Dupouy-Camet, J., Pujol, F., Nassif, X., Ferradini, L., Choudat, L., de Bievre, C., Dupont, B., Drouhet, E., and Lapierre, J., Un cas de pénicilliose disséminée a *Penicillium marneffei* chez un malade atteint d'un syndrome immunodéficitaire acquis, *Presse Med.*, 17, 1095, 1988.

86. Supparatpinyo, K., Nelson, K. E., Merz, W. G., Breslin, B. J., Cooper, C. R., Jr., Kamwan, C., and Sirisanthana, T., Response to antifungal therapy by human immunodeficiency virus-infected patients with disseminated *Penicillium marneffei* infections and *in vitro* susceptibilities of isolates from clinical specimens, *Antimicrob. Agents Chemother.*, 37, 2407, 1993.

87. Sekhon, A. S., Padhye, A. A., and Garg, A. K., *In vitro* sensitivity of *Penicillium marneffei* and *Pythium insidiosum* to various antifungal agents, *Eur. J. Epidemiol.*, 8, 427, 1992.

88. Sekhon, A. S., Stein, L., Garg, A. K., Black, W. A., Glezos, J. D., and Wong, C., Pulmonary penicilliosis marneffei: report of the first imported case in Canada, *Mycopathologia*, 128, 3, 1994.

89. Ko, K. F., Retropharyngeal abscess caused by *Penicillium marneffei*: an unusual cause of upper airway obstruction, *Otolaryngol. Head Neck Surg.*, 110, 445, 1994.

37.11 *PAECILOMYCES* SPP.

37.11.1 INTRODUCTION

The genus *Paecilomyces* of the family Moniliaceae, order Moniliales, comprises saprophytic fungi that can be found worldwide in soil and decaying vegetation. They have also been isolated as contaminants of culture specimens (skin, sputum) and sterile solutions. *Paecilomyces* was first classified as a genus by Banier, in 1907, when he isolated and described *P. varioti*.[1]

Morphologically, the hyaline mycelia of *Paecilomyces* are 2.0 to 4.0 μm wide and septate. The conidiophores are well developed and branching. The phialides, propagated on conidiophores, are tapered and the conidia are smooth-walled, hyaline to yellow, oval, lemon-shaped, and produced in unbranched chains.[2] *Paecilomyces* species are closely related to the genus *Penicillium*. While the conidial structures closely resemble those of *Penicillium* spp., the phialides are swollen at the base and more abruptly tapered at the apex.[2,3]

The first isolation of *Paecilomyces* spp. from humans was reported in 1916 by Turesson, who isolated the fungus from human feces. Among the various *Paecilomyces* spp.,[4,5] *P. varioti*,[2,6-9] *P. lilacinus*,[10-12] *P. keratitis*, *P. javanicus*,[13] and *P. marquandii*,[14] although seldom, have also been implicated in human infections affecting both immunocompetent and immunocompromised patients.

The most common site of *Paecilomyces* infection is the eye and eye structures.[10,15-17] After the eye and heart, the lungs are the third organ most frequently affected by these fungi. Since *Paecilomyces* spp. have been implicated as the cause of allergic alveolitis in patients living in substandard urban dwellings in proximity to decaying wood, the possibility has been raised that inhalation of fungal spores into the lungs may be a likely route of parenchymal infection.[18] Cell-mediated granulomatous inflammation of the pulmonary parenchyma without pneumonia has resulted from chronic alveolitis.[19]

The *Paecilomyces* spp. are well known for their resistance to sterilization methods, leading to contamination of sterile solutions.[20-22] A major *P. lilacinus* endophthalmitis outbreak, which was registered in the U.S.,[23-27] has been ultimately traced to a contaminated batch of neutralizing solution used to rinse the lenses during surgery.[23,25]

Increasingly, however, *Paecilomyces* spp. are recognized as potential pathogens in immuno-compromised hosts,[8,10,12,28] such as in renal transplant recipients,[6,10,14] and patients with chronic granulomatous disease (CGD).[6,11] CGD is a heterogeneous group of disorders characterized by impaired ability of neutrophils to produce bactericidal and fungicidal oxygen metabolites (hydrogen peroxide, hypochlorous acid) necessary for killing catalase-positive organisms.[29-34]

Specifically, *Paecilomyces* spp. have been associated with often lethal endocarditis after valve replacement,[5,7,13,35-37] mycotic infections of the skin,[14,28,38-40] keratitis,[41] pleural effusion and pneumonia,[8,42-45] sinusitis,[46-49] a lacrimal sac infection,[50] pyelonephritis,[51] a fatal case of ventriculoperitoneal shunt,[52] peritonitis in patients receiving continuous ambulatory peritoneal dialysis,[9,53] and catheter-related fungemia.[2,12]

Suppression of cell-mediated immunity is one of the predisposing factors for infection.[8] In the case of patients with diabetes mellitus, the impaired activity and reduced concentration of the α-1 protease inhibitor (an endogenous lung antiprotease), may have a bearing on the ability of *Paecilomyces* spp., normally fungi with low pathogenicity, to infect the lung parenchyma.[54]

37.11.2 EVOLUTION OF THERAPIES AND TREATMENT OF *PAECILOMYCES* INFECTIONS

Most human *Paecilomyces*-associated infections have occurred in immunocompromised hosts.[55] As defined by Ajello and McGinnis[56] and Ajello,[57] hyalohyphomycosis is an opportunistic infection involving hyphomycetes, such as *Paecilomyces* spp., with hyaline or light-colored cell walls (see Section 37.9). In contrast, infection with opportunistic hyphomycetes having melanin in the cell wall has been known as phaeohyphomycosis (see Section 37.1).[58] The term hyalohyphomycosis is not intended to replace such well-established names as aspergillosis, but may be used in place of such terms as fusariosis, penicilliosis, or paecilomycosis.[10]

Results from *in vitro* susceptibility testing in animal models and humans[7,15,23,25,55,59] have clearly indicated certain susceptibility trends. Thus, some *Paecilomyces* spp. (*P. lilacinus* and *P. marquandii*) have been found to be highly resistant to polyene antibiotics (amphotericin B) and flucytosine, while *P. varioti* was sensitive to both amphotericin B and flucytosine.[15,55,59] Because of such different sensitivities, species identification is important for the clinical outcome of the disease.[55]

Amphotericin B has been widely used in the treatment of *Paecilomyces* spp. infections. However, results have been largely disappointing because of the poor outcome of fungal endocarditis.[6] While the *in vitro* susceptibilities of *Paecilomyces* spp. to various antifungal agents have been determined,[7,42] the lack of standardization and clinical correlation has markedly limited their usefulness.[60]

Williamson et al.[6] have reported the successful treatment of an 8-year-old child with chronic granulomatous disease who developed a soft tissue *P. varioti* infection. The therapy consisted of amphotericin B for 7 weeks (0.8 mg/kg daily, for a total dose of 40 mg/kg), followed by 1 year of oral itraconazole (100 mg, b.i.d.). Itraconazole has been shown to converge in soft tissue collections of pus, making it particularly useful in the treatment of soft tissue infections.[61] In an earlier case of a child with CGD, the patient developed two unusual abdominal wall abscesses caused by *P. lilacinus*, an organism which was found as a contaminant in sterile solutions[15,23,24,62,63] and not known to cause infections in patients with CGD.[11] Contrary to the previously reported resistance of *P. lilacinus* to amphotericin B, the patient responded well to a 2-month course of this antibiotic at initial daily doses of 0.5 mg/kg for 3 weeks, followed by 1.0 mg/kg dose given three times weekly (total dose, 825 mg).[11]

Shing et al.[2] have described a case of *P. varioti* catheter-related fungemia in an allogeneic bone marrow transplant recipient receiving antifungal prophylaxis with fluconazole (50 mg daily). Successful treatment was achieved by removal of the central venous catheter and intravenous infusion of amphotericin B (initially at 0.5 mg/kg [11 mg daily], then increased to 1.0 mg/kg [23 mg/kg daily] on day 14). Because of renal toxicity, amphotericin B was discontinued after 40 d of treatment and the therapy was switched to oral itraconazole at 100 mg daily for 3 months.

P. varioti-associated peritonitis in patients receiving continuous ambulatory peritoneal dialysis (CAPD) has also been reported.[9] Early removal of the dialysis catheter and intravenous amphotericin B or oral ketoconazole were used in the successful management of the infection.

Byrd et al.[8] have presented the first case of *P. varioti* pneumonia in a patient with diabetes mellitus as predisposing factor. The pneumonia responded poorly to oral ketoconazole (400 mg daily for 3 months), and the chronic infiltrating process required administration of amphotericin B via a Hickman catheter to resolve.

A case of *Paecilomyces* keratitis was treated successfully with a combination of topical natamycin, intravenous miconazole (400 mg daily, for a total of 9.6 g over a 24-d period), a temporary conjunctival flap, and penetrating keratoplasty.[41]

A *P. lilacinus*-associated hyalohyphomycosis in a renal transplant patient responded well to oral griseofulvin (500 mg daily) given for 45 d.[10] Oral griseofulvin has also been used successfully in an earlier case of skin infection by *P. lilacinus*.[38]

37.11.3 REFERENCES

1. Banier, G., Mycotheque de l'Ecole de Pharmacie. XI. *Paecilomyces*, genre nouveau de Mucedinees, *Bull. Soc. Mycol. Fr.*, 23, 26, 1907.
2. Shing, M. M. K., Ip, M., Li, C. K., Chik, K. W., and Yuen, P. M. P., *Paecilomyces varioti* fungemia in a bone marrow transplant patient, *Bone Marrow Transplant.*, 17, 281, 1996.
3. Kwon-Chung, K. J. and Bennett, J. E., *Medical Mycology*, Lea & Fabiger, Philadelphia, 1992, 747.
4. Raper, K. B. and Thom, C., *A Manual of the Penicillia*, Williams & Wilkins, Baltimore, 1949, 284.
5. Silver, M. D., Tuffinel, P. G., and Bigelow, W. G., Endocarditis caused by *Paecilomyces varioti* affecting an aortic valve allograft, *J. Thorac. Cardiovasc. Surg.*, 61, 278, 1971.
6. Williamson, P. R., Kwon-Chung, K. J., and Gallin, J. I., Successful treatment of *Paecilomyces varioti* infection in a patient with chronic granulomatous disease and a review of *Paecilomyces* species infections, *Clin. Infect. Dis.*, 14, 1023, 1992.
7. Kalish, S. B., Goldschmidt, R., Li, C., Knop, R., Cook, F. V., Wilner, G., and Victor, T. A., Infective endocarditis caused by *Paecilomyces varioti*, *Am. J. Clin. Pathol.*, 78, 249, 1982.
8. Byrd, R. P. J., Roy, T. M., Field, C. L., and Lynch, J. A., *Paecilomyces varioti*, pneumonia in a patient with diabetes mellitus, *J. Diab. Comp.*, 6, 150, 1992.
9. Marzec, A., Heron, L. G., Pritchard, R. C., Butcher, R. H., Powell, H. R., Disney, A. P. S., and Tosolini, F. A., *Paecilomyces varioti* in peritoneal dialysate, *J. Clin. Microbiol.*, 31, 2392, 1993.
10. Castro, L. G., Salebian, A., and Soto, M. N., Hyalohyphomycosis by *Paecilomyces lilacinus* in a renal transplant patient and a review of human *Paecilomyces* species infections, *J. Med. Vet. Mycol.*, 28, 15, 1990.
11. Silliman, C. C., Lawellin, D. W., Lohr, J. A., Rodgers, B. M., and Donowitz, L. G., *Paecilomyces lilacinus* infection in a child with chronic granulomatous disease, *J. Infect.*, 24, 191, 1992.

12. Tan, T. Q., Ogden, A. K., Tillman, J., Demmler, G. J., and Rinaldi, M. G., *Paecilomyces lilacinus* catheter-related fungemia in an immunocompromised pediatric patient, *J. Clin. Microbiol.*, 30, 2479, 1992.

13. Allevato, P. A., Ohorodnik, J. M., Mezger, E., and Eisses, J. F., *Paecilomyces javanicus* endocarditis of native and prosthetic aortic valve, *Am. J. Clin. Pathol.*, 82, 247, 1984.

14. Harris, L. F., Dan, B. M., Lefkowitz, L. B., Jr., and Alford, R. H., *Paecilomyces* cellulitis in a renal transplant patient: successful treatment with intravenous miconazole, *South. Med. J.*, 72, 897, 1979.

15. Gordon, M. A., *Paecilomyces lilacinus* (Thom) Samson, from systemic infection in an armadillo (*Dasypus novemcinctus*), *Sabouraudia*, 22, 109, 1984.

16. Chandler, F. W., Kaplan, W., and Ajello, L., *A Color Atlas and Textbook of the Histopathology of Mycotic Diseases*, Wolf Medical, London, 1980, 102.

17. Rodrigues, M. M. and McLeod, D., Exogenous fungal endophthalmitis caused by *Paecilomyces*, *Am. J. Ophthalmol.*, 79, 687, 1980.

18. Bryant, D. H. and Rogers, P., Allergic alveolitis due to wood-rot fungi, *Allergy Proc.*, 12, 89, 1991.

19. Akhunova, A. M. and Shustova, V. I., *Paecilomyces* infection, *Probl. Tuberk.*, 8, 38, 1989.

20. Halde, C. and Okumoto, M., Ocular mycosis: a study of 82 cases, *Proc. 20th Int. Congr. Ophthalmol., Munich*, Excerpta Medica International Congresses Series, 146, 705, 1966.

21. Rippon, J. W., *Medical Mycology: The Pathogenic Fungi and the Pathogenic Actinomycetes*, 3rd ed., W. B. Saunders, Philadelphia, 1988, 728.

22. Volna, F. and Maderova, E., *Paecilomyces lilacinus*-sensitivity to disinfectants, *Cesk. Epidemiol. Mikrobiol. Imunol.*, 39, 315, 1990.

23. O'Day, D. M., Fungal endophthalmitis caused by *Paecilomyces lilacinus* after intraocular lens implantation, *Am. J. Ophthalmol.*, 83, 130, 1977.

24. Miller, G. R., Rebell, G., Magoon, R. C., Kulvin, S. M., and Forster, R. K., Intravitreal antimycotic therapy and the cure of mycotic endophthalmitis caused by a *Paecilomyces lilacinus* contaminated pseudophakos, *Ophthalmic Surg.*, 9, 54, 1978.

25. Pettit, T. H., Olson, R. J., Foos, R. Y., and Martin, W. J., Fungal endophthalmitis following intraocular lens implantation: a surgical epidemic, *Arch. Ophthalmol.*, 98, 1025, 1980.

26. Mosier, M., Lusk, B., Pettit, T. H., Howard, D. H., and Rhodes, J., Fungal endophthalmitis following intraocular lens implantation, *Am. J. Ophthalmol.*, 83, 1, 1977.

27. Webster, R. G., Jr., Martin, W. J., Pettit, T. H., Rhodes, J., Boni, B., Midura, T., and Skinner, M. D., Eye infection after plastic lens implantation, *Morbid. Mortal. Wkly. Rep.*, 24, 437, 1975.

28. Jade, K. B., Lyons, M. F., and Gnann, J. W., Jr., *Paecilomyces lilacinus* cellulitis in an immuno-compromised patient, *Arch. Dermatol.*, 122, 1169, 1986.

29. Tauber, A. I., Borregaard, N., Simons, E., and Wright, J., Chronic granulomatous disease: a syndrome of phagocyte oxidase deficiencies, *Medicine (Baltimore)*, 62, 286, 1983.

30. Gallin, J. I. and Malech, H. L., Update on chronic granulomatous disease of childhood: immunotherapy and potential for gene therapy, *JAMA*, 263, 1533, 1990.

31. Gallin, J. I., Malech, H. L., Weening, R. S., Curnutte, J. T., Quie, P. G., Jaffe, H. S., Ezekowitz, R. A. B., and the International Chronic Granulomatous Disease Cooperative Study Group, A controlled trial of interferon gamma to prevent infection in chronic granulomatous disease, *N. Engl. J. Med.*, 324, 509, 1991.

32. Hendrickson, D. H. and Krenz, M. M., Reagents and stains, in *Manual of Clinical Microbiology*, Balows, A., Ed., American Society for Microbiology, Washington, D.C., 1991, 1290.

33. Mandell, G. L. and Hook, E. W., Leukocyte bactericidal activity in chronic granulomatous disease: correlation of bactericidal hydrogen peroxide production and susceptibility to intracellular killing, *J. Bacteriol.*, 100, 531, 1969.

34. Gallin, J. I., Buescher, E. S., Seligmann, B. E., Nath, J., Gaither, T., and Katz, P., Recent advances in chronic granulomatous disease, *Ann. Intern. Med.*, 99, 675, 1983.

35. Uys, C. J., Don, P. A., Schrire, V., and Barnard, C. N., Endocarditis following cardiac surgery due to the fungus *Paecilomyces*, *S. Afr. Med. J.*, 37, 1276, 1963.

36. McClellan, J. R., Hamilton, J. D., Alexander, J. A., Wolfe, W. G., and Reed, J. B., *Paecilomyces varioti* endocarditis on a prosthetic aortic valve, *J. Thorac. Cardiovasc. Surg.*, 71, 472, 1976.

37. Haldane, E. V., MacDonald, J. L., Gittens, W. O., Yuce, K., and van Rooyen, C. E., Prosthetic valvular endocarditis due to the fungus *Paecilomyces*, *Can. Med. Assoc. J.*, 111, 963, 1974.

38. Takayatsu, S., Akagi, M., and Shimizu, Y., Cutaneous mycosis caused by *Paecilomyces lilacinus*, *Arch. Dermatol.*, 113, 1687, 1977.

39. Harris, L. F., Dan, B. M., Lefhowitz, L. B., Jr., and Alford, R. H., *Paecilomyces* cellulitis in a renal transplant patient: successful treatment with intravenous miconazole, *South. Med. J.*, 72, 897, 1979.

40. Arai, H. and Endo, T., A case of deep mycosis (*Fonsecaea pedrosoi* and *Paecilomyces lilacinus*) following renal transplant, *Hifuka*, 31, 481, 1977.

41. Mizunoya, S. and Watanabe, Y., *Paecilomyces* keratitis with corneal perforation salvaged by a conjunctival flap and delayed keratoplasty, *Br. J. Ophthalmol.*, 78, 157, 1994.

42. Dharmasena, F. M. C., Davies, G. S. R., and Catovsky, D., *Paecilomyces varioti* pneumonia complicating hairy cell leukaemia, *Br. Med. J.*, 290, 967, 1985.

43. French, F. F. and Mallia, C. P., Pleural effusion caused by *Paecilomyces lilacinus*, *Br. J. Dis. Chest*, 66, 284, 1972.

44. Dekhkan-Khodzhaeva, N. A., Shamsiev, S. Sh., Shakirova, R. Yu., Macarova, G. I., and Mingbaeva, Sh. N., The role of *Paecilomyces* in the etiology of prolonged and recurrent bronchopulmonary diseases in children, *Pediatryia*, 9, 12, 1982.

45. Mormede, M., Texier, J., Gomez, F., Couprie, B., Fourche, J., and Martigne, C., Isolement d'un *Paecilomyces* (*P. lilacinus*) a partir d'un épanchement pleural, *Med. Malad. Infect.*, 14, 76, 1984.

46. Otcenasek, M., Jirousek, Z., Nozicka, Z., and Mencl, K., Paecilomycosis of the maxillary sinus, *Mykosen*, 27, 242, 1984.

47. Thompson, R. F., Bode, R. B., Rhodes, J. C., and Gluckman, J. L., *Paecilomyces varioti*: an unusual cause of isolated sphenoid sinusitis, *Arch. Otolaryngol. Head Neck Surg.*, 114, 567, 1988.

48. Rockhill, R. C. and Klein, M. D., *Paecilomyces lilacinus* as the cause of chronic maxillary sinusitis, *J. Clin. Microbiol.*, 11, 737, 1980.

49. Rowley, S. D. and Strom, C. G., *Paecilomyces* fungus infection of the maxillary sinus, *Laryngoscope*, 92, 332, 1982.

50. Henig, F. E., Lehrer, N., Gabbay, A., and Kurz, O., Paecilomycosis of the lacrimal sac, *Mykosen*, 16, 25, 1973.

51. Sherwood, J. A. and Dansky, A. S., Paecilomyces pyelonephritis complicating nephrolithiasis and review of *Paecilomyces* infections, *J. Urol.*, 130, 526, 1983.

52. Fagerburg, R., Suh, B., Buchley, H. R., Lorber, B., and Karian, J., Cerebrospinal fluid shunt colonisation and obstruction by *Paecilomyces varioti*: case report, *J. Neurosurg.*, 54, 257, 1981.

53. Crompton, C. H., Summerbell, R. C., and Silver, M. M., Peritonitis with *Paecilomyces* complicating peritoneal dialysis, *Pediatr. Infect. Dis. J.*, 10, 869, 1991.

54. Sandler, M., Gemperli, B. M., Hanekom, C., and Kuhn, S. H., Serum alpha 1-protease inhibitor in diabetes mellitus: reduced concentration and impaired activity, *Diabetes Res. Clin. Pract.*, 5, 249, 1988.

55. Weitzmann, I., Saprophytic molds as agents of cutaneous and subcutaneous infection in the immuno-compromised host, *Arch. Dermatol.*, 122, 1161, 1986.

56. Ajello, L. and McGinnis, M., Nomenclature of human pathogenic fungi, in *Grundlagen der Antiseptik Band I, Teil 4*, Weuffen, W., Berencsi, G., Gröschel, D., Kenter, B., Kramer, A., and Krasilnikow, A. P., Eds., Volk und Gesundheit, Berlin, 1984, 365.

57. Ajello, L., Hyalohyphomycosis and phaeohyphomycosis: two global disease entities of public health importance, *Eur. J. Epidemiol.*, 2, 243, 1986.

58. Rippon, J. W., Larson, R. A., Rosenthal, D. M., and Clayman, J., Disseminated cutaneous and peritoneal hyalohyphomycosis caused by *Fusarium* species: three cases and review of the literature, *Mycopathologia*, 101, 105, 1988.

59. Gordon, M. A. and Norton, S. W., Corneal transplant infection by *Paecilomyces lilacinus*, *Sabouraudia*, 23, 295, 1985.

60. Galgiani, J. N., Progress in standardizing antifungal susceptibility tests, *Clin. Lab. Med.*, 9, 269, 1989.

61. Neijens, H. J., Frenkel, J., de Muinck Keizer-Schrama, S. M. P. F., Dzoljic-Danilovic, G., Meradji, M., and van Dongen, J. J. M., Invasive *Aspergillus* infection in chronic granulomatous disease: treatment with itraconazole, *J. Pediatr.*, 115, 1016, 1989.

62. Barron, G. L., *The Genera of Hyphomycetes From Soil*, Williams & Wilkins, Baltimore, 1978, 54.

63. Samson, R. A., *Paecilomyces* and some allied hyphomycetes, in *Studies in Mycology. No. 6. Baarn*, Centraalbureau voor Schimmelcultures, The Netherlands, 1974, 119.

38 Zygomycota

38.1 ZYGOMYCOSIS (MUCORMYCOSIS, PHYCOMYCOSIS)

38.1.1 INTRODUCTION

Zygomycosis is an umbrella term describing acute (rarely chronic) and often fatal opportunistic infections occurring mainly in patients with specific predisposing conditions such as chronic debilitating disease (diabetic ketoacidosis, leukemia, lymphoma), malnutrition, and immuno-suppression (liver transplant recipients, burns).[1-3] The etiologic agents of the disease are fungi belonging to the class Zygomycetes which are further subdivided into two orders: Entomophthorales and Mucorales. The latter includes such genera as *Absidia*, *Mucor*, and especially *Rhizopus* (*R. rhizopodiformis*, *R. arrhizus*, and *R. oryzae*),[4-6] which are ubiquitous saprophytic molds residing in decaying matter and soil.[7] The infection most often originates in the upper respiratory tract or lungs, in which spores germinate and from which mycelial growth metastasize to other organs.

Zygomycosis (the terms phycomycosis and mucormycosis have also been in use) is one of the most acute and fulminant fungal infections known.[8] It presents as a spectrum of diseases dependent on the portal of entry of the pathogen and the kind of predisposing debility of the patient. The infections are characterized by two distinct features: (1) an explicit predilection of the fungi to invade major blood vessels resulting in ischemia and necrosis of adjacent tissue (infarction), and (2) the production of "black pus."[8] Zygomycotic infections are divided into six major categories: rhinocerebral, pulmonary, gastrointesinal, primary cutaneous, disseminated, and miscellaneous.[2,9-13]

Cases of chronic nasal zygomycosis in otherwise healthy patients, although rare, have been reported.[8]

38.1.1.1 Ketoacidosis and Pathogenicity of Zygomycosis

The apparent tendency of the infection to affect acidotic patients has been widely investigated.[10-12] *In vitro* growth of *Rhizopus* has been facilitated by the metabolic conditions seen in the ketoacidotic patient.[4] Serum from patients with diabetic ketoacidosis compared to normal serum, did not have the ability to inhibit *Rhizopus arrhizus*; the ability was restored after correction of acidosis.[10]

The mechanism by which ketoacidosis leads to increased pathogenicity of phycomycetes has been the subject of several studies. It has been shown that while acute ketotic alloxan diabetes in rabbits and mice facilitated the invasive growth of *Rhizopus* organisms,[14-17] chronic nonketotic diabetes and infusional hyperglycemia did not.[17,18] Furthermore, Bybee and Rogers[19] have observed a decreased phagocytic activity *in vitro* by polymorphonuclear leukocytes obtained from keto-acidotic patients. In addition, the local tissue accumulation of granulocytes[20] and fibroblasts[21] in response to infection has been delayed and diminished in uremic and diabetic acidosis,[20] but not in uncontrolled but nonketotic diabetic patients.

Polli[22] has found the presence in *Rhizopus* of an active reductase system which is highly adapted to a medium of high glucose content and reaches peak metabolic activity at acid pH levels.[23]

38.1.2   Zygomycetous Infections

38.1.2.1   Rhinocerebral Zygomycosis

First defined by Gregory et al.[24] in 1943, rhinocerebral zygomycosis is the most common and distinct form of the disease.[5,10,24-44] In the overwhelming majority of cases, it is caused by *R. arrhizus*.[4] The portal of entry of the fungus is the palate or mucous membrane of the nose or the paranasal sinuses. A direct transmission from the nose to the sinuses has also been observed.[45] From the paranasal sinuses the infection may progress either through the cribriform plate and into the frontal lobe of the brain, or into the retroorbital region and then through the apex of the orbit into the brain.[46] The term rhinocerebral zygomycosis is used in the context of documented brain involvement in addition to involvement of the paranasal sinuses and the orbit. It has been recommended that paranasal zygomycosis and rhinoorbital zygomycosis be used to define only disease involving the sinuses alone or both sinuses and orbit, respectively.[46]

Rhinocerebral zygomycosis is an acute and rapidly progressing infection most often affecting immunosuppressed hosts such as poorly controlled diabetic patients and organ transplant recipients,[47-50] although on rare occasions it may also affect healthy individuals.[9,13] Acidosis, impaired phagocytosis, and glucosteroid therapy of hematologic neoplasms are the major predisposition factors of rhinocerebral zygomycosis.[45] Hyperglycemia itself, however, is not a predisposing factor for zygomycosis.[9] As the disease progresses, the fungus shows propensity for invading large blood vessels.

38.1.2.2   Pulmonary Zygomycosis

Pulmonary zygomycosis is linked prodominantly with immunosuppressed patients (diabetic and renal transplant recipients), as well as patients with leukemia, lymphoma, severe neutropenia, or carcinoma.[5,9,13,27,46,51-57] In addition, pulmonary zygomycosis may occur as part of disseminated or rhinocerebral disease.[9,13] The fungus invades the respiratory tract by inhalation, causing pulmonary vascular thrombosis and infarction.[8] The infection usually progresses rapidly, but appearance of chronic pulmonary lesions have also been reported.[58] Although pulmonary zygomycosis may follow an indolent course in diabetic patients and those with renal insufficiency, it still can be serious and frequently fatal.[4,45]

Rothstein and Simon[59] have described cases of diabetic patients presenting a subacute form of pulmonary zygomycosis (lasting weeks to months) where pulmonary infiltrates continue to progress in spite of conventional therapy.

38.1.2.3   Gastrointestinal Zygomycosis

Intestinal zygomycosis strictly limited to the gastrointestinal tract is uncommon, with the possible exception of South Africa.[60-65] Usually it is caused by fungal ingestion by malnourished children suffering from kwashiorkor[66] or pellagra, or uremic individuals.[67] In addition, severe underlying diseases (amebic colitis, typhoid fever) of the gastrointestinal tract, glucosteroid therapy, and postoperative bacterial infections have been determined to be predisposing factors.[9,26,60,61,67-69] The stomach is most commonly affected, followed by the colon.[5,61-66,70-79] However, a widespread dissemination from a primary gastrointestinal site may also occur:[80] involvement of the colon, ileum, and by extension, gall bladder, liver, pancreas, and spleen have been observed.[8] The disease is manifested by erosive necrotic ulcers with thromboses and gangrene in the gastrointestinal tract from the esophagus to the colon. The lesions may often perforate the GI wall leading to peritonitis. Death usually is caused by shock from hemorrhage of the bowel resulting in peritonitis and bowel infarction.[81]

38.1.2.4 Cutaneous Zygomycosis

Zygomycosis of the skin and soft tissue is frequently associated with burn wounds or diabetes mellitus.[53,82-99] *R. rhizopodiformis* and *R. oryzae* are the etiologic agents of this form of zygomycosis. A survey of 28 cases reported in the U.S. since 1985 revealed that 25% of the patients were immunocompromised, and 39% had trauma.[1] Cutaneous mucormycosis has been found in nodular lesions with hematogenous seeding,[93,94] in association with elastic adhesive bandages,[89,91,97] in burn patients,[53,94,95] renal transplant recipients,[100] patients with leukemia and lymphoma,[4,92,93,101] and diabetes,[87,90,101-103] and in disseminated disease as cutaneous infarct resembling ecthyma gangrenosum.[92,93] It has been rarely diagnosed in immunocompetent patients.[104]

Clinical manifestations of cutaneous zygomycosis include necrotic lesions, cellulitis, and ulceration.[105,106] Similarly to other forms of zygomycosis, cutaneous zygomycosis is characterized by vessel invasion and black, necrotic debris.[85,107] Necrosis is usually the result of infarction caused by the invasion of the pathogen into blood vessel walls.[8] Zygomycotic gangrenous cellulitis should be included in the differential diagnosis of progressive necrotizing lesions of the skin,[108] especially in diabetic patients.[86] As with all forms of zygomycosis, primary cutaneous zygomycosis can become disseminated and cause death.[86]

Subcutaneous mucormycosis is a deep infection of subcutaneous tissue mostly seen in Africa, India, and Indonesia.[109] Primary cutaneous mycormycosis is rare.[110,111]

38.1.2.5 Disseminated Zygomycosis

Disseminated zygomycosis if left untreated is uniformly fatal.[46] Lungs are the main route of dissemination of zygomycosis which then spreads to the central nervous system to form infarcts and abscesses.[9,13,26,51,54,79,110,112-120] Dissemination from the GI tract or from burns is rare.[25,51,69,112] Tissue infection is characterized by vessel invasion with infarction of the surrounding parenchyma with the lungs being the most common organs involved.[8] Cerebral involvement associated with disseminated zygomycosis may also occur through hematogenous seeding followed by abscess formation and multiple infarctions.[13]

38.1.2.6 Miscellaneous Zygomycetous Infections

Zygomycetous endocarditis, although rare, has been diagnosed in association with cardiac surgery.[9,121,122] Other miscellaneous forms include burn infection, wound infection (particularly after abdominal surgery), isolated renal infection, and brain abscesses.[9,53,67,86,123,124] Vascular infections and thrombosis are also important aspects of these infections.[8]

In one interesting observation, Chandler et al.[3] described four cases of zygomycosis where chlamidoconidia were formed in tissues.

38.1.3 Evolution of Therapies and Treatment of Zygomycosis

Before the introduction of amphotericin B as therapy, zygomycosis was almost always fatal.[5,26] In general, without immediate and specific therapy, invasive zygomycosis involving craniofacial structures, lungs, or internal organs is usually fatal.[8] Because of its morbidity, the need for early diagnosis (especially in diabetic and other immunosuppressed patients) of zygomycosis as a prerequisite for effective treatment is extremely important.

In the pre-amphotericin B era, treatment of zygomycosis consisted of a combination of surgery and chemotherapy with iodides, nystatin, or cycloheximide.[12] Since the chemotherapy has been largely ineffective (based on poorly standardized *in vitro* susceptibility assays), the accompanying surgery was undoubtedly the major reason for any beneficial response.[8]

The azole antimycotics (both imidazoles and triazoles) and 5-fluorocytozine have shown inconsistent *in vitro* and *in vivo* activities and have little clinical value as monotherapy for zygomycosis.[125-127] Oral nystatin therapy has also been unsuccessful.[60,110]

Intravenous amphotericin B is currently the only recommended antifungal agent for treatment of zygomycoses. Along with more efficient premortem diagnosis, the aggressive therapy with amphotericin B has been credited for the dramatically improved prognosis of zygomycosis in recent years.[128-131] Since the optimal duration and total amount of the antibiotic are still not well determined, the therapy should be individualized according to the patient's clinical response and the rate of clearing of the infection.[8] In most studies, a cumulative dose of 2.0 to 2.5 g of amphotericin B has been recommended, although in some patients as much as 4.0 g of the antibiotic was needed to complete the therapy.[9,10,25,132] The rate of administration of amphotericin B is determined by the clinical severity of the disease and the patient's overall condition.[8] It has been recommended that an initial subtherapeutic 1.0-mg dose in 5% glucose solution is administered during the first day of therapy, followed by incremental daily dose increases of 5.0 mg until a daily dose of 1.0 mg/kg is reached.[132,133] However, in seriously ill patients with fulminant zygomycosis, such gradual progression in dose schedule may cost valuable time. Instead, the 1.0-mg dose may be followed by larger increments of 10 to 12 mg every 12 h until a daily dose of 0.7 to 1.0 mg/kg is achieved.[133] Following clinical stabilization, doses of 0.7 to 1.0 mg/kg may be applied every other day.[25] In another therapeutic approach, the 1.0-mg subtherapeutic dose is avoided altogether; treatment is initiated at 0.25 mg/kg amphotericin B on day 1, followed by a 0.5-mg/kg dose on the second day, and 0.75 mg/kg on the third day of treatment, with a shift to alternate-day administration of 1.0 mg/kg thereafter.[133] Each dose, which is injected over a period of 60 min, is adjusted to produce a peak concentration of 2.0 to 3.0 µg/ml at 5 min after termination of the 60-min injection period of administration.[8] Abramson et al.[10] used a dose schedule in which the initial dose of 5.0 mg of amphotericin B was increased by 10 mg daily until the patient was receiving 100 mg daily (approximately 1.25 mg/kg); the antibiotic was administered intravenously over a 6-h period. Premedication with 600 mg chlorpromazine and 50 mg of diphenylhydramine helped eliminate side effects (chills and fever).[10] Battock et al.[25] have supported alternate-day amphotericin B therapy at 1.2 mg/kg which produced at 48 h post-administration adequate serum levels of the antibiotic (0.16 to 0.69 µg/ml) while reducing its adverse renal side effects as compared to daily treatment.

The therapy of rhinocerebral zygomycosis involved treatment to correct metabolic acidosis, discontinuation of immunosuppressive therapy if possible, adequate dose regimens of amphotericin B, and careful monitoring by computer-assisted tomography (CAT) scanning of brain involvement combined with successive biopsies to determine the adequacy of treatment.[8,84,134] In addition to systemic treatment with amphotericin B, drainage of the sinuses and thorough debridement of infarcted tissue, are usually necessary for successful treatment.[9,25-27,135-137] Two reports[9,28] have described successful outcome in patients with intracranial zygomycosis.

Amphotericin B therapy of pulmonary zygomycosis in immunosuppressed patients may be initiated on an empirical basis before diagnosis has been established.[8] Alongside amphotericin B therapy, surgical removal of extensive infected tissue has been recommended.[9,138,139]

Treatment of cutaneous zygomycosis includes therapy with amphotericin B,[53,90,106] surgical debridement, and control of the underlying risk factors or disease,[1,2,140] especially in diabetic patients.[8,84,141] Hall et al.[142] presented a rare case of cutaneous mucormycosis in a heart transplant recipient; successful treatment with amphotericin B was started with 50 mg daily, then gradually increased to reach a total dose of 2.4 g.

Woods and Elewski[1] treated a patient with cutaneous zygomycosis resembling herpes zoster infection (zosteriform zygomycosis) with a combination of amphotericin B and fluconazole. The patient was started with intravenous amphotericin B (60 mg daily) and topical amphotericin B lotion (three times daily) for 3 months. Only moderate improvement led to the addition of fluconazole (200 mg daily) to the treatment regimen. After 6 months of combined therapy (100 g total amphotericin B, and 360 g total of fluconazole), there was significant resolution of lesions; areas of persistent fungal granulomas were excised with no recurrence of lesions at 1-year follow-up examination. It is postulated that by binding to the fungal membrane and compromising its integrity, amphotericin B allows for a better uptake of fluconazole. When internalized, fluconazole inhibits the cytochrome P-450 system and prevents ergosterol biosynthesis and cytochrome respiration necessary for repair of the fungal cell wall.[1]

In addition to antifungal chemotherapy, surgical excision alone was reported efficient to cure cutaneous zygomycosis.[53,84] However, in cases of more widespread infection, surgery should be combined with amphotericin B therapy.[1,4]

38.1.4 REFERENCES

1. Woods, S. G. and Elewski, B. E., Zosteriform zygomycosis, *J. Am. Acad. Dermatol.*, 32, 357, 1995.
2. Lehrer, R. I., Mucormycosis, *Ann. Intern. Med.*, 93, 93, 1980.
3. Chandler, F. W., Watts, J. C., Kaplan, W., Hendry, A. T., McGinnis, M. R., and Ajello, L., Zygomycosis: report of four cases with formation of chlamydoconidia in tissue, *Am. J. Clin. Pathol.*, 84, 99, 1985.
4. Rippon, J. W., Jr., *Medical Mycology. The Pathogenic Fungi and the Pathogenic Actinomycetes*, 2nd ed., W. B. Saunders, Philadelphia, 1982, 615.
5. Baker, R. D., Mucormycosis (opportunistic phycomycosis), in *Human Infection With Fungi, Actinomycetes and Algae*, Baker, R. D., Ed., Springer-Verlag, New York, 1971, 832.
6. Lehrer, R. I., Howard, D. H., Sypherd, P. S., Edwards, J. E., Segal, G. P., and Winston, D. J., Mucormycosis, *Ann. Intern. Med.*, 93, 93, 1980.
7. Prevoo, P. L. M. A., Starink, T. M., and de Haan, P., Primary cutaneous mucormycosis in a healthy young girl, *J. Am. Acad. Dermatol.*, 24, 882, 1991.
8. Rinaldi, M. G., Zygomycosis, *Infect. Dis. Clin. North Am.*, 3, 19, 1989.
9. Mayer, R. D. and Armstrong, D., Mucormycosis — changing status, *Crit. Rev. Clin. Lab. Sci.*, 4, 412, 1973.
10. Abramson, E., Wilson, D., and Arky, R. A., Rhinocerebral phycomycosis in association with diabetic ketoacidosis: report of two cases and a review of clinical and experimental experience with amphotericin B therapy, *Ann. Intern. Med.*, 66, 735, 1967.
11. Deweese, D. D. and Schleuning, A. J., Mucormycosis of the nose and paranasal sinuses, *Laryngoscope*, 75, 1398, 1965.
12. Landau, J. W. and Newcomer, V. D., Acute cerebral phycomycosis (mucormycosis), *J. Pediatr.*, 61, 363, 1962.
13. Mayer, R. D., Rosen, P., and Armstrong, D., Phycomycosis complicating leukemia and lymphoma, *Ann. Intern. Med.*, 77, 871, 1972.
14. Sheldon, W. H. and Bauer, H., Activation of quiescent mucormycotic granulomata in rabbits by induction of acute alloxan diabetes, *J. Exp. Med.*, 108, 171, 1958.
15. Bauer, H., Flanagan, J. F., and Sheldon, W. H., Experimental cerebral mucormycosis in rabbits with alloxan diabetes, *Yale J. Biol. Med.*, 28, 29, 1955.
16. Elder, T. D. and Baker, R. D., Pulmonary mucormycosis in rabbits with alloxan diabetes, *Arch. Pathol. (Chicago)*, 61, 159, 1956.
17. Schofield, R. A. and Baker, R. D., Experimental mucormycosis in mice, *Arch. Pathol. (Chicago)*, 61, 407, 1956.
18. Bauer, H., Flanagan, J. F., and Sheldon, W. H., The effects of metabolic alterations on experimental *Rhizopus oryzae* (mucormycosis) infection, *Yale J. Biol. Med.*, 29, 23, 1956.
19. Bybee, J. D. and Rogers, D. E., The phagocytic activity of polymorphonuclear leukocytes obtained from patients with diabetes mellitus, *J. Lab. Clin. Med.*, 64, 1, 1964.
20. Perillie, P. E., Nolan, J. P., and Finch, S. C., Studies of the resistance to infection in diabetes mellitus: local exudative cellular response, *J. Lab. Clin. Med.*, 59, 1008, 1962.
21. Sheldon, W. H. and Bauer, H., The development of the acute inflammatory response to experimental cutaneous mucormycosis in normal and diabetic rabbits, *J. Exp. Med.*, 110, 845, 1959.

22. Polli, C., On the incidence of ketone reductase in microorganisms, *Pathol. Microbiol. (Basel)*, 28, 93, 1965.
23. Gale, G. R., Gas exchange in *Rhizopus oryzae*, *J. Infect. Dis.*, 106, 149, 1960.
24. Gregory, J. E., Golden, A., and Haymaker, W., Mucormycosis of the central nervous system: a report of three cases, *Bull. Johns Hopkins Hosp.*, 73, 405, 1943.
25. Battock, D. J., Grausz, H., Bobrowsky, M., and Littman, M. L., Alternate-day amphotericin B therapy in the treatment of rhinocerebral phycomycosis (mucormycosis), *Ann. Intern. Med.*, 68, 122, 1968.
26. Straatsma, B. R., Zimmerman, L. E., and Gass, J. D. M., Phycomycosis: a clinical pathologic study of fifty-one cases, *Lab. Invest.*, 11, 963, 1962.
27. Brown, J. F., Jr., Gottlieb, L. S., and McCormick, R. A., Pulmonary and rhinocerebral mucormycosis: successful outcome with amphotericin B and griseofulvin therapy, *Arch. Intern. Med.*, 137, 936, 1977.
28. Lowe, J. T., Jr. and Hudson, W. R., Rhinocerebral phycomycosis and internal carotid artery thrombosis, *Arch. Otolaryngol.*, 101, 100, 1975.
29. Addelstone, R. B. and Baylin, G. J., Rhinocerebral mucormycosis, *Radiology*, 115, 113, 1975.
30. Artis, W. M., Fountain, J. A., Delcher, H. K., and Jones, H. E., A mechanism of susceptibility to mucormycosis in diabetic ketoacidosis: transferrin and iron availability, *Diabetes*, 31, 1109, 1982.
31. Bauer, H., Ajello, L., Adams, E., and Hernandez, D., Cerebral mucormycosis: pathogenesis of the disease, *Am. J. Med.*, 18, 822, 1955.
32. Eisenberg, L., Wood, T., and Boles, R., Mucormycosis, *Laryngoscope*, 87, 347, 1977.
33. England, A. C., Weinstein, M., Ellner, J. J., and Ajello, L., Two cases of rhinocerebral zygomycosis (mucormycosis) with common epidemiologic and environmental features, *Am. Rev. Respir. Dis.*, 124, 497, 1981.
34. Gunson, H. H. and Bowden, D. H., Cerebral mucormycosis: report of a case, *Arch. Pathol.*, 60, 440, 1955.
35. Kurrein, P., Cerebral mucormycosis, *J. Clin. Pathol.*, 7, 141, 1954.
36. Latouche, C. J., Sutherland, T. W., and Telling, M., Rhinocerebral mucormycosis, *Lancet*, 2, 811, 1963.
37. Lecompte, P. M. and Meissner, W. A., Mucormycosis of the central nervous system associated with hemochromatosis, *Am. J. Pathol.*, 23, 673, 1947.
38. Maniglia, A. J., Mintz, D. H., and Novak, S., Cephalic phycomycosis: a report of eight cases, *Laryngoscope*, 92, 755, 1982.
39. Martin, F. P., Lukeman, J. M., Ranson, R. F., and Geppert, L. J., Mucormycosis of the central nervous system associated with thrombosis of the internal carotid artery, *J. Pediatr.*, 44, 437, 1954.
40. McNulty, J. S., Rhinocerebral mucormycosis, predisposing factors, *Laryngoscope*, 92, 1140, 1982.
41. Stratemeier, W. P., Mucormycosis of central nervous system: report of a case, *Arch. Neurol. Psychiat.*, 63, 179, 1950.
42. Succar, M. B., Nichols, R. D., and Burch, K. H., Rhinocerebral mucormycosis, *Arch. Otolaryngol.*, 105, 212, 1979.
43. Tanphaichitra, D., Rhinocerebral mucormycosis with emphasis on clinical diagnosis, altered host defensive mechanisms and management, *Postgrad. Med. J.*, 55, 622, 1979.
44. Yanagisawa, E., Friedman, S., Kundargi, R. S., and Smith, H. W., Rhinocerebral phycomycosis, *Laryngoscope*, 87, 1319, 1977.
45. Mayer, R. D., Agents of mucormycosis and related species, in *Principles and Practice of Infectious Diseases*, Mandell, G. L., Douglas, R. G., and Bennett, J. E., Eds., 2nd ed., John Wiley & Sons, New York, 1985, 1452.
46. Parfrey, N. A., Improved diagnosis and prognosis of mucormycosis: a clinico-pathologic study, *Medicine (Baltimore)*, 65, 113, 1986.
47. Gribetz, A. R., Chuang, M. T., Burrows, L., and Teirstein, A. S., Rhizopus lung abscess in renal transplant patient successfully treated by lobectomy, *Chest*, 77, 102, 1980.
48. Haim, S., Better, O. S., Lichtig, C., Erlik, D., and Barzilai, A., Rhinocerebral mucormycosis following kidney transplantation, *Isr. J. Med. Sci.*, 6, 646, 1970.
49. Hammer, G. S., Bottone, E. J., and Hirschman, S. Z., Mucormycosis in a transplant recipient, *Am. J. Clin. Pathol.*, 64, 389, 1975.
50. Kolbeck, P. C., Makhoul, R. G., Bollinger, R. R., and Sanfillipo, F., Widely disseminated Cunninghamella mucormycosis in an adult renal transplant patient: case report and review of the literature, *Am. J. Clin. Pathol.*, 83, 747, 1985.

51. Kline, M. W., Mucormycosis in children: review of the literature and report of cases, *Pediatr. Infect. Dis. J.*, 4, 762, 1985.
52. Meyer, R. D., Young, L. S., Armstrong, D., and Yu, B., Aspergillosis complicating neoplastic disease, *Am. J. Med.*, 54, 6, 1973.
53. Bruck, H. M., Nash, G., Foley, F. D., and Pruitt, B. A. J., Opportunistic fungal infection of the burn wound with Phycomycetes and *Aspergillus*: a clinical-pathogenic review, *Arch. Surg.*, 102, 476, 1971.
54. Baker, R. D., Pulmonary mucormycosis, *Am. J. Pathol.*, 32, 287, 1956.
55. Marchevsky, A. M., Bottone, E. J., Geller, S. A., and Giger, D. K., The changing spectrum of disease, etiology, and diagnosis of mucormycosis, *Hum. Pathol.*, 11, 457, 1980.
56. Matsushima, T., Soejima, R., and Nakashima, T., Solitary pulmonary nodule caused by phycomycosis in a patient without obvious predisposing factors, *Thorax*, 35, 877, 1980.
57. Medoff, G. and Kobayashi, G. S., Pulmonary mucormycosis, *N. Engl. J. Med.*, 286, 86, 1972.
58. Gale, A. M. and Kleitsch, W. P., Solitary pulmonary nodule due to phycomycosis (mucormycosis), *Chest*, 62, 752, 1972.
59. Rothstein, R. D. and Simon, G. L., Subacute pulmonary mucormycosis, *J. Med. Vet. Mycol.*, 24, 391, 1986.
60. Neame, P. and Raynor, D., Mucormycosis — a report of twenty-two cases, *Arch. Pathol.*, 70, 261, 1960.
61. Abramowitz, I., Fatal perforations of the stomach due to mucormycosis of the gastrointestinal tract, *S. Afr. Med. J.*, 38, 93, 1964.
62. Kahn, L. B., Gastric mucormycosis: report of a case with review of the literature, *S. Afr. Med. J.*, 37, 1265, 1963.
63. Levin, S. and Isaacson, C., Spontaneous perforation of the colon in the newborn infant, *Arch. Dis. Child.*, 35, 378, 1960.
64. Stein, A. and Schmaman, A., Rupture of the stomach due to mucormycosis, *S. Afr. J. Surg.*, 3, 123, 1965.
65. Sutherland, J. C. and Jones, T. H., Gastric mucormycosis: report of a case in a Swazi, *S. Afr. Med. J.*, 34, 161, 1960.
66. Watson, K. C., Gastric perforation due to the fungus Mucor in a child with kwashiorkor, *S. Afr. Med. J.*, 31, 99, 1957.
67. Mullens, J. E., Leers, W. D., and Smith, G. W., Phycomycosis involving the intestine and anterior abdominal wall: a case report, *J. Clin. Pathol.*, 13, 303, 1960.
68. Horowitz, A., Dinbar, A., and Tulcinsky, D. B., Isolated primary intestinal mucormycosis: a case report, *Isr. J. Med. Sci.*, 10, 1143, 1974.
69. McBride, R. A., Corson, J. M., and Dammin, G. J., Mucormycosis. Two cases of disseminated disease with cultural identification of *Rhizopus*: review of the literature, *Am. J. Med.*, 28, 832, 1960.
70. Deal, W. B. and Johnson, J. E., Gastric phycomycosis: report of a case and review of the literature, *Gastroenterology*, 57, 579, 1969.
71. Baker, R. D., Bassert, D. E., and Ferrington, E., Mucormycosis of the digestive tract, *Arch. Pathol.*, 63, 176, 1957.
72. Calle, S. and Klatsky, S., Intestinal phycomycosis (mucormycosis), *Am. J. Clin. Pathol.*, 45, 264, 1966.
73. Dannheimer, I. P., Fouche, W., and Nel, C., Gastric mucormycosis in a diabetic patient, *S. Afr. Med. J.*, 48, 838, 1974.
74. Deal, W. B. and Johnson, J. E., Gastric phycomycosis: report of a case and review of the literature, *Gastroenterology*, 57, 579, 1969.
75. Defeo, E., Mucormycosis of the colon, *Am. J. Roentgenol.*, 86, 86, 1961.
76. Gatling, R. R., Gastric mucormycosis in a newborn infant, *Arch. Pathol.*, 67, 249, 1959.
77. Lawson, H. H. and Schmaman, A., Gastric phycomycosis, *Br. J. Surg.*, 61, 743, 1974.
78. Moore, M., Anderson, W. A. D., and Everett, H. H., Mucormycosis of large bowel, *Am. J. Pathol.*, 25, 559, 1949.
79. Torack, R. M., Fungus infection associated with antibiotic and steroid therapy, *Am. J. Med.*, 22, 872, 1957.
80. Satin, A. A., Alla, M. D., Mahgoub, E. S., and Musa, A. R., Systemic phycomycosis, *Br. Med. J.*, 1, 440, 1971.
81. Fienberg, R. and Reisley, T. S., Mucormycotic infection of an arteriosclerotic thrombosis of the abdominal aorta, *N. Engl. J. Med.*, 260, 626, 1959.
82. Umbert, I. L. and Daniel Su, W. D., Cutaneous mucormycosis, *J. Am. Acad. Dermatol.*, 21, 1232, 1989.

83. Baker, R. D., The epidemiology of mucormycoses, in *The Epidemiology of Human Mycotic Disease*, Yousef, A. D., Ed., Charles C. Thomas, Springfield, IL, 1975, 197.

84. Tomford, J. W., Whittlesey, D., Ellner, J. J., and Tomaschefski, J. F., Invasive primary cutaneous phycomycosis in diabetic leg ulcers, *Arch. Surg.*, 115, 770, 1980.

85. Josefiak, E. J., Foushee, J. H. S., and Smith, L. C., Cutaneous mucormycosis, *Am. J. Clin. Pathol.*, 30, 547, 1958.

86. Wilson, C. B., Siber, G. R., O'Brien, T. F., and Morgan, A. P., Phycomycotic gangrenous cellulitis: a report of two cases and a review of the literature, *Arch. Surg.*, 111, 532, 1976.

87. Baker, R. D., Seabury, J. H., and Schneidan, J. D., Jr., Subcutaneous and cutaneous mucormycosis and subcutaneous phycomycosis, *Lab. Invest.*, 11, 1091, 1962.

88. Foley, F. D. and Schuck, J. M., Burn-wound infection with phycomycetes requiring amputation of hand, *JAMA*, 203, 596, 1968.

89. Gartenberg, G., Bottone, E. J., Keusch, G. T., and Weitzman, I., Hospital-acquired mucormycosis (*Rhizopus rhizopodiformis*) of skin and subcutaneous tissue: epidemiology, mycology and treatment, *N. Engl. J. Med.*, 299, 1115, 1978.

90. Jain, J. D., Markowitz, A., Khilanani, P. V., and Lauter, C. B., Localized mucormycosis following intramuscular corticosteroids: case report and review of the literature, *Am. J. Med. Sci.*, 275, 209, 1978.

91. Keys, T. F., Haldorson, A. M., Rhodes, K. H., Roberts, G. D., and Fifer, E. Z., Nosocomial outbreak of Rhizopus infections associated with elastoplast wound dressings — Minnesota, *Morbid. Mortal. Wkly. Rep.*, 27, 33, 1978.

92. Kramer, B. S., Hernandez, A. D., Reddick, R. L., and Levine, A. S., Cutaneous infarction: manifestation of disseminated mucormycosis, *Arch. Dermatol.*, 113, 1075, 1977.

93. Meyer, R. D., Kaplan, M. H., Ong, M., and Armstrong, D., Cutaneous lesions in disseminated mucormycosis, *JAMA*, 225, 737, 1973.

94. Nash, G., Foley, F. D., Goodwin, M. N., Jr., Bruck, H. M., Greenwald, K. A., and Pruitt, B. A., Jr., Fungal burn wound infection, *JAMA*, 215, 1664, 1971.

95. Rabin, E. R., Lundberg, G. D., and Mitchell, E. T., Mucormycosis in severely burned patients: report of two cases with extensive destruction of face and nasal cavity, *N. Engl. J. Med.*, 264, 1286, 1961.

96. Roberts, H. J., Cutaneous mucormycosis: report of a case with survival, *Arch. Intern. Med.*, 110, 108, 1962.

97. Sheldon, D. L. and Johnson, W. C., Cutaneous mucormycosis: two documented cases of suspected nosocomial cause, *JAMA*, 241, 1032, 1979.

98. Symmers, W. St. C., Silicon mastitis in "topless" waitresses and some other varieties of foreign body-mastitis, *Br. Med. J.*, 3, 19, 1968.

99. Veliath, A. J., Rao, R., Prabhu, M. R., and Aurora, A. L., Cutaneous phycomycosis (mucormycosis) with fatal pulmonary dissemination, *Arch. Dermatol.*, 112, 509, 1976.

100. Fisher, J., Tuazon, C. U., and Geelhoed, G. W., Mucormycosis in transplant patients, *Am. J. Surg.*, 46, 315, 1980.

101. Wong, B. D. and Armstrong, D., Clinical manifestations and management of mucormycosis in the compromised patient, in *Fungal Infections in the Compromised Patient*, Warnock, D. W. and Richardson, M. D., Eds., John Wiley & Sons, New York,. 1982, 155.

102. Boyce, J. M., Lawson, L. A., Lockwood, W. R., and Hughes, J. L., *Cunnughamella bertholletiae* wound infection of portable nosocomial origin, *South. Med. J.*, 74, 1132, 1981.

103. West, B. C., Kwong-Chung, K. J., King, J. W., Grafton, W. D., and Rohr, M. S., Inguinal abscess caused by *Rhizopus rhizopodiformis*: successful treatment with surgery and amphotericin B, *J. Clin. Microbiol.*, 18, 1384, 1983.

104. Patino, J. F., Mora, R., and Guzman, M. A., Mucormycosis: a fatal case by *Saksenaea vasiformis*, *World J. Surg.*, 8, 419, 1984.

105. Radentz, W. H., Opportunistic fungal infections in immunocompromised hosts, *J. Am. Acad. Dermatol.*, 20, 989, 1989.

106. Bateman, C. P., Umland, E. T., and Backer, L. E., Cutaneous zygomycosis in a patient with lymphoma, *J. Am. Acad. Dermatol.*, 8, 890, 1983.

107. Roberts, H. J., Cutaneous mucormycosis, *Arch. Intern. Med.*, 110, 146, 1962.

108. Dennis, J. E., Rhodes, K. H., Cooney, D. R., and Roberts, G. D., Nosocomial *Rhizopus* infection (zygomycosis) in children, *J. Pediatr.*, 96, 824, 1980.
109. Harahap, M., Subcutaneous phycomycosis, *Int. J. Dermatol.*, 25, 200, 1986.
110. Hutter, R. V. P., Phycomycetous infection (mucormycosis) in cancer patients: a complication of therapy, *Cancer*, 12, 330, 1959.
111. Baker, R. D., The epidemiology of mucormycosis, in *The Epidemiology of Human Mycotic Disease*, Aldoory, Y., Ed., Charles C. Thomas, Springfield, IL, 1975, 197.
112. Mamlok, V., Cowan, W. T., and Schnadig, V., Unusual histopathology of mucormycosis in acute myelogenous leukemia, *Am. J. Clin. Pathol.*, 88, 117, 1987.
113. Baker, R. D., Leukopenia and therapy in leukemia as factors predisposing to fatal mycosis: mucormycosis, aspergillosis, and cryptococcosis, *Am. J. Clin. Pathol.*, 37, 358, 1962.
114. Craig, J. M. and Farber, S., Development of disseminated visceral mucormycosis during therapy for acute leukemia, *Am. J. Pathol.*, 29, 601, 1953.
115. Cussen, L. J., Primary hypopituitary dwarfism with Fanconi's hypoplastic anemia syndrome, renal hypertension and phycomycosis: report of a case, *Med. J. Aust.*, 2, 367, 1965.
116. Gruhn, J. G. and Sanson, J., Mycotic infections in leukemic patients at autopsy, *Cancer*, 16, 61, 1963.
117. McBride, R. A., Corson, J. M., and Dammin, G. J., Two cases of disseminated disease with cultural identification of Rhizopus: review of the literature, *Am. J. Med.*, 28, 832, 1960.
118. Paltauf, A., Mycosis mucorina, *Virchows Arch. Pathol. Anat.*, 102, 543, 1885.
119. Parkhurst, G. F. and Vlahides, G. D., Fatal opportunistic fungus disease, *JAMA*, 202, 279, 1967.
120. Zimmerman, L. E., Fatal fungus infections complicating other disease, *Am. J. Clin. Pathol.*, 25, 46, 1955.
121. Khica, G. J., Berroya, R. B., Escano, F. B., and Lee, C. S., Mucormycosis in a mitral prosthesis, *J. Thorac. Cardiovasc. Surg.*, 63, 903, 1972.
122. Merchant, R. K., Louria, D. B., Geisler, P. H., Edgcomb, J. H., and Utz, J. P., Fungal endocarditis: review of the literature and report of three cases, *Ann. Intern. Med.*, 48, 242, 1958.
123. Caraveo, J., Trowbridge, A. A., Amaral, B., Green, J. B. III, Cain, P. T., and Hurley, D. L., Bone marrow necrosis associated with *Mucor* infection, *Am. J. Med.*, 62, 404, 1977.
124. Langston, C., Roberts, D. A., Porter, G. A., and Bennett, W. M., Renal phycomycosis, *J. Urol.*, 109, 941, 1973.
125. Hammer, G. S., Bottone, E. J., and Hirschman, S. Z., Mucormycosis in a transplant recipient, *Am. J. Clin. Pathol.*, 64, 389, 1975.
126. Bennett, J. E., Chemotherapy of systemic mycosis, *N. Engl. J. Med.*, 290, 30, 1974.
127. Stevens, D. A., Miconazole in the treatment of systemic fungal infections, *Am. Rev. Respir. Dis.*, 116, 801, 1977.
128. Meyers, B. R., Wormser, G., Hirschman, S. Z., and Blitzer, A., Rhinocerebral mucormycosis: premortem diagnosis and therapy, *Arch. Intern. Med.*, 139, 557, 1979.
129. Pastore, P. N., Mucormycosis of the maxillary sinus and diabetes mellitus: report of case with recovery, *South. Med. J.*, 60, 1164, 1967.
130. Pollock, R. A., Pratt, R. C., Shulman, J. A., and Turner, J. S., Nasal mucormycosis: early detection and treatment without radical surgery, or amphotericin B, *South. Med. J.*, 68, 1279, 1979.
131. Sandler, R., Tallman, C. B., Keamy, D. G., and Irving, W. R., Successfully treated rhinocerebral phycomycosis in well controlled diabetes, *N. Engl. J. Med.*, 285, 1180, 1971.
132. Pillsbury, H. C. and Fischer, N. D., Rhinocerebral mucormycosis, *Arch. Otolaryngol.*, 103, 600, 1977.
133. Hoeprich, P. D., *Infectious Diseases. A Treatise of Infectious Processes*, 3rd ed., Harper & Row, New York, 1983, 436.
134. Hamill, R., Oney, L. A., and Crane, L. R., Successful therapy for rhinocerebral mucormycosis with associated bilateral brain abscesses, *Arch. Intern. Med.*, 143, 581, 1983.
135. Berger, C. S., Disque, F. C., and Tapazian, R. G., Rhinocerebral zygomycosis: diagnosis and treatment, *Oral Surg.*, 40, 27, 1975.
136. Ferstenfeld, J. E., Cohen, S. H., and Rytel, M. W., Chronic rhinocerebral phycomycosis in association with diabetes, *Postgrad. Med. J.*, 53, 337, 1977.
137. Halderman, J. H., Cooper, H. S., and Mann, L., Chronic phycomycosis in a controlled diabetic, *Ann. Intern. Med.*, 80, 419, 1974.

138. DeSouza, R., MacKinnon, S., Spagnola, S. V., and Fossieck, B. E., Jr., Treatment of localized pulmonary phycomycosis, *South. Med. J.*, 72, 609, 1979.

139. Record, N. B., Jr. and Grinder, G. B., Pulmonary phycomycosis without obvious predisposing factors, *JAMA*, 235, 1256, 1976.

140. Ryan, M. E. and Ochs, J., Primary cutaneous mucormycosis: superficial and gangrenous infections, *Pediatr. Infect. Dis. J.*, 1, 110, 1982.

141. Baker, R. D., Mucormycosis — a new disease, *JAMA*, 163, 805, 1957.

142. Hall, J. C., Brewer, J. H., Reed, W. A., Steinhaus, D. M., and Watson, K. R., Cutaneous mucormycosis in a heart transplant patient, *Cutis*, 42, 183, 1988.

39 *Pneumocystis carinii*

39.1 INTRODUCTION

The taxonomy of *Pneumocystis carinii*, the causative agent of a highly contagious, epidemic, interstitial plasma cell pneumonia, particularly in infants, young children, and severely immuno-compromised patients, can be best described as uncertain.[1,2] Until recently, *Pneumocystis* was considered to be a unicellular parasite and classified as Protozoa based on various morphologic and ultrastructural studies,[3-5] chemical composition[6] (such as the lack of ergosterol in the plasma membrane), insensitivity to amphotericin B,[7] and responsiveness to antiprotozoal drugs.[8] Subsequently, Stringer et al.[9] and Edman et al.[10] have demonstrated that the 18S ribosomal gene sequence of *Pneumocystis* was more closely related to that of fungi rather than Protozoa, and have tentatively classified these organisms as Ascomycota. Further evidence to support such consideration came from the analysis and comparison of other *Pneumocystis* genes, including those of thymidylate synthase,[11] dihydrofolate reductase,[12] a P-type ATPase,[13] and a fungus-specific translation elongation factor 3 gene.[14]

As predicted earlier by electron microscopy of polyene antibiotic complexes[15] and the relative insensitivity of the pathogen to amphotericin B, results from studies on the sterol contents of *Pneumocystis* have confirmed that cholesterol has been its major sterol.[16] The lack of ergosterol in the *Pneumocystis* cell membrane would suggest a close relationships with the unique sterol and lipid compositions of the rust (*Cronartiium ribicola* and *Peridermium harkenessia*)[17,18] and smut fungi. Another important development in the sterol characterization of *Pneumocystis* was the presence of a Δ^7-double bond in the molecule of some C-24-alkylated sterols.[16] This latter capability is similar to that of rust fungi which are dominated by Δ^7-C-24-alkylated sterols.[19-21] However, the fact that contrary to other fungi which may have as many as 100 copies of their ribosomal locus, the phylogenetic analysis of *Pneumocystis* has revealed the presence of only one single ribosomal gene locus,[22] brings a certain degree of uncertainty about the correct taxonomy of this enigmatic pathogen and whether it should be considered as a diverse group of exotic fungi.[2,23,24]

The natural habitat of *P. carinii* is a variety of animals, including rats, mice, hares, dogs, cats, farm animals, as well as large and small primates. In addition to acutely and chronically ill animals, the *P. carinii* has been harbored by healthy animals.[25] *P. carinii* is thought to be transmitted by air, but soil must also be considered as a potential route of transmission.

As a pathogen, *P. carinii* was likely described for the first time by Chagas in 1909,[26] but it was not until 1951[27] when the organism was associated with several epidemics of intestinal plasma cell pneumonia among premature or malnourished infants. For many years afterwards, *Pneumocystis carinii* pneumonia (PCP, pneumocystic pneumonia) was primarily considered to be a disease of immunocompromised children,[28-33] especially those with severe combined immunodeficiency.[30,31] Parasitologic and serologic studies of *Pneumocystis* infection in healthy children have shown the presence of antibodies to *P. carinii* in most people by age 2 years,[34,35] indicating that primary infection is asymptomatic and that most clinical cases of pneumocystic pneumonia may be the result of reactivation of latent primary infection.[25] However, clusters of cases of interstitial plasma cell pneumonitis in infants[36-38] and PCP in cancer patients[34,39,40] have implied the possibility that patient-to-patient transmission may also occur.[25]

In humans, *P. carinii* exists in the lungs either as a small pleomorphic form (trophozoite) or a thick-walled cystic form (sporozoite). The latter carries up to eight daughter forms.[41] The organism propagates in the alveoli of some patients, causing acellular, eosinophilic, proteinaceous material containing cysts and trophozoites to accumulate, and damaging in the process the type I pneumocytes.[41] Most children are exposed to the pathogen by age 3 or 4 years.

With the advent of the AIDS pandemic in the last 15 years or so, the number of PCP cases has risen dramatically,[42-46] establishing *P. carinii* pneumonia as the first life-threatening opportunistic infection recognized in AIDS,[44-47] occurring as the initial manifestation in 50% to 60% of cases.[25,48,49] It has been estimated that as many as 80% of the AIDS patients may develop PCP at least once.[50,51] In addition, the incidence of PCP in patients with malignancies and other immunosuppressive diseases has also been on the rise.[52,53] Other underlying diseases predisposing to *P. carinii* pneumonia include organ transplantations, immunodeficiency disorders (affecting either cell-mediated or humoral immunity, or both),[29-33] malnutrition,[54,55] and collagen-vascular diseases.[56]

39.2   *PNEUMOCYSTIS CARINII* PNEUMONIA

The predominant and most important clinical manifestation of *P. carinii* infection is pneumonia.[57] Epidemic pneumocystic pneumonia in infants is generally insidious in onset.[25] Among the characteristic symptoms of the disease, restlessness and poor feeding have been observed at the earliest stage of the illness, followed by cyanosis and tachypnea.[58-60] Usually, the infection is presented with the same symptoms whether complicating cancer[61-63] or immunodeficiency states.[64-70] However, Kingsmore and Schwab[71] presented a case of subacute PCP in a transplant recipient with normal arterial oxygen tension and alveolar-arterial oxygen gradient, and normal findings on serial radiographs.

Studies by Epstein et al.[72] in AIDS patients have suggested that recurrences of PCP were more likely the result of new infection than to a relapse of prior disease.

In AIDS patients with pneumocystic pneumonia,[43,73,74] the clinical syndrome has an insidious onset with nonspecific symptoms (low-grade fever, chills, shortness of breath, mild, nonproductive cough, and dyspnea on exertion).[25] Additional symptoms may also include weight loss, malaise, and lymphadenopathy.[75] Compared to non-AIDS patients, the duration of symptoms in AIDS patients was on average longer (median: 28 d vs. 5 d).[73,76] There have been high mortality rates (as high as 50% to no survivors) among HIV-infected patients requiring mechanical ventilation for acute respiratory failure secondary to PCP.[77]

Several investigators[78,79] have shown that patients with Wagener's granulomatosis undergoing immunosuppressive therapy have an increased risk of developing PCP. In one of the studies,[78] the patients, who were all HIV-seronegative, were on a daily medication consisting of glucocorticosteroids and a second immunosuppressive therapy; consequently, lymphocytopenia appeared in all patients. Lymphocytopenia, coupled with lymphocyte and monocyte functional abnormalities caused by the glucocorticoids[80] may have been the most likely factor predisposing to PCP. This observation, which highlights the risk of opportunistic infections secondary to corticosteroid treatment, would make chemoprophylaxis against *P. carinii* exceedingly important.

There has been also a notable increase in the incidence of PCP in cancer patients, with potential for transmissibility of the infection.[61,62] The level of immunosuppression has played a critical role, especially the long-term (over 2 months) corticosteroid therapy.

39.2.1   SUBCLINICAL *P. CARINII* INFECTION

Over the years, subclinical infections, even though rare, have been well documented.[81-83] As demonstrated by several studies,[34,35,84] most adults and children have shown serologic evidence of occult infections with *P. carinii*.

39.2.2 Atypical Pulmonary Disease

Atypical pneumocystic pneumonia[73,85,86] may also present without chest X-ray abnormalities, dyspnea, or hypoxia, and cough being the only symptom,[73] or with subtle respiratory symptoms and resting or exercise-induced hypoxia but a normal chest X-ray.[25,85,86] Some of the more unusual radiologic findings[87] associated with atypical PCP include pleural effusion,[88] cavitating and noncavitating pulmonary nodules,[89-92] lobar pneumonia,[93] unilateral hyperlucent lung,[94] and bilateral upper lobe infiltrates.[95]

Atypical pulmonary manifestations of *P. carinii* infections in HIV-positive patients have also been associated with long-term prophylactic treatment with aerosolized pentamidine.[96,97]

39.2.3 Extrapulmonary *P. carinii* Infection

Extrapulmonary disease, usually as a complication of PCP,[29,98-121] has been well documented.[25] In non-AIDS patients, disseminated pneumocystic infections have been reported to involve lymph nodes, blood vessels, liver, spleen, heart, pericardium, thyroid, thymus, colon, small intestine, stomach, pancreas, kidney, adrenals, hard plate, and the retroperitoneum.[29,73,83,85,86,98-102,105-107] Occasionally, dissemination may afflict the bone marrow[99,110] and peripheral blood,[103] or present as disseminated granulomatous infection.[104] Eye involvement due to *P. carinii* has been rarely observed.[114,122-127]

In AIDS patients, PCP may very often disseminate to affect virtually all major organs.[25,112] Thus, pneumocystic infections complicating AIDS have been associated with otic polyps, otitis media, and mastoiditis,[111,113,119,128-130] retina[108] and choroiditis,[131,132] duodenum, esophagus, stomach, heart, pancreas, kidney, appendix, renal gland, and bone marrow,[11] temporal bone osteomyelitis,[120] thyroiditis,[118,133] and lesions involving the spleen,[115] liver, lymph nodes,[114] and the skin.[111] However, pleural effusions in PCP have been extremely rare.[134] There has been one report[135] of pleural pneumocystosis in an AIDS patient with PCP and bilateral pneumothorax, and another report[136] of an AIDS patient presenting with bilateral pleural effusions and no pneumothorax.

As reported on several occasions,[137-140] extrapulmonary *P. carinii* infection may often occur in those AIDS patients who receive aerosolized pentamidine prophylaxis because of its lack of systemic effect. As expected, dissemination has been strongly associated with severe immunosuppression.[141,142] Still unexplained low serum albumin levels have been observed in cases of hepatic *C. carinii* involvement.[143-145]

39.2.4 *P. carinii* Pneumonia Secondary to Methotrexate-Treated Rheumatoid Arthritis

Low-dose methotrexate has become an important treatment for rheumatoid and psoriatic arthritis.[146] In 1983, Perruquet et al.[147] have described the first case of *P. carinii* pneumonia in the setting of a low-dose weekly methotrexate therapy of rheumatoid arthritis. While other corroborating reports followed,[146,148-153] the exact pathophysiologic mechanism of this complication is still not known. Subsequently, Wallis et al.[154] have diagnosed *P. carinii* pneumonia complicating low-dose methotrexate treatment of psoriatic arthropathy.

Kane et al.[150] have reported a case of pneumocystic pneumonia associated with weekly parenteral methotrexate therapy (20 mg for 20 weeks for a total of 500 mg). The patient, who was HIV-negative, had a very low CD4+ count due to stage III squamous cell carcinoma of the larynx. Based on these and other studies,[147,151,152,154,155] it has been suggested that in patients with rheumatoid and psoriatic arthritis who receive low-dose (7.5 to 22.5 mg) weekly methotrexate medication, the possibility of developing PCP exists only when the total dose exceeds 400 mg.[150]

The first report of PCP secondary to cyclosporin A and methotrexate treatment of rheumatoid arthritis appeared in 1992.[156] Earlier,[157] it was suggested that in patients with chronic plaque psoriasis, some cyclosporin A metabolites may be synergistic to the side effects of the parent drug, and in patients with methotrexate-associated impairment of liver functions,[158,159] treatment with cyclosporin A would likely increase the likelihood of toxicity. However, the latter, although important in some patients, had not been necessarily the case in patients with no prior methotrexate-induced liver abnormalities.[156]

Apparently, methotrexate has the potential to parley more immunosuppressive activity than currently assumed, including effects on certain T lymphocyte subsets which may result in alterations of immune responses and increased susceptibility to opportunistic pathogens. Thus, Calabrese et al.[160] have examined peripheral lymphocyte subsets in 15 patients with active rheumatoid arthritis who were not receiving remittive therapy, as well as 33 controls. The results have demonstrated that patients with rheumatoid arthritis not only had a reduced percentage and number of CD4+/CD45RA naive T lymphocytes, but also a reduced percentage and number of CD8+ cells coexpressing the CD1 1b marker (suppressor/effector cells). Remarkably, the total number of CD8+ T lymphocytes was significantly lower in patients with rheumatoid arthritis treated for 8 weeks with methotrexate than untreated patients ($p < .05$). In another study, Houtman et al.[161] have determined the T lymphocyte subsets in a patient with rheumatoid arthritis who developed PCP while receiving treatment with low-dose methotrexate (7.5 to 15 mg weekly) in addition to D-penicillamine (750 mg daily for persistent high disease activity) and indomethacin (150 mg daily). While the percentage of total T cells (CD3+) and T helper/inducer cells (CD4+) did not differ from that of healthy controls, the number and percentage of naive T lymphocytes (CD4+ cells coexpressing CD45RA) and suppressor/effector T cells (CD8+ coexpressing CD1 1b), were clearly decreased as compared to controls (45 and 17/mm³, respectively, compared to 483 and 214/mm³, respectively, in normal controls). In addition, a significant decrease of the CD8+ subset titer was also observed (95 cells/mm³ vs. 524 cells/mm³ in normal controls).[161]

Sohen et al.[162] have also noted a decreased percentage of CD8+/CD45RA cells in the peripheral blood of patients with rheumatoid arthritis, even more pronounced in the synovial fluid.

The aforementioned findings have been corroborated in a mouse model where low-dose methotrexate treatment selectively inhibited Lyt-2+ cells in graft-versus-host reactions.[163]

39.3   STUDIES ON THERAPEUTICS

39.3.1   TRIMETHOPRIM–SULFAMETHOXAZOLE (CO-TRIMOXAZOLE, TMP-SMX)

Blaser et al.[164] have studied the serum pharmacokinetics of TMP-SMX in 23 patients during oral and intravenous treatment of PCP after daily doses of 15 to 22 mg/kg trimethoprim and 75 to 110 mg/kg sulfamethoxazole were given each every 6 h. Despite administration of a loading dose of twice the regular dose, serum trough concentrations continuously rose from 12 h to 96 h by 63% for trimethoprim and 102% for sulfamethoxazole. There was no difference in drug serum levels after oral or intravenous administration. However, large interindividual variability was observed despite weight-specific dosing.[164] Sulfamethoxazole levels of 100 to 150 µg/ml and trimethoprim levels of 5.0 to 8.0 µg/ml have been associated with successful therapy in non-AIDS patients.[165] Maintaining sulfamethoxazole levels below 200 µg/ml may reduce the incidence of leukopenia.[25]

Carr et al.[166] have examined a number of clinical, immunologic, and virologic variables to determine whether any of them will predict the development of hypersensitivity to TMP-SMX during treatment of pneumocystic pneumonia in AIDS patients. Results have shown that in 27% of patients, hypersensitivity occurred in those with significantly higher total lymphocyte and CD4+ and CD8+ cell counts, and CD4+:CD8+ ratios.

Lecuit et al.[140] have reported a case of an AIDS patient with hepatosplenic pneumocystosis who did not respond to treatment with TMP-SMX, most likely because of a drug-resistant strain.

39.3.1.1 Toxicity of Trimethoprim–Sulfamethoxazole

While co-trimoxazole has been the preferred agent for therapy and prophylaxis of PCP in HIV-infected patients, its frequent adverse side effects and greater incidence of hypersensitivity reactions[167-173] among HIV-infected patients may limit its usefulness.[174,175]

Adverse reactions to TMP-SMX have occurred in 50% to 100% of patients with AIDS,[176-180] especially among patients who received TMP-SMX both as treatment[168,177-186] and during prophylaxis,[159,176,187-191] prompting changes of therapy in as many as 57% of them.[178,179,181,183] However, in a prospective study of 1121 patients who received TMP-SMX, Jick[192] found that only 91 (8%) patients had developed adverse reactions. It has been noted in several other studies that patients in Zaire, Haiti, and among African-Americans had relatively lower incidence of adverse reactions,[193-195] whereas patients with CD4+ counts of less than 250 cells/mm^3 had a reduced risk of developing TMP-SMX hypersensitivity.[166] Some investigators have also found that patients receiving corticosteroids developed fewer adverse reactions to co-trimoxazole.[166,196-199]

As part of the adverse side effects of TMP-SMX, cutaneous eruptions occurred in 24% to 50% of the patients. They were characterized as generalized, maculopapular, and often intensely pruritic rashes which will develop 8 to 12 d after initiation of treatment, then reach maximal intensity 1 to 2 d later, and in some cases disappearing after 3 to 5 d despite continued treatment.[176-180] Severe rashes (mucous membrane-forming bullae, or intolerable pruritis) will require discontinuation of TMP-SMX therapy; the incidence of severe rashes has been between 0% and 20%.[159,176-179,182,184,188] Fever, which usually develops in conjunction with cutaneous eruptions, frequently resolves shortly thereafter despite continued therapy.[179]

Kelly et al.[169] have described a severe and unusual reaction in HIV patients, involving sudden fever and hypotension immediately after the administration of co-trimoxazole. The mechanism of this reaction, which occurred within approximately 2 weeks after completion of a previous course of the drug, may be associated with IgE-mediated anaphylaxis and cytokine (tumor necrosis factor-α)-mediated effects. Although the immunochemistry of allergic reactions to sulfonamides has not been fully understood, there has been evidence suggesting IgE mediation.[200-202] Marinac and Stanford[203] have reported a similar case in which an HIV-infected patient had received high doses of parenteral TMP-SMX approximately 5 weeks before rechallenge with oral TMP-SMX. On rechallenge, the patient experienced a progressively severe hypersensitivity reaction (facial and truncal rash) despite administration of antihistamines, corticosteroids, and epinephrine — nevertheless, there was rapid resolution of symptoms with no apparent sequalae.[173] Even though sulfonamide desensitization has been used successfully in HIV-positive patients,[204,205] severe reactions have still occurred during TMP-SMX desensitization.[206]

Additional side effects caused by TMP-SMX include nausea, vomiting, neutropenia, anemia, thrombocytopenia, and elevation in the aminotransferase level.[181] Less commonly observed toxicities have been hyponatremia, hyperkalemia,[207-209] azotemia, altered taste, resting tremor,[159,176,177,179-184,210] as well as toxic epidermal necrolysis,[211-213] and in AIDS patients, a severe, sepsis-like syndrome (hypotension, fever, rash, and pulmonary infiltrates on chest radiograms).[167,203,214-216]

Velazquez et al.[217] have examined the incidence and severity of hyperkalemia during trimethoprim therapy in AIDS patients, and found that trimethoprim acted in a fashion similar to that of amiloride, by blocking the apical membrane sodium channels in the mammalian distal nephron. As a result, the transepithelial voltage was reduced and the potassium secretion was inhibited. Decreased renal potassium excretion secondary to such direct effects on kidney tubules led to hyperkalemia in a substantial number of patients receiving trimethoprim-containing combinations.[217] In a particular example, Greenberg et al.[218] found that in HIV-infected patients treated for PCP, high daily doses of TMP-SMX (20 mg of TMP and 100 mg/kg of SMX) led to increase in the serum potassium concentrations and hyperkalemia. Malnutrition or cachexia, which are common in patients with advanced HIV infection, led to low rates of urea excretion, and according to Schreiber and Halperin,[219] one reason which may explain the trimethoprim-induced hyperkalemia is a low urea excretion rate that might diminish the delivery of tubular fluid to K+ secretory sites, thereby exacerbating the impact of the trimethoprim-mediated blockade of K+ secretion. In addition to AIDS patients, trimethoprim-induced hyperkalemia has also been seen in elderly patients receiving standard co-trimoxazole therapy.[220-222]

Several options exist for managing adverse reactions to TMP-SMX, namely continuous treatment through adverse reactions,[176,178,179,223-227] rechallenge, and desensitization.[181]

One example of continuous treatment through adverse reaction is to modify the TMP-SMX dose regimens in order to maintain drug serum levels considered to be safe (5.0 to 8.0 mg/l).[178] Other options, in particular to manage the hypersensitivity reactions, include changing the route of administration from intravenous to oral (despite prior occurrence of hypersensitivity reactions).[223]

Early administration of antihistamines[227] and antipyretics have also been used occasionally[223-225] — for example, concurrent therapy with diphenhydramine (25 mg orally, four times daily),[223,227] and acetaminophen.[223] In an open pilot trial, Gompels et al.[228] evaluated the safety and efficacy of ondansetron (8.0 mg orally, every 8 h) in blocking the nausea and vomiting in AIDS patients receiving co-trimoxazole. Good control of emesis and nausea was achieved in 69% and 47% of patients, respectively.

In the experience of some investigators, a high percentage of patients who have had and recovered from TMP-SMX adverse reaction can be successfully rechallenged without having recurrent adverse reactions.[181,185,188,226,229] However, there have been several reports of severe hypersensitivity reactions producing sepsis-like syndrome during rechallenge with TMP-SMX.[167,170,171,185,192,203,214-216]

One alternative option to rechallenge is for drug desensitization[181] by using gradually increasing doses of co-trimoxazole.[230-235] However, the current experience has been limited to small groups, and the many differences in the available desensitization protocols make interpretation of results difficult. In one such study,[229] 31 patients with a history of non-life-threatening hypersensitivity to TMP-SMX were treated with TMP (300 mg, twice a week, for 2 weeks), and if no major reaction occurred, continued on TMP-SMX medication (160 mg of TMP and 800 mg of SMX per tablet; one tablet, b.i.d.) twice a week. In patients where significant and persistent hypersensitivity had developed, the SMX was ceased and the patients were subsequently challenged with TMP-dapsone (300 mg and 100 mg, respectively) given twice weekly.[229] Sher et al.[234] have described a patient who developed anaphylactic shock during desensitization.

Intermittent dosing and supplementation with leucovorin (folinic acid) have been tried in attempts to improve patient tolerance towards co-trimoxazole. Bozzette et al.[236] have evaluated the value of intermittent prophylaxis with TMP-SMX and the effects of leucovorin in a randomized trial of 107 patients with advanced HIV disease (CD4+ counts of <200 cells/mm^3) and no history of pneumocystic pneumonia. The patients were given TMP-SMX either two or three times daily, with some of them also receiving leucovorin with each dose. All patients took zidovudine concurrently. The overall results suggested that intermittent therapy with TMP-SMX b.i.d., three times weekly was better tolerated than twice-daily regimen, and that leucovorin did not improve the tolerance for chronic TMP-SMX dosing in AIDS (even in AIDS patients receiving TMP-SMX daily). In another randomized, double-blind, placebo-controlled trial, 92 AIDS patients were given leucovorin in conjunction with TMP-SMX therapy.[237] Neither the frequency of dose-limiting toxicity (26% vs. 37%; $p = .4$) nor time to occurrence ($p = .7$) was linked to the leucovorin use. Surprisingly, the latter was associated with a higher rate of both therapeutic failure and death.

39.3.2 PENTAMIDINE

Pentamidine isethionate is an aromatic diamidine derivative structurally similar to some antiprotozoal agents, such as stilbamidine and propamidine. The mechanism of action of pentamidine isethionate is not precisely understood. However, experimental evidence provided strong indication that binding to DNA is the mode of action involved in its antiprotozoal activity.[238,239] Pentamidine has also the capacity to inhibit the release of cytokines from macrophages through a post-translational processing event.[240] Furthermore, in a murine model of endotoxemia (a disease with a pathophysiology that is clearly linked to host-produced cytokines), pentamidine was found to block the host inflammatory cytokine (TNF-α, IL-6) release.[241]

The ability to control the *Pneumocystis*-induced inflammation within the lung tissue may be one mechanism associated with the therapeutic activity of pentamidine against pneumocystic infection since both the pathogen and the inflammatory response it provokes probably contributed to acute reversible lung damage and eventually to the irrreversible distruction observed in some patients.[242,243]

Pentamidine isethionate when administered by the tracheal route to immunosuppressed rats with PCP showed higher serum concentrations than the control animals (309 ng/ml vs. 71 ng/ml at 20 min postadministration). The more rapid diffusion of pentamidine from the alveolar lumen to the pulmonary circulation may be explained by increased alveolocapillary permeability as the result of pneumocystosis.[244] Vinet et al.[245] have developed a clinically useful high-pressure liquid chromatographic procedure to determine serum pentamidine levels in AIDS patients.

39.3.2.1 Toxicity of Pentamidine

Common adverse reactions associated with pentamidine include azotemia, renal failure, leukopenia, thrombocytopenia, nausea, orthostatic hypotension, hyperglycemia (which may be irreversible and will require insulin), and hypoglycemia (more common in patients with renal dysfunction, or those receiving higher total dose).[25,246]

The frequent occurrence of bronchospasm due to aerosolized pentamidine may reduce its delivery to distal airways and produce therapy-limiting symptoms. To circumvent this unwarranted side effect, McSharry et al.[247] have successfully treated HIV-positive patients prophylactically with β-agonist aerosol before ensuing aerosolized pentamidine application; the bronchodilating prophylaxis eliminated the pentamidine-induced symptoms. In another study, Renzi et al.[248] have observed accelerated mortality following bilateral pneumothoraces in AIDS patients receiving secondary prophylaxis with aerosolized pentamidine.

TABLE 39.1
Drug Therapies for *P. carinii* Infections

Drug	Dose (Daily)	Route of Administration
Trimethoprim–sulfamethoxazole	TMP: 15–20 mg/kg SMX: 100 mg/kg	Intravenous or oral (divided into 3–4 doses)
Pentamidine isethionate	3.0–4.0 mg/kg 600 mg	Intravenously[a] or aerosol
Atovaquone	750 mg, t.i.d.	Oral
Dapsone–trimethoprim[b]	Dapsone: 100 mg TMP: 15–20 mg/kg	Oral (TMP divided into 3–4 doses)
Clindamycin–primaquine[b]	Clindamycin: 600 mg, t.i.d. Primaquine: 30 mg (as base)	Oral
Trimetrexate–leucovorin	Trimetrexate: 45 mg/m² Leucovorin: 80 mg/m²	Intravenous

[a] Intramuscular administration may be painful and associated with sterile abscess formation. Higher total doses of parenteral pentamidine may lead to hypoglycemia.[453]

[b] Recommended for patients intolerant to TMP-SMX.

Gearhart and Bhutani[249] have reported intravenous pentamidine-induced bronchospasm in an AIDS patient which required antihistamine and aerosolized β-agonist therapy. Intravenous pentamidine was also reported to cause fasting hypoglycemia and azotemia, most likely resulting from high pentamidine serum concentrations,[250,251] as well as localized cutaneous reactions.[252] Other side effects associated with intravenous pentamidine isethionate included gastrointestinal discomfort, pancreatitis,[253-255] cardiotoxicity,[256,257] and nephro- and hepatotoxicities.[258]

Treatment with pentamidine isethionate has also been associated with ventricular tachyarrhythmias, including *torsades de pointes*.[259-266] The latter term (from French, "fringe of pointed tips") refers to an unusual ventricular arrhythmia described as a sinusoidal rhythm of ventricular complexes that were twist around the isoelectric line with irregular beat-to-beat cycle lengths.[267,268] Most frequently, *torsades de pointes* is drug-induced either as idiosyncrasy or as a toxic effect. Other causes include electrolyte abnormalities (hypokalemia, hypomagnesemia, hypocalcemia), cardiac disease,[269] autonomic and central nervous system disorders, hypothermia, and toxins. *Torsades de pointes*, which may occur on average 10 d after the pentamidine treatment (either intravenous[261,263,264] or inhaled) was commenced, may be related to serum magnesium levels where hypomagnesemia may synergistically induce torsades. Accordingly, early magnesium supplementation may be helpful.[270] Associated hypokalemia or hypocalcemia may also be a cause or exacerbating factor in the development of *torsades de pointes*. In addition, it was also suggested that pentamidine may induce *torsades de pointes* by triggering early after-depolarizations, especially in the context of bradycardia and a long QT interval.[266,271]

Pentamidine has an extremely long serum half-life and may be detected 6 to 8 weeks after discontinuation of therapy.[261] Renal failure may prolong its half-life even further. If myocardial elimination of the drug parallels that of the liver and kidney, it can explain the persistence of electrophysiologic abnormalities for long periods (days and even weeks) after pentamidine therapy has ceased.[261,262]

Pais et al.[272] reported a case of an AIDS patient who, following treatment with intravenous pentamidine, suffered a massive spontaneous hemorrhage caused by a rupture of a pancreatic pseudocyst after pentamidine-induced pancreatitis. The patient presented with symptomatic hypoglycemia, severe nephrotoxicity, and hyperkalemia while not receiving any other drug but pentamidine.

39.3.3 PENTAMIDINE ANALOGS

A number of pentamidine-related analogs have shown antipneumocystic activity in a rat model of PCP.[239,273] One of the more active compounds, the 1,3-di[4-(2-imidazolinyl)-2-methoxy-phenoxy]propane, was found to be nearly 10-fold more potent than pentamidine, as well as orally active.[274,275] Further evidence was presented to indicate correlation of antimicrobial activity with the ability to bind to AT-rich regions in the minor groove of DNA.[276,277]

A series of structurally related dicationically substituted bis-benzimidazoles, also known for their potent DNA-binding properties,[278,279] were studied for activity in a rat model of pneumocystic pneumonia. One of the compounds, the 1,4-bis[5-(2-imidazolinyl)-2-benzimidazolyl]butane, when given at daily oral doses of 25 mg/kg was found to be more potent than pentamidine (no antipneumocystic activity was discerned at doses of up to 40 mg/kg).[280] Toxicity consistent with acute hypotension, as well as vascular damage near the injection site and necrosis of the surrounding tissue (upon intravenous administration) may be potential problems.

39.3.4 ATOVAQUONE

Initially developed as an antimalarial drug, the hydroxynaphthoquinone derivative atovaquone (BW 566C80) has also shown activity against other protozoans, as well as *P. carinii*.[238,239,281-283] The drug is highly lipophilic and, therefore, with low water solubility. In *Plasmodium* species, the mechanism of action of atovaquone was associated with its ability to block the electron transport at the cytochrome$_{bc\ 1}$ complex (complex III) resulting in inhibition of nucleic acids and ATP synthesis, and, ultimately, cell death.[284]

For still unexplained reasons, the steady-state plasma concentrations of atovaquone in AIDS patients were approximately one third to one half the levels in asymptomatic HIV-infected individuals.[285] The plasma concentration-time profile of atovaquone, which is double-peaked (the first peak occurring at 1 to 8 h and the second peak at 24 to 96 h after ingestion), suggested enterohepatic cycling. The drug seemed not to be metabolized in humans, and its mean half-life in normal volunteers was 2.9 d, and 2.2 d in AIDS patients.[285]

An immunosuppressed rat model was used to compare the therapeutic efficacies of atovaquone (at daily doses of 25, 50, and 100 mg/kg by gavage) and TMP-SMX (50 mg/kg TMP and 250 mg/kg SMX, daily).[286] After 3 weeks of treatment, histologic examination of the lung showed the presence of pneumocystic pneumonia in 20% of rats treated with TMP-SMX but none in animals treated with 100 mg/kg daily of atovaquone.

To date, only erythromycin has been shown to interfere with the activity of atovaquone. Thus, in an immunosuppressed rat model, a combination therapy of erythromycin (100 mg/kg daily) and atovaquone (10 mg/kg daily) provided only 30% protection of animals, compared with 100% of atovaquone alone, and 100% incidence of PCP with erythromycin alone.[287]

Pharmacokinetic and safety studies of atovaquone in patients with AIDS have demonstrated that at doses as high as 2.0 g daily, the drug was well tolerated with only erythematous maculopapular rash observed occasionally.[288]

39.3.5 COMPOUND PS-15

Compound PS-15, a new biguanide dihydrofolate reductase inhibitor, was evaluated for its antipneumocystic activity in an immunosuppressed rat model.[289] PS-15 when given orally for 7 weeks at daily doses of 5.0 and 25 mg/kg, prevented *P. carinii* infection in all (100%) animals; the same 100% prevention was observed when the drug was administered at a single weekly dose of 50 mg/kg. When PC-15 was given orally for 3 weeks to immunosuppressed rats with *P. carinii* pneumonia at daily doses of 25, 5.0, and 1.0 mg/kg, complete resolution of infection occurred in 100%, 67%, and 75% of rats, respectively. The drug was well tolerated at all dose regimens.

39.3.6 SULFONAMIDES

Alder et al.[290] have observed therapeutic synergy with combined use of clarithromycin and sulfamethoxazole in the treatment of experimental *P. carinii* infection in immunosuppressed rats.

39.3.7 TRIMETREXATE

Trimetrexate is a highly lipophilic analog of methotrexate, and a new nonclassic antifolate known for its strong binding to parasite dihydrofolate reductase. Because of its lipid solubility, it has the ability to readily cross both the mammalian and protozoan cell membranes independent of the folate membrane transport system.[291] Since *P. carinii* lacks this transport system, it is not susceptible to the classic folate agents, such as methotrexate and leucovorin.

Allegra et al.[292] evaluated trimetrexate by assessing the concentrations needed to inhibit the reaction catalyzed by *P. carinii* dihydrofolate reductase in specimens collected from homogenized rat lung. Trimetrexate and methotrexate were 1,500- and 28,000-fold more potent than trimethoprim, showing IC$_{50}$ values of 26.1 and 1.4 nmol, respectively.

In the host, trimetrexate is metabolized by oxidative demethylation and conjugation with glucuronic acid. The glucuronide metabolite is then excreted into the bile to account for 75% of the dose determined in isolated, perfused rat liver.[291] The pharmacokinetic profile of trimetrexate has been studied in both AIDS[291] and cancer[293-297] patients. All pharmacokinetic parameters, although highly variable in different patients, appeared to correlate well in both groups and fit a multicompartmental model with terminal half-life of up to 12 h. The drug was cleared both hepatically and renally with up to 41% of it excreted unchanged in the urine. Smit et al.[298] have studied the trimetrexate efficacy and pharmacokinetics during treatment of refractory *Pneumocystis carinii* in an infant with severe combined immunodeficiency syndrome.

39.3.8 BILOBALIDE

Bilobalide, a sesquiterpene isolated from leaves of *Gingko biloba,* has inhibited *in vitro* and *in vivo* the growth of *P. carinii.*[299] The compound was as effective as trimethoprim–sulfamethoxazole in suppressing *P. carinii* cultured on human embryonic lung fibroblasts. In an immunosuppressed rat model, intraperitoneal administration of bilobalide at 10 mg/kg for 8 d, lowered the number of organisms by 99% (approximately 2 logs) with no apparent toxicity.

39.3.9 8-AMINOQUINOLINE DERIVATIVES

A number of 8-aminoquinoline analogs (primaquine, WR6026, and WR238605) were found effective in the therapy or prophylaxis of PCP in rat models following either intermittent or continuous administration.[300] For treatment of PCP these drugs have shown detectable effects when administered once every 4 d (primaquine and WR6026 at doses greater than 8.0 mg/kg, and WR238605 at doses of over 2.0 mg/kg). For prophylaxis, WR6026 and WR238605 were effective given alone daily (WR6026 at doses greater than 0.25 mg/kg, and WR238605 at doses greater than 0.57 mg/kg). Intermittent administration of WR6026 and WR238605 at 4.0 mg/kg (once every 4 d) as prophylaxis for PCP was as effective as daily administration of co-trimoxazole.[300]

39.3.10 SYNERGISTIC ANTI-*P. CARINII* ACTIVITY

Drug synergism has been a significant factor in the development of antimicrobial therapies against PCP, although the cellular, biochemical, and molecular mechanisms for the synergistic effects are still unknown. For example, studies by Kluge et al.[301] in rats have demonstrated that while trimethoprim had no discernible anti-*P. carinii* effect and sulfamethoxazole had only a modest effect, the combination of these drugs was synergistic and highly effective in the treatment and prevention of pneumocystic pneumonia.[302]

Combination of trimethoprim and dapsone (which itself was only moderately effective against *P. carinii*) was also synergistic.[303] Similarly, pyrimethamine was inactive when given alone, but its combination with a sulfonamide drug has shown therapeutic value.[304]

Queener et al.[305] have reported another example of synergistic activity involving clindamycin and primaquine; while, respectively, inactive and weakly active, the combination of these two drugs was active in both *in vitro* and *in vivo* experiments in a rat model *P. carinii* infection. In another example, in AIDS patients with *P. carinii pneumonia,* trimetrexate plus sulfadiazine was more active than trimetrexate alone.[306]

Hughes and Killmar[307] have effectively prevented PCP in 90% of immunosuppressed rats following daily oral administration of 100 mg erythromycin and 300 mg/kg of sulfisoxazole. All of the untreated controls and erythromycin-treated animals developed the infection, and 80% of rats given sulfisoxazole alone had the pneumonitis. The erythromycin–sulfisoxazole ratio of 1:3 was the most effective of several dose combinations tested. No data available can explain the synergistic effect of erythromycin, although its neutrophil-motility-enhancing capability may play a role in augmenting the host response and clearance of the pathogen.[307]

Walzer et al.[308] have described synergistic combinations against *P. carinii* consisting of high-dose (100 mg/kg daily) dihydrofolate reductase inhibitors (Ro 11-8958, trimethoprim, diaveridine) and fixed low-dose dapsone (25 mg/kg daily) or sulfamethoxazole (3.0 mg/kg daily). For example, when Ro 11-8958 (a trimethoprim analog with improved antimicrobial and pharmacokinetic properties) was administered with dapsone, the combination reduced the cyst count over 1000-fold. The combination of Ro 11-8958 at 20 mg/kg daily with dapsone (25 mg/kg daily) lowered the cyst count by only 100- to 200-fold.

39.4 EVOLUTION OF THERAPIES AND TREATMENT OF *PNEUMOCYSTIS CARINII* PNEUMONIA

In spite of the wide use of various antiretroviral agents[309] and PCP prophylaxis,[176,310,311] *P. carinii* pneumonia still remains an important opportunistic infection in HIV-positive patients.[242] It is often characterized with high morbidity and mortality rates, especially in patients with rapidly progressive respiratory failure.[312-314] *P. carinii* organisms have been shown to persist throughout therapy for pneumocystic pneumonia.

Trimethoprim–sulfamethoxazole and parenteral pentamidine isethionate have been the two drugs considered to be most important for the therapy and prophylaxis of *P. carinii* infections in both AIDS and non-AIDS patients (Table 39.1).[73,74,315-317] Even though TMP-SMX is associated with side effects in a remarkably high number of AIDS patients (60% to 100%), the observed toxicity is often not severe, allowing for the drug therapy to be continued.[73,177,226,316,318-320] Hughes et al.[321,322] and others[323-326] have found that trimethoprim–sulfamethoxazole was also effective against pneumocystic pneumonia in immunocompromised children.

Trimethoprim (TMP), an inhibitor of dihydrofolate reductase, and sulfamethoxazole (SMX), an inhibitor of dihydropteroate synthetase, are administered concurrently either intravenously or orally at daily total doses of 20 mg/kg of TMP and 100 mg/kg of SMX divided in three or four doses. Intravenous administration is preferable as initial treatment of more severe cases of pneumonitis, but oral therapy is feasible after several days as well as in mild cases where there is no gastrointestinal dysfunction to interfere with drug absorption.[318,319,327] The adverse effect may be less severe or less frequent when dosage is decreased to 15 mg/kg of TMP and 75 mg/kg of SMX without reducing efficacy.[318]

Based on the initial classification of *P. carinii* as a protozoan, pentamidine, an established antitrypanosomal and antileishmanial agent, was the first successful drug used to treat pneumocystic pneumonia.[328] The drug can be safely administered by slow intravenous infusion over 60 min.[329,330] Aerosolized pentamidine has been another route of administration that is better tolerated than TMP-SMX but may not be as effective as parenteral treatment in cases of extensive airspace consolidation.[331,332] Intramuscular injection, which is painful and may cause sterile abscess formation, is not usually necessary and should be avoided.[25,333] The recommended total daily dose of pentamidine is 4.0 mg/kg, given once daily. However, in patients with mild pneumocystic pneumonia, doses of 3.0 mg/kg could be equally effective and less toxic.[330]

Aerosolized pentamidine seems to be effective in cases of mild cases of pneumocystic pneumonia because of reduced toxicity compared to parenteral administration.[25] However, there has been considerable difference in the recommended total daily dose regimens — 4.0 mg/kg in one report,[330] and 600 mg daily in another.[334] The response rates to these two regimens were also different — 70% (9 of 13 patients) and 87% (13 of 15 patients) for the 4.0-mg/kg and 600-mg daily regimens, respectively. Furthermore, there were three relapses for the 4.0-mg/kg dose, and none for the 600-mg daily dose. In terms of toxicity, with the exception of bronchospasm (especially in smokers), the aerosolized pentamidine seemed to be devoid of adverse side effects usually associated with parenteral pentamidine therapy.[25] The mode of drug delivery appears to be critically important for therapeutic efficacy since nebulizers that did not produce droplet particles of 2 to 3 μm in size were unable to deliver adequate drug concentrations to the pulmonary parenchyma.[335] In addition, the optimal pentamidine dose may also vary with the nebulizer.[145] Finally, there have been concerns that aerosolization may increase the incidence of atypical pulmonary disease[95] due to *P. carinii* or extrapulmonary pneumocytosis.[318,336]

With the exception of one report,[114] all other cases of *P. carinii*-induced choroiditis[122-127] have developed in the setting of aerosolized pentamidine prophylaxis following PCP. The recommended treatment of pneumocystic choroiditis consisted of intravenous administration of trimethoprim (20 mg/kg daily) together with either sulfamethoxazole (100 mg/kg daily) or pentamidine (4.0 mg/kg daily).[124,125] In most cases, the choroidal lesions gradually decreased in size.

The clinical efficacies and safety of TMP-SMX and pentamidine have been compared in a large prospective, randomized trial in AIDS patients.[337] Daily doses of TMP-SMX (20 mg/kg of TMP and 100 mg/kg of SMX) and pentamidine (4.0 mg/kg) were administered intravenously for 3 weeks. Failure to complete therapy was common, and survival rates were similar in both groups.

Lentino and Brooks[338] have described a rare case of an HIV-seronegative patient with tuberculosis who developed pneumocystic pneumonia but with no evidence of idiopathic CD4+ T lymphopenia syndrome. The latter immune disorder has been identified in several other patients, who in the absence of HIV infection had developed PCP as a consequence of their lymphopenia.[339-342] The patient was successfully treated with TMP-SMX (320 and 1600 mg, respectively, intravenously every 6 h) concurrently with antituberculosis therapy, and remained well 10 years after the initial presentation with pneumocystic pneumonia.[338]

While extrapulmonary pneumocystosis has been reported in a number of tissues (most often in patients receiving aerosolized pentamidine prophylaxis), Jayes et al.[343] have reported a unique case of disseminated pneumocystosis presenting as a pleural effusion without apparent lung involvement. The patient was successfully treated with a combination therapy consisting of chest tube drainage, intravenous (4.0 mg/kg daily) and inhaled (600 mg daily) pentamidine, dapsone (100 mg daily, orally), and trimethoprim. The addition of inhaled pentamidine to intravenously administered pentamidine may have increased the pleural fluid levels substantially by transfer across the inflamed pleural membrane, or through air leak of the hydropneumothorax, thus coinciding with the patient's improvement.[343]

Price et al.[344] have observed a dramatic response within 48 h (resolution of X-ray changes and improvement in gas exchange) in an AIDS patient given combined therapy of clarithromycin (500 mg, b.i.d.) and high-dose co-trimoxazole; initial treatment for 2 weeks with oxygen, intravenous co-trimoxazole, and steroids provided little objective clinical improvement.

Atovaquone has been approved by the U.S. Food and Drug Administration as a second-line therapeutic for use in the treatment of mild to moderate pneumocystic pneumonia in patients intolerant to TMP-SMX.[281] An open-label dose-escalation phase I/II study has confirmed that atovaquone is effective in treating mild to moderate PCP in AIDS patients.[345] After a 2-week therapy, improvement was observed in 85% of patients, and in 79% of them the treatment was considered a success, as defined by successful completion of therapy, improvements in all abnormal signs and symptoms, and no requirement for anti-PCP agent other than atovaquone.

In a multicenter, randomized, double-blind study of 408 AIDS patients lasting for 3 weeks, the activity of atovaquone was compared with that of TMP-SMX.[184] The patients received either 750 mg of oral atovaquone or oral TMP-SMX (320 and 1600 mg, respectively; two double-strength tablets, t.i.d.). The rates of therapeutic success did not differ substantially between the two drug regimens (62% and 64% for atovaquone and TMP-SMX, respectively); the corresponding failure rates were 20% and 7%, respectively ($p = .002$). It is important to note that the therapeutic efficacy of atovaquone was closely related to its steady-state concentrations: 98% success rate in patients with plasma concentrations of over 15 µg/ml, and 89% in those with drug levels exceeding 10 µg/ml (79% of the total patient population), as compared with only 69% success rate in patients with drug plasma concentrations of less than 15 µg/ml, and 50% in those with less than 10 µg/ml. It should be emphasized that the best way to achieve maximum bioavailability of atovaquone is to administer the drug with food and in the absence of underlying conditions (diarrhea) that may undermine its absorption. The most common side effects seen with atovaquone include rash, nausea, and diarrhea. Whereas atovaquone was less effective than TMP-SMX, it has been associated with fewer treatment-limiting adverse effects.[184]

The therapeutic efficacies of oral atovaquone (750 mg, t.i.d.) and intravenous pentamidine (3.0 to 4.0 mg/kg, once daily) were compared in a 3-week multicenter, randomized, open-label trial involving a small number of AIDS patients with mild to moderate pneumocystic pneumonia.[346] The results have shown that the therapeutic efficacies of the two drugs were similar, but atovaquone elicited significantly fewer treatment-limiting adverse side effects. Nevertheless, some investigators[347] strongly disagreed with the conclusion that both drugs are comparable because of the relatively small number of patients involved, and perceived flaws in determining the failure rate of atovaquone treatment.

In addition to atovaquone and pentamidine, other alternative therapies to treat pneumocystic pneumonia in patients with history of intolerance to TMP-SMX included trimethoprim-dapsone, clindamycin-primaquine, and rechallenge or desensitization (or both) with TMP-SMX.[348,349]

Trimethoprim combined with dapsone (an inhibitor of dihydropteroate synthetase) was also found to be effective as conventional therapy of AIDS patients with mild to moderate *P. carinii* pneumonia.[317,350] The enzyme dihydropteroate synthetase has been specifically associated with the *Pneumocystis* organism by blocking the incorporation of *p*-aminobenzoic acid during the first step of folate biosynthesis.[351,352] Although at doses of 25 and 125 mg/kg dapsone showed total efficacy in eradicating extensive pneumonitis in a rat model of pneumocystosis,[353] it was ineffective in treating pneumocystic pneumonia in AIDS patients when administered alone.[354] However, there has been an excellent clinical response rate of 100% when it was combined with trimethoprim.[317]

In a more recent double-blind, randomized study,[179] a combination of dapsone (100 mg daily) and trimethoprim (20 mg/kg daily), while as effective as daily administration of TMP (20 mg/kg)–SMX (100 mg/kg) in treating mild to moderate first episodes of PCP, was much better tolerated. Nonetheless, dapsone-associated methemoglobulinemia has been observed in most patients.[179] The toxicity of dapsone has been dose-related.[317] Daily dapsone doses of 100 mg in otherwise normal patients and 50 mg in those patients with glucose-6-phosphate dehydrogenase deficiency did not cause hemolysis, as compared to larger doses which have been frequently associated with this abnormality.[355] Less common side effects of dapsone include leukopenia, dermatitis, an infectious mononucleosis-like syndrome, abnormal liver function, peripheral neuropathy, and renal papillary necrosis.[353] Metroka et al.[356] have described a successful (13 out of 14 HIV-infected patients) desensitization protocol carried over 42 d.

The antipneumocystic activity of clindamycin in combination with primaquine was first documented by Queener et al.[305] In subsequent trials, the clinical efficacy and the response rate in initial and salvage therapy of PCP have been excellent (78% to 93%).[357-359] Adverse side effects associated with clindamycin–primaquine therapy included bone marrow depression, maculopapular rashes, increased liver enzyme levels (serum aspartate transaminase, alanine transaminase, alkaline phosphatase, bilirubin), gastrointestinal disorders, and methemoglobulinemia (usually at daily doses of 30 mg).[360-362] The most serious toxicity of primaquine has been associated with intravascular hemolytic anemia in patients with glucose-6-phosphate dehydrogenase deficiency — it was observed at daily doses of ≥15 mg (primaquine base).[361] The side effects of clindamycin were usually associated with diarrhea.[363]

In a randomized, double-blind pilot trial, Toma et al.[364] evaluated the toxicity and tolerability of clindamycin–primaquine combination vs. TMP-SMX as primary therapy for pneumocystic pneumonia in AIDS patients. Because of the small number of patients (n = 65) studied, the clinical efficacy was not the primary focus of the trial. No significant differences were documented in the outcome, duration of survival, length of the PCP-free interval, and the relapse rate. The overall toxicity of the clindamycin–primaquine combination was less than that of TMP-SMX.[364]

Noskin et al.[365] did a retrospective review of 26 patients who received clindamycin–primaquine therapy for PCP after conventional treatment had failed or was not tolerated; clindamycin (800 mg every 8 h) was administered intravenously after which oral primaquine (30 mg) was instituted on alternate days. The success rate was 86%, with erythematous rash being the most common adverse effect.

The combination of pyrimethamine and sulfadiazine has also been used in the therapy of PCP based on previously observed activity in a rat model.[366] However, the response was not encouraging, with only 31% of treated patients surviving.[367-372]

Trimetrexate, one of several inhibitors of *P. carinii* dihydrofolate reductase,[351,373,374] elicited a 63% to 71% response with or without sulfadiazine as initial or salvage therapy in AIDS patients with pneumocystic pneumonia.[306] Because of its ability to enter and harm host cells, trimetrexate needs to be administered with calcium leucovorin. The latter, being a reduced folate, is taken preferentially by the host cells, thereby countering the effect of trimetrexate.[25] The preferred therapeutic daily regimen of trimetrexate that is currently under investigation is 30 to 45 mg/m^3 administered intravenously as a single dose for up to 21 d.[41] There has been no specific direction for the dosing of leucovorin but current protocols recommend 30 mg/m^3 IV or orally for 24 d when patients are receiving trimetrexate for 21 d. According to Sattler et al.,[375] a 45-mg/m^2 daily dose of trimetrexate with 80 mg/m^2 daily of leucovorin resulted in the least dosage-modifying toxicity and excellent efficacy.

Among the side effects of trimetrexate, transient neutropenia or thrombocytopenia, and mild elevation of serum aminotransferase levels have been observed in approximately 25% of patients. When used alone as initial therapy for PCP, trimetrexate was associated with high relapse rate (60%).[25] During phase II trials in cancer patients, Grem et al.[376] have observed hypersensitivity reactions to trimetrexate. Immediate hypotension with loss of consciousness occurred in only one patient, but immediate systemic effects (facial flushing, fever, shaking, pruritis, bronchospasm, periorbital edema, and difficulty in swallowing) were more common.

α-Difluoromethylornithine (DFMO, eflornithine), a specific inhibitor of ornithine decarboxylase, was found to be moderately effective as salvage therapy against pneumocystic pneumonia in several studies of AIDS patients.[377-380] In a compassionate treatment of AIDS patients who were intolerant to and/or unresponsive to conventional TMP-SMX or pentamidine therapy,[381] a full course of treatment consisted of daily intravenous administration of 400 mg/kg of eflornithine (but no more than 30 g daily) in four divided doses for 10 d, followed by 4 d of oral administration at 300 mg/kg daily (in four divided doses), and then up to 6 weeks at 300 mg/kg daily in four divided oral doses where tolerated. Of the 33 patient-episodes, 15 patients were discharged without need of supplemental oxygen after receiving 10 or more days of parenteral therapy. The most serious side effects of eflornithine were leukopenia, thrombocytopenia (in 12 of 19 patients), as well as anorexia, nausea, and diarrhea.[317,381]

In a prospective, open-labeled trial, co-trimoxazole (3.84 g intravenously, b.i.d.) and eflornithine (400 mg/kg daily as a continuous intravenous infusion) were compared as primary treatment for first-episode PCP in AIDS patients.[382] Only 39% of patients treated with eflornithine and 40% of those receiving co-trimoxazole successfully completed therapy; overall, eflornithine was the less effective of the two drugs.

39.4.1 ADJUNCTIVE CORTICOSTEROID THERAPY FOR *P. CARINII* PNEUMONIA

Even though the exact mechanism of the potential therapeutic effect of corticosteroids has not been elucidated,[383] data from various case reports, small series, and several randomized trials[197,198,384-398] have indicated beneficial effects (lower number of respiratory failures and mortality rates[198,392-394]) after using corticosteroids as adjunctive therapy for pneumocystic pneumonia in AIDS patients with moderate to severe pulmonary dysfunctions (initial arterial oxygen partial pressure of less than 70 mmHg, or an alveolar-arterial gradient greater than 35 mmHg on room air). Thus, in a prospective, double-blind, placebo-controlled trial in AIDS patients with first episode of mild PCP, Montaner et al.[399] have assessed the effect of oral prednisone given at 60 mg/kg daily dose for 1 week, followed by a progressive tapering over 14 d. The oral corticosteroid therapy prevented early deterioration and increased the exercise tolerance of the patients as defined by pulse oximetry.

Studies on the pathogenesis of PCP have suggested the presence of an intense inflammatory component in the disease,[400] which may be reduced by the modulatory effects of corticosteroids. The mechanism by which corticosteroids improve the outcome of AIDS patients with severe PCP is still not elucidated. To this end, Huang and Eden[401] found that lipopolysaccharide-stimulated alveolar macrophages from patients receiving corticosteroids released significantly less IL-1β and TNF-α than alveolar macrophages from nontreated AIDS patients.

A consensus report[402] has been issued backing the use of corticosteroids as adjunctive therapy to pneumocystic pneumonia. However, this recommendation has not been universally accepted and doubts still persist whether adjunctive corticosteroid therapy should be applied to all patients.[403-405] The expressed reluctance to use adjunctive corticosteroid therapy has arisen from findings indicating that the known immunosuppressive properties of corticosteroids (reducing the T lymphocyte population by cytokine suppression) has the potential of causing more harm than benefits in already immunocompromised patients, thereby becoming risk factors for pneumocystis pneumonia,[406-408] other opportunistic pathogens,[403-405] and infections.[198] Theoretically, steroids could exacerbate non-PCP pulmonary infections, so it is important to confirm the diagnosis if they are to be used.[196] For example, with the increased incidence of multidrug-resistant tuberculosis in HIV-infected patients,[409] the empiric use of corticosteroids for undifferentiated pulmonary disease may eventually mask and delay treatment of pulmonary disorders caused by other pathogens, thereby increasing the risk to patients. In addition, corticosteroids have been known to cause malignancies,[410,411] as well as to precipitate PCP in animal models.[412-414] Additional side effects of corticosteroids include gastrointestinal hemorrhages, hyperglycemia, and neuropsychiatric abnormalities.[196]

Walmsley et al.[196] have presented results from a multicenter, randomized, double-blind, and placebo-controlled trial of AIDS patients with pneumocystic pneumonia that contradicted the aforementioned consensus report.[402] The results of this study indicated that corticosteroids (40 mg of parenteral methylprednisolone, b.i.d.) when used as an adjunctive therapy, did not significantly affect the outcome of pneumocystic pneumonia in HIV-positive patients, although they might have lowered the incidence of hypersensitivity reactions (fever and rash) that eventually will require discontinuation of TMP-SMX therapy.

In the majority of studies in which beneficial effects (prevention of death and respiratory failure) have been demonstrated, adjunctive corticosteroid therapy was evaluated in the early treatment of moderate to severe cases of pneumocystic pneumonia.[198,392,394] The one study that evaluated the late application of corticosteroids failed to demonstrate meaningful benefit.[415] After reexamination of the data obtained in the study by Walmsley et al.,[196] Bozzette and Morton[416] concluded that, while the suggested therapy may have narrowed the scope of potential benefits from early adjunctive corticosteroid treatment in acute pneumocystic pneumonia, it did not provide convincing new evidence suggesting harm from corticosteroids either.

In addition to different dose regimens, duration, and timing of corticosteroid therapy, other factors, such as the differences in study populations, entry criteria applied, protocol procedures (blinded vs. unblinded[198,394]), and the medical care of patients at different hospitals and at different times,[417,418] may have influenced the effectiveness of the corticosteroids, thereby explaining the differences in clinical outcome. Furthermore, as demonstrated by univariate and multivariate analyses, specific characteristics of patients may also be important in determining the response of PCP to antimicrobial therapy.[196]

Infants with congenitally acquired HIV infection who presented with acute respiratory failure (ARF) secondary to pneumocystic pneumonia were reported to have high morbidity and mortality rates (50% to 90%).[419-422] At present, there is no consensus regarding the use of corticosteroids in infants with pneumocystic pneumonia.[402] In two studies by Sleasman et al.[423] and Barone et al.,[424] the use of early adjunctive corticosteroid therapy did reduce the morbidity and mortality in HIV-infected infants with PCP and ARF. In the study by Barone et al.,[424] the four infants (CD4$^+$ counts ranging from 148 cells/mm^3 to 918 cells/mm^3) started to receive adjunctive methyl-prednisolone therapy (2 mg/kg daily, divided into four doses) immediately after the diagnosis of PCP was confirmed.[424] Three of the infants who completed a 21-d course of TMP-SMX, received high-dose corticosteroid for 5 d; the dosage was then tapered over the next 3 weeks. The fourth child's treatment was switched to pentamidine (4.0 mg/kg daily) after 9 d because of the clinical failure of treatment with TMP-SMX; the severely ill infant received high-dose corticosteroid for 10 d, followed by a tapered dose over the next 3 weeks. No apparent side effects of corticosteroid therapy (gastrointestinal hemorrhage, hyperglycemia) was observed in any of these patients, and all infants from both studies[423,424] have survived.

39.4.2 Prophylaxis For *P. carinii* Pneumonia

Prophylactic treatment of HIV-infected patients against *P. carinii* pneumonia with either TMP-SMX or aerosolized pentamidine should start when the CD4$^+$ cell counts fall below 200 cells/mm^3.[425-428] It has been suggested that appropriate antiretroviral therapy when combined with PCP prophylaxis will prolong the survival of HIV-infected patients in addition to slowing the progression to AIDS.[429,430] However, several issues related to the progress of the HIV infection (survival bias, validity of confidence interval, and comparison with previous results[431]) still remain controversial.[432-434]

The efficacy of trimethoprim–sulfamethoxazole as the preferred choice for prophylaxis of pneumocystic pneumonia has been well documented.[159,176,187,188,435] One recommended treatment consisted of trimethoprim at 160 mg daily plus sulfamethoxazole at 800 mg daily.[425] Other regimens, such as 80 mg of TMP and 400 mg of SMX,[436] have also been applied successfully.

MacGregor et al.[437] have investigated the efficacy and tolerance of intermittent (three times weekly) vs. daily co-trimoxazole prophylaxis for PCP in HIV-infected patients with CD4$^+$ counts of less than 200 cells/mm.^{3} Double-strength co-trimoxazole tablets (160 mg and 800 mg of TMP and SMX, respectively) were administered orally once or twice daily, three times weekly, or 7 d a week in a nonrandomized manner based on physician preference. In the thrice-weekly group, an equal number of patients received once- or twice-daily dosing. Most patients received concomitant zidovudine (500 to 1200 mg daily). The results of the trial confirmed that while both drug regimens were equavalent, the intermittent thrice-weekly co-trimoxazole prophylaxis may lower the cost and reduce dose-related toxicity.[437]

Metroka et al.[438] reported that prophylaxis with oral dapsone (25 mg, four times daily) was equally effective as daily TMP-SMX regimen in preventing pneumocystic pneumonia; only 10% of patients receiving dapsone experienced adverse reactions, as compared to 38% of those on TMP-SMX prophylaxis. Other studies[439,440] have also corroborated the efficacy of dapsone prophylaxis.

In a prospective, randomized, open-label study conducted by Blum et al.,[441] dapsone (100 mg daily) and TMP-SMX (160 and 800 mg/kg of TMP and SMX, respectively, daily) were administered orally to AIDS patients (CD4$^+$ counts of <200 cells/mm^3) as primary prophylaxis. Both therapies were found to be efficacious, but each was associated with significant toxicity.

The clinical efficacy and safety of two intermittent regimens (co-trimoxazole and dapsone–pyrimethamine) for simultaneous primary prevention of *P. carinii* pneumonia and toxoplasmosis in AIDS patients was studied in a prospective, randomized, and open trial by Podzamczer et al.[442] The patients (CD4 counts of <200 cells/mm^3) were randomized to receive either co-trimoxazole (160 mg TMP and 800 mg SMX, b.i.d., three times weekly) or dapsone (100 mg) plus pyrimethamine (25 mg) once weekly. Data from clinical and biological evaluation confirmed that at the doses given, dapsone–pyrimethamine was inferior to TMP-SMX in preventing the first episodes of pneumocystic pneumonia; both regimens prevented toxoplasmosis equally well.[442]

Two other studies were designed to compare the efficacy of primary prophylaxis against both PCP and toxoplasmosis in AIDS patients. Girard et al.[443] evaluated the effects of dapsone (50 mg daily)–pyrimethamine (50 mg weekly) combination and aerosolized pentamidine (300 mg per month). The data have shown that for primary prevention of PCP, dapsone–pyrimethamine was as effective (though not as well tolerated) as aerosolized pentamidine. Dapsone–pyrimethamine also prevented the first episodes of toxoplasmosis.[443] In the other study, Koppen et al.[444] assessed the effects of aerosolized pentamidine vs. fansidar (pyrimethamine–sulfadoxine), both regimens applied for either primary or secondary prophylaxis. Fansidar prophylaxis was recommended over aerosolized pentamidine for patients with history of pneumocystic pneumonia or toxoplasmosis, as well as for all HIV-infected patients with CD4$^+$ counts of <100 cells/μl; in patients with CD4$^+$ lymphocyte counts between 100 cells/μl and 200 cells/μl, aerosolized pentamidine prophylaxis appeared to be more beneficial.[444]

In an open, controlled, randomized trial, Jensen et al.[445] have evaluated the efficacy of a biweekly dose regimen of 60 mg aerosolized pentamidine (used with System 22 nebulizer) as primary prophylaxis for pneumocystic pneumonia. While the treatment was beneficial in reducing the impact on morbidity, there was no difference in the survival rates. In another study, Ong et al.[446] assessed the efficacy and effects on pulmonary function tests of once-weekly 600-mg doses of aerosolized pentamidine against primary and secondary (previously proven episodes of infection) prophylaxis for PCP. The treatment was well tolerated and effective in both settings.

Tullis et al.[447] have studied the long-term effects of aerosolized pentamidine on the pulmonary function. Their data, although collected from a small sample size, suggested that there was no clinically significant change of pulmonary function associated with the use of aerosolized pentamidine for up to 76 weeks.

Prophylaxis with oral co-trimoxazole or inhaled pentamidine successfully prevented *P. carinii* pneumonia in HIV-infected children.[448,449] Thus, a retrospective chart review of HIV-infected infants revealed that primary prophylaxis with TMP-SMX in the first year of life (median age, 3 months; median duration, 5.5 months) was highly effective in preventing PCP and prolonging the survival rate.[450] Aerosolized pentamidine as prophylaxis therapy against pneumocystic pneumonia in children with leukemia was well tolerated even by very young patients and may be of benefit to all immunosuppressed children unable to use TMP-SMX prophylaxis.[448]

Mallolas et al.[191] have conducted an open randomized trial in HIV-infected patients to compare the efficacy and tolerance of aerosolized pentamidine (300 mg every 4 weeks), co-trimoxazole (160 and 800 mg for TMP and SMX, respectively, three times weekly), and dapsone–pyrimethamine (100 and 25 mg, respectively, twice weekly) as primary prophylaxis for initial episodes of *P. carinii* pneumonia. While both co-trimoxazole and dapsone–pyrimethamine regimens were nearly as effective as the aerosolized pentamidine in preventing the first episode of PCP, the aerosolized pentamidine was better tolerated.[191]

In an immunosuppressed rat model, atovaquone given prophylactically at 100 mg/kg daily by gavage, completely prevented *P. carinii* pneumonia.[284,286,287]

The issue of prophylaxis against PCP in patients with refractory rheumatoid arthritis receiving cyclosporin A in combination with other immunosuppressive drugs (methotrexate) should be approached with caution because of potentially increased susceptibility to opportunistic infection.[156,161]

Murphy et al.[451] reported a fatal case of *P. carinii* pneumonia in a child with nephrotic syndrome secondary to focal segmental glomerulosclerosis who was treated with pulse methylprednisolone and chlorambucil, raising the issue of harm-vs.-benefit of PCP prophylaxis for these patients.

Yet another setting where effective prophylaxis against PCP should be viewed with caution is for patients with intracranial neoplasms receiving long-term corticosteroid therapy.[452]

39.5 REFERENCES

1. Kovacs, J. A. and Masur, H., Advances in the biology and immunology of *Pneumocystis carinii*, in *Parasitic Diseases*, Leech, J. H., Sande, M. A., and Root, R. K., Eds., Churchill Livingstone, New York, 1988, 177.
2. Yoshida, Y., Ultrastructural studies of *Pneumocystis carinii*, *J. Protozool.*, 36, 53, 1989.
3. Balachandran, I. M., Jones, D. B., and Humphrey, D. M., A case of *Pneumocystis carinii* in pleural fluid with cytologic, histologic, and ultrastructural documentation, *Acta Cytol.*, 34, 486, 1990.
4. Bouton, C., Kernbaum, S., Christol, D., Trinh Dinh, H., Vezinet, F., Gutman, L., Seman, M., and Bastin, R., Diagnostic morphologique de *Pneumocystis carinii*, *Pathol. Biol.*, 25, 153, 1977.
5. Vossen, M. E. M. H., Beckers, P. J. A., Meuwissen, J. E. H. T., and Stadhouders, A. M., Developmental biology of *Pneumocystis carinii*, an alternative view on the life cycle of the parasite, *Z. Parasitenkd.*, 55, 101, 1978.
6. Kaneshiro, E. S. and Sleight, R. G., Biochemistry of *Pneumocystis carinii*, in *Lung Biology in Health and Disease:* Pneumocystis carinii *Pneumonia*, 2nd ed., Walzer, P. D., Ed., Marcel Dekker, New York, 1994, 69.
7. Walzer, P. D., Development of new anti-*Pneumocystis carinii* drugs: cumulative experience at a single institution, in *Lung Biology in Health* and *Disease:* Pneumocystis carinii *Pneumonia*, 2nd ed., Walzer, P. D., Ed., Marcel Dekker, New York, 1994, 511.
8. Barton, E. G. and Campbell, W. G., *Pneumocystis carinii* in lungs of rats treated with cortisone acetate, *Am. J. Pathol.*, 54, 209, 1969.
9. Stringer, S. L., Stringer, J. R., Blase, M. A., Walzer, P. D., and Cushion, M. T., *Pneumocystis carinii*: sequence from ribosomal RNA implies a close relationship with fungi, *Exp. Parasitol.*, 68, 450, 1989.
10. Edman, J. C., Kovacs, J. A., Mansur, H., Santi, D., Elwood, J., and Sogin, M. L., Ribosomal RNA genes of *Pneumocystis carinii*, *J. Protozool.*, 36, 18S, 1989.
11. Edman, U., Edman, J. C., and Santi, D., Isolation and expression of the *Pneumocystis carinii* thymidate synthase gene, *Proc. Natl. Acad. Sci. U.S.A.*, 86, 6503, 1989.
12. Edman, J. C., Edman, U., Cao, M., Lungren, J. D., and Kovacs, J. A., Isolation and expression of the *Pneumocystis carinii* dihydrofolate reductase gene, *Proc. Natl. Acad. Sci. U.S.A.*, 86, 8625, 1989.
13. Meade, J. C., Smulian, A. G., Stringer, S. L., and Stringer, J. R., Characterization of TF IID and ATPase from isolates of *Pneumocystis*, *J. Protozool.*, 38, 69S, 1991.
14. Ypma-Wong, M. F., Fonz, A., and Buck, G. A., Fungus specific translation elongation factor 3 gene present in *Pneumocystis carinii*, *Infect. Immun.*, 60, 4140, 1992.
15. Yoshikawa, H., Morioka, H., and Yoshida, Y., Freeze-fracture localization of filipin-sterol complexes in plasma- and cyto-membranes of *Pneumocystis carinii*, *J. Protozool.*, 34, 131, 1987.
16. Kaneshiro, E. S., Jayasimhulu, K., Ellis, J. E., and Beach, D. H., Evidence for the presence of "metabolic sterols" in *Pneumocystis*: identification and initial characterization of *Pneumocystis carinii* sterols, *J. Eukaryot. Microbiol.*, 41, 78, 1994.
17. Bruns, T. D., Vigalys, R., Barns, S. M., Gonzalez, D., Hibbett, D. S., Lane, D. J., Simon, L., Stickel, S., Szaro, T. M., Weisberg, W. G., and Sogin, M. L., Evolutionary relationship within the fungi: analysis of nuclear small subunit rRNA sequences, *Mol. Phys. Evol.*, 1, 231, 1992.
18. Wilmotte, A., van de Peer, Y., Goris, A., Chapelle, S., de Baere, R., R., Nelissen, B., Neefs, J.-M., Hennebert, G. L., and de Wachter, R., Evolutionary relationship among higher fungi inferred from small ribosomal subunit RNA sequence analysis, *J. Syst. Appl. Microbiol.*, 16, 436, 1993.
19. Lin, H.-K., Langenbach, R. J., and Knoche, H. W., Sterols of *Uromyces phaseoli* uredospores, *Phytochemistry*, 11, 2319, 1972.
20. Nowak, R., Kim, W. K., and Rohringer, R., Sterols of healthy and rust-infected primary leaves of wheat and of non-germinated and germinated uredospores of wheat stem rust, *Can. J. Bot.*, 50, 185, 1972.
21. Weete, J. D., Structure and function of sterol in fungi, *Adv. Lipid Res.*, 23, 115, 1989.
22. Giuntoli, D., Stringer, S. L., and Stringer, J. R., Extraordinarily low number of ribosomal RNA genes in *P. carinii*, *J. Eukaryote Microbiol.*, 41, 88S, 1994.
23. Stringer, J. R., The identity of *Pneumocystis carinii*: not a single protozoan, but a diverse group of fungi, *Infect. Agents Dis.*, 2, 109, 1993.

24. Proceedings of the First International Symposium and Workshop on *Pneumocystis carinii*, Richards, F. F., Walzer, P. D., and Kaneshiro, E. S., Organizers, *J. Protozool.*, 36, 2S, 1989.

25. Lipschik, G. Y. and Masur, H., *Pneumocystis carinii* pneumonia (PCP), in *Progress in Clinical Parasitology*, Vol. 2, Sun, T., Ed., Field and Wood, New York, 1991, 27.

26. Chagas, C., Nova tripanomiazeae humana: ueber eine neve trypanomiasis de menschen, *Mem. Inst. Oswaldo Cruz*, 1, 159, 1909.

27. Vanek, J., Atypical interstitial pneumonia of infants produced by *Pneumocystis carinii*, *Cas. Lek. Cesk.*, 90, 1121, 1951.

28. Walzer, P. D., Krogstad, D. J., Rawson, P. G., and Schultz, M. G., *Pneumocystis carinii* pneumonia in the United States: epidemiologic, diagnostic, and clinical features, *Ann. Intern. Med.*, 80, 83, 1974.

29. Burke, B. A. and Good, R. A., *Pneumocystis carinii* infection, *Medicine (Baltimore)*, 52, 23, 1973.

30. Walzer, P. D., Schultz, M. G., Western, K. A., and Robbins, J. B., *Pneumocystis carinii* pneumonia and primary immune deficiency diseases of infancy and childhood, *J. Pediatr.*, 82, 416, 1973.

31. Leggiadro, R. J., Winkelstein, J. A., and Hughes, W. T., Prevalence of *Pneumocystis carinii* pneumonitis in severe combined immunodeficiency, *J. Pediatr.*, 99, 96, 1981.

32. Rao, C. P. and Gelfand, E. W., *Pneumocystis carinii* pneumonitis in patients with hypogamma-globulinemia and intact T cell immunity, *J. Pediatr.*, 103, 410, 1983.

33. Lederman, H. and Winkelstein, J. A., Congenital agammaglobulinemia: the clinical course of 88 patients, *Pediatr. Res.*, 17, 254A, 1983.

34. Meuwissen, J. H., Tauber, I., Leeuwenberg, A. D., Beckers, P. J., and Sieben, M., Parasitologic and serologic observations of infection with pneumocystis in humans, *J. Infect. Dis.*, 136, 43, 1977.

35. Pifer, L. L., Hughes, W. T., Stagno, S., and Woods, D., *Pneumocystis carinii* infection: evidence for high prevalence in normal and immunosuppressed children, *Pediatrics*, 61, 35, 1978.

36. Ammich, O., Uber de nichtsyphilitische pneumonie des ersten kindesalters, *Virchows Arch. Pathol. Anat.*, 302, 539, 1938.

37. Benecke, F., Eigenartige bronchioleherkraukung im ersten lebensjahr, *Verh. Dtsch. Ges. Pathol.*, 31, 402, 1938.

38. Feyrter, E., Uber eine eigenartige form interstitieller lungenentzundung beim säugling und kleinkind, *Munch. Med. Wochenschr.*, 86, 835, 1939.

39. Singer, C., Armstrong, D., Rosen, P. P., and Schottenfeld, D., *Pneumocystis carinii* pneumonia: a cluster of eleven cases, *Ann. Intern. Med.*, 82, 772, 1975.

40. Ruebush, T. K., Weinstein, R. A., Baehner, R. L., Wolff, D., Bartlett, M., Gonzales-Crussi, F., Sulzer, A. J., and Schultz, M. G., An outbreak of pneumocystis pneumonia in children with acute lymphocytic leukemia, *Am. J. Dis. Child.*, 132, 143, 1978.

41. Amsden, G. W., Kowalsky, S. F., and Morse, G. D., Trimetrexate for *Pneumocystis carinii* pneumonia in patients with AIDS, *Ann. Pharmacother.*, 26, 218, 1992.

42. Coolfont Report, A PHS plan for prevention and control of AIDS and the AIDS virus, *Public Health Rep.*, 101, 341, 1986.

43. Hopewell, P. C., *Pneumocystis carinii* pneumonia: diagnosis, *J. Infect. Dis.*, 137, 1115, 1988.

44. Gottlieb, M. S., Schroff, R., Schanker, H. M., Weisman, J. D., Fan, P. T., Wolf, E. A., and Saxon, A., *Pneumocystis carinii* pneumonia and mucosal candiasis in previously healthy homosexual men: evidence of a new acquired cellular immunodeficiency, *N. Engl. J. Med.*, 305, 1425, 1981.

45. Masur, H., Michelis, M. A., Greene, J. B., Onorato, I., Vande Stouwe, R. A., Holzman, R. S., Wormser, G., Brettman, L., Lange, M., Murray, H. W., and Cunningham-Rundles, S., An outbreak of community-acquired *Pneumocystis carinii* pneumonia: initial manifestation of cellular immune dysfunction, *N. Engl. J. Med.*, 305, 1431, 1981.

46. Centers for Disease Control, Pneumocystic pneumonia — Los Angeles, *Morbid. Mortal. Wkly. Rep.*, 30, 250, 1981.

47. Centers for Disease Control, Kaposi's sarcoma and pneumocystic pneumonia among homosexual men — New York City and California, *Morbid. Mortal. Wkly. Rep.*, 30, 305, 1981.

48. Curran, J. W., Morgan, W. M., Hardy, A. M., Jaffe, H. W., Darrow, W. W., and Dowdle, W. R., The epidemiology of AIDS: current status and future prospects, *Science*, 229, 1352, 1985.

49. Centers for Disease Control, Update: acquired immunodeficiency syndrome — United States, *Morbid. Mortal. Wkly. Rep.*, 34, 245, 1985.

50. Centers for Disease Control, Update: acquired immunodeficiency syndrome — United States, *Morbid. Mortal. Wkly. Rep.*, 35, 542, 1986.
51. Murray, J. F., Garay, S. M., Hopewell, P. C., Mills, J., Snider, G. L., and Stover, D. G., NHLBI workshop summary: pulmonary complications of the acquired immune deficiency syndrome: an update, *Am. Rev. Respir. Dis.*, 135, 504, 1987.
52. Hughes, W. T., *Pneumocystis carinii* pneumonitis, *N. Engl. J. Med.*, 317, 1021, 1987.
53. Haron, E., Bodey, G. P., Luna, M. A., Dekmezian, R., and Elting, L., Has the incidence of *Pneumocystis carinii* pneumonia in cancer patients increased with the AIDS epidemic? *Lancet*, 2, 904, 1988.
54. Dutz, W., Post, C., Vessal, K., and Kohout, E., Endemic infantile *Pneumocystis carinii* infection: the Shiraz study, *Natl. Cancer Inst. Monogr.*, 43, 31, 1976.
55. Hughes, W. T., Price, R. A., Sisko, F., Havron, W. S., Kafatos, A. G., Schonland, M., and Smythe, P. M., Protein-calorie malnutrition: a host determinant for *Pneumocystis carinii* pneumonia, *Am. J. Dis. Child.*, 128, 44, 1974.
56. Hughes, W. T., *Pneumocystis carinii* pneumonia, in *Infections and the Compromised Host: Clinical Correlations and Therapeutic Approaches*, 2nd ed., Allen, J. C., Ed., Williams & Wilkins, Baltimore, 1981, 91.
57. Hughes, W. T., Pneumocystis carinii *Pneumonitis*, CRC Press, Boca Raton, 1987.
58. Gajdusek, D. C., *Pneumocystis carinii* — etiologic agent of interstitial plasma cell pneumonia of premature and young infants, *Pediatrics*, 19, 543, 1957.
59. Dutz, W., Jennings-Khodadad, E., Post, C., Kohout, E., Nazarian, I., and Esmaili, H., Marasmus and *Pneumocystis carinii* pneumonia in institutionalized infants, *Z. Kinderheilkd.*, 117, 241, 1974.
60. Gleason, W. A., Roden, V. J., and Decastro, E., Pneumocystis pneumonia in Vietnamese infants, *J. Pediatr.*, 87, 1001, 1975.
61. Varthalitis, I. and Meunier, F., *Pneumocystis carinii* pneumonia in cancer patients, *Cancer Treat. Rev.*, 19, 387, 1993.
62. Varthalitis, I., Aoun, M., Daneau, D., and Meunier, F., *Pneumocystis carinii* pneumonia in patients with cancer: an increasing incidence, *Cancer*, 71, 481, 1993.
63. Sepkowitz, K. A., *Pneumocystis carinii* pneumonia among patients with neoplastic disease, *Semin. Respir. Dis.*, 7, 114, 1992.
64. Hughes, W. T., Sanyal, S. K., and Price, R. A., Signs, symptoms, and pathophysiology of *Pneumocystis carinii*, *Natl. Cancer Inst. Monogr.*, 43, 77, 1976.
65. Lipson, A., Marshall, W. C., and Hayward, A. R., Treatment of *Pneumocystis carinii* in children, *Arch. Dis. Child.*, 52, 314, 1977.
66. Bernstein, C. N., Kolodny, M., Block, E., and Shanahan, F., *Pneumocystis carinii* pneumonia in patients with ulcerative colitis treated with corticosteroids, *Am. J. Gastroenterol.*, 88, 574, 1993.
67. Liam, C. K. and Wang, F., *Pneumocystis carinii* pneumonia in patients with systemic lupus erythematosus, *Lupus*, 1, 379, 1992.
68. Tuan, I. Z., Dennison, D., and Weisdorf, D. J., *Pneumocystis carinii* pneumonitis followed bone marrow transplantation, *Bone Marrow Transplant.*, 10, 267, 1992.
69. Lim, K. L., Powell, R. J., and Johnston, I. D., *Pneumocystis carinii* pneumonia following immuno-suppressive therapy in systemic lupus erythematosus, *Br. J. Rheumatol.*, 31, 643, 1992.
70. Porter, D. R., Marshall, D. A. S., Madhok, R., Capell, H., and Sturrock, R. D., *Pneumocystis carinii* infection complicating cytotoxic therapy in two patients with lymphopenia, but a normal total white cell count, *Br. J. Rheumatol.*, 31, 71, 1992.
71. Kingsmore, S. F. and Schwab, S. J., Pneumonia due to *Pneumocystis carinii* in a transplant recipient with normal arterial oxygen tension and normal radiographic findings, *South. Med. J.*, 86, 1052, 1993.
72. Epstein, L. J., Meyer, R. D., Antonson, S., Strigle, S. M., and Mohsenifar, Z., Persistence of *Pneumocystis carinii* in patients with AIDS receiving chemoprophylaxis, *Am. J. Respir. Crit. Care Med.*, 150 (5 part 1), 1456, 1994.
73. Kovacs, J. A., Hiemenz, J. W., Macher, A. M., Stover, D., Murray, H. W., Shelhamer, J., Lane, H. C., Urmacher, C., Honig, C., Longo, D. L., Parker, M. M., Natanson, C., Parrillo, J. E., Fauci, A. S., Pizzo, P. A., and Masur, H., *Pneumocystis carinii* pneumonia: a comparison between patients with the acquired immunodeficiency syndrome and patients with other immunodeficiencies, *Ann. Intern. Med.*, 100, 663, 1984.

74. Safrin, S., *Pneumocystis carinii* pneumonia in patients with the acquired immunodeficiency syndrome, *Semin. Respir. Med.*, 8, 96, 1993.

75. Sterling, R. P., Bradley, B. B., Khalil, K. G., Kerman, R. H., and Conklin, R. H., Comparison of biopsy-proven *Pneumocystis carinii* pneumonia in acquired immune deficiency syndrome patients and renal allograft recipients, *Ann. Thorac. Surg.*, 38, 494, 1984.

76. Haverkos, H. W., Assessment of therapy for *Pneumocystis carinii* pneumonia: PCP therapy project group, *Am. J. Med.*, 76, 501, 1984.

77. Staikowsky, F., Lafon, B., Guidet, B., Denis, M., Mayaud, C., and Offenstadt, G., Mechanical ventilation for *Pneumocystis carinii* pneumonia in patients with the acquired immunodeficiency syndrome, *Chest*, 104, 756, 1993.

78. Ognibene, F. P., Shelhamer, J. H., Hoffman, G. S., Kerr, G. S., Reda, D., Fauci, A. S., and Leavitt, R. Y., *Pneumocystis carinii* pneumonia: a major complication of immunosuppressive therapy in patients with Wegener's granulomatosis, *Am. J. Respir. Crit. Care Med.*, 151(3 part 1), 795, 1995.

79. Jarrousse, B., Guillevin, L., Bindi, P., Hachulla, E., Leclerc, P., Nilson, B., Rémy, P., Rossert, J., Jacquot, C., and Nilson, B. (corrected to Gilson, B.), Increased risk of *Pneumocystis carinii* pneumonia in patients with Wegener's granulomatosis, *Clin. Exp. Rheumatol.*, 11, 615, 1993 (published erratum appeared in *Clin. Exp. Rheumatol.*, 12, 117, 1994).

80. Abernathy-Carver, K. J., Fan, L. L., Boguniewicz, M., Larsen, G. L., and Leung, D. Y., Legionella and Pneumocystis pneumonias in asthmatic children on high doses of systemic steroids, *Pediatr. Pulmonol.*, 18, 135, 1994.

81. Woodward, S. C. and Sheldon, W. H., Subclinical *Pneumocystis carinii* pneumonitis in adults, *Bull. Johns Hopkins Hosp.*, 109, 148, 1961.

82. Hamlin, W. B., *Pneumocystis carinii*, *JAMA*, 204, 171, 1968.

83. Esterly, J. A., *Pneumocystis carinii* in lungs of adults at autopsy, *Am. Rev. Respir. Dis.*, 97, 935, 1968.

84. Kovacs, J. A., Halpern, J. L., Swan, J. C., Moss, J., Parrillo, J. E., and Masur, H., Identification of antigens and antibodies specific for *Pneumocystis carinii*, *J. Immunol.*, 140, 2023, 1988.

85. Smith, D. E., McLuckie, A., Wyatt, J., and Gazzard, B., Severe exercise hypoxaemia with normal or near-normal x-rays: a feature of *Pneumocystis carinii* infection, *Lancet*, 2, 1049, 1988.

86. Israel, H. L., Gottlieb, J. E., and Schulman, E. S., Hypoxemia with normal chest roentgenogram due to *Pneumocystis carinii* pneumonia: diagnostic errors due to a low suspicion of AIDS, *Chest*, 92, 857, 1987.

87. Kennedy, C. A. and Goetz, M. B., Atypical roentgenographic manifestations of *Pneumocystis carinii* pneumonia, *Arch. Intern. Med.*, 152, 1390, 1992.

88. Peters, J. W. and Sattler, F. R., Atypical *Pneumocystis carinii* pneumonia: the potential hazards of empiric treatment, *South. Med. J.*, 76, 800, 1983.

89. Cross, A. S. and Steigbigel, R. T., *Pneumocystis carinii* pneumonia presenting as localized nodular densities, *N. Engl. J. Med.*, 291, 831, 1974.

90. Hartz, J. W., Geisinger, K. R., Scharyj, M., and Muss, H. B., Granulomatous pneumocystosis presenting as a solitary pulmonary nodule, *Arch. Pathol. Lab. Med.*, 109, 466, 1985.

91. Barrio, J. L., Suarez, M., Rodriguez, J. L., Saldana, M. J., and Pitchenik, A. E., *Pneumocystis carinii* pneumonia presenting as cavitating and noncavitating solitary pulmonary nodules in patients with the acquired immunodeficiency syndrome, *Am. Rev. Respir. Dis.*, 134, 1094, 1986.

92. Bleiweiss, I. J., Jagirdar, J. S., Klein, M. J., Siegel, J. L., Krellenstein, D. J., Gribetz, A. R., and Strauchen, J. A., Granulomatous *Pneumocystis carinii* pneumonia in three patients with the acquired immune deficiency syndrome, *Chest*, 94, 580, 1986.

93. Byrd, R. B. and Horn, B. R., Infection due to *Pneumocystis carinii* stimulating lobar bacterial pneumonia, *Chest*, 70, 91, 1976.

94. Stokes, D. C., Shenep, J. L., Horowitz, M. E., and Hughes, W. T., Presentation of *Pneumocystis carinii* pneumonia as unilateral hyperlucent lung, *Chest*, 94, 201, 1988.

95. Abd, A. G., Nierman, D. M., Ilowite, J. S., Pierson, R. N., Jr., and Bell, A. L., Jr., Bilateral upper lobe *Pneumocystis carinii* pneumonia in a patient receiving inhaled pentamidine prophylaxis, *Chest*, 94, 329, 1988.

96. Albrecht, H., Stellbrink, H. J., Fenske, S., Koch, J., and Greten, H., A novel variety of atypical *Pneumocystis carinii* infection after long-term prophylactic pentamidine inhalation in an AIDS patient, *Clin. Invest.*, 71, 310, 1993.

97. Srivatsa, S. S., Burger, C. D., and Douglas, W. W., Upper lobe pulmonary parenchymal calcification in a patient with AIDS and *Pneumocystis carinii* pneumonia receiving aerosolized pentamidine, *Chest*, 101, 266, 1992.

98. Anderson, C. D. and Barrie, B. M., Fatal pneumocystis pneumonia in an adult, *Am. J. Clin. Pathol.*, 34, 365, 1960.

99. Livingstone, C. B., Pneumocystis pneumonia occurring in a family with agammaglobulinemia, *Can. Med. Assoc. J.*, 90, 1223, 1964.

100. Jarnum, S., Rasmussen, E. F., Ohlsen, A. S., and Sorensen, A. W. S., Generalized *Pneumocystis carinii* infection with severe idiopathic hypoproteinuria, *Ann. Intern. Med.*, 68, 138, 1968.

101. Barnett, R. N., Hull, J. G., Vortel, V., and Schwartz, J., *Pneumocystis carinii* in lymph nodes and spleen, *Arch. Pathol.*, 88, 175, 1969.

102. Awen, C. F. and Baltzan, M. A., Systemic dissemination of *Pneumocystis carinii* pneumonia, *Can. Med. Assoc. J.*, 104, 809, 1971.

103. Roder, V. H. and Kleine-Natrop, H. E., Morphologischer zufallsbefund von *Pneumocystis carinii* in stromenden blut bei erythema nodosum, *Derm. Mschr.*, 157, 678, 1971.

104. LeGolvan, D. P. and Heidelberger, K. P., Disseminated granulomatous *Pneumocystis carinii* pneumonia, *Arch. Pathol.*, 95, 344, 1973.

105. Price, R. A. and Hughes, W. T., Histopathology of *Pneumocystis carinii* infestation and infection in malignant disease in childhood, *Hum. Pathol.*, 5, 737, 1974.

106. Rahimi, S. A., Disseminated *Pneumocystis carinii* in thymic alymphoplasia, *Arch. Pathol.*, 97, 162, 1974.

107. Henderson, D. W., Humeniuk, V., Meadows, R., and Forbes, I. J., *Pneumocystis carinii* pneumonia with vascular and lymph nodal involvement, *Pathology*, 6, 235, 1974.

108. Kwok, S., O'Donnell, J. J., and Wood, I. S., Retinal cotton-wool spots in a patient with *Pneumocystis carinii* infection, *N. Engl. J. Med.*, 307, 184, 1982.

109. Rossi, J. F., Dubois, A., Bengler, C., Arich, C., Gervais, C., Delage, A., and Janbon, C., *Pneumocystis carinii* in bone marrow, *Ann. Intern. Med.*, 102, 868, 1985.

110. Delage, A., Bengler, C., Ross, J. F., Marin, J., and Lauraine, M. C., *Pneumocystis carinii* dans la moelle osseuse, *Bull. Soc. Path. E*, 78, 478, 1985.

111. Coulman, C. U., Greene, I., and Archibald, R. W., Cutaneous pneumocystosis, *Ann. Intern. Med.*, 106, 396, 1987.

112. Grimes, M. M., LaPook, J. D., Bar, M. H., Wasserman, H. S., and Dwork, A., Disseminated *Pneumocystis carinii* infection in a patient with acquired immunodeficiency syndrome, *Hum. Pathol.*, 18, 307, 1987.

113. Schinella, R. A., Breda, S. D., and Hammerschlag, P. E., Otic infection due to *Pneumocystis carinii* in an apparently healthy man with antibody to the human immunodeficiency virus, *Ann. Intern. Med.*, 106, 399, 1987.

114. Macher, A. M., Bardenstein, D. S., Zimmerman, L. E., Steigman, C. K., Pastore, L., Poretz, D. M., and Eron, L. J., *Pneumocystis carinii* chorioditis in a male homosexual with AIDS and disseminated pulmonary and extrapulmonary *P. carinii* infection, *N. Engl. J. Med.*, 316, 1092, 1987.

115. Pilon, V. A., Echols, R. M., Celo, J. S., and Elmendorf, S. L., Disseminated *Pneumocystis carinii* infection in AIDS, *N. Engl. J. Med.*, 316, 1410, 1987.

116. Steigman, C. K., Pastore, L., Park, C. H., Fox, C. H., De Vinatea, M. L., Connor, D. H., and Macher, A. M., Case for diagnosis: AIDS, *Milit. Med.*, 152, M1, 1987.

117. Carter, T. R., Cooper, P. H., Petri, W. A., Jr., Kim, C. K., Walzer, P. D., and Guerrant, R. L., *Pneumocystis carinii* infection of the small intestine in a patient with acquired immune deficiency, *Am. J. Clin. Pathol.*, 89, 79, 1988.

118. Gallant, J. E., Enriquez, R. E., Cohen, K. L., and Hammers, L. W., *Pneumocystis carinii* thyroiditis, *Am. J. Med.*, 84, 303, 1988.

119. Gherman, C. R., Ward, R. R., and Bassis, M. L., *Pneumocystis carinii* otitis and mastoiditis as the initial manifestation of the acquired immunodeficiency syndrome, *Am. J. Med.*, 85, 250, 1988.

120. Breda, S. D., Hammerschlag, P. E., Gigliotti, F., and Schinella, R., *Pneumocystis carinii* in the temporal bone as a primary manifestation of the acquired immunodeficiency syndrome, *Ann. Otol. Rhinol. Laryngol.*, 97, 427, 1988.

121. Unger, P. D., Rosenblum, M., and Krown, S. E., Disseminated *Pneumocystis carinii* infection in a patient with acquired immunodeficiency syndrome, *Hum. Pathol.*, 19, 113, 1988.

122. Dugel, P. V., Rao, N. A., Forster, D. J., Chong, L. P., Frangieh, G. T., and Sattler, F., *Pneumocystis carinii* choroiditis after long-term aerosolized pentamidine therapy, *Am. J. Ophthalmol.*, 110, 113, 1990.

123. Rao, N. A., Zimmerman, P. L., Boyer, D., Biswas, J., Causey, D., Beniz, J., and Nichols, P. W., A clinical, histopathologic and electron microscopic study of *Pneumocystis carinii* choroiditis, *Am. J. Ophthalmol.*, 107, 218, 1989.

124. Lalonde, L., Allaire, G. S., Sebag, M., Lamer, L., Marcil, G., and Gervais, A., *Pneumocystis carinii* choroidopathy and aerosolized pentamidine prophylaxis in a patient with AIDS, *Can. J. Ophthalmol.*, 28, 291, 1993.

125. Freeman, W. R., Gross, J. G., Labelle, J., Oteken, K., Katz, B., and Wiley, C. A., *Pneumocystis carinii* choroidopathy, a new clinical entry, *Arch. Ophthalmol.*, 107, 863, 1989.

126. Armstrong, D. and Bernard, E., Aerosol pentamidine, *Ann. Intern. Med.*, 109, 852, 1988.

127. Hagopian, W. A. and Huseby, J. S., *Pneumocystis* hepatitis and choroiditis despite successful aerosolized pentamidine pulmonary prophylaxis, *Chest*, 96, 949, 1989.

128. Smith, M. A., Hirschfield, L. S., Zahtz, G., and Siejal, F. P., Pneumocystis carinii otitis media, *Am. J. Med.*, 85, 745, 1988.

129. Breda, S. D., Gigliotti, F., Hammerschlag, P. E., and Schinella, R., Pneumocystis carinii in the temporal bone as a primary manifestation to the acquired immunodeficiency syndrome, *Ann. Otol. Rhinol. Laryngol.*, 97, 427, 1988.

130. Sandler, E. D., Sandler, J. M., LeBoit, P. E., Wenig, B. M., and Mortensen, N., *Pneumocystis carinii* otitis media in AIDS: a case report and review of the literature regarding extrapulmonary pneumocystosis, *Otolaryngol. Head Neck Surg.*, 103, 817, 1990.

131. Patey, O., Salvanet, A., Serrhini, A., and Lafaix, C., *Pneumocystis carinii* in AIDS patients, *AIDS*, 7, 1015, 1993.

132. Sha, B. E., Benson, C. A., Deutsch, T., Noskin, G. A., Murphy, R. L., Pottage, J. C., Jr., Finn, W. G., Roth, S. I., and Kessler, H. A., *Pneumocystis carinii* chorioditis in patients with AIDS: clinical features, response to therapy, and outcome, *J. Acquir. Immune Defic. Syndr.*, 5, 1051, 1992.

133. Drucker, D. J., Bailey, D., and Rotstein, L., Thyroiditis as the presenting manifestation of disseminated extrapulmonary *Pneumocystis carinii* infection, *J. Clin. Endocrinol. Metab.*, 71, 1663, 1990.

134. Delorenzo, L. J., Huang, C. T., Maguire, G. P., and Stone, D. J., Roentgenographic patterns of *Pneumocystis carinii* pneumonia in 104 patients with AIDS, *Chest*, 91, 323, 1987.

135. Dyner, T. S., Lang, W., Busch, D. F., and Gordon, P. R., Intravascular and pleural involvement by *Pneumocystis carinii* in a patient with AIDS, *Ann. Intern. Med.*, 111, 94, 1989.

136. Mariuz, P., Raviglione, M. C., Gould, I. A., and Mullen, M. P., Pleural *Pneumocystis carinii* infection, *Chest*, 99, 774, 1991.

137. Telzak, E. E., Cote, R. J., Gold, J. W. M., Campbell, S. W., and Armstrong, D., Extrapulmonary *Pneumocystis carinii* infections, *Rev. Infect. Dis.*, 12, 380, 1990.

138. Witt, K., Nielsen, T. N., and Junge, J., Dissemination of *Pneumocystis carinii* in patients with AIDS, *Scand. J. Infect. Dis.*, 23, 691, 1991.

139. Hennessey, N. P., Parro, E. L., and Cockerell, C. J., Cutaneous *Pneumocystis carinii* infection in patients with acquired immunodeficiency syndrome, *Arch. Dermatol.*, 127, 1699, 1991.

140. Lecuit, M., Livartowski, J., Vons, C., Goujard, C., Lemaigre, G., Delfraissy, J.-F., and Dormont, J., Resistance to trimethoprim-sulfamethoxazole and sensitivity to pentamidine therapy in an AIDS patient with hepatosplenic pneumocystosis, *AIDS*, 8, 1506, 1994.

141. Northfelt, D., Michael, J., and Safrin, J., Extrapulmonary pneumocystosis: clinical features in human immunodeficiency infection, *Medicine (Baltimore)*, 89, 392, 1990.

142. Bazin, C., Hazera, P., Greder, A., Cren, P., Lechevalier, B., Gallet, E., and Charbonneau, P., Extrapulmonary disseminated pneumocystosis in HIV infection, *Presse Med.*, 22, 161, 1993.

143. Raviglione, M. C., Extrapulmonary pneumocystosis: the first 50 years, *Rev. Infect. Dis.*, 12, 1127, 1990.

144. Poblete, R. B., Rodriguez, K., Foust, R. T., Reddy, K. R., and Saldana, M. J., *Pneumocystis carinii* hepatitis in the acquired immunodeficiency syndrome (AIDS), *Ann. Intern. Med.*, 110, 737, 1989.

145. Jarnum, S., Rasmussen, E. F., Ohlsen, A. S., and Sorensen, A. W., Generalized *Pneumocystis carinii* infection with severe idiopathic hypoproteinemia, *Ann. Intern. Med.*, 68, 138, 1968.

146. Tugwell, P., Bennett, K., and Gent, M., Methotrexate in rheumatoid arthritis, *Ann. Intern. Med.*, 107, 418, 1987.

147. Perruquet, J. L., Harrington, T. M., and Davis, D. E., *Pneumocystis carinii* pneumonia following methotrexate therapy for rheumatoid arthritis, *Arthritis Rheum.*, 26, 1291, 1983.

148. Seideman, P., Müller-Suur, R., and Ekman, E., Renal effect of low dose methotrexate in rheumatoid arthritis, *J. Rheumatol.*, 20, 1126, 1993.

149. Marshall, D., Sturrock, R. D., Porter, D., and Capell, H. A., *Pneumocystis carinii* complicating low dose methotrexate treatment for rheumatoid arthritis, *Thorax*, 47, 67, 1992.

150. Kane, G. C., Troshinsky, M. B., Peters, S. P., and Israel, H. L., *Pneumocystis carinii* pneumonia associated with weekly methotrexate: cumulative dose of methotrexate and low CD_4 cell count may predict this complication, *Respir. Med.*, 87, 153, 1993.

151. Wollner, A., Mohle-Boetani, J., Lambert, R. E., Perruquet, J. L., Raffin, T. A., and McGuire, J. L., *Pneumocystis carinii* pneumonia complicating low dose methotrexate treatment for rheumatoid arthritis, *Thorax*, 46, 205, 1991.

152. Leff, R. L., Case, J. P., and McKenzie, R., Rheumatoid arthritis, methotrexate therapy, and *Pneumocystis carinii*, *Ann. Intern. Med.*, 112, 716, 1990.

153. Wollner, A., Mohle-Boetani, J., Lambert, R. E., Perruquet, J. L., Raffin, T. A., and Mcguire, J. L., *Pneumocystis carinii* pneumonia complicating low dose methotrexate treatment for rheumatoid arthritis, *Thorax*, 46, 205, 1991.

154. Wallis, P. J. W., Ryatt, K. S., and Constable, T. J., *Pneumocystis carinii* pneumonia complicating low dose methotrexate treatment for psoriatic arthropathy, *Ann. Rheum. Dis.*, 48, 247, 1989.

155. Olson, N. J., Callahan, L. F., and Pincus, T., Immunologic studies of rheumatoid arthritis patients treated with methotrexate, *Arthritis Rheum.*, 30, 481, 1987.

156. Dawson, T., Ryan, P. F. J., Findeisen, J. M., and Scheinkestel, C. D., *Pneumocystis carinii* pneumonia following cyclosporine A and methotrexate treated rheumatoid arthritis, *J. Rheumatol.*, 19, 997, 1992.

157. Powles, A. V., Baker, B. S., and Fry, L., Cyclosporine toxicity, *Lancet*, 335, 610, 1990.

158. Hammoudeh, M., Siam, A.-R., and Khanjar, I., Renal effect of low dose methotrexate in rheumatoid arthritis, *J. Rheumatol.*, 21, 1168, 1994.

159. Schneider, M. M. E., Hoepelman, A. I. M., Eeftinck Schattenkerk, J. K., Nielsen, T. L., van der Graaf, Y., Frissen, J. P. H. J., van der Ende, I. M. E., Kolsterss, A. F. P., Borleffs, J. C. C., and the Dutch AIDS Treatment Group, A controlled trial of aerosolized pentamidine or trimethoprim-sulfamethoxazole as primary prophylaxis against *Pneumocystis carinii* pneumonia in patients with human immunodeficiency virus infection, *N. Engl. J. Med.*, 327, 1836, 1992.

160. Calabrese, L. H., Taylor, J. V., Wilke, W. S., Segal, A. M., Valenzuela, R., and Clough, J. D., Response of immunoregulatory lymphocyte subsets to methotrexate in rheumatoid arthritis, *Cleve. Clin. J. Med.*, 57, 232, 1990.

161. Houtman, P. M., Stenger, A. A. M. E., Bruyn, G. A. W., and Mulder, J., Methotrexate may affect certain T lymphocyte subsets in rheumatoid arthritis resulting in susceptibility to *Pneumocystis carinii* infection, *J. Rheumatol.*, 21, 1168, 1994.

162. Sohen, S., Kita, H., and Tanaka, S., Abnormalities in bone marrow mononuclear cells in patients with rheumatoid arthritis, *J. Rheumatol.*, 20, 12, 1993.

163. Gibbons, J. J. and Lucas, J., Immunomodulation by low dose methotrexate. I. Methotrexate selectively inhibits Lyt-2+ cells in murine graft-versus-host reactions, *J. Immunol.*, 142, 1867, 1989.

164. Blaser, J., Joos, B., Opravil, M., and Luthy, R., Variability of serum concentrations of trimethoprim and sulfamethoxazole during high dose therapy, *Infection*, 21, 206, 1993.

165. Winston, D. J., Lau, W. K., Gale, R. P., and Young, L. S., Trimethoprim-sulfamethoxazole for the treatment of *Pneumocystis carinii*, *Ann. Intern. Med.*, 92, 762, 1980.

166. Carr, A., Swanson, C., Penny, R., and Cooper, D. A., Clinical and laboratory markers of hypersensitivity to trimethoprim-sulfamethoxazole in patients with *Pneumocystis carinii* pneumonia and AIDS, *J. Infect. Dis.*, 167, 180, 1993.

167. Silvestri, R. C., Jensen, W. A., Zibrak, J. D., Alexander, R. C., and Rose, R. M., Pulmonary infiltrates and hypoxemia in patients with the acquired immunodeficiency syndrome re-exposed to trimethoprim–sulfamethoxazole, *Am. Rev. Respir. Dis.*, 136, 1003, 1987.

168. Colm, D. L., Penley, K. A., Judson, F. N., Kirkpatrick, C. H., Horsburgh, C. R., and Davis, K. C., The acquired immunodeficiency syndrome and a trimethoprim-sulfamethoxazole adverse reaction, *Ann. Intern. Med.*, 100, 311, 1984.

169. Kelly, J. W., Dooley, D. P., Lattuada, C. P., and Smith, C. E., A severe unusual reaction to trimethoprim–sulfamethoxazole in patients infected with human immunodeficiency syndrome, *Clin. Infect. Dis.*, 14, 1034, 1992.

170. Ulstad, D. R., Ampel, N. M., Shon, B. Y., Galgiani, J. N., and Cutcher, A. B., Reaction after re-exposure to trimethoprim–sulfamethoxazole, *Chest*, 95, 937, 1989.

171. Arnold, P. A., Guglielmo, J., and Hollander, H., Severe hypersensitivity reaction upon rechallenge with trimethoprim–sulfamethoxazole in a patient with AIDS, *Drug Intell. Clin. Pharm.*, 22, 43, 1988.

172. Martin, G. J., Paparello, S. F., and Decker, C. F., A severe systemic reaction to trimethoprim–sulfamethoxazole in a patient infected with the human immunodeficiency virus, *Clin. Infect. Dis.*, 16, 175, 1993.

173. Johnson, M. P., Goodwin, S. D., and Shands, J. W., Trimethoprim–sulfamethoxazole anaphylactoid reactions in patients with AIDS: case reports and literature review, *Pharmacotherapy*, 10, 41, 1990.

174. Roudier, C., Caumes, E., Rogeaux, O., Bricaire, F., and Gentilini, M., Adverse cutaneous reactions to trimethoprim-sulfamethoxazole in patients with the acquired immunodeficiency syndrome and *Pneumocystis carinii* pneumonia, *Arch. Dermatol.*, 130, 1383, 1994.

175. Peters, B. S., Carlin, E., Weston, R. J., Loveless, S. J., Sweaney, J., Weber, J., and Main, J., Adverse effects of drugs used in the management of opportunistic infections associated with HIV infection, *Drug Safety*, 10, 439, 1994.

176. Fischl, M. A., Dickinson, G. M., and La Voie, L., Safety and efficacy of sulfamethoxazole and trimethoprim chemoprophylaxis for *Pneumocystis carinii* pneumonia in AIDS, *JAMA*, 259, 1185, 1988.

177. Wharton, J. M., Coleman, D. L., Wofsy, C. B., Luce, M., Blumenfeld, W., Hadley, W. K., Ingram-Drake, L., Volberding, P. A., and Hopewell, P. C., Trimethoprim–sulfamethoxazole or pentamidine for *Pneumocystis carinii* pneumonia in the acquired immunodeficiency syndrome, *Ann. Intern. Med.*, 105, 37, 1986.

178. Sattler, F. R., Cowen, R., Nielsen, D. M., and Ruskin, J., Trimethoprim–sulfamethoxazole compared with pentamidine for treatment of *Pneumocystis carinii* pneumonia in the acquired immunodeficiency syndrome, *Ann. Intern. Med.*, 109, 280, 1988.

179. Medina, I., Mills, J., Leoung, G., Hopewell, P. C., Lee, B., Hopewell, P. C., Lee, B., Modin, G., Benowitz, N., and Wofsy, C. B., Oral therapy for *Pneumocystis carinii* pneumonia in the acquired immunodeficiency syndrome: a controlled trial for trimethoprim–sulfamethoxazole vs. trimethoprim–dapsone, *N. Engl. J. Med.*, 323, 776, 1990.

180. Small, C. B., Harris, C. A., Friedland, G. H., and Klein, R. S., The treatment of *Pneumocystis carinii* pneumonia in the acquired immunodeficiency syndrome, *Arch. Intern. Dis.*, 145, 837, 1985.

181. Jung, A. C. and Paauw, D. S., Management of adverse reactions to trimethoprim–sulfamethoxazole in human immunodeficiency virus-infected patients, *Arch. Intern. Med.*, 154, 2402, 1994.

182. Lidman, C., Ortqvist, A., Lundbergh, P., Julander, I., and Bergdahl, S., *Pneumocystis carinii* in Stockholm, Sweden: treatment, outcome, one-year follow-up and pyrimethamine prophylaxis, *Scand. J. Infect. Dis.*, 21, 381, 1989.

183. Kovacs, J. A., Hiemenz, J. W., Macher, A. M., Stover, D., Murray, H. W., Shelhamer, J., Lane, H. C., Urmacher, C., Honig, C., Longo, D. L., Parker, M. M., Natanson, C., Parrillo, J. E., Fauci, A. S., Pizzo, P. A., and Masur, H., *Pneumocystis carinii* pneumonia: a comparison between patients with the acquired immunodeficiency syndrome and patients with other immunodeficiencies, *Ann. Intern. Med.*, 100, 663, 1984.

184. Hughes, W., Leoung, G., Kramer, F., Bozzette, S. A., Safrin, S., Frame, P., Clumeck, N., Masur, H., Lancaster, D., Chan, C., Lavelle, J., Rosenstock, J., Falloon, J., Feinberg, J., LaFon, S., Rogers, M., and Sattler, F., Comparison of atovaquone (566C80) with trimethoprim–sulfamethoxazole to treat *Pneumocystis carinii* pneumonia in patients with AIDS, *N. Engl. J. Med.*, 328, 1521, 1993.

185. Jaffe, H. S., Abrams, D. I., Ammann, A. J., Lewis, B. J., and Golden, J. A., Complications of co-trimoxazole in treatment of AIDS-associated *Pneumocystis carinii* pneumonia in homosexual men, *Lancet*, 2, 1109, 1983.

186. Mitsuyasu, R., Groopman, J., and Volberding, P., Cutaneous reaction to trimethoprim–sulfamethoxazole in patients with AIDS and Kaposi's sarcoma, *N. Engl. J. Med.*, 3, 1535, 1983.

187. U.S. Public Health Service Task Force on anti-pneumocystis prophylaxis in patients with human immunodeficiency virus infection: recommendation for prophylaxis against *Pneumocystis carinii* pneumonia for persons infected with human immunodeficiency virus, *J. Acquir. Immune Defic. Syndr.*, 6, 46, 1993.

188. Hardy, W. D., Feinberg, J., Finkelstein, D. M., Power, M. E., He, W., Kaczka, C., Frame, P. T., Holmes, M., Hetty Waskin, P. A.-C., Fass, R., Powderly, W. G., Steigbigel, R. T., Zuger, A., and Holzman, R. S., A controlled trial of trimethoprim–sulfamethoxazole or aerosolized pentamidine for secondary prophylaxis of *Pneumocystis carinii* pneumonia in patients with acquired immunodeficiency syndrome (AIDS clinical trial group protocol 021), *N. Engl. J. Med.*, 327, 1842, 1992.

189. Ruskin, J. and LaRiviere, M., Low-dose co-trimoxazole for prevention of *Pneumocystis carinii* pneumonia in human immunodeficiency virus disease, *Lancet*, 337, 468, 1991.

190. Wormser, G. P., Horowitz, H. W., Duncanson, F. P., Forseter, G., Javaly, K., Alanpur, S. K., Gilroy, S. A., Lenox, T., Rappaport, A., and Nedleman, R. B., Low-dose intermittent trimethoprim–sulfamethoxazole for prevention of *Pneumocystis carinii* pneumonia in patients with human immunodeficiency virus infection, *Arch. Intern. Med.*, 151, 688, 1991.

191. Mallolas, J., Zamora, L., Gatell, J. M., Miró, J. M., Vernet, E., Valls, M. E., Soriano, E., and SanMiguel, J. G., Primary prophylaxis for *Pneumocystis carinii* pneumonia: a randomized trial comparing cotrimoxazole, aerosolized pentamidine and dapsone plus pyrimethamine, *AIDS*, 7, 59, 1993.

192. Jick, H., Adverse reactions to trimethoprim–sulfamethoxazole in hospitalized patients, *Rev. Infect. Dis.*, 4, 426, 1982.

193. Colebunders, R., Izaley, L., Bila, K., Kabumpangi, K., Melameka, N., Nyst, M., Francis, H., Curran, J. W., Ryder, R., and Piot, P., Cutaneous reactions to trimethoprim–sulfamethoxazole in African patients with the acquired immunodeficiency syndrome, *Ann. Intern. Med.*, 107, 599, 1987.

194. DeHovitz, J. A., Johnson, W. D., and Pape, J. W., Cutaneous reactions to trimethoprim–sulfamethoxazole in Haitians, *Ann. Intern. Med.*, 103, 479, 1985.

195. Hazel, E., Sethi, N., Jacquette, G., and Dobkin, J., Diminished sulfa-trimethoprim toxicity in blacks treated for *Pneumocystis carinii*. Read before the International Conference on AIDS, June 5, 1987, Washington, D.C.

196. Walmsley, S., Levinton, C., Brunton, J., Muradali, D., Rappaport, D., Bast, M., Spence, D., and Salit, I., A multicenter randomized double-blind placebo-controlled trial of adjunctive corticosteroids in the treatment of *Pneumocystis carinii* pneumonia complicating the acquired immune deficiency syndrome, *J. Acquir. Immune Defic. Syndr. Hum. Retrovirol.*, 8, 348, 1995.

197. Walmsley, S., Salit, I. E., and Brunton, J., The possible role of corticosteroid therapy for *Pneumocystis carinii* in the acquired immune deficiency syndrome (AIDS), *J. Acquir. Immune Defic. Syndr.*, 1, 354, 1988.

198. Bozzette, S. A., Sattler, F. R., Chiu, J., Wu, A. W., Gluckstein, D., Kemper, C., Bartok, A., Niosi, J., Abramson, I., Coffman, J., Hughlett, C., Loya, R., Cassens, B., Akil, B., Meng, T.-C., Boylen, C. T., Nielsen, D., Richman, D. D., Tilles, J. G., Leedom, J., McCutchan, J. A., and the California Collaborative Treatment Group, A controlled trial of early adjunctive treatment with corticosteroids for *Pneumocystis carinii* pneumonia in the acquired immunodeficiency syndrome, *N. Engl. J. Med.*, 323, 1451, 1990.

199. Aguilar, X., Ruiz, J., Clotet, B., and Roig, J., The use of corticosteroids in the control of adverse reactions to cotrimoxazole in AIDS patients suffering from PCP, *AIDS*, 5, 777, 1991.

200. Carrington, D. M., Earl, H. S., and Sullivan, T. J., Studies of human IgE to a sulfonamide determinant, *J. Allergy Clin. Immunol.*, 79, 442, 1987.

201. Gruchalla, R. S. and Sullivan, T. J., *In vitro* and *in vivo* studies of immunologic reactivity to sulfamethoxazole, *J. Allergy Clin. Immunol.*, 85, 157, 1990.

202. Gruchalla, R. S. and Sullivan, T. J., Detection of human IgE to sulfamethoxazole by skin testing with sulfamethoxazole-poly-L-tyrosine, *Ann. Intern. Med.*, 106, 335, 1987.

203. Marinac, J. S. and Stanford, J. F., A severe hypersensitive reaction to trimethoprim–sulfamethoxazole in a patient infected with human immunodeficiency virus, *Clin. Infect. Dis.*, 16, 178, 1993.

204. Smith, R. M., Iwamoto, G. K., Richerson, H. B., and Flaherty, J. P., Trimethoprim–sulfamethoxazole desensitization in the acquired immunodeficiency syndrome, *Ann. Intern. Med.*, 106, 335, 1987.

205. Finegold, I., Oral desensitization to trimethoprim–sulfamethoxazole in a patient with acquired immunodeficiency syndrome, *J. Allergy Clin. Immunol.*, 78, 905, 1986.

206. Sher, M. R., Suchar, C., and Lockey, R. F., Anaphylactic shock induced by oral desensitization to trimethoprim–sulfamethoxazole, *J. Allergy Clin. Immunol.*, 77, 133, 1986.

207. Funai, N., Shimamoto, Y., Matsuzaki, M., Watanabe, M., Tokioka, T., Sueoka, E., Suga, K., Ono, K., Sano, M., and Yamaguchi, M., Hyperkaelemia with renal tubular dysfunction by sulfamethoxazole–trimethoprim for *Pneumocystis carinii* pneumonia in patients with lymphoid malignancy, *Haematologia (Budapest)*, 25, 137, 1993.

208. Greenberg, S., Reiser, I. W., and Chou, S. Y., Hyperkalemia with high-dose trimethoprim–sulfamethoxazole therapy, *Am. J. Kidney Dis.*, 22, 603, 1993.

209. Choi, M. J., Fernandez, P. C., Patnaik, A., Coupaye-Gerard, B., D'Andrea, D., Szerlip, H., and Kleyman, T. R., Brief report: trimethoprim-induced hyperkalemia in a patient with AIDS, *N. Engl. J. Med.*, 328, 703, 1993.

210. Borucki, M. J., Matzc, D. S., and Pollard, R. B., Tremor induced by trimethoprim–sulfamethoxazole in patients with the acquired immunodeficiency syndrome (AIDS), *Ann. Intern. Med.*, 148, 77, 1988.

211. Kimura, S., Oka, S., Mohri. H., Mitamura, K., and Shimada, K., Three cases of acquired immunodeficiency syndrome complicated with toxic epidermal necrolysis, *Jpn. J. Med.*, 30, 553, 1991.

212. Sonneville, E., Lecocq, P., Ajana, F., Chidiac, C., and Mouton, Y., Co-trimoxazole for toxic epidermal necrolysis in AIDS, *Lancet*, 337, 919, 1991.

213. Porteous, D. M. and Berger, T. G., Severe cutaneous drug reactions (Stevens-Johnson syndrome and toxic epidermal necrolysis) in human immunodeficiency virus infection, *Acta Dermatol.*, 127, 740, 1991.

214. Johnson, M. P., Goodwin, S. D., and Shands, J. W., Trimethoprim–sulfamethoxazole anaphylactoid reactions in patients with AIDS: case reports and literature review, *Pharmacotherapy*, 10, 413, 1990.

215. Kelly, J. W., Dooley, D. P., Lattuada, C. P., and Smith, C. E., A severe, unusual reaction to trimethoprim–sulfamethoxazole in patients with human immunodeficiency virus, *Clin. Infect. Dis.*, 14, 1034, 1992.

216. Martin, G. J., Paparello, S. F., and Decker, C. F., A severe systemic reaction to trimethoprim–sulfamethoxazole in a patient infected with the human immunodeficiency virus, *Clin. Infect. Dis.*, 16, 175, 1993.

217. Velazquez, H., Perazella, M. A., Wright, F. S., and Ellison, D. H., Renal mechanism of trimethoprim-induced hyperkalemia, *Ann. Intern. Med.*, 119, 296, 1993.

218. Greenberg, S., Reiser, I. W., Chou, S. Y., and Porush, J. G., Trimethoprim–sulfamethoxazole induces reversible hyperkalemia, *Ann. Intern. Med.*, 119, 291, 1993.

219. Schreiber, M. and Halperin, M. L., Urea excretion rate as a contributor to trimethoprim-induced hyperkalemia, *Ann. Intern. Med.*, 120, 166, 1994.

220. Modest, G. A., Price, B., and Macoli, N., Hyperkalemia in elderly patients receiving standard doses of trimethoprim–sulfamethoxazole, *Ann. Intern. Med.*, 120, 437, 1994.

221. Pennypacker, L. C., Mintzer, J., and Pitner, J., Hyperkalemia in elderly patients receiving standard doses of trimethoprim–sulfamethoxazole, *Ann. Intern. Med.*, 120, 437, 1994.

222. Canaday, D. H. and Johnson, J. R., Hyperkalemia in elderly patients receiving standard doses of trimethoprim–sulfamethoxazole, *Ann. Intern. Med.*, 120, 438, 1994.

223. Shafer, R. W., Seitzman, P. A., and Tapper, M. L., Successful prophylaxis of *Pneumocystis carinii* pneumonia with trimethoprim–sulfamethoxazole in AIDS patients with previous allergic reactions, *J. Acquir. Immune Defic. Syndr.*, 2, 389, 1989.

224. Gibbons, R. B. and Lindauer, J. A., Successful treatment of *Pneumocystis carinii* pneumonia with trimethoprim–sulfamethoxazole in hypersensitive AIDS patients, *JAMA*, 253, 1259, 1985.

225. Putterman, C., Rahav, G., Shalit, M., and Rubinow, A., Treating through hypersensitivity to co-trimoxazole in AIDS patients, *Lancet*, 336, 52, 1990.

226. Gordin, F. M., Simon, G. L., Wofsy, C. B., and Mills, J., Adverse reactions to trimethoprim–sulfamethoxazole in patients with the acquired immunodeficiency syndrome, *Ann. Intern. Med.*, 100, 495, 1984.

227. Toma, E. and Fournier, S., Adverse reactions to co-trimoxazole in HIV infection, *Lancet*, 338, 954, 1991.

228. Gompels, M., McWilliams, S., O'Hare, M., Harris, J. R., Pinching, A. J., and Main, J., Ondansetron usage in HIV positive patients: a pilot study on the control of nausea and vomiting in patients on high dose co-trimoxazole for *Pneumocystis carinii* pneumonia, *Int. J. STD AIDS*, 4, 293, 1993.

229. Carr, A., Penny, R., and Cooper, D. A., Efficacy and safety of rechallenge with low-dose trimethoprim–sulfamethoxazole in previously hypersensitive HIV-infected patients, *AIDS*, 7, 65, 1993.

230. Papakonstantinou, G., Fuessle, H., and Hehlmann, R., Trimethoprim–sulfamethoxazole desensitization in AIDS, *Klin. Wochenschr.*, 66, 351, 1988.

231. Papakonstantinou, G., Fuessle, H., and Hehlmann, R., Therapy of *Pneumocystis carinii* pneumonia after trimethoprim–sulfamethoxazole desensitization, *Klin. Wochenschr.*, 67, 316, 1989.

232. White, M. V., Haddad, Z. H., Brunner, E., and Saintz, C., Desensitization to trimethoprim–sulfamethoxazole in patients with acquired immunodeficiency syndrome and *Pneumocystis carinii*, *Ann. Allergy*, 62, 177, 1989.

233. Kreuz, W., Güngör, T., Lotz, C. H. R., and Kornhuber, B., "Treating through" hypersensitivity to co-trimoxazole in children with HIV infection, *Lancet*, 336, 508, 1990.

234. Sher, M. R., Suchar, C., and Lockey, R. F., Anaphylactic shock induced by oral desensitization to trimethoprim–sulfamethoxazole (TMP-SMZ), *J. Allergy Clin. Immunol.*, 77, 133, 1986.

235. Smith, R. M., Iwamoto, G. K., Richerson, H. B., and Flaherty, J. P., Trimethoprim–sulfamethoxazole desensitization in the acquired immunodeficiency syndrome, *Ann. Intern. Med.*, 106, 335, 1987.

236. Bozzette, S. A., Forthal, D., Sattler, F. R., Kemper, C., Richman, D. D., Tillis, J. G., Leedom, J., McCutchan, J. A., and the California Collaborative Treatment Group, The tolerance for zidovudine plus thrice weekly or daily trimethoprim–sulfamethoxazole with and without leucovorin for primary prophylaxis in advanced HIV disease, *Am. J. Med.*, 98, 177, 1995.

237. Safrin, S., Lee, B. L., and Sande, M. A., Adjunctive folinic acid with trimethoprim–sulfamethoxazole for *Pneumocystis carinii* pneumonia in AIDS patients is associated with an increased risk of therapeutic failure and death, *J. Infect. Dis.*, 170, 912, 1994.

238. Bell, C. A., Cory, M., Fairley, T. A., Hall, J. E., and Tidwell, R. R., Structure-activity relationships of pentamidine analogs against *Giardia lamblia* and correlation of antigiardial activity with DNA-binding affinity, *Antimicrob. Agents Chemother.*, 35, 1099, 1991.

239. Tidwell, R. R., Jones, S. K., Geratz, J. D., Ohemeng, K. A., Bell, C. A., Berger, B. J., and Hall, J. E., Development of pentamidine analogs as new agents for the treatment of *Pneumocystis carinii* pneumonia, *Ann. NY Acad. Sci.*, 616, 421, 1990.

240. Rosenthal, G. J., Corsini, E., Craig, W. A., Comment, C. E., and Luster, M. I., Pentamidine: an inhibitor of interleukin-1 that acts via a post-translational event, *Toxicol. Appl. Pharmacol.*, 107, 555, 1991.

241. Rosenthal, G. J., Craig, W. A., Corsini, E., Taylor, M., and Luster, M. I., Pentamidine blocks the pathophysiologic effects of endotoxemia through inhibition of cytokine release, *Toxicol. Appl. Pharmacol.*, 112, 222, 1992.

242. Masur, H., Lane, C., Kovacs, J. A., Allegra, C. J., and Edman, J. C., *Pneumocystis carinii* pneumonia: from bench to clinic, *Ann. Intern. Med.*, 111, 813, 1989.

243. Travis, W., Lack, E., Ognibene, F. P., Suffredini, A. F., and Shelhamer, J., Lung biopsy interpretation in the acquired immunodeficiency syndrome: experience of the National Institutes of Health with literature review, *Prog. AIDS Pathol.*, 6, 51, 1989.

244. Mordelet-Dambrine, M., Danel, C., Farinotti, R., Urzua, G., Barritauld, L., and Huchon, G. J., Influence of *Pneumocystis carinii* pneumonia on serum and tissue concentrations of pentamidine administered to rats by tracheal injections, *Am. Rev. Respir. Dis.*, 146, 735, 1992.

245. Vinet, B., Comtois, R., Gervais, A., and Lemieux, C., Clinical usefulness of high-pressure liquid chromatographic determination of serum pentamidine in AIDS patients, *Clin. Biochem.*, 25, 93, 1992.

246. Waskin, H., Stehr-Green, J. K., Helmick, C. G., and Sattler, F. R., Risk factors for hypoglycemia associated with pentamidine therapy for Pneumocystis pneumonia, *JAMA*, 260, 345, 1988.

247. McSharry, R. J., Kirsch, C. M., Jensen, W. A., and Kagawa, F. T., Prophylaxis of aerosolized pentamidine-induced bronchospasm: a symptom-based approach, *Am. J. Med. Sci.*, 306, 20, 1993.

248. Renzi, P. M., Corbeil, C., Chasse, M., Braidy, J., and Matar, N., Bilateral pneumothoraces hasten mortality in AIDS patients receiving secondary prophylaxis with aerosolized pentamidine: association with a lower Dco prior to receiving aerosolized pentamidine, *Chest*, 102, 491, 1992.

249. Gearhart, M. O. and Bhutani, M. S., Intravenous pentamidine-induced bronchospasm, *Chest*, 102, 1891, 1992.

250. Comtois, R., Pouliot, J., Gervais, A., Vinet, B., and Lemieux, C., High pentamidine levels associated with hypoglycemia and azotemia in a patient with *Pneumocystis carinii* pneumonia, *Diagn. Microbiol. Infect. Dis.*, 15, 523, 1992.

251. Comtois, R., Pouliot, J., Vinet, B., Gervais, A., and Lemieux, C., Higher pentamidine levels in AIDS patients with hypoglycemia and azotemia during treatment of *Pneumocystis carinii* pneumonia, *Am. Rev. Respir. Dis.*, 146, 740, 1992.

252. Jones, R. S., Jr., Collier-Brown, C., and Suh, B., Localized cutaneous reaction to intravenous pentamidine, *Clin. Infect. Dis.*, 15, 561, 1992.

253. Klatt, E. C., Pathology of pentamidine-induced pancreatitis, *Arch. Pathol. Lab. Med.*, 116, 162, 1992.

254. Pouwels, A., Eliaszewicz, M., Larrey, D., Lacassin, F., Poirier, J. M., Meyohas, M. C., and Frottier, J., Pentamidine-induced acute pancreatitis in a patient with AIDS, *J. Clin. Gastroenterol.*, 12, 457, 1990.

255. Murphy, R. L., Noskin, G. A., and Ehrenpreis, E. D., Acute pancreatitis associated with aerosolized pentamidine, *Am. J. Med.*, 88(5N), 53N, 1990.

256. Balslev, U., Berild, D., and Nielsen, T. L., Cardiac arrest during treatment of *Pneumocystis carinii* pneumonia with intravenous pentamidine isethionate, *Scand. J. Infect. Dis.*, 24, 111, 1992.

257. Quadrel, M. A., Atkin, S. H., and Jaker, M. A., Delayed cardiotoxicity during treatment with intravenous pentamidine: two case reports and a review of the literature, *Am. Heart J.*, 123, 1377, 1992.

258. Balslev, U. and Nielsen, T. L., Adverse effects associated with intravenous pentamidine isethionate as treatment of *Pneumocystis carinii* pneumonia, *Dan. Med. Bull.*, 39, 366, 1992.

259. Mani, S., Kocheril, A. G., and Andriole, V. T., Case report: pentamidine and polymorphic ventricular tachycardia revisited, *Am. J. Med. Sci.*, 305, 236, 1993.

260. Cortese, L. M., Gasser, R. A., Jr., Bjornson, D. C., Dacey, M. J., and Oster, C. N., Prolonged recurrence of pentamidine-induced torsades de pointes, *Ann. Pharmacother.*, 26, 1365, 1992.

261. Warton, J. M., Demopulos, P. A., and Goldschlager, N., Torsades de pointes during administration of pentamidine isethionate, *Am. J. Med.*, 83, 571, 1987

262. Harel, Y., Scott, W. A., Szeinberg, A., and Barzilay, Z., Pentamidine-induced torsades de pointes, *Pediatr. Infect. Dis. J.*, 12, 692, 1993.

263. Green, P. T., Reents, S., Harman, F., and Curtis, A. B, Pentamidine-induced torsades de pointes in a renal transplant recipient with *Pneumocystis carinii* pneumonia, *South. Med. J.*, 83, 481, 1990.

264. Mitchell, P., Dodek, P., Lawson, L., Kiess, M., and Russell, J., Torsades de pointes during intravenous pentamidine isethionate therapy, *Can. Med. Assoc. J.*, 140, 173, 1989.

265. Hancock, E. W., Possible torsade in a patient with AIDS, *Hosp. Pract.*, 25, 132, 1990.

266. Engrav, M. B., Coodley, G., and Magnusson, A. R., Torsades de pointes after inhaled pentamidine, *Ann. Emerg. Med.*, 21, 1404, 1992.

267. Vukmir, R. B., Torsades de pointes: a review, *Am. J. Emerg. Med.*, 9, 250, 1991.

268. Stein, K. M., Haronian, H., Mensah, G. A., Acosta, A., Jacobs, J., and Kligfield, P., Ventricular tachycardia and torsades de pointes complicating pentamidine therapy of *Pneumocystis carinii* pneumonia in the acquired immunodeficiency syndrome, *Am. J. Cardiol.*, 66, 888, 1990.

269. Miller, H. C., Cardiac arrest after intravenous pentamidine in an infant, *Pediatr. Infect. Dis. J.*, 12, 694, 1993.

270. Tzivoni, D., Keren, A., Cohen, A. M., Loebel, H., Zahavi, I., Chenzbraun, A., and Stern, S., Magnesium therapy for torsades de pointes, *Am. J. Cardiol.*, 53, 528, 1984.

271. Sasyniuk, B. I., Valois, M., and Toy, W., Recent advances in understanding the mechanisms of drug-induced torsades de pointes arrhythmias, *Am. J. Cardiol.*, 64, 29J, 1989.

272. Pais, J. R., Cazorla, C., Novo, E., and Viana, A., Massive haemorrhage from rupture of a pancreatic pseudocyst after pentamidine-associated pancreatitis, *Eur. J. Med.*, 1, 251, 1992.

273. Tidwell, R. R., Jones, S. K., Geratz, J. D., Ohemeng, K. A., Cory, M., and Hall, J. E., Analogues of 1,5-bis(4-amidinophenoxy)pentane (pentamidine) in the treatment of experimental *Pneumocystis carinii* pneumonia, *J. Med. Chem.*, 33, 1252, 1990.

274. Jones, S. K., Hall, J. E., Allen, M. A., Morrison, S. D., Ohemeng, K. A., Reddy, V. V., Geratz, J. D., and Tidwell, R. R., Novel pentamidine analogs in the treatment of experimental *Pneumocystis carinii* pneumonia, *Antimicrob. Agents Chemother.*, 34, 1026, 1990.

275. Tidwell, R. R., Jones, S. K., Dykstra, C. C., Gorton, L., and Hall, J. E., Treatment of experimental *Pneumocystis carinii* pneumonia with 1,3-di(4-imidazolino-2-methoxyphenoxy)propane lactate, *J. Protozool.*, 6, 148S, 1991.

276. Bell, C. A., Cory, M., Fairley, T. A., Hall, J. E., and Tidwell, R. R., Structure-activity relationships of pentamidine analogs against *Giardia lamblia* and correlation of antigiardial activity with DNA-binding affinity, *Antimicrob. Agents Chemother.*, 35, 1099, 1991.

277. Cory, M., Tidwell, R. R., and Fairley, T. A., Structure and DNA binding activity of analogs of 1,5-di(4-amidinophenoxy)pentane (pentamidine), *J. Med. Chem.*, 35, 431, 1992.

278. Fairley, T. A., Tidwell, R. R., Donkor, I., Naiman, N., Ohemeng, K., Lombardy, R., Bentley, J., and Cory, M., Structure, DNA minor groove binding, and base pair specificity of alkyl- and aryl-linked bis(amidinobenzimidazoles) and bis(amidinoindoles), *J. Med. Chem.*, 36, 1746, 1993.

279. Tidwell, R. R., Geratz, J. D., Dann, O., Volz, G., Zeh, D., and Loewe, H., Diarylamidine derivatives with one or both of the aryl moieties consisting of an indole or indole-like ring: inhibitors of arginine-specific esteroproteases, *J. Med. Chem.*, 21, 613, 1978.

280. Tidwell, R. R., Jones, S. K., Naiman, N. A., Berger, L. C., Brake, W. B., Dykstra, C. C., and Hall, J. E., Activity of cationically substituted bis-benzimidazoles against experimental *Pneumocystis carinii* pneumonia, *Antimicrob. Agents Chemother.*, 37, 1713, 1993.

281. Hughes, W. T., The role of atovaquone tablets in treating *Pneumocystis carinii* pneumonia, *J. Acquir. Immune Defic. Syndr. Hum. Retrovirol.*, 8, 247, 1995.

282. Haile, L. G. and Flaherty, J. F., Atovaquone: a review, *Ann. Pharmacother.*, 27, 1488, 1993.

283. Artymowicz, R. J. and James, V. E., Atovaquone: a new antipneumocystis agent, *Clin. Pharm.*, 12, 563, 1993.

284. Gutteridge, W. E., 556C80, an antimalarial hydroxynaphthoquinone with broad spectrum: experimental activity against opportunistic parasitic infections of AIDS patients, *J. Protozool.*, 38, 1418, 1991.

285. Burroughs Wellcome Co., Information for investigators: mepron brand atovaquone tablet, intravenous and oral suspension formulations, August 31, 1992.

286. Hudson, A. T., Dickins, M., Ginger, C. D., Gutteridge, W. E., Holdich, T., Hutchinson, D. B. A., Pudney, M., Randal, A. W., and Latter, V. S., 566C80: a potent broad spectrum anti-infective agent with activity against malaria and opportunistic infections in AIDS patients, *Drugs Exp. Clin. Res.*, 17, 427, 1991.

287. Hughes, W. T., Gray, V. L., Gutteridge, W. E., Latter, V. S., and Pudney, M., Efficacy of a hydroxy-naphthoquinone, 566C80, in experimental *Pneumocystis carinii* pneumonitis, *Antimicrob. Agents Chemother.*, 34, 225, 1990.

288. Hughes, W. T., Kennedy, W., Shenep, J. L., Flynn, P. M., Hetherington, S. V., Fullen, G., Lancaster, D. J., Stein, D. S., Palte, S., Rosenbaum, D., Liao, S. H. T., Blum, M. R., and Rogers, M. D., Safety and pharmacokinetics of 566C80, a hydroxynaphthoquinone with anti-*Pneumocystis carinii* activity: a phase I study in human immunodeficiency virus, *J. Infect. Dis.*, 163, 843, 1991.

289. Hughes, W. T., Jacobus, D. P., Canfield, C., and Killmar, J., Anti-*Pneumocystis carinii* activity of PS-15, a new biguanide folate antagonist, *Antimicrob. Agents Chemother.*, 37, 1417, 1993.

290. Alder, J., Mitten, M., Shipkowitz, N., Hernandez, L., Yu-hua, H., Marsh, K., and Clement, J., Treatment of experimental *Pneumocystis carinii* infection by combination of clarithromycin and sulfamethoxazole, *J. Antimicrob. Chemother.*, 33, 253, 1994.

291. Rogers, P., Allegra, C. J., Murphy, R. F., Drake, J. C., Masur, H., Poplack, D. G., Chabner, B. A., Parrillo, J. E., Lane, H. C., and Balis, F. M., Bioavailability of oral trimetrexate in patients with acquired immunodeficiency syndrome, *Antimicrob. Agents Chemother.*, 32, 324, 1988.

292. Allegra, C. J., Kovacs, J. A., Drake, J. C., Swan, J. C., Chabner, B. A., and Masur, H., Activity of antifolates against *Pneumocystis carinii* dihydrofolate reductase and identification of a potent new agent, *J. Exp. Med.*, 165, 926, 1987.

293. Reece, P. A., Morris, R. G., Bishop, J. F., Olver, I. N., and Raghaven, D., Pharmacokinetics of trimetrexate administered by five-day continuous infusion to patients with advanced cancer, *Cancer Res.*, 47, 2996, 1987.

294. Lin, J. T., Cashmore, A. R., Baker, M., Dreyer, R. N., Ernstoff, M., Marsh, J. C., Bertino, J. R., Whitfield, L. R., Delap, R., and Grillo-Lopez, A., Phase I studies with trimetrexate: clinical pharmacology, analytical methodology, and pharmacokinetics, *Cancer Res.*, 47, 609, 1987.

295. Stewart, J. A., McCormack, J. J., Tong, W., Low, J. B., Roberts, J. D., Blow, A., Whitfield, L. R., Haugh, L. D., Grove, W. R., Grillo-Lopez, A. J., and Delap, R. J., Phase I clinical and pharmacokinetic study of trimetrexate using a daily ×5 schedule, *Cancer Res.*, 48, 5029, 1988.

296. Ho, D. H. W., Covington, W. P., Legha, S. S., Newman, R. A., and Krakoff, I. H., Clinical pharmacology of trimetrexate, *Clin. Pharmacol. Ther.*, 42, 351, 1987.

297. Balis, F. M., Patel, R., Luks, E., Doherty, K. M., Holcenberg, J. S., Tan, C., Reaman, G. H., Belasco, J., Ettinger, L. J., Zimm, S., and Poplack, D. G., Pediatric phase I trial and pharmacokinetic study of trimetrexate, *Cancer Res.*, 47, 4973, 1987.

298. Smit, M. J. M., De Groot, R., Van Dongen, J. J. M., Van der Voort, E., Neijens, H. J., and Whitfield, L. R., Trimetrexate efficacy and pharmacokinetics during treatment of refractory *Pneumocystis carinii* pneumonia in an infant with severe combined immunodeficiency syndrome, *Pediatr. Infect. Dis. J.*, 9, 212, 1990.

299. Atzori, C., Bruno, A., Chichino, G., Bombardelli, E., Scaglia, M., and Ghione, M., Activity of bilobalide, a sesquiterpene from *Ginkgo biloba* in *Pneumocystis carinii*, *Antimicrob. Agents Chemother.*, 37, 1492, 1993.

300. Queener, S. F., Dean, R. A., Bartlett, M. S., Milhous, W. K., Berman, R. L., Ellis, W. Y., and Smith, J. W., Efficacy of intermittent dosage of 8-aminoquinolines for therapy or prophylaxis of *Pneumocystis* pneumonia in rats, *J. Infect. Dis.*, 165, 764, 1992.

301. Kluge, R. M., Spaulding, D. M., and Spain, A. J., Combination of pentamidine and trimethoprim–sulfamethoxazole in the therapy of *Pneumocystis carinii* pneumonia in rats, *Antimicrob. Agents Chemother.*, 13, 975, 1978.

302. Hughes, W. T., McNabb, P. C., Makres, T. D., and Feldman, S., Efficacy of trimethoprim and sulfamethoxazole in the prevention and treatment of *Pneumocystis carinii* pneumonitis, *Antimicrob. Agents Chemother.*, 5, 289, 1974.

303. Hughes, W. T. and Smith, B. L., Efficacy of diaminodiphenylsulfone and other drugs in murine *Pneumocystis carinii* pneumonitis, *Antimicrob. Agents Chemother.*, 26, 436, 1984.

304. Frenkel, J. K., Good, J. T., and Shultz, J. A., Latent pneumocystis infection of rats, relapse and chemotherapy, *Lab. Invest.*, 15, 1559, 1966.

305. Queener, S. F., Bartlett, M. S., Durkin, M. M., Jay, M. A., and Smith, J. W., Activity of clindamycin with primaquine toward *Pneumocystis carinii in vitro* and *in vivo*, *Proc. 27th Intersci. Conf. Antimicrob. Agents Chemother.*, American Society for Microbiology, Washington, D.C., Abstr. 574, 1987.

306. Allegra, C. J., Chabner, B. A., Tuazon, C. U., Ogata-Arakaki, D., Baird, B., Drake, J. C., Simmons, J. T., Lack, E. E., Shelhamer, J. H., Balis, F., Walker, R., Kovacs, J. A., Lane, H. C., and Masur, H., Trimetrexate for the treatment of *Pneumocystis carinii* pneumonia in patients with AIDS, *N. Engl. J. Med.*, 317, 978, 1987.

307. Hughes, W. T. and Killmar, J. T., Synergistic anti-*Pneumocystis carinii* effects of erythromycin and sulfisoxazole, *J. Acquir. Immune Defic. Syndr.*, 4, 523, 1991.

308. Walzer, P. D., Foy, J., Steele, P., and White, M., Synergistic combinations of Ro 11-8958 and other dihydrofolate reductase inhibitors with sulfamethoxazole and dapsone for therapy of experimental pneumocystosis, *Antimicrob. Agents Chemother.*, 37, 1436, 1993.

309. Fischl, M. A., Richman, D. D., Grieco, M. H., Gottlieb, M. S., Volberding, P. A., Laskin, O. L., Leedom, J. M., Groopman, J. E., Mildvan, D., Schooley, R. T., Jackson, G. G., Durack, D. T., King, D., and the AZT Collaborative Working Group, The efficacy of azidothymidine (AZT) in the treatment of patients with AIDS and AIDS-related complex: a double-blind, placebo-controlled trial, *N. Engl. J. Med.*, 317, 185, 1987.

310. Davey, R. T. and Masur, H., Recent advances in the diagnosis, treatment and prevention of *Pneumocystis carinii* pneumonia, *Antimicrob. Agents Chemother.*, 34, 499, 1990.

311. Graham, N. M., Zeger, S. L., Park, L. P., Phair, J. P., Detels, R., Vermund, S. H., Ho, M., and Saah, A. J., Effect of zidovudine and *Pneumocystis carinii* prophylaxis on progression of HIV-1 infection to AIDS, *Lancet*, 338, 265, 1991.

312. Efferen, L. S., Nabarajah, D., and Palat, D. S., Survival following mechanical ventilation for *Pneumocystis carinii* pneumonia in patients with the acquired immunodeficiency syndrome: a different perspective, *Am. J. Med.*, 87, 401, 1989.

313. El-Sadr, W. and Simberkoff, M. S., Survival and prognostic factors in severe *Pneumocystis carinii* pneumonia requiring mechanical ventilation, *Am. Rev. Respir. Dis.*, 137, 1264, 1988.

314. Brenner, M., Ognibene, F. P., Lack, E. E., Simmons, J. T., Suffredini, A. F., Lane, H. C., Fauci, A. S,, Parrillo, J. E., Shelhamer, J. H., and Masur, H., Prognostic factors and life expectancy of patients with acquired immunodeficiency syndrome and *Pneumocystis carinii* pneumonia, *Am. Rev. Respir. Dis.*, 136, 1199, 1987.

315. Thibert, J., Gasparini, A., Diaz-Mitoma, F. et al., Tolerance of oral trimethoprim–sulfamethoxazole (TMP-SMX) prophylaxis of *Pneumocystis carinii* pneumonia (PCP), *Proc. 9th Int. Conf. AIDS, Berlin*, Abstr. PO-B09-1397, 1993, p. 368.

316. Siegel, S. E., Wolff, L. J., Baehner, R. L., and Hammond, D., Treatment of *Pneumocystis carinii* pneumonitis: a comparative trial of sulfamethoxazole–trimethoprim vs. pentamidine in pediatric patients with cancer: report from the Children's Cancer Study Center, *Am. J. Dis. Child.*, 138, 1051, 1984.

317. Vöhringer, H.-F. and Arastéh, K., Pharmacokinetic optimisation in the treatment of *Pneumocystis carinii* pneumonia, *Clin. Pharmacokinet.*, 24, 388, 1993.

318. Masur, H. and Kovacs, J. A., Treatment and prophylaxis of *Pneumocystis carinii* pneumonia, *Infect. Dis. Clin. North Am.*, 2, 419, 1988.

319. Hughes, W. T., Feldman, S., Chaudhary, S. C., Ossi, M. J., Cox, F., and Sanyal, S. K., Comparison of pentamidine isethionate and trimethoprim–sulfamethoxazole in the treatment of *Pneumocystis carinii* pneumonia, *J. Pediatr.*, 92, 285, 1978.

320. Jaffe, H. S., Abrams, D. I., Ammann, A. J., Lewis, B. J., and Golden, J. A., Complications of co-trimoxazole in treatment of AIDS-associated *Pneumocystis carinii* pneumonia in homosexual men, *Lancet*, 2, 1109, 1983.

321. Hughes, W. T., Feldman, S., and Sanyal, S. K., Treatment of *Pneumocystis carinii* pneumonitis with trimethoprim–sulfamethoxazole, *Can. Med. Assoc. J.*, 112, 47, 1975.

322. Hughes, W. T., Kuhn, S., Chaudhary, S., Feldman, S., Verzosa, M., Aur, R. J. A., Pratt, C., and George, S. L., Successful chemoprophylaxis for *Pneumocystis carinii* pneumonia, *N. Engl. J. Med.*, 297, 1419, 1977.

323. Wolff, L. J. and Baehner, R. L., Delayed development of pneumocystis pneumonia following administration of short-term high-dose trimethoprim–sulfamethoxazole, *Am. J. Dis. Child.*, 132, 525, 1978.

324. Chusid, M. J. and Heyrman, B. A., An outbreak of *Pneumocystis carinii* pneumonia at a pediatric hospital, *Pediatrics*, 62, 1031, 1978.

325. Harris, R. E., McCallister, J. A., Allen, S. A., Barton, A. S., and Baehner, R. L., Prevention of pneumocystis pneumonia: use of continuous sulfamethoxazole–trimethoprim therapy, *Am. J. Dis. Child.*, 134, 35, 1980.

326. Wilber, R. B., Feldman, S., Malone, W. J., Ryan, M., Aur, R. J., and Hughes, W. T., Chemoprophylaxis for *Pneumocystis carinii*: outcome of unstructured delivery, *Am. J. Dis. Child.*, 134, 643, 1980.

327. Kovacs, J. A. and Masur, H., *Pneumocystis carinii* pneumonia: therapy and prophylaxis, *J. Infect. Dis.*, 158, 254, 1988.

328. Ivady, G. and Paldy, L., Ein neves behandlungsverfahren der interstitiellen plasmazelligen pneumonie fruhgeborener mit fünfwerigen stibium und aromatischen diamidien, *Monatsschr. Kinderheilkd.*, 106, 10, 1958.

329. Mallory, D. L., Parrillo, J. E., Bailey, K. R., Akin, G. L., Brenner, M., Lane, H. C., Fauci, A. S., and Masur, H., Cardiovascular effects and safety of intravenous and intramuscular pentamidine isethionate, *Crit. Care Med.*, 15, 503, 1987.

330. Conte, J. E., Hollander, H., and Golden, J., Inhaled or reduced-dose intravenous pentamidine for *Pneumocystis carinii* pneumonia, *Ann. Intern. Med.*, 107, 495, 1987.

331. Sattler, F. R. and Feinberg, J., New development in the treatment of *Pneumocystis carinii* pneumonia, *Chest*, 101, 451, 1992.

332. Monk, J. P. and Benfield, P., Inhaled pentamidine: an overview of its properties and a review of its therapeutic use in *Pneumocystis carinii* pneumonia, *Drugs*, 39, 741, 1990.

333. Navin, T. R. and Fontaine, R. E., Intravenous versus intramuscular administration of pentamidine, *N. Engl. J. Med.*, 311, 1701, 1984.

334. Montgomery, A. B., Debs, R. J., Luce, J. M., Corkery, K. J., Turner, J., Brunette, E. N., Lin, E. T., and Hopewell, P. C., Aerosolized pentamidine as sole therapy for *Pneumocystis carinii* pneumonia in patients with acquired immunodeficiency syndrome, *Lancet*, 2, 480, 1987.

335. O'Doherty, M. J., Thomas, S., Page, C., Barlow, D., Bradbeer, C., Nunan, T. O., and Bateman, N. T., Differences in relative efficacy of nebulizers for pentamidine administration, *Lancet*, 2, 1283, 1988.

336. Armstrong, D. and Bernard, E., Aerosol pentamidine, *Ann. Intern. Med.*, 109, 852, 1988.

337. Klein, N. C., Duncanson, F. P., Lenox, T. H., Forszpaniak, C., Sherer, C. B., Quentzel, H., Nunez, M., Suarez, M., Kawwaff, O., Pitta-Alvarez, A., Freeman, K., and Wormser, G. P., Trimethoprim–sulfamethoxazole versus pentamidine for *Pneumocystis carinii* pneumonia in AIDS patients: results of a large prospective randomized treatment trial, *AIDS*, 6, 301, 1992.

338. Lentino, J. R. and Brooks, D., *Pneumocystis carinii* pneumonia and tuberculosis in a human immuno-deficiency virus-seronegative patient without evidence of the idiopathic CD4+ T lymphopenia syndrome, *Clin. Infect. Dis.*, 18, 470, 1994.

339. Smith, D. K., Neal, J. J., and Holinberg, S. D., Unexplained opportunistic infections and CD4+ T-lymphocytopenia without HIV infection: an investigation of cases in the United States. The Centers for Disease Control Idiopathic CD4+ T-lymphocytopenia Task Force, *N. Engl. J. Med.*, 328, 373, 1993.

340. Tijhuis, G. J., Huisman, H. G., and Kauffmann, R. H., AIDS without detectable HIV: a case report, *Am. J. Med.*, 94, 442, 1993.

341. Lawrence, J., T-cell subsets in health, infectious disease, and idiopathic CD4+ T lymphopenia, *Ann. Intern. Med.*, 119, 55, 1993.

342. World Health Organization, Unexplained severe immunosuppression without incidence of HIV infection, *WHO Wkly. Epidem. Rec.*, 42, 309, 1992.

343. Jayes, R. L., Kamerow, H. N., Hasselquist, S. M., Delaney, M. D., and Parenti, D. M., Disseminated pneumocystosis presenting as a pleural effusion, *Chest*, 103, 306, 1993.

344. Price, D. A., Hollings, N. P., Janes, S. M., Main, J., and Coker, R. J., Clinical response to the addition of clarithromycin in *Pneumocystis carinii* pneumonia refractory to high dose co-trimoxazole, *J. Antimicrob. Chemother.*, 34, 303, 1994.

345. Falloon, J., Kovacs, J., Hughes, W., O'Neill, D., Polis, M., Davey, R. T., Jr., Rogers, M., LaFon, S., Feuerstein, I., Lancaster, D., Land, M., Tuazon, C., Dohn, M., Greenberg, S., Lane, H. C., and Masur, H., A preliminary evaluation of 566C80 for the treatment of *Pneumocystis* pneumonia in patients with the acquired immunodeficiency syndrome, *N. Engl. J. Med.*, 325, 1534, 1991.

346. Dohn, M. N., Weinberg, W. G., Torres, R. A., Follansbee, S. E., Caldwell, P. T., Scott, J. D., Gathe, J. C., Jr., Haghighat, D. P., Sampson, J. H., Spotkov, J., Deresinski, S. C., Meyer, R. D., Lancaster, D. J., and the Atovaquone Study Group, Oral atovaquone compared with intravenous pentamidine for *Pneumocystis carinii* pneumonia in patients with AIDS, *Ann. Intern. Med.*, 121, 174, 1994.

347. Lieberman, M. M., van der Horst, C., Stoeckle, M., and Tennenberg, A., Atovaquone for *Pneumocystis carinii* pneumonia, *Ann. Intern. Med.*, 122, 314, 1995.

348. Masur, H., Prevention and treatment of *Pneumocystis carinii*, *N. Engl. J. Med.*, 327, 1853, 1992.

349. Ashar, N., Daneshvar, H., and Beall, G., Desensitization to trimethoprim–sulfamethoxazole in HIV-infected patients, *J. Allergy Clin. Immunol.*, 93, 1001, 1994.

350. Leoung, G. S., Mills, J., Hopewell, P. C., Hughes, W., and Wofsy, C., Dapsone–trimethoprim for *Pneumocystis carinii* pneumonia in the acquired immunodeficency syndrome, *Ann. Intern. Med.*, 105, 45, 1986.

351. Kovacs, J. A., Allegra, C. J., Beaver, J., Boarman, D., and Lewis, M., Characterization of de novo folate synthesis in *Pneumocystis carinii* and *Toxoplasma gondii*: potential for screening therapeutic agents, *J. Infect. Dis.*, 160, 312, 1989.

352. Kovacs, J. A., Powell, F., Voeller, D., and Allegra, C. J., Inhibition of *Pneumocystis carinii* dihydropteroate synthetase by para-acetamidobenzoic acid: possible mechanism of action of isoprinosine in human immunodeficiency virus infection, *Antimicrob. Agents Chemother.*, 37, 1227, 1993.

353. Hughes, W. T. and Smith, B. L., Efficacy of diaminodiphenylsulfone and other drugs in murine *Pneumocystis carinii* pneumonia, *Antimicrob. Agents Chemother.*, 26, 436, 1984.

354. Mills, J., Leoung, G., Medina, I., Hughes, W., Hopewell, P., and Wofsy, C., Dapsone is ineffective therapy for pneumocystis pneumonia in patients with AIDS, *Clin. Res.*, 34, 101A, 1986.

355. DeGowin, R. L., Eppes, B., Powell, R. D., and Carson, P. E., The haemolytic effects of diphenylsulfone (DDS) in normal subjects and in those with glucose-6-phosphate-dehydrogenase deficiency, *Bull. WHO*, 35, 165, 1966.

356. Metroka, C. E., Lewis, N. J., and Jacobus, D. P., Desensitization to dapsone in HIV-positive patients, *JAMA*, 267, 512, 1992.

357. Kay, R. and Dubois, R. E., Clindamycin/primaquine therapy and secondary prophylaxis against *Pneumocystis carinii* pneumonia in patients with AIDS, *South. Med. J.*, 83, 403, 1990.

358. Toma, E., Clindamycin/primaquine for treatment of *Pneumocystis carinii* in AIDS, *Eur. J. Clin. Microbiol. Infect. Dis.*, 10, 210, 1991.

359. Black, J. R., Feinberg, J., Murphy, R. L., Fass, R. J., Carey, J., and Sattler, F. R., Clindamycin and primaquine as primary treatment for mild and moderately severe *Pneumocystis carinii* pneumonia in patients with AIDS, *Eur. J. Clin. Microbiol. Infect. Dis.*, 10, 204, 1991.

360. Ruf, B., Rohde, I., and Pohle, H. D., Efficacy of clindamycin/sulfamethoxazole in primary treatment of *Pneumocystis carinii* pneumonia, *Eur. J. Clin. Microbiol. Infect. Dis.*, 10, 207, 1991.

361. Panisko, D. M. and Keystone, J. S., Treatment of malaria — 1990, *Drugs*, 39, 160, 1990.

362. Smith, N., Blanshard, C., Smith, D., and Gazzard, B., Toxicity of clindamycin and primaquine treatment of AIDS-related *Pneumocystis carinii* pneumonia, *AIDS*, 7, 749, 1993.

363. Zambrano, D., Clindamycin in the treatment of obstetric and gynecologic infections: a review, *Clin. Ther.*, 13, 58, 1991.

364. Toma, E., Fournier, S., Dumont, M., Bolduc, P., and Deschamps, H., Clindamycin/primaquine versus trimethoprim–sulfamethoxazole as primary therapy for *Pneumocystis carinii* pneumonia in AIDS: a randomized, double-blind pilot trial, *Clin. Infect. Dis.*, 17, 178, 1993.

365. Noskin, G. A., Murphy, R. L., Black, J. R., and Phair, J. P., Salvage therapy with clindamycin/primaquine for *Pneumocystis carinii* pneumonia, *Clin. Infect. Dis.*, 14, 183, 1992.

366. Frenkel, J. K., Good, J. T., and Shultz, J. A., Latent Pneumocystis infection of rats, relapse, and chemotherapy, *Lab. Invest.*, 15, 1559, 1966.

367. Rifkind, D., Faris, T. D., and Hill, R. B., Jr., *Pneumocystis carinii* pneumonia: studies on the diagnosis and treatment, *Ann. Intern. Med.*, 65, 943, 1966.

368. Ruskin, J. and Remington, J. S., The immunocompromised host and infection. I. *Pneumocystis carinii* pneumonia, *JAMA*, 202, 96, 1967.

369. Kirby, H. B., Kenamore, B., and Guckian, J. C., *Pneumocystis carinii* pneumonia treated with pyrimethamine and sulfadiazine, *Ann. Intern. Med.*, 75, 505, 1971.

370. Farinas, E. and Quel, J. A., Hypertension and duodenal ulcer associated with *Pneumocystis carinii* pneumonitis and dysgammaglobulinemia, *Ill. J. Med.*, 139, 138, 1971.

371. Whisnant, J. K. and Buckley, R. H., Successful therapy of *Pneumocystis carinii* pneumonia in infants with x-linked immunodeficiency with hyper-IgM, *Natl. Cancer Inst. Monogr.*, 43, 211, 1976.

372. Young, R. C. and Devita, V. T., Jr., Treatment of *Pneumocystis carinii* pneumonia: current status of the regimens of pentamidine isethionate and pyrimethamine–sulfadiazine, *Natl. Cancer Inst. Monogr.*, 43, 193, 1976.

373. Allegra, C. J., Kovacs, J. A., Drake, J. C., Swan, J. C., Chabner, B. A., and Masur, H., Activity of antifolates against *Pneumocystis carinii* dihydrofolate reductase and identification of a potent new agent, *J. Exp. Med.*, 165, 926, 1987.

374. Queener, S. F., Bartlett, M. S., Jay, M. A., Durkin, M. M., and Smith, J. W., Activity of lipid-soluble inhibitors of dihydrofolate reductase against *Pneumocystis carinii* in culture and in rat model of infection, *Antimicrob. Agents Chemother.*, 31, 1323, 1987.

375. Sattler, F. R., Allegra, C. J., Vergedem, T. D., Akil, B., Tuazon, C. U., Highlett, C., Ogata-Arakaki, D., Feinberg, J., Shelhamer, J., Lane, H. C., Davis, R., Boylen, C. T., Leedom, J. M., and Masur, H., Trimetrexate–leucovorin dosage evaluation study for treatment of *Pneumocystis carinii* pneumonia, *J. Infect. Dis.*, 161, 91, 1990.

376. Grem, J. L., King, S. A., Costanza, M. E., and Brown, T. D., Hypersensitivity reactions to trimetrexate, *Invest. New Drugs*, 8, 211, 1990.

377. Golden, J. A., Sjoerdsma, A., and Santi, D. A., *Pneumocystis carinii* pneumonia treated with alpha-difluoromethylornithine: a prospective study among patients with the acquired immunodeficiency syndrome, *West. J. Med.*, 141, 613, 1984.

378. Neibart, E., Sacks, H. S., Hammer, G., and Hirschman, S. Z., Difluoromethylornithine in the treatment of pneumocystis pneumonia, *Proc. 28th Intersci. Conf. Antimicrob. Agents Chemother.*, American Society for Microbiology, Washington, D.C., Abstr. 224, 1986.

379. Paulson, Y. J., Gilrian, T. M., Boyle, C. T., Sharma, O. P., and Haseltine, P. N. R., Eflornithine treatment of *Pneumocystis carinii* pneumonia in patients failing other therapy, *Proc. 28th Intersci. Conf. Antimicrob. Agents Chemother.*, American Society for Microbiology, Washington, D.C., Abstr. 225, 1986.

380. Smith, D., Davies, S., Nelson, M., Youle, M., Gleeson, J., and Gazzard, B., *Pneumocystis carinii* pneumonia treated with eflornithine in AIDS patients resistant to conventional therapy, *AIDS*, 4, 1019, 1990.

381. Paulson, Y. J., Gilman, T. M., Heseltine, P. N., Sharma, O. P., and Boylen, C. T., Eflornithine treatment of refractory *Pneumocystis carinii* pneumonia in patients with acquired immunodeficiency syndrome, *Chest*, 101, 67, 1992.

382. Smith, D. E., Davies, S., Smithson, J., Harding, I., and Gazzard, B. G., Eflornithine versus cotrimoxazole in the treatment of *Pneumocystis carinii* pneumonia in AIDS patients, *AIDS*, 6, 1489, 1992.

383. Bozzette, S. A., The use of corticosteroids in *Pneumocystis carinii* pneumonia, *J. Infect. Dis.*, 162, 1365, 1990.

384. MacFadden, D. K., Edelson, J. D., and Rebuck, A. S., *Pneumocystis carinii* pneumonia in the acquired immune deficiency syndrome: response to inadvertent steroid therapy, *Can. Med. Assoc. J.*, 132, 1161, 1985.

385. Hurley, P., Weikel, C., Temeles, D., Rosenburg, S., and Pearson, R., Unusual remission of *Pneumocystis carinii* pneumonia in a patient with the acquired immune deficiency syndrome, *Am. J. Med.*, 82, 645, 1987.

386. Foltzer, M. A., Hannan, S. E., and Kozak, A. J., *Pneumocystis* pneumonia: response to corticosteroids, *JAMA*, 253, 979, 1985.

387. Rankin, J. A. and Pella, J. A., Radiographic resolution of *Pneumocystis carinii* pneumonia in response to corticosteroids therapy, *Am. Rev. Respir. Dis.*, 136, 182, 1987.

388. El-Sadr, W., Sudhu, G., Diamond, G., Zuger, A., Berman, D., Simberkoff, M. S., and Rahal, J. J., High-dose corticosteroids as adjunct therapy in severe *Pneumocystis carinii* pneumonia, *AIDS Res.*, 2, 349, 1986.

389. Admundson, D. E., Murray, K. M., Brodine, S., and Oldfield, E. C., High-dose corticosteroid therapy for *Pneumocystis carinii* pneumonia in patients with acquired immunodeficiency syndrome, *South. Med. J.*, 82, 711, 1989.

390. MacFadden, D. K., Hyland, R. H., Inouye, T., Edelson, J. D., Rodriguez, C. H., and Rebuck, A. S., Corticosteroids as adjunctive therapy in treatment of *Pneumocystis carinii* pneumonia in patients with acquired immunodeficiency syndrome, *Lancet*, 1, 1477, 1987.

391. Mottin, D., Denis, M., Dombret, H., Rossert, J., Mayaud, C. H., and Akoun, G., Role for steroids in treatment of *Pneumocystis* pneumonia in AIDS, *Lancet*, 2, 519, 1987.

392. Montaner, J. S. G. and Ruedy, J., Corticosteroids prevent early deterioration in patients with moderately severe *Pneumocystis carinii* pneumonia and the acquired immunodeficiency syndrome (AIDS), *Ann. Intern. Med.*, 113, 14, 1990.

393. Gagnon, S., Boota, A. M., Fischl, M. A., Baier, H., Kirksey, O. W., and La Voie, L., Corticosteroids as adjunctive therapy for severe *Pneumocystis carinii* pneumonia in the acquired immunodeficiency syndrome: a double-blind placebo-controlled trial, *N. Engl. J. Med.*, 323, 1440, 1990.

394. Nielsen, T. L., Eeftinck Schattenkerk, J. K., Jensen, B.N., Lundgren, J. D., Gerstaft, J., van Steenwijk, R. P., Bentsen, K., Frissen, P. H., Gaub, J., Orholm, M., Hansen, J.-E., Mathiesen, L., Skinhoj, P., Danner, S. A., and Nielsen, J. O., Adjunctive corticosteroids therapy for *Pneumocystis carinii* pneumonia in AIDS: a randomized European multicenter open label study, *J. Acquir. Immune Defic. Syndr.*, 5, 726, 1992.

395. Jeantils, V., Nguyen, G., Bacle, F., and Thomas, M., Adjunctive treatment with corticosteroids for *Pneumocystis carinii* pneumonia in AIDS, *Therapie*, 48, 70, 1993.

396. Sistek, C. J., Wordell, C. J., and Hauptman, S. P., Adjuvant corticosteroid therapy for *Pneumocystis carinii* pneumonia in AIDS patients, *Ann. Pharmacother.*, 26, 1127, 1992.

397. LaRocco, A., Jr., Amundson, D. E., Wallace, M. R., Malone, J. L., and Oldfield, E. C. III, Corticosteroids for *Pneumocystis carinii* pneumonia with acute respiratory failure: experience with rescue therapy, *Chest*, 102, 892, 1992.

398. Kaufman, M. B. and DeMuria, D., Corticosteroids in AIDS patients with *Pneumocystis carinii* pneumonia, *Ann. Pharmacother.*, 26, 932, 1992.

399. Montaner, J. S., Guillemi, S., Quieffin, J., Lawson, L., Le, T., O'Shaugnessy, M., Ruedy, J., Schechter, C., and Offenstadt, G., Oral corticosteroids in patients with mild *Pneumocystis carinii* pneumonia and the acquired immune deficiency syndrome (AIDS), *Tuberc. Lung Dis.*, 74, 173, 1993.

400. Bentsen, K. D., Nielsen, T. L., Eaftinck Schattenkerk, J. K., Jensen, B. N., and Lundgren, J. D., Serum type III procollagen peptide in patients with *Pneumocystis carinii* infection: the Copenhagen-Amsterdam PCP-Prednisolone Study Group, *Am. Rev. Respir. Dis.*, 148 (6 Part 1), 1558, 1993.

401. Huang, Z. B. and Eden, E., Effect of corticosteroids on IL-1 beta and TNF by alveolar macrophages from patients with AIDS and *Pneumocystis carinii* pneumonia, *Chest*, 104, 751, 1993.

402. The National Institute of Health-University of California Expert Panel for Corticosteroids as Adjunctive Therapy for *Pneumocystis carinii* Pneumonia, Consensus statement on the use of corticosteroids as adjunctive therapy for *Pneumocystis* pneumonia in the acquired immunodeficiency syndrome, *N. Engl. J. Med.*, 323, 1500, 1990.

403. Clumeck, N. and Hermans, P., Corticosteroids as adjunctive therapy for *Pneumocystis* pneumonia in patients with AIDS, *N. Engl. J. Med.*, 324, 1666, 1991.

404. El-Sadr, W., Milder, J., Capps, L., and Sivapalan, V., Corticosteroids as adjunctive therapy for *Pneumocystis* pneumonia in patients with AIDS, *N. Engl. J. Med.*, 324, 1667, 1991.

405. Rahal, J. J., Corticosteroids as adjunctive therapy for *Pneumocystis* pneumonia in patients with AIDS, *N. Engl. J. Med.*, 324, 1666, 1991.

406. Hardy, A. M., Wajszczuk, C. P., Suffredini, A. F., Hakala, T. R., and Ho, M., *Pneumocystis carinii* pneumonia in renal-transplant recipients treated with cyclosporine and steroids, *J. Infect. Dis.*, 149, 143, 1984.

407. Browne, M. J., Hubbard, S. M., Longo, D. L., Fisher, R., Wesley, R., Ihde, D. C., Young, R. C., and Pizzo, P. A., Excess prevalence of *Pneumocystis carinii* pneumonia in patients treated for lymphoma with combination chemotherapy, *Ann. Intern. Med.*, 104, 338, 1986.

408. Farr, R. W., *Pneumocystis carinii* pneumonia to corticosteroids, *South. Med. J.*, 85, 52, 1992.

409. Fischl, M. A., Uttamchandani, R. B., Daikos, G. L., Poblete, R. B., Moreno, J. N., Reyes, R. R., Boota, A. M., Thompson, L. M., Cleary, T. J., and Lai, S., An outbreak of tuberculosis caused by multiple-drug-resistant tuberculosis bacilli among patients with HIV infection, *Ann. Intern. Med.*, 117, 177, 1992.

410. Gill, P. S., Loureiro, C., Bernstein-Singer, M., Rarick, M. U., Sattler, F., and Levine, A. M., Clinical effect of glucocorticoids on Kaposi's sarcoma related to the acquired immunodeficiency syndrome (AIDS), *Ann. Intern. Med.*, 110, 937, 1989.

411. Schulhafer, E. P., Grossman, M. E., Fagin, G., and Bell, K. E., Steroid-induced Kaposi's sarcoma in a patient with pre-AIDS, *Am. J. Med.*, 82, 313, 1987.

412. Ueda, K., Goto, Y., Yamazaki, S., and Fujisawa, K., Chronic fatal pneumocystosis in nude mice, *Jpn. J. Exp. Med.*, 47, 475, 1977.

413. Walzer, P. D., Schnelle, V., Armstrong, D., and Rosen, P. P., Nude mouse: a new experimental model for *Pneumocystis carinii* infection, *Science*, 197, 177, 1987.

414. Waltzer, P. D., LaBine, M., Redington, T. J., and Cushion, M. T., Predisposing factors in *Pneumocystis carinii* pneumonia: effect of tetracycline, protein malnutrition, and corticosteroids on hosts, *Infect. Immun.*, 46, 747, 1984.

415. Clement, M., Edison, R., Turner, R., Montgomery, B., Luce, J., Feigal, D., and Hopewell, P., Corticosteroid as adjunctive therapy in severe *Pneumocystis carinii* pneumonia: a prospective, placebo-controlled trial, *Am. Rev. Respir. Dis.*, 139, A250, 1989.

416. Bozzette, S. A. and Morton, S. C., Reconsidering the use of adjunctive corticosteroids in Pneumocystis pneumonia? *J. Acquir. Immune Defic. Syndr. Hum. Retrovirol.*, 8, 348, 1995.

417. Harris, J. E., Improved short-term survival of AIDS patients initially diagnosed with *Pneumocystis carinii* pneumonia 1984 through 1987, *JAMA*, 263, 397, 1990.

418. Friedman, Y., Franklin, C., Rackow, E. C., and Weil, M. H., Improved survival in patients with AIDS, *Pneumocystis carinii* pneumonia, and severe respiratory failure, *Chest*, 96, 862, 1989.

419. Marolda, J., Pace, B., Bonforte, R. J., Kotin, N., and Kattan, M., Outcome of mechanical ventilation in children with acquired immunodeficiency syndrome, *Pediatr. Pulmonol.*, 7, 230, 1989.

420. Bye, M. R., Berstein, L. J., Glaser, J., and Kleid, D., *Pneumocystis carinii* pneumonia in young children with AIDS, *Pediatr. Pulmonol.*, 9, 251, 1990.

421. Notterman, D. A., Greenwald, B. M., Di Maio-Hunter, A., Wilkinson, J. D., Krasinski, K., and Borkowsky, W., Outcome after assisted ventilation in children with acquired immunodeficiency syndrome, *Crit. Care Med.*, 18, 18, 1990.

422. Vernon, D. D., Holzman, B. H., Lewis, P., Scott, G. B., Birriel, J. A., and Scott, M. B., Respiratory failure in children with acquired immunodeficiency syndrome and acquired immunodeficiency syndrome-related complex, *Pediatrics*, 82, 223, 1988.

423. Sleasman, J. W., Hemenway, C., Klein, A. S., and Barrett, D. J., Corticosteroids improve survival of children with AIDS and *Pneumocystis carinii* pneumonia, *Am. J. Dis. Child.*, 147, 30, 1993.

424. Barone, S. R., Aiuto, L. T., and Krilov, L. R., Increased survival of young infants with *Pneumocystis carinii* pneumonia and acute respiratory failure with early steroid administration, *Clin. Infect. Dis.*, 19, 212, 1994.

425. Stearn, B. F. and Polis, M. A., Prophylaxis of opportunistic infections in persons with HIV infection, *Cleve. Clin. J. Med.*, 61, 187, 1994.

426. Gifford, A. L., McPhee, S. J., and Fordham, D., Preventive care among HIV-positive patients in a general medicine practice, *Am. J. Prevent. Med.*, 10, 5, 1994.

427. Longini, I. M., Jr., Clark, W. S., and Karon, J. M., Effect of routine use of therapy in slowing the clinical course of human immunodeficiency virus (HIV) infection in a population-based cohort, *Am. J. Epidemiol.*, 137, 1229, 1993.

428. Chaisson, R. E., Keruly, J., Richman, D. D., and Moore, R. D., Pneumocystis prophylaxis and survival in patients with advanced human immunodeficiency virus infection treated with zidovudine, *Arch. Intern. Med.*, 152, 2009, 1992.

429. Graham, N. M., Zeger, S. L., Park, L. P., Vermund, S. H., Detels, R., Rinaldo, C. R., and Phair, J., The effects on survival of early treatment of human immunodeficiency virus infection, *N. Engl. J. Med.*, 326, 1037, 1992.

430. Mazur, H., Prophylaxis and therapy for *Pneumocystis* pneumonia — where are we? *Infect. Agents Dis.*, 1, 270, 1992.

431. Hamilton, J. D., Hartigan, P. M., Simberkoff, M. S., Day, P. L., Diamond, G. R., Dickinson, G. M., Drusano, G. L., Egorin, M. J., George, W. L., Gordin, F. M., Hawkes, C. A., Jensen, P. C., Klimas, N. G., Labriola, A. M., Lahart, C. J., O'Brien, W. A., Oster, C. N., Weinhold, K. J., Wray, N. P., Zolla-Pazner, S. B., and the Veterans Affairs Cooperative Study Group on AIDS Treatment, A controlled trial of early versus late treatment with zidovudine in symptomatic human immunodeficiency virus infection — results of the Veteran Affairs Cooperative Study, *N. Engl. J. Med.*, 326, 437, 1992.

432. Hirschel, B., Early zidovudine and survival in HIV infection, *N. Engl. J. Med.*, 327, 814, 1992.

433. Hartigan, P. M., Hamilton, J. D., and Simberkoff, M. S., Early zidovudine and survival in HIV patients, *N. Engl. J. Med.*, 327, 815, 1992.

434. Gail, M. H. and Mark, S. D., Early zidovudine and survival in HIV infection, *N. Engl. J. Med.*, 327, 815, 1992.

435. Arico, M., Molinari, E., Bacchella, L., DeAmici, M., Raiteri, E., and Burgio, G. R., Prospective randomized comparison of toxicity of two prophylactic regimens of cotrimoxazole in leukemic children, *Pediatr. Hematol. Oncol.*, 9, 35, 1992.

436. Nielsen, T. L., Jensen, B. N., Nelsing, S., Pedersen, C., Mathiesen, L. R., Skinhoj, P., and Nielsen, J. O., Prevention of *Pneumocystis carinii* pneumonia relapse in AIDS patients: the efficacy and tolerability of low-dose sulfamethoxazole-trimethoprim, *Dan. Med. Bull.*, 40, 503, 1993.

437. MacGregor, R. R., Morgan, A. S., Graziani, A. L., Pietroski, N. A., Frank, I., Braffman, M. N., Stern, J. J., and Buckley, R. M., Efficacy and tolerance of intermittent versus daily cotrimoxazole for PCP prophylaxis in HIV-positive patients, *Am. J. Med.*, 92, 227, 1992.

438. Metroka, C. E., Jacobus, D. P., and Lewis, N. J., Successful chemoprophylaxis for pneumocystis with dapsone or bactrim, *Proc. 5th Int. Conf. AIDS, Montreal*, Abstr. TB04, 1989.

439. Kemper, C. A., Tucker, R. M., Lang, O. S., Kessinger, J. M., Greene, S. I., Deresinski, S. C., and Stevens, D. A., Low-dose dapsone prophylaxis of *Pneumocystis carinii* pneumonia in AIDS and AIDS-related complex, *AIDS*, 4, 1145, 1990.

440. Hughes, W. T., Kennedy, W., Dugdale, M., Land, M. A., Stein, D. S., Weems, J. J., Jr., Palte, S., Lancaster, D., Gidan-Kovnar, S., and Morrison, R. E., Prevention of *Pneumocystis carinii* pneumonitis in AIDS patients with weekly dapsone, *Lancet*, 336, 1066, 1990.

441. Blum, R. N., Miller, L. A., Gaggini, L. C., and Cohn, D. L., Comparative trial of dapsone versus trimethoprim/sulfamethoxazole for primary prophylaxis of *Pneumocystis carinii* pneumonia, *J. Acquir. Immune Defic. Syndr.*, 5, 341, 1992.

442. Podzamczer, D., Santin, M., Jimenez, J., Casanova, A., Bolao, F., and Guidol, G. P., Thrice-weekly cotrimoxazole is better than weekly dapsone–pyrimethamine for the primary prevention of *Pneumocystis carinii* pneumonia in HIV-infected patients, *AIDS*, 7, 501, 1993.

443. Girard, P. M., Landman, R., Gaudebout, C., Olivares, R., Saimot, A. G., Jelazko, P., Gaudebout, C., Certain, A., Boué, F., Bouvet, E., Lecompte, T., Coulaud, J.-P., and the PRIO Study Group, Dapsone–pyrimethamine compared with aerosolized pentamidine as primary prophylaxis against *Pneumocystis carinii* pneumonia and toxoplasmosis in HIV infection, *N. Engl. J. Med.*, 328, 1514, 1993.

444. Koppen, S., Grunewald, T., Jautzke, G., Gottschalk, J., Pohle, A. D., and Ruf, B., Prevention of *Pneumocystis carinii* pneumonia and toxoplasmic encephalitis in human immunodeficiency virus infected patients: a clinical approach comparing aerosolized pentamidine and pyrimethamine/sulfadoxine, *Clin. Invest.*, 70, 508, 1992.

445. Jensen, B. N., Nielsen, T. L., Backer, V., Nelsung, S., Simonsen, L., Flaschs, H., Gaub, J., Hojlyng, N., Nielsen, J. O., Mathiesen, L., and Skinhoj, P., Aerosolized pentamidine for primary prophylaxis of *Pneumocystis carinii* pneumonia: a controlled, randomized trial, *J. Acquir. Immune Defic. Syndr.*, 6, 472, 1993.

446. Ong, E. L., Dunbar, E. M., and Mandal, B. K., Efficacy and effects on pulmonary function tests of weekly 600 mg aerosol pentamidine as prophylaxis against *Pneumocystis carinii* pneumonia, *Infection*, 20, 136, 1992.

447. Tullis, E., Yu, D. G., Rawji, M., Rachlis, A., Hyland, R., and Chan, C. K., The long-term effects of aerosol pentamidine on pulmonary function: the Toronto Aerosolized Pentamidine Study (TAPS) Group, *Clin. Invest. Med.*, 15, 42, 1992.

448. O'Sullivan, B. P. and Spaulding, R., The use of aerosolized pentamidine for prophylaxis of *Pneumocystis carinii* pneumonia in children with leukemia, *Pediatr. Pulmonol.*, 18, 228, 1994.

449. Güngör, T., Funk, M., Linde, R., Kynast, I., Allendorf, A., Lotz, C., Ehrenforth, S., Hofmann, D., Kornhuber, B., and Kreuz, W., Combined therapy in human immunodeficiency virus-infected children — a 4-year experience, *Eur. J. Pediatr.*, 152, 650, 1993.

450. Rigaud, M., Pollack, H., Leibovitz, E., Kim, M., Persaud, D., Kaul, A., Lawrence, R., Di John, D., Borkowsky, W., and Krasinski, K., Efficacy of primary chemoprophylaxis against *Pneumocystis carinii* pneumonia during the first year of life in infants affected with human immunodeficiency virus type 1, *J. Pediatr.*, 125, 476, 1994.

451. Murphy, J. L., Kano, H. L., Chenaille, P. J., and Makker, S. P., Fatal *Pneumocystis* pneumonia in a child treated for focal segmental glomerulosclerosis, *Pediatr. Nephrol.*, 7, 444, 1993.

452. Slivka, A., Wen, P. Y., Shea, W. M., and Loeffler, J. S., *Pneumocystis carinii* pneumonia during steroid taper in patients with primary brain tumors, *Am. J. Med.*, 94, 216, 1993.

453. Perrone, C., Bricaire, F., Leport, C., Assan, D., Vildé, J. L., and Assan, R., Hypoglycaemia and diabetes mellitus following parenteral pentamidine mesylate treatment in AIDS patients, *Diabetes Med.*, 7, 585, 1990.

Index

A

C